Neuropsychiatry and Behavioral Neurology

Principles and Practice

Neuropsychiatry and Behavioral Neurology

Principles and Practice

Editors

David A. Silbersweig, MD
Chairman, Department of Psychiatry
Co-Director, Center for the Neurosciences
Brigham and Women's Hospital
Stanley Cobb Professor of Psychiatry
Harvard Medical School
Boston, Massachusetts

Laura T. Safar, MD
Vice Chair of Psychiatry,
Lahey Hospital and Medical Center
Associate Neuropsychiatrist, Center for Brain/Mind Medicine
Brigham and Women's Hospital
Assistant Professor of Psychiatry
Harvard Medical School
Boston, Massachusetts

Kirk R. Daffner, MD, FAAN
Chief, Division of Cognitive and Behavioral Neurology
Director, Center for Brain/Mind Medicine
Stephen Muss Clinical Director of the Alzheimer Center
Brigham and Women's Hospital
J. David and Virginia Wimberly Professor of Neurology
Harvard Medical School
Boston, Massachusetts

New York Chicago San Francisco Athens London Madrid Mexico City
New Delhi Milan Singapore Sydney Toronto

Neuropsychiatry and Behavioral Neurology: Principles and Practice

1 2 3 4 5 6 7 8 9 DSS 25 24 23 22 21 20

ISBN 978-1-260-11710-3
MHID 1-260-11710-3

This book was set in MinionPro by MPS Limited.
The editors were Andrew Moyer and Kim J. Davis.
The production supervisor was Richard Ruzycka.
Project management was provided by Ishan Chaudhary and Jyoti Shaw, MPS Limited.

Library of Congress Cataloging-in-Publication Data

Names: Silbersweig, David, editor. | Safar, Laura T., editor. | Daffner,
    Kirk R., editor.
Title: Neuropsychiatry and behavioral neurology : principles and practice /
    editors, David Silbersweig, Laura T. Safar, Kirk R. Daffner.
Description: New York : McGraw Hill, [2020] | Includes bibliographical
    references and index. | Summary: "Neuropsychiatry and Behavioral
Neurology: Principles and Practice is a clinically oriented textbook
    that aims to link rapid advances in basic, cognitive, and affective
    neuroscience with the care of patients struggling with losses that often
    involve their most cherished human capacities"—Provided by publisher.
Identifiers: LCCN 2020015682 (print) | LCCN 2020015683 (ebook) | ISBN
    9781260117103 (paperback ; alk. paper) | ISBN 9781260117110 (ebook)
Subjects: MESH: Mental Disorders--therapy | Mental Disorders—diagnosis |
    Nervous System Diseases--therapy | Nervous System Diseases—diagnosis |
    Neuropsychiatry—methods
Classification: LCC RC467 (print) | LCC RC467 (ebook) | NLM WM 400 | DDC
    616.89—dc23
LC record available at https://lccn.loc.gov/2020015682
LC ebook record available at https://lccn.loc.gov/2020015683

For Arielle, Joshua, and Emily, with deepest love and appreciation.
David A. Silbersweig

For Juana and Chase, with love.
Laura T. Safar

For Lise, Molly, and Jesse, with love and gratitude.
Kirk R. Daffner

Contents

SECTION V
Special Topics in Neuropsychiatry

Contributors

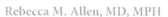

Rebecca M. Allen, MD, MPH
Partner, Director of Neuropsychiatry and Research
Seattle Neuropsychiatric Treatment Center
Seattle, Washington
Clinical Assistant Professor of Psychiatry
Department of Psychiatry and Behavioral Sciences
University of Washington
Seattle, Washington
15. Neuropsychiatry of Sleep and Sleep Disorders

Abby Altman, PhD
Associate Psychologist
Department of Psychiatry
Division of Geriatric Psychiatry
Psychology Lead, Behavioral Health
Program in Primary Care
Brigham and Women's Hospital
Instructor in Psychiatry
Harvard Medical School
Boston, Massachusetts
10. Psychosocial Interventions in Neuropsychiatry

Lindsay Barker, PhD, ABPP-CN
Clinical Neuropsychologist
Division of Cognitive and Behavioral Neurology
Partners Multiple Sclerosis Center
Brigham and Women's Hospital
Instructor in Psychiatry
Harvard Medical School
Boston, Massachusetts
27. Neuropsychiatry of Multiple Sclerosis

Gaston Baslet, MD
Chief, Division of Neuropsychiatry
Co-Director, Center for Brain/Mind Medicine
Brigham and Women's Hospital
Assistant Professor of Psychiatry
Harvard Medical School
Boston, Massachusetts
13. Functional Neurological Symptom Disorder
29. Neuropsychiatry of Epilepsy

Sheldon Benjamin, MD
Interim Chair of Psychiatry
Director of Neuropsychiatry and Residency Training
Professor of Psychiatry and Neurology
University of Massachusetts Medical School
Worcester, Massachusetts
5. Neuropsychiatric Assessment

Aaron L. Berkowitz, MD, PhD
Director of Global Health and Professor of Neurology
Kaiser Permanente Bernard J. Tyson School of Medicine
Pasadena, California
Past: Director, Global Neurology Program and
Associate Neurologist
Brigham and Women's Hospital
Boston, Massachusetts
38. Neuropsychiatry in Global Health

Kelsey D. Biddle, BA
Medical Student
Harvard Medical School
Boston, Massachusetts
Past: Clinical Research Assistant
Division of Geriatric Psychiatry
Department of Psychiatry
Brigham and Women's Hospital
Boston, Massachusetts
21. The Neuropsychiatry of Alzheimer's Disease

Katherine Brandt, MM
Director of the Caregiver Support Services and Public
Relations
MGH Frontotemporal Disorders Unit
Massachusetts General Hospital
Charlestown, Massachusetts
24. Frontotemporal Dementia

Montgomery C. Brower, MD
Department of Psychiatry
Saint Joseph Mercy Hospital
Ann Arbor, Michigan
34. Forensic Neuropsychiatry

Lorna Campbell, LICSW
Social Work Manager
Brigham Psychiatric Specialties,
Division of Cognitive and Behavioral Neurology,and
The Fish Center
Brigham and Women's Hospital
Boston, Massachusetts
10. Psychosocial Interventions in Neuropsychiatry

Kirk R. Daffner, MD, FAAN
Chief, Division of Cognitive and Behavioral Neurology
Director, Center for Brain/Mind Medicine
Stephen Muss Clinical Director of the Alzheimer Center
Brigham and Women's Hospital
J. David and Virginia Wimberly Professor of Neurology
Harvard Medical School
Boston, Massachusetts
Preface
*3. Functional Neurocircuitry of Cognition and Cognitive
Syndromes*
12. Focal Neurobehavioral Syndromes
39. Neuropsyciatry and Behavioral Neurology: Future Diredtions

Megan Dawson, MD
Psychiatrist
Massachusetts General Hospital
Past: Resident in Psychiatry
Harvard Longwood Psychiatry Residency Training Program
Brigham and Women's Hospital
Fellow in Geriartic Psychiatry, Partners Healthcare
Harvard Medical School
Boston, Massachusetts
31. Neuropsychiatry of Pain

Bradford C. Dickerson, MD
Director, MGH Frontotemporal Disorders Unit
Tom Rickles Chair in Primary Progressive Aphasia Research
Massachusetts General Hospital
Charlestown, Massachusetts
Professor of Neurology
Harvard Medical School
Boston, Massachusetts
24. Frontotemporal Dementia

Nancy J. Donovan, MD
Director, Division of Geriatric Psychiatry
Departments of Psychiatry and Neurology
Brigham and Women's Hospital
Associate Researcher, Department of Psychiatry
Massachusetts General Hospital
Assistant Professor of Medicine
Harvard Medical School
Boston, Massachusetts
21. The Neuropsychiatry of Alzheimer's Disease

Barbara A. Dworetzky, MD
Chief, Division of Epilepsy
Brigham and Women's Hospital
Professor of Neurology
Harvard Medical School
Boston, Massachusetts
13. Functional Neurological Symptom Disorder

Renana Eitan, MD
Senior Lecturer
The Hebrew University Hadassah Medical School
Director, Neuropsychiatry Unit
The Jerusalem Mental Health Center
Jerusalem, Israel
Visiting Researcher
Brigham and Women's Hospital
*11. Mood, Psychotic, Anxiety, and Obsessive-Compulsive
Disorders: A Neuropsychiatric Foundation*

Mark Eldaief, MD, MMSc
Associate Neurologist
Departments of Neurology and Psychiatry
Massachusetts General Hospital
Harvard University FAS Center for Brain Science
Cambridge, Massachusetts
Associate Professor of Neurology
Harvard Medical School
Boston, Massachusetts
9. Neurostimulation Therapies in Neuropsychiatry

Jane Erb, MD
Associate Psychiatrist
Brigham and Women's Hospital
Psychiatric Director, Behavioral Health Integration
Clinical Director, Brigham Depression Center
Assistant Professor of Psychiatry
Harvard Medical School
Boston, Massachusetts
8. Psychopharmacology in Neuropsychiatric Syndromes
*36. Integration of Neuropsychiatric Care in Primary Care and
Other Medical Settings*

Michael Erkkinen, MD
Medical Director, Memory and Aging Center
Assistant Professor of Clinical Neurology
University of California, San Francisco
San Francisco, CA
Past: Staff Neurologist, Center for Brain/Mind Medicine
Brigham and Women's Hospital
Boston, Massachusetts
*3. Functional Neurocircuitry of Cognition and Cognitive
Syndromes*
12. Focal Neurobehavioral Syndromes

Angela Essa, BS
Psychiatric and Neurodevelopmental Genetics Unit
Center for Genomic Medicine
Massachusetts General Hospital
Boston, Massachusetts
19. Tourette Syndrome and Related Neuropsychiatric Disorders

Nicole C. Feng, BA
Medical Student, Eastern Virginia Medical School
Norfolk, Virginia
Past:
Clinical Research Assistant
Laboratory of Healthy Cognitive Aging
Center for Brain/Mind Medicine
Brigham and Women's Hospital
Department of Neurology
Brigham and Women's Hospital
Boston, Massachusetts
27. Neuropsychiatry of Multiple Sclerosis

Barry S. Fogel, MD
Associate Neurologist and Psychiatrist
Center for Brain/Mind Medicine
Brigham and Women's Hospital
Professor of Psychiatry, Part-time
Harvard Medical School
Boston, Massachusetts
35. Holistic and Sustainable Management of Complex Neuropsychiatric Patients

Benjamin Fuchs, MD
Resident (PGY-4),
Departments of Neurology and Psychiatry
New York University School of Medicine
New York, New York
32. The Neuropsychiatry of Headache

Seth Gale, MD
Associate Neurologist
Division of Cognitive and Behavioral Neurology
Director, Program in Brain Health
Brigham and Women's Hospital
Instructor of Neurology
Department of Neurology
Center for Brain/Mind Medicine
Harvard Medical School
Boston, Massachusetts
8. Psychopharmacology in Neuropsychiatric Syndromes
16. ADHD and Executive Function Disorders

Anna E. Goodheart, MD
Clinical and Research Fellow
Department of Neurology
Brigham and Women's Hospital
Massachusetts General Hospital
Boston, Massachusetts
6. Neuroimaging in Clinical Neuropsychiatry

Deborah Green, PhD, ABPP
Clinical Neuropsychologist
Department of Neurology
Brigham and Women's Hospital
Instructor of Psychiatry
Harvard Medical School
Boston, Massachusetts
7. Neuropsychological Evaluation in Neuropsychiatry

Erica L. Greenberg, MD
Pediatric Psychiatry OCD and Tic Disorders Program
Department of Psychiatry
Massachusetts General Hospital
Instructor in Psychiatry
Harvard Medical School
Boston, Massachusetts
19. Tourette Syndrome and Related Neuropsychiatric Disorders

Rahul Gupta, MD
Associate Psychiatrist
Brigham and Women's Faulkner Hospital
Instructor in Psychiatry
Harvard Medical School
Boston, Massachusetts
28. Neuropsychiatric Complications of Cancer and Its Treatments

Jessica Harder, MD
Associate Psychiatrist
Division of Neuropsychiatry, Department of Psychiatry
Brigham and Women's Hospital
Instructor in Psychiatry
Harvard Medical School
Boston, Massachusetts
26. Neuropsychiatry of Inflammatory, Autoimmune, and Infectious Disorders

Aaron J. Hauptman, MD
Attending Psychiatrist, Department of Psychiatry
Boston Children's Hospital
Assistant Professor of Psychiatry
Harvard Medical School
Boston, Massachusetts
17. Neuropsychiatry of Autism Spectrum Disorder

Tamar Katz, MD, PhD
Boston Children's Hospital Department of Psychiatry
Brigham and Women's Hospital Division of Neuropsychiatry
Instructor in Psychiatry
Harvard Medical School
Boston, Massachusetts
26. Neuropsychiatry of Inflammatory, Autoimmune, and Infectious Disorders

Christopher J. Keary, MD
Behavioral Director, Angelman Syndrome Behavioral Clinic
Associate Program Director, Multidisciplinary Clinic
for Children,
Adolescents & Adults w/ Autism Spectrum Disorder
Staff Psychiatrist, Lurie Center for Autism Massachusetts
General Hospital for Children
Instructor in Psychiatry
Harvard Medical School
Boston, Massachusetts
18. Intellectual Developmental Disorders

Hema Kher, MD, MPH
Resident in Psychiatry
Brigham and Women's Hospital/Harvard Medical School
Psychiatry Residency Program
Brigham and Women's Hospital
Harvard Medical School
Boston, Massachusetts
21. The Neuropsychiatry of Alzheimer's Disease

Jung Won Kim, MD
Child and Adolescent Psychiatrist
Boston Children's Hospital
Boston, Massachusetts
18. Intellectual Developmental Disorders

Joshua P. Klein, MD, PhD
Vice Chair, Clinical Affairs
Chief, Division of Hospital Neurology
Department of Neurology
Brigham and Women's Hospital
Associate Professor of Neurology and Radiology
Harvard Medical School
Boston, Massachusetts
6. Neuroimaging in Clinical Neuropsychiatry

Nomi C. Levy-Carrick, MD, MPhil
Associate Vice Chair, Ambulatory Services
Associate Psychiatrist, Division of Medical Psychiatry
Department of Psychiatry
Brigham and Women's Hospital
Co-Chair, Mass General Brigham Trauma Informed Care Initiative
Assistant Professor of Psychiatry
Harvard Medical School
Boston, Massachusetts
25. Delirium and Catatonia
38. Neuropsychiatry in Global Health

Brady B. Lonergan, MD
Assistant Professor
University of Connecticut Health Center
Department of Psychiatry
Past: Consultation-Liason Psychiatry Fellow
Department of Psychiatry
Brigham and Women's Hospital
Boston, Massachusetts
8. Psychopharmacology in Neuropsychiatric Syndromes

Diane E. Lucente, MS, CGC
Genetic Counseling Manager
Center for Genomic Medicine
Department of Neurology
Massachusetts General Hospital
Boston, Massachusetts
24. Frontotemporal Dementia

Tatenda Mahlanza, BSc Hons
Clinical Research Assistant
Ann Romney Center for Neurologic Diseases
Department of Neurology
Brigham and Women's Hospital
Boston, Massachusetts
36. Integration of Neuropsychiatric Care in Primary Care and Other Medical Settings

Timothy Mariano, MD, PhD, MSc
Associate Investigator and Staff Psychiatrist
Center for Neurorestoration and Neurotechnology
Providence Veterans Affairs Medical Center
Providence, Rhode Island
Adjunct Assistant Professor of Psychiatry and
Human Behavior
Brown University
Providence, Rhode Island
Past: Department of Psychiatry
Brigham and Women's Hospital
Harvard Medical School
Boston, Massachusetts
9. Neurostimulation Therapies in Neuropsychiatry

Thomas W. McAllister, MD
Albert Eugene Sterne Professor and Chair
Department of Psychiatry
Indiana University School of Medicine
Indianapolis, Indiana
30. Neuropsychiatry of Traumatic Brain Injury

Christopher J. McDougle, MD
Director, Lurie Center for Autism
Massachusetts General Hospital
Nancy Lurie Marks Professor of Psychiatry
Harvard Medical School
Boston, Massachusetts
17. Neuropsychiatry of Autism Spectrum Disorder
18. Intellectual Developmental Disorders

Scott M. McGinnis, MD
Associate Neurologist
Center for Brain/Mind Medicine
and Center for Alzheimer Research and Treatment
Department of Neurology
Brigham & Women's Hospital
MGH Frontotemporal Disorders Unit
Department of Neurology
Massachusetts General Hospital
Associate Professor of Neurology
Harvard Medical School
Boston, Massachusetts
20. Approach to Neurocognitive Disorders

Fremonta L. Meyer, MD
Staff Psychiatrist
Brigham and Women's Hospital
Assistant Professor of Psychiatry
Harvard Medical School
Boston, Massachusetts
28. Neuropsychiatric Complications of Cancer and Its Treatments

Mia Minen, MD, MPH, FAHS
Chief of Headache Research
Department of Neurology
New York University School of Medicine
New York, New York
32. The Neuropsychiatry of Headache

Damien Miran, MD
Department of Psychosocial Oncology and Palliative Care
Dana-Farber Cancer Institute
Division of Medical Psychiatry
Brigham and Women's Hospital
Instructor in Psychiatry
Harvard Medical School
Boston, Massachusetts
31. Neuropsychiatry of Pain

Elizabeth Misasi, LICSW
Clinical Social Worker
Partners Multiple Sclerosis Center
Brigham and Women's Hospital
Boston, Massachusetts
27. Neuropsychiatry of Multiple Sclerosis

Leena Mittal, MD, FACLP
Director, Division of Women's Mental Health
Department of Psychiatry
Brigham and Women's Hospital
Instructor in Psychiatry
Harvard Medical School
Boston, Massachusetts
33. Women's Neuropsychiatry

Laura Morrissey, LICSW
Clinical Social Worker in Neuropsychiatry
Brigham and Women's Hospital
Boston, Massachusetts
10. Psychosocial Interventions in Neuropsychiatry

Margo Nathan, MD
Department of Psychiatry
Division of Women's Mental Health
Brigham and Women's Hospital
Instructor in Psychiatry
Harvard Medical School
Boston, Massachusetts
33. Women's Neuropsychiatry

Aaron P. Nelson, PhD, ABPP-CN
Retired Chief of Neuropsychology, Division of Cognitive and Behavioral Neurology, Brigham and Women's Hospital
Assistant Professor of Psychiatry, Harvard Medical School
Boston, Massachusetts
7. Neuropsychological Evaluation in Neuropsychiatry

Lisa Nowinski, PhD
Director of Clinical Services and Psychology Training
Lurie Center for Autism
Massachusetts General Hospital for Children
Instructor in Psychology in the Department of Psychiatry
Harvard Medical School
Boston, Massachusetts
18. Intellectual Developmental Disorders

Mary A. O'Neal, MD
Associate Neurologist
Brigham and Women's Hospital
Assistant Professor of Neurology
Harvard Medical School
Boston, Massachusetts
13. Functional Neurological Symptom Disorder
33. Women's Neuropsychiatry

Michelle L. Palumbo, MD
Assistant Pediatrician
Massachusetts General Hospital for Children
Instructor in Pediatrics
Harvard Medical School
Boston, Massachusetts
18. Intellectual Developmental Disorders

Palak Patel, MD
Departments of Neurology and Psychiatry
New York University School of Medicine
New York, New York
32. The Neuropsychiatry of Headache

Milena Pavlova, MD, FAASM
Medical Director, Faulkner Sleep Testing Center
Associate Neurologist, Department of Neurology
Brigham and Women's Hospital
Assistant Professor of Neurology
Harvard Medical School
Boston, Massachusetts
15. Neuropsychiatry of Sleep and Sleep Disorders

Ginger Polich, MD
Physical Medicine and Rehabilitation
Spaulding Rehabilitation Hospital
Charlestown, Massachusetts
Instructor in Physical Medicine and Rehabilitation
Harvard Medical School
Boston, Massachusetts
30. Neuropsychiatry of Traumatic Brain Injury

Laura C. Politte, MD
Associate Psychiatrist
Carolina Institute for Developmental Disabilities
Carborro, NC
Assistant Professor in Psychiatry
University of North Carolina
Carrboro, North Carolina
18. Intellectual Developmental Disorders

Deepti Putcha, PhD
Associate Neuropsychologist
Center for Brain/Mind Medicine
Brigham and Women's Hospital
MGH Frontotemporal Disorders Unit
Charlestown, Massachusetts
Instructor in Psychiatry
Harvard Medical School
Boston, Massachusetts
Frontotemporal Disorders Unit
Massachusetts General Hospital
Charlestown, Massachusetts
3. Functional Neurocircuitry of Cognition and Cognitive Syndromes
12. Focal Neurobehavioral Syndromes

Megan Quimby, MS, CCC-SLP
Director of the Speech-Language Program
MGH Frontotemporal Disorders Unit
Massachusetts General Hospital
Charlestown, Massachusetts
24. Frontotemporal Dementia

Shreya Raj, MD
Associate Psychiatrist
Division of Neuropsychiatry
Department of Psychiatry
Brigham and Women's Hospital
Instructor in Psychiatry
Harvard Medical School
Boston, Massachusetts
8. Psychopharmacology in Neuropsychiatric Syndromes

Katiuska J. Ramirez, MD
Associate Psychiatrist
Department of Psychiatry
Brigham and Women's Hospital
Instructor in Psychiatry
Harvard Medical School
Boston, Massachusetts
23. The Neuropsychiatry of Parkinson's Disease and Dementia with Lewy Bodies

Geoffrey Raynor, MD
Associate Neuropsychiatrist
Department of Psychiatry
Division of Neuropsychiatry
Brigham and Women's Hospital
Instructor in Psychiatry
Harvard Medical School
Boston, Massachusetts
2. Functional Neurocircuitry of Affective and Behavioral Processes and Neuropsychiatric Syndromes
16. ADHD and Executive Function Disorders

James O. Robbins
Medical Student
Warren Alpert Medical School of Brown University
Providence, Rhode Island
17. Neuropsychiatry of Autism Spectrum Disorder

Diana M. Robinson, MD
Associate Psychiatrist
Division of Consultation-Liaison Psychiatry
Parkland Memorial Hospital
Assistant Professor of Psychiatry
University of Texas Southwestern Medical School
Dallas, Texas
Past: Consultation-Liaison Psychiatry Fellow
Department of Psychiatry
Brigham and Women's Hospital
Boston, Massachusetts
38. Neuropsychiatry in Global Health

Claudia P. Rodriguez, MD
Director of Addiction Services
Brigham and Women's Faulkner Hospital
Associate Psychiatrist
Brigham and Women's Hospital
Instructor in Psychiatry
Harvard Medical School
Boston, Massachusetts
14. Addiction as a Neuropsychiatric Disease

Laura T. Safar, MD
Vice Chair of Psychiatry
Lahey Hospital and Medical Center
Associate Neuropsychiatrist, Brigham and Women's Hospital
Assistant Professor of Psychiatry
Harvard Medical School
Boston, Massachusetts
Preface
8. Psychopharmacology in Neuropsychiatric Syndromes
10. Psychosocial Interventions in Neuropsychiatry
22. The Neuropsychiatry of Stroke
27. Neuropsychiatry of Multiple Sclerosis
31. Neuropsychiatry of Pain
*36. Integration of Neuropsychiatric Care in Primary Care and
Other Medical Settings*
39. Neuropsychiatry and Behavioral Neurology: Future Directions

Kate Salama, MD
Staff Psychiatrist
Department of Psychiatry
Division of Women's Mental Health
Brigham and Women's Hospital
Instructor in Psychiatry
Harvard Medical School
Boston, Massachusetts
33. Women's Neuropsychiatry

Rani Sarkis, MD, MSc
Associate Neurologist, Division of Epilepsy
Department of Neurology
Brigham and Women's Hospital
Assistant Professor of Neurology,
Harvard Medical School
Boston, Massachusetts
29. Neuropsychiatry of Epilepsy

Jeremiah M. Scharf, MD, PhD
Tic Disorders Unit, Division of Movement Disorders
Psychiatric and Neurodevelopmental Genetics Unit
Center for Genomic Medicine
Departments of Neurology and Psychiatry
Massachusetts General Hospital
Center for Brain/Mind Medicine
Department of Neurology
Brigham & Women's Hospital
Assistant Professor of Neurology
Harvard Medical School
Boston, Massachusetts
*19. Tourette Syndrome and Related Neuropsychiatric
Disorders*

Barbara Schildkrout, MD, FANPA
Assistant Professor of Psychiatry, Part-time
Harvard Medical School
Brigham and Women's Hospital
Department of Psychiatry
Boston, Massachusetts
37. Individualized Psychotherapy with the Neuropsychiatric Patient

Jeremy D. Schmahmann, MD, FAAN, FANA, FANPA
Founding Director, Massachusetts General Hospital Ataxia Center
Director, Laboratory for Neuroanatomy and
Cerebellar Neurobiology
Cognitive Behavioral Neurology Unit
Department of Neurology,
Massachusetts General Hospital
Professor of Neurology,
Harvard Medical School
Boston, Massachusetts
*1. Neuroanatomical Foundations of Neuropsychiatry and
Behavioral Neurology*

Hope Schwartz, BS
Medical Student
University of California, San Francisco
San Francisco, CA
Past: Clinical Research Assistant, Laboratory of
Healthy Cognitive Aging
Center for Brain/Mind Medicine, Brigham and Women's Hospital
Department of Neurology, Brigham and Women's Hospital
Boston, Massachusetts
22. The Neuropsychiatry of Stroke
*36. Integration of Neuropsychiatric Care in Primary Care and
Other Medical Settings*

Meghan Searl, PhD
Clinical Neuropsychologist
Brigham and Women's Hospital
Instructor in Psychiatry
Harvard Medical School
Boston, Massachusetts
10. Psychosocial Interventions in Neuropsychiatry

Sejal B. Shah, MD
Chief, Division of Medical Psychiatry
Associate Vice Chair, Clinical Consultation Services
Brigham and Women's Hospital
Instructor in Psychiatry, Harvard Medical School
Boston, Massachusetts
25. Delirium and Catatonia

David A. Silbersweig, MD
Chairman, Department of Psychiatry
Co-Director, Center for the Neurosciences
Brigham and Women's Hospital
Stanley Cobb Professor of Psychiatry
Harvard Medical School
Boston, Massachusetts
Preface
*2. Functional Neurocircuitry of Affective and Behavioral
Processes and Neuropsychiatric Syndromes*
*4. The Value and Therapeutic Power of the Neuropsychiatric
Diagnostic Evaluation*
*11. Mood, Psychotic, Anxiety, and Obsessive-Compulsive Disor-
ders: A Neuropsychiatric Foundation*
*39. Neuropsychiatry and Behavioral Neurology: Future
Directions*

Tarun Singhal, MD
Director, PET Imaging Program in Beurologic Disease
Ann Romney Center for Neurologic Diseases
Associate Neurologist
Partners Multiple Sclerosis Center
Department of Neurology
Brigham and Women's Hospital
Assistant Professor of Neurology
Harvard Medical School
Boston, Massachusetts
27. Neuropsychiatry of Multiple Sclerosis

Irina A. Skylar-Scott, MD
Clinical Assistant Professor in Neurology
Center for Memory Disorders
Stanford University School of Medicine
Past: Cognitive and Behavioral Neurology Fellow
Center for Brain/Mind Medicine
Brigham and Women's Hospital
Harvard Medical School
Boston, Massachusetts
23. The Neuropsychiatry of Parkinson's Disease and Dementia
with Lewy Bodies
26. Neuropsychiatry of Inflammatory, Autoimmune, and
Infectious Disorders

Stephanie L. Smith, MD
Attending Psychiatrist
Division of Medical Psychiatry, Department of Psychiatry
Brigham and Women's Hospital
Associate Director, Mental Health
Partners In Health
Department of Global Health and Social Medicine
Instructor in Psychiatry
Harvard Medical School
Boston, Massachusetts
38. Neuropsychiatry in Global Health

Ian Steele, MD
Assistant Professor, Division of Consultation-Liaison
Psychiatry
Department of Psychiatry and Behavioral Medicine
Froedtert Hospital
Medical College of Wisconsin
Milwaukee, Wisconsin
25. Delirium and Catatonia

Emily Stern, MD
CEO, Ceretype Neuromedicine, Inc.
Departments of Radiology and Psychiatry
Brigham and Women's Hospital
Associate Professor of Radiology
Harvard Medical School
Boston, Massachusetts
2. Functional Neurocircuitry of Affective and Behavioral
Processes and Neuropsychiatric Syndromes

John Sullivan, MD
Medical Director, Adult Mental Health Unit
UMass Memorial Medical Center
Assistant Professor of Psychiatry and Neurology
University of Massachusetts Medical School
Worcester, Massachusetts
Past: Staff Psychiatrist, Brigham and Women's Hospital
22. The Neuropsychiatry of Stroke
23. The Neuropsychiatry of Parkinson's Disease and Dementia
with Lewy Bodies

Joji Suzuki, MD
Director, Division of Addiction Psychiatry
Department of Psychiatry
Brigham and Women's Hospital
Assistant Professor of Psychiatry, Harvard Medical School
Boston, Massachusetts
14. Addiction as a Neuropsychiatric Disease

Daniel Talmasov, MD
Resident in Neurology
Department of Neurology
New York University School of Medicine
New York, New York
Past: Resident in Psychiatry/DuPont-Warren Fellow
Department of Psychiatry
Brigham and Women's Hospital
Boston, Massachusetts
22. The Neuropsychiatry of Stroke

Adrienne D. Taylor, MD
Associate Director, Division of Medical Psychiatry
Department of Psychiatry
Brigham and Women's Hospital
Instructor in Psychiatry
Harvard Medical School
Boston, Massachusetts
23. The Neuropsychiatry of Parkinson's Disease and Dementia
with Lewy Bodies

Robyn Thom, MD
Child and Adolescent Psychiatry Fellow
Massachusetts General Hospital
Boston, Massachusetts
25. Delirium and Catatonia

Stephanie Tung, MD
Psychiatrist, Dana-Farber Cancer Institute, Brigham and
Women's Hospital
Instructor in Psychiatry, Harvard Medical School
Boston, Massachusetts
28. Neuropsychiatric Complications of Cancer and Its
Treatments

Mascha van't Wout-Frank, PhD
Center for Neurorestoration and Neurotechnology
Providence VA Medical Center
Associate Professor (Research)
Department of Psychiatry and Human Behavior
Alpert Medical School of Brown University
Providence, Rhode Island
9. Neurostimulation Therapies in Neuropsychiatry

Halyna Vitagliano, MD, MSci
Senior Physician
Department of Psychosocial Oncology and Palliative Care
Dana-Farber Cancer Institute
Attending Psychiatrist
Brigham and Women's Hospital
Assistant Professor of Psychiatry
Harvard Medical School
Boston, Massachusetts
28. Neuropsychiatric Complications of Cancer and Its Treatments

Victor Wang, MD, PhD
Division Chief, Pain Neurology
Medical Director, Brigham and Women's Milford Pain Center
Department of Neurology
Department of Anesthesia, Perioperative and Pain Medicine
Brigham and Women's Hospital
Instructor in Neurology
Harvard Medical School
Boston, Massachusetts
31. Neuropsychiatry of Pain

Daniel Weisholtz, MD
Associate Neurologist, Division of Epilepsy
Brigham and Women's Hospital
Instructor in Neurology, Harvard Medical School
Boston, Massachusetts
29. Neuropsychiatry of Epilepsy

Kim Willment, PhD, ABBP
Clinical Neuropsychologist
Brigham and Women's Hospital
Instructor in Psychiatry
Harvard Medical School
Boston, Massachusetts
10. Psychosocial Interventions in Neuropsychiatry

Bonnie Wong, PhD /ABPP-CN
Director of the Neuropsychology Program
MGH Frontotemporal Disorders Unit
Massachusetts General Hospital
Charlestown, Massachusetts
Instructor in Psychiatry
Harvard Medical School
Boston, Massachusetts
24. Frontotemporal Dementia

Preface

Neuropsychiatry and Behavioral Neurology: Principles and Practice is a clinically-oriented textbook that aims to link rapid advances in basic, cognitive, and affective neuroscience with the care of patients struggling with losses that often involve their most cherished human capacities. The work was inspired by an annual Harvard Medical School course on the same topic that the editors and their colleagues at Brigham and Women's Hospital initiated in 2014.

Neuropsychiatric and behavioral neurologic diseases are common, challenging, and extraordinarily fascinating. The symptoms of patients with these disorders can be puzzling to clinicians and result in individuals seeing numerous psychiatrists and neurologists before an appropriate diagnosis is made. The number of patients at risk for struggling with these disorders is rising, in part due to our increasingly aging population. At the same time, basic and translational research within the clinical neurosciences has been growing at exponential pace, which has important implications for the ways in which patients are and will be evaluated, diagnosed, treated, and followed. Given these converging trends, this is an opportune time to take stock of the field and provide guidance for understanding a rapidly expanding body of knowledge and the ways in which it can be meaningfully translated into clinical practice.

Our textbook relies on the perspective of authors who have a deep reservoir of clinical experience that helps them to synthesize and convey complex information about structural and functional neural networks most relevant to the practice of neuropsychiatry and behavioral neurology. These experts have utilized their experience caring for patients to refine their understanding of mechanisms underlying brain function and disease, and have endeavored to use their knowledge about underlying neural circuitry to inform their understanding of the emotional, cognitive, and behavioral difficulties facing their patients.

Several fundamental principles have served as guideposts for this textbook.

- First, given the complexity of the subject matter, inferences drawn about cerebral organization and function should be based on converging evidence from a variety of sources. These include experimental neuroanatomy, single cell recordings in awake behaving monkeys, depth electrode studies in humans, electrophysiologic, positron emission tomography (PET), and functional magnetic resonance imaging (fMRI) activity elicited while humans are participating in cognitive/experimental tasks, structural MRI delineating the distribution of changes in cortical volume, cortical thickness, and white matter integrity, resting state functional connectivity MRI (rs-fcMRI) characterizing intrinsic networks of the brain, and information derived from patients with focal lesions that disrupt specific neural networks.

- Second, given the complexity of clinical cases, a multidisciplinary approach is the most appropriate one for understanding the different contributions to the challenges facing our patients and delineating potential avenues for therapy, remediation, compensatory activity, and healing.

- Third, multidisciplinary work is most likely to be successful when efforts are made to foster an abiding respect for the knowledge and perspective offered by specialists outside of our own area of expertise and to work together to integrate approaches. Over the last 25 years, leaders of our group have endeavored to create an academic community that places a very high value on the process of listening to and learning from members with different subspecialty training and expertise. In keeping with this approach, the authors of chapters in this textbook represent the core disciplines of our Center for Brain/Mind Medicine, including neuropsychiatry, behavioral neurology, geriatric psychiatry, neuropsychology, clinical psychology, social work, and physiatry. In addition, chapters have been written by colleagues from related fields with whom we have close affiliations, including psychopharmacology, neuroradiology, child psychiatry, forensic psychiatry, speech and language pathology, sleep medicine, epilepsy, immunology, women's mental health, global health, and pain management.

- Fourth, the growing subspecialization and number of topics within the purview of neuropsychiatry and behavioral neurology, coupled with the explosion of information from the disciplines of cognitive and affective neuroscience, genetics, and psychotherapeutics, to name a few, make it difficult for individuals to have comprehensive knowledge about all these relevant fields. In this context, we are susceptible to getting lost in the myriad of details that are disseminated, losing sight of the big picture. It is more critical than ever to have access to an overview that can provide user-friendly frameworks for making sense of and accommodating new information. The editors have a deep appreciation for the value of chapters that distill large bodies of complex information. From our perspective, an outstanding chapter by experts can be viewed as a kind of gift to the rest of us.

■ Finally, this textbook was written with our colleagues and trainees in mind, who, like us, are passionate about understanding the principles and practice of neuropsychiatry and behavioral neurology. We have endeavored to provide our readers with comprehensive coverage of critical topics in the field to satisfy their (and our) thirst for knowledge and desire for improved clinical care, as well as the more pragmatic objective of preparing for the United Council of Neurologic Subspecialties (UCNS) board exam. Summary points, case vignettes, and multiple choice questions are included throughout the textbook to enhance its didactic quality.

It is very challenging to maintain uniformity in a textbook with many different authors. In an effort to enhance structural consistency and quality across chapters, each one underwent an elaborate, iterative editing and feedback process. Once a chapter was submitted by the authors, it was reviewed by at least three editors/co-editors. After each review by an editor, a version of the manuscript was returned to the authors for revisions, which upon being acceptable to that editor, was forwarded to the next editor. This elaborate system resulted in most chapters undergoing at least five revisions; some chapters had up to ten versions. We thank the authors for their patience and hard work. We believe that the process contributed to an outstanding finished product.

The textbook aims to be comprehensive, clinically relevant, and accessible to individuals with different training and academic backgrounds. **Section I** provides a foundation for understanding neuropsychiatry and behavioral neurology through a review of structural and functional neuroanatomy. Chapter 1, which masterfully ties together historical, phylogenetic, neurobiological and clinical perspectives, is devoted to the neuroanatomic basis of cognition, behavior, and emotion. We strongly anticipate that this chapter will serve as a definitive piece of work in our field. The following two chapters address the functional neurocircuitry of affective, behavioral and cognitive processing, and the neuropsychiatric and cognitive syndromes that arise from disruptions to these systems. **Section II** turns to an overview of different methods for conducting neuropsychiatric assessments. The topic is introduced with a discussion of how a thoughtful, engaging neuropsychiatric evaluation can both facilitate a more complete understanding of a patient's difficulties and serve as a powerful therapeutic tool (Chapter 4). Subsequent chapters address office assessments (based on the active generation and testing of hypotheses) (Chapter 5), neuroimaging techniques (Chapter 6), and neuropsychological evaluations (Chapter 7). **Section III** provides an overview of therapeutics for treating neuropsychiatric and cognitive disorders. Individual chapters are dedicated to psychopharmacological approaches (Chapter 8), neurostimulation (Chapter 9), and psychosocial interventions, including modifications in psychotherapy when working with neuropsychiatric patients, and cognitive rehabilitation (Chapter 10).

Section IV is the most extensive one in the textbook, which is comprised of 22 chapters. The first half of this section examines neurobehavioral and neuropsychiatric syndromes, and the second half tackles the neuropsychiatric aspects of different neurological and medical diseases. Chapter 11 offers a neuropsychiatric perspective on the mechanisms underlying core psychiatric disorders involving mood, anxiety, and psychosis. Chapter 12 reviews how injury to specific anatomical networks leads to common neurobehavioral syndromes. The next set of chapters addresses the growing number of the clinical entities that neuropsychiatrists and behavioral neurologists are being called upon to assess and manage. These include functional neurological disorders (Chapter 13), addiction disorders (Chapter 14), sleep disorders (Chapter 15), ADHD and executive function disorders (Chapter 16), autism spectrum disorder (Chapter 17), intellectual development disorders (Chapter 18), and Tourette syndrome and related neuropsychiatric disorders (Chapter 19).

The purpose of Chapter 20 is to introduce a practical approach for clinicians who assess patients with neurocognitive disorders. The chapters that follow review the neuropsychiatric manifestations of a range of common neurological and medical conditions, including Alzheimer's disease (Chapter 21), stroke (Chapter 22), Parkinson's disease and Dementia with Lewy Bodies (Chapter 23), frontotemporal dementia (Chapter 24), delirium and catatonia (Chapter 25), immune-mediated and infectious diseases (Chapter 26), multiple sclerosis (Chapter 27), cancer (Chapter 28), epilepsy (Chapter 29), traumatic brain injury (Chapter 30), pain (Chapter 31), and headache (Chapter 32).

In **Section V**, other critical issues involving our field are addressed. The topics examined include women's neuropsychiatry (Chapter 33), forensic neuropsychiatry (Chapter 34), a holistic and sustainable approach to caring for complex neuropsychiatric patients (Chapter 35), the integration of neuropsychiatric care in other medical settings like primary care (Chapter 36), a discussion of patient individuality as it pertains to neuropsychiatry and psychotherapy (Chapter 37), and the role of neuropsychiatry in global health (Chapter 38). The final chapter considers future directions for the fields of neuropsychiatry and behavioral neurology.

A major goal of this textbook is to help clinicians 1) link alterations in emotion, cognition, and behavior to their neurobiological origins, 2) place the unique aspects of a patient's illness within a broader context that emphasizes the role of underlying neurocircuitry, 3) develop informed differential diagnoses, and 4) plan and implement the most effective treatment strategies. At the same time, the textbook provides an opportunity for researchers to gain a more textured appreciation of clinical behavioral neuroscience and the different ways in which dysfunction of various neural networks impact the lives of patients. We hope to expand a common vocabulary across related disciplines to enhance communication and a greater sense of shared purpose between clinicians from different disciplines and with colleagues who primarily serve as investigators.

Given the breadth and complexity of the material, editing a textbook on neuropsychiatry and behavioral neurology is a daunting task. We are extremely grateful to the authors of each of the chapters. We set high standards and required more work than is typically asked of individuals preparing chapters for a textbook. Authors were remarkably receptive to the questions raised and feedback provided. All of us learned a lot in the process. Editors and authors alike feel indebted to our patients who help us refine our understanding of brain function and the impact of various interventions. We hope that one way to show our gratitude to patients is by promulgating information about neuropsychiatry and behavioral neurology that can improve clinical care.

We would like to thank our colleagues Gaston Baslet, Scott McGinnis, and Shreya Raj, who provided help in reviewing early drafts of several chapters. We would like to acknowledge the invaluable assistance we received from McGraw-Hill and its editorial staff, especially Andrew Moyer (senior editor) and Ishan Chaudhary (project manager). We are also thankful for the superb administrative help provided by Eva Maynard, Jayme Paynter, and Brittany McFeeley at Brigham and Women's Hospital.

The editors feel indebted to our mentors, who inspired us to enter the field and profoundly influenced our ways of thinking about it. In this context, Kirk Daffner offers special thanks to Marsel Mesulam, Sandra Weintraub, Martin Samuels, David Dawson, Michael Ronthal, Bruce Price, Kenneth Heilman, and the late Norman Geschwind. Laura Safar extends her appreciation to Jacinto Armando as a representative of her mentors in Buenos Aires; Boris Astrachan, Ovidio De Leon, and Laura Miller, as representatives of many mentors in Chicago; and Ben Liptzin, David Silbersweig and Kirk Daffner, as representatives of the many colleagues in Massachusetts who have further nurtured her love for clinical work and academic medicine. David Silbersweig acknowledges the important role that Fred Plum, Jerome Posner, Robert Michels, Jack Barchas, Richard Frackowiak, and Chris Frith played in the development of his career. In addition, we acknowledge the tremendous impact that our trainees have had on our approach to synthesizing and conveying the most essential components of neuropsychiatry, behavioral neurology, and neuropsychology. We also would like to thank our families for their ongoing support and wisdom, including Lise Bliss, Jesse Daffner, Molly Daffner-Deming, and Adam Daffner-Deming, Gregg Daffner, and the late Joseph and Adele Daffner (Dr. Daffner), Juana Martinez, Chase H. Harrison, Hugo Safar, Silvia Safar, Diego Safar, and the late Hector Safar (Dr. Safar), and Emily Stern, Arielle Silbersweig, Joshua Silbersweig, Martin Silbersweig, Jean Silbersweig, Susan Riedel, and Laurie Silbersweig. Finally, all of us recognize that given the rapid pace of change in our fields, some of the information in the textbook will not be fully up to date even as it is published. However, we hope that although components will require updating, the basic framework provided will endure, and continue to offer a guide for clinicians caring for patients with neuropsychiatric and behavioral neurologic symptoms. We look forward to the opportunity of revising the material in future editions of the textbook.

David A. Silbersweig
Laura T. Safar
Kirk R. Daffner
Brigham and Women's Hospital
Harvard Medical School
Boston, Massachusetts

Structural and Functional Neuroanatomy

I

Neuroanatomical Foundations of Neuropsychiatry and Behavioral Neurology

Jeremy D. Schmahmann

INTRODUCTION

The cerebral cortex contains ~20% of the approximately 100 billion neurons in the central nervous system,[1] arranged in multiple distinct areas characterized extensively with respect to their morphological and cellular specialization. The architecture of each of these cortical areas subserves functionally distinct domains of sensorimotor perception and action, complex reasoning, and emotional experience.

It is estimated that approximately 70% of the neurons in the central nervous system are located within the cerebellum, most of which are in the cerebellar granule cell layer. This underappreciated fact is consistent with the recognition that the cerebral cortex does not support nervous system function in isolation, and that all behaviors are subserved by distributed neural systems that comprise anatomic regions, or nodes, each displaying unique architectural properties, distributed geographically throughout cortical and subcortical areas, and linked anatomically and functionally in a precise and unique manner.[2–16] Neuropsychiatric/neurobehavioral syndromes following lesions of cerebral white matter and subcortical regions, and demonstration of abnormalities in subcortical as well as cortical areas in imaging studies of psychiatric disorders provide clinical correlates of these distributed neural circuits.

Understanding the neuroanatomy of cognition is essential to the evaluation and care of patients with neurobehavioral and neuropsychiatric disorders. Anatomical textbooks, focused monographs, review papers, and the primary literature, many of which are included here in the reference section and which informed this work, contain extensive information regarding each of the nervous system structures and their functions described here. This chapter aims to provide both an overview of, and detailed information regarding, the neural substrates of behavior, synthesized in a manner that combines principles of organization, descriptions of evolutionary and hierarchical development, and elaboration of structural organization and complexity, guided by their relevance to the clinical neuroscience of behavioral neurology and neuropsychiatry. It presents an overview of cerebral cortical organization, the essentials of the limbic circuitry subserving emotion, the anatomical organization of the white matter tracts linking different cerebral cortical areas with each other, the connections between the cerebral cortex and subcortical areas, a consideration of the anatomical features of basal ganglia, thalamus, and cerebellum, and the clinical manifestations of lesions in each of these major brain areas. Building on Norman Geschwind's (1926–1984) conceptualization of disconnection syndromes following lesions of cerebral cortical association areas and white matter structures[4,5] we view the behavioral neurology/neuropsychiatry of lesions of focal subcortical areas also as disconnection syndromes: disruptions of the subcortical nodes of the circuits that subserve neurologic function.

Caution is necessary when extrapolating from rodent, cat, and monkey studies to the human because of the comparative evolutionary complexity of the human brain. Nevertheless, the organizing principles derived from physiological, tract tracing, and behavioral studies in animal models have largely been validated in healthy humans using contemporary imaging techniques, and in patients in whom behavioral deficits have been correlated with the anatomical locations of the lesions and the networks they disrupt.

OUTLINE OF THE CHAPTER

We commence with a brief historical account, followed by an overview of the major divisions of the brain and the hierarchical organization of the cerebral cortex. We then consider the Papez circuit because it links neural structures critical to maintenance of the internal milieu with the emotional brain, which in turn is interconnected with circuits necessary for interaction with the external world. We next consider the major components of the circuits key to motivation, emotion, and drive, and upon which cognitive control and awareness are built to enable social and societal behaviors. These are the hypothalamus, corticoid structures of the basal forebrain and ventral and medial surfaces of the cerebral hemispheres, and the amygdala critical to emotion, fear, reward, and salience processing. Next, we consider the hippocampus and the pyriform/olfactory cortex from the perspectives of their roles in nervous system function and the key positions they occupy in the evolutionary development of the cerebral cortex. Hippocampus has a pivotal role in learning and memory, integral to the sense of past, present, and future self. The pyriform/olfactory cortex, the ancient smell brain, has direct access to emotional brain circuitry. We return to the cerebral cortex to consider its most pertinent neuronal elements, supporting structures and myelination patterns. We then review a schema of brain organization from the perspective of paralimbic, unimodal association cortex, multimodal or heteromodal association cortex, and specialized idiotypic/koniocortex of the primary sensory and motor regions. Cortical-cortical connections in the monkey provide the anatomical underpinning of the notion of distributed neural circuits. Understanding these pathways is key to unraveling the intricacies of brain behavior correlations. The foundational anatomical studies that initiated the modern area of brain behavior relationships are introduced and explained within the overarching frameworks of evolutionary theory (dual origin of the cerebral cortex) and the general and specific principles of organization of cerebral cortex. This is followed by more detailed exposition of the intrinsic and extrinsic connections of the major divisions of the cerebral hemispheres: parietal lobe, temporal lobe, occipital lobe, insula, and cingulate gyrus.

The connections of the cerebral cortex are considered within the framework of distributed neural circuits, first within the domain of attention, and then in a larger framework in which multimodal areas constitute transmodal epicenters of functionally specified neurocognitive/neuropsychiatric domains including language, spatial awareness, memory and emotion, and cognitive control. The notion of convergence zones is introduced for its focus on the neural basis of memory, creative thought, imagination, and consciousness. This segues into a consideration of the physiology proposed to solve the binding problem inherent in distributed neural circuits, namely, the challenge of determining how objects encoded by distinct brain circuits are combined for perception, decision, and action. This knowledge is translated into human brain through magnetic resonance imaging (MRI) technology using task-based functional MRI, and intrinsic connectivity networks using resting state functional connectivity MRI (rsfcMRI). We then briefly note the influence of neurochemistry/neurotransmitters (state functions) on the neural pathways (channel functions) of the nervous system.

Connections between cortical and subcortical areas are conveyed in white matter tracts, damage to which produces its own sets of neurobehavioral consequences ranging from disconnection syndromes to white matter dementia. The white matter tracts of the cerebral cortex are reviewed in some detail, focusing on the cingulum bundle (CB) and uncinate fasciculus (UF) that are most closely linked with emotion and affect, with other relevant pathways presented in outline.

Lesions and neurodegenerative disorders that target subcortical nuclei produce complex neurobehavioral phenomena which we regard as subcortical disconnection syndromes. In the ensuing sections we therefore provide both an overview and necessary detail regarding the anatomy and connections of the basal ganglia, thalamus, and cerebellum. We discuss the functional relevance for neurobehavior of these subcortical nodes which are integral to the distributed neural circuits subserving cognition, emotion, and sensorimotor processing. We end with a consideration of new and emerging information about the dynamics and functional implications of cerebrospinal fluid (CSF) in health and disease.

Throughout this chapter, links between neuroanatomy and clinically relevant information are discussed, which for easy identification are demarcated either by a green line before and after the pertinent text, or for lengthier material, by placing the section title in a green rectangle.

HISTORICAL BACKGROUND

Pythagoras (c. 572–490 BCE) is credited with introducing the idea that the brain is concerned with reasoning. Galen of Pergamon (CE 129/130–200/201) discarded the earlier idea of Hippocrates (c. 460–370 BCE) that the brain was a gland, and argued that it is the seat of intelligence, emotion, and sensation. He introduced anatomical localization in clinical neurological science, believed that brain function arose from natural spirits and placed great emphasis on the cerebral ventricles. The anatomical dissections of Andreas Vesalius (1514–1564) demarcated the beginning of the post-Galenic era, and Thomas Willis (1621–1675) introduced the idea that Galenic spirits were produced in the cerebral cortex, that the complexity of the cerebral cortical convolutions in humans was reflected in intelligence, and that the cerebral cortex was the originator of memories and the organ of thought.[15,17–19]

The idea that there are regions of the brain specialized for specific functions originated with Franz Joseph Gall (1758–1828) (Fig. 1-1). His doctrine of plurality of cerebral organs[20] concluded that brain function is based on the preeminence of the cerebral cortex; cerebral convolutions are the organs of mental activity necessary for intellectual functions; there is functional specialization of different parts of the cortex; the cortex is the originator of the connecting fibers of the white matter; there is specificity of the connections of the different regions of the cortex; association

fibers are intracerebral white matter tracts connecting the cortical gray matter regions, and these include short, arcuate fibers, and long fibers connecting parts of different cerebral lobes; commissural fibers link the two hemispheres, with topographical arrangement; and afferent and efferent projection fibers that link the cortex with subcortical regions, brainstem, and spinal cord and are related to sensation and movement.

The theories and investigations of Theodore Herman Meynert (1833–1892) into the association, commissural, and projection white matter systems provided the foundations of a more precise physiology of the nervous system. Paul Emil Flechsig (1847–1929) provided a comprehensive understanding of the development of the human brain and established the fundamental law of myelinogenesis which holds that the sequence of myelination of white matter pathways during development recapitulates their appearance during phylogeny. He also discovered the principle, Flechsig's rule, reintroduced by Geschwind[4,5] that primary sensory areas have cortical connections only with immediately adjacent unimodal sensory association areas within their particular somatosensory realm and they are not connected with each other or with higher order association areas, a fundamental concept that has "profoundly influenced the way that modern cognitive neuroscience thinks about cortical localization."[21] Clinical and anatomical investigations of, among others, Carl Wernicke (1848–1900) and Joseph Jules Déjerine (1849–1917) deepened the appreciation of the cerebral cortex and interconnecting pathways and underscored the clinical imperative for understanding the relationship between brain structure and mental function.

Pivotal histological studies of Santiago Ramón y Cajal (1852–1934) resulted in the neuron doctrine which opened the way to the discipline of cortical architectonics, exploring the anatomical basis of Gall's original idea that the cerebral cortex is anatomically and functionally heterogeneous. Investigations commencing in the early 1900s used the types of cells and their spatial distribution in different cortical regions (cytoarchitecture), and the pattern of myelin staining within different areas of the cortex (myeloarchitecture), as defining hallmarks of the anatomical subdivisions of the cerebral cortex, resulting in maps of the human and monkey brains illustrating cortical architectonic heterogeneity.[22–29] The introduction of chemoarchitectonics, immunohistochemistry, optical coherence tomography, and gene expression, as well as automated image analysis with 2D and 3D quantitative architectonics and high-performance computing using imaging modalities in postmortem human brain, has enabled a sophisticated understanding of cerebral cortical organization and the development of population-based probabilistic maps of cortical architecture.[30] These probabilistic maps quantify spatial consistency of architecture patterns across subjects by quantifying interindividual overlap for each voxel in stereotaxic reference space, and maximum probability maps that provide contiguous parcellation, enabling an objective anatomical reference and account for the structural variability of the human brain.[31] Contemporary online atlases provide readily approachable macroscopic and microscopic resources for analysis of normal cortical architecture and functional territories,[30,32] demonstration of normal anatomy on high-resolution brain MRI,[33,34] and radiological pathology.[862]

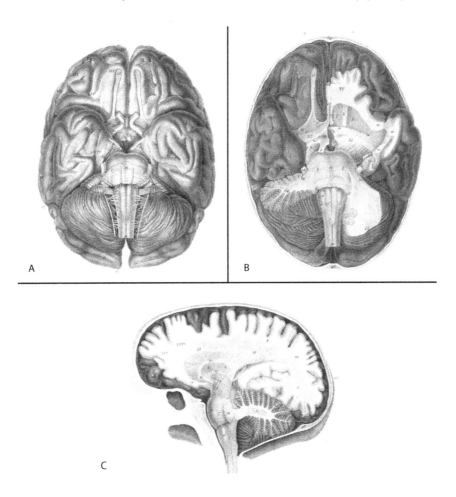

FIGURE 1-1. Images from the atlas of Franz Joseph Gall and Johann Kaspar Spurzheim (*Anatomie et Physiologie du Systeme Nerveux*[20]) showing cerebral convolutions, and dissections revealing differentiating features of cerebral cortex and white matter. **(A)** Plate IV; **(B)** Plate XIII; and **(C)** Plate X.

From the time of the gross brain dissections by investigators such as Johann Christian Reil (1859–1813), Karl Friedrich Burdach (1776–1847), and later Louis Pierre Gratiolet (1815–1865), it was apparent that different cortical areas are linked with each other by fiber tracts coursing through the cerebral white matter. The study of neural connections conveyed by these tracts commenced with methods such as lesion-degeneration studies[35-38] in which a focal cerebral cortical lesion would induce degeneration in an interconnected brain area, and strychnine neuronography[39] in which the excitatory neurotoxin strychnine applied to a point on the cerebral cortex would induce electrical potentials in a distant point, with the synchronously firing areas thus considered interconnected.[40] This was followed by important refinements in the lesion-degeneration method,[41,42] the introduction of anterograde axonal transport using the autoradiographic/isotope method,[43] retrograde axonal transport using horseradish peroxidase (HRP[44]) improved by tetramethyl benzidine histochemistry[45,46] and wheat germ agglutination of the HRP,[47] and the development of retrograde and anterograde axonal transport of fluorescent dyes[48] and anterograde transport of lectins[49] and biotinylated dextrans.[50] Trans-synaptic retrograde and anterograde tracing techniques using attenuated herpes and rabies viruses as tracers made it possible to define multisynaptic brain circuits through second- and third-order connections.[51,52] Optogenetic mapping has enabled the study of behavioral consequences of brain circuit manipulation in animal models in vivo.[53,54] Studies using task-based and functional connectivity MRI have made it possible to translate the knowledge derived from animal studies into the living human brain revealing new insights into the heterogeneity of cerebral cortical architecture,[55] connections,[56] and functions.[57]

GROSS DIVISIONS OF THE CEREBRAL HEMISPHERES

The cerebral hemispheres are traditionally divided into the lobes named by Gratiolet, with the central sulcus partitioning the hemispheres into pre- and post-Rolandic regions. The post-Rolandic cortex contains the parietal, temporal, and occipital lobes, whereas the pre-Rolandic area consists of precentral, premotor, and prefrontal cortices. The major subcortical nuclei are the basal ganglia, amygdala, thalamus, and hypothalamus. Anatomical nomenclature of these and many other brain areas has evolved over centuries of investigations in brain science, providing a rich, albeit sometimes challenging, heritage of insights into brain structure and function from the work of the early pioneers. The cerebellum is tightly interconnected with

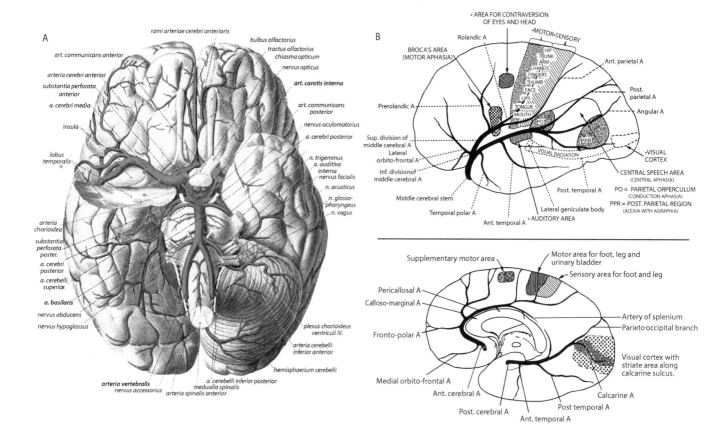

FIGURE 1-2. Cerebral vasculature. **(A)** The arteries at the base of the brain. On the right the tip of the temporal lobe, the cerebellum, and the optic nerves have been removed. (Figure and legend from Sobotta,[344] Fig. 682.) **(B)** Diagram of a cerebral hemisphere, lateral aspect, showing the branches and distribution of the middle cerebral artery and the principal regions of cerebral localization. **(C)** Diagram of a cerebral hemisphere, medial aspect, showing the branches and distribution of the anterior cerebral artery and the principal regions of cerebral localization. (Figures and legends in B and C from Adams and Victor.[860]) Central aphasia here refers to the language deficits resulting from stroke in Wernicke's area in the posterior superior temporal gyrus and/or in the inferior parietal lobule eponymously named Geschwind's area.[409]

the cerebral hemispheres via feedforward and feedback circuits. White matter tracts of the cerebral hemispheres comprise association tracts to the ipsilateral hemisphere, commissural projections to the contralateral hemisphere, striatal systems to the basal ganglia, and projection systems to thalamus, brainstem, and spinal cord. The intricacies of brainstem and spinal cord are not considered here, except for mention of selected brainstem nuclei, the neurotransmitter systems of which project widely throughout the cerebral hemispheres.

VASCULAR SUPPLY OF THE HUMAN BRAIN

A detailed understanding of the vasculature of the human brain is essential when considering stroke syndromes and their implications for behavioral neurology and neuropsychiatry. A thorough exposition of the topic is beyond the scope of this review. Published literature[58,59] and authoritative monographs[60,61] provide complete descriptions of the circle of Willis at the base of the brain; the arterial supply through the carotid arteries and its two main tributaries—the anterior and middle cerebral arteries that irrigate much of the cerebral cortex; the vertebrobasilar

circulation to the brainstem and cerebellum, and through posterior cerebral artery to the occipital and temporal lobe; and the perforating branches of these major vessels that supply the deep nuclei and white matter tracts of the cerebral hemispheres (Fig. 1-2). Later in the chapter we delve into the thalamic vasculature directly pertinent to behavioral neurology and neuropsychiatry,[62] a topic which has not been comprehensively covered in other syntheses.

APPROACH TO THE CONSIDERATION OF THE NEURAL SUBSTRATES OF COGNITION AND EMOTION

We adopt a hierarchical approach to the consideration of the neural circuits relevant to behavioral neurology and neuropsychiatry. The integrity of peripheral and autonomic nervous systems is essential for monitoring the internal milieu and external environment. Reflex responses to these types of stimuli are optimized to ensure the survival of the individual and society. The ability to experience and filter incoming information, sculpt responses to the internal and external environments, and monitor and develop long-range plans according to past events,

EXTRAPERSONAL SPACE

Primary sensory and motor areas
IDIOTYPIC CORTEX

modality-specific (unimodal) association areas
HOMOTYPICAL ISOCORTEX
high-order (heteromodal) association areas

temporal pole - caudal orbitofrontal anterior insula-cingulate-parahippocampal
PARALIMBIC AREAS

septum - substantia innominata- amygdala-piriform cortex-hippocampus
LIMBIC AREAS (CORTICOID + ALLOCORTEX)

HYPOTHALAMUS
INTERNAL MILIEU

FIGURE 1-3. Conceptual relationship of the cortical zones of human brain, reflecting hierarchical organization of cerebral cortical architecture. (From Mesulam.[63])

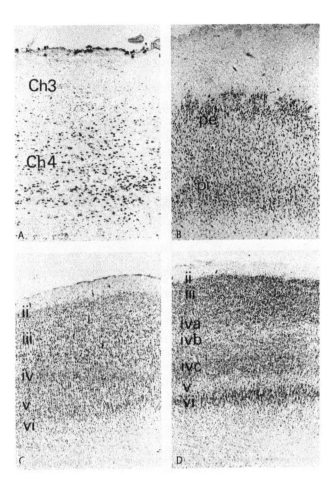

FIGURE 1-4. Four types of cortex in the human brain. The pial surface is at the top in all four photomicrographs. **(A)** Corticoid cortex: photomicrograph of the substantia innominata showing the nucleus basalis of Meynert (Ch4) and the more superficial horizontal limb nucleus of the diagonal band (Ch3). The lamination is incomplete, and there is no uniformity in the orientation of neurons. **(B)** Allocortex from the subicular portion of the hippocampal formation. There are two distinct layers, an external pyramidal (pe) and an internal pyramidal (pi). Dendrites within each layer have a relatively uniform orientation. **(C)** Homotypical isocortex from prefrontal heteromodal regions: six distinct layers include differentiated granularity in layers II and IV. **(D)** Idiotypic cortex from the striate visual area. There are at least seven layers, many strongly granular. From corticoid to idiotypic cortex there is a gradual increase of cell density and laminar differentiation. (Magnification ×10) (Image and legend reproduced from Mesulam.[63])

current environment, and future expectations is enabled by a progressively complex nervous system characterized by reciprocal feedforward and feedback interactions between the central nervous system's multiple levels of sensors, modifiers, and effectors.

The peripheral, visceral, and autonomic ganglia are not discussed here. The hypothalamus regulates the internal milieu; corticoid structures (see section below) are at the interface of the autonomic nervous system and the limbic system; and the cerebral cortex is built upon these lower centers.

CYTOARCHITECTURE AND HIERARCHICAL ORGANIZATION OF CEREBRAL CORTEX

(After Marsel Mesulam[63] and Schmahmann and Pandya[15])

Here we introduce the field of cytoarchitectonics and the terms that refer to the different types of cerebral cortex, from regions involved in autonomic regulation to those that provide substrates for emotional and cognitive control (Fig. 1-3).

Architectonics refers to the principles, as well as the study or character, of various types of architectural structures. In the nervous system, cytoarchitecture is defined by the histological appearance of a region based on the size, packing density, and special features of its constituent neurons and glia. In the cerebral cortex, there is a superimposed ordering of these cellular elements into identifiable layers (or laminae) and columns. Areas defined by cytoarchitectonic parcellation correlate well with cortical connectivity and with neurophysiologic mapping

methods, emphasizing their functional significance. Cerebral cortical parcellation can also be identified by staining methods for different constituents of the cortex including blood vessels, glia, chemoreceptors, and pigments.[64] Neurons in the neocortex are arranged in six layers; more primitive areas of the cerebral cortex have three layers (Fig. 1-4).

Corticoid Structures

Corticoid structures have features that are part cortical and part nuclear. Their organization is rudimentary, no consistent lamination can be discerned, and the orientation of their dendrites appears random and haphazard.

Allocortex

Allocortex is phylogenetically ancient, comprising about 10% of the cortical area. It is the most primitive, least well-differentiated type of cortex, with three layers, only one of which contains large pyramidal cells. Two types of allocortex are found in the primate brain: *archicortex* corresponds to the hippocampal formation, and *paleocortex* to the olfactory, or pyriform cortex. Allocortical cell layers extend into periallocortical components of the paralimbic region.

Periallocortex

Periallocortex surrounds allocortex and has neurons that are mostly randomly distributed.

Proisocortex

Proisocortex is characterized by a poorly defined IVth layer. Gradual cytoarchitectonic changes from the allocortical pole toward the isocortical side of the paralimbic region include progressive accumulation of small granule cells in layer IV and then layer II, sublamination and columnarization of layer III, differentiation of layer V from layer VI, and of layer VI from the underlying white matter, and an increase in the intracortical myelin, especially along the outer band of Baillarger in layer IV.

Isocortex or Neocortex

Isocortex or neocortex is more recently evolved, has six more or less distinct layers, and constitutes approximately 90% of the cerebral cortex.

Afferent Connections to the Cortical Laminae
Layer I of the cerebral cortex is sparsely populated with neurons and is thought to receive input from intralaminar thalamic nuclei and the reticular formation. This layer also receives feedback from precursor cortical areas. Layers II and IV receive intrinsic connections within the given cortical unit. Layers II, III, and IV receive feedforward input from adjacent cortical regions. Layers III and IV receive thalamic and commissural input. Layers V and VI receive intrinsic connections and some thalamic input.

Efferent Connections from the Cortical Laminae
Information received in layer I is transferred to the intrinsic circuitry of the cortical unit by providing contacts with the apical dendrites of supragranular (layers II and III) and infragranular neurons (layers V and VI). Layers II and IV provide information to the supra and infragranular neurons within a cortical module. Cells in layer III preferentially provide the long association axons, including commissural fibers. The efferents from layers V and VI participate in a feedback link to the first layer of the adjacent cortical area, and neurons in these layers also project to thalamus, basal ganglia, pons, and spinal cord.

Most of the isocortex consists of *association areas* that receive inputs from multiple other brain regions and which are engaged in complex functions. The different association areas have architectonic features that distinguish them from each other. Specialized areas of isocortex which subserve primary somatosensory, visual, and auditory senses are termed *koniocortex*, or *idiotypic isocortex*. These cortices have well-developed IVth layers, reflecting a disproportionately increased number of small granule neurons that are targets of input from the sensory nuclei of thalamus. The primary motor cortex, area 4, is also koniocortex and is characterized by giant pyramidal neurons, or Betz cells described by Vladimir Betz (1834–1894) in 1874,[65] that give rise to the corticospinal tract critical for motor function. The progressive elaboration of cerebral cortical maturation from allocortex to isocortex maps onto hierarchical levels of behavioral repertoires, from multidomain integration to single modality sensation, perception, and motor control. Anatomical and functional details of the isocortex are described in further detail below when we consider the schema of brain organization.

PAPEZ CIRCUIT

The Papez circuit serves as a bridge between the endocrine, visceral, emotional, and voluntary responses to the environment, because it includes many of the hierarchical levels of subcortical and cortical areas subserving emotion, and the intersection of autonomic function, affect, and cognitive control (Fig. 1-5).[66] The following is an overview of its circuitry; the details of its component parts are addressed in the following paragraphs.

Original Descriptions and Overview

Paul Broca (1824–1880) drew attention to a cortical region on the medial and ventral surface of the cerebral hemisphere, forming a border, or limbus, between the rest of the hemisphere and the diencephalon.[29] In his seminal 1937 paper, "A Proposed Mechanism of Emotion," James Papez (1883–1958)[67] proposed a neural pathway he believed to be involved in the cortical control of emotion. He hypothesized that the hippocampus, cingulate gyrus, hypothalamus, anterior thalamic nuclei, and their interconnections constituted a harmonious mechanism which elaborates the functions of emotions.[68] This notion was expanded upon by Paul MacLean (1913–2007)[69] who sought to account for sensations involved in the auras associated with seizures. He reasoned that there must be pathways connecting visual, auditory, and somatic neocortical areas with the hippocampus. He introduced the concept of a visceral brain and the term limbic system[70] to describe a circuit consisting of the limbic lobe and its major connections in the forebrain to the hypothalamus, amygdala, and septum.[71] The dorsal part of the septum, the septum pellucidum, is a thin membranous structure composed largely of glial cells and nerve fibers. The ventral part of the septum, the septum verum, contains the lateral septal nucleus; the medial septal complex includes the medial septal nucleus and the nucleus of the dorsal limb of the diagonal band of Broca.

The flow of information within the Papez circuit follows a sequence of fiber connections linking subcortical nuclei with corticoid and cortical areas, as follows. Each hippocampal formation sends information through the alveus of the hippocampus into the fornix which arches forward beneath the corpus

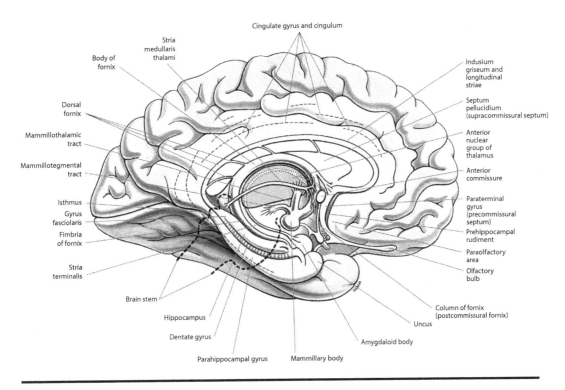

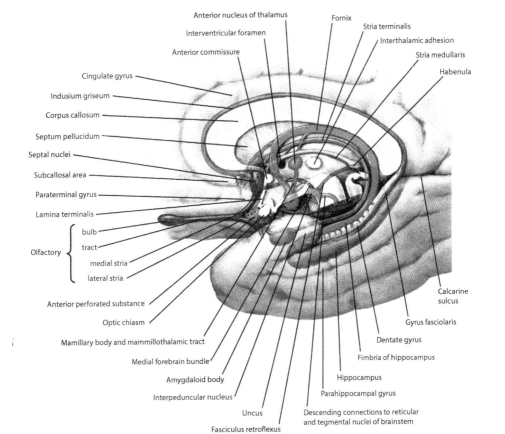

FIGURE 1-5. Papez circuit. **(A)** Viewed within the context of the medial wall of the cerebral hemisphere. (From *Gray's Anatomy*.[84]) **(B)** A closer view of the structures and tracts that link them, as illustrated by Frank H. Netter MD in Jones et al.[66]

callosum (CC), descending behind the anterior commissure (AC) as it reaches and terminates in the medial and lateral nuclei of the mammillary body (see the scholarly discussion by Jones[72] on the spelling through history of mamillary vs. mammillary). The mammillothalamic tract of Félix Vicq d'Azyr (1748–1794) links the mammillary body with the anterior thalamic nuclei: The medial mammillary nucleus projects ipsilaterally to the anteromedial and anteroventral thalamic nuclei, the lateral mammillary nucleus has bilateral projections to the anterodorsal thalamic nuclei.[73] The anterior thalamic nuclei in turn project to the cingulate cortex and other paralimbic areas of the cerebral cortex.

The amygdala, critical for emotion, behavior, and fear processing, sends information through the stria terminalis into the hypothalamus. The hypothalamus, along with the septal nuclei and the anterior thalamic nucleus, sends information through the stria medullaris to the habenula nucleus. The stria medullaris also conveys information into the habenula from limbic structures including the septum, diagonal band of Broca, bed nucleus of the stria terminalis (BNST), and lateral preoptic area.

Habenula

The medial habenula, which is intensely cholinergic, projects through the fasciculus retroflexus (also known as the habenulo-interpeduncular tract, Fig. 1-6) to the interpeduncular nucleus.[74] This pathway is implicated in the process of rapid eye movement (REM) sleep.[75] The lateral habenula, which is predominantly glutamatergic, receives input from the internal segment of the globus pallidus, and projects through the fasciculus retroflexus into the substantia nigra (SN) pars compact and the

limbic-midbrain ventral tegmental area, which are dopaminergic, and to the serotonergic dorsal and medial raphe nuclei. The medial and lateral habenula nuclei sit at the crossroads between the basal ganglia, brainstem monoaminergic nuclei, and the limbic system (Fig. 1-7).[76]

The connections of the habenula, lateral habenula in particular, confer upon it potential roles in the regulation of emotional behavior including emotional decision making. The lateral habenula has been termed the brain's antireward center.

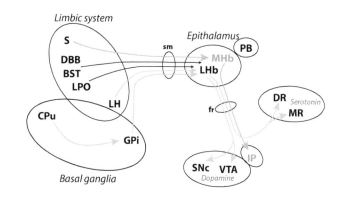

FIGURE 1-7. Connections of the habenula, according to Hikosaka et al.[76] BST, bed nucleus of stria terminalis; CPu, caudate and putamen; DBB, nucleus of diagonal band of Broca; DR, dorsal raphe; fr, fasciculus retroflexus; GPi, globus pallidus internal segment; IP, interpeduncular nucleus; LH, lateral hypothalamus; LHb, lateral habenula; LPO, lateral preoptic area; MHb, medial habenula; MR, medial raphe; PB, pineal body; S, septum; sm, stria medullaris; SNc, substantia nigra, pars compacta; VTA, ventral tegmental area.

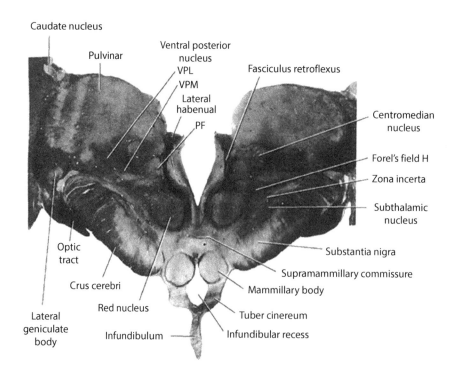

FIGURE 1-6. Myelin-stained section of the human diencephalon to show the location of the fasciculus retroflexus, also known as the habenulo-interpeduncular tract, and its relationship to structures in the region. It is surrounded by the parafascicular nucleus. PF, parafascicular nucleus; VPL, ventral posterolateral thalamic nucleus; VPM, ventral posteromedial thalamic nucleus. (From Carpenter.[89])

It plays a critical role in regulating negatively motivated behavior, is hyperactive in major depression, and has been implicated in schizophrenia and drug-induced psychosis.[77] There is increasing recognition of neuronal diversity within the lateral habenula, with physiologically distinct subclasses of neurons expressing parvalbumin or somatostatin which are markers of inhibitory neurons.[78] Potentiating inhibition of the lateral habenula has been proposed as a novel approach to antidepressant therapy. A more detailed exposition of the connections of the lateral habenula is therefore pertinent, as summarized in Hu et al.[77] The lateral habenula targets essentially all midbrain neuromodulatory systems, including the noradrenergic, serotonergic, and dopaminergic systems, serving as a hub that integrates value-based, sensory, and experience-dependent information to regulate motivational, cognitive, and motor processes.

Afferents

The lateral habenula receives inputs from limbic forebrain regions and the basal ganglia by way of the stria medullaris. Limbic inputs are derived from the hypothalamus—lateral hypothalamic area, lateral preoptic area, paraventricular nucleus, and suprachiasmatic nucleus (SCN); the central nucleus of the amygdala; and the basal forebrain including the nucleus accumbens (NAc), diagonal band nuclei/nucleus of the diagonal band of Broca, ventral pallidum (VP), lateral and medial septum, and BNST. Basal ganglia inputs are from the internal segment of the globus pallidus which receives cortical inputs through the striatum. It also receives direct cortical inputs from the medial prefrontal cortex, and reciprocal feedback from the monoaminergic ventral tegmental area (VTA, of Tsai[74]) and raphe nuclei.

Efferents

Lateral habenula projections through the fasciculus retroflexus target the gamma-aminobutyric acid (GABA)ergic rostromedial tegmental nucleus (RMTg) also known as the tail VTA. The RMTg, in turn, projects to the dopaminergic neurons in the VTA and SNc, inhibiting their activity. Activation of the lateral habenular-RMTg projections promotes active, passive, and conditioned behavioral avoidance, reduces effortful behaviors, and facilitates depressive-like behavior induced by a learned helplessness paradigm. The lateral habenula also provides direct glutamatergic projections to GABAergic and dopaminergic neurons in the VTA. Optogenetic activation of the direct lateral habenula–VTA pathway produces conditioned place avoidance and increases despair-like behaviors. Lateral habenula glutamatergic neurons project to GABAergic and serotonergic neurons in the raphe, suppressing neuronal activity in both the dorsal and medial raphe. Other lateral habenular targets include the noradrenergic locus coeruleus, the cholinergic lateral dorsal tegmental nucleus, thalamus (centromedian, medial dorsal, ventromedial [VM], and parafascicular nuclei), superior colliculus, and the dorsal tegmental region. Optogenetic activation of the lateral habenular glutamatergic terminals targeting the GABAergic interneurons in the lateral dorsal tegmental nucleus induces fear-like behavior in mice, mimicking the effect of predator odor (text adapted from Hu et al. [77]). The habenula commissure conveys substantial and topographically organized connections between the left and right habenulae, although their functional implications are unclear.

The Papez circuit is thus linked with monoaminergic nuclei in the brainstem that have widespread projections throughout the cerebral hemispheres. The cerebral cortical recruitment into the Papez circuit is through cingulate gyrus projections to the posterior parahippocampal gyrus and the perirhinal and entorhinal cortices which then send information into the hippocampus. The efferents from the hippocampus travel in the fornix back to the subcortical structures and then cerebral cortex.

We now transition to a more in-depth analysis of the structures that feed into, intersect with, and control the Papez circuit.

HYPOTHALAMUS

The hypothalamus is at the epicenter of the consideration of motivated behaviors that enable animals to enhance their own survival and promote that of their species. It is the head ganglion of the internal milieu, and one of the oldest structures in the brain. Its highly conserved neural circuitry controls the basic life functions of autonomic and instinctive behaviors. It regulates physiological homeostasis: energy metabolism—feeding, digestion, metabolic control, and energy expenditure; fluid and electrolyte balance—drinking, fluid absorption and excretion; thermoregulation—response to environment through heat production and conservation, and fever responses; and sleep-wake cycles. It contributes to social interactions concerned with individual security through emergency responses to stressors in the environment; and maintenance of the species through reproductive hormone control, mating, pregnancy, birth, and suckling.[79,80] Its interconnections link it to corticoid and primitive allocortical structures which lead in turn to the progressive elaboration of cerebral cortical connections, the basis of voluntary control of increasingly complex conscious behaviors. The hypothalamus and related structures in the limbic system are the nodal points of intersection between the awareness of and response to the internal milieu and to the external environment, based on mood state, memory of past events, current environment, and future expectation.

Anatomical Subdivisions

The hypothalamus is arranged in rostrocaudal and mediolateral zones containing nuclei of varying sizes (Fig. 1-8A, B).[80–86]

Rostrocaudal Groupings

These are from rostral to caudal: preoptic (chiasmatic), tuberal (including infundibular and retroinfundibular sectors), and mammillary.

The *preoptic* group lies above and anterior to the optic chiasm and includes the walls of the preoptic recess. The magnocellular neurosecretory nuclei define its posterior border.[83] It contains the rostral part of the paraventricular nucleus, the medial and ventrolateral preoptic nuclei, the medial and lateral preoptic areas, and the SCN, key integrative circuitry for thermoregulation, fever, electrolyte balance, sleep-wake, circadian rhythms, and sexual behavior.

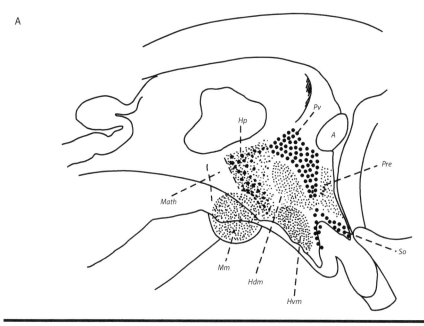

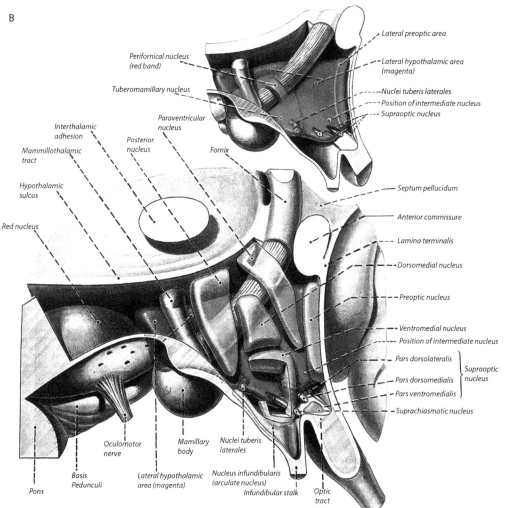

FIGURE 1-8. **(A)** Nuclei of the hypothalamus according to Le Gros Clark[81] showing the nuclei projected on to the lateral wall of the third ventricle. A, anterior commissure; Hdm, dorsomedial hypothalamic nucleus; Hp, posterior hypothalamic nucleus; Hvm, ventromedial hypothalamic nucleus; Mm, medial mammillary body; Mth, mammillo-thalamic tract; Pre, preoptic nucleus; Pv, paraventricular nucleus;

(Continued)

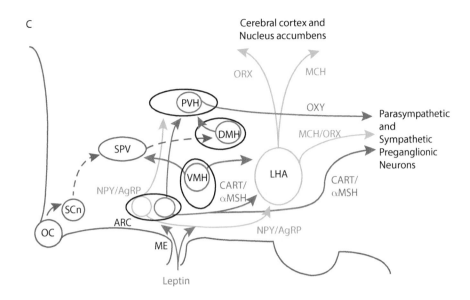

FIGURE 1-8. (*Continued*) So, supraoptic nucleus. **(B)** The hypothalamus is viewed from the medial aspect according to *Gray's Anatomy*.[84] This in turn is modified from Nauta and Haymaker.[85] In the upper diagram the medially placed nuclear groups are removed, in the lower diagram both the lateral and the medial nuclei are shown. The lower image has been edited by the author to add the SCN. **(C)** Schematic drawing of the rat hypothalamus in sagittal section illustrating the major pathways and neurotransmitters implicated in the regulation of feeding. Pathways activated by leptin that have an anorexic influence (inhibit feeding) are in red, those inhibited by leptin and that have a phagic influence (promote feeding) are in green. Circadian influences on feeding (inhibited at some times of the day and excited at other times) are illustrated by dashed blue pathways. Leptin enters the hypothalamus through the median eminence, where it diffuses to interact with neurons expressing high levels of leptin receptors in the arcuate (ARC), ventromedial, and dorsomedial hypothalamic nuclei. The ARC has two counterposed populations of neurons. Medially situated neurons express neuropeptide Y and agouti-related protein and are inhibited by systemic leptin. Neurons in the lateral ARC express α-melanocyte stimulating hormone (α-MSH) and CART and are activated by systemic leptin. Both populations of ARC neurons project to the paraventricular nucleus and the lateral hypothalamic area. The α-MSH/CART neurons also project to the sympathetic preganglionic cell column in the spinal cord. Ventral parvocellular neurons of the paraventricular nucleus containing oxytocin innervate vagal preganglionic parasympathetic neurons involved in gastrointestinal control. The caudal part of the dorsomedial nucleus provides the major leptin-activated input to the paraventricular nucleus. Leptin-activated cells in the ventromedial nucleus project to the subparaventricular zone, a region that also receives SCN inputs and is involved in the circadian regulation of feeding. The subparaventricular nucleus in turn innervates the leptin-activated part of the dorsomedial nucleus. Divergent projections from neurons in the lateral hypothalamus containing orexin (ORX) and melanin concentrating hormone (MCH) ascend to the cerebral cortex and the nucleus accumbens and descend to the brainstem and spinal cord. These neurons are activated during starvation or leptin deprivation. A lesion centered on the ventromedial nucleus and arcuate nucleus eliminates leptin influence, resulting in hyperphagia and obesity. A lesion in the lateral hypothalamus that destroys the ORX and MCH cells which promote feeding results in aphagia and inanition. α-MSH, α-melanocyte stimulating hormone; AgRP, agouti-related protein; ARC, arcuate nucleus; CART, cocaine and amphetamine regulated transcript; DMH, dorsomedial nucleus; LHA, lateral hypothalamic area; MCH, melanin concentrating hormone; ME, median eminence; NPY, neuropeptide Y; OC, optic chiasm; ORX, orexin; OXY, oxytocin; PVH, paraventricular nucleus; SCN, suprachiasmatic nucleus; SPV, subparaventricular zone; VMH, ventromedial nucleus. (Figure and legend from Elmquist[111] edited with permission [CB Saper, personal communication].)

The *middle group: The tuberal hypothalamus/tuber cinereum* lies between the optic chiasm anteriorly and the mammillary bodies posteriorly. It is cone-shaped, surrounds the infundibular recess, and extends to the neurohypophysis. It is a convex mass of gray matter, from which the hollow infundibulum becomes continuous ventrally with the posterior lobe of the pituitary. Around the base of the infundibulum is the median eminence demarcated by a shallow tuberoinfundibular sulcus. The tuber cinereum has a pair of lateral eminences which demarcate the lateral tuberal nuclei, and a small median postinfundibular eminence.

The *infundibular part* lies behind the optic chiasm and contains the caudal part of the paraventricular nucleus, the supraoptic, and arcuate (also, infundibular) nuclei, the VM and dorsomedial nuclei which lie close to the mid-line, and the more diffuse lateral hypothalamic area which lies more laterally.

The *retroinfundibular part* contains the posterior hypothalamic nucleus interposed between the VM hypothalamic nucleus in front and the mammillary body behind, extending upward and backward becoming continuous with the midbrain tegmental region. The tuberal hypothalamus contains integrative circuits for feeding, and output circuitry for sexual behavior, aggressiveness, and many autonomic and endocrine responses.

The *mammillary group* is dominated by the mammillary bodies: the large, parvicellular medial mammillary nucleus and the small, magnocellular lateral mammillary nucleus which are engaged in learning, memory, and emotion. It also contains the tuberomammillary nucleus which is the main source of histamine in the brain, necessary for the maintenance of wakefulness,[87] and the supramammillary nucleus, the neurons of which contain glutamate, GABA, and nitric oxide synthase, and which supports hippocampal theta rhythms and serves as a key node in the sleep-wake regulatory system.[88]

Mediolateral Groupings

The medial to lateral groupings are the periventricular, intermediate (medial), and lateral zones. Between the intermediate and lateral zones is a paramedian plane which contains the prominent myelinated fibers of the column of the fornix, the mammillothalamic tract, and the fasciculus retroflexus/habenulo-interpeduncular tract (Fig. 1-8B).[84,89]

The *periventricular* zone includes from rostral to caudal, the paraventricular preoptic nucleus, SCN, and paraventricular cell group that expands around the base of the third ventricle to form the arcuate nucleus.

The *intermediate or medial* zone contains the most well-differentiated nuclei: paraventricular, supraoptic, medial preoptic, VM, dorsomedial, posterior hypothalamic, and mammillary nuclei, and the anterior hypothalamic area.

The *lateral zone* includes the lateral preoptic nucleus, supraoptic nucleus, and the lateral hypothalamic area.

Braak and Braak[83] make the point that the basolateral portions of the tuber cinereum include the lateral tuberal nucleus and the tuberomammillary nucleus which considerably increase in size with phylogeny, contain neurons that are distinctly different from those in other hypothalamic nuclei, and should not be regarded as part of the lateral hypothalamic area. This is supported by the finding that the lateral tuberal nucleus together with the basolateral amygdaloid complex, the entorhinal cortex, and the CA1 subfield of the hippocampus bears the brunt of subcortical changes in dementia with argyrophilic grains,[90] a late-onset tauopathy dementia characterized by abundant spindle-shaped argyrophilic grains in neuronal processes and coiled bodies in oligodendrocytes.[91,92]

Fiber Tracts Traversing the Hypothalamus

(See Nieuwenhuys et al.[86] and Bear and Bollu[93])

Hypothalamo-Hypophyseal Pathway (Infundibulum/Pituitary Stalk)

Magnocellular neurons in the supraoptic and paraventricular nuclei express either oxytocin or vasopressin (also known as antidiuretic hormone [ADH]). Their axons traverse the pituitary stalk to end along blood vessels in the posterior pituitary gland (the neurohypophysis), transporting colloidal droplets of these hormones where they are released into the bloodstream and distributed systemically throughout the body (Fig. 1-9).[94]

Parvicellular neurons in the medial part of the paraventricular nucleus and the arcuate nucleus send axons to the floor of the third ventricle at the emergence of the *pituitary stalk*, and to the *median eminence* in the anterior wall of the infundibular stalk where they secrete hormones into the hypophyseal portal capillaries carrying blood to the anterior pituitary gland (adenohypophysis). The median eminence also receives neurosecretory fibers from the medial septal nucleus. These axonal projections either stimulate or inhibit release of the anterior

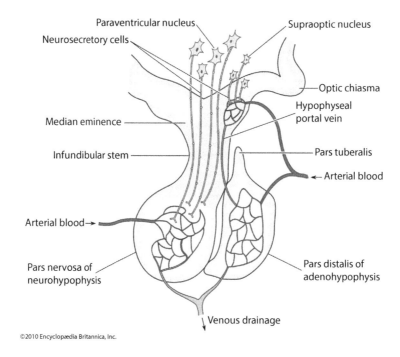

©2010 Encyclopædia Britannica, Inc.

FIGURE 1-9. Schematic illustration of the pituitary stalk/infundibular stem; the anterior pituitary (adenohypophysis) and posterior pituitary gland (neurohypophysis); the circulation within the pituitary gland; the parvicellular neurons (shown here in the supraoptic nucleus, but also in the arcuate, paraventricular, and periventricular nuclei) that provide releasing factors for the release of gonadotropins and other hormones from the anterior pituitary gland; and the magnocellular neurons in the paraventricular nucleus (and supraoptic nucleus) that express oxytocin and vasopressin which are released into the posterior pituitary gland. (Figure from Emerson.[94])

pituitary hormones—gonadotropins (luteinizing hormone and follicle-stimulating hormone), adrenocorticotropic hormone, thyroid-stimulating hormone, growth hormone, and prolactin.

The *fornix* descends through the hypothalamus, linking the hippocampus with the mammillary body. The *mammillothalamic tract* links the mammillary bodies with the anterior thalamic nuclei. The *stria terminalis* links the amygdala with the hypothalamus (see section "Amygdala").

The connections and functional relevance of these three tracts—the fornix, mammillothalamic tract, and stria terminalis are discussed in detail later in the chapter.

The *medial forebrain bundle* (MFB) courses through the lateral hypothalamic zone between the descending columns of the fornix medially and the cerebral peduncles laterally (Fig. 1-10). This tract is a key structure of the mesolimbic dopamine system for motivation and reward-seeking behavior. It links dopaminergic neurons of the VTA—the limbic region in the ventral aspect of the midbrain[95]—with the lateral and medial hypothalamus, lateral and medial preoptic region, ventral striatum, NAc, septal area, nucleus of the diagonal band of Broca, and ventral parts of the BNST.[96] Many of these nuclei in turn project to the olfactory bulb[81] and limbic-related regions in the orbitofrontal cortex and medial prefrontal cortices.[97] The MFB is bidirectional, containing both short and long ascending and descending components which enter and leave the bundle as small fascicles. It is particularly sizeable in animals with strong olfactory guidance of foraging behavior. In primates it consists of multiple distinct monoaminergic circuits including serotonin, norepinephrine, and orexin in addition to the dopaminergic system arising in the VTA. The VTA also appears to be

the origin of glutamatergic (excitatory) axons.[97-99] The MFB has reduced white matter integrity as revealed by reduced fractional anisotropy on diffusion weighted brain imaging in functional neurologic disorder (FND[100]). Other limbic bundles implicated in FND include the stria terminalis, fornix, UF, and CB. Through tract tracing diffusion imaging technology in living human brain a second, superolateral branch of the MFB has been proposed, thought to convey connections directly between the VTA and the paralimbic regions of the frontal lobe.[98] Deep brain stimulation of this superolateral branch produces rapid improvement in treatment refractory depression. The postulated mechanism includes recruitment of descending glutamatergic fibers from the medial prefrontal cortex to the VTA, regulating VTA dopaminergic firing which in turn modulates the upstream cortical regions.[101-103] Given the challenges inherent in anatomical mapping with diffusion tractography, this additional branch of the MFB remains to be confirmed. As discussed later in the chapter, there are strong reciprocal projections between the cerebellum (fastigial nucleus in particular) and the VTA from which the MFB originates, which has important implications for the cerebellar modulation of emotion and social cognition.

The *retinohypothalamic tract* links the retina with the hypothalamic SCN, a bilateral projection with a contralateral predominance. This pathway is the basis of circadian rhythm responses to light. Retinal ganglion cells also project via the retinohypothalamic tract to other hypothalamic nuclei involved in nonvisual photoreception, including the ventrolateral preoptic nucleus, a sleep-promoting area in the anterior hypothalamus, and the subparaventricular zone, the main efferent target of

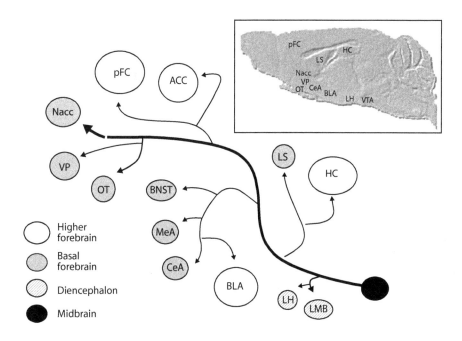

FIGURE 1-10. Schematic representation of the main forebrain areas in the rodent reached by the mesolimbic dopaminergic system, grouped into diencephalic, basal forebrain, and higher forebrain areas. Midbrain: VTA, ventral tegmental area. Diencephalon: LH, lateral hypothalamus, LMB, lateral mammillary body. Basal forebrain: NAc, nucleus accumbens, VP, ventral pallidum, OT, olfactory tubercle, CeA, central nucleus of amygdala, MeA, medial nucleus of the amygdala, BNST, bed nucleus of stria terminalis, LS, lateral septum. Higher forebrain: ACC, anterior cingulate cortex, BLA, basolateral amygdala, HC, hippocampal complex, pFC, prefrontal cortex. (Figure and legend from Alcaro et al.[96])

neural projections from the SCN, which is important for circadian regulation of sleep. Additionally, the retina projects to the olivary pretectal nucleus in the midbrain, part of the afferent pathway mediating the pupillary light reflex and engaged in light-evoked blinks, triggering of REM sleep, and modulating subcortical nuclei involved in circadian rhythms[104]; and to the intergeniculate leaflet, a subdivision between the dorsal and ventral components of the lateral geniculate complex that participates in the regulation of circadian function through its projections to the SCN.[105,106]

The *dorsal longitudinal fasciculus* (of Hugo Schütz [1859–1923][107,108]) is a diffuse bidirectional fiber system lying within the periaqueductal gray which interconnects the posterior part of the hypothalamus, particularly the dorsomedial nucleus[109] with visceral centers in the midbrain tegmentum, reticular formation, and medulla.[86,108]

Functional Specialization of Hypothalamic Nuclei

Saper and Lowell[80] view the role of the hypothalamus as integrative, bringing together sensory inputs necessary for decisions about basic life functions, and comparing the inputs to setpoints—ideal levels for parameters such as body temperature, blood sodium, glucose, and hormone levels. The hypothalamus activates autonomic, endocrine, and behavioral responses to maintain the body at the key setpoints (homeostasis) or to overcome a stressor (allostasis). Behavioral regulation is achieved through circuits that increase or decrease the likelihood that an animal will engage in certain behaviors.

Autonomic nervous system control by the hypothalamus resides mostly in the parvicellular part of the paraventricular nucleus, the adjacent lateral hypothalamic area, and the arcuate (infundibular) nucleus. The lateral hypothalamic area receives projections from the amygdala: In rat the central nucleus of the amygdala projects to its dorsal aspect, and the basal lateral nucleus of amygdala to its ventral aspect. These amygdalo-hypothalamic connections have functional relevance for the control of feeding and other motivated behaviors.[110]

Thermal regulation and fever are under the influence of the medial preoptic nucleus which integrates thermal inputs from the skin and thermosensitive neurons within the brain, such as neurons in the preoptic region that respond to brain temperature.

Feeding and energy metabolism are under the control of an extensive network of hypothalamic nuclei (Fig. 1-8C). These include the arcuate (infundibular), dorsomedial, VM, and premammillary hypothalamic nuclei which contain receptors for leptin (see Saper and Lowell,[80] Elmquist et al.,[111] and Bouret et al.[112]). Leptin is a peptide hormone made by white adipose cells during times of adequate metabolic substrate. It enters the hypothalamus through the median eminence and has an anorexic effect by inhibiting food intake and stimulating catabolic, autonomic, and neuroendocrine responses that direct nutrient stores away from the fat compartment. Leptin levels effect the expression of genes for transcription factors (c-fos), signaling molecules, and neurotransmitters including neuropeptide Y, agouti-related protein, cocaine and amphetamine

regulated transcript (CART), α-melanocyte stimulating hormone, melanin concentrating hormone (MCH), and orexin (also called hypocretin). Low levels of leptin increase hunger and reduce energy expenditure.[113] The arcuate nucleus is a key site in regulating feeding: leptin-receptive neurons in the arcuate nucleus project to the other hypothalamic sites implicated in the control of feeding including the paraventricular nucleus, dorsomedial nucleus, and the lateral hypothalamic area. The lateral hypothalamic area is the hypothalamic feeding center, containing the peptides MCH and orexin which promote eating. Lesions of the arcuate and VM nuclei eliminate leptin influence, resulting in hyperphagia and obesity; lesions of the lateral hypothalamic area destroy the MCH and orexin cells and result in aphagia and inanition.[111,114]

Sleep and wakefulness are regulated by neurons in the hypothalamus and brainstem.

Wakefulness is promoted by histaminergic neurons in the tuberomammillary nucleus, orexin/hypocretin neurons in the lateral hypothalamic area, and glutamatergic neurons in the supramammillary region which have extensive excitatory projections to the cerebral cortex. Arousal-promoting neurons in the brainstem send axons to the lateral hypothalamus on their way to the cerebral cortex. The neurotransmitters deployed by these systems are noradrenergic (locus coeruleus), serotonergic (dorsal and median raphe), dopaminergic (ventral periaqueductal gray), cholinergic (pedunculopontine and lateral dorsal tegmental nuclei), and glutamatergic (parabrachial nucleus).

Sleep-promoting neurons are in the ventrolateral preoptic and medial preoptic hypothalamic nuclei.

Saper[80,115,116] describes a mutually inhibitory system between the sleep-inducing ventrolateral preoptic nucleus and the awake-promoting hypothalamic/brainstem arousal systems as the basis of a flip-flop switch that is stable in either the fully on or fully off positions, enabling rapid transitions from one stage to the other. Orexin neurons in the lateral hypothalamus stabilize this switch system by exciting arousal regions during wakefulness, preventing unwanted transitions between wakefulness and sleep. The importance of this stabilizing role is apparent in narcolepsy, in which an absence of the orexin neurons causes numerous, unintended transitions in and out of sleep and allows fragments of REM sleep to intrude into wakefulness.

Endocrine regulation is by way of magnocellular, parvicellular, and endocrine gland pathways.

Axons of the neurosecretory magnocellular neurons in the supraoptic and paraventricular nuclei traverse the pituitary stalk to the posterior pituitary gland.

Vasopressin/ADH regulates thirst and water balance, inhibiting diuresis and promoting reabsorption of water from the kidney.

Oxytocin, a circular nonapeptide, is released into the circulation where it acts peripherally on reproductive physiologic processes to induce uterine contraction and stimulate milk ejection, and centrally where it influences social cognition, discussed below.

The regulation of thirst and drinking behavior is also under the control of two circumventricular organs characterized by extensive, highly permeable capillaries and no discernible blood-brain barrier: the subfornical organ lying on the ventral surface of the fornix, and the vascular organ of the lamina terminalis.

As described above, the axons arising from parvicellular neurons of the paraventricular and arcuate nucleus contribute to the portal system of the anterior pituitary gland. They secrete corticotropin-releasing hormone (CRH), which stimulates the anterior pituitary to produce adrenocorticotropin (ACTH), which acts on its target organ, the adrenal cortex, to secrete cortisol.

Hypothalamic innervation of the endocrine system is also by achieved by autonomic innervation of the pancreas (second-order neuron projections to pancreas arise from paraventricular, lateral, and retrochiasmatic nuclei of the hypothalamus[117]) which contribute to regulating secretion of insulin and glucagon.

The Stress Response and Social Behavior

In addition to its pivotal roles in homeostasis and energy metabolism, the hypothalamic-pituitary-adrenal axis is deeply influential in neuropsychiatric function. The field of psycho-neuro-endocrinology is firmly rooted in the neurobehavioral roles of the glands and hormones of the hypothalamus, and the receptors for these hormones.[118]

The stress response is dependent upon the hypothalamic-pituitary-adrenal axis control over cortisol production described above. Glucocorticoid receptors are found throughout the brain and directly affect cognition, memory, and mood. The hypothalamic-pituitary-adrenal axis plays a central role in all forms of stress and many neuropsychiatric conditions, and the CRH system is altered in depression.[118] Gold and Chrousos[119] note that stress precipitates depression and alters its natural history, and that major depression and the stress response share similar phenomena, mediators, and circuits. Activity of the CRH system appears to correlate with the nature of depression. In melancholic depression the stress response is hyperactive, patients are anxious, dread the future, lose responsiveness to the environment, have insomnia, lose their appetite, and exhibit diurnal variation with depression worst in the morning. In these patients, the CRH system is activated, together with the locus ceruleus-noradrenergic system, with diminished activities of the growth hormone and reproductive axes. In contrast, atypical depression presents with lethargy, fatigue, hyperphagia, hypersomnia, reactivity to the environment, and diurnal variation such that depression is least in the morning. This state is accompanied by a downregulated hypothalamic-pituitary adrenal axis and CRH deficiency of central origin.

The medial preoptic nucleus, the ventrolateral part of the VM nucleus, and the centrally projecting oxytocin neurons of the paraventricular nucleus are key to the hypothalamic contributions to regulating *social behavior*.

The *medial preoptic nucleus* contains neurons that are responsive to sex steroids. It is sexually dimorphic, larger, and with more neurons in males than in female rodents. Its neurons fire during sexual stimulation, and lesions of this area in rodents disrupt both male and female sexual behavior. It projects to the ventrolateral part of the VM nucleus, lesions of which prevent male (mounting) and female (lordosis) sexual behavior. The medial preoptic and VM nuclei have strong projections to the lateral periaqueductal gray matter thought to mediate motor and autonomic patterns associated with sexual behavior.

The *ventromedial nucleus* is important in coordinating aggressive attack behavior, leading to the conclusion that VM nucleus neurons, which gate two opposite types of social interactions, share many of the same inputs but likely have distinct and different sets of output pathways that remain to be elucidated.[80] Aggression and rage are commonly reported following lesions or stimulation of the VM hypothalamus. Hypothalamic rage is a characteristic feature of the rare hypothalamic hamartoma of childhood. In the largest series to date, epilepsy (mostly gelastic in nature), precocious puberty, and intellectual disability were common. Psychiatric disorders were present in more than half the affected individuals, including attention-deficit/hyperactivity disorder, conduct and oppositional defiant disorders; rage attacks were characterized as explosive episodes secondary to poor frustration tolerance and affective aggression.[120] Stimulation of the hypothalamus in animal models has long been known to produce aggression, or a syndrome of uncontrolled rage. Philip Bard (1898–1977)[121] who localized this relationship to the diencephalon reasoned that "behavior attending the major emotions, fear and rage, is called forth by the urgency of certain definite circumstances and it is plainly directed toward the preservation of the individual. It constitutes a reaction which is primitive, energetically purposive and common to the divergent members of the vertebrate series. This consideration certainly suggests that the reaction is dependent upon older divisions of the nervous system." Bard noted that the decorticate cats of Walter Bradford Cannon (1871–1945) and Britton exhibited "a group of remarkable activities such as are usually associated with emotional excitement—a sort of sham rage,"[122] and concluded that the behavior following decortication "simulates the expression of anger as seen in the normal cat and is best described as a sham rage." [121] Lesions of the hypothalamus in adults also produce aggression as a central component of the constellation,[123] and in one case of craniopharyngioma involved the VM hypothalamus as well as the anterior, paraventricular, dorsomedial, supraoptic, lateral, tuberal, and posterior hypothalamic nuclei.[124] The hypothalamic attack area defined in rats is distinct from the hypothalamic structures involved in defense. Areas implicated in defense include the anterior hypothalamic nucleus, dorsomedial part of the VM hypothalamic nucleus, and the dorsal premammillary nucleus, all of which are highly interconnected.[125] The attack areas also include the anterior hypothalamic nucleus, in addition to the lateral anterior hypothalamic nucleus, retrochiasmatic area, ventrolateral part of the VM hypothalamic nucleus, and tuber cinereum dorsolateral to the VM nucleus. Three neuronal phenotypes in these structures are involved in the induction of attacks: glutamatergic neurons expressing vesicular glutamate transporter 2 mRNA (VGLUT2), glutamatergic neurons that coexpress TRH, and GABAergic neurons dispersed among the glutamatergic cells.[126]

The *centrally projecting oxytocin neurons originating in the paraventricular nucleus* are directed to extrahypothalamic regions including the amygdala, hippocampus, NAc, and VTA. The VTA and mesocorticolimbic dopamine system conveyed in the MFB are crucial not only for reward and motivated behavior but also for the expression of affiliative behaviors. There are oxytocin receptors throughout the mesocorticolimbic dopamine system, indicating that oxytocin interacts closely with neural pathways responsible for a wide range of motivated behaviors, enhancing motivational salience attributions toward social stimuli and provoking shifts in motivational value. Oxytocin is therefore a complex neuromodulator with the capacity to shape human social activities including parental behavior, pair bonding, selective aggression, sexual behavior, affiliative preferences, and social cognition.[127]

The hypothalamus exerts its effects on a wide range of social behaviors through the hormones of the anterior pituitary. *Gonadotropin-releasing hormone* (GnRH) neurons in the pre-optic-hypothalamic region project to the median eminence where they control the synthesis and release of luteinizing hormone and follicle-stimulating hormone in the anterior pituitary gland, which stimulates sex steroid secretion and gametogenesis in the gonads, thereby regulating reproductive behaviors. GnRH release is modulated by other hypothalamic neuropeptides, neurotransmitters, and steroid hormones which together influence social behaviors such as grooming, courtship, mating, and aggression, with roles also in food intake, and mood disorders including anxiety and depression.[128] *Thyrotropin-releasing hormone* (TRH) promotes the release in the anterior pituitary gland of thyrotropin (thyroid-stimulating hormone), prolactin, and growth hormone, and it inhibits somatostatin release. In the CNS, TRH stimulates neuronal excitability, enhances amine and cholinergic transmitter turnover, and promotes wakefulness and arousal in part through the hypocretin/orexin system,[129] as well as by stimulating respiration, inducing hyperthermia and hyperglycemia, increasing cerebral blood flow, and increasing heart rate and blood pressure. TRH and its analogs possess locomotor stimulant, anorectic, antinociceptive, and anticonvulsant effects.[130]

CORTICOID STRUCTURES

As conceptualized by Mesulam,[63] the corticoid structures are at the interface between the hypothalamic regulation of the internal milieu, and the phylogenetically ancient, limbic areas of the cerebral cortex. *Corticoid* regions include the basal forebrain on the ventral and medial surfaces of the hemisphere. These include the *septal region*, *substantia innominata*, and parts of the *amygdaloid complex* which contain the simplest, most undifferentiated type of cortex in the entire forebrain. The amygdaloid complex is considered a corticoid structure even though substantial parts of it have a subcortical nuclear appearance.

The septal nuclei contain cholinergic neurons that innervate the entire cerebral cortex. They include the *medial septal nucleus* (designated Ch1), the *vertical limb nucleus of the diagonal band of Broca* (Ch2), the *horizontal limb nucleus of the diagonal band of Broca* (Ch3), and the *nucleus basalis of Meynert* (Ch4). According to Engelhardt[131] the *substantia innominata* was named by Reil in 1809, the ansa peduncularis by Gratiolet in 1857, and the neurons within this area that Meynert described in 1872 were called the nucleus basalis of Meynert by Albert von Koelliker (1817–1905) in 1896. The *substantia*

innominata refers to an area now known to include three identified structures: the ventral striatopallidal system, the BNST of the extended amygdala, and the nucleus basalis of Meynert.[132] The substantia innominata is divided into a primarily rostral, subcommissural part which is the ventral extension of the pallidum, and a posterior, sublenticular portion that is associated with the extended amygdala.[132,133]

Cholinergic projections from the medial septal nucleus and the vertical limb nucleus (Ch1 and Ch2) are directed to the hippocampus; those from the horizontal limb (Ch3) to olfactory structures; and from the nucleus basalis of Meynert (Ch4) to all other cortical zones and the amygdala.[63] The acetylcholinesterase (AChE)-rich fibers arising from the nucleus basalis are more concentrated in limbic and paralimbic cortical areas in human brain than in immediately adjacent neocortical association areas.[134] The cortical input to the Ch4 neurons is derived from prepyriform cortex, orbitofrontal cortex, the anterior insula, the temporal pole, entorhinal cortex, and the medial temporal cortex, and from septal nuclei, the NAc-VP complex, and the hypothalamus. The Ch4 complex therefore provides cholinergic relay, transmitting predominantly limbic and paralimbic information to the neocortex.[135] Loss of cholinergic neurons in the nucleus basalis is one of the hallmark pathologic features in Alzheimer's disease, and the pathophysiological basis for the treatment of Alzheimer's disease with cholinesterase inhibitors, both for amnestic dementia as well as for its primary progressive aphasia variant.[136]

AMYGDALA

The amygdala (synonymous with the term *amygdaloid complex*) is an almond-shaped nuclear complex situated in the dorsomedial portion of the temporal lobe, rostral to the hippocampus. Together with the extended amygdala (below), it is implicated in emotionally salient functions: experience and expression of fear, modulation of implicit information processing and unconscious memory, mediation of social communication, reward learning and motivation, and emotional states associated with aggressive, maternal, sexual, and ingestive (eating and drinking) behaviors.[132,137–139] This multiplicity of functions is subserved by its intrinsic and extrinsic connections.

Nuclei of the Amygdala

The nuclei of the amygdala are conceptualized as conforming to an evolutionarily primitive division associated with the olfactory system (cortical, medial, and central nuclei), and an evolutionarily newer division associated with the neocortex (lateral, basal, and accessory basal nuclei) (Fig. 1-11A,B). The areas of the older division are sometimes grouped as the corticomedial region (cortical and medial nuclei) and sometimes as the centromedial region (the central and medial nuclei). In contrast, the newer structures related to the neocortex are often referred to as the basolateral region.[86,139,140]

The *cortical nucleus* and the *medial nucleus* both have three cell layers: a cell-poor superficial or molecular layer, a middle cell-dense layer, and a deep layer consisting of less densely distributed neurons.

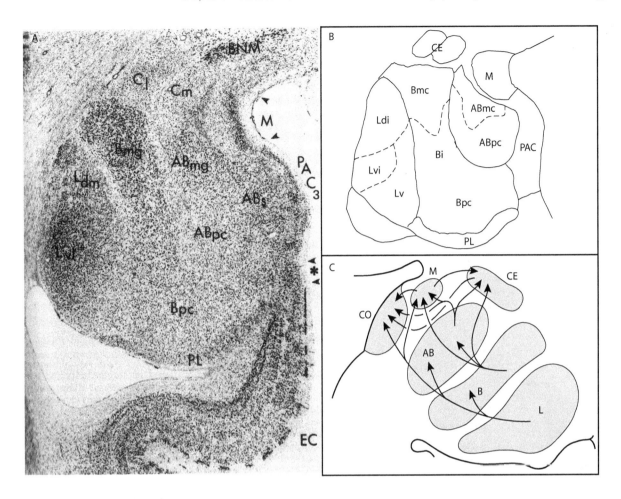

FIGURE 1-11. (A) Amygdaloid complex in monkeys, Nissl stain. (From *Gray's Anatomy*,[84] Fig. 8.246, as provided by David Amaral.) **(B)** Schematic of amygdaloid nuclei. (Adapted from Freese and Amaral,[146] Fig. 1.5.) **(C)** Intrinsic connections of amygdaloid nuclei. (From Nieuwenhuys et al.,[86] Fig. 13.5.) AB, accessory basal nucleus; ABmg/ABmc, accessory basal nucleus, magnocellular subdivision; ABpc, accessory basal nucleus, parvicellular subdivision; Abs, basal nucleus, superficial subdivision; B, basal nucleus; Bmg/Bmc, basal nucleus, magnocellular subdivision; Bi, basal nucleus, intermediate division; BNM, nucleus basalis of Meynert; Bpc, basal nucleus, parvicellular subdivision; CE, central nucleus; Cl, central nucleus, lateral subdivision; Cm, central nucleus, medial subdivision; CO, cortical nucleus; EC, entorhinal cortex; L, lateral nucleus; Ldi, lateral nucleus, dorsal intermediate division; Ldm, lateral nucleus, dorsomedial subdivision; Lv, lateral nucleus, ventral division; Lvl, lateral nucleus, ventrolateral subdivision; M, medial nucleus; PAC/PAC3, cortical nucleus or periamygdaloid complex (third subdivision); PL, basal nucleus, paralaminar subdivision.

The *central nucleus* has medial magnocellular and lateral magnocellular sectors, and its neurons resemble the medium spiny neurons (MSNs) of the striatum.

The *lateral nucleus* is the largest nucleus in the human amygdala and the principal recipient of sensory information from the neocortex. It is divided into three subnuclei: dorsal magnocellular, intermediate parvicellular, and a ventral paralaminar component.

The *basal nucleus* has a dorsal, magnocellular part, an intermediate parvicellular part, both of which have pyramidal-like projection neurons and smaller non-pyramidal local circuit neurons, and a ventral paralaminar basal nucleus that borders the white matter ventral to the amygdaloid complex. The basal nucleus has strong reciprocal connections with the adjacent temporal lobe and orbitofrontal neocortex.

The *accessory basal nucleus* has a dorsal magnocellular and ventral parvicellular part.

Extended Amygdala

The central and medial nuclei of the amygdala extend across the basal forebrain and within the stria terminalis, merging with the BNST. As conceptualized by Lennart Heimer (1930–2007) this expansive nuclear complex is the extended amygdala (Fig. 1-12), a macrostructure formed by the centromedial amygdaloid complex (medial nucleus, medial and lateral parts of the central nucleus), the BNST, and the cell columns traversing the sublenticular substantia innominata between them.[84] The extended amygdala has highly organized reciprocal pathways with the hypothalamus and brainstem.

The *bed nucleus of the stria terminalis* is located ventral to the septum, above and below the AC, and anterior to the hypothalamus, expanding caudally into the central and medial nuclei of the amygdala.[141] It is a cluster of between 12 and 18 subnuclei that surround the caudal part of the AC, located at the rostral extremity of the stria terminalis through which it connects

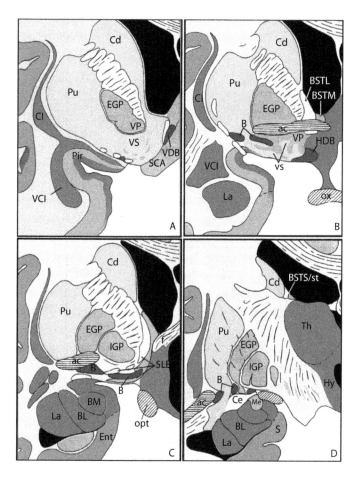

FIGURE 1-12. Extended amygdala and ventral striatum according to Heimer. Drawings showing the ventral striatum of the human basal forebrain. **(A)** Coronal schematic at the level of the nucleus accumbens. **(B)** The ventral pallidum (VP) extends downward into the region recognized as the substantia innominata. **(C)** The sublenticular portion of the substantia innominata is associated with the extended amygdala. In this concept of the substantia innominata, the basal nucleus of Meynert (B) is a relatively small third component. **(D)** Central (Ce) and medial (Me) nuclei of the amygdala are apparent with their corresponding projections along the stria terminalis and the superior component of the bed nucleus of the stria terminalis. ac, anterior commissure; BL, basolateral nucleus of amygdala; BM, basomedial nucleus of amygdala; BSTL, bed nucleus of stria terminalis, lateral division; BSTM, BST, medial division; BSTS, BST, superior division; Cd, caudate; Cl, claustrum; EGP, external segment of the globus pallidus; Ent, entorhinal cortex; f, fornix; HDB, diagonal band; Hy, hypothalamus; IGP, internal segment of GP; La, lateral nucleus of the amygdala; opt, optic track; ox, optic chiasm; Pir, piriform cortex; Pu, putamen; SLEA, sublenticular component of extended amygdala; st, stria terminalis; Th, thalamus; VDB, diagonal band; VS, ventral striatum. (Figure and legend reproduced from Elias et al.[133] Originally published in Heimer et al.[142])

receptors, neurotransmitters, transporters, and proteins. The anterior group specializes in energy balance, the posterior group contributes more to reproduction and defense. The anterior and posterior groups are highly interconnected, minimizing the likelihood of distinct or unrelated functions for the two divisions.[143] Anatomical studies of its connectivity indicate that the BNST is a coordinating and relay center where descending cerebral cortical information meets ascending interoceptive and exteroceptive information regarding homeostatic states or potential changes in homeostasis. Information flows into the BNST from all central nervous system levels—spinal cord, brainstem, and cerebral cortex. Exteroceptive inputs are derived from the main and accessory olfactory, touch and nociception, and gustatory sources; interoceptive inputs convey information regarding energy and fluid levels, tissue damage, and sex hormones. The BNST has widespread descending projections to effector regions of the hindbrain.[143] It has been proposed as a center of integration for limbic information and valence monitoring, regulating emotional state, arousal, motivation for social behavior, and social attachment. It is sexually dimorphic and is engaged in social attachment behaviors including initiation of mating and offspring and parental bonding. It is implicated in psychiatric states of sustained fear, generalized anxiety disorder, posttraumatic stress disorder, antisocial behavior, and aggression.[144]

Connections of the Amygdala

Intrinsic Connections

There are extensive intrinsic connections within the amygdala (Fig. 1-11C). The major flow of information is unidirectional, from lateral to medial. The intra-amygdaloid connections arise mostly in the lateral and basal nuclei and terminate particularly in the central and medial nuclei. Further details may be found in primary sources and reviews.[84,86,145-148]

Extrinsic Connections

(Approach adapted from Nieuwenhuys et al.[86])

There are three fiber tracts that convey the afferent and efferent connections of the amygdala.

The lateral olfactory stria carries secondary olfactory fibers to the cortical and medial amygdala nuclei. The *ventral amygdalofugal pathway* courses through the sublenticular region of the substantia innominata. It is a bidirectional pathway that links the dorsal medial part of the amygdala with the lateral preoptic hypothalamic area, medial dorsal thalamic nucleus, and medial prefrontal cortex. *The stria terminalis* is the dorsal amygdalofugal pathway. It emerges from the caudal aspect of the amygdala, runs a long, curved course along the medial border of the caudate nucleus to the AC, splits up into precommissural, commissural, and postcommissural components, and terminates in the hypothalamus.

Afferents to the Amygdala
Olfactory

Secondary olfactory fibers from the olfactory bulb course in the lateral olfactory tract to the cortical nucleus. Prepyriform cortex sends fibers to the basolateral complex. Olfactory recipient

with the amygdala. The exact number of BNST nuclei varies depending on the morphological criteria used. It is roughly divided into anterior and posterior subdivisions identified by their projection pattern and neurochemical identity, with different nuclei containing distinct neuronal subpopulations of

parts of the entorhinal cortex project to central, basolateral, and cortical nuclei.

Basomedial Telencephalon and Hypothalamus

The medial and central nuclei receive information from the BNST and the horizontal limb of the diagonal band of Broca, as well as from the periventricular, VM, and arcuate nuclei of the hypothalamus. The basal and accessory basal nuclei inputs are derived from the substantia innominata.

Thalamus

Midline thalamic nuclei and the parafascicular nucleus project to the central amygdala nucleus. The parvocellular part of the thalamic ventral posterior medial nucleus which receives visceral and gustatory information projects to the lateral nucleus of the amygdala that receives similar information. The medial geniculate nucleus (auditory recipient) sends projections to the lateral, accessory basal, and central nuclei.

Brainstem

The ventral amygdalofugal pathway conveys brainstem afferents to the central nucleus, arising from the periaqueductal gray, SNc, VTA, dorsal raphe nucleus, locus ceruleus, lateral parabrachial nucleus, nucleus of the solitary tract, and the ventrolateral medulla.

Hippocampus

The presubiculum and CA1 fields project to the lateral, basal, and central nuclei.

Cerebral Cortex

There are extensive, topographically precisely arranged cerebral cortical projections to the nuclei of the amygdala.[15,149–152] Sensory association cortices subserving vision, somatic sensation, and taste target separate areas within the lateral nucleus. Temporal lobe projections to the lateral nucleus arise from auditory association cortex in the anterior half of the superior temporal gyrus, visual association areas in the inferior part of the temporal lobe, medial temporal structures including the perirhinal areas, temporal pole, and the polymodal cortex in the upper back of the superior temporal sulcus (STS). Insula projections to the lateral nucleus are derived from the rostral, agranular insula involved in visceral and gustatory functions, and the posterior, granular cortex involved in somatosensory association functions including the processing of nociceptive information. The visual and auditory association areas, insula, and orbitofrontal cortex also project to the central nucleus. Medial prefrontal, and rostral and anterior cingulate projections target the basal and accessory basal nuclei. Caudal orbitofrontal areas project to the medial olfactory related nuclei.

Efferents from the Amygdala
Hypothalamus, Septum, and Preoptic Region

The cortical and medial nuclei send information through the stria terminalis to the hypothalamus, the precommissural fibers terminating in the medial preoptic nucleus, anterior hypothalamic area, paraventricular, VM, and premammillary nuclei. The cortical, medial, and central nuclei also send postcommissural fibers to the BNST. The ventral amygdalofugal pathway links the basal, accessory basal, and central nuclei to the lateral hypothalamic area and to the basal septal region: nucleus basalis of Meynert, nucleus of the horizontal limb of the diagonal band, and BNST.

Hippocampus

There are extensive projections from the amygdala to the hippocampus.[153] The accessory basal, lateral basal, and medial basal nuclei project to fields CA1–3, the heaviest termination in CA3, with additional projections from the basal nuclei to the subiculum (prosubiculum, presubiculum, and parasubiculum). Accessory basal and lateral nuclei project to entorhinal cortex (area 28) and the prorhinal cortex. The lateral basal nucleus projects to the perirhinal cortex. These amygdalo-hippocampal connections provide a neural substrate for the linkage of emotional experience with memory and affective response. In human imaging studies, the processing of emotionally salient events engages the amygdalo-hippocampal network, the amygdala influencing hippocampal dynamics during fear processing.[154]

Thalamus

The lateral basal nuclei project to the medial magnocellular part of the medial dorsal thalamic nucleus. The central and medial nuclei project to thalamic midline nuclei.

Brainstem

The central nucleus that sends fibers through the ventral amygdalofugal pathway into the lateral part of the hypothalamus also targets multiple nuclei in the midbrain tegmentum including those engaged in autonomic control.

Striatum

The basal and accessory basal nuclei send efferents through the stria terminalis to the ventral striatum including the NAc and striatal-like portions of the olfactory tubercle, as well as topographically arranged projections to the caudate nucleus and putamen, preferentially in the AChE-poor striosomes. These striatal projections overlap those from the cingulate cortex, VTA, and mesencephalic raphe nuclei.

Cerebral Cortex

There are extensive projections from the amygdala to the frontal, insular, temporal, and occipital cortices.[146,155–158]

Basal and accessory basal nuclei project to temporal and occipital visual association areas; lateral and accessory basal nuclei project to temporal auditory association cortices; basal and accessory basal nuclei project to the perirhinal cortex, as well as to the insular cortex which receives input also from the medial and cortical nuclei. The basal and accessory basal nuclei project widely to the cingulate gyrus, and throughout the medial, orbital, and dorsolateral prefrontal cortices. In the amygdalo-frontal circuity, cingulate areas 24 and 25 send comparatively more projections to the amygdala than they receive, whereas caudal orbitofrontal areas receive more input from the amygdala than they send. This has relevance for the pathways underlying the sequence of information processing for emotions.[159] The connections linking the posterior orbitofrontal cortex, anterior temporal sensory association areas, and the amygdala have a key role in emotion processing, and the laminar-specific details of their interactions suggest that they are engaged in sequential and collaborative interactions in evaluating sensory information and emotional milieu for decision and action in complex behavior.[160]

Further Functional Considerations

The structural boundaries of the amygdala remain a matter of debate, particularly with respect to the anatomy and functions of the extended amygdala. Nevertheless, generally accepted views are that (i) the amygdala receives input from many cortical and subcortical structures; (ii) it serves an important role in integrating and evaluating interoceptive and exteroceptive sensory stimuli, and thus in permitting an individual to ascribe emotional meaning to events; (iii) it coordinates adaptive behavioral responses to emotion elicitors; and (iv) it modulates cognitive processing in other brain regions. Further, the amygdala is the most densely interconnected region of the primate forebrain leading to the conclusion that its scope of influence must be wide ranging.[161]

Freese and Amaral[146] view the amygdala as a danger detector. Sensory information, particularly relating to vision and hearing, is evaluated after arriving in the lateral nucleus. If danger is detected, it orchestrates a whole-body response in the form of escape via connections to the neocortex enabling selective attention to the danger stimulus, via projections to the cholinergic basal forebrain that enhance generalized arousal, and projections to hypothalamus and brainstem from the central nucleus that mobilize visceral and autonomic components of the escape response. The lateral nucleus projections to the effector central nucleus is by way of the basal nucleus, which also receives input from the orbital cortex, thereby potentially acting as a coincidence detector engaged in context evaluation: A stimulus that may be fearful in one context may be benign in another.

Amygdala projections to all levels of the ventral stream visual pathway including the primary visual cortex, area V1, suggest that the amygdala has modulatory control over sensory processing at all stages of the ventral-stream visual cortical hierarchy.[157] This pathway, among others, has relevance for the phenomenon of motivated perception, seeing what we want to see, and of attentionally modulated salience perception, seeing what we need to see. Visual and other perceptions can be biased, selective, and malleable, even at the earliest stages of sensory experience.[162]

HIPPOCAMPUS

The hippocampus is critical for learning and memory, especially anterograde episodic and contextual memory. This is exemplified clinically by the case of HM who developed profound, permanent, anterograde amnesia following bilateral removal of the anterior temporal lobes and hippocampal formations to treat epilepsy.[163] Degree of hippocampal atrophy is a marker of the stage and severity of Alzheimer's disease,[164,165] and paradoxically increased hippocampal activity is an early indicator of Alzheimer's disease-related neurodegeneration.[166]

Gross Anatomy

The hippocampus lies in the floor of the inferior horn of the lateral ventricle of each cerebral hemisphere, deep to the parahippocampal gyrus, along the ventromedial edge of the temporal lobe. It has an elongated, curvilinear shape, broader at its anterior aspect in the temporal lobe and narrower further caudally (Fig. 1-5). At its most caudal end it becomes continuous with the rudimentary indusium griseum, a strand of hippocampal tissue lying on the superior surface of the CC, extending rostrally throughout its length (Fig. 1-5B). There are two small fiber bundles, the medial and lateral longitudinal striae of Lancisi (after Giovanni Maria Lancisi, 1654−1720[167]) embedded in the indusium griseum, that represent a small supracallosal component of the fornix. The indusium griseum and longitudinal striae, both dorsal remnants of the archicortex of the hippocampus and fornix, are minor components of the limbic system.

Historical Vignettes

The hippocampus and the pyriform/olfactory cortex are allocortical structures. Together with the periallocortical entorhinal and cingulate cortices and the amygdaloid and septal nuclei they comprise the phylogenetically oldest structures of the mammalian telencephalon.[168] The term hippocampus was introduced by Giulio Cesare Aranzio (Arantius) (1530–1589) in 1587[169] because when dissected free from the temporal lobe he found that it resembles the shape of a seahorse (hippocampus in Latin, hippokampos in Greek).[170] The etymology of the CA1 through CA4 fields of the hippocampus originates in the description by Jacques Bénigne Winslow (1669–1760) in 1732 of the coronal section of the hippocampus having the appearance of a ram's horn.[170,171] Rene de Garengeot (1688–1759)[170,172] called this horn-like appearance the Cornu Ammonis in recognition of the horns depicted in images of Amun/Ammon, the Egyptian god of sun and air.[173] In 1934 Rafael Lorente de Nó (1902–1990) coined the designation CA for the fields of the hippocampus.[168,174,175]

Definition of Terms

The term *hippocampus proper* is reserved for the pyramidal subfields CA1 through CA4, differentiated from each other by the size and packing density of their pyramidal cells; *hippocampus* refers to the pyramidal subfields plus the dentate gyrus (also known as the *fascia dentata*); *hippocampal formation* includes the hippocampus, subiculum, and the prosubiculum lying between the CA1 field and the subiculum (Fig. 1-13A,B). The parahippocampal gyrus contains the presubiculum and parasubiculum which are progressively lateral to the subiculum, and the entorhinal cortex adjacent to the parasubiculum and lying at the medial boundary of the ventral temporal lobe.

Histological Identifying Features

Four histologic features characterize the hippocampal formation (dentate gyrus, CA1–CA4 fields, subiculum, and prosubiculum)[168]:

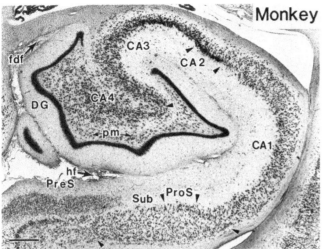

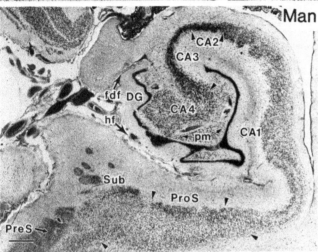

FIGURE 1-13. Coronal sections through the hippocampal formation in monkey and human (Nissl-stained). Bars, 0.5 mm in monkey, 1 mm in human. Approximate boundaries of cytoarchitectonic subdivisions marked by arrowheads. CA1, 2, 3, 4, Cornu Ammonis 1, 2, 3, 4, subfields of Lorente de Nó[174]; DG, dentate gyrus; fdf, fimbriodentate fissure; Hf, hippocampal fissure; Pm, polymorph cell layer of the dentate gyrus; PreS, presubiculum; ProS, prosubiculum; Sub, subiculum. (From Rosene and Van Hoesen[168] Fig. 4B,C.)

1. Three-layered allocortex:
   i. A superficial plexiform layer of dendrites, axons, glia, and a few scattered neurons.
   ii. A deeper prominent cellular layer composed of predominantly one cell type: granule cells in the dentate gyrus, pyramidal cells in the hippocampus and subiculum.
   iii. An underlying polymorph layer of dendrites, axons, and scattered polymorphic neurons.
2. Major source of direct input is from the adjacent periallocortical entorhinal cortex, terminating in the most superficial part of the molecular layer.
3. Tightly linked together by a serial set of intrinsic connections beginning in the dentate gyrus and terminating in the subiculum at the transition with the adjacent periallocortex of the presubiculum.

4. Highly segregated laminar organization of both extrinsic and intrinsic afferents.

Intrinsic Circuitry of the Hippocampus

Information enters the hippocampal formation from the entorhinal cortex and exits via the subiculum (Fig. 1-14A,B). The internal relay of information within the hippocampus is conveyed predominantly via a trisynaptic circuit described by Cajal.[176–179]

1. *The entorhinal cortex projects via the perforant pathway to the dentate gyrus*: Axons of the large stellate cells in layer II of entorhinal cortex perforate through the subiculum and the zone of the obliterated hippocampal fissure and ramify through the outer two-thirds of the molecular layer of the dentate gyrus forming excitatory synapses on dendritic spines of the granule cells.
2. *Dentate gyrus projects via mossy fibers to CA3*: The granule cells of the dentate gyrus send mossy fibers to the CA3 field and form a separate sublayer, participating in sizeable synaptic complexes with large CA3 pyramidal cells.
3. *CA3 projects via Schaffer collaterals to CA1*: The axons of the CA3 pyramidal neurons course to the alveus of the hippocampus, and in so doing issue Schaffer collaterals (after Károly Schaffer, 1864–1939) which synapse with apical and basal dendrites of pyramidal neurons in CA1.
4. *Information exits the hippocampal formation from CA1 and the subiculum*: The pyramidal cells of CA1 project extensively to the subiculum, and more lightly to the entorhinal cortex. The subiculum conveys efferents from the hippocampal formation, projecting to the presubiculum, parasubiculum, and entorhinal cortex.

Some fibers in the perforant pathway originating in layer II of the entorhinal cortex terminate in the CA3 field directly, and some originating in layer III of the entorhinal cortex course directly to CA1 and the subiculum.

Hippocampal area CA2 is a small zone lying between CA1 and CA3. Its hippocampal afferents are from granule cells of the dentate gyrus, CA3 neurons via Schaffer collaterals, and layer II pyramidal neurons of the medial and lateral entorhinal cortex. Extrahippocampal inputs to CA2 are from the vasopressin neurons in the paraventricular nucleus, the supramammillary nucleus of the hypothalamus, the median raphe, and diagonal band of Broca. Its projections target CA1 and the medial entorhinal cortex.[180] The pyramidal neurons in CA2 are molecularly distinct from those in neighboring CA1 and CA3,[181] and the Schaffer collaterals that synapse on CA2 neurons exhibit "a perplexing lack" of synaptic long-term potentiation.[182] This is consistent with the observation that, compared to other CA regions, CA2 pyramidal neurons are normally resistant to the induction of synaptic plasticity.[181] CA2 neurons are also relatively resistant to hypoxia.

In sum, the entorhinal cortex provides afferents into the hippocampus, and the subicular complex is the source of efferents from the hippocampal formation. These arrangements form a closed circuit consisting of a series of unidirectional, excitatory projections.[86]

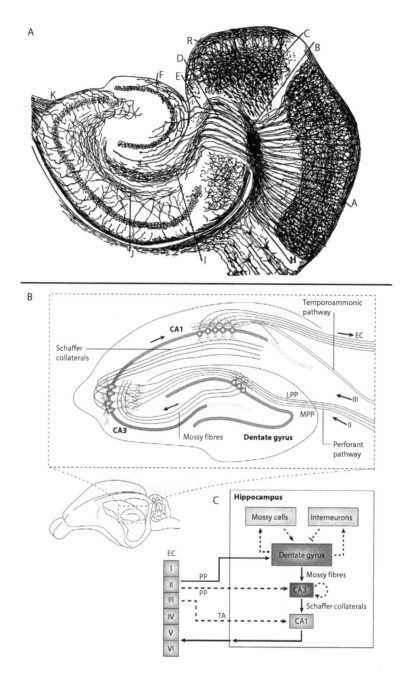

FIGURE 1-14. (A) Cajal's illustration of the mouse hippocampus, shown here to highlight the perforant pathway. (From Cajal,[177] Fig. 55.) A, spheno-occipital ganglion (entorhinal cortex); B, point of concurrence of the inferior perforating spheno-cornual bundles (perforant pathway conveying entorhinal cortex projections to Ammon's horn CA3 and to dentate gyrus); D, perforating fibres (perforant pathway); E, fibers destined for the fascia dentata (perforant pathway fibers to dentate gyrus); alvear spheno-cornual pathway (entorhinal-Ammon's horn) and the plexus that it forms in the subiculum; I, distribution of the perforating fibres in the stratum lacunosum of the horn (entorhinal cortex afferents to CA3); J, plexus of collaterals of the horn (Schaffer collaterals from CA3 to CA1). **(B)** Illustration and **(C)** schematic of the intrinsic circuitry of the mouse hippocampus. The traditional excitatory trisynaptic pathway (entorhinal cortex (EC)–dentate gyrus–CA3–CA1–EC) is depicted by solid arrows. The axons of layer II neurons in the entorhinal cortex project to the dentate gyrus through the perforant pathway (PP), including the lateral perforant pathway (LPP) and medial perforant pathway (MPP). The dentate gyrus sends projections to the pyramidal cells in CA3 through mossy fibers. CA3 pyramidal neurons relay the information to CA1 pyramidal neurons through Schaffer collaterals. CA1 pyramidal neurons send back-projections into deep-layer neurons of the EC. CA3 also receives direct projections from EC layer II neurons through the PP. CA1 receives direct input from EC layer III neurons through the temporoammonic pathway (TA). The dentate granule cells also project to the mossy cells in the hilus and hilar interneurons, which send excitatory and inhibitory projections, respectively, back to the granule cells. (Figure and legend from Deng et al.[179])

Extrinsic Connections of the Hippocampus

(Styled after Nieuwenhuys et al.[86])

Afferents to the Hippocampus
Cerebral Cortex

Many of these connections are mentioned later with discussion of the projections conveyed by the long association fiber pathways to the entorhinal cortex. They are derived from the inferotemporal regions in the perirhinal and parahippocampal areas, agranular insula, temporal pole, caudal orbitofrontal cortex, superior temporal gyrus, and the entire rostral to caudal extent of the cingulate gyrus from the pregenual to the retrosplenial cortex.[29,150,183–187] Association areas in prefrontal, posterior parietal, temporal, and occipital areas project to the hippocampus indirectly through multisynaptic inputs to the entorhinal cortex. Projections directly to the subicular complex are derived from perirhinal, posterior parahippocampal, posterior cingulate, and caudal inferior parietal regions. This multiplicity of cortical areas provides the hippocampus with a broad spectrum of sensory-specific and multimodal information with topographic arrangement such that limbic-related cortical and subcortical inputs are directed predominantly to the anterior hippocampus, whereas exteroceptive sensory information is preferentially available to the posterior hippocampus.[150,183]

Amygdala

The lateral basal and accessory basal nuclei of the amygdala project to the entorhinal cortex; the basal nuclei project also to the subicular complex.

Medial Septal—Diagonal Band Complex

Cholinergic projections from the medial septal nucleus and the nucleus of the diagonal band of Broca pass through the fornix-fimbria and the MFB, terminating principally in the dentate gyrus.[188] These septo-hippocampal projections underlie the hippocampal theta rhythm important for normal hippocampal function.[189]

Supramammillary Region

Neurons situated above the mammillary body have projections via the fornix to the dentate gyrus and CA3 and are involved in the regulation of theta activity.[190]

Thalamus

Thalamic fibers to the hippocampus course through the CB. Projections from the anterior thalamic nuclei terminate in the presubiculum, those from the midline reuniens and paraventricular nuclei terminate in the entorhinal cortex, subiculum, and CA1. The reuniens nucleus receives visceral information from the periphery through its brainstem afferents and transmits this information to limbic structures.

Monoaminergic Brainstem Nuclei

Afferents from modulatory neurotransmitter systems include serotonergic projections from the mesencephalic raphe nuclei, noradrenergic from the locus ceruleus, and dopaminergic from the VTA. Serotonin innovation is principally in the deep zone of the dentate gyrus plexiform layer and layer III of the entorhinal cortex. Noradrenergic fibers are seen throughout the dentate gyrus plexiform layer, and in CA3. These inputs complement the cholinergic inputs from the medial septum.

Efferents from the Hippocampal Formation

Efferents from the hippocampal formation exit either by way of the fornix or the subiculum, with minor efferents from the hippocampus proper.

Efferents Conveyed in the Fornix

The fornix carries axons arising from the subiculum, as well as those of the CA3 axons that gave rise to the Schaffer collaterals. Together they continue their course into the alveus of the hippocampus, a white layer of myelinated fibers on the ventricular surface of Ammon's horn (the hippocampus proper). They converge as the fimbria along the medial aspect of the hippocampus, run posteriorly and superiorly to enter the crus of the fornix, a flattened structure that arches upwards and medially under the splenium of the CC. Some fibers decussate to the opposite hemisphere, forming the hippocampal commissure. The two crura of the fornix join and course anteriorly beneath the CC, separate again at the anterior pole of the thalamus as the columns of the fornix, curve ventrally in front of the intraventricular foramen of Monro (Alexander Monro, Secundus [1733–1817][191]) and caudal to the AC, and descend through the hypothalamus. The fornix terminates either as precommissural fibers or postcommissural fibers. Precommissural fornix fibers terminate in the septum (lateral septal nucleus) and basal forebrain (NAc), caudate nucleus and putamen, anterior olfactory cortex, precommissural hypothalamus, medial part of the frontal cortex, and gyrus rectus. The postcommissural fornix fibers, a major highway in the Papez circuit involved in episodic memory and emotional processing, terminate in the mammillary bodies. Some fibers distribute directly also to the anterior thalamic nucleus, the BNST, and the zone around the VM hypothalamic nucleus.

Efferents Directly from the Subicular Complex/Hippocampus Proper

Projections to the lateral septal nucleus are derived from hippocampal CA1–CA4 fields. The multiple association and paralimbic areas of the cortex that project to the entorhinal cortex before entering the hippocampal formation, reviewed above, receive projections back from the hippocampal formation by way of the subicular complex, entorhinal cortex, and the perirhinal-posterior parahippocampal complex.

Functional Relevance

The discovery of place cells in the CA1 field of the hippocampus encoding spatial location prompted a general theory of hippocampal function called the cognitive map theory.[192] Confirmatory evidence was provided by a paradigmatic imaging experiment showing larger posterior hippocampal volumes in London cabdrivers.[193] The CA3 field is also engaged in spatial memory as it contains an autoassociative network in which synaptic connections between CA3 neurons that represent different components of a memory are strengthened via recurrent collateral connections, supporting multiple processes including the formation of spatial arbitrary associations, temporary maintenance of spatial working memory, spatial pattern completion, and spatial pattern separation.[194] In contrast to the spatial memory functions of the CA1 and CA3 fields, the CA2 field is a critical hub for sociocognitive memory processing.[195] This observation has clinical relevance because CA2 has a high concentration of inhibitory neurons preferentially affected in schizophrenia and neurodegenerative diseases including Parkinson's disease and Lewy body disease.[196,197]

Alzheimer's disease is characterized by progressive and massive focal neuropathology that isolates the hippocampal formation from much of its input and output.[198] Cell loss, neurofibrillary tangles, and neuritic plaques affect only certain subfields of the hippocampal formation, while adjacent, anatomically distinct subfields are relatively spared. The portions of the hippocampal formation most crucial for both cortical and subcortical efferent projections are severely affected. Neurofibrillary tangles are most notable in the subiculum and CA1 subfields, and layer IV of the entorhinal cortex. Hippocampal input is also compromised by severe neurofibrillary changes in layer II of entorhinal cortex, which gives rise to the perforant pathway hippocampal afferents. Neuritic plaques appear in a distinct layer in the terminal zone of the perforant pathway, which carries the majority of corticohippocampal afferents. Plaques are also common in a zone that receives serotonergic projections from the raphe complex, thus compromising another hippocampal afferent. These changes disrupt intrinsic and extrinsic hippocampal circuitry at multiple levels, and the pathological dissection deprives the hippocampal formation of many of its efferent and afferent connections with cortical and subcortical structures important in memory-related neural systems. These changes contribute to the memory impairment and intellectual decline that characterize Alzheimer's disease.[199]

PYRIFORM/OLFACTORY CORTEX

The two types of allocortex are archicortex (the hippocampal formation discussed above) and paleocortex, the pyriform/olfactory cortex. The olfactory cortices includes the *anterior olfactory cortex* (previously termed the anterior olfactory nucleus[200]), the *olfactory tubercle* (immediately behind the bifurcation of the medial and lateral olfactory striae forming part of the anterior perforated substance), and the *pyriform cortex*, as well as the *olfactory amygdala* (cortical amygdala and nucleus of the lateral olfactory tract) and the *part of the lateral entorhinal cortex which receives direct projections from the olfactory bulb.*[86,200–203]

The pyriform cortex (Fig. 1-15) receives inputs from the olfactory bulb and other regions of the olfactory cortex. It sends feedback projections to the olfactory bulb, the anterior olfactory cortex, olfactory tubercle, cortical amygdala, and the lateral entorhinal cortex, as well as the mediodorsal nucleus of thalamus, and caudal orbitofrontal and agranular insular cortices. According to Haberly,[200] the olfactory bulb serves as the primary olfactory cortex by encoding "molecular features" (structural components common to many odorant molecules) as a patchy mosaic reminiscent of the representation of simple features in primary visual cortex. The anterior olfactory cortex detects and

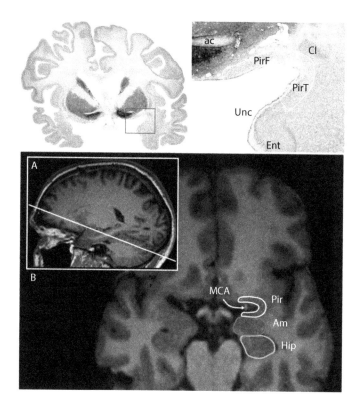

FIGURE 1-15. (A) Anatomical location of the pyriform cortex. Nissl-stained coronal brain slice at the level of the anterior commissure of a 65-year-old woman, from the BigBrain dataset.[32] ac, anterior commissure; Cl, claustrum; Ent, entorhinal cortex; PirF, frontal pyriform cortex; PirT, temporal pyriform cortex; Unc, uncus. **(B)** T1-weighted MPRAGE image of a 37-year-old man, displayed in a (A) para-sagittal and (B) oblique-axial orientation, approximately +20° relative to the anterior commissure-posterior commissure axis. This orientation allows the relationship between the pyriform cortex (Pir), amygdala (Am), and hippocampus (Hip) to be seen. The arrow indicates the position of the middle cerebral artery within the entorhinal sulcus. (Images and legend from Vaughan and Jackson.[202])

stores correlations between olfactory features, creating representations (gestalts) for odorants and odorant mixtures. This function places anterior olfactory cortex at the level of secondary visual cortex. The pyriform cortex participates in odor discrimination, association, and learning.[204] It enables object recognition in a sensory landscape, the relevant perceptual dimensions of which are dynamically shaped by sensory experience.[205] Pyriform cortex therefore carries out functions that define association cortex. It detects and learns correlations between olfactory gestalts formed in anterior olfactory cortex, and a large repertoire of behavioral, cognitive, and contextual information to which it has access through reciprocal connections with prefrontal, entorhinal, perirhinal, and amygdaloid areas.

The direct and strong interconnections between pyriform cortex subserving odor detection, and other structures of the limbic circuitry including the amygdala, thalamus, and entorhinal cortex, as well as insular and orbitofrontal cortices explain the importance of smell for eliciting powerful and emotionally valent memories. According to Vaughan and Jackson,[202] the pyriform cortex is highly relevant to the understanding of human

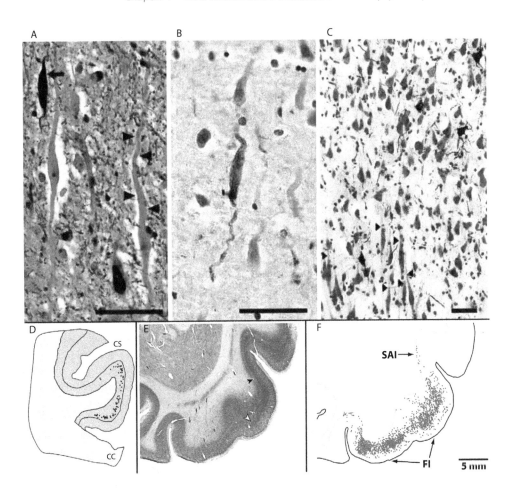

FIGURE 1-16. Von Economo neurons (VENs). **(A)** VENs in Pick's disease, possibly representing distinct stages of degeneration. VENs show dense argyrophilic deposits, at times obscuring nearly the entire neuron (arrow). Others show bloating and undulation of proximal dendrites (arrowheads). A VEN with normal morphology (directly below arrow) provides a comparison. Modified Bielschowsky silver stain. **(B)** VENs in Pick's disease show hyperphosphorylated tau deposition in proximal apical and basal dendrites. CP-13 antibody/hematoxylin counterstain. **(C)** In Alzheimer's disease, normal VEN clusters persist despite extensive anterior cingulate cortex (ACC) neurofibrillary pathology. Arrowheads point to VEN apical dendrites. CP-13 antibody/cresyl violet counterstain. Scale bars = 50 microns. Photomicrographs oriented with pial surface at the top. From Seeley et al.[210] **(D)** Computer-generated map of distribution of spindle neurons in the human anterior cingulate cortex at the level of the genu of the corpus callosum.[207] **(E, F)** Photomicrograph of frontal section through frontoinsular cortex (FI) in a 1.6-year-old male human, with a corresponding section in which the location was plotted of the 2415 VENs identified. SAI, superior insular cortex. (Figure and legend from Allman et al.[206])

focal epilepsy arising from the temporal or frontal lobes. It is a common node of discharge spread, can be injured and kindled by seizure activity, and may be involved in the facilitation and distribution of epileptic discharges throughout limbic and cortical networks. It is also a potential target for invasive therapies, including EEG recording and surgical resection.

CONSTITUENTS OF THE CEREBRAL CORTEX

The cerebral cortex consists of neurons, glial cells, and fibers.

Cortical neurons belong to two general types: pyramidal and non-pyramidal (including stellate, bitufted, and bipolar) cells. The fibers of the cerebral cortex are oriented either parallel (horizontal) or perpendicular (vertical) to the pial surface. Cells and fibers are organized in laminae. A specific subtype of cerebral cortical neuron, the *von Economo neuron* (VEN; Constantin von Economo 1876–1931)[206] was described by von Economo and

Koskinas.[27] These large, bipolar, projection neurons have shapes variously described as spindle, rod, or corkscrew (Fig. 1-16). They are present in the human brain in regions associated with social cognition, intuition, and emotional processing: layer V of the frontoinsular cortex, cortex of the pregenual, rostral, and anterior cingulate gyrus up to the midcingulate region, the entorhinal cortex, hippocampal formation, dorsomedial Brodmann's area 9, and frontopolar area 10.[207,208] VENs have also been identified in monkeys, great apes, whales, and elephants, suggesting that they have evolved along with the social brain, correlating with human-like social cognitive abilities and self-awareness.[209] VENs are selectively degenerated in frontotemporal dementia/Pick disease, which is characterized by loss of empathy, social awareness, and self-control, with the few surviving VENs showing dysmorphic appearance with pathological accumulation of tau protein.[210] They are also implicated in the neuropathology of schizophrenia[211] and autism.[212]

Glial cells (derived from the Greek word for glue) include astrocytes, oligodendrocytes, microglia, and NG2 glia—polydendrocytes identified by the expression of the proteoglycan nerve/glial antigen 2 (NG2).[213,214] The human brain consists roughly of 50% neuronal and 50% nonneuronal cells, although the overall proportion of glial cells in the brain varies in different species.[215,216] Glial cells do not participate directly in synaptic interactions or electrical signaling and were previously considered support cells for nervous system function.

Astrocytes have elaborate local processes that give them a star-like appearance. They have multiple functions including maintaining the ionic milieu of nerve cells, modulating the rate of nerve signal propagation, modulating synaptic action by controlling the uptake of neurotransmitters, providing a scaffold for neural development, and aiding in or preventing recovery from neural injury.[217] Single-cell RNA sequencing has revealed that astrocytes with different gene expression patterns have a laminar arrangement in superficial, mid, and deep layers of the cortex. These patterns are established in early postnatal brain and persist into adulthood, show areal organization, and are distinct from the laminar patterns of the cortical neurons.[218]

Oligodendroglia are central nervous system equivalents of the peripheral nervous system Schwann cell, manufacturing myelin critical for the speed of conduction of the action potential.

Microglia are the resident immune cells of the brain. They are derived from hematopoietic stem cells and colonize the brain early during embryonic development, or they arise directly from neural stem cells (NSCs). Like tissue macrophages, they have been regarded primarily as scavenger cells, migrating to injured areas to remove cellular debris from sites of injury or normal cell turnover. In addition, they express and secrete immune-related signaling molecules, and in the absence of inflammation are implicated in sculpting the wiring of the developing brain, pruning developing synapses and regulating synaptic plasticity and function.[219] Region-specific loss of synaptic integrity and aberrant neuronal networks have been observed in developmental disorders as well as in neurodegenerative disorders like Alzheimer's disease, one of the cardinal features of which is the presence of reactive microglia surrounding senile Aβ plaques. This has led to the hypothesis that microglia are involved in the pathophysiology of neurodegenerative diseases like Alzheimer's disease through synaptic loss and impairment, potentially opening a new avenue for targeted therapies.[220]

TYPES OF CEREBRAL CORTEX

A fundamental morphological feature of the cerebral cortex is the arrangement of its cell types in different layers, the variations in cytoarchitecture allowing it to be parcellated into multiple areas. This is the basis of the field of cortical cytoarchitectonics. The different cortical areas have varying proportions of pyramidal and non-pyramidal cells, which also vary with respect to their patterns of horizontal and vertical fibers. Most cortical areas have six layers beneath the pial surface; more primitive areas have fewer layers. Both the upper and lower cortical laminae are heavily myelinated, as seen on coronal sections of brain tissue as horizontal, myelinated bands. The best known are the bands of Baillarger (Jules Baillarger, 1809–1890), the external/outer band of Baillarger in layer IV and the internal/inner band of Baillarger in layer V of the cortex (Fig. 1-17). The outer band is particularly prominent in the primary visual cortex, area 17, which has markedly thickened horizontal fibers described "on February 2, 1776" by Francesco Gennari (1750–1797) as a white line (*lineola albidior*). Other myelinated bands are

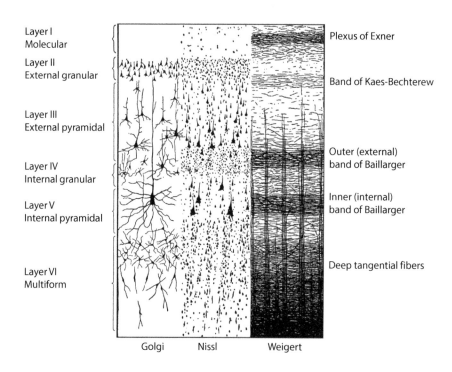

FIGURE 1-17. Cytoarchitecture of the neocortex with three staining methods showing intracortical horizontal myelin bands. (Modified from *Gray's Anatomy*,[84] Fig. 8.253.)

the plexus of Exner (Sigmund Exner, 1846–1926), horizontal myelinated fibers in the molecular layer,[221] and the stria of Kaes-Bechterew[222] (Theodor Kaes, 1852–1913; Vladimir Mikhailovic Bekhterev/W. Bekhterew, 1857–1927) in the most superficial part of layer III.

A SCHEMA OF BRAIN ORGANIZATION

(After Mesulam[63])

The following notions of brain organization are based on decades of investigation into connectional neuroanatomy in animal models, behavioral studies in animals, and structure-function correlations in patients with focal or diffuse injury. These patterns of cytoarchitectonic, connectional, and behavioral specialization in the cortex emerge from the dual origin theory of the cerebral cortex, discussed later, in which evolutionary principles of cerebral cortical development and organization follow a progressive elaboration of cortex and related functions from the limbic areas (corticoid and allocortical regions) to the paralimbic regions, homotopical isocortex, and idiotypic isocortex (Figs. 1-3, 1-18 through 1-20).

Paralimbic formations in the primate brain are cortical regions with cytoarchitectonic transitions from allocortex to

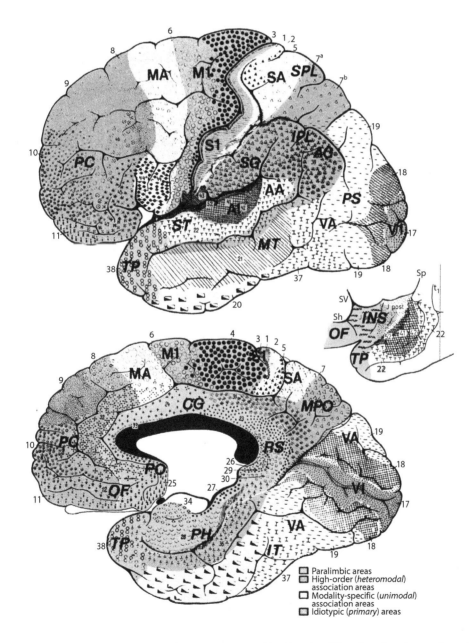

FIGURE 1-18. Brodmann's[22] map of cerebral cortical architecture arranged by Mesulam[63] into functional zones based on experimental evidence in animal models. AA, auditory association cortex; AG, angular gyrus; A1, primary auditory cortex; CG, cingulate gyrus; INS, insula; IPL, inferior parietal lobule; IT, inferior temporal gyrus; MA, motor association cortex; MPO, medial parieto-occipital area; MT, middle temporal gyrus; M1, primary motor area; OF, orbitofrontal region; PC, prefrontal cortex; PH, parahippocampal region; PO, parolfactory area; PS, peristriate cortex; RS, retrosplenial area; SA, somatosensory association cortex; SG, supramarginal gyrus; SPL, superior parietal lobule; ST, superior temporal gyrus; S1, primary somatosensory cortex; TP, temporopolar cortex; VA, visual association cortex; V1, primary visual cortex.

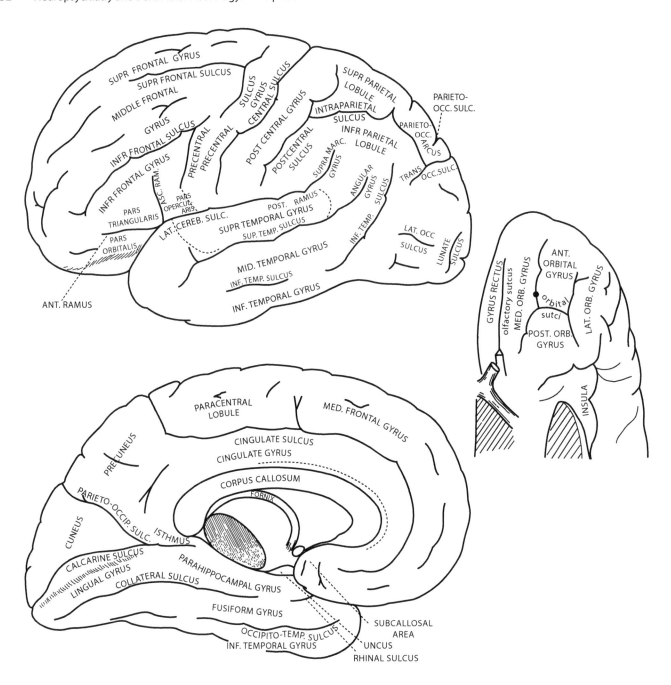

FIGURE 1-19. Nomenclature of cerebral gyri on the lateral, medial, and orbital surfaces of the human brain. (From *Gray's Anatomy*,[84] Figs. 8.219, 8.224, and 8.227.)

granular isocortex. The five major paralimbic regions are the *caudal orbitofrontal cortex, insula, temporal pole, parahippocampal gyrus* (entorhinal, prorhinal, perirhinal, presubicular, and parasubicular areas), and the *cingulate complex* (retrosplenial, cingulate, and parolfactory areas). These five paralimbic regions form an uninterrupted girdle surrounding the medial and basal cerebral hemispheres and subserve the integration of extrapersonal stimuli with the internal milieu.[63,223]

As described in Pandya et al.[29] and further considered below with the discussion of the dual origin of the cerebral cortex, the *paralimbic proisocortical areas in the olfactory/pyriform trend (the ventral trend)* are situated in the caudal orbitofrontal cortex, temporal pole, rostral Sylvian operculum, insula, perirhinal cortex, and rostral parahippocampal gyrus. Orbital proisocortex (area Pro) is situated in the caudal orbitofrontal region; area 13 is slightly more rostral and has incipient layer IV granule cells. Orbital proisocortex is continuous with proisocortex in the rostral operculum of the Sylvian fissure, rostral insula, and the temporal pole, all of which have an essentially uniform architectonic appearance. This opercular-insular component is the precursor of gustatory and vestibular cortex, insular paralimbic cortex, and isocortical ventral motor and somatosensory trends. The ventral paralimbic trend in the rostral parahippocampal gyrus includes two proisocortical areas, rostral agranular perirhinal cortex (area 35) and rostral area 36, also known as area TLr, that has a thin incipient layer IV.

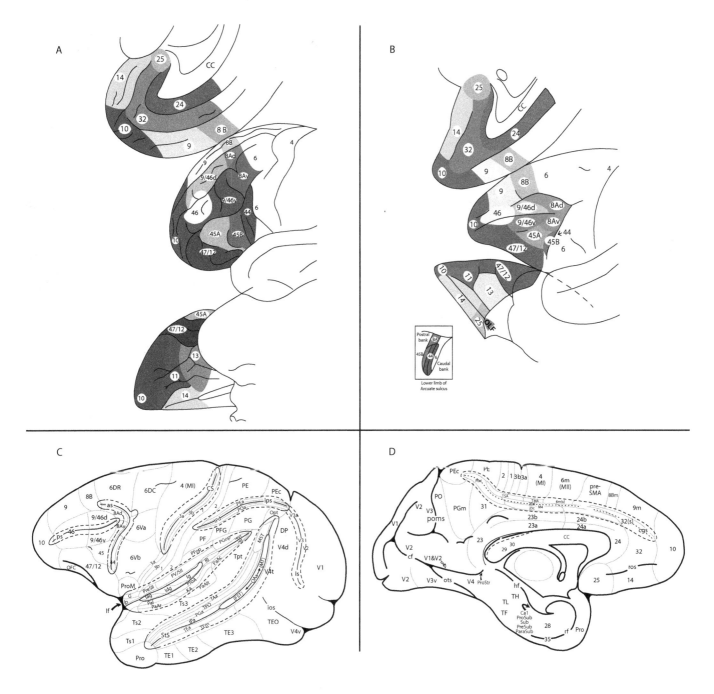

FIGURE 1-20. Cytoarchitecture of the frontal lobe in humans **(A)** and monkeys **(B)** according to Petrides and Pandya.[335] Architecture of the monkey brain at the **(C)** lateral and **(D)** medial surfaces with the sulci opened to reveal hidden architectonic areas according to Morecraft et al.[347]

Paralimbic areas in the parahippocampal trend (the dorsal trend) "consist of a ring of proisocortex on the medial surface of the hemisphere that encircles the corpus callosum and extends caudally to the calcarine sulcus and into the caudal parahippocampal gyrus. It consists of parahippocampal cortex (areas TH, TL, and TF), area prostriata, the caudal cingulate-retrosplenial region (areas 23a, 29, and 30), and the rostral cingulate and perigenual region (areas 24, 25, and 32). The first two components, namely the caudal parahippocampal gyrus and area prostriata, stem from the hippocampus proper by way of surrounding periallocortex in the ventromedial temporal region. The caudal

and rostral cingulate components of the dorsal paralimbic trend originate in the caudodorsal portion of the hippocampus via the adjacent periallocortex lying over the corpus callosum at the rostrocaudal level of the medial parietal and frontal region" (in Pandya et al.[29]).[224]

Homotypical association isocortex has six layers and occupies the great extent of the cortical surface of the human brain. It is divided into two major types: modality-specific or unimodal association cortex, and higher order or heteromodal association cortex. The unimodal association areas have a more differentiated organization than the heteromodal/multimodal association cortex: greater sublamination in layers III and V, columnarization in layer III, and more extensive granularization in layers IV and especially in layer II. On these architectonic grounds, heteromodal cortex is thus closer in structure to paralimbic cortex, an intercalated step between paralimbic and unimodal areas.

Unimodal association isocortex has three defining characteristics. The constituent neurons are almost exclusively responsive to stimulation in a single sensory modality; the predominant cortical inputs are provided by the primary sensory cortex or by other unimodal regions in the same modality; damage to these areas produces modality-specific deficits confined to tasks within that modality. The unimodal association areas for the three major sensory domains are in the superior temporal gyrus for the auditory modality, superior parietal lobule (SPL) for somatic sensation, and the peristriate mid-temporal and infratemporal regions for vision. This is exemplified for somatic sensation by the unimodal or intradomain somatosensory association cortex receiving information about different properties of touch, namely vibration, position sense, pressure, and two-point discrimination. Damage to these areas produces the phenomenon of cortical sensory loss, with impairment of graphesthesia, stereognosis, and loss of simultaneous bilateral or hierarchical two-point tactile discrimination.

Heteromodal association isocortex, also known as high-order, multimodal, or supramodal association cortex, is defined by the following characteristics: Even within relatively small areas of cortex neuronal responses are not confined to any single sensory modality, and some neurons respond to stimulation in more than one modality, indicating direct multimodal convergence. Damage to heteromodal association cortex leads to behavioral deficits that are not modality specific, and the cortical inputs originate from unimodal areas in more than one modality, and/ or from other heteromodal areas. These heteromodal association cortices are in the prefrontal region including the orbitofrontal cortex, ventromedial prefrontal cortex, and dorsolateral frontal cortex, the inferior parietal lobule (IPL) extending into the bank of the STS, and the posterior part of the ventral temporal lobe.

Idiotypic koniocortex defines areas with unique and highly specialized architecture: these are the primary sensory cortices for somatic sensation, vision, and hearing, and the primary motor cortex. The gradual trend of architectonic elaboration toward granularization and increased lamination reaches its maximal extent in idiotypic koniocortex, exemplified best in the primary visual cortex at the occipital pole and banks of the calcarine sulcus. The primary auditory cortex is in Heschl's gyrus in the superotemporal plane, the primary somatosensory cortex is in the postcentral gyrus, and the primary motor area is located within the precentral gyrus. As laid out in the theory of the dual origin of the cerebral cortex, idiotypic cortex is viewed as the most advanced and highly differentiated component of the cortical mantle.

CORTICOCORTICAL CONNECTIONS: FOUNDATIONAL STUDIES

The study of corticocortical connections aims to understand how the brain interacts with itself to subserve sensation, perception,

motor control, and higher order behavior. In a landmark anatomical study in rhesus monkeys, Pandya and Kupers[6] used the lesion degeneration method and the Nauta silver impregnation technique that afforded more accuracy than the earlier work using the Marchi degeneration technique.[225] In line with Flechsig's rule, the premotor area, pre- and postcentral gyri and adjacent sector of the parietal lobule projected to their immediate surroundings and to their counterparts across the central sulcus. The pre- and postcentral gyri, the supplementary motor cortex, and the secondary sensory cortex were interconnected in a topographically organized fashion. These connections across the central sulcus formed a cortical somatosensory-motor loop in parallel with similar connections at subcortical and spinal levels, thought to guide activity throughout the frontal motor area on the basis of somatosensory information. Striate cortex projected to a peristriate belt which in turn projected to the caudal parts of the IPL, the middle and inferior temporal gyri, and the premotor area rostrally adjoining the precentral gyrus. The middle and inferior temporal gyri projected to the prefrontal areas. The temporal pole projected to adjacent temporal areas, the insula, orbitofrontal cortex and adjoining prefrontal areas on the medial and lateral surfaces of the frontal lobe, the subcallosal part of the cingulate gyrus, and the indusium griseum and the caudal parts of the hippocampus, and it received projections from the amygdaloid complex. The superior temporal gyrus projected to the prefrontal areas and the premotor area rostrally adjoining the precentral gyrus. Higher order association areas within the prefrontal cortex and the IPL projected to the cingulate gyrus. The orbitofrontal cortex projected to ventral parts of the cingulate gyrus, the retrosplenial area, caudal parts of the parahippocampal gyrus, and the temporal pole. The dorsolateral prefrontal cortex projected to dorsal parts of the cingulate gyrus, and the rostral two-thirds of the lateral aspect of the temporal lobe. Prefrontal areas above and below the principal sulcus projected above and below the STS, respectively.

This seminal work was complemented by the similarly influential study of Jones and Powell[7] of converging sensory pathways within the cerebral cortex of the rhesus monkey. Their study was designed to evaluate the anatomical basis of the clinical and experimental observation that lesions of the posterior parietal lobe produce "defects of somatic as well as visual function … [that] would presuppose an element of convergence of the two sensory systems and probably, within a single sensory system, convergence of information relevant to the several topographic subdivisions of the body or visual fields."[7] They argued that whereas within a primary cortical area of a single sensory system there are intrinsic connections that link all parts of the representation of one topographic subdivision, such as the leg area or the superior quadrant of the retina, there are no connections with other subdivisions, such as between the leg and the arm area. Thus, the convergence within a system must occur at some point beyond the primary sensory area. They identified sequences of association connections passing outwards from the primary sensory cortex, areas SI and SII of Woolsey (Clinton Woolsey, 1904–1993[226]) situated respectively in the postcentral gyrus and the upper back of the lateral sulcus in the vicinity of the parietal operculum, as well as from the visual cortex in Brodmann areas 17, 18, and 19, and from auditory cortex in areas 41 and 42 (Fig. 1-18). As in Pandya and Kuypers,[6] they showed orderly sequences of projections directed from the single modality koniocortical sensory systems to unimodal association and then higher order association areas in the frontal, parietal, and temporal lobes. Convergence zones were identified in the depths of the STS (the homologue of areas 39 and 40 in man), the frontal pole, and the orbitofrontal cortex, all of which were interconnected with one another, and had connections with limbic/paralimbic structures in the cingulate gyrus, parahippocampal gyrus, and amygdala.

These early anatomical studies were performed in large part to understand the neural basis of higher order deficits exemplified by the apraxias, agnosias, and aphasias as well as amnestic syndromes following anterior/medial temporal lobectomy,[163] and were important in guiding the development of the field of behavioral neurology/neuropsychiatry reignited by the Geschwind 1965 papers.

THE DUAL ORIGIN OF THE CEREBRAL CORTEX (THE THEORY OF DART-ABIE-SANIDES-PANDYA)

A fundamental question posed at the outset of the resurgent field of connectional anatomy was whether there was an organizing principle underlying the apparent hierarchical arrangement of the architecture and connections of the different cerebral cortical areas. The answer to this question appears to lie in the theory of the dual origin of the cerebral cortex.

The theory arose from investigations into the evolutionary biology of the cerebral cortex by Raymond Arthur Dart (1893–1988) and Andrew Arthur Abbie (1905–1976), and it was expanded and elaborated upon by Friedrich Sanides (1914–1984) and Deepak Pandya (1932-2020).

Dart[863] studied the relatively simple cortex of South African reptiles (lizards, chameleons, geckos) to gain an overview of the cellular composition of the different parts of these brains. He observed that in the reptile brain the *primordium neopallii*, that is, the earliest recognizable structure that can be considered true cerebral cortex, lies between the hippocampal and pyriform cortical formations, and has two architectonically distinct divisions: a *parahippocampal* and a *parapyriform* region (Fig. 1-21). The realization that there were in fact two separate neopallial rudiments led Dart to propose that the cerebral cortex originated from these two prime entities—the *archicortical* or *hippocampal* moiety (as well as the indusium griseum, retrosplenial cingulate cortex, and periallocortex in the callosal sulcus), and the *paleocortical* or *pyriform/olfactory* moiety (and orbitoinsular cortex). Abbie's observations in monotremes, primitive egg-laying mammals found in Australia,[227] and in marsupials (*Perameles nasuta*, the Australian long-nosed bandicoot),[228] reinforced Dart's conclusions. The neocortex appeared to consist of two *trends* of progressively differentiating cortical architectonic areas. These trends, a dorsal trend arising from the archicortical or hippocampal moiety of the primitive three-layered allocortex, and a ventral trend arising from the paleocortical or pyriform/olfactory moiety, each lead to the highly arranged six-layered proisocortex and then isocortex. This was consistent with Ramón y Cajal's view that the intricacies of human

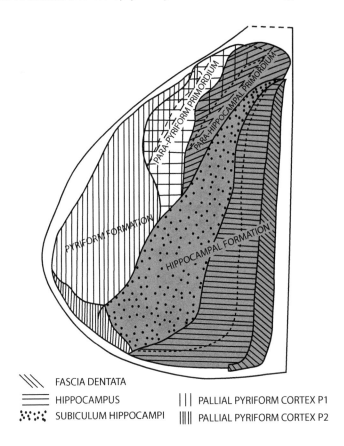

FASCIA DENTATA
HIPPOCAMPUS ||| **PALLIAL PYRIFORM CORTEX P1**
SUBICULUM HIPPOCAMPI |||| **PALLIAL PYRIFORM CORTEX P2**

FIGURE 1-21. Dorsal view of a reptilian brain *Agama nigricollis* (South African lizard) showing the two allocortical moieties: pyriform formation (blue) and hippocampal formation (pink). Adjoining the pyriform and hippocampal formations are the para-pyriform and para-hippocampal primordia. (Figure from Dart,[863] modified in Pandya et al.,[29] Fig. 1.1.)

functions were heralded by the arrival of the small granule cells in the fourth layer.[29]

Sanides[229] then studied cyto- and myeloarchitectonic features of the human frontal lobe, concluding that frontal cortex could also be arranged into two distinct sequences of cortical areas with progressive laminar differentiation stemming from either of the two primordial moieties into the dorsal and ventral trends. He identified the two trends in other species as well, noting parallel streams of cortical areas beginning in allocortex (either hippocampus or pyriform cortex) and passing through periallocortex to reach proisocortex. He went beyond proisocortex and described further stages of laminar differentiation within isocortex itself. He interpreted his findings to conclude that during evolution growth rings emerge from the two primordial moieties in a step-wise change of cortical architectonic laminar differentiation and lead to the different areas of the cerebral cortex.

Deepak Pandya, commencing in the early 1970s with Sanides[230] and then with collaborators through the years,[29] discovered and synthesized new data and notions concerning the organization of the cerebral cortex. Based on their study in the rhesus monkey of the progressively differentiating architecture and connections of the different cortical laminae of the two trends, they arrived at insights into and conclusions

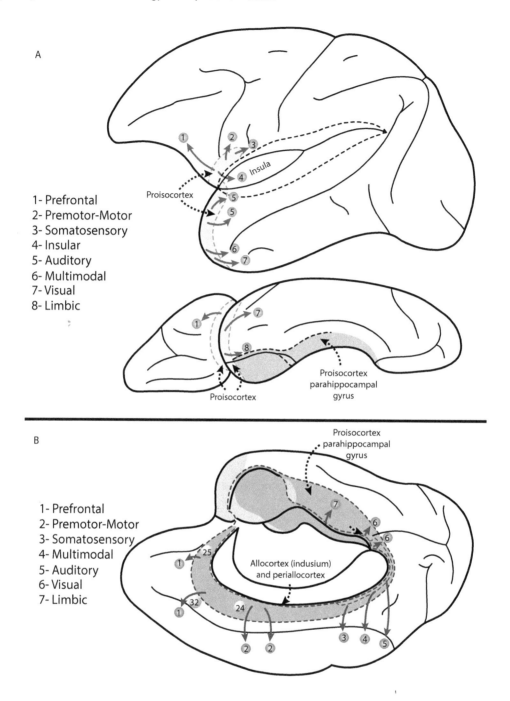

1- Prefrontal
2- Premotor-Motor
3- Somatosensory
4- Insular
5- Auditory
6- Multimodal
7- Visual
8- Limbic

1- Prefrontal
2- Premotor-Motor
3- Somatosensory
4- Multimodal
5- Auditory
6- Visual
7- Limbic

FIGURE 1-22. (A) Branches of the ventral trend proisocortical areas shown on a schematic of the lateral and basal surfaces of the monkey cerebral hemisphere. **(B)** Branches of the dorsal trend proisocortical areas on a schematic of the medial surface of the monkey cerebral hemisphere. (From Pandya et al., Fig. 3.11.[29])

regarding evolutionary biology (Fig. 1-22). They recognized another major feature of cortical organization in the context of laminar differentiation, namely, that each modality-specific, that is, auditory, somatosensory-motor, and visual branch of both the dorsal and ventral trends can be subdivided into three parallel lines of cortical architectonic areas: the core line, root line, and belt line, each with its own functional significance.

The core line is a succession of progressively differentiating areas that leads to the primary sensory or motor area of a given branch. The root line, adjacent to the core, consists of cortical zones including second or supplementary sensory and motor

areas. The belt line includes unimodal sensory and motor association cortical regions. Certain architectonic features characterize core, root, and belt line areas across modality. Core line areas of cortical sensory systems are characterized by a successive accumulation of IVth layer granule cells, whereas in root line areas the emphasis is on the infragranular cell layers. Belt line areas of sensory-related regions emphasize the progressive development of neurons in layer III (which give rise to the long association axons) and layer IV, while the belt line areas of motor cortex show progressive emphasis on pyramidal neurons in layers V and VI. The multimodal, prefrontal, and paralimbic branches of the dorsal and ventral trends also show

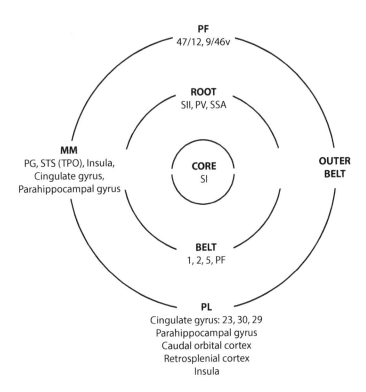

FIGURE 1-23. Summary diagram showing the link between the core (inner circle) and root and belt (middle circle) somatosensory areas. The root and belt areas, in turn, are linked with the outer belt regions: prefrontal (PF), multimodal (MM), and paralimbic (PL) areas. These connections suggest that core, root, and belt, as well as outer belt areas of the somatosensory region are interconnected and act together in somatosensory related functions. (Figure and legend from Pandya et al.,[29] Fig. 3.11.)

progressive laminar differentiation as one moves from proiso-cortex through different stages of isocortical development. Based on their locations with respect to modality-specific cortex and their cortical connections, these areas may be considered outer belts of auditory, somatosensory-motor, and visual cortex (Fig. 1-23).

The dual origin of cortex theory provided a coherent conceptual underpinning regarding the details and patterning of cortical architectonics, the arrangement of cerebral cortical areas throughout the hemispheres, and the guiding principles of the connections that link these different cortical areas to each other. Connections between the different cortical areas link the progressively differentiating core, root, and belt lines in a predictable intralinear and interlinear manner, and conform to the notion of duality, that is, the dorsal and ventral trends.[29,231]

Outline of the Dual Origin Concept

Allocortex is the most primitive and least well-differentiated type of cortex. It has three layers, one of which contains large pyramidal cells.

There are two allocortical regions in the primate brain, archicortex and paleocortex.

Archicortex (the hippocampal moiety/dorsal trend) corresponds to the dentate gyrus and caudal hippocampus.

Paleocortex (the pyriform moiety/ventral trend) consists of caudal orbital and rostral temporal (pyriform and prepyriform) cortex and the rostral hippocampus.

Periallocortex, adjacent to and surrounding both allocortical regions, has additional layers but no definite laminar organization. Periallocortical regions include the presubiculum, entorhinal cortex, and parapyriform cortex. Periallocortex lies at the interface of the more primitive allocortical areas and the more recently evolved proisocortical areas, with connections to cortices in both these developmental stages.

Proisocortex lies adjacent to the periallocortical regions and has a transitional cortical structure between periallocortex and isocortex, with a six-layered pattern typical of isocortex but without appreciable development of layer IV.

Proisocortex of the *archicortical/dorsal trend* lies in the *posterior parahippocampal gyrus, area prostriata, retrosplenial region, cingulate gyrus,* and *medial prefrontal cortex.* Although the cingulate-retrosplenial region appears to be far displaced from the hippocampus, which lies in the ventromedial temporal lobe, cingulate-retrosplenial proisocortex and hippocampal archicortex are related to each other by way of a vestigial hippocampal (allocortical) structure, the indusium griseum, and adjacent rudimentary periallocortex in the callosal sulcus.[12,29,232]

Proisocortex of the *paleocortical/ventral trend* is in the caudal orbitofrontal region, rostral Sylvian operculum, rostral insula, temporal pole, and rostral perirhinal cortex.

The proisocortical regions are the precursors of full, six-layered isocortex, and include the areas that comprise both the dorsal and ventral trends. According to the dual origin concept, the proisocortical areas of both the dorsal and ventral trends lead to the full complement of sensory and motor-specific, multimodal, prefrontal, and paralimbic cortical areas.

ANATOMICAL COMPONENTS OF THE DORSAL AND VENTRAL TRENDS (IN MACAQUE MONKEY)

(After Pandya et al., [29], Fig. 1-22)

The Dorsal Trend

The dorsal/archicortical trend originates in the three-layered allocortex of the hippocampus, and consists of multiple sequences of progressively differentiated areas transitioning away from proisocortex in the medial prefrontal cortex and the cingulate-retrosplenial region.

Prefrontal Branch

The prefrontal branch emerges from rostral proisocortical areas 24, 25, and 32. It includes a succession of cortical areas lying on the medial surface of the frontal lobe and on the dorsolateral surface up to the principal sulcus and dorsal concavity of the arcuate sulcus.

Somatosensory-Motor Branch

The somatosensory-motor branch arises from proisocortex of the mid-cingulate region and extends into medial and dorsolateral portions of the frontal and parietal lobes. This branch relates to sensory and motor function of the trunk and lower limbs.

Multimodal Branch

The multimodal branch begins on the medial surface of the hemisphere in caudal cingulate and retrosplenial proisocortical areas and extends onto the dorsolateral surface of the parietal lobe as far as the intraparietal sulcus and caudal IPL.

Auditory Branch

The auditory branch stems from the caudal cingulate-retrosplenial region and is linked with the caudal superior temporal region.[233] This is involved mainly with the spatial processing of sound.

Visual Branch

The visual branch arises from the most caudal sector of the dorsal proisocortex. It comprises a succession of areas emanating from the retrosplenial region and area prostriata, culminating in medial and dorsal occipital cortex,[234] areas of striate and pre-occipital cortex that serve visuospatial functions.

The Ventral Trend

The ventral/paleocortical trend originates in the three-layered allocortex of the olfactory/pyriform cortex. Branches of isocortical zones can be traced from ventral trend proisocortical areas (caudal orbitofrontal region, rostral Sylvian operculum, rostral insula, temporal pole, and rostral perirhinal cortex). Each branch consists of a sequence of interconnected cortical areas showing progressive laminar differentiation characterized by successive development of neurons in the upper strata (layers II, III, and IV) and diminished emphasis on the lower strata (layers V and VI).

Prefrontal Branch

The prefrontal branch is the most rostral and emerges from the orbital proisocortex directed to the caudal orbital prefrontal region. It encompasses the orbitofrontal and ventral prefrontal cortex up to the level of the principal sulcus and ventral arcuate concavity cortex.

Somatosensory-Motor Branch

The somatosensory-motor branch begins in the proisocortex of the frontal operculum and upper bank of the Sylvian fissure and extends into the ventral precentral gyrus, cortex of the ventral central sulcus, ventral postcentral gyrus, and rostral IPL. It consists of motor- and somatosensory-related areas pertaining to the head, face, and neck. It includes in the dorsal Sylvian operculum the second somatosensory area SII, the ventral parietal area PV, and the gustatory area, rostrally; and the vestibular area, caudally.

Multimodal and Paralimbic Branch

The multimodal and paralimbic branch is located immediately inferior to the somatosensory-motor branch. It consists of insular cortex hidden within the Sylvian fissure.

The multimodal branch corresponds to a stepwise series of differentiating cortical areas stemming from temporal polar proisocortex, including the cortex of the adjacent upper bank and depth of the STS. Neurons in this region respond to stimuli in more than one sensory modality.

The paralimbic branch, the most ventral, emerges from temporal polar proisocortex and encompasses paralimbic areas of the rostral perirhinal and parahippocampal region.

Auditory Branch

The auditory branch consists of a succession of progressively differentiating cortical areas emerging from the proisocortex of the temporal pole. It is a large region of cortex serving the modality of hearing, occupying the rostral lower bank of the Sylvian fissure (supratemporal plane) and adjacent superior temporal gyrus.

Visual Branch

The visual branch is situated further ventrally in the inferotemporal region including the lower bank of the STS and the ventral occipital lobe. These zones comprise progressively differentiating areas and can be traced from proisocortex of the temporal pole to the ventral occipital lobe. In functional terms, they deal with visual object recognition and visual memory.[11]

A NOTE ON THE PERIRHINAL CORTEX

The perirhinal cortex is a proisocortical region that lies on the ventral-medial surface of the temporal lobe surrounding the amygdala and anterior hippocampus, at the boundary between the medial temporal lobe and the ventral visual pathway (Fig. 1-24).[238] It includes a large, laterally situated area 36 and a smaller, medially situated area 35 (area TLr[29,239]). As mentioned throughout this chapter, the perirhinal cortex has major connections with adjacent regions of the medial temporal lobe, namely, the entorhinal cortex, parahippocampal cortex, amygdala, and

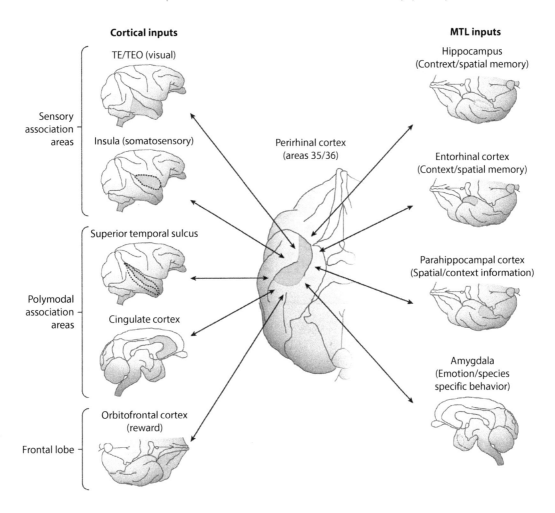

FIGURE 1-24. Schematic illustration of the cortical and medial temporal lobe (MTL) connections of the monkey perirhinal cortex, areas 35 and 36. (Figure and legend from Suzuki and Naya.[238])

hippocampus, as well as prominent and convergent projections from multiple sensory, polymodal, and reward-related cortical areas.[6,7,186,240–243] Neurophysiological studies report that the perirhinal cortex is activated by visual familiarity, and it has been considered a polymodal area for visual recognition memory. It appears to be a multifaceted memory area that conveys information about stimulus familiarity, as well as within- and between-domain associative learning, memory, and recall, and it can synergize with the amygdala to modulate information flow to the hippocampus relative to emotional salience of the situation.[238]

LAMINAR SPECIFICITY OF CORTICOCORTICAL CONNECTIONS

The dual origin concept is supported by the empiric observation that the intrinsic and long association connections of the different areas within the primary, unimodal association, heteromodal association, and limbic cortices are arranged with laminar specificity. The columnar corticocortical projections from the upper, supragranular layers to lower, granular layers of the cerebral cortex reflect a feedforward system directed from

the most highly developed cortex of each line (primary sensory regions) conveying information from the external world toward the proisocortex. In contrast, the feedback projections arise from infragranular layers of the proisocortex and are conveyed back to the first layer of the highly differentiated cortex (Fig. 1-25).[244] This sets up a consideration of bottom-up versus top-down information processing, the means whereby prior knowledge and perception may inform and shape (or distort) current sensation and experience.

PRINCIPLES OF CEREBRAL CORTICAL ORGANIZATION

From the study of white matter pathways of the cerebral hemispheres that carry efferents from the cerebral cortex, Schmahmann and Pandya[15] recognized the following general and specific principles of cerebral cortical organization.

General Principle of Cerebral Cortical Connections

The general principle is that every cerebral cortical area gives rise to efferent fibers arranged with topographic precision and

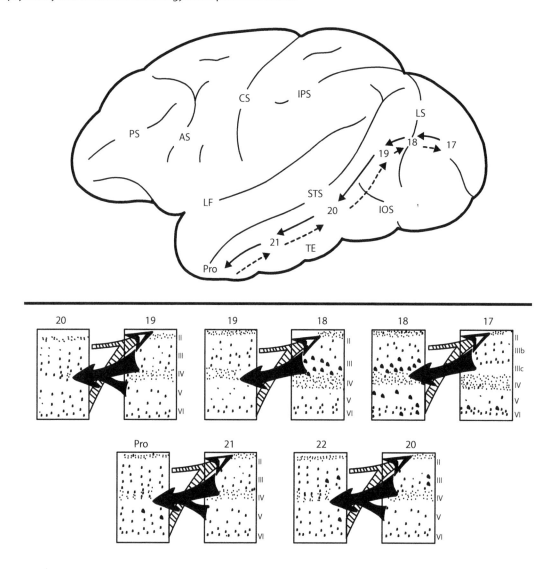

FIGURE 1-25. Diagram showing the common pattern of laminar origins and terminations of intrinsic connections of the visual association areas. (From Pandya and Yeterian.[244])

projecting to five sets of targets (Fig. 1-26): (a) association fiber tracts terminate in cerebral cortical areas in the same hemisphere. (b) Corticostriate fibers in the external capsule or the subcallosal fascicle of Muratoff terminate in the caudate nucleus, putamen, or claustrum. (c) Commissural fibers in the CC or AC terminate in the opposite cerebral hemisphere. A dense cord of fibers emanates from each cortical area and divides into (d) a subcortical, or projection, bundle which conveys fibers to the thalamus and diencephalon, and (e) a pontine fiber bundle that descends into and terminates in the brainstem, including the basis pontis, or continues into the spinal cord.

This general principle of cerebral cortical organization is integral to understanding the roles of both the cerebral cortical and subcortical areas in the genesis of aberrant behaviors. It also sets up two other conclusions.

First, no cortical region is an island, isolated from other areas of the nervous system. Therefore, a lesion in a focal cortical area is not focal in its effects, but rather disrupts the connections of that cortical nidus with other cortical and subcortical sites. The disconnection syndromes that Geschwind[4,5] described arise not only from lesions of white matter tracts linking association areas, but from focal lesions of the heteromodal association cortices themselves. The general principle is the anatomical basis of this notion of cortical disconnection syndromes.

The second, related conclusion, is that the neural circuits are anatomically hardwired to be highly interconnected and functionally coupled. This is exemplified by lesion network analysis using locations of lesions in many individuals translated onto healthy human functional connectivity brain maps. This makes it possible to test the von Monakow diaschisis hypothesis (Constantin von Monakow 1853–1930[245]) that symptoms emerge from sites functionally connected to a lesion location, not only from the lesion location itself. This approach reveals that whereas neurobehavioral symptoms can be induced by focal lesions in geographically distributed cortical and subcortical sites, they can be identified as belonging to an interconnected functionally coupled network linked to one or several cerebral cortical regions relevant for the complex function under consideration. This has been studied in peduncular hallucinosis (extrastriate visual cortex[246]), prosopagnosia (right

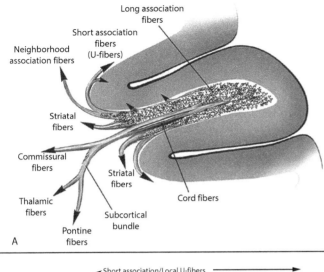

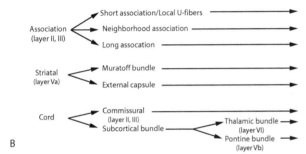

FIGURE 1-26. **(A)** Diagram and **(B)** schema of the principles of organization of white matter fiber pathways emanating from the cerebral cortex. Long association fibers are seen end-on as the stippled area within the white matter of the gyrus. In their course, these fibers either remain confined to the white matter of the gyrus, or they travel deeper in the white matter of the hemisphere. Short association fibers, or U-fibers, link adjacent gyri. Neighborhood association fibers link nearby regions usually within the same lobe. Striatal fibers intermingle with the association fibers early in their course, before coursing in the subcallosal fascicle of Muratoff or in the external capsule. Cord fibers segregate into commissural fibers that arise in cortical layers II and III, and the subcortical bundle, which further divides into fibers destined for thalamus arising from cortical layer VI, and those to brainstem and spinal cord in the pontine bundle arising from cortical layer V. (From Schmahmann and Pandya.[15,16])

fusiform face area, left frontal regions[247]), complex decision making (somatosensory, motor, and insula cortices[248]), criminality (orbitofrontal cortex, ventromedial prefrontal cortex, anterior temporal lobes[249]), and delusional misidentification/ Capgras syndrome (left retrosplenial cortex and right ventral frontal cortex/anterior insula[250]).

Specific Principle of Cerebral Cortical Connections

Using a reductionist approach and derived in part from Schmahmann's dysmetria of thought theory relating to cerebellar function,[251,252] Schmahmann and Pandya[16] further proposed the specific principle of organization which holds that (a) the connections of the cerebral cortical areas are arranged with

great topographic precision, (b) cortical areas can be defined by their patterns of subcortical and cortical connections, and (c) cerebral cortical connections obey the following rules:

(i) *Architecture determines the transform.* Each architectonically distinct cortical and subcortical area contributes a unique computation, or transform, to information processing.

(ii) *Architecture drives connections.* Evolutionary architectonics and connectional studies in monkeys show the interdependence of a cerebral cortical area and its connections.[29] Whether the architecture of a cerebral cortical area determines its connections, or the architecture and connections are a result of the same genetic influence, has not yet been established.[231]

(iii) *Connections define behavior.* Connections enable the different nodes within the distributed neural circuits to communicate with each other. These anatomically precise and segregated connections between each of the computationally unique nodes in the cortex and subcortical regions facilitate the network integration of the different transforms, and are the anatomical basis of sensorimotor, cognitive, and limbic domains within subcortical structures such as the basal ganglia and cerebellum. What makes cerebral cortex unique is that cross modal integration is exclusively the provenance of the cerebral cortex, enabled by association fiber tracts which are themselves exclusive to the cerebral cortex. Association fiber tracts are necessary for cross-modal integration required for evolved complex behaviors, because they link together different cortical areas with their different transforms. Thus, for example, posterior parietal cortical areas involved in spatial perception are interconnected with effector regions in the premotor or prefrontal cortices, and superior temporal region language areas interact with inferotemporal memory relevant areas, because of association fiber pathways linking these different cerebral cortical regions. Behavior is thus an emergent property of the interaction between the unique transforms of the interconnected cortical and subcortical nodes of the distributed neural circuits.

Clinical Implications of the General and Specific Principles

Clinical manifestations of brain lesions are determined by which node is damaged and which subpopulation of neurons within that node or its connecting axons are destroyed. Lesions of subcortical structures, discussed later in this chapter, can mimic deficits resulting from lesions of the cerebral cortex, but there are qualitative differences between the manifestations of lesions in functionally related areas.[16] In the motor system, whereas cerebral cortical or cerebral white matter lesions result in weakness or spasticity, basal ganglia lesions produce hypokinetic or hyperkinetic movement disorders, and cerebellar lesions cause ataxia. The same is predicted to hold true for cognitive and emotional disorders. This is the basis of the dysmetria of thought theory that underlies and accounts for the cerebellar cognitive affective syndrome, resulting from lesions of the cognitive and limbic cerebellum in the cerebellar posterior lobe.[251–256]

CORTICAL AREAS, CONNECTIONS, AND FUNCTIONS OF THE LOBES OF THE CEREBRAL HEMISPHERES

Parietal Lobe

The human parietal lobe houses the primary somatosensory cortex in the postcentral gyrus, and the unimodal and multimodal sensory areas in the posterior parietal lobe at the convexity of the hemisphere (supramarginal and angular gyri) and the precuneus at the medial convexity (Figs. 1-18 and 1-19). In monkeys, the somatic sensory association areas of both the SPL (areas PE and PEc) and IPL (areas PF and PFG) (Fig. 1-20C) are engaged in sequential processing of somatotopically organized information received from the adjacent primary somatosensory cortices.[7,257-260] Their architecture and connections provide insights into their functional specialization and clinical relevance.

There are two principal rostrocaudal architectonic gradients leading from the postcentral gyrus to the posterior parietal region, which can be understood within the concept of the dorsal versus ventral trends discussed above.[29] (i) One architectonic trend begins in the dorsal part of the postcentral gyrus (areas 3, 1, and 2) where the trunk and lower limb are represented in the primary somatic sensory cortex. The architecture then changes successively through areas PE and PEc of the SPL, ending at the medial surface of the parietal lobe, area PGm. (ii) The other trend begins in the more ventral part of the primary somatic sensory cortex containing the head, neck, and arm representations, located in the ventral postcentral gyrus. The architectonic features in this trend undergo progressive elaboration through the rostral and midsectors of the IPL, namely, areas PF, PFG, and rostral PG, leading to the most caudal regions of the IPL, areas PG and Opt.[261]

Paralleling these architectonic trends are two distinct rostrocaudal connectional sequences.[7,261] The cortex in the upper bank of the intraparietal sulcus, area PEa, is somatic sensory association area receiving topographically organized input from the rostral and caudal SPL.[261,262] Cortex in the lower bank of the intraparietal sulcus, area POa, receives multimodal inputs; from somatosensory-related cortex in the rostral IPL, from visual-related areas in the peristriate belt,[263] and from cortex at the rostral tip of the intraparietal sulcus known to contain a vestibular representation.[264,265] Area POa is therefore multimodal, dealing with somatosensory, visual, and vestibular information.[263,266-269]

The most caudal regions of the SPL (PGm) and IPL (PG and Opt) are multimodal association areas by virtue of their connections and functional properties. Area PGm in the caudal-medial part of the SPL is a site of convergence of somatosensory,[261] kinesthetic,[261] visual,[270] and auditory information[6,7] and it has long connections with the prefrontal cortex[6,7,271-274] and the cingulate gyrus.[151,261,275] Areas PG and Opt in the caudal IPL have prominent reciprocal connections with paralimbic cortices (parahippocampal gyrus, presubiculum, perirhinal cortex, and cingulate gyrus) and multimodal zones in the temporal and frontal lobes.[7,12,184,187,275-277] In contrast to the rostral part of the SPL and IPL which are connected with modality-specific thalamic nuclei, areas PGm and PG/Opt have thalamic connections predominantly with associative thalamic nuclei.[275,278-282] Area Opt

alone has connections with the lateral dorsal nucleus, as well as with the anterior nuclei of thalamus[280-282] which are part of the limbic system circuitry.[283,284] These caudally located multimodal zones in PG/Opt, and to a lesser degree in PGm, subserve highly complex, nonmodality-specific functions which are invested with emotional and motivational significance.[8,187,259,276,285,286]

Parietal lobe syndromes of cortical sensory loss (agraphesthesia, stereognosis, amorphosynthesis) are explained by lesions of the intramodality somatosensory association areas. High-level perceptual disruptions including hemispatial neglect, visual-spatial disorientation, and anosognosia (denial of illness) can be understood in the context of the anatomical organization of the multimodal areas in the posterior parietal association cortices.

Temporal Lobe

In monkeys, anatomical[6,7,287] and physiological observations[235-237,288-290] show that the temporal lobe contains unimodal and multimodal areas, which appear to contribute differentially to the organization of behavior (Fig. 1-20C). The superior temporal gyrus is an association area confined to the auditory realm.[291-294] The inferotemporal area and the inferior bank of the STS are unimodal visual association areas,[237,287,288,295,296] and the depth of the STS, area IPa, is an important association area in the somatosensory modality.[7,287,297] In contrast, the architectonic areas TPO and PGa in the upper bank of the STS are association areas concerned with multiple sensory modalities, namely, vision, somatic sensation, and audition.[7,235-237,287,297] These areas in the upper bank of the STS have connections with association areas of the frontal and parietal cortices, as well as with limbic-related structures at the medial and inferior frontal convexity and parahippocampal and cingulate gyri.[7,151,183,184,187,287,297-299] They contain neurons that respond preferentially to more than one modality, as well as to complex stimuli such as faces.[235-237,289] The posterior parahippocampal gyrus is concerned with visuospatial memory,[300] and connectional and behavioral studies reveal its importance in affect, memory, and motivation.[183]

The human temporal lobe includes the superior, middle, and inferior temporal gyri on the lateral convexity, and on the ventral surface the fusiform gyrus, adjacent to the more medially situated lingual and then parahippocampal gyrus (Figs. 1-18 and 1-19). The primary auditory area is in the transverse temporal gyrus, Heschl's gyrus (Richard L. Heschl, 1824−1881). Auditory association areas are adjacent to it in the superior temporal gyrus and supratemporal plane. This includes the planum temporale caudally adjacent to Heschl's gyrus that is markedly asymmetric, left side greater than right,[301] consistent with language dominance in the left hemisphere. Wernicke's area, corresponding to cytoarchitectonic area Tpt in the midposterior part of the superior temporal gyrus, critical for language processing, also demonstrates a size laterality, left greater than right.[302] The hippocampus critical for learning and memory and the rostrally adjacent amygdala engaged in processing emotional stimuli are at the ventromedial aspect of the temporal lobe. The laterality of the temporal lobe is reflected in the predominance of the left hemisphere for language processing and the right hemisphere for spatial processing, recall, and associated valence of visually presented information. The ventral regions of the left temporal lobe are anatomical substrates for semantic knowledge—the meaning of different kinds of words,[303] exemplified also by the task of retrieving names for unique persons and landmarks.[304] The right ventral temporal region, notably the fusiform face area, is the locus for recognition of objects, and particularly faces. Lesions of this region result in prosopagnosia, the inability to recognize faces (e.g., Barton et al.[305]). The lingual gyrus is important for visual information processing, and the posterior parahippocampal region for spatial memory. Visual hallucinations of elaborate scenes as auras of epilepsy described originally by John Hughling Jackson (1835–1911)[306] arise from visual association areas in the ventral visual stream of the inferotemporal cortex. In the neurodegenerative synucleinopathy Lewy body disease, neuropathologic study reveals that patients with well-formed visual hallucinations have high densities of Lewy bodies in the amygdala and parahippocampus, with early hallucinations relating to higher densities in parahippocampal and inferior temporal cortices.[307]

The connections of the ventral and rostral temporal lobe with orbital and medial prefrontal regions and with limbic and paralimbic structures are relevant when considering selected major neurobehavioral disorders. Patients with frontotemporal dementia in which the anterior temporal and inferior and medial prefrontal cortices bear the brunt of the neuropathology demonstrate alterations in comportment, social behavior, language, and executive control.[308] Monkeys subjected to removal of both temporal lobes including the uncus and the greater part of the hippocampus develop the syndrome described by Heinrich Klüver (1897–1979) and Paul Bucy (1904–1992)[309] including psychic blindness, hyperorality—strong oral tendencies in examining available objects, a tendency to attend and react to every visual stimulus ("hypermetamorphosis"), marked changes in emotional behavior or absence of emotional reactions in the sense that the motor and vocal reactions generally associated with anger and fear are not exhibited, and an increase in sexual activity. In patients with temporal lobe epilepsy Geschwind described a syndrome of interictal psychosis (Geschwind syndrome[310]), characterized by hyperemotionality, increased religious interests, hypergraphia, aggression, increased moral and philosophical concerns, viscosity, seriousness (lack of humor) and hyposexuality.[310,311]

Occipital Lobe

The occipital lobe has the primary visual cortex at its medial wall in the banks of the calcarine sulcus, and visual association areas processing progressively complex visual information in the parastriate cortices at the lateral and medial convexities (Figs. 1-18 and 1-19). The dorsal and visual streams of visual information processing originate in the peristriate cortex of the occipital lobe, as demonstrated in anatomical and physiological studies (for reviews, see Felleman and Van Essen[312] and Desimone and Ungerleider[313]). A dorsal visual stream is

directed into the parietal lobe and includes dorsal area V3; areas MT, MST, and FST in the caudal STS; and area V4 in the dorsal prelunate gyrus, terminating in the caudal IPL (Fig. 1-20C). This dorsal stream is concerned principally with the visuospatial attributes of events occurring in the peripheral visual field, including the speed and direction of stimulus motion. A ventral visual, or occipitotemporal, stream passes through the ventral aspect of areas V3 and V4, architectonic area TEO, and the subdivisions of area TE in the inferior temporal gyrus and the rostral lower bank of the STS (Fig. 1-25). Neurons in the ventral stream are principally concerned with object recognition, such as the perception of form, color, orientation, and size, and they are activated by stimuli occurring within the central 5–10 degrees of the visual field.[11,296,314] Area prostriata is a paralimbic region in the occipital lobe that lies at the fundus of the calcarine sulcus,[315] (Fig. 1-20D). It has connections with area V5/MT that responds to visual motion, as well as with the cingulate motor cortex, auditory cortex, orbitofrontal cortex, and frontal polar cortices. It responds to fast motion and events particularly in the peripheral visual field.[316]

Higher order visual deficits, including Balint syndrome (Rezső Bálint, 1874–1929), of optic ataxia, optic apraxia, and simultanagnosia result from damage to the visual association cortices and dorsal parieto-occipital stream of visual processing.[11] Anton syndrome/Anton-Babinski syndrome (Gabriel Anton, 1858–1933; Joseph Jules Babinski, 1857–1932) is characterized by anosognosia (denial) or unawareness of cortical blindness which develops following damage to the occipital cortices and visual association areas. Charles Bonnet syndrome (Charles Bonnet, 1720–1793) is characterized by complex, non-threatening visual scenes and people, occurring in individuals with impaired vision, as in macular degeneration,[317] often in the setting of suboptimal cognitive function, and following focal damage to the occipital lobe or extrastriate visual cortex.[318,319] Manford and Andermann[318] postulated that visual hallucinations share a release of visual association cortex, acting by loss of corticocortical inputs, and alteration of activity via effects on the reticular activating system, especially serotonergic inputs, explaining how such strikingly similar hallucinations may be produced by various pathologies at different sites. This idea received empirical support from lesion-network analysis in peduncular hallucinosis in which lesions of the pons, midbrain, or thalamus produce vivid, dynamic, and well-formed visual hallucinations; the disrupted network extended to extrastriate visual cortex.[246]

Frontal Lobe

The major gyri of the human frontal lobe are the vertically oriented precentral gyrus which is the representation of the motor cortex, more rostrally situated premotor region, and the three mostly horizontal convolutions of the superior, middle, and inferior frontal gyri (Fig. 1-19). It includes the supplementary motor area (SMA) at the dorsum and medial premotor region of the hemisphere, the frontal eye fields, and the prefrontal cortex which includes the dorsolateral, ventrolateral, dorsomedial,

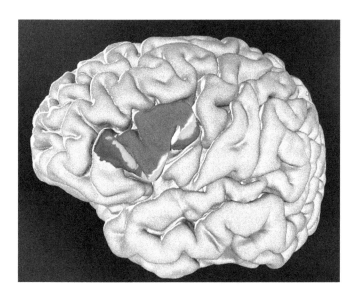

FIGURE 1-27. The location of area 45 in a probabilistic map of 1000 human brains, according to the JuBrain Cytoarchitectonic Atlas Viewer, http://www.jubrain.fz-juelich.de.[30]

ventromedial, orbitofrontal, and frontal polar cortices. The opercular region of the frontal lobe includes the pars opercularis, pars triangularis, and pars orbitalis. Broca's complex includes the pars opercularis important for word sounds (phonemics) and the pars triangularis important for the meaning of words (semantics) and expressive language production (Fig. 1-27).

The motor cortical homunculus identified both in the non-human primate (Clinton Woolsey)[320] and the human brain (Wilder Penfield, 1891–1976)[321,322] indicated an ordered topography from ventromedial precentral gyrus representation of the leg, to ventrolateral precentral gyrus cortex containing the representation of the tongue, mouth, and hand. Subsequent investigations have revealed multiple topographically arranged representations of the motor system in the precentral gyrus, as well as supplementary motor and secondary motor representations in precentral and premotor cortices, and in the third and fourth motor representations in cingulate gyrus areas 24c and 23c, respectively.[323–325]

The architecture and connections of the prefrontal cortical areas are the substrates for the multiple higher order functions of the prefrontal cortex and the neurobehavioral syndromes that result from frontal lobe damage. The human frontal lobe has undergone the greatest expansion during evolution, occupies nearly one-third of the totality of the neocortex,[326] and has been the subject of intensive study since the mid-1800s following the tamping rod accident that inflicted damage to the frontal lobe in Phineas Gage.[327]

The prefrontal cortex is an essential component of the normal integration of higher order behavior including attention, motivation, planning, and judgment. Based on behavioral studies in monkeys, different functions have been ascribed to orbital, medial, periprincipalis, and periarcuate prefrontal regions. This multiplicity of functional processes is matched by a connectional heterogeneity such that each of the prefrontal subdivisions

has a different set of connections with cortical as well as with subcortical structures.[274,314,328–332] The dorsolateral and medial prefrontal convexities, areas 8Ad, 8B, 9 (lateral and medial), 10, 9/46d, 9/46v, and 32 are important for spatial memory, as well as executive functions such as initiative, planning, execution, and verification of willed actions and thoughts.[3,13,333,334] Area 45B is homologous with the language area of humans (Figs 1-20 A, B).[335] The ventrolateral and orbitofrontal cortices including areas 11, 47/12, 14, and 9/46v have been shown to subserve object memory and recognition as well as autonomic and emotional response inhibition.[336–338] The dual streams of information processing in the visual system extend beyond the occipitotemporal/parietal regions into the frontal lobe, as predicted from the dual origin of the cortex hypothesis. Cortical areas in the dorsal visual stream concerned with events in the periphery of the visual field, including the dorsal prelunate, posterior parietal, superior temporal, and posterior parahippocampal regions, are interconnected with the dorsolateral and dorsomedial prefrontal cortices which constitute the dorsal stream areas of the prefrontal cortex (PFC). Cortical areas in the ventral visual stream including the inferotemporal and ventral prelunate regions have connections with the ventrolateral prefrontal and orbitofrontal convexities which constitute the ventral stream of the PFC.[330]

The *orbitofrontal and ventromedial prefrontal* cortex play a role in the expression and control of social and emotional processing and instinctual behaviors; *ventrolateral* prefrontal cortex is important for response inhibition and selective memory retrieval; and *dorsolateral* prefrontal cortex is critical for executive functions including working memory and the temporal organization of goal-directed actions for behavior, cognition, and language.[29,329,339] The medial prefrontal cortex can also be divided into three rostral to caudal functional zones, as shown in a meta-analytic data-driven approach to nearly 10,000 fMRI studies. The posterior zone was associated preferentially with motor function, the middle zone with cognitive control, pain, and affect, and the anterior with reward, social processing, and episodic memory. Within each zone, the more fine-grained subregions showed distinct, but subtler, variations in psychological function.[340] Many excellent sources are available for detailed analysis and review.[3,341–343]

INSULA

The insula, or Island of Reil (identified in 1809), lies deep within the lateral/Sylvian fissure, covered by the overlying parietal, frontal, and temporal opercula. The central sulcus of the human insula divides it into an anterior lobe with three gyri and a posterior lobe with two gyri (Fig. 1-28).[344] There are three architectonic sectors in the insula, with progressive elaboration moving from rostral to caudal. In monkeys and humans, the rostrally situated *periallocortical-agranular* sector is continuous with the insular extension of prepyriform cortex, has three layers, and lacks granule cells. Further caudally, *dysgranular* cortex has five or six cortical laminae, with a granular IVth layer and gradual differentiation of layer II. *Granular* cortex in the posterior

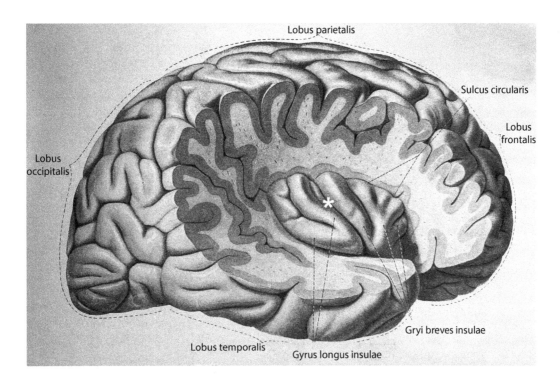

FIGURE 1-28. Insula cortex. The asterisk denotes the insular central sulcus. The Latin terms indicate the three short gyri anteriorly and the two long gyri posteriorly. The circular sulcus surrounds the insular distinguishing it from the surrounding opercular cortices. (Modified from Sobotta,[344] Fig. 696.)

dorsal aspect of the insula has well-demarcated granular layers IV and II, incipient sublamination of layer III, and increased cortical myelin with an outer band of Baillarger. The cortex of the insula, lateral orbitofrontal cortex, and the dorsal temporopolar areas share many architectonic features, to the extent that the insulo-orbital cortex is considered a single entity.[345] Note that the anterior insula contains the VENs implicated in social-emotional functions.

In monkeys the insula has bidirectional connections with adjacent orbital, temporopolar, and supratemporal regions as well as with the prefrontal cortex, lateral orbital region, frontoparietal operculum, cingulate gyrus and adjacent medial cortex, prepyriform olfactory cortex, amygdala, cortex of the STS, rhinal cortex, supratemporal plane, and the posterior parietal lobe. Frontal lobe projections arise from granular prefrontal cortex (areas 46 and lateral 12), lateral orbitofrontal cortex, frontal operculum, and ventral area 6. Cingulate projections are derived from areas 23 and 24 and from the adjacent sulcal cortex corresponding to area MII.[346] Parietal lobe projections originate in postcentral gyrus primary somatosensory cortex, area SI; second sensory area in the parietal operculum, area SII; the rostral IPL, area PF; and area 5 at the rostral SPL and anterior intraparietal sulcus. Temporal lobe connections are with the temporal pole, inferior temporal gyrus, parainsular, retroinsular, postauditory area, the supratemporal plane and cortex of the STS, and prorhinal, perirhinal, and entorhinal regions. There are widespread reciprocal connections between the insular cortex and almost all subnuclei of the amygdaloid complex. Only the anterior insula has connections with the prepyriform olfactory cortex and frontal operculum, and the lateral orbital

and rhinal cortex projections are mostly directed to the anterior insula. The posterior insula has substantial connections with the parietal lobe areas SI, SII, area PF, and area 5, and receives projections preferentially from the cingulate gyrus.[29,149,150,223,347]

The subcortical connections of the insula include the striatum, NAc, hypothalamus, and amygdala. The thalamic connections of the anterior insula are the ventroposterior medial complex, the medial dorsal nucleus, the centromedian-parafasicularis nuclei, and some midline nuclei. The posterior insula is linked with the ventroposterior inferior nucleus, the oral and medial pulvinar nuclei, and the suprageniculate nucleus.[135]

Diffusion-weighted MRI in humans demonstrates anterior-posterior differences in insular structural connections similar to those found in the macaque. Anterior insula connections are with the anterior cingulate, frontal, orbitofrontal, and anterior temporal areas; the posterior insula has connections with posterior temporal, parietal, and sensorimotor areas. A mid-insula transitional area demonstrates structural connections like those of the anterior and posterior insula cortices (reviewed in Uddin et al.[348]).

These architectonic and connectional features of the insula provide the anatomic underpinnings of the wide-ranging functions of the insula at the intersection of the internal milieu and the external world. The anterior insula with its agranular cortex is related to olfactory, gustatory, and viscero-autonomic behavior (sensory and motor) and is involved in social emotional processing. The posterior insula with its granular cortex is engaged in auditory, somesthetic, and skeletomotor function.[348]

CINGULATE GYRUS

The cingulate gyrus arches around the CC from the ventral prefrontal region rostrally to the retrosplenial region caudally (Figs. 1-5A, 1-18 through 1-19). The architecture, connections, and functions of the cingulate cortex at the medial wall of the hemisphere and that within the upper and lower banks of the cingulate sulcus are distinctly different.

The cingulate gyrus is implicated in emotion, motivation, drive, attention, and memory as well as control of autonomic functions, the direction of attention toward sensory stimuli, and the motivational-affective response to noxious stimuli.

Architectonic Subdivisions

The rostral limit of the cingulate gyrus in monkeys extends beyond the genu of the CC, merging with area 10 dorsally and area 14 ventrally (architecture of Walker[25]); its caudal limit extends beyond the splenium of the CC and merges with Brodmann area 7 dorsally and area 19 ventrally (Fig. 1-18).[150,349] The subgenual cingulate area 25 and the pregenual cingulate area 32 are architectonically similar with darkly stained neurons in layers V and VI, a sparsely populated layer III, and poorly developed layer IV, with minor differences between the two areas. The remaining cingulate gyrus is parcellated into three major subdivisions (each further divided into three cytoarchitectonic areas, as in Vogt et al.[350]). The rostral division, area 24, has large darkly stained neurons in layers V and VI, a cell sparse layer III, and no layer IV. This contrasts with the more caudally situated area 23 in which layer IV is quite distinct. The most caudal and ventral part of the cingulate gyrus is the retrosplenial cortex, a periallocortical structure including granular area 29 and dysgranular area 30, which extends to the splenium of the CC and ends in proximity to the anterior tip of the calcarine sulcus.

Corticocortical Connections

Considerable detail is available regarding the connections of the cingulate gyrus in monkeys,[15,150,151,275,351–356] summarized here.

Area 25

Subgenual cingulate area 25 is engaged in emotional expression and equilibrium, has a key role in affective networks, and its disruption is linked to mood disorders.[357] It is densely connected with other ventromedial and posterior orbitofrontal areas associated with emotions and homeostasis,[151] including connections with frontopolar area 10 thought to regulate emotions and dampen negative affect, auditory association areas and memory-related medial temporal cortices, the interoceptive-related anterior insula, and the entorhinal cortex.[358] Diffusion tractography in humans is consistent with the connectional neuroanatomy, showing strong connections between the subgenual region corresponding to the location of area 25 with orbitofrontal cortex, NAc, amygdala, and hypothalamus.[359]

Area 32

The connections of the most rostral part of the cingulate gyrus (area 32) are restricted to the lateral prefrontal and mid-orbitofrontal cortex and the rostral portion of the superior temporal gyrus.[150] The pathways from mostly upper layers of area 32 target excitatory neurons in the middle-deep layers of the orbitofrontal cortex, which is consistent with feedforward communication. The area 32-orbitofrontal terminations overlap with output pathways to thalamus and the amygdala, likely influencing emotional and cognitive processes which are disrupted in psychiatric disorders.[360] Tractography in humans reveals connections linking this pregenual region with anterior midcingulate cortex and medial prefrontal regions.[359]

Area 24

Situated in the rostral part of the cingulate gyrus, area 24 projects to the premotor region (areas 6 and 8), fronto-orbital cortex (area 12), rostral part of the IPL, anterior insular cortex, perirhinal area, and laterobasal nucleus of amygdala.

Area 23

The more caudally situated area 23 has connections with the dorsal prefrontal cortex (areas 9 and 10), rostral orbital cortex (area 11), parietotemporal cortex (posterior part of the IPL and the STS), parahippocampal gyrus (areas TH and TF), retrosplenial region, and presubiculum.[150] The area 23 projections to the hippocampal formation are much stronger from the ventral than from the dorsal portion of area 23. These anatomical features are relevant in the phenomena of retrosplenial amnesia and topographic disorientation that occur in patients with lesions of the caudoventral portions of the retrosplenial and posterior cingulate cortices.[361,362]

Cingulate Motor Areas 23 and 24

The dorsal and ventral banks of the cingulate sulcus can be parcellated in a ventrodorsal dimension[27] into three distinct types of cortex, rostral (CMAr), dorsal (CMAd), and ventral (CMAv) cingulate motor areas, involved in planning, preparing, and executing motor acts.[150,349,363] The primary motor cortex (M1) receives input from each of these three cingulate motor areas and from the SMA at the dorsomedial wall of the hemisphere. All four premotor areas have maps of the body containing proximal and distal somatomotor representations.

Retrosplenial Cortex Areas 29 and 30

These areas have extensive local connections to cingulate gyrus areas 23 and 24 and the areas 19 and PGm on the medial wall of the hemisphere, and major projections to frontal lobe areas 8AD, 46, 9, 10, 11, and 14, entorhinal cortex, subiculum, presubiculum, and parasubiculum of the hippocampal formation, areas TL, TH, and TF of the parahippocampal cortex, and to a lesser extent parastriate area V4, the dorsal bank of the STS, and area PG in the IPL. These connections with the hippocampal formation, parahippocampal region, and limbic thalamic nuclei emphasize the inclusion of the retrosplenial cortex in networks subserving learning, memory, spatial processing, emotional modulation, imagination, and planning.[15,233,354,362,364,365] The retrosplenial cortex is one of the earliest sites to reflect metabolic decline in Alzheimer's disease.[366]

Thalamic Connections

The thalamic connections of the cingulate gyrus are a core component of cingulate interactions with subcortical, allocortical, and periallocortical components within Papez circuit.

Areas 23 and 24 are both linked with the limbic thalamic nuclei—AM and AV, as well as with LD.[283,350,352,354,367,368] Area 24 also receives thalamic inputs from midline and intralaminar thalamic nuclei including paraventricular, reuniens, parafascicular, central superior lateral, and central densocellular nuclei, and from medial dorsal nucleus and nucleus limitans. Nonthalamic inputs to area 24 arise from the substantia innominata and claustrum.

The reciprocal efferent projections to thalamus from area 24 are with a similar set of nuclei: thalamic reticular nucleus, midline nuclei, AV and AD, MDdc, and VA.[15]

The posterior cingulate cortex area 23 thalamic afferents arise from all divisions of the anterior thalamic nucleus (AM, AV, AD), LD, and the medial pulvinar, and only minimally from midline and intralaminar nuclei. Both anterior and posterior sectors of the cingulate gyrus are similarly connected with MDdc, dorsal and median raphe nuclei, and the locus ceruleus.

The retrosplenial cortex area 30 receives heavy projections from the anterior thalamic nuclei, LD, and the lateral posterior (LP) nuclei. The reciprocal projections to thalamus from area 23 and area 30 are to the same dorsal, ventral, and medial divisions of the anterior thalamic nucleus, and the LD from which the thalamocortical projection arise. There are also projections to the CL, and midline nuclei including reuniens, the reticular nucleus of thalamus, the pulvinar nucleus (pulvinar oralis, lateralis, and medialis), LP, and limitans nucleus.[15,364,369,370]

Amygdala, Striatum, Pons Connections

The cingulate gyrus has reciprocal connections with the amygdala,[150] and topographically arranged projections to the striatum and pons, discussed below with the CB.

Human Connectivity Studies

Connectivity-based parcellation of the cingulate cortex in humans using probabilistic diffusion tractography complements the anatomical studies in monkeys of the cortical and subcortical connections of the cingulate gyrus.[371]

Clusters within the cingulate can be grouped into pregenual cingulate cortex area 25 involved in depression; areas 32 and 24 linked with the amygdala, hippocampus, hypothalamus, orbitofrontal cortex, and involved in emotion, motivation, inhibition, empathy, and social cognition; and area 23 engaged in memory and spatial processing.

THE CONCEPT OF DISTRIBUTED NEURAL CIRCUITS

Association Areas: Geschwind's Conceptual Framework of Neuroanatomy and Brain Localization in Clinical Neuroscience

At this point in our consideration of the association areas of the cerebral cortex, it may be helpful to pause and review the conceptual underpinnings of these neural circuits and how they are integrated into higher order brain function. The enduring impact of Norman Geschwind's 1965 papers "Disconnexion Syndromes in Animals and Man"[4,5] was summarized by Devinsky[372]: Geschwind resurrected the late 19th and early 20th century German and French literature, united the forgotten masters with recent anatomic, physiological, and clinical data, and rediscovered that neuronal masses and fiber pathways are essential to deciphering the mechanisms of behavior. He applied the term disconnection syndrome to lesions of the association pathways, emphasizing that humans have well-developed connections between different cortical association areas. In his original report, Geschwind[4] noted that whereas "in sub-human forms the only readily established sensory-sensory associations are those between a non-limbic (i.e., visual, tactile or auditory) stimulus and a limbic stimulus, it is only in man that associations between two non-limbic stimuli are readily formed and it is this ability which underlies the learning of names of objects."

The Distributed Neural Circuits Subserving Attention

Together with Ken Heilman and Deepak Pandya, Geschwind studied the phenomenon of trimodal neglect—somatosensory, visual. and auditory[373]—that occurs following damage to the right posterior parietal region.[374,375] Heilman et al.[376] summarize neglect as a failure to report, respond, or orient to contralateral stimuli that is not caused by an elemental sensorimotor deficit. Subtypes of neglect are distinguished by input (attentional) or output (intentional) demands, the distribution (personal, spatial, and representational), and the means of eliciting the signs (unilateral or bilateral stimuli).

The neuroanatomical basis of unilateral neglect and its different manifestations were explored by Mesulam in an influential paper[8] grounded in the anatomical principles discussed here. He concluded from a "review of unilateral neglect syndromes in monkeys and humans that four cerebral regions provide an integrated network for the modulation of directed attention within extrapersonal space. Each component region has a unique functional role that reflects its profile of anatomical connectivity, and each gives rise to a different clinical type of unilateral neglect when damaged. A posterior parietal component provides an internal sensory map and perhaps also a mechanism for modifying the extent of synaptic space devoted to specific portions of the external world; a limbic component in the cingulate gyrus regulates the spatial distribution of motivational valence; a frontal component coordinates the motor programs for exploration, scanning, reaching, and fixating; and a reticular component provides the underlying level of arousal and vigilance (Fig. 1-29A). This hypothetical network requires at least three complementary and interacting representations of extrapersonal space: a sensory representation in posterior parietal cortex, a schema for distributing exploratory movements in frontal cortex, and a motivational map in the cingulate cortex. Lesions in only one component of this network yield partial unilateral neglect syndromes, while those that encompass all the components result in profound deficits that transcend the mass effect of the larger lesion" (Fig. 1-29B).[8]

This network approach to the localization of complex functions emerges from the theoretical formulation that focal lesions within a network produce deficits that uniquely correspond to the lesion location. This approach is a cornerstone of the contemporary understanding of behavioral neurology and neuropsychiatry. It informs the discipline of subcortical behavioral neurology and neuropsychiatry as discussed in the remainder of this chapter, lesion network analysis, targeted therapeutic neuromodulation of focal nodes of distributed neural circuits, and the search for the neurobiology of neuropsychiatric disorders that do not have overtly manifesting brain structural lesions.

Transmodal Epicenters

In expanding the notion of the distributed neural circuits subserving cognitive processing, Mesulam[10] further proposed the notion of transmodal areas including Wernicke's area, hippocampal formation, and posterior parietal cortex, the functions of which are to bind multiple unimodal and other transmodal areas into distributed but integrated multimodal representations. These interconnected sets of transmodal nodes are then viewed as the anatomical and computational epicenters for large-scale neurocognitive networks.

The network for spatial awareness is based on transmodal epicenters in the posterior parietal cortex and frontal eye fields; the language network on epicenters in Wernicke's and Broca's areas; the explicit memory/emotion network on epicenters in the hippocampal-entorhinal complex and the amygdala; the face-object recognition network on epicenters in the midtemporal and temporopolar cortices; and the working memory-executive function network on epicenters in the lateral prefrontal cortex and posterior parietal cortex. The implication of this idea for clinical practice is that the destruction of transmodal epicenters causes global impairments such as multimodal anomia, neglect,

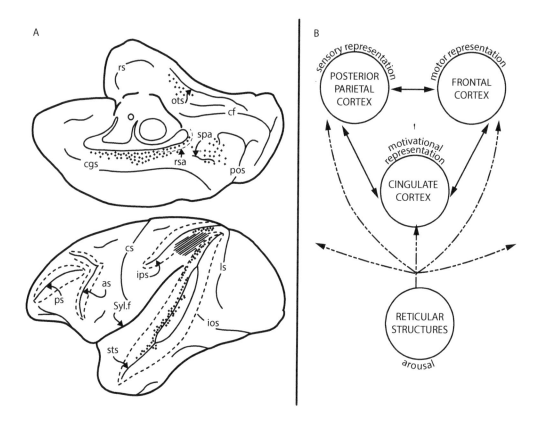

FIGURE 1-29. Cortical network for directed attention and unilateral neglect.[8] **(A)** The multimodal caudal part of the inferior parietal lobule in a rhesus monkey (dorsolateral area PG, shaded area) receives projections (identified with black dots) from neurons in the cortex of the upper bank of the superior temporal sulcus, mid-dorsolateral prefrontal cortex, cingulate gyrus, retrosplenial area, and parahippocampal gyrus, as demonstrated by Mesulam, Van Hoesen, Pandya and Geschwind in 1977.[187] **(B)** These connections underling the proposal for discrete, functionally specialized components of a neural network involved in modulating attention. as, arcuate sulcus; cf, calcarine fissure; cgs, cingulate sulcus; cs, central sulcus; ios, inferior occipital sulcus; ips, intraparietal sulcus; ls, lunate sulcus; ots, occipitotemporal sulcus; pos, parieto-occipital sulcus; ps, principal sulcus; rs, rhinal sulcus; rsa, retrosplenial area; sps, subparietal sulcus; Syl. f, Sylvian fissure.

and amnesia, whereas their selective disconnection from relevant unimodal areas elicits modality-specific impairments such as prosopagnosia, pure word blindness, and category-specific anomias.

The idea is further formulated to encompass an overarching evolutionary perspective: The ability to communicate abstract concepts, the critical pacemaker for human cognitive development, has shifted from the extremely slow process of structural brain evolution to the much more rapid one of distributed computations where each individual intelligence can become incorporated into an interactive lattice that promotes the transgenerational transfer and accumulation of knowledge.[10]

There is a remarkable resonance between these ideas and those of Franz Joseph Gall. This is best captured in the commentary by Flourens in what was intended as a "'pulverizing blow' upon on the doctrines of phrenology which are liable to impart, or are founded upon, manifestly erroneous conceptions of free-will, of the conscience, of the judgment and the perceptive powers…,"[377] but which in retrospect have the opposite effect. Flourens notes that "Gall's philosophy consists holy in the substitution of *multiplicity* for *unity*. In place of one general and single brain, he substitutes a number of small brains: Instead of one general sole understanding, he substitutes several individual understandings. These pretended *individual understandings* are the *faculties*. Now, Gall admits the existence of twenty-seven of these faculties, each one of them (since each one is a peculiar understanding) endowed with its perceptive faculty, its memory, its judgment, its imagination; etc." (italics original).[378] Gall's *individual understandings* and Mesulam's *individual intelligence(s)* are wholly compatible with the contemporary notion of association areas and distributed neural circuits.

Transmodal epicenters for large-scale neurocognitive networks are not confined to the cerebral cortex. They recruit subcortical regions which are incorporated into the distributed neural circuits subserving neurological function. The theory of the general and specific principles of cerebral cortical organization recognizes that subcortical centers and white matter tracts are integral to the distributed neural circuits, and that destruction of these subcortical nodes has clinically meaningful implications.

Convergence Zones

Antonio Damasio[379] outlined a theoretical framework for the understanding of the neural basis of memory and consciousness. He drew on a systems-based approach arising out of the connectional neuroanatomy and evolutionary principles of brain development summarized in this chapter. He summarized this arrangement as follows: Brain architecture is constituted by (i) neuron ensembles located in multiple and separate regions of primary and first-order sensory association cortices ("early cortices") and motor cortices; they contain representations of feature fragments inscribed as patterns of activity originally engaged by perceptuomotor interactions; (ii) neuron ensembles located downstream from the former throughout single modality cortices (local convergence zones); they inscribe amodal records of the combinatorial arrangement of feature fragments

that occurred synchronously during the experience of entities or events in sector (i); (iii) neuron ensembles located downstream from the former throughout higher order association cortices (non-local convergence zones), which inscribe amodal records of the synchronous combinatorial arrangements of local convergence zones during the experience of entities and events in sector (i); (iv) feedforward and feedback projections interlocking reciprocally the neuron ensembles in (i) with those in (ii) according to a many-to-one (feedforward) and one-to-many (feedback) principle. Drawing on these established critical anatomic underpinnings of behavior, Damasio proposed that (a) recall of entities and events occurs when the neuron ensembles in (i) are activated in time-locked fashion; (b) the synchronous activations are directed from convergence zones in (ii) and (iii); and (c) the process of reactivation is triggered from firing in convergence zones and mediated by feedback projections. This proposal rejects a single anatomical site for the integration of memory and motor processes and a single store for the meaning of entities of events. Rather, meaning is reached by time-locked multiregional retroactivation of widespread fragment records, thereby constituting the contents of consciousness.[379] Experimental support for this approach is derived from functional imaging experiments such as one that explored the neural basis of the representation of an object's unique feature-convergence. A pattern-classification algorithm decoded a visually presented object's shape in lateral occipital cortex and its color in right visual association area V4, whereas information about the identity of the object was in the left anterior temporal lobe, an area that was specifically predicted by the temporal convergence of shape and color codes in early visual regions. This fulfilled three key requirements for a neural convergence zone: a convergence result (object identity), ingredients (color and shape), and the link between them.[380]

Brain Oscillations—A Note on the Physiology of Neurons and Neural Circuits

The notion of convergence zones segues into brain physiology. The challenge of determining how objects encoded by distinct brain circuits are combined for perception, decision, and action is known as the binding problem,[381] and it is true for object identification as well as for issues relating to the emergence of consciousness.[382-384] In the visual realm, how is an image integrated by the brain when multiple specialized cortical visual areas respond to different features including orientation, depth, form, motion, and color? These areas are connected in parallel with each other and reciprocally with primary visual areas, but when they project to a common cortical area the inputs are largely distinct. Multiple local circuits in separate areas must therefore be integrated for the perception of a unified image.[372] The correlation theory of brain function was introduced to address this problem.[381] It proposed the existence of synaptic modulation, according to which synapses switch between a conducting and a nonconducting state, the dynamics of which are controlled on a fast time scale by correlations in the temporal fine structure of cellular signals. In this view, synaptic modulation and plasticity form the basis for short-term and long-term memory, respectively, and signal correlations, shaped by the variable network, express structure and relationships within objects. The basic idea of this spatiotemporal binding is that distributed sets of neurons that are grouped together are correlated in time.[385] Visually related activities are therefore transiently labeled by a temporal code that signalizes their momentary association.[386] Perceptual awareness of visual input, and perhaps consciousness of such input, may thus rely on synchronously linked activity in multiple areas.

Crick and Koch[382] proposed that the way to impose temporary unity on the activities of all neurons that are relevant at a particular moment is by a fast attentional mechanism, with the relevant neurons firing together in semi-synchrony, probably at a frequency in the 40–70 Hz range, activating the appropriate parts of the working memory system through transient alteration of synaptic strengths. Contemporary views of large-scale brain function now focus on spontaneous neuronal activity and neural synchrony as a key binding mechanism, and as the source of cognitive abilities. Self-emerged oscillatory timing is viewed as the brain's fundamental organizer of neuronal information.[387]

Rhythmic fluctuations in activity of neuronal populations are characterized by their frequency, amplitude, and phase,[388] each type of oscillation generated by a unique set of intrinsic neuronal currents, synaptic interactions, and extracellular factors.[389] Gamma oscillations (30–80 Hz) are generated by the synchronous activity of fast-spiking GABAergic interneurons in the cerebral cortex which express the Ca^{2+}-binding protein parvalbumin and receive N-methyl-D-aspartate (NMDA)-dependent excitatory input from pyramidal cells. They also regulate the activity of neural networks through GABAergic inhibition of local excitatory neurons. The gamma oscillations correlate with performance on cognitive tasks including the allocation of attention and working memory; they are thought to underlie cognitive disturbances in psychiatric disorders[390] and notably in schizophrenia in which impaired GABAergic neurotransmission is correlated with gamma band activity.[391]

Llinás and Paré[392] studied wakefulness and paradoxical sleep and determined that the main difference between them lies in the weight given to sensory afferents in cognitive images during wakefulness; otherwise, they concluded, wakefulness and paradoxical sleep are fundamentally equivalent brain states probably subserved by intrinsic thalamocortical loops. This assertion was predicated on the recognition that thalamic connectivity is mostly geared to the generation of internal functional modes which operate in the presence or absence of sensory activation (i.e., corticothalamic connections of the intralaminar, associative, and limbic thalamic nuclei discussed later in the chapter), whereas only a minor part of thalamic connectivity is devoted to the transfer of direct sensorimotor input (i.e., the motor-related and specific sensory thalamic nuclei). They further proposed that since most thalamic connectivity generates internal functional modes, consciousness is fundamentally a closed-loop property in which the ability of cells to be intrinsically active plays a central role, and that spatial and temporal mapping of electrical activity in the brain is key to the elaboration of cognitive and perceptual constructs. Subsequent studies reveal that thalamic oscillations are generated by sets of intrinsic neuronal currents, synaptic interactions, and extracellular factors

with frequencies ranging from infra-slow (<0.1 Hz) to ultra-fast (100–600 Hz).[389,393] Different corticothalamic modules are tuned to oscillate at their own characteristic rates, with dominant alpha-band oscillations (8–12 Hz) in area 19 of extrastriate occipital cortex, beta-band oscillations (13–20 Hz) in SPL area 7, and fast beta/gamma-band oscillations (21–50 Hz) in premotor cortex area 6.[394]

INTRINSIC CONNECTIVITY NETWORKS

The development and refinement of functional MRI has made it possible to translate the anatomy from the tract tracing studies of the nonhuman primate into the imaging investigations of the functioning human brain. The circuits that have been defined in the monkey translate in the human brain to intrinsic functional connectivity networks using rsfcMRI. The fluctuation of blood oxygen level dependent (BOLD) signal in functional MRI is used to infer anatomical connectivity in the human brain.[56,395]

The results of the rsfcMRI studies demonstrate that the brain forms local hierarchical relations, segregating into distinct neural networks within sensory and motor cortices, and within distributed networks of association regions. These include sensorimotor, dorsal and ventral attention, frontoparietal, salience, and default networks (Fig. 1-30A). The default network is engaged when a subject is not actively performing identifiable task activity, and it has been linked with creativity and with reflective and analytical thought.[396] Definition of these networks initially at the cortical level has been extended to demonstrations of these networks using a range of imaging techniques in the cerebellar cortex (Figs. 1-30 and 1-59D),[397,398] deep cerebellar nuclei,[399] thalamus,[400,401] and basal ganglia.[402]

CHANNEL AND STATE FUNCTIONS

Therapy in behavioral neurology and neuropsychiatry relies heavily on psychoneuropharmacology, and less often but increasingly important, on neurostimulation. This reflects the dichotomy, framed by Mesulam,[8] as channel functions versus state functions. *Channel functions* refer to anatomical structures, pathways, and connections. These are similar across individuals, but not invariant, as they respond dynamically to experience and learning. This is true at the level of gross morphometric analysis, exemplified in the posterior hippocampal morphometric imaging study of London cabdrivers cited above,[193] as well as at the level of the synapse. Long-term memories are stored by changes in synapses that involve activation of gene expression, new protein synthesis, and the formation of new connections[403]; and synaptic integrity and plasticity are induced by exercise in a mouse model of a neurodegenerative disease (spinocerebellar ataxia type 1).[404]

State functions refer to the chemical milieu superimposed upon the anatomical-physiological systems. Monoaminergic neurotransmitter systems that arise primarily from brainstem and

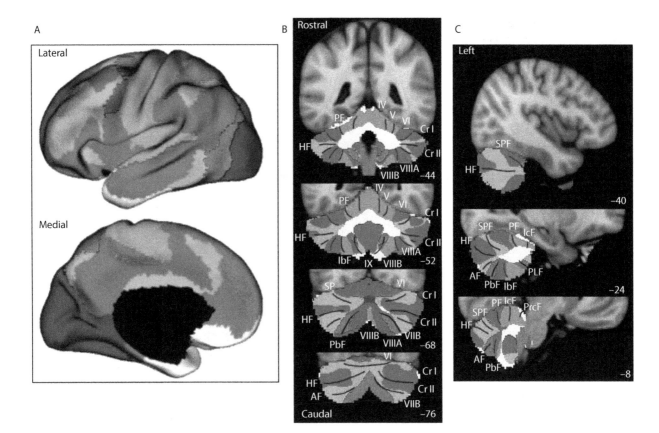

FIGURE 1-30. Resting state functional connectivity maps of the human cerebral hemisphere and cerebellum. **(A)** A seven-network parcellation of the human cerebral cortex based on 1000 subjects. Color coding: blue, somatomotor; green, dorsal attention; violet, ventral attention; orange, frontoparietal; red, default; purple, visual; cream, limbic/salience. (From Yeo et al.[56]) **(B)** Coronal and **(C)** sagittal views of the cerebellum based on functional connectivity to the seven major networks in the cerebrum. The coordinates at bottom right of each panel represent the section level in the MNI atlas space. Major fissures are demarcated on the left hemisphere, and lobules are labeled on the right hemisphere. AF, ansoparamedian fissure; HF, horizontal fissure; IbF, intrabiventer fissure; IcF, intraculminate fissure; PbF, prepyramidal/prebiventer fissure; PF, primary fissure; PLF, posterolateral fissure; PrcF, preculminate fissure; SF, secondary fissure; SPF, superior posterior fissure. (Modified from Buckner et al.[397])

basal forebrain nuclei (catecholaminergic, noradrenergic, dopaminergic, and serotonergic) project widely throughout the cerebral hemispheres as referenced throughout this chapter. These and other neurotransmitters and chemical and hormonal modulators act on arousal, attention, mood, and social cognition, and influence the interpretation of brain behavior correlations. They also provide opportunities for therapeutic intervention.

WHITE MATTER TRACTS OF THE CEREBRAL HEMISPHERES

We now bring into focus the intricacies of the white matter tracts that link the cortical and subcortical nodes of the distributed neural circuits in this section adapted from Schmahmann and Pandya.[15] These tracts and the areas that they connect are relevant to cognition, emotion, and social cognition.

An interesting feature of these white matter tracts at the level of microscopic analysis, as discovered in diffusion tractography MRI[405] and confirmed with histological study,[406] is that it appears that fibers branch by making right angle turns. It is not yet clear whether this is a ubiquitous feature of white matter organization, or indeed whether it has clinical relevance, but it may transpire that this is an important anatomical feature of white matter organization and development. As outlined above in the discussion of the general principles of organization of cerebral cortical connections, neurons within any cortical area give rise to groups of efferent fibers that can be identified within the white matter immediately beneath the gyrus (Fig. 1-26).

Association Fibers

Association fibers comprise local, neighborhood, and long association fibers. Local, or U-fibers, are closely adjacent to the undersurface of the sixth layer and are directed to cortical regions in the same or adjacent gyri. Neighborhood association fibers are distinct from local U-fibers and are directed to nearby cortical regions; for example, the fibers that connect the IPL to the medial parietal cortex. Long association fibers are the named fiber tracts that travel within the central part of the white matter of the core of the gyrus and link distant cortical areas within the same hemisphere.

Corticostriate Fibers

Corticostriate fibers course initially with the long association fibers before separating from them, then travel within one of two major fiber bundles. Fibers in the subcallosal fasciculus of Muratoff lead mainly to the caudate nucleus and putamen. Fibers in the external capsule target the ventral part of the caudate nucleus, the putamen, and claustrum.

The Cord of Fibers

The cord of fibers comprises a dense aggregation of fibers occupying the central core of the white matter of the gyrus and contains *commissural* fibers and the *subcortical projection* bundle. The commissural bundle travels to the opposite hemisphere via the CC or the AC. The subcortical bundle travels within the internal capsule (anterior or posterior limb) or the sagittal stratum (SS), and segregates into *thalamic* fibers that travel via thalamic peduncles to the thalamus, and a *pontine* fiber bundle that courses via the cerebral peduncle to the pons. The subcortical bundle also gives rise to fibers that travel to other diencephalic and brainstem structures.

Knowledge of these tracts and their putative functional properties is useful when considering the clinical consequence of white matter diseases, and in understanding the neurobehavioral consequence of subcortical lesions that affect white matter tracts. The tract tracing histological observations in monkeys are supported by diffusion spectrum MRI findings in monkeys,[407] and they closely match those in the human brain as determined using diffusion tensor imaging (DTI),[408-412] probabilistic tractography,[413-415] and resting-state functional connectivity mapping.[416-418] There are a few notable exceptions, however, exemplified by the finding of an inferior fronto-occipital fascicle in humans[419] that has not been identified in nonhuman primate tract tracing studies.[15,420] It possible that the extreme capsule (EmC) in monkeys which links the temporal lobe with prefrontal cortices has expanded in humans to the inferior fronto-occipital fascicle, because these two tracts occupy similar positions in relation to the insular cortex and inferior aspect of the claustrum.

LONG ASSOCIATION FIBER TRACTS

The long association fiber tracts are the essential anatomic substrates for communication between cortical areas that subserve different behaviors (Fig. 1-31).[15,421] The tracts most directly pertinent to neuropsychiatry are the dorsal limbic bundle, namely the CB, and the ventral limbic bundle, the UF. These tracts and their connections are presented here in greater detail.

The development of diffusion tractography has made it possible to visualize these pathways in humans in vivo and in animal models (Fig. 1-32).[407,411,412,422]

CINGULUM BUNDLE

Papez[67] proposed that the cingulate gyrus and CB were integral components of the circuitry subserving emotion, and MacLean[69] incorporated them into his conception of the visceral brain.

The CB was among the first of the major fiber systems of the brain to be recognized and depicted, and its precise anatomy and functional significance have long sparked interest and speculation.[15,19,421] It stretches from the frontal lobe around the rostrum and genu of the CC, lies above the CC nestled within the white matter of the cingulate gyrus, curves ventrally around the splenium, and then occupies a position in the white matter of the parahippocampal gyrus in the ventral part of the temporal lobe (Figs. 1-31C, 1-32B, C, and 1-33). It is a composite fiber bundle that contains association fibers arising from the cingulate gyrus itself as well as from other cortical regions, and fibers linking the cingulate gyrus with subcortical structures including thalamus, striatum, and pons, and commissural fibers to the opposite hemisphere. The association fibers generally course through the periphery of the CB, whereas the subcortical (commissural and subcortical) fibers are more ventral and central. The subcortical, commissural, striatal, and some association fibers that emanate from the cingulate gyrus have a characteristic radiating appearance in the coronal plane.[15,150,151,350–353,355,368,423,424]

Fibers Conveyed in the Cingulum Bundle

Corticocortical Fibers

The efferent long association fibers of the CB originate from the rostral cingulate cortex area 24, the caudal cingulate cortex area 23, and retrosplenial cortex areas 29 and 30, and they course to their destinations in the periphery of the CB. They are directed to periallocortical or limbic regions in the presubiculum and the entorhinal cortex; proisocortical or paralimbic cortices in the retrosplenial cortex, parahippocampal gyrus, and perirhinal area; and isocortical areas that include the prefrontal, posterior parietal, and temporal lobe association cortices.[63] Fibers directed rostrally terminate in mid-dorsolateral prefrontal cortex areas 8, 9, and 46, frontal polar area 10, orbitofrontal cortex area 11, and area 32 on the medial surface of the frontal lobe. Caudally directed CB fibers lead to the parietal cortex (area PG/Opt), retrosplenial cortex, and ventral temporal lobe (presubiculum, parahippocampal gyrus, and entorhinal cortex). Afferent fibers coursing to the cingulate gyrus in the CB arise from the same prefrontal, parietal, and temporal regions to which the efferent fibers from the cingulate gyrus are relayed. Some long association fibers arising from the cingulate gyrus penetrate laterally through the CB and collect in the fronto-occipital fasciculus (FOF) located above the subcallosal fasciculus of Muratoff, coursing rostrally and terminating in dorsal premotor area 6, dorsal area 8, and area 9.[15,356,425]

The cortical connections of the cingulate gyrus that run in the CB may thus be grouped into three broad categories based on their functional affiliations. These are to (i) periallocortical or limbic regions (presubiculum and entorhinal cortex);

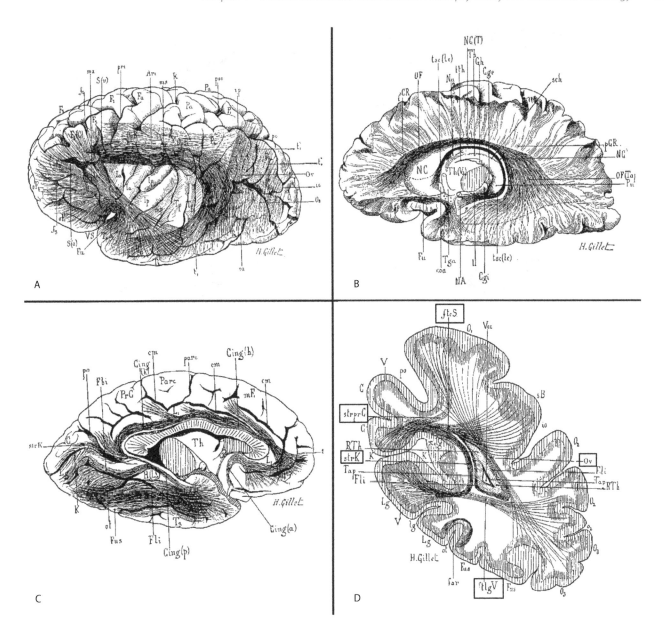

FIGURE 1-31. Diagrams from Déjerine's *Anatomie des centres nerveux* in 1895[421] summarizing some of the major pathways of the human brain discussed. **(A)** Déjerine's notion of the arcuate and uncinate fasciculi, and the vertical occipital fibers in Fig. 377; **(B)** the uncinate fasciculus, fronto-occipital fasciculus and the corona radiata are diagrammed in his Fig. 381; **(C)** the cingulum bundle and inferior longitudinal fascicles are represented in his Fig. 374; **(D)** this schematic coronal section depicts the intrinsic fibers of the occipital lobe including the occipito-vertical fascicle, or perpendicular occipital fascicle of Wernicke (Ov), the occipital transverse fascicle of the cuneus of Sachs (ftcS), the occipital transverse fascicle of the lingual lobule of Vialet (ftlgV), stratum proprium of the cuneus (strprC), and the stratum calcarinum (strK) or U-fiber layer of the calcarine fissure in Fig. 389. (Composite figure and legend from Schmahmann and Pandya.[15])

(ii) proisocortical or paralimbic cortices (retrosplenial cortex, parahippocampal gyrus, perirhinal cortex) that are linked with cortical association areas as well as limbic structures such as amygdala and hippocampal formation; and (iii) isocortical areas including the multimodal association areas in the frontal, parietal, and temporal regions that receive input from parasensory association cortices for vision, hearing, and somatic sensation.[63] These isocortical connections are with dorsolateral areas 8, 9/46, and 10, orbitofrontal area 11, medial prefrontal area 32, and premotor area 6; parietal lobe area PG/Opt laterally and area PGm medially; and with the caudal superior temporal gyrus area Tpt, area TPO in the upper bank of the STS, and the parahippocampal gyrus. The cingulate motor areas thought to engage in motivation and higher order planning of motor programming[323,324] have widespread connections not only with sensorimotor regions (like the primary motor cortex), but they also have connections with cortical association areas.

Striatal Fibers

A component of fibers courses laterally through the CB relaying projections from the cingulate gyrus and retrosplenial area into a compact fiber bundle above the head and body of the

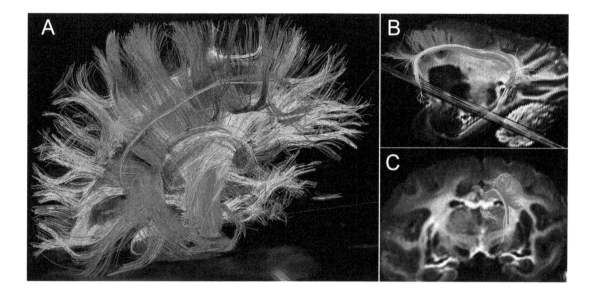

FIGURE 1-32. Diffusion spectrum imaging (a form of diffusion tractography) identifies white matter tracts in intact brain. **(A)** Human brain pathways. (From Wedeen et al.[422]). **(B)** Sagittal plane view and **(C)** coronal plane view of the cingulum bundle in rhesus monkey. (From Schmahmann et al.[407])

caudate nucleus, the subcallosal fasciculus of Muratoff, or the Muratoff bundle (MB). The MB fibers distribute to the caudate nucleus, NAc, and putamen. Some of the striatal fibers move further laterally, either directly from the CB or via the MB, cross the corona radiata or the internal capsule, and then descend in the external capsule before terminating in the claustrum and putamen.

The caudate nucleus is implicated in the pathophysiology of obsessive-compulsive disorder and decreases in size in patients following cingulotomy.[426] It is possible, therefore, that fibers passing through the CB are linked with striatal regions that play a role in initiating the expression of affective behavior and motor responses.

Commissural and Projection Fibers
A group of fibers originating from the cingulate gyrus aggregates in a dense cord, moves laterally through the CB, and divides into two components, commissural and subcortical. The commissural fibers course ventrally to become incorporated into the callosal fibers that pass to the opposite hemisphere. The subcortical fibers progress laterally into the corona radiata and enter the internal capsule. One group of fibers terminates in thalamus, and the other continues into the cerebral peduncle as it courses to the pons.

Thalamic Fibers
The cingulate cortex has bidirectional connections with the limbic thalamic nuclei (AV, AM, AD, LD, and intralaminar) as well as limbic regions of the PM, MDdc, and the VA. The thalamus provides a specific alerting response,[427,428] increasing input to memory of category-specific material while simultaneously inhibiting retrieval from memory. Crosson[429] proposed that thalamus contributes a selective engagement mechanism to

cortical areas required to perform a cognitive task, while maintaining other areas in a state of relative disengagement.

The defects of emotional expression and affective regulation that occur following lesions of the limbic thalamus[62] may result in part from destruction of these thalamo-cingulate projections that travel in the CB. The role of the thalamic connections of the cingulate gyrus in the modulation of emotion and memory by the Papez circuit was discussed above.

Pontine Fibers
The contingent of fibers that penetrates laterally through the CB and contributes to the feedforward limb of the cerebrocerebellar pathway links the cingulate gyrus with nuclei in the basis pontis.[430] Cingulopontine projections have been implicated in the investigations of patients who demonstrate impairments of cognitive and affective behaviors following cerebellar lesions.[256,431] Likewise, patients with selective infarction of the rostral basis pontis have been described who display emotional blunting and pathologic laughter and crying.[432,433] It is therefore likely that cingulate gyrus projections coursing through the CB to the basis pontis are relevant in the modulation of the experience and expression of emotion, memory, and motivation.

Functional Correlates
The connections conveyed in the CB facilitate the behavioral properties attributed to it in disease states in people and in behavioral studies in animals. This includes autonomic phenomena,[369,434] complex motor behaviors,[369,434] the emotional coloring of sensation and nociception,[69] attention toward sensory stimuli with affective valence and visual spatial attention,[435] facial movements that convey emotional expression,[315,369] avoidance behavior, motivation, drive, will and exploratory behavior,[341]

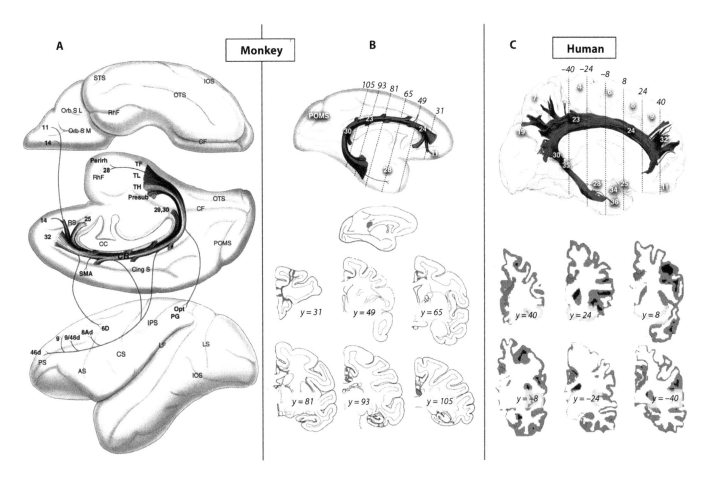

FIGURE 1-33. Cingulum bundle. **(A)** The cingulum bundle in monkeys determined through isotope tract tracing, with the findings represented in an artist's rendition.[15] **(B)** Colorization of the Schmahmann and Pandya[15] findings, for comparison with **(C)** diffusion tensor imaging observations in the human brain, by Thiebaut de Schotten et al.[411]

and working memory and self-regulation.[354,424] The CB may contribute to mnemonic processing: Declarative memory invokes the hippocampal connections,[436] spatial memory and spatial attention draw on parietal and hippocampal systems,[300] working memory is supported by its links with the dorsolateral prefrontal cortex,[13,150,364] and episodic memory may be dependent upon connections with area 10 in the frontal pole.[437] By linking the retrosplenial cortex, medial prefrontal cortex, and medial temporal lobe, the CB is implicated in the default mode network, likely playing a role in inner thought and creativity including autobiographical memory retrieval, envisioning the future, and conceiving the perspectives of others.[396]

Clinical Implications

The role of the CB in the regulation of emotional processing is underscored by behavioral changes in monkeys following ablation of the anterior cingulate region, including tameness and loss of fear.[438,439] Autonomic phenomena in monkeys[369,438] and humans[434] are elicited by electrical stimulation of the anterior cingulate cortex, and more complex behavioral responses including fear, anxiety, and pleasure have been recorded in humans following stimulation of the CB itself.[440]

Cingulotomy was introduced as a treatment for depression and psychosis[441,442] based largely on the theory of Papez[67] and

experimental observations in monkeys.[443] Glees et al.[439] noted little change following localized ablation of this area in patients with advanced psychosis, but there was considerable improvement in those with obsessive-compulsive behaviors. Adey and Meyer[444] believed that the therapeutic effect of prefrontal leucotomy lay in its interruption of fibers in the cingulum arising from prefrontal areas 9 and 10. Cingulectomy[445] and subsequent bilateral stereotaxic cingulotomy are again in use for neuropsychiatric illness such as obsessive-compulsive disorder and for intractable pain.[446-452] The heterogeneous composition of the CB, containing association, commissural, subcortical, and striatal fibers, indicates that disrupting the CB, whether for clinical or experimental purposes, must necessarily involve extensive disconnections among various cortical, subcortical, and limbic structures.[364]

UNCINATE FASCICULUS

The UF has long been recognized through gross dissection.[453-456] Anatomical mapping methods reveal that it is a bidirectional pathway linking rostral temporal lobe, insula, and amygdala with the inferior, orbital, and medial prefrontal regions (Figs. 1, 1-31A, and 1-34).[2,15,298,457] Fibers from the rostral part of the

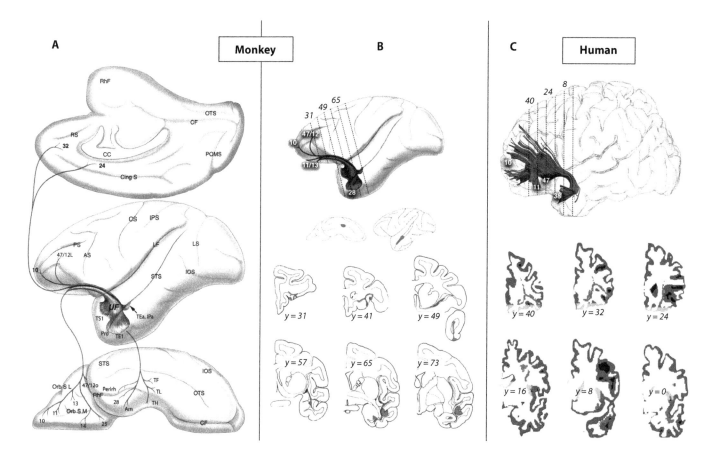

FIGURE 1-34. Uncinate fasciculus. **(A)** The uncinate fasciculus in monkeys determined through isotope tract tracing, with the findings represented in an artist's rendition.[15] **(B)** Colorization of the Schmahmann and Pandya findings in 2006,[15] for comparison with **(C)** diffusion tensor imaging observations in the human brain, by Thiebaut de Schotten et al.[411]

superior temporal gyrus (temporal proisocortex and area TS1) and the inferotemporal region (areas TE1 and TEa) ascend in the temporal stem where they are positioned rostral to the most anteriorly situated fibers of the inferior longitudinal fasciculus (ILF). The uncinate fibers then aggregate lateral to the ventral part of the claustrum, situated medial to the insular cortex, and below and medial to the fibers of the EmC. They move medially through the limen insula into the white matter of the orbital cortex where they assume a plate-like formation as they move rostrally and medially in the frontal lobe. These fibers terminate in ventral prefrontal area 12/47 and in the orbital cortex in areas 11, 13, and the orbital proisocortex. Some fibers move medially and ascend at the medial wall of the prefrontal cortex, terminating in areas 14 and 32, while others terminate in the rostral cingulate gyrus, area 24. The fibers in the UF also originate from the rostral parts of the STS (areas TEa and Ipa) and the parahippocampal gyrus (areas TF, TL, and TH), course to the frontal lobe, and terminate first in basal forebrain areas, and then in areas 47/12, 13, 14, 10, and 25. As the UF courses from all these temporal lobe areas through the temporal stem toward the frontal lobe, it contributes projections also to the amygdala and to the temporal polar proisocortex and perirhinal region.

The UF conveys reciprocal fibers leading from these orbital, ventrolateral, and medial prefrontal lobe areas back to the temporal lobes. They lead to the rostral parts of the superior temporal gyrus, STS, and inferotemporal region, as well as to the parahippocampal gyrus and the amygdala.

Functional Correlations

Whereas the CB is a dorsal limbic pathway connecting the frontal, parietal, cingulate, and ventral temporal cortices, the UF is a ventral limbic pathway connecting the rostral temporal, inferotemporal, and ventral temporal regions with the medial and orbital frontal cortices. It appears that there is no direct link between these two fiber tracts. Further, both the CB and UF are limbic pathways at the medial border of the hemisphere, and both are strongly cholinergic,[458] but they appear to have different functions. The roles to which the CB contributes include spatial and working memory, motivation, pain perception, avoidance behavior, response selection, and error detection. The putative functions of the UF, in contrast, appear to be somewhat different as may be inferred from a consideration of the cortical areas that it links.

The rostral part of the superior temporal gyrus and superior temporal proisocortex are involved in sound recognition and in memory for acoustic information.[459] These areas give rise to fibers that run in the UF and terminate in areas 13, 12/47, and 11 in the orbitofrontal cortex that are important for behavioral responses to emotionally salient stimuli,[460] and in areas 14, 25, and 32 in the medial prefrontal cortex. The UF, therefore, that connects these temporal and prefrontal areas, may be a crucial component of the system that regulates emotional responses to auditory stimuli.

The UF also conveys fibers to the frontal lobe from regions of the rostral part of the inferotemporal cortex (area TE1 and the ventral part of inferotemporal proisocortex) that are concerned with object-related visual information, to orbitofrontal cortex areas 12/47 and area 11. By transmitting object-related visual information from the temporal lobe to the orbitofrontal cortex, the UF makes it possible to attach emotional valence to visual information and to facilitate appropriate responses.

A contingent of fibers within the UF leads from the parahippocampal region (entorhinal, perirhinal, parahippocampal gyrus, areas TF, TH, and TL) to the orbitofrontal cortex. Some of these fibers terminate in medial forebrain areas, while the major component of the fibers terminates in areas 13, 12/47, 11, and 10. Some fibers from the posterior parahippocampal gyrus terminate also in the rostral cingulate cortex area 24. The parahippocampal gyrus receives input from modality-specific association areas, multimodal regions of the parietotemporal cortices, the prefrontal cortex, and the cingulate gyrus. Recognition memory has been shown to be dependent upon the medial temporal region[436,461] as well as the orbitofrontal cortex.[338] By linking these two cortical regions, the UF is likely to be an important component of the circuit underlying recognition memory.

Thus, the UF links temporal lobe areas that contain highly processed modality-specific information, multimodal information, and limbic/emotional processing, with frontal lobe areas that regulate behaviors and emotions. The modality-specific inputs are auditory—rostral superior temporal gyrus; visual—rostral inferotemporal region; and somatosensory and gustatory—rostral insular opercular cortex. The multimodal information in the UF is derived from the rostral STS, and mnemonic information from parahippocampal areas. The amygdala connections with the medial prefrontal and caudal orbital regions[155,462] that are carried by the UF have relevance for the processing of information about the emotional significance of stimuli and the generation of emotional expression.

The orbitofrontal regions that are linked by the UF with these temporal cortices are involved in aversive and aggressive behaviors in monkeys,[463] self-regulation,[464] recognition memory,[338] and decision making.[465] The UF also links the amygdala with the temporal pole and the inferior temporal cortices. It may therefore facilitate optimal responses to the prevailing external as well as internal milieu, and consequently play a role enabling what Nauta[466] regarded as the nervous system's need to ensure stability of complex goal-directed forms of behavior in time and space. Further, this tract appears to be essential for what Barbas regards as a triadic network, consisting of the orbitofrontal cortex, anterior temporal visual and auditory association cortices, and the amygdala, which may be recruited in cognitive tasks that are inextricably linked with emotional associations.[462]

The functional anatomy of the UF also sets up the hypothesis of Von Der Heide et al.[467] that the tract enables mnemonic associations in the temporal lobe to modify behavior through interactions with the lateral orbitofrontal cortex which provides valence-based biasing of decisions. Because of the bidirectionality of information flow within the tract, orbital frontal cortex-based reward and punishment history can modulate temporal lobe-based mnemonic representation.

Clinical Correlations

The UF is clinically relevant in disorders of social and moral cognition, such as psychopathy and sociopathy.[468,469] It is implicated as the anatomical correlate of impaired emotional empathy—the ability to share in and make inferences about how other people feel, for the reason that it links the structures that underlie this ability, namely, the orbitofrontal cortex, anterior insula, anterior cingulate, temporal pole, and amygdala.[470] DTI studies point to a role in schizophrenia, with greater anisotropy in the left UF compared to the right indicating a higher number and/or density of fibers on the left,[471] and decreased fractional anisotropy bilaterally in early stage schizophrenia indicative of altered white matter integrity.[472]

The UF may be relevant in the interictal personality disorder of temporal lobe epilepsy. Temporal lobectomy lowers seizure frequency by excision of the epileptic focus.[473] It also improves psychosocial outcome, and aggressive and antisocial behavior in some children and adults.[474] This may represent the beneficial effect of a temporal-frontal disconnection syndrome because components of the UF are removed during the anterior temporal lobectomy,[475] and therefore they are no longer able to convey pathologic information from the temporal lobe to the decision-making regions of the medial and orbitofrontal cortex. This would be analogous to the beneficial effects of cingulotomy.[448,452]

SUPERIOR LONGITUDINAL FASCICULUS (SLF)

The SLF links the frontal and parietal lobes, and has three subcomponents.

SLF I lies medially situated in the white matter of the SPL and the superior frontal gyrus (Fig. 1-35A). It links the superior parietal region and adjacent medial parietal cortex in a reciprocal manner with the frontal lobe supplementary and premotor areas. It is thought to play a role in the regulation of higher order motor behavior requiring information about body part location, and it may contribute to the initiation of motor activity.

SLF II is more laterally situated and occupies a position in the central core of the hemisphere white matter, lateral to the corona radiata and above the Sylvian fissure (Fig. 1-35B). It links the caudal IPL (equivalent in humans to the angular gyrus) and the parieto-occipital areas, with the posterior part of the dorsolateral and mid-dorsolateral prefrontal cortex. It is thought to serve as the conduit for the neural system subserving visual awareness, the maintenance of attention, and engagement in the environment. It provides a means whereby the prefrontal cortex can regulate the focusing of attention within different parts of space.

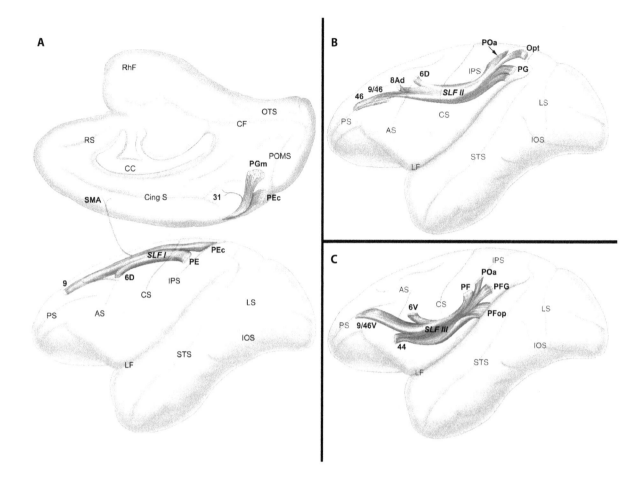

FIGURE 1-35. Summary diagrams of the course and composition of the superior longitudinal fasciculus (SLF) in the rhesus monkey. **(A)** SLF I; **(B)** SLF II; and **(C)** SLF III. The lateral and medial views of the cerebral hemispheres show the trajectory of the three components of the SLF and the cortical areas that contribute axons to these fiber pathways. (Adapted from Schmahmann and Pandya.[15])

SLF III is further lateral and ventral, and it is located in the white matter of the parietal and frontal operculum (Fig. 1-35C). It provides the ventral premotor region and pars opercularis with higher order somatosensory input, it may be crucial for monitoring orofacial and hand actions, and in the humans it is important for articulation and the phonemic aspects of language.

ARCUATE FASCICULUS (AF)

The AF runs in the white matter of the superior temporal gyrus and deep to the upper shoulder of the Sylvian fissure (Figs. 1-31A and 1-36A). By linking the caudal temporal lobe with the dorsolateral prefrontal cortex, it may be viewed as an auditory spatial bundle, important for the spatial features of acoustic stimuli and auditory-related processing. The AF has historically been regarded as linking the posterior (Wernicke) and anterior (Broca) language areas in the human brain, and to be involved in conduction aphasia. The connectional studies in monkeys are consistent with the evolving notion that the AF subserves a dorsal stream of linguistic processing.[476,477] Together with the SLF III, it appears that the AF is engaged in the phonemic aspects of language (sound appreciation and production).

EXTREME CAPSULE

The EmC is situated between the claustrum and the insular cortex caudally, and between the claustrum and the orbital frontal cortex rostrally (Figs. 1-36B and 1-38). In monkeys, the EmC is the principal association pathway linking the middle superior temporal region with the caudal parts of the orbital cortex and the ventral-lateral prefrontal cortex, including area 45. These areas are homologous to the Wernicke and Broca language cortices in humans. The EmC, together with the middle longitudinal fasciculus (MdLF), is implicated in ventral stream processing of language, concerned with the semantic aspects of communication, namely, the meanings of words.[478] An inferior FOF identified in humans but not monkeys[15,411] may be homologous to the EmC, extending further caudally into the occipital lobe.

MIDDLE LONGITUDINAL FASCICULUS

The MdLF is situated within the white matter of the caudal IPL and extends into the white matter of the superior temporal gyrus (Fig. 1-36C). It links high-level association and paralimbic cortical areas, including the IPL, caudal cingulate gyrus,

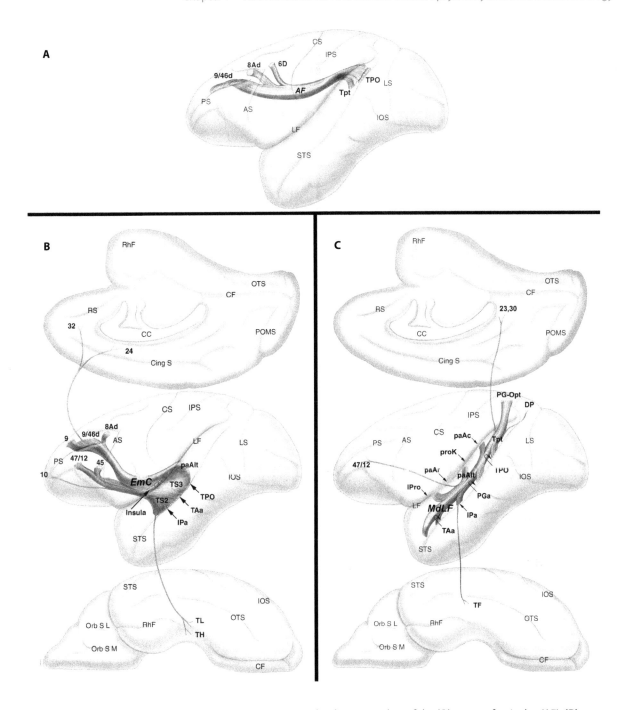

FIGURE 1-36. Summary diagrams of the course and composition in the rhesus monkey of the **(A)** arcuate fasciculus (AF); **(B)** extreme capsule (EmC); and **(C)** middle longitudinal fasciculus (MdLF). The lateral and medial views of the cerebral hemispheres show the trajectory of the three components of the SLF and the cortical areas that contribute axons to these fiber pathways. (Adapted from Schmahmann and Pandya.[15])

parahippocampal gyrus, and prefrontal cortex. In humans the MdLF may play a role in language, possibly imbuing linguistic processing with information dealing with spatial organization, memory, and motivational valence.

FRONTO-OCCIPITAL FASCICULUS

The FOF travels above the body and head of the caudate nucleus and the subcallosal fasciculus of Muratoff (MB), lateral

to the CC, and medial to the corona radiata (Fig. 1-37A). It links the parieto-occipital region with dorsal premotor and prefrontal cortices. The FOF is the long association system of the dorsomedial part of the dorsal visual stream, and it appears to be an important component of the anatomical substrates involved in peripheral vision and the processing of visual spatial information. The FOF is distinct from the inferior FOF described in humans but not in monkeys (see EmC above).

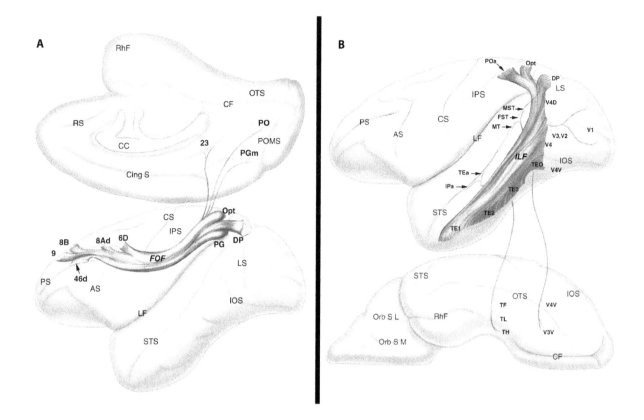

FIGURE 1-37. Summary diagrams of the course and composition in the rhesus monkey of the **(A)** fronto-occipital fasciculus (FOF); and **(B)** inferior longitudinal fasciculus (ILF). The lateral, medial, and basal views of the hemisphere show the trajectory of these fiber pathways and the cortical areas that contribute axons to them. (Adapted from Schmahmann and Pandya.[15])

INFERIOR LONGITUDINAL FASCICULUS

The ILF lies in the white matter between the sagittal stratum medially and the parieto-occipital and temporal cortices laterally (Fig. 1-37B). It has a vertical limb in the parietal and occipital lobes, and a horizontal component contained within the temporal lobe. The ILF is the long association system of the ventral visual pathways in the occipitotemporal cortices. Visual agnosia and prosopagnosia are two clinical syndromes that may arise from ILF damage.

NEIGHBORHOOD ASSOCIATION FIBER TRACTS

Fibers that arise from a cortical area directed to nearby cortical regions usually within the same lobe are termed neighborhood association fibers.[15] These are distinct from local U-fibers linking adjacent cerebral gyri, and from long association fiber tracts, described above, that link different lobes of the cerebral hemispheres.

A **frontal lobe** neighborhood fiber tract that links the dorsomedial prefrontal cortex with the inferior frontal gyrus in monkeys[15] has also been identified in human brain and named the *frontal aslant tract*.[411]

It has been suggested that the frontal aslant tract plays a role in the planning, timing, and coordination of sequential motor movements through the resolution of competition among potential motor plans, with hemisphere specialization such

that the left frontal aslant tract is engaged in speech initiation, stuttering, and verbal fluency,[479,480] and the right is specialized for general action control of the organism, especially in the visuospatial domain.[479]

Neighborhood connections in monkeys link the orbital part of area 47/12 with more rostral orbital cortex area 11 and the ventral parts of areas 10 and 46.[15] In humans this corresponds to an *orbitopolar tract* which connects the posterior orbital gyrus, including the olfactory cortex, with the anterior orbitofrontal gyrus and inferior frontal pole.[411]

The orbitopolar tract links orbital cortices implicated in motivation and reward with prefrontal cortices concerned with working memory and long-range planning. The orbitopolar tract is therefore likely to be engaged in awareness of potential consequences of one's actions, an insight which is impaired following lesions of the orbitofrontal cortex in both monkeys and humans.[336,465]

In the **parietal lobe** of monkeys neighborhood association fibers link the IPL to the medial parietal cortex. These connections are likely important for higher order spatial processing particularly when imbued with motivational valence.

In the **occipital lobe** of humans, Déjerine[421] identified five neighborhood association fiber tracts (Fig. 1-31D), which Schmahmann and Pandya[15] also observed in monkeys.

(i) The *vertical occipital fascicle of Wernicke*, also called the stratum proprium of the convexity of Sachs (Heinrich

Sachs, 1863–1928), connects the superior aspect of the occipital lobe to its inferior surface.

(ii) A superiorly situated *transverse fascicle of the cuneus of Sachs* in humans connects the cuneus to the convexity of the occipital lobe and to its inferior lateral aspect. In monkeys this is the dorsal occipital bundle which links the medial and lateral parts of the dorsal occipital lobe.

(iii) The ventrally situated *transverse occipital fascicle of Vialet* (Vialet was a student of Déjerine; described in humans by Sachs and further studied by Vialet) links the inferior lip of the calcarine fissure with the cortex of the occipital convexity and its inferior lateral aspect. In monkeys, the transverse fibers in the ILF that lie within the ventral parts of the occipital and temporal lobe and that link the lateral cortices with the medial cortices are equivalent to this transverse fascicle of the lingual lobule of Vialet.

(iv) The *stratum proprium of the cuneus of Sachs* is a layer of short associative fibers intrinsic to the cuneus, comprising vertical fibers that take their origin from within the superior lip of the calcarine fissure, radiating in the cortex of the superior aspect of the hemisphere. In monkeys the fibers within the SPL and dorsal occipital white matter caudal to the SLF I that link areas PGm and PO are likely equivalent to this intrinsic fascicle of the cuneus of Sachs.

(v) The *stratum calcarinum (fringed blade) of the cuneus of Brissaud* (Édouard Brissaud, 1852–1909) is a thick U-fiber layer of the calcarine fissure connecting the superior and inferior lips of the calcarine fissure. This U-fiber tract is identifiable also in the calcarine sulcus of the monkeys and is not a true neighborhood association system.

The functions of these intrinsic occipital lobe fiber systems, and the clinical manifestations of damage to any of these tracts individually or to the intrinsic occipital lobe fiber tracts collectively remain unclear. It is likely, however, that they are relevant in the evolving understanding of cerebral visual impairment in children with perinatal injury that often includes or may be concentrated in cerebral white matter fiber systems.[481] This includes decreased visual acuity, impaired oculomotor control, variable visual attention and inattention (particularly in unfamiliar or complex environments), supplementing vision with touch, looking away while reaching for objects, close viewing in the absence of refractive errors, objects that are moving are attended better than when static, attraction to colored objects, light gazing, photophobia, and difficulties in higher order visuospatial processing (object recognition, face recognition, visual memory, orientation, visual spatial perception, motion perception, and simultaneous perception[482]). These all can lead to functional limitations that impact a child's learning, mobility, and development.[481,483]

STRIATAL FIBERS

Corticostriatal fibers to the caudate nucleus, putamen, and claustrum are conveyed mainly by the subcallosal fasciculus of Muratoff and the external capsule (Fig. 1-38).

Muratoff Bundle (Subcallosal Fasciculus of Muratoff)

The MB is a semilunar condensed fiber system situated immediately above the head and body of the caudate nucleus. It conveys axons to the striatum principally from association and limbic areas, with some fibers also from the dorsal part of the motor cortex.

External Capsule

The external capsule (EC) lies between the putamen medially and the claustrum laterally. It conveys fibers from the ventral and medial prefrontal cortex, ventral premotor cortex, precentral gyrus, the rostral superior temporal region, and the inferotemporal and preoccipital regions. Projections from primary sensorimotor cortices are directed to the putamen; those from the SMA and association cortices terminate also in the caudate nucleus.

The MB and external capsule thus convey fibers from sensorimotor, cognitive, and limbic regions of the cerebral cortex to areas within the striatum in a topographically arranged manner. These corticostriatal pathways provide the critical links that enable different regions with the basal ganglia to contribute to motor control, cognition, and emotion.

A striatal bundle (StB) from the inferior temporal region is directed to the most ventral part of the putamen situated above the tail of the caudate nucleus. This sector of the putamen also receives fibers via the external capsule from the ventral prefrontal cortex.

CORD FIBER SYSTEM

In addition to association and corticostriatal systems, every cortical region in monkeys gives rise to a dense aggregation of fibers, termed the cord, which occupies the central core of the white matter of the gyrus. The fibers in the cord separate into two distinct segments: commissural fibers and projection fibers in the subcortical bundle.

Commissural Fibers

Corpus Callosum

The CC is divisible into five equal sectors conveying fibers across the hemispheres from the following locations: (1) the rostrum and genu contain fibers from the prefrontal cortex, rostral cingulate region, and SMA; (2) premotor cortex; (3) ventral premotor region and the motor cortex (face representation most rostral, followed by the hand and the leg, and postcentral gyrus fibers behind the motor fibers); (4) posterior parietal cortex; and (5) the splenium contains superior temporal fibers rostrally, and inferotemporal and preoccipital fibers caudally. These comments regarding CC topography apply to the midsagittal plane. The topographic arrangement of fibers in the CC in humans, determined using diffusion tractography,[484,485] reflects observations in the monkeys defined with tract tracing techniques (Fig. 1-39).[15,486]

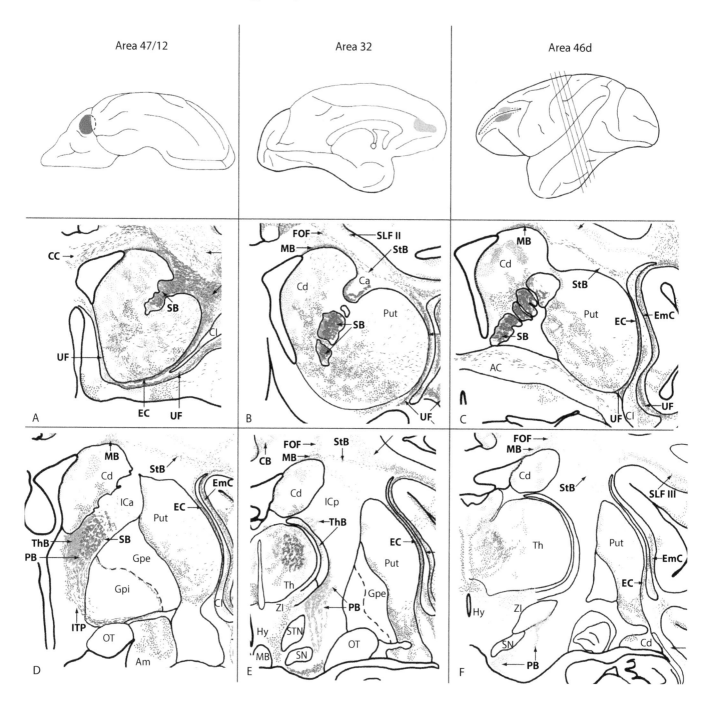

FIGURE 1-38. Diagrams illustrating the principle of topographic arrangement of cerebral cortical projections to the caudate nucleus (Cd) and putamen (Put) from prefrontal cortex in the rhesus monkey. Injections of anterogradely transported isotope tracer were placed in the prefrontal cortex. From left to right—orbital prefrontal cortex area 47/12 encroaching posteriorly on the insular proisocortex; medial prefrontal convexity area 32; and area 46d above the midportion of the principal sulcus. Coronal images through the striatum are shown in the columns below, from rostral above to caudal at the bottom. Black dots represent terminations in the striatum. The amygdala (Am), anterior commissure (AC), claustrum (Cl), hypothalamus (Hy), and thalamus (Th) are shown for orientation. (Adapted from Schmahmann and Pandya.[15])

Studies of the CC have led to novel understanding of the anatomic underpinnings of perception, attention, memory, language, and reasoning and have provided insights into consciousness, self-awareness, and creativity.[487–490] Knowledge of the CC topography is relevant in the clinical context of callosal section for control of seizures.

Anterior Commissure

The AC traverses the midline in front of the anterior columns of the fornix, above the basal forebrain, and beneath the medial and ventral aspect of the anterior limb of the internal capsule. Its fibers link the caudal part of the orbital frontal cortex, the temporal pole, the rostral superior temporal region, the major

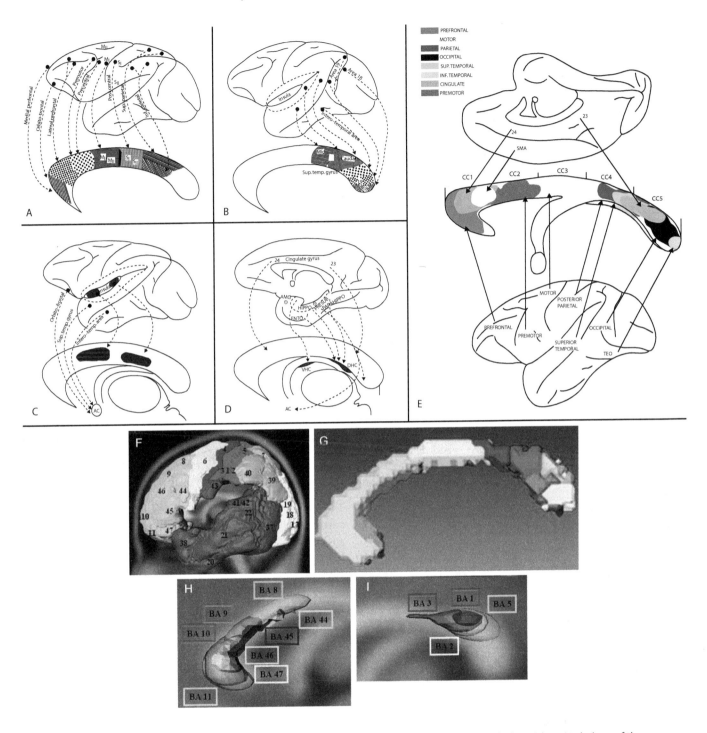

FIGURE 1-39. Schematic diagrams of the cortical origins of interhemispheric fibers passing through the mid-sagittal plane of the corpus callosum, anterior commissure, and hippocampal commissures. **(A)** Frontal and parietal areas. **(B)** Superior and inferior temporal gyri and parastriate areas. **(C)** Insula, anterior temporal, and orbitofrontal cortices. **(D)** Paralimbic cortices in cingulate gyrus, amygdala, and medial temporal lobe of rhesus monkey. (From Pandya and Rosene.[486]) **(E)** Composite summary diagram of the topography in the mid-sagittal plane of the corpus callosum of axons derived from the major lobar regions of the cerebral hemisphere of the rhesus monkey. The lateral view of the cerebral hemisphere (shown below) and the medial view (above) are shown to depict the region of origin of the fibers traversing the corpus callosum, color coded according to the legend top left. The designations CC1 through CC5 refer to the five rostral to caudal sectors of the corpus callosum. (Figure and legend from Schmahmann and Pandya.[15]) Results of probabilistic diffusion MRI tractography in human brain: Segmentation of the midsagittal human corpus callosum in one representative individual **(G)** showing topographic arrangement of fibers from **(F)** the frontal cortex (green), premotor and supplementary motor areas (light blue), primary motor cortex (dark blue), primary sensory cortex (red), parietal lobe (orange), occipital lobe (yellow), and temporal lobe (violet). Sagittal views of 3D reconstruction of major callosal distributions of fibers connected to the selected areas in **(H)**, the human prefrontal cortex, Brodmann areas 8, 9, 10, and 11, and areas 44, 45, 46, and 47; and **(I)**, the parietal lobe areas 3, 1, 2 and area 5. (Figures F through I and edited legend are from Chao et al.[485])

part of the inferotemporal area, and the parahippocampal gyrus with their counterparts in the opposite hemisphere. In the non-human primates the AC is concerned with functional coordination across the hemispheres of highly processed information in the auditory and visual domains, particularly when imbued with mnemonic and limbic valence.[491–493]

Hippocampal Commissures

Three fiber systems link the ventral limbic and paralimbic regions across the hemispheres.

Anterior (uncal and genual) hippocampal fibers are conveyed in the *ventral hippocampal commissure.*

Fibers from the presubiculum, entorhinal cortex, and posterior parahippocampal gyrus are conveyed in the *dorsal hippocampal commissure.*

The *hippocampal decussation* conveys fibers from the body of the hippocampal formation to the contralateral septum.[494]

Damage to the hippocampal commissures in patients with lesions of the splenium of the CC may be responsible in part for the amnesia that occurs in this setting along with damage to the fornix that links the frontal and temporal lobes.[361,495]

Projection Fibers

Projection (cortico-subcortical) fibers in the subcortical bundle are conveyed to their destinations via the anterior and posterior limbs of the internal capsule, and in the SS. Each fiber system differentiates further as it progresses in the white matter into two principal systems: one destined for thalamus, and the other destined for brainstem and/or spinal cord.

Internal Capsule

The anterior limb of the internal capsule (ICa) is a bidirectional tract conveying fibers from the prefrontal cortex, rostral cingulate region, and SMA (coursing through the genu of the capsule), principally to the thalamus, hypothalamus, and basis pontis. The ICa carries information between the anterior thalamic nuclei and the prefrontal cortex, as well as extensive connections between the different subdivisions of the medial dorsal thalamic nucleus and all sectors of the prefrontal cortex.

The ICa thus conveys both the anterior thalamic radiation that has been linked to negative feelings such as sadness. The recently identified superolateral branch of the MFB associated with motivation and reward that runs with the ICa has been targeted successfully with deep brain stimulation or focal lesion induction for treatment of depression and other psychiatric disorders.[98] Deep brain stimulation has been successfully applied to the ICa in some patients with obsessive-compulsive disorder[496] and intractable pain.[497]

The posterior limb of the internal capsule (ICp) is also bidirectional. It conveys descending fibers from the premotor and motor cortices: face, hand, arm, and leg fibers are arranged in a progressively caudal position.[15,498–500] In addition, the ICp

conveys descending fibers from the parietal, temporal, and occipital lobes and the caudal cingulate gyrus, and reciprocal thalamic projections to all these cortical areas, topographically arranged within the capsule in the rostral-caudal and superior-inferior dimensions.

Focal motor and sensory deficits follow infarction of the ICp,[501] and complex behavioral syndromes result from lesions of the genu of the ICa and genu.[502–504] Deficits include fluctuating alertness, inattention, memory loss, apathy, abulia, and psychomotor retardation, with neglect of contralateral space and visual-spatial impairment from lesions of the genu in the right hemisphere, and severe verbal memory loss following genu lesions on the left.

Sagittal Stratum

The SS is a major cortico-subcortical white matter bundle that conveys fibers from the parietal, occipital, cingulate, and temporal regions to thalamus, basis pontis, and other brainstem structures. It also conveys afferents principally from thalamus to cortex. The SS comprises an internal segment conveying corticofugal fibers efferent from the cortex and an external segment that contains corticopetal fibers to the cortex. The rostral sector of the SS corresponds to the anteriorly reflected fibers of the Flechsig-Meyer loop, while the ventral parts of the midsection of the SS contain the optic radiations and thalamic fibers of the caudal inferior temporal and occipitotemporal areas.

The SS is the equivalent of the internal capsule of the posterior part of the hemispheres. The functional implications are also analogous to those of the ICa and ICp. Whereas damage to the optic radiations in the ventral sector of the SS can lead to hemianopsia, damage to the dorsal part of the SS may result in distortion of high-level visual information.

Thalamic Peduncles

Cortico-subcortical fibers enter the thalamus in locations determined by their site of origin. The afferent and efferent fibers between thalamus and cerebral cortex are arrayed around the thalamus, and they are collectively termed thalamic peduncles.

The mammillothalamic tract that links the mammillary bodies with the anterior thalamic nuclei is particularly pertinent to the memory system; when damaged by lesions of thalamus, it can produce a profound amnestic syndrome.

Clinical Features of White Matter Lesions

Lesions of white matter fiber pathways themselves produce clinical consequences. Neuropsychiatric disturbances or dementia occur in the setting of disseminated white matter damage from a large number of diseases, including small vessel cerebrovascular disease and multiple sclerosis.[505,506] Some neurodegenerative diseases, particularly tauopathy forms of frontotemporal lobar degeneration, are associated with primary neurodegenerative pathology within the frontotemporal white matter subjacent to frontotemporal cortex. Poststroke language recovery depends on involvement of the subcallosal fasciculus of Muratoff,[507] parietal pseudothalamic pain results from white matter lesions that disconnect second somatosensory (SII) cortex from thalamus,[508] and deficits in executive dysfunction and episodic memory are associated with white matter hyperintensities in aging.[509] Focal white matter lesions result in aphasia, apraxia, and agnosia,[4,5,505] hemispatial neglect occurs with lesions in the anterior limb and genu of the internal capsule,[15,503,504] frontal behavioral disturbances are noted in Marchiafava-Bignami disease of the CC,[510] fornix lesions impair memory,[511,512] and alexia without agraphia is seen with dual lesions in the splenium of the CC and the left occipital pole[513] as well as from a single subcortical lesion undercutting Wernicke's area.[15]

The clinical deficits from loss of the white matter tracts linking different nodes may differ from those following lesions of the cortex or subcortical nodes for many reasons. White matter lesions may disrupt information destined for more than one node; they may involve association, projection, and striatal fibers; and they may affect more than one functional domain. Involvement of afferent versus efferent fibers may have clinical significance—striatal fibers are unidirectional from cortex to caudate-putamen; the middle cerebellar peduncle (MCP) is essentially exclusively afferent from pons to cerebellum, whereas the superior cerebellar peduncle is predominantly efferent from cerebellum to the cerebral hemispheres; and the thalamic peduncles are bidirectional. Fiber tract disruptions are often incomplete by virtue of the anatomical arrangement of the pathways and the pathologic conditions that affect white matter, and the effects of partial versus complete disconnection are likely to be pertinent.

BASAL GANGLIA

The basal ganglia are the largest group of subcortical nuclei in the forebrain, consisting of the caudate nucleus, putamen, and globus pallidus (Fig. 1-40). Related nuclei are the subthalamic nucleus (STN) in the diencephalon, the SN in the midbrain, and the pedunculopontine nucleus in the pons.

The caudate nucleus and putamen are collectively termed the striatum, because of the striated appearance of the anterior limb of the internal capsule as it courses between the head of the caudate nucleus and the adjacent putamen. The ventral striatum includes the NAc (its lateral core region and medial shell region), the septum, and olfactory tubercle. The globus pallidus, named for its pale appearance on fresh-cut section of the brain, has an external segment—the globus pallidus externa (GPe), an internal segment—the globus pallidus interna (GPi), and a ventral pallidum—VP, which lies ventral and anterior to the AC. The STN in the diencephalon lies medial and ventral to the zona incerta (ZI). In the midbrain the SN has a dense section, the pars compacta—SNc with dopamine-containing neuromelanin neurons, and a more sparsely populated region, the pars reticulata—SNr. The pedunculopontine nucleus lies medially at the junction of the midbrain and pons and contains dopaminergic neurons.

Histology of the Striatum

There are two types of neurons in the striatum. Projection neurons are MSNs and account for approximately 90%, interneurons the remaining 10%. The MSNs are multipolar neurons with small to medium cellular somata (20 microns in diameter), and dendritic processes covered by postsynaptic spines. All striatal MSNs are inhibitory and use GABA as their neurotransmitter.

The cytoarchitecture of the striatum appears homogeneous throughout, but immunohistochemical staining with AChE reveals two subdivisions each with distinct chemoarchitecture and connections: a background matrix and embedded striosomes.[514,515]

Matrix stains intensely with AChE. It has weak expression of mu opioid receptors and is enriched with calcium-binding proteins parvalbumin and calbindin. *Striosomes* have weak AChE activity and high mu opioid receptor expression, as well as enkephalin, substance P, GABA, and neurotensin. Different types of striosomes can be identified based on their patterns of immunoreactivity. MSN dendrites remain confined to their compartment—dendrites from matrix MSNs do not enter the striosomes, and striosomal MSN dendrites do not enter the matrix.

The NAc lies at the most ventral and medial aspect of the striatum, surrounding the AC. Together with the olfactory tubercle,[516] it comprises the ventral striatum. The NAc extends dorsolaterally into the putamen and dorsomedially into the caudate nucleus but lacks any sharp demarcation between the two areas. The accumbens has the typical matrix-striosome organization: the matrix is innervated by sensorimotor and prefrontal cortices and projects to the SNr, whereas the striosomes receive projections from paralimbic cortices and SN and project to the SNc. Unlike the rest of the striatum, the NAc can be divided into a central core and a shell region which surrounds it medially, ventrally, and laterally. The AC courses through the core region. The core and the shell have different cellular composition, histochemical, electrophysiological and connectional properties, and functions, as discussed below.

Basal Ganglia Circuitry: Cortical-Basal Ganglionic Loops

The nuclei of the basal ganglia participate in cortical-subcortical loops of information processing by way of input, intrinsic, and output nuclei.

Input Nuclei

Afferents to the basal ganglia from the cerebral cortex, thalamus, and SN target the striatum, namely, the caudate nucleus, putamen, and NAc. Tract tracing reveals multiple parallel loops, or circuits, in the corticostriatal system, each of which comprises a parent cerebral cortical area (motor, association, or limbic cortex) that projects topographically to nuclei of the basal ganglia, and then via thalamus back to the cortical region of origin (Fig. 1-41).[14,517-519] The concept that the basal ganglia are

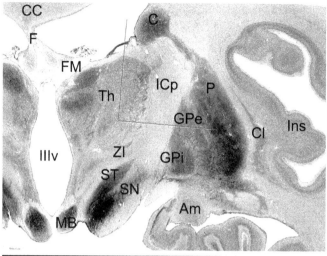

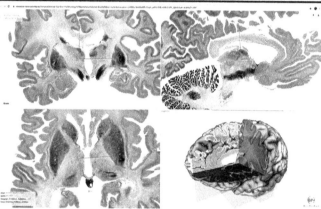

FIGURE 1-40. Images derived from the BigBrain high-resolution human brain model of the Human Brain Project (Amunts et al.[32]). Above, a close view of deep structures of the cerebral hemisphere in the coronal plane at the level of the basal ganglia and thalamus, and below, the three cardinal planes (coronal, sagittal, and axial), along with a three-dimensional view of the hemisphere with the planes of section identified. This high-resolution interactive atlas magnifies to show cytoarchitecture within these gross morphological structures. Am, amygdala; C, caudate nucleus body; CC, corpus callosum; Cl, claustrum; F, fornix; FM, foramen of Monroe; GPe, globus pallidus, external part; GPi, globus pallidus, internal part; ICp, posterior limb of the internal capsule; IIIv, third ventricle; Ins, insula; MB, mammillary body; P, putamen; SN, substantia nigra; ST, subthalamic nucleus; Th, thalamus; ZI, zona incerta.

linked by segregated loops to different cerebral cortical areas, each loop supporting distinct domains of behavior, is fundamental to understanding the differential effects of basal ganglia lesions.

Corticostriatal projections are glutamatergic and excitatory, and derived from almost all regions of the cerebral cortex. They terminate on the MSNs and are arranged with a high degree of topographic specificity. Cortical areas that project to adjacent areas within the striatum are themselves likely to share corticocortical connections. A given region of the caudate nucleus therefore receives input not only from a focal area of cortex, but

also from other cortical areas reciprocally interconnected with that cortical area.[520]

Motor, primary somatosensory, and parietal intramodality sensory association cortices project predominantly to the dorsal and midsectors of the putamen.

Association areas in the prefrontal, posterior parietal, and superior temporal polymodal cortices send their efferents preferentially to the caudate nucleus.

Orbital and medial prefrontal cortices and the cingulate gyrus target the ventral striatum (Fig. 1-38).

Rostral and inferior temporal and parahippocampal cortex output is directed to the ventral striatum as well as to the ventral part of the putamen.[15,521–523]

The corticostriate projections are conveyed by the subcallosal fasciculus of Muratoff and/or the external capsule, depending on their site of origin in the cortex. Motor areas project to the caudate via the MB, and the putamen via the external capsule. The MB conveys fibers predominantly from dorsal association areas to the head, body, and genu of the caudate nucleus. The external capsule, on the other hand, conveys fibers mostly from ventral association areas to the putamen and tail of the caudate nucleus. There is some interchange of fibers between these two striatal tracts, and the fibers from all areas reach the claustrum at least in part by way of the external capsule. The cortical afferents in the striatum are arranged in multiple discrete patches, each cortical area giving rise to a unique set of terminations. There appears to be interdigitation of projections from the different cortical areas, but some overlap is noted as well.[15]

Intrinsic Nuclei

The GPe, STN, and SNc and pedunculopontine nucleus participate in the internal circuity of the basal ganglia, functionally situated between the input and output nuclei.

Output Nuclei

Information flows from the basal ganglia by way of the internal segment of the globus pallidus (GPi), SNr, and VP. The GPi is organized into functionally specific divisions: the dorsal part is associative, the ventrolateral is sensorimotor, and the rostromedial region is limbic.[524]

Recurring spiral projections link the ventromedial part of SNc with the striatum (the striato-nigrostriatal system), leading to the suggestion that the ventral striatum (limbic) is able to influence dorsal (associative) striatal areas.[525]

Direct and Indirect Pathways

The output from the striatum is the anatomical-connectional basis of two complementary basal ganglia circuits which compete functionally: a direct pathway that releases movement/action, and an indirect pathway that inhibits movement/action (Fig. 1-42).[526]

The *direct, striatopallidal pathway* is a monosynaptic GABAergic projection from the striatum to the GPi or the SNr (striatum-GPi-thalamus-cortex). Its MSNs have high levels of substance P and dynorphin and contain dopamine receptor subtype 1 (D1R) which activates intracellular adenylcyclase signaling (D1-containing neurons).

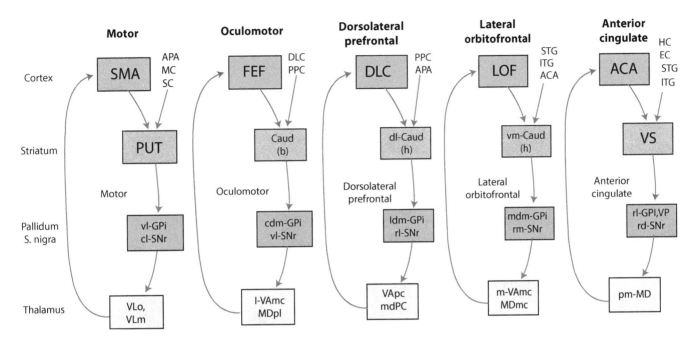

FIGURE 1-41. Parallel organization of the five basal ganglia-thalamocortical circuits according to Alexander, DeLong, and Strick.[517] Each circuit engages specific regions of the cerebral cortex, striatum, pallidum, substantia nigra, and thalamus. ACA, anterior cingulate area; APA, arcuate premotor area; CAUD, caudate, (b) body (h) head; DLC, dorsolateral prefrontal cortex; EC, entorhinal cortex; FEF, frontal eye fields; GPi, internal segment of globus pallidus; HC, hippocampal cortex; ITG, inferior temporal gyrus; LOF, lateral orbitofrontal cortex; MC, motor cortex; MDpl, medial dorsal thalamic nucleus pars paralamellaris; MDmc, medial dorsal thalamic nucleus pars magnocellularis; MDpc, medial dorsal thalamic nucleus pars parvocellularis; PPC, posterior parietal cortex; PUT, putamen; SC, somatosensory cortex; SMA, supplementary motor area; SNr, substantia nigra pars reticulata; STG, superior temporal gyrus; VAmc, ventral anterior thalamic nucleus pars magnocellularis; VApc: ventral anterior thalamic nucleus pars parvocellularis; VLm, ventral lateral thalamic nucleus pars medialis; VLo, ventral lateral thalamic nucleus pars oralis; VP, ventral pallidum; VS, ventral striatum; c1-, caudolateral; cdm-, caudal dorsomedial; dl-, dorsolateral; l-, lateral; ldm-, lateral dorsomedial; m-, medial; mdm-, medial dorsomedial; pm, posteromedial; rd-, rostrodorsal; rl-, rostrolateral; rm-, rostromedial; vm-, ventromedial; vl-, ventrolateral. (Figure originated in Alexander et al.,[517] modified by Mink,[861] Fig. 31.5, and further modified here.)

The *indirect pathway* involves GABAergic projections from the striatum to GPe and from GPe to the STN, and excitatory glutamatergic projections from the STN to GPi and SNr (striatum-GPe-STN-GPi/SNr-thalamus-cortex). The striatal MSNs in the indirect pathway contain enkephalin, and dopamine receptor subtype 2 (D2R) which inhibits intracellular adenylcyclase through G-protein signaling (D2-containing neurons).

Dopamine therefore has different effects on the direct and indirect pathways, but because the MSNs in both these circuits utilize GABA to inhibit their targets, the net effect of activation of the direct and indirect pathways in the presence of normal amounts of dopamine is that cortical excitation of the striatum leads to less inhibition of thalamus and increased activity in the circuit.

As conceptualized by Ann Graybiel,[527] the competing pathways act like the accelerator and brake in a car. Release/disinhibition of the thalamus by the direct pathway (the accelerator) is opposed by the indirect pathway (the brake), which inhibits the thalamus via the additional, excitatory, subthalamic projection to the internal pallidum. Optogenetics studies in rats[528] show that selective stimulation of striatal MSNs expressing D1R leads to movement activation, whereas stimulation of MSNs expressing D2R provokes movement arrest, confirming the model of direct and indirect circuits in functional equilibrium.

Matrix and Striosome Connectional Specificity

Matrix

Inputs from the sensory, motor, and association areas of the cerebral cortex, together with thalamostriatal projections and dopaminergic neurons from the SNc, mainly innervate the acetylcholine-rich MSNs in the matrix region. The matrix MSNs participate either in the direct striatopallidal pathway through the GPi/SNr, or the indirect pathway through the GPe.

Striosomes

Posterior orbitofrontal/anterior insular cortex, mediofrontal prelimbic/anterior cingulate, temporal limbic cortices, the basolateral amygdala, and ventral parts of the SNc target MSNs in the striosomes that are low in acetylcholine.[332] These striosomal MSNs preferentially project to the SNc, with axon collaterals targeting the GPi/SNr, and the GPe (Fig. 1-43) (for reviews, see Ragsdaler and Graybiel,[514] Lanciego et al.,[515] and Graybiel[529]).

Thalamic Connections of the Basal Ganglia

Efferents from the basal ganglia via the GPi and SNr target different nuclei of thalamus according to the parent cerebral cortical area of origin of the corticobasal-ganglionic loop. Motor circuit output from the GPi and SNr reaches the anterior portion of the

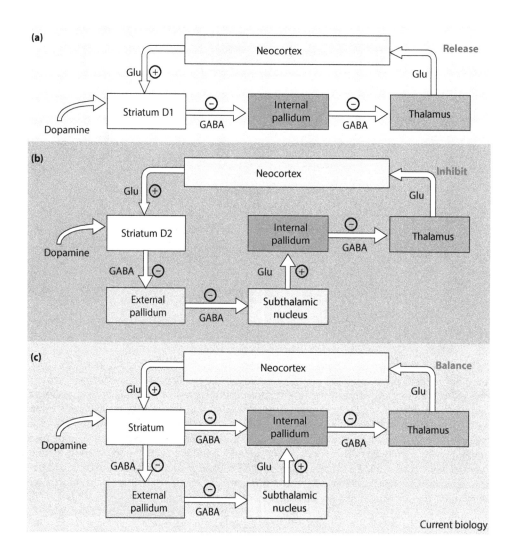

FIGURE 1-42. The brake-accelerator model for basal ganglia motor disorders. **(A)** The direct pathway (leading to release of movement) consists of two successive GABAergic connections, from the striatum to the internal pallidum and from the internal pallidum to the thalamus. This flow diagram suggests that excitatory (glutamate; Glu) inputs from the neocortex to the striatum would disinhibit thalamic neurons. Dopamine modulates the system mainly in the striatum, where it activates D1-class and D2-class dopamine receptors. **(B)** In the indirect pathway (leading to inhibition of movement), there is an extra step after the external pallidum, so that the subthalamic nucleus excites the internal pallidum. **(C)** Balance is achieved when these antagonistic systems are combined under normal circumstances. (Figure and legend from Graybiel,[52] based on the model of Penney and Young.[526])

ventrolateral thalamic nucleus (VLa), which then projects back to motor areas of the frontal cortex completing the cortical-basal ganglia-thalamocortical circuit. In contrast, associative circuit output from the SNr and GPi reaches the thalamic ventral anterior (VA) nucleus, which sends efferents to the dorsolateral prefrontal cortex and the lateral orbitofrontal cortices.[530] Collaterals of the GPi/SNr projection to the ventral thalamus reach the intralaminar thalamic centromedian and parafascicular nuclei (CM/Pf), as well as brainstem targets such as the pedunculopontine nucleus, and the reticular formation.[531] These thalamic intralaminar nuclei have strong reciprocal projections back to the striatum which are arranged in a topographically precise manner[531,532] allowing the CM/Pf to influence widespread striatal regions involved in processing functionally segregated information: The rostral Pf is mainly related to the limbic striatum,

the dorsolateral Pf is preferentially connected with associative striatal territories, and the medial part of the CM is the main source of inputs to sensorimotor striatal regions. In addition, thalamostriatal projections also arise from midline and specific thalamic nuclei.[531]

The Ventral Striatum and Ventral Striatopallidal System

Corticostriato-pallidal projections are as characteristic for limbic cortex as they are for neocortex.[132] Ventral parts of the basal ganglia, that is, the ventral striatum (NAc and olfactory tubercle) and VP (ventral part of the globus pallidus) (Fig. 1-12) are reciprocally interconnected with the allocortex, namely, the hippocampus and olfactory/prepyriform cortex. This finding

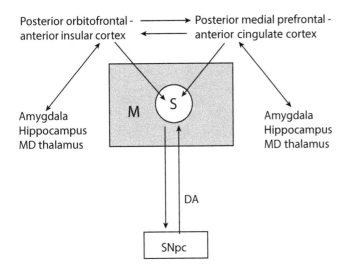

FIGURE 1-43. Diagram summarizing the main prefrontal subsystems targeting the striosomes in the monkey caudate nucleus which have reciprocal connections with structures in the limbic system. Striosomes target the SNc. Diagrams summarize main prefrontal inputs to the anterior striosomal compartment. DA, dopamine; M, matrix compartment of striatum; MD, medial dorsal thalamic nucleus; S, striosomal compartment of striatum; SNpc, pars compacta of substantia nigra. (Figure and modified legend from Eblen and Graybiel.[332])

that both the neocortex and allocortex are related to the basal ganglia is consistent with the general principles of organization of cerebral cortical connections.[15,16]

Neurons that respond to different types of reward such as anticipation and value are found throughout the brain. They constitute a network which includes the orbitofrontal cortex and anterior cingulate cortex, as well as the ventral striatum, VP, and midbrain dopamine neurons as crucial components of the reward circuit.

The basal ganglia work in concert with cerebral cortex to execute motivated, well-planned behaviors, and the reward circuit is a key driver of the development and monitoring of these behaviors.[533] As conceptualized by Suzanne Haber,[533] goal-directed behaviors rely on the combined interplay of sensory inputs, emotional information, and memories of prior outcomes. The anatomy of the reward system is uniquely adapted to this task which relies on sensory inputs, that is, conditioned stimuli eliciting goal-directed responses, gaining access to the basal ganglia. The ventral striatum receives its primary inputs from the cingulate cortex, from the insula and orbital prefrontal cortex which receive sensory information from all modalities, from the amygdala which is tightly linked to sensory processing, the superior colliculus which has direct basal ganglia connections via inputs to the SN, and from the olfactory bulb providing direct olfactory input to the olfactory tubercle. Many of the brain's reward systems converge on the NAc, which is richly innervated by excitatory, inhibitory, and modulatory afferents representing the circuitry necessary for selecting adaptive motivated behaviors. The ventral subiculum of the hippocampus

provides contextual and spatial information, the basolateral amygdala conveys affective influence, and the prefrontal cortex provides an integrative impact on goal-directed behavior.

Integration occurs at the cellular level, with individual NAc MSNs receiving convergent glutamatergic projections from ventral hippocampus, medial prefrontal cortex, and basolateral amygdala, in addition to other regions such as the thalamus. The balance of these afferents is under the modulatory influence of dopamine neurons in the VTA.[534,535]

In monkeys, the efferent projections from the ventral striatum are directed to the VP (the subcommissural part of the globus pallidus), rostral pole of the GPe, and rostromedial portion of GPi. This ventral striatal output is segregated from the dorsal striatal efferent projections to the pallidum. Fibers from the ventral striatum project widely throughout the SN, indicating that they may contribute to the integration of limbic and other output systems of the striatum. The ventral striatum projects to the pedunculopontine nucleus, and to non-extrapyramidal regions including the BNST, nucleus basalis, lateral hypothalamus, and medial thalamus.[536]

The core and shell regions of the NAc have different connections and functions. An anatomical gradient moves from the more sensorimotor-/cognitive-related core to the limbic shell. The shell receives converging limbic inputs from the basolateral amygdala and from the ventral subiculum, the major output region of the hippocampus: it is implicated in the control of reward- or drug-seeking behavior by spatial/contextual information. The core receives inputs from the basolateral amygdala and parahippocampal regions and is engaged in control over these behaviors by discrete cues.[537] In rats, projections from the core are to the dorsolateral compartment of the entopeduncular nucleus (equivalent to the GPi in primates) which is more engaged with sensorimotor and cognitive processing. The shell projects to ventromedial part of the VP concerned with limbic valance. The core projects to the dorsolateral part of the VP; the shell to the medial part of the subcommissural VP. Mesencephalic projections of the NAc from the core are directed to the motor-related SN, those from the shell to the limbically relevant VTA. And whereas the hypothalamic projections of the NAc core are directed primarily to the entopeduncular nucleus (~GPi) including a part that invades the lateral hypothalamus, the shell projects diffusely throughout the rostrocaudal extent of the lateral hypothalamus as well as to the extended amygdala, especially its sublenticular part.[538,539]

By virtue of its inputs from limbic forebrain structures, either directly or indirectly via the VTA, and its efferents to the motor system via the globus pallidus, the NAc serves as a limbic–motor interface where learned associations of motivational significance are converted into goal-directed behavior.[537,540]

Zona Incerta

Other nuclei and circuits of the basal ganglia are critical nodes and hubs for motivation, reward, emotional processing, mating behavior, and internal homeostasis in addition to their roles in motor control. These include the ZI, STN, SN, and pedunculopontine nucleus, in addition to the VTA discussed earlier.

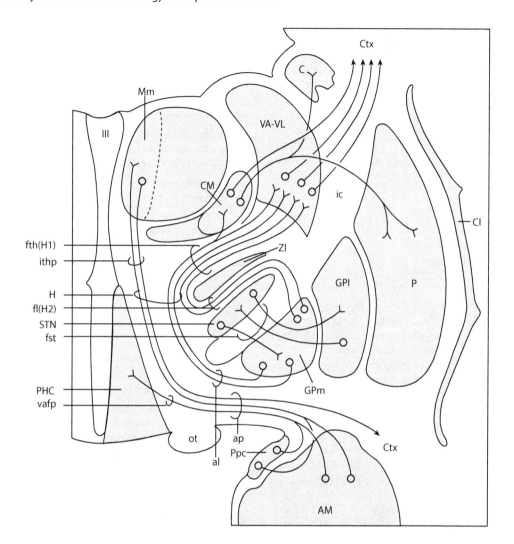

FIGURE 1-44. Some fiber bundles interconnecting telencephalic and diencephalic structures, semi-diagrammatically represented in the coronal plane. AM, amygdaloid complex; al, ansa lenticularis; ap, ansa peduncularis; C, caudate nucleus; Cl, claustrum; CM, centromedian thalamic nucleus; Ctx, cerebral cortex; Ppc fl, fasciculus lenticularis; fst, fasciculus subthalamicus; fth, fasciculus thalamicus; GPl, globus pallidus, lateral (external) segment; GPm, globus pallidus, medial (internal) segment; H, H1, H2, tegmental fields of Forel; ic, internal capsule; ithp, inferior thalamic peduncle; Mm, magnocellular part of mediodorsal thalamic nucleus; ot, optic tract; P, putamen; PHC, preopticohypothalamic continuum; Ppc, prepyriform cortex; STN, subthalamic nucleus; VA, ventral anterior thalamic nucleus; VL, ventral lateral thalamic nucleus; vafp, ventral amygdalofugal projection; ZI, zona incerta; III, third ventricle. (Figure and legend adapted from Niewenhuys et al.,[86] Fig. 9.1)

The ZI lies medially adjacent to the thalamic reticular nucleus, situated ventral to the thalamus and above the STN (Figs. 1-38 and 1-40). It is composed of loosely arranged cell groups and has been regarded as a rostral continuation of the brainstem reticular formation. The ZI is surrounded by the efferents from the globus pallidus which pass through the H fields of Forel on their way to the thalamus, namely the fasciculus lenticularis ventrally and medially, the ansa lenticularis medially, and the thalamic fasciculus dorsally comprising the fibers of both the ansa and fasciculus lenticularis and including inputs from the cerebellum via the brachium conjunctivum and from the spinal cord via the medial lemniscus (Fig. 1-44).[86,541]

The widespread connections of the ZI imbue this region with roles in visceral regulatory functions such as eating, drinking, and sexual behavior; motor control including posture, locomotion, and eye movements; nociception, arousal, and attention; and high-level processing in the visual, somatosensory, and limbic domains.

Its inputs are derived from prefrontal and cingulate cortices in addition to the somatosensory regions, amygdala, basal forebrain, basal ganglia, brainstem, and cerebellum; and its efferents are directed to the intra-laminar and associative thalamic nuclei, hypothalamus, brainstem, cerebellum via the inferior olivary nuclear complex, and spinal cord.

Studies in rats identify four different sectors within the ZI each of which has relatively distinct cytoarchitectonic characteristics, immunohistochemical staining, and connections. The rostral sector contains tyrosine hydroxylase cells, the dorsal sector nitric oxide synthase, the ventral sector parvalbumin cells, and the caudal sector stains for calbindin D 28k along with the remainder of the ZI.[542] There is evidence within the ZI of somatotopic organization[543] and its connectional details reveal that there are auditory[544] and visual subsectors.[545] It therefore appears that each subsector of the nucleus contributes differentially to the range of behaviors with which the ZI has been linked. Emerging data have reintroduced the suggestion[546] that targeting the motor regions of the ZI with deep brain stimulation can be useful in the treatment of Parkinson's disease producing improvements in rigidity, bradykinesia, tremor, and axial features.[547-549]

Subthalamic Nucleus

The STN lies in the caudal part of the diencephalon, below the ZI, and above the posterior limb of the internal capsule where it transitions into the cerebral peduncle (Figs. 1-38E, 1-40, and 1-44). It is an intrinsic node in the basal ganglia circuitry, receiving inhibitory GABAergic input from the external part of the globus pallidus (GPe) and the pedunculopontine nucleus in the tegmentum of the midbrain. It also receives excitatory glutamatergic projections from the CM/Pf of the thalamus, and from the cerebral cortex. Cerebral cortical projections to the STN, regarded as part of a hyperdirect pathway (as opposed to the direct and indirect pathways of the basal ganglia circuitry), are derived from the primary motor cortex, SMA, premotor cortices, frontal eye field area, and supplementary eye field of the frontal lobe. The STN projects to the globus pallidus and the SNr: its topographically organized projections to both pallidal segments in monkeys and cats are "truly massive,"[550] and its projections to the SNr are prominent but not as intense as those to the pallidum. The STN also projects to the VA and ventral lateral (VL) motor-related nuclei of the thalamus, and to the pedunculopontine nucleus of the mesencephalic tegmentum.[86,550]

The STN has been shown to be topographically arranged into three main regions in both monkeys[551,552] and humans[553]: a large dorsolateral motor region, a ventromedial associative area, and a limbic region at the medial tip.[554] These different territories receive functionally organized projections from the cerebral cortex and GPe, and the projections to the GPi and thalamus in turn arise from different subpopulations of STN neurons (Fig. 1-45).[515,555]

The *motor territory* in the dorsolateral region of the STN receives somatotopically organized inputs from the primary motor cortex, and projects to both the GPe and the GPi. In Parkinson's disease oscillatory activity in the beta (12–30 Hz) band is associated with akinetic-rigid Parkinson's disease (PD) symptoms and is observed exclusively in this dorsolateral motor region.[556]

The STN forms part of the indirect basal ganglia circuitry whereby the striatum, via GABAergic inputs to the GPe, disinhibits the STN which then, by way of its glutamatergic excitatory neurons increases activity of the two output structures of the basal ganglia, the GPi and the SNr. This pathway inhibits motor programs (Graybiel's brake system) that may interfere with the execution of a selected motor program activated via the direct striatal projection to the GPi/SNr. Most of the inputs to the STN from the GPe and from the motor cortex target STN neurons that provide powerful excitatory projections back to the GPe, underscoring

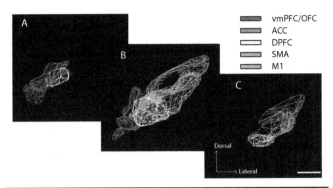

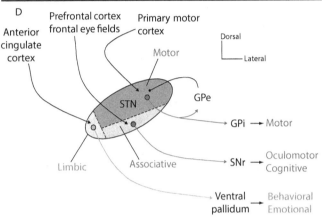

FIGURE 1-45. Cortical projections to the subthalamic nucleus of monkeys shown in coronal plane in A–C. **(A)** anterior, **(B)** central, and **(C)** posterior thirds of a 3D model. Colored meshes represent the outer surface of the combined dense projections from each cortical area. Overlaps occur mainly between projections from functionally close cortical regions. Scale bar, 1 mm. (Figure and edited legend from Haynes and Haber.[552]) **(D)** Functional territories of the STN: large dorsolateral motor territory, ventromedial associative territory, and medial limbic territory. Each territory receives inputs from different areas of the cerebral cortex and provides output to different target nuclei, including the internal segment (GPi) and external segment (GPe) of the globus pallidus, substantia nigra pars reticulata (SNr), and ventral pallidum. These input-output interactions provide for parallel control of motor, oculomotor, cognitive, and emotional functions independently of "indirect" pathways via the striatum and GPe. (Figure and legend from Benarroch.[554])

the importance of the reciprocal STN-GPe connection in normal motor control and in pathologic basal ganglia activity.

The *associative territory* situated ventromedially in the STN receives inputs from the dorsolateral prefrontal cortex and frontal eye fields. Its neurons project to the SNr which is involved in oculomotor control and cognitive aspects of motor behavior.

The *limbic territory at the medial tip of the STN* receives inputs from the medial prefrontal and anterior cingulate cortices. Its neurons project to the GPi and the VP which control motivational and emotional aspects of motor behavior.

At the boundaries between these functional territories there appears to be integration of information between the different modalities. The STN thus acts as a second, independent input area through which the cerebral cortex controls motor function and behavior. The excitatory influence of the STN on the basal ganglia output nuclei, GPI and SNr, which exert a tonic inhibitory influence on thalamic relay neurons and brainstem targets confers on the STN a pivotal role in controlling activity within each corticobasal ganglia-thalamocortical network (see Benarroch[554]).

Abnormal activity in the indirect pathway in the setting of dopamine deficiency in Parkinson's disease is the basis for the use of deep brain stimulation of the STN for treatment of the motor manifestations of PD. The existence of cognitive and limbic zones of the STN account for the behavioral and cognitive consequences of STN stimulation and provide rationale for the potential application of this procedure to other disorders, including epilepsy and psychiatric disorders.[554] The anatomical and physiological details of the STN drive these considerations. This is exemplified by the finding of hemispheric asymmetry in the oscillation properties of STN neurons in humans: emotive auditory stimulation evoked activity in the ventral non-oscillatory region of the right STN but not in the left ventral STN or in the dorsolateral motor region of either side, suggesting that DBS of the right ventral STN may be associated with either beneficial or adverse emotional effects observed in PD patients, and may relieve mental symptoms in other neurological and psychiatric diseases.[557]

Substantia Nigra

The two largest midbrain dopamine-containing nuclei essential for controlling key functions of the brain such as voluntary movement, reward processing, and working memory are the VTA, discussed earlier, and the neighboring SN.

The SN lies in the midbrain dorsal to the cerebral peduncle (Figs. 1-38 E,F and 1-40). It consists of the closely packed, densely melanin-pigmented, dopamine-containing neurons of the SNc, and the more ventrally situated pars reticulata (SNr) with its scattered, nonpigmented neurons. The neurons of the SNr utilize GABA as their inhibitory neurotransmitter, project to the thalamus, superior colliculus, and reticular formation, and as output nuclei of the basal ganglia are key elements in the circuitry and function of the basal ganglia as discussed above.

The nigrostriatal pathway is the conduit of the reciprocal connections that link the SNc with the caudate nucleus and putamen. A summarized by Grofová,[558] some neurons in the pars reticulata of the substantia nigra and paranigral cell groups in the ventral and ventrolateral tegmental areas also contribute to this projection. Nigrostriatal fibers ascend along the dorsomedial border of the SN to the prerubral area and lateral hypothalamus, enter the medial part of the internal capsule, and run in a dorsorostral direction to reach the head of the caudate nucleus and the rostral part of the putamen. Fibers destined for the posterior parts of putamen and caudate nucleus leave the main bundle in Forel's field, course laterally, dorsal to the STN, and penetrate through the posterior part of the internal capsule and through the globus pallidus. This projection is topographically organized in anteroposterior, mediolateral, and dorsoventral directions, matching the reciprocal striatonigral connection. There is a mediolateral organization of nigrostriatal fibers; the projection is overwhelmingly ipsilateral, but some contralateral projections have been reported.

The SNc neurons are the critical focus of neurodegeneration in Parkinson's disease. In Huntington's disease, the brunt of the neuropathology is in the striatum and whereas the SNr has decreased numbers of neurons,[559] differing observations have been offered concerning the degree to which the SNc is either spared[559] or demonstrates neuronal loss.[560]

Pedunculopontine Nucleus

The pedunculopontine tegmental nucleus (PPN) is the caudalmost cell mass clearly integrated in the circuitry of the basal ganglia, with an important role in controlling motor pattern generators including those involved in gait (Fig. 1-46).[561] It is a neurochemically and functionally heterogeneous structure that occupies a strategic position in the dorsal tegmentum of the midbrain and upper pons. The PPN has been regarded as synonymous with the cholinergic cell group Ch5, a rostral brainstem structure regarded as part of the ascending reticular activating system because of its ascending cholinergic projections to thalamus that modulate cortical activation.[562,563] Cholinergic neurons represent about 50% of the total cell population of the nucleus, the remainder containing GABAergic, dopaminergic, glutamatergic, and peptidergic neurons.[563] The basal ganglia and PPN have a similar pattern of inputs and outputs including cerebral cortex, thalamus, superior colliculus, amygdala, and motor areas of the brainstem and spinal cord. The PPN is reciprocally connected with other basal ganglia structures including the STN. Via these connections, the PPN is involved in locomotion and muscle tone, and in the mechanisms of cortical arousal, behavioral reinforcement, learning, and attention. It is a crucial element in the generation and maintenance of the rapid rhythms in the cortex associated with wakefulness and REM sleep.[563] The PPN is affected in PD and atypical parkinsonian syndromes such as progressive supranuclear palsy and multiple system atrophy, in which REM sleep behavior disorders often appear early in the disease predating the motor manifestations.[564] These clinical features may reflect neurodegeneration of the PPN in these disorders. Deep brain stimulation is now being applied to the PPN for relief of the motor phenomena in parkinsonian syndromes.[86,554,565,566]

Red Nucleus

The red nucleus (RN) is not part of the basal ganglia, but its proximity to the other basal ganglia nuclei discussed above (Fig. 1-46) warrants its consideration here. The RN is a large round cell group in the mesencephalon dorsomedial to the SN. It consists of a magnocellular division, RNm, and a parvocellular part, RNp. The RN evolved along with the development of limbs and limb-like structures,[567] and in rodents and cats it consists mainly of the RNm which projects to the contralateral spinal cord via the rubrospinal tract. In humans the RNm is very small and occupies only the caudal pole of the nucleus. The RNp is situated rostrally and projects to the ipsilateral inferior olivary nuclei in the medulla via the central tegmental tract. The neurons of the spinal projecting RNm and olivary projecting RNp are mutually exclusive, although both cell populations receive input from the cerebellar nuclei and from the cerebral cortex.

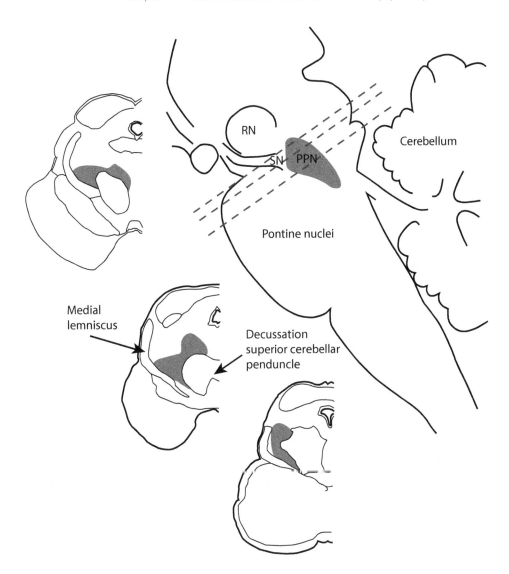

FIGURE 1-46. Three axial sections through the human brainstem showing the position of the pedunculopontine nucleus. The level of the three sections is indicated by the dashed lines in the para-sagittal cartoon of the brainstem and midbrain. RN, red nucleus; PPN, pedunculopontine nucleus; SN, substantia nigra. (Figure and legend from Jenkinson et al.[561])

The RN is integrally involved in motor control. The reticulospinal system is part of the lateral motor system[568,569] concerned with the control of appendicular or distal movements of the extremity such as reaching and grasping. This contrasts with the medial motor system involved in the control of the head, trunk, and limb girdle with its contributions from brainstem nuclei by way of the vestibulospinal, reticulospinal, interstitiospinal, and tectospinal tracts. The RN interconnects with the cerebellum by way of the central tegmental tract to the inferior olive (that provides climbing fibers to the cerebellum), and the RN inputs from the cerebellar deep nuclei, particularly the interpositus nuclei, are relevant in the RN role in motor control. These RN afferent and efferent connections with the cerebellum constitute the Guillain-Mollaret triangle (George Guillain, 1876–1961; Pierre Mollaret, 1898–1987; RNpc-inferior olive-cerebellum), lesions to any part of which lead to the clinical phenomenon of palatal tremor and which may be associated with cerebellar ataxia.[570]

Behavioral Correlates of Basal Ganglia Function and Disorders

The basal ganglia were long known to play a major role in the initiation and control of movement.[571] Anatomical studies that revealed new insights into the complexity of basal ganglia circuitry[572,573] were followed by investigations showing disruption of complex behaviors in the animal model and in patients with basal ganglia lesions. This included the syndrome of the dorsolateral frontal cortex following lesions of the anterodorsal head of the caudate nucleus in monkeys, the orbitofrontal syndrome following lesions of the ventrolateral caudate nucleus with impaired response inhibition, and symptoms resembling the syndrome of the inferotemporal cortex with impaired visual discrimination learning following lesions of the tail of the caudate nucleus[574]; and impairments in perception of personal and extrapersonal space were found to be impaired in patients with Parkinson's disease.[575] The basal ganglia are now recognized as essential substrates for movement as well as affect and cognitive processing, with the different cortical-basal ganglia-thalamic circuits enabling initiation or inhibition of action programs in these different domains. The modular corticostriatal loops interconnecting the cortex, striatum, and dopamine-containing cell groups in the midbrain are critical for reward-based learning and memory, particularly procedural or implicit learning that underlies automatized responses that characterize habits.[527]

The marked degree of topography within the pattern of corticostriate projections helped advance the realization that there are important functional divisions within the striatum, and that the striatum is a critical node in the distributed neural systems that participate not only in sensorimotor functions[571] but also in the domains of cognition and emotion.[517,519,576–579] Further, the specificity of the corticostriate projections indicates that different regions of the striatum have behavioral specializations that are similar to those of the cortical areas from which they receive their major cortical input.[63] An early indicator of differential contributions of striatum to cognitive operations was derived from maze-learning studies in rats, in which the nature of the learning impairments differed according to the location of the lesion in the caudate nucleus.[580] It is now apparent that the striatum is involved in the acquisition and retention of procedural knowledge, or habit learning, that is acquired incrementally and dependent upon stimulus-response associations, and this differentiates it from medial temporal lobe structures that support declarative knowledge.[461,581–585] The caudate nucleus is important for motor skill learning in humans,[586] and the tail of the caudate that is anatomically linked with the inferior temporal lobe is necessary for visual habit formation in monkeys.[587] The differential connectivity of the caudate nucleus is reflected also in different kinds of working memory, such that the head of the caudate, preferentially interconnected with the dorsolateral prefrontal cortex, participates in spatial working memory tasks in humans as determined by positron emission tomography, whereas the caudate body, more strongly interconnected with the temporal lobe, is activated in tasks of delayed object alternation.[588]

A fundamental functional dichotomy has been suggested by anatomical studies of striatal connections with the cerebral cortex as well as with subcortical structures. This distinction is between the dorsal striatum that is linked with the dorsolateral prefrontal and posterior parietal cortices, and the ventral striatum, or NAc, which is linked with limbic and paralimbic regions including the orbitofrontal cortex, hippocampal formation, and amygdala, and is more involved in emotionally relevant behaviors. The notion that the striatum is involved with repetitive behaviors or habits that take place without true conscious awareness assumes a significance when these habits are emotionally charged. This has been shown to be relevant in rats in which infusions of dopamine into the ventral striatum enhance conditioned reinforcement of formerly motivationally neutral stimuli,[589] and lesions of the accumbens impair response control related to affective feedback.[590] In monkeys, tonically active striatal neurons are involved in detecting motivationally relevant stimuli.[591] Studies of the role of the ventral striatum in reward, motivation, and addiction in humans have revealed new insights into the functions of the basal ganglia and the pathophysiology of major addictive behaviors.[592–594] The behaviors that characterize obsessive-compulsive disorder have also been shown to reflect dysfunction of the striatum, and particularly its ventral component,[595,596] and patients with this disorder can improve clinically following deep brain stimulation applied to the ventral striatum.[597] The role of dopamine in motor control regions of the basal ganglia is well understood from the study of Parkinson's disease and related disorders, and it appears that dopamine plays an important role also in these affective behaviors possibly through associative binding of reward to cue salience and response sequences.[579]

The precise nature of the striatal contribution to learning is a matter of ongoing study. It has been suggested that it is involved in attentional control used to guide the early stages of reinforcement-based learning and encoding strategies in explicit paradigms.[579] Miller[598] elucidated the problem that the span of immediate memory imposes severe limitations on the amount of information that we are able to receive, process, and remember, whereas by organizing the stimulus input simultaneously into several dimensions and successively into a sequence of chunks, we manage to break (or at least stretch) this informational bottleneck. Graybiel[527,599] built on this theory and proposed that the striatum is responsible for performing this chunking of motor or cognitive information into performance units, providing a mechanism for the acquisition and expression of action repertoires that would otherwise be biologically unwieldy or difficult to implement. Chunking of representations of motor and cognitive action sequences allows them to be implemented more efficiently as performance units. Learning and memory functions are thus seen as core features of the basal ganglia influence on motor and cognitive pattern generators.[599]

The associative functions of the striatum have direct clinical relevance. Observations in patients with extrapyramidal disorders such as Parkinson's disease, Tourette syndrome, Huntington's disease, and progressive supranuclear palsy in whom the burden of disease is in the basal ganglia, led to the notion of subcortical dementias,[595,600–604] and focal lesions from stroke further emphasized the role of the caudate nucleus in language, neglect, and attention.[605] Subcortical dementia as a clinical entity was first recognized in progressive supranuclear palsy and Huntington's disease,[600] characterized by slowness of mental processing, forgetfulness, apathy, and depression. This notion was later expanded when it became apparent that focal subcortical lesions play a role in arousal, attention, mood, motivation, language, memory, abstraction, and visuospatial skills.[606] Patients with Parkinson's disease experience apathy with diminished emotional responsiveness[607] and cognitive decline, including impairment of concentration (bradyphrenia[608]), loss of mental and behavioral flexibility with impaired strategic planning, sequential organization, constructional praxis, verbal fluency, working memory, attentional set shifting, initial encoding of information, procedural learning and spontaneous recall, and language functions that rely on procedural memory.[601,609–613] These deficits are thought to reflect damage to frontostriatal interactions, and interference with the role of basal ganglia in the cognitive processes that lead to habit formation[599,614] and goal-directed behaviors.[615] The consequence of basal ganglia lesions on the motor system include hypokinetic movement disorders such as Parkinson's disease, and hyperkinetic movement disorders such as Huntington's disease and hemiballism. This is consistent with the accelerator-brake model, which applies to neuropsychiatry in the same way that it applies to motor control.

Neurologic/neuropsychiatric phenomena reflect the modular organization of cortical-basal ganglionic circuits

1. *Putamen.* Lesions of the dorsal and midregions of the putamen that receive afferents from motor cortices lead to extrapyramidal motor syndromes and akinesia, and apathy and unconcern can follow damage to the dorsolateral striatum.[616] Hypophonic dysarthria is common in Parkinson's disease, reflecting involvement of the putamen.

2. *Caudate nucleus.* Deficits in executive function and spatial cognition follow lesions of the head of the caudate which is connected with the dorsolateral prefrontal cortex concerned with attention and executive functions, and the posterior parietal cortex attending to personal and extrapersonal space. Caudate head lesions can result in impaired working memory, strategy formation, and cognitive flexibility. Focal lesions are associated with impairments true to hemisphere—hemineglect and visual-spatial disorientation following right caudate lesions, aphasia after left caudate stroke.[605,617] The precisely arranged topography of the associative projections to the striatum likely accounts for the observation that different regions of striatum engage in different domains of cognition

3. *Ventral striatum.* Lesions of the ventral striatum produce disinhibited, irritable, and labile behaviors, and they are implicated in the neurobiology of addiction[618] and obsessive-compulsive disorder,[619] which can be conceptualized as the neuropsychiatric/neurocognitive manifestations of disordered habit formation and control. These disturbances of social and emotional function (behaviors with limbic valence) are congruent with the ventral striatal connections of the orbital and medial prefrontal cortices concerned with drive, motivation, emotional attributes of performance, inhibition of inappropriate responses, and reward-guided behaviors. Apathy most likely is a consequence of involvement of the limbic ventral striatopallidal system, but it can also occur following damage to dorsolateral striatum which has connections with the medial prefrontal and anterior cingulate regions.

4. *Globus pallidus.* Motor and behavioral consequences of pallidotomy are determined by lesion location. Posterior and ventrolateral regions (linked to motor cortical areas) have a beneficial impact on bradykinesia but no influence on cognitive performance.[620] Rostral and dorsomedial GPi lesions (linked to prefrontal cortical areas 9 and 46) produce impaired semantic fluency, mathematical ability, and memory under conditions of proactive interference. Left-sided lesions produce deficits in verbal fluency and verbal encoding.[621] Bilateral pallidotomy, while generally effective at reducing the disabling features of Parkinson's disease,[622] can result in prominent behavioral changes, disinhibition, reckless and socially inappropriate behaviors, apathy, poor judgment, and lack of insight.[623]

A NOTE ON THE CLAUSTRUM

The claustrum is a subcortical gray matter structure deep to the insular cortex, sandwiched between the EmC laterally and the external capsule medially (Fig. 1-47).[624] It is phylogenetically ancient with a homologue in lizards and turtles.[625] It has reciprocal connections with extensive areas of the cerebral cortex[15,223] and receives inputs from subcortical structures including the hypothalamus and monoaminergic systems in the midbrain and pons.[625] The fiber tracts that lead to the claustrum travel with the striatal fibers in the external capsule,[15] but this gray matter structure cannot be considered either truly cortical, or truly a component of the basal ganglia. The claustrum and insula have a close topographic relationship, but they do not share the same origin; the claustrum develops independently of the cortical plate, and they have different functional specializations.[223]

Many functional properties have been assigned to the claustrum. It is thought to play a role in setting and controlling behavioral states such as sleep.[625,626] By participating as a node in the default mode and salience networks, with connections to medial prefrontal cortex, medial dorsal thalamus, and basolateral amygdala it directs attention toward relevant sensory events including novel sensory stimuli.[626,627] It is engaged in cross-modal transfer of information.[628] Crick and Koch[629] suggested

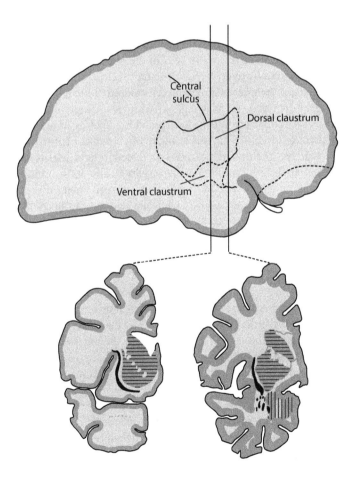

FIGURE 1-47. The human claustrum according to Rae,[624] modified by Crick and Koch[629] and further modified here.

that the neuroanatomy of the claustrum is compatible with a global role in integrating information at a fast time schedule, and that it plays a key role in consciousness.

EPITHALAMUS

Older anatomical terms describing the thalamus can be explained simply with current nomenclature, as follows.

The ventral thalamus refers to the STN.

The dorsal thalamus is the thalamus proper.

The metathalamus incorporates the lateral and medial geniculate nuclei.

The epithalamus includes the habenula (discussed above) and the pineal gland, as well as the habenular commissure and the stria medullaris.

Pineal Gland

The pineal gland achieved notoriety because René du Perron Descartes (1596–1650) believed it was the seat of the soul. Lancisi, in contrast, considered the pineal body to have a reinforcing effect, giving propulsive force to the animal spirits streaming out of the CC.[15,17]

The pineal gland has the dual functions of secreting melatonin and sensing light. Light reaches the pineal gland through a circuitous route: it is sensed by the retina, travels through the retinohypothalamic tract to the SCN of the hypothalamus, which sends projections to the paraventricular nucleus, with efferents traveling in the intermediolateral cell column of the spinal cord to the superior cervical ganglion, with post-ganglionic neurons ascending back to the pineal gland modulating its activity. Melatonin levels are highest at night when pineal neurons are most active. Their activity can be suppressed by light. Melatonin promotes sleep by inhibiting the activity of the SCN, inhibits memory, and is decreased in aging and in Alzheimer's disease and Parkinson's disease, likely clinically relevant in the altered sleep patterns in these conditions.[630]

THALAMUS

The thalamus is a large nucleated subcortical structure, bounded medially by the third ventricle, laterally by the posterior limb of the internal capsule, and extending from the anterior nuclear group at the level of the genu of the internal capsule rostrally to the pulvinar nucleus caudally (Fig. 1-40). It conveys somatosensory, visual, auditory, and gustatory afferents to the cerebral cortex as well as those from the brainstem and cerebellum and is engaged in extensive reciprocal interactions with all areas of the cerebral cortex as well as the hypothalamus, hippocampus, amygdala, and basal ganglia.

Neurobehavioral syndromes resulting from thalamic lesions may be understood by considering the functional properties of the thalamic nuclei deduced from tract-tracing investigations in monkeys, and physiological and clinical studies in patients. In addition to the reticular nucleus surrounding thalamus, the thalamic nuclei have been grouped into five broad functional classes: midline and intralaminar nuclei that subserve arousal, awareness, and nociception; limbic nuclei concerned with mood and motivation; specific sensory nuclei; effector nuclei concerned with movement and language; and associative nuclei participating in high-level cognition (Fig. 1-48; Table 1-1).[62]

Anatomical Features and Connections

(After Schmahmann[62])

Reticular Thalamic Nucleus

This nuclear shell surrounds thalamus and conveys afferents from cerebral cortex. It contributes to synchrony and rhythms of thalamic neuronal activity and is relevant in the pathophysiology of epilepsy[631] and neural substrates of consciousness.[632]

Intralaminar and Midline Thalamic Nuclei

The paracentral (Pcn), central lateral (CL), centromedian (CM), parafascicular (Pf), and midline nuclei such as paraventricular, rhomboid, and reuniens play a role in autonomic drive. They receive afferents from brainstem, spinal cord, and cerebellum and have reciprocal connections with cerebral hemispheres. The CM/Pf nuclei are linked with the basal ganglia in tightly connected functional circuits. A sensorimotor circuit links putamen with CM through the ventrolateral part of the internal segment of the globus pallidus (GPi). Cognitive circuits link the caudate with Pf through the dorsal GPi and through the SNr.[633] A limbic circuit links the ventral striatum with the Pf through the rostromedial GPi, and midline nuclei receiving input from the periaqueductal gray and spinothalamic tract are involved in processing the motivational-affective components of pain.[634–636] As discussed above, there are strong bidirectional thalamic connections with the amygdala: Midline and parafascicular thalamic nuclei project to the central amygdaloid nucleus; the part of the VPM that receives visceral and gustatory information projects to the lateral nucleus; and the medial geniculate nucleus sends projections to the lateral, accessory basal, and central nuclei. Projections from the amygdala link the basal lateral nucleus to MDmc (medial dorsal nucleus, magnocellular part); the central and medial amygdaloid nuclei target thalamic midline nuclei.

Van der Werf et al.[637] studied the intralaminar and midline nuclei in rats, clustered them into four groups based on their patterns of cortical and subcortical afferent and efferent projections, and proposed functional relationships for each: (i) a dorsal group, consisting of the paraventricular, parataenial, and intermediodorsal nuclei, involved in viscero-limbic functions; (ii) a lateral group, comprising the CL and Pcn nuclei and the anterior part of the central medial nucleus, involved in cognitive functions; (iii) a ventral group, made up of the reuniens and rhomboid nucleus and the posterior part of the central medial nucleus, involved in multimodal sensory processing; and (iv) a posterior group, consisting of the central median and parafascicular nuclei, involved in limbic motor functions.

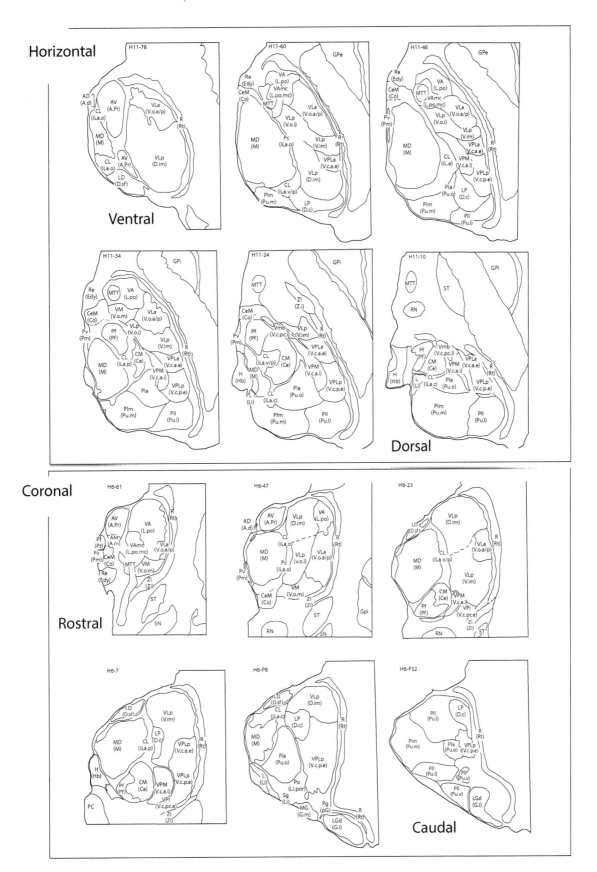

FIGURE 1-48. Diagram illustrating the nuclei of the human thalamus. Horizontal sections are seen above, from ventral to dorsal. Coronal sections below proceed from rostral to caudal. The revised nomenclature correlates with terminology used in the monkeys. An earlier nomenclature is shown in parentheses. (Adapted from Jones[648]; figure reproduced from Schmahmann and Pandya.[16])

TABLE 1-1. Behavioral Roles of Thalamic Nuclei.

Major Functional Grouping	Thalamic Nuclei	Putative Functional Attributes
Reticular	Reticular	Arousal, rhythmicity, role in epileptogenesis
Intralaminar	CM, Pf, CL, Pcn, midline (reuniens, paraventricular, rhomboid)	Arousal, attention, motivation, affective components of pain
Limbic	Anterior nuclear group (AD, AM, AV), lateral dorsal nucleus	Learning, memory, emotional experience and expression, drive, motivation
	Other—MDmc, medial pulvinar, ventral anterior	
Specific sensory	Medial geniculate	Auditory
	Lateral geniculate	Visual
	Ventroposterior—lateral (VPL)	Somatosensory body and limbs
	—medial (VPM)	Somatosensory head and neck
	—medial, parvicellular (VPMpc)	Gustatory
	—inferior (VPI)	Vestibular
Effector	Ventral anterior—reticulata recipient	Complex behaviors
	—pallidal recipient	Motor programming
	Ventral medial	Motor
	Ventral lateral—ventral part	Motor
	—dorsal part	Language (dominant hemisphere)
Associative	Lateral posterior	High-order somatosensory and visuospatial integration—spatial cognition
	Medial dorsal—medial, magnocellular (MDmc)	Drive, motivation, inhibition, emotion
	—intermediate, parvicellular (MDpc)	Executive functions, working memory
	—lateral, multiform (MDmf)	Attention, horizontal gaze
	Pulvinar—medial	Supramodal, high-level association region across multiple domains
	—Lateral	Somatosensory, visual association
	—Inferior	Visual association
	—Anterior (pulvinar oralis)	Intramodality somatosensory association, pain appreciation

Source: From Schmahmann.[62]

Limbic Thalamic Nuclei

The functions of the anterior nuclear group—ventral, medial, and dorsal (AV, AM, and AD nuclei), and the lateral dorsal (LD) nucleus are determined by their reciprocal anatomic connections with limbic structures in the cingulate gyrus, hippocampus, parahippocampal formation, entorhinal cortex, retrosplenial cortex, orbitofrontal and medial prefrontal cortices, and with subcortical structures, including the mammillary bodies and amygdala.[283,367,370,638]

The magnocellular part of the medial dorsal nucleus (MDmc), parts of the medial pulvinar, and parts of the VA nucleus are reciprocally interconnected with the cingulate gyrus and other components of the limbic system and thus may also be considered limbic. Like their cortical and subcortical counterparts,[63,639] limbic thalamic nuclei are likely to be essential for learning and memory, emotional experience and expression, drive, and motivation. The tuberothalamic artery irrigates these nuclei as well as the mammillothalamic and ventral amygdalofugal tracts that link the anterior thalamic nuclei with other nodes in the Papez circuit, accounting for the profound amnestic and limbic deficits resulting from tuberothalamic stroke.

The key role played by the anterior thalamic nuclei in memory, cognition, and spatial navigation and a review of their connections are to be found in Jankowski et al.[640]

Specific Sensory Thalamic Nuclei

The specific sensory nuclei include the medial geniculate nucleus (MGN), lateral geniculate nucleus (LGN), and ventroposterior nuclei (lateral, medial, and inferior—VPL, VPM, and VPI).

Medial geniculate nucleus connections with primary and association auditory cortices underscore the role of the MGN in higher level auditory processing as well as in elementary audition.[294,641,642]

The *lateral geniculate nucleus* projects to primary and secondary visual cortices.[643] It also receives projections back from visual areas,[644] indicating that higher order processing can influence visual perception at an early stage.

The *VPL* and *VPM nuclei* are reciprocally interconnected with primary somatosensory cortices; VPL serves body and limbs, and VPM serves head and neck.[7] Gustatory function is subserved by the parvicellular division of VPM.[645] The somatotopy of these nuclei is precise, and lacunar infarcts of the inferolateral artery produce focal sensory deficits. The VPI nucleus is linked with the rostral IPL and the second somatosensory area in the parietal operculum (SII)[281,282] and with the frontal operculum engaged in vestibular functions.[646]

Spinothalamic and trigeminothalamic inputs, and topographically organized wide dynamic neurons and nociceptive-specific neurons in the ventroposterior nuclei facilitate their role in the specific component of the pain system.[636] Disruption of SII cortex connections with these nuclei has been postulated to cause the parietal pseudothalamic pain syndrome.[508]

Effector Thalamic Nuclei

Motor nuclei include the VA, VM, and VL nuclei. Subregions within VA receive afferents from the GPi,[647] are linked with premotor cortices,[648] and may be responsible for dystonia in rostral thalamic lesions. Neurons in VA receive afferents from the SNr[649,650]; are linked with premotor, supplementary motor,[651] prefrontal,[652] caudal parts of the posterior parietal,[282] and rostral cingulate cortices[350]; and may account for complex behavioral syndromes following lesions of the VA thalamus.

The ventral sector of the posterior part of VL is linked with the motor cortex[653] and causes ataxia and mild motor weakness following thalamic stroke.[654–656] The dorsal part is linked with the posterior parietal,[282] prefrontal,[657–659] and superior temporal cortices[660] and has a role in articulation and language. Perseveration results from electrical stimulation of left medial VL; misnaming and omissions with stimulation of left posterior VL. It is also responsible for encoding and retrieval of verbal (left) and nonverbal information (right).[428,661–663]

Associative Thalamic Nuclei

The lateral posterior, medial dorsal, and pulvinar nuclei are interconnected with cerebral association areas and have no peripheral afferents or links with primary sensorimotor cortices.

The *lateral posterior (LP) nucleus* is reciprocally linked with the posterior parietal,[280–282] medial and dorsolateral extrastriate,[664] and posterior cingulate and medial parahippocampal cortices.[638] It integrates intramodal and multimodal associative somatosensory and visual information, and it is likely engaged in spatial functions, goal-directed reaching,[665] and in conceptual and analytical thinking.

The *medial dorsal (MD) nucleus* has reciprocal connections with the prefrontal cortex.[652,666–670] The laterally placed multiformis part (MDmf) is linked with the area 8 in the arcuate concavity, and lesions produce impairments of horizontal gaze and attention. The intermediate part of MD (the parvicellular MDpc) is linked with dorsolateral and dorsomedial prefrontal cortices, areas 9 and 46, possibly accounting for poor working memory and perseveration resulting from MD lesions. The medial part (magnocellular MDmc) is linked with paralimbic regions—medial and orbital prefrontal cortices, amygdala, basal forebrain, and olfactory and entorhinal cortices.[671,672] Apathy, abulia, disinhibition, and failure

to inhibit inappropriate behaviors are likely to result from MDmc lesions, along with memory[673] and language deficits.[674] The densocellular region (MDdc) projects to cingulate cortex area 24[350] and in the posterior parietal cortex it projects to the rostral and most caudal parts of the SPL (areas PE and PGm) and the caudal, multimodal parts of the IPL, areas PG and Opt.[282] In the parietal lobe, the MDdc projections resemble those of the intralaminar nuclei, consistent with the view that it is not truly a part of the medial dorsal nucleus, both because of its architecture as well as its cortical connections.[650,675] Neuronal loss in the MD nucleus is confined to the MDdc and MDpc nuclei in schizophrenia, which may account for the hypoactivity of dorsolateral prefrontal cortex seen in this disorder on imaging studies.[676]

Different subregions within *medial pulvinar (PM)* are topographically linked with prefrontal,[638,677,678] posterior parietal,[281,282,677] and auditory-related[642] and multimodal superior temporal cortices,[578] and with the cingulate, parahippocampal,[638] and insula cortices.[679] Aphasia,[662] spatial neglect,[680] and psychosis[681] may result from PM lesions. The lateral pulvinar (PL) is linked with posterior parietal,[282,677] superior temporal,[578] and medial and dorsolateral extrastriate cortices,[664] and the superior colliculus.[682] It is engaged in the integration of somatosensory and visual information. Inferior pulvinar (PI) is linked with temporal lobe areas concerned with visual feature discrimination, and with ventrolateral and ventromedial extrastriate areas concerned with visual motion.[664,683] It also receives input from retinal ganglion cells[684] and visual neurons of the superior colliculus.[682] The anterior pulvinar (pulvinar oralis, PO) is interconnected with intramodality somatosensory association cortices in the rostral part of the inferior parietal region, and with the second somatosensory area (SII).[281,282,665,677] The PO nucleus may be important in the appreciation of pain, as are the suprageniculate, limitans, and posterior nuclei.[650]

Sensorimotor, effector, limbic, and associative regions of cerebral cortex are therefore linked with distinctly different sets of thalamic nuclei. Thalamic projections to the posterior parietal lobe exemplify this concept.[282] Connections become progressively elaborated as one moves from rostral to caudal within both the superior and the inferior parietal lobules (Fig. 1-49). Rostral areas concerned with intramodality somatosensory processing are related to modality-specific thalamic nuclei, whereas caudal regions, concerned with complex functions, derive their input from multimodal and limbic nuclei. This rostral-caudal cortical topography is represented within the LP and PO nuclei that project to both superior and inferior parietal lobules. Rostral parietal subdivisions receive projections from ventral regions within these thalamic nuclei, caudal parietal afferents arise from the dorsal parts of these nuclei, and the intervening cortical levels receive projections from intermediate positions within the nuclei. A similar topographic arrangement is present also in the medial pulvinar projections to the IPL (Fig. 1-50).

This concept of intranuclear topographic specificity of connections is not confined to thalamus. A similar pattern is evident also in the lateral nucleus of the amygdala, each sector within it contributing topographically organized projections to other amygdala areas, terminating in distinct parts of the target regions.[685]

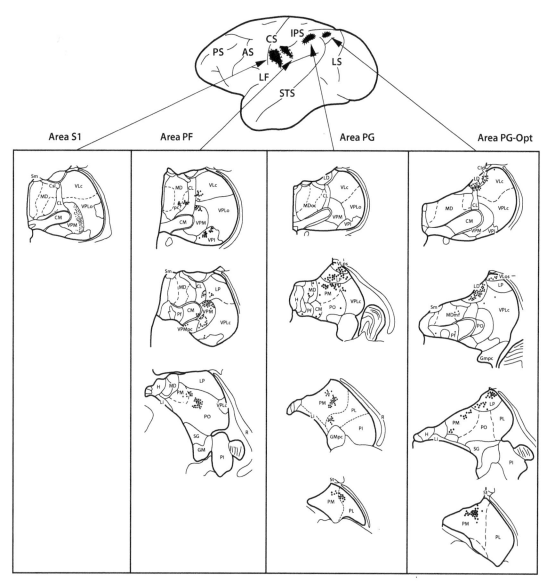

PARIETAL CORTICAL REGION	S1	Area PF	Area PG	Area PG-Opt
PRINCIPAL THALAMIC NUCLEAR AFFERENTS	<u>Sensory</u> Ventral posterior medial (VPM)	<u>Sensory</u> VPM Ventral posterior inferior (VPI) <u>Associative</u> Pulvinar oralis Lateral posterior Pulvinar medialis	<u>Associative</u> Pulvinar medialis Lateral posterior <u>Effector</u> Ventral lateral (caudal and pars postrema)	<u>Associative</u> Pulvinar medialis Lateral posterior <u>Effector</u> Ventral lateral (pars postrema) <u>Intralaminar</u> Paracentralis <u>Limbic</u> Lateral dorsal Anterior nuclei
PUTATIVE FUNCTIONAL PROPERTIES	Primary unimodal somatosensory	Intramodality association within somatosensory domain: for graphesthesia, stereognosis	Multimodal somatosensory and visual: for integration of visual and cutaneo-kinesthetic spatial information	Multimodal associative and paralimbic: visual spatial and somesthetic stimuli invested wit emotional and motivational valence

FIGURE 1-49. Diagrammatic representation of projections from thalamus (black dots) to primary somatosensory cortex S1, area PF, area PG, and area PG-Opt of the parietal lobe in rhesus monkey following cortical injections (blackened areas) of wheat germ agglutinated horseradish peroxidase. Representative rostral to caudal levels of thalamus are shown. Thalamic nomenclature according to Olszewski.[675] Parietal lobe nomenclature according to Pandya and Seltzer.[261] The table summarizes the areas injected with tracer, the principal thalamic nuclei demonstrating retrogradely labeled neurons, and the putative functional attributes of the cortical areas studied. (Derived from Schmahmann and Pandya[282]; figure reproduced from Schmahmann and Pandya.[16])

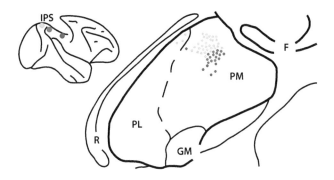

FIGURE 1-50. Diagrammatic representation of the projections from the medial pulvinar nucleus of thalamus (PM) to the inferior parietal lobule in rhesus monkey. Fluorescent retrograde tracers were placed in area PF (blue), area PG (red), and area PG-Opt (green) in a rhesus monkey, and the resulting retrogradely labeled neurons were identified in the PM nucleus. Color-coding of labeled neurons was according to the injection site in each case. (Adapted from Schmahmann and Pandya.[282])

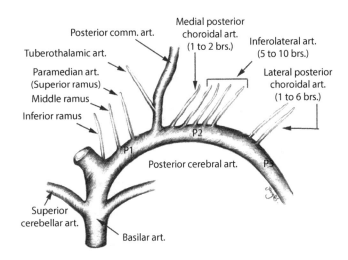

FIGURE 1-51. Artist's rendition of origin of arteries to thalamus arising from the vertebrobasilar system. Note that the medial posterior choroidal artery (art.) may arise before (P1) or after (P2) the origin of the posterior communicating artery. The inferolateral arteries may arise individually or from a common pedicle. brs., branches (Figure and legend from Schmahmann.[62])

CLINICAL FEATURES OF THALAMIC LESIONS

C. Miller Fisher (1913–2012) first described neglect (modified anosognosia and hemiasomatognosia), global dysphasia, confusion, and visual hallucinations in patients with thalamic hemorrhage.[686] Accounts followed of thalamic dementia from prion diseases[687] and behavioral changes in patients with thalamic tumors,[688,689] but these lesions are seldom confined to thalamus. Focal lesions in thalamus occur in the setting of ischemic infarction. There are four main vascular syndromes of the thalamus. A review of these vascular syndromes illustrates the behavioral roles of the different thalamic nuclei and highlights the clinical relevance of the thalamic afferent and efferent connections (Figs. 1-51 and 1-52; Table 1-2).[62,690,691]

Tuberothalamic Artery Infarction

The tuberothalamic artery originates from the middle third of the posterior communicating artery. Within thalamus it follows the course of the mammillothalamic tract (MMT). It is absent in approximately one-third of the normal population, in which case its territory is supplied by the paramedian artery.[692] The tuberothalamic artery irrigates the reticular nucleus, VA, rostral part of VL, ventral pole of MD, the MMT, the ventral amygdalofugal pathway, the ventral part of the internal medullary lamina, and the anterior thalamic nuclei—AM, AV, and AD. Percheron[693] concludes that the anterior nuclear group is not supplied by this tuberothalamic artery, but rather by the posterior choroidal artery, an assertion reflected in the discussion of von Cramon et al.[690] This relationship is uncertain, however, given the anatomic proximity of the tuberothalamic artery and the MMT to the AM/AV/AD nuclei, and by the demonstration[694,695] of involvement of the anterior nuclei along with the VA, VL, MMT, and internal medullary lamina that are known to be supplied by the tuberothalamic artery.

Patients with tuberothalamic artery infarction (Fig. 1-53A,B) demonstrate fluctuating levels of consciousness, disorientation in time and place, and personality changes, including euphoria, lack of insight, apathy, lack of spontaneity, and emotional unconcern.[674,692,696,697] New learning and verbal and visual memory are impaired. Amnesia is greater following left thalamic lesions, along with anomia, impaired comprehension, fluent and meaningless discourse with semantic and phonemic paraphasic errors, neologisms, and perseveration. In contrast, repetition and reading aloud are preserved. Acalculia, buccofacial apraxia, and limb apraxia may occur.[698] Right thalamic lesions produce the amnestic syndrome along with impairments in visual processing and visual memory, and hemispatial neglect. Lesions on either side produce emotional central facial paralysis (good facial movement with volition, but facial asymmetry during emotional display) and constructional apraxia. Motor findings are mild, and sensory disturbances are rare.

Stroke confined to the anterior/polar branch of the tuberothalamic artery affects memory and personality. Autobiographic memory and newly acquired information are disorganized with respect to temporal order, with patients displaying superimposition of temporally unrelated information (palipsychism). Apathy, inattention, disorientation, impaired sequencing, and perseveration are prominent. Dysarthria, hypophonia, anomia, and decreased verbal fluency are noted, but comprehension, writing, reading, and repetition are preserved.[694,695]

Paramedian Artery Infarction

According to Percheron[693] the paramedian arteries represent a special differentiation of the highest of the group of paramedian arteries which can be found all along the neuraxis. They arise from the P1 section of the posterior cerebral artery, the mesencephalic artery, the proximal stretch of the posterior cerebral

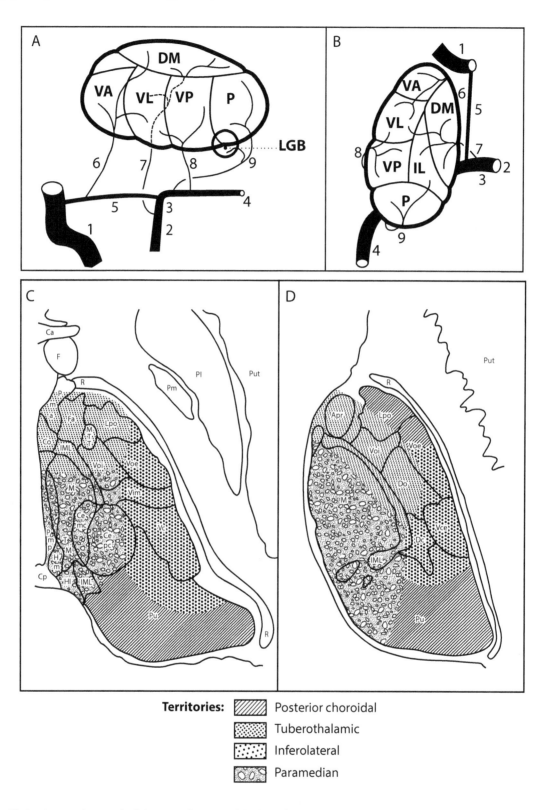

Territories:

- ▨ Posterior choroidal
- ▨ Tuberothalamic
- ▨ Inferolateral
- ▨ Paramedian

FIGURE 1-52. Thalamic vascular supply. Schematic diagram of the lateral **(A)** and dorsal **(B)** views of the four major thalamic arteries, and the nuclei they irrigate, according to Bogousslavsky et al.[674] 1, carotid artery; 2, basilar artery; 3, P1 region of the posterior cerebral artery (mesencephalic artery); 4, posterior cerebral artery; 5, posterior communicating artery; 6, tuberothalamic artery; 7, paramedian artery; 8, inferolateral artery; 9, posterior choroidal artery; DM, dorsomedial nucleus; IL, intralaminar nuclear complex; P, pulvinar; VP, ventral posterior complex. The illustrations in **(C)** and **(D)** from De Freitas and Bogousslavsky[691] are an adapted version of the conclusions of Von Cramon et al.[690] regarding the patterns of irrigation by the thalamic arterial supply to the thalamic nuclei. (Composite image from Schmahmann.[62])

TABLE 1-2. Thalamic Arterial Supply and Principal Clinical Features of Focal Infarction.		
Thalamic Blood Vessel	**Nuclei Irrigated**	**Clinical Features Reported**
Tuberothalamic artery (arises from middle third of posterior communicating artery)	Reticular, intralaminar, VA, rostral VL, ventral pole of MD, anterior nuclei—AD, AM, AV, ventral internal medullary lamina, ventral amygdalofugal pathway, mammillothalamic tract	Confusion; memory, emotion, and behavior changes Fluctuating arousal and orientation Impaired learning, memory, autobiographical memory Superimposition of temporally unrelated information Personality changes, apathy, abulia Executive failure, perseveration True to hemisphere—language if VL involved on left; hemispatial neglect if right sided Emotional facial expression, acalculia, apraxia
Paramedian artery (arises from P1)	MD, intralaminar—CM, Pf, CL, posteromedial VL, ventromedial pulvinar, paraventricular, LD, dorsal internal medullary lamina	Confusion; memory, language, and behavior changes Decreased arousal (coma vigil if bilateral) Impaired learning and memory, confabulation, temporal disorientation, poor autobiographical memory Aphasia if left sided, spatial deficits if right sided Altered social skills and personality, including apathy, aggression, agitation
Inferolateral artery (arises from P2)		
Principal inferolateral branch	Ventroposterior complex—VPM, VPL, VPI Ventral lateral nucleus, ventral (motor) part	Variable elements of a triad—hemisensory loss, hemiataxia, and hemiparesis Sensory loss (variable extent, all modalities) Hemiataxia Hemiparesis Post-lesion pain syndrome (Déjerine-Roussy)—right hemisphere predominant
Medial branch	Medial geniculate	Auditory consequences
Inferolateral pulvinar branches	Rostral and lateral pulvinar, LD nucleus	Behavioral consequences
Posterior choroidal artery (arises from P2)		
Lateral branches	LGN, LD, LP, inferolateral parts of pulvinar	Visual field loss (hemianopsia, quadrantanopsia)
Medial branches	MGN, posterior parts of CM and CL, pulvinar	Variable sensory loss, weakness, aphasia, memory impairment, dystonia, hand tremor

Source: From Schmahmann.[62]

artery from the bifurcation of the basilar to its junction with the posterior communicating artery.[699] Tatu et al.[59] adopt a useful approach of grouping the interpeduncular branches that arise from the mesencephalic, or P1 artery, into inferior, middle, and superior rami. The inferior ramus of the interpeduncular arteries that arises from the basilar bifurcation, and the middle ramus, that Percheron[693] together called the paramedian mesencephalic pedicle, irrigate the pons and midbrain[59,700] and can produce the locked-in component of the top of the basilar stroke.[701] The superior ramus that irrigates the thalamus, corresponds to the posterior thalamo-subthalamic paramedian artery of Percheron,[693] or in the nomenclature adopted here, the paramedian artery. The paramedian arteries can arise as a pair from each P1, but they may equally arise from a common trunk off one P1, thus supplying thalamus bilaterally.

The paramedian artery ascends within thalamus from its medial and ventral aspect to its lateral and dorsal part. It supplies a variable extent of thalamus, but principally MD, the internal medullary lamina, and intralaminar nuclei—CL, CM, and Pf. The paraventricular nuclei, posteromedial part of VL, and VM part of the pulvinar may also be supplied along with the LD, LP, and VA. When the tuberothalamic artery is absent, the paramedian artery may assume that territory and therefore the consequence of infarction can be greater.

Unilateral thalamic infarction in the territory of the paramedian artery (Fig. 1-53C) produces neuropsychological disturbances predominantly in the areas of arousal and memory. A left-right asymmetry is evident in language versus visual-spatial deficits.

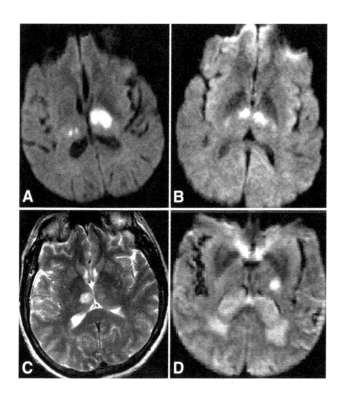

FIGURE 1-53. **(A)** Diffusion weighted image (DWI) of left tuberothalamic artery territory infarction (right of diagram). **(B)** DWI showing infarction bilaterally in the territory of the polar branch of the tuberothalamic artery, likely representing an example of the paramedian artery irrigating both the paramedian and tuberothalamic territories. **(C)** Right paramedian artery territory infarction, seen on T2-weighted magnetic resonance imaging. **(D)** Acute infarction in the left inferolateral artery territory on DWI. (From Schmahmann and Pandya.[16])

Impairment of arousal with decreased and fluctuating level of consciousness is a conspicuous early feature, lasting hours to days. Confusion, agitation, aggression, and apathy may persist.[674,696,700] Speech and language impairments are characterized by hypophonia and dysprosodies, with frequent perseveration and reduced verbal fluency, but generally preserved syntactic structure with occasional paraphasic errors and normal repetition—the adynamic aphasia of Guberman and Stuss.[702]

Bilateral infarction in the paramedian artery territory results in an acutely ill and severely impaired patient. Disorientation, confusion, hypersomnolence, deep coma, coma vigil or akinetic mutism (awake unresponsiveness), and severe memory impairment with perseveration and confabulation are prominent behavioral features,[696,700,703] often accompanied by eye movement abnormalities because of damage to descending pathways to vertical gaze centers in the midbrain (see section "Thalamic Fiber Systems"). The anterograde and retrograde memory deficit and the apathy can be severe and persistent. The syndrome may be accompanied in the late stages by inappropriate social behaviors, impulsive aggressive outbursts, emotional blunting, loss of initiative, and a reported absence of spontaneous thoughts or mental activities,[702] conceptualized as loss of psychic self-activation.[704,705] Severe and systematic distortion of personally relevant autobiographical

memory but relative sparing of knowledge of famous people and public events has been described,[706] suggesting a thematic retrieval memory disorder resulting from disconnection of frontal and medial temporal memory systems. Prominent disorientation in time, chronotaraxis,[707] may occur,[671,700] and apraxia and dysgraphia are noted in some.[700] Complete recovery from bilateral paramedian thalamic infarction has been described.[708]

The amnestic syndrome resulting from paramedian territory infarction is like the thiamine-deficient Korsakoff syndrome which destroys MD along with the mammillary bodies,[673] but the addition of the other behavioral features produces thalamic dementia,[699] seen also in the behavioral and cognitive consequences of thalamic involvement in Creutzfeldt-Jakob disease and fatal familial insomnia.[687] Transient global amnesia is thought to be related to transient ischemia in the paramedian thalamus.[709]

Elementary neurologic signs from stroke in the territory of the paramedian artery include asterixis, complete or partial vertical gaze paresis, loss of convergence, pseudo-sixth nerve palsies, bilateral internuclear opthalmoplegia, miosis, and photophobia.[674,702] These are among the findings reported by Fisher[686] in cases of medially situated thalamic hemorrhage and likely result from lesions involving midbrain nuclei supplied by the inferior and middle rami of the interpeduncular arteries arising from P1 medial to the paramedian artery.

Inferolateral Artery Infarction

The inferolateral arteries[674,693] are comprised of 5–10 arteries that arise from the P2 branch of the posterior cerebral artery, that is, after the level of the posterior communicating artery. There are three main groups—the medial geniculate, the principal inferolateral arteries, and the inferolateral pulvinar arteries.

(i) The medial branch supplies the external half of the MGN.
(ii) The principal inferolateral arteries are large, vertically oriented short branches of the posterior cerebral artery which penetrate between the geniculate bodies, ascend in the lateral medullary lamina, and supply most of the ventral posterior nuclei—lateral (VPL), medial (VPM), and inferior (VPI), as well as the ventral and lateral parts of the VL nucleus more rostrally. In Percheron's material, the CM nucleus is not supplied by these vessels, as suggested by Foix and Hillemand[710] and Plets et al.[711]
(iii) The inferolateral pulvinar branches are situated posteriorly in the inferolateral arterial group, and supply dorsal and posterolateral regions, including the rostral and lateral parts of the pulvinar, and the LD nucleus.[59,674,693,712]

Patients with inferolateral artery infarction (Fig. 1-53D) present with the thalamic syndrome described by Déjerine and Roussy[713]: variable sensory loss to touch, temperature, pin, position, and vibration; impaired extremity movement; and sometimes with post-lesion pain when the lesion is on the right side.[674,712,714–717]

Ataxia with hemiparesis can occur in this group.[654,710,712,713,718] The combination of sensory loss with ataxic hemiparesis points to a thalamic lesion, although it is not pathognomonic because midbrain lesions produce a similar constellation. The thalamic hand[710] produced by lesions of the inferolateral artery, is flexed and pronated, with the thumb buried beneath the other fingers.

The complexity of the penetrating arteries that constitute the inferolateral arteries explains why small vessel disease can have distinctly different presentations. Pure sensory stroke affecting face, arm, and leg in whole or in part results from variable involvement of the VPM (head and neck) or VPL nuclei (trunk and extremities). Infarction in those VL regions that convey cerebellar fibers to the motor-related cortices adds an ataxic component to the presentation. Cognitive and psychiatric presentations are notably missing from the descriptions of infarction restricted to the ventral posterior nuclei. The pulvinar is strongly associative, and LD is related to limbic cortices, but reports of the clinical manifestations of infarction in the inferolateral pulvinar vessels restricted to, or predominantly involving, these nuclei have yet to appear. Similarly, whereas the VL nucleus receives some supply from the inferolateral arteries, it is mostly supplied by the tuberothalamic artery territory. Incoordination is noted in patients with inferolateral territory infarction when it involves the VL. Language disturbances after VL lesions in tuberothalamic artery infarction are not commonly seen following stroke in the inferolateral artery territory. Occasional reports describe impaired fluency, comprehension, and naming.[696,719]

Posterior Choroidal Artery Infarction

The posterior choroidal arteries, like the inferolateral, arise from the P2 segment of the posterior cerebral artery, and are made up of several branches. One to two medially placed branches arise adjacent to the take-off of the posterior communicating artery (i.e., at the distal P1 or proximal P2 segment of the posterior cerebral artery). These supply the STN and midbrain, the medial half of the MGN, the posterior parts of the intralaminar nuclei CM and CL (densocellular part of MD in the terminology of Olszewski, CL in the terminology of Jones), and the pulvinar nuclei.[59,674,693,700] Percheron's[693] conclusion that it also supplies the AD, AV, and AM components of the anterior nuclear group is not universally shared.[59] In the lateral group of posterior choroidal arteries, one to six branches arise from the distal P2 segment of the posterior cerebral artery. Some of these supply medial temporal structures. The thalamic branches irrigate the LGN, the inferolateral region of the pulvinar, the lateral dorsal nucleus, and the LP nucleus. The LGN may also receive supply from the anterior choroidal artery,[59] although Percheron[693] could not confirm this in his material, and thalamus was not involved in the series of anterior choroidal artery infarcts reported by Decroix et al.[720]

Limited information on the clinical manifestations of infarction confined to thalamus in the distribution of the posterior choroidal arteries reveals visual field deficits, eye movement abnormalities, sensory impairments,[674,721] and a "jerky, dystonic, unsteady hand."[864]

Thalamic Fiber Systems

Damage to thalamic fiber pathways has clinical consequences. The MMT and fornix bind the anterior thalamic nuclei into the neural system for learning and memory. The ventral amygdalofugal pathway links amygdala with the medial part of MD, and damage contributes to amnesia and emotional dysregulation.[671]

Lesions of the superior, medial and inferior, and lateral thalamic peduncles and of the anterior limb of the internal capsule (conveying prefrontal and anterior cingulate interactions)[15] can produce corticothalamic disconnection and complex behavioral syndromes.[502–504]

Disorders of eye movement result from medial thalamic lesions destroying descending tracts from motor and premotor cortices to the midbrain nuclei of Darkschewitz and the interstitial nucleus of Cajal (upgaze and downgaze), and the rostral nucleus of the medial longitudinal fasciculus in the tectum (downgaze).[674,686,702,722]

Further Functional Considerations Regarding the Thalamus

It has been proposed that the fundamental role of the thalamic nuclei is related to its specific alerting response that directs attention to information in the external environment while simultaneously blocking retrieval from memory.[427] Four putative mechanisms of the specific alerting response derived from the study of its involvement in language are as follows[723]: (i) selective engagement of task-relevant cortical areas in a heightened state of responsiveness in part through the nucleus reticularis, (ii) passing information from one cortical area to another through corticothalamo-cortical mechanisms, (iii) sharpening the focus on task-relevant information through corticothalamo-cortical feedback mechanisms, and (iv) selection of one language (or other functional) unit over another in the expression of a concept, accomplished in concert with basal ganglia loops. The precise nature of the transform is expected to vary across thalamic nuclei because of their individual unique architectural characteristics but all are thought to share common underlying principles reflecting the anatomical features that govern thalamic connections.

CEREBELLUM

The cerebellum is subcortical only in the sense that it is distinct from cerebral cortex (Fig. 1-54). The now-historical view that cerebellar function is confined to the coordination of voluntary motor activity is no longer tenable.[251,252,255,724] Evidence from anatomical and imaging studies and from patients with cerebellar damage has made it plain that cerebellar pathology is related to intellectual and emotional deficits in addition to motor incoordination. Knowledge of the cerebellum is now essential for understanding the neural substrates of higher order behavior and neuropsychiatric disorders.

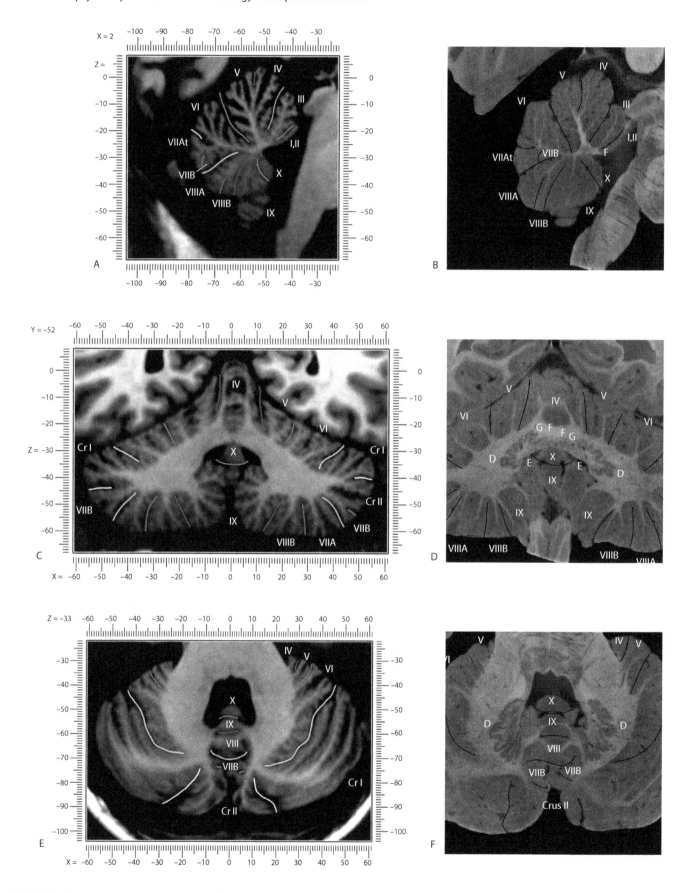

FIGURE 1-54. Images of the human cerebellum on magnetic resonance imaging (left) and postmortem cryosection (right). The cerebellum is sectioned in the sagittal plane 2 mm to the right of midline in **(A)** and **(B)**; in the coronal plane 52 mm behind the anterior commissure—posterior commissure (AC-PC) line in **(C)** and **(D)**; and in the transverse plane 33 mm below the AC-PC line in **(E)** and **(F)**. Cerebellar fissures are demarcated and the lobules are designated. Deep cerebellar nuclei are identified in the cryosection brain: D, dentate nucleus; E, emboliform nucleus; F, fastigial nucleus; G, globose nucleus. (From *MRI Atlas of the Human Cerebellum*, Schmahmann et al.[728,729])

Gross Anatomy

The cerebellum is in the posterior cranial fossa, beneath the tentorium cerebelli, and behind the brainstem. It is linked with the spinal cord, brainstem, and cerebral hemispheres by three major fiber tracts: the inferior, middle, and superior cerebellar peduncles. The *inferior cerebellar peduncle* contains the large restiform body that conveys afferents from spinal cord and inferior olivary nuclei, and the smaller juxtarestiform body that conveys afferent and efferent vestibular fibers.[725] The *middle cerebellar peduncle* is a massive tract carrying axons from the pontine nuclei in the opposite side of the pons to the cerebellar hemispheres. The *superior cerebellar peduncle*, or brachium conjunctivum, which transmits efferent fibers from cerebellum, decussates in the midbrain and ascends to the thalamus. Nucleo-olivary projections from cerebellum to the inferior olivary nucleus are located ventral to the superior cerebellar peduncle and descend into the medulla. Some fibers from the spinal cord and brainstem enter the cerebellum by way of the superior cerebellar peduncle.

The cerebellum has three lobes: anterior, posterior, and flocculonodular. There are 10 cerebellar lobules, equivalent to cerebral hemispheric gyri, and 11 major cerebellar fissures equivalent to the cerebral hemispheric sulci that separate the lobules and their principal subdivisions. The designations are according to Olof Larsell (1886–1964)[726] and Lodewijk 'Louis' Bolk (1866–1930),[727] adapted and modified in Schmahmann et al.[728,729] (Fig. 1-55). Lobules I through V comprise the anterior lobe. Lobules I and II are closely apposed to the superior medullary velum, and usually joined, as lobule I is vestigial in the human brain. The anterior lobe is separated from the posterior lobe by the primary fissure. Lobules VI through IX are the

posterior lobe. Lobule VIIA includes crus I and crus II, which together with lobule VI occupies the great extent of the human cerebellum. The horizontal fissure separates crus I from crus II. Lobule X is the flocculonodular lobe, separated from lobule IX by the posterolateral fissure (Fig. 1-55). Note that the term tonsil used in clinical neurology is an older anatomical term that includes parts of both lobules VIII and IX.

The white matter of the cerebellum contains the four deep cerebellar nuclei, from medial to lateral, fastigial, globose, emboliform, and dentate. The fastigial nucleus has multiple roles: balance and gait, oculomotor function, autonomic control, and limbic valence. The globose and emboliform nuclei (homologous with the posterior and anterior interposed nuclei in lower species) are heavily engaged in motor control. The dentate nucleus has expanded massively through evolution; its dorsal microgyric part is phylogenetically older and related to sensorimotor function; its ventral macrogyric part has expanded in concert with the cerebral hemisphere association areas with which it is interconnected, and it is connectionally and functionally related to the cognitive cerebellum in the posterior lobe. The lateral vestibular nucleus in the medulla is regarded as an extracerebellar deep nucleus, because its connections follow the same principles as the other cerebellar nuclei.

Histology

The histology of the cerebellar cortex differs fundamentally from the cerebral cortex.[176,730] It has a repeating architecture throughout that gives it the appearance of a paracrystalline structure. It has a three-layered cortex, entirely different in organization and concept from the primitive three-layered allocortex of the

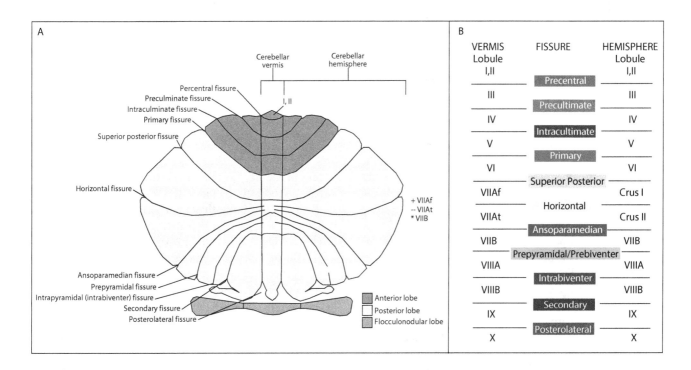

FIGURE 1-55. **(A)** Schematic of a flattened and unfolded view of the human cerebellum developed in Makris et al.[410] identifies the major lobes designated by color code, lobules labeled according to our[728,729] modification of earlier nomenclatures,[726,727] and fissures as identified in the *MRI Atlas of the Human Cerebellum*.[728,729] **(B)** Relationship of the fissures to the cerebellar lobules in the vermis and hemispheres. (From *MRI Atlas of the Human Cerebellum*, Schmahmann et al.[728,729])

cerebral hemisphere (Fig. 1-56). It consists of a monolayer of Purkinje cells sandwiched between the granule cell layer below, and the molecular layer above. The cortex of each cerebellar folium surrounds a white matter lamella conveying afferents to the cerebellar cortex, and Purkinje cell axons from the cortex to the nuclei.

The *Purkinje cell (PC) layer* is a monolayer of Purkinje neurons (Jan Evangelista Purkyně, 1787–1869). These defining neuronal elements of the cerebellum have large pear-shaped somata, and extensive dendritic trees oriented in a flattened plate perpendicular to the long axis of the folium. They are GABAergic, and the only neurons that send axons out of the cerebellar cortex to the cerebellar nuclei.

The *granule cell layer* contains most of the neurons in the nervous system. These tiny glutamatergic neurons have four to five short, claw-like dendrites that participate in a granule cell glomerulus with the axons of other neuronal elements. Granule cells emit their axons into the molecular layer where they branch perpendicularly to form parallel fibers traveling in opposite directions for ~5–6 mm, providing excitatory synapses on the distal dendritic spines of up to 300 PCs. Also in the granule cell layer are the Golgi cells (Camillo Golgi 1843–1926) the axons of which provide inhibitory input to the granule cell glomerulus.

The *molecular layer* contains the ascending axons of the granule cells, the parallel fibers, dendritic arborizations of PCs and Golgi interneurons, cell bodies of the inhibitory basket and stellate cells, and the supporting glial cells.

Cerebellar Corticonuclear Circuitry

The cerebellar cortex is organized into zones identified by AChE and monoclonal antibody staining, and microzones which share common afferent and efferent projections.[731–736]

Cerebellar inputs are conveyed via three major afferents, all of which are excitatory (Fig. 1-56A,B).

Mossy fibers (MFs) arise from all non-olivary cerebellar afferents, including the spinal cord[737–739] and most heavily from the neurons of the basis pontis. They terminate in the granule cell glomerulus and give off collaterals to the deep cerebellar nuclei. The granule cell axon ascends to the molecular layer, dividing to form the parallel fibers. Mossy fiber excitatory input via the parallel fibers to the PCs induces a repetitive simple spike with a frequency between 50 and 150 spikes per second. The parallel fiber input is thought to provide information about incoming signals, such as direction and speed of limb movement. In the cognitive domain the parallel fibers provide the PC with the context in which specific behaviors occur.

Climbing fibers (CFs) arise exclusively from the inferior olivary nuclei. The axons of olivary neurons course in the medulla to the contralateral inferior cerebellar peduncle and cerebellar hemisphere. The axon provides collateral input to the cerebellar nuclei and reaches the PC layer where each of its branches provides extensive excitatory synaptic contact with the proximal dendritic tree of a single PC. Olivary neurons receive inhibitory feedback projections from the neurons in the cerebellar nuclei to which they project, forming a closed loop system. The PC generates a very different action potential in response to the climbing fiber input: a complex spike with a low frequency of 0.5–2 spikes per second, the same rate of firing as the olivary neurons from which the climbing fiber originates. The climbing fiber input to the Purkinje cell is thought to signal the occurrence of errors.

Monoaminergic inputs to all levels of the cerebellar cortex arise from brainstem noradrenergic, catecholaminergic, serotonergic, and dopaminergic nuclei. These are relatively minor, but nevertheless important.

The output from the cerebellar cortex is derived exclusively from PCs, precisely organized, and directed toward the DCN and precerebellar nuclei. PCs in each lobule project to those parts of the deep cerebellar nuclei closest to them. The vermis projects to the fastigial nucleus, the intermediate cortex to the globose and emboliform nuclei, and much of the lateral hemispheres project to the dentate nucleus.

There is an exquisitely precise topographic relationship between subsectors of the olivary nuclei, deep cerebellar nuclei, and parasagittal zones of the cerebellar cortex.[732,735] These are linked together in multiple repeating anatomic microcircuits, corticonuclear-olivary microcomplexes, that serve as the essential functional unit of the cerebellum. Whereas inputs to the cerebellum are excitatory, output from the cerebellar cortex to the deep nuclei via the PC is inhibitory. Output from the cerebellum via the cerebellar nuclei is excitatory to thalamus and brainstem but inhibitory to the inferior olive.

The cerebellar nuclear projections to the spinal cord, brainstem, diencephalon, and cerebral cortex are the basis of the cerebellar incorporation into the neural circuits subserving autonomic function, motor control, emotion, and cognition.

Cerebellar Connections with the Cerebral Hemispheres

Corticopontine projections originate from layer V pyramidal neurons of the cerebral cortex and descend to the ipsilateral pons where they synapse on the dendrites of neurons in the basis pontis (Fig. 1-57).[740–742] The pontine neurons send their axons (pontocerebellar projection) through the contralateral MCP to the opposite cerebellar hemisphere.[743] This is the feedforward limb of the cerebrocerebellar system. The feedback limb arises in the cerebellar cortex, the Purkinje neurons projecting to the deep cerebellar nuclei, from where the cerebellothalamic projections target the contralateral thalamus. After synapsing in thalamus, they return to the cerebral cortex as the thalamocortical projection, where the circuit originated. These cerebrocerebellar loops tend to originate and return to the same cortical areas, but they are not strictly closed.

Cerebrocerebellar projections arise from motor cortices, target the motor regions of the cerebellum (see below), and return to the motor cortex via the ventrolateral nucleus of the thalamus. The association and paralimbic regions of the cerebral cortex participate heavily in topographically organized reciprocal circuits with the cerebellum. Association cortex projections arise from the prefrontal, posterior parietal, superior temporal polymodal regions, and dorsal parastriate cortices.[742,744–748] Paralimbic projections arise from the posterior parahippocampal cortex, limbic regions of the cingulate gyrus, and the anterior

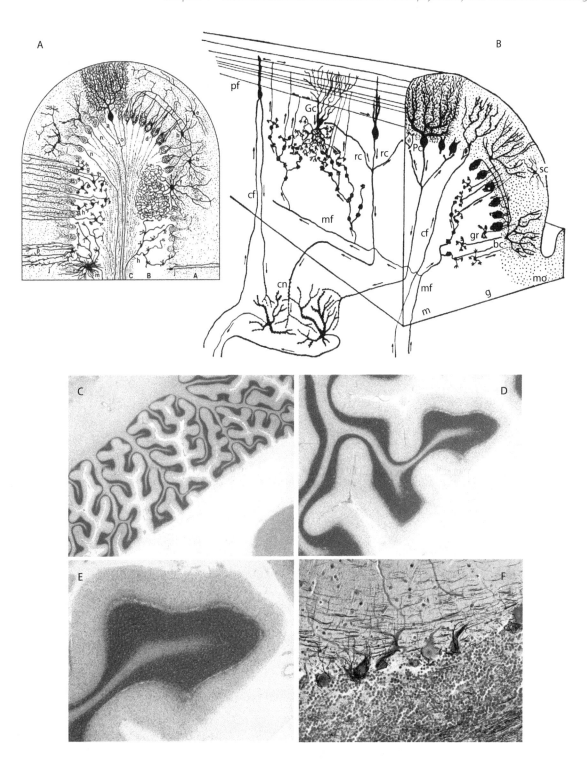

FIGURE 1-56. Cerebellar cortical elements and circuitry. **(A)** Cajal's depiction of the cerebellar cortex.[176] **(B)** Cerebellar cortex by Sir John Eccles, 1973. Schematic diagram showing in perspective drawing the various neurons and neuronal connexions of the cerebellar cortex. bc, basket cell; cf, climbing fibre; cn, cerebellar nucleus; g, granular layer; Gc, Golgi cell; gr, granule cell; mf, mossy fibre; Pc, Purkyne cell; pf, parallel fibre; mo, molecular layer; sc, stellate cell. (Figure and legend from Eccles.[730]) **(C)** 0.5×, **(D)** 2×, and **(E)** 4× magnification of cerebellar cortex showing cerebellar folia and subfolia, and trilaminar cortex with Purkinje cell layer interleaved between the molecular layer above and the granule cell layer below. (Schmahmann laboratory in Schmahmann.[760]) **(F)** Cerebellar cortex studied with Bielschowsky silver stain (20×) showing Purkinje cell somata surrounded by the axonic pinceau of basket cells. (Schmahmann laboratory, courtesy of Dr. Matthew Frosch, in Schmahmann.[760])

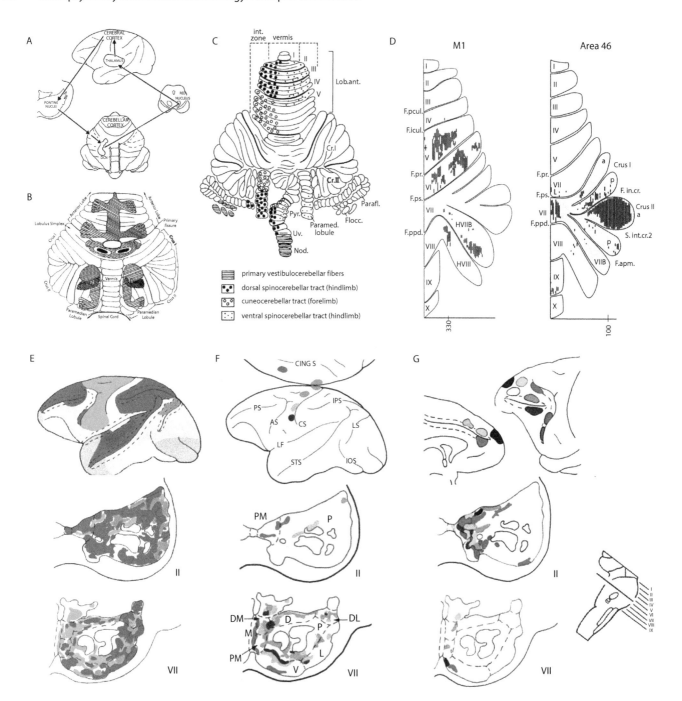

FIGURE 1-57. Essential systems neuroanatomy of the cerebellum. **(A)** The cerebrocerebellar circuit. (From Schmahmann.[749]) **(B)** Somatotopy identified by physiological mapping in monkeys. Note the silence of lobule VII (the hemispheric extensions of which are crus I and II). (Adapted from Snider and Eldred.[797]) **(C)** Somatotopy in cat with fibers from the dorsal and ventral spinocerebellar tracts and external cuneate nucleus[737,738] and primary vestibular fibers (Brodal and Hoivik[725]), all avoiding crus I and II. (Adapted from Brodal.[739]) **(D)** Reciprocal cerebrocerebellar connections between primary motor cerebral cortex (M1) cerebellar lobules V, VI, and some in lobule VIIIB contrasted with connections of dorsolateral prefrontal cortex area 46 with crus I and II and some in lobule IX. (Adapted from Kelly and Strick.[752]) **(E)** Corticopontine projections to pontine levels II and VII from multiple cerebral cortical areas showing regional heterogeneity and interdigitation of terminations. (Adapted from Schmahmann.[749]) **(F)** Motor cortex projections to the basis pontis topographically arranged in the caudal pontine nuclei. Note the relative abundance of projections in level VII compared to level II. (Adapted from Schmahmann et al.[750]) **(G)** Prefrontal cortex projections to the basis pontis topographically arranged and interdigitated in the rostral pontine nuclei. Note the relative abundance of projections in level II compared to level VII. (Adapted from Schmahmann and Pandya.[747]) AS, arcuate sulcus; CING S, cingulate sulcus; CS, central sulcus; D, dorsal pontine nucleus; DCN, deep cerebellar nuclei; DL, dorsolateral pontine nucleus; DM, dorsomedial pontine nucleus; F.apm., ansoparamedian fissure; F.icul., intraculminate fissure; F.in.cr., intracrural fissure; Flocc., flocculus; F.pcul., preculminate fissure; F. ppd., prepyramidal fissure; F.pr., primary fissure; F.ps., posterior superior fissure; int., intermediate; IOS, inferior occipital sulcus; IPS, intraparietal sulcus; L, lateral pontine nucleus; LF, lateral fissure; LS, lunate sulcus; M, median pontine nucleus; Nod., nodulus; P, peduncular pontine nucleus; PM, paramedian pontine nucleus; PS, principal sulcus; Pyr., pyramis; R, reticular pontine nucleus; S.int.cr.2, second intracrural sulcus; Uv, uvula; V, ventral pontine nucleus. (Figure and legend from Schmahmann et al.[252])

insular cortex involved in autonomic and pain modulation systems.[430,748,749] These associative corticopontine pathways are funneled through the cerebrocerebellar circuit within multiple parallel but partially overlapping loops converging with topographic ordering throughout the pons. The motor corticopontine projections are mostly in the caudal half of the pons.[740,748,750]

The pontine projections to the cerebellar cortex respect topographic specificity. The cerebellar anterior lobe and the adjacent part of lobule VI as well as lobule VIII are the motor cerebellum, linked with the motor and premotor cortices. In contrast, association areas in the prefrontal and posterior parietal cortices are linked with crus I and crus II of the posterior lobe.[751,752] These streams of information are acted upon by the cerebellar corticonuclear microcomplexes[732] and then transmitted via the deep cerebellar nuclei to thalamus before returning to the cerebral cortex.

Cerebellar projections to thalamus arise from fastigial and interpositus nuclei as well as from the dentate nucleus, and they are directed not only to the cerebellar recipient VL but also to CL, Pcn, the CM-Pf complex, and MD that have efferent projections to association cortices.

The cerebellar vermis, interconnected with the fastigial nucleus, is implicated in the control of posture, gait, and oculomotor control. It also influences the autonomic nervous system and is a critical node in the circuitry underlying neurobehavioral phenomena in animal models and in neuropsychiatric phenomena resulting from cerebellar lesions in patients.[251–253,256,753–755]

The vermis and fastigial nucleus have been proposed as the cerebellar representation of the limbic system.[251,753,755] Using the techniques of single-cell gene expression profiling, neuronal morphology, and anatomical circuit analyses of vermis output neurons in the mouse fastigial (medial cerebellar) nucleus, Fujita et al.[756] identified five major classes of fastigial nucleus glutamatergic projection neurons. Each fastigial cell type is connected with a specific set of Purkinje cells and inferior olive neurons, and in turn innervates a distinct collection of downstream targets that comprise cognitive, affective, and motor forebrain circuits. In the mouse model, the diverse cerebellar vermis functions are therefore mediated by modular synaptic connections of distinct fastigial cell types which differentially coordinate posturomotor, oromotor, positional-autonomic, orienting, and vigilance circuits.

The cerebellar dentate nucleus sends projections through thalamus to different areas of the frontal lobe in the monkeys.[757] The dorsomedial part of the dentate nucleus sends its projections to the motor cortex, whereas the ventrolateral and ventromedial parts of the dentate nucleus are connected with the prefrontal cortex, including area 9/46.[752,758] Further anatomical details of the cerebrocerebellar linkage and of the olivary inputs to cerebellum may be found elsewhere.[736,748,749,759–762]

Pathways linking the cerebellum with subcortical regions relevant to neuropsychiatry include reciprocal cerebellar connections with multiple hypothalamic nuclei (Fig. 1-58)[763–765] and the projections from the mammillary body to the pontocerebellar circuit.[766] *Direct hypothalamocerebellar projections* are derived primarily from the lateral, posterior, and dorsal hypothalamic areas; the supramammillary, tuberomammillary, and lateral mammillary nuclei; the dorsomedial and ventromedial nuclei; and the periventricular zone. They terminate in all layers of the cerebellar cortex, as histaminergic and occasionally as GABAergic fibers. *Hypothalamo-ponto-cerebellar projections* fibers originate in similar areas, mostly in the posterior hypothalamus.

The mammillary bodies have projections to the nucleus reticularis tegmenti pontis and to the medial pontine nuclei, both of which are important waystations between cerebral hemispheres and the cerebellum.[766] The *cerebello-hypothalamic projections* leave the deep cerebellar nuclei (fastigial, globose, emboliform, and dentate) via the superior cerebellar peduncle and are directed mostly to the contralateral hypothalamus, terminating in lateral, posterior, and dorsal hypothalamic areas and in the dorsomedial and paraventricular nuclei.[763–765] The connections of these subcortical regions are part of the critical neural substrates enabling the cerebellar modulation of autonomic function, limbic valence, and emotional control.[251,255]

The hypothalamocerebellar connections are relevant when considering that hypothalamic rage is evoked in cats by stimulation of the rostral and central parts of the fastigial nucleus of the cerebellum,[767] accompanied by elevated arterial pressure, tachypnea, mydriasis, and retraction of the nictitating membrane.[768,769] Social and appetitive behaviors under the control of the hypothalamus are also influenced by fastigial nucleus stimulation, including self-stimulation, eating, and grooming. These behaviors respond to changes in the availability of goal objects[770,771] consistent with the view that the fastigial nucleus functions as a modulator of emotional and visceral reaction patterns. These and other physiological, anatomical, and clinical observations of autonomic phenomena, grooming, feeding, and predatory behavior have been the impetus for considering the cerebellar fastigial nucleus and its interconnected vermis cortex as the cerebellar representation of the limbic system.[251,255,753,755]

Cerebellum has bidirectional connections with the hippocampus and these pathways have functional significance. Fastigial nucleus stimulation evokes discharges in the hippocampus,[772,773] with stimulation of the posterior vermis, fastigial nucleus, and intervening midline folia of the cerebellum evoking facilitation in the septal region, and inhibition in the hippocampus.[772] Stimulation of the hippocampus produces cerebellar responses in lobule VI.[773] Robert G. Heath's (1915–1999) physiological and lesion-degeneration anatomical studies in monkeys and cats concluded that fastigial nuclei are directly connected to the hippocampus (CA3, dentate gyrus, subiculum), amygdaloid complex, and cortical sites in the temporal lobe.[774] Contemporary anterograde and retrograde viral tracers in mouse brain indicate that the fastigial nucleus projects to the LD and VL thalamic nuclei which then project to retrosplenial cortex, rhinal cortex, and subiculum before terminating in the CA1 neurons and dentate gyrus of the hippocampus.[775] Task-based and functional connectivity MRI in humans reveals that the hippocampus and cerebellum are co-activated during tasks that require spatio-temporal prediction of movements on the basis of visuomotor integration.[776] Further, cognitive attributes of navigation recruit targeted cerebello-hippocampal circuits: *place-based* navigation is supported by coherent activity

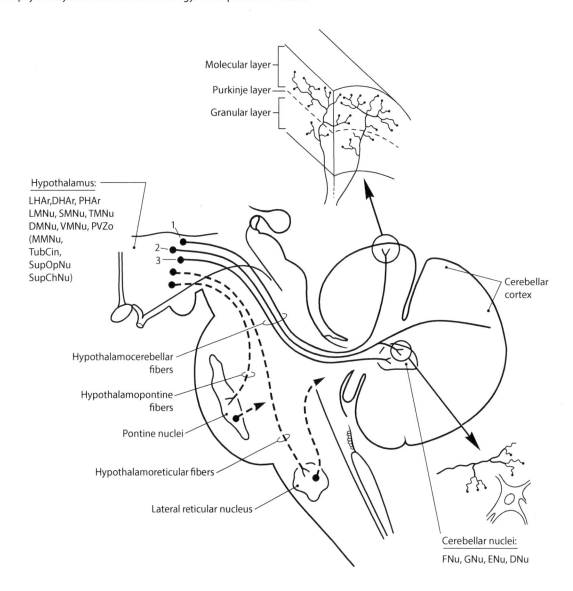

FIGURE 1-58. Diagrammatic representation of the different projections of the hypothalamus to the cerebellum and to the pontine nuclei and to the lateral reticular nucleus. Those cell groups listed under hypothalamus and out of parentheses are the prime source of hypothalamocerebellar fibers; those listed in parentheses give rise to fewer projections. Cell numbers 1, 2, and 3 are indicative of (1) hypothalamic cells that project only to the cortex, (2) hypothalamic cells that project to the cortex and send collaterals into the cerebellar nuclei, and (3) hypothalamic cells that project only to the cerebellar nuclei. Hypothalamus spinal fibers are not shown. (Figure and legend from Haines et al.[765])

between left cerebellar lobule VIIA crus I and medial parietal cortex along with right hippocampus activity, while *sequence-based* navigation is supported by coherent activity between right lobule VIIA crus I, medial prefrontal cortex, and left hippocampus.[777]

Amygdala-cerebellar interactions have also been identified. Inactivating or lesioning the central nucleus of the amygdala slows the acquisition rate of eyeblink conditioning, an associative learning paradigm known to be dependent on cerebellar lobule VI and the interpositus nucleus.[778,779] A model of amygdala-cerebellum interactions has been proposed whereby amygdala gates conditioned stimulus inputs to the cerebellum through a direct projection from the medial central nucleus to the basilar pontine nucleus, providing an attention-like mechanism that facilitates cerebellar learning as well as retrieval of cerebellar memory after learning has been established.[779]

Of great importance in the consideration of the cerebellar contribution to social-emotional processing is the optogenetic confirmation[780] of earlier findings that there are direct cerebellar fastigial nucleus projections to the VTA in the midbrain,[781,782] which in turn projects back to the cerebellum.[783,784] The VTA is the source of axons in the mesolimbic dopaminergic pathway conveyed by the MFB, described above with the hypothalamus, and the strong cerebellar contribution to the VTA, also seen with diffusion imaging tractography in humans,[98] is powerful evidence for the cerebellar role in this circuit. The functional relevance of this bidirectional fastigial nucleus-VTA communication is confirmed by the optogenetic technique which reveals that the cerebellar-VTA projection enables dynamic encoding and modulation of social-related signals.[780]

Cerebellar granule cell activity represents motor and sensory context as well as nonmotor properties of contextual information such as expectation of reward.[785] Studies are commencing on the likely role of the granule cells in the cerebellar encoding of a diverse array of functions that allows it to participate in motor, cognitive, and emotional processing. The importance of this approach is underscored by the recognition of the behavioral consequences of cerebellar disorders ranging from ataxia, dystonia, and tremor to neuropsychiatric conditions including autism spectrum disorders, schizophrenia, and attention-deficit/hyperactivity disorder.[256,786–789]

Imaging Studies of Functional Organization in the Human Cerebellum

rsfcMRI extends the anatomical investigations to humans using the physiological feature of fluctuating BOLD signal to infer anatomical connectivity. These studies show that activity in the cerebellar anterior lobe (most notably in lobules III through V), the adjacent part of lobules VI, and lobule VIII correlates with sensorimotor regions of the cerebral cortex. In contrast, activity in the cerebellar posterior lobe (mostly crus I and II of lobule VII) correlates with prefrontal, parietal, and temporal association areas and the cingulate gyrus (Figs. 1-30B,C and 1-59D).[398,790–793] Further, cerebellar correlations with intrinsic functional connectivity networks in the cerebral hemispheres reveal that lobules VI, crus I and crus II, and lobule IX correlate with the executive control network; lobule VI with the salience network; and lobule IX with the default network.[397]

A more complete notion of the sensorimotor and cognitive representations in the cerebellum emerges from the results of rsfcMRI[397,398] and task-based functional MRI[398,794–796] revealing two motor and three nonmotor representations in the cerebellar cortex. Building on earlier work of Snider and colleagues,[797] sensorimotor processing is represented twice in the cortex of each cerebellar hemisphere; first representation in lobules I–VI; second representation in lobule VIII. Further, cognitive functions in the domains of attentional/executive and default-mode processing has a triple representation: the first representation is in lobules VI–crus I; the second in lobules crus II–VIIB; and the third in lobules IX–X. rsfcMRI studies of the dentate nucleus extends the anatomical connectional data from monkeys to the different compartments of the nucleus in humans (Fig. 1-59D).[399]

Task-based functional MRI indicates that the cerebellar anterior lobe, adjacent parts of lobule VI, and lobule VIII are activated in sensorimotor tasks; lobules VI and VII in the posterior lobe are active during language, spatial, and executive function tasks; and affective processing engages the posterior lobes, including the vermis (Fig. 1-59A,B,D).[398,794,795] Working memory and executive functions engage lobules VI and VII, language recruits posterolateral cerebellum on the right, and spatial tasks recruit it on the left. Affective/emotional processing and pain and autonomic functions involve lobules VI and VII in the vermis more than the hemispheres.[798] Task paradigms in cerebellum are becoming more nuanced, and it is apparent that in the domain of spatial attentional, encoding is medially situated in lobule VIIB whereas attentional load is more lateral.[799]

The anterior lobe is not engaged in cognitive tasks; the posterior lobe is not involved in motor tasks except for rostral parts of lobule VI and the second sensorimotor representation in lobule VIII.[794,795,800,801] Sensorimotor control is therefore topographically separate and distinct from cognitive and emotional regulation in the cerebellum. In sum, the cerebellar anterior lobe (lobules I through V) and parts of medial lobule VI, together with lobule VIII of the posterior lobe and the globose and emboliform nuclei (or, more accurately the interpositus nucleus in the experimental animal), constitute the sensorimotor cerebellum. Lobule VII (that includes crus I and crus II of lobule VIIA, and lobule VIIB), more posterior parts of lobule VI, and the ventral part of the dentate nucleus constitute the anatomical substrate of the cognitive cerebellum. The limbic cerebellum corresponds to the fastigial nucleus and the cerebellar vermis, particularly the posterior vermis. Lobule IX is likely part of the default mode network, and lobule X is an essential node in the vestibular system, also with a role in cognition, having been identified recently as the location of a third cognitive representation.

Little is known about which parts of the cerebellar white matter convey afferent and efferent fibers to which specific cerebellar lobules. Nuclei in the rostral part of the basis pontis project via the MCP to the posterior lobe of the cerebellum, and those in the caudal basis pontis project to the anterior cerebellum,[802,803] but more precise information concerning MCP organization remains to be elucidated. The degree to which there is anatomical and functional differentiation within the superior cerebellar peduncle efferents to thalamus is also not presently known. The topographical organization of motor, cognitive, and affective domains in cerebellum[251,254] suggests that defining the arrangement of the cerebellar white matter pathways that connect with extracerebellar structures will be important. This has potential clinically relevance, exemplified by the finding that in relapsing remitting multiple sclerosis which attacks white matter pathways, patients with cognitive impairment have greater pathology involving the MCPs, the main source of input to cerebellum from sensorimotor, multimodal association, and paralimbic regions of the cerebral cortex.[804]

Clinical Features of Cerebellar Lesions

There are three principal clinical syndromes that arise following cerebellar lesions.

The cerebellar motor syndrome of gait ataxia, appendicular dysmetria, dysarthric speech, and oculomotor abnormalities results from lesions that affect the anterior lobe of the cerebellum, notably lobules I through V, with lobule VI (Fig. 1-59C) likely engaged in motor control in a manner possibly equivalent to premotor regions of the cerebral cortex.[252,794,795,805] Lesions in the second sensorimotor area in lobule VIII at the medial part of the posterior lobe[797,806] produce only minimal cerebellar motor signs.[805,807]

The vestibulocerebellar syndrome incudes prominent vestibular symptoms (vertigo, nausea, emesis) together with oculomotor abnormalities, arising from lesions that involve lobules IX and X of the posterior and flocculonodular lobes.[808,809]

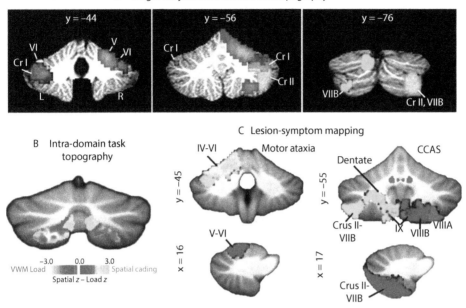

FIGURE 1-59. Human cerebellar functional topography. (A) Intraindividual topography of task-based activations in the cerebellum for finger tapping (red), working memory (purple), verb generation (blue), and mental rotation (green). (From Stoodley et al.[801]) **(B)** Spatial gradients within the dorsal attention network in lobule VIIB on a working memory task. The locus of spatial attention encoding is medially situated; attentional load content is more lateral. This gradient of activity also exists within the cortical dorsal attention network (not shown). (Adapted from Brissenden et al.[799]) **(C)** Lesions of lobules IV–V of the anterior lobe extending into adjacent lobule VI produce the cerebellar motor syndrome of ataxia in patients with stroke. Lesions confined to posterior lobe lobules crus II through lobule IX produce the cerebellar cognitive affective/Schmahmann syndrome but no motor ataxia. (Adapted from Stoodley et al.[807]) **(D)** Task and resting-state activation reveal topography in motor and nonmotor domains. Task activation (top row) reveals a pattern of two motor (first column) and three nonmotor representations (second and third columns). An overlapping pattern is observed when calculating resting-state functional connectivity from cerebral cortical activation peaks for each corresponding task activity contrast (bottom row). First motor (lobules I–VI) or first nonmotor representation (VI/crus I) (green arrows), second motor (VIII) or second nonmotor representation (crus II/lobule VIIB) (yellow arrows), and third nonmotor representation (IX/X) (red arrows) are shown. First and second nonmotor representations can be contiguous (as in story listening) or separate (as in working memory). (Adapted from Guell et al.[398]) CCAS, cerebellar cognitive affective syndrome; Cr, crus; L, left; R, right; VWM, verbal working memory. (Composite figure and legend from Schmahmann et al.[252])

TABLE 1-3. Neuropsychiatric Manifestations in Cerebellar Disorders.

	Positive (Exaggerated) Symptoms	Negative (Diminished) Symptoms
Attentional control	Inattentiveness	Ruminativeness
	Distractibility	Perseveration
	Hyperactivity	Difficulty shifting focus of attention
	Compulsive and ritualistic behaviors	Obsessional thoughts
Emotional control	Impulsiveness, disinhibition	Anergy, anhedonia
	Lability, unpredictability	Sadness, hopelessness
	Incongruous feelings, pathological laughing/crying	Dysphoria
	Anxiety, agitation, panic	Depression
Autism spectrum	Stereotypical behaviors	Avoidant behaviors, tactile defensiveness
	Self-stimulation behaviors	Easy sensory overload
Psychosis spectrum	Illogical thought	Lack of empathy
	Paranoia	Muted affect, emotional blunting, apathy
Social skill set	Anger, aggression	Passivity, immaturity, childishness
	Irritability	Difficulty with social cues and interactions
	Overly territorial	Unawareness of social boundaries
	Oppositional behavior	Overly gullible and trusting

Source: From Schmahmann et al.[813]

The cerebellar cognitive affective syndrome (CCAS),[256] now Schmahmann syndrome,[810,011] occurs following lesions of the major expansion of the cerebellar hemispheres, that is, lobules crus I and II and lobule VIIB in the posterior lobe.[256,788,805,807,812] The CCAS is characterized by deficits in executive function, visual spatial performance, linguistic processing, and affective dysregulation. Executive impairments include deficits in working memory, motor or ideational set shifting, and perseveration. Verbal fluency is impaired to the point of telegraphic speech or mutism. Visuospatial disintegration impairs attempts to draw or copy a diagram, conceptualization of figures can be disorganized, and some patients display simultanagnosia. Anomia, agrammatic speech, and abnormal syntactic structure are observed, with abnormal prosody characterized by high-pitched, hypophonic whining. Abnormal modulation of behavior and personality is notable with posterior lobe lesions that involve the vermis and fastigial nucleus. This manifests as flattening of affect alternating or coexistent with disinhibited behaviors such as overfamiliarity, flamboyant and impulsive actions, and humorous but inappropriate and flippant comments. Regressive, childlike behaviors and obsessive-compulsive traits can be observed. Autonomic changes are noted following lesions of the fastigial nucleus and vermis, manifesting as bradycardia and syncope, or tachycardia in the setting of acquired panic disorder.[256,813] The principal features and clinical relevance of the CCAS have been replicated in adults with stroke,[814,815] in children who have undergone excision of cerebellar tumors,[431,816,817] and in other acquired and developmental disorders of the cerebellum.[786,788,811,818–825] Deficits in social cognition[826] and emotional expression in patients with strokes and neurodegenerative lesions have been linked to involvement of the cerebellar system.[827,828] The range of neuropsychiatric

impairments in the setting of cerebellar lesions falls into five major behavioral domains: attentional control, emotional control, social skill set, autism spectrum disorders, and psychosis spectrum disorders (Table 1-3).[813]

The postoperative pediatric cerebellar mutism syndrome (previously, posterior fossa syndrome) represents a particularly acute form of the CCAS.[431,816,829–831] Within 48 hours following surgical resection of midline tumors of the cerebellum, children develop mutism, buccal and lingual apraxia, apathy, and poverty of spontaneous movement. Emotional lability is marked by rapid fluctuation from irritability and agitation to giggling and easy distractibility. In a structure-function analysis of this phenomenon using contemporary imaging methodology[832] the CCAS was present in ~25% of patients, and the responsible damage was in the cerebellar outflow system (cerebellar cortex, nuclei, superior cerebellar peduncle) to cognitively relevant MD thalamic nucleus and limbically valent anterior thalamic nuclei as well as the left temporal region important for language. Damage to the fastigial nucleus and vermal lobules IX and X is in accord with the notion that fastigial nucleus and vermis are the limbic cerebellum,[251,252,833] and with the observation that these vermal lobules are substrates for the third representation of cognitive processing.[397,398] Damage to the dentate nucleus is consistent with convergent evidence that the ventral part of the dentate nucleus is anatomically and functionally linked to cognitive systems.[758]

The cerebrocerebellar system is thus defined by the duality of (i) a unique, lattice-like cerebellar cytoarchitecture with repeating corticonuclear microcomplexes enabling a consistent cerebellar computation, set against (ii) the modular organization of cerebellar connections with cerebral cortex within the framework of the feedforward connections through pons and the feedback connections through thalamus. This anatomical organization is the substrate for the theories of dysmetria of thought[251,252,255,256,749] and the universal cerebellar transform.[252,254,255,755,834] This idea holds that the cerebellum plays an essential role in automatization and in optimizing the full range of behaviors around a homeostatic baseline, preventing overshoot or undershoot, and doing so according to the context of the internal and external environment; that the cerebellum modulates cognition and emotion in the same way that it coordinates motor control; and that disruption of the neural circuitry linking the cerebellum with the association and paralimbic cerebral regions prevents the cerebellar modulation of functions subserved by the affected subsystems, thereby impairing the regulation of movement, cognition, and emotion. This loss of the universal cerebellar transform leads to gait and appendicular ataxia, dysarthria, and oculomotor abnormalities when the motor cerebellum is involved, and the CCAS when the cognitive and limbic cerebellar regions are damaged.[251,252,254–256,749,755,834] The theories of dysmetria of thought and the universal cerebellar transform were foundational in the subsequent development of the specific principles of organization of cerebral cortical connections discussed earlier.

CEREBROSPINAL FLUID AND CEREBRAL VENTRICLES

Historical Note

(Adapted from Schmahmann and Pandya[15])

The earliest notions of brain function revolved around the chambers that form the brain's ventricles. At the center of Galen's physiological conceptions was the notion that natural spirit, a mysterious substance indispensable for life and originating in the liver, transforms into vital spirit conveyed by the heart to the brain, and this in turn transforms into the more refined animal spirit. A necessary ingredient for this brain process was air inspired into the cerebral ventricles. Whereas Galen proposed that mental faculties were localized in the brain, Herophilus of Chalcedon (c. 330–260 BCE) and medieval writers such as Nemesius, Bishop of Emesa (c.A.D. 390, published manuscript 1512), and St. Augustine (4th century) believed that mental faculties resided in the cerebral ventricles. Albert von Bollstädt (Albertus Magnus, 1193–1280) first depicted the cerebral ventricles in *Philosophia Naturalis* (published 1496), in which he localized common sense in the frontal lobes, imagination in the midbrain, and memory in the cerebellum or in the four ventricles. Mondino dei Luzzi (Mundinus, 1275–1326) wrote his *Anothomia* in 1316 (first printed in 1478) and ascribed fantasy and retention to the anterior compartment of the lateral ventricles, special senses in the middle compartment, imagination and the ability to combine separate things in the posterior compartment. The third ventricle was endowed with the power of cognition and prognostication, and the fourth ventricle was concerned with the reception of impressions and memory (Clarke and O'Malley).[18] The drawings of Gregor Reisch (c. 1467–1525) in *Margarita Philosophica* (1503) further perpetuated the notion

that complex functions reside in the ventricles, with functional specialization according to the different parts of the ventricular system. Leonardo da Vinci (1452–1519) successfully made the first wax casts of the cerebral ventricles, although his anatomical drawings did not become available until 1784.

The renaissance in neuroscience commenced in 1543 with Andreas Vesalius' (1514–1564) *De Humani Corporis Fabrica* (*On the Structure of the Human Body*), and the scientific method arguably began with Thomas Willis (1621–1675) and Nicolaus Steno (Niels Stensen, 1638–1686). CSF thereafter became progressively relegated to the role of a shock absorber cushioning the central nervous system from trauma against the inner table of the skull or spinal cord, and together with the ventricles notable mostly for clinical relevance in hydrocephalus and as diagnostic markers in neurological/neurosurgical diseases.

Current Understanding of Cerebrospinal Fluid

The long-held view about CSF production and absorption was that it emanates exclusively from the choroid plexus, circulates through the ventricular system, makes its way to the cerebral convexities, and is reabsorbed by the arachnoid granulations back into the systemic circulation. The system appears to be more nuanced and complex.

CSF Constituents

CSF is an active secretion, clear, and colorless, 99% water compared to 92% water of plasma. It has a lower concentration than plasma of protein, potassium, and urea, and a higher concentration of chloride and magnesium. It also has lower levels of protein and most amino acids, except for glutamine which has a higher concentration in CSF than in plasma.[835] Red blood cells are not typically present in CSF and there are less than five white blood cells per mm^3. Glucose levels are between 45 and 80 mg/dl, protein level is 20–40 mg/dl.[836]

Production

Most of the CSF (66–75%) is secreted by the choroid plexuses,[837,838] which are expansions of the ependymal epithelium lining the lateral, third, and fourth ventricles. The choroid plexuses are highly folded and vascularized structures consisting of a single-layered cuboidal or low cylindrical epithelium residing on a basement membrane. The luminal surface area of the choroid plexus epithelial cells is densely covered by microvilli and possess either one primary cilia or small tufts of motile cilia. CSF production at the choroid plexus is mediated by exchange and transport of ions (especially chloride, sodium, and bicarbonate) across the epithelial cells, which generates an osmotic gradient that drives the movement of water from the blood to the ventricle lumen.[839] A novel view holds that the rest of the CSF formation occurs by filtration and flux of fluid through the capillary walls, and that the respective volumes of CSF and interstitial fluid mainly depend on hydrostatic and osmotic forces between the CSF and brain parenchyma created by gradients of proteins and inorganic ions across the capillary membrane.[840] The daily production of CSF in adults is 500–600 mL. CSF pressure in adults is about 100 mm H_2O, with a pulsatile flow depending upon arterial hemodynamics in the choroid plexus.[837,841] Total CSF space in young adults is about 160 mL, comprising more than half the brain interstitial fluid volume. The ratio of CSF volume to brain volume increases in aging and neurodegeneration. Clearance of brain metabolites depends on rate of CSF renewal, which is totally replaced about four times each day.

Flow

Flow is from the lateral ventricles through the paired foramina of Monro into the IIIrd ventricle, traveling down the aqueduct of Sylvius (Franciscus de le Boë, or Sylvius [1614–1672]) to the IVth ventricle, where it escapes through the laterally placed foramina of Luschka (Hubert von Luschka [1820–1875]) and the midline foramen of Magendie (François Magendie [1783–1855]) into the basal cisterns, and is then convected into the spinal and cortical subarachnoid spaces. From the cortical subarachnoid space, it penetrates the brain parenchyma perivascularly and bathes the brain before it exits the CNS and drains into the lymphatic system.[18,191,839]

Return

The teaching has been that CSF is absorbed by arachnoid villi into the cerebral venous sinuses and veins via a valve-like mechanism called bulk flow, with a minor portion of the CSF absorbed into the cerebral vessels by simple diffusion, and another small portion likely absorbed via the lymphatics of the cribriform plate region to the nasal submucosa.[838] There is general agreement that CSF returns from the subarachnoid space to the macrocirculation by multiple routes, but the results of investigations over the past two decades have indicated that CSF does not return to the venous circulation primarily via the arachnoid granulations. It has been suggested, rather, that CSF passes through ventriculo-subarachnoid spaces, by bulk flow into Virchow-Robin perivascular spaces and the sleeves of the subarachnoid space surrounding cranial nerves that enter the nose and eyes, and through the cribriform plate (via the glymphatic system) where it reaches the nasal submucosa and downstream cervical lymphatics, along spinal nerves (Fig. 1-60).[837,839,842]

Glymphatic System

(Adapted from Jessen et al.[839])

The glymphatic system is a recently discovered waste clearance system that utilizes a unique system of perivascular channels, formed by astroglial cells, to promote efficient elimination of soluble proteins and metabolites from the central nervous system. It was named the glymphatic system based on its functional similarity to the lymphatic system in peripheral tissue, and the important role of glial aquaporin-4 channels in convective fluid transport. Aquaporin-4 is a water channel protein that belongs to the aquaporin family of integral membrane proteins that conduct water through the cell membrane; it is localized to astrocytic endfeet and plays a central role in facilitating the exchange of CSF and interstitial fluid along periarterial influx pathways as well as interstitial solute clearance through perivascular drainage pathways. Besides waste elimination, the glymphatic system may also function to help distribute non-waste compounds in the brain, such as glucose, lipids, amino acids, and neurotransmitters related to volume transmission.

CSF is driven into the perivascular space by pulse waves created by smooth muscle cells of the penetrating leptomeningeal arteries diving into the brain from the cortical surface. Glymphatic transport of CSF along the periarterial spaces is followed by convective flow through the brain parenchyma and exit of interstitial fluid along the perivenous space to the cervical lymph system. Constant production of CSF by the choroid plexus creates pressure that dictates the direction of the fluid flow through the ventricular system to the subarachnoid space. Respiration is also instrumental in movement of CSF in this system.

The glymphatic system functions mainly during sleep and is largely disengaged during wakefulness. This may have relevance for the role of sleep in eliminating potentially neurotoxic waste products including β-amyloid. Activity of the glymphatic system declines sharply with age, and it is suppressed in some neurodegenerative diseases including Alzheimer's disease, vascular dementia, stroke, and following traumatic brain injury.

Neural Stem Cells

CSF plays a central role in the maintenance and transport of neural stem cells (NSCs) both in the developing brain and in adult life. Neurogenesis persists in two regions in the postnatal brain: the ventricular subventricular zone located in the walls of the lateral ventricles, and the subgranular zone in the dentate gyrus of the hippocampus. NSCs originating in the ventricular-subventricular zone migrate a long way into the olfactory bulb where they differentiate into local circuit interneurons. In embryonic life, direct contact between NSCs and CSF is necessary for survival, replication, and neural differentiation. In the adult brain CSF also appears to be necessary for NSC migratory guidance.[843–845]

Clinical Relevance

Analysis of CSF has long been used clinically for diagnosing a comprehensive range of infections, inflammatory conditions, and immunologically based illnesses such as multiple sclerosis, and paraneoplastic and non-paraneoplastic autoimmune brain disorders. The use of CSF mechanisms of entry into the nervous system for the delivery of chemotherapeutic agents serves as a model for the delivery of novel therapies on the horizon including antisense oligonucleotides and other viral vector-mediated treatments for previously intractable genetic disorders.

Obstructive hydrocephalus as a complication of space-occupying lesions or aqueductal stenosis may be a neurosurgical emergency. The more slowly evolving normal pressure hydrocephalus with its clinical triad of cognitive and neuropsychiatric decline, gait impairment, and urinary incontinence[846–848] is diagnosed by the combination of clinical and imaging features together with the removal of a large volume of CSF (~40 cc) and is treated usually by ventriculoperitoneal drainage. Ventriculomegaly is frequently seen in aging populations and

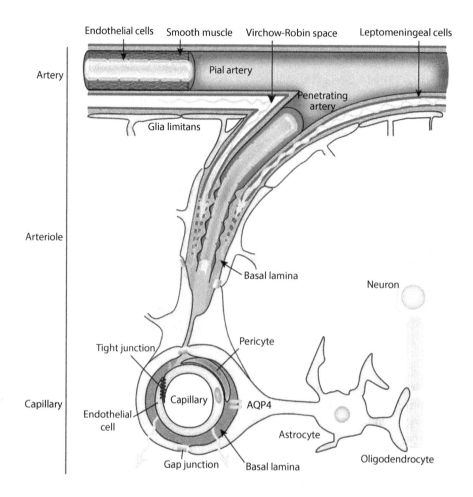

FIGURE 1-60. The cerebrospinal fluid neurovascular unit. The structure and function of the neurovascular unit allow bidirectional communication between the microvasculature and neurons, with astrocytes playing intermediary roles. Pial arteries in the subarachnoid space bathed in CSF become penetrating arteries upon diving into the brain parenchyma. The perivascular space around penetrating arteries is termed the Virchow-Robin space. As the penetrating arteries branch into arterioles and capillaries the CSF-containing Virchow-Robin spaces narrow and finally disappear. However, the perivascular space extends to arterioles and capillaries to venules where it is made up by the basal lamina's extracellular matrix that provides a continuity of the fluid space between arterioles and venules. Astrocytic vascular endfeet expressing aquaporin-4 (AQP4) surround the entire vasculature and form the boundary of the perivascular spaces. (Figure and legend from Jessen et al.[839])

in neurodegenerative disorders, and ongoing investigations are focused on determining whether this is a result of *ex vacuo* dilatation of the ventricles because of primary loss of cerebral volume, or whether the enlarged ventricles have a pathophysiological role in the neurodegenerative disorder.

Slow leakage of CSF out of the subarachnoid space leads to CSF hypotension syndrome, presenting principally with headache when standing and relieved by recumbency, and often with prominent enhancement of the leptomeninges on brain imaging.[838] A less common but striking constellation resulting from CSF leakage is the sagging brain syndrome, the clinical manifestations of which can resemble the neuropsychiatric phenomena seen in frontotemporal dementia including obsessive-compulsive behaviors, often accompanied by impairments of gait and motor control.[849] The sunken flap syndrome is a similar and marked consequence seen in patients who have undergone craniectomy, often accompanied also by cognitive and motor manifestations.[850]

Elevated intracranial pressure may be a presenting sign of a space-occupying lesion, with headache, vomiting, and papilledema. It is also seen in communicating hydrocephalus, and in idiopathic intracranial hypertension or pseudotumor cerebri, previously known as benign intracranial hypertension but which is not always benign because it can be accompanied by progressive visual loss with only tunnel vision preserved.

In patients with intracerebral or subarachnoid hemorrhage, when the ventricle is breached the prognosis is substantially worse.[851] Even in patients in whom there is primary intraventricular hemorrhage, the clinical constellation includes a marked confusional state which does not always recover even after the hemorrhage has resolved, for reasons that have not yet adequately been explained but that may be related to neurotoxic effect of iron and hemoglobin on periventricular organs.[851,852]

Impaired dynamics of CSF flow are present in Chiari malformations as well as the often accompanying syringomyelia,[853,854] relevant for neuropsychiatry because of the increasing awareness of neuropsychiatric presentations in the setting of Chiari I malformation.[855]

CONCLUSIONS

The premise of this chapter is that the theory and practice of behavioral neurology/neuropsychiatry are fundamentally predicated on a deep understanding of the structures within the nervous system and the connections that link these structures together with topographical precision in geographically distributed, functionally interdependent neural circuits. Integrated with these channels that comprise the anatomical hard wiring of the brain are the neurotransmitters that influence the state of the organism, and the physiology of both the individual neural components and the interconnected dynamic systems. We have considered how the brain is constructed in a hierarchical and interdependent manner to enable feeling states—autonomic imperatives related to the internal milieu, emotional tone salient to individual survival, and altruistic drives related to societal well-being, woven together with perception, language, memory, reasoning, and judgement in order to sense, respond to, and exert control over inner state, motivations, and actions. Increasingly hierarchical levels of behavior are defined by their distance from the automatic stimulus-response bond, matched by the progressive differentiation of cerebral cortical cytoarchitecture according to the theory of the dual origin of the cerebral cortex and the evolution of the cortical areas upon which the theory is predicated.

We considered the general and specific principles of organization of the connections of the cerebral cortex to conceptualize in a reductionistic manner how complex neural systems enable the emergent properties of drive, motivation, emotion, sensorimotor processing, and cognitive operations—from such seemingly simple pastimes as daydreaming to the highest forms of deductive reasoning, reflective thought and human accomplishment

(John Dewey, 1859–1952[856,857]). The "inextricable interwovenness of the cognitive, emotional, visceral, and somatic realms of human experience"[858] is the basis of neuropsychiatry. Behavioral neurology and neuropsychiatry are among the most demanding and challenging disciplines in the clinical neurological sciences precisely because the details of the evolution and dissolution of the nervous system[859] are as nuanced and complex as the individuals and societies to which these fields are devoted. Sensorimotor systems that are the basis of traditional neurology provide additional clues to diagnosis and to anatomical or system localization, but the principal challenge for behavioral neurology/neuropsychiatry is to understand how the neural systems that support complex behaviors are organized, how they disintegrate, and how to use that information for diagnostic and therapeutic purposes. This makes it possible for the increasingly sophisticated field of clinical cognitive neuroscience to accept the challenge and improve the human condition one patient at a time. To accomplish this goal, the practitioner must be versed in the neuroanatomical foundations detailed in this chapter.

ACKNOWLEDGMENTS

Supported in part by the National Ataxia Foundation, the MINDlink Foundation, and Mrs Mary Jo Reston. The assistance of Jason MacMore, BA, is gratefully acknowledged. The author thanks the editors for their detailed critique and helpful suggestions as the manuscript evolved. This chapter is dedicated to Professor Deepak N. Pandya, my teacher, mentor, and friend who recently passed away. He is widely regarded as one of our greatest neuroanatomists whose brilliant ideas and meticulous investigations changed the way we understand the architecture, connections, origins and functions of the brain. He was the epitome of a gentleman and a scholar, he was devoted to his family and his students, and his humility, kindness and generosity inspired me and generations of colleagues.

References

1. Pakkenberg B, Gundersen HJ. Neocortical neuron number in humans: effect of sex and age. *J Comp Neurol.* 1997;384(2):312-320.
2. Nauta W. Some efferent connections of the prefrontal cortex in the monkey. In: Warren JM, Akert K, eds. *The Frontal Granular Cortex and Behavior.* New York, NY: McGraw-Hill; 1964:397-409.
3. Luria AR. Higher cortical functions in man. Prefaces to the English edition by Hans-Lukas Teuber and Karl H. Pribram. Authorized translation from the Russian by Basil Haigh. New York, NY: Basic Books; 1966.
4. Geschwind N. Disconnexion syndromes in animals and man. I. *Brain.* 1965;88(2):237-294.
5. Geschwind N. Disconnexion syndromes in animals and man. II. *Brain.* 1965;88(3):585-644.
6. Pandya DN, Kuypers HG. Cortico-cortical connections in the rhesus monkey. *Brain Res.* 1969;13(1):13-36.
7. Jones EG, Powell TP. An anatomical study of converging sensory pathways within the cerebral cortex of the monkey. *Brain.* 1970;93(4):793-820.

8. Mesulam MM. A cortical network for directed attention and unilateral neglect. *Ann. Neurol.* 1981;10(4):309-325.
9. Mesulam MM. Large-scale neurocognitive networks and distributed processing for attention, language, and memory. *Annals of Neurology.* 1990;28(5):597-613.
10. Mesulam MM. From sensation to cognition. *Brain.* 1998;121 (pt 6):1013-1052.
11. Ungerleider LG, Mishkin M. Two cortical visual systems. In: Ingle DJ, Goodale MA, Mansfield RJW, eds. *Analysis of Visual Behavior.* Cambridge, MA: MIT Press; 1982:549-586.
12. Pandya DN, Yeterian EH. Architecture and connections of cortical association areas. In: Peters A, Jones EG, eds. *Cerebral Cortex.* Vol 4. New York, NY: Plenum Press; 1985:3-61.
13. Goldman-Rakic PS. Topography of cognition: parallel distributed networks in primate association cortex. *Annu Rev Neurosci.* 1988;11:137-156.
14. Selemon LD, Goldman-Rakic PS. Topographic intermingling of striatonigral and striatopallidal neurons in the rhesus monkey. *J Comp Neurol.* 1990;297(3):359-376.

15. Schmahmann JD, Pandya DN. *Fiber Pathways of the Brain*. New York, NY: Oxford University Press; 2006.

16. Schmahmann JD, Pandya DN. Disconnection syndromes of basal ganglia, thalamus, and cerebrocerebellar systems. *Cortex*. 2008;44(8):1037-1066.

17. Neuburger M. Die historische Entwicklung der experimentellen Gehirn-und Rückenmarksphysiologie vor Flourens. Ferdinand Enke Verlag, Stuttgart, 1897. Translated and edited, with additional material, by Edwin Clarke. *The Historical Development of Experimental Brain and Spinal Cord Physiology Before Flourens*. Baltimore, MD: Johns Hopkins University Press; 1981.

18. Clarke E, O'Malley CD. *The Human Brain and Spinal Cord. A Historical Study Illustrated by Writings from Antiquity to the Twentieth Century*. 2nd ed. San Francisco, CA: Norman Publishing; 1996.

19. Schmahmann JD, Pandya DN. Cerebral white matter—historical evolution of facts and notions concerning the organization of the fiber pathways of the brain. *J Hist Neurosci*. 2007;16(3):237-267.

20. Gall FJ, Spurzheim G. *Anatomie et Physiologie du Systeme Nerveux en general, et du Cerveau en particulier*. Paris: Chez F. Schoell; 1810.

21. Milner BL. A commentary on "disconnexion syndromes in animals and man". *Neuropsychol Rev*. 2010;20(2):126-127.

22. Brodmann K. *Vergleichende Lokalisationslehre der Grosshirnrinde*. Leipzig: Barth; 1909.

23. Campbell AW. *Histological Studies on the Localisation of Cerebral Function*. Cambridge: University Press; 1905.

24. Vogt C, Vogt O. Allgemeinere Ergebnisse unserer Hirnforschung. *J Psych Neurol*. 1919;24:279-462.

25. Walker A. A cytoarchitectural study of the prefrontal area of the macaque monkey. *J Comp Neurol*. 1940;73:59-86.

26. Bonin G von, Bailey P. *The Neocortex of Macaca mulatta*. Urbana, IL: University of Illinois Press; 1947.

27. von Economo C, Koskinas G. *Die cytoarchitektonik der Hirnrinde des erwachsenen Menschen*. Berlin: Springer; 1925.

28. Sarkisov SA. Atlas tsitoarkhitektoniki kory bol'shogo mozga cheloveka. Institut mozga (Akademiia meditsinskikh nauk SSSR). 1955.

29. Pandya DN, Seltzer B, Petrides M, Cipolloni PB. *Cerebral Cortex: Architecture, Connections, and the Dual Origin Concept*. New York, NY: Oxford University Press; 2015.

30. Amunts K, Zilles K. Architectonic mapping of the human brain beyond Brodmann. *Neuron*. 2015;88:1086-1107. JuBrain Cytoarchitectonic Atlas Viewer. 0. Institute of Neuroscience and Medicine. Structural and functional organization of the brain (INM-1). Available at www.jubrain.fz-juelich.de.

31. Scheperjans F, Eickhoff SB, Hömke L, et al. Probabilistic maps, morphometry, and variability of cytoarchitectonic areas in the human superior parietal cortex. *Cereb Cortex*. 2008;18(9):2141-2157.

32. Amunts K, Lepage C, Borgeat L, et al. BigBrain: an ultrahigh-resolution 3D human brain model. *Science*. 2013;340(6139):1472-1475. Available at www.humanbrainproject.eu/en/explore-the-brain/atlases/#bigbrain.

33. Hoch MJ, Bruno MT, Faustin A, et al. 3T MRI whole-brain microscopy discrimination of subcortical anatomy, part 1: brain stem. *AJNR Am J Neuroradiol*. 2019;40(3):401--407.

34. Hoch MJ, Bruno MT, Faustin A, et al. 3T MRI whole-brain microscopy discrimination of subcortical anatomy, part 2: basal forebrain. *AJNR Am J Neuroradiol*. 2019;40(7):1095--1105.

35. Gudden B von. Experimentaluntersuchungen über das peripherische und centrale Nervensystem. *Archiv für Psychiatrie und Nervenkrankheiten*. 1870;2:693-723.

36. von Monakow C. Über einige durch Extirpation circumscripter Hirnrinden regionen bedingte Entwickelungshemmungen des Kanninchengehirns. *Archiv für Psychiatrie und Nervenkrankheiten*. 1882;12:141-156.

37. Marchi V, Algeri G. Sulle degenerazioni discendenti consecutive a lesioni della corteccia cerebrale. *Riv Sper d freniat*. 1885;11:492-494.

38. Bielschowsky M. Die Silberimprägnation der Achsencylinder. *Neurologisches Zentralblatt*. 1902;21:579-584.

39. Dusser de Barenne JG. Experimental researches on sensory localizations in the cerebral cortex. *Quart J Exp Physiol*. 1916;9:355-390.

40. Mendelow H, Wright MK. A critique of strychnine neuronography as a method of defining area 4s in the monkey. *Brain*. 1955;78(3): 433-440.

41. Nauta WJ, Gygax PA. Silver impregnation of degenerating axon terminals in the central nervous system: (1) technic. (2) Chemical notes. *Stain Technol*. 1951;26:5-11.

42. Nauta WJ, Gygax PA. Silver impregnation of degenerating axons in the central nervous system: a modified technic. *Stain Technol*. 1954;29:91-93.

43. Cowan WM, Gottlieb DI, Hendrickson AE, Price JL, Woolsey TA. The autoradiographic demonstration of axonal connections in the central nervous system. *Brain Res*. 1972;37:21-51.

44. LaVail JH, LaVail MM. Retrograde axonal transport in the central nervous system. *Science*. 1972;176:1416-1417.

45. Mesulam MM. The blue reaction product in horseradish peroxidase neurohistochemistry: incubation parameters and visibility. *J Histochem Cytochem*. 1976;24:1273-1280.

46. Mesulam MM. Tetramethyl benzidine for horseradish peroxidase neurohistochemistry: a non-carcinogenic blue reaction product with superior sensitivity for visualizing neural afferents and efferents. *J Histochem Cytochem*. 1978;26:106-117.

47. Harper CG, Gonatas JO, Stieber A, Gonatas NK. In vivo uptake of wheat germ agglutinin-horseradish peroxidase conjugates into neuronal GERL and lysosomes. *Brain Res*. 1980;188:465-472.

48. Kuypers HG, Bentivoglio M, Catsman-Berrevoets CE, Bharos AT. Double retrograde neuronal labeling through divergent axon collaterals, using two fluorescent tracers with the same excitation wavelength which label different features of the cell. *Exp Brain Res*. 1980;40:383-392.

49. Gerfen CR, Sawchenko PE. An anterograde neuroanatomical tracing method that shows the detailed morphology of neurons, their axons and terminals: immunohistochemical localization of an axonally transported plant lectin, *Phaseolus vulgaris* leucoagglutinin (PHA-L). *Brain Res*. 1984;290:219-238.

50. Veenman CL, Reiner A, Honig MG. Biotinylated dextran amine as an anterograde tracer for single- and double-labeling studies. *J Neurosci Methods*. 1992;41:239-254.

51. Ugolini G, Kuypers HG, Strick PL. Transneuronal transfer of herpes virus from peripheral nerves to cortex and brainstem. *Science*. 1989;243(4887):89-91.

52. Dum RP, Strick PL. Transneuronal tracing with neurotropic viruses reveals network macroarchitecture. *Curr Opin Neurobiol*. 2013;23(2):245-249.

53. Boyden ES, Zhang F, Bamberg E, Nagel G, Deisseroth K. Millisecond-timescale, genetically targeted optical control of neural activity. *Nat Neurosci*. 2005;8(9):1263-1268.

54. Kim CK, Adhikari A, Deisseroth K. Integration of optogenetics with complementary methodologies in systems neuroscience. *Nat Rev Neurosci*. 2017;18(4):222-235.

55. Glasser MF, Coalson TS, Robinson EC, et al. A multi-modal parcellation of human cerebral cortex. *Nature*. 2016;536(7615):171-178.

56. Yeo BT, Krienen FM, Sepulcre J, et al. The organization of the human cerebral cortex estimated by intrinsic functional connectivity. *J Neurophysiol.* 2011;106(3):1125-1165.
57. Huth AG, de Heer WA, Griffiths TL, Theunissen FE, Gallant JL. Natural speech reveals the semantic maps that tile human cerebral cortex. *Nature.* 2016;532(7600):453-458.
58. Tatu L, Moulin T, Bogousslavsky J, Duvernoy H. Arterial territories of human brain: brainstem and cerebellum. *Neurology.* 1996;47(5):1125-1135.
59. Tatu L, Moulin T, Bogousslavsky J, Duvernoy H. Arterial territories of the human brain: cerebral hemispheres. *Neurology.* 1998;50:1699-1708.
60. Salamon G. *Atlas of the Arteries of the Human Brain.* Paris: Sandoz; 1973.
61. Caplan LR, van Gijn J. *Stroke Syndromes.* 3rd ed. New York, NY: Cambridge University Press; 2012.
62. Schmahmann JD. Vascular syndromes of the thalamus. *Stroke.* 2003;34(9):2264-2278.
63. Mesulam MM. Patterns in behavioral neuroanatomy: association areas, the limbic system, and hemispheric specialization. In: Mesulam M, ed. *Principles of Behavioral Neurology.* Philadelphia, PA: FA Davis; 1988.
64. Galaburda AM, Pandya DN. Role of architectonics and connections in the study of primate brain evolution. In: Armstrong E, Falk D, eds. *Primate Brain Evolution.* Boston, MA: Springer; 1982:203-216.
65. Betz W. Anatomischer Nachweis zweier Gehirncentra. *Centralblatt für die medizinischen Wissenschaften.* 1874;12:578-580, 595-599.
66. Jones HR, Burns TM, Aminoff MJ, Pomeroy SL. The Netter collection of medical illustrations. In: Frank H, Netter MD, eds. *Nervous System Part 1, Brain.* Vol 7. 2nd ed. Philadelphia, PA: Elsevier/Saunders; 2013.
67. Papez JW. A proposed mechanism of emotion. *Arch Neurol Psychiatry.* 1937;38:725-743.
68. Livingston KE, James W. *Papez Oral History Collection.* U.S. National Library of Medicine; 1981.
69. MacLean PD. Psychosomatic disease and the visceral brain; recent developments bearing on the Papez theory of emotion. *Psychosom Med.* 1949;11(6):338-353.
70. MacLean PD. Some psychiatric implications of physiological studies on frontotemporal portion of limbic system (visceral brain). *Electroencephalogr Clin Neurophysiol.* 1952;4:407-418.
71. Newman JD, Harris JC. The scientific contributions of Paul D. MacLean (1913-2007). *J Nerv Ment Dis.* 2009;197(1):3-5.
72. Jones EG. Mamillary or mammillary? What's an "m"? *J Hist Neurosci.* 2011;20(2):152-159.
73. Vann SD, Saunders RC, Aggleton JP. Distinct, parallel pathways link the medial mammillary bodies to the anterior thalamus in macaque monkeys. *Eur J Neurosci.* 2007;26(6):1575-1586.
74. Tsai C. The descending tracts of the thalamus and midbrain of the opossum, *Didelphis virginiana. J Comp Neurol.* 1925;39(2):217-248.
75. Valjakka A, Vartiainen J, Tuomisto L, Tuomisto JT, Olkkonen H, Airaksinen MM. The fasciculus retroflexus controls the integrity of REM sleep by supporting the generation of hippocampal theta rhythm and rapid eye movements in rats. *Brain Res Bull.* 1998;47(2):171-184.
76. Hikosaka O, Sesack SR, Lecourtier L, Shepard PD. Habenula: crossroad between the basal ganglia and the limbic system. *J Neurosci.* 2008;28(46):11825-11829.
77. Hu H, Cui Y, Yang Y. Circuits and functions of the lateral habenula in health and in disease. *Nat Rev Neurosci.* 2020;21(5):277-295.
78. Webster JF, Vroman R, Balueva K, Wulff P, Sakata S, Wozny C. Disentangling neuronal inhibition and inhibitory pathways in the lateral habenula. *Sci Rep.* 2020;10(1):8490.
79. Hahn JD, Fink G, Kruk MR, Stanley BG. Editorial: current views of hypothalamic contributions to the control of motivated behaviors. *Front Syst Neurosci.* 2019;13:32.
80. Saper CB, Lowell BB. The hypothalamus. *Curr Biol.* 2014;24(23):R1111--R1116.
81. Le Gros Clark WE. The topography and homologies of the hypothalamic nuclei in man. *J Anat.* 1936;70(pt 2):203-214.3.
82. Crosby EC, Woodburne RT. The comparative anatomy of the preoptic area and the hypothalamus. *Res Publ Assoc Nerv Ment Dis.* 1940;20:52-169.
83. Braak H, Braak E. Anatomy of the human hypothalamus (chiasmatic and tuberal region). In: Swaab DF, Hofman MA, Mirmiran M, Ravid R, Van Leeuwen FW, eds. *The Human Hypothalamus in Health and Disease. Progress in Brain Research.* 1992;93:3-16.
84. *Gray's Anatomy.* 38th ed. New York, NY: Churchill Livingston; 1995.
85. Nauta WJH, Haymaker W. Hypothalamic nuclei and fiber connections. In: Haymaker W, Anderson E, Nauta WJH, eds. *The Hypothalamus.* Springfield, IL: Thomas Books; 1969:136-209.
86. Nieuwenhuys R, Voogd J, van Huijzen C. *The Human Central Nervous System.* 4th ed. New York, NY: Springer; 2008.
87. Fujita A, Bonnavion P, Wilson MH, et al. Hypothalamic tuberomammillary nucleus neurons: electrophysiological diversity and essential role in arousal stability. *J Neurosci.* 2017;37(39):9574-9592.
88. Pedersen NP, Ferrari L, Venner A, et al. Supramammillary glutamate neurons are a key node of the arousal system. *Nat Commun.* 2017;8(1):1405.
89. Carpenter MB. *Human Neuroanatomy.* 7th ed. Baltimore, MD: Williams & Wilkins; 1976.
90. Braak H, Braak E. Cortical and subcortical argyrophilic grains characterize a disease associated with adult onset dementia. *Neuropathol Appl Neurobiol.* 1989;15(1):13-26.
91. Probst A, Tolnay M. La maladie des grains argyrophiles: une cause fréquente mais encore largement méconnue de démence chez les personnes âgées [Argyrophilic grain disease (AgD), a frequent and largely underestimated cause of dementia in old patients]. *Rev Neurol (Paris).* 2002;158(2):155-165.
92. Tolnay M, Clavaguera F. Argyrophilic grain disease: a late-onset dementia with distinctive features among tauopathies. *Neuropathology.* 2004;24(4):269-283.
93. Bear MH, Bollu PC. Neuroanatomy, hypothalamus. In: *StatPearls.* Treasure Island, FL: StatPearls Publishing; 2020. Available at https://www.ncbi.nlm.nih.gov/books/NBK525993/. Accessed January 13, 2019.
94. Emerson CH. Pituitary gland anatomy. *Encyclopedia Britannica.* 2010. Available at britannica.com/science/pituitary-gland.
95. Nauta WJ. Hippocampal projections and related neural pathways to the midbrain in the cat. *Brain.* 1958;81(3):319-340.
96. Alcaro A, Huber R, Panksepp J. Behavioral functions of the mesolimbic dopaminergic system: an affective neuroethological perspective. *Brain Res Rev.* 2007;56(2):283--321.
97. Zahm DS. The evolving theory of basal forebrain functional-anatomical 'macrosystems'. *Neurosci Biobehav Rev.* 2006;30(2):148-172.
98. Coenen VA, Panksepp J, Hurwitz TA, Urbach H, Mädler B. Human medial forebrain bundle (MFB) and anterior thalamic radiation (ATR): imaging of two major subcortical pathways and the dynamic balance of opposite affects in understanding depression. *J Neuropsychiatry Clin Neurosci.* 2012;24(2):223-236.

99. Barbano MF, Wang HL, Zhang S, et al. VTA glutamatergic neurons mediate innate defensive behaviors. *Neuron*. 2020;107(2):368.e8-382.e8. [Epub ahead of print, May 12, 2020].

100. Diez I, Williams B, Kubicki MR, Makris N, Perez DL. Reduced limbic microstructural integrity in functional neurological disorder. *Psychol Med*. 2019;1-9. [Epub ahead of print].

101. Schlaepfer TE, Bewernick BH, Kayser S, Mädler B, Coenen VA. Rapid effects of deep brain stimulation for treatment-resistant major depression. *Biol Psychiatry*. 2013;73(12):1204-1212.

102. Fenoy AJ, Schulz PE, Selvaraj S, et al. A longitudinal study on deep brain stimulation of the medial forebrain bundle for treatment-resistant depression. *Transl Psychiatry*. 2018;8(1):111.

103. Coenen VA, Bewernick BH, Kayser S, et al. Superolateral medial forebrain bundle deep brain stimulation in major depression: a gateway trial. *Neuropsychopharmacology*. 2019;44(7):1224-1232.

104. Gamlin PD. The pretectum: connections and oculomotor-related roles. *Prog Brain Res*. 2006;151:379-340.

105. Moore RY, Card JP. Intergeniculate leaflet: an anatomically and functionally distinct subdivision of the lateral geniculate complex. *J Comp Neurol*. 1994;344(3):403-430.

106. Gooley JJ, Saper CB. Anatomy of the mammalian circadian system. In: Kryger MH, Roth T, Dement WC, eds. *Principles and Practice of Sleep Medicine*. 6th ed. New York, NY: Elsevier; 2017:343-350.

107. Schütz H. Anatomische Untersuchungen über den Faserverlauf im centralen Höhlengrau und den Nervenfaserschwund in demselben bei der Paralyse der Irren. *Archiv für Psychiatrie und Nervenkrnakheiten*. 1891;22:527-587 (cited in Swanson LW, 2015).

108. Swanson LW. *Neuroanatomical Terminology. A Lexicon of Classical Origins and Historical Foundations*. New York, NY: Oxford University Press; 2015.

109. Bernardis LL. The dorsomedial hypothalamic nucleus in autonomic and neuroendocrine homeostasis. *Can J Neurol Sci*. 1975;2(1):45-60.

110. Reppucci CJ, Petrovich GD. Organization of connections between the amygdala, medial prefrontal cortex, and lateral hypothalamus: a single and double retrograde tracing study in rats. *Brain Struct Funct*. 2016;221(6):2937-2962.

111. Elmquist JK, Elias CF, Saper CB. From lesions to leptin: hypothalamic control of food intake and body weight. *Neuron*. 1999;22(2):221-232.

112. Bouret SG, Draper SJ, Simerly RB. Formation of projection pathways from the arcuate nucleus of the hypothalamus to hypothalamic regions implicated in the neural control of feeding behavior in mice. *J Neurosci*. 2004;24(11):2797-2805.

113. Klok MD, Jakobsdottir S, Drent ML. The role of leptin and ghrelin in the regulation of food intake and body weight in humans: a review. *Obes Rev*. 2007;8(1):21-34.

114. Lee CH, Suk K, Yu R, Kim MS. Cellular contributors to hypothalamic inflammation in obesity. *Mol Cells*. 2020;43(5):431-437.

115. Saper CB, Cano G, Scammell TE. Homeostatic, circadian, and emotional regulation of sleep. *J Comp Neurol*. 2005;493(1):92-98.

116. Lu J, Sherman D, Devor M, Saper CB. A putative flip-flop switch for control of REM sleep. *Nature*. 2006;441(7093):589-594.

117. Babic T, Travagli RA. Neural control of the pancreas. *Pancreapedia: Exocrine Pancreas Knowledge Base*. September 22, 2016.

118. Miller WL. The hypothalamic-pituitary-adrenal axis: a brief history. *Horm Res Paediatr*. 2018;89(4):212-223.

119. Gold PW, Chrousos GP. Organization of the stress system and its dysregulation in melancholic and atypical depression: high vs low CRH/NE states. *Mol Psychiatry*. 2002;7(3):254-275.

120. Corbet Burcher G, Liang H, Lancaster R, et al. Neuropsychiatric profile of paediatric hypothalamic hamartoma: systematic review and case series. *Dev Med Child Neurol*. 2019;61(12):1377-1385.

121. Bard P. A diencephalic mechanism for the expression of rage with special reference to the sympathetic nervous system. *Am J Physiol*. 1928;84:490-515.

122. Cannon WB, Britton SW. Studies on the conditions of activity in endocrine glands. XV. Pseudaffective medulliadrenal secretion. *Am J Physiol*. 1925;72 (2):283-294.

123. Bauer HG. Endocrine and other clinical manifestations of hypothalamic disease; a survey of 60 cases, with autopsies. *J Clin Endocrinol Metab*. 1954;14(1):13-31.

124. Flynn FG, Cummings JL, Tomiyasu U. Altered behavior associated with damage to the ventromedial hypothalamus: a distinctive syndrome. *Behav Neurol*. 1988;1(1):49-58.

125. Thompson RH, Swanson LW. Structural characterization of a hypothalamic visceromotor pattern generator network. *Brain Res Rev*. 2003; 41:153-202.

126. Hrabovszky E, Halász J, Meelis W, Kruk MR, Liposits Z, Haller J. Neurochemical characterization of hypothalamic neurons involved in attack behavior: glutamatergic dominance and co-expression of thyrotropin-releasing hormone in a subset of glutamatergic neurons. *Neuroscience*. 2005;133(3):657-666.

127. Love TM. Oxytocin, motivation and the role of dopamine. *Pharmacol Biochem Behav*. 2014;119:49-60.

128. Parhar IS, Ogawa S, Ubuka T. Reproductive neuroendocrine pathways of social behavior. *Front Endocrinol (Lausanne)*. 2016;7:28.

129. Hara J, Gerashchenko D, Wisor JP, Sakurai T, Xie X, Kilduff TS. Thyrotropin-releasing hormone increases behavioral arousal through modulation of hypocretin/orexin neurons. *J Neurosci*. 2009;29(12):3705-3714.

130. Sharif NA. Thyrotropin-releasing hormone: analogs and receptors. *Methods Neurosci*. 1993;13:199-219.

131. Engelhardt E. Meynert and the basal nucleus. *Dement Neuropsychol*. 2013;7(4):435-438.

132. de Olmos JS, Heimer L. The concepts of the ventral striatopallidal system and extended amygdala. *Ann N Y Acad Sci*. 1999; 877:1-32.

133. Elias WJ, Ray DK, Jane JA. Lennart Heimer: concepts of the ventral striatum and extended amygdala. *Neurosurg Focus*. 2008;25(1):E8.

134. Mesulam MM, Geula C. Nucleus basalis (Ch4) and cortical cholinergic innervation in the human brain: observations based on the distribution of acetylcholinesterase and choline acetyltransferase. *J Comp Neurol*. 1988;275(2):216-240.

135. Mesulam MM, Mufson EJ. Neural inputs into the nucleus basalis of the substantia innominata (Ch4) in the rhesus monkey. *Brain*. 1984;107(pt 1):253-274.

136. Mesulam MM, Lalehzari N, Rahmani F, et al. Cortical cholinergic denervation in primary progressive aphasia with Alzheimer pathology. *Neurology*. 2019;92(14):e1580-e1588.

137. Amaral DG. The amygdala, social behavior, and danger detection. *Ann NY Acad Sci*. 2003;1000:337-347.

138. Heimer L. A new anatomical framework for neuropsychiatric disorders and drug abuse. *Am J Psychiatry*. 2003;160:1726-1739.

139. Le Doux JE. Amygdala. *Scholarpedia*. 2008;3(4):2698.

140. Crosby EC, Humphrey T. Studies of the vertebrate telencephalon. II. The nuclear pattern of the anterior olfactory nucleus, tuberculum olfactorium and the amygdaloid complex in adult man. *J Comp Neurol*. 1941;47:309-352.

141. Johnston JB. Further contributions to the study of the evolution of the forebrain. *J Comp Neurol*. 1923;35:337-481.

142. Heimer L, de Olmos JS, Alheid GF, Pearson J, Sakamoto N. The human basal forebrain part II. In: Bloom FE, Björklund A, Hökflet T, eds. *Handbook of Chemical Neuroanatomy.* Amsterdam: Elsevier; 1999:57-226.

143. Dumont EC. What is the bed nucleus of the stria terminalis? *Prog Neuro-Psychopharmacol Biol Psychiatry.* 2009;33(8):1289-1290.

144. Lebow M, Chen A. Overshadowed by the amygdala: the bed nucleus of the stria terminalis emerges as key to psychiatric disorders. *Mol Psychiatry.* 2016;21:450-463.

145. Amaral DG. Memory: anatomical organization of candidate brain regions. In: Plum F, ed. *Handbook of Physiology—The Nervous System.* Vol V, Part 2. Washington, DC: American Physiological Society; 1987:211-294.

146. Freese JL, Amaral DG. Neuroanatomy of the primate amygdala. In: Whalen PJ, Phelps EA, eds. *The Human Amygdala.* New York, NY: Guilford Press; 2009:3-42.

147. Whalen PJ, Phelps EA, eds. *The Human Amygdala.* New York, NY: Guilford Press; 2009.

148. Benarroch EE. The amygdala: functional organization and involvement in neurologic disorders. *Neurology.* 2015;84(3):313-324.

149. Mufson EJ, Mesulam MM, Pandya DN. Insular interconnections with the amygdala in the rhesus monkey. *Neuroscience.* 1981;6(7):1231-1248.

150. Pandya DN, Van Hoesen GW, Mesulam MM. Efferent connections of the cingulate gyrus in the rhesus monkey. *Exp Brain Res.* 1981;42(3-4):319-330.

151. Vogt BA, Pandya DN. Cingulate cortex of the rhesus monkey: II. Cortical afferents. *J Comp Neurol.* 1987;262(2):271-289.

152. Petrides M, Pandya DN. Efferent association pathways from the rostral prefrontal cortex in the macaque monkey. *J Neurosci.* 2007;27(43):11573-11586.

153. Aggleton JP. A description of the amygdalo-hippocampal interconnections in the macaque monkey. *Exp Brain Res.* 1986;64:515-526.

154. Zheng J, Anderson KL, Leal SL, et al. Amygdala-hippocampal dynamics during salient information processing. *Nat Commun.* 2017;8:14413.

155. Barbas H, De Olmos J. Projections from the amygdala to basoventral and mediodorsal prefrontal regions in the rhesus monkey. *J Comp Neurol.* 1990;300(4):549-571.

156. Stefanacci L, Suzuki WA, Amaral DG. Organization of connections between the amygdaloid complex and the perirhinal and parahippocampal cortices in macaque monkeys. *J Comp Neurol.* 1996;375(4):552-582.

157. Amaral DG, Behniea H, Kelly JL. Topographic organization of projections from the amygdala to the visual cortex in the macaque monkey. *Neuroscience.* 2003;118(4):1099-1120.

158. Pitkänen A, Kelly JL, Amaral DG. Projections from the lateral, basal, and accessory basal nuclei of the amygdala to the entorhinal cortex in the macaque monkey. *Hippocampus.* 2002;12(2):186-205.

159. Ghashghaei HT, Hilgetag CC, Barbas H. Sequence of information processing for emotions based on the anatomic dialogue between prefrontal cortex and amygdala. *NeuroImage.* 2007;34(3):905-923.

160. Barbas H. Flow of information for emotions through temporal and orbitofrontal pathways. *J Anat.* 2007;211(2):237-249.

161. LaBar KS, Warren LH. Methodological approaches to studying the human amygdala. In: Whalen PJ, Phelps EA, eds. *The Human Amygdala.* New York, NY: Guilford Press; 2009:155-176.

162. Leong YC, Hughes BL, Wang Y, Zaki J. Neurocomputational mechanisms underlying motivated seeing. *Nat Hum Behav.* 2019;3(9):962-973.

163. Scoville WB, Milner B. Loss of recent memory after bilateral hippocampal lesions. *J Neurol Neurosurg Psychiatry.* 1957;20(1):11-21.

164. Jack CRJr, Dickson DW, Parisi JE, et al. Antemortem MRI findings correlate with hippocampal neuropathology in typical aging and dementia. *Neurology.* 2002;58(5):750-757.

165. Killiany RJ, Hyman BT, Gomez-Isla T, et al. MRI measures of entorhinal cortex vs hippocampus in preclinical AD. *Neurology.* 2002;58(8):1188-1196.

166. Putcha D, Brickhouse M, O'Keefe K, et al. Hippocampal hyperactivation associated with cortical thinning in Alzheimer's disease signature regions in non-demented elderly adults. *J Neurosci.* 2011;31(48):17680-17688.

167. Di Ieva A, Fathalla H, Cusimano MD, Tschabitscher M. The indusium griseum and the longitudinal striae of the corpus callosum. *Cortex.* 2015;62:34-40.

168. Rosene DL, Van Hoesen GW. The hippocampal formation of the primate brain: a review of some comparative aspects of cytoarchitecture and connections. In: Jones EG, Peters A, eds. *Cerebral Cortex.* Vol. 6. New York, NY: Plenum Press; 1987:345-456.

169. Gurunluoglu R, Shafighi M, Gurunluoglu A, Cavdar S. Giulio Cesare Aranzio (Arantius) (1530-89) in the pageant of anatomy and surgery. *J Med Biogr.* 2011;19(2):63-69.

170. Lewis FT. The significance of the term hippocampus. *J Comp Neurol.* 1923;35:213-230.

171. Winslow JB. Exposition anatomique de la structure du corps humain. Paris; 1732:619 (cited in Lewis, 1923).

172. de Garengeot RJC. *Splanchnologie ou l'anatomie des visceres.* Paris. 1742;(2):250-251 (cited in Lewis, 1923).

173. Mark JJ. Amun. Ancient History Encyclopedia. Available at https://www.ancient.eu/amun/. Accessed July 29, 2016.

174. Lorente de Nó R. Studies of the structure of the cerebral cortex. II. Continuation of the study of the ammonic system. *J Psychol Neurol.* 1934;46:113-177.

175. Olry R, Haines DE. Cerebral mythology: a skull stuffed with gods. (Neurowords 3). *Hist Neurosci.* 1998;7(1):82-83.

176. Cajal S Ramón y. *Histologie du système nerveux de l'homme et des vertébrés.* Translated into French by L. Azoulay. 1909-1910. Paris: Maloine. Translated into English by Swanson N, Swanson LW. *Histology of the Nervous System of Man and Vertebrates.* New York, NY: Oxford University Press; 1995.

177. Cajal S Ramón y. *Studies on the Cerebral Cortex. Limbic Structures.* Kraft LM, trans-ed. Chicago, IL: Year Book; 1955.

178. Leichnetz G. Available at ecurriculum.som.vcu.edu/portal/resources/2009/neuro/LimbicSystem/lecture.pdf.

179. Deng W, Aimone JB, Gage FH. New neurons and new memories: how does adult hippocampal neurogenesis affect learning and memory? *Nat Rev Neurosci.* 2010;11(5):339-350.

180. Dudek SM, Alexander GM, Farris S. Rediscovering area CA2: unique properties and functions. *Nat Rev Neurosci.* 2016;17(2):89-102.

181. Carstens KE, Dudek SM. Regulation of synaptic plasticity in hippocampal area CA2. *Curr Opin Neurobiol.* 2019;54:194-199.

182. Lee SE, Simons SB, Heldt SA, et al. RGS14 is a natural suppressor of both synaptic plasticity in CA2 neurons and hippocampal-based learning and memory. *Proc Natl Acad Sci U S A.* 2010;107(39):16994-16998.

183. Van Hoesen GW. The parahippocampal gyrus: new observations regarding its cortical connections in the monkey. *Trends Neurosci.* 1982;5:345-350.

184. Van Hoesen GW, Pandya DN, Butters N. Cortical afferents to the entorhinal cortex of the Rhesus monkey. *Science.* 1972;175(4029):1471-1473.

185. Van Hoesen G, Pandya DN, Butters N. Some connections of the entorhinal (area 28) and perirhinal (area 35) cortices of the rhesus monkey. II. Frontal lobe afferents. *Brain Res.* 1975;95(1):25-38.

186. Van Hoesen G, Pandya DN. Some connections of the entorhinal (area 28) and perirhinal (area 35) cortices of the rhesus monkey. I. Temporal lobe afferents. *Brain Res.* 1975;95(1):1-24.

187. Mesulam MM, Van Hoesen GW, Pandya DN, Geschwind N. Limbic and sensory connections of the inferior parietal lobule (area PG) in the rhesus monkey: a study with a new method for horseradish peroxidase histochemistry. *Brain Res.* 1977;136(3):393-414.

188. Swanson LW, Cowan WM. The connections of the septal region in the rat. *J Comp Neurol.* 1979;186(4):621-655.

189. Mitchell SJ, Rawlins JN, Steward O, Olton DS. Medial septal area lesions disrupt theta rhythm and cholinergic staining in medial entorhinal cortex and produce impaired radial arm maze behavior in rats. *J Neurosci.* 1982;2(3):292-302.

190. Kocsis B, Vertes RP. Characterization of neurons of the supramammillary nucleus and mammillary body that discharge rhythmically with the hippocampal theta rhythm in the rat. *J Neurosci.* 1994;14(11 pt 2):7040–7052.

191. Garrison FH. History of neurology. Revised and enlarged with a bibliography of classical, original, and standard works in neurology, by Lawrence C. McHenry, Jr. With a foreword by Derek E. Denny-Brown. Springfield, IL: Thomas; 1969.

192. O'Keefe J. Place units in the hippocampus of the freely moving rat. *Exp Neurol.* 1976;51(1):78-109.

193. Maguire EA, Gadian DG, Johnsrude IS, Good CD, Ashburner J, Frackowiak RS, Frith CD. Navigation-related structural change in the hippocampi of taxi drivers. *Proc Natl Acad Sci U S A.* 2000;97(8):4398-4403.

194. Gilbert PE, Brushfield AM. The role of the CA3 hippocampal subregion in spatial memory: a process oriented behavioral assessment. *Prog Neuropsychopharmacol Biol Psychiatry.* 2009;33(5):774-781.

195. Hitti FL, Siegelbaum SA. The hippocampal CA2 region is essential for social memory. *Nature.* 2014;508(7494):88-92.

196. Chevaleyre V, Piskorowski RA. Hippocampal area CA2: an overlooked but promising therapeutic target. *Trends Mol Med.* 2016;22(8):645-655.

197. Pang CC, Kiecker C, O'Brien JT, Noble W, Chang RC. Ammon's horn 2 (CA2) of the hippocampus: a long-known region with a new potential role in neurodegeneration. *Neuroscientist.* 2019;25(2):167-180.

198. Hyman BT, Van Hoesen GW, Damasio AR, Barnes CL. Alzheimer's disease: cell-specific pathology isolates the hippocampal formation. *Science.* 1984;225(4667):1168-1170.

199. Van Hoesen GW, Hyman BT. Hippocampal formation: anatomy and the patterns of pathology in Alzheimer's disease. *Prog Brain Res.* 1990;83:445-457.

200. Haberly LB. Parallel-distributed processing in olfactory cortex: new insights from morphological and physiological analysis of neuronal circuitry. *Chem Senses.* 2001;26(5):551-576.

201. Sanchez-Andrade G, Kendrick KM. The main olfactory system and social learning in mammals. *Behav Brain Res.* 2009;200(2):323-335.

202. Vaughan DN, Jackson GD. The piriform cortex and human focal epilepsy. *Front Neurol.* 2014;5:259.

203. Klingler E. Development and organization of the evolutionarily conserved three-layered olfactory cortex. *eNeuro.* 2017;4(1):ENEURO.0193-16.2016.

204. Bekkers JM, Suzuki N. Neurons and circuits for odor processing in the piriform cortex. *Trends Neurosci.* 2013;36(7):429-438.

205. Fournier J, Müller CM, Laurent G. Looking for the roots of cortical sensory computation in three-layered cortices. *Curr Opin Neurobiol.* 2015;31:119-126.

206. Allman JM, Tetreault NA, Hakeem AY, et al. The von Economo neurons in the frontoinsular and anterior cingulate cortex. *Ann N Y Acad Sci.* 2011;1225:59-71.

207. Nimchinsky EA, Gilissen E, Allman JM, Perl DP, Erwin JM, Hof PR. A neuronal morphologic type unique to humans and great apes. *Proc Natl Acad Sci U S A.* 1999;96(9):5268-5273.

208. González-Acosta CA, Escobar MI, Casanova MF, Pimienta HJ, Buriticá E. Von Economo neurons in the human medial frontopolar cortex. *Front Neuroanat.* 2018;12:64.

209. Cauda F, Geminiani GC, Vercelli A. Evolutionary appearance of von Economo's neurons in the mammalian cerebral cortex. *Front Hum Neurosci.* 2014;8:104.

210. Seeley WW, Carlin DA, Allman JM, et al. Early frontotemporal dementia targets neurons unique to apes and humans. *Ann Neurol.* 2006;60(6):660-667.

211. Brüne M, Schöbel A, Karau R, et al. Von Economo neuron density in the anterior cingulate cortex is reduced in early onset schizophrenia. *Acta Neuropathol.* 2010;119(6):771-778.

212. Santos M, Uppal N, Butti C, et al. Von Economo neurons in autism: a stereologic study of the frontoinsular cortex in children. *Brain Res.* 2011;1380:206-217.

213. Nishiyama A, Komitova M, Suzuki R, Zhu X. Polydendrocytes (NG2 cells): multifunctional cells with lineage plasticity. *Nat Rev Neurosci.* 2009;10(1):9-22.

214. Jäkel S, Dimou L. Glial cells and their function in the adult brain: a journey through the history of their ablation. *Front Cell Neurosci.* 2017;11:24.

215. Azevedo FA, Carvalho LR, Grinberg LT, et al. Equal numbers of neuronal and nonneuronal cells make the human brain an isometrically scaled-up primate brain. *J Comp Neurol.* 2009;513(5):532-541.

216. Herculano-Houzel S. The glia/neuron ratio: how it varies uniformly across brain structures and species and what that means for brain physiology and evolution. *Glia.* 2014;62(9):1377-1391.

217. Purves D, Augustine GJ, Fitzpatrick D, et al., eds. *Neuroscience.* 2nd ed. Sunderland, MA: Sinauer Associates; 2001.

218. Bayraktar OA, Bartels T, Holmqvist S, et al. Astrocyte layers in the mammalian cerebral cortex revealed by a single-cell in situ transcriptomic map. *Nat Neurosci.* 2020;23(4):500-509.

219. Wu Y, Dissing-Olesen L, MacVicar BA, Stevens B. Microglia: dynamic mediators of synapse development and plasticity. *Trends Immunol.* 2015;36(10):605-613.

220. Hong S, Dissing-Olesen L, Stevens B. New insights on the role of microglia in synaptic pruning in health and disease. *Curr Opin Neurobiol.* 2016;36:128-134.

221. Gray H. *Anatomy of the Human Body.* Philadelphia, PA: Lea and Febiger; 1918.

222. Hofer H, Schultz AH, Starck D. *Primatologia: Handbuch der Primatenkunde/Handbook of Primatology. Vol 2, Part 2. Pattern of the Cerebral Isocortex.* New York, NY: S. Karger; 1961.

223. Mufson EJ, Mesulam MM. Insula of the old world monkey. II: afferent cortical input and comments on the claustrum. *J Comp Neurol.* 1982;212(1):23-37.

224. Vogt BA, Palomero-Gallagher N. Cingulate cortex. In: Mai JK, Paxinos G, eds. *The Human Nervous System.* 3rd ed. Amsterdam: Elsevier; 2012:943-987.

225. Mettler R. Corticofugal fiber connections of the cortex of *Macaca mulatta.* The frontal region. *J Comp Neurol.* 1935;61:509-542.

226. Woolsey CN. Patterns of sensory representation in the cerebral cortex. *Fed Proc.* 1947;6(2):437-441.

227. Abbie AA. Cortical lamination in the Monotremata. *J Comp Neurol.* 1940;72:429-467.

228. Abbie AA. Cortical lamination in a polyprotodont marsupial, *Perameles nasuta. J Comp Neurol.* 1942;76:509-536.

229. Sanides F. Architectonics of the human frontal lobe of the brain. With a demonstration of the principles of its formation as a reflection of phylogenetic differentiation of the cerebral cortex. *Monogr Gesamtgeb Neurol Psychiatr.* 1962;98:1-201. [German].

230. Pandya DN, Sanides F. Architectonic parcellation of the temporal operculum in rhesus monkey and its projection pattern. *Z Anat Entwickl Gesch.* 1973;139:127-161.

231. Schmahmann JD. Foreword. In: Pandya DN, Seltzer B, Petrides M, Cipolloni PB, eds. *Cerebral Cortex: Architecture, Connections, and the Dual Origin Concept.* New York, NY: Oxford University Press; 2015:xv-xx.

232. Sanides F. Comparative architectonics of the neocortex of mammals and their evolutionary interpretation. *Ann N Y Acad Sci.* 1969;167:404-423.

233. Seltzer B, Pandya DN. Posterior cingulate and retrosplenial cortex connections of the caudal superior temporal region in the rhesus monkey. *Exp Brain Res.* 2009;195(2):325-334.

234. Yeterian EH, Pandya DN. Fiber pathways and cortical connections of preoccipital areas in rhesus monkeys. *J Comp Neurol.* 2010;518(18):3725-3751.

235. Desimone R, Gross CG. Visual areas in the temporal cortex of the macaque. *Brain Res.* 1979;178(2-3):363-380.

236. Bruce C, Desimone R, Gross CG. Visual properties of neurons in a polysensory area in superior temporal sulcus of the macaque. *J Neurophysiol.* 1981;46(2):369-384

237. Baylis GC, Rolls ET, Leonard CM. Functional subdivisions of the temporal lobe neocortex. *J Neurosci.* 1987;7(2):330-342.

238. Suzuki WA, Naya Y. The perirhinal cortex. *Ann Rev Neurosci.* 2014;37:39-53.

239. Blatt GJ, Pandya DN, Rosene DL. Parcellation of cortical afferents to three distinct sectors in the parahippocampal gyrus of the rhesus monkey: an anatomical and neurophysiological study. *J Comp Neurol.* 2003;466(2):161-179.

240. Van Hoesen GW, Pandya DN. Some connections of the entorhinal (area 28) and perirhinal (area 35) cortices of the rhesus monkey. III. Efferent connections. *Brain Res.* 1975;95(1):39-59.

241. Suzuki WA, Amaral DG. Perirhinal and parahippocampal cortices of the macaque monkey: cortical afferents. *J Comp Neurol.* 1994;350:497-533.

242. Lavenex P, Suzuki WA, Amaral DG. Perirhinal and parahippocampal cortices of the macaque monkey: projections to the neocortex. *J Comp Neurol.* 2002;447(4):394-420.

243. Lavenex P, Suzuki WA, Amaral DG. Perirhinal and parahippocampal cortices of the macaque monkey: intrinsic projections and interconnections. *J Comp Neurol.* 2004;472(3):371-394.

244. Pandya DN, Yeterian EH. Architecture and connections of cerebral cortex: implications for brain evolution and function. In: Scheible AB, Wechsler AF, eds. *Neurobiology of Higher Cognitive Function.* New York, NY: Guilford Press; 1990:53-84.

245. von Monakow C. *Die Lokalisation im Grosshirn und der Abbau der function durch kortikale Herde.* Wiesbaden: J. F. Bergmann; 1914.

246. Boes AD, Prasad S, Liu H, et al. Network localization of neurological symptoms from focal brain lesions. *Brain.* 2015;138 (pt 10):3061-3075.

247. Cohen AL, Soussand L, Corrow SL, Martinaud O, Barton JJS, Fox MD. Looking beyond the face area: lesion network mapping of prosopagnosia. *Brain.* 2019;142(12):3975-3990.

248. Sutterer MJ, Bruss J, Boes AD, Voss MW, Bechara A, Tranel D. Canceled connections: lesion-derived network mapping helps explain differences in performance on a complex decision-making task. *Cortex.* 2016;78:31-43.

249. Darby RR, Horn A, Cushman F, Fox MD. Lesion network localization of criminal behavior. *Proc Natl Acad Sci U S A.* 2018;115(3):601-606.

250. Darby RR, Laganiere S, Pascual-Leone A, Prasad S, Fox MD. Finding the imposter: brain connectivity of lesions causing delusional misidentifications. *Brain.* 2017;140(2):497-507.

251. Schmahmann JD. An emerging concept. The cerebellar contribution to higher function. *Arch Neurol.* 1991;48(11):1178-1187.

252. Schmahmann JD, Guell X, Stoodley CJ, Halko MA. The theory and neuroscience of cerebellar cognition. *Annu Rev Neurosci.* 2019;42:337-364.

253. Schmahmann JD. Dysmetria of thought: clinical consequences of cerebellar dysfunction on cognition and affect. *Trends Cogn Sci.* 1998;2(9):362-371.

254. Schmahmann JD. Disorders of the cerebellum: ataxia, dysmetria of thought, and the cerebellar cognitive affective syndrome. *J Neuropsychiatry Clin Neurosci.* 2004;16(3):367-378.

255. Schmahmann JD. The role of the cerebellum in cognition and emotion: personal reflections since 1982 on the dysmetria of thought hypothesis, and its historical evolution from theory to therapy. *Neuropsychol Rev.* 2010;20(3):236-260.

256. Schmahmann JD, Sherman JC. The cerebellar cognitive affective syndrome. *Brain.* 1998;121(pt 4):561-579.

257. Duffy FH, Burchfiel JL. Somatosensory system: organizational hierarchy from single units in monkey area 5. *Science.* 1971;172:273-275.

258. Sakata H, Takaoka Y, Kawarasaki A, Shibutani H. Somatosensory properties of neurons in the superior parietal cortex (area 5) of the rhesus monkey. *Brain Res.* 1973;64:85-102.

259. Mountcastle VB, Lynch JC, Georgopoulos A, Sakata H, Acuna C. Posterior parietal association cortex of the monkey: command functions for operations within extrapersonal space. *J Neurophysiol.* 1975;38:871-908.

260. Leinonen L, Hyvärinen J, Nyman G, Linnankoski I. Functional properties of neurons in lateral part of associative area 7 in awake monkeys. *Exp Brain Res.* 1979;34(2):299-320.

261. Pandya DN, Seltzer B. Intrinsic connections and architectonics of posterior parietal cortex in the rhesus monkey. *J Comp Neurol.* 1982;204(2):196-210.

262. Seltzer B, Pandya DN. Posterior parietal projections to the intraparietal sulcus of rhesus monkey. *Exp Brain Res.* 1986;62:459-469.

263. Seltzer B, Pandya DN. Converging visual and somatic sensory cortical input to the intraparietal sulcus of the rhesus monkey. *Brain Res.* 1980;192:339-351.

264. Fredrickson JM, Scheid P, Figge U, Kornhuber HH. Vestibular nerve projection to the cerebral cortex of the rhesus monkey. *Exp Brain Res.* 1966;2(4):318-327.

265. Buttner U, Lang W. The vestibulocortical pathway: neurophysiological and anatomical studies in the monkey. In: Granit R, Pompeiano 0, eds. *Reflex Control of Posture and Movement.* Amsterdam: Elsevier; 1979:581-588.

266. Lynch JC, Mountcastle VB, Talbot WH, Yin TC. Parietal lobe mechanisms for directed visual attention. *J Neurophysiol.* 1977;40(2):362-389.

267. Hyvarinen J. *The Parietal Cortex of Monkey and Man.* Berlin: Springer-Verlag; 1982.

268. Blatt GJ, Andersen RA, Stoner GR. Visual receptive field organization and cortico-cortical connections of the lateral

intraparietal area (area LIP) in the macaque. *J Comp Neurol.* 1990;299(4):421-445.

269. Colby CL, Duhamel JR, Goldberg ME. Ventral intraparietal area of the macaque: anatomic location and visual response properties. *J Neurophysiol.* 1993;69(3):902-914.

270. Mishkin M, Lewis ME, Ungerleider LG. Equivalence of parieto-preoccipital subareas for visuospatial ability in monkeys. *Behav Brain Res.* 1982;6(1):41-55.

271. Nauta WJH. Neural associations of the frontal cortex. *Acta Neurobiol Exp (Warsz).* 1972;32:125-140.

272. Murray EA, Coulter JD. Supplementary sensory area: the medial parietal cortex in the monkey. In: Woolsey CN, ed. *Cortical Sensory Organization. Vol 1. Multiple Somatic Areas.* Clifton, NJ: Humana Press; 1981:167-196.

273. Petrides M, Pandya DN. Projections to the frontal cortex from the posterior parietal region in the rhesus monkey. *J Comp Neurol.* 1984;228(1):105-116.

274. Barbas H, Mesulam MM. Cortical afferent input to the principalis region of the rhesus monkey. *Neuroscience.* 1985;15(3):619-637.

275. Baleydier C, Mauguiere F. Network organization of the connectivity between parietal area 7, posterior cingulate cortex and medial pulvinar nucleus: a double fluorescent tracer study in monkey. *Exp Brain Res.* 1987;66:385-393.

276. Seltzer B, Pandya DN. Some cortical projections to the parahippocampal area in the rhesus monkey. *Exp Neurol.* 1976;50:146-160.

277. Pandya DN, Seltzer B. Association areas of the cerebral cortex. *Trends Neurosci.* 1982;5:386-390.

278. Kasdon DL, Jacobson S. The thalamic afferents to the inferior parietal lobule of the rhesus monkey. *J Comp Neurol.* 1978;177:685-705.

279. Jones EG, Wise SP, Coulter JD. Differential thalamic relationships of sensory-motor and parietal cortical fields in monkeys. *J Comp Neurol.* 1979;183(4):833-881.

280. Weber JT, Yin TC. Subcortical projections of the inferior parietal cortex (area 7) in the stump-tailed monkey. *J Comp Neurol.* 1984;224(2):206-230.

281. Yeterian EH, Pandya DN. Corticothalamic connections of the posterior parietal cortex in the rhesus monkey. *J Comp Neurol.* 1985;237(3):408-426.

282. Schmahmann JD, Pandya DN. Anatomical investigation of projections from thalamus to posterior parietal cortex in the rhesus monkey: a WGA-HRP and fluorescent tracer study. *J. Comp Neurol.* 1990;295(2):299-326.

283. Yakovlev PI, Locke S, Koskoff DY, Patton RA. Limbic nuclei of thalamus and connections of limbic cortex. *Arch Neurol.* 1960;3:620-641.

284. Locke S, Angevine JBJr, Yakovlev PI. Limbic nuclei of thalamus and connections of limbic cortex; thalamocortical projections of lateral dorsal nucleus in cat and monkey. *Arch Neurol.* 1964;11:1-12.

285. Yin TC, Mountcastle VB. Mechanisms of neural integration in the parietal lobe for visual attention. *Fed Proc.* 1978;37(9):2251-2257.

286. Rolls ET, Perrett D, Thorpe SJ, Puerto A, Roper-Hall A, Maddison S. Responses of neurons in area 7 of the parietal cortex to objects of different significance. *Brain Res.* 1979;169(1):194-198.

287. Seltzer B, Pandya DN. Afferent cortical connections and architectonics of the superior temporal sulcus and surrounding cortex in the rhesus monkey. *Brain Res.* 1978;149:1-24.

288. Desimone R, Ungerleider LG. Multiple visual areas in the caudal superior temporal sulcus of the macaque. *J Comp Neurol.* 1986;248(2):164-189.

289. Perrett DI, Mistlin AJ, Chitty AJ. Visual neurons responsive to faces. *Trends Neurosci.* 1987;10:358-364.

290. Van Essen DC, Maunsell JHR. Hierarchical organization and functional streams in the visual cortex. *Trends Neurosci.* 1983;6:370-375.

291. Colombo M, D'Amato MR, Rodman HR, Gross CG. Auditory association cortex lesions impair auditory short-term memory in monkeys. *Science.* 1990;247(4940):336-338.

292. Galaburda AM, Pandya DN. The intrinsic architectonic and connectional organization of the superior temporal region of the rhesus monkey. *J Comp Neurol.* 1983;221(2):169-184.

293. Merzenich MM, Brugge JF. Representation of the cochlear partition of the superior temporal plane of the macaque monkey. *Brain Res.* 1973;50(2):275-296.

294. Mesulam MM, Pandya DN. The projections of the medial geniculate complex within the Sylvian fissure of the rhesus monkey. *Brain Res.* 1973;60(2):315-333.

295. Gattass R, Gross CG. Visual topography of striate projection zone (MT) in posterior superior temporal sulcus of the macaque. *J Neurophysiol.* 1981;46(3):621-638.

296. Zeki SM. Functional organization of a visual area in the posterior bank of the superior temporal sulcus of the rhesus monkey. *J Physiol.* 1974;236:549-573.

297. Seltzer B, Pandya DN. Further observations on parietotemporal connections in the rhesus monkey. *Exp Brain Res.* 1984;55:301-312.

298. Moran MA, Mufson EJ, Mesulam MM. Neural inputs into the temporopolar cortex of the rhesus monkey. *J Comp Neurol.* 1987;256:88-103.

299. Seltzer B, Pandya DN. Frontal lobe connections of the superior temporal sulcus in the rhesus monkey. *J Comp Neurol.* 1989;281:97-113.

300. Nadel L. The hippocampus and space revisited. *Hippocampus.* 1991;1:221-229.

301. Geschwind N, Levitsky W. Human brain: left-right asymmetries in temporal speech region. *Science.* 1968;161(3837):186-187.

302. Galaburda AM, Sanides F, Geschwind N. Human brain. Cytoarchitectonic left-right asymmetries in the temporal speech region. *Arch Neurol.* 1978;35(12):812-817.

303. Damasio H, Grabowski TJ, Tranel D, Hichwa RD, Damasio AR. A neural basis for lexical retrieval. *Nature.* 1996;380(6574):499-505.

304. Grabowski TJ, Damasio H, Tranel D, Ponto LL, Hichwa RD, Damasio AR. A role for left temporal pole in the retrieval of words for unique entities. *Hum Brain Mapp.* 2001;13(4):199-212.

305. Barton JJ, Press DZ, Keenan JP, O'Connor M. Lesions of the fusiform face area impair perception of facial configuration in prosopagnosia. *Neurology.* 2002;58(1):71-78.

306. Jackson JH. In: Taylor J, ed. *Selected Writings of John Hughlings Jackson, Volume I: On Epilepsy and Epileptiform Convulsions.* New York, Basic Books; 1958.

307. Harding AJ, Broe GA, Halliday GM. Visual hallucinations in Lewy body disease relate to Lewy bodies in the temporal lobe. *Brain.* 2002;125(pt 2):391-403.

308. Olney NT, Spina S, Miller BL. Frontotemporal dementia. *Neurol Clin.* 2017;35(2):339-374.

309. Klüver H, Bucy PC. Preliminary analysis of functions of the temporal lobes in monkeys. *Arch Neurol Psychiatry.* 1939;42:979-1000.

310. Benson DF. The Geschwind syndrome. *Adv Neurol.* 1991;55:411-421.

311. Devinsky J, Schachter S. Norman Geschwind's contribution to the understanding of behavioral changes in temporal lobe epilepsy: the February 1974 lecture. *Epilepsy Behav.* 2009;15(4):417-424.

312. Felleman DJ, Van Essen DC. Distributed hierarchical processing in the primate cerebral cortex. *Cereb Cortex.* 1991;1(1):1-47.

313. Desimone H, Ungerleider LG. Neural mechanisms of visual processing in monkeys. In: Boller F, Grafman J, eds. *Handbook of Neurophysiology*. Vol. 2. 1989:267-299.

314. Boussaoud D, Desimone R, Ungerleider LG. Visual topography of area TEO in the macaque. *J Comp Neurol*. 1991;306:554-575.

315. Morecraft RJ, Rockland KS, Van Hoesen GW. Localization of area prostriata and its projection to the cingulate motor cortex in the rhesus monkey. *Cereb Cortex*. 2000;10(2):192-203.

316. Mikellidou K, Kurzawski JW, Frijia F, et al. Area prostriata in the human brain. *Curr Biol*. 2017;27(19):3056.e3-3060.e3.

317. Teunisse RJ, Cruysberg JR, Hoefnagels WH, Verbeek AL, Zitman FG. Visual hallucinations in psychologically normal people: Charles Bonnet's syndrome. *Lancet*. 1996;347(9004):794--797.

318. Manford M, Andermann F. Complex visual hallucinations. Clinical and neurobiological insights. *Brain*. 1998;121(pt 10):1819-1840.

319. Choi EJ, Lee JK, Kang JK, Lee SA. Complex visual hallucinations after occipital cortical resection in a patient with epilepsy due to cortical dysplasia. *Arch Neurol*. 2005;62(3):481-484.

320. Woolsey CN, Settlage PH, Meyer DR, et al. Patterns of localization in precentral and "supplementary" motor areas and their relation to the concept of a premotor area. Association for Research in Nervous and Mental Disease. New York, NY: Raven Press; 1952;30:238-264.

321. Penfield W, Boldrey E. Somatic motor and sensory representation in the cerebral cortex of man as studied by electrical stimulation. *Brain*. 1937;60:389-443.

322. Schott GD. Penfield's homunculus: a note on cerebral cartography. *J Neurol Neurosurg Psychiatry*. 1993;56(4):329-333.

323. Morecraft RJ, Van Hoesen GW. Cingulate input to the primary and supplementary motor cortices in the rhesus monkey: evidence for somatotopy in areas 24c and 23c. *J Comp Neurol*. 1992;322(4):471-489.

324. Picard N, Strick PL. Motor areas of the medial wall: a review of their location and functional activation. *Cereb Cortex*. 1996;6(3):342-353.

325. Morecraft RJ, Schroeder CM, Keifer J. Organization of face representation in the cingulate cortex of the rhesus monkey. *Neuroreport*. 1996;7(8):1343-1348.

326. Fuster JM. Frontal lobe and cognitive development. *J Neurocytol*. 2002;31(3-5):373-385.

327. Harlow JM. Passage of an iron rod through the head. *Boston Med Surg J*. 1848;39:389-393.

328. Milner B. Some effects of frontal lobectomy in man. In: Warren JM, Akert K, eds. *The Frontal Granular Cortex and Behavior*. New York, NY: McGraw Hill; 1964:313-334.

329. Fuster JM. *The Prefrontal Cortex: Anatomy, Physiology and Neuropsychology of the Frontal Lobe*. New York, NY: Raven Press; 1980.

330. Pandya DN, Yeterian EH. Prefrontal cortex in relation to other cortical areas in rhesus monkey: architecture and connections. *Prog Brain Res*. 1991;85:63-94.

331. Cavada C, Goldman-Rakic PS. Posterior parietal cortex in rhesus monkey. I. Parcellation of areas based on distinctive limbic and sensory corticocortical connections. *J Comp Neurol*. 1989;287:393-421.

332. Eblen F, Graybiel AM. Highly restricted origin of prefrontal cortical inputs to striosomes in the macaque monkey. *J Neurosci*. 1995;15:5999-6013.

333. Eslinger PJ, Damasio AR. Severe disturbance of higher cognition after bilateral frontal lobe ablation: patient EVR. *Neurology*. 1985;35(12):1731-1741.

334. Shallice T, Burgess P. Higher-order cognitive impairments and frontal lobe lesions in man. In: Levin HS, Eisenberg HM, Benton AL, eds. *Frontal Lobe Function and Dysfunction*. New York, NY: Oxford University Press; 1991:125-138.

335. Petrides M, Pandya DN. Comparative architectonic analysis of the human and the macaque frontal cortex. In: Boller F, Grafman J, eds. *Handbook of Neuropsychology*. Vol. 9. Amsterdam: Elsevier; 1994:17-57.

336. Iversen SD, Mishkin M. Perseverative interference in monkeys following selective lesions of the inferior prefrontal convexity. *Exp Brain Res*. 1970;11(4):376-386.

337. Rosvold HE. The frontal lobe system: cortical-subcortical interrelationships. *Acta Neurobiol Exp (Warsz)*. 1972;32:439-460.

338. Bachevalier JB, Mishkin M. Visual recognition impairment follows ventromedial but not dorsolateral prefrontal lesions in monkeys. *Behav Brain Res*. 1986;20:249-261.

339. Tranel D, Bechara A, Denburg NL. Asymmetric functional roles of right and left ventromedial prefrontal cortices in social conduct, decision-making, and emotional processing. *Cortex*. 2002;38(4):589-612.

340. de la Vega A, Chang LJ, Banich MT, Wager TD, Yarkoni T. Large-scale meta-analysis of human medial frontal cortex reveals tripartite functional organization. *J Neurosci*. 2016;36(24):6553-6562.

341. Stuss DT, Benson DF. Neuropsychological studies of the frontal lobes. *Psychol Bull*. 1984;95(1):3-28.

342. Stuss DT, Knight RT, eds. *Principles of Frontal Lobe Function*. New York, NY: Oxford University Press; 2002.

343. D'Esposito M, Grafman J, eds. *The Frontal Lobes. Handbook of Clinical Neurology*. Vol. 163. 2019.

344. Sobotta J. *Atlas of Human Anatomy*. Vol. III. New York, NY: G.E. Stechert and Co.; 1928.

345. Mesulam MM, Mufson EJ. Insula of the old world monkey. I. Architectonics in the insulo-orbito-temporal component of the paralimbic brain. *J Comp Neurol*. 1982;212(1):1-22.

346. Woolsey CN. Organization of sensory and motor areas. In: Harlow HF, Woolsey CN, eds. *Biological and Biochemical Bases of Behavior*. Madison, WI: University of Wisconsin Press; 1958:63-81.

347. Morecraft RJ, Stilwell-Morecraft KS, Ge J, Cipolloni PB, Pandya DN. Cytoarchitecture and cortical connections of the anterior insula and adjacent frontal motor fields in the rhesus monkey. *Brain Res Bull*. 2015;119(pt A):52-72.

348. Uddin LQ, Nomi JS, Hébert-Seropian B, Ghaziri J, Boucher O. Structure and function of the human insula. *J Clin Neurophysiol*. 2017;34(4):300-306.

349. Vogt BA. *Cingulate Neurobiology and Disease*. New York, NY: Oxford University Press; 2009.

350. Vogt BA, Pandya DN, Rosene DL. Cingulate cortex of the rhesus monkey: I. Cytoarchitecture and thalamic afferents. *J Comp Neurol*. 1987;262(2):256-270.

351. Yakovlev PI, Locke S. Corticocortical connections of the anterior cingulate gyrus; the cingulum and subcallosal bundle. *Trans Am Neurol Assoc*. 1961;86:252-256.

352. Vogt B, Rosene D, Pandya DN. Thalamic and cortical afferents differentiate anterior from posterior cingulate cortex in the monkey. *Science*. 1979;204(4389):205-207.

353. Morecraft RJ, Van Hoesen GW. Convergence of limbic input to the cingulate motor cortex in the rhesus monkey. *Brain Res Bull*. 1998;45(2):209-232.

354. Morris R, Petrides M, Pandya DN. Architecture and connections of retrosplenial area 30 in the rhesus monkey (*Macaca mulatta*). *Eur J Neurosci*. 1999;11:2506-2518.

355. Morecraft RJ, Cipolloni PB, Stilwell-Morecraft KS, Gedney MT, Pandya DN. Cytoarchitecture and cortical connections of the posterior cingulate and adjacent somatosensory fields in the rhesus monkey. *J Comp Neurol.* 2004;469(1):37-69.

356. Morecraft RJ, Tanji J. Cingulofrontal interactions and the cingulate motor areas. In: Vogt B, ed. *Cingulate Neurobiology and Disease.* New York, NY: Oxford University Press; 2009:114-144.

357. Mayberg HS, Lozano AM, Voon V, et al. Deep brain stimulation for treatment-resistant depression. *Neuron.* 2005;45(5):651-660.

358. Joyce MKP, Barbas H. Cortical connections position primate area 25 as a keystone for interoception, emotion, and memory. *J Neurosci.* 2018;38(7):1677-1698.

359. Johansen-Berg H, Gutman DA, Behrens TE, et al. Anatomical connectivity of the subgenual cingulate region targeted with deep brain stimulation for treatment-resistant depression. *Cereb Cortex.* 2008;18(6):1374-1383.

360. García-Cabezas MÁ, Barbas H. Anterior cingulate pathways may affect emotions through orbitofrontal cortex. *Cereb Cortex.* 2017;27(10):4891-4910.

361. Valenstein E, Bowers D, Verfaellie M, Heilman KM, Day A, Watson RT. Retrosplenial amnesia. *Brain.* 1987;110(pt 6):1631-1646.

362. Kobayashi Y, Amaral DG. Macaque monkey retrosplenial cortex: III. Cortical efferents. *J Comp Neurol.* 2007;502(5):810-833.

363. Dum RP, Strick PL. Cingulate motor areas. In: Vogt BA, Gabriel M, eds. *Neurobiology of Cingulate Cortex and Limbic Thalamus.* Boston, MA: Birkhäuser; 1993.

364. Mufson EJ, Pandya DN. Some observations on the course and composition of the cingulum bundle in the rhesus monkey. *J Comp Neurol.* 1984;225(1):31-43.

365. Vann SD, Aggleton JP, Maguire EA. What does the retrosplenial cortex do? *Nat Rev Neurosci.* 2009;10(11):792-802.

366. Minoshima S, Giordani B, Berent S, Frey KA, Foster NL, Kuhl DE. Metabolic reduction in the posterior cingulate cortex in very early Alzheimer's disease. *Ann Neurol.* 1997;42(1):85-94.

367. Locke S, Angevine JB Jr, Yakovlev PI. Limbic nuclei of thalamus and connections of limbic cortex. II. Thalamocortical projection of the lateral dorsal nucleus in man. *Arch Neurol.* 1961;4:355-364.

368. Baleydier C, Mauguiere F. The duality of the cingulate gyrus in monkey. Neuroanatomical study and functional hypothesis. *Brain.* 1980;103(3):525-554.

369. Showers MJ. The cingulate gyrus: additional motor area and cortical autonomic regulator. *J Comp Neurol.* 1959;112:231-301.

370. Yakovlev PI, Locke S. Limbic nuclei of thalamus and connections of limbic cortex. III. Corticocortical connections of the anterior cingulate gyrus, the cingulum, and the subcallosal bundle in monkey. *Arch Neurol.* 1961;5:364-400.

371. Beckmann M, Johansen-Berg H, Rushworth MF. Connectivity-based parcellation of human cingulate cortex and its relation to functional specialization. *J Neurosci.* 2009;29(4):1175-1190.

372. Devinsky O. Disconnexion syndromes. In: Devinsky O, Schachter SC, eds. *Behavioral Neurology and the Legacy of Norman Geschwind.* Philadelphia, PA: Lippincott-Raven; 1997:115-126.

373. Critchley M. *The Parietal Lobes.* London: E. Arnold; 1953.

374. Heilman KM, Pandya DN, Geschwind N. Trimodal inattention following parietal lobe ablations. *Trans Am Neurol Assoc.* 1970;95:259-261.

375. Heilman KM, Pandya DN, Karol EA, Geschwind N. Auditory inattention. *Arch Neurol.* 1971;24(4):323-325.

376. Heilman KM, Valenstein E, Watson RT. Neglect and related disorders. *Semin Neurol.* 2000;20(4):463-470.

377. CRK. Book review. Brodie's clinical lectures. *Am J Med Sci.* 1846;11:347.

378. Flourens P. *Phrenology Examined.* de Lucena Meigs C, trans-ed. Philadelphia, PA: Hogan and Thompson; 1846.

379. Damasio AR. Time-locked multiregional retroactivation: a systems-level proposal for the neural substrates of recall and recognition. *Cognition.* 1989;33(1-2):25-62.

380. Coutanche MN, Thompson-Schill SL. Creating concepts from converging features in human cortex. *Cereb Cortex.* 2015;25(9):2584-2593.

381. von der Malsburg C. The correlation theory of brain function. Internal Report 81-2, Department of Neurobiology, Max-Planck-Institute for Biophysical Chemistry, 1981.

382. Crick F, Koch C. Towards a neurobiological theory of consciousness. *Semin Neurosci.* 1990;2:263-275.

383. Chalmers D. *The Conscious Mind: In Search of a Fundamental Theory.* Oxford: Oxford University Press; 1996.

384. Feldman J. The neural binding problem(s). *Cogn Neurodyn.* 2013;7(1):1-11.

385. von der Malsburg C. The what and why of binding: the modeler's perspective. *Neuron.* 1999;24(1):95-125.

386. Eckhorn R, Bauer R, Jordan W, et al. Coherent oscillations: a mechanism of feature linking in the visual cortex? Multiple electrode and correlation analyses in the cat. *Biol Cybern.* 1988;60(2):121-130.

387. Buzsáki G. *Rhythms of the Brain.* New York, NY: Oxford University Press; 2006.

388. Gallotto S, Sack AT, Schuhmann T, de Graaf TA. Oscillatory correlates of visual consciousness. *Front Psychol.* 2017;8:1147.

389. Bazhenov M, Timofeev I. Thalamocortical oscillations. *Scholarpedia.* 2006;1(6):1319.

390. Carlén M, Meletis K, Siegle JH, et al. A critical role for NMDA receptors in parvalbumin interneurons for gamma rhythm induction and behavior. *Mol Psychiatry.* 2012;17(5):537-548.

391. McNally JM, McCarley RW. Gamma band oscillations: a key to understanding schizophrenia symptoms and neural circuit abnormalities. *Curr Opin Psychiatry.* 2016;29(3):202-210.

392. Llinás RR, Paré D. Of dreaming and wakefulness. *Neuroscience.* 1991;44(3):521-535.

393. Neske GT. The slow oscillation in cortical and thalamic networks: mechanisms and functions. *Front Neural Circuits.* 2016;9:88.

394. Rosanova M, Casali A, Bellina V, Resta F, Mariotti M, Massimini M. Natural frequencies of human corticothalamic circuits. *J Neurosci.* 2009;29(24):7679-7685.

395. Fox MD, Zhang D, Snyder AZ, Raichle ME. The global signal and observed anticorrelated resting state brain networks. *J Neurophysiol.* 2009;101(6):3270-3283.

396. Buckner RL, Andrews-Hanna JR, Schacter DL. The brain's default network: anatomy, function, and relevance to disease. *Ann N Y Acad Sci.* 2008;1124:1-3.

397. Buckner RL, Krienen FM, Castellanos A, Diaz JC, Yeo BT. The organization of the human cerebellum estimated by intrinsic functional connectivity. *J Neurophysiol.* 2011;106(5):2322-2345.

398. Guell X, Gabrieli JDE, Schmahmann JD. Triple representation of language, working memory, social and emotion processing in the cerebellum: convergent evidence from task and seed-based resting-state fMRI analyses in a single large cohort. *NeuroImage.* 2018;172:437-449.

399. Guell X, D'Mello AM, Hubbard NA, et al. Functional territories of human dentate nucleus. *Cereb Cortex.* 2020;30(4):2401-2417.

400. Behrens TE, Johansen-Berg H, Woolrich MW, et al. Non-invasive mapping of connections between human thalamus and cortex using diffusion imaging. *Nat Neurosci.* 2003;6(7):750-757.

401. Hwang K, Bertolero MA, Liu WB, D'Esposito M. The human thalamus is an integrative hub for functional brain networks. *J Neurosci.* 2017;37(23):5594-5607.

402. Szewczyk-Krolikowski K, Menke RA, Rolinski M, et al. Functional connectivity in the basal ganglia network differentiates PD patients from controls. *Neurology.* 2014;83(3):208-214.

403. Kandel ER. The molecular biology of memory storage: a dialogue between genes and synapses. *Science.* 2001;294(5544):1030-1038.

404. Fryer JD, Yu P, Kang H, et al. Exercise and genetic rescue of SCA1 via the transcriptional repressor Capicua. *Science.* 2011;334(6056):690-693.

405. Wedeen VJ, Rosene DL, Wang R, et al. The geometric structure of the brain fiber pathways. *Science.* 2012;335(6076):1628-1634.

406. Mortazavi F, Oblak AL, Morrison WZ et al. Geometric navigation of axons in a cerebral pathway: comparing dMRI with tract tracing and immunohistochemistry. *Cereb Cortex.* 2018;28(4):1219-1232.

407. Schmahmann JD, Pandya DN, Wang R, et al. Association fibre pathways of the brain: parallel observations from diffusion spectrum imaging and autoradiography. *Brain.* 2007;130(pt 3):630-653.

408. Catani M, Howard RJ, Pajevic S, Jones DK. Virtual in vivo interactive dissection of white matter fasciculi in the human brain. *NeuroImage.* 2002;17(1):77-94.

409. Catani M, Jones DK, ffytche DH. Perisylvian language networks of the human brain. *Ann Neurol.* 2005;57(1):8-16.

410. Makris N, Schlerf JE, Hodge SM, et al. MRI-based surface-assisted parcellation of human cerebellar cortex: an anatomically specified method with estimate of reliability. *NeuroImage.* 2005;25(4):1146-1160.

411. Thiebaut de Schotten M, Dell'Acqua F, Valabregue R, Catani M. Monkey to human comparative anatomy of the frontal lobe association tracts. *Cortex.* 2012;48(1):82-96.

412. Wedeen VJ, Wang RP, Schmahmann JD, et al. Diffusion spectrum magnetic resonance imaging (DSI) tractography of crossing fibers. *NeuroImage.* 2008;41(4):1267-1277.

413. Johansen-Berg H, Behrens TE, Sillery E, et al. Functional-anatomical validation and individual variation of diffusion tractography-based segmentation of the human thalamus. *Cereb Cortex.* 2005;15(1):31-39.

414. Lehéricy S, Ducros M, Krainik A, et al. 3-D diffusion tensor axonal tracking shows distinct SMA and pre-SMA projections to the human striatum. *Cereb Cortex.* 2004;14(12):1302-1309.

415. Lehéricy S, Ducros M, Van de Moortele PF, et al. Diffusion tensor fiber tracking shows distinct corticostriatal circuits in humans. *Ann Neurol.* 2004;55(4):522-529.

416. Fox MD, Snyder AZ, Vincent JL, Corbetta M, Van Essen DC, Raichle ME. The human brain is intrinsically organized into dynamic, anticorrelated functional networks. *Proc Natl Acad Sci U S A.* 2005;102(27):9673-9678.

417. Greicius MD, Supekar K, Menon V, Dougherty RF. Resting-state functional connectivity reflects structural connectivity in the default mode network. *Cereb Cortex.* 2009;19(1):72-78.

418. Raichle ME, MacLeod AM, Snyder AZ, Powers WJ, Gusnard DA, Shulman GL. A default mode of brain function. *Proc Natl Acad Sci U S A.* 2001;98(2),676-682.

419. Forkel SJ, Thiebaut de Schotten M, Kawadler JM, Dell'Acqua F, Danek A, Catani M. The anatomy of fronto-occipital connections from early blunt dissections to contemporary tractography. *Cortex.* 2014;56:73-84.

420. Schmahmann JD, Pandya DN. The complex history of the fronto-occipital fasciculus. *J Hist Neurosc.* 2007;16(4):362-377.

421. Déjerine JJ. *Anatomie des centres nerveux.* Paris: Rueff et Cie; 1895.

422. Wedeen VJ, Wang R, Schmahmann JD, et al. Diffusion spectrum MRI in three mammals—rat, monkey and human. *Frontiers in Neuroscience.* 2009;3(1):74-77.

423. Pandya DN, Van Hoesen GW, Domesick VB. A cingulo-amygdaloid projection in the rhesus monkey. *Brain Res.* 1973;61:369-373.

424. Morris R, Pandya DN, Petrides M. Fiber system linking the mid-dorsolateral frontal cortex with the retrosplenial/presubicular region in the rhesus monkey. *J Comp Neurol.* 1999;407:183-192.

425. Bubb EJ, Metzler-Baddeley C, Aggleton JP. The cingulum bundle: anatomy, function, and dysfunction. *Neurosci Biobehav Rev.* 2018;92:104-127.

426. Rauch SL, Kim H, Makris N, et al. Volume reduction in the caudate nucleus following stereotactic placement of lesions in the anterior cingulate cortex in humans: a morphometric magnetic resonance imaging study. *J Neurosurg.* 2000;93:1019-1025.

427. Ojemann GA. Language and the thalamus: object naming and recall during and after thalamic stimulation. *Brain Lang.* 1975;2(1):101-120.

428. Johnson MD, Ojemann GA. The role of the human thalamus in language and memory: evidence from electrophysiological studies. *Brain Cogn.* 2000;42(2):218-230.

429. Crosson B. Subcortical aphasia: a working model. *Brain Lang.* 1985;25:257-292.

430. Vilensky JA, van Hoesen GW. Corticopontine projections from the cingulate cortex in the rhesus monkey. *Brain Res.* 1981;205(2):391-395.

431. Levisohn L, Cronin-Golomb A, Schmahmann JD. Neuropsychological consequences of cerebellar tumour resection in children: cerebellar cognitive affective syndrome in a paediatric population. *Brain.* 2000;123(pt 5):1041-1050.

432. Kim JS, Lee JH, Lee MC, Lee SD. Transient abnormal behavior after pontine infarction. (Letter). *Stroke.* 1994;25:2295-2296.

433. Schmahmann JD, Ko R, MacMore J. The human basis pontis: motor syndromes and topographic organization. *Brain.* 2004;127(pt 6):1269-1291.

434. Talairach J, Bancaud J, Geier S, et al. The cingulate gyrus and human behaviour. *Electroencephalogr Clin Neurophysiol.* 1973;34:45-52.

435. Watson RT, Heilman KM, Cauthien JC, King FA. Neglect after cingulectomy. *Neurology.* 1973;23:1003-1007.

436. Squire LR, Zola-Morgan S. The medial temporal lobe memory system. *Science.* 1991;253:1380-1386.

437. Lepage M, Ghaffar O, Nyberg L, Tulving E. Prefrontal cortex and episodic memory retrieval mode. *Proc Natl Acad Sci U S A.* 2000;97:506-511.

438. Smith WK. The functional significance of the rostral cingular cortex as revealed by its responses to electrical excitation. *J Neurophysiol.* 1945;8:241-255.

439. Glees P, Cole J, Whitty CWM, Cairns HWB. The effects of lesions in the cingular gyrus and adjacent areas in monkeys. *J Neurol Neurosurg Psychiatry.* 1950;13:178-190.

440. Meyer G, MacElhaney M, Martin W, MacGraw CP. Stereotaxic cingulotomy with results of acute stimulation and serial psychological testing. In: Laitinen LV, Livingston KE, eds. *Surgical Approaches in Psychiatry.* Lancaster, UK: Medical and Technical Publishing; 1973:38-58.

441. Moniz E. Prefrontal leucotomy in the treatment of mental disorders. *J Psychiatry.* 1937;93:1379-1385.

442. Freeman W, Watts J. *Psychosurgery: Intelligence, Emotion and Social Behavior Following Prefrontal Lobotomy for Mental Disorders.* Springfield, IL: Charles C. Thomas; 1942.

443. Fulton JF. *Functional Localization in Relation to Frontal Lobotomy.* New York, NY: Oxford University Press; 1949.

444. Adey WR, Meyer M. An experimental study of hippocampal afferent pathways from prefrontal and cingulate areas in the monkey. *J Anat.* 1952;86:58-74.

445. LeBeau J. Anterior cingulectomy in man. *J Neurosurg.* 1954;11:268-276.

446. Foltz EL, White LE Jr. Pain "relief" by frontal cingulumotomy. *J Neurosurg.* 1962;19:89-100.

447. Ballantine HT Jr, Cassidy WL, Flanagan NB, Marino R Jr. Stereotaxic anterior cingulotomy for neuropsychiatric illness and intractable pain. *J Neurosurg.* 1967;26(5):488-495.

448. Ballantine HT Jr, Bouckoms AJ, Thomas EK, Giriunas IE. Treatment of psychiatric illness by stereotactic cingulotomy. *Biol Psychiatry.* 1987;22(7):807-819.

449. Jenike MA, Baer L, Ballantine T, et al. Cingulotomy for refractory obsessive-compulsive disorder. A long-term follow-up of 33 patients. *Arch Gen Psychiatry.* 1991;48(6):548-555.

450. Spangler WJ, Cosgrove GR, Ballantine HT Jr, et al. Magnetic resonance image-guided stereotactic cingulotomy for intractable psychiatric disease. *Neurosurgery.* 1996;38(6):1071-1078.

451. Price BH, Baral I, Cosgrove GR, et al. Improvement in severe self-mutilation following limbic leucotomy: a series of 5 consecutive cases. *J Clin Psychiatry.* 2001;62(12):925-932.

452. Cosgrove GR, Rauch SL. Stereotactic cingulotomy. *Neurosurg Clin North Am.* 2003;14(2):225-235.

453. Reil JC. Untersuchungen über den Bau des großen Gehirns im Menschen. Archiv für die Physiologie. Halle: Curtschen Buchhandlung. 1809;9:136-146.

454. Burdach KF (CF). *Vom Baue und Leben des Gehirns. Zweyter Band.* Leipzig: In der Dyk'schen Buchhandlung; 1822.

455. Klingler J, Gloor P. The connections of the amygdala and of the anterior temporal cortex in the human brain. *J Comp Neurol.* 1960;115:333-369.

456. Ebeling U, von Cramon D. Topography of the uncinate fascicle and adjacent temporal fiber tracts. *Acta Neurochir.* 1992;115:143-148.

457. Pribram KH, Lenox MA, Dunsmore RH. Some connections of the orbito-fronto-temporal, limbic and hippocampal areas of *Macaca mulatta. J Neurophysiol.* 1950;13:127-135.

458. Selden NR, Gitelman DR, Salamon-Murayama N, Parrish TB, Mesulam MM. Trajectories of cholinergic pathways within the cerebral hemispheres of the human brain. *Brain.* 1998;121:2249-2257.

459. Colombo M, Rodman HR, Gross CG. The effects of superior temporal cortex lesions on the processing and retention of auditory information in monkeys (*Cebus apella*). *J Neurosci.* 1996;16 4501-4517.

460. Frey S, Kostopoulos P, Petrides M. Orbitofrontal involvement in the processing of unpleasant auditory information. *Eur J Neurosci.* 2000;12:3709-3712.

461. Mishkin M. A memory system in the monkey. *Phil Trans R Soc Lond Series B.* 1982;298:85-95.

462. Ghashghaei HT, Barbas H. Pathways for emotion: interactions of prefrontal and anterior temporal pathways in the amygdala of the rhesus monkey. *Neuroscience.* 2002;115(4):1261-1279.

463. Butter CM, Snyder DR, McDonald JA. Effects of orbital frontal lesions on aversive and aggressive behaviors in rhesus monkeys. *J Comp Physiol Psychol.* 1970;72(1):132-144.

464. Levine B, Katz DI, Dade L, Black SE. Novel approaches to the assessment of frontal damage and executive deficits in traumatic brain injury. In: Stuss DT, Knight RT, eds. *Principles of Frontal Lobe Function.* Oxford: Oxford University Press; 2002:448-465.

465. Bechara A, Damasio AR, Damasio H, Anderson SW. Insensitivity to future consequences following damage to human prefrontal cortex. *Cognition.* 1994;50:7-15.

466. Nauta WJ. The problem of the frontal lobe: a reinterpretation. *J Psychiatr Res.* 1971;8(3):167-187.

467. Von Der Heide RJ, Skipper LM, Klobusicky E, Olson IR. Dissecting the uncinate fasciculus: disorders, controversies and a hypothesis. *Brain.* 2013;136(pt 6):1692-1707.

468. Motzkin JC, Newman JP, Kiehl KA, Koenigs M. Reduced prefrontal connectivity in psychopathy. *J Neurosci.* 2011;31(48):17348-17357.

469. Sarkar S, Craig MC, Catani M, et al. Frontotemporal white-matter microstructural abnormalities in adolescents with conduct disorder: a diffusion tensor imaging study. *Psychol Med.* 2013;43(2):401-411.

470. Oishi K, Faria AV, Hsu J, Tippett D, Mori S, Hillis AE. Critical role of the right uncinate fasciculus in emotional empathy. *Ann Neurol.* 2015;77(1):68-74.

471. Kubicki M, Westin CF, Maier SE, et al. Uncinate fasciculus findings in schizophrenia: a magnetic resonance diffusion tensor imaging study. *Am J Psychiatry.* 2002;159(5):813-820.

472. Kawashima T, Nakamura M, Bouix S, et al. Uncinate fasciculus abnormalities in recent onset schizophrenia and affective psychosis: a diffusion tensor imaging study. *Schizophr Res.* 2009;110(1-3):119-126.

473. Glaser GH. Treatment of intractable temporal lobe-limbic epilepsy (complex partial seizures) by temporal lobectomy. *Ann Neurol.* 1980;8:455-459.

474. Hill D, Pond DA, Mitchell W, Falconer MA. Personality changes following temporal lobectomy for epilepsy. *J Ment Sci.* 1957;103:18-27.

475. Sindou M, Guenot M. Surgical anatomy of the temporal lobe for epilepsy surgery. *Adv Tech Stand Neurosurg.* 2003;28:315-343.

476. Saur D, Kreher BW, Schnell S, et al. Ventral and dorsal pathways for language. *Proc Natl Acad Sci U S A.* 2008;105(46):18035-18040.

477. Petrides M, Pandya DN. Distinct parietal and temporal pathways to the homologues of Broca's area in the monkey. *PLoS Biol.* 2009;7(8):e1000170.

478. Weiller C, Bormann T, Saur D, Musso M, Rijntjes M. How the ventral pathway got lost: and what its recovery might mean. *Brain Lang.* 2011;118(1-2):29-39.

479. Dick AS, Garic D, Graziano P, Tremblay P. The frontal aslant tract (FAT) and its role in speech, language and executive function. *Cortex.* 2019;111:148-163.

480. Kemerdere R, de Champfleur NM, Deverdun J, et al. Role of the left frontal aslant tract in stuttering: a brain stimulation and tractographic study. *J Neurol.* 2016;263(1):157-167.

481. Merabet LB, Mayer DL, Bauer CM, Wright D, Kran BS. Disentangling how the brain is "wired" in cortical (cerebral) visual impairment. *Semin Pediatr Neurol.* 2017;24(2):83-91.

482. Boot FH, Pel JJ, van der Steen J, Evenhuis HM. Cerebral visual impairment: which perceptive visual dysfunctions can be expected in children with brain damage? A systematic review. *Res Dev Disabil.* 2010;31(6):1149-1159.

483. Jan JE, Groenveld M, Sykanda AM, Hoyt CS. Behavioural characteristics of children with permanent cortical visual impairment. *Dev Med Child Neurol.* 1987;29(5):571-576.

484. Hofer S, Frahm J. Topography of the human corpus callosum revisited—comprehensive fiber tractography using diffusion tensor magnetic resonance imaging. *NeuroImage.* 2006;32(3):989-994.

485. Chao YP, Cho KH, Yeh CH, Chou KH, Chen JH, Lin CP. Probabilistic topography of human corpus callosum using

cytoarchitectural parcellation and high angular resolution diffusion imaging tractography. *Hum Brain Mapp.* 2009;30(10): 3172-3187.

486. Pandya DN, Rosene DL. Some observations on trajectories and topography of commissural fibers. In: Reeves AG, ed. *Epilepsy and the Corpus Callosum.* New York, NY: Plenum Publishing; 1985:21-39.

487. Bogen JE, Bogen GM. Creativity and the corpus callosum. *Psychiatr Clin N Am.* 1988;11(3):293-301.

488. Gazzaniga MS. The human brain is actually two brains, each capable of advanced mental functions. When the cerebrum is divided surgically, it is as if the cranium contained two separate spheres of consciousness. *Sci Am.* 1967;217(2):24-29.

489. Gazzaniga MS. Cerebral specialization and interhemispheric communication: does the corpus callosum enable the human condition? *Brain.* 2000;123(pt 7):1293-1326.

490. Sperry RW. The great cerebral commissure. *Sci Am.* 1964;210:42-52.

491. Heath CJ, Jones EG. Interhemispheric pathways in the absence of a corpus callosum. An experimental study of commissural connexions in the marsupial phalanger. *J Anat.* 1971;109: 253-270.

492. Sullivan MV, Hamilton CR. Memory establishment via the anterior commissure of monkeys. *Physiol Behav.* 1973;11:873-879.

493. Sullivan MV, Hamilton CR. Interocular transfer of reversed and nonreversed discrimination via the anterior commissure in monkeys. *Physiol Behav.* 1973;10:355-359.

494. Demeter S, Rosene DL, Van Hoesen GW. Interhemispheric pathways of the hippocampal formation, presubiculum, and entorhinal and posterior parahippocampal cortices in the rhesus monkey: the structure and organization of the hippocampal commissures. *J Comp Neurol.* 1985;233(1):30-47.

495. Rudge P, Warrington EK. Selective impairment of memory and visual perception in splenial tumours. *Brain.* 1991;114 (pt 1B):349-360.

496. Anderson D, Ahmed, A. Treatment of patients with intractable obsessive-compulsive disorder with anterior capsular stimulation. Case report. *J Neurosurg.* 2003;98(5):1104-1108.

497. Kumar K, Toth C, Nath RK. Deep brain stimulation for intractable pain: a 15-year experience. *Neurosurgery.* 1997;40(4):736-747.

498. Beevor CE, Horsley V. An experimental investigation into the arrangement of the excitable fibres of the internal capsule of the bonnet monkey (*Macacus sinicus*). *Phil Trans Roy Soc Lond Series B.* 1890;181:49-88.

499. Ross ED. Localization of the pyramidal tract in the internal capsule by whole brain dissection. *Neurology.* 1980;30:59-64.

500. Morecraft RJ, Herrick JL, Stilwell-Morecraft KS, Louie JL, et al. Localization of arm representation in the corona radiata and internal capsule in the non-human primate. *Brain.* 2002;125:176-198.

501. Fisher CM, Cole M. Homolateral ataxia and crural paresis: a vascular syndrome. *J Neurol Neurosurg Psychiatry.* 1965;28:48-55.

502. Chukwudelunzu FE, Meschia JF, Graff-Radford NR, Lucas JA. Extensive metabolic and neuropsychological abnormalities associated with discrete infarction of the genu of the internal capsule. *J Neurol Neurosurg Psychiatry.* 2001;71(5):658-662.

503. Schmahmann JD. *Hemi-Inattention from Right Hemisphere Subcortical Infarction.* Boston, MA: Society of Neurology and Psychiatry; 1984.

504. Tatemichi TK, Desmond DW, Prohovnik I, et al. Confusion and memory loss from capsular genu infarction: a thalamocortical disconnection syndrome? *Neurology.* 1992;42(10):1966-1979.

505. Filley CM. *Behavioral Neurology of White Matter.* 2nd ed. New York, NY: Oxford University Press; 2012.

506. Schmahmann JD, Smith EE, Eichler FS, Filley CM. Cerebral white matter: neuroanatomy, clinical neurology, and neurobehavioral correlates. *Ann N Y Acad Sci.* 2008;1142:266-309.

507. Naeser MA, Palumbo CL, Helm-Estabrooks N, Stiassny-Eder D, Albert ML. Severe nonfluency in aphasia. Role of the medial subcallosal fasciculus and other white matter pathways in recovery of spontaneous speech. *Brain.* 1989;112(pt 1):1-38.

508. Schmahmann JD, Leifer D. Parietal pseudothalamic pain syndrome. Clinical features and anatomic correlates. *Arch Neurol.* 1992;49(10):1032-1037.

509. Smith EE, Salat DH, Jeng J, et al. Correlations between MRI white matter lesion location and executive function and episodic memory. *Neurology.* 2011;76(17):1492-1499.

510. Leventhal CM, Baringer JR, Arnason BG, Fisher CM. A case of Marchiafava Bignami disease with clinical recovery. *Trans Am Neurol Assoc.* 1965;90:87-91.

511. D'Esposito M, Verfaellie M, Alexander MP, Katz DI. Amnesia following traumatic bilateral fornix transection. *Neurology.* 1995;45(8):1546-1550.

512. Heilman KM, Sypert GW. Korsakoff's syndrome resulting from bilateral fornix lesions. *Neurology.* 1977;27(5):490-493.

513. Déjerine JJ. Contribution à l'étude anatomo-pathologique et clinique des différentes variétés de cécité verbale. *Mémoires de la Société de Biologie.* 1892;4:61-90.

514. Ragsdale CW Jr, Graybiel AM. Fibers from the basolateral nucleus of the amygdala selectively innervate striosomes in the caudate nucleus of the cat. *J Comp Neurol.* 1988;269(4):506-522.

515. Lanciego JL, Luquin N, Obeso JA. Functional neuroanatomy of the basal ganglia. *Cold Spring Harb Perspect Med.* 2012;2(12):a009621.

516. Xiong A, Wesson DW. Illustrated review of the ventral striatum's olfactory tubercle. *Chem Senses.* 2016;41(7):549-555.

517. Alexander GE, DeLong MR, Strick PL. Parallel organization of functionally segregated circuits linking basal ganglia and cortex. *Annu Rev Neurosci.* 1986;9:357-381.

518. Mega MS, Cummings JL. Frontal-subcortical circuits and neuropsychiatric disorders. *J Neuropsychiatry Clin Neurosci.* 1994;6(4):358-370.

519. Nauta WJ, Domesick VB. Afferent and efferent relationships of the basal ganglia. *Ciba Foundation Symposium.* 1984;107:3-29.

520. Yeterian EH, Van Hoesen GW. Cortico-striate projections in the rhesus monkey: the organization of certain cortico-caudate connections. *Brain Res.* 1978;139(1):43-63.

521. Yeterian EH, Pandya DN. Striatal connections of the parietal association cortices in rhesus monkeys. *J Comp Neurol.* 1993;332(2):175-197.

522. Yeterian EH, Pandya DN. Laminar origin of striatal and thalamic projections of the prefrontal cortex in rhesus monkeys. *Exp Brain Res.* 1994;99(3):383-398.

523. Yeterian EH, Pandya DN. Corticostriatal connections of the superior temporal region in rhesus monkeys. *J Comp Neurol.* 1998;399(3):384-402.

524. Shink E, Bevan MD, Bolam JP, Smith Y. The subthalamic nucleus and the external pallidum: two tightly interconnected structures that control the output of the basal ganglia in the monkey. *Neuroscience.* 1996;73:335-357.

525. Haber SN, Fudge JL, McFarland NR. Striatonigrostriatal pathways in primates form an ascending spiral from the shell to the dorsolateral striatum. *J Neurosci.* 2000;20(6):2369-2382.

526. Penney JB Jr, Young AB. Speculations on the functional anatomy of basal ganglia disorders. *Annu Rev Neurosci.* 1983;6:73-94.

527. Graybiel AM. The basal ganglia. *Curr Biol.* 2000;10(14): R509-11.

528. Kravitz AV, Freeze BS, Parker PR, et al. Regulation of parkinsonian motor behaviours by optogenetic control of basal ganglia circuitry. *Nature.* 2010;466(7306):622-626.

529. Graybiel AM. Correspondence between the dopamine islands and striosomes of the mammalian striatum. *Neuroscience.* 1984;13(4):1157-1187.

530. Rommelfanger KS, Wichmann T. Extrastriatal dopaminergic circuits of the basal ganglia. *Front Neuroanat.* 2010;4:139.

531. Smith Y, Raju D, Nanda B, Pare JF, Galvan A, Wichmann T. The thalamostriatal systems: anatomical and functional organization in normal and parkinsonian states. *Brain Res Bull.* 2009;78(2-3):60-68.

532. Giménez-Amaya JM, McFarland NR, de las Heras S, Haber SN. Organization of thalamic projections to the ventral striatum in the primate. *J Comp Neurol.* 1995;354(1):127-149.

533. Haber SN. Neuroanatomy of reward: a view from the ventral striatum. In: Gottfried JA, ed. *Neurobiology of Sensation and Reward.* Boca Raton, FL: CRC Press/Taylor and Francis; 2011.

534. Sesack SR, Grace AA. Cortico-basal ganglia reward network: microcircuitry. *Neuropsychopharmacology.* 2010;35(1):27-47.

535. Bagot RC, Parise EM, Peña CJ, et al. Ventral hippocampal afferents to the nucleus accumbens regulate susceptibility to depression. *Nat Commun.* 2015;6:7062.

536. Haber SN, Lynd E, Klein C, Groenewegen HJ. Topographic organization of the ventral striatal efferent projections in the rhesus monkey: an anterograde tracing study. *J Comp Neurol.* 1990;293(2):282-298.

537. Ito R, Hayen A. Opposing roles of nucleus accumbens core and shell dopamine in the modulation of limbic information processing. *J Neurosci.* 2011;31(16):6001-6007.

538. Heimer L, Zahm DS, Churchill L, Kalivas PW, Wohltmann C. Specificity in the projection patterns of accumbal core and shell in the rat. *Neuroscience.* 1991;41(1):89-125.

539. Root DH, Melendez RI, Zaborszky L, Napier TC. The ventral pallidum: subregion-specific functional anatomy and roles in motivated behaviors. *Prog Neurobiol.* 2015;130:29-70.

540. Mogenson GJ, Jones DL, Yim CY. From motivation to action: functional interface between the limbic system and the motor system. *Prog Neurobiol.* 1980;14(2-3):69-97.

541. Neudorfer C, Maarouf M. Neuroanatomical background and functional considerations for stereotactic interventions in the H fields of Forel. *Brain Struct Funct.* 2018;223(1):17-30.

542. Mitrofanis J, Ashkan K, Wallace BA, Benabid AL. Chemoarchitectonic heterogeneities in the primate zona incerta: clinical and functional implications. *J Neurocytol.* 2004;33(4):429-440.

543. Shaw V, Mitrofanis J. Anatomical evidence for somatotopic maps in the zona incerta of rats. *Anat Embryol (Berl).* 2002;206(1-2):119-130.

544. Mitrofanis J. Evidence for an auditory subsector within the zona incerta of rats. *Anat Embryol (Berl).* 2002;205(5-6):453-462.

545. Power BD, Leamey CA, Mitrofanis J. Evidence for a visual subsector within the zona incerta. *Vis Neurosci.* 2001;18(2):179-186.

546. Mundinger F. Stereotaxic interventions on the zona incerta area for treatment of extrapyramidal motor disturbances and their results. *Confin Neurol.* 1965;26(3):222-230.

547. Blomstedt P, Stenmark Persson R, Hariz GM, et al. Deep brain stimulation in the caudal zona incerta versus best medical treatment in patients with Parkinson's disease: a randomised blinded evaluation. *J Neurol Neurosurg Psychiatry.* 2018;89(7):710-716.

548. Mostofi A, Evans JM, Partington-Smith L, et al. Outcomes from deep brain stimulation targeting subthalamic nucleus and caudal zona incerta for Parkinson's disease. *NPJ Parkinsons Dis.* 2019;5:17.

549. Ossowska K. Zona incerta as a therapeutic target in Parkinson's disease. *J Neurol.* 2020;267:591-606.

550. Nauta HJ, Cole M. Efferent projections of the subthalamic nucleus: an autoradiographic study in monkey and cat. *J Comp Neurol.* 1978;180(1):1-16.

551. Hartmann-von Monakow K, Akert K, Künzle H. Projections of the precentral motor cortex and other cortical areas of the frontal lobe to the subthalamic nucleus in the monkey. *Exp Brain Res.* 1978;33:395-403.

552. Haynes WI, Haber SN. The organization of prefrontal-subthalamic inputs in primates provides an anatomical substrate for both functional specificity and integration: implications for basal ganglia models and deep brain stimulation. *J Neurosci.* 2013;33(11):4804-4814.

553. Lambert C, Zrinzo L, Nagy Z, et al. Confirmation of functional zones within the human subthalamic nucleus: patterns of connectivity and sub-parcellation using diffusion weighted imaging. *NeuroImage.* 2012;60(1):83-94.

554. Benarroch EE. Subthalamic nucleus and its connections: anatomic substrate for the network effects of deep brain stimulation. *Neurology.* 2008;70(21):1991-1995.

555. Rico AJ, Barroso-Chinea P, Conte-Perales L, et al. A direct projection from the subthalamic nucleus to the ventral thalamus in monkeys. *Neurobiol Dis.* 2010;39(3):381-392.

556. Zaidel A, Spivak A, Grieb B, Bergman H, Israel Z. Subthalamic span of beta oscillations predicts deep brain stimulation efficacy for patients with Parkinson's disease. *Brain.* 2010;133(pt 7):2007-2021.

557. Eitan R, Shamir RR, Linetsky E, et al. Asymmetric right/left encoding of emotions in the human subthalamic nucleus. *Front Syst Neurosci.* 2013;7:69.

558. Grofová I. Extrinsic connections of the neostriatum. In: *The Neostriatum. Proceedings of a Workshop Sponsored by the European Brain and Behaviour Society,* Denmark; 1979:37-51.

559. Vonsattel JP. Huntington disease models and human neuropathology: similarities and differences. *Acta Neuropathol.* 2008;115(1):55-69.

560. Oyanagi K, Takeda S, Takahashi H, Ohama E, Ikuta F. A quantitative investigation of the substantia nigra in Huntington's disease. *Ann Neurol.* 1989;26(1):13-19.

561. Jenkinson N, Nandi D, Muthusamy K, et al. Anatomy, physiology, and pathophysiology of the pedunculopontine nucleus. *Mov Disord.* 2009;24(3):319--328.

562. Mesulam MM, Mufson EJ, Levey AI, Wainer BH. Cholinergic innervation of cortex by the basal forebrain: cytochemistry and cortical connections of the septal area, diagonal band nuclei, nucleus basalis (substantia innominata), and hypothalamus in the rhesus monkey. *J Comp Neurol.* 1983;214(2):170-197.

563. Mena-Segovia J, Bolam JP, Magill PJ. Pedunculopontine nucleus and basal ganglia: distant relatives or part of the same family? *Trends Neurosci.* 2004;27(10):585-588.

564. Lin DJ, Hermann KL, Schmahmann JD. The diagnosis and natural history of multiple system atrophy, cerebellar type. *Cerebellum.* 2016;15(6):663-679.

565. Benarroch EE. Pedunculopontine nucleus: functional organization and clinical implications. *Neurology.* 2013;80(12):1148-1155.

566. Goetz L, Bhattacharjee M, Ferraye MU, et al. Deep brain stimulation of the pedunculopontine nucleus area in Parkinson disease: MRI-based anatomoclinical correlations and optimal target. *Neurosurgery.* 2019;84(2):506-518.

567. ten Donkelaar HJ. Evolution of the red nucleus and rubrospinal tract. *Behav Brain Res.* 1988;28(1-2):9-20.

568. Lawrence DG, Kuypers HG. The functional organization of the motor system in the monkey. I. The effects of bilateral pyramidal lesions. *Brain.* 1968;91(1):1-14.

569. Lawrence DG, Kuypers HG. The functional organization of the motor system in the monkey. II. The effects of lesions of the descending brain-stem pathways. *Brain.* 1968;91(1):15-36.

570. Guillain G, Mollaret P. Deux cas de myoclonies synchrones et rythmées vélo-pliaryngo-oculo-diaphragmatiques. Le problème anatomique et physio-pathologique de ce syndrome. *Rev Neurol (Paris).* 1931;2:545-566.

571. Denny-Brown D. *The Basal Ganglia and Their Relation to Disorders of Movement.* London: Oxford University Press; 1962.

572. Nauta WJ, Mehler WR. Projections of the lentiform nucleus in the monkey. *Brain Res.* 1966;1(1):3-42.

573. Haber S. Perspective on basal ganglia connections as described by Nauta and Mehler in 1966: where we were and how this paper effected where we are now. *Brain Res.* 2016;1645:4-7.

574. Teuber H-L. Complex functions of basal ganglia. In: Yahr MD, ed. *The Basal Ganglia.* New York, NY: Raven Press; 1976:151-168.

575. Bowen FP. Behavioral alterations in patients with basal ganglia lesions. In: Yahr MD, ed. *The Basal Ganglia.* New York, NY: Raven Press; 1976:169-180.

576. Alexander GE, Crutcher MD, DeLong MR. Basal ganglia-thalamocortical circuits: parallel substrates for motor, oculomotor, "prefrontal" and "limbic" functions. *Prog Brain Res.* 1990;85:119-146.

577. Goldman-Rakic PS, Selemon LD. New frontiers in basal ganglia research. Introduction. *Trends Neurosci.* 1990;13(7):241-244.

578. Yeterian EH, Pandya DN. Corticothalamic connections of the superior temporal sulcus in rhesus monkeys. *Exp Brain Res.* 1991;83(2):268-284.

579. Saint-Cyr JA. Frontal-striatal circuit functions: context, sequence, and consequence. *J Int Neuropsychol Soc.* 2003;9:103-127.

580. Dunnett SB, Iversen SD. Learning impairments following selective kainic acid-induced lesions within the neostriatum of rats. *Behav Brain Res.* 1981;2:189-209.

581. Phillips AG, Carr GD. Cognition and the basal ganglia: a possible substrate for procedural knowledge. *Can J Neurol Sci.* 1987;14(3 suppl):381-385.

582. Knowlton BJ, Mangels JA, Squire LR. A neostriatal habit learning system in humans. *Science.* 1996;273:1399-1402.

583. Packard MG, Knowlton BJ. Learning and memory functions of the basal ganglia. *Ann Rev Neurosci.* 2002;25:563-593.

584. Squire LR. Mechanisms of memory. *Science.* 1986;232:1612-1619.

585. Squire LR. Memory systems. *CR Acad Sci III.* 1998;321:153-156.

586. Doyon J, Penhune V, Ungerleider LG. Distinct contribution of the cortico-striatal and cortico-cerebellar systems to motor skill learning. *Neuropsychologia.* 2003;41:252-262.

587. Fernandez-Ruiz J, Wang J, Aigner TG, Mishkin M. Visual habit formation in monkeys with neurotoxic lesions of the ventrocaudal neostriatum. *Proc Natl Acad Sci U S A.* 2001;98:4196-4201.

588. Levy R, Friedman HR, Davachi L, Goldman-Rakic PS. Differential activation of the caudate nucleus in primates performing spatial and nonspatial working memory tasks. *J Neurosci.* 1997;17:3870-3882.

589. Robbins TW, Cador M, Taylor JR, Everitt BJ. Limbic-striatal interactions in reward-related processes. *Neurosci Biobehav Rev.* 1989;13:155-162.

590. Christakou A, Robbins TW, Everitt BJ. Prefrontal cortical-ventral striatal interactions involved in affective modulation of attentional performance: implications for corticostriatal circuit function. *J Neurosci.* 2004;24:773-780.

591. Ravel S. Reward unpredictability inside and outside of a task context as a determinant of the responses of tonically active neurons in the monkey striatum. *J Neurosci.* 2001;21:5730-5739.

592. Koob GF. The role of the striatopallidal and extended amygdala systems in drug addiction. *Ann N Y Acad Sci.* 1999;877:445-460.

593. Everitt BJ, Parkinson JA, Olmstead MC, Arroyo M, Robledo P, Robbins TW. Associative processes in addiction and reward. The role of amygdala-ventral striatal subsystems. *Ann N Y Acad Sci.* 1999;877:412-438.

594. Gerdeman GL, Partridge JG, Lupica CR, Lovinger DM. It could be habit forming: drugs of abuse and striatal synaptic plasticity. *Trends Neurosci.* 2003;26:184-192.

595. Rauch SL, Savage CR, Alpert NM, et al. Probing striatal function in obsessive-compulsive disorder: a PET study of implicit sequence learning. *J Neuropsychiatry Clin Neurosci.* 1997;9:568-573.

596. Stein DJ, Goodman WK, Rauch SL. The cognitive-affective neuroscience of obsessive-compulsive disorder. *Curr Psychiatry Rep.* 2000;2:341-346.

597. Aouizerate B, Cuny E, Martin-Guehl C, et al. Deep brain stimulation of the ventral caudate nucleus in the treatment of obsessive-compulsive disorder and major depression. Case report. *J Neurosurg.* 2004;101:682-686.

598. Miller GA. The magical number seven, plus or minus two: some limits on our capacity for processing information. *Psychol Rev.* 1956;63(2):81-97.

599. Graybiel AM. The basal ganglia and chunking of action repertoires. *Neurobiol Learn Mem.* 1998;70(1-2):119-136.

600. Albert ML, Feldman RG, Willis AL. The 'subcortical dementia' of progressive supranuclear palsy. *J Neurol Neurosurg Psychiatry.* 1974;37(2):121-130.

601. Growdon JH, Corkin S. Cognitive impairments in Parkinson's disease. *Adv Neurol.* 1987;45:383-392.

602. Heilman KM, Gilmore RL. Cortical influences in emotion. *J Clin Neurophysiol.* 1998;15:409-423.

603. Savage CR. Neuropsychology of subcortical dementias. *Psychiatr Clin North Am.* 1997;20:911-931.

604. Turner MA, Moran NF, Kopelman MD. Subcortical dementia. *Br J Psychiatry.* 2002;180:148-151.

605. Caplan LR, Schmahmann JD, Kase CS, et al. Caudate infarcts. *Arch Neurol.* 1990;47(2):133-143.

606. Cummings JL, Benson DF. Subcortical dementia. Review of an emerging concept. *Arch Neurol.* 1984;41(8):874-879.

607. Dujardin K, Sockeel P, Devos D, et al. Characteristics of apathy in Parkinson's disease. *Mov Disord.* 2007;22(6):778-784.

608. Naville F. Etudes sur les complications et les sequelles mentales de l'encephalite epidemique. La bradyphrenie. *Encephale.* 1922;17:369-375, 423-436.

609. Cronin-Golomb A, Corkin S, Growdon JH. Impaired problem solving in Parkinson's disease: impact of a set-shifting deficit. *Neuropsychologia.* 1994;32(5):579-593.

610. Muslimovic D, Post B, Speelman JD, Schmand B. Motor procedural learning in Parkinson's disease. *Brain.* 2007;130(pt 11):2887-2897.

611. Owen AM, James M, Leigh PN, et al. Fronto-striatal cognitive deficits at different stages of Parkinson's disease. *Brain.* 1992;115(pt 6):1727-1751.

612. Smith JG, McDowall J. When artificial grammar acquisition in Parkinson's disease is impaired: the case of learning via trial-by-trial feedback. *Brain Res.* 2006;1067(1):216-228.

613. Williams-Gray CH, Foltynie T, Brayne CE, Robbins TW, Barker RA. Evolution of cognitive dysfunction in an incident Parkinson's disease cohort. *Brain.* 2007;130(pt 7):1787-1798.

614. Barnes TD, Kubota Y, Hu D, Jin DZ, Graybiel AM. Activity of striatal neurons reflects dynamic encoding and recoding of procedural memories. *Nature*. 2005;437(7062):1158-1161.

615. Delgado MR. Reward-related responses in the human striatum. *Ann N Y Acad Sci*. 2007;1104:70-88.

616. Levy R, Dubois B. Apathy and the functional anatomy of the prefrontal cortex-basal ganglia circuits. *Cereb Cortex*. 2006;16(7):916-928.

617. Kumral E, Evyapan D, Balkir K. Acute caudate vascular lesions. *Stroke*. 1999;30(1):100-108.

618. Peoples LL, Kravitz AV, Guillem K. The role of accumbal hypoactivity in cocaine addiction. *Sci World J*. 2007;7:22-45

619. Remijnse PL, Nielen MM, van Balkom AJ, et al. Reduced orbitofrontal-striatal activity on a reversal learning task in obsessive-compulsive disorder. *Arch Gen Psychiatry*. 2006;63(11):1225-1236.

620. Lombardi WJ, Gross RE, Trepanier LL, Lang AE, Lozano AM, Saint-Cyr JA. Relationship of lesion location to cognitive outcome following microelectrode-guided pallidotomy for Parkinson's disease: support for the existence of cognitive circuits in the human pallidum. *Brain*. 2000;123(pt 4):746-758.

621. Trépanier LL, Saint-Cyr JA, Lozano AM, Lang AE. Neuropsychological consequences of posteroventral pallidotomy for the treatment of Parkinson's disease. *Neurology*. 1998;51(1):207-215.

622. Scott R, Gregory R, Hines N, et al. Neuropsychological, neurological and functional outcome following pallidotomy for Parkinson's disease. A consecutive series of eight simultaneous bilateral and twelve unilateral procedures. *Brain*. 1998;121(pt 4):659-675.

623. Ghika J, Ghika-Schmid F, Fankhauser H, et al. Bilateral contemporaneous posteroventral pallidotomy for the treatment of Parkinson's disease: neuropsychological and neurological side effects. Report of four cases and review of the literature. *J Neurosurg*. 1999;91(2):313-321.

624. Rae AS. The form and structure of the human claustrum. *J Comp Neurol*. 1954;100(1):15-39.

625. Norimoto H, Fenk LA, Li HH, et al. A claustrum in reptiles and its role in slow-wave sleep. *Nature*. 2020;578(7795):413-418.

626. Brown SP, Mathur BN, Olsen SR, Luppi PH, Bickford ME, Citri A. New breakthroughs in understanding the role of functional interactions between the neocortex and the claustrum. *J. Neurosci*. 2017;37(45):10877-10881.

627. Smith JB, Watson GDR, Liang Z, Liu Y, Zhang N, Alloway KD. A role for the claustrum in salience processing? *Front Neuroanat*. 2019;13:64

628. Hadjikhani N, Roland PE. Cross-modal transfer of information between the tactile and the visual representations in the human brain: a positron emission tomographic study. *J Neurosci*. 1998;18(3):1072-1084.

629. Crick FC, Koch C. What is the function of the claustrum? *Philos Trans R Soc Lond B Biol Sci*. 2005;360(1458):1271-1279.

630. Sapède D, Cau E. The pineal gland from development to function. *Curr Top Dev Biol*. 2013;106:171-215.

631. Huguenard J, Prince D. Basic mechanisms of epileptic discharges in the thalamus. In: Steriade M, Jones EG, McCormick DA, eds. *Thalamus, Vol 2. Experimental and Clinical Aspects*. New York, NY: Elsevier; 1997:295-330.

632. Llinás R, Ribary U. Consciousness and the brain. The thalamocortical dialogue in health and disease. *Ann N Y Acad Sci*. 2001;929:166-175.

633. Sidibé M, Paré JF, Smith Y. Nigral and pallidal inputs to functionally segregated thalamostriatal neurons in the centromedian/parafascicular intralaminar nuclear complex in monkey. *J Comp Neurol*. 2002;447(3):286-299.

634. Bentivoglio M, Kultas-Ilinsky K, Ilinsky I. Limbic thalamus: structure, intrinsic organization, and connections. In: Vogt BA, Gabriel M, eds. *Neurobiology of Cingulate Cortex and Limbic Thalamus*. Boston, MA: Birkhäuser; 1993:71-122.

635. Lenz F, Dougherty P. Pain processing in the human thalamus. In: Steriade M, Jones EG, McCormick DA, eds. *Thalamus, Vol 2. Experimental and Clinical Aspects*. New York, NY: Elsevier; 1997:617-651.

636. Willis WJ. Nociceptive functions of thalamic neurons. In: Steriade M, Jones EG, McCormick DA, eds. *Thalamus, Vol 2. Experimental and Clinical Aspects*. New York, NY: Elsevier; 1997:373-424.

637. Van der Werf YD, Witter MP, Groenewegen HJ. The intralaminar and midline nuclei of the thalamus. Anatomical and functional evidence for participation in processes of arousal and awareness. *Brain Res Brain Res Rev*. 2002;39(2-3):107-140.

638. Yeterian EH, Pandya DN. Corticothalamic connections of paralimbic regions in the rhesus monkey. *J Comp Neurol*. 1988;269(1):130-146.

639. Devinsky O, Luciano D. The contributions of cingulate cortex to human behavior. In: Vogt B, Gabriel M, eds. *Neurobiology of Cingulate Cortex and Limbic Thalamus*. Boston, MA: Birkhäuser; 1997:527-556.

640. Jankowski MM, Ronnqvist KC, Tsanov M, et al. The anterior thalamus provides a subcortical circuit supporting memory and spatial navigation. *Front Syst Neurosci*. 2013;7:45.

641. Hackett TA, Stepniewska I, Kaas JH. Thalamocortical connections of the parabelt auditory cortex in macaque monkeys. *J Comp Neurol*. 1998;400(2):271-286.

642. Pandya DN, Rosene DL, Doolittle AM. Corticothalamic connections of auditory-related areas of the temporal lobe in the rhesus monkey. *J Comp Neurol*. 1994;345(3):447-471.

643. Kennedy H, Bullier J. A double-labeling investigation of the afferent connectivity to cortical areas V1 and V2 of the macaque monkey. *J Neurosci*. 1985;5(10):2815-2830.

644. Shatz CJ, Rakic P. The genesis of efferent connections from the visual cortex of the fetal rhesus monkey. *J Comp Neurol*. 1981;196(2):287-307.

645. Pritchard TC, Hamilton RB, Morse JR, Norgren R. Projections of thalamic gustatory and lingual areas in the monkey, *Macaca fascicularis. J Comp Neurol*. 1986;244(2):213-228.

646. Deecke L, Schwarz DW, Fredrickson JM. Vestibular responses in the rhesus monkey ventroposterior thalamus. II. Vestibulo-proprioceptive convergence at thalamic neurons. *Exp Brain Res*. 1977;30(2-3):219-232.

647. Ilinsky IA, Kultas-Ilinsky K. Sagittal cytoarchitectonic maps of the *Macaca mulatta* thalamus with a revised nomenclature of the motor-related nuclei validated by observations on their connectivity. *J Comp Neurol*. 1987;262(3):331-364.

648. Jones E. A description of the human thalamus. In: Steriade M, Jones EG, McCormick DA, eds. *Thalamus, Vol 2. Experimental and Clinical Aspects*. New York, NY: Elsevier; 1997: 425-499.

649. François C, Tande D, Yelnik J, Hirsch EC. Distribution and morphology of nigral axons projecting to the thalamus in primates. *J Comp Neurol*. 2002;447(3):249-260.

650. Jones E. *The Thalamus*. New York, NY: Plenum Press; 1985.

651. Schell GR, Strick PL. The origin of thalamic inputs to the arcuate premotor and supplementary motor areas. *J Neurosci*. 1984;4(2):539-560.

652. Goldman-Rakic PS, Porrino LJ. The primate mediodorsal (MD) nucleus and its projection to the frontal lobe. *J Comp Neurol*. 1985;242(4):535-560.

653. Strick PL. Anatomical analysis of ventrolateral thalamic input to primate motor cortex. *J. Neurophysiol.* 1976;39(5):1020-1031.

654. Gutrecht JA, Zamani AA, Pandya DN. Lacunar thalamic stroke with pure cerebellar and proprioceptive deficits. *J Neurol Neurosurg Psychiatry.* 1992;55(9):854-856.

655. Murthy JM. Ataxic hemiparesis—ventrolateral nucleus of the thalamus: yet another site of lesion. *Stroke.* 1988;19(1):122.

656. Solomon DH, Barohn RJ, Bazan C, Grissom J. The thalamic ataxia syndrome. *Neurology.* 1994;44(5):810-814.

657. Kievit J, Kuypers HG. Organization of the thalamo-cortical connexions to the frontal lobe in the rhesus monkey. *Exp Brain Res.* 1977;29(3-4):299-322.

658. Künzle H, Akert K. Efferent connections of cortical, area 8 (frontal eye field) in *Macaca fascicularis.* A reinvestigation using the autoradiographic technique. *J Comp Neurol.* 1977;173(1):147-164.

659. Middleton FA, Strick PL. Anatomical evidence for cerebellar and basal ganglia involvement in higher cognitive function. *Science.* 1994;266(5184):458-461.

660. Yeterian EH, Pandya DN. Thalamic connections of the cortex of the superior temporal sulcus in the rhesus monkey. *J Comp Neurol.* 1989;282(1):80-97.

661. Hugdahl K, Wester K. Neurocognitive correlates of stereotactic thalamotomy and thalamic stimulation in Parkinsonian patients. *Brain Cogn.* 2000;42(2):231-252.

662. Ojemann GA, Fedio P, Van Buren JM. Anomia from pulvinar and subcortical parietal stimulation. *Brain.* 1968;91(1):99-116.

663. Ojemann GA, Ward AAJr. Speech representation in ventrolateral thalamus. *Brain.* 1971;94(4):669-680.

664. Yeterian EH, Pandya DN. Corticothalamic connections of extrastriate visual areas in rhesus monkeys. *J Comp Neurol.* 1997;378(4):562-585.

665. Acuña C, Cudeiro J, Gonzalez F, Alonso JM, Perez R. Lateral-posterior and pulvinar reaching cells—comparison with parietal area 5a: a study in behaving *Macaca nemestrina* monkeys. *Exp Brain Res.* 1990;82(1):158-166.

666. Tobias TJ. Afferents to prefrontal cortex from the thalamic mediodorsal nucleus in the rhesus monkey. *Brain Res.* 1975;83(2):191-212.

667. Giguere M, Goldman-Rakic PS. Mediodorsal nucleus: areal, laminar, and tangential distribution of afferents and efferents in the frontal lobe of rhesus monkeys. *J Comp Neurol.* 1988;277(2):195-213.

668. Barbas H, Henion TH, Dermon CR. Diverse thalamic projections to the prefrontal cortex in the rhesus monkey. *J Comp Neurol.* 1991;313(1):65-94.

669. Siwek DF, Pandya DN. Prefrontal projections to the mediodorsal nucleus of the thalamus in the rhesus monkey. *J Comp Neurol.* 1991;312(4):509-524.

670. Ray JP, Price JL. The organization of projections from the mediodorsal nucleus of the thalamus to orbital and medial prefrontal cortex in macaque monkeys. *J Comp Neurol.* 1993;337(1):1-31.

671. Graff-Radford NR, Tranel D, Van Hoesen GW, Brandt JP. Diencephalic amnesia. *Brain.* 1990;113(pt 1):1-25.

672. Russchen FT, Amaral DG, Price JL. The afferent input to the magnocellular division of the mediodorsal thalamic nucleus in the monkey, *Macaca fascicularis. J Comp Neurol.* 1987;256(2):175-210.

673. Victor M, Adams RD, Collins GH. The Wernicke-Korsakoff syndrome. A clinical and pathological study of 245 patients, 82 with post-mortem examinations. *Contemp Neurol Ser.* 1971;7:1-206.

674. Bogousslavsky J, Regli F, Uske A. Thalamic infarcts: clinical syndromes, etiology, and prognosis. *Neurology.* 1988;38(6):837-848.

675. Olszewski J. *The Thalamus of the Macaca mulatta: An Atlas for Use with the Stereotaxic Instrument.* Basel, Switzerland: S. Karger; 1952.

676. Popken GJ, Bunney WEJr, Potkin SG, Jones EG. Subnucleus-specific loss of neurons in medial thalamus of schizophrenics. *Proc Natl Acad Sci U S A.* 2000;97(16):9276-9280.

677. Asanuma C, Andersen RA, Cowan WM. The thalamic relations of the caudal inferior parietal lobule and the lateral prefrontal cortex in monkeys: divergent cortical projections from cell clusters in the medial pulvinar nucleus. *J Comp Neurol.* 1985;241(3):357-381.

678. Romanski LM, Giguere M, Bates JF, Goldman-Rakic PS. Topographic organization of medial pulvinar connections with the prefrontal cortex in the rhesus monkey. *J Comp Neurol.* 1997;379(3):313-332.

679. Mufson EJ, Mesulam MM. Thalamic connections of the insula in the rhesus monkey and comments on the paralimbic connectivity of the medial pulvinar nucleus. *J Comp Neurol.* 1984;227(1):109-120.

680. Karnath HO, Himmelbach M, Rorden C. The subcortical anatomy of human spatial neglect: putamen, caudate nucleus and pulvinar. *Brain.* 2002;125(pt 2):350-360.

681. Guard O, Bellis F, Mabille JP, Dumas R, Boisson D, Devic M. Démence thalamique après lésion hémorragique unilatérale du pulvinar droit [Thalamic dementia after a unilateral hemorrhagic lesion of the right pulvinar]. *Rev Neurol (Paris).* 1986;142(10):759-765.

682. Robinson D, Cowie R. The primate pulvinar: structural, functional and behavioral components of visual salience. In: Steriade M, Jones EG, McCormick DA, eds. *Thalamus, Vol 2. Experimental and Clinical Aspects.* New York, NY: Elsevier; 1997:53-92.

683. Cusick CG, Scripter JL, Darensbourg JG, Weber JT. Chemoarchitectonic subdivisions of the visual pulvinar in monkeys and their connectional relations with the middle temporal and rostral dorsolateral visual areas, MT and DLr. *J Comp Neurol.* 1993;336(1):1-30.

684. Cowey A, Stoerig P, Bannister M. Retinal ganglion cells labelled from the pulvinar nucleus in macaque monkeys. *Neuroscience.* 1994;61(3):691-705.

685. Pitkänen A, Amaral DG. Organization of the intrinsic connections of the monkey amygdaloid complex: projections originating in the lateral nucleus. *J Comp Neurol.* 1998;398(3):431-458.

686. Fisher CM. The pathologic and clinical aspects of thalamic hemorrhage. *Transac Am Neurol Assoc.* 1959;84:56-59.

687. Martin J. Degenerative diseases of the human thalamus. In: Steriade M, Jones EG, McCormick DA, eds. *Thalamus, Vol 2. Experimental and Clinical Aspects.* New York, NY: Elsevier; 1997:653-687.

688. Nass R, Boyce L, Leventhal F, et al. Acquired aphasia in children after surgical resection of left-thalamic tumors. *Dev Med Child Neurol.* 2000;42(9):580-590.

689. Ziegler DK, Kaufman A, Marshall HE. Abrupt memory loss associated with thalamic tumor. *Arch Neurol.* 1977;34(9):545-548.

690. von Cramon DY, Hebel N, Schuri U. A contribution to the anatomical basis of thalamic amnesia. *Brain.* 1985;108(pt 4):993-1008.

691. De Freitas GR, Bogousslavsky J. Thalamic infarcts. In: Donnan G, Norving B, Bamford J, Bogousslavsky J, eds. *Subcortical Stroke.* London: Oxford University Press; 2002:255-285.

692. Bogousslavsky J, Regli F, Assal G. The syndrome of unilateral tuberothalamic artery territory infarction. *Stroke.* 1986;17(3):434-441.

693. Percheron G. The anatomy of the arterial supply of the human thalamus and its use for the interpretation of the thalamic vascular pathology. *Z Neurol.* 1973;205:1-13.

694. Clarke S, Assal G, Bogousslavsky J, et al. Pure amnesia after unilateral left polar thalamic infarct: topographic and sequential neuropsychological and metabolic (PET) correlations. *J. Neurol Neurosurg Psychiatry.* 1994;57(1):27-34.

695. Ghika-Schmid F, Bogousslavsky J. The acute behavioral syndrome of anterior thalamic infarction: a prospective study of 12 cases. *Ann Neurol.* 2000;48(2):220-227.

696. Graff-Radford NR, Damasio H, Yamada T, Eslinger PJ, Damasio AR. Nonhaemorrhagic thalamic infarction. Clinical, neuropsychological and electrophysiological findings in four anatomical groups defined by computerized tomography. *Brain.* 1985;108(pt 2):485-516.

697. Lisovoski F, Koskas P, Dubard T, Dessarts I, Dehen H, Cambier J. Left tuberothalamic artery territory infarction: neuropsychological and MRI features. *Eur Neurol.* 1993;33(2):181-184.

698. Warren JD, Thompson PD, Thompson PD. Diencephalic amnesia and apraxia after left thalamic infarction. *J Neurol Neurosurg Psychiatry.* 2000;68(2):248.

699. Segarra JM. Cerebral vascular disease and behavior, I: the syndrome of the mesencephalic artery (basilar artery bifurcation). *Arch Neurol.* 1970;22:408-418.

700. Castaigne P, Lhermitte F, Buge A, Escourolle R, Hauw JJ, Lyon-Caen O. Paramedian thalamic and midbrain infarct: clinical and neuropathological study. *Ann Neurol.* 1981;10(2):127-148.

701. Caplan LR. "Top of the basilar" syndrome. *Neurology.* 1980;30:72-79.

702. Guberman A, Stuss D. The syndrome of bilateral paramedian thalamic infarction. *Neurology.* 1983;33(5):540-546.

703. Reilly M, Connolly S, Stack J, Martin EA, Hutchinson M. Bilateral paramedian thalamic infarction: a distinct but poorly recognized stroke syndrome. *Q J Med.* 1992;82(297):63-70.

704. Bogousslavsky J, Regli F, Delaloye B, Delaloye-Bischof A, Assal G, Uske A. Loss of psychic self-activation with bithalamic infarction. Neurobehavioural, CT, MRI and SPECT correlates. *Acta Neurol Scand.* 1991;83(5):309-316.

705. Engelborghs S, Marien P, Pickut BA, Verstraeten S, De Deyn PP. Loss of psychic self-activation after paramedian bithalamic infarction. *Stroke.* 2000;31(7):1762-1765.

706. Hodges JR, McCarthy RA. Autobiographical amnesia resulting from bilateral paramedian thalamic infarction. A case study in cognitive neurobiology. *Brain.* 1993;116(pt 4):921-940.

707. Spiegel EA, Wycis HT, Orchinik C, Freed H. Thalamic chronotaraxis. *Am J Psychiatry.* 1956;113(2):97-105.

708. Krolak-Salmon P, Croisile B, Houzard C, Setiey A, Girard-Madoux P, Vighetto A. Total recovery after bilateral paramedian thalamic infarct. *Eur Neurol.* 2000;44:216-218.

709. Goldenberg G, Podreka I, Pfaffelmeyer N, Wessely P, Deecke L. Thalamic ischemia in transient global amnesia: a SPECT study. *Neurology.* 1991;41:1748-1752.

710. Foix C, Hillemand P. Les artères de l'axe encèphalique jusqu'au diencèphale inclusivement. *Revue Neurologique (Paris).* 1925;2:705-739.

711. Plets C, De Reuck J, Vander Eecken H, Van den Bergh R. The vascularization of the human thalamus. *Acta Neurol Belg.* 1970;70:687-770.

712. Caplan LR, DeWitt LD, Pessin MS, Gorelick PB, Adelman LS. Lateral thalamic infarcts. *Arch Neurol.* 1988;45(9):959-964.

713. Déjerine JJ, Roussy G. Le syndrome thalamique. *Revue Neurologique (Paris).* 1906;14:521-532.

714. Garcin R, Lapresle J. Sensory syndrome of the thalamic type and with hand-mouth topography due to localized lesions of the thalamus. *Revue Neurologique (Paris).* 1954;90(2):124-129.

715. Fisher CM. Thalamic pure sensory stroke: a pathologic study. *Neurology.* 1978;28(11):1141-1144.

716. Lapresle J, Haguenau M. Anatomico-chemical correlation in focal thalamic lesions. *Zeitschrift für Neurologie.* 1973;205(1):29-46.

717. Nasreddine ZS, Saver JL. Pain after thalamic stroke: right diencephalic predominance and clinical features in 180 patients. *Neurology.* 1997;48(5):1196-1199.

718. Garcin R. Cerebello-thalamic syndrome caused by localized lesion of the thalamus; sign of so-called main creuse and its symptomatologic value. *Revue Neurologique (Paris).* 1955;93(1):143-149.

719. Karussis D, Leker RR, Abarmsky O. Cognitive dysfunction following thalamic stroke: a study of 16 cases and review of the literature. *J Neurol Sci.* 2000;172:25-29.

720. Decroix JP, Graveleau P, Masson M, Cambier J. Infarction in the territory of the anterior choroidal artery: a clinical and computerized tomographic study of 16 cases. *Brain.* 1986;109:1071-1085.

721. Neau JP, Bogousslavsky J. The syndrome of posterior choroidal artery territory infarction. *Ann Neurol.* 1996;39(6):779-788.

722. Leigh R, Zee D. *The Neurology of Eye Movements.* Philadelphia, PA: FA Davis; 1983.

723. Crosson B. Thalamic mechanisms in language: a reconsideration based on recent findings and concepts. *Brain Lang.* 2013;126(1):73-88.

724. Schmahmann JD, ed. *The Cerebellum and Cognition. International Review of Neurobiology.* Vol 47. San Diego, CA: Academic Press; 1997.

725. Brodal A, Hoivik B. Site and termination of primary vestibulocerebellar fibres in the cat. An experimental study with silver impregnation methods. *Arch Ital Biol.* 1964;102:1-21.

726. Larsell O, Jansen J. *The Comparative Anatomy and Histology of the Cerebellum. The Human Cerebellum, Cerebellar Connections, and Cerebellar Cortex.* Minneapolis, MN: University of Minnesota Press; 1972.

727. Bolk L. *Das Cerebellum der Säugetiere.* Haarlem: Fischer; 1906.

728. Schmahmann JD, Doyon J, McDonald D, et al. Three-dimensional MRI atlas of the human cerebellum in proportional stereotaxic space. *NeuroImage.* 1999;10(3, pt 1):233-260.

729. Schmahmann JD, Doyon J, Toga A, Evans A, Petrides M. *MRI Atlas of the Human Cerebellum.* San Diego, CA: Academic Press; 2000.

730. Eccles JC. The cerebellum as a computer: patterns in space and time. *J Physiol.* 1973;229(1):1-32.

731. Oscarsson O. Functional organization of the spino- and cuneocerebellar tracts. *Physiol Rev.* 1965;45:495-522.

732. Ito M. *The Cerebellum and Neural Control.* New York, NY: Raven Press; 1984.

733. Napper RM, Harvey RJ. Number of parallel fiber synapses on an individual Purkinje cell in the cerebellum of the rat. *J Comp Neurol.* 1988;274(2):168-177.

734. Hawkes R, Gravel C. The modular cerebellum. *Prog Neurobiol.* 1991;36(4):309-327.

735. Sugihara I, Wu H-S, Shinoda Y. The entire trajectories of single olivocerebellar axons in the cerebellar cortex and their contribution to cerebellar compartmentalization. *J Neurosci.* 2001;21(19):7715-7723.

736. Voogd J, Ruigrok TJH. Cerebellum and precerebellar nuclei. In: May J, Paxinos G, eds. *The Human Nervous System.* Amsterdam: Elsevier; 2012:471-547.

737. Grant G. Spinal course and somatotopically localized termination of the spinocerebellar tracts. An experimental study in the cat. *Acta Physiol Scand Suppl.* 1962;56(193):1-61.

738. Grant G. Projection of the external cuneate nucleus onto the cerebellum in the cat: an experimental study using silver methods. *Exp Neurol.* 1962;5:179-195.

739. Brodal A. *Neurological Anatomy in Relation to Clinical Medicine.* 2nd ed. New York, NY: Oxford; 1981.

740. Brodal P. The corticopontine projection in the rhesus monkey. Origin and principles of organization. *Brain.* 1978;101(2): 251-283.

741. Glickstein M, May JG3rd, Mercier BE. Corticopontine projection in the macaque: the distribution of labelled cortical cells after large injections of horseradish peroxidase in the pontine nuclei. *J Comp Neurol.* 1985;235(3):343-359.

742. Schmahmann JD, Pandya DN. Course of the fiber pathways to pons from parasensory association areas in the rhesus monkey. *J Comp Neurol.* 1992;326(2):159-179.

743. Schmahmann JD, Rosene DL, Pandya DN. Ataxia after pontine stroke: insights from pontocerebellar fibers in monkey. *Ann Neurol.* 2004;55(4):585-589.

744. Schmahmann JD, Pandya DN. Anatomical investigation of projections to the basis pontis from posterior parietal association cortices in rhesus monkey. *J Comp Neurol.* 1989;289(1):53-73.

745. Schmahmann JD, Pandya DN. Projections to the basis pontis from the superior temporal sulcus and superior temporal region in the rhesus monkey. *J Comp Neurol.* 1991;308(2):224-248.

746. Schmahmann JD, Pandya DN. Prelunate, occipitotemporal, and parahippocampal projections to the basis pontis in rhesus monkey. *J Comp Neurol.* 1993;337(1):94-112.

747. Schmahmann JD, Pandya DN. Anatomic organization of the basilar pontine projections from prefrontal cortices in rhesus monkey. *J Neurosci.* 1997;17(1):438-458.

748. Schmahmann JD, Pandya DN. The cerebrocerebellar system. *Int Rev Neurobiol.* 1997;41:31-60.

749. Schmahmann JD. From movement to thought: anatomic substrates of the cerebellar contribution to cognitive processing. *Human Brain Mapp.* 1996;4:174-198.

750. Schmahmann JD, Rosene DL, Pandya DN. Motor projections to the basis pontis in rhesus monkey. *J Comp Neurol.* 2004;478(3):248-268.

751. Allen GI, Tsukahara N. Cerebrocerebellar communication systems. *Physiol Rev.* 1974;54(4):957-1006.

752. Kelly RM, Strick PL. Cerebellar loops with motor cortex and prefrontal cortex of a nonhuman primate. *J Neurosci.* 2003;23(23):8432-8444.

753. Heath RJ. Modulation of emotion with a brain pacemaker. *J Nerv Ment Dis.* 1977;165:300-317.

754. Berman AF, Berman D, Prescott JW. The effect of cerebellar lesions on emotional behavior in the rhesus monkey. In: Cooper IS, Riklan M, Snider RS, eds. *The Cerebellum, Epilepsy and Behavior.* New York, NY: Plenum Press; 1978:277-284.

755. Schmahmann JD. The role of the cerebellum in affect and psychosis. *J Neurolinguistics.* 2000;13:189-214.

756. Fujita H, Kodama T, du Lac S. Modular output circuits of the fastigial nucleus mediate diverse motor and nonmotor functions of the cerebellar vermis. *bioRxiv.* 2020. doi:https://doi.org/10.1101/2020.04.23.047100.

757. Middleton FA, Strick PL. Cerebellar output channels. *Int Rev Neurobiol.* 1997;41:61-82.

758. Dum RP, Li C, Strick PL. Motor and nonmotor domains in the monkey dentate. *Ann N Y Acad Sci.* 2002;978:289-301.

759. Schmahmann JD. Cerebellum and spinal cord—principles of development, anatomical organization, and functional relevance. In: Brice A, Pulst S, eds. *Spinocerebellar Degenerations: The Ataxias and Spastic Paraplegias.* New York, NY: Elsevier; 2006:1-60.

760. Schmahmann JD. Cerebellum and ataxia. In: Jones HR, Burns TM, Aminoff MJ, Pomeroy SL, eds. *The Netter Collection of Medical Illustrations, Frank H. Netter, MD, Vol 7. Nervous System*

Part 1, Brain. 2nd ed. Philadelphia, PA: Elsevier/Saunders; 2013:177-197.

761. Voogd J, Glickstein M. The anatomy of the cerebellum. *Trends Neurosci.* 1998;21(9):370-375.

762. *Gray's Anatomy.* 42nd ed. London: Elsevier; 2020.

763. Haines DE, Dietrichs E, Sowa TE. Hypothalamo-cerebellar and cerebello-hypothalamic pathways: a review and hypothesis concerning cerebellar circuits which may influence autonomic centers affective behavior. *Brain Behav Evol.* 1984;24(4):198-220.

764. Dietrichs E, Haines DE. Interconnections between hypothalamus and cerebellum. *Anat Embryol (Berl).* 1989;179(3):207-220.

765. Haines DE, Dietrichs E, Mihailoff GA, McDonald EF. The cerebellar-hypothalamic axis: basic circuits and clinical observations. *Int Rev Neurobiol.* 1997;41:8-107.

766. Allen GV, Hopkins DA. Topography and synaptology of mammillary body projections to the mesencephalon and pons in the rat. *J Comp Neurol.* 1990;301(2):214-231.

767. Reis DJ, Doba N, Nathan MA. Predatory attack, grooming and consummatory behaviors evoked by electrical stimulation of cat cerebellar nuclei. *Science.* 1973;182:845-847.

768. Moruzzi G. Sham rage and localized autonomic responses elicited by cerebellar stimulation in the acute thalamic cat. *Proc XVII Int Congr Physiol Oxford.* 1947:114-115.

769. Zanchetti A, Zoccolini A. Autonomic hypothalamic outbursts elicited by cerebellar stimulation. *J Neurophysiol.* 1954;17:473-483.

770. Berntson G, Potolicchio SJr, Miller N. Evidence for higher functions of the cerebellum. Eating and grooming elicited by cerebellar stimulation in cats. *Proc Natl Acad Sci U S A.* 1973;70: 2497-2499.

771. Ball G, Micco DJr, Berntson G. Cerebellar stimulation in the rat. Complex stimulation bound oral behaviors and self-stimulation. *Physiol Behav.* 1974;13:123-127.

772. Heath RG, Dempesy CW, Fontana CJ, Myers WA. Cerebellar stimulation: effects on septal region, hippocampus, and amygdala of cats and rats. *Biol Psychiatry.* 1978;13(5):501-529.

773. Newman PP, Reza H. Functional relationships between the hippocampus and the cerebellum: an electrophysiological study of the cat. *J Physiol.* 1979;287:405-426.

774. Heath RG, Harper JW. Ascending projections of the cerebellar fastigial nucleus to the hippocampus amygdala and other temporal lobe sites. Evoked potential and histological studies in monkeys and cats. *Exp Neurol.* 1974;45:2682-2687.

775. Bohne P, Schwarz MK, Herlitze S, Mark MD. A new projection from the deep cerebellar nuclei to the hippocampus via the ventrolateral and laterodorsal thalamus in mice. *Front Neural Circuits.* 2019;13:51.

776. Onuki Y, Van Someren EJ, De Zeeuw CI, Van der Werf YD. Hippocampal-cerebellar interaction during spatio-temporal prediction. *Cereb Cortex.* 2015;25(2):313-321.

777. Iglói K, Doeller CF, Paradis AL, et al. Interaction between hippocampus and cerebellum crus I in sequence-based but not place-based navigation. *Cereb Cortex.* 2015;25(11):4146-4154.

778. McCormick DA, Thompson RF. Cerebellum. Essential involvement in the classically conditioned eyelid response. *Science.* 1984;223:296-299.

779. Farley SJ, Radley JJ, Freeman JH. Amygdala modulation of cerebellar learning. *J Neurosci.* 2016;36(7):2190-2201.

780. Carta I, Chen CH, Schott AL, Dorizan S, Khodakhah K. Cerebellar modulation of the reward circuitry and social behavior. *Science.* 2019;363(6424):eaav0581.

781. Snider RS, Maiti A. Snider SR. Cerebellar pathways to ventral midbrain and nigra. *Exp Neurol.* 1976;53(3):714-728.

782. Snider RS, Maiti A. Cerebellar contributions to the Papez circuit. *J Neurosci Res.* 1976;2(2):133-146.

783. Simon H, Le Moal M, Calas A. Efferents and afferents of the ventral tegmental-A10 region studied after local injection of [3H]leucine and horseradish peroxidase. *Brain Res*. 1979;178(1):17-40.

784. Oades RD, Halliday GM. Ventral tegmental (A10) system: neurobiology. 1. Anatomy and connectivity. *Brain Res*. 1987;434(2):117-165.

785. Wagner MJ, Kim TH, Savall J, Schnitzer MJ, Luo L. Cerebellar granule cells encode the expectation of reward. *Nature*. 2017;544(7648):96-100.

786. Koziol LF, Budding D, Andreasen N, et al. Consensus paper: the cerebellum's role in movement and cognition. *Cerebellum*. 2014;13(1):151-177.

787. Adamaszek M, D'Agata F, Ferrucci R, et al. Consensus paper: cerebellum and emotion. *Cerebellum*. 2017;16(2):552-576.

788. Hoche F, Guell X, Vangel MG, Sherman JC, Schmahmann JD. The cerebellar cognitive affective/Schmahmann syndrome scale. *Brain*. 2018;141(1):248-270.

789. Lackey EP, Heck DH, Sillitoe RV. Recent advances in understanding the mechanisms of cerebellar granule cell development and function and their contribution to behavior. *F1000Res*. 2018;7:F1000 Faculty Rev-1142.

790. Habas C, Kamdar N, Nguyen D, et al. Distinct cerebellar contributions to intrinsic connectivity networks. *J Neurosci*. 2009;29(26):8586-8594.

791. Krienen FM, Buckner RL. Segregated fronto-cerebellar circuits revealed by intrinsic functional connectivity. *Cereb Cortex*. 2009;19(10):2485-2497.

792. O'Reilly JX, Beckmann CF, Tomassini V, Ramnani N, Johansen-Berg H. Distinct and overlapping functional zones in the cerebellum defined by resting state functional connectivity. *Cereb Cortex*. 2010;20(4):953-965.

793. Guell X, Schmahmann J. Cerebellar functional anatomy: a didactic summary based on human fMRI evidence. *Cerebellum*. 2020;19(1):1-5.

794. Stoodley CJ, Schmahmann JD. Functional topography in the human cerebellum: a meta-analysis of neuroimaging studies. *NeuroImage*. 2009;44(2):489-501.

795. Stoodley CJ, Valera EM, Schmahmann JD. Functional topography of the cerebellum for motor and cognitive tasks: an fMRI study. *NeuroImage*. 2012;59(2):1560-1570.

796. Keren-Happuch E, Chen SH, Ho MH, Desmond JE. A meta-analysis of cerebellar contributions to higher cognition from PET and fMRI studies. *Hum Brain Mapp*. 2014;35(2):593-615.

797. Snider RS, Eldred E. Cerebrocerebellar relationships in the monkey. *J Neurophysiol*. 1952;15(1):27-40.

798. Moulton EA, Elman I, Pendse G, Schmahmann J, Becerra L, Borsook D. Aversion-related circuitry in the cerebellum: responses to noxious heat and unpleasant images. *J Neurosci*. 2011;31(10):3795-3804.

799. Brissenden JA, Tobyne SM, Osher DE, Levin EJ, Halko MA, Somers DC. Topographic cortico-cerebellar networks revealed by visual attention and working memory. *Curr Biol*. 2018;28:3364-3372.

800. Stoodley CJ, Schmahmann JD. Evidence for topographic organization in the cerebellum of motor control versus cognitive and affective processing. *Cortex*. 2010;46(7):831-844.

801. Stoodley CJ, Valera EM, Schmahmann JD. An fMRI study of intra-individual functional topography in the human cerebellum. *Behav Neurol*. 2010;23(1-2):65-79.

802. Bechterew W. Zur Anatomie der Schenkel des Kleinhirns, insbesondere der Brückenarme. *Neurologisches Centralblatt*. 1885;4:121-125.

803. Takahashi E, Song JW, Folkerth RD, Grant PE, Schmahmann JD. Detection of postmortem human cerebellar cortex and white matter pathways using high angular resolution diffusion tractography: a feasibility study. *NeuroImage*. 2013;68:105-111.

804. Tobyne SM, Ochoa WB, Bireley JD, et al. Cognitive impairment and the regional distribution of cerebellar lesions in multiple sclerosis. *Mult Scler*. 2018;24(13):1687-1695.

805. Schmahmann JD, Macmore J, Vangel M. Cerebellar stroke without motor deficit: clinical evidence for motor and non-motor domains within the human cerebellum. *Neuroscience*. 2009;162(3):852-861.

806. Grodd W, Hülsmann E, Lotze M, Wildgruber D, Erb M. Sensorimotor mapping of the human cerebellum: fMRI evidence of somatotopic organization. *Hum Brain Mapp*. 2001;13(2):55-73.

807. Stoodley CJ, MacMore JP, Makris N, Sherman JC, Schmahmann JD. Location of lesion determines motor vs. cognitive consequences in patients with cerebellar stroke. *NeuroImage Clin*. 2016;12:765-775.

808. Duncan GW, Parker SW, Fisher CM. Acute cerebellar infarction in the PICA territory. *Arch Neurol*. 1975;32(6):364-368.

809. Lee H, Sohn SI, Cho YW, et al. Cerebellar infarction presenting isolated vertigo: frequency and vascular topographical patterns. *Neurology*. 2006;67(7):1178-1183.

810. Manto M, Mariën P. Schmahmann's syndrome—identification of the third cornerstone of clinical ataxiology. *Cerebellum Ataxias*. 2015;2:2.

811. Argyropoulos GPD, van Dun K, Adamaszek M, et al. The cerebellar cognitive affective/Schmahmann syndrome: a task force paper. *Cerebellum*. 2020;19(1):102-125.

812. Exner C, Weniger G, Irle E. Cerebellar lesions in the PICA but not SCA territory impair cognition. *Neurology*. 2004;63(11):2132-2135.

813. Schmahmann JD, Weilburg JB, Sherman JC. The neuropsychiatry of the cerebellum—insights from the clinic. *Cerebellum*. 2007;6(3):254-267.

814. Malm J, Kristensen B, Karlsson T, Carlberg B, Fagerlund M, Olsson T. Cognitive impairment in young adults with infratentorial infarcts. *Neurology*. 1998;51(2):433-440.

815. Neau JP, Arroyo-Anllo E, Bonnaud V, Ingrand P, Gil R. Neuropsychological disturbances in cerebellar infarcts. *Acta Neurol Scand*. 2000;102(6):363-370.

816. Riva D, Giorgi C. The cerebellum contributes to higher functions during development: evidence from a series of children surgically treated for posterior fossa tumours. *Brain*. 2000;123 (pt 5):1051-1061.

817. Scott RB, Stoodley CJ, Anslow P, et al. Lateralized cognitive deficits in children following cerebellar lesions. *Dev Med Child Neurol*. 2001;43(10):685-691.

818. Allin M, Matsumoto H, Santhouse AM, et al. Cognitive and motor function and the size of the cerebellum in adolescents born very pre-term. *Brain*. 2001;124(pt 1):60-66.

819. Poretti A, Boltshauser E, Schmahmann JD. Cerebellar agenesis. In: Boltshauser E, Schmahmann JD, eds. *Cerebellar Disorders in Children*. London: MacKeith Press; 2012:117-121.

820. van Harskamp NJ, Rudge P, Cipolotti L. Cognitive and social impairments in patients with superficial siderosis. *Brain*. 2005;128(pt 5):1082-1092.

821. Limperopoulos C, Robertson RL, Estroff JA, et al. Diagnosis of inferior vermian hypoplasia by fetal magnetic resonance imaging: potential pitfalls and neurodevelopmental outcome. *Am J Obstet Gynecol*. 2006;194(4):1070-1076.

822. Tavano A, Grasso R, Gagliardi C, et al. Disorders of cognitive and affective development in cerebellar malformations. *Brain.* 2007;130(pt 10):2646-2660.

823. Tedesco AM, Chiricozzi FR, Clausi S, Lupo M, Molinari M, Leggio MG. The cerebellar cognitive profile. *Brain.* 2011;134 (pt 12):3672-3686.

824. Schmahmann JD. The cerebellum and cognition. *Neurosci Lett.* 2019;688:62-75.

825. Schmahmann JD. Pediatric post-operative cerebellar mutism syndrome, cerebellar cognitive affective syndrome, and posterior fossa syndrome: historical review and proposed resolution to guide future study. *Childs Nerv Syst.* 2020;36(6):1205-1214.

826. Hoche F, Guell X, Sherman JC, Vangel MG, Schmahmann JD. Cerebellar contribution to social cognition. *Cerebellum.* 2016;15(6):732-743.

827. Parvizi J, Anderson SW, Martin CO, Damasio H, Damasio AR. Pathological laughter and crying: a link to the cerebellum. *Brain.* 2001;124(pt 9):1708-1719.

828. Parvizi J, Joseph J, Press DZ, Schmahmann JD. Pathological laughter and crying in patients with multiple system atrophy-cerebellar type. *Mov Disord.* 2007;22(6):798-803.

829. Wisoff JH, Epstein FJ. Pseudobulbar palsy after posterior fossa operation in children. *Neurosurgery.* 1984;15(5):707-709.

830. Pollack IF. Posterior fossa syndrome. *Int Rev Neurobiol.* 1997;41:411-432.

831. Gudrunardottir T, Morgan AT, Lux AL, et al. Consensus paper on post-operative pediatric cerebellar mutism syndrome: the Iceland Delphi results. *Childs Nerv Syst.* 2016;32(7):1195-1203.

832. Albazron FM, Bruss J, Jones RM, et al. Pediatric postoperative cerebellar cognitive affective syndrome follows outflow pathway lesions. *Neurology.* 2019;93(16):e1561-e1571.

833. Schmahmann JD. Neuroanatomy of pediatric postoperative cerebellar cognitive affective syndrome and mutism. *Neurology.* 2019;93(16):693-694.

834. Guell X, Hoche F, Schmahmann JD. Metalinguistic deficits in patients with cerebellar dysfunction: empirical support for the dysmetria of thought theory. *Cerebellum.* 2015;14(1): 50-58.

835. Jurado R, Walker HK. Cerebrospinal fluid. In: Walker HK, Hall WD, Hurst JW, eds. *Clinical Methods: The History, Physical, and Laboratory Examinations.* 3rd ed. Boston, MA, Butterworths, 1990:chap. 74.

836. Sofronescu AG. Cerebrospinal fluid analysis. 2015. Available at medscape.com/article/2093316-overview.

837. Johanson CE, Duncan JA, Klinge PM, et al. Multiplicity of cerebrospinal fluid functions: new challenges in health and disease. *Cerebrospinal Fluid Res.* 2008;14(5):10.

838. Mokri B. Spontaneous intracranial hypotension. *Continuum (Minneap Minn).* 2015;21(4 Headache):1086-1108.

839. Jessen NA, Munk AS, Lundgaard I, Nedergaard M. The glymphatic system: a beginner's guide. *Neurochem Res.* 2015;40(12):2583-2599.

840. Orešković D, Klarica M. The formation of cerebrospinal fluid: nearly a hundred years of interpretations and misinterpretations. *Brain Res Rev.* 2010;64(2):241-262.

841. Mestre H, Tithof J, Du T, et al. Flow of cerebrospinal fluid is driven by arterial pulsations and is reduced in hypertension. *Nat Commun.* 2018;9(1):4878.

842. Johnston M, Zakharov A, Papaiconomou C, Salmasi G, Armstrong D. Evidence of connections between cerebrospinal fluid and nasal lymphatic vessels in humans, non-human primates and other mammalian species. *Cerebrospinal Fluid Res.* 2004;1(1):2.

843. Lacar B, Young SZ, Platel JC, Bordey A. Imaging and recording subventricular zone progenitor cells in live tissue of postnatal mice. *Front Neurosci.* 2010;4:43.

844. Lim DA, Alvarez-Buylla A. The adult ventricular-subventricular zone (V-SVZ) and olfactory bulb (OB) neurogenesis. *Cold Spring Harb Perspect Biol.* 2016;8(5):a018820.

845. Alonso MI, Gato A. Cerebrospinal fluid and neural stem cell niche control. *Neural Regen Res.* 2018;13(9):1546-1547.

846. Adams RD, Fisher CM, Hakim S, Ojemann RG, Sweet WH. Symptomatic occult hydrocephalus with "normal" cerebrospinal fluid pressure. A treatable syndrome. *N Engl J Med.* 1965;273:117-126.

847. Schwarzschild M, Rordorf G, Bekken K, Buonanno F, Schmahmann JD. Normal-pressure hydrocephalus with misleading features of irreversible dementias: a case report. *J Geriatr Psychiatry Neurol.* 1997;10(2):51-54.

848. Halperin JJ, Kurlan R, Schwalb JM, Cusimano MD, Gronseth G, Gloss D. Practice guideline: idiopathic normal pressure hydrocephalus: response to shunting and predictors of response: report of the Guideline Development, Dissemination, and Implementation Subcommittee of the American Academy of Neurology. *Neurology.* 2015;85(23):2063-2071.

849. Wicklund MR, Mokri B, Drubach DA, Boeve BF, Parisi JE, Josephs KA. Frontotemporal brain sagging syndrome: an SIH-like presentation mimicking FTD. *Neurology.* 2011;76(16):1377-1382.

850. Ashayeri K, Jackson EM, Huang J, Brem H, Gordon CR. Syndrome of the trephined: a systematic review. *Neurosurgery.* 2016;79(4):525-534.

851. Zanaty M, Nakagawa D, Starke RM, et al. Intraventricular extension of an aneurysmal subarachnoid hemorrhage is an independent predictor of a worse functional outcome. *Clin Neurol Neurosurg.* 2018;170:67-72.

852. Weinstein R, Ess K, Sirdar B, Song S, Cutting S. Primary intraventricular hemorrhage: clinical characteristics and outcomes. *J Stroke Cerebrovasc Dis.* 2017;26(5):995-999.

853. Dolar MT, Haughton VM, Iskandar BJ, Quigley M. Effect of craniocervical decompression on peak CSF velocities in symptomatic patients with Chiari I malformation. *Am J Neuroradiol.* 2004;25(1):142-145.

854. McGirt MJ, Atiba A, Attenello FJ, et al. Correlation of hindbrain CSF flow and outcome after surgical decompression for Chiari I malformation. *Childs Nerv Syst.* 2008;24(7):833-840.

855. Allen PA, Houston JR, Pollock JW, et al. Task-specific and general cognitive effects in Chiari malformation type I. *PLoS One.* 2014;9(4):e94844.

856. Dewey J. *How We Think.* London: D.C. Heath; 1909.

857. Schmahmann JD. How we think: A consideration of the neural substrates of cognition. American Society for Neuroradiology, 51st Annual Meeting, May 22, 2013. Available at https://www.ajnrblog.org/2013/06/28/how-does-the-brain-think/.

858. Zahm DS, Trimble M, Van Hoesen GW. Preface. In: Heimer L, Van Hoesen GW, Trimble M, Zahm DS, eds. *Anatomy of Neuropsychiatry. The New Anatomy of the Basal Forebrain and Its Implications for Neuropsychiatric Illness.* Amsterdam: Elsevier; 2008:xiv.

859. Jackson JH. Remarks on evolution and dissolution of the nervous system. 1887. In: Taylor J, ed. *Selected Writings of John Hughlings Jackson, Volume II: Evolution and Dissolution of the Nervous System Speech, Various Papers, Addresses and Lectures.* New York, NY: Basic Books, 1958:76-91.

860. Adams RD, Victor M. *Principles of Neurology.* 2nd ed. New York, NY: McGraw-Hill; 1981.

861. Mink J. The basal ganglia. In: Squire LR, Bloom FE, McConnell, et al., eds. *Fundamental Neuroscience*. New York, NY: Academic Press; 2003:815-839.
862. Johnson KA, Becker JA. The whole brain atlas. Available at www.med.harvard.edu/AANLIB/.
863. Dart RA. The dual structure of the neopallium: its history and significance. *J Anat*. 1934;69(pt 1):3-19.
864. Ghika J, Bogousslavsky J, Henderson J, Maeder P, Regli F. The "jerky dystonic unsteady hand": a delayed motor syndrome in posterior thalamic infarctions. *J Neurol*. 1994;241:537-542.

FIGURE CREDITS

FIGURE 1-1. Gall FJ, Spurzheim G: *Anatomie et Physiologie du Systeme Nerveux en general, et du Cerveau en particulier*. Paris, Chez F. Schoell. 1810.

FIGURE 1-2. Part A: Sobotta J: *Atlas of Human Anatomy* (*Volume III*). New York, G.E. Stechert and Co., 1928, figure 682, page 607.

Parts B,C: Reproduced with permission from Adams RD, Victor M. *Principles of Neurology*. 2nd ed. Copyright © McGraw Hill LLC. All rights reserved.

FIGURE 1-3. Mesulam MM: *Principles of Behavioral and Cognitive Neurology*, 2nd ed. Copyright © 2000 by Oxford University Press, Inc. Reproduced with permission of Oxford Publishing Ltd. through PLSclear.

FIGURE 1-4. Mesulam MM: *Principles of Behavioral and Cognitive Neurology*, 2nd ed. Copyright © 2000 by Oxford University Press, Inc. Reproduced with permission of Oxford Publishing Ltd. through PLSclear.

FIGURE 1-5. Part A: Gray HL, Williams PL, Bannister LH. *Gray's Anatomy: The Anatomical Basis of Medicine and Surgery*, 38th ed. New York. Copyright © 1995 Churchill Livingstone, an imprint of Elsevier Ltd. All rights reserved.

Part B: Jones HR, Burns TM, Aminoff MJ, Pomeroy SL: *The Netter collection of medical illustrations, Frank H. Netter, MD, Vol. 7. Nervous system Part 1, Brain* (2nd ed.), Philadelphia, PA, Elsevier/Saunders, 2013. Copyright © Elsevier. All rights reserved.

FIGURE 1-6. Carpenter MB. *Human Neuroanatomy*, 7th ed. Baltimore, Lippincott Williams & Wilkins. 1976.

FIGURE 1-7. Hikosaka O, Sesack SR, Lecourtier L, Shepard PD: Habenula: Crossroad between the basal ganglia and the limbic system. *J. Neurosci*. 2008(Nov12);28(46):11825-11829. Copyright © 2008 Society for Neuroscience. https://www.jneurosci.org/content/28/46/11825.

FIGURE 1-8. Part A: Le Gros Clark WE: The Topography and Homologies of the Hypothalamic Nuclei in Man. *J. Anat*. 1936;70 (Pt 2):203-214. https://www.ncbi.nlm.nih.gov/pmc/articles/PMC1249116. National Center for Biotechnology Information, U.S. National Library of Medicine.

Part B: Modified from Haymaker W, Anderson E, Nauta WJH. *The Hypothalamus*. 1969. Courtesy of Charles C. Thomas Publisher Ltd., Springfield, Illinois.

Part C: Elmquist JK, Elias CF, Saper CB: From lesions to leptin: Hypothalamic control of food intake and body weight. *Neuron*. 1999;22(2):221-232. Copyright © 1999 Cell Press. All rights reserved. https://www.sciencedirect.com/science/article/pii/S0896627300810843.

FIGURE 1-9. Emerson CH: Pituitary gland anatomy. *Encyclopedia Brittanica*, 2010. https://www.britannica.com/science/pituitary-gland.

FIGURE 1-10. Alcaro A, Huber R, Panksepp J: Behavioral functions of the mesolimbic dopaminergic system: An affective neuroethological perspective. *Brain Res Rev*. 2007;56(2):283-321. Copyright © 2007 Elsevier B.V. All rights reserved. https://www.sciencedirect.com/science/article/abs/pii/S0165017307001373?via%3Dihub.

FIGURE 1-11. Part A: Gray HL, Williams PL, Bannister LH. *Gray's Anatomy: The Anatomical Basis of Medicine and Surgery*, 38th ed. New York. Copyright © 1995 Churchill Livingstone, an imprint of Elsevier Ltd. All rights reserved.

Part B: Freese JL, Amaral DG. Neuroanatomy of the primate amygdala. In: *The Human Amygdala*, edited by PJ Whalen, EA Phelps. The Guilford Press, 2009. Reproduced with permission of Guilford Publications, Inc.; permission conveyed through Copyright Clearance Center, Inc

Part C: Nieuwenhuys R, Voogd J, van Huijzen C. Telencephalon: Amygdala and Claustrum. In: *The Human Central Nervous System*. © Springer Nature 2008. https://doi.org/10.1007/978-3-540-34686-9_13.

FIGURE 1-12. Heimer L, de' Olmos JS, Alheid GF, Pearson J, Sakamoto N: The human basal forebrain part II. In: *Handbook of Chemical Neuroanatomy*, edited by FE Bloom, A Björklund, T Hökflet T. Amsterdam. Copyright © 1999 Elsevier Science B.V. All rights reserved. https://www.sciencedirect.com/science/article/pii/S0924819699800244.

FIGURE 1-13. Rosene DL, Van Hoesen GW: The hippocampal formation of the primate brain: A review of some comparative aspects of cytoarchitecture and connections. In: Jones EG, Peters A (eds), *Cerebral Cortex* (Vol. 6). © Plenum Press, New York 1987.

FIGURE 1-14. Part A: Cajal S. Ramón y: *Studies on the Cerebral Cortex. Limbic Structures*. Translated by Kraft LM. Chicago, Year Book. 1955.

Part B: Deng W, Aimone JB, Gage FH: New neurons and new memories: how does adult hippocampal neurogenesis affect learning and memory? *Nat. Rev. Neurosci*. 2010;11(5):339-350. https://www.nature.com/nrn/.

FIGURE 1-15. Vaughan DN, Jackson GD: The piriform cortex and human focal epilepsy. *Front Neurol*. 2014;5:259. Copyright: © Vaughan and Jackson. https://www.frontiersin.org/articles/10.3389/fneur.2014.00259/full. https://bigbrainproject.org.

FIGURE 1-16. Parts A–C: Seeley WW, Carlin DA, Allman JM, et al: Early frontotemporal dementia targets neurons unique to apes and humans. *Ann. Neurol.* 2006;60(6):660-667. Copyright © American Neurological Association.

Part D: Nimchinsky EA, Gilissen E, Allman JM, et al: A neuronal morphologic type unique to humans and great apes. *Proc. Natl. Acad. Sci.* USA. 1999;96(9):5268-5273. Copyright © 1999 National Academy of Sciences, U.S.A.

Parts E,F: Allman JM, Tetreault NA, Hakeem AY, et al: The von Economo neurons in the frontoinsular and anterior cingulate cortex. *Ann. N. Y. Acad.* Sci. 2011;1225: 59–71. © 2011 New York Academy of Sciences. All rights reserved.

FIGURE 1-17. Gray HL, Williams PL, Bannister LH. *Gray's Anatomy: The Anatomical Basis of Medicine and Surgery*, 38th ed. New York. Copyright © 1995 Churchill Livingstone, an imprint of Elsevier Ltd. All rights reserved.

FIGURE 1-18. Mesulam MM: *Principles of Behavioral and Cognitive Neurology*, 2nd ed. Copyright © 2000 by Oxford University Press, Inc. Reproduced with permission of Oxford Publishing Ltd. through PLSclear.

FIGURE 1-19. Gray HL, Williams PL, Bannister LH. *Gray's Anatomy: The Anatomical Basis of Medicine and Surgery*, 38th ed. New York. Copyright © 1995 Churchill Livingstone, an imprint of Elsevier Ltd. All rights reserved.

FIGURE 1-20. Parts A,B: Petrides M, Pandya DN: Comparative architectonic analysis of the human and the macaque frontal cortex, in *Handbook of Neuropsychology* (Vol 9), edited by F Boller, J Grafman, H Spinnler. Amsterdam. Copyright © 1994 Elsevier. All rights reserved.

Parts C,D: Morecraft RJ, Stilwell-Morecraft KS, Ge J, et al: Cytoarchitecture and cortical connections of the anterior insula and adjacent frontal motor fields in the rhesus monkey. *Brain Res. Bull.* 2015;119(Pt A):52-72. Copyright © 2015 Elsevier Inc. Published by Elsevier Inc. All rights reserved.

FIGURE 1-21. Dart RA: The Dual Structure of the Neopallium: Its History and Significance. *J. Anat.* 1934;69(Pt 1):3-19. Blackwell Publishing Ltd. Copyright © John Wiley & Sons - Books, permission conveyed through Copyright Clearance Center, Inc.

FIGURE 1-22. Pandya DN, Seltzer B, Petrides M, Cipolloni PB: *Cerebral Cortex: Architecture, Connections, and the Dual Origin Concept*. New York, Oxford University Press, 2015. Reproduced with permission of Oxford Publishing Ltd. through PLSclear.

FIGURE 1-23. Pandya DN, Seltzer B, Petrides M, Cipolloni PB: *Cerebral Cortex: Architecture, Connections, and the Dual Origin Concept*. New York, Oxford University Press, 2015. Reproduced with permission of the Oxford Publishing Ltd. through PLSclear.

FIGURE 1-24. Suzuki WA, Naya Y: The Perirhinal Cortex. *Annual Review of Neuroscience.* 2014;37:39–53. Republished with permission of Annual Reviews, Inc., permission conveyed through Copyright Clearance Center, Inc.

FIGURE 1-25. Pandya DN, Yeterian, EH: Architecture and connections of cerebral cortex: Implications for brain evolution and function. In: *Neurobiology of Higher Cognitive Function: UCLA Forum in Medical Sciences, Number 29*, edited by AB Scheible AB, AF Wechsler AF, Adam F. New York, Guilford Press, 1990, pp. 53-84.

Republished with permission of Guilford Publications, Inc; permission conveyed through Copyright Clearance Center, Inc.

FIGURE 1-26. Schmahmann JD, Pandya DN: Disconnection syndromes of basal ganglia, thalamus, and cerebrocerebellar systems. *Cortex.* 2008;44(8):1037-1066. Copyright © 2008. Published by Elsevier Srl. All rights reserved.

FIGURE 1-27. Amunts K, Zilles K: Architectonic mapping of the human brain beyond Brodmann. *Neuron.* 2015;88:1086-1107. Copyright © 2015 Elsevier Inc. All rights reserved.

FIGURE 1-28. Sobotta J: *Atlas of Human Anatomy (Volume III)*. New York, G.E. Stechert and Co., 1928.

FIGURE 1-29. Part A: Mesulam MM: A cortical network for directed attention and unilateral neglect. *Ann. Neurol.* 1981;10(4):309-325. Copyright © 1981 American Neurological Association. Copyright © John Wiley and Sons. All rights reserved.

Part B: Mesulam MM, Van Hoesen GW, Pandya DN, Geschwind N: Limbic and sensory connections of the inferior parietal lobule (area PG) in the rhesus monkey: a study with a new method for horseradish peroxidase histochemistry. *Brain Res.* 1977(Nov18);136(3):393-414. Copyright © 1977. Published by Elsevier B.V.

FIGURE 1-30. Part A: Yeo BT, Krienen FM, Sepulcre J, et al: The organization of the human cerebral cortex estimated by intrinsic functional connectivity. *J. Neurophysiol.* 2011;106(3):1125-1165. Reproduced with permission of the American Physiological Society; permission conveyed through Copyright Clearance Center, Inc.

Parts B,C: Buckner RL, Krienen FM, Castellanos A, et al: The organization of the human cerebellum estimated by intrinsic functional connectivity. *J. Neurophysiol.* 2011;106(5):2322-2345. Reproduced with permission of the American Physiological Society; permission conveyed through Copyright Clearance Center, Inc.

FIGURE 1-31. Déjerine JJ: *Anatomie des centres nerveux*. Paris, Rueff et Cie, 1895.

FIGURE 1-32. Part A: Wedeen VJ, Wang R, Schmahmann JD, et al: Diffusion Spectrum MRI in Three Mammals - Rat, Monkey and Human. *Frontiers in Neuroscience.* 2009;3(1):74-77. © Copyright 2007-2020 Frontiers Media SA. All rights reserved.

Parts B,C: Schmahmann JD, Pandya DN, Wang R, et al: Association fibre pathways of the brain: parallel observations from diffusion spectrum imaging and autoradiography. *Brain.* 2007;130(Pt 3): 630-653, by permission of Oxford University Press.

FIGURE 1-33. Part A: Schmahmann JD, Pandya DN: *Fiber pathways of the brain*. New York, NY, Oxford University Press, 2006.

Part B: Thiebaut de Schotten M, Dell'Acqua F, Valabregue R, Catani M: Monkey to human comparative anatomy of the frontal lobe association tracts. *Cortex.* 2012;48(1):82-96. Copyright © 2011 Elsevier Srl. All rights reserved.

FIGURE 1-34. Part A: Schmahmann JD, Pandya DN: *Fiber pathways of the brain*. New York, NY, Oxford University Press, 2006.

Part B: Thiebaut de Schotten M, Dell' Acqua F, Valabregue R, Catani M: Monkey to human comparative anatomy of the frontal lobe association tracts. *Cortex.* 2012;48(1):82-96. Copyright © 2011 Elsevier Srl. All rights reserved.

FIGURE 1-35. Schmahmann JD, Pandya DN: *Fiber pathways of the brain*. New York, NY, Oxford University Press, 2006. Reproduced with permission of the Oxford Publishing Ltd. through PLSclear.

FIGURE 1-36. Schmahmann JD, Pandya DN: *Fiber pathways of the brain*. New York, NY, Oxford University Press, 2006. Reproduced with permission of the Oxford Publishing Ltd. through PLSclear.

FIGURE 1-37. Schmahmann JD, Pandya DN: *Fiber pathways of the brain*. New York, NY, Oxford University Press, 2006. Reproduced with permission of the Oxford Publishing Ltd. through PLSclear.

FIGURE 1-38. Schmahmann JD, Pandya DN: *Fiber pathways of the brain*. New York, NY, Oxford University Press, 2006. Reproduced with permission of the Oxford Publishing Ltd. through PLSclear.

FIGURE 1-39. Parts A–D: Pandya D.N., Rosene D.L. (1985) Some Observations on Trajectories and Topography of Commissural Fibers. In: *Epilepsy and the Corpus Callosum*, edited by AG Reeves. Copyright © 1985, Springer-Verlag US. https://doi.org/10.1007/978-1-4613-2419-5_2.

Part E: Schmahmann JD, Pandya DN: *Fiber pathways of the brain*. New York, NY, Oxford University Press, 2006. Reproduced with permission of the Oxford Publishing Ltd. through PLSclear.

Parts F–I: Chao YP, Cho KH, Yeh CH, Chou KH, Chen JH, Lin CP: Probabilistic topography of human corpus callosum using cytoarchitectural parcellation and high angular resolution diffusion imaging tractography. *Hum Brain Mapp*. 2009;30(10):3172-3187. Copyright © John Wiley and Sons.

FIGURE 1-40. Amunts K, Lepage C, Borgeat L, et al. BigBrain: An ultrahigh-resolution 3D human brain model. *Science*. 2013; 340(6139):1472-1475. doi: 10.1126/science.1235381. PMID: 23788795. Reprinted with permission from AAAS. https://bigbrainproject.org

FIGURE 1-41. Alexander GE, DeLong MR, Strick PL: Parallel organization of functionally segregated circuits linking basal ganglia and cortex. *Annu. Rev. Neurosci*. 1986;9:357-381. Reproduced with permission of Annual Reviews, Inc.; permission conveyed through Copyright Clearance Center, Inc.

FIGURE 1-42. Graybiel AM: The basal ganglia. *Curr. Biol*. 2000;10(14):R509-11. Copyright © 2000 Elsevier Science Ltd. All rights reserved.

FIGURE 1-43. Eblen F, Graybiel AM: Highly restricted origin of prefrontal cortical inputs to striosomes in the macaque monkey. *J. Neurosci*. 1995;15:5999-6013. Copyright © Society for Neuroscience. https://www.jneurosci.org/content/15/9/5999.

FIGURE 1-44. Nieuwenhuys R, Voogd J, van Huijzen C. Diencephalon: Ventral Thalamus or Subthalamus. In: *The Human Central Nervous System*. Copyright © 2008 Springer Berlin Heidelberg.

FIGURE 1-45. Parts A–C: Haynes WI, Haber SN: The organization of prefrontal-subthalamic inputs in primates provides an anatomical substrate for both functional specificity and integration: implications for Basal Ganglia models and deep brain stimulation. *J. Neurosci*. 2013;33(11):4804-4814. https://www.jneurosci.org/content/33/11/4804.

Part D: Benarroch EE: Subthalamic nucleus and its connections: Anatomic substrate for the network effects of deep brain stimulation. *Neurology*. 2008;70(21):1991-1995. Copyright © American Academy of Neurology. https://n.neurology.org/content/70/21/1991.

FIGURE 1-46. Jenkinson N, Nandi D, Muthusamy K, et al. Anatomy, physiology, and pathophysiology of the pedunculopontine nucleus. *Mov Disord*. 2009;24(3):319-328. Copyright © John Wiley and Sons. All rights reserved.

FIGURE 1-47. Crick FC, Koch C: What is the function of the claustrum? *Philos. Trans. R. Soc. Lond. B. Biol. Sci*. 2005;360(1458):1271-1279. Reproduced with permission of the Royal Society (U.K.); permission conveyed through Copyright Clearance Center, Inc.

FIGURE 1-48. Jones E: A description of the human thalamus. In: *Thalamus, Vol. 2. Experimental and Clinical Aspects*, edited by M Steriade, EG Jones, DA McCormick. New York, NY, Elsevier, 1997 pp. 425-499. Copyright © 1998 Elsevier Science Ltd. All rights reserved.

FIGURE 1-49. Schmahmann JD, Pandya DN: Disconnection syndromes of basal ganglia, thalamus, and cerebrocerebellar systems. *Cortex*. 2008;44(8):1037-1066. Copyright © 2008. Published by Elsevier Srl. All rights reserved.

FIGURE 1-50. Schmahmann JD, Pandya DN: Anatomical investigation of projections from thalamus to posterior parietal cortex in the rhesus monkey: a WGA-HRP and fluorescent tracer study. *J. Comp. Neurol*. 1990;295(2):299-326. Copyright © John Wiley and Sons. All rights reserved.

FIGURE 1-51. Schmahmann JD: Vascular syndromes of the thalamus. *Stroke*. 2003;34(9):2264-2278. Copyright © American Heart Association, Inc. All rights reserved. www.ahajournals.org/journal/str.

FIGURE 1-52. Parts A,B: Bogousslavsky J, Regli F, Uske A: Thalamic infarcts: Clinical syndromes, etiology, and prognosis. *Neurology*. 1988; 38(6): 837-48. Copyright © American Academy of Neurology. https://n.neurology.org/.

Parts C,D: von Cramon DY, Hebel N, Schuri U: A contribution to the anatomical basis of thalamic amnesia. *Brain*. 1985;108(Pt 4):993-1008, by permission of Oxford University Press.

FIGURE 1-53. Schmahmann JD, Pandya DN: Disconnection syndromes of basal ganglia, thalamus, and cerebrocerebellar systems. *Cortex*. 2008;44(8):1037-1066. Copyright © Published by Elsevier Srl. All rights reserved.

FIGURE 1-54. Schmahmann JD, Doyon J, McDonald D, et al: Three-dimensional MRI atlas of the human cerebellum in proportional stereotaxic space. *Neuroimage*. 1999(Sep);10(3, Pt 1):233-260. Copyright © Academic Press. All rights reserved.

FIGURE 1-55. Part A: Makris N, Schlerf JE, Hodge SM et al: MRI-based surface-assisted parcellation of human cerebellar cortex: an anatomically specified method with estimate of reliability. *Neuroimage*. 2005;25(4):1146-1160. Copyright © Elsevier Inc. All rights reserved.

Functional Neurocircuitry of Affective and Behavioral Processes and Neuropsychiatric Syndromes

2

David A. Silbersweig · Geoffrey Raynor · Emily Stern

INTRODUCTION

And men ought to know that from nothing else but thence [from the brain] come joys, delights, laughter and sports, and sorrows, griefs, despondency, and lamentations. And by this, in an especial manner, we acquire wisdom and knowledge, and see and hear, and know what are foul and what are fair, what are bad and what are good, what are sweet, and what unsavory... And by the same organ we become mad and delirious, and fears and terrors assail us... All these things we endure from the brain, when it is not healthy... In these ways I am of the opinion that the brain exercises the greatest power in the man. This is the interpreter to us of those things which emanate from the air, when it [the brain] happens to be in a sound state.

—Hippocrates (460–370 BC)[1]

Since ancient times, humans have tried to understand what accounts for thoughts and feelings. Alcmaeon of Croton (5th century BC) believed sense organs were connected to the brain via vessels and that the brain was the seat of consciousness.[2] Hippocrates (460–370 BC) was prescient in his realization that not only perception, cognition, emotion, and behavior are governed by the brain, but that disorders of these functions also arise in the brain. Alternatively, Aristotle (384–322 BC) later believed that the heart was the center of thought and emotions.[3,4] Across the ensuing centuries, artists and scientists (such as DaVinci and Rembrandt) gradually learned more about the nervous system through detailed (neuro)anatomic studies with careful dissection. By the 19th century, studies of brain lesions associated with specific behavioral manifestations (such as the pioneering work of Paul Broca) helped to bridge the gap between anatomy and functional specialization. In the 20th century, work by Kluver and Bucy demonstrated the link between emotional function and medial temporal lobe structures in primate models, and Papez and MacLean made important contributions to our understanding of how the limbic system is associated with emotions in humans.[3]

With the advent of modern scientific methods, there has been an explosion of knowledge pertaining to neural function and its link to emotion, cognition, and behavior. Animal models, from rodents though nonhuman primates, have provided detailed information ranging from molecular to cellular to systems-level insights. These models have greatly informed our understanding of how human brain organization can be linked to human experiences. However, there are limitations to animal models, both in examining normal brain function (such as complex language, a uniquely human function) and especially in studying brain disorders that affect complex, higher-order functions, such as psychiatric disorders, for which accurate animal models often do not exist. And while human post-mortem studies can yield important information regarding anatomy, physiology, and even molecular processes, by definition, the autopsied brain is not in a state that can reflect active, functional processes.

The advent of functional neuroimaging methods in the 1980s allowed, for the first time, the examination, in vivo, of human neuronal activity associated with specific mental states, traits, or tasks. This technology has revolutionized our ability to begin to understand the complex neural circuitry that underlies normal and abnormal perception, cognition, and emotion—those functions that were first recognized by Hippocrates as arising from this most complex organ of the human body.

This chapter will examine the higher-order functional neurocircuitry associated with affective and behavioral function (Chapter 11 will follow-up with further detail on the neuroscience of mood, anxiety, and psychosis). Affective and behavioral functions will refer to processes involved in emotion and motivation, and associated behaviors, such as approach or avoidance. The distinction between these functions and cognition (discussed in Chapter 3) can be difficult to segregate, as they both integrate functions of perception, salience detection, and goal-oriented behaviors with the ultimate objective of ensuring homeostasis and survival.

Given the importance of imaging technologies for the study of brain function, a brief introduction to functional neuroimaging methods will be presented. The neurocircuitry associated with the functional domains of anxiety/fear/threat and stress, reward and motivation, executive control/modulation, and the sense of self/others will then be reviewed. Next, examples that illustrate how convergent abnormal phenotypes/symptoms are associated with common underlying neurocircuit dysfunction will be presented. Finally, an integrated brain circuit model of emotion and behavior will be proposed.

THE ROLE OF NEUROIMAGING: A WINDOW ONTO BRAIN FUNCTION

With the emergence of advanced imaging techniques, including magnetic resonance imaging (MRI) and positron emission tomography (PET), detailed examination of brain structure and function has become possible. MRI uses powerful, superconducting magnets to produce a strong magnetic field. When protons, found most abundantly in water within body tissue, are placed in this magnetic field, they will align with it. If a radiofrequency pulse is administered, the protons will be perturbed, and when the radiofrequency pulse is turned off, energy is released, and measured, as the protons realign with the magnetic field. The chemical environment of the proton affects the time it takes for the protons to realign as well as the amount of energy released, enabling the distinction of subtle differences between tissues. MRI uses no ionizing radiation.

PET is a nuclear medicine imaging technique in which a molecule with specific biochemical activity is labeled with a positron-emitting (radioactive) atom. A wide range of physiological processes in both normal and pathological states can be examined by labeling their relevant biologically active molecules. For example, in the brain, metabolic function, blood flow, neurotransmitter receptor density, and amyloid burden can all be measured. To perform a scan, a small amount of the radioligand is injected into the subject. When the radioisotope decays, a positron is emitted which then combines with and annihilates an electron, producing two 511 keV gamma photons at 180° in relation to each other. These gamma rays are detected by rows of detectors within the PET scanner. Coincidence detection takes advantage of the fact that the two photons will arrive at opposite detectors at nearly the same time, and this information is used to determine where the annihilation event occurred, allowing for the localization of the physiological activity. While a small amount of ionizing radiation is used in PET, the high chemical specificity, and sensitivity in the subnanomolar range, enable the study of in vivo functions that can't be assessed in any other way.

Functional neuroimaging, which includes a number of techniques that measure parameters indirectly reflective of neuronal activity, has revolutionized the study of in vivo brain function. It is based on the principle that when neurons become focally more active, cell body metabolic activity is locally increased. Within 200–400 ms, blood flow increases via neurovascular coupling mechanisms to supply oxygen and nutrients/glucose to the cells, and to take away metabolic waste products.[5] There is also an accompanying increase in blood volume, which, together with the increased flow, results in increased delivery of oxygenated blood. By measuring any of these parameters, one can indirectly infer changes in neuronal activity (Figure 2-1).

The most commonly used measure for brain mapping is blood oxygenation level dependent (BOLD) MRI, which takes advantage of the paramagnetic susceptibility of deoxyhemoglobin (vs. oxyhemoglobin which is diamagnetic).[6] When focal neuronal activity increases, there is an increase in oxygen consumption; however, the increase in blood flow and volume overcompensates, resulting in a relative decrease in deoxyhemoglobin, predominantly in post-capillary vessels, with an associated increase in MRI signal that occurs approximately 4–6 s after the initiation of the increased brain activity. It is important to note that because the BOLD signal results from a combination of changing parameters (blood flow, volume, and deoxyhemoglobin concentration), it is relatively farther removed from neuronal activity, in both time and space, compared to other methods. However, the ability to use differences in endogenous contrast to noninvasively monitor brain activity, without the use of ionizing radiation, has resulted in a wealth of new information related to both normal and pathological brain function.

Functional neuroimaging techniques can be used to measure brain activity both at rest and during the performance of specific mental tasks that can probe perception, cognition, emotion, or behavior. After preprocessing of images, a variety of analytic techniques, including univariate and multivariate statistical approaches, can be applied to extract meaningful information. Covariance patterns of activity are reflected in the form of interregional correlation matrices.

By examining interregional correlations between fluctuations of BOLD signal across the brain (often via multivariate techniques), functional connectivity can be assessed. While this type of analysis cannot yield information regarding absolute directionality or causality, effective connectivity analyses, using, for example, structural equation modeling or path analyses, can incorporate a hypothesized model that includes directional interactions between regions. Unbiased, data-driven approaches can also be used to identify and classify neural profiles of translational interest.[7]

Functional imaging provides helpful data to bridge the gap between basic neuroscience, on a molecular and cellular level, and human behavior. It focuses across systems, where brain states can be correlated with mental states directly, in health and disease. Fear conditioning and threat processing demonstrate how a translational approach, using multiple study techniques, can support a more complete conceptualization of the link between anatomy and behavior. Through molecular studies with animal models we are able to understand that fear conditioning in rodents leads to changes in synapse strength between neurons within the lateral amygdala, a key area of fear processing.[8] That same area can then be studied with functional imaging in vivo to confirm and elaborate upon types of threat (e.g., danger elicited by language) that lead to its activation.[9]

NEUROCIRCUITRY OF INTEREST

To understand psychiatric conditions, one may begin with the more evolutionarily and phylogenetically preserved limbic and subcortical regions (see Figure 2-2). These more primitive

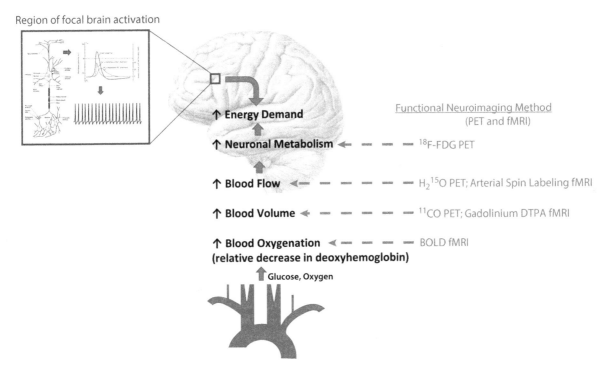

FIGURE 2-1. Functional brain imaging methods as indices of neuronal activity. When neuronal activity increases focally, there is an accompanying increase in energy demand and neuronal metabolism. Through neurovascular coupling, an increase in blood flow and blood volume provides the necessary increase in glucose and oxygen delivery. Specific functional neuroimaging methods measure specific components of this cascade of physiological events, each of which can serve as a proxy for neuronal activity. (Background brain surface drawing adapted with permission from Martin J. Neuroanatomy Text and Atlas. 4th ed. https://neurology.mhmedical.com. Copyright © McGraw Hill LLC. All rights reserved. Axon figure (boxed) reproduced with permission from Nestler EJ, Nyman SE, Holtzman DM, Malenka RC. Molecular Neuropharmacology: A Foundation for Clinical Neuroscience. 3rd ed. https://neurology.mhmedical.com. Copyright © McGraw Hill LLC. All rights reserved. Action potential and neuronal firing figure (boxed) adapted with permission from Huxley AF, Hodgkin AL. A quantitative description of membrane current and its application to conduction and excitation in nerve. *J. Physiol.* 1952;117:500-544. Copyright © John Wiley & Sons, Inc. All rights reserved.)

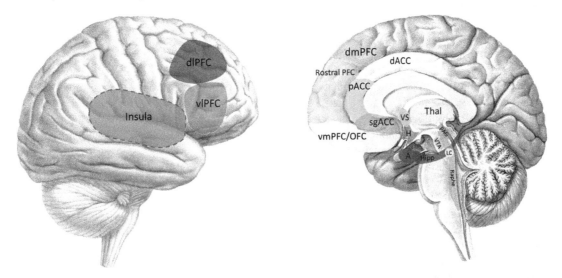

FIGURE 2-2. Brain areas of interest. The figure illustrates key brain regions (network nodes) discussed in this chapter. These regions are associated with emotion, motivation, behavior, and social functions, and their regulation. Neuroanatomy of these regions is discussed in Chapter 1. Neurochemistry associated with these regions is discussed in Chapter 11. Brainstem areas include the locus coeruleus (LC), raphe, ventral tegmental area (VTA), and periaqueductal gray (PAG). Subcortical areas include the thalamus (Thal), ventral striatum (VS), and hypothalamus (H). Limbic areas include the amygdala (A) and hippocampus (Hipp). Paralimbic areas include the insula. Prefrontal areas include the rostral prefrontal cortex (rostral PFC), dorsolateral prefrontal cortex (dlPFC), dorsomedial prefrontal cortex (dmPFC), ventrolateral prefrontal cortex (vlPFC), ventromedial prefrontal cortex (vmPFC), orbitofrontal cortex (oFC), dorsal anterior cingulate cortex (dACC), pregenual anterior cingulate cortex (pACC), and subgenual anterior cingulate cortex (sgACC). (Background brain drawings adapted with permission from Martin J. Neuroanatomy Text and Atlas. 4th ed. https://neurology.mhmedical.com. © McGraw Hill LLC. All rights reserved.)

systems involve lower level, stereotyped, emotional-behavioral phenomena. Psychiatric syndromes may arise through a disruption or misallocation of these preserved drives or responses. Over millions of years of evolution the size of the human brain increased and expanded into now familiar areas of prefrontal, posterior parietal, lateral temporal, and insular regions, which interact bidirectionally with the limbic system.[10] When reflecting upon a depressed patient from this perspective, one can appreciate the more primitive, hypothalamic disruption on sleep, appetite, and sexual drive as well as the higher-order association cortex contributions that may lead to an existential crisis.

To develop a model of brain-behavior processing, one can move dorsally and rostrally in the brain from the deep, evolutionarily preserved regions, which mediate more automatic/unconscious, reflexive, stereotyped behaviors, toward neocortical, higher-order processing that is more conscious, voluntary and flexible. The major functional domains that will be highlighted in this chapter include (1) threat detection and defensive responses and their relation to limbic circuitry, (2) reward and motivational processing and the ventral striatum and associated regions, (3) appraisal and top-down modulation by prefrontal regions, and (4) systems related to subjective feeling states, and sense of self and others, including social awareness. Though these systems share complex bidirectional interactions with significant overlap, distinguishing among them is a meaningful heuristic exercise. One can then conceptualize each structure-function relationship as a potential area of circuit dysfunction underlying the spectrum of psychiatric disease.

Threat Detection and Response

Detection of threat, defensive behaviors, and conscious states of fear and anxiety are essential factors for survival, explaining its preservation through evolution. For clarification, discussion of nonconscious threat detection and associated defensive responses associated with amygdala circuitry will be referred to as the defensive survival circuit, whereas the emotions of fear and anxiety will refer to subjective feeling states mediated by neocortical (including frontal) systems.[11] Essential brain areas including the amygdala, ventral hippocampus, bed nucleus of the stria terminalis (BNST), and hypothalamic pituitary axis assist in recognizing danger, whether internal (concerning memories or predictions for the future) or external (environmental dangers), and mobilizing appropriate bodily responses.[12] The amygdala itself, located within the medial temporal lobe, is comprised of distinct nuclei that are functionally distinguishable. The lateral amygdala processes incoming sensory stimuli and may learn through conditioning to recognize specific stimuli as threats.[13] Information from the lateral amygdala may then lead to the central amygdala and associated freezing pathways or to the basal amygdala and more goal-oriented avoidance behaviors.[14] While the amygdala is typically associated with immediate threat detected by sensory modalities, more distant or uncertain threats are associated with the BNST,[14,15] a structure involved in modulating trait anxiety and more chronic threat processing.[16]

The limbic system has vast connections to other brain regions that are worthy of a textbook of its own, though here a few important relationships will be mentioned. Threats may trigger reflexive behaviors (including flight, fight, or freezing) or may lead to more complex and deliberate defensive actions with greater involvement of cortical areas. The limbic and orbito-medial prefrontal systems are involved in fear conditioning, salience attribution, emotional evaluation, valence assignment, and behavioral response generation. An anterior-to-posterior gradient exists along medial temporal lobe with greater connectivity of anterior components to the amygdala and salience network.[17] Ventral hippocampal/parahippocampal systems help to mediate the contextual aspects of affective memories.[18,19] The BNST has greater connectivity to hippocampus rather than sensory systems, which would be consistent with its role in processing chronic and uncertain threats.[14] Medial prefrontal/anterior cingulate regions are involved in attention and action selection, and in extinction learning (a process in which an individual learns a stimulus is no longer associated with the feared outcome).[20,21] It may be noted that the sensory and language cortices themselves can be modulated in their activity via the processing of emotional stimuli.[22] The hypothalamic-pituitary-adrenal axis contributes to neuroendocrine signaling, leading to autonomic activation and behavior associated with persistent stress and anxiety states.[12,23] The neuromodulatory effect of stress hormones on medial temporal memory regions also leads to greater long-term memory for such emotional or stressful events compared to neutral ones.[24] Early life stress, such as physical abuse or neglect, has been associated with increased amygdala and decreased hippocampal and ventromedial prefrontal volumes[25] and may make this system hyperresponsive to cues perceived as associated with potential threat.[26]

Indeed, it may be helpful to conceptualize this process in ways that can ultimately be modeled and quantified. Each person, through a confluence of factors (see Figure 2-8), has a baseline level of activity, associated with the balance of these aversive/avoidance systems and approach systems (reward and motivation, discussed below), and the degree of top-down control/modulation (executive functions, reviewed below).[27,28] Cortisol fluctuations and autonomic tone (sympathetic/parasympathetic balance) are associated with these states. Some individuals may have higher or lower baseline or trait levels, and positive or negative emotional processing biases, with differing amounts of fluctuation or variance.[27,29] A stressor results in varying degrees of reactivity within the population, and each individual has different thresholds of activation for varying types of stress responses. Some people will react to relatively minor stressors, while others may only respond to major trauma. The presence of past trauma, particularly in developmentally sensitive periods, and the net risk-resilience diathesis may influence the threshold, as well as the duration of sustained reactivity before returning to baseline. Additionally, one's basal level of arousal and reactivity may be changed in the context of chronic stressors, depending upon epigenetic and neuroplastic processes, such as priming, inhibition, habituation, or extinction learning.[27] Specific therapeutic interventions, such as pharmacologically mediated emotional memory reconsolidation (e.g., propranolol's effect impairing emotional memory consolidation) or cognitive behavioral therapy-based exposure and response prevention, may be targeted at particular elements of this model.[29-32]

Reward and Motivation

The reward domain reflects the importance of evaluating salient stimuli to the well-being of the individual and associated goal-directed behaviors.[33] Reward circuitry assists in detection of salient stimuli, assigning value, and balancing approach motivation with threat detection networks that facilitate avoidance. By taking into account past experiences, a prediction regarding potential outcomes is made, and if the benefits considerably outweigh risks, the influence of threat circuitry is reduced.[12] Thus, one can conceptualize avoidance and approach behaviors as reflecting the activity of reciprocal systems in the brain. Figure 2-3 outlines the contributing factors that lead to goal attainment. That said, it should be noted that the amygdalocentric and ventral striatal systems are broadly salience detection and response systems. Each may respond to both positive and negative stimuli under various circumstances with different degrees of arousal.

The nucleus accumbens (NAcc) in the ventral striatum is most classically associated with motivation and regularly implicated in disorders of motivational dysfunction.[33] The NAcc receives dopaminergic neuron projections from the ventral tegmental area which are involved in encoding reward prediction errors, critical to reinforcement learning.[34] Dopamine reward processing is thought to have two sequential components, first broadly assessing sensory input across modalities, and then identifying more specifically items of value and utility.[35] In the initial detection phase, greater dopamine activation is associated with stimuli similar to previously rewarded objects (generalization),

involvement in reward-related contexts, or stimuli identified as novel.[35] The stimulus is then further identified and valued based on perceived subjective value (balancing reward, risk, delay, etc.) and utility.[35] The second dopamine response persists until the predicted reward can be compared to the outcome, allowing for learning and updating value predictions.[35] Unexpected positive outcomes (positive prediction errors) lead to greater dopamine reward signal, and unexpected negative outcomes (negative prediction errors) lead to depressed activity.[36]

The NAcc itself can be subdivided into a core and shell component. The core is related to the dorsal striatum and approach behavior; the shell is associated with limbic structures and aversion to nonrewarding stimuli.[33,37,38] The most basic drives, such as thirst and hunger, are mediated by the hypothalamus which may contribute to increasing salience of objects needed for survival.[39] The prefrontal cortex, particularly orbitofrontal, ventromedial, and anterior cingulate cortices,[33,40] assist in appraising potential rewards or outcomes. The lateral prefrontal cortex also assists in directing attention to salient stimuli and encodes and tracks histories of choices and their outcomes.[33] Additionally, the habenula (a brain region that together with the pineal gland form the epithalamus) is implicated in negative reward prediction error. It is activated by unexpected negative or nonrewarding events, leading to inhibiting the response of dopamine neurons.[41] This complex valuation system assists with mediating motor activity that occur in areas such as the posterior mid-cingulate cortex, anterior cingulate cortex (ACC), supplementary motor cortex, and dorsal striatum, to produce the necessary behavior to reach a goal.[42]

Prefrontal Cortex, Evaluation, and Regulation

Higher-order brain regions allow for responses to stimuli to be adjusted depending on the context and circumstances in which they emerge.[43] The prefrontal cortices allow for monitoring, planning, sustaining goal-directed activity, and modifying behavior based on feedback and changing contingencies.[33] One suggested unifying theme of the prefrontal cortex's role in emotion is appraisal (assigning value) and evaluation of emotion in the setting of its surrounding context.[44] Importantly, this domain of control and modulation has reciprocal feedback with the lower-order brain regions. There are many ways to parcellate the prefrontal cortex, though here it will be divided into orbitofrontal, medial, lateral, and cingulate cortices.

The orbitofrontal cortex (oFC) can be grossly subdivided into medial and lateral aspects based on connectivity patterns.[45] The lateral oFC, which has direct input from sensory modalities as well as the limbic system, is thought to contribute to evaluation of external stimuli in the context of current goals.[44] It assists in learning the inferred associations of initially neutral environmental cues to reward or aversive outcomes. There is evidence that the medial oFC, coactivated with limbic and default mode network areas, appraises internal stimuli, such as imagined future events and episodic memories.[44]

The medial prefrontal cortex is often divided into dorsal and ventral aspects (dmPFC and vmPFC, respectively). The dmPFC is associated with the appraisal of others' mental states, involved in intuiting others' anticipated mental states to guide choices.[44,46]

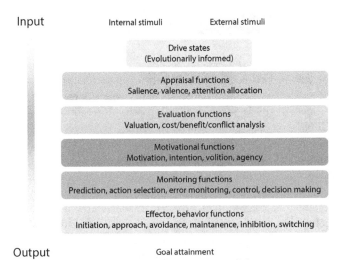

Input   Internal stimuli   External stimuli

Drive states
(Evolutionarily informed)

Appraisal functions
Salience, valence, attention allocation

Evaluation functions
Valuation, cost/benefit/conflict analysis

Motivational functions
Motivation, intention, volition, agency

Monitoring functions
Prediction, action selection, error monitoring, control, decision making

Effector, behavior functions
Initiation, approach, avoidance, maintenance, inhibition, switching

Output   Goal attainment

FIGURE 2-3. Emotional/motivational processing. A schematic illustrating steps in the processing of internal and external stimuli, their integration with drive states, the ascription of salience, the appraisal of emotional significance, the triggering of reactions, the evaluation and valuation with context, the engagement of motivational functions, and the initiation and execution of associated behavior. This is a functional simplification that maps onto the brain regions and circuits discussed in the sections of this chapter. Note that such processes, involving different levels of the neuraxis as discussed, have elements that are both automatic and conscious, parallel and serial, and feed-forward and feedback/hierarchical.

The most rostral portion of the medial PFC may mediate the appraisal of one's own mental state and self-related information.[44] In addition to performing value estimation to inform decision making, the vmPFC is implicated in emotion regulation and altering behavior in response to environmental changes.[47]

The lateral prefrontal cortex is similarly divided into the dorsolateral prefrontal cortex (dlPFC) and ventrolateral prefrontal cortex (vlPFC). Impulsive reward selection, associated with lower-order subcortical systems, can be contrasted with the ability to defer gratification and value future opportunities, associated with lateral prefrontal cortices.[48] Goal values are assessed and integrated within the vmPFC, while the dlPFC provides cognitive control to assist in guiding behavior (e.g., dlPFC activity is increased when a dieter's active maintenance of long-term goals allows for greater reflection and self-control in making food choices).[49] Reappraisal of initial negative reactions to a situation is associated with increased lateral prefrontal cortex activation and decreased amygdala activation, while fear extinction suggests an inhibitory role of medial prefrontal cortex on amygdala activation.[21] A study of psychodynamic therapy, for example, associated clinical improvement in borderline personality disorder (BPD) patients with greater activation of dorsal anterior cingulate and dorsolateral prefrontal cortices, thought to reflect improvement in top-down behavioral restraint.[50]

The cingulate cortex can be divided into anterior, middle, posterior, and retrosplenial cortices, with its anterior division functionally subserving emotion, and middle and posterior regions typically subserving skeletomotor and sensory processes.[51] The anterior cingulate cortex (ACC) is further subdivided into subgenual and pregenual subregions involved in emotion, and a cognitively/behaviorally oriented dorsal ACC (at times referred to as the anterior midcingulate cortex).[52] Dixon et al.[44] suggested the subgenual ACC is involved in anticipating future physiological needs by top-down control of brain circuits mediating autonomic responses. The pregenual ACC (closely associated but a separate structure from the ventromedial prefrontal cortex) is thought to assist in the value determination of interoceptive sensation, along with the medial oFC and the anterior insula,[44] and is considered a key region involved in somatoform disorders.[53] The anterior midcingulate is proposed to appraise actions and behaviors and potential future outcomes.[44]

Awareness of Self, Feeling States, and Others

Much behavioral and affective processing occurs outside of one's awareness. Individuals, though, can also describe conscious feeling states, such as happiness, anger, sadness, disgust, or love. The anterior insular cortex is considered to be an important region involved in subjective feeling states via the re-representation of interoceptive information (heartrate, visceral distension, dyspnea, sensual touch, etc.).[54] The insula itself contains a posterior-to-anterior gradient in which interception becomes integrated along with environmental and motivational context to develop an emotional awareness.[54] Reflecting on classical antiquity, Aristotle's assertion that the heart was the source of emotion can be appreciated if we consider the interoceptive contribution of the sympathetic system and its processing into

emotional awareness by the insular cortex. The anterior insular cortex is frequently coactivated with the ACC (subgenual, pregenual, and dorsal components), which can be regarded as probable sites for awareness of emotion (as an extension of sensorially organized networks) and initiation of behaviors and desire to act (as an extension of motorically organized networks) respectively.[44,55,56] There are also higher-order centers of emotional awareness monitoring and modulation in prefrontal cortices, which may be engaged with cognitive emotional reappraisal as used in cognitive-behavioral therapy.[57]

Awareness of self may include an unconscious recognition of the body as belonging to itself, the more conscious awareness of first-person perspective in the moment of task-engagement, or a reflective, narrative version of oneself as a person.[58] All these processes are associated with their own functional and anatomical substrates. The brainstem, subcortical, and insula regions are involved in the embodied sense of self, and the hippocampal systems play an integral role in autobiographical sense of self. Extending self-recognition to distinction of self from other is critical for social development, with overlap between neural substrates mediating "self" and those mediating "other."[59] Mirror neurons are activated when an individual performs an action, but also when an individual passively observes another person performing a similar action, suggesting a relationship in which one's own motor circuitry is utilized to interpret others' actions.[60,61] Mentalizing/theory of mind and related social cognition are mediated by dorsomedial prefrontal and specific temporoparietal regions. Medial frontal cortex is involved with determining future behavior and anticipated value, with the more anterior medial frontal cortex associated with metacognitive representations of abstract outcomes and the mediation of social cognition.[62]

Large-Scale Networks

Functional imaging techniques have allowed for consistent correlation between activity of various neuroanatomical areas recognized as neural networks. Large-scale networks include the default mode network (DMN), central executive network (CEN), and salience network. The DMN is active during the resting state, when the individual is not engaged in task-oriented activities (at times referred to as "task-negative" network). It is divided into three main subdivisions: the ventromedial prefrontal, dorsomedial prefrontal, and posterior cingulate and adjacent precuneus cortices.[63] It is involved in self-referential thoughts including reflecting on past experiences or envisioning the future, and contributes to emotional processing.[63,64] The DMN is at times divided into an anterior component involved more specifically in self-reflection and emotion and a posterior component involved in episodic memory and perceptual processing.[65] The CEN, with nodes in dorsolateral prefrontal and posterior parietal cortices, is task-focused and involved in the attention to and manipulation of information and decision making.[66] The salience network, with key nodes in the anterior insular cortex, dorsal ACC, and subcortical (thalamus, hypothalamus, amygdala, periaqueductal gray) regions, assists in detecting behaviorally relevant internal and external stimuli and assists in toggling between task-negative and task-positive (i.e., CEN) networks.[66,67]

Atypical connectivity among the default mode, salience, and executive control networks is thought to be reflective of the pathological changes present in a variety of neuropsychiatric disorders.[68] For example, in major depressive disorder there is an increase in DMN activity with increase connectivity to salience network and decreased connectivity to CEN[69]; this may be conceptualized as the salience network (including amygdala threat detection) selecting focus on self-reflective ruminations with diminished balance of CEN task-focus and decision making, overall leading to depressive symptoms. Depressive and anxiety symptom scores tend to have greater correlation with anterior components of the DMN and negative correlation to posterior components, raising selectivity within this network in certain pathological states.[65,69] Mapping of abnormalities in connectivity demonstrates overlapping, as well as distinct patterns of dysfunction. This makes sense, given the overlapping phenomenology across psychiatric disorders. Symptom-specific, syndrome-specific, and disorder-specific patterns are emerging. And within disorders, subtypes are being identified, providing a mechanistic underpinning for the clinical heterogeneity.[70]

SELECTED EXAMPLES: CONVERGENT SYMPTOMS AND BRAIN CIRCUIT ABNORMALITIES ACROSS PSYCHIATRY AND NEUROLOGY

Psychiatric and neurological disorders share common underlying substrates in the central nervous system. Functional neuroimaging localization of emotional-behavioral disorders observed in "psychiatric" disease converge with localized emotional-behavioral disorders resulting from "neurological" disease, further eroding the distinction between the fields. Below are several examples to demonstrate these common pathways.

Stress Reactions and Anxiety

As noted above, abnormal fear responses typically involve limbic circuitry. In post-traumatic stress disorder (PTSD), patients demonstrate exaggerated amygdala activation to external threat-related stimuli, especially trauma-related threats, with a limited ability to habituate to threatening conditions over time.[71] Similarly, amygdala hyperactivation to threat has been demonstrated in panic disorder and social anxiety disorder with hyperawareness of internal cues.[72,73] Depressive subtypes characterized by high levels of anxiety have decreased frontoamygdalar connectivity and top-down regulation of amygdala activation.[70] Schizophrenic patients with paranoid ideation and adolescents experiencing psychotic symptoms also have greater amygdala hyperactivation, even in response to cues that should be neutral,[74–76] demonstrating the heightened threat response in the paranoid state (see Figure 2-4 for functional neuroimaging example). In mesial temporal epilepsy, complex partial seizure semiology involving the amygdala is often described by patients as a perception of fear,[77] and is significantly associated with autonomic features such as dyspnea, palpitations, and chest tightness.[78]

Psychosis

Psychosis may also be seen across a range of psychiatric and neurological disorders and is generally thought of as a failure of reality testing. When electrically stimulating aspects of the

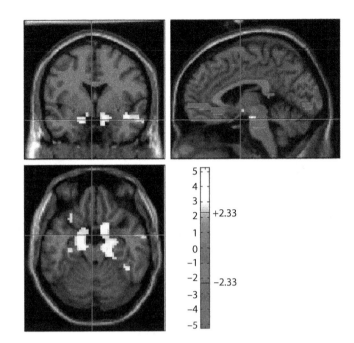

FIGURE 2-4. Fear/threat circuitry involved in paranoid delusions. Profile of neural activity associated with paranoid delusions in patients with schizophrenia, in the context of a threat paradigm. Note increased activity in bilateral amygdalar/ventral hippocampal, right anterior insular, and midline midbrain regions, in the setting of decreased activity in subgenual and pregenual anterior cingulate regions. This pattern is consistent with increased threat reactivity and decreased top-down control and modulation in this critical brain circuitry. (Figure courtesy of D. Silbersweig and E. Stern.)

temporal lobe during epilepsy surgery, patients' auditory hallucinations are able to be recreated, with a "crude sensation" moving to a more experiential response (a voice, voices, or music) as the electrode is moved from the primary auditory cortex toward the adjacent interpretive cortex of the first transverse temporal gyrus. They generally acknowledged the experiences were not real and sometimes described them like a dream state or "like I go into a daze."[79] In schizophrenia, hallucinations and delusions are also hypothesized to be related to hyperdopaminergic state with dysregulation of salience networks. In this model, patients attempt to make sense of misattributed assignment of salience of experiences or internal representations which lead to symptoms of delusions and hallucinations, respectively.[66] Additionally, there is an associated failure of prefrontal monitoring and modulation of posterior and ventral regions that leads to symptom formation.[80] Patients undergoing epilepsy surgery and individuals with schizophrenia likely share similar activation of their auditory cortices when experiencing auditory hallucinations. However, the lack of insight in the psychotic schizophrenic state implies further deficits in error monitoring and reality testing. Corollary discharge, also known as reafferent signaling, is a mechanism involved in the identification of self-generated actions. Failure of this mechanism has also been implicated in psychotic symptom formation,[81] resulting from a disruption of connectivity between anterior (initiation of a thought or internal vocalization) and posterior (receive the sensory consequence of that activity) regions. This produces a misinterpretation of agency and the conclusion that the internally generated representation is coming from an external source.[81,82]

Affect and Motivation

Abnormalities in the processing of positive emotion and motivation also may span psychiatric and neurological conditions. Compared to controls, depressed patients have shown significantly less activation in bilateral ventral striatal regions in anticipation of reward, suggesting dysfunction in reward pathways, leading to anhedonic characteristics of depression.[83,84] Parkinson's disease patients frequently experience symptoms of depression, and degree of apathy is inversely correlated to dopamine transporter binding in the ventral striatum.[85] Patients with major depression have failure to segregate activity in regions of emotional processing (ventral striatum, anterior cingulate, and insula) from activity in sensory, linguistic, and motor functions. This is consistent with the depressive phenomenology of experiencing affective bias coloring one's cognition and behavior (see Figure 2-5).[86] Due to the subgenual cingulate cortex association with depressed mood states, it has been studied as the target of deep brain stimulation for treatment-refractory depression.[87,88]

The syndrome of apathy is characterized by diminished motivation that can be subdivided into goal-directed cognitive, affective/emotional, and behavioral components. Patients suffering from apathy may have goal-directed cognitive changes associated with decreases in assigned value to stimuli or experiences that had once held greater influences. Emotional changes are demonstrated by decreased affective responsivity or flat affect; and behavioral changes are exemplified by decrease in effort, initiation, or productivity.[89] A goal must be decidedly valuable enough to act toward it as well as sustain effort accomplishing it.[42] Apathetic patients may be hypersensitive or overestimate effort to reach a goal while underestimating the reward itself.[42] The negative symptoms of schizophrenia (anhedonia, apathy, asociality) are theorized to represent motivational abnormalities, with hypotheses including potentially overestimating effort and underestimating reward or deficits in orienting to salient stimuli associated with reward.[90]

The reward system can also become imbalanced in pathology of addiction, in which the increasing motivation to acquire a reinforcing stimulus (i.e., drugs) leads to downregulation of dopaminergic response to other natural rewards and diminished ability to consider alternative behaviors via higher-order brain areas.[91] Previously neutral stimuli paired to the drug become conditioned to become reward predictors and act

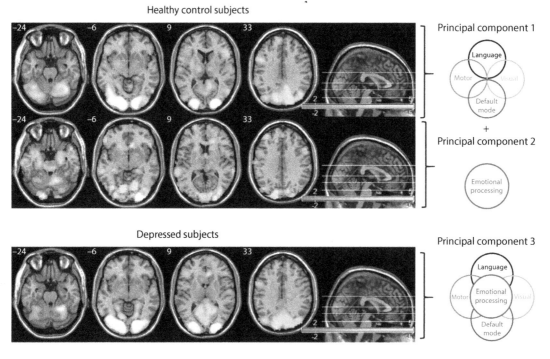

FIGURE 2-5. Depression circuitry. Functional circuitry associated with emotional and cognitive processing, and associated abnormalities in patients with major depression. Subjects were scanned with fMRI while reading positive emotional words and pressing a button, and a principal components analysis was performed. Healthy subjects show two uncorrelated profiles of activity: one (top row of axial brain images) highlights brain circuits associated with the task—visual, language, and motor functions (yellow), anti-correlated with default mode network regions (blue); and another one (second row) highlights ventral striatal and hippocampal regions (yellow), anti-correlated with amygdalar regions (blue). In patients with major depression, the task, default, and emotional processing regions are all part of one set of positively and negatively correlated activations, with decreased ventral striatal (reward/motivation circuitry) activation to the positive stimuli, and failure to demonstrate the negatively correlated amygdalar activity. These abnormalities represent plausible neural substrates for the failure to segregate emotional, resting, and cognitive processing in depressed patients, and the failure to react to positive emotional stimuli. (Figure adapted with permission from Epstein J, Perez DL, Ervin K, et al. Failure to segregate emotional processing from cognitive and sensorimotor processing in major depression. *Psychiatry Res Neuroimaging.* 2011;193(3):144-150. https://www.sciencedirect.com/journal/psychiatry-research-neuroimaging.)

as cues associated with promotion of drug-seeking behavior.[92] Parkinson's disease patients may develop excessive desire and overuse of their dopamine replacement medication despite negative side effects, similar to addiction, leading to what is characterized as dopamine dysregulation syndrome.[93]

Impulsivity and Compulsivity

Impulsivity suggests a diminished degree of constraint, with behavior influenced by immediate drives and cues rather than social context or long-term goals. It is a core component of BPD, along with negative emotion, fear of abandonment, and absence of coherent sense of self and others.[94] An emotional linguistic go/no-go task with BPD patients demonstrated decreased constraint correlated with decreased ventromedial prefrontal activity and increased negative emotion correlated with increased extended amygdala-ventral striatal activation (see Figure 2-6).[95] Impulsivity can also be seen in traumatic brain injury with damage to the orbito-medial prefrontal cortex. One of the most famous neuropsychiatric patients, Phineas Gage, demonstrated profound disinhibition and planning failures after his traumatic brain injury involving the right and left prefrontal cortices that included orbitofrontal regions.[96,97] In bipolar patients, mania is associated with hyperactivity of approach motivation (wanting, liking, and predicting positive outcomes) with great effort expended in reward pursuit.[33] Even in the euthymic state, bipolar patients display greater activation in ventral striatum, and oFC in anticipation of reward.[33] These abnormalities across different components of motivation and control circuitry are conducive to impulsivity and reinforce the role of these key regions in producing such symptomatology across a range of pathophysiological processes.

Similarly, compulsivity represents an urge to act in response to an obsession or rigid thought pattern and can be seen across a number of psychiatric disorders, including obsessive-compulsive disorder (OCD), eating disorders, or addiction.[98] A popular model of OCD involves dysfunction within cortico-striatal-thalamic-cortical loops, which leads to greater urge to engage in compulsive behaviors.[99]

Agency and Volition

Disorders of volition generally refer to deficits of desire to act or dysfunction in feelings of agency (responsibility for one's actions).[56] This may include a range of disorders, including brain lesions leading to akinetic mutism or alien limb phenomena, tic disorder, catatonia, and functional neurological disorders. Tics in Tourette syndrome are defined as involuntary, brief stereotyped motor behaviors, often associated with irresistible urges. Tic occurrence has been associated with abnormality within a variety of brain regions including medial and lateral premotor, anterior cingulate, dorsolateral-rostral, and inferior parietal cortices as well as putamen, caudate, and primary motor cortex.[100] On the more extreme end of the avolitional spectrum, akinetic mutism describes a state of apathy without initiative, spontaneous movement, or speech. It has been associated with bilateral lesions of the ACC (despite intact speech and movement cortices).[101] Functional neurological disorders present with a wide range of neurological symptoms ranging from functional tremor to psychogenic non-epileptic seizures (PNES) in which patients experience little to no control over their movements. In PNES, decreased metabolism in ACC and right parietal cortex may suggest dysfunction in emotion regulation and processes involving self- and environmental-awareness.[102,103] Within functional movement disorders, decreased activity in the angular gyrus of the temporoparietal junction is thought to reflect diminished subjective control over one's movements.[103] Overall, brain lesions leading to disorders of volition and agency are quite heterogenous, though network mapping demonstrated distinct networks with disruptions of volition defined by connectivity to the anterior cingulate and disruptions of agency defined by connectivity to the precuneus.[56]

Social Cognition

Social cognition involves the perception and processing of social information (including theory of mind) to effectively guide interpersonal behaviors. Psychiatric conditions such as autism spectrum disorder (ASD) and schizophrenia share deficits in social cognition.[104] Both ASD and schizophrenia patients shared abnormal activation within the temporoparietal junction during tasks involving theory of mind.[105,106] Patients with behavioral variant frontotemporal dementia can present with personality changes and are characterized as often having a loss of interpersonal warmth, which has been linked to decreases in salience network connectivity.[107] The associated loss of empathic responses in frontotemporal dementia may reflect impairments in theory of mind,[108] or a decreased awareness and attendance to interpersonal details due to an associated diminished interoceptive response to social cues.[107]

SYNTHESIS: INTEGRATED BRAIN CIRCUIT MODEL OF EMOTION, BEHAVIOR

A circuit-based approach assists in understanding the neural underpinnings of perception, cognition, emotion, behavior,

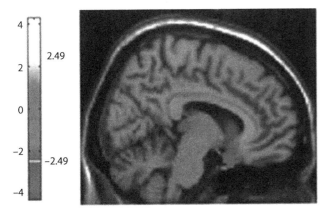

FIGURE 2-6. Behavioral inhibition in the setting of negative emotion is a challenge for many individuals, including those with borderline personality disorder. This figure shows decreased activation of medial orbitofrontal cortex under such conditions in patients versus health control subjects.[95] As discussed in the text, lesions or dysfunction in this region are associated with impulsive behavior across a number of psychiatric and neurological conditions.

social interactions, and how disorders thereof can be mapped to disruptions of these systems and processes. Behavioral neural systems lie along hierarchical gradients from primitive to higher order. They have homeostatic balances, with feed-forward and feedback processing, in the context of serial and parallel processing. Disease dysfunction lies along a spectrum, though some categorical elements can be ascertained.

As noted above, phylogenetically older ventral-medial systems involve the brainstem, hypothalamus, amygdala, ventral hippocampus, ventral striatum, medial oFC, insula, and subgenual anterior cingulate. These brain regions themselves lie along a cytoarchitectural, connective, and functional gradient through limbic, paralimbic, and neocortical dimensions. They involve past and present self-associated feelings that are informed by the internal body/drive state and external experience, are relatively stereotyped, involve

pervasive behavioral sets and relatively simple-concrete representations, are often involuntary, and often unconscious or with partial awareness by the individual. These ventral-medial systems interact with dorsal-lateral neocortical systems involving the dorsolateral prefrontal cortices, temporal and parietal association cortices. These systems are associated with future predictions, appraisal of others and the external world, flexibility, decision making, and complex-abstract representations, and are conscious and under more volitional control.[33,44] Emotional-behavioral gradients include positive affect and approach, such as drives, urges, motivation, volition, and planning, which are countered by negative affects and avoidance/withdrawal, such as fear, anxiety, threat, frustration, inhibition, rumination, and concern. The degree of salience and meaning the brain ascribes to stimuli reflects a spectrum. There is also a gradient between self- and other-awareness.[108] Figure 2-7 represents a simplified diagram of the described gradients.

There is spatio-temporal coordination among the gradients and connections that constitute the networks of brain activity. Modulation of these systems by ascending neurotransmitters and neuromodulators, and connectivity of activity via subcortically controlled oscillations are important elements to consider as well. The regulation of emotion and behavior are associated with dynamic modulation in the modular, hierarchical, and

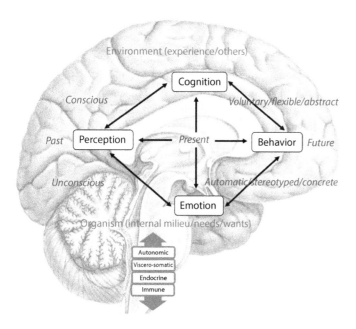

FIGURE 2-7. The figure is a simplified, heuristic representation displaying general processes and gradients that can help to understand brain function. The brain is the highest order orchestrator of internal body functions, through bidirectional interactions involving the peripheral nervous system (somatic, including sensorial and motor nerve fibers, and autonomic, including sympathetic and parasympathetic), endocrine system (hormones, releasing factors), and immune system (innate, adaptive). The brain also mediates changing interactions between the organism (with its physiological and drive states) and the environment. In general, functions in phylogenetically older ventromedial regions are more automatic, stereotyped, and concrete, while functions in more recently evolved, dorsolateral/rostral neocortical regions are more voluntary, flexible and abstract, and conscious. The interaction of broad domains of perception, cognition, emotion, and behavior allow the person to process and integrate salient present information, in the context of past experience, to produce adaptive behavior, in the context of future goals. Chapters 3 also describes cognitive (including linguistic), perceptual, and executive systems in detail. (Background brain drawing adapted with permission from Martin J. Neuroanatomy Text and Atlas. 4th ed. https://neurology.mhmedical.com. Copyright © McGraw Hill LLC. All rights reserved.)

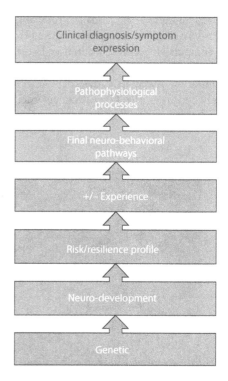

FIGURE 2-8. Factors associated with neuropsychiatric symptom expression: simplified flow diagram of factors that interact to influence the expression of neuropsychiatric symptomatology. A patient's presentation can be seen as a result of numerous biological and environmental factors that combine to produce the clinical phenomenology, through the final common neurobehavioral pathways discussed.

bidirectional systems. Disorders are associated with distinct patterns of abnormal activity and connectivity in frontolimbic, neocortical, and subcortical regions, both in small-scale neuronal circuits within regional nodes as well as large in scale distributed networks.

These final common pathways of disease expression illustrate the need to transcend the traditional distinction between psychiatry and neurology. Disruption of a particular node or network will result in dysfunction, regardless of whether the cause is genetic, environmental (or both; epigenetic), neurochemical, or due to a stroke, seizure, or tumor (see Figure 2-8). This is a helpful model to explain to patients and families when discussing the biological accounts of their suffering (and explaining that the patient may not be aware of, or able to control, his or her actions). To explain symptoms and affect states through a neurobiological lens helps to remove excessive self-blame and stigmatization of psychological suffering. However, if the emphasis shifts too much to the neurobiological, it

may remove the patient from a personal sense of responsibility and locus of control over his/her fate, which may result in excessive externalization that also counters potential for self-development.

Increasingly, and ultimately, a greater understanding of the functional neuroanatomy of neuropsychiatric disorders will allow a biological classification and taxonomy of these conditions, based upon neural systems mechanisms. Mechanism-based subtypes of neuropsychiatric dysfunction will be identified. This will help to characterize and explain heterogeneity within current psychiatric diagnoses, as well as common "comorbidities" among them. This ongoing process will be supplemented by advances in cellular and molecular neuroscience (including optogenetics), to allow the development and personalized application of more targeted neuromodulatory therapeutics (including brain stimulation, pharmacology, psychotherapy), and improved prognostication, with the hope of early intervention and prevention (see Figure 2-9).

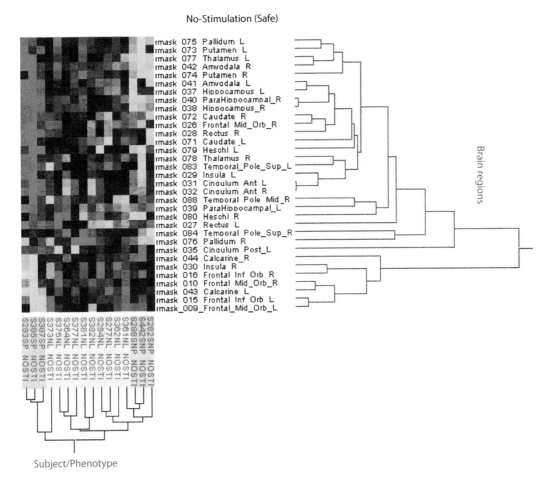

FIGURE 2-9. Visualization of a data-driven cluster analysis showing differing patterns of brain region/circuit activity for patients with schizophrenia and psychosis, patients with schizophrenia without psychosis, and healthy control subjects. Each column is an individual patient, each row represents significance of activation in a particular brain region. The clinical and neurobiological clustering can be seen in the lines connecting rows and columns, beside the matrix. Such approaches, with multivariate analytics, have the potential to identify mechanistic subtypes of patients within and across diagnostic groups, and potentially across treatment groups, with clinical correlation. This can provide a foundation for brain circuit-based tools in neuropsychiatry. (Figure courtesy of D. Silbersweig and E. Stern.)

Summary and Key Points

- Advances in technology, which include functional magnetic resonance imaging and positron emission topography, have allowed for measuring levels of brain activation. These tools combined with sophisticated scientific methods allow for association of behavior and affect with specific regions of brain activity.
- Brain networks guiding behavior and affect are complex and distributed. It is a helpful heuristic to consider neural networks involved across four domains: threat detection and avoidance, motivation and approach, higher-order appraisal and regulation, and awareness of feeling states.
- Important limbic regions comprising circuitry processing threat and defense include the amygdala, responsible for the detection of immediate threats, and the bed nucleus of the stria terminalis, which is active in response to uncertain future or chronic stressors.
- Motivational circuitry includes appraisal by lower-order subcortical circuitry such as the ventral striatum, and further modulation by prefrontal cortical areas.
- Higher-order, neocortical, top-down regulation facilitates manipulation of more primitive responses by utilizing information from memory, environmental context, and current goals to guide behavior.
- Awareness of emotions and self-states includes important contributions from the insular cortex representation of interoceptive stimuli as well as hippocampus and prefrontal areas guiding narrative self-representation; mid-line frontal and parietal structures are involved with default mode network and the process of self-reflection.
- Psychiatric and neurological disorders with emotional and behavioral symptoms share common pathways that cross diagnostic boundaries. Exploring similar phenotypes arising from separate pathologies allows one to identify common underlying mechanisms and to reduce stigma associated with psychiatric conditions by demonstrating biological causes.
- Heightened activation of circuitry involved in threat detection (including the amygdala) may be implicated in anxiety disorders, depressive disorders with high anxiety traits, or psychotic paranoia.
- Motivational network dysfunction can be seen in depressive phenotypes, spanning psychiatric depressive disorders in anhedonic depressive phenotypes, the depressed affect associated with Parkinson's disease, and negative symptoms of schizophrenia.
- Impulsivity reflects failure of inhibitory control mechanisms and often prioritizes immediate rather than long-term rewards, with inappropriate social-emotional behavior. Types of impulsivity can be associated with orbitofrontal dysfunction and may be seen across a range of disorders including borderline personality disorder, bipolar disorder, or traumatic brain injury.
- An understanding of the complex and distributed networks involved in affective and behavioral circuitry allows appreciation of the intricate systems contributing to psychiatric and neurological presentations, as well as guidance in the development of potential novel treatments.

Multiple Choice Questions

1. Functional neuroimaging is most commonly accomplished with BOLD MRI, characterized by
   a. detection of gamma photons with coincidence detection
   b. immediate detection of brain metabolic states
   c. detection of electrical activity
   d. detection of changes in blood flow, volume, and oxygenation
   e. injection of contrast

2. The amygdala is a subcortical structure within the limbic system and
   a. is responsible for the conscious feeling of fear and anxiety
   b. is associated in detection of immediate threat
   c. is associated in evaluation of uncertain threat
   d. has diminished activity in post-traumatic stress disorder
   e. extended amygdala includes prefrontal systems such as the dorsolateral prefrontal cortex.

3. Functional imaging allows for detection of large-scale neural networks. Please select the correct pairing of network and associated brain regions.
   a. Default mode network—posterior parietal and dorsolateral prefrontal cortices
   b. Executive control network—medial prefrontal and posterior cingulate cortices
   c. Salience network—anterior insular, dorsal anterior cingulate cortex, and subcortical (thalamus, hypothalamus, amygdala) regions
   d. Defensive survival circuit—lateral temporal and ventrolateral prefrontal cortices
   e. Language network—medial temporal cortex and subcortical regions

4. Which of the following statements are correct?
   a. The anterior insular cortex is involved in the subjective feeling of emotions.
   b. The nucleus accumbens of the ventral striatum is involved in reward circuitry.
   c. Prefrontal cortices allow for monitoring, planning, and sustaining of goal-directed behavior.
   d. Anterior cingulate cortex is involved in initiation of behaviors.
   e. All of the above.

Multiple Choice Answers

1. Answer: d

BOLD MRI detects changes in blood flow via magnetic characteristics of deoxyhemoglobin. It is not immediate, occurring about 4–6 s after initiation of increased brain activity. PET imaging detects gamma photons released after a positron emitted by decay of injected radioligand combines with a positron. MRI indirectly detects neuronal electrical activity, whereas electroencephalography (EEG) more directly detects electrical activity, though with poorer spatial resolution compared to MRI.

2. Answer: b

The amygdala is involved in the detection of immediate threat, whereas the bed nucleus of the stria terminalis is more closely associated with evaluation of uncertain, distant, or chronic threats. The amygdala is a subcortical structure and an important part of the defensive survival circuit, though the conscious awareness of fear and anxiety states is mediated via neocortical systems. PTSD is an example of pathological state involving amygdala hyperactivation.

3. Answer: c

The salience network is involved in detecting relevant internal and external stimuli and assists in activating either task-positive or task-negative networks. The default mode network involves medial prefrontal and posterior cingulate cortices, while the executive control network involves posterior parietal and dorsolateral prefrontal cortices. The defensive survival circuit involves subcortical limbic structures including the amygdala.

4. Answer: e

All of the above statements are correct.

References

1. Adams F. *Genuine Works of Hippocrates*. Vol 2. William Wood & Co; 1886.
2. Lloyd G. Alcmaeon and the early history of dissection. *Sudhoff's Archiv*. 1975;59(2):113-147.
3. Roxo MR, Franceschini PR, Zubaran C, Kleber FD, Sander JW. The limbic system conception and its historical evolution. *Sci World J*. 2011;11:2427-2440.
4. Smith CUM. Cardiocentric neurophysiology: the persistence of a delusion. *J Hist Neurosci*. 2013;22(1):6-13.
5. Iadecola C. The neurovascular unit coming of age: a journey through neurovascular coupling in health and disease. *Neuron*. 2017;96(1):17-42.
6. Ogawa S, Lee TM, Kay AR, Tank DW. Brain magnetic resonance imaging with contrast dependent on blood oxygenation. *Proc Natl Acad Sci U S A*. 1990;87(24):9868-9872.
7. Pan H, Epstein J, Silbersweig DA, Stern E. New and emerging imaging techniques for mapping brain circuitry. *Brain Res Rev*. 2011;67(1-2):226-251.
8. Ostroff LE, Cain CK, Bedont J, Monfils MH, LeDoux JE. Fear and safety learning differentially affect synapse size and dendritic translation in the lateral amygdala. *Proc Natl Acad Sci U S A*. 2010;107(20):9418-9423.
9. Isenberg N, Silbersweig D, Engelien A, et al. Linguistic threat activates the human amygdala. *Proc Natl Acad Sci U S A*. 1999;96(18):10456-10459.
10. Kaas JH. The evolution of brains from early mammals to humans: evolution of brains from early mammals to humans. *Wiley Interdiscip Rev Cogn Sci*. 2013;4(1):33-45.
11. LeDoux JE. Semantics, surplus meaning, and the science of fear. *Trends Cogn Sci*. 2017;21(5):303-306.
12. Calhoon GG, Tye KM. Resolving the neural circuits of anxiety. *Nat Neurosci*. 2015;18(10):1394-1404.
13. Johansen JP, Cain CK, Ostroff LE, LeDoux JE. Molecular mechanisms of fear learning and memory. *Cell*. 2011;147(3):509-524.
14. LeDoux JE, Pine DS. Using neuroscience to help understand fear and anxiety: a two-system framework. *Am J Psychiatry*. 2016;173(11):1083-1093.
15. Yassa MA, Hazlett RL, Stark CEL, Hoehn-Saric R. Functional MRI of the amygdala and bed nucleus of the stria terminalis during conditions of uncertainty in generalized anxiety disorder. *J Psychiatr Res*. 2012;46(8):1045-1052.
16. Daniel SE, Rainnie DG. Stress modulation of opposing circuits in the bed nucleus of the stria terminalis. *Neuropsychopharmacology*. 2016;41(1):103-125.
17. Ruiz-Rizzo AL, Beissner F, Finke K, et al. Human subsystems of medial temporal lobes extend locally to amygdala nuclei and globally to an allostatic-interoceptive system. *NeuroImage*. 2019;207:116404.
18. Fanselow MS, Dong H-W. Are the dorsal and ventral hippocampus functionally distinct structures? *Neuron*. 2010;65(1):7-19.
19. Sekeres MJ, Winocur G, Moscovitch M. The hippocampus and related neocortical structures in memory transformation. *Neurosci Lett*. 2018;680:39-53.
20. LeDoux J, Daw ND. Surviving threats: neural circuit and computational implications of a new taxonomy of defensive behaviour. *Nat Rev Neurosci*. 2018;19(5):269-282.
21. Phelps EA. Emotion and cognition: insights from studies of the human amygdala. *Annu Rev Psychol*. 2006;57(1):27-53.
22. Weisholtz DS, Root JC, Butler T, et al. Beyond the amygdala: linguistic threat modulates peri-sylvian semantic access cortices. *Brain Lang*. 2015;151:12-22.
23. Tovote P, Fadok JP, Lüthi A. Neuronal circuits for fear and anxiety. *Nat Rev Neurosci*. 2015;16(6):317-331.
24. LaBar KS, Cabeza R. Cognitive neuroscience of emotional memory. *Nat Rev Neurosci*. 2006;7(1):54-64.
25. Hanson JL, Nacewicz BM, Sutterer MJ, et al. Behavioral problems after early life stress: contributions of the hippocampus and amygdala. *Biol Psychiatry*. 2015;77(4):314-323.
26. Grant MM, Cannistraci C, Hollon SD, Gore J, Shelton R. Childhood trauma history differentiates amygdala response to sad faces within MDD. *J Psychiatr Res*. 2011;45(7):886-895.
27. Osório C, Probert T, Jones E, Young AH, Robbins I. Adapting to stress: understanding the neurobiology of resilience. *Behav Med*. 2017;43(4):307-322.

28. Southwick SM, Charney DS. The science of resilience: implications for the prevention and treatment of depression. *Science.* 2012;338(6103):79-82.

29. Robinson OJ, Krimsky M, Lieberman L, Vytal K, Ernst M, Grillon C. Anxiety-potentiated amygdala–medial frontal coupling and attentional control. *Transl Psychiatry.* 2016;6(6):e833.

30. Watkins LE, Sprang KR, Rothbaum BO. Treating PTSD: a review of evidence-based psychotherapy interventions. *Front Behav Neurosci.* 2018;12:258.

31. Hoskins M, Pearce J, Bethell A, et al. Pharmacotherapy for post-traumatic stress disorder: systematic review and meta-analysis. *Br J Psychiatry.* 2015;206(2):93-100.

32. Thomas É, Saumier D, Pitman RK, Tremblay J, Brunet A. Consolidation and reconsolidation are impaired by oral propranolol administered before but not after memory (re)activation in humans. *Neurobiol Learn Mem.* 2017;142:118-125.

33. Epstein J, Silbersweig D. The neuropsychiatric spectrum of motivational disorders. *J Neuropsychiatry Clin Neurosci.* 2015; 27(1):7-18.

34. Cox J, Witten IB. Striatal circuits for reward learning and decision-making. *Nat Rev Neurosci.* 2019;20(8):482-494.

35. Schultz W. Dopamine reward prediction-error signalling: a two-component response. *Nat Rev Neurosci.* 2016;17(3):183-195.

36. Schultz W. Dopamine reward prediction error coding. *Dialogues Clin Neurosci.* 2016;18(1):10.

37. Xia X, Fan L, Cheng C, et al. Multimodal connectivity-based parcellation reveals a shell-core dichotomy of the human nucleus accumbens: multimodal parcellation of the human NAc. *Hum Brain Mapp.* 2017;38(8):3878-3898.

38. Floresco SB. The nucleus accumbens: an interface between cognition, emotion, and action. *Annu Rev Psychol.* 2015;66(1):25-52.

39. Allen WE, Chen MZ, Pichamoorthy N, Tien RH, Pachitariu M, Luo L, et al. Thirst regulates motivated behavior through modulation of brainwide neural population dynamics. 2019;364(6437):253.

40. Kennerley SW, Walton ME. Decision making and reward in frontal cortex: complementary evidence from neurophysiological and neuropsychological studies. *Behav Neurosci.* 2011;125(3):297-317.

41. Proulx CD, Hikosaka O, Malinow R. Reward processing by the lateral habenula in normal and depressive behaviors. *Nat Neurosci.* 2014;17(9):1146-1152.

42. Le Heron C, Holroyd CB, Salamone J, Husain M. Brain mechanisms underlying apathy. *J Neurol Neurosurg Psychiatry.* 2019; 90(3):302-312.

43. Mesulam M. From sensation to cognition. *Brain.* 1998;121(6): 1013-1052.

44. Dixon ML, Thiruchselvam R, Todd R, Christoff K. Emotion and the prefrontal cortex: an integrative review. *Psychol Bull.* 2017;143(10):1033-1081.

45. Zald DH, McHugo M, Ray KL, Glahn DC, Eickhoff SB, Laird AR. Meta-analytic connectivity modeling reveals differential functional connectivity of the medial and lateral orbitofrontal cortex. *Cereb Cortex.* 2014;24(1):232-248.

46. Hampton AN, Bossaerts P, O'Doherty JP. Neural correlates of mentalizing-related computations during strategic interactions in humans. *Proc Natl Acad Sci U S A.* 2008;105(18):6741-6746.

47. Delgado MR, Beer JS, Fellows LK, et al. Viewpoints: dialogues on the functional role of the ventromedial prefrontal cortex. *Nat Neurosci.* 2016;19(12):1545-1552.

48. McClure SM. Separate neural systems value immediate and delayed monetary rewards. *Science.* 2004;306(5695):503-507.

49. Hare TA, Camerer CF, Rangel A. Self-control in decision-making involves modulation of the vmPFC valuation system. 2009;324:4.

50. Perez DL, Vago DR, Pan H, Root J, Tuescher O, Fuchs BH, et al. Frontolimbic neural circuit changes in emotional processing and inhibitory control associated with clinical improvement following transference-focused psychotherapy in borderline personality disorder: neural mechanisms of psychotherapy. *Psychiatry Clin Neurosci.* 2016;70(1):51-61.

51. Palomero-Gallagher N, Vogt BA, Schleicher A, Mayberg HS, Zilles K. Receptor architecture of human cingulate cortex: evaluation of the four-region neurobiological model. *Hum Brain Mapp.* 2009;30(8):2336-2355.

52. Vogt BA. Pain and emotion interactions in subregions of the cingulate gyrus. *Nat Rev Neurosci.* 2005;6(7):533-544.

53. Perez DL, Barsky AJ, Vago DR, Baslet G, Silbersweig DA. A neural circuit framework for somatosensory amplification in somatoform disorders. *J Neuropsychiatry Clin Neurosci.* 2015;27(1): e40-e50.

54. Craig AD. How do you feel—now? The anterior insula and human awareness. *Nat Rev Neurosci.* 2009;10(1):59-70.

55. Craig AD. How do you feel? Interoception: the sense of the physiological condition of the body. *Nat Rev Neurosci.* 2002;3(8): 655-666.

56. Darby RR, Joutsa J, Burke MJ, Fox MD. Lesion network localization of free will. *Proc Natl Acad Sci U S A.* 2018;115(42):10792-10797.

57. Buhle JT, Silvers JA, Wager TD, et al. Cognitive reappraisal of emotion: a meta-analysis of human neuroimaging studies. *Cereb Cortex.* 2014;24(11):2981-2990.

58. Damasio A. *Self Comes to Mind: Constructing the Conscious Brain.* New York, NY: Pantheon Books; 2010:384.

59. Vago DR, Silbersweig DA. Self-awareness, self-regulation, and self-transcendence (S-ART): a framework for understanding the neurobiological mechanisms of mindfulness. *Front Hum Neurosci.* 2012;6. Available at http://journal.frontiersin.org/article/10.3389/fnhum.2012.00296/abstract. Accessed September 28, 2019.

60. Cook R, Bird G, Catmur C, Press C, Heyes C. Mirror neurons: from origin to function. *Behav Brain Sci.* 37(2):177-192.

61. Kilner JM, Lemon RN. What we know currently about mirror neurons. *Curr Biol.* 2013;23(23):R1057-R1062.

62. Amodio DM, Frith CD. Meeting of minds: the medial frontal cortex and social cognition. *Nat Rev Neurosci.* 2006;7(4):268-277.

63. Raichle ME. The brain's default mode network. *Annu Rev Neurosci.* 2015;38(1):433-447.

64. Buckner RL, DiNicola LM. The brain's default network: updated anatomy, physiology and evolving insights. *Nat Rev Neurosci.* 2019;20(10):593-608.

65. Coutinho JF, Fernandesl SV, Soares JM, Maia L, Gonçalves ÓF, Sampaio A. Default mode network dissociation in depressive and anxiety states. *Brain Imaging Behav.* 2016;10(1):147-157.

66. Uddin LQ. Salience processing and insular cortical function and dysfunction. *Nat Rev Neurosci.* 2015;16(1):55-61.

67. Seeley WW, Menon V, Schatzberg AF, et al. Dissociable intrinsic connectivity networks for salience processing and executive control. *J Neurosci.* 2007;27(9):2349-2356.

68. van den Heuvel MP, Sporns O. A cross-disorder connectome landscape of brain dysconnectivity. *Nat Rev Neurosci.* 2019;20(7):435-446.

69. Mulders PC, van Eijndhoven PF, Schene AH, Beckmann CF, Tendolkar I. Resting-state functional connectivity in major depressive disorder: a review. *Neurosci Biobehav Rev.* 2015;56:330-344.

70. Drysdale AT, Grosenick L, Downar J, et al. Resting-state connectivity biomarkers define neurophysiological subtypes of depression. *Nat Med.* 2017;23(1):28-38.

71. Protopopescu X, Pan H, Tuescher O, et al. Differential time courses and specificity of amygdala activity in posttraumatic

stress disorder subjects and normal control subjects. *Biol Psychiatry*. 2005;57(5):464-473.

72. Liberzon I, Duval E, Javanbakht A. Neural circuits in anxiety and stress disorders: a focused review. *Ther Clin Risk Manag*. 2015;11:115-126.

73. Tuescher O, Protopopescu X, Pan H, et al. Differential activity of subgenual cingulate and brainstem in panic disorder and PTSD. *J Anxiety Disord*. 2011;25(2):251-257.

74. Pinkham AE, Liu P, Lu H, Kriegsman M, Simpson C, Tamminga C. Amygdala hyperactivity at rest in paranoid individuals with schizophrenia. *Am J Psychiatry*. 2015;172(8):784-792.

75. Bourque J, Spechler PA, Potvin S, et al. Functional neuroimaging predictors of self-reported psychotic symptoms in adolescents. *Am J Psychiatry*. 2017;174(6):566-575.

76. Perez DL, Pan H, Weisholtz DS, et al. Altered threat and safety neural processing linked to persecutory delusions in schizophrenia: a two-task fMRI study. *Psychiatry Res*. 2015;233(3):352-366.

77. Urbanic PT, Zaar K, Eder H, Gruber-Cichocky L, Feichtinger M. Ictal fear auras after selective amygdalohippocampectomy: the use of ictal SPECT and scalp EEG in the presurgical reevaluation. *Epilepsy Behav*. 2011;22(3):577-580.

78. Chong DJ, Dugan P. Ictal fear: associations with age, gender, and other experiential phenomena. *Epilepsy Behav*. 2016;62:153-158.

79. Penfield W, Perot P. The brain's record of auditory and visual experience: a final summary and discussion. *Brain*. 1963;86(4):595-696.

80. Garrison JR, Fernandez-Egea E, Zaman R, Agius M, Simons JS. Reality monitoring impairment in schizophrenia reflects specific prefrontal cortex dysfunction. *Neuroimage Clin*. 2017;14:260-268.

81. Parlikar R, Bose A, Venkatasubramanian G. Schizophrenia and corollary discharge: a neuroscientific overview and translational implications. *Clin Psychopharmacol Neurosci*. 2019;17(2):170-182.

82. Silbersweig D, Stern E. Functional neuroimaging of hallucinations in schizophrenia: toward an integration of bottom-up and top-down approaches. *Mol Psychiatry*. 1996;1(5):367-375.

83. Keren H, O'Callaghan G, Vidal-Ribas P, et al. Reward processing in depression: a conceptual and meta-analytic review across fMRI and EEG studies. *Am J Psychiatry*. 2018;175(11):1111-1120.

84. Epstein J, Pan H, Kocsis JH, et al. Lack of ventral striatal response to positive stimuli in depressed versus normal subjects. *Am J Psychiatry*. 2006;163(10):1784-1790.

85. Remy P, Doder M, Lees A, Turjanski N, Brooks D. Depression in Parkinson's disease: loss of dopamine and noradrenaline innervation in the limbic system. *Brain*. 2005;128(6):1314-1322.

86. Epstein J, Perez DL, Ervin K, et al. Failure to segregate emotional processing from cognitive and sensorimotor processing in major depression. *Psychiatry Res Neuroimaging*. 2011;193(3):144-150.

87. Crowell AL, Riva-Posse P, Holtzheimer PE, et al. Long-term outcomes of subcallosal cingulate deep brain stimulation for treatment-resistant depression. *Am J Psychiatry*. 2019;176(11):949-956.

88. Riva-Posse P, Holtzheimer PE, Mayberg HS. Cingulate-mediated depressive symptoms in neurologic disease and therapeutics. In: *Handbook of Clinical Neurology*. Elsevier; 2019:371–379. Available at https://linkinghub.elsevier.com/retrieve/pii/B978044 4641960000212. Accessed January 11, 2020.

89. Marin R. Apathy: a neuropsychiatric syndrome. *J Neuropsychiatry Clin Neurosci*. 1991;3:12.

90. Galderisi S, Mucci A, Buchanan RW, Arango C. Negative symptoms of schizophrenia: new developments and unanswered research questions. *Lancet Psychiatry*. 2018;5(8):664-677.

91. Volkow ND, Wise RA, Baler R. The dopamine motive system: implications for drug and food addiction. *Nat Rev Neurosci*. 2017;18(12):741-752.

92. Koob GF, Volkow ND. Neurobiology of addiction: a neurocircuitry analysis. *Lancet Psychiatry*. 2016;3(8):760-773.

93. Warren N, O'Gorman C, Lehn A, Siskind D. Dopamine dysregulation syndrome in Parkinson's disease: a systematic review of published cases. *J Neurol Neurosurg Psychiatry*. 2017;88(12):1060-1064.

94. American Psychiatric Association. *Diagnostic and Statistical Manual of Mental Disorders*: DSM-5. 5th ed. Arlington, VA: American Psychiatric Association.

95. Silbersweig D, Clarkin JF, Goldstein M, et al. Failure of frontolimbic inhibitory function in the context of negative emotion in borderline personality disorder. *Am J Psychiatry*. 2007;164(12):1832-1841.

96. Van Horn JD, Irimia A, Torgerson CM, Chambers MC, Kikinis R, Toga AW. Mapping connectivity damage in the case of Phineas Gage. *PLoS One*. 2012;7(5):e37454.

97. Damasio H, Grabowski T, Frank R, Galaburda A, Damasio A. The return of Phineas Gage: clues about the brain from the skull of a famous patient. *Science*. 1994;264(5162):1102-1105.

98. Gillan CM, Fineberg NA, Robbins TW. A trans-diagnostic perspective on obsessive-compulsive disorder. *Psychol Med*. 2017;47(9):1528-1548.

99. Dougherty DD, Brennan BP, Stewart SE, Wilhelm S, Widge AS, Rauch SL. Neuroscientifically informed formulation and treatment planning for patients with obsessive-compulsive disorder: a review. *JAMA Psychiatry*. 2018;75(10):1081.

100. Stern E, Silbersweig DA, Chee KY, et al. A functional neuroanatomy of tics in Tourette syndrome. *Arch Gen Psychiatry*. 2000;57(8):741-748.

101. Bonelli RM, Cummings JL. Frontal-subcortical circuitry and behavior. *Transl Res*. 2007;9(2):11.

102. Baslet G, Seshadri A, Bermeo-Ovalle A, Willment K, Myers L. Psychogenic non-epileptic seizures: an updated primer. *Psychosomatics*. 2016;57(1):1-17.

103. Baizabal-Carvallo JF, Hallett M, Jankovic J. Pathogenesis and pathophysiology of functional (psychogenic) movement disorders. *Neurobiol Dis*. 2019;127:32-44.

104. Fernandes JM, Cajão R, Lopes R, Jerónimo R, Barahona-Corrêa JB. Social cognition in schizophrenia and autism spectrum disorders: a systematic review and meta-analysis of direct comparisons. *Front Psychiatry*. 2018;9:504.

105. Kana RK, Libero LE, Hu CP, Deshpande HD, Colburn JS. Functional brain networks and white matter underlying theory-of-mind in autism. *Soc Cogn Affect Neurosci*. 2014;9(1):98-105.

106. Kronbichler L, Tschernegg M, Martin AI, Schurz M, Kronbichler M. Abnormal brain activation during theory of mind tasks in schizophrenia: a meta-analysis. *Schizophr Bull*. 2017;43(6):1240-1250.

107. Toller G, Yang WFZ, Brown JA, et al. Divergent patterns of loss of interpersonal warmth in frontotemporal dementia syndromes are predicted by altered intrinsic network connectivity. *NeuroImage Clin*. 2019;22:101729.

108. Strikwerda-Brown C, Ramanan S, Irish M. Neurocognitive mechanisms of theory of mind impairment in neurodegeneration: a transdiagnostic approach. *Neuropsychiatr Dis Treat*. 2019;15:557-573.

109. Martin J. *Neuroanatomy Text and Atlas*. 4th ed. New York, NY: The McGraw-Hill Companies, Inc.; 2012.

110. Nestler E, Human S, Holtzman D, Malenka R. *Molecular Neuropharmacology: A Foundation for Clinical Neuroscience*. 3rd ed. New York, NY: The McGraw-Hill Companies, Inc.; 2015.

111. Kandel E, Schwartz J, Jessell T, Siegelbaum S, Hudspeth A. *Principles of Neural Science*. 5th ed. New York, NY: The McGraw-Hill Companies, Inc.; 2013.

3

Functional Neurocircuitry of Cognition and Cognitive Syndromes

Deepti Putcha · Michael Erkkinen · Kirk R. Daffner

INTRODUCTION

To maintain our survival and well-being, the nervous systems must carry out a number of critical operations that comprise cognition. We need to process information about the external environment (sensory-perceptual representations and visuospatial cognition) and be able to prepare and execute actions (motor planning and output). We rely on information that allows us to communicate with others (language), and encode, store, and retrieve information (learning and memory). Importantly, we must be able to select, control, and monitor these complex operations as internal and external demands shift (executive control functions). This chapter will explore the neural circuitry underlying these varied cognitive processes. In our companion chapter (Chapter 12), we will illustrate how disruption of these operations can impact patients, and outline an approach to localization providing a series of clinical cases as examples. Of note, behavioral neurology and cognitive neuroscience are dynamically changing fields. We present a brief snapshot of the state of our discipline, and fully acknowledge the ongoing debate about which proposed frameworks provide the best account of the relevant data. In some of the "boxes" included throughout the chapter, we briefly highlight differences between classical and emerging theories, and touch upon some unresolved controversies. Other boxes will provide a summary of the neural circuitry subserving each of the major cognitive realms discussed.

Virtually all aspects of cognition arise from the dynamic interactions of distributed brain regions conceptualized as large-scale neural networks.[1,2] Brain networks fall into two different categories: *structural* networks, which represent anatomical wiring, and *functional* networks, which are derived from estimates of correlated neural activity among brain regions that are connected by underlying mono- or polysynaptic neuronal connections.[3] Functional networks are interconnected ensembles of cortical and subcortical neurons that are coactivated to mediate a cognitive or behavioral function. A wealth of evidence from anatomical, neuroimaging, and physiological studies supports the idea that individual brain regions are functionally specialized

and make specific contributions to cognition, and further, that these functionally specific regions comprise networks that mediate cognitive and behavioral functions. Some investigators have described a network's functional connectivity as represented by temporal coherence in activity across different neurons or neuronal ensembles.[4] Such work is increasingly informed by network or graph theoretical approaches that define nodes and edges (or paired relationships) between nodes.[2,5] Functional network connectivity can reflect both direct and indirect underlying anatomical connections via other cortical or subcortical regions, and the dynamic modulation of specialized brain networks are critical for the specialized cognitive functions of memory, language, attention, visual/spatial functioning, and executive control.[6] Cognition and behavior are considered broadly to be emergent phenomena of large-scale neural networks and their subcomponent networks, while critical network centers, or nodes, are thought to constitute relay or integration centers.[7] Lesions to the circuit can lead to the inability to transfer information from one node to another.[8,9] Recent work has focused on identifying the breakdown in dynamic connectivity within and between these large-scale networks, as these approaches provide new insight into cognitive dysfunction observed in psychopathology and neurodegenerative disease.[10,11]

Neuroimaging techniques have made vital contributions to our understanding of functional neurocircuitry of the human brain. Decades of task-related positron emission tomography (PET) and functional magnetic resonance imaging (fMRI) experiments have revealed that groups of brain regions functionally coactivate during certain tasks. More recently, fMRI advances in delineating functional connectivity between brain regions have helped researchers better understand the human brain's intrinsic functional network architecture.[11-14] These studies have shown a high degree of temporal correlation across spatially distinct, but functionally related brain regions in the resting state, or task-free condition. Further, resting state functional connectivity is also observable during task-related conditions, suggesting that functional networks coupled at rest are also systematically engaged during cognition, and vice versa,[15] reminiscent of the Hebbian adage, "*neurons that fire together, wire together.*" Efforts to integrate these findings with studies of structural connectivity (e.g., diffusion tensor imaging) and findings from lesion studies and depth electrode recordings have created a framework for understanding the neural basis of cognition. For example, knowing which brain areas are connected via white matter tracts, and the network properties of these structural connections, allow us to know which functional interactions are possible.[1] Lastly, a critical concept to understanding neurodegenerative disorders of cognition is the theory that structural abnormalities (e.g., abnormally folded proteins) propagate across regions of a given network over time, and may lead to reductions in synchronized neuronal activity, or reduced functional connectivity.[10] There is now increasing evidence that disorders such as frontotemporal dementia and Alzheimer's disease,[11,16,17] as well as psychopathologies like schizophrenia,[10,18,19] initially arise from focal structural abnormalities that may then propagate to the other nodes within a functionally defined network.[5,11] A useful mnemonic describing this phenomenon is "*neurons that wire together, expire together.*"

In this chapter, we will summarize the current understanding of how cognition is supported in the human brain, as well as the impact of neurological disease on the dynamic functioning of core neurocircuitry. A simplified framework for cognitive processing is sketched in Figure 3-1. The base of Figure 3-1 suggests that information processing is influenced by ascending systems originating in brainstem and thalamus. The ascending reticular activating system along with the intralaminar thalamic nuclei and their cortical projections are central for pacing EEG activity, the regulation of wakefulness and arousal, and the tonic

aspects of attention. Recent evidence has highlighted the crucial role of the left parabrachial region in the rostral dorsolateral pontine tegmentum and the integrity of its connections with left anterior insula and pregenual anterior cingulate cortex (ACC) in the maintenance of arousal and consciousness.[20]

Ascending systems in brainstem and basal forebrain serve as a major source of neurotransmitters (norepinephrine, acetylcholine, dopamine, and serotonin), which innervate widely distributed parts of the brain and can modulate levels of arousal, attention, motivation, and mood. Norepinephrine from the locus coeruleus in the pons helps to mediate alertness and improve signal-to-noise ratio during information transfer. Acetylcholine from the basal forebrain and brainstem reticular systems modulates excitability of the thalamus and cortex, influences overall information processing capacity, and facilitates the orienting of attention.[21] Dopamine from the ventral tegmental area of the midbrain promotes working memory functions[22,23] and helps to regulate motivational states and reward systems.[24,25] For example, evidence in animals suggests that there is an "optimal" amount of dopamine, which follows an inverted "u-shaped" curve. Too much or too little dopamine is detrimental to working memory performance.[26] Serotonin from brainstem raphe nuclei plays an important role in the regulation of mood, appetite, and a range of behaviors. Abnormalities of serotonin have been associated with disruptive, repetitive, aggressive, and impulsive behaviors.

Figure 3-1 also illustrates the hemispheric lateralization of cognitive functions in the human brain: the left hemisphere has specialization in most of us for language processing, for verbal semantic knowledge, and for the execution of complex, learned motor movements (i.e., praxis), whereas the right hemisphere

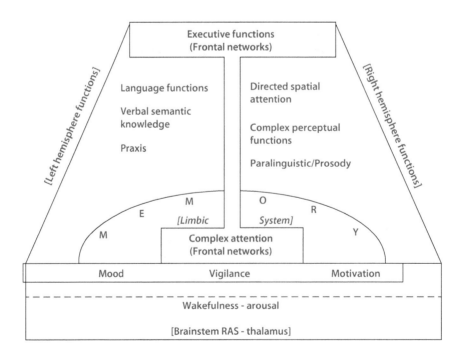

FIGURE 3-1. A simplified framework for cognitive processing. The base of this framework suggests that information processing is influenced by ascending systems originating in the brainstem and thalamus, which give rise to supporting complex attention and motivation. Illustrated here is also the hemispheric lateralization of cognitive functions in the human brain: typically, the left hemisphere is specialized for language, verbal semantic knowledge, and learned motor movements (praxis), while the right hemisphere is specialized for directed spatial attention, complex perceptual functions, and prosody.

has specialized networks for directed spatial attention, complex perceptual functions, and paralinguistic activities (e.g., prosody). This typical organization is true for approximately 95–99% of right-handers, and approximately 80% of left-handers. The limbic system, which will be delineated elsewhere in this chapter, mediates memory functions and affective processing. And lastly, complex attention and executive functions are subserved by frontal systems and connections to subcortical and parietal cortical regions. The chapter will be organized by broad cognitive domains, with the caveat that some cognitive functions are not purely domain-specific (e.g., attention is a critical component of executive functions, language, spatial cognition, and memory).

ATTENTION AND WORKING MEMORY

Attention refers to a set of processes that are necessary to engage in any higher-order cognitive function, and includes arousal, orienting, selectivity, and the capacity to sustain vigilance. Attention also reflects mechanisms involved in disengaging and shifting focus and dividing resources among tasks. Although attention and working memory have some conceptual overlap with executive functions, discussed below, here we will present networks critical for orientating and monitoring of attention as well as the maintenance, manipulation, and sequencing functions considered broadly as working memory. Spatial attention has historically been attributed to four cerebral regions that work in a unified fashion for the modulation of directed attention to extrapersonal space (Figure 3-2A): *the posterior parietal cortex*, which provides an internal sensory-perceptual map, the

limbic-cingulate gyrus component which regulates the spatial distribution of motivational valence, a *frontal component*, which coordinates the motor programs for exploration, scanning, reaching, and fixating, and lastly, *a reticular component*, which provides the underlying arousal/vigilance.[27] This initial conceptualization evolved into a description of a large-scale attention network that included the three monosynaptically interconnected frontal, parietal, and cingulate regions noted. Early fMRI experiments of spatial attention also emphasized subcortical regions including the basal ganglia and thalamic regions, and regions of the posterior temporo-occipital cortex and anterior insula.[28] Further work has refined these regions to include specialized attention control networks for both cognitive (top-down) factors such as knowledge, expectation, and goals, as well as bottom-up factors that reflect sensory stimulation.[29] Corbetta and Shulman[29] proposed that the visual attention system is controlled by two partially segregated neural systems, each supporting top-down (or goal-driven) and bottom-up (or stimulus-driven) attention control. The *top-down attention* system is centered on the dorsal frontal and posterior parietal cortices (later termed the **dorsal attention network** [DAN]), and the *bottom-up attention system* is centered on the right-hemisphere temporoparietal and ventral frontal cortex (later termed the **ventral attention network** [VAN]) (see Figure 3-2B).

Anatomically, the DAN is largely bilateral and anchored in intraparietal sulcus (IPS) and frontal eye fields (FEF), as well as the middle temporal complex (MT+). Some frontal and parietal regions within this system partially overlap with regions of the executive control network discussed in the next section on executive functions, though there is ample evidence that they

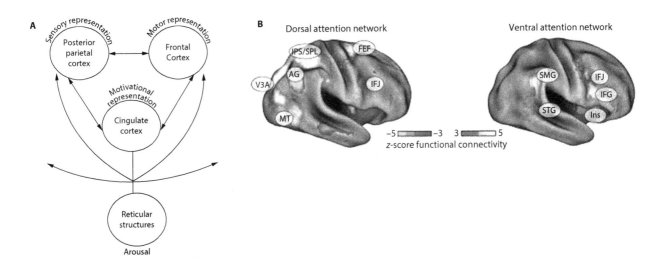

FIGURE 3-2. The evolution of attention networks. **Panel A** depicts spatial attention as it has historically been conceptualized, as four cerebral regions working in a unified fashion for the modulation of directed attention to extrapersonal space: *the posterior parietal cortex*, which provides an internal sensory-perceptual map; the *limbic-cingulate gyrus*, which regulates the spatial distribution of motivational valence; the *frontal cortex*, which coordinates the motor programs for exploration, scanning, reaching, and fixating; and lastly, *a reticular component*, which provides the underlying arousal/vigilance. (Adapted with permission from Mesulam MM. A cortical network for directed attention and unilateral neglect. *Ann Neurol.* 1981;10(4):309-325. https://onlinelibrary.wiley.com/journal/15318249. Copyright © John Wiley & Sons, Inc.) **Panel B** depicts a current conceptualization of the visual attention system which has been built upon the historical framework depicted in Panel A. This model shows a two-part system, with the *dorsal attention network* supporting top-down, goal-oriented attentional control, and *ventral attention network* supporting bottom-up, stimulus-driven attention. (Reproduced with permission from Annual Reviews, Inc., from Corbetta M, Shulman GL. Spatial neglect and attention networks. *Annu Rev Neurosci.* 2011;34:569-599; permission conveyed through Copyright Clearance, Inc.)

are two distinct networks.[13,30–32] The DAN has been specifically implicated in the cognitive selection of sensory information and response. That is, activity colocalizes to regions of the DAN when focusing on an object or task, or reorienting to goal-directed activity in the contralateral hemispace.[29,33] The VAN is anchored in right-hemisphere temporoparietal junction (TPJ) and inferior frontal gyrus/middle frontal gyrus (IFG/MFG). In contrast to the functional specificity of the DAN, the VAN is thought to serve as a kind of "circuit breaker" to current cognitive activities in response to salient, potentially relevant external environmental stimuli. These two attentional systems dynamically interact with each other during the processing of environmental stimuli to determine where and what we attend to. Specifically, the DAN is thought to send top-down filtering signals to visual areas and the VAN, thus modulating ventral activation in response to behaviorally important stimuli and coordinating stimulus-response selection.[29,33] Conversely, when a salient stimulus occurs during stimulus-driven reorienting, the VAN sends an attention reorientation signal to the dorsal network.[33] Though some have considered the VAN and the salience network (discussed further in the next section on executive functions) to be overlapping, both functionally and anatomically,[34] it is generally accepted these networks are distinct entities.[4,35,36]

Implications for Unilateral Stroke and Neglect

Patients with unilateral injury to the brain tend to neglect events that occur within the contralateral half of space. In severe cases, patients may shave, groom, and dress only one side of the body, or eat food placed on only one side of the tray, while in less severe cases, neglect may not be obvious during spontaneous behavior but can be elicited in the form of unilateral extinction during bilateral simultaneous stimulation. Since primary sensorimotor deficits are not necessary for these symptoms, it is thought that unilateral neglect reflects an underlying attentional deficit for segments of extrapersonal space.[27] Unilateral neglect syndromes are more frequent and severe after lesions to the right hemisphere. The right hemisphere has neural processors that can represent and shift attention to both the contralateral (left) and the ipsilateral (right) hemispace. In contrast, the left hemisphere has the capacity to represent only the contralateral (right) hemispace. Thus, lesions to the left hemisphere usually do not produce dramatic neglect symptoms because the right hemisphere can function as a kind of "backup" system for attending to ipsilateral (right) hemispace. Patients with left-sided neglect are particularly drawn toward stimuli on their right side, as if attention were "stickier" on the right side of space. They tend to have problems in directing actions (eye movements or arm movements) toward the left side of space, and have reduced vigilance, which exacerbates these deficits in spatial attention processing.[29,37,38]

Unilateral spatial neglect was initially attributed to right-hemisphere posterior parietal lobes, cingulate cortex, and FEF,[27] and later to the interactions between the right- and left-hemisphere localized DAN networks. To illustrate this point, Koch et al.[39] demonstrated baseline hyperexcitability of the circuits between left PPC and left primary motor cortex in right-hemisphere stroke patients with neglect, compared to the controls. This observation provided evidence for previously hypothesized "hemispheric rivalry" theories positing that some circuits in the left hemisphere may become disinhibited in right-hemisphere neglect patients, presumably due to release from a mutual inhibition stemming from the right hemispheric PPC lesion in the neglect group.[39] These results underscore the observation that pathological hyperactivity of contralesional brain regions may be a critical mechanism in impaired visual attention.[40] A newer framework of dual orienting networks suggests that the VAN, and the interactions between the VAN and DAN, may be playing an important role in this clinical phenomenon. This claim is based upon evidence showing that lesions that cause unilateral neglect frequently involve the right TPJ, and specifically, the right superior temporal gyrus, in cases without a visual field deficit.[41,42] Taken together with work demonstrating that the spatial bias of neglect depends on a functional imbalance between the left- and right-hemisphere DANs, this framework proposes that the syndrome of unilateral neglect arises as a result of lesions to the right VAN, which lead to impaired ability to shift attention to the left, as well as hypoarousal of the right DAN, disrupting the balance between right and left DAN activity.[29,33,43,44] Notably, the critical node of interaction between the DAN and VAN is identified as the right MFG, as well as the white matter fibers connecting MFG to the dorsal parietal cortex.[45]

Working Memory

Working memory describes a system, traditionally thought of as having limited capacity, where information is temporarily stored and manipulated, and ultimately used for guiding cognition and behavior.[46] Like attention, working memory is considered a critical building block to enable widespread cognitive functions from language comprehension, learning, planning and reasoning to visual/spatial cognition.[47,48] The contemporary understanding of working memory processes finds its roots in the observation that individual neurons of the prefrontal cortex (PFC) in monkeys demonstrated sustained activity throughout the delay period of a delayed-response task,[49] suggesting that the activity in response to initially presented information was maintained in the brain after the initial stimuli were taken away. Following this proposal, a multiple component model of working memory was developed by Baddeley and colleagues, which described a dynamic, tripartite "blackboard of the mind" with a central executive process managing two independent "buffers" for the storage of verbal and visuospatial information, and a more recently proposed buffer for episodic memory.[46,50] These two cross-species hypotheses across humans and nonhuman primates were integrated by Goldman-Rakic and her colleagues,[51–53] who offered a modified multiple component model of working memory which included a model of cortical specialization for representing object ("what") and spatial ("where") information, respectively. This standard model proposing that working memory storage functions are the product of specialized systems that are anchored in the PFC represents the idea that working memory for different domains of information is accomplished by PFC nodes that receive direct projections from specific posterior perceptual information processing areas. That is, the dorsolateral PFC carries out working memory processing

---

BOX 3-1 The Neuroanatomical Basis of Working Memory

Several empirical dissociations have emerged in regards to the circuitry underlying working memory that cannot be explained by the standard model of independent storage buffers. These include, but are not limited to, working memory for both visual/spatial information, manipulatable versus non-manipulatable objects,[58] faces versus outdoor scenes,[59] as well as for verbal information such as phonological versus semantic versus syntactic information[60]; see Postle[54] for a detailed review. In other words, it is unlikely that different parts of the PFC are specialized for each one of these dissociable aspects of working memory. Furthermore, results from human neuropsychological and fMRI studies showing the lack of one-to-one concordance between PFC lesions and working memory impairment call into question the unifying standard model of working memory circuitry.[61,62]

An alternative view has been put forth that working memory is an emergent property of a nervous system that is capable of representing many different kinds of information (sensory representation- or action-related), functioning together with flexible deployment of attention.[54] The "two-stage model" of working memory, originally proposed by Petrides and Owen et al. suggests that there are two executive processing systems: *the ventral PFC* [Brodmann areas (BA) 45/47] is where information is initially received from posterior association areas and actively held in working memory ("maintenance") while *the dorsal PFC* (BA 9/46) is where "manipulation" and "monitoring" is supported.[63–65] Some newer frameworks of working memory focus on process rather than content, and suggest that there is a further dissociation between *prefrontal* and *posterior* nodes (described in more detail below in the section on executive functions). The PFC nodes implicated in working memory tasks are responsible generally for both task monitoring and manipulation, while the posterior nodes—functionally connected to those PFC nodes—are selectively responsive for the "manipulation" and retrieval of nonverbal[66] and verbal[67] information. There is further evidence of hemispheric lateralization among spatial versus nonspatial working memory tasks, with spatial working memory tasks eliciting greater activation in the right hemisphere and nonspatial studies exhibiting bilateral activation patterns, but greater activation in the left hemisphere.[63,66] The role of the posterior parietal cortex in working memory has garnered support over the last decade but remains controversial. Reviews of the neural circuitry underlying spatial, object, and verbal working memory will be presented in the visual/spatial and language sections to follow.

BOX 3-2 Summary Box of Attention and Working Memory Circuitry

- Sustained attention relies on the coordinated activity between a set of large-scale attention networks critical for processing information that reflect both *top-down* factors such as knowledge, expectation, and goals, as well as *bottom-up* factors in response to sensory stimulation.
- The *top-down attention* system is centered on the dorsal frontal and posterior parietal cortices (**dorsal attention network**), and the *bottom-up attention system* is centered on the right-hemisphere temporoparietal and ventral frontal cortex (**ventral attention network**).
- Working memory is an emergent property of a nervous system that is capable of representing many different kinds of information (sensory representation- or action-related), working together with flexible deployment of attention. **The "two-stage model" of working memory** suggests that there are two executive processing systems: the *ventral PFC*, where information is initially received from posterior association areas and where information is actively held ("maintenance"), and the *dorsal PFC* where "manipulation" and "monitoring" abilities are supported.
- Some newer frameworks suggest that there is a further dissociation between prefrontal and posterior nodes such that the PFC nodes implicated in working memory tasks are responsible generally for both task monitoring and manipulation, while the posterior nodes that are functionally connected to those PFC nodes are selectively responsive for the "manipulation" and retrieval of nonverbal and verbal information.
- There is further evidence of hemispheric lateralization among spatial versus nonspatial working memory tasks, with **spatial working memory tasks eliciting greater activation in the right hemisphere** and **nonspatial tasks eliciting bilateral activation patterns, but greater activation in the left hemisphere**.

---

of information from the posterior dorsal stream, and ventrolateral PFC performs the same function for information processed by the posterior ventral stream of the visual system.[54,55] While many working memory experiments have focused on visual stimuli, neuroimaging studies of verbal working memory

have implicated left-hemisphere localized regions. The "phonological loop," was initially localized to the left supramarginal gyrus,[68] but since then several other neuroimaging studies have identified a network of regions implicated in verbal working memory, including the DLPFC, premotor areas, IPS, posterior parietal lobule, and superior temporal gyrus.[50] Recent consensus seems to argue for a "sylvian-parietal-temporal" region, sitting at the nexus of the anterior supramarginal gyrus and the posterior superior temporal lobe, as the best candidate for the phonological store, critical for mediating between acoustic and articulatory representations of speech as well as for nonlexically mediated phonological encoding (e.g., ordered recall of lists of letters, words, or digits).[50,56,57]

EXECUTIVE FUNCTIONS

The term "executive functions" refers to a complex set of cerebral processes that exert top-down, volitional control over sensory-perceptual input, cognition, emotion, and motor output, thus allowing individuals to carry out goal-directed behaviors. A "goal" is defined as a cognitive representation of an objective that one is committed or motivated to accomplish via directed behavioral or mental activity. A wide range of goal-directed behaviors fall under the rubric of executive functions, including but not limited to sustained and selective attention, anticipation and monitoring of outcomes/rewards (motivation and salience), response inhibition, mental manipulation and task-switching, initiation, abstract reasoning, problem-solving, and social cognition. One major difficulty in defining distinct executive functions is the relative interrelatedness of these constructs, and the variability in observed deficits in patients with similar lesion locations. Executive dysfunction often leads to deficits in other cognitive domains, including memory, language, and visuospatial functioning that rely heavily on executive control (e.g., strategic aspects of encoding new information). The process of executive control can be divided broadly into three classes of operations: *working memory* (which includes attentional control as described in the previous section of this chapter), as well as *task setting/planning* (including organization, reward monitoring, coding conflict, and internal updating), and *response/behavioral selection* (including initiating activity, task switching, and inhibiting activity[69]).

The so-called "frontal systems" underlying executive functions include coordinated activity of the prefrontal and orbitofrontal cortices, frontal-subcortical circuitry, and distributed frontoparietal networks. PFC can be divided into two major divisions based on cytoarchitecture and connectivity: the paralimbic and heteromodal association cortices.[70] The paralimbic regions of the frontal lobe include the paraolfactory, orbitofrontal, anterior cingulate regions, and frontoinsular (FI)) cortex. They receive extensive direct input from limbic regions, including the amygdala which is centrally involved in the mediation of emotional and experiential phenomena. Paralimbic structures also receive major input from frontal heteromodal association cortex to which they also send extensive projections. The largest part of the PFC consists of granular heteromodal association cortex, located in the lateral part of the frontal lobe. The major cortical inputs to this part of the brain come from (1) modality-specific association areas dedicated to the processing of information in only one sensory modality, such as visual or auditory, (2) other heteromodal association areas (e.g., parts of the posterior parietal lobes and superior temporal region that are involved in the multimodal integration of sensory information, and (3) paralimbic regions such as ACC and orbitofrontal cortex (OFC). See Daffner and Willment[69] for more details on these circuits.

Executive dysfunction can arise from not only direct insult to prefrontal cortices, but also from damage to subcortical regions or white matter connections between critical nodes within distributed frontal-subcortical systems. The PFC is connected to the parietal cortex, temporal lobes, and basal ganglia by the white matter tracts comprising the cingulum, superior longitudinal fasciculus, arcuate fasciculus, and internal capsule.[71–73] Based on converging evidence from multisynaptic circuit tracing techniques in nonhuman primates and human brain imaging studies, seven major circuits ("frontostriatal loops") that connect the frontal cortices with the basal ganglia and thalamus have been characterized[74,75]: (1) dorsolateral prefrontal, (2) lateral orbitofrontal, (3) anterior cingulate, (4) motor, (5) oculomotor, (6) medial orbitofrontal, and (7) inferotemporal/posterior parietal circuits. Lesions at any point within these circuits can lead to dysexecutive symptoms with relative domain specificity. For example, lesions in the "oculomotor" circuit, connecting the FEF (BA 8) to the central portion of the caudate body, which also receives projections from dorsolateral prefrontal cortex (DLPFC) and posterior parietal cortex (BA 7), will interfere with voluntary saccadic eye movements or ability to maintain visual fixation.

Dorsal regions of ACC (dACC) and connected regions have been associated with a range of executive functions, including the coding of conflict between competing responses, response selection, performance/reward monitoring, and task initiation. Thus, the *dACC* plays an important role in the brain's decision-making monitoring system. An outcome that deviates from what was expected elicits an error signal from the ACC, which impacts how the next event is handled. An outcome that is better than what was predicted leads to the release of dopamine within the brain's reward system, which facilitates learning. Medial frontal structures, including the *ventral ACC* (BA 24, 25, 32), the *supplementary motor area* (BA 6), and *pre-supplementary motor area* (BA 6), are thought to play an important role in drive, motivation, and the initiation of behavior.[76,77] The ventral ACC (vACC) mediates the anticipation of the reward value of potential actions (which could be understood as an operational definition of motivation).

There is growing evidence that the *lateral prefrontal cortex*, especially in the right hemisphere, is active during the inhibition or stopping of behavioral responses, for example during the no-go part of a motor go/no-go task. Functional imaging studies show that the inferior lateral PFC is recruited when a person's cognitive set needs to be shifted, for example during the Wisconsin Card Sorting Task. The OFC appears to mediate top down regulation of the amygdala, critical for affective processing, and activity of the OFC often is inversely correlated with the activity of the amygdala. Patients who have damaged the OFC frequently exhibit poor emotional regulation and disinhibited behaviors.

Functional neuroimaging studies utilizing intrinsic functional connectivity mapping techniques have expanded our understanding of the frontal systems, and particularly the connectivity of the PFC and other nodes within large-scale functional networks.[1] Both dACC and lateral PFC are consistently coactivated by cognitively demanding tasks,[78-80] and have been frequently interpreted as constituting a unitary network with regions of the lateral parietal cortex, variably termed the frontoparietal control network, executive control network, or the **central executive network (CEN)**, as it will be referred to here.[31] Other work has distinguished a specialized set of regions within the medial frontal cortex, including the ACC and orbital FI, which also activate in response to pain, uncertainty, and other threats to homeostasis.[81-83] It has been suggested that these medial regions, conceptualized as a separate **salience network (SN**; discussed further below), are perhaps responding to homeostatic significance and signaling whether a change in response is required.[82,84]

While the number of distinct intrinsic brain networks and the complexity of their interactions have not been fully delineated,[31,85,86] a complex network model of cognitive control has been proposed by Seeley and colleagues,[13] and expanded upon by Menon and colleagues.[10,87] In the initial model, the dACC and anterior insular (AI) cortices comprise the SN, while regions of the prefrontal heteromodal cortex, including DLPFC and superior parietal cortices, constitute the previously described CEN (Figure 3-3). The primary function of the SN is to identify the most homeostatically relevant stimuli for the rapid integration of sensory, visceral, autonomic, and hedonic signals. In this way, the SN can provide ongoing surveillance of internal (and external) events or activity that is homeostatically relevant.[87,88] In doing so, the SN helps to allocate, and may even compete for, resources with the CEN, in order to account for emotional factors that influence goal-directed processes.[13,88]

Regions of the ACC, which are functionally connected to the paralimbic OFC and ventral striatum, are also thought to play a critical role in anticipating outcomes and consequences of actions and have been associated with coding conflict between competing responses.[68,89] Though some consider these regions to be overlapping with the portion of the ACC comprising the "cognitive control SN," other conceptualize the paralimbic ventral/pregenual ACC to be the critical region important for affective and motivational processing. A separate "affective SN" has been dissociated from the more dorsally located "cognitive control SN" and found to be integral to performance on affective salience tasks.[13,90] In addition to the SN and CEN, intrinsic networks responsible for attentional control[29] and internally focused, self-referential operations, such as reexperiencing one's past and imagining one's future,[14,45,74,91-93] also play important roles in goal-directed behavior. This latter network has been referred to broadly as the **default mode network (DMN)**, which has a high level of functional interaction with the CEN.

Menon and colleagues have developed a unifying theory of *core neurocognitive networks* that describes cognitive dysfunction as arising from aberrant salience mapping and resulting in impaired modulation across three core networks: one specialized in high-level cognitive control (CEN), one specialized in self-monitoring and self-referential activity (DMN), and one responsible for detecting and dynamically orienting to salient external stimuli or internal events (SN). The theory suggests that deficits in the engagement and disengagement of these three core neurocognitive networks play a significant role in many neurological and psychiatric disorders; it is the dynamic interaction between these large-scale networks that are thought

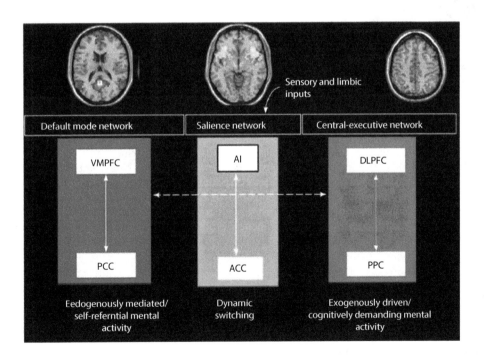

FIGURE 3-3. The core neurocognitive networks. It is hypothesized that the salience network (SN) initiates dynamic switching between the central executive network (CEN) and default mode network (DMN), and mediates between attention to internal and external events. In this way, the SN initiates the appropriate neurocognitive signals to regulate behavior. (Adapted with permission from Bressler SL, Menon V. Large-scale brain networks in cognition: emerging methods and principles. *Trends Cogn Sci*. 2010;14(6):277-290. https://www.sciencedirect.com/journal/trends-in-cognitive-sciences.)

BOX 3-3   The Default Mode Network (DMN)

The regions that compose the DMN, as measured by resting state functional connectivity (RSFC) analyses include the medial PFC, the superior lateral frontal cortex, the inferior frontal gyrus, medial parietal cortex (posterior cingulate and retrosplenial cortex), medial temporal lobe (the hippocampus and parahippocampal cortices), lateral parietal cortex (spanning the angular gyrus and posterior supramarginal gyrus/temporoparietal junction [TPJ]), and lateral temporal cortex. These regions are thought to play an important role in internally driven thought. However, since the early observations of the deactivation of the DMN in response to externally oriented tasks and activation in response to internally driven thought,[14] converging evidence in the last decade has suggested that the DMN is composed of distinct, interacting subsystems. Using hierarchical clustering analyses to interrogate RSFC and task-related fMRI data, two subsystems in addition to a "core" DMN were identified. A *medial temporal subsystem* comprised the hippocampus, parahippocampal cortex, retrosplenial cortex, posterior IPL, and vmPFC, while a *dorsal medial subsystem* comprised the dmPFC, TPJ, lateral temporal cortex, and temporal pole. A *core* DMN comprising the anterior medial portions of the PFC and posterior cingulate cortex (PCC) along the cortical midline is strongly functionally coherent with both subsystems and is hypothesized to act as a functional hub, allowing transfer of information between the DMN subsystems (Figure 3-4).

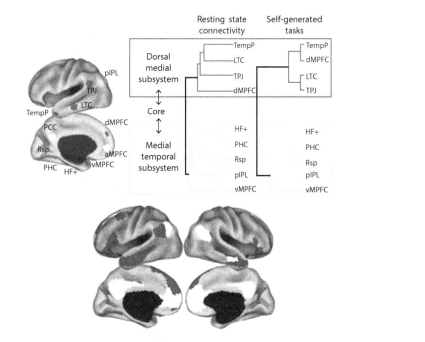
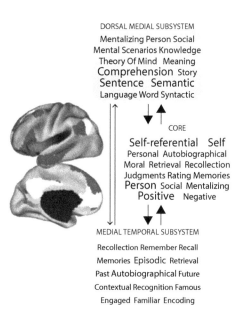

FIGURE 3-4. Subsystems of the default mode network (DMN). Using hierarchical clustering analyses, three DMN subsystems have been delineated: a "*core DMN*" (in yellow) comprising medial prefrontal cortex (PFC) and posterior cingulate cortex (PCC) acts as a functional hub responsible for self-referential and autobiographical cognition, a "*dorsal medial DMN*" (in blue) comprising the dorsal medial PFC, temporoparietal junction (TPJ), lateral temporal cortex, and temporal pole supports semantic language processing and theory of mind, and a "*medial temporal DMN*" (in green) comprising the medial temporal lobes, hippocampus, retrosplenial cortex, angular gyrus, and ventromedial PFC, is critical for episodic encoding and recollection. (Reproduced with permission from Andrews-Hanna JR, Smallwood J, Spreng RN. The default network and self-generated thought: component processes, dynamic control, and clinical relevance. *Ann NY Acad Sci.* 2014;1316:29-52. © 2014 New York Academy of Sciences.)

to be critical for higher cognitive processes (Figure 3-3). These investigators and others have shown that the CEN and SN typically show increases in activation during stimulus-driven cognitive and affective information processing, respectively, whereas the DMN shows increases in activation during self-referential processing.[10,30] Furthermore, the observation that activation of the SN precedes activation of the CEN and deactivation of the DMN offers support for the overarching framework that the SN plays a dynamic causal role modulating large-scale networks engaging the brain's attentional, working memory, and other higher-order cognitive control processes, while disengaging other systems that are not task-relevant.[30] See Box 3-2 for a more detailed discussion of the DMN.

LANGUAGE

The neuroanatomical basis of speech and language has been studied for more than 150 years, with new advances to our understanding of the neural mechanisms underlying these complex cognitive processes emerging every decade. Dating

BOX 3-4 Social Cognition and Theory of Mind

Social cognition is another domain that relies, in part, on networks subserving executive functions, and is often undermined due to injury to the frontal networks. Theory of mind (ToM) is a construct that falls under the umbrella of social cognition; it allows individuals to ascribe a variety of psychological states (i.e., intentions, emotions) to others to understand and predict behavior.[95-96] Recent neuroimaging evidence supports a tripartite model that distinguishes between cognitive, affective, and conative or complex ToM.[97,98] *Cognitive ToM* refers to perspective taking, or the understanding of another's belief set. *Affective ToM* refers to understanding of facial expressions that are socially modulated to communicate emotions.[97] Lastly, *Complex ToM* is the ability to understand how indirect speech acts involving irony and empathy are used to influence the mental or affective state of the listener.[100] This skill tends to reflect an extended maturation period through late childhood and adolescence,[101,102] thought to coincide with the protracted development of frontotemporal association areas.

Complex social-affective processes such as ToM are likely supported by the coordinated activity of the three large-scale, domain-general neural systems described above—the DMN, the SN, and the CEN.[100] Specifically, the DMN is activated by self-referential cognitive processes that likely support inferences about others' beliefs, intentions, and emotional states.[91,103] The affective component of the SN (ventral/pregenual ACC and frontoinsular cortex) is critical for motivation, valuation/context appraisal and deficits within this network lead to disinhibited or apathetic behavior. Connectivity between the SN and DMN helps guide attention to the emotional cues relevant to interpreting the social cognitive aspects of the moment; inter-network disruptions impair the typically anticorrelated modulations between the DMN and SN activity, and can cause abnormal autonomic responses, intensified feeling states, and inappropriate/inaccurate interpretations of emotional cues.[104] The connectivity between the SN and CEN have been linked with recruitment of executive resources for task set maintenance, and dysfunction within these circuits can lead to distractibility, reduced task engagement, and problem-solving difficulties.

The CEN is thought to support ToM via cognitive control mechanisms that preferentially engage domain-specific neural networks thought to process task-relevant social cues, such as the putative *mirror-neuron/empathy network*, comprising the premotor and parietal regions of the brain,[105,106] and the *cerebro-cerebellar mentalizing network*, comprising the medial PFC, superior temporal sulcus, temporal pole, and temporoparietal junction (TPJ) and the cerebellum.[107,108] Studies of empathy have highlighted distinct regions of the frontal cortices that are hypothesized to be involved in the cognitive aspects of empathy (i.e., medial frontal cortex) versus emotional empathy processes, which are hypothesized to rely on the frontoinsular cortices, amygdala, ACC, and OFC. *Affect sharing* in particular, also referred to as emotional contagion, involves taking on and resonating with the emotional state of another and relies on the frontoinsular cortices and the amygdala.[109] Empathy involves self-regulatory mechanisms which allow the establishment of boundaries between the self and others, and as such, the brain regions responsible for regulating emotional reactivity (i.e., the prefrontal and cingulate systems) play a key role in the empathic process by establishing a distinction between other- and self-related feelings.[110,111]

BOX 3-5 Summary Box of Executive Function Circuitry

■ **A wide range of goal-directed behaviors fall under the rubric of executive functions,** including but not limited to sustained and selective attention, anticipation and monitoring of outcomes/rewards (motivation and salience), response inhibition, mental manipulation and task-switching, initiation, abstract reasoning, problem-solving, and social cognition.

■ **The so-called "frontal systems" supporting executive functions include the coordinated activity of the prefrontal and orbitofrontal cortices, frontal-subcortical circuitry, and distributed frontoparietal networks.** Executive dysfunction can also be related to network disruptions of white matter connectivity between the PFC and subcortical regions, or to damage to critical nodes within distributed frontal-subcortical systems. Seven major circuits ("frontostriatal loops") that connect the frontal cortices with the basal ganglia and thalamus have been characterized.

■ Regions of the **ventral/pregenual ACC** which are functionally connected to the paralimbic OFC and ventral striatum are thought to play a critical role in anticipating the reward value of outcomes and consequences of actions. In contrast, **dorsal ACC** regions have been associated with processing conflict between competing responses.

■ **A unifying theory of** *core neurocognitive networks* **describes cognitive dysfunction as arising from aberrant salience mapping and dysfunctional modulation across three core neurocognitive networks: the frontoparietal or central executive network (CEN), the default mode network (DMN), and the salience network (SN),** which is responsible for detecting and dynamically orienting to salient external stimuli or internal events. The SN modulates the anticorrelated activity between the CEN and the DMN. Deficits in the engagement and disengagement of these three core neurocognitive networks play a significant role in many neurological and psychiatric disorders.

back to 1861, when Ernest Auburtin applied a light pressure to the frontal lobe of a patient and noted how the precise location of pressure caused cessation of speech production, clinico-anatomical localizations have been proposed for the different components of speech and language. Paul Broca was among those in the audience at Auburtin's lecture, and published an account of left inferior frontal lesion in a patient who lost the use of speech the following year (1862). Twelve years later, Carl Wernicke (1874) described the brain region critical for "understanding words," and in the following two decades, Sigmund Exner (1881) and Joseph Jules Dejerine (1892) described brain regions responsible for writing and reading, respectively.[112] Though the localizations of these regions have been finessed over time and conceptualized as important nodes of coordinated language networks, the study of the neuroscience of speech and language owes its beginnings to these landmark lesion cases (Figure 3-5).

The classic language model based on the observations of Broca and Wernicke, and elaborated on by Geschwind,[113-115] postulated two major interconnected cortical regions involved in the processing of spoken language: Broca's area in the IFG and Wernicke's area in the superior temporal region. These regions are connected by the arcuate fasciculus, serving to transfer information between these regions. According to this model, damage to Broca's area yields a nonfluent, agrammatical aphasia with relatively preserved comprehension, whereas damage to Wernicke's area results in aphasia characterized by fluent, nonsensical speech and impaired comprehension. Although studies generally have supported these hypotheses over time, some cases have been reported that challenge this classic aphasiology model.

Since then, these seminal findings have been the object of vigorous scientific debate. For example, some have argued that damage to Broca's area impairs speech rather than language, whereas others have linked damage in this region to fundamental disruptions of grammar, lexical retrieval, and sentence comprehension.[116-118] Indeed, Broca's area, along with regions in

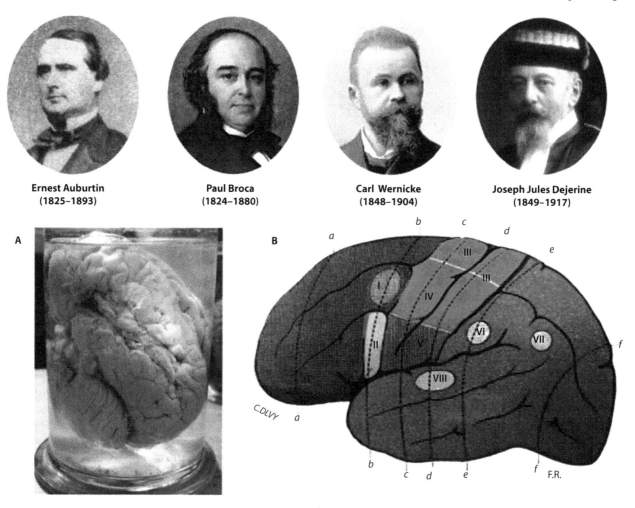

FIGURE 3-5. Classical language models. The top panel depicts the pioneers of the clinical-anatomical correlation method that led to our traditional understanding of aphasiology. **Panel A** depicts the brain of Monsieur Leborgne, the first patient of Paul Broca who presented with speech difficulties due to a lesion in the left inferior frontal gyrus. **Panel B** shows the cortical representations from lesion studies of where higher cognitive-motor functions are supported: (I) writing center of Exner, (II) Broca's center for speech production, (III) motor center, lower limb, (IV) motor center, upper limb, (V) motor center for face and tongue control, (VI–VII) Dejerine's center for reading, (VIII) Wernicke's center for verbal comprehension. The red area depicts primary motor and sensory cortices, blue and purple are posterior and anterior zones of association cortex, respectively. (Reproduced with permission from Catani M, Dell'Acqua F, Bizzi A, et al. Beyond cortical localization in clinico-anatomical correlation. *Cortex.* 2012;48(10):1262-1287. https://www.sciencedirect.com/journal/cortex.)

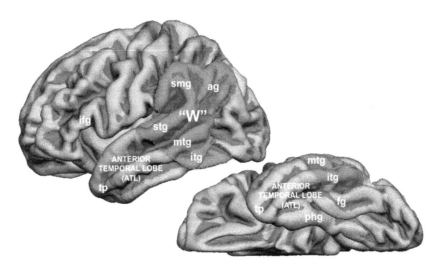

FIGURE 3-6. Wernicke's area. Mesulam and colleagues[125] offer an aggregate map of localizations of language processing and comprehension referring to as Wernicke's area, which includes large portions of the lateral temporal cortices as well as inferior parietal cortex. (Reproduced with permission from Mesulam MM, Thompson CK, Weintraub S, Rogalski EJ. The Wernicke conundrum and the anatomy of language comprehension in primary progressive aphasia. *Brain*. 2015;138(8):2423-2437. Published by Oxford University Press on behalf of the Guarantors of Brain. All rights reserved.)

the medial frontal cortex, including the ACC, supplementary motor area, and pre-supplementary motor area, are thought to play an important role in the speech planning and initiation, or *energization* of speech. Although there has been general consensus regarding the function of Wernicke's area as contributing to language processing, there is great debate regarding where it might be located.[119,120] Mesulam and colleagues offer an aggregate map of localizations subsumed under the term "Wernicke's area," which includes the supramarginal and angular gyri of the inferior parietal lobule, as well as the posterior regions of the superior, middle, and inferior temporal gyri (Figure 3-6). By capitalizing on the neuropathological heterogeneity of primary progressive aphasias (PPA), the precise aspects of language comprehension supported by Wernicke's area were further elucidated. These studies revealed that the posterior temporal/inferior parietal nodes comprising Wernicke's area were critical for sentence comprehension, though others argue that this relationship is mediated by phonological processing deficits rather than sentence comprehension deficits.[50,121–124] Single-word comprehension, previously within the purview of Wernicke's area and subsumed under sentence comprehension, is instead understood to be related to the left-hemisphere anterior temporal lobe, as clarified in studies of semantic variant PPA.[11,125]

The role of the anterior temporal lobe warrants more in-depth discussion, as this region has been the focus of controversy regarding its role as the "semantic processing" hub of the brain, with some arguing that semantic concepts are represented throughout heteromodal association cortex, and others describing a "hub and spoke" model, whereby core, amodal (i.e., abstract, symbolic, not modality-specific) generalized semantic processing regions are initially activated, shortly followed by category-specific processing regions (e.g., the dorsolateral motor subsystem for processing action words, and the ventral visual subsystem for processing object words).[126–128] These function as semantic circuits, as they link information about the word form to category-specific meaning. These semantic

circuits have been shown to have different distributions across extra-sylvian, modality-specific areas.[128] The anterior temporal lobes, together with the PFC and angular gyrus, have been proposed as the main amodal connector hub regions of the semantic language network.

A dual stream model of speech production and comprehension has been proposed by Hickok and Poeppel,[129] which aimed to follow the logic laid out in previously accepted models of dual stream auditory processing (Figure 3-7B).[115,130,131] These streams identify specific interconnected regions comprising language networks, keeping in mind that the task of speech perception also involves some degree of executive control and working memory, and therefore association with frontal systems.[132–134] Similar to previous hypotheses regarding the auditory "what" stream,[130] this model proposes that a **ventral stream of processing** is specifically involved in processing speech signals for language comprehension (**"sound to meaning" pathway**). This ventral stream involves bilateral mid-posterior superior temporal sulcus and dorsal superior temporal gyrus (hubs of the phonological network), bilateral posterior middle temporal and inferior temporal gyri (dubbed the "lexical interface"), and the left-dominant anterior middle temporal gyrus and anterior inferior temporal sulcus (dubbed the "combinatorial network" to describe syntactic and semantic integration). A parallel **dorsal stream** is also proposed, which supports the perception and recognition of speech and allows for sensorimotor integration supporting speech production (**"sound to action" pathway**). The functional role of the dorsal stream, like that of the ventral stream, is still a matter of active debate, with some suggesting a role as interface to the motor system involved in speech production.[135–137] The proposed dorsal stream of speech is again rooted in the phonological network (mid-posterior superior temporal sulcus), but also includes a sensorimotor interface in the parieto-temporal junction (also called "Area Spt" in the literature[50,56]) and an articulatory network rooted in the posterior IFG and anterior insula (left-hemisphere dominant). The articulatory

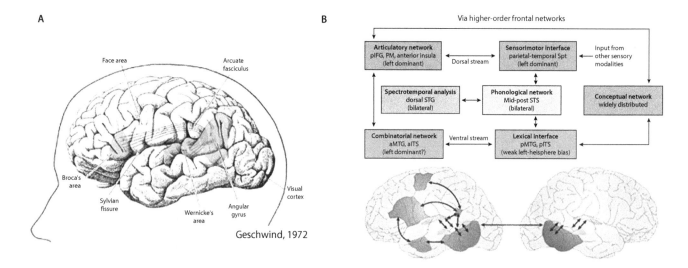

FIGURE 3-7. Contrasting models of speech and language. **Panel A** depicts the classical language model, centered on two major interconnected left-hemisphere cortical regions involved in processing spoken language: Broca's area in the inferior frontal gyrus and Wernicke's area in the temporal-parietal junction. (Reproduced from Geschwind N. Language and the brain. *Sci Am*. 1972; 226:76-83. Used with permission from the estate of Bunji Tagawa.) **Panel B** shows the more recently posited dual-stream model of speech processing, which distinguishes a *ventral stream* important for processing speech signals for language comprehension from a *dorsal stream* which allows for sensorimotor integration supporting speech production. (Reproduced with permission from Hickok G, Poeppel D. The cortical organization of speech processing. *Nat Rev Neurosci*. 2007;8(5):393-402. https://www.nature.com/nrn.)

BOX 3-6 Comparing the Classical Language Model to the Dual-Stream Model for Speech Processing

The classical language model is centered on two major interconnected cortical regions involved in the processing of spoken language: Broca's area in the inferior frontal gyrus and Wernicke's area in the temporal-parietal region. These regions are connected by the arcuate fasciculus, serving to transfer information between these regions (Figure 3-7A). According to this model, damage to Broca's area yields a nonfluent, agrammatical aphasia with relatively preserved comprehension, whereas damage to Wernicke's area results in aphasia characterized by fluent, nonsensical speech and impaired comprehension. Although studies generally have supported these hypotheses over time, some cases have been reported that challenge this classic aphasiology model.

The classic aphasiology model has been elaborated upon in several important ways, to include not just meaningful speech production, but other higher-level cognitive and linguistic functions. Work focusing on prefrontal cortex (PFC) contributions to speech and language have identified a further specialization of regions that may have initially been construed as "Broca's area." Specifically, regions of the posterior and dorsal part of the ventrolateral PFC (BA 44/6) are thought to be important for processing **phonological information**, while the anterior and ventral portions (BA 47) are thought to be specialized for processing **semantic information**, and the intermediate regions (BA 44/45) have been linked to processing **syntax and grammar**.[141] These findings are consistent with known connectivity between the posterior and frontal brain regions in the macaque monkey,[142] and provide the foundation for the more recently posited **dual-stream model of speech processing** (Figure 3-7B). This dual-stream model proposes that a **ventral stream of processing** is specifically involved in processing speech signals for language comprehension (**"sound to meaning" pathway**), while a parallel **dorsal stream** supports the perception and recognition of speech and allows for sensorimotor integration supporting speech production (**"sound to action" pathway**). In this way, the acoustic/phonological speech networks interface with the conceptual systems in one route (ventral), and with the motor-articulatory systems in the other route (dorsal), thus giving rise to speech functions.

---

network is described as translating acoustic speech signals into articulatory representations in the frontal lobe, which is essential for speech development and normal speech production.[56] The auditory-motor integration function differs from earlier presentations of a dorsal auditory "where" system,[130] but is closer to conceptualizations of a dorsal visual stream, and has gained support from converging evidence.[131,137,138] This model proposes

that *speech perception* tasks (i.e., distinguishing phonological elements of speech) rely to a greater extent on dorsal stream circuitry, whereas *speech recognition* tasks rely more on ventral stream circuitry (with a shared neural substrate in the left superior temporal gyrus). With regard to hemispheric laterality, this model suggests that the ventral stream is bilaterally organized with important computational differences between the

BOX 3-7   Summary Box for Language Circuitry

- The classic language model based on the observations of Broca and Wernicke, and elaborated on by Geschwind, postulated two major interconnected cortical regions involved in the processing of spoken language: **Broca's area** in the inferior frontal gyrus, the center of fluent, grammatical speech, and **Wernicke's area** in the temporal-parietal region, the center of speech comprehension.

- The **anterior temporal lobes**, together with the prefrontal cortex and angular gyrus, have been proposed as the main amodal (i.e., abstract, symbolic, not modality-specific) connector hub regions of the semantic language network.

- Regions of the posterior and dorsal part of the ventrolateral PFC (BA 44/6) are thought to be important for *processing phonological information*, while the anterior and ventral portions (BA 47) are believed to be specialized for *processing semantic information*, and the intermediate regions (BA 44/45) have been linked to processing syntax and grammar.

- The **dual-stream model of speech processing** proposes that a *ventral stream* of processing is specifically involved in processing speech signals for language comprehension (**"sound to meaning" pathway**), while a parallel *dorsal stream* supports the perception and recognition of speech and allows for sensorimotor integration supporting speech production (**"sound to action" pathway**).

two hemispheres, a hypothesis that is proposed to explain the lack of speech recognition deficits following unilateral temporal lobe damage. The dorsal stream, however, is strongly left-hemisphere dominant, consistent with observations of speech production deficit arising from dorsal temporal and frontal lesions, and why left-hemisphere injury alone can substantially impair performance in speech perception.[56] Patients with lesions in the superior temporal gyrus show a severe impairment in verbal short-term memory in the auditory modality,[139] while activity in the posterior ventral temporal cortex, a region known to be involved in orthographic stimulus perception (i.e., reading), is linked to working memory for visually presented verbal information.[140] Reading and writing are additional language skills that interface with visual perceptual systems, and as such will be discussed in the following section on visuospatial cognition.

MEMORY

Memory refers broadly to a collection of cognitive processes that facilitate encoding, storage, and retrieval of information that helps us to understand ourselves and interact meaningfully with our environment. These varied processes are subserved by several interacting neural systems. Research into the functional

neurocircuitry supporting various aspects of memory began with neuropsychological studies of patients with focal lesions and provided an invaluable foundation for our understanding of concepts such as anterograde versus retrograde memory, and explicit versus implicit memory. Since then, neurophysiological models in animals and neuroimaging techniques in humans have afforded us a refined understanding of memory systems. The focus of this discussion is on *explicit* (declarative) memory, as deficits in this domain are more commonly seen in neurological illness compared to *implicit* (procedural) memory, though we will broadly cover neurocircuitry of both types of memory systems. To define these terms further, *explicit* memory is conceptualized as two overarching constructs: **episodic memory**, which refers to the capacity to remember events that are related to a specific temporal or spatial context, and **semantic memory**, which refers to the capacity to recall "fact-based" information in more permanent stores without reference to the specific learning context, and is inclusive of the ability to process conceptual knowledge from experience. For example, remembering a short story, or what you did on your last birthday are examples of episodic memory. Knowing who was the first president of the United States or what is the color of a lion are examples of semantic memory. In contrast, *implicit* memory refers to procedural, automatic, or subconscious learning, such as what happens in classical conditioning or priming. Examples of implicit memory include learning how to tie your shoes or drive a car (procedural), correctly completing word-stem completion tasks (priming), or associating your friend with the taste of beer because the only time you see him is when you go out for drinks (classical conditioning).

Episodic memory itself represents a set of cognitive processes, including ones that are engaged when an event is experienced and a new memory representation is being formed (encoding), storage of this new learning into long-term repositories (consolidation), and the recollection of the new information at a later time (retrieval processes). Recollection refers to detailed recall ("remembering"), while familiarity, a related concept often tested in recognition memory paradigms, describes the general gist knowledge of a concept ("knowing"). The episodic memory system is thought to be dependent upon the medial temporal lobes (MTL) including the hippocampus, perirhinal cortex, and parahippocampal cortex,[143,144] as episodic memory has historically been characterized based on patients with MTL lesions.[144] Other critical structures in the memory system comprise regions involving the Papez circuit, which include the basal forebrain with the medial septum and diagonal band of Broca's area, the retrosplenial cortex, the presubiculum, the fornix, mammillary bodies, the mammillary tract, and the anterior nucleus of the thalamus.[6] A lesion in any of these structures or the connections between them can cause episodic memory dysfunction (see Figure 3-8).[145]

Here we have outlined only cursorily how the MTL system encodes, stores, and facilitates the retrieval of new memories; further details are available from other sources.[146] When an individual experiences an event (i.e., has an "episode"), the cortically distributed patterns of neural activity representing the various pieces of information in the environment (sights, sounds, tastes, thoughts, etc.) are transferred first to the parahippocampal

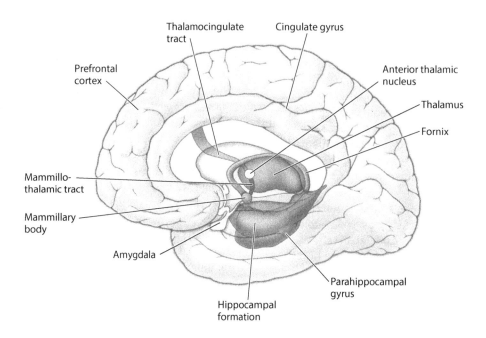

FIGURE 3-8. The episodic memory system. The medial temporal lobes, including the hippocampus and parahippocampal cortex, form the core of the episodic memory system. Other critical structures in the episodic memory system comprise regions of the Papez circuit, the retrosplenial cortex, the presubiculum, the fornix, mammillary bodies, the medial prefrontal cortex, and the anterior nucleus of the thalamus.

region, which includes the perirhinal and parahippocampal cortex, then to the entorhinal cortex, and finally to the dentate gyrus region of the hippocampus proper, where all of these disparate threads of experience are bound together as a single memory.[147] This information is then transferred to the CA3 region of the hippocampus where it is "tagged" with a hippocampal index, allowing the memory to be stored in a unique way for later recall. Typically, memories are retrieved when a cue from the environment matches a part of the stored memory. This sensory cue is transferred from sensory cortex to the parahippocampal region to the hippocampus, where the "index" is retrieved and a unique pattern of activity is transferred to other regions of the hippocampus (CA1, subiculum) and the back out to association cortex via the entorhinal cortex to actively recreate all of the components of the original memory. Importantly, the hippocampus remains critical for memory retrieval until consolidation occurs, after which it is thought that the memory can be retrieved directly from cortical-cortical connections without the need for retrieving the hippocampal index.[146]

Neuroimaging studies of episodic memory over the last decade have suggested that memory function is subserved by a distributed network that includes not only the MTL memory system, but also subsystems of the DMN including medial and lateral parietal regions and medial prefrontal regions.[91,148] fMRI studies in healthy, young subjects have shown that the DMN can be specifically modulated during memory processing, demonstrating activation during memory retrieval and deactivation during successful encoding.[149,150] The ability to flexibly modulate activity from encoding deactivation to retrieval activation in the precuneus and posterior cingulate cortex is thought to be critical to memory success.[151,152] It is precisely this modulation within

the DMN and between the DMN and MTL memory systems that becomes dysfunctional in early stages of Alzheimer's disease.[153–155]

Episodic memory loss attributable to dysfunction of this system follows a predictable pattern known as Ribot's law: that events encoded closest to the onset of the injury (including memories encoded shortly after the injury) are more vulnerable to dissolution while remote memories are most resistant. Thus, in cases of episodic memory dysfunction, the ability to learn new information is impaired (anterograde amnesia), recently learned information cannot be retrieved (retrograde amnesia), and remotely learned information is usually spared.[156] Memories are not recorded like a photograph, but rather encoded in a fragmented, distributed manner which then reconstitutes during recollection. In the model put forth by Eichenbaum and colleagues,[157] neocortical input regarding features of objects ("what" pathway) converges on the perirhinal cortex and the lateral entorhinal area, while information about the location of object ("where" pathway) converges on the parahippocampal cortex and medial entorhinal area (Figure 3-9). These streams of processing are ultimately integrated and "bound" in the hippocampus. Subsequently, when a previously encountered stimulus is processed, perirhinal and lateral entorhinal areas can signal its match to a preexisting item representation and this match signal is propagated back to neocortical areas which is sufficient to generate a sense of familiarity.[157]

In the past few decades, an extensive body of research has shown that the frontal lobes have important contributions to episodic memory distinct from the role of the MTL. Specifically, the frontal lobes are important for organizing, evaluating, and monitoring the encoding and retrieval operations of the MTL.[158] As a result, damage to the frontal lobes leads to deficits

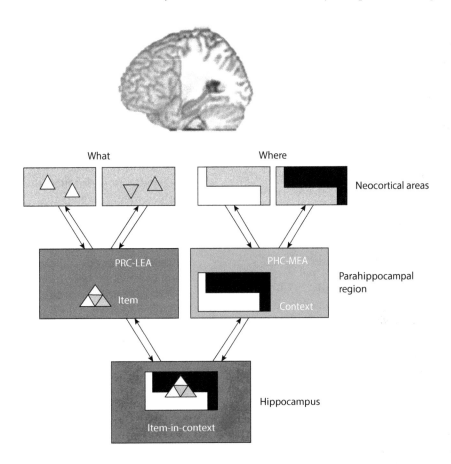

FIGURE 3-9. Functional organization of the medial temporal lobe (MTL) system. Neocortical input regarding object features "what" converges in the perirhinal cortex (PRC) and lateral entorhinal area (LEA), while details about location ("where") of objects converge in the parahippocampal cortex (PHC) and medial entorhinal area (MEA). These streams converge in the hippocampus, which encodes items as embedded in the context in which they were experienced. Back projections to the PHC-MEA may support recall of context, whereas back projections to the PRC-LEA may support recall of item associations. (Reproduced with permission from Eichenbaum H, Yonelinas AR, Ranganath C. The medial temporal lobe and recognition memory. *Annu Rev Neurosci.* 2007;30:123-152; permission conveyed through Copyright Clearance, Inc.)

on a variety of memory tasks that put demands on effortful or strategic encoding and/or retrieval, such as for list learning tasks.[159] Further, though familiarity is often thought of as a more automatic process than recollection and referable to MTL systems, frontal lesion patients may have particular difficulty on item recognition tasks because the familiarity signal is inherently more ambiguous and thus requires more careful retrieval monitoring than does recollection.[159] In addition to frontal lobe contributions, dysfunction within the DMN, anchored in the medial PFC and precuneus (including MTL regions), has been well-established as giving rise to episodic memory deficits as well as to deficits in *prospective memory*, a form of memory that involves remembering to perform a planned action or intention at some future time, relying heavily on self-referential episodic memory function.[45,91,153]

There is also considerable debate regarding the role of the lateral parietal cortices in episodic memory retrieval. Some argue that the parietal cortices hold retrieved information in a form accessible to decision-making processes, similar to Baddeley's working memory buffers, while others suggest that parietal regions shift attention to, or maintain attention on, internally generated mnemonic representations.[150] Building on Corbetta

and Shulman's description of posterior nodes in the DAN and VAN,[29,33,157] Cabeza and colleagues presented a dual attention process for episodic memory retrieval, suggesting that the dorsal (superior) parietal cortex contributes top-down attentional processing guided by retrieval goals, while the ventral (inferior) parietal cortex contributes bottom-up attentional processing triggered by retrieval of information, and that the two processes interact to determine the relevance of incoming information that may alter behavioral goals.[161] For a unifying theory on the role of ventral parietal cortex in attentional contributions underlying memory deficits ("Attention to Memory" model), see Cabeza et al.[162]

Semantic memory refers to our store of factual and conceptual knowledge that is not related to any specific episode in time. Like episodic memory, semantic memory is an explicit, declarative form of memory. Evidence that semantic and episodic memory are separate memory systems has emerged from both neuroimaging studies[127,163] and the fact that previously acquired semantic memory can be spared in patients who have severe impairment of the episodic memory system.[164] Semantic memory includes all of our knowledge of the world not related to any specific episodic memory. Therefore, it could be argued that semantic memory resides in multiple cortical areas throughout the brain. For example, there is evidence that visual images are stored in the visual association areas.[165] A more contemporary view of semantic memory is based on findings from naming and categorization tasks, by which semantic knowledge is usually tested, which highlights the critical importance of the inferolateral temporal lobes and connected regions to semantic memory as was described above in the discussion on language.[166–168] The role of the inferolateral temporal lobe as the "semantic processing" hub of the brain has been the focus of controversy, with some arguing that semantic concepts are represented throughout heteromodal association cortex, and others describing semantic processing regions in the inferotemporal and anterior temporal cortex that are initially activated, shortly followed by category-specific processing regions (e.g., the dorsolateral motor subsystem for processing action words, and the ventral visual subsystem for processing object words).[126–128] Lesion studies including those with progressive semantic dementia syndromes,[169,170] herpes simplex virus encephalitis,[171] as well as other, stable lesions[166] support the view that the **left-hemisphere anterior temporal lobe (ATL)**, including temporal pole, is a critical hub for semantic processing. The most common clinical disorder undermining semantic memory is Alzheimer's disease,[172,173] in which the disruption of semantic memory systems has been linked to pathology in the inferolateral temporal lobes[174] or pathology in the frontal cortex.[175–177]

Implicit, non-declarative memory can take the form of *classical conditioning*, in which an unconditioned stimulus and a conditioned stimulus are paired together; *procedural memory*, the ability to learn cognitive and behavioral skills that operate an automatic, subconscious level; and *priming*, when a prior encounter with a particular item changes the response to the current item.[146] Though disorders of classical conditioning do not often present to clinical attention, patients with bilateral amygdala damage have been reported to show classical conditioning impairment in the absence of episodic memory dysfunction.[178] This type of learning is thought to be supported by amygdala and related structures in the basolateral limbic system, including the dorsomedial thalamic nuclei, subcallosal area, and the stria terminalis.[179] Examples of procedural memory include knowing how to tie your shoelaces, how to ride a bike, or how to play an instrument. It is clear that procedural memory systems are distinct from episodic memory systems from observations of patients who have procedural learning deficits but intact episodic memory, and vice versa.[164,180] Neuroimaging work has implicated a number of brain regions, with the most converging evidence presented for the roles of the basal ganglia, supplementary motor area, and cerebellum.[181,182] Patients with selective lesions in these regions, including Parkinson's disease, tumors, strokes, and hemorrhages, may also demonstrate disrupted procedural memory.[146] Lastly, priming is a phenomenon that occurs unconsciously, and can be divided into perceptual (modality specific) and conceptual priming (not modality specific, shows enhancement with more successful learning). Converging evidence suggests that posterior cortical regions involved in processing of sensory information are important for perceptual priming, while changes in the left prefrontal regions have been linked with conceptual priming.[183,184]

BOX 3-8　Summary Box for Memory Circuitry

- **Explicit memory** refers to **episodic memory**, the capacity to remember events that are related to a specific temporal or spatial context, and **semantic memory**, the capacity to recall "fact-based" information in more permanent stores without reference to the specific learning context, and is inclusive of the ability to form conceptual knowledge from experience.

- **Implicit memory** refers to *procedural*, automatic, or subconscious learning, such as what happens in *classical conditioning* or *priming*. Examples of implicit memory include learning how to tie your shoes or drive a car (procedural), correctly completing word-stem completion tasks (priming), or associating your friend with the taste of beer because the only time you see him is when you go out for drinks (classical conditioning).

- **Episodic memory** function is subserved by a distributed network that includes not only the *hippocampal-medial temporal lobe (MTL) memory system*, but also the *"core default mode network (DMN)"* subsystem which includes medial frontal and parietal regions, as well as *lateral prefrontal and parietal cortical regions* critical for goal-directed retrieval.

- **Semantic memory** is supported by a "hub and spoke" model, whereby *core, generalized semantic processing regions* (anterior temporal and inferotemporal cortices) are initially activated, shortly followed by *category-specific processing regions* (e.g., the dorsolateral motor subsystem for processing action words, and the ventral visual subsystem for processing object words). These function as semantic circuits, as they link information about the word form to category-specific meaning.

- Some forms of **implicit memory** (e.g., *classical conditioning*) are thought to be supported by amygdala and related structures in the basolateral limbic system, including the dorsomedial thalamic nuclei, subcallosal area, and the stria terminalis.

- *Procedural memory* is supported by the basal ganglia, supplementary motor area, and cerebellum. Lastly, *priming* is a phenomenon that occurs unconsciously; posterior cortical regions involved in processing of sensory information are important for *perceptual priming*, while left prefrontal cortical regions have been linked with *conceptual priming*.

VISUAL/SPATIAL COGNITION

Studies of WWII patients with gunshot wounds and macaque monkeys[185] with lesions to parietal or temporal cortex, led to a model suggesting two major visual pathways or streams originating from occipital cortex, the dorsal "where" pathway and the ventral "what" pathway. The ventral pathway is viewed as a processing route running from the primary visual area coursing through the occipitotemporal cortex to the ATL and possibly extending to the ventrolateral PFC.[186] This processing pathway is responsible for conscious visual perception, visual recognition, and visual memory. The ventral stream reflects a serial, hierarchical processing model, suggesting that features or components that were processed separately in previous stages are integrated in subsequent stages into more complex representations. Color, orientation, and brightness are examples of basic features that are integrated during later stages to create higher-order categories, such as objects, places, faces, and text. Nodes along the ventral pathway connect perceptual representations to distributed neural activity in the temporal cortex that link object forms to their meaning, allowing for recognition and the activation of relevant associations. Modifications of this model have emphasized that in addition to bottom-up processing, there is top-down activity that facilitates perceptual processing and recognition. For example, when an individual recognizes letters and integrates adjacent letter combinations into words, contextually relevant prior semantic knowledge of words in a given language may help the ATL carry out top-down operations to guide word representations from generic to increasingly specific word forms. The hierarchical pathway model assumes that the complexity of the information that is processed in a particular pathway increases progressively and systematically. Furthermore, regions of the MTL (perirhinal cortex) are heavily connected with temporal lobe areas lying at the apex of the ventral visual processing stream, facilitating object-specific memory.[187]

Aspects of visuospatial processing are also critical to language functions of reading and writing. The left posterior occipitotemporal sulcus is a key region in the neural circuitry of reading, including a focal region referred to as the visual word form area (VWFA).[188] It is consistently activated by visual words across various written language systems,[189] shows adaptations to repeated presentation of written words,[190] and activates in response to orthographic similarity among words along a posterior-to-anterior axis.[191] Incidentally, the right-hemisphere homologue of the VWFA is the fusiform face area (FFA), located in the right posterior occipitotemporal cortex and specialized in early processing of faces. In contrast to consistent findings localizing the VWFA and FFA, the functional neurocircuitry supporting writing is much more heavily debated. Historically, writing was attributed to a specific region of the MFG[28] called "Exner's area," and later conceptualized as premotor cortex. However, more recent fMRI studies suggest that while the MFG is important for grapheme representation and motor program generation, the posterior segment of the superior frontal gyrus, and the left supramarginal gyrus, left superior parietal gyrus (disrupted in the case of apractic agraphia), left posterior inferior temporal gyrus (spelling), and bilateral mid-cingulate cortices support the ability to write meaningful language.[192–195] From a theoretical perspective, it is unlikely that a specific region in the brain is responsible for writing ability,[196] and the fact that pure agraphia is very rare suggests that the ability to write is a complex task relying on several interacting neural networks, perhaps comprising an integrated writing network.[197]

The dorsal stream was thought originally to mediate conscious space perception (e.g., "where?"), allowing us to navigate from one place to another and search for things in the environment. More recent accounts suggest that the dorsal pathway also serves nonconscious visually guided action, fulfilling an additional "how" function.[186] The seminal observation that led to this frame shift was in the patient D.F., who had a large bilateral lesion of the occipitotemporal cortex (ventral stream) and a smaller left-sided lesion of the occipitoparietal cortex (dorsal stream).[198,199] She was found to have impaired object perception (ventral stream) but intact ability to reach to objects, including shaping her grasping hand to reflect the size, shape, and orientation of objects (dorsal stream). However, she could not accurately adjust the orientation of her hand to match the orientation of a distant slot in which to place an envelope, but was accurate in orienting her hand when reaching toward that same slot.[200] Her ability to reach accurately for an object to which she could not consciously orient led to the hypothesis that the dorsal stream was concerned with automatic, nonconscious, visually guided action, rather than the traditional view of conscious space perception. Of course, information between these dorsal and ventral streams interact continually to help us complete visual/spatial cognitive tasks.

Kravitz and colleagues[186] presented a more detailed characterization of the dorsal stream of visual processing by describing not one, but three pathways that consist of projections from the posterior parietal cortices to prefrontal, premotor, and MTL, that support both conscious and nonconscious visuospatial processing, including spatial working memory, visually guided action, and navigation, respectively (see Figure 3-10). All three pathways share source neurocircuitry in occipitoparietal regions. Initial visual representations are entirely retinotopic, and portions of the primary visual cortex (V1) project to area V6 in the anterior wall of the parietooccipital sulcus, which also receives projections from other visual areas (V2, V3, V3A), and project both medially and laterally, to ultimately integrate information from central and peripheral visual fields representing space largely in egocentric frames of reference. "Egocentric" here is an umbrella term for maps and/or patterns of activity that can be defined in relation to some point on the observer (e.g., head- or eye-centered maps). In humans, egocentric hemispatial neglect most commonly arises from damage to the IPL, whereas allocentric neglect (i.e., hemispatial neglect relative to objects) is primarily associated with damage to ventral occipitotemporal cortical areas. Bilateral disruption to this occipitoparietal circuit can lead to simultanagnosia. Patients with simultanagnosia have a restricted spatial window of visual attention and cannot process more than one object at a time in a scene that contains many objects. The egocentric maps of space formed in this circuit are the functional antecedents of the three specialized dorsal stream pathways described here.

The *parieto-prefrontal pathway* is strongly involved in the control of eye movements, and is crucial for spatial working memory.[201] This pathway provides input to PFC necessary for top-down executive control of visuospatial processing. Findings in both humans and monkeys demonstrate that regions of the

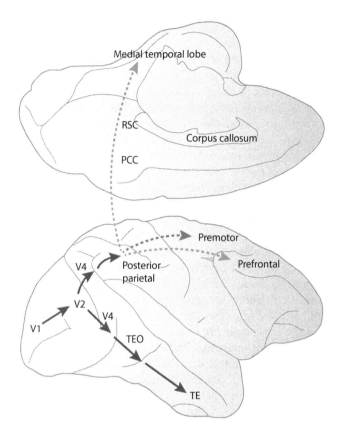

FIGURE 3-10. Beyond where/how: a new framework for dorsal stream function. At least three distinct pathways emanate from the occipitoparietal cortex: *the parieto-prefrontal pathway* that supports spatial working memory (shown by a dashed green arrow), *the parieto-premotor pathway* that supports visually guided actions (shown by a dashed red arrow), and *the parieto-medial temporal pathway* that supports navigation (shown by a dashed blue arrow). Shown in dark gray is the traditional ventral "what" stream that represents a multisynaptic pathway projecting from the striate cortex to the inferior temporal cortex and supports object/feature identification. (Reproduced with permission from Kravitz DJ, Saleem KS, Baker CI, Mishkin M. A new neural framework for visuospatial processing. *Nat Rev Neurosci.* 2011;12(4):217-230. https://www.nature.com/nrn.)

IPS coactivate with posterolateral prefrontal areas during spatial working memory tasks,[202,203] consistent with description of the DAN (reviewed above in the section Attention and Working Memory). The *parieto-premotor* pathway is responsible for maintaining coordinated maps of space and body position to facilitate visually guided action in egocentric space. The superior parietal lobule (SPL) contains head-centered maps of somatosensory and visual space, the IPS has been found to maintain hand- and arm-centered visual maps, the "middle temporal visual processing complex (MT+) integrates change in observer motion, and the rostral IPL is specialized for guiding action. Together, these regions allow the "how" functions inherent to visually guided reaching and grasping that have been referable to the dorsal visual stream. Lastly, the *parieto-medial temporal pathway* defines a subregion of the caudal IPL that is specialized for processing distant space[204] and less involved in guiding actions of the body. Neurons in this region are also sensitive to encoding visual motion during navigation (together with area

BOX 3-9   Summary Box for Visuospatial Circuitry

- The **ventral (or "what") pathway** is responsible for conscious visual perception, visual recognition, and visual memory. The ventral stream reflects a serial, hierarchical processing model suggesting that features or components that were processed separately in previous stages are integrated in subsequent stages into more complex representations. Color, orientation, and brightness are examples of basic features that are integrated during later stages to create higher-order categories, such as objects, places, faces, and text. This route runs from the primary visual area coursing through the occipitotemporal cortex to the anterior temporal lobe and possibly extending to the ventrolateral PFC.

- The **dorsal (or "where/how") pathway** mediates conscious space perception, allowing us to navigate from one place to another and search for objects in the environment, and allows for visually guided reach. More recent accounts of the dorsal stream suggest that there are in fact **three dorsal pathways** that project from the posterior parietal cortices to prefrontal, premotor, and medial temporal lobes, respectively, that support both conscious and nonconscious visuospatial processing, including spatial working memory, visually guided action, and navigation, respectively.

- **All three dorsal pathways share source neurocircuitry in occipitoparietal regions.** Initial visual representations are entirely retinotopic, and portions of the primary visual cortex (V1) project to area V6 in the anterior wall of the parietooccipital sulcus, which also receives projections from other visual areas (V2, V3, V3A), and project both medially and laterally to integrate information from central and peripheral visual fields to represent space largely in egocentric frames of reference. Injury to this "occipitoparietal" circuitry gives rise to simultanagnosia.

- The ***parieto-prefrontal pathway*** is strongly involved in the control of eye movements, and is crucial for spatial working memory. The ***parieto-premotor pathway*** is responsible for maintaining coordinated maps of space and body position to facilitate visually guided action in egocentric space. Lastly, the ***parieto-medial temporal pathway*** is specialized for processing distant space and lesions in this circuitry can lead to impairments of egocentric depth perception and disorientation, and disruption of navigation.

V3A and V6). These projections connect from caudal IPL to the hippocampus and parahippocampal areas of the MTL both directly and indirectly through medial parietal regions of the posterior cingulate and retrosplenial cortices. Lesions in this circuitry can lead to impairments of egocentric depth perception and disorientation, and disruption of navigation.[205,206]

Summary and Key Points

- Virtually all aspects of cognition arise from the dynamic interactions of distributed brain regions conceptualized as large-scale neural networks. A wealth of evidence from anatomical, neuroimaging, and physiological studies supports the idea that individual brain regions are functionally specialized and make specific contributions to cognition, and further, that these functionally specific regions comprise networks that mediate cognitive and behavioral functions. Recent work has focused on identifying the breakdown in dynamic connectivity within and between these large-scale networks, as these approaches provide new insight into cognitive dysfunction observed in psychopathology and neurodegenerative disease.

- A **unifying theory of *core neurocognitive networks*** describes cognitive dysfunction as arising from aberrant salience mapping and dysfunctional modulation across *three core neurocognitive networks*: **the frontoparietal or central executive network (CEN), the default mode network (DMN), and the salience network (SN).** The SN modulates the anticorrelated activity between the CEN and the DMN. Deficits in the engagement and disengagement of these three core neurocognitive networks play a significant role in many neurological and psychiatric disorders.

- **Spatial attention** relies on the coordinated activity between a set of large-scale attention networks critical for processing information for both *top-down* factors such as knowledge, expectation, and goals, as well as *bottom-up* factors that reflect sensory stimulation. The *top-down attention* system is centered on the dorsal frontal and posterior parietal cortices (**dorsal attention network**), and the *bottom-up attention system* is centered on the right-hemisphere temporoparietal and ventral frontal cortex (VAN). These two attentional systems dynamically interact with each other during the processing of environmental stimuli to determine where and what we attend to. Specifically, the DAN is thought to send top-down filtering signals to visual areas and the VAN, thus modulating ventral activation in response to behaviorally important stimuli and coordinating stimulus-response selection. Conversely, when a salient event occurs during stimulus-driven reorienting, the VAN sends an attention reorientation signal to the dorsal network.

- **Working memory** is an emergent property of a nervous system that is capable of representing many different kinds of information (sensory representation- or action-related), working together with flexible deployment of attention. The **"two-stage model" of working memory** suggests that there are two executive processing systems: the *ventral PFC*, where information is initially received from posterior association areas and where information is actively held ("maintenance"), and the *dorsal PFC* where "manipulation" and "monitoring" abilities are supported.

- **Executive functions are supported by the coordinated activity of the prefrontal and orbitofrontal cortices, frontal-subcortical circuitry, and distributed frontoparietal networks.** Executive dysfunction can also be related to network disruptions of white matter connectivity between the PFC and subcortical regions, or damage to critical nodes within distributed frontal-subcortical systems. Seven major circuits ("frontostriatal loops") that connect the frontal cortices with the basal ganglia and thalamus have been characterized. Regions of the ventral/pregenual ACC, which are functionally connected to the paralimbic OFC and ventral striatum, are thought to play a critical role in anticipating outcomes and consequences of actions and dorsal regions of ACC have been associated with processing conflict between competing responses.[69,89]

- **Spoken language** has historically been thought to be supported by two major interconnected cortical regions: **Broca's area** in the inferior frontal gyrus, the center for fluent, grammatical speech, and **Wernicke's area** in the temporal-parietal region, the center for speech comprehension. Regions of the posterior and dorsal part of the ventrolateral PFC (BA 44/6) are thought to be important for *processing phonological information*, while the anterior and ventral portions (BA 47) are thought to be specialized for *processing semantic information*, and the intermediate regions (BA 44/45) have been linked to processing syntax and grammar. The **dual-stream model of speech processing** proposes that a *ventral stream* of processing is specifically involved in processing speech signals for language comprehension (**"sound to meaning" pathway**), while a parallel *dorsal stream* supports the perception and recognition of speech and allows for sensorimotor integration supporting speech production (**"sound to action" pathway**). The **anterior temporal lobes**, together with the prefrontal cortex and angular gyrus, have been proposed as the main hub region of the semantic language network.

- **Episodic memory** is subserved by a distributed network that includes not only the *hippocampal-MTL memory system*, but also the *"core DMN"* subsystem which includes medial frontal and parietal regions, as well as *lateral prefrontal and parietal cortical regions* critical for goal-directed retrieval.

- **Semantic memory** is supported by a "hub and spoke" model, whereby *core, generalized semantic processing regions* (anterior temporal and inferotemporal cortices) are initially activated, shortly followed by *category-specific processing regions* (e.g., the dorsolateral motor subsystem for processing action words, and the ventral visual subsystem for processing object words). These function as semantic circuits, as they link information about the word form to category-specific meaning.

- **Implicit memory** (e.g., **classical conditioning**) is thought to be supported by amygdala and related structures in the basolateral limbic system, including the dorsomedial thalamic nuclei, subcallosal area, and the stria terminalis.[179] *Procedural memory* is supported by the basal ganglia, supplementary motor area, and cerebellum. *Priming* is a phenomenon that occurs unconsciously; posterior cortical regions involved in processing of sensory information are important for *perceptual priming*, while left prefrontal cortical regions have been linked with *conceptual priming*.

■ **Visual/Spatial cognition** is generally divided into ventral and dorsal streams of information processing. The **ventral (or "what") pathway** is responsible for conscious visual perception, visual recognition, and visual memory. This route runs from the primary visual area coursing through the occipito-temporal cortex to the anterior temporal lobe and possibly extending to the ventrolateral PFC. The **dorsal (or "where/how") pathway** mediates conscious space perception, allowing us to navigate from one place to another and search for objects in the environment, and mediates visually guided reaching. **The dorsal stream is purported to consist of three pathways** that project from the occipitoparietal cortices to prefrontal, premotor, and medial temporal lobes, respectively, that support both conscious and nonconscious visuospatial processing, including spatial working memory, visually guided action, and navigation, respectively.

Multiple Choice Questions

1. Which of the following is true regarding networks supporting spatial attention?
   a. Bottom-up attention relies on the dorsal attention network.
   b. Top-down attention relies on the ventral attention network.
   c. Top-down attention relies on the dorsal attention network.
   d. Spatial attention relies on the coordinated activity between both dorsal attention network and ventral attention network.
   e. Both c and d are true regarding spatial attention networks.

2. Semantic knowledge is supported by a distributed network of regions described by a "hub and spoke" model. Which left-hemisphere brain regions are frequently considered to represent the conceptual "hub"?
   a. Medial PFC and posterior cingulate cortex
   b. Inferolateral temporal cortex and anterior temporal lobe
   c. Angular gyrus and temporo-parietal junction
   d. Medial temporal lobes and hippocampus
   e. Thalamus and mammillary body

3. Which of the following brain regions is not implicated in supporting episodic memory encoding, storage, or retrieval?
   a. Hippocampus
   b. Lateral parietal cortex
   c. Medial prefrontal cortex
   d. Mammillary bodies
   e. None of the above; all of these brain regions serve an important role in supporting episodic memory.

4. A patient is able to identify the color and shape of a common household object, but is unable to reach out and grab the object from you. She also has difficulty showing you how the object is used. She most likely has damage to which of the following visual processing pathways?
   a. Perirhinal-lateral entorhinal area of the MTL
   b. Ventral stream pathway
   c. Parieto-medial temporal pathway
   d. Parieto-premotor pathway
   e. Parieto-prefrontal pathway

Multiple Choice Answers

1. **Answer: e**
   Spatial attention relies on the coordinated activity between a set of large-scale attention networks critical for processing information for both *top-down* factors such as knowledge, expectation, and goals, as well as *bottom-up* factors that reflect sensory stimulation. The *top-down attention* system is centered on the dorsal frontal and posterior parietal cortices (**dorsal attention network**), and the *bottom-up attention system* is centered on the right-hemisphere temporoparietal and ventral frontal cortex (**ventral attention network**). These two attentional systems dynamically interact with each other during the processing of environmental stimuli to determine where and what we attend to. Specifically, the DAN is thought to send top-down filtering signals to visual areas and the VAN, thus modulating ventral activation in response to behaviorally important stimuli and coordinating stimulus-response selection.[29,33] Conversely, when a salient event occurs during stimulus-driven reorienting, the VAN sends an attention reorientation signal to the dorsal network.

2. **Answer: b**
   Semantic knowledge is supported by a "hub and spoke" model, whereby *core, generalized semantic processing regions* that are considered to be the conceptual "hub" (anterior temporal and inferolateral temporal cortices) are initially activated, shortly followed by *category-specific processing regions* which are considered to be the "spokes" (e.g., the dorsolateral motor subsystem for processing action words, and the ventral visual subsystem for processing object words). These function as semantic circuits, as they link information about the word form to category-specific meaning.

3. **Answer: e**
   The medial temporal lobes, including the hippocampus and parahippocampal cortex, form the core of the episodic memory system. Other critical structures in the episodic memory

system comprise regions of the Papez circuit (fornix, mammillary bodies, anterior thalamic nucleus, cingulum), the retrosplenial cortex, and the medial prefrontal cortex. The lateral parietal cortices are also critical to guiding attention to goal-directed retrieval of previously encoded information.

4. Answer: d

Visual/spatial cognition is generally divided into ventral and dorsal streams of information processing. The ventral (or "what") pathway that allows for object/feature identification is responsible for conscious visual perception, visual recognition, and visual memory. This route runs from the primary visual area coursing through the occipitotemporal cortex to the anterior temporal lobe and possibly extending to the ventrolateral PFC. The dorsal (or "where/how") pathway mediates conscious space perception, allowing us to navigate from one place to another and search for things in the environment, and mediates visually guided reaching. The dorsal stream is purported to consist of three pathways that project from the posterior parietal cortices to prefrontal, premotor, and medial temporal lobes, respectively, that support both conscious and nonconscious visuospatial processing, including spatial working memory, visually guided action, and navigation, respectively. Deficits in visually guided reach in the setting of intact object recognition suggests that there is a dorsal stream deficit with intact ventral stream processing. More specifically, the deficit is likely in the parieto-premotor pathway.

REFERENCES

1. Bressler SL, Menon V. Large-scale brain networks in cognition: emerging methods and principles. *Trends Cogn Sci.* 2010;14(6):277-290.
2. van den Heuvel MP, Sporns O. Network hubs in the human brain. *Trends Cogn Sci.* 2013;17(12):683-696.
3. Sporns O. Contributions and challenges for network models in cognitive neuroscience. *Nat Neurosci.* 2014;17(5):652-660.
4. Power JD, Cohen AL, Nelson SM, et al. Functional network organization of the human brain. *Neuron.* 2011;72(4):665-678.
5. Cao M, Wang JH, Dai ZJ, et al. Topological organization of the human brain functional connectome across the lifespan. *Dev Cogn Neurosci.* 2014;7:76-93.
6. Mesulam M. Behavioural neuroanatomy: large-scale networks, association cortex, frontal syndromes, the limbic system, and the hemispheric specializations. In: Mesulam M, ed. *Principles of Behavioral and Cognitive Neurology.* Oxford: Oxford University Press; 2000.
7. Catani M, Mesulam M. What is a disconnection syndrome? *Cortex.* 2008;44(8):911-913.
8. Ross ED. Cerebral localization of functions and the neurology of language: fact versus fiction or is it something else? *Neuroscientist.* 2010;16(3):222-243.
9. Bartolomeo P. The quest for the 'critical lesion site' in cognitive deficits: problems and perspectives. *Cortex.* 2011;47(8):1010-1012.
10. Menon V. Large-scale brain networks and psychopathology: a unifying triple network model. *Trends Cogn Sci.* 2011;15(10):483-506.
11. Seeley WW, Crawford RK, Zhou J, Miller BL, Greicius MD. Neurodegenerative diseases target large-scale human brain networks. *Neuron.* 2009;62(1):42-52.
12. Fox MD, Snyder AZ, Vincent JL, Corbetta M, van Essen DC, Raichle ME. The human brain is intrinsically organized into dynamic, anticorrelated functional networks. *Proc Natl Acad Sci U S A.* 2005;102(27):9673-9678.
13. Seeley WW, Menon V, Schatzberg AF, et al. Dissociable intrinsic connectivity networks for salience processing and executive control. *J Neurosci.* 2007;27(9):2349-2356.
14. Raichle ME, MacLeod AM, Snyder AZ, Powers WJ, Gusnard DA, Shulman GL. A default mode of brain function. *Proc Natl Acad Sci U S A.* 2001;98(2):676-682.
15. Smith SM, Fox PT, Miller KL, et al. Correspondence of the brain's functional architecture during activation and rest. *Proc Natl Acad Sci U S A.* 2009;106(31):13040-13045.
16. Ewers M, Sperling RA, Klunk WE, Weiner MW, Hampel H. Neuroimaging markers for the prediction and early diagnosis of Alzheimer's disease dementia. *Trends Neurosci.* 2011;34(8):430-442.
17. Zhou J, Greicius MD, Gennatas ED, et al. Divergent network connectivity changes in behavioural variant frontotemporal dementia and Alzheimer's disease. *Brain.* 2010;133(pt 5):1352-1367.
18. Volk DW, Lewis DA. Prefrontal cortical circuits in schizophrenia. *Curr Top Behav Neurosci.* 2010;4:485-508.
19. van den Heuvel MP, Mandl RC, Stam CJ, Kahn RS, Hulshoff Pol HE. Aberrant frontal and temporal complex network structure in schizophrenia: a graph theoretical analysis. *J Neurosci.* 2010;30(47):15915-15926.
20. Fischer DB, Boes AD, Demertzi A, et al. A human brain network derived from coma-causing brainstem lesions. *Neurology.* 2016;87(23):2427-2434.
21. Posner MI, Rothbart MK. Toward a physical basis of attention and self regulation. *Phys Life Rev.* 2009;6(2):103-120.
22. Goldman-Rakic PS. Regional and cellular fractionation of working memory. *Proc Natl Acad Sci U S A.* 1996;93(24):13473-13480.
23. Williams GV, Goldman-Rakic PS. Modulation of memory fields by dopamine D1 receptors in prefrontal cortex. *Nature.* 1995;376(6541):572-575.
24. Horvitz JC, Stewart T, Jacobs BL. Burst activity of ventral tegmental dopamine neurons is elicited by sensory stimuli in the awake cat. *Brain Res.* 1997;759(2):251-258.
25. Schultz W. Dopamine neurons and their role in reward mechanisms. *Curr Opin Neurobiol.* 1997;7(2):191-197.
26. Arnsten AF. Catecholamine regulation of the prefrontal cortex. *J Psychopharmacol.* 1997;11(2):151-162.
27. Mesulam MM. A cortical network for directed attention and unilateral neglect. *Ann Neurol.* 1981;10(4):309-325.
28. Gitelman DR, Nobre AC, Parrish TB, et al. A large-scale distributed network for covert spatial attention: further anatomical delineation based on stringent behavioural and cognitive controls. *Brain.* 1999;122(pt 6):1093-1106.
29. Corbetta M, Shulman GL. Control of goal-directed and stimulus-driven attention in the brain. *Nat Rev Neurosci.* 2002;3(3):201-215.
30. Sridharan D, Levitin DJ, Menon V. A critical role for the right fronto-insular cortex in switching between central-executive and default-mode networks. *Proc Natl Acad Sci U S A.* 2008;105(34):12569-12574.

31. Vincent JL, Kahn I, Snyder AZ, Raichle ME, Buckner RL. Evidence for a frontoparietal control system revealed by intrinsic functional connectivity. *J Neurophysiol.* 2008;100(6):3328-3342.

32. Spreng RN, Sepulcre J, Turner GR, Stevens WD, Schacter DL. Intrinsic architecture underlying the relations among the default, dorsal attention, and frontoparietal control networks of the human brain. *J Cogn Neurosci.* 2013;25(1):74-86.

33. Corbetta M, Patel G, Shulman GL. The reorienting system of the human brain: from environment to theory of mind. *Neuron.* 2008;58(3):306-324.

34. Kucyi A, Hodaie M, Davis KD. Lateralization in intrinsic functional connectivity of the temporoparietal junction with salience- and attention-related brain networks. *J Neurophysiol.* 2012;108(12):3382-3392.

35. Cole MW, Reynolds JR, Power JD, Repovs G, Anticevic A, Braver TS. Multi-task connectivity reveals flexible hubs for adaptive task control. *Nat Neurosci.* 2013;16(9):1348-1355.

36. Uddin LQ. Salience processing and insular cortical function and dysfunction. *Nat Rev Neurosci.* 2015;16(1):55-61.

37. Mesulam MM. Spatial attention and neglect: parietal, frontal and cingulate contributions to the mental representation and attentional targeting of salient extrapersonal events. *Philos Trans R Soc Lond B Biol Sci.* 1999;354(1387):1325-1346.

38. Robertson IH, Mattingley JB, Rorden C, Driver J. Phasic alerting of neglect patients overcomes their spatial deficit in visual awareness. *Nature.* 1998;395(6698):169-172.

39. Koch G, Oliveri M, Cheeran B, et al. Hyperexcitability of parietal-motor functional connections in the intact left-hemisphere of patients with neglect. *Brain.* 2008;131(pt 12):3147-3155.

40. Cazzoli D, Muri RM, Hess CW, Nyffeler T. Treatment of hemispatial neglect by means of rTMS—a review. *Restor Neurol Neurosci.* 2010;28(4):499-510.

41. Karnath HO, Ferber S, Himmelbach M. Spatial awareness is a function of the temporal not the posterior parietal lobe. *Nature.* 2001;411(6840):950-953.

42. Karnath HO, Fruhmann Berger M, Kuker W, Rorden C. The anatomy of spatial neglect based on voxelwise statistical analysis: a study of 140 patients. *Cereb Cortex.* 2004;14(10):1164-1172.

43. Corbetta M, Kincade MJ, Lewis C, Snyder AZ, Sapir A. Neural basis and recovery of spatial attention deficits in spatial neglect. *Nat Neurosci.* 2005;8(11):1603-1610.

44. He BJ, Snyder AZ, Vincent JL, Epstein A, Shulman GL, Corbetta M. Breakdown of functional connectivity in frontoparietal networks underlies behavioral deficits in spatial neglect. *Neuron.* 2007;53(6):905-918.

45. Gusnard DA, Akbudak E, Shulman GL, Raichle ME. Medial prefrontal cortex and self-referential mental activity: relation to a default mode of brain function. *Proc Natl Acad Sci U S A.* 2001;98(7):4259-4264.

46. Baddeley A. Working memory: looking back and looking forward. *Nat Rev Neurosci.* 2003;4(10):829-839.

47. Baddeley A. Working memory and language: an overview. *J Commun Disord.* 2003;36(3):189-208.

48. Wilhelm O, Hildebrandt A, Oberauer K. What is working memory capacity, and how can we measure it? *Front Psychol.* 2013;4:433.

49. Fuster JM, Alexander GE. Neuron activity related to short-term memory. *Science.* 1971;173(3997):652-654.

50. Buchsbaum BR, D'Esposito M. The search for the phonological store: from loop to convolution. *J Cogn Neurosci.* 2008;20(5):762-778.

51. Goldman-Rakic P. Localization of function all over again. *NeuroImage.* 2000;(5 pt 1):451-457.

52. Goldman-Rakic PS. Circuitry of the frontal association cortex and its relevance to dementia. *Arch Gerontol Geriatr.* 1987;6(3):299-309.

53. Goldman-Rakic PS. Cellular and circuit basis of working memory in prefrontal cortex of nonhuman primates. *Prog Brain Res.* 1990;85:325-335; discussion 335-336.

54. Postle BR. Working memory as an emergent property of the mind and brain. *Neuroscience.* 2006;139(1):23-38.

55. Courtney SM. Attention and cognitive control as emergent properties of information representation in working memory. *Cogn Affect Behav Neurosci.* 2004;4(4):501-516.

56. Hickock G, Poeppel D. The cortical organization of speech processing. *Nat Rev Neurosci.* 2007;8(5):393-402.

57. Jonides J, Schumacher EH, Smith EE, et al. The role of the parietal cortex in verbal working memory. *J Neurosci.* 1998;18(13):5026-5034.

58. Mecklinger A, Muller N. Dissociations in the processing of "what" and "where" information in working memory: an event-related potential analysis. *J Cogn Neurosci.* 1996;8(5):453-473.

59. Ranganath C, DeGutis J, D'Esposito M. Category-specific modulation of inferior temporal activity during working memory encoding and maintenance. *Brain Res Cogn Brain Res.* 2004;20(1):37-45.

60. Shivde G, Thompson-Schill SL. Dissociating semantic and phonological maintenance using fMRI. *Cogn Affect Behav Neurosci.* 2004;4(1):10-19.

61. D'Esposito M, Postle BR. The dependence of span and delayed-response performance on prefrontal cortex. *Neuropsychologia.* 1999;37(11):1303-1315.

62. Arnott SR, Grady CL, Hevenor SJ, Graham S, Alain C. The functional organization of auditory working memory as revealed by fMRI. *J Cogn Neurosci.* 2005;17(5):819-831.

63. D'Esposito M, Aguirre GK, Zarahn E, Ballard D, Shin RK, Lease J. Functional MRI studies of spatial and nonspatial working memory. *Cogn Brain Res.* 1998;7:1-13.

64. Owen AM, Evans AC, Petrides M. Evidence for a two-stage model of spatial working memory processing within the lateral frontal cortex: a positron emission tomography study. *Cereb Cortex.* 1996;6(1):31-38.

65. Petrides M. Lateral frontal cortical contribution to memory. *Semin Neurosci.* 1996;8:57-63.

66. Champod AS, Petrides M. Dissociable roles of the posterior parietal and the prefrontal cortex in manipulation and monitoring processes. *Proc Natl Acad Sci U S A.* 2007;104(37):14837-14842.

67. Champod AS, Petrides M. Dissociation within the fronto-parietal network in verbal working memory: a parametric functional magnetic resonance imaging study. *J Neurosci.* 2010;30(10):3849-3856.

68. Paulesu, E., Frith, CD., Frackowiak, RS. The neural correlates of the verbal component of working memory. *Nature.* 1993;362(6418):342-5.

69. Daffner KR, Willment KC. Executive control, the regulation of goal-directed behaviors, and the impact of dementing illness. In: Dickerson BC, Atri A, eds. *Dementia: Comprehensive Principles and Practice.* New York, NY: Oxford University Press; 2014.

70. Mesulam MM. Frontal cortex and behavior. *Ann Neurol.* 1986;19(4):320-325.

71. Yeterian EH, Pandya DN, Tomaiuolo F, Petrides M. The cortical connectivity of the prefrontal cortex in the monkey brain. *Cortex.* 2012;48(1):58-81.

72. Krause M, Mahant N, Kotschet K, et al. Dysexecutive behaviour following deep brain lesions—a different type of disconnection syndrome? *Cortex.* 2012;48(1):97-119.

73. Catani M, Dell'acqua F, Vergani F, et al. Short frontal lobe connections of the human brain. *Cortex.* 2012;48(2):273-291.

74. Middleton FA, Strick PL. Basal ganglia and cerebellar loops; motor and cognitive circuits. *Brain Res Rev.* 2000;31:236-250.

75. Alexander GE, DeLong MR, Strick PL. Parallel organization of functionally segregated circuits linking basal ganglia and cortex. *Ann Rev Neurosci.* 1986;9:357-381.

76. Paus T. Primate anterior cingulate cortex: where motor control, drive and cognition interface. *Nat Rev Neurosci.* 2001;2(6):417-424.

77. Ridderinkhof KR, van den Wildenberg WP, Segalowitz SJ, Carter CS. Neurocognitive mechanisms of cognitive control: the role of prefrontal cortex in action selection, response inhibition, performance monitoring, and reward-based learning. *Brain Cogn.* 2004;56(2):129-140.

78. Curtis CE, D'Esposito M. Persistent activity in the prefrontal cortex during working memory. *Trends Cogn Sci.* 2003;7(9):415-423.

79. Kerns JG, Cohen JD, MacDonald AW3rd, Cho RY, Stenger VA, Carter CS. Anterior cingulate conflict monitoring and adjustments in control. *Science.* 2004;303(5660):1023-1026.

80. Menon V, Adleman NE, White CD, Glover GH, Reiss AL. Error-related brain activation during a Go/NoGo response inhibition task. *Hum Brain Mapp.* 2001;12(3):131-143.

81. Craig AD. How do you feel? Interoception: the sense of the physiological condition of the body. *Nat Rev Neurosci.* 2002;3(8):655-666.

82. Craig AD. How do you feel—now? The anterior insula and human awareness. *Nat Rev Neurosci.* 2009;10(1):59-70.

83. Grinband J, Hirsch J, Ferrera VP. A neural representation of categorization uncertainty in the human brain. *Neuron.* 2006;49(5):757-763.

84. Critchley HD. Neural mechanisms of autonomic, affective, and cognitive integration. *J Comp Neurol.* 2005;493(1):154-166.

85. van den Heuvel MP, Sporns O. An anatomical substrate for integration among functional networks in human cortex. *J Neurosci.* 2013;33(36):14489-14500.

86. Yeo BT, Krienen FM, Eickhoff SB, et al. Functional specialization and flexibility in human association cortex. *Cereb Cortex.* 2015;25(10):3654-3672.

87. Menon V, Uddin LQ. Saliency, switching, attention and control: a network model of insula function. *Brain Struct Funct.* 2010;214(5-6):655-667.

88. Dosenbach NU, Fair DA, Miezin FM, et al. Distinct brain networks for adaptive and stable task control in humans. *Proc Natl Acad Sci U S A.* 2007;104(26):11073-11078.

89. Botvinick MM, Braver TS, Barch DM, Carter CS, Cohen JD. Conflict monitoring and cognitive control. *Psychol Rev.* 2001;108(3):624-652.

90. Touroutoglou A, Hollenbeck M, Dickerson BC, Feldman Barrett L. Dissociable large-scale networks anchored in the right anterior insula subserve affective experience and attention. *NeuroImage.* 2012;60(4):1947-1958.

91. Buckner RL, Andrews-Hanna JR, Schacter DL. The brain's default network: anatomy, function, and relevance to disease. *Ann N Y Acad Sci.* 2008;1124:1-38.

92. Christoff K, Irving ZC, Fox KC, Spreng RN, Andrews-Hanna JR. Mind-wandering as spontaneous thought: a dynamic framework. *Nat Rev Neurosci.* 2016;17(11):718-731.

93. Schacter DL, Addis DR, Buckner RL. Remembering the past to imagine the future: the prospective brain. *Nat Rev Neurosci.* 2007;8(9):657-661.

94. Andrews-Hanna JR., Smallwood J, Spreng RN. The default network and self-generated thought: component processes, dynamic control, and clinical relevance. *Ann N Y Acad Sci.* 2014;1316:29-52.

95. Blakemore SJ. The social brain in adolescence. *Nat Rev Neurosci.* 2008;9(4):267-277.

96. Herbet G, Lafargue G, Bonnetblanc F, Moritz-Gasser S, Duffau H. Is the right frontal cortex really crucial in the mentalizing network? A longitudinal study in patients with a slow-growing lesion. *Cortex.* 2013;49(10):2711-2727.

97. Dennis M, Agostino A, Taylor HG, et al. Emotional expression and socially modulated emotive communication in children with traumatic brain injury. *J Int Neuropsychol Soc.* 2013;19(1):34-43.

98. Dennis M, Simic N, Bigler ED, et al. Cognitive, affective, and conative theory of mind (ToM) in children with traumatic brain injury. *Dev Cogn Neurosci.* 2013;5:25-39.

99. Hein G, Singer T. I feel how you feel but not always: the empathic brain and its modulation. *Curr Opin Neurobiol.* 2008;18(2):153-158.

100. Ryan NP, Catroppa C, Beare R, et al. Uncovering the neuroanatomical correlates of cognitive, affective and conative theory of mind in paediatric traumatic brain injury: a neural systems perspective. *Soc Cogn Affect Neurosci.* 2017;12(9):1414-1427.

101. Dumontheil I, Apperly IA, Blakemore SJ. Online usage of theory of mind continues to develop in late adolescence. *Dev Sci.* 2010;13(2):331-338.

102. Sebastian CL, Fontaine NM, Bird G, et al. Neural processing associated with cognitive and affective Theory of Mind in adolescents and adults. *Soc Cogn Affect Neurosci.* 2012;7(1):53-63.

103. Ahmed RM, Devenney EM, Irish M, et al. Neuronal network disintegration: common pathways linking neurodegenerative diseases. *J Neurol Neurosurg Psychiatry.* 2016;87(11): 1234-1241.

104. Seeley WW, Zhou J, Kim EJ. Frontotemporal dementia: what can the behavioral variant teach us about human brain organization? *Neuroscientist.* 2012;18(4):373-385.

105. Iacoboni M, Dapretto M. The mirror neuron system and the consequences of its dysfunction. *Nat Rev Neurosci.* 2006;7(12):942-951.

106. Molenberghs P, Cunnington R, Mattingley JB. Is the mirror neuron system involved in imitation? A short review and meta-analysis. *Neurosci Biobehav Rev.* 2009;33(7):975-980.

107. Van Overwalle F, Baetens K, Marien P, Vandekerckhove M. Cerebellar areas dedicated to social cognition? A comparison of meta-analytic and connectivity results. *Soc Neurosci.* 2015;10(4):337-344.

108. Van Overwalle F, Marien P. Functional connectivity between the cerebrum and cerebellum in social cognition: a multi-study analysis. *NeuroImage.* 2016;124(pt A):248-255.

109. Shdo SM, Ranasinghe KG, Gola KA, et al. Deconstructing empathy: neuroanatomical dissociations between affect sharing and prosocial motivation using a patient lesion model. *Neuropsychologia.* 2018;116(pt A):126-135.

110. Decety J, Svetlova M. Putting together phylogenetic and ontogenetic perspectives on empathy. *Dev Cogn Neurosci.* 2012;2(1):1-24.

111. Ochsner KN, Gross JJ. The cognitive control of emotion. *Trends Cogn Sci.* 2005;9(5):242-249.

112. Catani M, Dell'acqua F, Bizzi A, et al. Beyond cortical localization in clinico-anatomical correlation. *Cortex.* 2012;48(10): 1262-1287.

113. Broca P. Remarques sur le siege de la faculte du langage articule, suivies d'une observation d'aphemie. *Bull Soc Anat.* 1861;2:330-357.

114. Geschwind N. Disconnexion syndromes in animals and man. I. *Brain.* 1965;88(2):237-294.

115. Wernicke C. Der aphasische Symptomencomplex. In: Cohen RS, Wartofsky MW, eds. *Boston Studies in the Philosophy of Science.* Dordrecht, NL: D. Reidel; 1874:34-97.

116. Benson F, Geschwind N. Aphasia and related disorders: a clinical approach. In: Mesulam M, ed. *Principles of Behavioral Neurology.* Philadelphia, PA: F.A. Davis; 1985:193-238.

117. Caplan D. Why is Broca's area involved in syntax? *Cortex.* 2006;42(4):469-471.

118. Thompson CK, Meltzer-Asscher A, Cho S, et al. Syntactic and morphosyntactic processing in stroke-induced and primary progressive aphasia. *Behav Neurol.* 2013;26(1-2):35-54.

119. Bogen JE, Bogen GM. Wernicke's region—where is it? *Ann N Y Acad Sci.* 1976;280:834-843.

120. DeWitt I, Rauschecker JP. Wernicke's area revisited: parallel streams and word processing. *Brain Lang.* 2013;127(2):181-191.

121. Gorno-Tempini ML, Brambati SM, Ginex V, et al. The logopenic/phonological variant of primary progressive aphasia. *Neurology.* 2008;71(16):1227-1234.

122. Pillay SB, Stengel BC, Humphries C, Book DS, Binder JR. Cerebral localization of impaired phonological retrieval during rhyme judgment. *Ann Neurol.* 2014;76(5):738-746.

123. Robson H, Grube M, Lambon Ralph MA, Griffiths TD, Sage K. Fundamental deficits of auditory perception in Wernicke's aphasia. *Cortex.* 2013;49(7):1808-1822.

124. Rogalski E, Cobia D, Harrison TM, et al. Anatomy of language impairments in primary progressive aphasia. *J Neurosci.* 2011;31(9):3344-3350.

125. Mesulam MM, Thompson CK, Weintraub S, Rogalski EJ. The Wernicke conundrum and the anatomy of language comprehension in primary progressive aphasia. *Brain.* 2015;138(pt 8):2423-2437.

126. Binder JR, Desai RH, Graves WW, Conant LL. Where is the semantic system? A critical review and meta-analysis of 120 functional neuroimaging studies. *Cereb Cortex.* 2009;19(12):2767-2796.

127. Patterson K, Nestor PJ, Rogers TT. Where do you know what you know? The representation of semantic knowledge in the human brain. *Nat Rev Neurosci.* 2007;8(12):976-987.

128. Tomasello R, Garagnani M, Wennekers T, Pulvermuller F. Brain connections of words, perceptions and actions: a neurobiological model of spatio-temporal semantic activation in the human cortex. *Neuropsychologia.* 2017;98:111-129.

129. Hickok G, Poeppel D. The cortical organization of speech processing. *Nat Rev Neurosci.* 2007;8(5):393-402.

130. Rauschecker JP. Cortical processing of complex sounds. *Curr Opin Neurobiol.* 1998;8(4):516-521.

131. Scott SK, Johnsrude IS. The neuroanatomical and functional organization of speech perception. *Trends Neurosci.* 2003;26(2):100-107.

132. Blumstein SE, Baker E, Goodglass H. Phonological factors in auditory comprehension in aphasia. *Neuropsychologia.* 1977;15(1):19-30.

133. Demonet JF, Chollet F, Ramsay S, et al. The anatomy of phonological and semantic processing in normal subjects. *Brain.* 1992;115(pt 6):1753-1768.

134. Price CJ, Wise RJ, Warburton EA, et al. Hearing and saying. The functional neuro-anatomy of auditory word processing. *Brain.* 1996;119(pt 3):919-931.

135. Hickok G, Poeppel D. Towards a functional neuroanatomy of speech perception. *Trends Cogn Sci.* 2000;4(4):131-138.

136. Hickok G, Poeppel D. Dorsal and ventral streams: a framework for understanding aspects of the functional anatomy of language. *Cognition.* 2004;92(1-2):67-99.

137. Wise RJ, Scott SK, Blank SC, Mummery CJ, Murphy K, Warburton EA. Separate neural subsystems within 'Wernicke's area'. *Brain.* 2001;124(pt 1):83-95.

138. Warren JE, Wise RJ, Warren JD. Sounds do-able: auditory-motor transformations and the posterior temporal plane. *Trends Neurosci.* 2005;28(12):636-643.

139. Takayama Y, Kinomoto K, Nakamura K. Selective impairment of the auditory-verbal short-term memory due to a lesion of the superior temporal gyrus. *Eur Neurol.* 2004;51(2):115-117.

140. Fiebach CJ, Rissman J, D'Esposito M. Modulation of inferotemporal cortex activation during verbal working memory maintenance. *Neuron.* 2006;51(2):251-261.

141. Bookheimer S. Functional MRI of language: new approaches to understanding the cortical organization of semantic processing. *Annu Rev Neurosci.* 2002;25:151-188.

142. Petrides M, Pandya DN. Distinct parietal and temporal pathways to the homologues of Broca's area in the monkey. *PLoS Biol.* 2009;7(8):e1000170.

143. Squire LR, Stark CE, Clark RE. The medial temporal lobe. *Annu Rev Neurosci.* 2004;27:279-306.

144. Scoville WB, Milner B. Loss of recent memory after bilateral hippocampal lesions. *J Neurol Neurosurg Psychiatry.* 1957;20(1):11-21.

145. Budson AE, Price BH. Memory dysfunction. *N Engl J Med.* 2005;352:692-699.

146. Budson AE. Memory systems in dementia. In: Dickerson B, Atri A, ed. *Dementia: Comprehensive Principles and Practice.* New York, NY: Oxford University Press; 2014:108-125.

147. Wolosin SM, Zeithamova D, Preston AR. Reward modulation of hippocampal subfield activation during successful associative encoding and retrieval. *J Cogn Neurosci.* 2012;24(7):1532-1547.

148. Spreng RN, Mar RA, Kim AS. The common neural basis of autobiographical memory, prospection, navigation, theory of mind, and the default mode: a quantitative meta-analysis. *J Cogn Neurosci.* 2009;21(3):489-510.

149. Daselaar SM, Prince SE, Cabeza R. When less means more: deactivations during encoding that predict subsequent memory. *NeuroImage.* 2004;23(3):921-927.

150. Wagner AD, Shannon BJ, Kahn I, Buckner RL. Parietal lobe contributions to episodic memory retrieval. *Trends Cogn Sci.* 2005;9(9):445-453.

151. Daselaar SM, Prince SE, Dennis NA, Hayes SM, Kim H, Cabeza R. Posterior midline and ventral parietal activity is associated with retrieval success and encoding failure. *Front Hum Neurosci.* 2009;3:13.

152. Kim H, Daselaar SM, Cabeza R. Overlapping brain activity between episodic memory encoding and retrieval: roles of the task-positive and task-negative networks. *NeuroImage.* 2010;49(1):1045-1054.

153. Greicius MD, Srivastava G, Reiss AL, Menon V. Default-mode network activity distinguishes Alzheimer's disease from healthy aging: evidence from functional MRI. *Proc Natl Acad Sci U S A.* 2004;101(13):4637-4642.

154. Troxler T, Hoyer D, Langenegger D, et al. Identification and SAR of potent and selective non-peptide obeline somatostatin sst1 receptor antagonists. *Bioorg Med Chem Lett.* 2007;17(14):3983-3987.

155. Wang L, Laviolette P, O'Keefe K, et al. Intrinsic connectivity between the hippocampus and posteromedial cortex predicts memory performance in cognitively intact older individuals. *NeuroImage.* 2010;51(2):910-917.

156. Ribot T. Diseases of memory: an essay in the positive psychology. In: Smith WH, trans-ed. *The International Scientific Series*. New York, NY: Appleton; 1882.

157. Eichenbaum H, Yonelinas AR, Ranganath C. The medial temporal lobe and recognition memory. *Annu Rev Neurosci*. 2007;30:123-152.

158. Simons JS, Spiers HJ. Prefrontal and medial temporal lobe interactions in long-term memory. *Nat Rev Neurosci*. 2003;4(8):637-648.

159. Aly M, Yonelinas AP, Kishiyama MM, Knight RT. Damage to the lateral prefrontal cortex impairs familiarity but not recollection. *Behav Brain Res*. 2011;225(1):297-304.

160. Corbetta M, Shulman GL. Spatial neglect and attention networks. *Annu Rev Neurosci*. 2011;34:569-599.

161. Cabeza R. Role of parietal regions in episodic memory retrieval: the dual attentional processes hypothesis. *Neuropsychologia*. 2008;46(7):1813-1827.

162. Cabeza R, Ciaramelli E, Moscovitch M. Cognitive contributions of the ventral parietal cortex: an integrative theoretical account. *Trends Cogn Sci*. 2012;16(6):338-352.

163. Schacter DL, Wagner AD, Bucker R. Memory systems of 1999. In: Tulving E, Craik FIM, eds. *The Oxford Handbook of Memory*. New York, NY: Oxford University Press; 2000:627-643.

164. Corkin S. Lasting consequences of bilateral medial temporal lobectomy: clinical course and experimental findings in H.M. *Semin Neurol*. 1984;4:249-259.

165. Vaidya CJ, Zhao M, Desmond JE, Gabrieli JD. Evidence for cortical encoding specificity in episodic memory: memory-induced re-activation of picture processing areas. *Neuropsychologia*. 2002;40(12):2136-2143.

166. Damasio H, Grabowski TJ, Tranel D, Hichwa RD, Damasio AR. A neural basis for lexical retrieval. *Nature*. 1996;380(6574):499-505.

167. Levy DA, Bayley PJ, Squire LR. The anatomy of semantic knowledge: medial vs. lateral temporal lobe. *Proc Natl Acad Sci U S A*. 2004;101(17):6710-6715.

168. Schmidt CSM, Schumacher LV, Romer P, et al. Are semantic and phonological fluency based on the same or distinct sets of cognitive processes? Insights from factor analyses in healthy adults and stroke patients. *Neuropsychologia*. 2017;99:148-155.

169. Gorno-Tempini ML, Dronkers NF, Rankin KP, et al. Cognition and anatomy in three variants of primary progressive aphasia. *Ann Neurol*. 2004;55(3):335-346.

170. Warrington EK. The selective impairment of semantic memory. *Q J Exp Psychol*. 1975;27(4):635-657.

171. Noppeney U, Patterson K, Tyler LK, et al. Temporal lobe lesions and semantic impairment: a comparison of herpes simplex virus encephalitis and semantic dementia. *Brain*. 2007;130(pt 4):1138-1147.

172. Gardini S, Cuetos F, Fasano F, et al. Brain structural substrates of semantic memory decline in mild cognitive impairment. *Curr Alzheimer Res*. 2013;10(4):373-389.

173. Papp KV, Mormino EC, Amariglio RE, et al. Biomarker validation of a decline in semantic processing in preclinical Alzheimer's disease. *Neuropsychology*. 2016;30(5):624-630.

174. Price JL, Morris JC. Tangles and plaques in nondemented aging and "preclinical" Alzheimer's disease. *Ann Neurol*. 1999;45(3):358-368.

175. Bakkour A, Morris JC, Dickerson BC. The cortical signature of prodromal AD: regional thinning predicts mild AD dementia. *Neurology*. 2009;72(12):1048-1055.

176. Dickerson BC, Bakkour A, Salat DH, et al. The cortical signature of Alzheimer's disease: regionally specific cortical thinning relates to symptom severity in very mild to mild AD dementia and is detectable in asymptomatic amyloid-positive individuals. *Cereb Cortex*. 2009;19(3):497-510.

177. Lidstrom AM, Bogdanovic N, Hesse C, Volkman I, Davidsson P, Blennow K. Clusterin (apolipoprotein J) protein levels are increased in hippocampus and in frontal cortex in Alzheimer's disease. *Exp Neurol*. 1998;154(2):511-521.

178. Bechara A, Tranel D, Damasio H, Adolphs R, Rockland C, Damasio AR. Double dissociation of conditioning and declarative knowledge relative to the amygdala and hippocampus in humans. *Science*. 1995;269(5227):1115-1118.

179. Markowitsch HJ. Anatomical basis of memory disorders. In: Gazzangia MS, ed. *The Cognitive Neurosciences*. Cambridge, MA: MIT Press; 1995:765-779.

180. Heindel WC, Salmon DP, Shults CW, Walicke PA, Butters N. Neuropsychological evidence for multiple implicit memory systems: a comparison of Alzheimer's, Huntington's, and Parkinson's disease patients. *J Neurosci*. 1989;9(2):582-587.

181. Daselaar SM, Rombouts SA, Veltman DJ, Raaijmakers JG, Jonker C. Similar network activated by young and old adults during the acquisition of a motor sequence. *Neurobiol Aging*. 2003;24(7):1013-1019.

182. Exner C, Koschack J, Irle E. The differential role of premotor frontal cortex and basal ganglia in motor sequence learning: evidence from focal basal ganglia lesions. *Learn Mem*. 2002;9(6):376-386.

183. Keane MM, Gabrieli JD, Mapstone HC, Johnson KA, Corkin S. Double dissociation of memory capacities after bilateral occipital-lobe or medial temporal-lobe lesions. *Brain*. 1995;118(pt 5):1129-1148.

184. Schacter DL, Buckner RL. Priming and the brain. *Neuron*. 1998;20(2):185-195.

185. Mishikin M, Ungerleider LG, Macko K. Object vision and spatial vision: two cortical pathways. *Trends Neurosci*. 1983;6:414-417.

186. Kravitz DJ, Saleem KS, Baker CI, Mishkin M. A new neural framework for visuospatial processing. *Nat Rev Neurosci*. 2011;12(4):217-230.

187. Ranganath C, Ritchey M. Two cortical systems for memory-guided behaviour. *Nat Rev Neurosci*. 2012;13(10):713-726.

188. Cohen L, Dehaene S, Naccache L, et al. The visual word form area: spatial and temporal characterization of an initial stage of reading in normal subjects and posterior split-brain patients. *Brain*. 2000;123(pt 2):291-307.

189. Bolger DJ, Perfetti CA, Schneider W. Cross-cultural effect on the brain revisited: universal structures plus writing system variation. *Hum Brain Mapp*. 2005;25(1):92-104.

190. Glezer LS, Jiang X, Riesenhuber M. Evidence for highly selective neuronal tuning to whole words in the "visual word form area". *Neuron*. 2009;62(2):199-204.

191. Zhao L, Chen C, Shao L, et al. Orthographic and phonological representations in the fusiform cortex. *Cereb Cortex*. 2017;27(11):5197-5210.

192. Menon V, Desmond JE. Left superior parietal cortex involvement in writing: integrating fMRI with lesion evidence. *Brain Res Cogn Brain Res*. 2001;12(2):337-340.

193. Nakamura K, Honda M, Okada T, et al. Participation of the left posterior inferior temporal cortex in writing and mental recall of kanji orthography: a functional MRI study. *Brain*. 2000;123(pt 5):954-967.

194. Sugihara G, Kaminaga T, Sugishita M. Interindividual uniformity and variety of the "writing center": a functional MRI study. *NeuroImage*. 2006;32(4):1837-1849.

195. Rapcsak SZ, Beeson PM. The role of left posterior inferior temporal cortex in spelling. *Neurology.* 2004;62(12):2221-2229.

196. Dehaene S, Cohen L, Sigman M, Vinckier F. The neural code for written words: a proposal. *Trends Cogn Sci.* 2005;9(7):335-341.

197. Potgieser AR, van der Hoorn A, de Jong BM. Cerebral activations related to writing and drawing with each hand. *PLoS One.* 2015;10(5):e0126723.

198. Milner AD, Perrett DI, Johnston RS, et al. Perception and action in 'visual form agnosia'. *Brain.* 1991;114(pt 1B):405-428.

199. James TW, Culham J, Humphrey GK, Milner AD, Goodale MA. Ventral occipital lesions impair object recognition but not object-directed grasping: an fMRI study. *Brain.* 2003;126(pt 11):2463-2475.

200. Goodale MA, Milner AD, Jakobson LS, Carey DP. A neurological dissociation between perceiving objects and grasping them. *Nature.* 1991;349(6305):154-156.

201. Konen CS, Kastner S. Representation of eye movements and stimulus motion in topographically organized areas of human posterior parietal cortex. *J Neurosci.* 2008;28(33):8361-8375.

202. Friedman HR, Goldman-Rakic PS. Coactivation of prefrontal cortex and inferior parietal cortex in working memory tasks revealed by 2DG functional mapping in the rhesus monkey. *J Neurosci.* 1994;14(5 pt 1):2775-2788.

203. Todd JJ, Marois R. Capacity limit of visual short-term memory in human posterior parietal cortex. *Nature.* 2004;428(6984):751-754.

204. Chafee MV, Crowe DA, Averbeck BB, Georgopoulos AP. Neural correlates of spatial judgement during object construction in parietal cortex. *Cereb Cortex.* 2005;15(9):1393-1413.

205. Aguirre GK, D'Esposito M. Topographical disorientation: a synthesis and taxonomy. *Brain.* 1999;122(pt 9):1613-1628.

206. Stark RE, Heinz JM. Vowel perception in children with and without language impairment. *J Speech Hear Res.* 1996;39(4):860-869.

Neuropsychiatric Assessment

The Value and Therapeutic Power of the Neuropsychiatric Diagnostic Evaluation

4

David A. Silbersweig

Contemporary neuropsychiatry has come of age. After a flourish at the interface of neurology and psychopathology in the late 19th century, a decline during the era of psychoanalysis, and precursors in the forms of psychopharmacology and biological psychiatry, a substantial neuropsychiatric evidence and experience base has accrued, and the field has been defined. Localization of brain functions has extended beyond sensory-motor and even cognitive processes to emotional, social, and complex behavioral processes. The interactions among nodes within brain networks that mediate higher-order human mental function are being elucidated. Interdisciplinary clinical teams, like that of the Center for Brain/Mind Medicine at Brigham and Women's Hospital, are being formed. The American Neuropsychiatric Association and the *Journal of Neuropsychiatry and Clinical Neurosciences* have played a major role in bringing together the neuropsychiatric community and advancing the field. Specialized training programs have been developed.

These developments have resulted in a convergent, evolving understanding of the neurobiology of psychiatric conditions and the psychiatric aspects of neurologic conditions. Systems-level functional and structural neuroimaging is identifying brain circuits as final common pathways of clinical phenotypic expression of psychiatric phenomena. This work is elucidating the brain regions, circuits, and connectivity underlying the full range of human experience and behavior (including social interactions). Such findings are often consistent with the brain-behavior, structure-function relationships that had been identified through case studies of patients with focal neurologic lesions. This convergence reinforces our confidence in a fundamental neuropsychiatric knowledge base. At the same time, cellular and molecular research is identifying pathophysiological mechanisms that disrupt signaling pathways within the implicated circuits across a range of disease processes.

A neuropsychiatrist combines this knowledge with clinical acumen in both psychiatry and neurology. This integration occurs through combined residency training in psychiatry and neurology, or through a UCNS-approved fellowship in behavioral neurology and neuropsychiatry after a single residency in

either field. The neuropsychiatrist is thus ideally suited to evaluate and treat patients who have abnormalities in perception, cognition, emotion, and/or behavior due to a known psychiatric or neurologic disorder; due to the simultaneous presence of, or interaction between, psychiatric and neurologic disorders (or their treatments, and associated psychosocial elements); or due to an unknown underlying brain condition.

Patients who come to, or are referred to, a neuropsychiatrist have often seen multiple psychiatrists and neurologists (and internists) and have received multiple diagnoses or continue to suffer despite treatment prescribed. Psychiatrists or neurologists may feel uncomfortable ruling in or out a diagnosis that is outside of their core expertise, or may not know what they don't know within the vast span of neurobehavioral medicine. In some cases, patients and families may be reluctant to see a psychiatrist due to stigma, misunderstanding, and residual dualism in society. In all these instances, the neuropsychiatrist can provide a synthetic, "buck-stops-here," "one-stop-shopping" evaluation of tremendous value to all concerned.

Indeed, in many cases a comprehensive neuropsychiatric evaluation may itself have significant therapeutic effects. While any excellent patient encounter builds a therapeutic alliance, and while the establishment of a clear diagnosis can be a relief for the patient and guide subsequent treatment, neuropsychiatric content and context provide some unique opportunities in these regards.

The principal task is arriving at a sophisticated understanding of the patient's condition, and conveying that in a manner that the patient and significant others can assimilate. This requires confidence and expertise across the entire neurologic-psychiatric spectrum, in addition to empathy and communication skills.

The differential diagnosis and formulation are central to this process, and rely upon a careful neuropsychiatric interview, record review, exam, and testing. Limitations in the patient's cognition or insight need to be assessed, noted, and compensated for through additional sources of information. Previous diagnoses or labels are not accepted uncritically. Previous tests are not repeated unless an updated assessment is needed. The full spectrum of neurologic, psychiatric, and medical conditions must be considered in the context of the patient's psychological state, demographics, psychosocial stressors, and circumstance.

In the interview, the timing (acute, subacute, chronic) and progression (rate, fluctuation, stepwise, or gradual) of signs and symptoms provide important information about the underlying disease. Sometimes a single, cross-sectional assessment does not provide sufficient diagnostic clarity, which can only come with the way the condition progresses or declares itself with time. Whether signs and symptoms are "neighborhood" localizing (e.g., brainstem, vascular territory) or syndrome-clustering (e.g., bipolar manic, Parkinsonian) provides critical information as well. Atypicality of age of onset, presentation, or treatment response is an important clue in neuropsychiatric diagnosis. So too are changes in personality or comportment. Being open to the unexpected (e.g., a patient's ingestion of mothballs, or poisoning) or to indirect effects (e.g., of malabsorption nutritional deficiencies after bariatric surgery) is vital.

Familiarity with the brain lesion and functional neuroimaging literature greatly aids the determination of whether the clinical problem may be focal, multifocal, nonfocal, or diffuse. A strong knowledge of the neuraxis, functional/behavioral neuroanatomy, and pathophysiology is essential as the history and exam are being assessed and combined into diagnostic hypotheses that direct the workup. The ability to perform a thorough, yet targeted, and flexible neuropsychiatric exam is invaluable. The neuropsychiatric exam, including full psychiatric and neurologic elements as well as integrated elements, are described in this textbook, as are indications for phased neuropsychological testing, brain imaging studies, EEG, blood, and cerebrospinal fluid tests.

Neuropsychiatric conditions are frequently multidetermined, so consideration of complexity as well as parsimony is required in the case formulation. This process entails identifying, separating, and integrating (interactions among) the full set of psychopathophysiological possibilities: neurological, medical, developmental, psychiatric, psychological, psychosocial, iatrogenic, functional, single underlying uniting etiology/mechanism, or simultaneous presence of, and bi- or multidirectional interaction among, more than one condition.

Accordingly, therapeutic recommendations in neuropsychiatry are often multifaceted, involving pharmacology, psychotherapy, brain stimulation, rehabilitation, social work, and legal advice, to address the full range of symptomatic and life-function issues. Being familiar with all of these modalities, and being part of (or being able to access) a coordinated, multidisciplinary team, is essential.

The importance of such a team cannot be overstated, though resources may not always permit it. The close, simultaneous evaluation and treatment of these complex cases often involve neuropsychiatrists, cognitive-behavioral neurologists, neuropsychologists, social workers, occupational therapists, and physical therapists.

The role, perspective, and specialized expertise of the neuropsychiatrist enables the assessment and recommendations to be conveyed in a therapeutic manner. The explanatory model of neuropsychiatry is powerful, and can help patients and families to frame, understand, and accept difficult news. The definitive nature of the evaluation can help to establish what is and (importantly) isn't known about the patient's condition; can tie together hitherto disparate elements; can distinguish unrelated findings ("red herrings," such as an arteriovenous malformation in a location that isn't responsible for the symptoms, versus one that is, whether anatomically, physiologically, or epileptically); can reassure or reduce uncertainty (e.g., the relevance of past head trauma); and can preclude further unnecessary workups or doctor shopping.

For example, the neuropsychiatrist can help patients and caregivers realize that the patient's change in behavior is due to an orbitofrontal brain tumor or frontotemporal dementia, and is not within the awareness of or under the control of the patient, or the patient's "fault" (marriages have been saved with this single intervention). In a patient with multiple sclerosis, the neuropsychiatrist can distinguish lesion-associated affective dysregulation, from reactive depression, from steroid-induced emotional effects. The neuropsychiatrist has expertise to distinguish between tics and seizures, with major differential treatment implications and new management approaches. The neuropsychiatrist is also well positioned to help a patient (who wouldn't go to a psychiatrist due to perceived stigma) accept and legitimize a primary psychiatric diagnosis in a brain-mind-body context. Functional neurologic (conversion) conditions can sometimes even be acutely mitigated in such a setting, with explanation and suggestion, or referral for specialized cognitive behavioral interventions.

The patient's confidence and expectation, the doctor-patient relationship, the experienced physician's confidence, and the role of the neuropsychiatrist as a healer and comforter are all relevant in this context. As always, the patient's beliefs, values, socioeconomic circumstances, and culture need to be taken into account. It is not uncommon for the debriefing with patients and family members at the conclusion of the neuropsychiatric evaluation to bring about relief and hope (even if there is challenging news without a definitive intervention).

Finally, the neuropsychiatrist's synopsis and recommendations, and availability for follow-up or reconsultation, can be of great value to the referring physicians. For instance, the neuropsychiatrist can provide vital guidance for psychiatrists, neurologists, or internal medicine colleagues in cases of neuropsychiatric systemic lupus erythematosus or cancer-related paraneoplastic limbic encephalitis. If the patient has a severe, complex, or refractory set of neuropsychiatric difficulties, the neuropsychiatrist may play a critical role as an ongoing care provider, with the rest of the clinical team.

The value of this neuropsychiatric approach, as reflected throughout this textbook, is becoming more widely appreciated as the field evolves, as the population ages, and as health care is redesigned. The comprehensive neuropsychiatric evaluation remains at its core, and its therapeutic as well as diagnostic benefits can be profound.

5

Neuropsychiatric Assessment

Sheldon Benjamin

INTRODUCTION

Neuropsychiatric assessment proceeds from history to examination to formulation in a manner similar to that used in other fields of medicine but adapted to demonstrate brain-behavior relationships. Findings from the patient history, physical, mental status examination, and available laboratory, neuroimaging, neuropsychological evaluation, and other ancillary data are synthesized to create the neuropsychiatric formulation. This chapter offers an approach to neuropsychiatric assessment that includes both the details and the thought process of the neuropsychiatrist as the examination is conducted. For each major section discussed (history gathering, general physical examination, neurological examination, mental status examination, cognitive examination), please review the corresponding textbox that invites the clinician to maintain an active thinking process, analyzing and synthesizing each section's information with the aim of reaching an accurate and comprehensive assessment.

HISTORY

The common approach to psychiatric examination, involving phenomenology and descriptive psychopathology emphasizing the patient's subjective experience, has changed little since it was conceptualized by Karl Jaspers in the early years of the 20th century.[1] The neurological examination used today, though expanded by a host of subsequent investigators,[2] still follows the form laid down by John Hughlings Jackson in the late 19th century.[3] The neuropsychiatric examination combines elements of both methods, in use for over a century.

APPROACH TO NEUROPSYCHIATRIC ASSESSMENT

The neuropsychiatrist dynamically adapts the examination according to the purpose of the assessment, the cognitive capacity of the patient, and the evolving diagnostic hypothesis being considered by the examiner. It is helpful for the examiner to develop a series of different adapted approaches for patients who are, for example, uncooperative, demented, unresponsive, acutely ill, highly intelligent, intellectually disabled, autistic, violent, or catatonic. A different examination approach is required for young children, adolescents, or young adults. The examination is also adapted if it is being done for forensic purposes, risk assessment, rehabilitation planning, or vocational assessment. Just as one would not evaluate calculation deficits by asking a math professor to perform single digit addition, one would not ask an intellectually disabled individual to interpret a complex proverb. When performing a dementia evaluation, one might include a cue to help the patient remember the examiner's name when introducing oneself.

The neuropsychiatric examination serves several purposes in addition to gathering data for neuropsychiatric formulation. Precisely delineating the patient's symptoms not only yields useful diagnostic information but also serves to increase the alliance between clinician and patient by demonstrating the clinician's intention to try to understand the patient's experience. The examiner formulates a diagnostic hypothesis at the outset of the interaction with the patient and uses the examination to refine the hypothesis in real time. While refining the hypothesis, the clinician mentally plans for ancillary testing, rehabilitation, and treatment.

Neuropsychiatry is occasionally described as a search for "zebra" diagnoses. This is not the case. The neuropsychiatric examination leads to the differential diagnosis of common conditions such as dementia, epilepsy, traumatic brain injury, stroke sequelae, demyelinating diseases, brain tumors, encephalitides, and neurodevelopmental disabilities. It underlies the diagnosis of psychiatric comorbidities of common neurologic disease and neurologic comorbidities of common psychiatric disorders.

Although it is true that conditions included in a neuropsychiatric differential diagnosis are often less common than the major mental and neurological disorders, even when one considers the numerous rare disorders that can cause neuropsychiatric symptoms, these rare disorders are not at all rare. Rare diseases affect 1 in 15 people or about 400 million people worldwide[4] and should be considered in neuropsychiatric evaluation. Features common to rare disorders as causes for neuropsychiatric symptoms include: first presentation of a major psychiatric disorder outside the usual age of onset of that disorder; major personality change; sudden symptom onset in a previously asymptomatic individual; new psychiatric symptoms in context of a steep decline in cognitive or functional level, especially in adolescence or young adulthood; stereotyped behavioral episodes; onset in proximity to or in context of a medical or neurological condition; presence of dysmorphic features, birthmarks, or focal signs on neurological examination; and family history of a rare disease.[5] If one considers the many risk factor genes that have been identified for major mental illnesses and the large number of copy number variants and microdeletions identified using genetic microarrays, the idiopathic psychiatric disorders themselves can be seen as a collection of rare diseases.

THE NEUROPSYCHIATRIC HISTORY

Gather the neuropsychiatric history in a manner conducive to building an alliance. Sitting so that the examiner is at eye level with the patient is preferable to standing. If the patient is known to have hemianopia, hemineglect, or hemi-inattention, the examiner should take a position in the patient's "good" hemifield. Although the history begins with the patient's chief complaint or the referring clinician's consultation question as in other areas of medicine, there are a number of additional areas in the patient's history that are emphasized in neuropsychiatric assessment, enumerated in Table 5-1. The Neuropsychiatric Review of Systems includes inquiry into a number of behaviors such as those enumerated in Table 5-2.

While gathering the history, the examiner should take pains to understand the patient's subjective experience of their symptoms. The examiner forms a hypothesis as to the cause of the symptoms, informed by whether they are acquired versus preexisting, single episode or recurrent, or progressive versus static. Any well-known patterns of behavior are noted, and evidence of neurological, medical, or psychiatric causes of the chief complaint or consultation question is used to further refine the history. Any hint of risk to self or others in the past is followed up with detailed inquiry. While still gathering the history, the examiner considers whether there are any aspects of the history that would not fit the hypothesis being considered and inquires further as appropriate to the situation. At the same time the examiner considers which, if any, rating scales might be appropriate to this particular evaluation. It is helpful for neuropsychiatric clinicians to have available ready differential diagnoses of neuropsychiatric presentations such as those listed in Table 5-3. Box 5-1 contains a list of questions to consider while gathering the history.

TABLE 5-1 • Areas of Inquiry in Gathering the Neuropsychiatric History.
Psychiatric/Behavioral history
Psychiatric disorders (hospitalizations; psychopharmacologic treatment history; psychotherapy history)
Aggressive behavior (age at onset; description/type; episode length; time of day; presence of clear onset/offset; prodrome; precipitant; pattern; purpose; environmental factors)
Past danger to self or others
Past medical and surgical history
Neurological history
Traumatic brain injuries (length of loss of consciousness, retrograde amnesia, anterograde amnesia, initial Glasgow Coma Scale, deficits)
Seizures (cause if known; age at onset; frequency; longest seizure-free interval; details of semiology including aura, automatisms, peri-ictal, post-ictal and interictal behaviors; incontinence; injuries; EEG and MRI findings; anticonvulsant history)
Stroke (age, etiology, location, sequelae)
CNS infection/HIV-associated neurocognitive disorder
Intellectual disability/learning disorder
Preexisting neurological deficits
Dementia history (onset; rate of progression; risk factors; cognitive/personality deficits; motor involvement; contributions from sensory deprivation; genes/biomarkers)
Demyelinating disease history
Sleep disorders
Pain syndromes
Family History of Psychiatric or Neurological Disorders
Neurodevelopmental history
Birth
Known congenital or developmental syndromes
Handedness
Developmental milestones
Social history
Substance use history
Education (best and worst subjects in HS, grades, support needed)
Occupational history (description, longest held jobs, environmental exposures)
Special skills
ADLs/iADLs
Household members
Means of support, disability income
Legal history (arrests; lawsuits; incarceration)
Military history (years of service; highest rank; combat exposure; injuries; service-connected disability)

TABLE 5-2 • Areas of Inquiry in the Neuropsychiatric Review of Systems.
Behavior change
Motor symptoms and involuntary movements
Paroxysmal and periodic symptoms
Sleep symptoms
Cognitive symptoms
Neurovegetative functions
Endocrine symptoms
Rheumatologic symptoms
ADLs, iADLs

TABLE 5-3 • Common Neuropsychiatric Presentations.	
Delirium	Dementia with prominent
Catatonia	behavioral changes
Catatonic excitement	Dementia with prominent
Neuroleptic malignant	language changes
syndrome	Dementia with seizures
Serotonin syndrome	Stereotyped paroxysmal
Autoimmune limbic	phenomena
encephalitis	Alcohol-related conditions
Aggressive behavior	Sleep disorders: insomnia,
New onset aggression in	hypersomnia, parasomnia
nonverbal individuals	Frontal/dysexecutive syndromes
Self-injurious behavior	Multiple CNS deficits
Aggression related to	Autism or autistic features
cognitive deficits	Intellectual disability with
Post-traumatic brain injury	dysmorphic features
syndromes	
Dementia	
Dementia with	
extrapyramidal	
features	
Dementia with weakness	
or incoordination	

TABLE 5-4 • Body Areas to Check for Dysmorphic Features.
Stature
Hair growth pattern
Ear structure, size, placement
Nose size
Face size and structure
Philtrum
Mouth and lips
Teeth
Hand size
Fingers and thumbs
Nails
Feet structure and size

BOX 5-1   Questions to Ask Yourself While Gathering the History

What is the patient's subjective experience of the symptoms?

Do the symptoms fit a familiar pattern?

Is the problem newly acquired or recurrent?

Is the condition progressive or static?

Could the symptoms be explained by an undiagnosed medical, neurological, or psychiatric condition?

What aspects of the history don't fit my diagnostic hypothesis?

What risks does this patient present to self or others?

Which rating scales might I want to use in this case?

TABLE 5-5 • Common Dysmorphic Syndromes in Intellectual Disability.	
Down syndrome	*Fragile X syndrome*
Microcephaly	Macrocephaly
Short stature	High forehead
Hypotonia	Long narrow face
Flat face	Prognathism
Epicanthic folds	Thickened nasal bridge
Upslanting palpebral	Large ears/soft cartilage
fissures	Pale blue irides
Small ears	Epicanthic folds
Small mouth	High arched palate
Short neck	Dental crowding
Short fingers	Hyperextensible finger joints
Brushfield spots (grayish	Flat feet
brown spots at	Pectus excavatum
periphery of iris)	Macro-orchidism
Fetal Alcohol Syndrome	*Velocardiofacial syndrome (22 q11.2 deletion)*
Short stature	Short stature
Microcephaly	Microcephaly
Narrow face	Upslanted palpebral fissures
Telecanthus	Hooded eyelids
Short palpebral fissures	Palatal abnormalities
Smooth philtrum/upper lip	Micrognathia
	Small mouth
	Round ears

THE NEUROPSYCHIATRIC EXAMINATION

General Exam

After checking vital signs, the examination may take different forms depending on the individual being examined. It is helpful to have a rough outline of examination approaches one might use for any of the types of evaluation discussed in the "Approach to the Patient" section above.

Note any asymmetry or abnormally large or small head size. In the setting of intellectual disability (ID) or autistic spectrum disorder, the clinician notes dysmorphic features that may serve as clues to associated syndromes. A list of body areas to observe for these features is found in Table 5-4. Certain features may be associated with abnormal brain development. Midline defects such as hypertelorism, for instance, are occasionally found in partial agenesis of the corpus callosum. With the advent of readily available genetic testing, there is a burgeoning amount of data relating to behaviorally relevant phenotypes. A suite of phenotyping apps is available from Face2Gene.com to aid in identifying less common syndromes. Several other printed and online resources can help the consultant identify developmental syndromes.[6-8] Familiarity with the Fragile X syndrome (FrX), fetal alcohol syndrome (FAS), Down syndrome, and velocardiofacial syndrome phenotypes, the most common dysmorphic syndromes that occur in ID, is helpful (Table 5-5).

A common reason for neuropsychiatric consultation is the evaluation for possible causative factors in the differential diagnosis of psychotic symptoms. In addition to a search for neurologic or cognitive signs that could be caused by pathology in a given circuit, a knowledge of the more common congenital, genetic, and metabolic syndromes that have been associated with the development of psychosis in children or young adults is helpful. A list of these syndromes is provided in Table 5-6.[9]

TABLE 5-6 • Syndromes Associated with Psychosis in Children and Young Adults.

Acute intermittent porphyria	Huntington's disease
Autism spectrum disorder	Klinefelter syndrome XXY
Down syndrome	Marfan syndrome
Fragile X syndrome	Neurofibromatosis type 1
Gilbert syndrome	Oculocutaneous albinism
Glucose-6-phosphate dehydrogenase deficiency	Phenylketonuria
	Turner syndrome
XXX Karyotype	22q11.2 deletion (velocardiofacial syndrome)

TABLE 5-7 • Cutaneous Features of Four Common Neurocutaneous Syndromes.

Tuberous sclerosis	*Sturge-Weber syndrome*
Hypomelanotic macules (ash leaf spots)	Port wine stain in trigeminal nerve territories
Shagreen patches	
Subungual fibromas	*Ataxia-telangiectasia*
Angiofibromas	Telangiectasias on ears, cheeks, trunk
Adenoma sebaceum	Premature graying of hair
	Progeric facies
Neurofibromatosis type 1	Hypopigmented macules
	Café au lait spots
Axillary and inguinal freckling	
Café au lait spots (≥6 spots, ≥1 cm each)	
Cutaneous neurofibromas	
Plexiform neurofibromas	

Alopecia, hirsutism, rashes, and birthmarks are noted on general examination. Examination of the skin also affords a unique opportunity to learn about the embryologic development of the nervous system since skin and brain share a common ectodermal origin. The examination is of increased importance in the presence of seizures and learning disorder, common features of the neurocutaneous syndromes. Although a large number of neurocutaneous syndromes are known to exist, the four most common of these are tuberous sclerosis, neurofibromatosis type 1 (NF1), Sturge-Weber syndrome, and ataxia-telangiectasia. The cutaneous features of these syndromes are listed in Table 5-7. Psychiatric abnormalities occur most often in NF1 and tuberous sclerosis, with tuberous sclerosis frequently associated with ASD. Neurocutaneous syndromes may also be consistent with normal development and absence of neurologic symptoms, especially in the carrier state.

The clinician should observe for risk factors for obstructive sleep apnea, including small oropharyngeal opening, and large neck and upper torso size. The tongue should be inspected for signs of atrophic glossitis seen in B_{12} deficiency. Arrhythmias or cardiac murmurs on cardiovascular examination may indicate an increased risk for stroke or vascular dementia. The combination of rash and joint pain, swelling, or deformity indicates a need to consider rheumatologic disease. See Box 5-2 for questions to consider while performing the general medical examination.

BOX 5-2 Questions to Ask Yourself During the General Physical Examination

Are there any signs of a congenital disorder (especially if intellectually disabled or autistic spectrum)?

Could the symptoms be consistent with an inherited metabolic disorder?

Could a medical condition either be the cause of or share the same cause as the neurobehavioral symptoms?

Which findings on general physical examination are related to one another?

Are any findings on physical examination related to the chief neurobehavioral complaint?

BOX 5-3 Questions to Ask Yourself While Performing the Neurological Examination

Are the findings consistent with upper motor neuron pathology?

Are the findings consistent with lower motor neuron pathology?

Are the findings consistent with neuromuscular disease?

Are the findings consistent with myopathy?

Are the findings consistent with neuropathy?

Are the findings consistent with basal ganglia disease?

Are the findings consistent with cerebellar disease?

What cognitive deficits might be associated with these neurological findings?

What is the relationship of the neurological deficits to the neurobehavioral chief complaint?

Neurological Examination

The neurological examination consists of cranial nerve, motor, sensory, and gait examinations. A discussion of neurodevelopmental "soft" signs and the detection of embellishment and malingering follows the basic neurological examination sections. See Box 5-3 for questions the clinician may consider while conducting the neurological exam.

Cranial Nerve Examination

Abnormalities of cranial nerve function are often seen in neuropsychiatric disorders. Diminished olfaction in absence of cigarette smoking or chronic rhinitis may be seen in traumatic brain injury of any severity, in neurodegenerative diseases such as Alzheimer's or Parkinson's disease, in demyelinating disease, and orbitofrontal tumors. The combination of diminished vision and anosmia is seen in the Foster-Kennedy syndrome associated with unilateral compressive frontal tumors. Olfaction may be tested with a tube of scented lip balm or "scratch and sniff" olfactory testing cards.[10]

The optic nerve is inspected directly by fundoscopy. Visual acuity is customarily assessed with a Snellen card at 14 inches. Visual fields may be estimated at the bedside by confrontation.

The examiner moves a wiggling finger in from the periphery approximately 14 inches from the patient in each of the quadrants while asking the patient to indicate the location of the movements with their finger. Double simultaneous stimulation is included to test for extinction. To determine whether the macula has been spared in a visual field cut, the examiner holds a stimulus with a red point at the end (a pen top or red painted hat pin) behind a white stimulus (such as a hat pin) and moves the red stimulus laterally just outside the edge of the white stimulus. Failure to detect the red stimulus indicates macular involvement. An Amsler grid for detection of macular degeneration is included with the OKN strips app mentioned below. Color blindness can be assessed using a smartphone app (PseudoChromatic ColorTest app) containing the pseudochromatic color test stimuli. Light perception by the optic nerve is tested by shining a flashlight first at one pupil than the other while observing for direct and consensual pupillary responses. In the presence of an afferent pupillary defect the affected pupil, which constricts when the light is shined in the opposite eye, will dilate when the light swings over it. Shining a light at both eyes simultaneously affords a quick check for dysconjugate gaze, indicated by failure of the light to align on both pupils at the same "o'clock." Pupillary diameters should be recorded for future comparison. This can be done by replacing the "E" in "PERRLA" with the pupillary diameters in mm recording the right on top and the left on the bottom. A comment may be added indicating whether the examination was done in bright light, ambient light, or a darkened room.

Ocular motility is assessed by instructing the patient to follow the examiner's finger as the shape of an H is traced in the air to isolate functions of the ocular muscles. The patient's eyes should smoothly follow the examiner's finger. Presence of saccadic pursuits or square wave jerks may indicate cerebellar dysfunction but can also be seen in parkinsonian syndromes. Supranuclear gaze is assessed by having the patient move his/her eyes to command. Inability to move the eyes vertically to command in the setting of preserved doll's eyes phenomenon with passive head movement is consistent with supranuclear gaze palsy. Supranuclear gaze palsy is seen in progressive supranuclear palsy, most common in middle-aged males, and in Niemann-Pick type C disease, commonly presenting in young people. It can also be seen in Whipple's disease, a less common but treatable disorder caused by *Tropheryma whipplei* that typically includes GI symptoms and arthritis as well. Internuclear ophthalmoplegia (INO), most commonly seen in demyelinating disease, is diagnosed when the patient is directed to look quickly from one of the examiner's laterally outstretched hands to the other and back. In the presence of an INO, the adducting eye does not move beyond the midline while the abducting eye develops nystagmus. Onset of ptosis with prolonged upgaze, known as the fatigue phenomenon, occurs in myasthenic syndromes. Ptosis is described in relation to the pupil (e.g., ptosis to mid-pupil). Gaze-evoked nystagmus is seen in a variety of metabolic disorders and medication toxicities but may also occur in brainstem and cerebellar lesions. Optokinetic nystagmus or OKN testing is accomplished by horizontally passing a cloth with wide vertical stripes in front of the patient's eyes while instructing the patient to count the stripes silently as they pass by. Failure to direct one's gaze to the approaching stripe may indicate frontal dysfunction

while failure to follow the moving stripe is indicative of more posterior dysfunction. OKN's may also be tested with a rotating OKN drum or an app for smartphones or tablets. One such app is called "OKN strips." Additional information about frontal function may be easily obtained while testing ocular motility. Inability to move the eyes in the direction opposite the movement of the examiner's finger, a task known as anti-saccades, may indicate stimulus bound behavior. Prolonged visual fixation on a target may represent the "visual grasp" of posterior cortical atrophy or occasionally Alzheimer's disease.

Facial sensation is assessed by light touch (as opposed to stroking) in each of the three trigeminal dermatomes. In an unresponsive or delirious patient V1 can be assessed by testing the corneal reflex, V2 by tickling the inner nares, and V3 by eliciting the jaw jerk. The afferent arcs of all three reflexes are trigeminal. In upper motor neuron lesions, the jaw jerk may be exaggerated. Palpation of the temporalis and masseter muscles while the patient clenches the jaw or grinds side to side is used to test trigeminal motor fibers. Facial strength is tested both in the upper and lower face since the upper face receives bilateral facial nerve innervation and the lower face receives crossed unilateral innervation. The upper division of the facial nerve is tested by having the patient raise their eyebrows, observable while testing vertical gaze to command, and shut their eyes tightly. The lower division of the facial nerve is tested by having the patient puff out their cheeks and eliciting both a spontaneous smile (this may require the telling of a joke) and a smile to command. An intact smile to command coupled with an asymmetric spontaneous smile has been associated with lesions in the contralateral limbic system, basal ganglia, or supplementary motor area (SMA).[11] Lower motor neuron facial weakness may have many causes including prior Bell's palsy, typically resulting in a widened palpebral fissure and drooping of the corner of the mouth on the affected side.

The auditory nerve is customarily tested by finger rubbing near the auditory meatus, by detection of the sound of a 256 Hz tuning fork, or by whispering in the patient's ear. To differentiate whether apparent hearing loss is conductive or sensorineural, the examiner can perform the Weber test in which a ringing 256 Hz tuning fork is touched to the top of the head. The sound appears louder on the side with conductive hearing loss. If the sound appears louder in the opposite ear the defective ear may have sensorineural hearing loss.

If the patient's speech is dysarthric the affected muscle group can be identified by having the patient repeat the sounds "pa," "ta," and "ka" over and over separately and together as "pa-ta-ka." These sounds stress labial, lingual, and guttural muscles respectively. Scanning speech due to cerebellar dysfunction may be elicited by having the patient say a prolonged "ahh" and listening for variability in volume and pitch. Although the gag reflex is commonly used to test the ninth and tenth cranial nerves, a more useful test is watching the patient drink a full tumbler of water without pause. Dysphagia due to movement disorders is a common source of morbidity in patients with neuropsychiatric disorders.

The spinal accessory nerve is tested by shoulder shrug and head turn against resistance. The hypoglossal nerve is tested by observing the tongue at rest within the mouth and performing lateral movements while extended. A lower motor neuron hypoglossal lesion causes tongue deviation toward the side of the lesion when observed in the mouth and away from the lesion when protruded. Such a lesion may also result in fasciculations and lateralized atrophy. Upper motor neuron hypoglossal weakness is seen in bulbar ALS.

Bilateral corticobulbar lesions can result in pseudobulbar palsy, which can seem as if the cranial nerve nuclei themselves had been damaged. Pseudobulbar palsy includes dysarthria, dysphagia, hyperactive jaw jerk and gag reflex, and affective lability. The affective lability of pseudobulbar palsy is also known as pseudobulbar affect, pathological laughing and crying, or emotional incontinence. Pseudobulbar palsy is commonly seen in ALS, demyelinating disease, traumatic brain injury, and stroke. For further information on pseudobulbar affect, see Chapter 7.

Motor Examination

After examining the extremities for bulk, muscle tone, strength to resistive testing, deep tendon reflexes, and fine finger movements, the clinician attempts to elicit pathological reflexes that can indicate upper motor neuron involvement. If the plantar response is equivocal the examiner may utilize the Gordon (squeeze calf muscle), Chaddock (stroke lateral malleolus with a sharp stimulus similar to that used to elicit Babinski), or Oppenheim (stroke tibia between two knuckles) responses as alternatives. A positive response consists of an upgoing toe similar to the Babinski sign. Primitive reflexes, including the glabella tap, forced grasping, palmomental, snout, and suck may also be elicited. Inability to suppress eye blinking after five glabella taps (tapping from above and remaining outside the visual field) is known as Myerson's sign, and may be seen in Parkinson's disease or diffuse frontal dysfunction.[12] Forced grasping, and the related groping response toward objects within the visual field, has been associated with dysfunction of the medial prefrontal and SMAs. The grasp response is elicited by upward stroking of the outstretched palm while reminding the patient not to hold on. Forced grasping is diagnosed when the patient grasps ever more tightly on to the examiner's fingers as the examiner attempts to pull away. An analogous pathological reflex in the lower extremity, the forced foot grasp, may be elicited by stroking the sole of the foot of the seated patient with the side of the reflex hammer and then holding the hammer in front of the patient's foot. A positive response consists of the foot extending toward the hammer and the toes curling as if to grasp it.[13] The palmomental reflex, elicited by stroking the thenar eminence and observing for ipsilateral mentalis contraction, is more nonspecific and can be seen in both normal and abnormal brains.[14] The snout reflex, elicited by tapping the philtrum with the reflex hammer, and the suck reflex, elicited by touching an object to the lips, are also nonspecific indicators of brain dysfunction. Gegenhalten rigidity or paratonia, a release sign seen in catatonia and dementia, refers to variably increasing muscle resistance in proportion to the force or speed with which the examiner moves the patient's limb. Paraplegia in flexion, the posture seen in the end stage of dementia, is an extreme form of gegenhalten.[15]

Cerebellar dysfunction can be associated with mood and cognitive abnormalities that have been called the cerebellar cognitive affective syndrome or Schmahmann syndrome.[16] Signs of cerebellar dysfunction include saccadic intrusions and square wave jerks when assessing oculomotor movement, scanning speech, dysarthria on the "pa-ta-ka" test, decreased muscle tone, decreased check response during pronator drift and reflex testing, irregular performance on rapidly alternating movements, end of movement dysmetria when reaching toward an object, and difficulty smoothly following a target with a finger.[16] The cerebellar cognitive affective syndrome, featuring cognitive equivalents of motor abnormalities (e.g., cognitive dysmetria), should be considered in neuropsychiatric patients with cerebellar motor findings.[17]

During the motor examination, the patient is assessed for the presence of hypokinetic and hyperkinetic movement disorders commonly seen in neuropsychiatric conditions. Decreased movement may be due to depression, delirium, catatonia, stroke or other basal ganglia lesions, metabolic disorders, drug side effects, or extrapyramidal disorders. Increased movement may be seen in mania, ADHD, Gilles de la Tourette syndrome, OCD (tics), delirium, catatonia, stroke or other focal basal ganglia lesions, metabolic disorders, drug side effects, or extrapyramidal disorders. The most common hypokinetic movement disorder, parkinsonism, includes a triad of akinesia, rigidity, and resting tremor. When examining a patient for parkinsonism, supranuclear gaze, cerebellar function, orthostatic vital signs, observation for arm swing, and *en bloc* turning during gait examination are included to facilitate diagnosis of Parkinson plus syndromes. The contralateral limb is activated during the muscle tone exam to bring out latent upper extremity rigidity. Axial rigidity and akinesia form the core of the atypical parkinsonian syndromes such as PSP, corticobasal degeneration, and some frontotemporal dementias. The applause sign can be seen in patients with PSP who have difficulty accurately stopping when asked to quickly clap three times.[18] The alien hand sign, seen in corticobasal degeneration and callosal disconnection, refers to the feeling that one hand is foreign or has a "mind of its own," often associated with involuntary hand movements.[19] When following a patient for tremor a smartphone seismometer app can serve as an adjunct in recording tremor severity. Tic, tremor, dystonia, choreoathetosis, hemiballismus, and myoclonus are hyperkinetic movements. Choreoathetoid movements, such as those seen in tardive dyskinesia, may be assessed using the Abnormal Involuntary Movement Scale (AIMS).[20] The AIMS exam begins with the patient seated with arms at rest to observe for adventitious movements, which can be the earliest sign of a choreoathetoid movement disorder. Distracting maneuvers are done to accentuate movements with arms outstretched (piano playing fingers), and during mouth opening, tongue protrusion, fine finger movement, standing, and walking. The patient's face, arms, trunk, and legs are observed during each distraction maneuver. The patient is observed for evidence of glottal movement or exploratory tongue movement with mouth closed (the "bonbon sign"), and sudden inhalation while speaking that may indicate diaphragmatic dyskinesia, a risk factor for aspiration. The milkmaid grip, elicited by having the patient sustain a steady grasp of the examiner's forefinger, is another sign of choreoathetosis. The presence of abnormal involuntary movements does not prove the patient has tardive dyskinesia. Two common neuropsychiatric disorders with hyperkinetic involuntary movements are Gilles de la Tourette syndrome and Huntington's disease. Dystonia refers to an involuntary muscle contraction associated with repetitive or twisting movements that can occur spontaneously or during a specific action like writing or eating. Dystonia commonly occurs in the eyelids, neck, oromandibular area, vocal cords, and upper extremities. Cervical dystonia may be accompanied by a *geste antagoniste* or sensory trick (more recently known as an alleviating maneuver) in which the patient knows a place to touch that temporarily alleviates the dystonia. This feature, once thought to be evidence of psychogenic origin, is now known to bolster the diagnosis of dystonia. Tics are abrupt, non-rhythmic repetitive movements which involve discrete muscle groups. Tics mimic normal coordinated movements, vary in intensity, and can be temporarily suppressed voluntarily. Gilles de la Tourette syndrome involves both motor and vocal tics and typically includes aspects of OCD as well. Motor tics are seen in OCD and in first-degree relatives of patients with OCD or Gilles de la Tourette syndrome. Abnormal involuntary movements were also known to occur in individuals with schizophrenia before the neuroleptic era.[21]

The catatonic syndrome, though typically hypokinetic, may also take the form of catatonic excitement with hyperkinesis. Components of the catatonic syndrome from the Bush-Francis Catatonia Scale are listed in Table 5-8.[22] Catatonia should be treated as a neuropsychiatric emergency. Combined with seizures, anterograde amnesia, or hippocampal FLAIR hyperintensities on MRI, catatonia may be a presentation of autoimmune limbic encephalitis. Elements of the syndrome may also occur in neuroleptic malignant syndrome, serotonin syndrome, and so-called lethal catatonia.

Sensory Examination

Following primary sensory assessment, test for cortical sensory loss due to contralateral parietal dysfunction by assessing graphesthesia, 2-point discrimination, stereognosis, and double simultaneous stimulation. Graphesthesia is tested by asking the patient to identify numbers traced on the fingertip or palm with an applicator stick. The 2-point discrimination threshold may be assessed with metal calipers graduated in millimeters or with a note card in which pinholes have been made 5, 7, and 10 mm apart. Stereognosis is tested by asking the patient to close their eyes and name a small object placed in their hand. Inability to name objects placed in the left hand with preserved ability on the right is also seen in callosal disconnection. Double simultaneous stimulation is used to test for hemineglect in the visual, somatosensory, or auditory spheres. In the visual sphere, the patient is asked to indicate the finger that is moving when the examiner moves fingers in both hemifields simultaneously. Somatosensory hemineglect is assessed by lightly touching both limbs at once and asking the patient to indicate the side being touched. Auditory hemi-inattention can be assessed at the bedside by simultaneously making different sounds in each ear (e.g., crinkling paper in one hand and jingling keys in the other) and asking the patient to identify the sound.

Gait Examination

When observing gait, note ease of gait initiation, stride length, step height, any aids or appliances used, gait-evoked involuntary movements, and arm swing. Observe the normal gait, then ask the patient to walk on heels, toes, and in tandem. Note any

TABLE 5-8 • Components of the Catatonic Syndrome from the Bush-Francis Catatonia Scale.	
Excitement	Waxy flexibility
Immobility/stupor	Withdrawal
Mutism	Impulsivity
Staring	Automatic obedience
Posturing/catalepsy	Mitgehen
Grimacing	Gegenhalten
Echopraxia/echolalia	Ambitendency
Stereotypy	Grasp reflex
Mannerisms	Perseveration
Verbigeration	Combativeness
Rigidity	Autonomic abnormality
Negativism	

TABLE 5-9 • Neurodevelopmental Soft Signs (NSS).[24,25]	
Non-lateralizing	*Potentially lateralizing*
Dysarthria	Dystonic posturing
Inability to move eyes without moving head	Hemiparesis
	Hyperreflexia, unsustained clonus
Clumsiness, incoordination	Reflex asymmetry
Drooling	Slow or irregular fine finger movements
Ataxia	
Dysphagia	Asymmetric size of face or extremities
Nystagmus	
Slow or irregular rapid alternating movements	Asterognosis
	Agraphesthesia
Bradykinesia	Motor impersistence
Synkinesia (overflow/mirror movements)	Extinction to visual/tactile double simultaneous stimulation

Note: These signs are known in the literature as neurological or neurodevelopmental "soft signs" because they are frequently seen in patients with developmental or psychiatric disorders in the absence of neurodiagnostic evidence of a focal lesion. For a more comprehensive listing see Tupper[24] and Chen et al.[25]

circumduction or antalgic gait. If signs of parkinsonism are present ask the patient to arise from a chair without using their hands, have them do an "about face" turn to observe for *en bloc* turning, and include a "pull test" from behind for retropulsion. When testing for Romberg's sign, the examiner can observe for signs of motor impersistence, seen in right frontal dysfunction.[23] Asked to stand with feet together, eyes closed, and arms outstretched, the patient with motor impersistence will require repeated reminders to continue doing each of the three parts of the command.

Neurological "Soft" Signs

Neurodevelopmental or neurological "soft" signs (NSS) are seen with increased frequency in individuals with neurodevelopmental disorders, schizophrenia, bipolar disorder, substance use disorders, obsessive compulsive disorder, antisocial personality disorder, as well as in prematurity, low birth weight, and malnutrition.[21] A list of NSS is given in Table 5-9. This term refers to signs that are not associated with demonstrable abnormalities on brain imaging but may well represent subtle brain dysfunction in the above conditions. Those signs that are potentially lateralizing may reflect early CNS damage not seen on conventional imaging. NSS should therefore be considered a diagnosis of exclusion.

Embellishment and Malingering

Neuropsychiatrists often examine people in whom there may be a question of symptom embellishment or malingering. A few additions to the neurological examination can be helpful in these cases. When examining someone with complaint of field cut or tunnel vision, simply test visual fields to confrontation at 14 inches, 3 feet, and 15 feet. Since visual fields expand in a conical fashion, the field cut should not be identical at all distances. Similarly, hemisensory deficits to pinprick or light touch that precisely split the midline on the face or trunk or a hemivibratory loss on the skull are also physiologically inconsistent. Another technique that may be used to test for embellished or malingered hemisensory loss is to ask the patient to hold their hands out with thumbs down, then clasp, interdigitate and rotate their hands upward before testing primary sensation. This makes it difficult for the patient to quickly track which of the interdigitated fingers are from the right versus left hands. The Hoover sign is used to assess malingered or embellished leg weakness. With the patient supine, the examiner places his/her hands under the patient's heels and instructs the patient to raise the hemiparetic leg. Failure of the normal heel to press down on the examiner's hand is physiologically inconsistent with effort at straight leg raising. Additional evidence of feigned unilateral leg weakness may be obtained by having the patient walk around a chair with the weak leg out while using the chair back for support. Then have the patient switch hands on the chair back and walk the opposite way around the chair while observing for inconsistency in the gait circumduction.

Mental Status Examination

General Observations

Mental status assessment includes both mental status and cognitive status examinations. The traditional mental status examination is a collection of observations and subjective descriptions in the areas listed in Table 5-10. Questions for the clinician to consider while conducting the mental state examination are listed in Box 5-4. Level of consciousness is described as alert, lethargic, stuporous, or comatose. Arousal is also described in terms of response to verbal command or to pain. Peculiarities in appearance or style of dress are noted. Idiosyncrasies, unusual preoccupations or traits, and particular triggers of irritability (e.g., misophonia) are noted. The ability to anticipate, plan, and self-monitor for errors is an indicator of executive function. In the presence of prefrontal dysfunction, patients may be unaware of their own behavior, and unable to appropriately match their behavior to the environment or situation, missing social cues and failing to respect personal space. Denial of symptoms or deficits may be related to right hemisphere dysfunction. The examiner notes eye contact, cooperation, engagement, relatedness, degree of apathy or interest, attitude toward symptoms, and the degree of effort on cognitive tasks.

TABLE 5-10 • Behavioral Observations in the Mental Status Examination.

Level of consciousness/Arousal	Verbal production
Appearance	Thought form
Idiosyncrasies	Thought process
Awareness, self-monitoring, planning	Thought content
Attitude and demeanor	Self-destructive or homicidal thoughts
Relatedness and empathy	Abnormal perceptions
Motor activity	Agnosias
Affect	Insight
Mood	Judgment

BOX 5-4 Questions to Ask Yourself While Performing the Mental Status Examination

Are the mental status changes typical for a general psychiatric disorder?

Could the mental status changes be caused by a medical or neurological condition?

What are the risks of harm to self or others?

What is the patient's rehabilitation potential?

Which rating scales might be appropriate to use in this case?

Motor Activity

Observation of motor activity and general behavior begins from the very first contact with the patient. Note is made of fluidity of movements and gait as the patient walks into the room. Psychomotor agitation or slowing becomes apparent as the interview proceeds. Hypokinetic and hyperkinetic movements should be described along with any observed compulsions, rituals, or stereotypies (repetitive, purposeless movements).

Affect and Mood

Affect, the external manifestations of one's internal mood state, is reflected in posture, facial expression, prosody, and gesture. The apparent emotion, range, amplitude, stability, and appropriateness are reported when describing affect. Mood is described according to the subjective emotion reported by the patient, though it must sometimes be inferred from affective cues in nonverbal individuals. Common descriptors include depressed, dysphoric, euphoric, expansive, elated, anxious, hostile, and euthymic.

Verbal Production

In observing verbal output, the examiner notes the overall fluency, phrase length, melodic line, and prosody of speech. Emotional prosody, which may have more of a right hemisphere contribution than linguistic prosody, can be noted separately. Word-finding pauses, circumlocution, hesitation, paraphasic errors, pronunciation, and rhythm of speech are noted. Other important components of verbal production include volume, quantity, and rate of speech from mutism to tachyphemia (speech cluttering). Pressured speech is seen in mania. Foreign accent syndrome is a particular type of dysprosody in which a person's pronunciation makes them sound as if they come from a foreign country. Foreign accent syndrome can be neurogenic and involuntary, due to stroke, traumatic brain injury, or migraine; or psychogenic and voluntary. Neurogenic cases have typically been reported following damage to left hemisphere sites including Broca's area, the insula, the SMA, and motor cortex; but have also been reported as congenital abnormalities and following cerebellar lesions.[26]

Dysarthria refers to a motor speech disorder as opposed to a language disorder. Dysarthria may be flaccid in neuromuscular or lower motor neuron disorders; spastic in bilateral upper motor neuron and extrapyramidal disorders; ataxic in cerebellar disorders; hypokinetic in basal ganglia and parkinsonian disorders; hyperkinetic in basal ganglia disorders with abnormal involuntary movements; or mixed as in amyotrophic lateral sclerosis with upper and lower motor neuron involvement. Apraxia of speech, typically seen accompanying Broca aphasia, describes problems correctly sequencing phonemic components resulting in effortful, poorly modulated speech, often with difficulty initiating responses. Stuttering, the involuntary repetition of sounds or syllables, is more often developmental than acquired and appears to run in families. Acquired stuttering in adulthood is more commonly psychogenic but can rarely occur after TBI or stroke. In neurogenic cases, the stuttering is less likely to be limited to initial sounds, less likely to attenuate with adaptation to the situation, and more likely to occur across all types of speech output including oral reading, repetition, conversation, and explanation.[27] Palilalia, the involuntary repetition of words, phrases, or even sentences, occurs in Tourette syndrome, neurodegenerative disorders, and hypodopaminergic states. Verbigeration refers to obsessive repetition of words.

In addition to the motor aspects of verbal production, the examiner attends to any unusual word production. Excessive punning or rhyming may be seen in psychotic disorders, mania, or frontotemporal dementia.[28] When the only connection between subsequent thoughts is that they contain rhyming words, a phenomenon seen in mania, the term clang association is applied. Witzelsucht or excessive and pathological joking may be seen in individuals with frontal dysfunction.[29] The well-known phenomenon of coprolalia, seen in individuals with Gilles de la Tourette syndrome, actually occurs in less than 10% of cases.[30] The presence of malapropisms, the inappropriate use of a word that sounds similar to the intended word, may be an indicator of limited education or mania. Neologisms or made-up words are seen in psychosis, but also occur in fluent jargon aphasia and occasionally in partial seizures. One way to differentiate psychotic from aphasic neologisms is simply to ask the patient why they used that word. The aphasic neologism is unintentional while the psychotic neologism is used for a reason unique to that individual's thought process. Another language idiosyncrasy that may occur in schizophrenia is metonymy, the use of one word as a substitute for another, such as saying "I've lost the bus of my thoughts" instead of "I've lost my train of thought." The mere presence of a language disorder does not signify neurogenic origin. Non-neurogenic language disorders such as non-aphasic misnaming are sometimes confused with neurogenic disorders.[31]

Thought Process and Content

The term "thought process" refers to the quantity, rate, organization, and connectedness of one's thoughts and is typically used in the description of psychotic behavior. Formal thought disorder refers to disorganized, impoverished, or abnormally connected thoughts including loose associations, derailment, thought blocking, circumstantiality, tangentiality, speaking in word salad, non-sequitur speech, and perseveration. The examiner attempts to understand whether the person's thoughts appear to flow logically from one another. The term "knight's move" refers to a discernable but unstated connection between loosely associated thoughts similar to the way in which a knight moves on a chessboard. Ganser syndrome refers to the syndrome of approximate answers (e.g., being consistently off by 1 on the day, date, or year) seen in individuals embellishing their condition. Thought content refers to the description of abnormal thoughts including delusions, preoccupations, overvalued ideas, obsessions, phobias, depressive thoughts, and dangerousness to oneself or others.

Agnosias

Agnosias are the loss of ability to recognize sounds, shapes, objects, or smells despite having intact primary sensory perception. Apperceptive agnosia describes the inability to recognize, discriminate among, or copy objects. Associative agnosia refers to the inability to recognize objects despite intact primary sensory perception and ability to describe and copy them. Individuals with lateralized parietal damage may develop anosognosia (denial of deficit) or anosodiaphoria (denial of the seriousness of the deficit). Bilateral occipital strokes, such as in tip-of-the-basilar syndrome, can cause Anton's syndrome, with cortical blindness, confabulation, and denial of blindness. Some patients during multiple sclerosis exacerbations are described as having eutonia, or denial of the seriousness of their demyelinating symptoms. Specific agnosias are listed in Table 5-11.

Delusional misidentification and reduplicative phenomena are particular delusions that can be seen in both psychiatric and neurological disorders. Delusional misidentification syndromes include the Capgras delusion that a familiar person has been replaced by an imposter, the Fregoli delusion that a persecutor is taking on the form of familiars, and the intermetamorphosis delusion that people are swapping identities without changing outward appearance. Reduplicative paramnesia, the delusional belief that a place, event, or time has been duplicated or relocated, is seen in psychiatric disorders, following traumatic brain injury, in delirium, partial seizures, encephalopathy, and other causes.

Perceptions

The examiner inquires about the presence of dissociative symptoms, illusions, hallucinations, and pseudohallucinations—the latter being hallucinations recognized as hallucinations by the patient. Derealization and depersonalization are dissociative symptoms that can be seen in post-traumatic stress disorder (PTSD) as well as partial seizures or migraine. Hallucinations and illusions are common in neuropsychiatric conditions including stroke, tumor, migraine, and partial seizures. Autoscopic hallucinations, the perception of seeing

TABLE 5-11 • Specific Agnosias.

Agnosia	Definition
Akinetopsia	Inability to perceive motion despite intact ability to perceive objects
Alexia	Inability to read despite intact vision, writing, and language
Amusia	Loss of ability to recognize familiar melodies, read music, or identify notes
Anosodiaphoria	Minimization of importance of deficit despite acknowledgment of its existence
Anosognosia	Denial of deficit
Astereognosis	Inability to recognize objects by feel (tactile agnosia)
Auditory agnosia	Inability to discriminate speech from non-speech sounds
Autotopagnosia	Inability to recognize or point to parts of one's own body, an examiner's, or a visual representation of a body. Anosognosia may include corresponding hemi-autotopagnosia.
Color agnosia	Inability to recognize colors despite intact ability to match or group them
Environmental agnosia	Inability to recognize or give directions to familiar places
Finger agnosia	Inability to recognize fingers
Form agnosia	Inability to recognize objects despite ability to recognize their parts
Phonagnosia	Inability to recognize familiar voices despite intact ability to understand language
Prosopagnosia	Inability to recognize familiar faces
Pure word deafness	Inability to understand spoken language despite intact hearing and otherwise intact language
Simultanagnosia	Inability to recognize the whole of a picture or complex object despite ability to pick out some details
Social-emotional agnosia	Inability to understand body language, facial expressions, or emotional prosody (some overlap with emotional aprosodia and alexithymia) resulting in socially awkward interactions
Visual agnosia	Inability to recognize objects despite otherwise intact vision

oneself, have been associated with migraine and partial seizures. Formication, the tactile hallucination that feels like insects are crawling over one's skin, is seen in stimulant intoxication, substance withdrawal delirium, menopause, Parkinson's disease, and occasionally in B_{12} or folate deficiency states. Olfactory hallucinations are seen in depression and partial seizures, though olfactory hallucinations that last longer than about 3 minutes are unlikely to be seizures. Hypnogogic and hypnopompic hallucinations, representing dysregulated REM sleep, are seen in narcolepsy. Peduncular hallucinosis, in which the patient sees vivid, well-formed images, mostly at night, also tend to occur in the context of sleep disorders that include insomnia and daytime sleepiness. The Lilliputian hallucinations of the so-called Alice in Wonderland syndrome are a form of peduncular hallucinosis. Peduncular hallucinosis occurs in context of thalamic, midbrain, or pontine pathology. The Charles Bonnet syndrome refers to complex visual release hallucinations associated with diminishing vision, often in the elderly. Simple auditory hallucinations of machine like noises are more likely of neurologic origin than are complex hallucinations of voices. Musical hallucinations can be seen in temporal lobe pathology, seizures, migraines, psychiatric disorders, or as release phenomena with diminishing hearing, especially in the elderly. Commentary and command auditory hallucinations are experienced by people with schizophrenia.

Illusions (the misperception of sensory stimuli) are common in migraine sufferers but are also seen in encephalopathy of any etiology. Allochiria, sometimes called allesthesia, the perception of a sensory stimulus applied to one side of the body on the contralateral side, occurs in right parietal lesions. A number of visual illusions, including micropsia, macropsia, teleopsia (illusion of distance), pelopsia (illusion of nearness), metamorphopsia, and chromatopsia, that have been described in migraine also occur in other neurological conditions. Palinopsia refers to visual perseveration or afterimages. The trailing phenomenon is a related visual illusion reported by psychedelic drug users. Hypoacusis and hyperacusis, the perception of auditory stimuli as softer or louder than they are, are common auditory illusions seen in migraine and other disorders. Certain illusions occur in normal individuals. Synesthesia, for example, the involuntary perception of a sensory or cognitive phenomenon when a different sense is stimulated, occurs in roughly 2% of the population.[32] Pareidolia, another common illusion, refers to the perception of a familiar pattern, shape, or sound when looking at or listening to an unfamiliar or ambiguous stimulus.

Insight and Judgment

Insight is best assessed by a person's awareness of their own symptoms and their effect on others. Judgment may be reflected in a patient's approach to their medical treatment, their social behavior, and their ability to appreciate gray areas as opposed to black and white thinking about problems.

Cognitive Status Examination

General Approach to Cognitive Testing

The goal of the "bedside" cognitive examination is for the examiner to form an opinion as to the patient's attention, memory, language, visuospatial, executive, and other related cognitive functions in support of the neuropsychiatric formulation. The examiner forms this opinion based on what has been learned from other aspects of the interview combined with a series of cognitive tasks. In addition, the examiner seeks evidence in the cognitive testing to support hypotheses as to the cause of particular behaviors. For example, a mental health inpatient who always becomes agitated and raises her voice when other patients are agitated and yelling near her may be found to have stimulus bound behavior related to frontal dysfunction or have sensory hypersensitivity related to autism spectrum disorder. A demented patient who gets caught touching things in other people's rooms may have elements of the Klüver-Bucy syndrome. A person with delusional misidentification may be found on visual recall testing to focus on and distort particular details in the diagram. See Box 5-5 for questions the clinician may consider while conducting the cognitive status examination.

It is common practice for psychiatrists and neurologists to substitute a general mental status rating scale for interactive cognitive assessment. General cognitive rating scales such as the Mini-Mental State Examination (MMSE) or the Montreal Cognitive Assessment (MoCA) certainly have their place, as they allow for comparison of findings over time, at different venues, and as a tool in research. However, they are not sufficient to determine the cognitive basis for a patient's complaint or to reach a precise neuropsychiatric diagnosis. Rating scales are covered in more detail later in this chapter.

"Bedside" cognitive assessment refers to interactive testing done by the clinician during any patient encounter. Although not a substitute for formal neuropsychological assessment (see Chapter 6), it is a way to quickly test diagnostic hypotheses during a medical evaluation. It also allows the examiner to ask more focused questions in the referral for neuropsychological testing.

It is incumbent upon the examiner to flexibly apply bedside cognitive status tasks to determine whether there are cognitive deficits related to a patient's complaint. The examiner adapts the tasks to the patient's educational level and to the cognitive complaint. Utilizing a "screen and metric" approach increases examination efficiency, allowing less time to be spent on areas of relative strength and more time on areas of relative deficiency.

BOX 5-5 Questions to Ask Yourself While Performing the Cognitive Examination

Is the patient making a good effort at the tasks?

Are the cognitive deficits consistent?

What are the sources of the patient's errors on cognitive tasks?

Could the psychiatric disorder or the medication be causing the errors?

How strong is the patient's executive function?

What was the patient's executive function prior to the current episode?

What is the cognitive rehabilitation potential of the patient?

For example, a patient who can readily solve a screening shopping problem may not need as much attention to metrics for auditory attention span, executive function, or arithmetic skills. Examples of cognitive screening tasks are given in Table 5-12.

When presenting written tasks to the patient, it is recommended that plain, unlined paper presented in landscape mode be used and that a clean sheet of paper be presented for each task to minimize perseverative errors and errors due to stimulus-bound behavior. When giving a patient oral instructions for any cognitive task the examiner first assures that the patient has "established set" (understands the instructions and that they are expected to do the task). This will minimize misinterpretation of performance errors. Cognitive status assessment is not merely a search for deficits. The examiner not only notes the patient's response to each task, but the nature of the prompts needed to assist the patient in performing the task. These prompts may form the basis of instructions the examiner will later give to the clinical staff who work with the patient.

Convergent findings from different areas of the neurological and cognitive examinations increase the likelihood of dysfunction in the network or anatomic location implicated. For example, poor performance on a construction task does not necessarily indicate right parietal dysfunction. In combination with a left inferior quadrantanopia, however, a compelling case may be made.

Attention

The examiner should determine the subject's level of arousal and attention before proceeding with more complex cognitive tasks in order to avoid findings that mimic specific neurocognitive abnormalities but are solely due to arousal or attention dysfunction. Degree of distractibility should be noted. Perseveration, classically associated with prefrontal dysfunction, may be seen with most other causes of brain dysfunction as well. It is a frequent concomitant of aphasia and can make the language exam difficult. The examiner observes for perseveration during the interview and during all cognitive tasks. Perseverance may be assessed with the "ramparts" task, the "mn" task, or the "multiple loops" task (Figure 5-1).[33] The "mn" and "ramparts" tasks are reciprocal motor programs that emphasize language and visual spatial functions respectively. All three tasks should be presented by the examiner first drawing the target stimuli twice to indicate they are to be repeated. The patient should be instructed to make a copy of the target stimulus beneath it and then continue across the paper without stopping. For the "mn" and "ramparts" tasks the patient should be instructed not to lift the pen from the paper. Observation of the patient's performance may yield additional information about prefrontal function. In the setting of severely stimulus-bound behavior, the patient's pen may be magnetically drawn upward to actually trace the target stimulus or may incorporate a copy of whatever else is above the area of the page on which the drawing is being done. On the multiple loops task, the stimulus-bound patient may draw the number "3" instead of the multiple loops. Some patients with right anterior dysfunction will produce drawings of increasing size or sloping diagonally as they proceed. Perseveration may be continuous, if the patient fails to stop performing the task; stuck in set, if the patient is unable to switch from the last command

TABLE 5-12 • Examples of Bedside Cognitive Screening Tasks.

Task	Instruction	Cognitive Domains Assessed
Complex problem solving (shopping problem)	"How much change should you expect from $5 if you buy 4 packets of nuts at 89¢ per pack?"	Planning, error checking, working memory, arithmetic functions, cognitive estimation, sequencing
2-Finger test	"Hold up the number of fingers on your left hand equal to the order in the alphabet of the first letter of the capital of China."	Attention span, working memory, right/left orientation, auditory comprehension, mental control, general knowledge, praxis
Draw-a-clock task	"Draw a big circle and put in the numbers so it looks like a clock. Then draw the hands so the time is 10 past 11."	Spatial attention, constructional praxis, behavioral independence (freedom from stimulus-bound behavior), working memory, planning
Complex figure task	Copy a complex asymmetric figure. Remove drawings and then draw the figure from memory immediately. Remove drawing and draw from memory again at 15 minutes. (Reproduced with permission from Benjamin S, Lauterbach M. *The Brain Card*®. 3rd ed. Newton, MA: Brain Educators LLC; 2016.)	Nonverbal recall, spatial attention, constructional praxis, behavioral independence
Brooks E	Show the patient a block capital letter E with an x and upward arrow at lower left as in the drawing below. Remove the drawing and ask the subject to indicate each right or left turn needed to return to the starting point. Correct response: R R R L L R R L L R R R (R=right; L=left) (Reproduced with permission from Benjamin S, Lauterbach M. *The Brain Card*®. 3rd ed. Newton, MA: Brain Educators LLC; 2016.)	Visual-spatial memory, right/left orientation, mental rotation, visual-spatial working memory

to the new command; or recurrent, if the patient returns to a task command given earlier in the examination.[34] If perseveration is noted, the examiner may need to adjust the order of the examination or change to a different type of task (e.g., change from written to oral responses) to "deblock" the patient in order to obtain the best response, especially for the aphasia exam.

There are several ways to assess for hemispatial inattention, which can result in poor performance on the affected side. One can simply ask the patient to look straight ahead and describe the things she sees around her in the room, noting if fewer details are noticed on one side. The line bisection task is another simple method of assessing hemispatial attention. Draw a horizontal line across an entire sheet of paper presented in landscape mode and ask the patient to bisect it.

Displacement of the bisection point to one side of the paper may indicate contralateral hemianopia or hemineglect. The Albert line bisection task assesses spatial attention in more detail.[35] Forty straight 2.5 cm lines are drawn at random angles on a piece of plain white paper in landscape orientation. The examiner demonstrates how to cross a single horizontal line placed in the middle of the paper and the patient is asked to place a short line through the middle of each of the other lines. Quadrantic or hemi-inattention may both be detected with this method.

Attention span is a determinant of how much information the examiner can convey to the patient at once. In non-aphasic individuals it may be assessed by determining the number of digits a person can repeat. In intellectually neurotypical

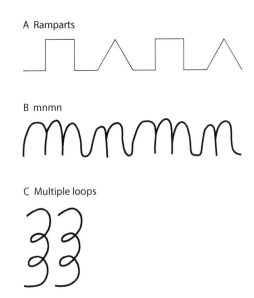

A Ramparts

B mnmn

C Multiple loops

FIGURE 5-1. **Perseverance tasks.** Present unlined paper in landscape mode. Instruct patient to copy the drawing below the example then continue drawing it over and over without removing pen from paper (**A, B**) or until told to stop (**A, B, C**). (Reproduced with permission from Benjamin S, Lauterbach M. *The Brain Card*®. 3rd ed. Newton, MA: Brain Educators LLC; 2016.)

J R G A T A X D K H I A O L J E A A U S P M B A Z
C T A V E N A T E D S R A Y U E K L S I E H A W L

FIGURE 5-2. **Auditory continuous performance task.** The examiner reads the following list of letters at an even pace instructing the patient to tap the table whenever the letter, A, is heard.

Memory

Memory impairment may be caused by deficient memory storage or recall, impaired attention, or psychological factors. Impaired attention may be due to a large number of factors including brain dysfunction, sleep disorders, metabolic disorders, substance or medication use, psychiatric disorders, or other causes. Therefore, comprehensive cognitive assessment is indicated for memory complaints. Memory assessment begins from the moment the examiner encounters the patient. If memory problems are suspected, the examiner may introduce herself by associating her name with a phonemic or category cue to facilitate later inquiry as to whether the patient remembers the examiner's name. The examiner will have already compared the history related by the patient to that in the chart and will know if the patient can recall things said earlier in the interview. Difficulty recalling recent personal or news events may indicate problems with either memory or attention. Recall tasks should be adjusted to estimated intellect and, if appropriate, may be associated with category cues when words for later recall are given. For example, the examiner could tell the patient, "I'd like you to remember the flower, daisy; the address, 50 Belmont Street; and the color, teal." Verbal and nonverbal recall are assessed with both immediate and delayed recall conditions to assess both verbal and visual-spatial memory networks and to help separate inattention from memory deficits. Verbal recall may be done with three, four, or five stimuli. I typically use four, avoiding the use of easily visualized objects for more than one of the stimuli. For example, one can include a color, a member of an object category (e.g., a particular type of flower), an address (with both number and street name), and an intangible word, such as a feeling or value. The number of repetitions required for the subject to register the four items and repeat them back correctly is noted. After teaching the stimuli to this criterion, the number recalled spontaneously at 5 and 15 minutes, and the number produced when given category cues or phonemic cues (if necessary) are noted. If cued recall is incorrect, the patient may be read or shown a list of 10 words and asked to select the ones that were in the original list. Poor spontaneous recall with improved performance on selecting from a word list is seen in frontal-subcortical retrieval-type memory deficits. Perseveration, intrusions, confabulation, or inconsistency is also noted when testing recall.

Nonverbal recall is tested by having the patient copy an asymmetric figure containing distinct external shape and internal details (e.g., see Table 5-12), then removing the stimulus and

individuals begin with seven digits forward and add or subtract digits as needed. Then ask the patient to recite the digits provided by the examiner in reverse order. Reversed digit span is typically about two digits less than forward digit span. In the presence of aphasia or other language impairment, an object pointing span may be used as a measure of attention span. Place five objects (e.g., pen, paperclip, key, comb, coin) on a table and verify that the patient can identify them. Cover the objects with a piece of plain paper and say (or indicate) "when I take away the paper point to the objects in the order I say them" and establish how many objects the person can point to.

Reverse digit span is one measure of working memory, the temporary storage of information needed to complete a task. Other working memory tasks in order from simple to more complex include counting backward from 20, reciting the days of the week in reverse, reciting the months of the year in reverse, alphabetizing the letters in EARTH, or reciting the alphabet backward. The Oral Trails B task, in which the subject is asked to orally alternate letters and numbers beginning with A-1 until reaching the number 13, is another measure of working memory.[36] A more complex working memory task that includes elements of vigilance and executive function is to ask the patient to recite all of the letters of the alphabet that rhyme with "key" or all of the capital block letters that have curves in them, if a visual spatial element is desired.

Auditory vigilance is assessed with a continuous performance task. The examiner reads a long list of letters such as that in Figure 5-2 and instructs the patient to tap the table whenever she hears the letter, A. Decreased auditory vigilance may occur in decreased attention due to a number of causes including metabolic, drug-induced, disorders of excessive daytime sleepiness, delirium, and others.

having the patient draw the figure from immediate recall and at 5 and 15 minutes. The productions are compared to determine whether missing details were already missing at immediate recall implying an attention problem, or whether the details were only lost on later recall, implying a memory problem. If a person is unable to copy or draw, nonverbal recall may be assessed by the hidden objects task. The examiner "hides" three objects within or under items in the patient's immediate surroundings in full view of the patient, and then asks the patient what has been hidden and where. Immediate and delayed recall are again assessed.

Assuming intact arousal and attention, reciting the names of presidents of the country in reverse order gives a rough estimate of the temporal gradient of a patient's recall. In Korsakoff's psychosis, an abrupt falloff in memory may be traced to a particular era with further inquiry concerning historical events in past decades. People with Alzheimer's disease may have some recall of distant historical facts but fewer and fewer approaching the present day.

More detailed bedside assessment of learning and retention can be done with a supraspan word list learning task.[33] The patient is read a list of 12 words at a rate of about one per second. The patient is asked to recall the words immediately while the examiner notes the order in which they are recalled by placing numbers on a chart (Figure 5-3). The list is read three more times in succession, each time noting the patient's responses on the chart. Delayed recall is assessed 15 minutes later following distraction. By choosing words from three categories, later memory consolidation may be assessed. Normal individuals can recall about six words on initial presentation. Most neurologically impaired individuals, with the exception of people with Korsakoff psychosis or other complete anterograde amnesia, demonstrate at least some learning over the four trials. Normal individuals have a primacy and recency effect, recalling the initial and final words of a list most easily. Memory impaired individuals do not show the primacy effect. People with attention deficit may recall different words on each trial. People with Alzheimer's disease recall few words on the first trial and improve only modestly over all trials, with little word recall after the 15-minute filled delay. Demonstration of a verbal learning curve (the ability to recall an increased number of words over the four trials) at the bedside, regardless of the degree of brain dysfunction, indicates that the patient may be able to benefit from psychotherapy or cognitive rehabilitation strategies. To further explore a memory complaint, the examiner may employ a paired associate learning task or a story recall task. Paired associate learning involves presenting the patient with several "easy" word pairs (e.g., book-page) and several "hard" word pairs (e.g., cabbage-elephant). The examiner then gives one word and the patient is asked to recall the paired associate word. Story recall involves reading the patient a few sentence "story" containing a known number of facts. The patient is asked to recall the story and the number of facts correctly recalled is recorded.

Fund of Knowledge

Fund of knowledge is a measure of crystallized intelligence, composed of facts, understanding, and experience that a person has accumulated through life. Examples include the freezing or

Name_____

Record Number_____

Date_____

Supraspan Auditory Learning Curve

Read these words at about one word/second and ask the patient to recall as many words as possible. Repeat the list 4 times, and again at 15 minutes. Note the order of words recalled by putting numbers (1–12) in the boxes. For 15 minute recall, offer category cues only if needed.

	Trial 1	Trial 2	Trial 3	Trial 4	15 min delay
Violet					
Saxophone					
Airplane					
Train					
Piano					
Orange					
Crimson					
Helicopter					
Steamship					
Flute					
Silver					
Trombone					
TOTAL					

FIGURE 5-3. 12-Word supraspan learning task. (Reproduced with permission from Benjamin S, Lauterbach M. *The Brain Card®*. 3rd ed. Newton, MA: Brain Educators LLC; 2016.)

boiling points of water, the number of cards in a deck, the reason white clothing is cooler than dark clothing in the summer, and how rust forms.

Language

The language examination is undertaken to determine if aphasia is present and to ascertain that delirium, dysarthria, or psychiatric disorders are not the cause of the language abnormality. The examiner should form an initial opinion as to the presence of aphasia based on conversation with the patient. Note is made of melodic line, phrase length, vocabulary, word finding problems, and paraphasic errors in spontaneous speech. The eight most frequently occurring aphasias can be specified by observing three parameters: fluency, auditory comprehension, and repetition (Figure 5-4). Short phrase length, effortful quality, and difficulty in articulation characterize nonfluent aphasias, while superficially intact sentence structure, ease of production, and normal articulation are seen in fluent aphasias. Paraphasic errors are described as verbal or semantic, when a real word is substituted for the intended word; and literal or phonemic, when the substitution is a non-sense word often beginning with the same phoneme as the intended word. Apraxia of speech refers to slow,

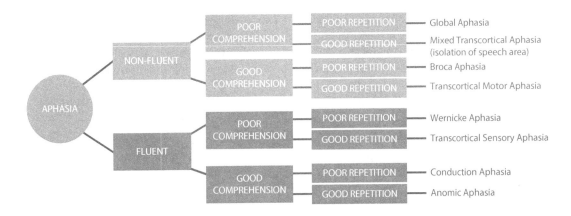

FIGURE 5-4. **The aphasias.**

poorly articulated, dysprosodic, or distorted speech due to brain damage. The script generation task can help elicit a sample of spontaneous speech to assess language function. In script generation, the patient is asked to describe all of the steps in a common task (e.g., changing a tire or making scrambled eggs). The examiner may also note evidence of executive dysfunction manifested as listing steps in incorrect order during script generation.

Auditory comprehension may be assessed by giving a three-step crossed command, such as "close your eyes and touch your left shoulder twice with your right hand." The Marie 3 Paper task also assesses auditory comprehension with additional stress on attention span and working memory. The patient is given three pieces of paper and told, "crumple the large piece and toss it on the floor, hand me the medium sized piece, and place the small piece in your pocket."

Word finding problems are assessed using naming and verbal fluency tasks. Confrontation naming consists of pointing to the relevant item and asking the patient to name body parts, objects, parts of objects, colors, and actions that occur at high and low frequency in language. Responsive naming involves the examiner describing an object and asking the patient to name it. Word list generation is a measure of verbal fluency. Phonemic or letter fluency is assessed by asking the patient to name all of the words they can think of in 1 minute that begin with a given letter of the alphabet. Avoiding the letters f, a, and s may be helpful since verbal fluency is assessed using these letters in formal neuropsychological testing. Using the letter "b" with the instruction to avoid using names that begin with a capital B works well. To assess category fluency, ask the patient to name all of the members of a given category he can think of (e.g., animals, items in a grocery store, etc.). It is helpful to specify they can begin with any letter if phonemic fluency was recently assessed. When recording the generated word lists, the examiner writes down the words listed by the patient marking 15-second intervals. Frontal-subcortical pathology may result in a patient exhausting his/her ability to list words in the first 15 or 20 seconds. A patient with executive dysfunction might benefit from the increased structure of the category fluency task compared to phonemic fluency. Word list generation also provides information on self-monitoring (repeated words), rule following, and use of creative strategies. A high school graduate

of average intelligence can usually produce 12 words in a phonemic task and 18 words in a category task.

Repetition ability is assessed by having the patient repeat progressively more complex phrases, including tongue twisters (e.g., "seventy-seven benevolent elephants") and sentences laden with functor words that express syntactic relationships, connections, or modify nouns or verbs (e.g., "no ifs, ands, or buts about it"). These types of sentences are particularly challenging for people with non-fluent aphasias. Oral reading and reading comprehension are best assessed by having the patient read a paragraph (e.g., from a magazine) and explain what they read. Gathering a writing sample allows the examiner to assess for aphasia by looking for similar deficits to those in running speech, with the addition of noting spelling errors. Suggesting the patient focus her sentence on something related to her treatment can be helpful.

Paralinguistic Functions

The paralinguistic functions of emotional prosody; and comprehension of idiom, pun, and sarcasm require intact right hemisphere networks in addition to left hemisphere language functions. Gestural, intrinsic (the rhythm of speech such as that indicated by punctuation), and guttural (nonverbal sounds that convey meaning) prosody are left hemisphere functions. To assess spontaneous emotional prosody, ask the patient to say an intrinsically neutral sentence (e.g., "I am going to the movies") as if they are angry, sad, happy, and surprised. Then the examiner stands out of sight of the patient and asks the patient to identify the examiner's emotion as he/she says a neutral sentence as if angry, sad, happy, or surprised. Emotional prosodic repetition can also be tested. Assessment of comprehension of idiom, pun, and sarcasm requires culturally appropriate stimuli and are difficult to assess in someone of a different culture or who requires an interpreter. For native English speakers, idiomatic comprehension can be assessed by asking what is meant by expressions such as "back seat driver," "cry wolf," or "go cold turkey." The ability to decode pun, sarcasm, and double-entendre is an aspect of lexical processing that relates to humor comprehension. The examiner can ask the patient to explain a joke such as: "What did the mayonnaise jar say to the refrigerator?" "Shut the door, I'm dressing"; or "Did you hear about the fellow who swallowed the spoon?" "He didn't stir." The ability to decode sarcasm requires analysis of context in addition to denotative meaning. The examiner might, for example, tell the patient: "I told my partner I would have to miss our daughter's birthday party due to being on-call for the hospital," and he said, "Great, you're missing another family event." "How did my partner feel about my being on call that day?" Failure to comprehend the paralinguistic aspects of language places one at a tremendous disadvantage. The paralinguistic functions are components of pragmatics, the use of language in social context. Pragmatic deficits can occur in the setting of right hemisphere dysfunction, intellectual disability, autism spectrum disorder, and other conditions. In some cases, they can lead to reinforcement of paranoid ideas in addition to causing social dysfunction.

Praxis

Apraxia refers to the inability to plan and carry out a motor command despite intact comprehension, muscle strength, and coordination. Patients with ideomotor apraxia can explain a movement but cannot act it out or pretend they are doing it. In ideational apraxia, the patient cannot perform a complex motor act in correct sequence despite being able to perform parts of the task correctly in isolation. Praxis is assessed with buccofacial, axial, and limb commands. Buccofacial commands include asking the patient to pretend to blow out a match, sniff a flower, or cough. Axial commands include asking the patient to assume a boxing stance or pretend to swing a golf club. Limb praxis commands may be gestural ("pretend to stop traffic" or "wave goodbye") or transitive (pretend to use a tool such as screwdriver, toothbrush, or comb). A common error in ideomotor apraxia is to use a body part as the object (e.g., pretend to brush teeth with finger instead of an imaginary toothbrush). Apraxia tends to occur in left hemisphere lesions, especially in association with aphasia.

Constructional Praxis

Like other apraxias, constructional apraxia involves the inability to draw simple shapes despite intact comprehension and motor function. Common bedside tests of constructional praxis include figure copying, clock drawing, drawing a three-dimensional cube or a simple house in perspective (showing the front and one side), and design fluency. Copying an asymmetric figure (Table 5-12) for assessment of nonverbal recall (above) also yields information about constructional praxis, hemiattention, and learning style. The clock drawing task (Table 5-12) is an excellent screen not only for construction ability, but for hemispatial attention and executive function as well. Design fluency is also a measure of constructional ability and executive function. Similar to verbal fluency, there is an unstructured and a structured version. The patient is instructed to draw as many simple objects as possible in 1 minute in the unstructured task (normally three to four). For the structured task, the patient is asked to make as many designs as possible in 1 minute using four straight lines (normally five).[37]

Calculation

Orally presented arithmetic problems are not as straightforward as they might seem. Attention, recall, and working memory as well as arithmetic skills are required to solve oral problems. Doing simple arithmetic problems on paper avoids some of these issues. Spatial acalculia may impair oral or written performance when the patient must align digits, carry, or maintain the structure of a problem to solve it. Arithmetic functions per se are generally localized to the left hemisphere. Spatial acalculia, however, implies right hemisphere dysfunction. Working memory and attention may be affected in a variety of conditions. To assess for spatial acalculia, the examiner asks the patient to add, subtract, multiply, or divide two- to four-digit numbers using unlined paper.

Right/Left, Spatial and Topographic Orientation, Finger Gnosis

After establishing that the patient knows their own right and left hands, the examiner gives a crossed command as part of an auditory comprehension test, such as "Tap your left shoulder twice with your right hand," or "point to my right hand." Topographic orientation requires familiarity by both examiner and patient of a topographic area being visualized. In a hospitalized patient, for example, the examiner may establish topographic orientation by asking for directions from the patient's bedroom to the nursing station. Alternatively, the patient may be asked to draw a rough floor plan of their home if a partner can provide their own drawing for comparison. Another approach to assessment of topographic localization is to present the patient with an outline of a map of the country, ask them to label the compass directions, then to locate major cities or geographic features, including cities in all four quadrants. The patient may then be asked to indicate what direction one would travel to go from one labeled city to another. For this and other tasks, it is important to remember that the patient's educational background and fund of knowledge may impact her/his performance. A more complex screening test of spatial orientation involving right/left sense, mental rotation, visual recall, and visual-spatial working memory is the Brooks E task (Table 5-12).[38] The patient is shown a block capital letter B with an x and a short upward arrow at the lower left corner. The drawing is then taken away and the patient is asked to list all of the turns necessary (there are 12) to return to the starting point, by saying R, R, R, L, etc. as shown in Table 5-12. In the event of difficulty with this screening task, the examiner follows up with tests of visual recall, right/left orientation, and working memory as needed. Finger orientation is the most frequently disturbed body part orientation symptom. Finger orientation is assessed by naming the finger being pointed to and pointing to the finger being named. Finger agnosia, a component of Gerstmann's syndrome, is diagnosed only if both hands are affected and a unilateral sensory deficit is absent. It may be due to dysfunction in either hemisphere but occurs most often in left hemisphere dysfunction.

Prefrontal and Executive Functions

The complex problem solving or shopping problem task (Table 5-12) may be used as a screening test for prefrontal executive function. Solving it requires planning, working memory, sequencing, cognitive estimation, error checking, and basic arithmetic. If the patient is unable to solve the problem orally the examiner proceeds to assess its component functions to determine the source of error. Individual components of prefrontal and executive functions are easily examined at the bedside. Cognitive estimation may be assessed by asking the patient to guess the height of the examination room ceiling or the length of the average person's spine. Inhibition and motor regulation may be tested using reciprocal motor programs and the go/no-go task. After establishing set for an imitation task in which the patient is asked to copy the examiner by holding up either one or two fingers when the examiner does, the examiner instructs the patient to do the opposite of what she/he does, holding up two fingers if the examiner holds up one and one finger if the examiner holds up two. Once set is established for this reciprocal motor program, the examiner converts to the go/no-go task by explaining that the patient should continue to hold up two fingers when the examiner holds up one, but refrain from holding up any fingers at all when the examiner holds up two fingers ("no-go"). Errors of omission and commission are noted.

Cognitive flexibility, which is associated with empathy and creativity,[39] can be assessed with the alternate uses, inferential reasoning, and headline tasks. The alternate uses task is an indicator of divergent thinking or the ability to come up with novel solutions to real-life problems, such as being locked out of one's apartment. The patient is asked to name all of the uses they can think of for a common object (e.g., a paper clip or a toothpick). Normal individuals can generate at least 10 uses in 3 minutes.[40] Inferential reasoning and conceptual flexibility may also be assessed by telling the patient: "Sally took pen and spiral notebook to meet the famous athlete. What do you think she planned to do?" After the patient responds the examiner may then say: "The article was to include the opinions of famous people about global warming. Now what do you think was Sally's plan?" Another approach to the assessment of cognitive flexibility that also gets at connotative reasoning is the "Headline Test" in which the examiner presents the patient with a double-entendre headline such as "Red Tape Holds Up New Bridge" or "Thief Gets Two Years in Violin Case" and asks the patient to explain the story that might have gone with that headline.[41] A patient who immediately comprehends the double-entendre will generally smile and explain that the headline is funny because of the double-meaning, while a person who relies primarily on left hemisphere strategies will work through the meaning in serial order before realizing the humor in it. A related task is conceptual series completion, in which the patient is asked to fill in the blank to complete a series ranging from simple to difficult. An example of a simple conceptual series problem is: AZ BY CX D__.

The capacity for abstract reasoning is typically assessed with the proverbs and similarities tasks, though the headline task and the assessment of paralinguistic functions (above) assess related areas of cognitive flexibility and connotative reasoning. Like all cognitive tasks the examiner ascertains that the patient has established set before proceeding with the task. This can be accomplished by saying: "We sometimes use expressions to teach lessons. For instance, have you ever heard the expression, don't cry over spilled milk?" Having established that the patient is able to provide an abstract explanation for simple proverbs, the examiner then asks for an interpretation of a more difficult proverb, such as: "One swallow doesn't make a summer" or "The golden hammer breaks the iron door." Since proverbs are dependent upon language fluency and cultural reference, this task is best used with native English speakers. However, common proverbs from other countries may be found on creativeproverbs.com. In the similarities task the patient is asked how two things are alike, beginning with simpler concepts (e.g., apple and orange) and moving to more abstract associations (e.g., watch and ruler, tree and fly). If the patient is slow to grasp what is meant by the task command, the examiner can say: "Into what category could the following items be placed?"

Sequencing is a basic function of the prefrontal cortex. Motor sequencing is assessed using the Luria-3-Step task, in which the patient is asked to mimic the examiner in performing three hand positions: fist, side, flat. The examiner demonstrates the move three times and then asks the patient to do it with their right then left hands. If the patient is unable, the examiner can describe the three positions using action words while demonstrating them: "knock, chop, slap." If three positions appear too complex for the patient, the examiner decreases to two positions by asking the patient to alternately make a fist and then a ring with their thumb and third finger. Verbal sequencing can be assessed by presenting the patient with cards containing the words: right, hand, change, the, him; or: police, car, found, the, alert; and asking them to unscramble the sentence. (If you've not yet solved it, the answers are "Hand him the right change" and "Alert police found the car.") Nonverbal sequencing can be assessed at the bedside as well if one has a series of picture cards that tell a story if arranged correctly.

Another basic prefrontal function is the capacity for independent behavior. Behavior that is entirely dictated by the most salient stimulus to which a person is exposed is called stimulus-bound behavior. Failure of behavioral independence may manifest in echopraxia or utilization behavior. If the examiner suspects echopraxia he/she first places a finger over closed lips to indicate silence, then extends his/her hands above the head, crosses arms, or assumes other postures to see if the patient mimics the examiner. The examination for utilization behavior is a bit more nuanced. The examiner places various objects on the table between examiner and patient prior to bringing the patient into the room. The most salient objects would be those related to the patient's occupation, though common objects like notebook and pen, glasses, or smartphone could be used. Utilization behavior describes the situation that occurs if the patient picks up the objects and starts to use them unbidden during the interview.

Rating Scales

Rating scales, typically employed in clinical trials, are also useful in generating objective data for comparison of symptoms and signs across multiple examinations. A very large number of such scales exist. It is helpful, however, to become familiar with an exemplar for the common disorders examined by neuropsychiatrists. A list of commonly used scales is given in Table 5-13. When utilizing rating scales in the medical record the examiner should select those readily available in the medical literature or freely available without royalty.

TABLE 5-13 • Useful Rating Scales for Neuropsychiatric Assessment.	
Disorder	Rating Scale
ADHD	Adult ADHD Self-Report Scale[42]
ADHD	Conners Scale[43]
Aggression	Overt Aggression Scale (OAS)[44]
Anxiety	Hamilton Anxiety Scale (HAM-A)[45]
Catatonia	Bush-Francis Catatonia Rating Scale (BFCRS)[22]
Dementia	Blessed Dementia Scale[46]
Dementia	Dementia Severity Rating Scale[47]
Dementia/MCI screen	Montreal Cognitive Assessment (MoCA)[48]
Depression	Hamilton Depression Scale (HAM-D)[49]
Depression	Patient Health Questionnaire (PHQ-9)[50]
Drug-induced dyskinesia	Abnormal Involuntary Movement Scale (AIMS)[20]
Excessive daytime sleepiness	Epworth Sleepiness Scale[51]
Frontal lobe dysfunction	Frontal Assessment Battery (FAB)[52]
Multiple sclerosis	Expanded Disability Status Scale (EDSS)[53]
Obsessive compulsive disorder	Yale-Brown Obsessive-Compulsive Scale (Y-BOCS)[54]
Parkinson's disease	Unified Parkinson's Disease Rating Scale (UPDRS)[55]
Psychiatric symptoms in dementia	Neuropsychiatric Inventory (NPI)[56]
Psychosis	Brief Psychiatric Rating Scale (BPRS)[57]
Traumatic brain injury	Rancho Los Amigos Scale[58]

ANCILLARY DIAGNOSTIC TESTING

Having completed the relevant parts of the neuropsychiatric examination, the examiner plans a relevant and targeted evaluation with selected ancillary tests. These may include structural neuroimaging, functional neuroimaging, neurovascular imaging, electrophysiologic testing, routine blood, urine and/or cerebrospinal fluid testing, autoantibody testing, genetic testing, and/or neuropsychological testing. With the wealth of modalities readily available to most clinicians, it becomes increasingly important to practice cost-effective medicine. Unless the testing is being ordered to follow the progress of a known condition, the neuropsychiatrist should always have a diagnostic hypothesis and preferably have reduced the differential diagnosis to a binary decision before ordering specialized testing. To minimize the chances of the patient being unable to complete the desired testing, it is imperative to prepare the patient in advance by providing a detailed explanation of the procedure. A brief guide to the use of ancillary tests in neuropsychiatry follows. Detailed discussion of each modality is beyond the scope of this chapter. Please see Chapter 6 for further information about the use of neuroimaging in clinical neuropsychiatry.

Structural Neuroimaging

Structural brain imaging techniques commonly used include computed tomography (CT) and magnetic resonance imaging (MRI). Selection of the appropriate modality flows directly from the diagnostic question. A list of frequent clinical presentations, diagnostic questions, and usual structural imaging modality is given in Table 5-14. Cranial CT imaging is adequate for ruling out bleeding, cerebral calcifications, or skull fracture, is typically used in acute stroke and TBI, and is the preferred structural imaging modality for patients who are unable to remain motionless in an MRI scanner for at least 30 minutes. A quick CT image that gives a reasonable view of the anatomy may be preferred over an MRI image severely degraded by patient movement. However, assuming a patient is able to remain motionless in the scanner, MRI imaging is the preferred modality for most neuropsychiatric questions, and especially for posterior fossa, temporal lobe, and inferior frontal pathology where the proximity of bony surfaces results in artifacts that can obscure small lesions on CT. In addition, careful consideration should be given to the use of iodine contrast, taking allergies, renal function, and hydration status into account. MRI imaging is also strongly preferred for diagnosis of white matter pathology, and in women of child-bearing age since no ionizing radiation is used. In an acute or emergent situation, consider using sedation to obtain the MRI if the patient is uncooperative. The American College of Radiology Appropriateness Criteria provides a helpful guide to imaging modality selection.[59] Following a 1-year pilot, by January 2021 Medicare payment for imaging will be contingent upon compliance with these criteria. It is always a good idea to speak with the neuroradiologist when ordering neuroimaging if there are any questions.

CT and MR images are generated quite differently. The CT scanner contains a rotating x-ray source and an array of gamma detectors 180 degrees opposite. A number of images are obtained as the source and detectors rotate around the patient's head, and the x-y coordinates of each imaging voxel along with the amount of attenuation with each detection are used to construct the CT image. Iodine contrast is used to find interruptions in the blood-brain barrier. The MR image is obtained by placing the patient in a very strong magnetic field (the reason one must not take ferro-metallic objects into the scanner room) that causes protons to align with the field, then using a radio frequency pulse generator to excite the protons and move them perpendicular to the magnetic field. The MR image is a map of the energy released by the protons as they relax back into a state parallel to the magnetic field. Gadolinium contrast is used to identify recent ischemic deficits, and to evaluate pathology such as brain tumor and demyelination. There are many different types of MR images created by measuring the energy released after exciting the protons. The T1 image is similar to a CT image in that water is black. Water appears white in T2 images. The T1 image is best suited for defining anatomy while the T2 image is best for showing pathology since this typically involves abnormal water distribution. Many other image

TABLE 5-14 • Selection of Clinical Neuroimaging Method.

Clinical Presentation	Diagnostic Question	Neuroimaging Method
Acute symptoms		
Acute traumatic brain injury (TBI)	Are there fractures, subdural or epidural hematomas, intracerebral hemorrhages, subarachnoid hemorrhages, or contusions?	I⁻ CT
Recent TBI with loss of consciousness and focal neurobehavioral syndrome but normal initial CT/MRI	Is there evidence of diffuse (traumatic) axonal injury (DAI)?	MRI with GRE, SWAN, or SWI images to facilitate detection of iron in blood breakdown products from axonal injury
Delirium with focal signs	Rule out mass lesion, vascular pathology, hemorrhagic lesions, increased intracranial pressure	I⁻ CT if acute MRI (G⁺) if chronic
Acute onset seizures or movement disorder, with amnestic syndrome	Rule out autoimmune limbic encephalitis (hippocampal enhancement on FLAIR images)	MRI with dedicated seizure protocol
Acute febrile illness with seizures, amnestic syndrome	Rule out herpes (or other) encephalitis	MRI with dedicated seizure protocol
Acute cortical neurologic deficits	Rule out stroke or metastasis and evaluate for TPA treatment	CT (I⁻) and CTA. CT perfusion if penumbra assessment is needed (for delayed endovascular treatment). MRI for best stroke assessment and lesion identification Abbreviated hyperacute stroke MRI if needed
Remote or chronic symptoms		
Remote head injury	Is there focal atrophy or arachnoid cyst suggestive of prior hemorrhage?	MRI
Remote head injury with deterioration	Has hydrocephalus developed?	MRI or CT (MRI offers better visualization of the aqueduct)
Frontal lobe syndrome of unknown etiology	Rule out focal frontal pathology (vascular, remote trauma, tumor, FTD)	MRI (G⁺ if deterioration has occurred) If unable to lie still, I⁺ CT
Partial seizures	Rule out focal cortical pathology, evidence of past temporal lobe damage (focal atrophy), mesial temporal sclerosis, or heterotopias	MRI with dedicated seizure protocol (including coronal T1, T2, FLAIR images), preferably on a 3T magnet
Dementia with history of stroke	Rule out vascular dementia, small vessel disease (white matter), or combined AD and vascular dementia	MRI If unable to lie still, CT
Dementia of unknown origin	Rule out hydrocephalus, basal ganglia disease, vascular disease, tumor, focal atrophy consistent with FTD or AD, white matter diseases	MRI If unable to lie still, I⁺ CT
Multiple lesions in time and space	Rule out demyelinating disease, vasculitides, etc.	MRI with gadolinium
Dyskinesia	Rule out Huntington's or other basal ganglia disease	MRI or CT (MRI better for degenerative basal ganglia diseases with metal deposition)
Specific (focal) learning disorder	Rule out congenital hemispheric damage (also see developmental disability)	MRI If unable to lie still, CT
Developmental disability with seizures, developmental regression, microcephaly, macrocephaly, dysmorphic features, or neurocutaneous signs	Rule out agenesis of the corpus callosum, pachygyria, polymicrogyria, Dandy-Walker syndrome, cortical dysplasia, hydrocephalus, aqueductal stenosis, Arnold-Chiari malformation, neurocutaneous syndromes, arachnoid cysts, vascular malformations, evidence of congenital stroke, leukodystrophies	MRI
Pseudobulbar palsy	Rule out bilateral lesions of brainstem and/or hemispheres	MRI

(continued)

TABLE 5-14 • Selection of Clinical Neuroimaging Method. (*continued*)

Clinical Presentation	Diagnostic Question	Neuroimaging Method
AIDS with neurological deterioration	Rule out focal abscess, tumor, progressive multifocal leukoencephalopathy (PML)	MRI (G$^+$)
Psychosis with signs of neurodevelopmental disorder or dysmorphic features	See developmental disability above	MRI

CT, Computed tomography; CTA, CT angiogram; FLAIR, fluid attenuated inversion recovery; G$^+$, gadolinium enhanced; GRE, gradient recalled echo; I$^-$, non-contrast; MRI, magnetic resonance imaging; SWAN, 3D T2 star weighted angiography method used in GE scanners; SWI, susceptibility weighted imaging used in Siemens scanners.

sequences are commonly used, with fluid attenuated inversion recovery (FLAIR) being the most common as it represents a compromise between demonstrating pathology while preserving anatomy. CT angiography and MR angiography are often used in the evaluation of acute stroke, vasculitis, and as part of planning for endovascular treatment. Detailed discussion of vascular imaging is beyond the scope of this chapter, however. Patients must be carefully screened for metallic objects prior to MR imaging and the referring clinician must provide the exact make and model of any indwelling cerebral implants.

Diffusion tensor imaging (DTI) is an MRI technique that exploits the behavior of the hydrogen protons in water to allow imaging of white matter. DTI creates images of white matter by determining the protons that are aligned in nerve fibers (anisotropy) versus those randomly positioned in the extracellular space (isotropy). DTI images are readily available and are studied extensively in traumatic axonal injury, ischemia, demyelination, and other white matter diseases. However, DTI is not yet a standard clinical diagnostic modality. The clinician should be wary that DTI and MRI methodology used in neurobehavioral research may be associated with methodological issues that could result in false positive and false negative studies.[60]

Functional Neuroimaging

Functional images may be obtained by using radioactive tracers (SPECT and PET imaging) or exploiting the natural difference between oxygenated and deoxygenated blood to obtain BOLD (blood oxygen level determination) images. BOLD fMRI images are used either to demonstrate areas of increased or decreased blood flow during cognitive or motor tasks, or to obtain resting state functional data, and are used mainly in behavioral and cognitive research paradigms. Currently, the only clinically approved uses for fMRI are in presurgical evaluation of epileptic foci and brain tumors.

Single photon emission computed tomography (SPECT) and positron emission tomography (PET) are often used in the differential diagnosis of dementia since early AD presents with decreased posterior blood flow on SPECT or posterior hypometabolism on FDG-PET, while a patient with FTD would be expected to show anterior hypoperfusion or hypometabolism. These techniques may be useful in differentiating early AD from depression since depression may cause decreased frontal perfusion if it does affect the image. They would not be as useful for differentiating FTD from depression, however, for this reason.

Functional imaging is also used in preoperative localization of partial complex seizures in the temporal lobe. The combination of interictal hypometabolism or hypoperfusion and ictal hypermetabolism or hyperperfusion provides presumptive localization data. Cerebral PET is also used to assess tumor activity. Though not formally recognized as a clinical indication, the identification of focal hypoperfusion (SPECT) or hypometabolism (PET) may provide anatomic correlation of clinically identified focal neurobehavioral syndromes.

Electrophysiologic Testing

Common electrophysiologic testing modalities used in neuropsychiatric evaluation include electroencephalography (EEG), long-term EEG monitoring with video EEG telemetry (LTM), magnetoencephalography (MEG), evoked potentials (EPs), polysomnography (PSG), and the multiple sleep latency test (MSLT). Electronystagmography (ENG), electromyography (EMG), and nerve conduction velocity (NCV) are beyond the scope of this chapter.

EEG is primarily used to assess encephalopathies and seizure disorders. It can aid in the differential diagnosis of paroxysmal neurological disorders, in distinguishing partial from generalized epilepsies, and in helping determine the safety of stopping an anti-epileptic medication. In the case of seizure disorders, an EEG positive for interictal epileptiform discharges (IEDs) is suggestive but may not be diagnostic since ultimately it is the tendency to have recurrent seizures that defines epilepsy, and a small percentage of normal individuals may have IEDs. Similarly, the absence of seizures during an EEG recording does not rule out seizure disorder. EEG has relatively low sensitivity in epilepsy but higher specificity. Sleep deprivation prior to the EEG increases the likelihood of seizure detection during transition to sleep. Three sleep-deprived EEGs are sufficient to identify most seizure disorders but 10% of seizures will remain EEG negative. IEDs are found in about half of people with epilepsy on the first EEG. IED's include interictal spikes, polyspikes, sharp waves, and paroxysmal sharp and slow waves.

The gold standard for diagnosing psychogenic nonepileptic seizures (PNES) is LTM with video EEG monitoring. Observation of an EEG-negative convulsive event may indicate PNES, assuming other causes such as arrhythmia are eliminated. The presence of a normal resting alpha rhythm immediately after a convulsive seizure is also suggestive of PNES. Another frequently available form of LTM, ambulatory EEG monitoring, may be helpful in detecting events that occur only once or twice a week.

Evaluation of encephalopathy is accomplished with waking EEG (sleep deprivation not needed). Presence of bilateral theta and delta slowing combined with absence of the normal posterior resting alpha rhythm occurs in toxic-metabolic encephalopathies. A completely normal EEG usually eliminates delirium from the differential diagnosis. In early Alzheimer's disease, the usual resting posterior 8–13 Hz alpha rhythm slows to less than 8 Hz with the degree of slowing and disorganization roughly proportional to the severity of the dementia. Specific abnormalities such as triphasic waves occur in hepatic and uremic encephalopathy though they may occasionally be seen in antipsychotic medication and lithium toxicity as well. Other specific patterns may be present in disorders such as herpes encephalitis, Creutzfeldt-Jakob disease, subacute sclerosing panencephalitis, and autoimmune limbic encephalitis. Benzodiazepines produce excessive beta activity. Taken together, these abnormalities explain why chloral hydrate or melatonin are the preferred agents if sedation is needed for an EEG.

Quantitative EEG or brain mapping involves the construction of a topographical map of various EEG frequencies found in an identified epoch of EEG. Although there are numerous claims of its use in clinical diagnosis, it remains a research tool at present. Though it is also primarily a research technique, MEG is used clinically in the presurgical evaluation of patients undergoing surgery for epilepsy and brain tumor resection. MEG uses superconducting quantum interference devices (SQUIDs) to detect the very subtle magnetic fields generated by neuronal currents in the brain. When co-registered with MRI data it can allow visualization of seizure propagation or brain activity during specific neurocognitive tasks. Currently, MEG is not used in clinical diagnosis apart from the above indications.

EP testing is used primarily in the diagnosis of demyelinating disease to demonstrate the presence of multiple lesions in the nervous system and in the diagnosis of other disorders affecting nerve conduction speed. The commonly used EPs are visual (VEP), brainstem auditory (BAEP), and somatosensory (SEP). In each case a stimulus is applied in the appropriate sensory domain and the time it takes to reach standard points in the scalp EEG is measured. Demyelination in that pathway results in delayed scalp signal detection. Other types of event-related potentials, such as the P300 which is related to cognitive priming, are used in neurocognitive research paradigms but at present have no clinical indications.

Neuropsychiatric assessment frequently includes evaluation for sleep disorders. PSG is helpful in the differential diagnosis of excessive daytime sleepiness. The PSG is typically done as an overnight study in a sleep laboratory and can be used to diagnose sleep-related breathing disorders, periodic limb movement disorder, insomnias, idiopathic hypersomnia, REM behavior disorder, and many other conditions. An apnea hypopnea index (AHI) calculated from the number of apneas and hypopneas occurring on average per hour during the PSG is calculated to see if the patient requires continuous positive airway pressure (CPAP). An AHI of 5–15 is considered mild apnea, 15–30 moderate, and greater than 30 reflects severe obstructive apnea. Many sleep laboratories also offer ambulatory sleep studies for

diagnosis of obstructive sleep apnea that include a chest belt to measure respiratory effort, a nasal canula for airflow and snore detection, a pulse oximeter, and an actigraphic motion sensor to measure movement during the night. PSG done in the sleep laboratory is more accurate than home sleep testing, but home testing may be sufficient if the history is clear and the differential diagnosis is minimal. If the patient requires CPAP titration, this is done in the laboratory. If narcolepsy or idiopathic hypersomnia are in the differential diagnosis, the patient should have a MSLT during the day following the PSG beginning about 90 minutes following conclusion of the PSG. For the MSLT, the patient is brought to the sleep lab every 2 hours during the day and asked to lay down and take a nap with lights off for a total of five sessions. If no sleep occurs the patient leaves after 20 minutes. If sleep occurs, the patient is awoken at 15 minutes. The time to sleep onset and time to REM onset are noted. Average sleep onset of 5 minutes or less combined with at least two episodes of sleep-onset REM are consistent with narcolepsy.

Blood and Urine Testing

The selection of appropriate blood or urine tests, like all laboratory testing, is hypothesis driven. The routine laboratory evaluation used in dementia diagnosis, for example, surveys for a number of diagnoses known to cause cognitive decline. A common panel for this evaluation includes, complete blood count, electrolytes, BUN, creatinine, glucose, liver function tests, thyroid stimulating hormone, calcium, B_{12}, and folate levels. In addition to testing for toxic-metabolic conditions, hepatic, renal, endocrine, and hematologic values, it is helpful for the neuropsychiatric consultant to be familiar with specific tests for some of the more common congenital and inherited disorders that can present with mental status changes, including psychosis (see also Table 5-6).[9] Included are some devastating early childhood disorders that have a milder adolescent or young adult form. A list of blood and urine studies for the diagnosis of some of these conditions with prevalence of at least 1 in 50,000 people is found in Table 5-15.

When patients present with the subacute onset (<3 months) of memory loss, confusion, psychosis, or mania, associated with seizures or movement disorders, a diagnosis of autoimmune limbic encephalitis is entertained. The presence of bilateral enhancement on FLAIR MRI of hippocampi or other limbic structures combined with either CSF pleocytosis or EEG consistent with seizures or encephalopathy is considered diagnostic pending return of antibody studies.[61] Some cases of autoimmune encephalitis are paraneoplastic, and the neuropsychiatric evaluation may lead directly to the discovery of a neoplasm. A growing number of antibodies have been associated with the syndrome of autoimmune limbic encephalitis. A list of these autoimmune syndromes is given in Table 5-16. Note that thyroid peroxidase antibody (TPO) and anti-nuclear antigen (ANA) are often positive but are nonspecific and nondiagnostic, and do not appear directly linked to autoimmune encephalitis.

Genetic testing has become more practical and cost effective in recent years, and clinicians are now able to directly test for the presence of abnormal genes, though it remains quite costly to test for all possible genes implicated in a given neuropsychiatric

TABLE 5-15 • Laboratory Diagnosis of Disorders Causing Psychosis in Adults.

Disease	Laboratory Evaluation
22q11.2 deficiency (velocardiofacial syndrome)	FISH test CGH (comparative genomic hybridization) SNP microarray
Acute intermittent porphyria	Increased porphobilinogen Increased δ-aminolevulinic acid
Adrenoleukodystrophy	Increased very long chain fatty acids
Alzheimer's disease (autosomal dominant form)	APP PSEN1 PSEN2
Cerebrotendinous xanthomatosis	Increased cholestanol
Fabry disease	Decreased α-galactosidase A
Fragile X Fragile X tremor ataxia syndrome (FXTAS)	>200 CGG repeats 55–200 CGG repeats (premutation)
Frontotemporal dementia (familial)	GRN C9orf72 MAPT
Gilbert syndrome	Increased indirect bilirubin (fluctuates)
Glucose-6-phosphate dehydrogenase (G6PD) deficiency	RBC G6PD test, fluorescent spot test
Huntington's disease	≥40 CAG repeats 36–39 CAG repeats indicate reduced penetrance state
Klinefelter syndrome	XXY karyotype
Metachromatic leukodystrophy	Decreased aryl sulfatase A in leukocytes or fibroblasts
Phenylketonuria	Increased phenylalanine
Porphyria variegata	Increased porphobilinogen Increased δ-aminolevulinic acid
Turner syndrome	XO karyotype
Wilson's disease	Decreased serum ceruloplasmin Increased urine copper excretion/24 hours Increased hepatic copper (biopsy)
XXX syndrome	XXX karyotype
XYY syndrome	XYY karyotype

TABLE 5-16 • Autoimmune Encephalitis Antigens.

Antigen	Associated Tumor*	Symptoms
AMPA	Thymoma, small cell lung CA	Memory loss, confusion
CASPR-2	Thymoma	Memory loss, sleep disorder, neuromyotonia
Dopamine 2	NA	Lethargy, movement disorder, psychosis
DPPX	Lymphoma	Diarrhea, weight loss, hyperekplexia, confusion
GABA$_A$	Thymoma	Memory loss, confusion
GABA$_B$	Small cell lung CA	Memory loss, seizures
IgLON5	NA	NREM and REM sleep disorder PSP-like, chorea, cognitive decline Brainstem dysfunction
LGI-1	Thymoma	Memory loss, seizures
mGluR5	Hodgkin's disease	Memory loss
Neurexin-3α	NA	Confusion, seizures
NMDA NR1	Teratoma	Psychosis, memory loss, dyskinesias, seizures

*Tumor type represents most frequent tumor associated with the antibody but may only be found in a minority of patients. NA, no tumor has been associated with syndrome. Data from Graus F, Titulaer MJ, Balu R, et al. A clinical approach to diagnosis of autoimmune encephalitis. *Lancet Neurol.* 2016;15(4):391-404. and Dalmau J, Geis C, Graus F. Autoantibodies to synaptic receptors and neuronal cell surface proteins in autoimmune diseases of the central nervous system. *Physiol Rev.* 2017;97(2):839-887.

possibilities before ordering specific genetic testing. Although a number of different genes may be employed in the diagnosis of other neurologic conditions, the most frequent applications of genetic testing in neuropsychiatry are in the differential diagnosis of dementia, pharmacogenomic testing, and in the evaluation of autism. The assessment of risk factor genes is generally confined to research applications. Before ordering genetic testing, it is incumbent upon the clinician to discuss the ramifications with the patient and/or family. A referral for genetic counseling is strongly recommended.

CSF Examination

Cerebrospinal fluid examination is an important component of the evaluation for CNS infection, inflammation, autoimmune disease, and certain neurodegenerative diseases. Any two of fever, new-onset headache, and nuchal rigidity is generally an indication for lumbar puncture (LP) to evaluate for infection or subarachnoid hemorrhage. Acute mental status change in the setting of fever with or without seizures also merits CSF examination. Opening pressure, color, cell count, protein, and glucose are always recorded with additional studies depending on the diagnostic question. Pleocytosis is the name given to elevated white blood cells in the CSF. CSF findings in various diseases are given in Table 5-17. Fundoscopy and cranial

syndrome. Currently there are no clinical indications for whole exome or whole genome sequencing and the performance of genetic testing without careful consideration could raise ethical issues.[63] Karyotyping remains useful for identification of chromosomal level abnormalities (XXY, trisomy 21, etc.). Disease-specific gene panels and microarray testing are used for specific syndromes. The neuropsychiatrist relies on careful examination to narrow the differential diagnosis to a small number of

TABLE 5-17 • Cerebrospinal Fluid Testing.	
Diagnosis	**CSF Abnormality**
Alzheimer's disease	Increased pTau Decreased A-beta-42 Amyloid/Tau ratio
Autoimmune limbic encephalitis	Elevated protein Pleocytosis NMDA-NR1, VGKC (LGI-1), CASPR antibodies
Bacterial meningitis	Elevated CSF pressure Granulocytic pleocytosis Elevated protein Decreased glucose Gram stain and/or culture
Creutzfeldt-Jakob disease	14-3-3 protein Neuron-specific enolase Cytology to rule out malignancy
Guillain-Barré syndrome	Albumino-cytologic dissociation (increased protein without pleocytosis)
Herpes simplex encephalitis	PCR for herpes simplex virus
Multiple sclerosis	Oligoclonal bands Myelin basic protein IgG index
Neurosyphilis	Lymphocytic pleocytosis Elevated protein VDRL T Pallidum antibody index
Progressive multifocal leukoencephalopathy (AIDS with cerebral lesion(s))	JC virus titer
SSPE (subacute sclerosing panencephalitis)	Anti-measles antibody
Subarachnoid hemorrhage	Bloody fluid Increased red and white blood cells in same proportion as blood (all tubes) Elevated protein Xanthochromic supernatant
TB and fungal meningitis	Lymphocytic pleocytosis Elevated protein Mildly decreased glucose Cryptococcal antigen
Viral meningitis	Lymphocytic pleocytosis Elevated protein PCR for enterovirus, herpes simplex, Epstein-Barr virus, CMV as indicated

TABLE 5-18 • Example of Neuropsychiatric Formulation.

Signs and symptoms: A 51-year-old previously healthy, successful businessman without prior family or personal neuropsychiatric history who became manic and paranoid 1 week after right frontal subarachnoid hemorrhage and aneurysm clipping (not a candidate for endovascular coiling). Normal elemental neurological examination. Normal cognitive examination except for difficulty comprehending pun, sarcasm, double-entendre, context, and idiom. Supportive spouse and daughter.

Localization/Network dysfunction: Paralinguistic deficits indicate right hemisphere dysfunction. Absence of motor findings indicates lack of involvement of frontal motor areas. Focal lesions causing manic behavior have been reported with right hemisphere or orbitofrontal dysfunction.

Differential diagnosis: Right frontal dysfunction may be due to hemorrhagic damage, surgical damage (e.g., postoperative subdural hematoma or contusion) or due to preexisting deficits. Rule out new onset mania despite absent family history.

Cognitive hypothesis for symptoms: Paralinguistic deficits and manic behavior could both be due to right hemisphere dysfunction plus or minus orbitofrontal dysfunction. Paranoia may be due to impaired inferential reasoning or difficulties decoding paralinguistic aspects of communication.

Potentially reversible symptoms: If subdural hematoma is present, it may be surgically evacuated or allowed to resorb over time in absence of critical mass effect. Given absence of family history and likely focal etiology of manic behavior this will most likely be a single manic episode. Paralinguistic deficits may improve with time if the cortex is not irreversibly damaged.

Treatment and rehabilitation plan: Cardiovascular risk factor mitigation, cranial MRI, neuropsychological testing to obtain a baseline functional assessment for later comparison, EEG, carbamazepine as both seizure prophylaxis and mood stabilizer for 1 year, then taper. Speech and language therapy. Psychoeducation for family regarding his cognitive deficits with suggestion to avoid pun, sarcasm, double-entendre, irony in everyday discourse and have the patient give his understanding of nuanced situations to be certain he correctly understands. Gradual return to work as cognitive symptoms improve. Neuropsychiatry follow-up until tapered from mood stabilizer.

Prognosis: Good, given age, psychosocial supports, treatable symptoms, and potentially reversible pathophysiology.

CT scanning are typically done first to rule out brain tumor or increased intracranial pressure, contraindications for LP. Other contraindications include coagulopathy, anticoagulation, and skin infection in the lumbosacral area.

Neuropsychological Testing

Please see Chapter 7 for detailed information on the use of neuropsychological testing in neuropsychiatric assessment.

NEUROPSYCHIATRIC FORMULATION

The history, behavior description, neuropsychiatric review of systems, combined with the findings on neurological, mental status and cognitive examination, and relevant ancillary tests findings become part of the neuropsychiatric formulation. The neuropsychiatric formulation includes a summary of the patient's signs and symptoms, the anatomic localization or network dysfunction causing the neurocognitive findings, the differential diagnosis of the symptoms, one or more cognitive hypotheses for the symptoms, a list of potentially reversible symptoms, a treatment and rehabilitation plan that addresses the symptoms and diagnoses in the context of the cognitive hypothesis, and a prognostic statement. When the data from all ancillary testing and neuropsychological evaluation are available, the formulation may be updated. An example of neuropsychiatric formulation is given in Table 5-18.

CONCLUSION

The neuropsychiatric examination remains the mainstay of neuropsychiatric assessment, and lays the groundwork for neuropsychiatric formulation, targeted laboratory, neuroimaging, and other ancillary assessment, and treatment planning.

Summary and Key Points

Neuropsychiatric assessment is the basis for comprehensive treatment planning and consists of:

- Gathering the history
- General physical examination
- Neurological examination
- Mental status examination
- Cognitive examination
- Ancillary testing (laboratory, neuroimaging, other)
- Neuropsychiatric formulation

Multiple Choice Questions

1. Which of the following tasks can be used to assess recall in a nonverbal individual?
   a. Clock drawing
   b. Hidden objects
   c. Ramparts
   d. Shopping problem
   e. Supraspan learning curve

2. A patient who smiles symmetrically when spontaneously laughing has decreased movement of the left corner of the mouth when smiling to command. Which of the following is the most likely site of the lesion?
   a. Right cerebral corticobulbar fibers
   b. Left cerebral corticobulbar fibers
   c. Right medial temporal lobe
   d. Left medial temporal lobe
   e. Medulla

3. Which of the following cognitive functions is best assessed by the alternate uses task?
   a. Auditory comprehension
   b. Behavioral independence
   c. Cognitive flexibility
   d. Set maintenance
   e. Working memory

Multiple Choice Answers

1. **Answer: b**
   In testing a nonverbal individual, the examiner must flexibly substitute tasks that do not rely on verbal instruction and are appropriate to the patient's cognitive level. The hidden objects task can be "acted out" by the examiner so that the patient gets the message that she is to find the hidden objects.

2. **Answer: a**
   The command to smile involves contralateral corticobulbar fibers as opposed to spontaneous or unconscious smiling which involves contralateral limbic structures in the medial temporal lobe.[11]

3. **Answer: c**
   The alternate uses task[40] is a measure of cognitive flexibility. Although any orally presented task relies on auditory comprehension, independence, and working memory, and continuing to produce responses on any task involves maintenance of set, the alternate uses task specifically assesses the flexibility of one's cognitive approach or one's ability to creatively solve problems.

References

1. Jablensky A. Karl Jaspers: psychiatrist, philosopher, humanist. *Schizophr Bull.* 2013;39(2):239-241.
2. Fine E, Darkhabani M. History of the development of the neurological examination. *Handb Clin Neurol.* 2010;95:213-233.
3. York G, Steinberg D. Hughlings Jackson's neurological ideas. *Brain.* 2011;134:3106-3113.
4. de Vrueh R, Baekelandt E, de Haan J. Background Paper 6.19 Rare Diseases. Priority medicines for Europe and the world: "A public health approach to innovation". Geneva 2013. http://www.who.int/medicines/areas/priority_medicines/BP6_19Rare.pdf. Accessed May 18, 2018.
5. Lauterbach MD, Schildkrout B, Benjamin S, Gregory MD. The importance of rare diseases for psychiatry. *Lancet Psychiatry.* 2016;3(12):1098-1100.
6. Firth HV, Hurst JA. *Clinical Genetics and Genomics (Oxford Desk Reference).* 2nd ed. Oxford, UK: Oxford University Press; 2017.
7. Hamosh A, Scott AF, Amberger JS, Bocchini CA, McKusick VA. Online Mendelian Inheritance in Man (OMIM), a knowledgebase of human genes and genetic disorders. *Nucleic Acids Res.* 2005;33(Database issue):D514-D517.
8. Jones KL, Jones MC, Campo MD. *Smith's Recognizable Patterns of Human Malformation.* 7th ed. Philadelphia, PA: Elsevier Saunders; 2013.
9. Benjamin S, Lauterbach M, Stanislawski A. Congenital and acquired disorders presenting as psychosis in children and young adults. *Child Psychiatry Clin N Amer.* 2013;22(4):581-608.
10. Doty R. Olfactory dysfunction and its measurement in the clinic. *World J Otorhinolaryngol-Head Neck Surg.* 2015;1:28-33.
11. Hopf H, Müller-Forell W, Hopf N. Localization of emotional and volitional facial paresis. *Neurology.* 1992;42:1918-1923.
12. Schott JM, Rossor MN. The grasp and other primitive reflexes. *J Neurol Neurosurg Psychiatry.* 2003;74(5):558-560.
13. Fradis A, Botez M. The groping phenomena of the foot. *Brain.* 1958;81(2):218-230.
14. Owen G, Mulley GP. The palmomental reflex: a useful clinical sign? *J Neurol Neurosurg Psychiatry.* 2002;73(2):113-115.
15. Siegler EL, Beck LH. Stiffness: a pathophysiologic approach to diagnosis and treatment. *J Gen Intern Med.* 1989;4(6):533-540.
16. Bodranghien F, Bastian A, Casali C, et al. Consensus paper: revisiting the symptoms and signs of cerebellar syndrome. *Cerebellum.* 2016;15(3):369-391.
17. Schmahmann JD, Weilburg JB, Sherman JC. The neuropsychiatry of the cerebellum—insights from the clinic. *Cerebellum.* 2007;6(3):254-267.
18. Dubois B, Slachevsky A, Pillon B, et al. "Applause sign" helps to discriminate PSP from FTD and PD. *Neurology.* 2005;64(12):2132-2133.
19. Doody RS, Jankovic J. The alien hand and related signs. *J Neurol Neurosurg Psychiatry.* 1992;55(9):806-810.
20. Munetz MR, Benjamin S. How to examine patients using the Abnormal Involuntary Movement Scale. *Hosp Community Psychiatry.* 1988;39(11):1172-1177.
21. Whitty PF, Owoeye O, Waddington JL. Neurological signs and involuntary movements in schizophrenia: intrinsic to and informative on systems pathobiology. *Schizophr Bull.* 2009;35(2):415-424.
22. Bush G, Fink M, Petrides G, Dowling F, Francis A: Catatonia. I. Rating scale and standardized examination. *Acta Psychiatr Scand.* 1996;93(2):129-136.
23. Kertesz A, Hooper P. Praxis and language: the extent and variety of apraxia in aphasia. *Neuropsychologia.* 1982;20(3):275-286.
24. Tupper DE. *Soft Neurological Signs.* Orlando, FL: Grune & Stratton, Inc.; 1987.
25. Chen EY, Shapleske J, Luque R, et al. The Cambridge Neurological Inventory: a clinical instrument for assessment of soft neurological signs in psychiatric patients. *Psychiatry Res.* 1995;56(2):183-204.
26. Keulen S, Marien P, van Dun K, et al. The posterior fossa and foreign accent syndrome: report of two new cases and review of the literature. *Cerebellum.* 2017;16(4):772-785.
27. Cruz C, Amorim H, Beca G, Nunes R. Neurogenic stuttering: a review of the literature. *Rev Neurol.* 2018;66(2):59-64.
28. Mendez MF, Carr AR, Paholpak P. Psychotic-like speech in frontotemporal dementia. *J Neuropsychiatry Clin Neurosci.* 2017;29(2):183-185.
29. Granadillo ED, Mendez MF. Pathological joking or witzelsucht revisited. *J Neuropsychiatry Clin Neurosci.* 2016;28(3):162-167.
30. Robertson MM, Eapen V, Singer HS, et al. Gilles de la Tourette syndrome. *Nat Rev Dis Primers.* 2017;3:16097.
31. Mendez MF. Non-neurogenic language disorders: a preliminary classification. *Psychosomatics.* 2018;59(1):28-35.
32. Ward J. Synesthesia. *Annu Rev Psychol.* 2013;64:49-75.
33. Benjamin S, Lauterbach M. *The Brain Card®.* 3rd ed. Newton, MA: Brain Educators LLC; 2016.
34. Sandson J, Albert ML. Perseveration in behavioral neurology. *Neurology.* 1987;37(11):1736-1741.
35. Albert ML. A simple test of visual neglect. *Neurology.* 1973;23(6):658-664.
36. Daffner KR, Gale SA, Barrett AM, et al. Improving clinical cognitive testing: report of the AAN Behavioral Neurology Section Workgroup. *Neurology.* 2015;85(10):910-918.
37. Jones-Gotman M, Milner B. Design fluency: the invention of nonsense drawings after focal cortical lesions. *Neuropsychologia.* 1977;15(4-5):653-674.
38. Brooks LR. Spatial and verbal components of the act of recall. *Can J Psychol.* 1968;22(5):349-368.
39. Grattan LM, Eslinger PJ. Higher cognition and social behavior: changes in cognitive flexibility and empathy after cerebral lesions. *Neuropsychology.* 1989;3:175-185.
40. Dippo C. Evaluating the alternative uses test of creativity. In: Proceedings of the National Conference on Undergraduate Research (NCUR). La Crosse, WI: University of Wisconsin; 2013.
41. Albert ML. *Personal communication.* 1985.
42. Ustun B, Adler LA, Rudin C, et al. The World Health Organization adult attention-deficit/hyperactivity disorder self-report screening scale for DSM-5. *JAMA Psychiatry.* 2017;74(5):520-526.
43. Conners CK, Sitarenios G, Parker JD, Epstein JN. The revised Conners' Parent Rating Scale (CPRS-R): factor structure, reliability, and criterion validity. *J Abnorm Child Psychol.* 1998;26(4):257-268.
44. Yudofsky SC, Silver JM, Jackson W, Endicott J, Williams D. The overt aggression scale for the objective rating of verbal and physical aggression. *Am J Psychiatry.* 1986;143(1):35-39.
45. Hamilton M. The assessment of anxiety states by rating. *Br J Med Psychol.* 1959;32(1):50-55.
46. Blessed G, Tomlinson BE, Roth M. The association between quantitative measures of dementia and of senile change in the cerebral grey matter of elderly subjects. *Br J Psychiatry.* 1968;114(512):797-811.
47. Hughes CP, Berg L, Danziger WL, Coben LA, Martin RL. A new clinical scale for the staging of dementia. *Br J Psychiatry.* 1982;140:566-572.
48. Nasreddine ZS, Phillips NA, Bedirian V, et al. The Montreal Cognitive Assessment, MoCA: a brief screening tool for mild cognitive impairment. *J Am Geriatr Soc.* 2005;53(4):695-699.
49. Rehm LP, O'Hara MW. Item characteristics of the Hamilton Rating Scale for depression. *J Psychiatr Res.* 1985;19(1):31-41.

50. Kroenke K, Spitzer RL, Williams JB. The PHQ-9: validity of a brief depression severity measure. *J Gen Intern Med.* 2001;16(9):606-613.

51. Johns MW. A new method for measuring daytime sleepiness: the Epworth sleepiness scale. *Sleep.* 1991;14(6):540-545.

52. Dubois B, Slachevsky A, Litvan I, Pillon B. The FAB: a frontal assessment battery at bedside. *Neurology.* 2000;55(11):1621-1626.

53. Kurtzke JF. Rating neurologic impairment in multiple sclerosis: an Expanded Disability Status Scale (EDSS). *Neurology.* 1983;33(11):1444-1452.

54. Goodman WK, Price LH, Rasmussen SA, et al. The Yale-Brown Obsessive Compulsive Scale. I. Development, use, and reliability. *Arch Gen Psychiatry.* 1989; 46(11):1006-1011.

55. Goetz CG, Tilley BC, Shaftman SR, et al. Movement Disorder Society-sponsored revision of the Unified Parkinson's Disease Rating Scale (MDS-UPDRS): scale presentation and clinimetric testing results. *Mov Disord.* 2008;23(15):2129-2170.

56. Cummings JL. The Neuropsychiatric Inventory: assessing psychopathology in dementia patients. *Neurology.* 1997;48(5 Suppl 6):S10-S16.

57. Overall J, Gorham DR. The Brief Psychiatric Rating Scale (BPRS): recent developments in ascertainment and scaling. *Psychopharmacol Bull.* 1988;24:97-99.

58. Hagen C, Malkmus D, Durham P. *Rancho Los Amigos Levels of Cognitive Functioning Scale.* Downey, CA: Professional Staff Association; 1972.

59. American College of Radiology. ACR Appropriateness Criteria®. https://acsearch.acr.org/list. Accessed August 10, 2019.

60. Weinberger DR, Radulescu E. Finding the elusive psychiatric "lesion" with 21st-century neuroanatomy: a note of caution. *Am J Psychiatry.* 2016;173(1):27-33.

61. Graus F, Titulaer MJ, Balu R, et al. A clinical approach to diagnosis of autoimmune encephalitis. *Lancet Neurol.* 2016;15(4):391-404.

62. Dalmau J, Geis C, Graus F. Autoantibodies to synaptic receptors and neuronal cell surface proteins in autoimmune diseases of the central nervous system. *Physiol Rev.* 2017;97(2):839-887.

63. Hoge SK, Appelbaum PS. Ethics and neuropsychiatric genetics: a review of major issues. *Int J Neuropsychopharmacol.* 2012;15(10):1547-1557.

6

Neuroimaging in Clinical Neuropsychiatry

Anna E. Goodheart · Joshua P. Klein

INTRODUCTION

When used in the appropriate clinical context, neuroimaging is a useful tool in the evaluation of patients with neuropsychiatric disease and behavioral neurologic problems. Although primary psychiatric disorders such as depression, bipolar disorder, and schizophrenia do not have specific or pathognomonic diagnostic imaging findings, neuroimaging remains helpful in evaluating for secondary underlying causes of psychiatric symptoms. These underlying causes can include focal lesions such as tumors, strokes, or demyelination.

Perhaps the most widely used implementation of neuroimaging in neuropsychiatry is its use in the evaluation of patients with dementia. Therefore, a major focus of this chapter will be the application of neuroimaging in the diagnosis of dementing disorders including Alzheimer's disease (AD), frontotemporal dementia (FTD), dementia with Lewy bodies (DLB), Parkinson's disease dementia (PDD), vascular dementia (VD), and normal pressure hydrocephalus (NPH).

An important concept in the use of neuroimaging is that imaging captures only a snapshot in time. Neuropsychiatric disorders, particularly those resulting from neurodegeneration, generally evolve insidiously over months to years, and imaging thereby offers only a glimpse at a particular time point in the course of disease. The key to the effective use of neuroimaging in the diagnosis of neuropsychiatric disease is to correlate the snapshot that the imaging provides with the clinical narrative of the patient. A hypothesis about the diagnosis and the localization of the disorder needs to be generated clinically, after which neuroimaging can be used as a supplement to help support or refute that hypothesis. And when available, comparison of current to prior imaging findings can be highly informative as subtle changes in brain volume, for example, can be difficult to discern on a single study and are much more easily visualized by side-by-side comparison of old and new images.

There are several major categories of neuroimaging that will be covered in this chapter: structural imaging, functional imaging, and molecular imaging. Structural imaging includes computed tomography (CT) and magnetic resonance (MR) imaging. Functional and molecular imaging includes magnetic resonance spectroscopy (MRS), magnetic resonance perfusion (sometimes referred to as "perfusion imaging"), functional magnetic resonance imaging (fMRI), diffusion tensor imaging (DTI), positron emission tomography (PET), and single photon emission computed tomography (SPECT). Each of these imaging modalities will be discussed, with greater weight given to the more commonly used modalities and their utility in common neuropsychiatric disorders. It is important to remember that in neuroimaging, images are presented in "radiographic orientation" meaning that on axial and coronal images, the right side of the image is the left side of the patient's brain, and vice versa.

CASE VIGNETTE 6.1

A 74-year-old woman with well-controlled hypertension presents to clinic with memory complaints that started a few years ago. Her family members report that she can remember past events but that she is having difficulty recalling conversations that happened earlier in the day. She sometimes asks the same question multiple times throughout the course of a conversation. Her mental status and cognitive testing reveal difficulties mainly with memory recall as well as some abnormalities in executive and visuospatial functioning. Her other cognitive domains, including language, are intact. Her general neurologic exam is normal. The clinician suspects that the patient may be suffering from early amnesic dementia due to AD. As we read through this chapter, we can think about which imaging modalities would be useful to confirm this hypothesis and what those images might show.

Lastly, while it is difficult to make generalizations about when an imaging study should be obtained for any given patient, the finding of a focal neurological deficit or aggregate of symptoms or signs that localize to a particular brain area should certainly prompt imaging evaluation.

STRUCTURAL NEUROIMAGING: CT AND MRI

Structural neuroimaging allows us to look at the architecture of the brain and to detect any distortions to its structure. Since the primary psychiatric disorders such as depression are not associated with specific imaging abnormalities, structural neuroimaging is mainly used to rule out lesions that may be producing psychiatric symptoms secondarily. When focal lesions are suspected based on the history or neurologic exam, structural imaging is used to evaluate for these lesions, which can include tumors, strokes, demyelination, or at times focal infectious or inflammatory lesions. Structural neuroimaging is also useful in the evaluation of neurodegenerative diseases, as the pattern of atrophy (i.e., focal, regional, lobar, diffuse) seen on structural neuroimaging can help point toward diagnoses of different types of dementing illnesses. The two mainstays of structural neuroimaging are CT and MR imaging.

Computed Tomography

CT uses x-rays to create two-dimensional images that are generally displayed as contiguous slices. Different tissues allow varying degrees of penetration of x-rays and therefore look either bright or dark on CT. Materials through which x-rays pass easily, such as air and fluid, appear dark (hypodense) on CT. Denser material, such as metal or bone, appears bright (hyperdense) on CT. The brain, and different structures within it, lie in the middle of this spectrum and appear in varying shades of gray. The degree of x-ray absorption of certain tissues and lesions can be quantified using the Hounsfield unit scale.

CT scans are acquired on the order of minutes and provide rapid visualization of brain structures and ventricles. These scans are therefore very useful in acute clinical scenarios, such as acute strokes, intracranial hemorrhages, or obstructive hydrocephalus. They are also useful for patients who cannot safely undergo MR, either because of metallic implants that are not MR-compatible or because of inability to tolerate the length of time it takes to undergo an MR.

CT is highly sensitive for detecting acute hemorrhage, which will appear hyperdense due to the x-ray absorption of iron within hemoglobin in blood (Figure 6-1). Subacute or chronic hemorrhage appears less hyperdense, due to degradation of hemoglobin and dispersion of iron. CT is also useful for general assessment of overall structure (global atrophy, hydrocephalus, etc.) and for detecting any major lesions, such as edema caused by large strokes or tumors. CT is thus useful in emergency room settings when a patient presents with an acute change in mental status. CT is particularly effective in ruling out hemorrhage as a cause of mental status change, especially in patients presenting with head trauma.

CT can be obtained with iodinated contrast, which is a radiopaque material injected intravenously. Lesions that cause

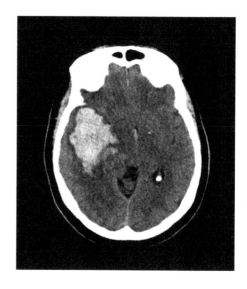

FIGURE 6-1. Axial CT of the head showing a large acute hemorrhage in the right hemisphere. The hemorrhage appears bright due to x-ray attenuation by iron in hemoglobin. Note that on axial and coronal images, the right side of the image shows the left side of the brain, and vice versa.

disruption or breakdown of the blood-brain barrier, such as tumors or abscesses, will allow extravasation of the contrast from the bloodstream into the brain parenchyma. The difference between the post-contrast and pre-contrast images is what is referred to as contrast enhancement. The presence and pattern of contrast enhancement can help refine a radiologic differential diagnosis, as different pathologies are associated with different enhancement patterns. CT scans with contrast can therefore be useful if enhancing lesions are suspected in a patient who is unable to undergo MR.

The major limitation of CT, compared to MR, is its relatively lower resolution. Other limitations of CT include the nephrotoxicity of iodinated contrast, which should be avoided in patients with impaired renal function, and the use of ionizing radiation. Because of the radiation exposure associated with CT, these scans are generally avoided as much as possible in children and pregnant women. MR imaging does not use ionizing radiation and provides higher resolution images compared to CT.

Magnetic Resonance

MR imaging uses a magnetic field and radiofrequency pulses that lead hydrogen atoms within tissues to align and then relax. The energy emitted by the hydrogen nuclei as they realign themselves is detected by the MR scanner and reconstructed into two-dimensional images that, like CT, are displayed as contiguous slices. Hydrogen atoms are abundant in the many water molecules in the brain, and the binding and microenvironments of these water molecules allow for distinction between different tissues and pathologies. MR imaging provides much higher resolution images of soft tissue than does CT and is therefore the preferred structural neuroimaging modality outside of the emergency setting. It is important to remember that images are presented in "radiographic orientation" meaning that on axial and coronal images, the right side of the image corresponds to the left side of the patient's brain, and vice versa. The main characteristics of the most commonly used structural MR sequences are outlined in Table 6-1.

The two main acquired MR sequences, T1 and T2, differ in the length of radiofrequency pulses applied. T1-weighted images are acquired using specific radiofrequency pulses to highlight hydrogen atoms in more hydrophobic environments such as the myelin found in the white matter of the brain. In T1-weighted imaging, white matter appears bright (hyperintense), and the more hydrophilic gray matter appears less bright (hypointense). Cerebrospinal fluid (CSF) appears even darker. T1-weighted images therefore provide a basic structural image of the brain and are useful in assessing overall anatomy and architecture (Figure 6-2). Lesions that produce or are associated with edema will appear dark (hypointense) on T1-weighted sequences.

T1-weighted images—particularly high-resolution three-dimensional T1-weighted sequences—are useful in assessing patterns of atrophy, as seen in different types of neurodegenerative diseases. In AD, atrophy may first be evident in the hippocampi of the medial temporal lobes, then spreading to involve more of the temporal lobes, the parietal, and then frontal lobes.[1] FTD, as the name suggests, involves degeneration and atrophy of the frontal and temporal lobes with less involvement of the hippocampus than in AD. There are various subtypes of FTD, which have different clinical symptomatology and patterns of atrophy (Figure 6-3). For example, the behavioral variant of FTD (bvFTD) is typically associated with atrophy of the frontal and temporal lobes, with relative sparing of the parietal lobes. The atrophy of bvFTD usually progresses from anterior to posterior and is often asymmetric, with right greater than left hemispheric atrophy. The primary progressive aphasia (PPA) variants of FTD, which clinically have more language symptoms, are more likely to be associated with atrophy of the left temporal lobe and left perisylvian region, areas typically involved in language. DLB may result in hippocampal atrophy that is milder than that seen in AD.[2] These patterns of atrophy can be assessed on T1 MR imaging and can help to support a clinical diagnosis of mild cognitive impairment or dementia due to a neurodegenerative condition.

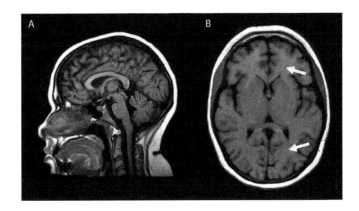

FIGURE 6-2. Sagittal **(A)** and axial **(B)** T1-weighted MRI showing relative hyperintensity of the white matter (arrows) compared to gray matter.

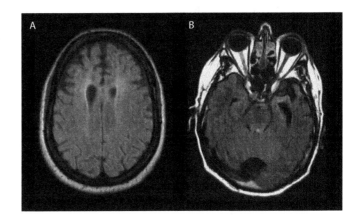

FIGURE 6-3. Axial MR images showing bifrontal lobar atrophy in a patient with behavioral variant frontotemporal dementia **(A)** and asymmetric (left greater than right) temporal lobar atrophy in a patient with an aphasic variant of frontotemporal dementia **(B)**.

TABLE 6-1 • Characteristics of the Most Commonly Used Structural MR Sequences.

	Characteristics	Useful For
T1	Gray matter is darker than white matter, CSF is black	Looking at structural anatomy, assessing for atrophy
T2	Gray matter is brighter than white matter, CSF is white	Looking for focal lesions/pathology, which generally appear bright
T2-FLAIR	Same as T2 but bright CSF signal is suppressed (black)	Same as T2, but better at assessing lesions close to CSF-containing spaces
Contrast	Areas of contrast extravasation will appear hyperintense on T1. "Enhancement" implies a comparison to a T1 pre-contrast image	Looking for lesions that involve breakdown of the blood-brain barrier including tumor, abscess, infection, inflammation, active demyelination
Diffusion (DWI)	Areas of reduced water diffusivity will appear hyperintense	Mainly used for acute ischemic stroke. Bacterial abscesses and densely cellular tumors also restrict diffusion
Susceptibility (SWI/GRE)	Blood products (hemosiderin) and mineralization appear dark	Looking for hemoglobin degradation products and foci of mineralization

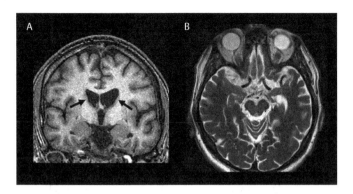

FIGURE 6-4. Coronal T1-weighted MRI of a patient with Huntington's disease showing atrophy of the caudate heads (arrows) adjacent to the lateral ventricles **(A)**. Axial T2-weighted MRI of a patient with PSP showing atrophy of the dorsal midbrain and reduction in the anteroposterior diameter of the midbrain **(B)**.

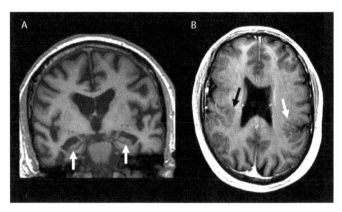

FIGURE 6-5. Coronal T1-weighted MRI of the patient with Alzheimer's disease showing atrophy of the medial temporal lobes, particularly the hippocampi **(A, arrows)**. Axial T1-weighted MRI of the patient with epilepsy and behavioral problems showing multifocal lesions resulting from abnormal neuronal migration, including a focus of polymicrogyria in the left parietal lobe (white arrow) and abnormal cortical folding in the right hemisphere (black arrow) **(B)**.

Some patterns of focal atrophy can be useful in diagnosing neuropsychiatric disease associated with movement disorders, including the atrophy of the striatum seen in Huntington's disease (HD) (Figure 6-4A) and the atrophy of the midbrain seen in progressive supranuclear palsy (PSP) (Figure 6-4B).[3,4] Focal areas of atrophy and encephalomalacia are commonly seen as sequela of traumatic brain injury or stroke. Depending on their location, these insults and their resultant focal atrophy can lead to neurological deficits and a wide variety of neuropsychiatric symptoms.

It can be helpful to look at T1 images in different orthogonal planes (i.e., axial, coronal, and sagittal) to get a sense of the three-dimensional pattern of atrophy. For example, coronal slices are particularly helpful in assessing the hippocampal atrophy that occurs in AD (Figure 6-5A). Volumetric analyses can provide quantification of the degree of atrophy, although these quantitative analyses are currently used more in research than in clinical practice. When ordering an MR for the purpose of detecting the presence or pattern of atrophy, it can be helpful to request high-resolution sequences that have thin (typically 1 mm) slices through the brain. Beyond atrophy, T1-weighted images are also useful for detecting structural malformations, such as developmental disorders of neuronal migration or mesial temporal sclerosis that may underlie neuropsychiatric symptoms or seizures (Figure 6-5B).

T2 imaging uses specific radiofrequency pulses to highlight structures containing water rather than lipid. On T2-weighted images gray matter appears brighter (hyperintense) than white matter, and CSF is brighter than both (Figure 6-6A). Most lesions in the brain, whether acute (with associated edema and swelling) or chronic (with associated gliosis and atrophy) appear bright on T2-weighted images, allowing them to stand out against the darker background of normal white matter. A modified T2 sequence called fluid attenuated inversion recovery (FLAIR) includes an additional radiofrequency pulse that suppresses the bright signal of free fluid. With suppression of the bright signal of CSF, lesions—particularly small ones near CSF-containing spaces—are more easily visualized. Examples of lesions that can be easily visualized with T2 and T2-FLAIR

images include microvascular disease and strokes (important in the evaluation of vascular cognitive impairment/dementia), tumors, demyelination (including the classic ovoid periventricular lesions of multiple sclerosis), infections, or inflammation (Figure 6-6B–D), all of which may produce neuropsychiatric symptomatology depending on their location.

Gadolinium contrast can be given during MR imaging to help further define pathology. Pathophysiologic processes that lead to disruption or breakdown of the blood-brain barrier, such as tumors, abscesses, and certain other infections, and some instances of acute demyelination, will lead to extravasation of contrast into the parenchyma. Extravasated contrast will appear as abnormal hyperintensity on post-contrast scans. Because gadolinium contrast appears hyperintense on T1-weighted images, the T1 sequence is obtained before and after contrast administration to determine the presence and pattern of enhancement (Figure 6-6E,F). Although used most typically to look at lesions within the brain parenchyma itself, contrast enhancement of the meninges can also be seen in certain disorders, such as infectious meningitis or leptomeningeal carcinomatosis. In general, if tumor, abscess, infection, active demyelination, or inflammation is suspected then a contrast-enhanced scan should be obtained. If one is interested only in the structure of the brain, in order to assess for atrophy of neurodegenerative dementia or for chronic vascular changes associated with VD, then a contrast-enhanced scan is not needed. Gadolinium contrast should generally be avoided in patients with renal failure and in pregnant or breastfeeding patients.

Two other commonly used MR sequences are diffusion-weighted and susceptibility-weighted images. Diffusion-weighted imaging (DWI) measures the freedom of movement of water molecules in brain tissue. DWI is most useful to detect acute ischemic stroke, in which the abrupt failure of cellular metabolism and cell membrane ion channel homeostasis causes cellular swelling, cytotoxic edema, and an overall restriction of

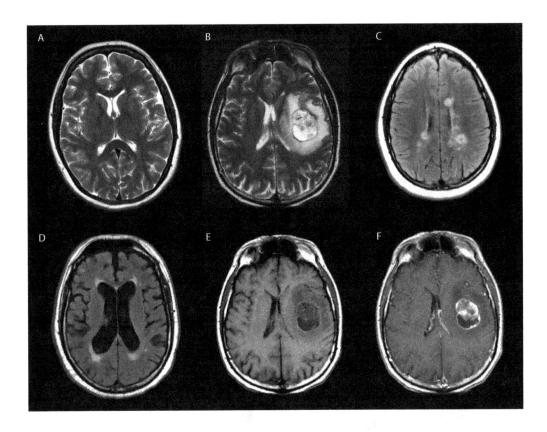

FIGURE 6-6. Axial T2-weighted MRI of a normal brain **(A)**. Axial T2-weighted MRI of a patient with a left frontal glioblastoma, with abnormal hyperintensity within the mass itself as well as the surrounding edematous brain **(B)**. Axial T2-FLAIR MRI of a patient with multiple sclerosis showing focal ovoid periventricular lesions **(C)**. Axial T2-FLAIR MRI of a patient with chronic microvascular changes affecting the periventricular white matter, with accompanying *ex vacuo* ventricular dilatation **(D)**. Axial T1 **(E)** and T1-post contrast **(F)** images of the patient shown in panel B, demonstrating abnormal enhancement of the core of the tumor, with a cystic rim-enhancing area at the posterior extent of the mass containing necrotic debris.

diffusion of water within the injured tissue. Some other lesions, including bacterial abscesses and certain highly cellular tumors, are also associated with abnormal restricted diffusion of water, and in fact this imaging feature can help differentiate these entities from other lesions that are not associated with restricted diffusion (Figure 6-7).

Susceptibility-weighted imaging (SWI) and the gradient echo (GRE) sequence both detect the deposition of metal or minerals in the brain. By far the most common use of SWI is in detecting hemosiderin deposition from prior hemorrhage. SWI imaging can also detect very small areas of bleeding, unlike CT or even T1 or T2 MRI. An example of the utility of SWI in neuropsychiatry is to detect the microhemorrhages and hemosiderosis characteristic of cerebral amyloid angiopathy (CAA) (Figure 6-8A,B).[5] The GRE and SWI sequences can also help detect subdural hematomas, which can occur in older people spontaneously or after falls, and in both cases, be associated with cognitive changes and neuropsychiatric symptoms (Figure 6-8C).

MR imaging is generally very safe and does not make use of ionizing radiation like CT. However, since MR utilizes strong electromagnetic fields, it is not safe for patients with certain types of metal-containing implants, shrapnel, or certain models of pacemakers and other devices. Patients must be carefully screened for the presence of anything magnetic prior to

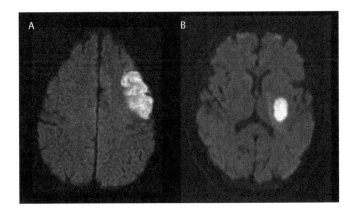

FIGURE 6-7. Axial diffusion weighted images showing restricted diffusion (abnormal hyperintensity) from an acute left middle cerebral artery territory ischemic infarction **(A)**, and a bacterial abscess in the left subinsular area **(B)**.

undergoing MR imaging. Another limitation of MR imaging, which is of particular relevance in the psychiatric population, is the lengthy time it takes to acquire an MR scan (which can be on the order of 20–40 minutes). Some patients, particularly those with dementia or those who are prone to claustrophobia or paranoia, are not able to tolerate being in the scanner for that

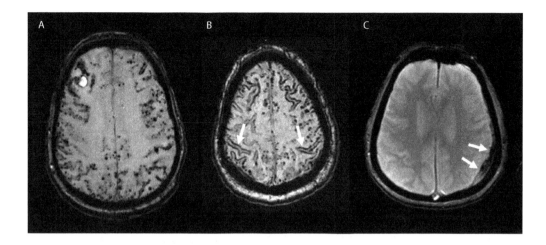

FIGURE 6-8. Axial susceptibility-weighted images of a patient with cerebral amyloid angiopathy. In **(A)**, innumerable chronic cortical and subcortical microhemorrhages are noted as hypointense spots, with a larger and more acute hyperintense hemorrhage in the right frontal lobe. In **(B)**, curvilinear hemosiderosis along the cortical surface is noted (arrows), in addition to cortical and subcortical microhemorrhages. In **(C)**, an axial gradient echo image shows a hypointense left convexity subdural hematoma (arrows).

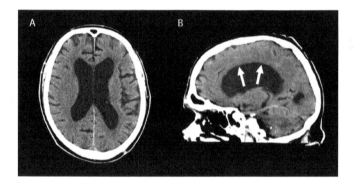

FIGURE 6-9. Axial **(A)** and sagittal **(B)** CT images of a patient with NPH. Ventriculosulcal disproportion is evident in A, and abnormal upward bowing of the corpus callosum is evident in B (arrows).

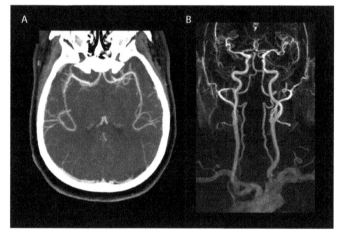

FIGURE 6-10. An axial CT angiogram at the level of the middle cerebral arteries is shown in **(A)**. A coronal MR angiogram showing the cerebral and cervical (neck) arteries is shown in **(B)**.

amount of time and may require sedatives in order to undergo these scans, or they may need to undergo a limited imaging protocol.

Another use of structural neuroimaging to highlight is in the diagnosis of NPH, a disease whose pathogenesis is poorly understood and remains controversial. The clinical hallmarks of NPH are cognitive impairment, gait abnormalities, and urinary incontinence, thought to be caused by disruption of frontal white matter tracts by transudation of CSF into the periventricular white matter and expansion of the lateral ventricles. The core imaging features of NPH include no evidence of obstruction of CSF flow (i.e., by a tumor or other mass lesion), ventricular enlargement out of proportion to sulcal atrophy ("ventriculo-sulcal disproportion"), and upward bowing of the corpus callosum (Figure 6-9). The ventriculomegaly in NPH is not caused by a lesion obstructing CSF outflow (obstructive hydrocephalus). Obstructive hydrocephalus, a setting in which ventriculomegaly is associated with elevated intraventricular pressure, is accompanied by effacement of the cortical sulcal spaces. Of note, many neurodegenerative diseases result in the imaging appearance of enlarged ventricles due to regional or diffuse brain atrophy ("hydrocephalus *ex vacuo*"), with concomitant widening of cortical sulcal spaces. In contrast, as stated above, in NPH the degree of ventriculomegaly is out of proportion to atrophy of the brain and widening of cortical sulcal spaces. The Evans index, calculated as the ratio of the maximum width of the frontal horns of the lateral ventricles to the maximum width of the inner table of the skull, can be used to quantify ventriculomegaly. An Evans index greater than 0.3 is suggestive of ventriculomegaly, although this criterion is somewhat controversial given its poor specificity for NPH.[6,7]

CT and MR Angiography

Both CT and MR can be used for angiography, which provides a detailed visualization of the cerebral vasculature (Figure 6-10). CT angiography (CTA) uses radiopaque iodinated contrast injected into a peripheral vein. MR angiography (MRA) uses gadolinium-based contrast that can display vessels on T1-weighted sequences. In patients with contraindications to contrast, such as contrast allergies or renal failure, MRA can be done using a "time of flight" (TOF) protocol which does not require administration of intravenous contrast. This method uses the properties of flowing materials (i.e., blood in a vessel) to map the cerebral vasculature. TOF imaging can produce high-resolution images of cerebral and cervical (neck) vasculature, but the technique is somewhat more susceptible to motion artifact than contrast-based angiography. Angiography is used to look for vascular malformations, aneurysms, atherosclerosis, vasculitis, or thrombosis of blood vessels. It is of course of great utility in stroke neurology and in neurosurgery but has somewhat less utility in routine neuropsychiatry.

In summary, structural neuroimaging including CT and MR can be invaluable in the diagnosis of neuropsychiatric disorders in correlating structural (focal, multifocal, or diffuse) changes and neuropsychiatric symptoms.

FUNCTIONAL AND MOLECULAR IMAGING: MRS, MR PERFUSION, FMRI, DTI, PET, AND SPECT

While CT and MR provide information about the structure of the brain, functional and molecular imaging provide details about its function. Functional neuroimaging can provide details about cerebral blood flow and perfusion, metabolic activity, and network connectivity. Molecular neuroimaging refers to the labeling and mapping of specific biomolecules. There are a variety of different modalities of functional and molecular imaging, and here we will briefly consider the principal ones including MRS, magnetic resonance perfusion (MR perfusion), fMRI, DTI, PET, and SPECT. Although these imaging techniques are mainly used in research, they can be useful clinically in selected circumstances. A summary of functional and molecular neuroimaging techniques is provided in Table 6-2.

MR Spectroscopy and MR Perfusion

MRS looks at different metabolites in brain tissue. MRS data is represented in the form of a waveform with peaks representing the presence and concentration of various molecules (Figure 6-11A). It is frequently used in neuro-oncology, since neoplastic tissue is metabolically different from normal brain tissue (Figure 6-11B). However, abnormal ratios of certain brain metabolites can become altered in neurodegenerative disease as well.[8] The clinical utility of MRS in neurodegenerative disorders is an emerging concept and has yet to become a standard clinical study in the workup of dementia.

MR perfusion measures cerebral blood volume and blood flow. The most common utilization of MR perfusion is in

TABLE 6-2 • Characteristics of the Most Commonly Used Functional and Molecular Imaging Techniques.

	Brief Description	Useful For (Examples)
MRS	Characterizes metabolites of brain tissue	Neuro-oncology
MR perfusion	Measures cerebral blood volume and blood flow	Vascular disorders of the brain
fMRI	Maps task-based activation of brain regions	Neurocognitive research
DTI	Maps white matter tracts	Neural circuits research
PET	Maps brain metabolism (FDG-PET) or molecular targets (e.g., amyloid-PET)	FDG-PET: Dementia
		Amyloid-PET: Alzheimer's disease
SPECT	Maps cerebral blood flow or molecular targets (e.g., DaT scans)	Parkinson's disease

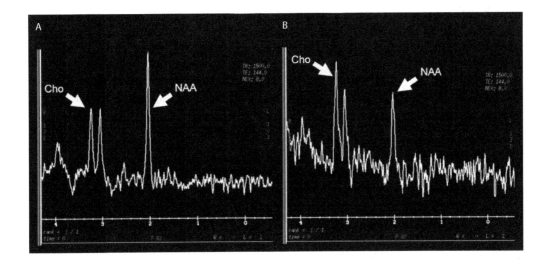

FIGURE 6-11. A normal MR spectrogram is shown in **(A)**; Cho = choline, NAA = *N*-acetyl aspartate. Note that the NAA peak is higher than the choline peak. The spectrogram from a patient with a glioma is shown in **(B)**. Note that the choline peak is now higher than the NAA peak. Choline is a marker of membrane turnover and NAA is a marker of neuronal integrity. In gliomas, there is elevated membrane turnover and dilution or destruction of neurons.

vascular disorders of the brain. While altered perfusion can also be detected in neurodegenerative diseases,[9] as with MRS, the utility in this setting is an emerging concept that has yet to be applied routinely in clinical settings. The specifics of MRS and MR perfusion are beyond the scope of this chapter, but these imaging modalities may become more mainstream in clinical neuropsychiatry in the future.

Functional Magnetic Resonance

fMRI, as the name suggests, is used to look at the function of areas of the brain. fMRI is also useful in understanding connectivity of brain structures and neural circuits. The basic concept behind fMRI is that of autoregulation of blood flow: neural activation leads to an increased oxygen requirement, which then leads to increased blood flow to the active area of the brain.

fMRI uses the differing magnetic properties of oxyhemoglobin and deoxyhemoglobin to create blood flow maps. This technique is known as blood-oxygen level dependent (BOLD) imaging.[10] BOLD-fMRI maps can be created in the resting state or during activation states, such as during the execution of various neurocognitive tasks. The blood flow maps created by fMRI are mapped onto structural MR images, providing a three-dimensional visualization of areas of brain activation. This technique is widely used in neurocognitive research to better understand which areas of the brain are involved in functions such as language, memory, motor planning and execution, and vision (Figure 6-12).[11] Some limitations of fMRI include blood flow artifact (such as that created by overlying veins) and the delay in hemodynamic response after a stimulus. Task-based fMRI also assumes that the subject has a certain level of mental status and attention necessary to participate in the testing and also

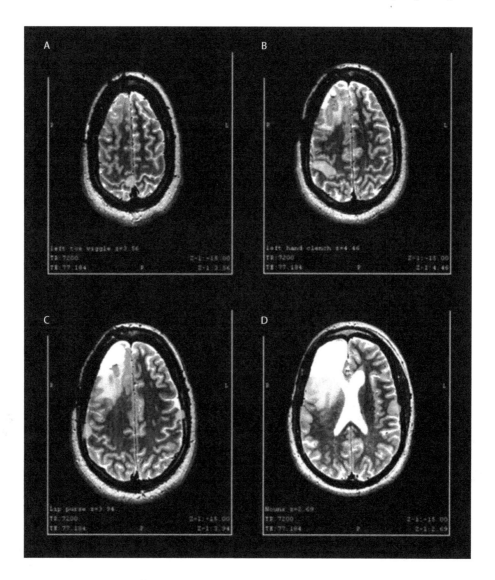

FIGURE 6-12. BOLD fMRI maps overlaid on axial T2-weighted images of a patient with a right frontal tumor. In **(A)**, the patient is asked to wiggle her left toe, resulting in focal activation (delineated in orange) of the right parasagittal precentral gyrus. In **(B)**, the patient is asked to clench her left hand, resulting in focal activation of the hand area of the right precentral gyrus. In **(C)**, the patient is asked to purse her lips, resulting in bilateral focal activation of the mouth area of the precentral gyrus. The posterior displacement of the focus of activation on the right is due to tumor-related edema. In **(D)**, the patient is asked to generate nouns, resulting in bilateral focal activation of the mouth area of the precentral gyrus, as well as focal activation of Broca's area anterior to the precentral gyrus in the left lateral frontal lobe.

assumes a healthy cerebrovascular system capable of adapting to changes in blood flow demands. The use of fMRI is largely restricted to neurocognitive research, with clinical applications currently limited to locating eloquent cortex prior to neurosurgery or stereotactic radiosurgery, so as to avoid it during procedures to remove tumors or other lesions.

Diffusion Tensor Imaging

DTI is a type of MR imaging that assesses the integrity of subcortical white matter pathways, which are disrupted in destructive lesions such as stroke and can also degrade in conditions such as AD.[12] DTI combines voxel-based measurements of diffusion with information about the directionality or vector of restricted diffusion to create probabilistic maps of expected locations of white matter pathways. Functional MRI and DTI can provide information on the functional and structural connectivity of neural circuits involved in a variety of neurocognitive tasks and are thus important tools in neuropsychiatric research.[13]

Positron Emission Tomography and Single Photon Emission Computed Tomography

PET and SPECT are two forms of molecular nuclear imaging. In nuclear imaging, a radioactive isotope is either used alone or is coupled to a molecule of interest, forming a compound known as a tracer. This tracer is injected into the bloodstream and crosses the blood-brain barrier into the brain. As the radioisotope decays, it emits radioactive particles that can be detected. In this way, the areas of the brain in which the tracer has accumulated can be mapped. PET and SPECT images are often co-registered to structural images (CT or MR) to provide an anatomical map of tracer uptake. Historically, PET has been used most frequently to detect brain metabolism and SPECT to detect brain perfusion, though both PET and SPECT radioisotopes can be coupled to a variety of molecules for other uses as well. Molecular neuroimaging is a rapidly evolving field with a recent explosion of research. Here, we will review the major highlights as they relate to neuropsychiatry.

In PET, decaying radioisotopes emit positrons that are detected by the scanner. The most commonly used radiomolecules in PET are radioactive fluorine (^{18}F) and carbon (^{11}C). ^{18}F-Fluorodeoxyglucose (FDG) is the most widely used PET tracer. FDG is a radioactive analog of glucose, taken up and utilized by metabolically active neurons and other cells. FDG-PET therefore provides a map of glucose utilization of the brain. In neuropsychiatry, FDG-PET is particularly useful in detecting patterns of hypometabolism seen in neurodegenerative diseases, as regions affected by a disease demonstrate reduced FDG-PET signal. AD is associated with characteristic hypometabolism in the medial temporal and parietal lobes, with early involvement of the posterior cingulate gyrus and precuneus. In DLB, the pattern may be similar to that seen in AD but with additional hypometabolism in the occipital lobes (seen less frequently in AD) and relative preservation of metabolism in the posterior cingulate cortex.[14] FTD is predictably associated with hypometabolism of the frontal and temporal lobes, with patterns varying depending on subtype and frequently a much greater degree of asymmetry than typically seen in AD or DLB.

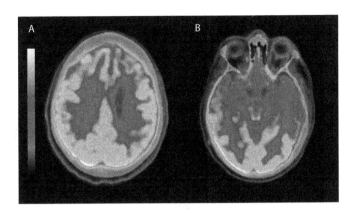

FIGURE 6-13. Axial ^{18}FDG-PET color maps overlaid on CT images of two patients with frontotemporal dementia. The color bar indicates decreasing FDG metabolism from top (white-orange) to bottom (blue-green). In **(A)**, there is marked cortical hypometabolism in the left greater than right frontal lobes in a patient with behavioral variant FTD, and in **(B)**, there is marked cortical hypometabolism in the left greater than right temporal lobes in a patient with an aphasic variant of FTD.

For example, in behavioral variant FTD, there is classically right frontal and/or temporal hypometabolism, whereas in PPA the hypometabolism is much more pronounced in the left frontal, temporal, and/or parietal lobes (Figure 6-13).[2,15] In Parkinson's disease (PD), FDG hypermetabolism is evident in the pallidum, posterior putamen, and pons,[16] whereas this finding is not seen in drug-induced parkinsonism, or in other parkinsonian conditions such as multiple system atrophy, PSP, or DLB. As metabolic changes typically precede the structural changes seen on CT or MRI, FDG-PET may be of particular use early in the course of a neurodegenerative disease, as it is for distinguishing between many neurodegenerative syndromes and, potentially, predicting underlying neuropathologies.[17]

More recently, PET tracers have been developed that bind to beta-amyloid and tau, the abnormal proteins that accumulate in AD. ^{11}C-Pittsburgh Compound-B (PiB) was the first such tracer, which uses radioactive carbon-11 coupled to a molecule that binds to beta-amyloid (Figure 6-14A,B).[18] In this way, deposition of beta-amyloid in the brain can be detected and quantified in vivo. Other beta-amyloid tracers have since been developed including ^{18}F-florbetapir, ^{18}F-florbetaben, and ^{18}F-flutemetamol, each of which has been approved for clinical use by the United States Food and Drug Administration (FDA). An Amyloid Imaging Taskforce (including members of the Alzheimer Association and the Society of Nuclear Medicine and Molecular Imaging) developed a set of guidelines for the appropriate clinical use of amyloid PET.[19] In general, amyloid PET scans are not helpful in older patients with presentations suggestive of typical (amnesic) AD dementia. However, they can be useful to establish whether or not AD neuropathology is present in scenarios of greater diagnostic uncertainty such as persistent unexplained mild cognitive impairment, or dementia with an atypical presentation due to either young age of onset (age <65) or primary impairment in a cognitive domain other than episodic memory.

Of note, while tracer uptake correlates well with amyloid plaque levels in the brain,[20] plaque levels themselves do not

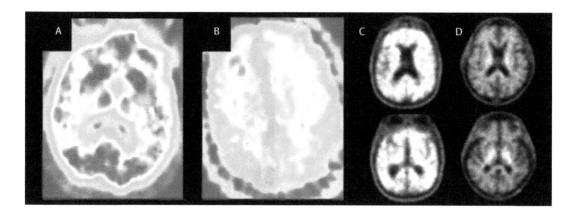

FIGURE 6-14. Axial PiB **(A, B)** and florbetapir **(C, D)** PET images showing elevated amyloid avidity in patients with Alzheimer's disease (A, C) compared to age-matched controls (B, D).

correlate well with disease severity in patients with AD. Given the lack of effective disease modifying therapies in AD and the fact that, despite their FDA-approved status amyloid PET scans are expensive and not currently reimbursed by insurers, their use has remained largely restricted to clinical research studies. However, given both the importance of establishing underlying AD neuropathology in studies investigating potential disease-modifying agents and the desire to conduct such studies at the earliest identifiable stages of disease, amyloid PET scans have transformed the world of AD research.[21]

The use of PET tracers for tau is restricted to research for the time being. There are numerous other PET tracers that are used in research settings including tracers that bind to neurotransmitters and other signaling molecules,[15] as well as tracers that serve as markers of neuroinflammation.

SPECT is similar in concept to PET, but is used to detect cerebral blood flow rather than cerebral metabolism. Most SPECT imaging uses the radiomolecule technetium, although sometimes iodine and other molecules are used. These radioactive molecules travel via the bloodstream to well-perfused areas and emit gamma rays as they decay. Using this technique, areas of increased and decreased perfusion can be mapped. In dementia, there is reduced blood flow to atrophic regions, similar to the areas of hypometabolism seen with FDG-PET.

SPECT tracers can also be used to target specific molecules. One example of relevance to neuropsychiatry is dopamine transporter imaging (DaT) with [123]Ioflupane. The decreased presence of dopamine transporters in the striatum and basal ganglia structures in PD (and other neurodegenerative conditions causing parkinsonism) is reflected in reduced tracer uptake in DaT scans, thus distinguishing neurodegenerative parkinsonism from parkinsonism due to nondegenerative etiologies.[22] This can be useful as an adjunct in the diagnosis of parkinsonian dementia, and to distinguish between neurodegenerative parkinsonism and drug-induced parkinsonism (in which a DaT scan should be normal).

There are several limitations to PET and SPECT imaging including the use of ionizing radiation and the poor spatial resolution of these techniques. One of the most prohibitive factors in the use of these technologies is their cost and limited accessibility. PET tracers in particular are by definition unstable molecules that are synthesized in a particle accelerator known as a cyclotron and must be used soon after synthesis.

In summary, functional and molecular neuroimaging are broad categories with many areas of active research. Though their clinical use is more limited, in the appropriate setting these techniques can aid in the diagnosis of neuropsychiatric disorders.

CASE VIGNETTE RESOLUTION

The most appropriate imaging modality for this patient is a non-contrast MR scan with diffusion, susceptibility, T2-FLAIR, and high-resolution three-dimensional T1-weighted sequences. The MR does not show any focal lesions (as suspected, based on the normal neurologic exam). It does show some mild microvascular ischemic changes in the white matter on the T2-FLAIR sequence, which are likely sequelae of the patient's hypertension but which are too mild to account for the degree of her symptoms on their own. On the T1 sequence, there is atrophy affecting the medial temporal lobes (including the hippocampi) and some atrophy in the parietal lobes as well. The medial temporal atrophy becomes particularly clear when looking at the

coronal T1 sequence. These findings support the clinical suspicion of a diagnosis of dementia due to AD. As this is a fairly straightforward case on clinical grounds, the clinician does not feel that PET imaging is necessary nor cost-effective. If PET imaging were to be pursued, it would likely show hypometabolism on FDG-PET in the temporal and parietal lobes. If the clinician were to order amyloid-PET, such as ^{18}F-florbetapir, there would likely be evidence of elevated amyloid deposition. Given the cost of PET and the confidence in the diagnosis of AD, the clinician decides not to order this test. Dementia is a clinical diagnosis, and imaging should be used as an adjunct to help support a hypothesis, generated from the history and neurologic exam.

Summary and Key Points

■ Structural neuroimaging includes CT and MR and is useful in assessing for focal lesions that may cause neuropsychiatric symptoms as well as for specific patterns of atrophy such as those seen in neurodegenerative disease.

■ Functional and molecular neuroimaging techniques include MRS, MR perfusion, fMRI, DTI, PET, and SPECT; these modalities are mainly used in research but can be helpful in the appropriate clinical settings.

■ In the near future, we will likely see more clinical use of functional and molecular neuroimaging, particularly PET. More research needs to be done before these techniques reach mainstream diagnostic use.

■ An imaging study shows only one snapshot in time and must be interpreted in the context of clinical symptomatology. Comparison to prior scans can be highly informative, particularly in recognizing subtle changes that occur over long time intervals.

Multiple Choice Questions

1. A 78-year-old woman with longstanding hypertension, hyperlipidemia, and a history of smoking presents with several years of memory complaints. You suspect that she may have vascular or mixed vascular/Alzheimer dementia given her vascular risk factors. Which MR sequence would be best to look for microvascular ischemic changes?
   a. T1
   b. T2
   c. T2-FLAIR
   d. SWI
   e. DWI

2. Ordering an MR WITH gadolinium contrast would be most useful in evaluation of which of the following conditions?
   a. Alzheimer dementia
   b. Normal pressure hydrocephalus
   c. Parkinson's disease
   d. Brain tumor
   e. Schizophrenia

3. A 64-year-old man presents with subacute behavioral changes including personality change, making offensive jokes, and engaging in socially inappropriate behavior, which is very different from his baseline. FDG-PET is likely to show hypometabolism most pronounced in which of the following areas?
   a. Temporal and parietal lobes
   b. Occipital lobes
   c. Pituitary gland
   d. Cerebellum
   e. Frontal and temporal lobes

4. A 72-year-old man presents with falls, worsening gait, cognitive decline, and urinary incontinence. You suspect he has NPH. Which of the following findings on structural imaging would be consistent with this diagnosis?
   a. Atrophy mainly of the temporal and parietal lobes
   b. A mass obstructing the fourth ventricle
   c. Ventricular enlargement out of proportion to sulcal widening without a clear obstructing lesion
   d. Acute blood in the ventricles
   e. A large arachnoid cyst

Multiple Choice Answers

1. **Answer: c**
   The best sequence to see microvascular changes is the T2-FLAIR sequence. On T2-weighted sequences, edema, inflammation, and gliosis appear as abnormal hyperintensity. Since microvascular changes most often accumulate in the subcortical and periventricular white matter, the suppression of CSF with FLAIR imaging increases the visibility of these lesions. T1-weighted imaging is more useful to look at global brain structure. SWI imaging is useful to look for blood products. DWI imaging is useful to look for acute ischemic strokes.

2. **Answer: d**
   Lesions that break down the blood-brain barrier will show enhancement on contrast scans. Examples of lesions that break down the blood-brain barrier include tumors, acute demyelination, and many infections. Contrast is not necessary in the routine workup of neurodegenerative diseases, normal pressure hydrocephalus, or primary psychiatric disorders.

3. **Answer: e**
   This patient is exhibiting symptoms consistent with behavioral variant frontotemporal dementia. FDG-PET would show hypometabolism in the frontal and temporal lobes. Other common patterns of hypometabolism on FDG-PET include temporal and parietal lobes (Alzheimer's disease) and occipital lobes (dementia with Lewy bodies).

4. **Answer: c**
   NPH is by definition a communicating hydrocephalus with normal intracranial pressure, meaning that there is not a lesion causing obstruction of CSF outflow (such as a tumor, blood, or an arachnoid cyst). Answer choice a is more consistent with Alzheimer's disease.

References

1. Whitwell JL, Przybelski SA, Weigand SD, et al. 3D maps from multiple MRI illustrate changing atrophy patterns as subjects progress from mild cognitive impairment to Alzheimer's disease. *Brain*. 2007;130(Pt 7):1777-1786.

2. Mortimer AM, Likeman M, Lewis TT. Neuroimaging in dementia: a practical guide. *Pract Neurol*. 2013;13(2):92-103.

3. Draganski B, Bhatia KP. Brain structure in movement disorders: a neuroimaging perspective. *Curr Opin Neurol*. 2010;23(4):413-419.

4. Oba H, Yagishita A, Terada H, et al. New and reliable MRI diagnosis for progressive supranuclear palsy. *Neurology*. 2005;64(12):2050-2055.

5. Biffi A, Greenberg SM. Cerebral amyloid angiopathy: a systematic review. *J Clin Neurol*. 2011;7(1):1-9.

6. Gallia GL, Rigamonti D, Williams MA. The diagnosis and treatment of idiopathic normal pressure hydrocephalus. *Nat Clin Pract Neurol*. 2006;2(7):375-381.

7. Toma AK, Holl E, Kitchen ND, Watkins LD. Evans' index revisited: the need for an alternative in normal pressure hydrocephalus. *Neurosurgery*. 2011;68(4):939-944.

8. Kantarci K. 1H magnetic resonance spectroscopy in dementia. *Br J Radiol*. 2007;80 Spec No 2:S146-S152.

9. Binnewijzend MA, Kuijer JP, van der Flier WM, et al. Distinct perfusion patterns in Alzheimer's disease, frontotemporal dementia and dementia with Lewy bodies. *Eur Radiol*. 2014;24(9):2326-2333.

10. Ogawa S, Lee TM, Kay AR, Tank DW. Brain magnetic resonance imaging with contrast dependent on blood oxygenation. *Proc Natl Acad Sci USA*. 1990;87(24):9868-9872.

11. van Heerden J, Desmond PM, Phal PM. Functional MRI in clinical practice: a pictorial essay. *J Med Imaging Radiat Oncol*. 2014;58(3):320-326.

12. Teipel SJ, Wegrzyn M, Meindl T, et al. Anatomical MRI and DTI in the diagnosis of Alzheimer's disease: a European multicenter study. *J Alzheimers Dis*. 2012;31(Suppl 3):S33-S47.

13. Khanna N, Altmeyer W, Zhuo J, Steven A. Functional neuroimaging: fundamental principles and clinical applications. *Neuroradiol J*. 2015;28(2):87-96.

14. Lim SM, Katsifis A, Villemagne VL, et al. The 18-F-FDG PET cingulate island sign and comparison to 123I-beta-CIT SPECT for diagnosis of dementia with Lewy bodies. *J Nucl Med*. 2009;50(10):1638-1645.

15. Nasrallah I, Dubroff J. An overview of PET neuroimaging. *Semin Nucl Med*. 2013;43(6):449-461.

16. Meles SK, Teune LK, de Jong BM, Dierckx RA, Leenders KL. Metabolic imaging in Parkinson disease. *J Nucl Med*. 2017;58(1):23-28.

17. Nobili F, Arbizu J, Bouwman F, et al. European Association of Nuclear Medicine and European Academy of Neurology recommendations for the use of brain 18-F-fluorodeoxyglucose positron emission tomography in neurodegenerative cognitive impairment and dementia: Delphi consensus. *Eur J Neurol*. 2018;25(10):1201-1217.

18. Klunk WE, Engler H, Nordberg A, et al. Imaging brain amyloid in Alzheimer's disease with Pittsburgh Compound-B. *Ann Neurol*. 2004;55(3):306-319.

19. Johnson KA, Minoshima S, Bohnen NI, et al. Appropriate use criteria for amyloid PET: a report of the Amyloid Imaging Task Force, the Society of Nuclear Medicine and Molecular Imaging, and the Alzheimer's Association. *J Nucl Med*. 2013;54(3):476-490.

20. Clark CM, Pontecorvo MJ, Beach TG, et al. Cerebral PET with florbetapir compared with neuropathology at autopsy for detection of neuritic amyloid-beta plaques: a prospective cohort study. *Lancet Neurol*. 2012;11(8):669-678.

21. Villemagne VL, Pike KE, Chetelat G, et al. Longitudinal assessment of Aβ and cognition in aging and Alzheimer's disease. *Ann Neurol*. 2011;69(1):181-192.

22. Kagi G, Bhatia KP, Tolosa E. The role of DAT-SPECT in movement disorders. *J Neurol Neurosurg Psychiatry*. 2010;81(1):5-12.

7

Neuropsychological Evaluation in Neuropsychiatry

Aaron P. Nelson · Deborah Green

INTRODUCTION

Clinical neuropsychology is an applied science of human behavior based on principles of brain–behavior relationships. Central to this approach is *neuropsychological assessment*, which involves gathering information about an individual's history, current symptoms and functioning, as well as administering a variety of behavioral measures designed to probe specific cognitive functions. A clinical neuropsychologist integrates objective data within a biopsychosocial context to evaluate and diagnose abnormalities in the realm of behavior and cognition. The assessment may address a variety of clinical questions, often to aid in diagnostic clarification and guide treatment planning.

HISTORICAL PERSPECTIVE

Neuropsychology emerged from a confluence of disciplines within psychology and clinical neuroscience, with its foundation primarily rooted in three areas: psychophysics, psychometrics, and behavioral neuroanatomy. Psychophysics, the branch of psychology that deals with the relationships between physical stimuli and mental phenomena, and psychometrics, the science of measuring mental processes, established that mental phenomenon could be measured with appropriate methods and test instruments to capture a construct of interest with accuracy and precision. Developing and interpreting neuropsychological tools has been rooted in this methodology and guided by ever-increasing knowledge of brain–behavior relationships. Early advancements in basic neuroscience and functional neuroanatomy helped elucidate the neural mechanisms of brain function and identify associations between brain lesions and resultant abnormalities in cognition and behavior. Spurred in large part by new methodologies in structural and functional imaging, our understanding of the complexity of these relationships expanded steeply, with experimental and clinical practice developing in tandem. The phenomenal growth of clinical neuropsychology over the past half century owes much to contemporaneous work in clinical neuroscience.

Although it is not possible to pinpoint the date of its establishment as a discipline, prior to 1960, there were no professional organizations, journals, or training programs in neuropsychology.[1] In its earliest form, neuropsychology was practiced in medical settings in association with departments of neurology and neurosurgery. Psychologists with expertise in psychological measurement and a special interest in behavioral effects of brain injury designed tests to assess various abilities in their patients.

The term "neuropsychology" came into use only relatively recently in the mid-20th century, although theories and cultural musings about the bases of human behavior can be traced back to the writings of the ancients. The Egyptians originally localized the seat of human thought in the heart. This concept remained largely unchallenged for 3000 years, when a student of Pythagoras argued that aspects of mental function were represented in specific regions of the brain. This approach to thinking about the brain was later termed *localization* and became the center of great controversy 2000 years later. Hippocrates, writing in the 4th century BC, posited that the brain was the organ of intellect, sensation, and emotion. While anomalous human behavior had been attributed to spiritual forces, he conceptualized mental illness as a product of abnormal brain function. Along this line, he advanced the hypothesis that epilepsy was not the result of demonic possession but rather an organic ailment.

Beginning in the middle of the 19th century, psychophysics comprised a refined approach to the precise measurement of various human attributes. Galton, Cattell, and their contemporaries assessed cognitive functions by measuring individual differences in the threshold for discriminating sensory stimuli and speed of psychomotor responses. The early work of Ebbinghaus on "individual memory curves of retention"[2] also epitomized this approach. At the beginning of the 20th century, Binet and Simon[3] and others introduced the revolutionary concept of measurable intelligence, a notion that continues to have a profound and controversial impact on human society.

Following the First World War, the necessity for diagnosing and treating brain injuries sustained by returning soldiers was a driving factor in the development of early assessment methodologies. Subsequent wars saw the implementation of screening methods and intelligence/ability assessments for military recruits. The psychometric method was employed to design and construct measurement tools possessing validity and reliability, that is, instruments capable of measuring the construct of interest with precision and consistency, which are crucial underpinnings of all psychological and neuropsychological tests. The routine application of these methods in the aftermath of the Second World War marked the establishment of modern clinical psychology with an emphasis on psychological testing. The expanded role of assessment in educational settings—particularly with regard to intelligence, aptitude, and achievement—further spurred the growth in development of neuropsychological methods.

Two schools of thought emerged in the 1950s: a primarily quantitative approach which emphasized well-normed, standardized procedures versus a more qualitative approach rooted in the tradition of European behavioral neurology epitomized by Alexander Luria, who is often regarded as the founder of modern clinical neuropsychology. The earliest codification of neuropsychological examination methods can be attributed to Dr. Ralph Reitan. Reitan and his colleagues developed a battery of test measures in which specific patterns of scores were correlated to dysfunction of associated brain regions.[4] Later assessment methods relied less on a fixed battery of tests and instead used a more dynamic "process" approach to neuropsychological assessment developed by Dr. Edith Kaplan in her work at the Boston Veterans Administration Hospital.[5] This method entails paying special attention to the qualitative aspects of a patient's test response to inform in situ hypothesis testing during the exam. Although quantitative data are also valuable, the patient's approach to completing a task or solving a particular cognitive problem reveals an underlying process that is presumed to reveal the functional integrity of brain regions. In contemporary neuropsychological practice, both the fixed and process approach rely on a vast body of knowledge about characteristic syndromes that are associated with underlying disease states.

Prior to the development of neuroimaging techniques, neuropsychological assessment provided evidence for the detection and localization of brain lesions. Lesion identification was predicated on knowledge of functional neuroanatomy, initially garnered through early case reports of acquired brain injury. The famous case of Phineas Gage in 1848 involved a railroad worker who survived a catastrophic injury in which an iron spike was blasted through his head, essentially disconnecting the anterior portion of his brain.[6] The resulting pattern of spared and affected functions in Gage gave rise to an early understanding of the functional role of the frontal lobes in human behavior. The pioneering work of Paul Broca, a French neurologist who described his patient "Tan" in 1861,[7] was instrumental in unveiling the role of the dominant hemisphere in human language function. In the 1950s, Scoville and Milner's studies of patient "HM" shed new light on the role of the medial temporal lobe and limbic system in anterograde memory function.[8] In contemporaneous applications, the orthodox lesion method has yielded to a more complex understanding of larger distributed networks underlying many aspects of cognitive function.

Knowledge of brain–behavior relationships and characteristic syndromes guides the evaluation for the purpose of understanding the functional integrity of the brain. The current practice of clinical neuropsychology, through the use of psychometrically sound test instruments interpreted within a biopsychosocial context, applies these methodologies in the diagnosis and treatment of brain-related injuries and illness.

FUNDAMENTAL ASSUMPTIONS

Clinical neuropsychology as a field is firmly rooted in the neurosciences and therefore shares the assumption that brain function gives rise to cognition and behavior. Conversely, inferences can be made about the integrity of the brain based on observable behavior. The ability to make accurate and meaningful inferences regarding brain integrity depends upon a thorough understanding of the functional neuroanatomy that underlies normal cognition as well as characteristic neurocognitive profiles and neurobehavioral syndromes.

Observable behavior is frequently the most sensitive manifestation of brain pathology. Such behavior can range from subtleties of social comportment to performance on a specific neuropsychological test. A competent neuropsychologist will sample multiple domains of behavior with attention to both spontaneous signs and symptoms (e.g., an anomic pause) as well as provoked responses on formal measures (e.g., semantic paraphasias on a naming task). Observable behavior, including "test behavior," reflects an interaction between the domains of person and environment. Consideration of multiple variables within and across domains is necessary to determine the clinical significance of a given behavior.

Cognitive domains and their respective parcellated component processes are sampled via performance on neuropsychological tests. Test construction along sound psychometric principles is essential to ensure their validity and reliability (i.e., their utility in measuring a construct of interest with accuracy and precision). Individual performance is interpreted relative to normative standards, which incorporate a range of demographic variables. The neuropsychologist relies on knowledge of test construction and standardization to select and interpret measures for a given clinical context. Importantly, test selection must consider using measures with normative data derived from subjects of similar age, education, language, and nationality to the patient currently being tested. Where possible, normative data may be referenced in peer-reviewed journal articles for groups who are not well-represented by test publisher norms, such as for individuals with limited education or from different nationalities.

Neuropsychological tests are not process pure and therefore the interpretation of test results depends on an understanding of the component processes involved in any given test response. For example, the ability to name an object to visual confrontation depends on multiple processes that are mediated by different brain systems. The individual must first orient and attend to the stimulus. Second, the stimulus must be accurately registered at the level of visual perception. Third, the neural pathway that links the visual percept to meaningful recognition must be patent. Fourth, the ability to assign a phonemic/lexical label to the object must be intact. Finally, the individual must be able to convey a response through speech. Because a complex cognitive action, such as naming an object, can be undermined by perturbation at any point within the network linking multiple functions, a neuropsychologist must understand the component processes involved in each behavior. By examining the patient's function in multiple domains with multiple measures, the neuropsychologist can determine which processes and associated neural circuits are functioning abnormally.

Performance on a single test is not sufficient to make a diagnostic inference. A common misconception is that a poor score on a particular test denotes an impairment in the domain that the test is nominally designed to assess. For example, if a patient performs poorly on a "memory" test, this does not necessarily signify impairment in memory but could indicate difficulties with attention or language. The neuropsychologist must also consider the effects of transient factors such as mood, motivation, pain, and fatigue. A degree of variability is expected in cognitively intact individuals who may exhibit a few spuriously low findings in an otherwise normal profile.[9] A neuropsychologist will evaluate a profile of test results in a dynamic, interactive fashion in order to arrive at a diagnostic formulation.

Neuropsychological testing is simply one means of obtaining a sample of behavior. A neuropsychologist must proceed with caution in using test data to predict behavior. The testing environment is, by necessity, contrived to promote a standard approach to test administration. This contrivance constitutes a challenge in understanding how test performance corresponds to "real life" behavior. For example, a patient who complains of difficulty with concentration and memory at work may perform quite normally in the context of the quiet, distraction-free examination room. Discrepancy between "test behavior" and "real-life" behavior is the source of ongoing challenge for the design of an ecologically valid assessment environment. Assessment recommendations often incorporate relevant information about the patient's life (e.g., the complexity of their work, details of social stressors, etc.) in order to mitigate some of these challenges.

CLINICAL APPLICATIONS

A neuropsychological evaluation yields a dynamic portrait of a patient's cognitive and psychological profile to address myriad clinical questions. Characterizing cognitive strengths and weaknesses is a fundamental goal of the neuropsychological evaluation, as this contributes to an understanding of the underlying etiology and elucidation of the differential diagnosis. Precise quantitative measurement of cognitive functions also yields data that can be useful for establishing a baseline of cognitive functioning against which to calibrate degree of change over time. This involves systematically monitoring cognitive functioning to determine response to a specific treatment intervention, or to characterize the course of a symptomatic pattern for the purpose of further clarifying a diagnosis or prognosis. For example, with objective quantitative data, neuropsychologists are in a unique position to evaluate the efficacy of treatment interventions (e.g., pharmacotherapy, electroconvulsive therapy, neurosurgery) by reevaluating after initiation of therapy—with the potential limitation, as

discussed above, that individuals' performance on testing may only partially reflect their functioning in real life. On the basis of neuropsychological findings, specific and detailed recommendations are made for rehabilitation in cases of brain injury, tumor, and stroke. Rehabilitation may involve remediation for skill acquisition or implementation of compensatory strategies.

Neuropsychological assessment is capable of detecting mild changes in older adults to differentiate normal aging from cognitive decline. Often these changes are subtle and may not be evident on casual observation or by a standard mental status examination or the use of brief screening measures (e.g., Mini Mental State Examination [MMSE],[10] Montreal Cognitive Assessment [MoCA][11]). For individuals with a high baseline level of functioning, detecting subtle impairment that reflects a relative decline can be quite challenging. A perfect score on the MMSE or MoCA, for example, would not rule out incipient changes that precede more overt impairment. As Americans live longer and become more aware of the relationship between aging and dementia, they are more likely to notice subtle changes in cognitive function in themselves and in family members. This awareness is particularly heightened in individuals with a family history of neurodegenerative disease.

Because of its knowledge base in behavioral neuroscience as well as psychological principles, neuropsychology has an important role in treatment planning. Enumeration of cognitive strengths and intact abilities can be used to design real-world adaptive or compensatory strategies that a patient may employ to circumvent deficits. Neuropsychologists help determine the potential impact of brain pathology on avenues of real-life functioning, ranging from the most rudimentary human activities (bathing and dressing) to work life and the complexities of intimate relationships. Sequelae of neurocognitive disorders, in addition to cognitive decline, may include changes in mood, personality, and behavior. Providing an explanatory context that these changes are not under voluntary control, but rather part of a disease process, may benefit family relationships. Shifting the attribution from willful control to a medical cause promotes an improved problem-solving approach.

Neuropsychological consultation is frequently pivotal in cases involving adjudication of criminal or civil matters. Neuropsychologists with special training and experience in forensics play an important role in determination of competency in matters ranging from criminal responsibility to financial capacity. There has been significant increased appreciation of the utility of neuropsychological knowledge for assisting the courts in understanding functional consequences of neurological disorder in personal injury cases ranging from product liability to accidental injury. Neuropsychology is becoming central to determination of competency and medical decision making in end-of-life care. Neuropsychologists have pioneered the development of free-standing and embedded measures of effort and symptom validity for use in cases in which motivational factors are important.[12]

The neuropsychological exam can be "negative" in a range of scenarios. The "worried well" may be relieved to learn that their occasional word-finding hesitancy does not bespeak the onset of a dementia; recommendations for maintaining optimal brain health going forward are often appreciated.

APPROACH TO NEUROPSYCHOLOGICAL ASSESSMENT

There have been three main approaches to neuropsychological assessment. The quantitative fixed battery, the more qualitative process approach, and a flexible blend which represents the majority practice of neuropsychologists today.

Fixed Battery Approach

Prior to the development of widely available neuroimaging, neuropsychological evaluation was a means of assessing the anatomical location, extent, and severity of impairment relating to a brain injury or disease. In this setting, the fixed-battery approach, developed primarily by Ralph Reitan and his colleagues, was formulated to be a comprehensive, first-line diagnostic method to capture the totality of brain dysfunction. The Halstead-Reitan battery that emerged utilized a standard set of tests tapping each major cognitive domain and relied on interpretation of quantitative scores. It was intended as a comprehensive assessment for the detection of deficits that might not be otherwise evident. In addition to its comprehensiveness, the use of a standardized, fixed test set promoted increased sensitivity to slight variations in performance of component tasks by its practitioners.

Process Approach

Another major approach to neuropsychological assessment is the Boston Process approach, developed by Edith Kaplan and colleagues.[13] This approach is hypothesis-driven and uses the patient's test performance to guide and inform an evolving and dynamic assessment strategy. Each evaluation is individually tailored to the patient with test selection focused to answer particular clinical questions. Test performance guides decision making in real time. As data emerges, the neuropsychologist moves through a series of decision points and probes certain cognitive areas for more information as necessary. The Boston Process approach utilizes quantitative data but differs substantively from the Fixed Battery approach given the former's equally strong emphasis on qualitative aspects of performance. The manner in which a patient arrives at a solution to a problem is emphasized, rather than exclusively relying on test scores. Task performance is analyzed across multiple measures to parse out component processes and identify specific cognitive deficits. While the tests are administered in a standardized fashion, this approach allows for modification to test the limits of cognitive function (e.g., the extent to which the patient benefits from cues/prompts) and produce richer qualitative data.

Flexible Battery Approach

In current practice, most neuropsychologists utilize the so-called "flexible battery" approach.[14] Just as the name implies, a select battery of tests may be the starting point for assessing a particular case type. For example, a specific set of test measures is used for evaluating elderly individuals referred with a question of dementia. However, the clinician can modify the battery either beforehand or during the course of the assessment, depending upon the specifics of the case. For instance, compared to a patient with suspected Lewy body dementia, the battery for a patient with prominent features of a temporal variant of frontotemporal dementia would call for incorporating more extensive testing of receptive and expressive language. This approach has the virtue of generating a substantial repository of core common data on similar cases that can be pooled for both clinical and scientific benefit, while allowing for latitude in the individual case.

CLINICAL METHOD

A neuropsychological assessment is ultimately a means of sampling behavior, gathering information, and incorporating various streams of data to inform differential diagnosis and treatment planning. This process is illustrated in Figure 7-1. Although test administration is the most time-consuming component of the process, it is often the case that some of the most valuable information emerges while discussing a patient's history and current life situation. The history gathered during the clinical interview and review of collateral documentation provides the framework and initial hypotheses which guide the remainder of the assessment.

Referral Question and Chief Complaint

The first task of a neuropsychological evaluation is to clarify the reason for the referral. Indications for neuropsychological evaluation include diagnostic clarification, elaboration of cognitive features of a clinical syndrome, assessment of treatment response (e.g., following surgery or initiation of medicine), and determination of rehabilitative needs and recommended treatment strategies. Specialized forensic referrals can include determination of disability in employment contexts, evaluation of competency/capacity in both criminal and civil litigation, and assessment of neuropsychological effects in personal injury actions. After information is gleaned from available records and other informants, the patient is interviewed and a chief complaint is elicited. This should include a clear description of the onset and course of the complaint (e.g., symptoms, concerns) as well as information regarding the medical and social context in which the problem(s) emerged. The patients' overall understanding of the rationale for the consultation and appreciation of his/her current circumstances also sheds light on their level of insight and current functioning.

History

A comprehensive history is gathered from various sources including the patient's self-report, information from the referring provider, and review of medical records, as well as any prior evaluations from medical, academic, or vocational settings. Obtaining collateral information from family members or close friends is particularly important in cases in which the patient's insight and/or memory is limited. A review of medical history includes current problems and past illnesses, injuries, surgeries and hospitalizations, medications and supplements, substance use history, and relevant family medical history. The psychiatric history spans a review of current and past symptoms, treatment

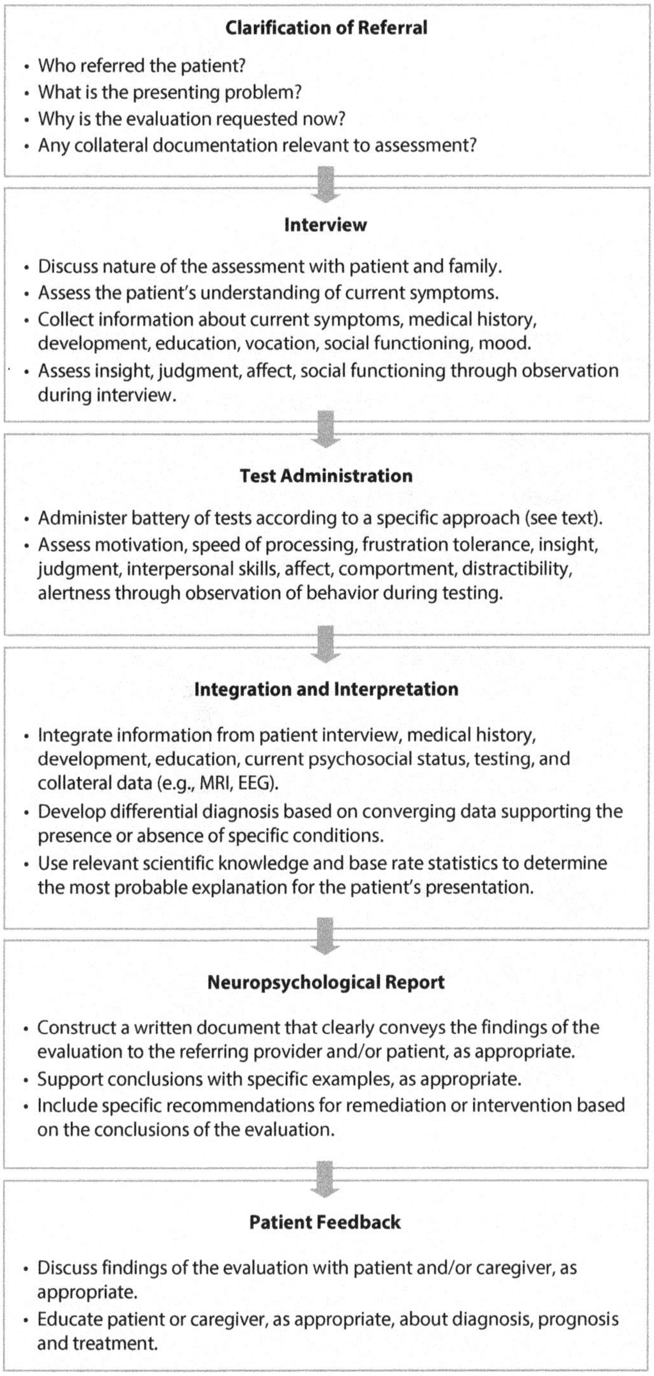

Clarification of Referral

- Who referred the patient?
- What is the presenting problem?
- Why is the evaluation requested now?
- Any collateral documentation relevant to assessment?

Interview

- Discuss nature of the assessment with patient and family.
- Assess the patient's understanding of current symptoms.
- Collect information about current symptoms, medical history, development, education, vocation, social functioning, mood.
- Assess insight, judgment, affect, social functioning through observation during interview.

Test Administration

- Administer battery of tests according to a specific approach (see text).
- Assess motivation, speed of processing, frustration tolerance, insight, judgment, interpersonal skills, affect, comportment, distractibility, alertness through observation of behavior during testing.

Integration and Interpretation

- Integrate information from patient interview, medical history, development, education, current psychosocial status, testing, and collateral data (e.g., MRI, EEG).
- Develop differential diagnosis based on converging data supporting the presence or absence of specific conditions.
- Use relevant scientific knowledge and base rate statistics to determine the most probable explanation for the patient's presentation.

Neuropsychological Report

- Construct a written document that clearly conveys the findings of the evaluation to the referring provider and/or patient, as appropriate.
- Support conclusions with specific examples, as appropriate.
- Include specific recommendations for remediation or intervention based on the conclusions of the evaluation.

Patient Feedback

- Discuss findings of the evaluation with patient and/or caregiver, as appropriate.
- Educate patient or caregiver, as appropriate, about diagnosis, prognosis and treatment.

FIGURE 7-1. Schematic of neuropsychological evaluation.

(e.g., psychotherapy, medication, ECT, TMS), and details regarding inpatient hospitalizations. The developmental history sheds light on whether there may be a congenital or longstanding vulnerability based on the circumstances of gestation, birth and delivery, acquisition of developmental milestones, and early socialization skills. The social history of the patient is clarified by surveying major autobiographical events, obtaining an understanding of the level of enrichment and support available in the childhood home, taking stock of the family system, and gaining a sense of the nature and quality of current interpersonal

relationships. Information regarding educational background includes early school experiences and academic performance during high school, college, postgraduate study, and other educational and technical training; the presence of a learning disability, developmental attention deficit, and behavioral problems should be assessed. Obtaining a good vocational history (jobs, relationships with colleagues and authority figures, work satisfaction) is important for gauging the patient's aspirations, ability to utilize innate and acquired skills in applied/practical pursuits, and as a marker of intelligence and general capacity. Lastly, an understanding of their recreational interests and hobbies provides a wealth of information that illuminates natural strengths and proclivities, and level of activity, motivation, and socialization in their community.

Behavioral Observations

Physical appearance is inspected including symmetry of anatomical features, possible syndromal stigmata, facial expression, manner of dress, and attention to personal hygiene. The patient is asked specific questions regarding unusual sensory or motor symptoms. Affect and mood are assessed with respect to range and modulation of felt and expressed emotions and their congruence with concurrent ideation and the contemporaneous situation. Interpersonal comportment is evaluated in the context of the interview. Specifically, attention is paid to whether the patient's behavior reflects a normal awareness of self and other in the interaction, along with whether the patient is motivated and compliant with examination requests, instructions, and test procedures. An appreciation of the patient's level of effort/motivation to participate in the evaluation and comply with examination instructions is crucial to gauging the validity of the test data. General level of arousal or alertness is determined by observing the patient's degree of drowsiness, tendency to yawn or fall asleep during the interview, level of interpersonal engagement, and speed of response in conversation. Environmental and diurnal factors can modify arousal, and an attempt should be made to assess whether these factors are relevant for a particular patient by inquiring about consistency of arousal level and any fluctuations that the patient or caregiver has observed.

Examination

A sufficiently broad range of neuropsychological functions is evaluated using tests and other assessment techniques. The major domains to be surveyed include general intellectual ability, attention, executive function and comportment, memory, language, visuospatial abilities, motor functioning, and mood/personality. As a prelude to test administration, it is imperative to establish the integrity of sensation and perception because impairments in these areas can invalidate the results of examination. For example, it would be incorrect to conclude that a patient has a receptive language impairment when, in fact, there is a primary hearing deficit.

Diagnostic Formulation

Data from the history, observation, and testing of the patient are analyzed collectively to produce a concise understanding of the patient's symptoms and neuropsychological diagnosis. The result is an in-depth characterization of each patient's abilities and limitations, for use both diagnostically and as a framework through which to address the goals of treatment. When possible, the diagnostic formulation should identify the neuropathological factors that could give rise to the patient's clinical presentation, including underlying anatomy and disease process.

Recommendations and Feedback

Consultation concludes with the process of feedback, through which the findings of the evaluation and treatment recommendations are reviewed with relevant individuals (i.e., referring physician, the patient, family, treatment team members). Treatment recommendations may include ongoing neurological care, psychiatric consultation, psychotherapy, cognitive/behavioral remediation, and vocational guidance. When working with school-aged children or college students, recommendations might include provision of in-class accommodations such as extended time allowances for testing, specific assistance to enhance comprehension of material, or environmental modifications to reduce distraction. Similar treatment strategies could be relevant for adults struggling with work/professional demands due to developmental factors or acquired injury. In all cases, recommendations should be pragmatic and individually tailored to each patient's specific needs. When possible, the clinician outlines concrete strategies to facilitate remediation of identified problems. Sensitivity to cultural norms, psychological factors (e.g., level of insight, motivation) and environmental resources (e.g., financial, family support) are crucial for successful care planning. Appropriate neuropsychological follow-up is also arranged when indicated.

Recommendations may include supplementary diagnostic procedures (e.g., imaging, electroencephalogram, polysomnography) and/or referral for additional specialty consultation (e.g., neurology, ophthalmology) in order to round out the diagnostic process and/or initiate treatment. Referral to psychiatry may be indicated for consideration of pharmacologic intervention (e.g., treatment with antidepressant, stimulant, cognitive-enhancing, or mood-stabilizing medication). A psychiatrist may also suggest psychotherapy, either as an adjunct to medication or as the sole treatment modality.

Treatment recommendations often include behavioral strategies aimed at circumventing or compensating for cognitive weaknesses. For example, behavioral strategies to enhance planning and organization can be implemented via post-evaluation consultation with the neuropsychologist or through the use of structured workbooks and guides (The Mindfulness Prescription for Adult ADHD[15]; The Harvard Medical School Guide to Achieving Optimal Memory[16]). Review of areas of cognitive strength are emphasized as they bear on development of compensatory cognitive strategies. If more intensive or ongoing treatment is indicated, a referral can be made to a clinician or program specializing in cognitive rehabilitation. For higher functioning patients, self-help books may be recommended to provide additional psychoeducation and skill development. Incorporating mindfulness-based activities may be recommended to address cognitive or emotional symptoms.

Mindfulness-based stress reduction may ease anxiety symptoms. Psychoeducation about mindfulness and developing a daily meditative practice may also help improve attention (via metacognition, i.e., bringing awareness to one's thoughts and attention). Lifestyle behavior modifications are recommended to optimize cognition and well-being. Aerobic exercise and a heart-healthy diet are empirically supported interventions to reduce risk of decline associated with chronic diseases. Examples of neuro-protective, heart-healthy diets include the Mediterranean and MIND Diets (**M**editerranean-DASH Diet **I**ntervention for **N**eurodegenerative **D**elay).[17] Patients with poor sleep quality would benefit from learning ways to promote sleep hygiene that can lead to improved, restorative sleep. Consistent treatment for obstructive sleep apnea (e.g., using a continuous positive airway pressure mask) may attenuate the white matter injury and cognitive sequelae which often accompany this disorder.[18,19]

Circumventing neurologic deficits may include assistive devices, such as eyeglasses affixed with prisms to help patients with spatial neglect perceive their environment. Modification of environmental factors can be effective for enhancing patient safety and caregiver confidence. Implementing fall precautions and using medical alert systems and tracking devices for wandering patients (e.g., GPS-enabled shoes and bracelets) can be practical solutions for common problems in elderly individuals with neurodegenerative illness.

Domains of Neuropsychological Function

The parsing of neuropsychological functions into specific domains is a somewhat arbitrary organizational contrivance. In reality, there is considerable overlap within and between cognitive domains. For example, working memory shares much common ground with aspects of attention and language.

General Intellectual Ability

Determining an individual's level of intellectual functioning is a fundamental component of the neuropsychological assessment because this serves as a point of reference from which to evaluate performance in other domains. Intelligence encompasses a broad range of capacities, many of which are not directly assessed in the traditional clinical setting. The estimate of general intellectual ability is based on both formal assessment methods and a survey of demographic factors and life accomplishments. Information regarding the patient's educational background and longstanding difficulties (e.g., learning disability, repeated grades), occupational history, and special abilities is used to establish an estimate of baseline intellectual functioning. Comparing cognitive test performances to this estimate is crucial in determining whether there has been a change or decline in level of functioning. However, it is important to note that an individual's profile of cognitive abilities can range considerably from domain to domain; variable capability across diverse neuropsychological functions is often the rule rather than the exception in normal human development.[20]

Measures of general intellectual functioning assess a broad range of abilities across verbal and nonverbal domains

TABLE 7-1 • General Intellectual Ability	
Test Name	**Description**
Wechsler Intelligence Scales	The Wechsler Adult Intelligence Scale-IV (WAIS-IV) is composed of 13 individual subtests. Administration of all subtests generates three Intellectual Quotients (IQs): Full-Scale IQ, Verbal IQ, and Performance IQ; and four different performance indices: Verbal Comprehension Index, Perceptual Organization Index, Working Memory Index, and Processing Speed Index.
	The Wechsler Abbreviated Scale of Intelligence (WASI) is designed to be a short and reliable measure of intelligence that produces VIQ, PIQ, and FSIQ scores that are similar to those obtained with the WAIS-III.
	The Wechsler Intelligence Scale for Children (WISC-IV) is used for testing children and adolescents ranging in age from 6 to 17 years.
	The Wechsler Preschool and Primary Scale of Intelligence (WPPSI-IV) is used for testing children ranging in age from 4 to 6.5 years.
Wechsler Test of Adult Reading (WTAR)	The WTAR is a measure of recognition vocabulary requiring oral reading of 50 phonetically "irregular" words. It is used to estimate premorbid baseline intellectual ability in patients with known or suspected dementia. Similar measures include the National Adult Reading Test, NART-Revised and American National Adult Reading Test (AmNART). Errors consist of word mispronunciations.
Raven's Standard and Colored Progressive Matrices	These are standardized measures of nonverbal analogical reasoning widely used both within and outside the United States as a "culture fair" measure of general intellectual ability. Both tests require the patient to demonstrate an understanding of the logic underlying visual patterns by selecting the missing component of the pattern from a series of choices. The Standard Matrices contain 60 black and white items ranging from simple to extremely difficult, while the Colored Matrices consist of 36 colored items that span a limited range of complexity. Errors consist of incorrect identification of the missing component of the visual pattern.

(e.g., Wechsler Adult Intelligence Scale [WAIS-IV],[21] Wechsler Intelligence Scale for Children [WISC-IV][22]) from which an "intelligence quotient (IQ)" and other indices are derived. Overall intellectual ability may be estimated using tests that are highly correlated with IQ measures (e.g., Ravens Progressive Matrices). Single-word reading tests (e.g., Wechsler Test of Adult Reading [WTAR],[23] the Test of Premorbid Functioning [TOPF][24]) provide reliable estimates of full-scale IQ, particularly with regard to verbal intelligence. These measures often serve a critical function estimating premorbid ability in individuals with known or suspected neurodegenerative conditions. Premorbid ability may also be surmised by using a "best performance" method approach, in which the patient's highest level of performance serves as a reference point for their maximal baseline capabilities (Table 7-1).

Attention and Executive Function

Attention

Attention to the surrounding environment is a foundational aspect of all cognitive function. For example, an individual cannot effectively name an object if the object is not first attended to and visually processed.[25] Attention should be assessed early in the evaluation as impairments in this domain will directly or indirectly affect performance in other areas of cognition (Table 7-2).

Attention is a general term that encompasses a number of different component processes. Attention span refers to the number of unrelated "bits" of information that can be held on line at a given moment in time. Assessment of attention span is typically accomplished through the recall of progressively longer series of information bits, such as numbers (digit span) or spatial locations (spatial span). Sustained attention, also called vigilance, refers to the capacity to maintain active attention over time. The most common method of assessing vigilance utilizes a target detection paradigm. Here the patient is instructed to respond to an infrequently occurring target stimulus. For example, on a measure of auditory vigilance, the patient hears a series of letters of the alphabet and must signal by pressing a response key each time a particular target letter is presented. Selective attention is similar to sustained attention but requires a response only to a particular class of stimuli and not to other stimuli. Set-shifting refers to the capacity to relinquish an existing procedural strategy in favor of a new response, based on recognition of a change in environmental contingencies. It is typically measured with tasks requiring the patient to shift focus among stimulus features of a test display (see Trail Making Test, Parts A and B, Wisconsin Card Sorting Test, Luria Graphomotor Sequences in Table 7-2). Resistance to interference, also called response inhibition, refers to the ability to sustain a given response even in the face of a salient distraction designed to obscure the target response. This is assessed with tasks requiring the patient to inhibit overlearned or automatized responses in the face of distractions contrived to undermine a desired response (e.g., Stroop Interference Test, Trail Making Test, Part B).

Executive Functioning

Executive functioning is a broad term to describe a varied set of processes involved in planning, organizing, strategizing, and managing one's actions and mental resources to achieve a goal in a contextually appropriate manner.[26,27] Formal tests of executive function assess a number of different capacities, including some functions mentioned above (set-shifting, overcoming interference, response inhibition) and also planning, perseverance, initiation, reasoning, and abstraction.[28,29] Planning involves thinking several steps ahead of one's current circumstances for the purpose of informing and altering a course of action.

TABLE 7-2 • Attention and Executive Functioning

Function	Test	Description
Attention span	Digit Span	The examiner reads increasingly long strings of numbers aloud. The examinee must repeat the numbers aloud in the same order, first forward and then in the reverse order.
	Spatial Span	The examiner taps a series of blocks in fixed locations. The examinee must repeat this series in the same order, and then in the reverse order.
Sustained attention and vigilance	Auditory and Visual Continuous Performance Test (CPT)	Basic auditory vigilance is tested by having the patient listen to a series of letters read serially and responding to a single target letter or series of letter configurations. Visual vigilance can be tested by showing a series of single numbers on a computer screen and requires responding to a target stimulus, but not to nontarget stimuli.
	Paced Auditory Serial Addition Test (PASAT)	The patient hears a tape-recorded voice reading numbers at various rates, ranging from every 2.4 seconds to every 1.2 seconds. The objective of the task is to sum the last two numbers heard and voice the sum aloud (e.g., if the numbers from the tape were "5, 2, 8, 4," the patients responses would be the following (in italics): "5, 2, *7*, 8, *10*, 4, *12*," etc. The process of voicing the sum aloud serves as interference, which must be overcome in order to attend to the following number. In total, 60 numbers are read in each of the four trials and every subsequent trial is faster than the one preceding it.
Set-shifting	Trail Making Test A and B	Measures of visual scanning, visuomotor tracking, and response set flexibility. Trails A involves connecting consecutively numbered circles, from 1 to 25. Trails B requires the patient to continually shift set, alternating between letters and numbers (i.e., 1, A, 2, B, etc.). Both tasks must be performed as quickly as possible and without lifting the writing utensil from the paper.
	Wisconsin Card Sorting Test	A measure of nonverbal concept formation, response set flexibility, sustained attention, and ability to integrate corrective feedback. The patient must sort cards according to underlying principles (color, form, number), which must be deduced, and which are shifted at set intervals.
	Luria Graphomotor Sequencing	Involves using a pencil to copy a series of patterns (i.e., m-n-m-n, peaks and plateaus, and multiple loops) without lifting the pencil. Errors consist of failing to alternate (i.e., m-n-m-m-m-m)
	Luria Motor Sequences	Involves performing repeated sequences of hand movements. Errors consist of failure to maintain the order of movements within each sequence.
Response inhibition	Stroop Color-Word Interference Test	Composed of three parts that require (1) reading a series of black and white color words (red, blue, green), (2) identifying the color of red, blue and green "Xs," and (3) identifying the ink color of incongruent color words (i.e., the correct response to the word "red" printed in blue ink would be "blue"). In all conditions the patient is asked to perform as quickly as possible.
	Motor Go-No-Go	Involves responding to a target signal (1 loud knock) by lifting a finger, but not to a second signal (2 loud knocks). The tendency to respond to the second signal must be inhibited. The examiner produces a series of one or two knocks and observes the patient's responses.
Planning	Delis-Kaplan Executive Function System (D-KEFS) Tower Test	Involves ordering four colored beads within a set of constraints. Only one bead may be moved at a time, and beads moved from their initial placement may not be returned. Similar tests include Tower of Hanoi and Tower of London.
Perseverance	Verbal and Design Fluency	Letters: the examinee must recite as many words as possible that start with a particular letter, with the exception of proper nouns, numbers, and more than one iteration of the same root word. This is repeated with three different letters in total. Categories: the examinee must recite as many words as possible from a particular category. This is repeated with three different categories in total. Design: the examinee must create as many unique designs as possible by connecting lines between dots laid out in a grid.

Tests measuring planning ability often require subjects to determine the correct series of steps needed to successfully reach a particular goal (e.g., Delis-Kaplan Executive Function System [D-KEFS] Tower Test[30]). Perseverance is the ability to sustain a particular course of action, even in the absence of an external prompt (e.g., D-KEFS Verbal and Design Fluency[30]). Measurement of perseverance often begins with both examiner and patient performing the same task, but involves the subject continuing the task even after the examiner has stopped (see Luria Motor Sequences). Initiation refers to the ability to spontaneously commence an action in the absence of a direct prompt from the external environment. This function is measured with presentation of a task followed by a period of time during which the subject is expected to respond independently (see Verbal Fluency, Go-No-Go). Reasoning involves using a system of logic to solve a particular problem or task. This can be measured in a variety of ways, including using visual puzzles and verbal analogies (see Ravens Progressive Matrices,[31] WAIS-IV Comprehension[32]). Abstraction is the ability to articulate and/or recognize shared attributes of seemingly dissimilar objects or concepts (e.g., WAIS-IV Similarities, Wisconsin Card Sorting Test) (Table 7-2).

Comportment, Insight, and Judgment

Although few tests probe these functions in a formal manner, they are important components of cognitive status and are frequently disturbed in cases of neurological and neuropsychiatric illness. Comportment refers to behavior in an interpersonal context. Disturbances often manifest as socially inappropriate behaviors that suggest insensitivity to accepted cultural norms. Examples include making offensive comments, crossing interpersonal boundaries, or interrupting during conversation. In the context of neuropsychological assessment, insight involves an accurate perception of one's mental and physical condition as well as appreciation of the impact of one's behavior on others. Cognitively impaired individuals often lack one or both of these components of insight. Judgment involves the capacity to make considered decisions that reflect sensitivity to preserving the safety and integrity of oneself, and appreciation of the likely outcomes of an action or plan.

A neuropsychologist can assess these functions informally through naturalistic observation, reports from individuals familiar with the patient, and also by inquiring about any accidents or legal infractions involving the patient. Formal measures to assess judgment may include presenting the patient with hypothetical circumstances to navigate in order to assess their understanding and decision making related to various health and safety situations (e.g., through tests like the Test of Practical Judgment[33] and the Judgment module of the Neuropsychological Assessment Battery[34]).

The Frontal Systems Behavior Scale (FrSBe)[35] comprises descriptions of various behaviors that are characteristic of patients with frontal systems damage. Each behavior is assigned a severity rating by the patient and by a family member, and the overall severity rating is thought to reflect the degree of behavioral disturbance present. The Neuropsychiatric Inventory (NPI)[36] is a rating scale that is completed by a family member or caregiver and surveys a range of potential problem areas, for example, cooperativeness, paranoia, aggression, and impulsivity. Both the extent of the patient's behavior and the degree of subsequent familial distress are rated.

Learning and Memory

The assessment of learning and memory function is perhaps the most complex endeavor of the neuropsychological examination. Memory is not a unitary construct. Neuropsychologists fractionate memory into multiple systems. Examples include declarative versus non-declarative memory, semantic versus episodic memory, etc. Memory is assessed with respect to modality of presentation (auditory vs. visual), material (linguistic vs. figural), and locus of reference (personal vs. nonpersonal). Also important is the time of initial exposure, namely whether information was learned before the onset of brain damage (retrograde memory; e.g., Boston Retrograde Memory Test, Transient Events Test) or after (anterograde memory; e.g., Wechsler Memory Scale-IV [WMS],[36] Rey Auditory Verbal Learning Test,[37] Bushke Selective Reminding Test,[38] Three Words Three Shapes,[39] Warrington Recognition Memory Test[40]).

With regard to formal neuropsychological assessment, the evaluation of memory should include measures that allow the dissociation of component processes entailed in the acquisition and later recall of information, namely encoding, consolidation, and retrieval. To this end, measures are used to assess performance with respect to length of interval between exposure to information and demand for recall (immediate vs. short vs. long delay) and extent of facilitation required to demonstrate retention (free recall vs. cued recall vs. recognition). The assessment of retrograde memory function poses a special problem insofar as it is difficult to know with certainty what information was previously registered in the remote memory of a particular patient. Although there are a number of formal tests that can be used for this purpose (e.g., Boston Remote Memory Battery,[41] Transient Events Test[42]), we also assess this aspect of memory function by asking for personal information which presumably is well known, or had been well known at one time, by the patient (e.g., names of family members, places of prior employment). In these instances, it is helpful to obtain confirmation of the accuracy of this information from family members or friends, if possible (see Table 7-3).

Working memory involves holding a stimulus or set of stimuli in mind in order to either produce it after a delay (e.g., looking up a telephone number and remembering it until it is successfully dialed) or use it in a mental procedure involving manipulation of information (e.g., carrying out mental arithmetic). The simpler aspect of working memory, also called maintenance of information, can be tested by requiring a subject to hold information in mind and reproduce it after a short delay (e.g., Digit Span Forward). The more complex components of working memory can be tested in a number of ways, all of which entail online maintenance and manipulation of information (e.g., WMS Tests of Mental Control, WAIS-IV Letter-Number Sequencing, WAIS-IV Arithmetic, PASAT).

Language

Language is the medium through which much of the neuropsychological examination is accomplished. Language function is assessed both opportunistically during the interview and via formal test instruments (Table 7-4). Conversational speech is observed with respect to fluency, articulation, rate, and prosody (i.e., the pattern of stress and intonation in speech). The patient's capacity to respond to interview questions and test instructions provides an informal index of receptive language ability or comprehension. Visual confrontation naming is carefully assessed so that word-finding problems and paraphasic errors may be elicited. Repetition is measured with phrases of varying length and phonemic complexity. Auditory comprehension is evaluated by asking the patient questions that range in length and grammatical complexity. Reading measures include identification of individual letters, common

TABLE 7-3 • Learning and Memory

Function	Test	Description
Working Memory	Tests of Mental Control	The examinee is asked to recite familiar sequences such as the alphabet, days of the week, months of the year, and numbers from 1 to 20 as quickly as possible. The examinee then must recite all sequences, except the alphabet, in reverse order. Serial subtractions involve subtracting a particular number until a predetermined point is reached.
	WAIS-IV Letter-Number Sequencing	The patient hears a series of alternating numbers and letters and is required to reconfigure them so that all of the numbers are recited first, in ascending order, and then letters in alphabetical order.
	WAIS-IV Arithmetic	Involves mental calculation of aurally presented arithmetic problems of increasing difficulty.
		See also Digit Span Forward and PASAT in Table 7-2.
Retrograde memory	Boston Retrograde Memory Test	Involves showing a series of black and white photos of famous persons from the 1920s to the 1980s. If the patient cannot spontaneously generate the correct name, the examiner can give a semantic cue (i.e., "he was a singer in the 1920s") and then a phonemic cue (i.e., first name). This test assumes that the patient has been exposed to the information in the first place.
	Transient Events Test (TET)	This is a measure of memory for popular news events from the 1950s through the 1990s. Items were selected by way of the *New York Times* index according to the criteria that they were mentioned at least 250 times during a particular year and less than five times over the subsequent 2 years. Hence, all items were of transient notoriety thereby minimizing confounding effects of overexposure. Free recall and recognition are tested.
Anterograde memory	Wechsler Memory Scale (WMS-IV)	This is a composite battery of tests assessing orientation, attention, learning, and memory for verbal and visual information across immediate and delayed intervals. It yields a series of index scores.
	Rey Auditory Verbal Learning Test	This measure of verbal encoding, learning, and retention involves drilling the examinee on a series of 15 unrelated words over five successive trials. Learning is followed by an interference trial, immediate recall, and 30-minute delayed recall and recognition. Various comparisons yield information regarding sensitivity to proactive and retroactive interference and rate of forgetting.
	Bushke Selective Reminding Test	This is a special type of list-learning test that is most helpful in cases where encoding is intact, but there may be a question of impairment at the level of consolidation or storage. A list of 12 words is read, and the patient must repeat as many words as possible. However, different from the previous list-learning tasks, the examiner then reads only the words that the patient did not recall. This continues across six trials, and each time the patient must try to recite as many words as possible but only hears the words not recalled on the preceding trial. There are immediate and delayed recall trials followed by visual multiple-choice recognition paradigms.
	Three Words Three Shapes Memory Test	The patient is instructed to copy three words and three shapes, after which incidental recall is tested. The patient is drilled on the words and shapes until criterion is reached, and recall is tested after intervals of 5, 15, and 30 minutes. Recognition is tested using distracter shapes and words.
	Warrington Recognition Memory Test	Involves the visual presentation of single words and faces at the rate of one every 3 seconds. The patient is instructed to reach each word silently and make and report a judgment regarding his association (pleasant or unpleasant) to it. Immediately afterward, the patient is shown a pair of words, each containing a target word and a distracter, with the instruction to identify the one presented previously. Memory for faces is tested in the same way.

words, irregularly spelled words, and nonwords, as well as measures of reading speed and comprehension. Spelling can be assessed in both visual and auditory modalities. A narrative handwriting sample can be obtained by instructing the patient to describe a standard stimulus scene.

Visuospatial Functions

After establishing the integrity of basic visual acuity, the spatial distribution of visual attention is evaluated. The presence of visual neglect is assessed through the use of tasks that require scanning across all quadrants of visual space. Assessment of left/right orientation involves directing patients to point to specific body parts, either on themselves or the examiner. Topographical orientation can be tested by instructing the patient to indicate well-known locales on a blank map. Graphic reproduction of designs and assembly of patterns using sticks, blocks, or other media are used to assess visual organization and constructional abilities. Facial recognition represents a special component perceptual process and can be measured using Benton's Facial Recognition Test.[43] The Judgment of Line Orientation Test[43] assesses perceptual accuracy in judging the angular displacement of lines. Warrington's Visual Object Space Perception Battery[44] is an example of a collection of measures designed to assess various aspects of perceptual function (see Table 7-5).

TABLE 7-4 • Language Function

Test Name	Description
Boston Diagnostic Aphasia Examination (BDAE)	This is composed of measures that assess all aspects of expressive and receptive language function including naming, comprehension, repetition, reading, writing, praxis, and prosody.
Boston Naming Test	One component of the BDAE, this measure of confrontation naming is often administered independently. It consists of a series of 60 black and white line drawings of objects. Naming difficulty increases as the objects progress from high frequency to low frequency. Stimulus cues are provided in the event of perceptual difficulty. Phonemic cues are used to distinguish between retrieval difficulties and lack of knowledge of a particular object name.
Nelson Denny Reading Test	This test contains two multiple-choice measures that assess vocabulary and reading comprehension. Reading speed is also computed. Reading comprehension can be scored on the basis of both a standard and extended length of time.
Wide Range Achievement Test-IV (WRAT-4)	This standardized battery of acquired scholastic skills includes measures of spelling, written arithmetic, and single word reading.
Wechsler Individual Achievement Test (WIAT)	This Wechsler test assesses the academic achievement of children, adolescents, and adults, aged 4 through 85 years. The test enables the assessment of a broad range of academic skills or only a particular area of need within the areas of reading, written language, oral language, and math.

TABLE 7-5 • Visuospatial Function

Test Name	Description
Benton Facial Recognition Test	This task is composed of two parts. The first involves matching a target face with one of six faces. The target stimulus is always identical to the correct answer. The second part of the task involves choosing the three photographs, out of the array of six, that contain the same face as the target photograph. Increasing use of camera angle and shadow contribute to the progressive difficulty of the task.
Benton Line Orientation Test	This task involves judging the spatial orientation of sets of line segments by comparing them to a grid composed of 11 radii. It is sensitive to visuoperceptual deficits associated with posterior right hemisphere lesions.
Visual Object Space Perception Battery	This battery contains eight individual tests that each probe a specific component of object or space perception. Individual subtests are untimed and can be given in isolation or within the context of the full battery. Normative data are based on healthy control subjects as well as patients with right- and left-hemisphere lesions.
Letter/Symbol Cancellation	The objective of this task is to circle each instance of a target letter or symbol from among a field of similar stimuli. There are a total of 60 targets evenly distributed among the four quadrants of the 8-1/2 × 11-inch page. Errors of omission involve failing to respond to the target stimulus. Errors of commission involve responding to stimuli other than the target stimulus.
Hooper Visual Organization Test	This task involves examining line drawings of objects that have been broken into fragments and rotated. The objective is to mentally reorganize each set of fragments and subsequently identify the corresponding coherent whole.
Complex Figure Drawing	This task involves copying a complex line drawing, usually the Rey-Osterreith complex figure or Taylor complex figure. Ability to reproduce the gestalt as well as the internal details of the design facilitate the detection of various perceptual deficits. Significant distortion of or failure to copy one side of the figure can indicate the presence of hemispatial neglect.

Motor Functions

Naturalistic observations of the patient's gait and upper and lower extremity coordination are an important part of the motor examination. Hand preference should be assessed either through direct inquiry or a formal handedness questionnaire (Table 7-6). Motor speed, dexterity, and programming are tested with timed tasks, some of which involve repetition of a specific motor act (e.g., finger tapping, peg placement) and others that involve more complex motor movements (e.g., finger sequencing, sequential hand positions). Manual grasp strength can be assessed with a hand dynamometer.

Affect, Mood, and Psychological Functioning

Standardized measures of mood, personality, and psychopathology can be used to assess the contribution of psychiatric illness to the patient's presentation and diagnosis (Table 7-7). However, it is important to understand that many neurological illnesses can cause disorders of affect and mood. In addition, certain neurological illnesses can produce symptoms that overlap with particular psychiatric disorders. Therefore, neuropsychologists must possess a thorough understanding of the psychiatric profiles associated with various neurobehavioral syndromes and proceed with caution when evaluating

TABLE 7-6 • Motor Functioning

Test Name	Description
Finger Oscillation Test	Finger tapping speed is measured by having the patient tap a key as quickly as possible over a period of 10 seconds, using the index finger. Each hand is tested a number of times and trial totals are averaged. Poor performance consists of slow tapping speed. Unilateral motor weakness can be assessed by comparing tapping speeds of each hand. Bilateral weakness is assessed through comparison with age-matched norms.
Hand Dynamometer	Grip strength in each hand is measured by having the patient squeeze a pressure-calibrated instrument. Unilateral motor weakness can be assessed by comparing performance with each hand. Bilateral weakness is assessed through comparison with age-matched norms.
Grooved Pegboard	Measures of fine motor speed and dexterity, entailing placement of pegs in a pegboard, are obtained with each hand separately. Poor performance consists of difficulty grasping and manipulating the pegs, resulting in slowed performance.
Reitan-Klove Sensory-Perceptual Examination	Collection of measures of tactile, auditory, and visual perception using unilateral and double simultaneous stimulation. Fingertip number writing, visual fields, and tactile finger recognition are tested.

TABLE 7-7 • Psychological Functioning and Mood

Test Name	Description
Beck Depression Inventory	This instrument is used to assess depression severity based on self-reported ratings of a number of different relevant symptoms. Higher scores indicate greater severity of symptoms.
Beck Anxiety Inventory	This instrument is used to assess anxiety severity based on self-reported ratings of a variety of somatic, cognitive, and psychological symptoms of anxiety. Higher scores indicate greater severity of symptoms.
Personality Assessment Inventory (PAI)	This test contains 344 statements to be rated according to how accurate they are as self-descriptors (i.e., false, slightly true; mainly true; very true). The items comprise 22 nonoverlapping scales that assess constructs relevant to personality and psychopathology. The test-taker's approach to the items is also assessed utilizing a number of validity scales and indicators.
Minnesota Multiphasic Personality Inventory-2 (MMPI-2)	This series of 537 true/false questions load on to a number of different subscales that correspond to various personality traits or types of psychopathology. Scores on each subscale are standardized. Combinations of high and low scores on individual subscales correspond differentially to the presence or absence of various psychopathologies. Careful interpretation of subscale scores is crucial to the accurate use of this measure.
Reading the Mind in the Eyes Test	An emotion recognition task to determine the mental state conveyed by pictures of eyes in isolation (rather than whole faces). Participants choose from four mental state descriptions.

psychiatric symptoms in the presence of neurological or medical illness.

Neuropsychiatric and neurologic disorders may also impact social cognition, undermining the perception, interpretation, and ability to respond appropriately to social information. Such deficits may arise from a neurodevelopmental condition (e.g., autism spectrum disorder), psychiatric illness, the sequelae of trauma (e.g., head injury or stroke), or the manifestation of a neurodegenerative disorder. Social cognitive skills are vital for communication and sound interpersonal relationships. As such, impairments in these areas may have negative effects on mental health and functional outcomes (e.g., ability to reintegrate in the work force) and should be considered during comprehensive neuropsychological evaluation and treatment planning (for review of clinical assessment of this domain, see Henry et al.[45]). Deficits may be evident in the perception of social stimuli, abnormal behavior (e.g., lack of adherence to social standards), reduced affective empathy, or problems taking another's perspective (poor theory of mind). One example of clinical measure is the Reading the Mind in The Eyes Test, an emotion recognition task to determine the mental state conveyed by subtle social cues (in the form of pictures of eyes in isolation vs. whole faces) (see Table 7-8).[46] The Advanced Clinical Solutions for WAIS-IV and WMS-IV contains several measures of social cognition, such as affect labeling, affect recognition from faces and prosody, identification of sarcasm, face recognition, and recall of names and pertinent information about a person from facial images.[47]

Effort and Motivation

Assessment of effort is important in evaluating the overall validity of the patient's examination. The degree of effort a patient exerts in responding to test items can be impacted by a wide range of factors including psychopathology, illness, cultural background, insight into the purpose of the referral, and secondary gain issues. Neuropsychologists rely on both embedded and free-standing measures in assessing effort (see Table 7-9). These tests are also known as symptom validity or performance validity tests. Embedded measures focus on analysis of performance

TABLE 7-8 • Social Cognition	
Test Name	**Description**
Advanced Clinical Solutions for WAIS-IV and WMS-IV	The social cognition subtests developed for ACS were designed to measure relevant components of social cognition, such as affect labeling, affect recognition from faces and prosody, identification of sarcasm, and the ability to verbalize intent of a speaker, and facial memory, such as face recognition and recall of names and pertinent information about a person from facial images.
Reading the Mind in the Eyes Test	An emotion recognition task to determine the mental state conveyed by pictures of eyes in isolation (rather than whole faces). Participants choose from four mental state descriptions.

TABLE 7-9 • Effort and Motivation	
Test Name	**Description**
Reliable Digit Span	A symptom validity test based on the standard Digit Span subtest of the WAIS based on improbably poor performance
Structured Inventory of Malingered Symptomatology (SIMS)	A 75-item true/false screening instrument that is sensitive to both malingered psychopathology and feigned neuropsychological symptoms
Test of Memory Malingering (TOMM)	A forced choice visual recognition test designed to distinguish bona fide memory impairment from poor performance based on weak effort or feigned deficit

TABLE 7-10 • Dementia Screening Tools	
Test Name	**Description**
Mini Mental Status Exam (MMSE)	This is a set of brief tasks that can be administered at the bedside and used to screen for obvious cognitive impairment. It includes items that assess attention, orientation, language, memory, and construction. Lower scores indicate greater severity of dementia. The MMSE score ranges between 0 and 30; recommended cut-off scores have ranged from 24 to 27 with various allowances for educational background.
Montreal Cognitive Assessment (MoCA)	This brief screening measure assesses multiple cognitive domains, including short-term and long-term memory recall, visuospatial abilities, language, attention and concentration, and aspects of executive functioning. Like the MMSE, the MoCA yields a score between 0 and 30, with recommended cut-off scores ranging between 23 and 26.
Mattis Dementia Rating Scale (DRS)	This scale assesses a wide range of neuropsychological domains including attention, initiation and perseverance, construction, conceptualization, and memory. It is used for grading and tracking overall degree of dementia. Lower scores indicate greater severity of dementia.

exaggerated/fabricated cognitive dysfunction. The interested reader is referred to Lippa's[53] recent paper for a comprehensive review of this topic.

Dementia Screening Tools

A significant role of neuropsychological evaluation is the detection of age-related cognitive impairment and dementia. As such, a number of specific screening tools have been developed for this purpose (Table 7-10). Many of these measures are designed to quickly assess gross level of functioning in major cognitive domains and can be administered in a matter of minutes (e.g., MMSE, MoCA). The Mattis Dementia Rating Scale[54] is a more comprehensive set of items designed to stage severity of impairment in patients with known dementia.

within standard clinical tests (e.g., Reliable Digit Span).[48] The Test of Memory Malingering (TOMM)[49,50] is an example of a free-standing memory performance validity measure based on statistical probability of response patterns in a forced choice format. The Structured Inventory of Malingered Symptomatology (SIMS)[51] is an instrument designed to detect feigned psychiatric disorder. Slick et al.[52] proposed an overall schema for detecting

CASE VIGNETTE 7.1

A 64-year-old man was referred for neuropsychological evaluation by his neurologist in the setting of subjective memory complaints. His medical history was significant for hypertension, type II diabetes, and untreated obstructive sleep apnea. He reported that his mood has been low after recently losing his wife of 35 years and he is worried about his finances.

The neuropsychologist gathered additional history to determine the nature and course of his memory complaints. These concerns manifested two years ago as he was

dealing with significant stressors related to his wife's illness and have remained stable over time. He had no difficulties at work or his day-to-day functioning in tasks at home. Indeed, he had been well organized, managing his wife's myriad medical appointments and complex medication regimen. He continued to work as a copy editor for a large publication. Other salient aspects of the history include the fact that his father exhibited cognitive impairment following a stroke in his 70s, while his mother and his siblings remain in reasonably good health. Socially, he had a few acquaintances but no children or close sources of emotional support. His PCP ordered basic screening labs for reversible causes of cognitive impairment (e.g., B12, TSH), which were normal. No neuroimaging was available for review.

Neuropsychological testing revealed a pattern of mild inefficiencies in memory encoding and retrieval. His memory storage for the material he learned was well preserved. He was mildly inattentive and slow on psychomotor tasks, bilaterally. His reasoning, problem solving, and other aspects of executive functioning were consistent with his estimated baseline intellectual abilities, which were in the average range. Language and visuospatial abilities were also found to be intact. On further evaluation, he endorsed sadness, problems with sleep quality and fatigue, and worrying about his future.

On the basis of the assessment, the neuropsychologist concluded the patient's mild cognitive changes were consistent with frontal systems dysfunction, and probably had multifactorial etiology. Contributory factors were thought to include prominent mood changes, poor sleep quality, and fatigue, as well as the possible contribution of multiple cerebrovascular risk factors. The exam findings and clinical history were not suggestive of the type of progressive decline that would be concerning for a neurodegenerative process. Further workup was recommended to include a brain MRI to determine the presence and extent of chronic microvascular disease. The patient was provided psychoeducation regarding the importance of healthy lifestyle behaviors, including appropriate management of medical conditions and the benefit of definitive treatment for sleep apnea. A brief follow-up consultation was scheduled to review these findings and recommendations, as well as go over cognitive compensatory strategies to enhance attention and everyday memory. He was additionally referred for psychotherapy to address his mood symptoms and also to build motivation for engaging in healthy behavioral changes. Neuropsychological re-evaluation was recommended as clinically indicated, with this exam serving as a baseline against which he may be monitored for possible improvement or decline.

CONTENDING WITH SPECIAL CIRCUMSTANCES

Examining the Patient with Sensory or Motor Deficits

Patients with limitations in primary sensory or motor function present special challenges for assessment. Visual problems are highly common within the aging population, including presbyopia, glaucoma, and cataracts. Since a considerable amount of typical testing entails visual processing of various stimuli and materials, patients should be examined while using their usual corrective lenses. Keeping several pairs of reading glasses of varying diopter strength on hand as part of testing equipment is always a good idea. In some instances, test stimuli can be modified (enlarged) to make viewing easier for the visually impaired. When evaluating the blind patient, tests requiring visual processing are simply excluded from the test battery.

Acquired visual impairment is often observed in individuals with traumatic brain injury, stroke, tumor, or different types of neurodegenerative disease. It is important to distinguish between peripheral and central causes of impaired performance in the neuropsychological examination, as these etiologies have different diagnostic significance and will respond to different types of treatment interventions. This determination can be difficult in some cases and require additional specialty evaluation by ophthalmology or neuro-ophthalmology.

Hearing loss is also an exceptionally common problem in the elderly patient. Interestingly, many older patients are either reluctant to acknowledge or unaware of problems with diminished hearing acuity. Furthermore, a significant number of patients with identified hearing loss are unwilling to utilize hearing aids. When examining the hearing-impaired patient, the clinician must speak clearly, slowly, and loudly. It can be helpful and informative to have the patient repeat back questions to ensure apprehension. It is essential for a neuropsychologist to consider the unique aspects of hearing loss for their individual patient, including the type and degree of hearing loss, age of onset and etiology, preferred mode of communication, and presence of additional disability. Ideally, patients with congenital or acquired deafness can be seen by a clinician with American Sign Language (ASL) expertise. As this is frequently not possible, the neuropsychologist will adapt testing methods to the situation. For example, instead of presenting a word list aurally, words to be remembered can be presented in written form.

Modification of response parameters is often useful when evaluating individuals with disorders of expressive speech or motor function. For example, a recognition paradigm can be utilized in place of open-ended, spoken responses and tasks that require a motor response. Rather than have the patient produce a verbal response, they may identify a response from a visual array. When assessing visual memory in motorically challenged patients, they may indicate a choice among design options instead of drawing the design. Various forms of assistive technology have been developed for use with both aphasic and paralyzed patients.

Lateralized sensory deficits can be partially accommodated by presenting information to the relatively spared side. For example, directing spoken instruction to the preferred ear or presenting visual information to the relatively spared hemifield. Using visual stimuli in vertical arrays can be helpful as well. Various authors have considered the sensory and/or motoric demands of many commonly used neuropsychological tests and proposed alternative administration approaches.[55]

Hill-Briggs et al.[56] provide a comprehensive review of issues pertaining to neuropsychological test administration, accommodations, modifications, specialized test development, and disability-related factors that influence test interpretation across the spectrum of disabled individuals. Bylsma and Doninger[57] review the assessment of individuals with significant visual loss.

Patients from Divergent Linguistic/Cultural Backgrounds

Neuropsychologists are increasingly involved in the evaluation of individuals from divergent cultural backgrounds and for whom English is not the primary language. Cultural competency is essential at all levels of the assessment, from building rapport and history taking, to accurate test interpretation and formulating diagnostic conclusions. Simply translating the examiner's instructions and test items from standard English to the native language of the examinee rarely overcomes the wide gulf in cultural experience and all that comes with it. People from different parts of the world are acculturated with widely varying attitudes toward the very notion of testing and assessment. For example, performance on measures of processing speed may be influenced by cultural norms regarding whether "best" performance sacrifices speed for accuracy or vice versa.[58] Neuropsychologists must be highly sensitive to these deeply ingrained and pervasive differences and take them into account when examining individuals from diverse backgrounds.

Ideally, patients from divergent backgrounds should be examined by clinicians who share their sociocultural heritage. Slowly but surely, test measures derived from divergent cultural/linguistic are being developed and disseminated for clinical use. Given realistic constraints extant in most health care settings, it is usually necessary to compromise by using professional interpreters and adopting a highly conservative approach to test data generated in this fashion. Although neuropsychology is making headway in this regard, we are truly only at the beginning of this work to address health care disparities and increase access to evaluation services. Continuing education for current practitioners to expand their cultural competency, establishing appropriate normative data for individuals from various cultures, and incorporating cultural neuropsychology as a component of training programs will help the field serve a wider array of individuals.

Summary and Key Points

- Drawing from the earliest studies of brain–behavior relationships in patients with naturally acquired lesions and the accumulating body of literature in cognitive neuroscience, neuropsychologists have created a diverse collection of test instruments and other assessment methods that permit the precise measurement of specific components of mental processes.
- Together with a comprehensive knowledge of neuropathologic syndromes and functional neuroanatomy, the results of neuropsychological examination provide both descriptive and diagnostic information regarding the condition of the brain.
- The fractionation of neuropsychological functions into specific domains is a somewhat arbitrary organizational contrivance. In reality, there is considerable overlap within and between cognitive domains. For example, working memory shares much common ground with aspects of attention and language.
- A competent neuropsychologist will sample multiple domains of behavior; variables from each domain must be considered in order to arrive at an understanding of the clinical significance of a given behavior.
- Variable capability across diverse neuropsychological functions is often the rule rather than the exception in normal human development.
- Test interpretation must consider all aspects of the patient history, observations of appearance and behavior, as well as transient "state" factors such as mood, fatigue, and pain.
- Information obtained during the initial interview is important for differential diagnosis and guides the remainder of the assessment.
- The Boston Process approach proceeds in a hypothesis-driven manner and uses the patient's test performance to guide and inform an evolving and dynamic assessment strategy. The process-oriented evaluation is individually tailored to each patient and uses specific tests for the purpose of answering particular questions, with test selection occurring in real time, that is, a Flexible Battery approach. This is in contrast to a Fixed Battery approach, which consists of a standard set of measurements administered to every patient regardless of presentation or referral question; the comprehensive nature of this approach is thought to reveal not only the pattern of deficits, but also subtle issues not readily apparent by observation or history alone.
- Neuropsychological consultation often concludes with the process of feedback, through which the findings of the evaluation and treatment recommendations are reviewed with relevant individuals (i.e., referring physician, the patient, family, treatment team members). Treatment recommendations should be pragmatic and individually tailored, with sensitivity to cultural norms and consideration of access to resources.
- Discrepancy between "test behavior" and "real-life" behavior is a major source of ongoing challenge for the design of ecologically valid assessment measures and environment.
- Neuropsychologists in the 21st century face the challenge of minimizing disparities in health care by increasing cultural competence throughout doctoral training and beyond and developing appropriate normative information and assessment methodologies suited to diverse patient populations.

Multiple Choice Questions

1. Interpretation of neuropsychological test results must occur in the context of sampling multiple cognitive domains because:
   a. Neuropsychological assessments by nature are comprehensive.
   b. It is important to employ a fixed battery approach.
   c. Increasing the number of tests administered increases diagnostic accuracy.
   d. Performance on any one measure relies on multiple cognitive processes.
   e. A global cognitive composite score should be derived from the test results.

2. Fundamental assumptions which underlie neuropsychological assessment include all but the following:
   a. Inferences about the integrity of the brain can be made based on observable behavior.
   b. Neuropsychological tests should be constructed according to sound psychometric principles.
   c. Performance on a single test is not sufficient to make a diagnostic inference.
   d. Performance on neuropsychological tests perfectly predicts real-world behavior.
   e. Observable behavior is frequently the most sensitive manifestation of brain pathology.

3. Neuropsychological assessment in current practice is best defined as:
   a. A means of assessing the extent and location of evolving CNS lesions.
   b. The utilization of standardized test methods to characterize brain function based on principles of brain–behavior relationships.
   c. Assessing psychological coping and adjustment in patients with neurologic disease.
   d. Assessing the impact of central nervous system integrity on personality characteristics.
   e. An alternative to neuroimaging in patients for whom it is contraindicated.

4. Clinical applications of neuropsychological assessment include:
   a. Establishing a cognitive baseline against which to measure change over time.
   b. Characterizing the nature and severity of cognitive impairment to inform treatment planning.
   c. Creating a differential diagnosis, for example, of dementia subtypes.
   d. Determining capacity, for example, for independent living or medical decision making.
   e. All of the above.

Multiple Choice Answers

1. **Answer: d**
   Neuropsychological tests are typically not "process pure" as they rely on integration of several component processes across multiple domains. For example, a low score on a verbal memory test may result from problems in attention, language, or even a hearing loss. By sampling multiple domains, a pattern of information emerges that reflects the functional integrity of underlying neural processes.

2. **Answer: d**
   Although it is true that performance on neuropsychological testing is strongly related to functioning in the outside world, this relationship is imperfect. The patient who has grossly impaired performance on memory tests will almost certainly have difficulty in everyday memory; the patient who performs extraordinarily well on tests of memory and retention will have a fair degree of success in everyday memory. However, a large number of patients fall into a "gray area" with regard to testing outcomes and it can be much more difficult to predict with precision how these patients will function in their day-to-day life.

3. **Answer: b**
   Neuropsychological assessment uses standardized assessment methodologies to characterize brain function, inform diagnosis, and design treatment. Clinical reasoning relies on a deep knowledge of brain–behavior relationships in normal development and disease. The combination of this knowledge and prototypic test profiles leads to the recognition of characteristic syndromes associated with known brain diseases and disorders.

4. **Answer: e**
   Neuropsychological assessment aids in diagnosis and treatment planning for a variety of clinical ends, including all those listed above.

References

1. Benton A. Clinical neuropsychology: 1960–1990. *J Clin Exp Neuropsychol*. 1992;14(3):407-417.

2. Ebbinghaus H. *Memory: A Contribution to Experimental Psychology*. Ruger H, Bussenius C, trans. New York, NY: Teachers College; 1913.

3. Binet A, Simon T. *The development of intelligence in children: The Binet-Simon Scale*. Publications of the Training School at Vineland New Jersey Department of Research No. 11. Kite ES, trans. Baltimore, MD: Williams & Wilkins; 1916.

4. Reitan RM, Wolfson D. *The Halstead-Reitan Neuropsychological Test Battery: Theory and Clinical Interpretation*. 2nd ed. Tucson, AZ: Neuropsychology Press; 1993.

5. Kaplan E. The process approach to neuropsychological assessment of psychiatric patients. *J Neuropsychiatry Clin Neurosci*. 1990;2(1):72-87.

6. Harlow JM. Recovery from the passage of an iron bar through the head. Published 1868 in *Bulletin of the Massachusetts Medical Society*. Reprinted in *History of Psychiatry*. 1993;4(14): 274-281.

7. Broca P. Perte de la parole, ramollissement chronique et destruction partielle du lobe antérieur gauche. *Bulletin de la Société d'Anthropologie*. 1861;2:235-238.

8. Scoville WB, Milner B. Loss of recent memory after bilateral hippocampal lesions. *J Neurol Neurosurg Psychiatry*. 1957;20(1): 11-21.

9. Binder LM, Iverson GL, Brooks BL. To err is human: "abnormal" neuropsychological scores and variability are common in healthy adults. *Arch Clin Neuropsychol*. 2009;24(1):31-46.

10. Folstein MF, Folstein SE, McHugh PR. Mini-Mental State (MMSE). *J Psychiatr Res*. 1975;12:189-198.

11. Roalf DR, Moberg PJ, Xie SX, Wolk DA, Moelter ST, Arnold SE. Comparative accuracies of two common screening instruments for classification of Alzheimer's disease, mild cognitive impairment, and healthy aging. *Alzheimers Dement*. 2013;9(5):29-37.

12. Bianchini KJ, Mathias CW, Greve KW. Symptom validity testing: a critical review. *Clin Neuropsychol*. 2001;15(1):19-45.

13. Milberg WP, Hebben NA, Kaplan E. The Boston Process approach to neuropsychological assessment. In: Grant I, Adams K, eds. *Neuropsychological Assessment of Neuropsychiatric Disorders*. New York, NY: Oxford University Press; 1986:58-80.

14. Sweet JJ, Moberg PJ, Suchy Y. Ten-year follow-up survey of clinical neuropsychologists: Part I. Practices and beliefs. *Clin Neuropsychol*. 2001;14(1):18-37.

15. Zylowska L. *The Mindfulness Prescription for Adult ADHD*. Boston, MA: Trumpeter Books; 2012.

16. Nelson A, Gilbert S. *The Harvard Medical School Guide to Achieving Optimal Memory*. New York, NY: McGraw-Hill Professional Publishing; 2005.

17. Morris MC, Tangney CC, Wang Y, Sacks FM, Barnes LL, Bennett DA, Aggarwal NT. MIND diet slows cognitive decline with aging. *Alzheimers Dement*. 2015;1(9):1015-1022.

18. Baker CA, Hurley RA, Taber K. Update on obstructive sleep apnea: implications for neuropsychiatry. *J Neuropsychiatry Clin Neurosci*. 2016;28(3):A6-A159.

19. Dalmases M, Solé-Padullés C, Torres M, et al. Effect of CPAP on cognition, brain function, and structure among elderly patients with OSA: a randomized pilot study. *Chest*. 2015;148(5):1214-1223.

20. Schretlen DJ, Munro CA, Anthony JC, Pearlson GD. Examining the range of intraindividual variability in neuropsychological test performance. *J Int Neuropsychol Soc*. 2003;9(6):864-870.

21. Wechsler D. *Wechsler Adult Intelligence Scale*. San Antonio, TX: NCS Pearson; 2008.

22. Kaufman AS, Flanagan DP, Alfonso VC, Mascolo JT. Test review: Wechsler Intelligence Scale for Children (WISC-IV). *J Psychoeduc Assess*. 2006;24(3):278-295.

23. Wechsler D. *Wechsler Test of Adult Reading: WTAR*. San Antonio, TX: The Psychological Corporation; 2001.

24. Wechsler D. *The Test of Premorbid Functioning (TOPF)*. San Antonio, TX: The Psychological Corporation; 2011.

25. Clarke ADF, Coco MI, Keller F. The impact of attentional, linguistic, and visual features during object naming. *Front Psychol*. 2013;4:927.

26. Vaughan L, Giovanello K. Executive function in daily life: age-related influences of executive processes on instrumental activities of daily living. *Psychol Aging*. 2010;25(2):343-355.

27. Shallice T. *From Neuropsychology to Mental Structure*. Cambridge, UK: Cambridge University Press; 1988.

28. Baddeley A. Fractionating the central executive. In: Knight RL, Stuss DT, eds. *Principles of Frontal Lobe Function*. Oxford [Oxfordshire]: Oxford University Press; 2002:246-260.

29. Alvarez JA, Emory E. Executive function and the frontal lobes: a meta-analytic review. *Neuropsychol Rev*. 2006;16(1):17-42.

30. Delis D, Kaplan E, Kramer J. Delis-Kaplan Executive Function System (D-KEFS). [Database record]. PsycTESTS. 2001. Available at https://doi.org/10.1037/t15082-000, last accessed on 04/11/2018.

31. Raven J. Manual for Raven's Progressive Matrices and Vocabulary Scales. Research Supplement No. 1: The 1979 British Standardisation of the Standard Progressive Matrices and Mill Hill Vocabulary Scales, Together with Comparative Data from Earlier Studies in the UK, US, Canada, Germany and Ireland. San Antonio, TX: Harcourt Assessment; 1981.

32. Rabin LA, Borgos MJ, Saykin AJ, Wishart HA, Crane PK, Nutter-Upham KE, Flashman LA. Judgment in older adults: development and psychometric evaluation of the Test of Practical Judgment (TOP-J). *J Clin Exp Neuropsychol*. 2007;29(7):752-767.

33. Stern RA, White T. *Neuropsychological Assessment Battery*. Lutz, FL: Psychological Assessment Resources; 2003.

34. Grace J, Malloy PF. *Frontal Systems Behavior Scale. Professional Manual*. Lutz, FL: Psychological Assessment Resources; 2001.

35. Cummings JL, Mega M, Gray K, Rosenberg-Thompson S, Carusi DA, Gornbein J. The Neuropsychiatric Inventory: comprehensive assessment of psychopathology in dementia. *Neurology*. 1994;44(12):2308-2308.

36. Wechsler D. *Wechsler Memory Scales—Fourth Edition (WMS-IV): Administration and Scoring Manual*. San Antonio, TX: Pearson Clinical Assessment; 2009.

37. Tierney MC. Use of the Rey Auditory Verbal Learning Test in differentiating normal aging from Alzheimer Parkinson's dementia. *Psychol Assess*. 1994;6(2):129-134.

38. Buschke H. Selective reminding for analysis of memory and learning. *J VL VB*. 1973;12:543-550.

39. Weintraub S, Peavy GM, O'Connor M, Johnson NA, Acar D, Sweeney J, Janssen I. Three words three shapes: a clinical test of memory. *J Clin Exp Neuropsychol*. 2000;22(2):267-278.

40. Warrington EK. *Recognition Memory Test: Manual*. Berkshire, UK: NFER-Nelson; 1984.

41. Albert MS, Butters N, Levin J. Temporal gradients in the retrograde amnesia of patients with alcoholic Korsakoff's disease. *Arch Neurol*. 1979;36:211-216.

42. O'Connor MG, Sieggreen MA, Bachna K, Kaplan B, Cermak LS, Ransil BJ. Long-term retention of transient news events. *J Int Neuropsychol Soc*. 2000;6(1):44-51.

43. Benton AL, Sivan AB, Hamsher K, Varney NR, Spreen O. *Contributions to Neuropsychological Assessment*. New York, NY: Oxford University Press; 1994.

44. Warrington EK, James M. *The Visual Object and Space Battery Perception*. Bury St Edmunds, UK: Thames Valley Company; 1991.

45. Henry JD, Von Hippel W, Molenberghs P, Lee T, Sachdev PS. Clinical assessment of social cognitive function in neurological disorders. *Nat Rev Neurol*. 2016;12(1):28.

46. Baron-Cohen S, Wheelwright S, Hill J, Raste Y, Plumb I. The "Reading the Mind in the Eyes" Test revised version: a study with normal adults, and adults with Asperger syndrome or high-functioning autism. *J Child Psychol Psychiatry*. 2001;42(2):241-251.

47. Wechsler D. *Advanced Clinical Solutions for the WAIS-IV and WMS-IV*. San Antonio, TX: The Psychological Corporation; 2009.

48. Greiffenstein MF, Baker WJ, Gola T. Validation of malingered amnesia measures with a large clinical sample. *Psychol Assess*. 1994;6(3):218-224.

49. Tombaugh TN. *TOMM, Test of Memory Malingering*. North Tonawanda, NY: Multi-Health Systems Inc; 1996.

50. Tombaugh TN. The Test of Memory Malingering (TOMM): normative data from cognitively intact and cognitively impaired individuals. *Psychol Assess*. 1997;9:260-268.

51. Smith GP, Burger GK. Detection of malingering: validation of the Structured Inventory of Malingered Symptomatology (SIMS). *J Am Acad Psychiatry Law*. 1997;25(2):183-189.

52. Slick DJ, Sherman EM, Iverson GL. Diagnostic criteria for malingered neurocognitive dysfunction: proposed standards for clinical practice and research. *Clin Neuropsychol*. 1999;13:545-561.

53. Lippa SM. Performance validity testing in neuropsychology: a clinical guide, critical review, and update on a rapidly evolving literature. *Clin Neuropsychol*. 2018;32(3):391-421.

54. Woodard JL, Salthouse TA, Godsall RE, Green RC. Confirmatory factor analysis of the Mattis Dementia Rating Scale in patients with Alzheimer's disease. *Psychol Assess*. 1996;8(1):85-91.

55. Caplan B, Schechter J. The role of nonstandard neuropsychological assessment in rehabilitation: history, rationale, and examples. In: Cushman L, Scherer M, eds. *Psychological Assessment in Medical Rehabilitation. Measurement and Instrumentation in Psychology*. Washington, DC: American Psychological Association; 1995:359-392.

56. Hill-Briggs F, Dial JG, Morere DA, Joyce A. Neuropsychological assessment of persons with physical disability, visual impairment or blindness, and hearing impairment or deafness. *Arch Clin Neuropsychol*. 2007;22(3):389-404.

57. Bylsma FD, Doninger N. Neuropsychological assessment in individuals with severe visual impairment. *Top Geriatr Rehabil*. 2004;20(3):196-203.

58. Agranovich AV, Panter AT, Puente AE, Touradji P. The culture of time in neuropsychological assessment: exploring the effects of culture-specific time attitudes on timed test performance in Russian and American samples. *J Int Neuropsychol Soc*. 2011;17(4):692-701.

Neuropsychiatric Therapeutics

Psychopharmacology in Neuropsychiatric Syndromes

Laura T. Safar · Seth Gale · Brady B. Lonergan · Shreya Raj · Jane Erb

INTRODUCTION: OVERALL PRINCIPLES

The focus of this chapter is the review of the pharmacological treatment of neuropsychiatric syndromes including depression, anxiety, psychosis, agitation, apathy, and pathological laughing and crying. The chapter also includes a discussion of cognitive disorders from a syndrome or domain-based perspective, and their pharmacological treatment. The details of the pharmacological treatment of each specific neuropsychiatric disorder are presented in the chapters devoted to each disorder, in Section IV of this textbook.

Pharmacotherapy is one of many available interventions to help alleviate suffering in neuropsychiatric disorders. Medications can be an effective and important tool when used in a thoughtful, stepwise approach, addressing syndromes as varied as cognitive impairment, psychosis, aggression, sleep, depression, and aberrant behavior, among others. It is usually the combination of pharmacotherapy and other interventions, such as environmental modification, cognitive rehabilitation, neurostimulation, and forms of behavioral therapy, that is more effective than any singular approach.[1-4] Because of the complex overlap between many neuropsychiatric syndromes, a prudent strategy is to conduct a careful clinical evaluation before treatment, to identify the presenting symptoms and syndromes to be targeted with drug regimens, and to consistently monitor their effect once treatment is initiated. The pharmacological intervention may target aberrations in a neurotransmitter system that is involved in the pathogenesis of several presenting disturbances. For example, a patient with anxiety, sleep disruption, and attention deficits, may respond to just one medication targeting anxiety, rather than necessarily one medication for each problem. This makes sense from a clinical and empirical standpoint in other disorders as well: A medication initiated for depression can have significant benefits for attention difficulties tied to the depression.

With neuropsychiatric pharmacotherapy, one is often navigating through clinical scenarios without the guidance of a robust evidence basis for any unique case. It is thus essential to prescribe medications in a stepwise manner, adding or discontinuing medications one at a time, titrating slowly, and carefully monitoring for efficacy and side effects. It is also helpful to use patient or caregiver feedback, including rating scales, as benchmark for treatment responses and to consistently track, challenge, or corroborate one's clinical impression. In neuropsychiatry, establishing a strong, therapeutic alliance and durable trust with neuropsychiatric patients and families leads to better outcomes, and is critical given that the wide variability of treatment responses necessitates frequent follow-ups and interactions.[5,6]

PSYCHOPHARMACOLOGY OF COGNITIVE DISORDERS: A DOMAIN-BASED APPROACH

An effective way to plan cognitive pharmacotherapy is to first determine what specific functional "domains" (e.g., arousal, attention, executive function, memory) are affected or seem most affected. This domain-based approach allows providers to most effectively and parsimoniously target overlapping symptoms. Many pharmacotherapy solutions are "off label" of typical neurologic or psychiatric indications. Combining a detailed clinical interview with a thorough review of neurocognitive or neuropsychological test results is very valuable, as affected domains can be challenging to identify or dissociate from each other.

The interview should try to elicit the essential phenomenology involved: What is it like to experience, or observe the patient experiencing, the cognitive symptoms? Are there certain settings, or other variables, that make the symptoms and the functioning better or worse? For example, the patient may be able to remember important, past milestone events but unable to learn new information from daily interactions (memory). She may be observed to have difficulty focusing long enough to complete a basic task or may seem "lost in thought" during conversations (attention). She may have difficulty with the organizing and basic planning needed to participate in several activities at different times on one day (executive function). Results from cognitive testing can serve to corroborate, challenge, or augment the identified domains that seem impaired from the interview.

With domains identified, providers can then consider the implicated anatomy, networks, and neurotransmitter systems. Ultimately, this leads to a narrowing down of the most promising pharmacology to treat the syndrome(s), even while acknowledging the inherent overlap in domains and the limitations of the domain-based framework. This section focuses on four broad cognitive domains (arousal, attention, executive functions, and memory) and the symptomatology, anatomy, and pharmacotherapy paradigms within each.

Disorders of Arousal

Disorders of arousal fall along a spectrum, from states of minimal or no experience of wakefulness/arousal to disorders of hyperarousal and hyperactivity. At one extreme, there are the disorders of consciousness, which include coma, the minimally conscious state (MCS), and persistent vegetative state (PVS). Each of these can arise from diverse etiologies. At the other extreme are disorders like mania, agitated delirium and hypervigilance, for instance as seen in post-traumatic stress disorder. Disorders of consciousness or arousal may arise from a multitude of causes, including hypoxic-ischemic brain injury, traumatic brain injury (TBI), and severe metabolic disturbances.[7] While impossible to access the experience of patients in extreme cases of hypoarousal, functional imaging evidence suggests that some patients who meet criteria for MCS or PVS are likely carrying out some mental functions, willfully.[8,9] With hyperarousal states, patients have the experience of feeling "on-edge" or being "easily startled."[10,11]

The neuroanatomic pathways typically implicated include the neurotransmitter-specific fiber tracts that make up the ascending reticular activating system (ARAS).[12] These include projections from noradrenergic neurons from the locus coeruleus, cholinergic neurons of the meso-pontine tract, dopaminergic neurons from the brainstem and hypothalamus to thalamus, and glutamatergic neurons from brainstem reticular nuclei to the thalamus and prefrontal cortex.[13] There is a dynamic interplay in the wakeful brain between these neural systems and their respective neurotransmitters. Disorders of consciousness likely arise when they are disrupted, whether from ischemia (e.g., from cardiac arrest), shearing effects (e.g., from TBI/axonal injury), compression (e.g., from hematoma expansion), or other processes.[14]

There are no regulatory agency-approved medications for disorders of consciousness, but the neurophysiology suggests possible benefits from cholinergic stimulation, catecholamine augmentation (i.e., dopamine, norepinephrine, epinephrine), or glutamate modulation. Amantadine has had replicated evidence of improving functional outcomes in altered consciousness following severe TBI.[15-17] These studies suggest amantadine may promote an earlier recovery of meaningful interactions and vocalizations. Amantadine is thought to enhance dopaminergic transmission through the neuroaxis by inhibiting its re-uptake and increasing the number of post-synaptic receptors.[18] Relatedly, some small series have shown that the dopaminergic

D1 or D2 agonists bromocriptine and apomorphine can accelerate return of normal arousal and improvement on some cognitive measures in the acute periods after severe TBI.[19-21] Zolpidem, which modulates GABA receptors and is normally used as a hypnotic, has shown, paradoxically, to promote restorative brain activity in PVS[22] and, in some series, to improve functional recovery from coma.[23] For states of hyperarousal, as is seen in PTSD, medications like propranolol[24] and prazosin[25] may have some benefit.

Disorders of Attention

Disorders of attention range from the neurodevelopmental attention-deficit hyperactivity disorder (ADHD), to those acquired due to stroke, TBI, or neurodegenerative disease, among others. Following an adequate level of arousal, a basic level of attention is the next necessary process for most other mental functions, and thus daily functioning, to take place. Attention involves a set of different processes. Multiple levels of complexity may be involved during any task, ranging from low-level "orienting" or shifting direction of the sensory organs (for hearing, seeing, or touching) to the higher level of "dividing" mental resources to process stimuli simultaneously.[26] Patients with attention dysfunction can experience a range of symptoms, including feeling "easily distracted" by interfering conversations, having trouble "holding on to" or learning what they hear or read, having trouble shifting attention efficiently when this is needed, or having difficulty sustaining "focus" on a task without distractibility, as seen in individuals with deficits in sustained attention or concentration. In patients with dementia, inattention is often under-recognized and can sometimes be observed as "lack of awareness of surroundings" or "staring off into space."[27]

The functional neuroanatomy of attention likely involves a large-scale network, with hubs in the dorsal posterior parietal cortex, the frontal eye fields, and the cingulate gyrus.[28] This frontoparietal-predominant network has dynamic interactions with prefrontal, premotor, and limbic cortices, as well as the arousal network, centered in the ARAS, all of which modulate the degree of attention.[28,29] Many neurotransmitter systems probably subserve attention and play roles in its dysfunction; gamma-aminobutyric (GABA), dopamine, acetylcholine, norepinephrine, and serotonin projections are all implicated.[30-33] In ADHD, there may be a disruption in neurotransmitter transporter systems, with identified genetic variants in some cases, that leads to depleted levels of dopamine and norepinephrine.[34] Catecholamines are responsible for modulating or regulating the attentional tone, where appropriate levels help improve the "signal" of processed information to attend to, while inhibiting potential distractors (i.e., "noise").[28,35] Dextroamphetamine, methylphenidate, atomoxetine, and other noradrenergic agents, like duloxetine and venlafaxine, can enhance this catecholaminergic tone.

Methylphenidate is thought to block the reuptake of norepinephrine and dopamine into presynaptic neurons and is used in ADHD and narcolepsy. Methylphenidate has been shown to ameliorate attention dysfunction and, variably, increase processing speed in TBI and dementia, among other disorders.[36-38]

Bupropion seems to weakly inhibit reuptake of dopamine and norepinephrine, and may help in ADHD and cognitive dysfunction in major depression.[39] See Chapter 16 on ADHD in this textbook for more details about ADHD-specific treatment.

Decreasing excessive glutamatergic transmission, like that which occurs in the prefrontal cortex in states of hyperarousal or hyperactivity, may also help improve attention. Therapeutic strategies for states of hyperarousal include using low-dose GABA agonists[40] or blocking glutamatergic NMDA-receptors with memantine or amantadine.[41,42] As discussed above in the section of disorders of arousal, amantadine also enhances dopaminergic neurotransmission. Perhaps related to this mechanism of action, in some cases this agent can cause anxiety and irritability as side effects. See Chapter 30 on TBI in this textbook for further information about the potential benefits and risks of amantadine use, in that clinical setting.

Central cholinergic transmission that flows throughout frontoparietal and visual cortices is also important in the "top-down" control of selective attention, among a broad spectrum of cognitive functions, supporting the use of cholinergic agonists or acetylcholinesterase inhibitors (AChIs), like galantamine.[43,44]

Disorders of Executive Functions

The impairment of executive functions can occur in many neuropsychiatric disorders, and highly correlates with disability and loss of autonomy in daily functioning.[45–48] Executive functions include "low-level" tasks, like inhibiting automatic motor responses and allocating attentional resources to more than one stimuli. They also involve "higher-level" functions, like planning future actions and deriving figurative meaning from texts.[28,49] To detect signs and symptoms of dysfunction, it can be helpful to divide executive dysfunction into several practical, clinically oriented constructs: working memory, inhibition, set-shifting, and fluency.[49] See Chapter 2 "Functional Neurocircuitry of Cognition and Cognitive Syndromes" in this textbook for additional discussion of executive functions.

Working memory is the ability to temporarily store and manipulate information, which in turn allows for longer-term information storage. This enables us to carry out more complicated, future actions. Working memory deficits can be experienced when someone "does not remember why they entered a room" or has difficulty "putting together" back-to-back sentences in a conversation. Inhibition is our evolution-primed, adaptive ability to control automatic or previously learned responses to certain stimuli in the service of a goal at hand. A failure of inhibitory control can manifest as someone interrupting others frequently in conversation or showing a loss of social decorum, such as making inappropriate comments. Set-shifting refers to adapting one's behavior or thoughts in response a changing environment. Patients with set-shifting difficulty may be "inflexible" in their thinking or have difficulty solving a problem that require multiple, different steps. Fluency is the ability to generate verbal and visual information. Fluency deficits can often manifest as word-retrieval problems or individuals feeling "slow" in their thinking or speech. An overarching construct which is often linked to the executive functions is processing speed, which reflects both the speed and efficiency of

---

CASE VIGNETTE 8.1

A 47-year-old librarian presents to Neuropsychiatry clinic for evaluation of cognitive complaints in the setting of his relapsing remitting multiple sclerosis (RRMS). He first had MS symptoms in his early 20s, with an episode of trigeminal neuralgia and right arm and leg tingling. He has had two other clear relapses: one at age 32 with fatigue and generalized weakness following a pneumonia and the second at age 44 with leg weakness, imbalance, and subsequent depression, and has used a cane since. His current cognitive complaints started about 6 months ago, when he noticed difficulty working with a software program at his job that required several complicated steps. He was unable to carry out the necessary keystrokes in the right order to be effective. He also noticed that he is about "50% slower" in many tasks at work, including scanning returned books and completing library research queries. He finds that he can "get these things done but it just takes him "twice as long." He also describes some word-finding difficulties in conversation. Along with his cognitive complaints, he reports intermittent fatigue with even light exertion. He is currently being treated with fingolimod for his RRMS. He asks about medications to improve his cognition.

Cognitive disorders are very common in MS. Although the severity of deficits often has direct correlation with the duration of illness, some patients have notable cognitive problems early on in the disease. This patient had the first symptoms of MS about 25 years prior to his cognitive complaints. His complaint of having difficulty with completing multiple steps of a software program in the right order should make clinicians think about what has been labelled as problems sequencing or shifting set, which are executive functions. His complaints of being slower in many of his tasks at work are typical for problems with "processing speed," which is often grouped with executive functions, but underlies all mental processes. Processing speed is a measure that reflects the speed and efficiency of information transfer in the brain. Given his complaints, the implicated anatomy likely involves the frontal cortex and/or white matter tracts that connect cortical-subcortical structures. Disruptions in GABA/glutamate, acetylcholine, serotonin, and the catecholamines have all been implicated in executive dysfunction. Given the evidence-basis of psychostimulants for executive function disorders, broadly, and some evidence of efficacy in MS to improve processing speed, executive function and fatigue, a trial of a medication like methylphenidate or lisdexamfetamine would be a reasonable first step.

information transfer in the brain. Clinically, it can also manifest as slowness in retrieving words, thinking, or speaking.

The neuroanatomy of executive functions is complex, and likely involves a large-scale distributed network, with nodes in prefrontal cortex, parietal areas, basal ganglia, and cerebellum.[28,50,51] Processing speed may be predominantly subserved by distributed white matter tracts in the brain, and can thus be slowed in diseases like multiple sclerosis, TBI, stroke, toxic exposures like carbon monoxide, and inflammatory conditions like SLE.[52] Injury to any of these brain regions and the resultant changes in their neurotransmitters systems, including GABA/glutamate, acetylcholine, serotonin, and the catecholamines, can be implicated in executive dysfunction. Examples of specific conditions and pharmacotherapy agents are as follows: Cholinesterase inhibitors have demonstrated marginal improvement of executive function in subcortical vascular dementia and Parkinson's disease (PD) dementia.[53,54] Psychostimulants, including lisdextroamphetamine and amphetamine salts, may help improve executive function performance (in addition to reducing overall symptom severity) in children and adults with ADHD.[55,56] And vortioxetine, a serotonin reuptake inhibitor and mixed serotonin agonist/antagonist, is able to improve executive function and other cognitive domains in patients with depression.[57-59]

Disorders of Memory

Disorders of memory are common in neuropsychiatric conditions and manifest with varied symptomatology. Broadly, patients with a memory disorder have some difficulty with learning, storing, or recalling information or experiences. Patients with Alzheimer's disease (AD), PD, dementia with Lewy bodies, schizophrenia, polypharmacy involving anti-cholinergic drugs, strokes or cerebrovascular conditions, and major depression, among others, commonly have memory complaints and objective deficits on testing.[60-63] Patients may demonstrate difficulty with declarative memory (the memory of "facts and events," or previously learned information) and/or procedural memory or skill learning (the memory of "how to do things," a component of longer-term memory), or sometimes both.

Memory function in the brain is likely mediated by a large-scale, distributed network. The circuit that subserves declarative memory is localized in the temporal lobe (hippocampus, entorhinal cortex, inferolateral cortex), thalamus, and cingulate cortex. The hubs that subserve procedural memory are localized in the basal ganglia, cerebellum, and prefrontal cortex (supplementary motor area).[28,64] The neural basis of memory relies on glutamatergic and cholinergic signaling of information, processed from an initial stream of sensory information, like sound, vision, and touch. This signaling leads to the strengthening of synapses (long-term potentiation [LTP]) throughout the network, which creates a representation or "store" of the information for later recall.[65] Disruption of frontal-subcortical structures, as is common in PD and major depression among others, can lead to impaired reactivation of this neural representation of memories, leading to retrieval or recall difficulty.[64,66]

The cholinergic system, which is widespread throughout the brain, seems to be the most effective drug target for memory disorders. AChIs, like galantamine, rivastigmine, and donepezil are the main agents used. These medications have shown marginal to modest benefit for memory, including a slower memory decline, in patients with various neuropsychiatric disorders, including AD, PD, schizophrenia, and vascular cognitive impairment/dementia.[67-70] Some small studies have also shown benefits of AChIs for memory in patients with minimally symptomatic bipolar disorder,[71] Korsakoff syndrome,[72] and primary brain tumors.[73] The glutamate system has also been an effective therapeutic target: non-competitive NMDA receptor antagonists, like memantine, may improve memory by blocking the uncontrolled, toxic signaling arising from dysfunctional glutamate-mediated receptors.[74] Memantine has a strong evidence-basis for small memory improvements either as monotherapy or adjunct to AChIs in moderate-to-severe AD.[75] While there is some evidence that catecholamine augmentation can improve memory performance, like with methylphenidate for adults with ADHD,[76] these results have been inconsistent overall.

PSYCHOPHARMACOLOGY OF DEPRESSION, ANXIETY, AND PSYCHOSIS IN NEUROPSYCHIATRY

This section provides a general review of the diagnosis and treatment of depression, and recommendations for managing depression in the context of neuropsychiatric disorders. It also presents clinical pearls to consider when addressing anxiety and psychosis in the context of a neurologic illness.

Review of Depression Diagnosis and Treatment

Depression can be a symptom of several psychiatric disorders, such as a depressive disorder due to a medical condition or substance use (see Figure 8-1). Thus, taking a comprehensive

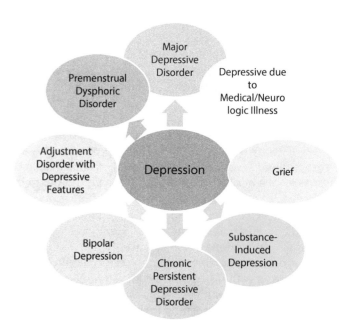

FIGURE 8-1. Conditions that may present as a depressive syndrome.

history is an important step in addition to determining the severity of the disorder and degree of distress and dysfunction the symptoms are causing in an individual's life. Only then can one properly establish an appropriate treatment plan. For example, an individual may have a major depressive disorder of moderate severity and an active alcohol use disorder in which case evidence suggests the best outcomes occur when one addresses both conditions simultaneously.

The Patient Health Questionnaire or PHQ-9 (see Figure 8-2) provides a validated quantitative measure of the frequency of the depressive symptoms over the past 2 weeks, in addition to a qualitative measure of impairment.[77] While there are many other evidence-based tools one can use to measure illness severity, the PHQ-9 is the most widely used one in clinical settings, is free, can be self- or clinician-administered, and is available in over 50 languages. The total score with cutoffs of 5, 10, and 15, represent mild, moderate, and severe depression respectively, and guide general treatment selection. Based on the work done by the MacArthur Foundation's Initiative on Depression and Primary Care and utilizing PHQ-9 severity definitions, mild depression requires "watchful waiting" and optimization of self-care, whereas in moderately severe depression or in chronic mild depression, active treatment involving medication and/or psychotherapy is suggested. In severe cases of depression, medication is viewed as an essential element. It is usually supplemented by supportive therapy, with more depression-specific

psychotherapeutic interventions incorporated as the patient improves and is able to more actively engage in the therapeutic process. In all cases, clinical judgment should be used in interpreting scores and implementing treatment. A very useful toolkit emerged from the MacArthur initiative and is available online.[78]

The specific medication selected very much depends on the specific symptoms of depression with which the individual presents, the subtype of depression (see Figure 8-1), and its comorbidities. Selecting a medication is also done by considering any previous medication treatment and its effects, the family history of treatment responses, the side-effect profile of the medication, and the potential interactions with other medications (see Table 8-1). One approach to selecting an antidepressant in treating non-bipolar, non-psychotic major depressive episode is provided in Figure 8-3. Once a medication is agreed upon by the patient, start with the lowest possible dose for at least a few days so that the individual's tolerability of the drug can be discerned. Once the initial tolerability is evident, titrate to the minimum therapeutic dose as rapidly as tolerated. Given the therapeutic mechanisms of antidepressant action in major depressive disorder are G-protein receptor mediated, continue the drug at a therapeutic dose for at least 4–6 weeks, potentially up to 8 weeks in order to provide a therapeutic trial on a medication.[79] Switching to a different antidepressant is usually advised if there is no evidence of response, versus augmenting

PATIENT HEALTH QUESTIONNAIRE-9				
Over the <u>last 2 weeks,</u> how often have you been bothered by any of the following problems?	Not at all	Several days	More than half the days	Nearly every day
1. Little interest or pleasure in doing things	0	1	2	3
2. Feeling down, depressed, or hopeless	0	1	2	3
3. Trouble falling or staying asleep, or sleeping too much	0	1	2	3
4. Feeling tired or having little energy	0	1	2	3
5. Poor appetite or overeating	0	1	2	3
6. Feeling bad about yourself — or that you are a failure or have let yourself or your family down	0	1	2	3
7. Trouble concentrating on things, such as reading the newspaper or watching television	0	1	2	3
8. Moving or speaking so slowly that other people could have noticed? Or the opposite — being so fidgety or restless that you have been moving around a lot more than usual	0	1	2	3
9. Thoughts that you would be better off dead or of hurting yourself in some way	0	1	2	3

FOR OFFICE CODING

_0_ + _____ + _____ + _____

=Total Score: _____

If you checked off <u>any</u> problems, how <u>dificult</u> have these problems made it for you to do your work, take care of things at home, or get along with other people?

Not difficult at all	Somewhat difficult	Very difficult	Extremely difficult
☐	☐	☐	☐

FIGURE 8-2. PHQ-9.

TABLE 8-1 • Some Antidepressant-CYP450 Drug Interactions.

Enzyme	Substrates	Inhibitors	Inducers
1A2	Tertiary amine tricyclic antidepressants (TCAs), duloxetine, theophylline, phenacetin, TCAs (demethylation), clozapine, diazepam, caffeine	Fluvoxamine, fluoxetine, moclobemide, ramelteon	Tobacco, omeprazole
2C19	TCAs, citalopram (partly), warfarin, tolbutamide, phenytoin, diazepam	Fluoxetine, fluvoxamine, sertraline, imipramine, ketoconozole, omeprazole	Rifampin
2D6	TCAs, benztropine, perphenazine, clozapine, haloperidol, codeine/oxycodone, risperidone, class Ic antiarrhythmics, β blockers, trazodone, paroxetine, maprotiline, amoxapine, duloxetine, mirtazapine (partly), venlafaxine, bupropion	Fluoxetine, paroxetine, duloxetine, hydroxybupropion, methadone, cimetidine, haloperidol, quinidine, ritonavir	Phenobarbital, rifampin
3A4	Citalopram, escitalopram, TCAs, glucocorticoids, androgens/estrogens, carbamazepine, erythromycin, Ca^{2+} channel blockers, levomilnacipran, protease inhibitors, sildenafil, alprazolam, triazolam, vincristine/vinblastine, tamoxifen, zolpidem	Fluvoxamine, nefazodone, sertraline, fluoxetine, cimetidine, fluconazole, erythromycin, protease inhibitors, ketoconazole, verapamil	Barbiturates, glucocorticoids, rifampin, modafinil, carbamazepine

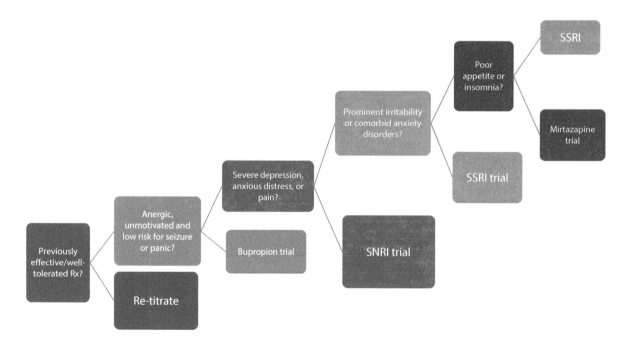

FIGURE 8-3. Selecting an antidepressant for non-bipolar, non-psychotic depression.

with a complementary antidepressant if there is an incomplete response (see Table 8-2 for examples of complementary antidepressants combinations). The goal of treatment is to achieve remission, which is defined as at least 75% improvement in the utilized measures' scores and/or returning to peak level of functioning. Incompletely treated depression leads to increased risk of recurrence. Once remission is achieved, continuation therapy for at least another 6–9 months is advised. After that remission is maintained, the individual is considered recovered. Slow tapering off the medication may be considered at that point, if there is minimal past depression. In patients with recurrent depressive illness there is a higher risk of increasingly more recurrent and often treatment-refractory episodes; for this

TABLE 8-2 • Complementary Antidepressant Combinations.

[SSRI or SNRI] and mirtazapine
[SSRI or SNRI] and bupropion
[SSRI or SNRI] and mirtazapine and bupropion
Mirtazapine and bupropion

reason, maintenance treatment on the regimen that allowed for remission is recommended.[80]

Incomplete adherence to treatment is the general rule and not the exception.[81] Understanding this is important as it allows the clinician to engage more productively with the patient when

---

Box 8-1   Reasons for Incomplete Adherence to Antidepressants

Forgetting to take

Side effects

Cost

Feel Rx is not necessary

Fear of side effects

Fear it will be hard to stop

Fear it will alter one's personality

Disbelief that medication is the correct solution or could help

Delayed onset of benefits

Inadequate education of the patient by the clinician

Certain personality styles, e.g., extroversion, Cluster B personality traits

Fear of addiction

Comorbid substance use disorder

Complicated titration or dosing schedule

Lower depression severity

Lack of follow-up with clinician

Low patient motivation

---

inquiring about "how often" not "are you" taking the medication, thereby leading to more honest answers. Research conducted to better understand poor adherence to treatment reveals that there are many different factors to consider (see Box 8-1).[82] A meaningful discussion with the patient about their specific reasons for not taking a medication as prescribed can then lead to viable solutions and thus improved adherence.

Treatment of Depression-Specific Considerations in Neuropsychiatry

Most antidepressants undermine sleep quality. For example, serotonergic reuptake inhibitors can induce or aggravate restless legs syndrome and/or periodic limb movements.[83] In addition, they suppress REM sleep and are associated with diminished slow wave sleep and microarousals.[84-86] Individuals with neuropsychiatric disorders are especially vulnerable to the effects of chronic sleep deprivation. Not only does the impaired sleep destabilize mood, but also attention and memory are impaired. Thus, it can be a challenging calculus to decide whether to use an antidepressant for treating a depression and/or anxiety disorder when patients are especially vulnerable to the effects of this sometimes subtle form of sleep disturbance. Certainly, the disorder itself can drive insomnia and so when treatment is initiated, tracking carefully to see if sleep is improving or worsening is important. Pharmacologic options worth considering that promote improved sleep include the off-label use of mirtazapine, nefazodone, or trazodone. Low-dose doxepin, which is FDA-approved for insomnia, is also a possible alternative but less preferred due to its anticholinergic activity. These medications appear to reduce sleep-latency and improve sleep continuity, while having limited REM-sleep suppression.[85,87,88] Bupropion has been identified as having no REM-sleep suppressant effects

and in fact might increase REM sleep.[89] There is also evidence that it might reduce restless legs symptoms at least in the short term and no evidence that it aggravates the condition[83] and so it is a preferred antidepressant for these individuals. While some individuals experience insomnia with bupropion, usually in the form of sleep maintenance difficulties, this is usually a short-term phenomenon that resolves within a few weeks of treatment. Insomnia aside, it is estimated that up to 6% of individuals taking antidepressants have REM-sleep behavior disorder (RBD). This includes, but is not limited to, individuals with RBD due to antidepressant medication. Since this sleep disorder is a predictor of PD, it is important to assess whether it is antidepressant-induced or a signal of increased risk for developing PD in the future.[90]

A commonly reported side effect of selective serotonergic reuptake inhibitors (SSRIs) is that of feeling emotionless or apathetic. As discussed elsewhere in this chapter, apathy is often seen in neuropsychiatric disorders. Alternative agents that carry less risk of apathy, such as bupropion or serotonin and norepinephrine reuptake inhibitors (SNRIs), should be considered.

While tricyclic antidepressants might be gentler on sleep and benefit any coexisting pain, their anticholinergic burden is likely to aggravate underlying cognitive difficulties so commonly seen in neuropsychiatric syndromes. Thus, minimizing exposure to this class of antidepressants or using cautiously with very low dosing is advised. Paroxetine is an SSRI that has significant anticholinergic effects, and can also worsen cognition.[91] Therefore, sparing use in neuropsychiatric syndromes is recommended.

Primary diseases involving the CNS do increase the risk for seizures and to varying degrees, antidepressant-class medications lower the seizure threshold. Bupropion, particularly at high doses and with the immediate release form, is most likely to do this. A more detailed review of this is covered in this textbook's Epilepsy chapter (Chapter 29).

Finally, the clinician should always consider the relationship between psychiatric symptoms such as depression and anxiety, and the comorbid neurologic disorder. Depression, for instance, can occur as a direct physiological consequence of the underlying neurological illness, such as in undertreated PD, or during a flare of multiple sclerosis. In this situation, treating the underlying neurologic disorder may be the best strategy for treating the psychiatric symptoms.

Treatment of Anxiety-Specific Considerations in Neuropsychiatry

Anxiety is extremely common in neurologic disorders and can be either a symptom of or a reaction to the disorder. Anxiety can also be the vehicle for expressing other discomfiting symptoms, for example, pain, or when the neurologic disorder renders the individual unable to properly communicate. Where there's anxiety, there's often depression given their high comorbidity. In assessing anxiety, it is also important to clarify its expression. For example, anxiety presenting as generalized anxiety disorder and phobias is extremely common in late life. Of the phobias, fear of falling and agoraphobia are the most common in older individuals. However, the late life new onset of panic disorder and obsessive-compulsive disorder (OCD) is much less frequent, and more likely associated with an underlying neurologic insult such as dementia, movement disorder, or stroke.

As untreated anxiety aggravates cognitive symptoms and typically leads to worse outcomes, it is important to treat, though to do so judiciously. One should avoid benzodiazepines and antihistamines not only because of the cognitive impairment they can cause, but also because diseased neural substrate increases the risk of paradoxical reactions such as increased anxiety. While there is very little research to guide treatment specifically of anxiety in the context of most neurologic disorders, SSRIs, SNRIs, and mirtazapine are considered the best options given their relatively more forgiving side-effect profiles. Weigh the potential side effects of these antidepressants as one would do in using them to treat depression. Buspirone is also worth considering for the treatment of generalized anxiety, given that is has no adverse cognitive effects. However, it does not treat OCD, panic attacks, or PTSD.

Treatment of Psychosis-Specific Considerations in Neuropsychiatry

Low-potency first-generation antipsychotics (FGAs) have very high anticholinergic activity and so are best avoided given their cognitive risks.

As high-potency FGAs and risperidone are especially apt to induce parkinsonism, quetiapine and clozapine are the second-generation antipsychotics (SGAs) recommended for the treatment of psychosis in the context of PD. Pimavanserin has a unique mechanism of action devoid of anti-dopaminergic activity and will be discussed in more detail in the PD chapter (Chapter 23). Patients with dementia with Lewy bodies are particularly sensitive to antipsychotics—they can precipitate prominent side effects including worsening of cognition, even at low doses.

Increased mortality in the elderly who were prescribed antipsychotics is a well-established risk. It is seen with both first- and second-generation agents, and is thought to occur due to a variety of factors including QTc prolongation, cardiovascular effects, and infectious processes.

Antipsychotics, particularly olanzapine and clozapine, significantly increase the risk for metabolic syndrome which then aggravates the risk of vascular insults. This should be considered in all populations, but especially in the case of patients who have other cerebrovascular risk factors.

Antipsychotics lower the seizure threshold. This is important to consider when treating patients with epilepsy, as well as when treating those individuals with other neurological disorders that also increase the risk of seizures.

AGITATION

Definition

As a not infrequent manifestation of neuropsychiatric disorders, agitation is likely a phenomenon most clinicians have encountered, regardless of practice setting. There is no consensus among experts on a single accepted definition of agitation.[92] It can be conceptualized as a single symptom, or a symptom complex that may include an internal experience of emotional distress, and outward manifestations consisting of excessive motor activity (i.e., rocking or pacing) and vocalizations, disruptive irritability, and disinhibition.[92] While it may include aggressive behaviors, it can occur without aggression. Agitation is typically considered to include behaviors that are disproportionate to the inciting stimulus, and to occur on a continuum that goes from increased verbal or physical activity, up to and including assault directed toward objects, others, and/or the self.[93]

Epidemiology

Agitation can occur in the setting of most or all neuropsychiatric disorders. This section will primarily focus on agitation in the setting of psychiatric illness (psychosis, bipolar disorder), major neurocognitive disorder, and TBI. Each year, there are approximately 900,000–1.7 million psychiatric emergency service visits or emergency department presentations related to agitation.[94] The prevalence of agitation in psychiatric emergency services range from 4.3% to 10%.[95-97] Agitation and its management lead to greater health care costs, longer length of stay, more frequent rehospitalization, and greater use of medication.[98-100] Patients with schizophrenia spectrum illness have a 20% lifetime prevalence of agitation,[101] and approximately 14% of hospitalized patients with schizophrenia present with agitation and violent behavior at some point during the course of admission.[102] The prevalence of agitation in major neurocognitive disorders ranges from 20% to 60%,[92] while 35–96% of individuals with TBI experience agitation during the acute phase of recovery, and 31–71% demonstrate agitation in the 1–15 years after severe TBI.[103,104]

Pathophysiology

While the pathophysiology of agitation is not fully understood,[105] several cortical and subcortical structures have been implicated in this phenomenon. The frontal lobes are considered the locus of behavioral inhibition and control, and the limbic system the locus of intense emotional states, including aggressive impulses. One hypothesis of the neurobiology of agitation entails the failure of one or both of two pathways. The first is a "bottom-up" failure, mediated by limbic overactivation of ascending input from the amygdala, insula, and anterior temporal lobes. The second is a failure in "top-down" control, and disruption in the capacity to monitor internal and external stimuli and to modulate behavior via the dorsolateral prefrontal (DLPFC), orbitofrontal (OFC), and anterior cingulate (ACC) cortical areas.[93,106,107] Catecholaminergic, cholinergic, glutamatergic, and GABAergic pathways play an important role within these circuits,[108] and so derangement of these neurotransmitter systems can be both a contributor to and a therapeutic target for agitation. More specifically, serotonergic pathways in the PFC, OFC, and ACC are felt to play an important role in the prefrontal inhibition of impulsivity and aggression, and 5-HT_{2a} antagonism and 5-HT_{2c} agonism have been found to decrease impulsivity in animal models. Increased glutamatergic and decreased GABAergic activity may enhance limbic reactivity predisposing to aggression; in this way, GABAergic stimulation can reduce this limbic overactivation.[107] Treatment strategies have been geared toward addressing these disruptions in neurotransmitter systems with glutamatergically and GABAergically active anticonvulsants to tamp down limbic activity, noradrenergic and dopaminergic antagonism with beta blockers and neuroleptics respectively to suppress monoaminergically mediated limbic drive, as well as pro-dopaminergic and serotonergic medications to enhance frontal cortical function.[93,107,108]

Clinical Presentation

Agitation exists on a spectrum, from a subjective experience of internal tension to objective motor and verbal activity that can take the form of psychomotor agitation and reach the level of physical aggression toward self, objects, and others. It can occur in different settings. In the inpatient medical setting, for instance, it can cause the individual to pull out the IV line or disrupt other medical treatments. Agitation can occur in a wide variety of psychiatric, neurological, and medical disorders, and thus the clinical presentation will vary according to the underlying disease. It can occur in the setting of delirium and catatonia (see Chapter 25 for further discussion of these two entities), endocrinopathy (e.g., Cushing's disease, thyrotoxicosis), immunologic/inflammatory/infectious conditions (e.g., meningoencephalitides, cysticercosis, multiple sclerosis, etc.), neoplastic processes, neurocognitive, and motor disorders (e.g., Alzheimer's, Parkinson's, Huntington's), toxic-metabolic disturbances (i.e., hyper/hypoglycemia, electrolyte abnormalities), vascular disease (e.g., stroke, myocardial ischemia), thought disorders (i.e., schizophrenia, schizoaffective disorder), mood disorders (e.g., major depression, bipolar spectrum illness), anxiety disorders (e.g., GAD, panic disorder, PTSD), substance/medication related disorders (e.g., intoxication, withdrawal, akathisia), neurodevelopmental disorders, intellectual disability disorders, TBI, seizure disorders, personality disorders as well as impulse control, ADHD and other learning disorders.[95,109–116]

Assessment and Differential Diagnosis

As outlined above, agitation may present as a symptom of several medical and neuropsychiatric disorders. As such, the differential is broad and warrants a thorough evaluation. In addition to history, physical, mental status, neurological and cognitive exams as well as vital signs, laboratory studies (complete blood count, electrolytes, renal function, liver function, toxicology, pregnancy test, etc.), and possibly brain imaging, collateral information from family/caretakers, providers and outside hospitals can be especially helpful to understand if the current presentation is a departure from the individual's baseline, and if previous similar episodes have taken place. Identifying the underlying pathological process can inform further diagnostic and therapeutic interventions.

With regard to standardized assessment, a number of validated agitation scales exist; becoming familiar with some of them may be helpful, as they are used frequently as outcome measures in research studies and clinical settings.

The Positive and Negative Syndrome Scale-Excited Component (PANSS-EC)[117] is often used to assess efficacy of pharmacotherapy in psychotic agitation treatment research trials.[118–120] It rates the severity of five items in a 1–7 range: hostility, uncooperativeness, impulsivity, tension, and excitability. Of note, a positive response in most studies requires a $\geq$40% decrease in severity within 2 hours. Although primarily a research tool, this scale possesses clinical utility and can be used when treating agitation in patients with schizophrenia.[121–123]

The Overt Aggression Scale (OAS) and the Overt Agitation Severity Scale (OASS) are less specific to the underlying diagnosis and may be useful when considering a heterogeneous clinical population. These scales emphasize observed rather than subjective phenomena. The OAS can be performed by family or staff, and rates agitation severity from 1 to 4 in four categories: verbal aggression, physical aggression toward objects, physical aggression toward self, and physical aggression toward others.[123] This scale has been validated in both pediatric and adult patient populations.[120] The OASS requires a 15-minute observation period. It focuses on observable items: A, vocalizations and oral/facial movements; B, upper torso and upper extremity movements; C, lower extremity movements and their intensity (I) 1–4 and frequency (F) 0–4. It can be corrected for baseline neuromuscular disorders.[124,125]

Treatment

While least invasive interventions such as environmental adjustment and verbal de-escalation remain the recommended first line of treatment for agitation, the focus of this chapter is on pharmacotherapy. As mentioned above, agitation can occur in the context of multiple disorders, and some aspects of treatment will vary according to the underlying etiology. It is always important to attempt to determine what are the contributing and potentially treatable factors. For instance, if agitation is a symptom of psychosis, antipsychotic medication will be the first line of treatment; if it is a manifestation of an underlying delirium, treatment should be directed toward the causative process precipitating that delirium. However, treatment of the underlying cause is not always sufficient or even possible, and so this section will discuss the symptomatic management of agitation within the hypothetical construct outlined above ("top-down" vs. "bottom-up" dysfunction). Among the pharmacological treatment options, oral (PO) and sublingual (SL) formulations should be considered prior to use of intramuscular (IM) or intravenous (IV) parenteral ones. As a rule, in the elderly and in individuals with neurological illnesses, the recommendation is always to start low and to go slow in terms of dosing. It is worth keeping in mind that while there is some evidence, albeit at times mixed, for the use of several medications in the setting of agitation, there is no clear consensus or singular set of guidelines.[120,126–133] The present section outlines the treatment options available that possess some support in the literature.

Antipsychotics and benzodiazepines remain the most frequently used and most effective medications for the treatment of acute agitation. The inhaled formulation of loxapine for agitation in the context of bipolar disorder type I or schizophrenia, and IM olanzapine, ziprasidone, and aripiprazole for agitation in bipolar mania, are the only medications specifically approved by the FDA for agitation. However, a variety of both FGAs and SGAs have proven efficacious for the treatment of agitation in these and other populations. In the short term, side effects of FGAs include extrapyramidal symptoms (EPS) and QTc prolongation particularly in IV formulations (e.g., haloperidol), which may necessitate telemetry. Akathisia as a side of effect of neuroleptics can also mimic worsening psychotic agitation and so can lead to a cycle of repeated dosing, worsening akathisia, and subsequent agitation, which highlights the importance of ongoing and thoughtful consideration of the possible pathophysiology of the agitation in question. Diphenhydramine or benztropine can be used to address dystonia, and benzodiazepines such as lorazepam can mitigate akathisia; however, all these medications run the risk of worsening mental status in the case of delirium or a preexisting poor neurological substrate. The SGAs are less likely to generate EPS, but more likely to cause metabolic syndrome in the long term. FGAs have a higher risk than SGAs of causing tardive dyskinesia (TD) in the long term. While FGAs like haloperidol have comparable efficacy to SGAs, most experts recommend using the latter to reduce the risk of EPS and neuroleptic malignant syndrome (NMS), both higher with FGAs.[120,134] In individuals with TBI, neuroleptics may have an adverse effect on neurocognitive recovery.[104,135]

With regard to benzodiazepines, there are no randomized controlled trials (RCTs) for the use of PO benzodiazepines as monotherapy; however, there is some evidence to support their use IM both alone and in combination with antipsychotic medication.[136,137] When using benzodiazepines, the general recommendation is for short to intermediate acting, renally cleared agents with fewer drug-drug interactions and active metabolites, like lorazepam and oxazepam.[93]

In terms of the hypothetical framework outlined above, both antidopaminergic and GABAergic medications within these classes may mediate their effect on agitation by inhibiting limbic activation. For chronic agitation, it can remain helpful to consider the pathophysiology predisposing to agitation. In this way, individuals with overactive catecholaminergic limbic activity and/or dysfunction of the PFC-mediated inhibition, may benefit from agents that produce noradrenergic blockade, dopaminergic blockade, GABAergic enhancement, or have anti-glutamatergic activity. Individuals with intact executive function may benefit from augmentation of those faculties via serotonergic and/or pro-dopaminergic medications.

Treatment of Agitation in the Setting of Major Neurocognitive Disorder

For the treatment of long-term agitation in individuals with major neurocognitive disorders, who typically present impairment of prefrontal inhibitory faculties, there is some evidence for the use of several medication classes beyond neuroleptics, which have an FDA black-box warning for increased risk of death in the elderly with dementia. For instance, the combination of dextromethorphan and quinidine has demonstrated evidence for its efficacy to treat agitation in the context of AD.[138] AChIs have not been found to be effective in this context.[139] NDMA receptor antagonists like memantine have shown some promise, although subsequent studies did not reinforce those initial findings.[140-142] Among serotonergic medications, citalopram has shown evidence for its efficacy in the treatment of chronic agitation in the setting of dementia.[143-146] Among the antiepileptic drugs (AEDs) or mood stabilizers, carbamazepine can be efficacious,[147,148] while valproic acid (VPA) has been found to possess limited efficacy and poor tolerability in this population.[149-153]

Lastly, among the neuroleptics, evidence supports the use of risperidone, and also aripiprazole and olanzapine[139,154] for this indication. With regard to IM formulations of SGA to treat acute agitation in patients with dementia, there is evidence for the efficacy of olanzapine[155] and aripiprazole.[156] For additional details including dosing parameters, see Table 8-3.

TABLE 8-3 • Treatment of Agitation in Neurocognitive Disorders.				
	Neurocognitive Disorders			
Route	**Class**	**Medication**	**Dose**	**Literature**
PO	SSRI	Citalopram	10–30 mg/d	Pollock et al.[143,144]; Seitz et al.[145]; Prosteinsson et al.[200]
PO	SGA	Risperidone	0.5–2 mg/d	Herrmann et al.[139]; Ballard et al.[154]
PO	SGA	Aripiprazole	5–15 mg/d	Herrmann et al.[139]; Ballard et al.[154]
PO	SGA	Olanzapine	5–10 mg/d	Herrmann et al.[139]; Ballard et al.[154]
PO	AED	Carbamazepine	400 mg/d	Olin et al.[147]; Tariot et al.[148]
PO	NMDAR antagonist	Memantine	20 mg/d	Gauthier et al.[140]
PO	Other	Dextromethorphan/Quinidine	20 mg/10 mg–60 mg/20 mg/d	Cummings et al.[138]
IM	SGA	Olanzapine	2.5–5 mg	Meehan et al.[155]
IM	SGA	Aripiprazole	10–15 mg	Rappaport et al.[156]

Abbreviations: AED, antiepileptic drug; NMDAR, N-methyl-d-aspartate receptor; SGA, second-generation antipsychotic; SSRI, selective serotonin reuptake inhibitor.

Treatment of Agitation in the Setting of TBI

Beta blockers such as propranolol and pindolol have demonstrated the greatest effectiveness for the treatment of agitation in TBI.[157–162] Alternatives such as serotonergic and dopaminergic medications, VPA and lithium remain as viable options based on the available data.[126] For beta blockers, if once daily dosing is required, the long-acting formulation of propranolol can be used in place of the immediate release. If propranolol causes symptomatic bradycardia, pindolol can be used instead given its sympathomimetic activity.[108] After beta blockers, serotonergic medications within the classes of selective serotonin reuptake inhibitors (SSRIs) and tricyclic antidepressants (TCAs) are typically next in line.[126,163–167] The serotonergic anxiolytic buspirone has also been found to be helpful in agitation.[168–172] After serotonergic agents, mood stabilizers such as lithium, VPA, and carbamazepine have the next best body of evidence.[128,173–176] Dopaminergic medications like methylphenidate and amantadine have also demonstrated some benefit in the treatment of chronic agitation. They have been hypothesized to augment executive function for those individuals with completely intact frontal circuitry.[177–181]

After the aforementioned medications, neuroleptics have also been found to be helpful in managing more chronic in addition to acute agitation in individuals with TBI. As in acute aggression, SGAs are preferred, given the reduced risk of cognitive and motor side effects as well as their serotonergic 5HT$_{2a}$ antagonism alongside dopaminergic antagonism. Haloperidol is the preferred FGA to use, if initial SGA trials are ineffective or poorly tolerated.[128] For additional details including dosing parameters, see Table 8-4.

Treatment of Agitation in the Setting of Psychosis and Bipolar Disorder

As outlined above, antipsychotics are typically first line of treatment for acute agitation in the context of psychosis; however, unlike in dementia and TBI, they are also the standard of care for chronic agitation in this setting. SGAs are preferred over FGAs given the lower risk of EPS and TD; however, efficacy is comparable between the two classes. Haloperidol is typically the FGA of choice in this population, and it is approved for both PO and IM use in schizophrenia. For acute agitation requiring IM medication, among FGAs, droperidol and haloperidol with or without concomitant lorazepam have the most evidence.[137,182–184] While the IV formulation of haloperidol can be used, it confers a greater risk of QTc prolongation and torsades de pointes (TdP) typically necessitating telemetry.[132,185,186] Another option and the only medication available in an inhaled form is the FGA loxapine, which has FDA approval for agitation in both bipolar mania and psychotic agitation and has been found effective in those populations despite the rare risk of bronchospasm.[187–189]

For moderate agitation, several of the PO forms of SGAs have been found effective including risperidone, olanzapine, quetiapine, aripiprazole, brexpiprazole, and asenapine. Risperidone PO and in orodispersible tablet (ODT) form has been shown to be effective and comparable to IM haloperidol, with or without lorazepam.[190–193] Although more commonly associated with orthostasis than the other agents mentioned, quetiapine has also been found to be beneficial.[194,195] Quetiapine also demonstrated efficacy in studies looking at agitation in bipolar mania, in addition to schizophrenia.[196–199] Olanzapine has also been found effective, and comparable to haloperidol[202]; a rapid dosing escalation has demonstrated greater efficacy.[203] Aripiprazole has been found to be effective in PO form versus placebo and to be noninferior to PO olanzapine for psychotic agitation.[204,205] Initial data for brexpiprazole and for SL asenapine suggest some benefit for agitation in schizophrenia as well.[206,207]

With regard to acute agitation requiring parenteral medications, the IM SGAs olanzapine, ziprasidone, and aripiprazole have all been found to be at least as effective as haloperidol.[208,209] Additionally, IM olanzapine, ziprasidone, and aripiprazole have all been approved for agitation associated with bipolar mania.[119] Ziprasidone was found to have comparable efficacy to olanzapine and haloperidol, as well as to droperidol.[210,211] IM olanzapine has been found to be superior to both placebo and lorazepam, and either comparable or superior to haloperidol.[192,208,212–215] IM

TABLE 8-4 • Treatment of Agitation in Traumatic Brain Injury.				
	TBI			
Route	Class	Medication	Dose	Literature
PO	BB	Propranolol	420–520 mg/d	Brooke et al.[157]; Mattes[158]; Greendyke et al.[159]; Silver et al.[160]; Alpert et al.[161]
PO	BB	Pindolol	40–100 mg/d	Greendyke et al.[159]; Greendyke et al.[162]
PO	SSRI	Sertraline	25–200 mg/d	Fann et al.[201]
PO	TCA	Amitriptyline/ Desipramine	≤150 mg/d	Mysiw et al.[135]; Mysiw et al.[164]; Jackson et al.[165]; Szlabowicz and Stewart[166]; Kant et al.[167]
PO	Serotonergic	Buspirone	10–60 mg/d	Gualtieri[168,169]; Ratey et al.[171]; Stanislav et al.[172]
PO	Other	Lithium	0.4–1.4 mEq/L	Bellus et al.[173]; Glenn et al.[174]
PO	AED	VPA	750–2250 mg/d	Wroblewski et al.[175]
PO	AED	Carbamazepine	400–800 mg/d	Azouvi et al.[176]
PO	Dopaminergic	Methylphenidate	30 mg/d	Mooney and Haas[177]
PO	Dopaminergic	Amantadine	≤400 mg/d	Nickels et al.[178]; Chandler et al.[179]; Hammond et al.[180,181]

Abbreviations: AED, antiepileptic drug; BB, beta-blocker; SSRI, selective serotonin reuptake inhibitor; TCA, tricyclic antidepressant.

TABLE 8-5 • Treatment of Agitation in Psychosis and Mania.

Route	Psychosis/Mania Class	Medication	Dose	Literature
PO	SGA	Risperidone	2–6 mg/d	Veser et al. [235]
PO	SGA	Olanzapine	10–40 mg/d	Baker et al.[203]; Kinon et al.[204]
PO	SGA	Quetiapine	150–800 mg/d	Currier et al.[194]; Chengappa et al.[195]; Yatham et al.[196]; Sachs et al.[197]; Bowden et al.[198] 2005; McIntyre et al.[199]
PO	SGA	Aripiprazole	10–30 mg/d	Kinon et al.[204]; Marder et al.[205]
PO	SGA	Brexpiprazole	2–4 mg/d	Das et al.[206]
PO	FGA	Haloperidol	5–20 mg/d	Villari et al.[134]
PO ODT	SGA	Risperidone	2–6 mg	Lim et al.[193]
PO ODT	SGA	Olanzapine	10 mg	Hsu et al.[192]
SL	SGA	Asenapine	10 mg	Pratts et al.[207]
INH	FGA	Loxapine	10 mg	Allen et al.[187]; Lesem et al.[188]; Kwentus et al.[189]
IM	SGA	Olanzapine	10 mg	Hsu et al.[192]; Breier et al.[208]; Katagiri et al.[212]; Meehan et al.[213]; Wright et al.[214]; Chan et al.[215]
IM	SGA	Ziprasidone	10–20 mg	Baldacara et al.[210]; Martel et al.[211]
IM	SGA	Aripiprazole	9.75–15 mg	Tran-Johnson et al.[216]; Andrezina et al.[217]; Daniel et al.[218]; Zimbroff et al.[219]
IM	FGA	Haloperidol/ Droperidol	5–10 mg	Battaglia et al.[137]; Resnick and Burton[182]; Chouinard et al.[183]; Nobay et al.[184]
IM	BDZ	Lorazepam	2–4 mg	Lenox et al.[136]; Battaglia et al.[137]
IV	FGA	Haloperidol/ Droperidol	2–5 mg	Knott et al.[221]; Richards et al.[222,223]; Rosen et al.[224]
IV	SGA	Olanzapine	5 mg	Chan et al.[225]
IV	AED	VPA	20 mg/kg	Asadollahi et al.[226]

Abbreviations: AED, antiepileptic drug; BDZ, benzodiazepine; FGA, first-generation antipsychotic; SGA, second-generation antipsychotic.

aripiprazole has been found to be superior to placebo, and comparable to lorazepam and to haloperidol, without causing oversedation.[216-219] A systematic review found IM aripiprazole to be less effective than IM ziprasidone and olanzapine for agitation.[220]

And finally, with regard to agitation requiring immediate intervention, IV formulations of a few medications have been studied. For undifferentiated, psychotic, and/or substance-related agitation occurring in the context of the emergency department, IV droperidol and olanzapine have both been found to be effective.[221-225] IV VPA and IV haloperidol were compared, for patients with undifferentiated agitation. No statistically significant difference in efficacy was found on two of three scales, while VPA caused a greater decrease in the Agitation and Calmness Evaluation Scale (ACES) score as compared to haloperidol.[226]

For additional details including dosing parameters, see Table 8-5.

APATHY

Apathy is a frequent and often debilitating syndrome found across a variety of neurological and psychiatric illnesses. It can arise from myriad etiologies, including primary psychiatric disease, stroke, TBI, PD, AD, and other neurodegenerative

illnesses. It can also be the result of a medication side effect. Apathy has been correlated with a worsened quality of life as well as greater caregiver distress.

Definition

Apathy is a neuropsychiatric syndrome that has been conceptualized as a deficit in motivation.[227] Evidence for motivational deficits include decline in goal-directed behaviors, diminished goal-directed cognition, and a decrease in the emotional concomitants of goal-directed behavior.[227] Some researchers have argued that defining apathy as a disorder of diminished motivation requires the observer to make a projective inference about an individual's inner psychological state and postulated instead that apathy should be objectively measurable.[228] A behaviorist view proposes that apathy should be defined by a "quantitative reduction of self-generated voluntary and purposeful behavior." These changes should be a departure from previous behavioral baselines and occur without causative environmental or physical factors.

Epidemiology

Apathy can be found across a wide range of brain-based diseases. There is considerable heterogeneity in prevalence studies due to differences in apathy scales utilized and the underlying

CASE VIGNETTE 8.2

Mr. Joseph is 68-year-old man who presents to psychiatry at the urging of his family. They have noticed that over the last year he has become more disengaged from his work and hobbies. Whereas previously he was an avid exerciser and active participant in his church's choir, he now prefers to spend most weekends at home in front of the television. He denies feeling depressed or anxious; rather, he says that he just prefers to "relax" at home. When pressed to go out with his family, he appears to enjoy himself. He presents no problems with his sleep or appetite, and denies being concerned with negatives thoughts about himself, his life, or other topics.

His wife also notes he has been slightly more forgetful over the past 6 months. He seems to repeat himself and needs frequent reminders to manage his appointments. He sometimes requires prompting to recall acquaintances' names. He has lost his house keys twice, which in the past would have been highly unusual for him, as he has always been a very organized and meticulous individual.

When interviewed directly, Mr. Joseph acknowledges his family's descriptions may be accurate; however, he has not noticed nor been particularly bothered by these changes. He is not particularly interested in further workup or treatment but came today as a courtesy to his wife and children. His medical history is benign. His weight is normal, he does not use alcohol or other substances, and he is not taking any medication.

Mr. Joseph seems to present with a syndrome of apathy, and, in addition, symptoms of cognitive dysfunction that are starting to impact his functioning. The next step in his management would involve a diagnostic workup, including neuropsychological evaluation and brain MRI with contrast, to understand the etiology of his behavioral and cognitive changes. His history raises concerns about a possible underlying neurodegenerative process, although structural lesions (e.g., strokes, tumor) need to be ruled out.

disease of the surveyed population. A study of young healthy subjects (ages 19–40) found apathy in 1.45% of subjects, independent of depression or medical illness.[229] In studies of cognitively normal older adults (ages 65 and older, or 70 and older, in different studies), prevalence of apathy has ranged from 2% to 4.8%.[230] Apathy is one of the most common symptoms in AD, with a mean prevalence of 49%.[231] Apathy rates in patients with PD can range from 25% in the earlier stages to 60% as disease severity progresses.[232,233] Apathy is a hallmark symptom of behavioral variant frontotemporal dementia, with prevalence rates ranging from 54% to 96%.[234]

Clinical Neurobehavioral Presentation

Individuals with apathy may present with a decrease in goal-directed activity, interest, emotional responsiveness to life events, and inability to experience pleasure (anhedonia). They are likely to have increased dependence on others for the fulfillment of daily activities. Often, individuals with apathy are not concerned about the changes in their behavior—their caregivers are the ones who express concern to the clinician. Levy and Dubois[228] proposed three subtypes of apathy, differentiated by the deficits underlying the behavioral change. The "emotional affective" subtype involves loss of ability to interpret affective context in order to guide behavior, to prospectively appraise consequences in terms of positive or negative outcome, and to associate emotion with behavior. Its hallmarks are emotional blunting and decreased reward sensitivity. This subtype may be related to lesions of the orbital-medial prefrontal cortex or to the related subregions within the basal ganglia (e.g., ventral striatum, ventral pallidum). The "cognitive inertia" subtype arises from difficulties in generating the cognitive programs underpinning complex voluntary actions. It may be related to lesions of the DLPFC and related subregions within the basal ganglia (e.g., dorsal caudate nucleus). Lastly, the "autoactivation" subtype involves a deficit in the internal drive to self-activate and carry out goal-directed behavior, but is able to perform the tasks when provided strong external motivation. This subtype may be related to direct, bilateral lesions of the basal ganglia, anterior cingulate, or to a nigro-striatal dopaminergic loss, as it occurs in PD.[228]

Assessment and Differential Diagnosis

The assessment of apathy is based on the clinical presentation. The change in activity and behavior should not be attributable to intellectual impairment or alterations in level of consciousness. Apathy can be considered a less severe entity along a spectrum of disorders of diminished motivation, followed by abulia and the most severe form, akinetic mutism.[236] Differentiating between apathy and depression is complicated by considerable overlap in key symptoms, such as loss of interest and diminished motivation.[237] Nevertheless, the two syndromes are dissociable. A negative mood is far more indicative of depression than apathy, whereas apathy is usually associated with emotional blunting.[238] Depression is more likely than apathy to present with anxiety, agitation, irritability, and agitation. Apathy is more likely to present with unusual motor behaviors.[239] Importantly, individuals can present with comorbid apathy and depression (Table 8-6).

A number of scales may assist the clinician in the assessment of apathy. Two commonly utilized instruments are the Apathy Evaluation Scale (AES) and the Neuropsychiatric Inventory (NPI). The AES involves ratings on 18 items, and each of those is assessed on a four-point scale. It can be administered as a self-rated scale, a caregiver scale, or a clinician rated semi-structured

TABLE 8-6 • Differentiating apathy from depression.

Apathy	Depression
Decreased initiative	Sadness
Diminished interest in environment	Guilt
Blunted emotional response	Hopelessness
Both	
Low social engagement	
Decreased enthusiasm for previously enjoyable activities	

inventory. The NPI was developed for use in patients with dementia and is based on responses from a structured interview with caregivers. It assesses 10 or 12 behavioral domains common in dementia, including apathy and depression. The apathy subscale (NPI-apathy) starts with a screening question, with a positive response leading to a request for more information about eight sub-items. The Lille Apathy Rating Scale (LARS) and the Unified Parkinson's Disease Rating Scale (UPDRS) are useful to assess apathy in patients with PD. The LARS has a particular focus on distinguishing between apathy and depression. The Frontal Systems Behavior Scale (FrSBe) is utilized when there is a known or suspected frontal lobe disorder. It assesses apathy, disinhibition, and executive functioning deficits.

Treatment

There is no gold standard treatment for apathy, as most studies evaluated the treatment of apathy in the setting of a particular disease (e.g., AD, frontotemporal dementia, PD, etc.).

Cholinesterase inhibitors have been shown to improve apathy, particularly in AD.[240,241] There is no one cholinesterase inhibitor that has demonstrated superior efficacy over the others. Studies have looked at donepezil, galantamine, and rivastigmine. A few studies of memantine in AD and vascular dementia showed improvement in apathy.[242,243] A small open label study of memantine in frontotemporal dementia patients failed to show any decrease in apathy scores.[244]

Psychostimulants have had some positive effects in patients with apathy in the setting of AD, vascular dementia, PD, and frontotemporal dementia. The majority of these studies have used methylphenidate, with dosing typically between 10 and 20 mg daily (usually in divided doses). A 2017 study found that methylphenidate improved apathy, cognition, functional status, and depression in a group of community-dwelling veterans with AD; there was also a measurable alleviation of caregiver burden.[245] In a 12-week study, Parkinson patients treated with piribedil, a D2/D3 agonist, showed significant improvement in apathy scores as compared to the placebo group.[246] Evidence from case reports suggests that other dopamine agonists such as pramipexole and ropinirole may be helpful.[247–250] It is important to monitor for the emergence of impulsive behaviors such as gambling addiction as an adverse effect from these medications. Modafinil was also found to be helpful in select cases.[251] Further work in this area is necessary.

Antidepressants can be tried in the treatment of an apathetic patient, especially if there is a question of a comorbid depression. They must be used with caution, as serotonergic medications can actually induce apathy as a side effect. Bupropion, an agent with dopaminergic and noradrenergic action, may be helpful for apathy. A case report series of three males with apathy showed "significant improvement" with bupropion, although it should be noted that depression may have been confounding.[252] There is currently a multicenter placebo-controlled trial underway looking at the effects of bupropion in AD-related apathy (https://clinicaltrials.gov/ct2/show/NCT01047254). Agomelatine is a novel antidepressant agent. It is a melatonin receptor agonist, and serotonin 5-HT2c and 5-HT2b antagonist; it appears to lead to an increase in dopaminergic and noradrenergic tone. In a study with behavioral variant frontotemporal dementia patients, apathy decreased after a 10-week trial of 50 mg.[253]

There has also been work in the area of neurostimulation treatments for apathy. A 2017 study of AD patients receiving 5 weeks of TMS and cognitive rehabilitation demonstrated an improvement in apathy that continued as far out as 6 months.[254]

PATHOLOGICAL LAUGHING AND CRYING

Pathological laughing and crying (PLC) is a syndrome characterized by frequent, brief, and intense bouts of uncontrollable crying and/or laughing, due to a neurological disorder.[255] Other names used for this presentation include pseudobulbar affect and emotional incontinence.

Epidemiology

PLC is commonly associated with several neurological conditions: AD, amyotrophic lateral sclerosis (ALS), multiple sclerosis (MS), PD, stroke, and TBI. The mean prevalence of PLC across these disorders is about 10%. The specific estimates in each of these conditions have varied widely, due to the different groups studied (e.g., clinic or population-based), definition of PLC used, and sensitivity/specificity of the instruments utilized. See Table 8-7 for the range of estimated PLC prevalence in each

TABLE 8-7 • Estimated PLC Prevalence in Different Neurological Conditions.[252,253]

Neurological Disorder	Lowest Estimated Prevalence	Highest Estimated Prevalence
Alzheimer's disease (AD)	10%	74%
Amyotrophic lateral sclerosis (ALS)	27%	50%
Multiple sclerosis (MS)	10%	46%
Parkinson's disease (PD)	3.6%	24%
Stroke	11%	34%
Traumatic brain injury (TBI)	5%	48%

of these conditions. It is highest for ALS, and lowest for PD.[255,256] In addition, PLC has been described in normal pressure hydrocephalus, corticobasal degeneration, Angelman syndrome, herpes encephalitis, brainstem arterio-venous malformation or aneurysm, cerebral tumors, CNS lipid storage diseases, progressive supranuclear palsy, neurosyphilis, frontotemporal dementia, and other disorders.[255]

Pathophysiology

PLC may result from lesions that disrupt the neurocircuitry involved in emotional regulation and expression.[257] Lesions of heterogeneous localization may precipitate PLC (frontal and parietal lobes, descending pathways to the brain stem, subcortical tracts involving the cerebellum),[257,258] in line with a model of an extended emotion and affect regulation neural network that can be affected at different points. A traditional view posits that the cerebral cortex is crucial for the appraisal of the contextual information of an emotional stimulus, and the modulation of the intensity, frequency, and duration of the emotional response. This top-down model proposes that emotional modulation is facilitated by cortico-bulbar pathways, and that PLC may occur due to lesions in cortex, or in these descending tracts.

A more specific description of this model[259] proposes a volitional system, involving frontoparietal (primary motor, premotor, supplementary motor, posterior insular, dorsal ACC), primary sensory, and related parietal) corticopontine projections, and emotional pathways, involving projections from OFC, ventral ACG, anterior insular, inferior temporal, and parahippocampal areas, that regulate the amygdala. The amygdala and hypothalamus, in turn, activate the periaqueductal gray (PAG)-dorsal tegmentum (dTg) complex, which activates the displays of laughing and crying. The volitional system inhibits the emotional pathway at multiple levels. Lesions of the volitional corticopontine projections (or of their feedback or processing circuits) can produce PLC.[259]

An alternative model contends that the cerebellum plays a significant role in modulating emotional expression, and thus lesions that impact the cerebro-ponto-cerebellar pathways responsible for adjusting the automatic execution of laughter or crying can provoke PLC.[257]

Monoaminergic neurotransmitter systems and specific receptors that may be implicated in PLC include glutamatergic NMDA, muscarinic M1-3, GABA-A, dopamine D2, norepinephrine alpha-1,2, serotonin 5HT1a, 5HT1b/d, and sigma-1 receptors. This helps to explain the efficacy of diverse pharmacological agents active in these systems in patients with PLC.[255,259,260]

Clinical Presentation

The individual presents uncontrollable episodes of crying and/or laughing that are mood-incongruent, thus not related to feelings of sadness or joy. Of note, pathological crying is more common than pathological laughter. In some individuals, there may be an underlying emotional state present (e.g., sad mood), but the affect displayed is clearly excessive with respect to the mood. Similarly, the intense affective display is incongruent with the context surrounding the individual, or a clearly exaggerated

response. For instance, a sad commercial may trigger profuse, disproportionate tearfulness. PLC may present as comorbid with other neuropsychiatric disorders including mood and cognitive disorders.[261]

Assessment and Differential Diagnosis

PLC tends to be underdiagnosed and undertreated. It is important to screen for it, and to educate patients, family members, and medical providers about this syndrome.[256] Clinicians may confuse it with depression or bipolar disorder. PLC can cause social distress and embarrassment, given its prominent and odd phenomenology. Family members may worry or be critical about this exaggerated affective expression. Obtaining a detailed history may be sufficient to assess the presence of this syndrome. However, given its overlap with other psychiatric manifestations, rating scales may be helpful for screening and diagnosis. The Center for Neurologic Study-Lability Scale (CNS-LS) is a self-report measure initially developed to assess affective lability in individuals with ALS,[262] later validated for other disorders. It includes an auxiliary subscale for episodes of anger/frustration. The presence of a mood disorder such as major depression may result in a high score in several of the scale's items, potentially producing a false positive.[261] Similarly, a proposed cutoff score of 13 is highly sensitive but not specific. A more conservative cutoff score of 21 appears to be more accurate.[256] The Pathological Laughter and Crying Scale (PLACS) is a clinician-administered instrument that measures the severity of PLC symptoms. It was developed for PLC in stroke patients.[263] A proposed cutoff of >13 renders a similar PLC prevalence as the CNS-LS cutoff of >21.[256]

In terms of differential diagnoses, it is important to assess if the individual presents with a mood disorder such as depression, or bipolar disorder and its spectrum. In mood disorders, mood and affect are congruent. However, mood disorders may co-exist with PLC. In rare cases where the bouts of laugher or crying are very stereotyped and present with alteration of consciousness, they may represent an episode of epilepsy (gelastic or dacrystic, respectively). Regular EEG, and in some cases video-monitoring EEG, may be indicated.[255]

Treatment

Treatment should be instituted when PLC is bothersome to the individual or results in social or occupational dysfunction.[255]

Multiple pharmacological agents have been shown to be effective for PLC.[255,264]

- **SSRIs** (fluoxetine, fluvoxamine, citalopram,[265] paroxetine, sertraline) may be effective for PLC in MS, ALS, TBI, and other illnesses. Evidence level includes case series, open-label trials, and double-blind trials. These medications tend to be used at low therapeutic doses, and the therapeutic response may be evident within the first few weeks, typically sooner than in depression.
- **TCAs** (nortriptyline, amitriptyline, imipramine) have demonstrated to be effective as well. Most studies have involved their use in PLC post-stroke, including a double-blind trial that showed effectiveness of nortriptyline for PLC

post-stroke.[263] A small (n=12) double-blind crossover study showed amitriptyline's effectiveness in treating PLA in MS.[266]

▨ **Dextromethorphan/Quinidine** has proven useful for treatment of PLC in ALS, MS[267] dementia, stroke, and TBI.[268] It can also treat symptoms of frustration and anger[269] which may represent the involvement of similar pathophysiological mechanisms, even if they do not strictly fit the clinical definition of PLC. Dextromethorphan is a weak, uncompetitive N-methyl-D-aspartate (NMDA) receptor antagonist, a sigma-1 receptor agonist, a serotonin and norepinephrine reuptake inhibitor, and an α3β4 neuronal nicotinic receptor antagonist. However, the mechanism whereby it exerts its clinical effects in PLC is not fully elucidated. Normally, dextromethorphan is rapidly metabolized through the cytochrome P450 2D6 (CYP2D6) isoenzyme, limiting its CNS bioavailability. Low-dose quinidine (10 mg) is a potent inhibitor of cytochrome P450 2D6 that substantially increases DM bioavailability. Quinidine prolongs the QT interval, although at the dose used in the dextromethorphan/quinidine combination the risk is considered minor.

▨ **Other agents:** Multiple agents have shown effectiveness to treat PLC in various neurological illnesses, as indicated in case reports. They include venlafaxine, duloxetine, reboxetine, mirtazapine, lamotrigine,[255,270] valproic acid,[271] agents that enhance dopaminergic activity (levodopa, methylphenidate), and amantadine, perhaps through its action as an NMDA receptor antagonist.[255] These medications should be reserved for cases where better-proven agents fail, or where added therapeutic benefits (e.g., dual action on mood and pain; mood stabilizing properties) are important.

Summary and Key Points

▨ A cognitive domain-based approach to pharmacotherapy, in which affected cognitive domains (e.g., memory, attention, level of arousal) are identified using both clinical phenomenology and cognitive testing, leads to the most precise, personalized, and effective treatment.

▨ For cognitive disorders in neuropsychiatric patients, linking the symptoms to the implicated neuroanatomy/neurotransmitter systems, and tracking treatment responses, are critical for choosing and adapting a drug regimen.

▨ Diseases involving the CNS present a high risk for developing psychiatric disorders, including depression, anxiety, psychosis, agitation, and others. Treating the psychiatric disorder generally improves neurologic outcomes.

▨ There is no perfect pill, and non-pharmacological interventions should always be optimized.

▨ Careful and ongoing evaluation of psychotropics side effects will optimize adherence and generate the best risk:benefit equation.

▨ Not all depression is treated the same way—clinicians should consider the depression subtype, comorbidities, severity, functional impact, and duration when designing the treatment plan.

▨ Agitation may be mediated at least in part by one of two mechanisms, either a "bottom-up" dysfunction due to limbic overactivation or a failure in "top-down" control, with disruption in the capacity to monitor internal and external stimuli and to modulate behavior.

▨ Glutamatergic antagonism, GABAergic agonism, and noradrenergic and dopaminergic antagonism tamping down monoaminergically mediated limbic drive may mediate the therapeutic anti-agitation effect of certain medications.

▨ Pro-dopaminergic and serotonergic modulation may exert a therapeutic effect by enhancing frontal cortical function in individuals with intact executive function at greater risk of agitation.

▨ Apathy is a frequent and debilitating syndrome that can arise from myriad etiologies, including psychiatric disorders, neurodegenerative disease, and traumatic brain injury.

▨ While there is considerable overlap between the symptoms of depression and apathy, they are dissociable and separate syndromes.

▨ Most treatment studies for apathy have had mixed results, and there is no medication with a specific indication for this syndrome; choice of agent should be guided by etiology of the syndrome and potential side-effect profile of the therapeutic agents considered.

▨ Pathological laughing and crying (PLC) is a syndrome characterized by frequent, brief, and intense bouts of uncontrollable crying and/or laughing that are mood-incongruent, or clearly excessive compared to the underlying mood.

▨ PLC is typically associated with a neurological condition. It has been described in individuals with Alzheimer's disease, amyotrophic lateral sclerosis, multiple sclerosis, Parkinson's disease, stroke, traumatic brain injury, and other neurological illnesses. It is thought to result from lesions that disrupt the neurocircuitry involved in emotional regulation and expression.

▨ Treatment should be instituted when PLC is bothersome to the individual or results in social or occupational dysfunction.

▨ Psychopharmacological agents shown to be effective in the treatment of PLC include SSRIs, TCAs, and the combination of dextromethorphan/quinidine, among other agents.

Multiple Choice Questions

1. The following class of medications has the most robust evidence-basis to treat memory disorders across a range of neuropsychiatric disorders:
   a. Serotonin- augmenting medications
   b. Pro-cholinergic medications, like acetylcholinesterase inhibitors
   c. GABA-receptor modulators
   d. Psychostimulants, like methylphenidate

2. A 61-year-old married female presents to her primary care doctor with new-onset anxiety. Aside from being moderately overweight and with hyperlipidemia, her only other health issue is hard-to-control blood pressure (BP). She describes her anxiety as a very uncomfortable sense of nervousness or agitation, with occasional palpitations. She reports she drinks at most one to two alcoholic beverages once per week, though finds it particularly tempting to drink more as it quells the agitation. She denies using cannabis in any form. An ECG is unremarkable. Her BP remains elevated (155/92) despite lisinopril and HCTZ. The most appropriate next step would be to:
   a. Prescribe lorazepam, given how effective alcohol is for her anxiety
   b. Start sertraline
   c. Administer an MoCA
   d. Add propranolol as her BP remains elevated
   e. Order a brain MRI

3. A 21-year-old male with no medical history except for a motor vehicle accident (MVA) at age 18 presents to an outpatient neuropsychiatry clinic with complaints of irritability and impulsive behaviors at home and at work. He explains that at the time of the MVA he lost consciousness for several minutes, and he was evaluated in the emergency department (ED). He was told at the ED that his non-contrast head CT and his neurological exam were both completely normal. However, over several months following the accident, he experienced intermittent headaches, dizziness, inattention, and sleep disturbance. He did not seek further medical attention and those symptoms largely resolved over subsequent months. He presents now at the behest of his family, as he was terminated from his most recent employment as a retail manager after getting into a physical altercation with a customer. He also describes frequent conflicts with his partner and family for the last couple of years, due to his ongoing agitation, as well as difficulty completing tasks at work and home. He denies any abuse of alcohol or substances. On cognitive testing he presents difficulties with attention and executive function. Laboratory tests, including toxicology screen and brain imaging, are otherwise normal. The patient was started on propranolol to address his chronic agitation. At his next follow-up visit, he reports marked improvement in irritability and impulsivity, but noted a side effect of light-headedness after up-titrating propranolol. On exam, he is found to be slightly bradycardic. What would be the next best course of action?
   a. Switch propranolol to methylphenidate
   b. Switch propranolol to desipramine
   c. Switch propranolol to pindolol
   d. Switch propranolol to amantadine
   e. Switch propranolol to carbamazepine

4. All of the following are true of apathy, EXCEPT:
   a. Depression and apathy have considerable overlap in terms of symptomatology but are separate and dissociable syndromes.
   b. Apathy can be a sequela of many different diseases, including neurodegenerative processes and psychiatric disorders.
   c. High-dose serotonergic medications are an effective treatment for apathy.
   d. Higher levels of patient apathy are correlated with increased caregiver distress.
   e. Some studies have shown prevalence of apathy in Alzheimer's disease to approach 50%.

5. Ms. V. is a 44-year-old woman with relapsing remitting multiple sclerosis (RRMS) who, for the past month, has been crying very often (once daily, or more) and for "silly" reasons, or for "no reason at all"—in her own words. She cries when she sees a sappy TV commercial, when her daughter calls to check-in, and when the cat jumps onto the couch. She cried, unexpectedly, at the opening of a new boutique in town. In addition, Ms. V. feels less interested in things. She is not calling her friends, and not going to yoga. Her house is in disarray. She is ordering delivery of meals more often, because she does not feel like cooking. She skips her shower about half the days in the week. She stays in bed until 10 AM, and her appetite is diminished. Her prior psychiatric history is fully benign. Her PHQ-9 score is 18, and her CNS-LS score is 18 (positive for PLC). At her neurological visit last week, her RRMS was assessed as stable; her MRI did not show any new lesions, and she has not started any new medication in the last few months. Which of the following pharmacological agents is the best next option to treat Ms. V.?
   a. Sertraline
   b. Dextromethorphan/Quinidine
   c. Methylphenidate
   d. Lamotrigine
   e. Valproic acid

Multiple Choice Answers

1. Answer: b

Pro-cholinergic medications. The cholinergic system, which is widespread throughout the brain, seems to be the most effective drug target for memory disorders. Acetylcholinesterase inhibitors, like galantamine, rivastigmine, and donepezil are the main agents used. While there is some evidence that catecholamine augmentation can improve memory performance, for example, methylphenidate for adults with ADHD, these results have been overall inconsistent. There is no evidence that serotonergic and GABA-A modulating medications are effective in the treatment of memory disorders.

2. Answer: d

Explanation: This case illustrates a common scenario involving a middle-aged individual presenting with new complaints of anxiety in the context of a metabolic syndrome. Adding propranolol is the best next step among the presented options, as it might not only normalize her BP but also help her anxiety. Should the propranolol not prove helpful to her anxiety then an SSRI such as sertraline would be an appropriate intervention, ideally combined with cognitive behavioral psychotherapy (CBT). CBT by itself, without the SSRI, would also be a reasonable treatment option. If possible, benzodiazepines should be avoided, given their short and potentially long-term cognitive risks. Once her BP is stabilized, it may be appropriate to conduct further cognitive screening and workup, if indicated. Given her risk factors of being overweight, with hard to treat hypertension, it is also important to get further information about her sleep, ideally with collateral from her partner, to assess if she exhibits signs of sleep apnea.

3. Answer: c

Explanation: For symptomatic bradycardia with propranolol, pindolol can be used instead, given its intrinsic sympathomimetic activity. Although pro-dopaminergic, serotonergic, and anticonvulsant medications, like the ones listed among the other answer options, can be used as second- and third-line agents, beta blockers remain first line in the treatment of chronic agitation in TBI. In addition, this patient showed benefit from the first agent tried within this class.

4. Answer: c

Explanation: While antidepressants with serotonergic action (e.g., SSRIs, SNRIs) can provide some benefit for patients with apathy, especially when it occurs in the context of depression, they can also induce apathy as a side effect, and especially at higher doses. When evaluating for apathy, medication lists should be carefully reviewed for medications that may be causing or exacerbating apathy.

5. Answer: a

Explanation: Ms. V. presents symptoms compatible with a major depressive episode. Comorbid with this diagnosis, she seems to present with PLC, given her frequent bouts of crying not related to sad mood or sad situations. SSRIs can treat both, major depression and PLC, thus sertraline is the agent of choice for this patient. Dextromethorphan/quinidine should be reserved for cases with PLC without a concurrent mood disorder. While methylphenidate could help some of Ms. V.'s symptoms, such as her low energy and motivation, it is not indicated as the sole treatment of major depression. Lamotrigine and valproic acid have mood stabilizing properties, but our patient has no history of bipolar disorder symptoms. While case reports indicate these two agents may help PLC, they are not the first line of treatment for this.

References

1. Medalia A, Opler LA, Saperstein AM. Integrating psychopharmacology and cognitive remediation to treat cognitive dysfunction in the psychotic disorders. *CNS Spectr.* 2014;19(2):115-120.
2. Culpepper L, Lam RW, McIntyre RS. Cognitive impairment in patients with depression: awareness, assessment, and management: (Academic Highlights). *J Clin Psychiatry.* 2017;78(9):1383-1394.
3. Furukawa TA, Efthimiou O, Weitz ES, et al. Cognitive-behavioral analysis system of psychotherapy, drug, or their combination for persistent depressive disorder: personalizing the treatment choice using individual participant data network metaregression. *Psychother Psychosom.* 2018;87(3):140-153.
4. Tuchman R, Alessandri M, Cuccaro M. Autism spectrum disorders and epilepsy: moving towards a comprehensive approach to treatment. *Brain Dev.* 2010;32(9):719-730.
5. Totura CMW, Fields SA, Karver MS. The role of the therapeutic relationship in psychopharmacological treatment outcomes: a meta-analytic review. *Psychiatr Serv.* 2018;69(1):41-47.
6. Webb CA, Beard C, Auerbach RP, Menninger E, Björgvinsson T. The therapeutic alliance in a naturalistic psychiatric setting: temporal relations with depressive symptom change. *Behav Res Ther.* 2014;61:70-77.
7. Schnakers C. *Coma and Disorders of Consciousness.* 2nd ed. Switzerland: Springer International Publishing; 2018.
8. Li Y, Pan J, He Y, et al. Detecting number processing and mental calculation in patients with disorders of consciousness using a hybrid brain-computer interface system. *BMC Neurol.* 2015 Dec;15(1) [cited July 26, 2019]. Available at http://bmcneurol.biomedcentral.com/articles/10.1186/s12883-015-0521-z.
9. Cruse D, Chennu S, Chatelle C, et al. Relationship between etiology and covert cognition in the minimally conscious state. *Neurology.* 2012;78(11):816-822.
10. Olff M, Sijbrandij M, Opmeer BC, Carlier IVE, Gersons BPR. The structure of acute posttraumatic stress symptoms: 'reexperiencing', 'active avoidance', 'sysphoria', and 'hyperarousal.' *J Anxiety Disord.* 2009;23(5):656-659.
11. Boettger S, Breitbart W. Phenomenology of the subtypes of delirium: phenomenological differences between hyperactive and hypoactive delirium. *Palliat Support Care.* 2011;9(2):129-135.
12. Edlow BL, Takahashi E, Wu O, et al. Neuroanatomic connectivity of the human ascending arousal system

critical to consciousness and its disorders. *J Neuropathol Exp Neurol*. 2012;71(6):531-546.

13. Lin J-S, Anaclet C, Sergeeva OA, Haas HL. The waking brain: an update. *Cell Mol Life Sci*. 2011;68(15):2499-2512.

14. McClenathan B, Thakor N, Hoesch R. Pathophysiology of acute coma and disorders of consciousness: considerations for diagnosis and management. *Semin Neurol*. 2013;33(02):91-109.

15. Saniova B, Drobny M, Kneslova L, Minarik M. The outcome of patients with severe head injuries treated with amantadine sulphate. *J Neural Transm*. 2004;111(4):511-514.

16. Schnakers C, Monti MM. Disorders of consciousness after severe brain injury: therapeutic options. *Curr Opin Neurol*. 2017;30(6):573-579.

17. Giacino JT, Whyte J, Bagiella E, et al. Placebo-controlled trial of amantadine for severe traumatic brain injury. *N Engl J Med*. 2012;366(9):819-826.

18. Ciurleo R, Bramanti P, Calabrò RS. Pharmacotherapy for disorders of consciousness: are 'awakening' drugs really a possibility? *Drugs*. 2013;73(17):1849-1862.

19. Fridman EA, Krimchansky BZ, Bonetto M, et al. Continuous subcutaneous apomorphine for severe disorders of consciousness after traumatic brain injury. *Brain Injury*. 2010;24(4):636-641.

20. Munakomi S, Bhattarai B, Mohan Kumar B. Role of bromocriptine in multi-spectral manifestations of traumatic brain injury. *Chin J Traumatol*. 2017;20(2):84-86.

21. Passler MA, Riggs RV. Positive outcomes in traumatic brain injury–vegetative state: patients treated with bromocriptine. *Arch Phys Med Rehabil*. 2001;82(3):311-315.

22. Du B, Shan A, Zhong X, Zhang Y, Chen D, Cai K. Zolpidem arouses patients in vegetative state after brain injury: quantitative evaluation and indications. *Am J Med Sci*. 2014;347(3):178-182.

23. Bomalaski MN, Claflin ES, Townsend W, Peterson MD. Zolpidem for the treatment of neurologic disorders: a systematic review. *JAMA Neurol*. 2017;74(9):1130.

24. Kassie GM, Nguyen TA, Kalisch Ellett LM, Pratt NL, Roughead EE. Preoperative medication use and postoperative delirium: a systematic review. *BMC Geriatr*. 2017 Dec;17(1) [cited July 26, 2019]. Available at https://bmcgeriatr.biomedcentral.com/articles/10.1186/s12877-017-0695-x.

25. Singh B, Hughes AJ, Mehta G, Erwin PJ, Parsaik AK. Efficacy of prazosin in posttraumatic stress disorder: a systematic review and meta-analysis. *Prim Care Companion CNS Disord*. July 28, 2016 [cited July 26, 2019]. Available at http://www.psychiatrist.com/PCC/article/Pages/2016/v18n04/16r01943.aspx.

26. Samuels MA, Ropper AH. *Samuels's Manual of Neurologic Therapeutics*. 9th ed. Philadelphia, PA: Wolters Kluwer; 2017.

27. Kolanowski AM, Fick DM, Yevchak AM, Hill NL, Mulhall PM, McDowell JA. Pay attention!: the critical importance of assessing attention in older adults with dementia. *J Gerontol Nurs*. 2012;38(11):23-27.

28. Mesulam M-M, ed. *Principles of Behavioral and Cognitive Neurology*. 2nd ed. New York, NY: Oxford University Press; 2000:540.

29. Chambers CD, Heinen K. TMS and the functional neuroanatomy of attention. *Cortex*. 2010;46(1):114-117.

30. Blum K, Chen AL-C, Braverman ER, et al. Attention-deficit-hyperactivity disorder and reward deficiency syndrome. *Neuropsychiatr Dis Treat*. 2008;4(5):893-918.

31. Faraone SV. The pharmacology of amphetamine and methylphenidate: relevance to the neurobiology of attention-deficit/hyperactivity disorder and other psychiatric comorbidities. *Neurosci Biobehav Rev*. 2018;87:255-270.

32. Ma S, Hangya B, Leonard CS, Wisden W, Gundlach AL. Dual-transmitter systems regulating arousal, attention, learning and memory. *Neurosci Biobehav Rev*. 2018;85:21-33.

33. Sarter M, Bruno JP, Turchi J. Basal forebrain afferent projections modulating cortical acetylcholine, attention, and implications for neuropsychiatric disorders. *Ann N Y Acad Sci*. 1999;877:368-382.

34. Faraone SV, Mick E. Molecular genetics of attention deficit hyperactivity disorder. *Psychiatr Clin N Am*. 2010;33(1):159-180.

35. Briggs F, Mangun GR, Usrey WM. Attention enhances synaptic efficacy and the signal-to-noise ratio in neural circuits. *Nature*. 2013;499(7459):476-480.

36. Lanctôt KL, Chau SA, Herrmann N, et al. Effect of methylphenidate on attention in apathetic AD patients in a randomized, placebo-controlled trial. *Int Psychogeriatr*. 2014;26(2):239-246.

37. Ruthirakuhan MT, Herrmann N, Abraham EH, Chan S, Lanctôt KL. Pharmacological interventions for apathy in Alzheimer's disease. Cochrane Dementia and Cognitive Improvement Group, editor. *Cochrane Database Syst Rev*. May 4, 2018 [cited July 26, 2019]. Available at http://doi.wiley.com/10.1002/14651858.CD012197.pub2.

38. Huang C-H, Huang C-C, Sun C-K, Lin G-H, Hou W-H. Methylphenidate on cognitive improvement in patients with traumatic brain injury: a meta-analysis. *Curr Neuropharmacol*. 2016;14(3):272-281.

39. Baune BT, Renger L. Pharmacological and non-pharmacological interventions to improve cognitive dysfunction and functional ability in clinical depression—a systematic review. *Psychiatry Res*. 2014;219(1):25-50.

40. Bast T, Pezze M, McGarrity S. Cognitive deficits caused by prefrontal cortical and hippocampal neural disinhibition: prefrontal and hippocampal GABA and cognition. *Br J Pharmacol*. 2017;174(19):3211-3225.

41. van Wageningen H, Jørgensen HA, Specht K, Hugdahl K. Evidence for glutamatergic neurotransmission in cognitive control in an auditory attention task. *Neurosci Lett*. 2009;454(3):171-175.

42. Wesnes KA, Aarsland D, Ballard C, Londos E. Memantine improves attention and episodic memory in Parkinson's disease dementia and dementia with Lewy bodies: memantine in Parkinson's dementia and dementia with Lewy bodies. *Int J Geriatr Psychiatry*. 2015;30(1):46-54.

43. Klinkenberg I, Sambeth A, Blokland A. Acetylcholine and attention. *Behav Brain Res*. 2011;221(2):430-442.

44. Bracco L, Bessi V, Padiglioni S, Marini S, Pepeu G. Do cholinesterase inhibitors act primarily on attention deficit? A naturalistic study in Alzheimer's disease patients. *J Alzheimers Dis*. 2014;40(3):737-742.

45. Roy S, Ficarro S, Duberstein P, et al. Executive function and personality predict instrumental activities of daily living in Alzheimer disease. *Am J Geriatr Psychiatry*. 2016;24(11):1074-1083.

46. Marshall GA, Rentz DM, Frey MT, Locascio JJ, Johnson KA, Sperling RA. Executive function and instrumental activities of daily living in mild cognitive impairment and Alzheimer's disease. *Alzheimer Dement*. 2011;7(3):300-308.

47. Middleton LE, Lam B, Fahmi H, et al. Frequency of domain-specific cognitive impairment in sub-acute and chronic stroke. *NeuroRehabilitation*. 2014;34(2):305-312.

48. Matias-Guiu JA, Cortés-Martínez A, Valles-Salgado M, et al. Functional components of cognitive impairment in multiple sclerosis: a cross-sectional investigation. *Front Neurol*. November 28, 2017;8 [cited July 26, 2019]. Available at http://journal.frontiersin.org/article/10.3389/fneur.2017.00643/full. Accessed on: August 2, 2019.

49. Rabinovici GD, Stephens ML, Possin KL. Executive dysfunction. *Continuum (Minneap Minn)*. 2015;21:646-659.

50. Molinari M, Masciullo M, Bulgheroni S, D'Arrigo S, Riva D. Cognitive aspects: sequencing, behavior, and executive functions. In: *Handbook of Clinical Neurology*. Elsevier; 2018:167–180 [cited July 26, 2019]. Available at https://linkinghub.elsevier.com/retrieve/pii/B9780444639561000102. Accessed on: July 30, 2019.

51. Florio TM, Scarnati E, Rosa I, et al. The basal ganglia: more than just a switching device. *CNS Neurosci Ther*. 2018;24(8):677-684.

52. Schmahmann JD, Smith EE, Eichler FS, Filley CM. Cerebral white matter. *Ann N Y Acad Sci*. 2008;1142(1):266-309.

53. Kandiah N, Pai M-C, Senanarong V, et al. Rivastigmine: the advantages of dual inhibition of acetylcholinesterase and butyrylcholinesterase and its role in subcortical vascular dementia and Parkinson's disease dementia. *Clin Interv Aging*. 2017;12:697-707.

54. Dubois B, Tolosa E, Katzenschlager R, et al. Donepezil in Parkinson's disease dementia: a randomized, double-blind efficacy and safety study. *Mov Disord*. 2012;27(10):1230-1238.

55. Maneeton B, Maneeton N, Suttajit S, Reungyos J, Srisurapanont M, Martin S. Exploratory meta-analysis on lisdexamfetamine versus placebo in adult ADHD. *Drug Des Dev Ther*. 2014;8:1685.

56. Roth RM, Saykin AJ. Executive dysfunction in attention-deficit/hyperactivity disorder: cognitive and neuroimaging findings. *Psychiatr Clin N Am*. 2004;27(1):83-96.

57. Smith J, Browning M, Conen S, et al. Vortioxetine reduces BOLD signal during performance of the N-back working memory task: a randomised neuroimaging trial in remitted depressed patients and healthy controls. *Mol Psychiatry*. 2018;23(5):1127-1133.

58. Harrison JE, Lophaven S, Olsen CK. Which cognitive domains are improved by treatment with Vortioxetine? *Int J Neuropsychopharmacol*. 2016;19(10):pyw054.

59. Frampton JE. Vortioxetine: a review in cognitive dysfunction in depression. *Drugs*. 2016;76(17):1675-1682.

60. Dillon DG, Pizzagalli DA. Mechanisms of memory disruption in depression. *Trends Neurosci*. 2018;41(3):137-149.

61. Berna F, Potheegadoo J, Aouadi I, et al. A meta-analysis of autobiographical memory studies in schizophrenia spectrum disorder. *Schizophr Bull*. 2015; 42:56-66.

62. Das T, Hwang JJ, Poston KL. Episodic recognition memory and the hippocampus in Parkinson's disease: a review. *Cortex*. 2019;113:191-209.

63. Lim C, Alexander MP. Stroke and episodic memory disorders. *Neuropsychologia*. 2009 Dec;47(14):3045-3058.

64. Budson AE, Price BH. Memory dysfunction. *N Engl J Med*. 2005;352(7):692-699.

65. Kandel ER, ed. *Principles of Neural Science*. 5th ed. New York, NY: McGraw-Hill; 2013:1709.

66. Bonelli RM, Cummings JL. Frontal-subcortical dementias: the neurologist. 2008;14(2):100-107.

67. Birks JS, Harvey RJ. Donepezil for dementia due to Alzheimer's disease. Cochrane Dementia and Cognitive Improvement Group, ed. *Cochrane Database Syst Rev*. June 18, 2018 [cited July 26, 2019]. Available at http://doi.wiley.com/10.1002/14651858.CD001190.pub3. Accessed on: August 15, 2019.

68. Pagano G, Rengo G, Pasqualetti G, et al. Cholinesterase inhibitors for Parkinson's disease: a systematic review and meta-analysis. *J Neurol Neurosurg Psychiatry*. 2015;86(7):767-773.

69. Singh J, Kour K, Jayaram MB. Acetylcholinesterase inhibitors for schizophrenia. Cochrane Schizophrenia Group, ed. *Cochrane Database Syst Rev*. January 18, 2012 [cited July 26, 2019]. Available at http://doi.wiley.com/10.1002/14651858.CD007967.pub2.

70. Farooq MU, Min J, Goshgarian C, Gorelick PB. Pharmacotherapy for vascular cognitive impairment. *CNS Drugs*. 2017;31(9):759-776.

71. Ghaemi SN, Gilmer WS, Dunn RT, et al. A double-blind, placebo-controlled pilot study of galantamine to improve cognitive dysfunction in minimally symptomatic bipolar disorder. *J Clin Psychopharmacol*. 2009;29(3):291-295.

72. Cochrane M, Cochrane A, Jauhar P, Ashton E. Acetylcholinesterase inhibitors for the treatment of Wernicke-Korsakoff syndrome—three further cases show response to donepezil. *Alcohol Alcohol*. 2005;40(2):151-154.

73. Shaw EG, Rosdhal R, D'Agostino RB, et al. Phase II study of donepezil in irradiated brain tumor patients: effect on cognitive function, mood, and quality of life. *J Clin Oncol*. 2006;24(9):1415-1420.

74. Newcomer JW, Farber NB, Olney JW. NMDA receptor function, memory, and brain aging. *Dialogues Clin Neurosci*. 2000;2(3):219-232.

75. McShane R, Westby MJ, Roberts E, et al. Memantine for dementia. Cochrane Dementia and Cognitive Improvement Group, ed. *Cochrane Database Syst Rev*. March 20, 2019 [cited July 26, 2019]. Available at http://doi.wiley.com/10.1002/14651858.CD003154.pub6.

76. Fuermaier ABM, Tucha L, Koerts J, et al. Effects of methylphenidate on memory functions of adults with ADHD. *Appl Neuropsychol Adult*. 2017;24(3):199-211.

77. Kroenke K, Spitzer RL, Williams JB. The PHQ-9: validity of a brief depression severity measure. *J Gen Intern Med*. 2001;16(9):606-613.

78. Depression Management Toolkit. The Macarthur Initiative on Depression and Primary Care; 2009. Available at www.depression-primarycare.org. Accessed on: February 6, 2020.

79. Trivedi MH, Rush AJ, Wisniewski SR, et al. Evaluation of outcomes with citalopram for depression using measurement-based care in STAR*D: implications for clinical practice. *AJP*. 2006;163(1):28-40.

80. Judd LL, Akiskal HS, Maser JD, et al. Major depressive disorder: a prospective study of residual subthreshold depressive symptoms as predictor of rapid relapse. *J Affect Disord*. 1998;50(2-3):97-108.

81. Martin LR, Williams SL, Haskard KB, Dimatteo MR. The challenge of patient adherence. *Ther Clin Risk Manag*. 2005;1(3):189-199.

82. Sansone RA, Sansone LA. Antidepressant adherence: are patients taking their medications? *Innov Clin Neurosci*. 2012;9(5-6):41-46.

83. Kolla BP, Mansukhani MP, Bostwick JM. The influence of antidepressants on restless legs syndrome and periodic limb movements: a systematic review. *Sleep Med Rev*. 2018;38:131-140.

84. DeMartinis NA, Winokur A. Effects of psychiatric medications on sleep and sleep disorders. *CNS Neurol Disord Drug Targets*. 2007;6(1):17-29.

85. Rush AJ, Armitage R, Gillin JC, et al. Comparative effects of nefazodone and fluoxetine on sleep in outpatients with major depressive disorder. *Biol Psychiatry*. 1998;44(1):3-14.

86. Sharpley AL, Williamson DJ, Attenburrow ME, Pearson G, Sargent P, Cowen PJ. The effects of paroxetine and nefazodone on sleep: a placebo controlled trial. *Psychopharmacology (Berl)*. 1996;126(1):50-54.

87. Mendelson WB. A review of the evidence for the efficacy and safety of trazodone in insomnia. *J Clin Psychiatry*. 2005;66(4):469-476.

88. Winokur A, DeMartinis NA, McNally DP, Gary EM, Cormier JL, Gary KA. Comparative effects of mirtazapine and fluoxetine on sleep physiology measures in patients with major depression and insomnia. *J Clin Psychiatry*. 2003;64(10):1224-1229.

89. Nofzinger EA, Reynolds CF, Thase ME, et al. REM sleep enhancement by bupropion in depressed men. *Am J Psychiatry*. 1995;152(2):274-276.

90. Postuma RB, Gagnon J-F, Tuineaig M, et al. Antidepressants and REM sleep behavior disorder: isolated side effect or neurodegenerative signal? *Sleep*. 2013;36(11):1579-1585.

91. Sanchez C, Reines EH, Montgomery SA. A comparative review of escitalopram, paroxetine, and sertraline: are they all alike? *Int Clin Psychopharmacol.* 2014;29(4):185-196.

92. Panza F, Solfrizzi V, Seripa D, et al. Progresses in treating agitation: a major clinical challenge in Alzheimer's disease. *Expert Opin Pharmacother.* 2015;16(17):2581-2588.

93. McAllister TW, Arciniegas DB. Pharmacotherapy of neuropsychiatric disturbances. In: Arciniegas DB, Anderson CA, Filley CM, eds. *Behavioral Neurology and Neuropsychiatry.* New York, NY: Cambridge University Press; 2013:566-586.

94. Piechniczek-Buczek J. Psychiatric emergencies in the elderly population. *Emerg Med Clin N Am.* 2006;24(2):467-490, viii.

95. San L, Marksteiner J, Zwanzger P, et al. State of acute agitation at psychiatric emergencies in Europe: the STAGE study. *Clin Pract Epidemiol Ment Health.* 2016;12:75-86.

96. PRIME PubMed. A naturalistic study: 100 consecutive episodes of acute agitation in a psychiatric emergency department [cited July 26, 2019]. Available at https://wwww.unboundmedicine. com/medline/citation/16823684/[A_naturalistic_study:_100_ consecutive_episodes_of_acute_agitation_in_a_psychiatric_ emergency_department]. Accessed on: July 26, 2019.

97. Pajonk F-G, Schmitt P, Biedler A, et al. Psychiatric emergencies in prehospital emergency medical systems: a prospective comparison of two urban settings. *Gen Hosp Psychiatry.* 2008;30(4):360-366.

98. Flood C, Bowers L, Parkin D. Estimating the costs of conflict and containment on adult acute inpatient psychiatric wards. *Nurs Econ.* 2008;26(5):324, 325-330.

99. Rubio-Valera M, Luciano JV, Ortiz JM, Salvador-Carulla L, Gracia A, Serrano-Blanco A. Health service use and costs associated with aggressiveness or agitation and containment in adult psychiatric care: a systematic review of the evidence. *BMC Psychiatry.* 2015;15:35.

100. Zhang J, Harvey C, Andrew C. Factors associated with length of stay and the risk of readmission in an acute psychiatric inpatient facility: a retrospective study. *Aust N Z J Psychiatry.* 2011;45(7):578-585.

101. Pilowsky LS, Ring H, Shine PJ, Battersby M, Lader M. Rapid tranquillisation. A survey of emergency prescribing in a general psychiatric hospital. *Br J Psychiatry.* 1992;160:831-835.

102. Soyka M. Aggression in schizophrenia: assessment and prevalence. *Br J Psychiatry.* 2002;180:278-279.

103. Levin HS, Grossman RG. Behavioral sequelae of closed head injury. A quantitative study. *Arch Neurol.* 1978;35(11):720-727.

104. Rao N, Jellinek HM, Woolston DC. Agitation in closed head injury: haloperidol effects on rehabilitation outcome. *Arch Phys Med Rehabil.* 1985;66(1):30-34.

105. Silver JM, Yudofsky SC. Aggressive disorders. In: Silver JM, Yudofsky SC, Hales RE, eds. *Neuropsychiatry of Traumatic Brain Injury.* Washington, DC: American Psychiatric Press; 1994:313-353.

106. Morrissette DA, Stahl SM. Treating the violent patient with psychosis or impulsivity utilizing antipsychotic polypharmacy and high-dose monotherapy. *CNS Spectr.* 2014;19(5):439-448.

107. Siever LJ. Neurobiology of aggression and violence. *Am J Psychiatry.* 2008 Apr;165(4):429-442.

108. Silver JM, Yudofsky SC. Aggressive disorders. In: Silver JM, McAllister TW, Yudofsky SC, eds. *Neuropsychiatry of Traumatic Brain Injury.* 2nd ed. Arlington, VA: American Psychiatric Publishing, Inc.; 2011.

109. Elliott FA. Violence. The neurologic contribution: an overview. *Arch Neurol.* 1992;49(6):595-603.

110. Ballard C, Corbett A. Agitation and aggression in people with Alzheimer's disease. *Curr Opin Psychiatry.* 2013;26(3):252-259.

111. Buckley PF, Noffsinger SG, Smith DA, Hrouda DR, Knoll JL4th. Treatment of the psychotic patient who is violent. *Psychiatr Clin N Am.* 2003;26(1):231-272.

112. Nordstrom K, Allen MH. Managing the acutely agitated and psychotic patient. *CNS Spectr.* 2007;12(10 Suppl 17):5-11.

113. Battaglia J. Pharmacological management of acute agitation. *Drugs.* 2005;65(9):1207-1222.

114. Lesser JM, Hughes S. Psychosis-related disturbances. Psychosis, agitation, and disinhibition in Alzheimer's disease: definitions and treatment options. *Geriatrics.* 2006;61(12):14-20.

115. Warren RE, Deary IJ, Frier BM. The symptoms of hyperglycaemia in people with insulin-treated diabetes: classification using principal components analysis. *Diabetes Metab Res Rev.* 2003;19(5):408-414.

116. Citrome L. New treatments for agitation. *Psychiatr Q.* 2004;75(3):197-213.

117. Montoya A, Valladares A, Lizán L, San L, Escobar R, Paz S. Validation of the Excited Component of the Positive and Negative Syndrome Scale (PANSS-EC) in a naturalistic sample of 278 patients with acute psychosis and agitation in a psychiatric emergency room. *Health Qual Life Outcomes.* 2011;9:18.

118. Kay SR, Fiszbein A, Opler LA. The Positive and Negative Syndrome Scale (PANSS) for schizophrenia. *Schizophr Bull.* 1987;13:261-276.

119. Citrome L, Volavka J. The psychopharmacology of violence: making sensible decisions. *CNS Spectr.* 2014;19(5):411-418.

120. Garriga M, Pacchiarotti I, Kasper S, et al. Assessment and management of agitation in psychiatry: expert consensus. *World J Biol Psychiatry.* 2016;17(2):86-128.

121. Zeller SL, Rhoades RW. Systematic reviews of assessment measures and pharmacologic treatments for agitation. *Clin Ther.* 2010;32(3):403-425.

122. Lindenmayer J-P, Bossie CA, Kujawa M, Zhu Y, Canuso CM. Dimensions of psychosis in patients with bipolar mania as measured by the positive and negative syndrome scale. *Psychopathology.* 2008;41(4):264-270.

123. Yudofsky SC, Silver JM, Jackson W, Endicott J, Williams D. The Overt Aggression Scale for the objective rating of verbal and physical aggression. *Am J Psychiatry.* 1986;143(1):35-39.

124. Yudofsky SC, Kopecky HJ, Kunik M, Silver JM, Endicott J. The Overt Agitation Severity Scale for the objective rating of agitation. *J Neuropsychiatry Clin Neurosci.* 1997;9(4):541-548.

125. Kopecky HJ, Kopecky CR, Yudofsky SC. Reliability and validity of the Overt Agitation Severity Scale in adult psychiatric inpatients. *Psychiatr Q.* 1998;69(4):301-323.

126. Neurobehavioral Guidelines Working Group, Warden DL, Gordon B, et al. Guidelines for the pharmacologic treatment of neurobehavioral sequelae of traumatic brain injury. *J Neurotrauma.* 2006;23(10):1468-1501.

127. Beaulieu C, Wertheimer JC, Pickett L, et al. Behavior management on an acute brain injury unit: evaluating the effectiveness of an interdisciplinary training program. *J Head Trauma Rehabil.* 2008;23(5):304-311.

128. Arciniegas DB, Silver JM. Pharmacotherapy of neuropsychiatric disturbances. In: Zasler N, Katz DI, Zafonte RD, eds. *Brain Injury Medicine: Principles and Practice.* 2nd ed. New York, NY: Demos Medical Publishing, LLC; 2012:1227-1244.

129. Hasan A, Falkai P, Wobrock T, et al. World Federation of Societies of Biological Psychiatry (WFSBP) guidelines for biological treatment of schizophrenia, part 1: update 2012 on the acute

treatment of schizophrenia and the management of treatment resistance. *World J Biol Psychiatry.* 2012;13(5):318-378.

130. Nordstrom K, Zun LS, Wilson MP, et al. Medical evaluation and triage of the agitated patient: consensus statement of the American Association for Emergency Psychiatry Project Beta Medical Evaluation Workgroup. *West J Emerg Med.* 2012;13(1):3-10.

131. Stowell KR, Florence P, Harman HJ, Glick RL. Psychiatric evaluation of the agitated patient: consensus statement of the American Association for Emergency Psychiatry Project Beta Psychiatric Evaluation Workgroup. *West J Emerg Med.* 2012;13(1):11-16.

132. Wilson MP, Pepper D, Currier GW, Holloman GH, Feifel D. The psychopharmacology of agitation: consensus statement of the American Association for Emergency Psychiatry Project BETA Psychopharmacology Workgroup. *West J Emerg Med.* 2012;13(1):26-34.

133. Lukens TW, Wolf SJ, Edlow JA, et al. Clinical policy: critical issues in the diagnosis and management of the adult psychiatric patient in the emergency department. *Ann Emerg Med.* 2006;47(1):79-99.

134. Villari V, Rocca P, Fonzo V, Montemagni C, Pandullo P, Bogetto F. Oral risperidone, olanzapine and quetiapine versus haloperidol in psychotic agitation. *Prog Neuropsychopharmacol Biol Psychiatry.* 2008;32(2):405-413.

135. Mysiw WJ, Bogner JA, Corrigan JD, Fugate LP, Clinchot DM, Kadyan V. The impact of acute care medications on rehabilitation outcome after traumatic brain injury. *Brain Injury.* 2006;20(9):905-911.

136. Lenox RH, Newhouse PA, Creelman WL, Whitaker TM. Adjunctive treatment of manic agitation with lorazepam versus haloperidol: a double-blind study. *J Clin Psychiatry.* 1992;53(2):47-52.

137. Battaglia J, Moss S, Rush J, et al. Haloperidol, lorazepam, or both for psychotic agitation? A multicenter, prospective, double-blind, emergency department study. *Am J Emerg Med.* 1997;15(4):335-340.

138. Cummings JL, Lyketsos CG, Peskind ER, et al. Effect of dextromethorphan-quinidine on agitation in patients with Alzheimer disease dementia: a randomized clinical trial. *JAMA.* 2015;314(12):1242-1254.

139. Herrmann N, Lanctôt KL, Hogan DB. Pharmacological recommendations for the symptomatic treatment of dementia: the Canadian Consensus Conference on the Diagnosis and Treatment of Dementia 2012. *Alzheimers Res Ther.* 2013;5(Suppl 1):S5.

140. Gauthier S, Loft H, Cummings J. Improvement in behavioural symptoms in patients with moderate to severe Alzheimer's disease by memantine: a pooled data analysis. *Int J Geriatr Psychiatry.* 2008;23(5):537-545.

141. Herrmann N, Gauthier S, Boneva N, Lemming OM; 10158 Investigators. A randomized, double-blind, placebo-controlled trial of memantine in a behaviorally enriched sample of patients with moderate-to-severe Alzheimer's disease. *Int Psychogeriatr.* 2013;25(6):919-927.

142. Fox C, Crugel M, Maidment I, et al. Efficacy of memantine for agitation in Alzheimer's dementia: a randomised double-blind placebo controlled trial. *PLoS One.* 2012;7(5):e35185.

143. Pollock BG, Mulsant BH, Rosen J, et al. Comparison of citalopram, perphenazine, and placebo for the acute treatment of psychosis and behavioral disturbances in hospitalized, demented patients. *Am J Psychiatry.* 2002;159(3):460-465.

144. Pollock BG, Mulsant BH, Rosen J, et al. A double-blind comparison of citalopram and risperidone for the treatment of behavioral and psychotic symptoms associated with dementia. *Am J Geriatr Psychiatry.* 2007;15(11):942-952.

145. Seitz DP, Adunuri N, Gill SS, Gruneir A, Herrmann N, Rochon P. Antidepressants for agitation and psychosis in dementia. *Cochrane Database Syst Rev.* 2011;(2):CD008191.

146. Porsteinsson AP, Drye LT, Pollock BG, et al. Effect of citalopram on agitation in Alzheimer disease: the CitAD randomized clinical trial. *JAMA.* 2014;311(7):682-691.

147. Olin JT, Fox FS, Pawluczyk S, Taggart NA, Schneider LS. A pilot randomized trial of carbamazepine for behavioral symptoms in treatment-resistant outpatients with Alzheimer disease. *Am J Geriatr Psychiatry.* 2001;9: 400-405.

148. Tariot PN, Erb R, Podgorski CA, et al. Efficacy and tolerability of carbamazepine for agitation and aggression in dementia. *Am J Psychiatry.* 1998;155(1):54-61.

149. Herrmann N, Lanctôt KL, Rothenburg LS, Eryavec G. A placebo-controlled trial of valproate for agitation and aggression in Alzheimer's disease. *Dement Geriatr Cogn Disord.* 2007;23(2):116-119.

150. Porsteinsson AP, Tariot PN, Erb R, et al. Placebo-controlled study of divalproex sodium for agitation in dementia. *Am J Geriatr Psychiatry.* 2001;9(1):58-66.

151. Tariot PN, Schneider LS, Mintzer JE, et al. Safety and tolerability of divalproex sodium in the treatment of signs and symptoms of mania in elderly patients with dementia: results of a double-blind, placebo-controlled trial. *Curr Ther Res.* 2001;62(1):51-67.

152. Tariot PN, Schneider LS, Cummings J, et al. Chronic divalproex sodium to attenuate agitation and clinical progression of Alzheimer disease. *Arch Gen Psychiatry.* 2011;68(8):853-861.

153. Tariot PN, Raman R, Jakimovich L, et al. Divalproex sodium in nursing home residents with possible or probable Alzheimer Disease complicated by agitation: a randomized, controlled trial. *Am J Geriatr Psychiatry.* 2005;13(11):942-949.

154. Ballard C, Corbett A, Chitramohan R, Aarsland D. Management of agitation and aggression associated with Alzheimer's disease: controversies and possible solutions. *Curr Opin Psychiatry.* 2009;22(6):532-540.

155. Meehan KM, Wang H, David SR, et al. Comparison of rapidly acting intramuscular olanzapine, lorazepam, and placebo: a double-blind, randomized study in acutely agitated patients with dementia. *Neuropsychopharmacology.* 2002;26(4):494-504.

156. Rappaport SA, Marcus RN, Manos G, McQuade RD, Oren DA. A randomized, double-blind, placebo-controlled tolerability study of intramuscular aripiprazole in acutely agitated patients with Alzheimer's, vascular, or mixed dementia. *J Am Med Dir Assoc.* 2009;10(1):21-27.

157. Brooke MM, Patterson DR, Questad KA, Cardenas D, Farrel-Roberts L. The treatment of agitation during initial hospitalization after traumatic brain injury. *Arch Phys Med Rehabil.* 1992;73(10):917-921.

158. Mattes JA. Comparative effectiveness of carbamazepine and propranolol for rage outbursts. *J Neuropsychiatry Clin Neurosci.* 1990;2(2):159-164.

159. Greendyke RM, Kanter DR, Schuster DB, Verstreate S, Wootton J. Propranolol treatment of assaultive patients with organic brain disease. A double-blind crossover, placebo-controlled study. *J Nerv Ment Dis.* 1986;174(5):290-294.

160. Silver JM, Yudofsky SC, Slater JA, et al. Propranolol treatment of chronically hospitalized aggressive patients. *J Neuropsychiatry Clin Neurosci.* 1999;11(3):328-335.

161. Alpert M, Allan ER, Citrome L, Laury G, Sison C, Sudilovsky A. A double-blind, placebo-controlled study of adjunctive nadolol in the management of violent psychiatric patients. *Psychopharmacol Bull.* 1990;26(3):367-371.

162. Greendyke RM, Berkner JP, Webster JC, Gulya A. Treatment of behavioral problems with pindolol. *Psychosomatics.* 1989;30(2):161-165.

163. Janowsky DS, Shetty M, Barnhill J, Elamir B, Davis JM. Serotonergic antidepressant effects on aggressive, self-injurious and destructive/disruptive behaviours in intellectually disabled adults: a retrospective, open-label, naturalistic trial. *Int J Neuropsychopharmacol.* 2005;8(1):37-48.

164. Mysiw WJ, Jackson RD, Corrigan JD. Amitriptyline for post-traumatic agitation. *Am J Phys Med Rehabil.* 1988;67(1):29-33.

165. Jackson RD, Corrigan JD, Arnett JA. Amitriptyline for agitation in head injury. *Arch Phys Med Rehabil.* 1985;66(3):180-181.

166. Szlabowicz JW, Stewart JT. Amitriptyline treatment of agitation associated with anoxic encephalopathy. *Arch Phys Med Rehabil.* 1990;71(8):612-613.

167. Kant R, Smith-Seemiller L, Zeiler D. Treatment of aggression and irritability after head injury. *Brain Injury.* 1998;12(8):661-666.

168. Gualtieri CT. Buspirone: neuropsychiatric effects. *J Head Trauma Rehabil.* 1991a;6(1):90-92.

169. Gualtieri CT. Buspirone for the behavior problems of patients with organic brain disorders. *J Clin Psychopharmacol.* 1991b;11(4):280-281.

170. Colella RF, Ratey JJ, Glaser AI. Paramenstrual aggression in mentally retarded adult ameliorated by buspirone. *Int J Psychiatry Med.* 1992;22(4):351-356.

171. Ratey JJ, Leveroni CL, Miller AC, Komry V, Gaffar K. Low-dose buspirone to treat agitation and maladaptive behavior in brain-injured patients: two case reports. *J Clin Psychopharmacol.* 1992;12(5):362-364.

172. Stanislav SW, Fabre T, Crismon ML, Childs A. Buspirone's efficacy in organic-induced aggression. *J Clin Psychopharmacol.* 1994;14(2):126-130.

173. Bellus SB, Stewart D, Vergo JG, Kost PP, Grace J, Barkstrom SR. The use of lithium in the treatment of aggressive behaviours with two brain-injured individuals in a state psychiatric hospital. *Brain Injury.* 1996;10(11):849-860.

174. Glenn MB, Wroblewski B, Parziale J, Levine L, Whyte J, Rosenthal M. Lithium carbonate for aggressive behavior or affective instability in ten brain-injured patients. *Am J Phys Med Rehabil.* 1989;68(5):221-226.

175. Wroblewski BA, Joseph AB, Kupfer J, Kalliel K. Effectiveness of valproic acid on destructive and aggressive behaviours in patients with acquired brain injury. *Brain Injury.* 1997;11(1):37-47.

176. Azouvi P, Jokic C, Attal N, Denys P, Markabi S, Bussel B. Carbamazepine in agitation and aggressive behaviour following severe closed-head injury: results of an open trial. *Brain Injury.* 1999 Oct;13(10):797-804.

177. Mooney GF, Haas LJ. Effect of methylphenidate on brain injury-related anger. *Arch Phys Med Rehabil.* 1993;74(2):153-160.

178. Nickels JL, Schneider WN, Dombovy ML, Wong TM. Clinical use of amantadine in brain injury rehabilitation. *Brain Injury.* 1994;8(8):709-718.

179. Chandler MC, Barnhill JL, Gualtieri CT. Amantadine for the agitated head-injury patient. *Brain Injury.* 1988;2(4):309-311.

180. Hammond FM, Bickett AK, Norton JH, Pershad R. Effectiveness of amantadine hydrochloride in the reduction of chronic traumatic brain injury irritability and aggression. *J Head Trauma Rehabil.* 2014;29(5):391-399.

181. Hammond FM, Malec JF, Zafonte RD, et al. Potential impact of amantadine on aggression in chronic traumatic brain injury. *J Head Trauma Rehabil.* 2017;32(5):308-318.

182. Resnick M, Burton BT. Droperidol vs. haloperidol in the initial management of acutely agitated patients. *J Clin Psychiatry.* 1984;45(7):298-299.

183. Chouinard G, Annable L, Turnier L, Holobow N, Szkrumelak N. A double-blind randomized clinical trial of rapid tranquilization with I.M. clonazepam and I.M. haloperidol in agitated psychotic patients with manic symptoms. *Can J Psychiatry.* 1993;38(Suppl 4):S114-S121.

184. Nobay F, Simon BC, Levitt MA, Dresden GM. A prospective, double-blind, randomized trial of midazolam versus haloperidol versus lorazepam in the chemical restraint of violent and severely agitated patients. *Acad Emerg Med.* 2004;11(7):744-749.

185. MacDonald K, Wilson MP, Minassian A, et al. A retrospective analysis of intramuscular haloperidol and intramuscular olanzapine in the treatment of agitation in drug- and alcohol-using patients. *Gen Hosp Psychiatry.* 2010;32(4):443-445.

186. Clinton JE, Sterner S, Stelmachers Z, Ruiz E. Haloperidol for sedation of disruptive emergency patients. *Ann Emerg Med.* 1987;16(3):319-322.

187. Allen MH, Feifel D, Lesem MD, et al. Efficacy and safety of loxapine for inhalation in the treatment of agitation in patients with schizophrenia: a randomized, double-blind, placebo-controlled trial. *J Clin Psychiatry.* 2011;72(10):1313-1321.

188. Lesem MD, Tran-Johnson TK, Riesenberg RA, et al. Rapid acute treatment of agitation in individuals with schizophrenia: multicentre, randomised, placebo-controlled study of inhaled loxapine. *Br J Psychiatry.* 2011;198(1):51-58.

189. Kwentus J, Riesenberg RA, Marandi M, et al. Rapid acute treatment of agitation in patients with bipolar I disorder: a multicenter, randomized, placebo-controlled clinical trial with inhaled loxapine. *Bipolar Disord.* 2012;14(1):31-40.

190. Currier GW, Simpson GM. Risperidone liquid concentrate and oral lorazepam versus intramuscular haloperidol and intramuscular lorazepam for treatment of psychotic agitation. *J Clin Psychiatry.* 2001;62(3):153-157.

191. Currier GW, Chou JC-Y, Feifel D, et al. Acute treatment of psychotic agitation: a randomized comparison of oral treatment with risperidone and lorazepam versus intramuscular treatment with haloperidol and lorazepam. *J Clin Psychiatry.* 2004;65(3):386-394.

192. Hsu W-Y, Huang S-S, Lee B-S, Chiu N-Y. Comparison of intramuscular olanzapine, orally disintegrating olanzapine tablets, oral risperidone solution, and intramuscular haloperidol in the management of acute agitation in an acute care psychiatric ward in Taiwan. *J Clin Psychopharmacol.* 2010;30(3):230-234.

193. Lim HK, Kim JJ, Pae CU, Lee CU, Lee C, Paik IH. Comparison of risperidone orodispersible tablet and intramuscular haloperidol in the treatment of acute psychotic agitation: a randomized open, prospective study. *Neuropsychobiology.* 2010;62(2):81-86.

194. Currier GW, Trenton AJ, Walsh PG, van Wijngaarden E. A pilot, open-label safety study of quetiapine for treatment of moderate psychotic agitation in the emergency setting. *J Psychiatr Pract.* 2006;12(4):223-228.

195. Chengappa KNR, Goldstein JM, Greenwood M, John V, Levine J. A post hoc analysis of the impact on hostility and agitation of quetiapine and haloperidol among patients with schizophrenia. *Clin Ther.* 2003;25(2):530-541.

196. Yatham LN, Paulsson B, Mullen J, Vågerö AM. Quetiapine versus placebo in combination with lithium or divalproex for the treatment of bipolar mania. *J Clin Psychopharmacol.* 2004;24(6):599-606.

197. Sachs G, Chengappa KNR, Suppes T, et al. Quetiapine with lithium or divalproex for the treatment of bipolar mania: a randomized, double-blind, placebo-controlled study. *Bipolar Disord.* 2004;6(3):213-223.

198. Bowden CL, Grunze H, Mullen J, et al. A randomized, double-blind, placebo-controlled efficacy and safety study of quetiapine or lithium as monotherapy for mania in bipolar disorder. *J Clin Psychiatry.* 2005;66(1):111-121.

199. McIntyre RS, Brecher M, Paulsson B, Huizar K, Mullen J. Quetiapine or haloperidol as monotherapy for bipolar mania—a 12-week, double-blind, randomised, parallel-group, placebo-controlled trial. *Eur Neuropsychopharmacol.* 2005;15(5):573-585.

200. Porsteinsson AP, Keltz MA, Smith JS. Role of citalopram in the treatment of agitation in Alzheimer's disease. *Neurodegener Dis Manag.* 2014;4:345-349.

201. Fann JR, Uomoto JM, Katon WJ. Sertraline in the treatment of major depression following mild traumatic brain injury. *J Neuropsychiatry Clin Neurosci.* 2000;12:226-232.

202. Kinon BJ, Ahl J, Rotelli MD, McMullen E. Efficacy of accelerated dose titration of olanzapine with adjunctive lorazepam to treat acute agitation in schizophrenia. *Am J Emerg Med.* 2004;22(3):181-186.

203. Baker RW, Kinon BJ, Maguire GA, Liu H, Hill AL. Effectiveness of rapid initial dose escalation of up to forty milligrams per day of oral olanzapine in acute agitation. *J Clin Psychopharmacol.* 2003;23(4):342-348.

204. Kinon BJ, Stauffer VL, Kollack-Walker S, Chen L, Sniadecki J. Olanzapine versus aripiprazole for the treatment of agitation in acutely ill patients with schizophrenia. *J Clin Psychopharmacol.* 2008;28(6):601-607.

205. Marder SR, West B, Lau GS, et al. Aripiprazole effects in patients with acute schizophrenia experiencing higher or lower agitation: a post hoc analysis of 4 randomized, placebo-controlled clinical trials. *J Clin Psychiatry.* 2007;68(5):662-668.

206. Das S, Barnwal P, Winston AB, Mondal S, Saha I. Brexpiprazole: so far so good. *Ther Adv Psychopharmacol.* 2016;6(1):39-54.

207. Pratts M, Citrome L, Grant W, Leso L, Opler LA. A single-dose, randomized, double-blind, placebo-controlled trial of sublingual asenapine for acute agitation. *Acta Psychiatr Scand.* 2014;130(1):61-68.

208. Breier A, Meehan K, Birkett M, et al. A double-blind, placebo-controlled dose-response comparison of intramuscular olanzapine and haloperidol in the treatment of acute agitation in schizophrenia. *Arch Gen Psychiatry.* 2002;59(5):441-448.

209. Brook S, Lucey JV, Gunn KP. Intramuscular ziprasidone compared with intramuscular haloperidol in the treatment of acute psychosis. Ziprasidone I.M. Study Group. *J Clin Psychiatry.* 2000; 61(12):933-941.

210. Baldaçara L, Sanches M, Cordeiro DC, Jackoswski AP. Rapid tranquilization for agitated patients in emergency psychiatric rooms: a randomized trial of olanzapine, ziprasidone, haloperidol plus promethazine, haloperidol plus midazolam and haloperidol alone. *Braz J Psychiatry.* 2011;33(1):30-39.

211. Martel M, Sterzinger A, Miner J, Clinton J, Biros M. Management of acute undifferentiated agitation in the emergency department: a randomized double-blind trial of droperidol, ziprasidone, and midazolam. *Acad Emerg Med.* 2005;12(12):1167-1172.

212. Katagiri H, Fujikoshi S, Suzuki T, et al. A randomized, double-blind, placebo-controlled study of rapid-acting intramuscular olanzapine in Japanese patients for schizophrenia with acute agitation. *BMC Psychiatry.* 2013;13:20.

213. Meehan K, Zhang F, David S, et al. A double-blind, randomized comparison of the efficacy and safety of intramuscular injections of olanzapine, lorazepam, or placebo in treating acutely agitated patients diagnosed with bipolar mania. *J Clin Psychopharmacol.* 2001;21(4):389-397.

214. Wright P, Birkett M, David SR, et al. Double-blind, placebo-controlled comparison of intramuscular olanzapine and intramuscular haloperidol in the treatment of acute agitation in schizophrenia. *Am J Psychiatry.* 2001;158(7):1149-1151.

215. Chan H-Y, Ree S-C, Su L-W, et al. A double-blind, randomized comparison study of efficacy and safety of intramuscular olanzapine and intramuscular haloperidol in patients with schizophrenia and acute agitated behavior. *J Clin Psychopharmacol.* 2014;34(3):355-358.

216. Tran-Johnson TK, Sack DA, Marcus RN, Auby P, McQuade RD, Oren DA. Efficacy and safety of intramuscular aripiprazole in patients with acute agitation: a randomized, double-blind, placebo-controlled trial. *J Clin Psychiatry.* 2007;68(1):111-119.

217. Andrezina R, Josiassen RC, Marcus RN, et al. Intramuscular aripiprazole for the treatment of acute agitation in patients with schizophrenia or schizoaffective disorder: a double-blind, placebo-controlled comparison with intramuscular haloperidol. *Psychopharmacology (Berl).* 2006;188(3):281-292.

218. Daniel DG, Currier GW, Zimbroff DL, et al. Efficacy and safety of oral aripiprazole compared with haloperidol in patients transitioning from acute treatment with intramuscular formulations. *J Psychiatr Pract.* 2007;13(3):170-177.

219. Zimbroff DL, Marcus RN, Manos G, et al. Management of acute agitation in patients with bipolar disorder: efficacy and safety of intramuscular aripiprazole. *J Clin Psychopharmacol.* 2007;27(2):171-176.

220. Citrome L. Comparison of intramuscular ziprasidone, olanzapine, or aripiprazole for agitation: a quantitative review of efficacy and safety. *J Clin Psychiatry.* 2007;68(12):1876-1885.

221. Knott JC, Taylor DM, Castle DJ. Randomized clinical trial comparing intravenous midazolam and droperidol for sedation of the acutely agitated patient in the emergency department. *Ann Emerg Med.* 2006;47(1):61-67.

222. Richards JR, Derlet RW, Duncan DR. Methamphetamine toxicity: treatment with a benzodiazepine versus a butyrophenone. *Eur J Emerg Med.* 1997;4(3):130-135.

223. Richards JR, Derlet RW, Duncan DR. Chemical restraint for the agitated patient in the emergency department: lorazepam versus droperidol. *J Emerg Med.* 1998;16(4):567-573.

224. Rosen CL, Ratliff AF, Wolfe RE, Branney SW, Roe EJ, Pons PT. The efficacy of intravenous droperidol in the prehospital setting. *J Emerg Med.* 1997;15(1):13-17.

225. Chan EW, Taylor DM, Knott JC, Phillips GA, Castle DJ, Kong DCM. Intravenous droperidol or olanzapine as an adjunct to midazolam for the acutely agitated patient: a multicenter, randomized, double-blind, placebo-controlled clinical trial. *Ann Emerg Med.* 2013;61(1):72-81.

226. Asadollahi S, Heidari K, Hatamabadi H, et al. Efficacy and safety of valproic acid versus haloperidol in patients with acute agitation: results of a randomized, double-blind, parallel-group trial. *Int Clin Psychopharmacol.* 2015;30(3):142-150.

227. Marin RS. Apathy: a neuropsychiatric syndrome. *J Neuropsychiatry Clin Neurosci.* 1991;3(3):243-254.

228. Levy R, Dubois B. Apathy and the functional anatomy of the prefrontal cortex-basal ganglia circuits. *Cereb Cortex.* 2006;16(7):916-928.

229. Pardini M, Cordano C, Guida S, et al. Prevalence and cognitive underpinnings of isolated apathy in young healthy subjects. *J Affect Disord.* 2016;189:272-275.

230. Lanctôt KL, Agüera-Ortiz L, Brodaty H, et al. Apathy associated with neurocognitive disorders: recent progress and future directions. *Alzheimer Dement.* 2017;13:84-100.

231. Zhao Q-F, Tan L, Wang H-F, et al. The prevalence of neuropsychiatric symptoms in Alzheimer's disease: systematic review and meta-analysis. *J Affect Disord.* 2016;190:264-271.

232. Pagonabarraga J, Kulisevsky J, Strafella AP, Krack P. Apathy in Parkinson's disease: clinical features, neural substrates, diagnosis, and treatment. *Lancet Neurol.* 2015;14(5):518-531.

233. Aarsland D, Brønnick K, Ehrt U, et al. Neuropsychiatric symptoms in patients with Parkinson's disease and dementia: frequency, profile and associated care giver stress. *J Neurol Neurosurg Psychiatry.* 2007;78(1):36-42.

234. Bang J, Spina S, Miller BL. Frontotemporal dementia. *Lancet.* 2015;386(10004):1672-1682.

235. Veser FH, Veser BD, McMullan JT, et al. Risperidone versus haloperidol, in combination with lorazepam, in the treatment of acute agitation and psychosis: a pilot, randomized, double-blind, placebo-controlled trial. *J Psychiatr Pract.* 2006;12:103-108.

236. Marin RS, Wilkosz PA. Disorders of diminished motivation. *J Head Trauma Rehabil.* 2005;20(4):377-388.

237. Tagariello P, Girardi P, Amore M. Depression and apathy in dementia: same syndrome or different constructs? A critical review. *Arch Gerontol Geriatr.* 2009;49(2):246-249.

238. Landes AM, Sperry SD, Strauss ME. Depression in relation to dementia severity in Alzheimer's disease. *J Neuropsychiatry.* 2005;342-349.

239. Levy ML, Cummings JL, Fairbanks LA, et al. Apathy is not depression. *J Neuropsychiatry Clin Neurosci.* 1998;10(3):314-319.

240. Feldman H, Gauthier S, Hecker J, et al. A 24-week, randomized, double-blind study of donepezil in moderate to severe Alzheimer's disease. *Neurology.* 2001;57(4):613-620.

241. Holmes C, Wilkinson D, Dean C, et al. The efficacy of donepezil in the treatment of neuropsychiatric symptoms in Alzheimer disease. *Neurology.* 2004;63(2):214-219.

242. Cummings JL, Schneider E, Tariot PN, Graham SM. Behavioral effects of memantine in Alzheimer disease patients receiving donepezil treatment. *Neurology.* 2006;67(1):57-63.

243. Diehl-Schmid J, Förstl H, Perneczky R, Pohl C, Kurz A. A 6-month, open-label study of memantine in patients with frontotemporal dementia. *Int J Geriatr Psychiatry.* 2008;23(7):754-759.

244. Berman K, Brodaty H, Withall A, Seeher K. Pharmacologic treatment of apathy in dementia. *Am J Geriatr Psychiatry.* 2012;20(2):104-122.

245. Padala PR, Padala KP, Lensing SY, et al. Methylphenidate for apathy in community-dwelling older veterans with mild Alzheimer's disease: a double-blind, randomized, placebo-controlled trial. *Am J Psychiatry.* 2018;175(2):159-168.

246. Thobois S, Lhommée E, Klinger H, et al. Parkinsonian apathy responds to dopaminergic stimulation of D2/D3 receptors with piribedil. *Brain.* 2013;136(5):1568-1577.

247. Blundo C, Gerace C. Dopamine agonists can improve pure apathy associated with lesions of the prefrontal-basal ganglia functional system. *Neurol Sci.* 2015;36(7):1197-1201.

248. Kohno N, Abe S, Toyoda G, Oguro H, Bokura H, Yamaguchi S. Successful treatment of post-stroke apathy by the dopamine receptor agonist ropinirole. *J Clin Neurosci.* 2010;17(6):804-806.

249. Kohno N, Nabika Y, Toyoda G, Bokura H, Nagata T, Yamaguchi S. The effect of ropinirole on apathy and depression after herpes encephalitis. *Cogn Behav Neurol.* 2012;25(2):98-102.

250. Adam R, Leff A, Sinha N, Turner C, et al. Dopamine reverses reward insensitivity in apathy following globus pallidus lesions. *Cortex.* 2013;49(5):1292-1303.

251. Camargos EF, Quintas JL. Apathy syndrome treated successfully with modafinil. *BMJ Case Rep.* 2011;2011.

252. Corcoran C, Wong ML, O'Keane V. Bupropion in the management of apathy. *J Psychopharmacol (Oxford).* 2004;18(1):133-135.

253. Callegari I, Mattei C, Benassi F, et al. Agomelatine improves apathy in frontotemporal dementia. *Neurodegener Dis.* 2016;16(5-6): 352-356.

254. Nguyen J-P, Suarez A, Kemoun G, et al. Repetitive transcranial magnetic stimulation combined with cognitive training for the treatment of Alzheimer's disease. *Clin Neurophysiol.* 2017;47(1):47-53.

255. Wortzel HS, Oster TJ, Anderson CA, Arciniegas DB. Pathological laughing and crying: epidemiology, pathophysiology and treatment. *CNS Drugs.* 2008;22(7):531-545.

256. Work SS, Colamonico JA, Bradley WG, Kaye RE. Pseudobulbar affect: an under-recognized and under-treated neurological disorder. *Adv Ther.* 2011;28(7):586-601.

257. Parvizi J, Coburn KL, Shillcutt SD, Coffey CE, Lauterbach EC, Mendez MF. Neuroanatomy of pathological laughing and crying: a report of the American Neuropsychiatric Association Committee on Research. *J Neuropsychiatry Clin Neurosci.* 2009; 21(1):75-87.

258. Ghaffar O, Chamelian L, Feinstein A. Neuroanatomy of pseudobulbar affect: a quantitative MRI study in multiple sclerosis. *J Neurol.* 2008;255(3):406-412.

259. Lauterbach EC, Cummings JL, Kuppuswamy PS. Toward a more precise, clinically informed pathophysiology of pathological laughing and crying. *Neurosci Biobehav Rev.* 2013;37(8): 1893-1916.

260. Stahl SM. Dextromethorphan-quinidine-responsive pseudobulbar affect (PBA): psychopharmacological model for wide-ranging disorders of emotional expression? *CNS Spectr.* 2016;21(6): 419-423.

261. Hanna J, Feinstein A, Morrow SA. The association of pathological laughing and crying and cognitive impairment in multiple sclerosis. *J Neurol Sci.* 2016;361:200-203.

262. Moore SR, Gresham LS, Bromberg MB, Kasarkis EJ, Smith RA. A self report measure of affective lability. *J Neurol Neurosurg Psychiatry.* 1997;63(1):89-93.

263. Robinson RG, Parikh RM, Lipsey JR, Starkstein SE, Price TR. Pathological laughing and crying following stroke: validation of a measurement scale and a double-blind treatment study. *Am J Psychiatry.* 1993;150(2):286-293.

264. Pioro EP. Current concepts in the pharmacotherapy of pseudobulbar affect. *Drugs.* 2011;71(9):1193-1207.

265. Andersen G, Vestergaard K, Riis JO. Citalopram for post-stroke pathological crying. *Lancet.* 1993;342(8875):837-839.

266. Schiffer RB, Herndon RM, Rudick RA. Treatment of pathologic laughing and weeping with amitriptyline. *N Engl J Med.* 1985;312(23):1480-1482.

267. Yang LPH, Deeks ED. Dextromethorphan/quinidine: a review of its use in adults with pseudobulbar affect. *Drugs.* 2015;75(1):83-90.

268. Hammond FM, Alexander DN, Cutler AJ, et al. PRISM II: an open-label study to assess effectiveness of dextromethorphan/quinidine for pseudobulbar affect in patients with dementia, stroke or traumatic brain injury. *BMC Neurol.* 2016;16:89.

269. Smith RA, Licht JM, Pope LE, Berg JE, Arnold R. Combination dextromethorphan and quinidine in the treatment of frustration and anger in patients with involuntary emotional expression disorder (IEED). *Ann Neurol.* 2006;60(S10):S50.

270. Ferentinos P, Paparrigopoulos T, Rentzos M, Evdokimidis I. Duloxetine for pathological laughing and crying. *Int J Neuropsychopharmacol.* 2009;12(10):1429-1430.

271. Johnson B, Nichols S. Crying and suicidal, but not depressed. Pseudobulbar affect in multiple sclerosis successfully treated with valproic acid: case report and literature review. *Palliat Support Care.* 2015;13(6):1797-1801.

Neurostimulation Therapies in Neuropsychiatry

Mark Eldaief · Timothy Mariano · Mascha van't Wout-Frank

INTRODUCTION

Neurostimulation modalities modulate activity in prespecified regions of the neuraxis or, through trans-synaptic propagation, in prespecified circuits. The exact mechanism by which electrical stimulation results in therapeutic gains is unknown. Possibilities include changes in neurotransmission, changes in synaptic plasticity (e.g., long-term potentiation [LTP] and long-term depression [LTD]), hippocampal neurogenesis or other regional structural changes, changes in gene expression (e.g., brain-derived neurotrophic factor [BDNF]), changes in second messenger systems, neuroendocrine changes, or most likely, some combination of these. Neurostimulation modalities can be broadly divided into invasive approaches (which involve neurosurgical hardware implantation) or noninvasive approaches. Noninvasive brain stimulation (NIBS) involves cortical stimulation through the skull, scalp, and meninges. NIBS modalities include electroconvulsive therapy (ECT), transcranial magnetic stimulation (TMS), transcranial direct current stimulation (tDCS), and newer technologies such as focused ultrasound and optically based strategies. Invasive approaches include deep brain stimulation (DBS) and vagal nerve stimulation (VNS). In this chapter we provide an overview of a select number of neurostimulation modalities, for example, TMS, tDCS, ECT, VNS, and DBS and briefly discuss focused ultrasound and optically based strategies. We recognize that some emerging modalities are not included (e.g., transcranial alternating current stimulation [tACS], low-field magnetic stimulation [LFMS]); our aim is to emphasize those modalities that, at the time of this writing, show the most promise for eventual clinical deployment. We review clinical applications of the main modalities, with special focus on their use in major depressive disorder, particularly in treatment-resistant depression (TRD).

NEUROSTIMULATION MODALITIES

Table 9-1 provides a quick reference about the various neurostimulation techniques.

Transcranial Magnetic Stimulation (TMS)

TMS operates on the principle of electromagnetic induction, discovered by Michael Faraday, wherein a rapidly changing magnetic field creates a current in a conductive medium. Developed in 1985 by Barker, the TMS apparatus consists of a stimulator which delivers a large current into an attached TMS coil—consisting of loops of copper wiring in a plastic case—which is placed on the scalp over the area to be stimulated. TMS coils are commonly configured in a figure-of-eight shape, allowing increasing focality of stimulation at the intersection of two loops of copper windings.[1] The magnetic field produced by the TMS coil (approximately 1.5–2.0 tesla in field strength) induces a perpendicularly oriented electric field in stimulated cortex (Figure 9-1). TMS results in direct neuronal depolarization under the coil, up to an estimated depth of 2 cm. The electrical field, or E-field, produced by TMS can be computationally modeled using realistically shaped element head models based on data about coil type, location, orientation, etc.[2] TMS dose is commonly calculated as a percentage of the total machine energy output (on a scale of 0–100%). This can either be a fixed number (e.g., 60% of total machine output), or a percentage of the motor threshold. The *resting* motor threshold (RMT) is typically calculated as the percentage of machine output which elicits, through single pulses delivered to the hand region of primary motor cortex, a motor evoked potential (MEP) in the contralateral, resting hand, of 50 μv amplitude or higher, on 50% of trials. An *active* motor threshold (AMT) is calculated in a similar manner, except that the stimulated hand is undergoing submaximal voluntary contraction and the minimum amplitude of the MEPs is 200 μv or higher. Sham TMS is an important control condition both for cognitive neuroscience and clinical studies. Sham stimulation is typically accomplished by mimicking the somatosensory effects of active TMS, without delivering actual pulses. For example, some TMS devices may include skin electrodes which superficially stimulate the scalp to simulate muscle contractions induced by TMS.

TABLE 9-1 • Summary of Neurostimulation Modalities.			
Modality	Invasiveness	FDA Indications	Comment
Transcranial magnetic stimulation (TMS)	Non-portable external coil and stimulator	TRD, OCD	Patient is conscious during treatment.
Transcranial direct current stimulation (tDCS)	Portable external electrodes and stimulator	None	Patient is conscious during treatment.
Electroconvulsive therapy (ECT)	External electrodes and stimulator	Grandfathered: FDA never required premarket approval. Most commonly used for TRD, bipolar depression, catatonia	Requires general anesthesia and paralytic agents to prevent injury to patient during treatment.
Vagus nerve stimulation (VNS)	Implanted vagal nerve electrode and stimulator	TRD, epilepsy (adjunctive)	Noninvasive experimental VNS devices are in development.
Deep brain stimulation (DBS)	Implanted cortical electrode and stimulator	Essential tremor, Parkinson's disease, Dystonia, OCD, epilepsy (adjunctive)	Able to provide both depth and focality of stimulation.
Low-intensity focused ultrasound (LIFUS)	External transducer(s) and equipment	None	Able to provide both depth and focality of stimulation.
Optogenetic stimulation	Implanted optrodes, external equipment	None	Preclinical use only.

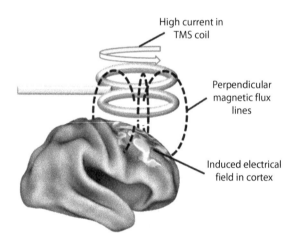

High current in TMS coil

Perpendicular magnetic flux lines

Induced electrical field in cortex

FIGURE 9-1. TMS works by passing a large current through a TMS coil (often figure-of-eight shaped). This current creates a rapidly changing perpendicular magnetic field of approximately 1.5 T which induces an electrical field in stimulated cortex, depolarizing neurons.

TMS Patterns

TMS can be delivered as single pulses, or as trains of pulses separated by fixed intervals at specific frequencies—referred to as repetitive TMS (rTMS) (Figure 9-2). rTMS can either be applied at low frequency (e.g., 1 Hz), or at high frequency (≥5 Hz). Low-frequency rTMS is associated with cortical inhibition, while high-frequency rTMS induces cortical excitation.[3] These principles are qualified by the fact that most studies establishing the effects of rTMS on cortical excitability have been performed in primary motor cortex, where output metrics of excitability are readily available in the form of MEPs. A more recent version

of rTMS, theta-burst stimulation (TBS), is delivered as triplets of 50 Hz stimulation, with these triplets occurring at a rate of 5 Hz (e.g., every 200 ms). TBS can either be delivered in intermittent (iTBS) or continuous (cTBS) patterns. iTBS is delivered as a 2-second train of TBS separated by an inter-train interval (ITI) of 10 seconds for a total of 190 seconds. As the name implies, cTBS is delivered continuously, often for 20 (300 total pulses) or 40 seconds (600 pulses). iTBS has been shown to increase cortical excitability, whereas cTBS decreases cortical excitability (with the same caveat that evidence for this being mostly restricted to experiments in motor cortex).[4,5] TBS is hypothesized to alter synaptic plasticity—with iTBS believed to induce LTP (Long-Term Potentiation) and cTBS believed to induce LTD (Long-Term Depression). This hypothesis is based on mathematical modeling[6] as well as through evidence that the effects of TBS are blocked by NMDA receptor antagonists.[5] Generally, the physiological effects of rTMS have been shown to outlast the duration of the stimulation by as much as several minutes,[7,8] and there is some evidence that the effects of TBS last longer than those of more traditional rTMS. Again, this finding has mostly been established in motor cortex.

TMS Safety Considerations

The most worrisome side effect of TMS is seizure provocation. Fortunately, this remains an exceedingly unlikely complication, with estimates of far less than 1% of stimulation sessions resulting in seizures in individuals who do not have intracranial pathology. Seizures are especially rare when established safety parameters are followed.[9] Other side effects of TMS include mild headaches (which tend to be transient and tend to respond to over-the-counter medications), neck pain, dental pain, hearing loss (if earplugs are not worn during treatment), or dizziness. While more common than seizures, the prevalence

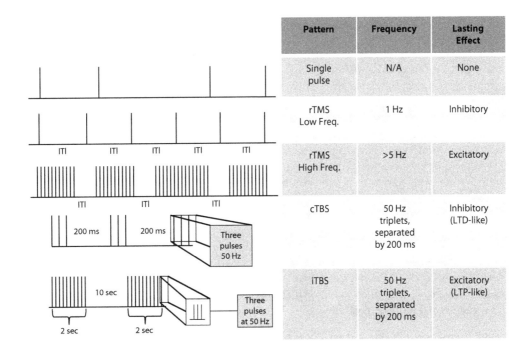

Pattern	Frequency	Lasting Effect
Single pulse	N/A	None
rTMS Low Freq.	1 Hz	Inhibitory
rTMS High Freq.	>5 Hz	Excitatory
cTBS	50 Hz triplets, separated by 200 ms	Inhibitory (LTD-like)
iTBS	50 Hz triplets, separated by 200 ms	Excitatory (LTP-like)

FIGURE 9-2. TMS can be delivered as single pulses or as patterned stimulation at specified frequencies (rTMS). Theta-burst stimulation (TBS) is a form of rTMS in which three pulses (triplets) are delivered at 50 Hz, with these triplets occurring at a rate of 5 Hz. The effects of rTMS outlast the duration of stimulation. High-frequency (HF) rTMS and intermittent TBS (iTBS) are excitatory; low frequency (LF) rTMS and continuous TBS (cTBS) are inhibitory. LTP, long-term potentiation; LTD, long-term depression.

of these symptoms are also very low, making TMS a well-tolerated modality. Due to the multi-tesla magnetic field strengths that TMS can generate, implanted metal or stimulation devices (e.g., aneurysm clips, pacemakers, cochlear implants, implanted pumps) in the head or neck are contraindications to performing TMS, and any metallic jewelry must be removed before treatment.

Transcranial Direct Current Stimulation (tDCS)

tDCS works by passing a weak direct electrical current, typically less than 2.5 milliamps (mA), between at least two electrodes, of which at least one is placed on the head (Figure 9-3). The application of such a weak electrical current alters cortical excitability via subthreshold modulation of neuronal resting membrane potentials, causing neuronal cells to be more or less likely to generate action potentials, depending on current direction.[10,11] Thus, in contrast to the suprathreshold stimulation of TMS, tDCS does not directly cause neurons to depolarize and "fire." Instead, tDCS changes the voltage across neuronal membranes, modulating the chance that an action potential is generated depending on how close the neuron is to threshold.[12]

tDCS electrodes come in many shapes, sizes, and configurations. They are typically placed on the scalp, often arranged according to the 10–20 system of electroencephalography (EEG) coordinates into a montage intended to pass current through the brain region or circuit of interest. There is no direct electron flow from the electrodes into the skin (or the brain), as biological tissues are not metallic conductors. Rather, electrodes establish an electric field,[14] resulting in a directional

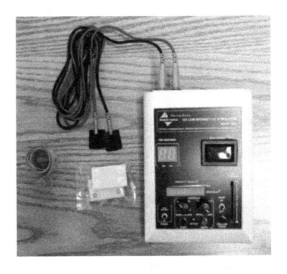

FIGURE 9-3. Most tDCS devices employ a battery-powered, microprocessor-controlled stimulator to produce the current-controlled output. The simplest tDCS montage uses two electrodes (bipolar stimulation). Current flows from the stimulator, through the red lead, to the anodal electrode. Current flows from the cathodal electrode, through the black lead, and back to the stimulator, completing the electrical circuit. An electric field is established between the anodal and cathodal electrodes, resulting in current flow through the brain. This photograph shows a Soterix Medical (New York, NY) 1X1 tDCS device, leads, carbon rubber electrodes, sponge pockets, and head strap (Reproduced with permission from Mariano TY, van't Wout M, Jacobson BL, et al. Effects of transcranial direct current stimulation (tDCS) on pain distress tolerance: a preliminary study. *Pain Med.* 2015;16(8):1580-1588. © Oxford University Press on behalf of American Academy of Pain Medicine. All Rights Reserved.)

current flow through intervening brain tissue. The electrode from which current flows into underlying tissue is termed the *anodal electrode* (or simply the *anode*). The electrode beneath which current exits tissue is the *cathodal electrode* (or the *cathode*). Neurons beneath the anodal electrode have an increased likelihood of "firing" action potentials if appropriately oriented relative to the current path.[12,15,16] Conversely, neurons beneath the cathodal electrode are considered to be less likely to "fire" action potentials if appropriately oriented. However, a recent review[17] highlights that this anodal versus cathodal tDCS terminology can be a deceptive oversimplification.[11,18] Specifically, it would be incorrect to conclude that anodal tDCS only produces excitatory effects on neuronal cells, whereas cathodal tDCS only produces inhibitory effects, as both excitatory and inhibitory effects can occur under either electrode depending on factors such as individual cortical folding and axonal orientation relative to the direction of current flow.[16,19] Moreover, effects of a particular polarity can be unexpected, or even opposite to what is expected, due to experimental and individual variability.[20,21]

tDCS Dosage and Considerations for Targeting

Research-grade tDCS devices typically allow for the following settings to be manipulated: stimulation duration (e.g., 1–30 minutes) and stimulation intensity expressed as current amplitude (e.g., 0.5–2.5 mA). These are important parameters of tDCS "dose." Waveform is not relevant to tDCS, as it is direct current and is simply "on" for the full duration of stimulation (apart from a brief typical ramp-up and ramp-down of current at the beginning and end of stimulation, respectively, to acclimate the individual receiving tDCS). Additionally, tDCS dose is also comprised of the total number of tDCS sessions, as well as the size, type, and location of all electrodes used.[17,22] Regarding electrode type and size, a main distinction can be made between flat rubber electrodes that are either covered in electrolyte gel/paste or inserted into a sponge moistened with saline; and smaller circular "high-definition" (HD) electrodes—comparable to EEG electrodes—that are embedded in electrode gel.[23] Some manufacturers also produce "dry" electrodes that do not require saline or electrolyte gel. Whereas sponge-based tDCS is typically "bipolar" in that it uses a total of two electrodes (one anode and one cathode), HD-tDCS often involves the application of more than two electrodes in various configurations, such as the electrode of interest being surrounded by a ring of four "return" electrodes in the opposite direction (e.g., one anode and four cathodes).[24,25]

Modeling of electrical current flow, "E-field modeling," has shown that HD electrode montages render a more focused stimulation area versus larger sponge-based electrodes,[26,27] which can result in a more variable and wider spread of current flow.[28] Whether larger sponge-based or HD electrodes are preferred depends on the desired effect of tDCS. Specifically, electrical current follows the path of least resistance between electrodes. Although this means that current shunting through the scalp is common, this also leverages the ability to shunt current through cerebrospinal fluid which is, relative to white and grey matter, a good conductor.[26,29] By placing larger electrodes further away from one another, scalp shunting is reduced and E-field modeling suggests that deeper brain structures can be reached. Indeed, using functional magnetic resonance imaging, multiple

studies have demonstrated neural effects of tDCS in brain areas, including subcortical areas, distal to the electrodes.[30,31] This finding has been buttressed by recent work that used implanted DBS electrodes to measure tDCS-induced effects in the subthalamic structures.[32] Using an array of multiple HD electrodes might be more suitable for focal targeting of neural regions that are closer to the scalp. Moreover, most studies use a fixed current amplitude (typically 0.5–2.5 mA) for all study participants. Given that current flow depends on individual cortical folding, a potentially better approach would be to perform individualized electrical field modeling to ensure that a similar current intensity in the brain region of interest is achieved for each individual, resulting in variable and customized current amplitudes for individual participants. Such an approach should reduce uncertainty as to whether a comparable amount of current has reached a particular brain target.[23]

Regarding the number of stimulation sessions, the conventional wisdom is that multiple sessions will result in stronger results than one stimulation session. However, it is not a simple dose-response relationship.[33] The time between multiple stimulation sessions affects outcomes. For instance, similar to rTMS, the effects of stimulation upon cortical excitability outlast the period of stimulation.[34,35] Applying a second tDCS session during this period of ongoing effects might change, abolish, or reverse the polarity-dependent effect of the original stimulation.[36] Moreover, recent clinical studies of tDCS have suggested a delayed or cumulative effect, such that changes in behavioral or clinical outcomes may not occur until *after* completion of the acute treatment phase.[23,37]

The ability to target a brain region focally with tDCS, also known as specificity, is an important topic in the scientific literature, because tDCS is considered a less focal neuromodulation technique when compared to other neuromodulation modalities, such as TMS. A distinction can be made between *anatomical specificity* or focusing on ensuring that current reaches a prespecified neural target, and *functional specificity* in which intrinsically active neuronal networks (i.e., those brain regions or networks engaged in a task-based process or pathology) are preferentially modulated by tDCS relative to nonactive networks.[38] *Functional* targeting is theoretically possible precisely because tDCS is a subthreshold modulatory technique, and thus only intrinsically active neurons (e.g., those neurons close to action potential threshold) will be impacted by tDCS. Thus, although current might flow through other neural regions, tDCS might have a greater net effect on regions that are critically engaged in the cognitive process being functionally targeted. Anatomical and functional specificity are critical components to consider when designing theoretically driven tDCS study protocols intended to influence a particular brain region or cognitive process.

tDCS Effects and Safety

Because tDCS is a subthreshold neuromodulatory technique, the low-intensity electric field on the skull can influence intrinsic neural plasticity.[39,40] As such, tDCS can "prime" the brain for subsequent responses and facilitate ongoing plasticity and cognitive processing, including learning, memory, and attention.[41] This also implies that it is vital to consider state-dependent effects during tDCS application[42]; the timing of tDCS in relation to a cognitive process of interest is thus equally important as the stimulation itself. For instance, there is preliminary evidence suggesting that combining tDCS with a relevant cognitive process or desired behavior, in a so-called "online" tDCS protocol, may increase efficacy.[11,12,42] Conversely in "offline" tDCS protocols, tDCS is delivered while the individual is at rest or prior to a cognitive process. The rationale for delivering offline tDCS prior to a cognitive task is based on the observation that tDCS induces after-effect excitability changes for up 5 minutes after 1 mA stimulation of 5-minutes' duration,[34] with duration of such after effects increasing with increasing tDCS dose (e.g., stimulation intensity and/or duration).[35]

Because tDCS involves subthreshold neuromodulation, the safety profile is quite favorable compared to other NIBS techniques, with a very low risk of tDCS-induced seizure—in epileptic participants, stimulation with a cathodal electrode placed over the epileptogenic focus has been studied as a means of suppressing seizure activity.[17] To date there is one case report of a seizure occurring 4 hours after a third daily tDCS session in a pediatric patient suffering from spastic tetraparesis and a history of seizures. The causal relationship between the occurrence of this seizure and tDCS is not known, as other factors—recent antiepileptic treatment regimen changes and/or premedication with escitalopram—might have contributed.[43] The most common side effects of tDCS tend to be mild and include local skin sensations at the electrode sites (tingling or itching) and temporary redness of the skin under the electrodes. Moderate fatigue and headache have also been reported.[44,45] Skin irritations can occur. In a small number of case reports, local skin burns where the electrodes are attached have been reported. In addition, three case studies report patients developing temporary hypomania during the course of a daily tDCS protocol (e.g., 10 sessions over the course of 2 weeks) for the treatment of depression targeting the dorsolateral prefrontal cortex.[46–48] In all cases, patients had experienced hypomanic periods prior to tDCS[46,48] or had received a diagnosis of bipolar II in the past.[47]

Electroconvulsive Therapy (ECT)

ECT involves the application of an electrical current with the expressed intent of inducing a generalized seizure. Patients require general anesthesia as well as paralytics to prevent injury (e.g., fractures and/or skeletal muscle injury). Atropine and glycopyrrolate may also be used for the prevention of bradycardia and drooling, respectively.[49] In light of this, patients must be thoroughly screened for their suitability to receive general anesthesia, as well as for medical or neurological conditions that may be exacerbated by a generalized seizure. Therefore, while there are no absolute contraindications to receiving ECT, relative contraindications include the presence of a space occupying intracranial mass or hemorrhage, increased intracranial pressure, a recent myocardial infarct, an unstable arrhythmia, or other contraindications to receiving general anesthesia.[49,50]

ECT can be administered with bilateral (bitemporal or less commonly bifrontal) or right unilaterally placed electrodes. ECT doses are expressed in millicoulombs, a unit of electric charge, with therapeutic dosing based on some percentage or multiplication factor of the dose needed for seizure induction. For example, 1.5–2 times the seizure threshold can be used for bilateral treatments and higher charges (e.g., 6–8 times the seizure threshold)[50] are often used for unilateral treatments. Another modifiable ECT parameter is pulse width: ECT can be administered with brief or ultrabrief pulses. Concomitant EEG recording is done to ensure that a seizure is achieved, and to record seizure duration. Seizure induction can also be confirmed by isolating blood flow (and thus paralytic delivery) to the foot with a tourniquet and observing motor contraction there.

ECT Safety Considerations

The most common cognitive side effects associated with ECT are anterograde and retrograde amnesia.[49] When anterograde amnesia occurs, loss of memories of events during or temporally adjacent to the induced seizures are common. Anterograde amnesia is often self-limited, resolving soon after treatment has ended. Retrograde amnesia can extend to memories up to several months, or less commonly, years before the treatment. The memory of autobiographical information is less likely to be affected. Preexisting cognitive impairment and older age increase the risk of cognitive side effects post-ECT. Variations in ECT technique (e.g., right unilateral electrode placement or ultrabrief pulse width) can reduce their incidence and severity. Brief postictal disorientation may occur. Prolonged seizures during ECT are rare. Other side effects of ECT include headache, muscle aches, nausea, and fatigue.[49]

Vagal Nerve Stimulation (VNS)

Originally approved for the treatment of epilepsy, VNS involves the electrical stimulation of the vagus nerve (specifically the left vagus nerve to limit effects on heart rate) via an implanted electrode. This electrode is connected to an implanted pulse generator, itself subcutaneously placed in the chest wall, and functions somewhat similarly to a pacemaker. The vagus nerve is part of the autonomic nervous system and modulates involuntary body functions such as breathing, the heartbeat, and digestive processes. VNS sends mild electrical pulses to the brain via the vagus nerve, which are typically not noticeable to patients. Stimulation parameters, which can be modified by the treating clinician through telemetry, include the duty cycle (i.e., the cycle of operation of a device that is turned on intermittently rather than continuously—often 30 seconds on and 300 seconds off), current (often starting at a low current of 0.25–0.75 mA), frequency (often 20–30 Hz), and pulse width (e.g., 250 μs).[42] VNS is thought to work by retrograde propagation of the electrical stimulation to the nucleus solitarius in the medulla, where it is believed to modulate activity in afferent projection areas such as the dorsal raphe, the locus coeruleus, the parabrachial nucleus, the hypothalamus, the amygdala, the insula and the bed nucleus of the stria terminalis.[51] VNS is also thought to enact its antidepressant effect through changes in monoaminergic transmission, neurotrophic effects, and even through modulation of neuroinflammation.[51]

VNS Safety Considerations

VNS side effects include hoarseness, dyspnea, and cough. Traditionally, VNS involves surgery and individuals who cannot tolerate general anesthesia are precluded. Infection of site implantation is a risk factor as well as other risks associated with surgery and general anesthesia. Other criteria that may make an individual unsuitable to get VNS are heart arrhythmias or other heart abnormalities, dysautonomias (abnormal functioning of the autonomic nervous system), lung diseases or disorders (shortness of breath, asthma, etc.), ulcers (gastric, duodenal, etc.), and vasovagal syncope. More recently, noninvasive VNS options are being developed and tested experimentally.

Deep Brain Stimulation (DBS)

DBS is an invasive neurostimulation procedure in which surgically implanted electrodes (a single electrode, or an electrode array or lead) delivers electrical stimulation to subcortical or deep cortical structures.[52] Electrode insertion is often performed under local anesthesia in an awake patient through a burr hole in a stereotactic, magnetic resonance imaging (MRI)-guided manner. In addition to the electrode, the DBS apparatus consists of a pulse generator which is implanted subcutaneously (often in the subclavicular region). An extension wire travels subcutaneously from the pulse generator to the electrode. Electrodes typically contain four contacts, each of which can deliver stimulation, thus allowing variable anatomical specificity of stimulation from a single electrode. Aside from the electrode contact(s) delivering stimulation, adjustable DBS parameters include pulse width (60–200 μs), frequency (typically 60–130 Hz), and amplitude/voltage (typically 2–10 volts).[52] These parameters are modulated by the clinician through remote communication with the pulse generator.[53] DBS works by interfering with ongoing activity in the brain through pulses sent from the pulse generator through the implanted electrode. For instance, in Parkinson's disease, DBS of the subthalamic nucleus blocks the abnormal neural activity that gives rise to unwanted motor symptoms typically observed in these patients.

DBS Safety Considerations

Adverse effects of DBS include hemorrhage, infection, negative mood or cognitive changes, or other surgical complications. Although some studies suggest DBS for Parkinson's disease to be safe in terms of cognitive effects,[54,55] other studies demonstrate the presence of cognitive deterioration, including impairments in verbal fluency and a transient increase in depression in 1.5–25% of patients, most likely due to postsurgery dopaminergic medication reduction.[56] These negative effects might be particularly pronounced in elderly patients.[57]

Focused Ultrasound (FUS)

Ultrasound is simply mechanical pressure waves in a medium (such as air or tissue) with a fundamental frequency above the upper limit of human hearing (20 kHz).[58] FUS is the use of one or several ultrasound transducers to focus the energy at a specific target which can be deep within the brain and not readily accessed by other NIBS modalities. FUS can be *high intensity* or *low intensity*. High-intensity focused ultrasound—or HIFUS—can be used to ablate specific brain targets, for example, for the treatment of essential tremor.[59] Low-intensity

focused ultrasound (LIFUS) on the other hand is being tested as a noninvasive and reversible neurostimulation technique able to inhibit or excite targeted regions.[60] The main benefit of LIFUS, as compared to other NIBS techniques such as TMS and tDCS, is that it offers superior spatial resolution (on the millimeter scale) and the ability to stimulate subcortical structures (deeper than 10 cm) noninvasively. Key sonication parameters are fundamental frequency, pulse repetition frequency (PRF), duty cycle, sonication duration, and intensity. Changes in these parameters impact the magnitude and direction of neuromodulation effects, as do mechanical aspects of the medium through which the LIFUS energy must propagate (e.g., attenuation and reflection by bone). A potential therapeutic application is the use of LIFUS to increase the permeability of the blood-brain barrier in order to better facilitate psychoactive drug delivery into the central nervous system, which has shown considerable promise in preclinical studies.[61] Still, at the time of this writing, LIFUS is an experimental technique for which research into feasibility and safety are active and rapidly evolving.[62] Computerized neuronavigation and virtual projection techniques are being developed to assist these efforts.[58,63]

Optically Based Strategies

Optically based neurostimulation techniques, such as optogenetic stimulation, allow both spatial as well as temporal precision in a noninvasive, reversible manner. Optogenetic stimulation is an experimental technique that uses light wavelengths emitted from an optrode to stimulate genetically targeted neurons that express a light-sensitive channel protein. Stimulation allows selectivity on the individual neuronal cell type and its spiking activity can be manipulated on a millisecond basis.[64] Subcellular manipulations are also possible with optogenetics. For example, it appears possible to control mitochondrial localization as well as ATP generation with this technique.[65] Given the need for genetically modified neurons to express light-sensitive ion channels, the technique is restricted to preclinical (animal) models of neuropsychiatric disorders.

CLINICAL APPLICATIONS OF NEUROSTIMULATION IN NEUROPSYCHIATRY

TMS

By far the most established clinical application for TMS is in treating major depressive disorder (MDD), and TMS is a commonly used neuromodulation strategy in treating TRD. For this indication, rTMS is delivered either to the left dorsolateral prefrontal cortex in a high-frequency, excitatory pattern; or to the right dorsolateral prefrontal cortex in a low-frequency, inhibitory pattern.

rTMS Clinical Trials in MDD

In 2007, a landmark multisite (23 sites) study establishing the clinical efficacy of rTMS in depression was conducted by O'Reardon et al.[66] A total of 301 medication-free (but not medication naïve, as at least one but no more than four failed adequate antidepressant trials were required) patients were randomized to receive either active (n = 155) or sham rTMS (n = 146) monotherapy daily for 4–6 weeks followed by a taper. rTMS parameters were as follows: 10 Hz rTMS, at 120% of the RMT, over 75 trains, 40 pulses per train, with an ITI of 26 seconds, for a total of 3000 pulses. These application parameters continue to be employed (with some modifications, such as shortening of the ITI to 11 seconds) as of this writing. Active rTMS was found to be superior to sham in response rates (defined as a ≥50% reduction in the Montgomery Asberg Depression Rating Scale [MADRS]) and remission rates (defined as a MADRS score ≤10). Following this study, the United States Food and Drug Administration (FDA) approved the use of the Neurostar™ TMS system (Neuronetics, Malvern, PA). Another pivotal multisite study established the clinical efficacy of "deep TMS" in treating depression. Compared to standard rTMS, deep TMS makes use of a different coil that allows greater intracranial penetration and thus stimulates a larger area of the brain that reaches deeper than the 2 cm attained by rTMS. Levkovitz et al.[67] recruited 212 MDD patients who were randomly assigned to rTMS monotherapy with either active or sham deep TMS. Patients received 4 weeks of deep TMS, followed by biweekly treatment for 12 weeks. Deep TMS was delivered at 18 Hz, at 120% of RMT, 36 pulses per train, with an ITI of 20 seconds for a total of 55 trains, or 1980 pulses. A deep TMS system, Brainsway™ (Jerusalem, Israel) was FDA approved in 2013. The efficacy of rTMS in depression has now been established by several randomized, sham-controlled trials, and is further supported by several meta-analyses.[68] At the time of this writing, seven TMS systems have been FDA approved in the United States for TRD: the aforementioned Neurostar™ and Brainsway™ devices, the MagVita™ device (Magventure, Denmark), the Magstim™ device (Wales, United Kingdom), the Nexstim™ system (Helsinki, Finland), the Cloud™ TMS system (New York, Boston, Los Angeles, CA), and the Apollo™ TMS system (Germany).

Importantly, Blumberger and colleagues[69] published a non-inferiority study comparing traditional high-frequency rTMS and intermittent TBS in TRD. These findings led to FDA approval for the use of iTBS in depression. This has significant ramifications for the future of depression treatment with TMS, as iTBS has a similar safety profile to traditional high-frequency rTMS[70] and can be administered over a much shorter duration (e.g., 190 seconds vs. 20–30 minutes). The latter attribute could pave the way for performing multiple treatment sessions in the same day with many fewer days of overall treatment, limiting the total time commitment imposed on patients.

Recent Improvements in rTMS Targeting in Depression

Traditional treatment paradigms use structural landmarks to establish the dorsolateral prefrontal target for rTMS. More specifically, targets are placed 5 cm anterior to the location in primary motor cortex where the RMT is determined. Recently, investigators have questioned whether this somewhat arbitrarily derived location is clinically optimal. This led to efforts to optimize dorsolateral prefrontal cortex (dlPFC) targeting based on established connectivity with limbic and paralimbic regions thought to be part of the neurocircuitry involved in the pathophysiology of depression (e.g., the subgenual anterior cingulate cortex, sgACC). Fox and colleagues used intrinsic

functional connectivity measures derived from a large dataset of healthy controls to establish regions within dlPFC whose blood oxygenation level dependent timecourses are the most negatively correlated to those of the sgACC. These regions are typically ventral and lateral to the traditional and lateral dlPFC targets. They then retrospectively showed that clinical courses of rTMS which targeted these regions were more likely to be clinically effective.[71] In a prospective clinical follow-up, Fox and colleagues demonstrated that using a patient's own intrinsic functional connectivity to select dlPFC targets most negatively correlated to the sgACC improved clinical outcomes.[72]

Treatment Algorithm for rTMS in MDD

rTMS treatment of MDD is now covered by several insurance companies in the United States. While requirements vary by payer, common features include (1) evidence that patients carry a diagnosis of moderate-to-severe unipolar MDD without psychotic features and (2) evidence that the patient has failed a number (e.g., 2–4) of antidepressant trials (either by demonstrating lack of efficacy after a sufficient dose and length of antidepressant use; or by demonstrating an inability to tolerate an antidepressant). Patients should also be prescreened for contraindications to rTMS, such as a history of epilepsy, a first-degree relative with epilepsy, a space-occupying lesion or other neurological pathology which may predispose to seizures, the presence of metallic implants or stimulators, particularly those in the head and neck, and the presence of medications that significantly lower seizure threshold (most psychotropics would not preclude rTMS except those which are particularly epileptogenic, e.g., clozapine and high doses of immediate release bupropion). Case vignette 9.1 illustrates considerations that clinicians should bear in mind when prescreening patients for TMS treatment eligibility.

Paralleling clinical trials, rTMS is often delivered in daily sessions, Monday through Friday, for several weeks, followed by a taper period. The choice between left-sided and right-sided treatment is often made an on individualized patient basis. Specifically, many practitioners will elect to use high-frequency, left-sided stimulation in the setting of significant anhedonia, melancholy, and anergia; whereas right-sided, inhibitory stimulation is often employed in the setting of predominant symptoms of anxiety (e.g., in the setting of generalized anxiety disorder or posttraumatic stress disorder [PTSD]), irritability, or mood lability (e.g., in the setting of bipolar disorder). Target location can be the traditional "5 cm" location as referenced above, the F3 position on a 10–20 system EEG montage, or based on individual MRI-guided metrics (e.g., individualized functional connectivity, as discussed above). Stimulation intensity (or strength) is expressed as a percentage of maximum output of the stimulator (0–100%), and can be based on either resting or active motor threshold (e.g., stimulation at 110% of an RMT of 40% would equal 44%). Finally, clinicians can now choose to employ traditional rTMS or TBS.

In the absence of a clinical effect within approximately the first 3 weeks, many of these parameters can be changed. For example, the number of pulses per session can be increased from 3000 to 4500 or 5500 (or in the case of TBS from 600 to 1200 or 1800 pulses), stimulation can be delivered at 120% of the *visual*

RMT (as opposed to that obtained through EMG), the RMT can be re-checked (particularly if known changes in medications expected to alter cortical excitability are being made during treatment), the side of stimulation can be switched (e.g., from left excitatory to right inhibitory, if the patient is becoming overly activated), the target can be moved more anterior and lateral in dlPFC, or bilateral treatments can be employed during each session, for example, 10 Hz rTMS on the left immediately followed by cTBS on the right. In partial responders, treatment courses can be extended, or a second full course of rTMS can be undertaken.

TMS for Other Neuropsychiatric Conditions

Other than major depression, evidence is strongest for the use of TMS in the treatment of obsessive-compulsive disorder (OCD). Therapeutic response is typically monitored through periodic administration of the Yale-Brown Obsessive-Compulsive Scale (Y-BOCS). Three cortical targets have emerged for the treatment of OCD: the dorsomedial prefrontal cortex (dmPFC), the orbitofrontal cortex, and the pre-supplementary motor area (pre-SMA). In 2018, the FDA approved the use of the Brainsway™ deep rTMS device for the treatment of OCD. With this system, stimulation is delivered at 20 Hz to dmPFC with the Brainsway deep H7-TMS coil™. Importantly, patients undergo OCD symptom provocation prior to each rTMS session, with provocation stimuli individually tailored to the patient.[73] The RMT used for calculating TMS dose is obtained in the *leg* (often in the anterior tibialis muscle), with the rationale being that recording the MT in medial motor cortex better approximates cortical excitability in dmPFC. In contrast to dmPFC stimulation, stimulation to pre-SMA is inhibitory (1 Hz rTMS), often delivered as 1200 pulses (20 minutes) in daily sessions.[74] Unlike deep rTMS to dmPFC, rTMS to pre-SMA has not been FDA approved for the treatment of OCD at the time of this writing.

While TMS has been explored for the treatment of other neuropsychiatric conditions, including bipolar affective disorder, addiction disorders, anxiety disorders, and psychotic disorders, there is currently insufficient clinical evidence to recommend its use in these contexts.

CASE VIGNETTE 9.1

A 45-year-old woman presents to the TMS clinic to evaluate the appropriateness of TMS as a treatment for her depression. The woman reports having chronic symptoms of depression that have significantly worsened in the past 2 years. Her complaints include profound dysphoria and tearfulness, hopelessness about the future, a significant inability to derive pleasure from activities she used to enjoy, and many neurovegetative symptoms with very low energy levels. She reports active suicidal ideation and has thought of how she may end her life, but does not have an imminent intent to do so—citing a concern about how it would affect her husband and children. She feels increasingly irritable, and has "snapped" at colleagues at work, placing her employment in danger. She is mildly anxious, but does not report hypervigilance, avoidance behaviors, panic attacks or derealization, and she does not feel that her anxiety is overwhelming. She denies ever having had manic/hypomanic or psychotic symptoms.

Her past psychiatric history is notable for having tried multiple psychotropic medications, including fluoxetine, paroxetine, venlafaxine, and bupropion. Fluoxetine, venlafaxine, and bupropion were all tried at adequate doses for at least 6 months over the past 2 years. Paroxetine could not be tolerated because it was too sedating, so this was stopped after 3 weeks. She is currently taking 200 mg of lamotrigine for depression, which she says is of limited efficacy. She has asked her psychiatrist to taper her off of this in the coming weeks/months. She is also taking meperidine as needed for recent back surgery. The woman has no history of implanted metal or stimulation devices (e.g., pacemaker, cochlear implant) in her head or neck and no personal or family history of epilepsy. She did have a "mild concussion" in high school while playing lacrosse and once passed out when she reports getting blood drawn.

This vignette highlights several considerations when evaluating a patient for TMS treatment of depression. First, we recommend that patients have a treating psychiatrist who knows them outside of the clinic. This enables the TMS clinic to maintain a dialogue about the patient's progress and concurrent medications, clarify diagnostic uncertainties and establish their overall suitability for TMS.

In terms of TMS eligibility, this patient seems to meet criteria for major depressive disorder of significant clinical severity. There are not obvious stigmata of other symptoms which might invoke other diagnostic considerations. The patient is also eligible to receive TMS based on her history of having failed five medications. Notably, paroxetine is included in this tally because she could not tolerate it, even though a sufficient trial duration was never reached. While the patient has active suicidal ideation, she does not pose an imminent danger to herself—in which case an ECT referral may be more appropriate.

As to contraindications to receiving TMS, the patient has no history of implanted pumps, stimulators, pacemakers, etc. She had a distant, mild concussion, but this would not be a strong contraindication. She has no history of seizures, and the report of syncope was likely a vasovagal episode. The patient takes meperidine as needed for pain, a medication which is highly epileptogenic. As such, there should be consultation with her prescribing provider about whether this can be stopped or can be replaced with another agent during her TMS treatment.

Finally, one should consider what TMS paradigm to use. This patient expresses profound dysphoria, anhedonia, and low energy, with limited anxiety. As such, left-sided, high-frequency rTMS would be appropriate.

tDCS

At the time of this writing, tDCS is not an FDA-approved treatment modality for any neuropsychiatric disorder and is considered for investigational/experimental use only. Successful application of tDCS requires an adequate understanding of how stimulation may result in neural and cognitive-behavioral change. As acknowledged in a recent review, there is a gap between scientific knowledge of transcranial electrical current stimulation and optimal implementation of tDCS to bring about neural, behavioral, and medical change.[11] Because tDCS, unlike TMS, is not FDA approved for any clinical indication, research-grade tDCS devices can only be purchased and utilized in humans with Institutional Review Board (IRB) approval that outlines the application of tDCS on human subjects and provides adequate protection against risks. There are manufacturers that sell commercial tDCS devices online, and there is an online community of "do-it-yourself" (DIY) tDCS users and device makers. Online comments include concerning stories regarding individuals who may have improperly used tDCS devices (e.g., with excessively high electrode-to-scalp impedance resulting in skin burns, stimulation parameters outside of typically accepted ranges, etc.). Furthermore, when applied without knowledge of the neurocircuitry to be modulated, tDCS may worsen cognition.[11] As such, tDCS should not be attempted without the direct supervision of fully trained medical or research personnel, in a safe and officially approved setting.

Most clinical trials compare active tDCS with a sham condition to allow testing for placebo effects. Sham stimulation often consists of ramping the tDCS device's current output up and then immediately back down to produce skin sensations without passing appreciable current through the brain. Some researchers have argued that such sham can be too easily distinguished from full stimulation, particularly at higher current amplitudes.[13,75] Furthermore, there is a growing understanding that "sham" may still modulate the cortical region of interest—especially over multiple sessions—due to small leakage currents from the stimulator, the amplitude of which can vary by device.[76] An active control condition during which tDCS is applied over a location or brain region not thought to be involved in the process under study might be superior for testing the functional specificity of tDCS effects. The downside of an active control condition is that current flow can be variable and broad, and it thus might impact the network under study, resulting in unanticipated observations. Unintentional unblinding is also possible, due to such parameters as impedance readouts from the device while operating, charge state of device batteries after a stimulation session, and degree of skin erythema after removing electrodes at the end of a session.[12,75] The topic of what is an appropriate sham condition and what is an adequate level of blinding remains an active area of study and debate.

Unfortunately, many of the early clinical studies suffered from deficiencies of design (very small sample size, inadequate or absent sham control, lack of double-blinding, etc.), and aggregate results are often unsatisfyingly mixed. Keeping this in mind, we present several of the larger areas of work investigating tDCS as a potential treatment modality.

tDCS has been tested for the reduction of depressive symptoms in individuals with MDD, mimicking the FDA-approved use of TMS. In these clinical trials, tDCS is applied multiple times over the course of 2–3 weeks, either with a research-grade stimulator or via "off-label" use of a commercial iontophoresis unit, usually *without* the participant performing a particular task.[77,78] Similar to rTMS, the left dlPFC is typically the target region over which an anodal electrode is placed. The intention is that "at rest" tDCS might favorably modulate a pathological process. Results have generally been mixed, although with better-designed studies in more recent years, the preponderance of evidence is beginning to support the potential clinical efficacy of tDCS in MDD.[11,79]

tDCS has also been tested for the reduction of anxiety-related symptoms. Specifically, tDCS has been tested for OCD,[80] social and generalized anxiety disorders,[81,82] and PTSD.[83–85] As expected, tDCS montages depend on the symptoms, neural network, or underlying cognitive process being targeted. For example, early research on the use of tDCS for PTSD specifically focuses on modulating fear memories and retention of safety memories that can inhibit fear memories,[85–91] as these processes are thought to underlie persistent PTSD symptoms and treatment success, respectively. Most of these early studies have not involved patients, with the exception of a few studies specifically testing the effects of tDCS combined with extinction or therapeutic habituation processes in PTSD patients.[84,85] Nonetheless, non-patient studies have aimed to understand underlying mechanisms by examining the effect of specific tDCS montages on the modulation of fear-related processes. Whereas studies focusing on modulating fear memories target the dlPFC,[86,88] studies focusing on augmenting safety memories tend to target the medial prefrontal cortex,[86,87,89] in line with neurobiological models of PTSD. However, further clinical studies are needed.

tDCS has been investigated as a potential treatment for chronic pain disorders. Pain is defined as having both sensory and emotional (affective) components.[92] Most existing chronic pain treatments (such as opioid or nonsteroidal anti-inflammatory drugs [NSAIDs]) treat the former via analgesic effects. Experimentally, tDCS has also been tested as a means of reducing the sensory component of chronic pain[93–97]; a recently updated *Cochrane Review* analysis suggests that there may be a small overall effect on chronic pain intensity and quality of life.[98] The emotional component, most often seen in chronic pain, has serious psychiatric sequelae including fear avoidance, anxiety, depression, and even suicide.[99,100] Preliminary work has attempted to modulate this component of chronic pain with tDCS[101,102]—this shows some promise, although larger replication randomized-controlled trials (RCTs) are needed.

tDCS has been explored to varying degrees in schizophrenia and motor or cognitive rehabilitation, although results to date do not support its routine clinical use in these areas.[11,102] There are slightly more promising results for treatment of substance use disorders, although rigorously designed RCTs are lacking and there is some evidence suggesting negative behavioral effects of the stimulation.[11]

It should again be noted that because tDCS is a subthreshold neuromodulation technique, the brain state during tDCS is a critical parameter[33] and combining tDCS with a desired behavior may increase efficacy.[11,12,42] Clinical studies frequently overlook these synergistic effects, although researchers are now considering multimodal approaches involving tDCS and psychotherapy such as cognitive behavioral therapy (CBT),[23,42] and this is expected to be a new frontier of NIBS-based treatment approaches. Due to tDCS's effects on synaptic plasticity that are still not fully understood, clinically meaningful effects may not manifest until some time *after* an acute tDCS treatment phase has finished.[23,37,103]

ECT

ECT is a highly efficacious treatment for TRD. Specific efficacy estimates vary, but some groups have found high response, and even remission rates. For example, one study of 230 patients found remission rates of over 60%,[104] and the Consortium for Research in ECT (CORE) reported a 75% remission rate among 217 patients.[105] There is evidence that bilateral treatment is more effective, and it is common for treaters to start with unilateral treatment in an effort to limit cognitive side effects, but then switch to bilateral treatment if there has not been a sufficient clinical response. Unlike TMS and tDCS, ECT is indicated in the treatment of bipolar affective disorder, and has been successfully used in manic, mixed, or depressive states.[106] Importantly, ECT is also indicated in the treatment of catatonia. ECT success in TRD is associated with shorter illness duration, older patient age, psychotic features, and in patients who have not failed many other treatments.[50] ECT is particularly indicated when a rapid clinical response is needed, for example, in MDD with psychotic features, in the setting of catatonia, or in the setting of acute suicidality.

ECT is often given three times a week for a total of 6–12 treatments, but specific treatment courses can be highly treater-specific. Relapse rates in ECT are unfortunately rather high. Pharmacotherapy is often used in relapse prevention, with particular support for the use of lithium and nortriptyline, and more recently, lithium and venlafaxine.[107] Maintenance ECT is an effective means to prevent and/or treat relapse. Maintenance ECT is done on a patient-specific basis, but some clinics will employ a prolonged taper after initial treatment (e.g., weekly, then bimonthly, then monthly).[50]

Two strategies have evolved to limit cognitive side effects from ECT. The first is to use right unilateral electrode placement. Bilateral treatments may still be used when right unilateral treatment is not expected to be suitable, or when right unilateral treatment has failed. For example, bilateral treatment may be chosen if a patient has failed unilateral treatment in the past, or if they are not responding to right unilateral therapy during the treatment period in question. In addition to electrode placement, pulse width can be shortened to brief or more recently, ultrabrief (approximately 0.25 ms) pulses, to limit cognitive side effects.

VNS

In 2005, the FDA approved the use of VNS as a long-term adjunct treatment for TRD. Evidence for the efficacy of VNS has been limited by a relative scarcity of RCTs. Still, many open-label clinical trials suggest a clinical benefit, with therapeutic improvements achieved approximately 3–12 months after treatment initiation.[51]

DBS

DBS has established clinical efficacy in neurologic patients—most prominently in Parkinson's disease, with other FDA-approved indications for dystonia and essential tremor. At the time of this writing, studies have shown mixed results in efficacy and further research is needed to understand the best way to implement DBS for TRD. Pioneered by Helen Mayberg and colleagues, much of the early work involving DBS for TRD used the sgACC/Brodmann Area 25 (or its surrounding white matter bundles) as a stimulation target. Encouraging results from open-label trials of DBS to the sgACC led to a multisite, randomized, sham-controlled clinical trial involving DBS of subcallosal white matter tracts. In this trial, 90 TRD patients were randomly assigned to receive either active or sham subcallosal DBS for 6 months, followed by an additional, 6-month open-label phase. The primary outcome measure was a 40% reduction in depression severity. Unfortunately, while generally well tolerated, active DBS was not statistically superior to sham (20% responders in the active group and 17% responders in the sham group).[108] Two other RCTs have explored the efficacy of DBS to the ventral capsule and ventral striatum.[53] The first involved 30 TRD patients randomized to active or sham DBS to the ventral capsule/ventral striatum for 16 weeks. The primary outcome measure was a 50% reduction on the MADRS from baseline.[109] This study also yielded negative results. However, a longer clinical trial of DBS in 25 TRD patients using a very similar target, the ventral anterior limb of the internal capsule, was positive.[110] Notably, the design of this trial was considerably different, with an initial open-label phase of 1 year, followed by a 12-week randomized-, double-blinded, sham-controlled treatment phase, which did show statistical superiority of active over sham DBS. Other DBS targets in TRD which have shown promise in open-label trials or in case reports include the lateral habenula, the nucleus accumbens, and the superolateral branch of the medial forebrain bundle.[111]

Dougherty[53] points out three shortcomings that may explain the relative lack of efficacy of DBS in TRD to date. First, it may be that DBS has a delayed clinical effect, explaining why the only positive controlled trial involved a prolonged initial open-label phase before primary outcome measures were assessed. Second, targeting based on stereotactic coordinates in standard space may be inferior to those derived by individualized tractography methods, given heterogeneity in anatomy across patients. Finally, given the heterogeneity of depression phenotypes (e.g., anxio-somatic vs. melancholic),[112] DBS targets may need to be tailored to circuits underlying a patient's specific symptom profile.

Other applications for DBS include its use for severe and highly refractory OCD, with a focus on targeting the ventral capsule/ventral striatum (VC/VS) or relatedly, the nucleus accumbens.[113,114] Available data are limited as only the most severe cases of intractable OCD were eligible, with four out of six patients reporting a ≥35% improvement in the Y-BOCS and end point Y-BOCS severity ≤16, classified as responders.[113] Another common target in OCD has been the subthalamic nucleus. In 2008, Mallet and colleagues[115] published a

randomized double-blind crossover study in which 16 OCD patients underwent bilateral subthalamic nucleus stimulation and found that Y-BOCS scores decreased significantly more with active versus sham stimulation.

Summary and Key Points

Neuromodulation continues to emerge as a powerful therapeutic tool in neuropsychiatry. It is often only employed when patients have proved refractory to medications and/or psychotherapy, due to the relative novelty, cost, and sometimes invasive nature of the techniques. However, safety profiles of many of these techniques are comparable to medications, and health insurance is increasingly covering neurostimulation treatments, raising the possibility of these treatments becoming more commonplace. At the time of this writing:

■ TMS, ECT, and VNS are the only FDA-approved neuromodulation treatments in the United States for treatment-resistant depression. Of these, ECT has the greatest therapeutic efficacy (but TMS efficacy is comparable). ECT should be especially considered when a rapid clinical response is needed, for example, in the case of catatonia or imminent

risk of suicide; as well as in MDD with psychotic features and in bipolar depression.

■ tDCS and DBS have both shown some possible effects in open-label and controlled trials, making both viable considerations for future research as potential TRD treatments. These two modalities are not yet FDA approved.

■ Researchers are currently exploring the importance of brain state during NIBS, and future multi-modal synergistic approaches may enhance efficacy—especially with subthreshold neuromodulation techniques such as tDCS.[10,11,23]

■ Finally, it is likely that all neuromodulation techniques will greatly benefit from a richer understanding of the neurobiology of depression, particularly with respect to which circuits are affected in different depression biotypes.[84] This would permit clinicians to target regions with greater anatomic specificity; and as many neuropsychiatric conditions are heterogeneous entities, to tailor stimulation to circuits most affected in a given patient.

Multiple Choice Questions

1. To what do the terms "anodal" and "cathodal" in tDCS refer?
   a. The two electrodes that form an electric field
   b. The direction of current, where anodal means excitatory tDCS and cathodal means inhibitory tDCS
   c. Anodal refers to the electrode through which electrons enter the brain, and cathodal refers to the electrode through which electrons exit the brain.
   d. Anodal refers to the "inhibiting" electrode, and cathodal refers to "exciting" electrode.
   e. Anodal refers to the electrode through which current exits the brain, and cathodal refers to the electrode through which current enters the brain.

2. Which of the following statements is *true*?
   a. tDCS directly causes neuronal depolarization, whereas TMS modulates resting membrane potential and thus the chances of depolarization.
   b. Both tDCS and TMS directly cause neuronal depolarization.
   c. Both tDCS and TMS can directly cause neuronal depolarization, but TMS is more likely than tDCS to do this.
   d. TMS directly causes neuronal depolarization, whereas tDCS modulates resting membrane potential and thus the chances of depolarization.
   e. Neither tDCS nor TMS can cause neuronal depolarization, but rather both modulate resting membrane potential and thus the chances of depolarization.

3. In which modality are pulse width, frequency, and location of the stimulation parameters modified while treating patients?
   a. TMS
   b. tDCS
   c. VNS
   d. ECT
   e. DBS

4. Which of the following is *least* likely to alter the effects of TMS stimulation?
   a. Orientation and angle of the TMS coil
   b. Cortical morphometry under the TMS coil
   c. Repetitive TMS delivered to the same area right before the stimulation
   d. A surgically implanted titanium hip replacement
   e. Benzodiazepine withdrawal during TMS

5. Clinical efficacy of TMS in major depressive disorder is most likely to be achieved in which two of the following?
   a. 1 Hz (low frequency) rTMS or cTBS to the right dorsolateral prefrontal cortex
   b. 10 Hz (high frequency) rTMS or cTBS to the left dorsolateral prefrontal cortex
   c. 10 Hz (high frequency) rTMS or cTBS to the right dorsolateral prefrontal cortex
   d. 1 Hz (low frequency) rTMS or iTBS to the left dorsolateral prefrontal cortex
   e. 10 Hz (high frequency) rTMS or iTBS to the right dorsolateral prefrontal cortex

6. Which of the following is *not* a strategy to consider if a depressed patient has not responded to their initial rTMS treatments?
   a. Increase the number of TMS pulses per session.
   b. Use bilateral treatments (e.g., rTMS on one side and TBS on the other side).
   c. Lower the frequency and/or intensity of rTMS if using high-frequency stimulation.
   d. Check to make sure the stimulation target is optimal and consider changing it.
   e. Re-check the patient's motor threshold if it is discovered that they have started taking lorazepam since their last motor threshold was assessed.

7. Which of the following statements is *false*?
   a. The effects of TMS can propagate to regions distal from, but interconnected to, the site of stimulation.
   b. tDCS and TMS have comparable rates of seizure induction.
   c. VNS has received FDA approval in the United States for the treatment of major depressive disorder.
   d. DBS has indications in neurological disorders.
   e. ECT is preferred over TMS in catatonia.

8. Which of the following statements is *true* regarding cognitive side effects associated with ECT?
   a. ECT is almost never associated with cognitive side effects.
   b. Memories for events during or surrounding the period of ECT are often the most preserved.
   c. Bilateral ECT treatment is slightly less effective than right unilateral ECT, but is less likely to induce memory loss.
   d. Brief and ultrabrief pulse width is associated with less cognitive side effects.
   e. Visuospatial impairment is the cognitive side effect most observed with ECT.

9. Which of the following is *true* about the use of DBS in major depression?
   a. DBS was among the first neurostimulation treatments approved by the US FDA for major depressive disorder.
   b. DBS studies have not suggested that it could be useful in major depressive disorder.
   c. Potential DBS targets for treating major depressive disorder include the subgenual cingulate cortex, the lateral habenula, and the subthalamic nucleus.
   d. B and C
   e. None of the above

10. Which of the following would significantly improve the use of neurostimulation as a treatment for major depressive disorder in the future?
   a. Coverage of TMS treatments by insurance companies
   b. Better knowledge of the neurocircuitry of depression, including how this circuitry differs among different depression biotypes
   c. Improvement of the safety profile of tDCS, so that it approaches that of antidepressants
   d. More standardized and less individualized locations for DBS electrode placement
   e. All of the above

Multiple Choice Answers

1. **Answer: a**
   There is no direct electron flow from the electrodes into the skin (or the brain), as biological tissues are not metallic conductors. Rather, electrodes establish an electric field, resulting in a directional current flow through intervening brain tissue. The electrode from which current flows into underlying tissue is termed the anodal electrode (or sometimes simply the anode). The electrode beneath which current exits tissue is the cathodal electrode (or sometimes simply the cathode).

2. **Answer: d**
   TMS directly causes neuronal depolarization, whereas tDCS modulates resting membrane potential and thus the chances of depolarization. Unlike TMS, tDCS does not cause neurons to reach their action potential.

3. **Answer: e**
   Pulse width is not a modifiable parameter in TMS or tDCS, but is with the other modalities. Frequency is modifiable in TMS, DBS, and VNS, but not in ECT or tDCS. Stimulation location is a modifiable factor in all modalities except VNS, where electrodes are placed on the left vagus nerve.

4. **Answer: d**
   All of the listed factors would significantly alter the effects of TMS by changing the electric field or altering cortical excitability (brain state) during stimulation. The exception is (d): a titanium hip replacement. Implanted hardware is generally a safety consideration for TMS, and not a determinant about its efficacy. Further, the hip is likely to be too far from the coil to be affected by the electric field, and titanium is not ferromagnetic.

5. **Answer: a**
   The clinical efficacy of rTMS in depression is most likely with "inhibitory" stimulation (1 Hz rTMS or cTBS) to the right dorsolateral prefrontal cortex, and "excitatory" stimulation (10 Hz rTMS or iTBS) to the left dorsolateral prefrontal cortex.

6. **Answer: c**
   All of the strategies listed are appropriate to consider if a depressed patient is not responding to rTMS except (c).

Lowering the frequency or intensity of high-frequency rTMS may make stimulation more tolerable but would not be expected to make it more effective.

7. **Answer: b**
TMS effects are thought to be instantiated not only through stimulation of the targeted region, but through propagation to regions connected to the stimulation site. VNS is an FDA-approved treatment for major depressive disorder. ECT is preferred over TMS in patients with bipolar depression, imminent threat of suicide and catatonia, or generally when a more rapid response is needed.

8. **Answer: d**
ECT cognitive side effects are most likely to be characterized by anterograde and retrograde memory loss, and memory loss for events surrounding therapy is most common. Bilateral ECT is often used if right unilateral has not been effective, but bilateral ECT is not necessarily less effective and is more likely than right unilateral or brief/ultrabrief pulse ECT to cause cognitive side effects.

9. **Answer: e**
As of 2018, DBS has not been FDA approved for use in major depression. DBS studies have suggested clinical utility, but thus far most of these have been open-label, and not controlled trials; thus far, two controlled trials were negative and one controlled trial was positive. Potential DBS targets that have been investigated in MDD include the subcallosal cortex and white matter tracts near the subgenual cingulate, the lateral habenula, the ventral anterior limb of the internal capsule, the nucleus accumbens, and the superolateral branch of the medial forebrain bundle. The subthalamic nucleus is typically a DBS target for Parkinson's disease.

10. **Answer: b**
Better knowledge of the neurocircuitry of depression, including how this circuitry differs among different depression biotypes is very likely to improve the clinical efficacy of neurostimulation techniques. TMS treatment for depression is already covered by many insurance companies. tDCS is arguably the safest of the neurostimulation modalities covered in this chapter. Finally, some have theorized that more individualized, and not more standardized, placement of DBS electrodes based on individual variations in cortical and white matter topography may improve the likelihood of a clinical response in TRD.

References

1. Hallett M. Plasticity of the human motor cortex and recovery from stroke. *Brain Res Rev.* 2001;36(2-3):169-174.
2. Nummenmaa A, Stenroos M, Ilmoniemi RJ, et al. Comparison of spherical and realistically shaped boundary element head models for transcranial magnetic stimulation navigation. *Clin Neurophysiol.* 2013;124(10):1995-2007.
3. Valero-Cabré A, Payne BR, Pacual-Leone A. Opposite impact on 14 C-2-deoxyglucose brain metabolism following patterns of high and low frequency repetitive transcranial magnetic stimulation in the posterior parietal cortex. *Exp Brain Res.* 2007;176(4):603-615.
4. Huang YZ, Edwards MJ, Rounis E, et al. Theta burst stimulation of the human motor cortex. *Neuron.* 2005;45(2):201-206.
5. Huang YZ, Chen RS, Rothwell JC, et al. The after-effect of human theta burst stimulation is NMDA receptor dependent. *Clin Neurophysiol.* 2007;118(5):1028-1032.
6. Huang YZ, Rothwell JC, Chen RS, et al. The theoretical model of theta burst form of repetitive transcranial magnetic stimulation. *Clin Neurophysiol.* 2011;122(5):1011-1018.
7. Siebner HR, Filipovic SR, Rowe JB, et al. Patients with focal arm dystonia have increased sensitivity to slow-frequency repetitive TMS of the dorsal premotor cortex. *Brain.* 2003;126(Pt 12):2710-2725.
8. Speer AM, Kimbrell TA, Wassermann EM, et al. Opposite effects of high and low frequency rTMS on regional brain activity in depressed patients. *Biol Psychiatry.* 2000;48(12):1133-1141.
9. Rossi S, Hallett M, Rossini PM, et al. Safety, ethical considerations, and application guidelines for the use of transcranial magnetic stimulation in clinical practice and research. *Clin Neurophysiol.* 2009;120(12):2008-2039.
10. Nitsche MA, Cohen LG, Wassermann EM, et al. Transcranial direct current stimulation: state of the art. *Brain Stimul.* 2008;1(3):206-223.
11. Philip NS, Nelson B, Frohlich F, et al. Low-intensity transcranial current stimulation in psychiatry. *Am J Psychiatry.* 2017;174(7):628-639.
12. Woods AJ, Antal A, Bikson M, et al. A technical guide to tDCS, and related non-invasive brain stimulation tools. *Clin Neurophysiol.* 2016;127(2):1031-1048.
13. O'Connell NE, Cossar J, Marston L, et al. Rethinking clinical trials of transcranial direct current stimulation: participant and assessor blinding is inadequate at intensities of 2 mA. *PLoS One.* 2012;7(10):e47514.
14. Rahman A, Reato D, Arlotti M, et al. Cellular effects of acute direct current stimulation: somatic and synaptic terminal effects. *J Physiol.* 2013;591(10):2563-2578.
15. Foerster A, Yavari F, Farnad L. Effects of electrode angle-orientation on the impact of transcranial direct current stimulation on motor cortex excitability. *Brain Stimul.* 2019;12(2):263-266.
16. Rawji V, Ciocca M, Zacharia A, et al. tDCS changes in motor excitability are specific to orientation of current flow. *Brain Stimul.* 2018;11(2):289-298.
17. Bikson M, Grossman P, Thomas C, et al. Safety of transcranial direct current stimulation: evidence based update. *Brain Stimul.* 2016;9(5):641-661.
18. Garnett EO, Malyutina S, Datta A, et al. On the use of the terms anodal and cathodal in high-definition transcranial direct current stimulation: a technical note. *Neuromodulation.* 2015;18(8):705-713.
19. Bikson M, Datta A, Rahman A, Scaturro J. Electrode montages for tDCS and weak transcranial electrical stimulation:

role of "return" electrode's position and size. *Clin Neurophysiol.* 2010;121(12):1976-1978.

20. Batsikadze G, Moliadze V, Paulus W, et al. Partially non-linear stimulation intensity-dependent effects of direct current stimulation on motor cortex excitability in humans. *J Physiol.* 2013;591(7):1987-2000.

21. Tremblay S, Lepage JF, Latulipe-Loiselle A, et al. The uncertain outcome of prefrontal tDCS. *Brain Stimul.* 2014;7(6):773-783.

22. Brunoni AR, Nitsche MA, Bolognini N, et al. Clinical research with transcranial direct current stimulation (tDCS): challenges and future directions. *Brain Stimul.* 2012;5(3):175-195.

23. Bikson M, Brunoni AR, Charvet LE, et al. Rigor and reproducibility in research with transcranial electrical stimulation: an NIMH-sponsored workshop. *Brain Stimul.* 2018;11(3):465-480.

24. Edwards D, Cortes M, Datta A, et al. Physiological and modeling evidence for focal transcranial electrical brain stimulation in humans: a basis for high-definition tDCS. *NeuroImage.* 2013;74:266-275.

25. Villamar MF, Wivatvongvana P, Patumanond J, et al. Focal modulation of the primary motor cortex in fibromyalgia using 4×1-ring high-definition transcranial direct current stimulation (HD-tDCS): immediate and delayed analgesic effects of cathodal and anodal stimulation. *J Pain.* 2013;14(4):371-383.

26. Faria P, Hallett M, Miranda PC. A finite element analysis of the effect of electrode area and inter-electrode distance on the spatial distribution of the current density in tDCS. *J Neural Eng.* 2011;8(6):066017.

27. Kuo HI, Bikson M, Datta A, et al. Comparing cortical plasticity induced by conventional and high-definition 4 × 1 ring tDCS: a neurophysiological study. *Brain Stimul.* 2013;6(4):644-648.

28. Datta A. Inter-individual variation during transcranial direct current stimulation and normalization of dose using MRI-derived computational models. *Front Psychiatry.* 2012;3:91.

29. Opitz A, Paulus W, Will S, et al. Determinants of the electric field during transcranial direct current stimulation. *NeuroImage.* 2015;109:140-150.

30. Weber MJ, Messing SB, Rao H, et al. Prefrontal transcranial direct current stimulation alters activation and connectivity in cortical and subcortical reward systems: a tDCS-fMRI study. *Human Brain Mapp.* 2014;35(8):3673-3686.

31. Polanía R, Paulus W, Nitsche MA. Modulating cortico-striatal and thalamo-cortical functional connectivity with transcranial direct current stimulation. *Human Brain Mapp.* 2012;33(10):2499-2508.

32. Chhatbar PY, Kautz SA, Takacs I, et al. Evidence of transcranial direct current stimulation-generated electric fields at subthalamic level in human brain in vivo. *Brain Stimul.* 2018;11(4):727-733.

33. Esmaeilpour Z, Marangolo P, Hampstead BM, et al. Incomplete evidence that increasing current intensity of tDCS boosts outcomes. *Brain Stimul.* 2018;11(2):310-321.

34. Nitsche MA, Paulus W. Excitability changes induced in the human motor cortex by weak transcranial direct current stimulation. *J Physiol.* 2000;527(3):633-639.

35. Nitsche MA, Paulus W. Sustained excitability elevations induced by transcranial DC motor cortex stimulation in humans. *Neurology.* 2001;57(10):1899-1901.

36. Monte-Silva K, Kuo MF, Hessenthaler S, et al. Induction of late LTP-like plasticity in the human motor cortex by repeated non-invasive brain stimulation. *Brain Stimul.* 2013;6(3):424-432.

37. Sampaio-Junior B, Tortella G, Borrione L, et al. Efficacy and safety of transcranial direct current stimulation as an add-on treatment for bipolar depression: a randomized clinical trial. *JAMA Psychiatry.* 2018;75(2):158-166.

38. Bikson M, Rahman A. Origins of specificity during tDCS: anatomical, activity-selective, and input-bias mechanisms. *Front Hum Neurosci.* 2013;7:688.

39. Reato D, Rahman A, Bikson M, et al. Low-intensity electrical stimulation affects network dynamics by modulating population rate and spike timing. *J Neurosci.* 2010;30(45):15067-15079.

40. Kronberg G, Bridi M, Abel T, et al. Direct current stimulation modulates LTP and LTD: activity dependence and dendritic effects. *Brain Stimul.* 2017;10(1):51-58.

41. Coffman BA, Clark VP, Parasuraman R. Battery powered thought: enhancement of attention, learning, and memory in healthy adults using transcranial direct current stimulation. *NeuroImage.* 2014;85(3):895-908.

42. Sathappan AV, Luber BM, Lisanby SH. The dynamic duo: combining noninvasive brain stimulation with cognitive interventions. *Prog Neuropsychopharmacol Biol Psychiatry.* 2019;89:347-360.

43. Ekici B. Transcranial direct current stimulation-induced seizure: analysis of a case. *Clin EEG Neurosci.* 2015;46(2):169.

44. Bikson M, Grossman P, Thomas C, et al. Safety of transcranial direct current stimulation: evidence based update 2016. *Brain Stimul.* 2016;9:641-661.

45. Poreisz C, Boros K, Antal A, et al. Safety aspects of transcranial direct current stimulation concerning healthy subjects and patients. *Brain Res Bull.* 2007;72:208-214.

46. Arul-Anandam AP, Loo C, Mitchell P. Induction of hypomanic episode with transcranial direct current stimulation. *J ECT.* 2010;26(1):68-69.

47. Gálvez V, Alonzo A, Martin D, et al. Hypomania induction in a patient with bipolar II disorder by transcranial direct current stimulation (tDCS). *J ECT.* 2011;27(3):256-258.

48. Baccaro A, Brunoni AR, Bensenor IM, Fregni F. Hypomanic episode in unipolar depression during transcranial direct current stimulation. *Acta Neuropsychiatr.* 2010;22(6):316-318.

49. Lisanby SH. Electroconvulsive therapy for depression. *N Engl J Med.* 2007;357(19):1939-1945.

50. Milev RV, Giacobbe P, Kennedy SH, et al. Canadian Network for Mood and Anxiety Treatments (CANMAT) 2016 clinical guidelines for the management of adults with major depressive disorder: Section 4. Neurostimulation treatments. *Can J Psychiatry.* 2016;61(9):561-575.

51. Carreno FR, Frazer A. Vagal nerve stimulation for treatment-resistant depression. *Neurotherapeutics.* 2017;14(3):716-727.

52. Holtzheimer P, Mayberg HS. Deep brain stimulation in psychiatric disorders. *Annu Rev Neurosci.* 2011;34:289-307.

53. Dougherty D. Deep brain stimulation: clinical applications. *Psychiatr Clin N Am.* 2018;41(3):385-394.

54. Ardouin C, Pillon B, Peiffer E, et al. Bilateral subthalamic or pallidal stimulation for Parkinson's disease affects neither memory nor executive functions: a consecutive series of 62 patients. *Ann Neurol.* 1999;46:217-223.

55. Pillon B, Ardouin C, Damier P, et al. Neuropsychological changes between "off" and "on" STN or GPi stimulation in Parkinson's disease. *Neurology.* 2000;55:411-418.

56. Witt K, Daniels C, Reiff J, et al. Neuropsychological and psychiatric changes after deep brain stimulation for Parkinson's disease: a randomised, multicentre study. *Lancet Neurol.* 2008;7(7):605-614.

57. Saint-Cyr JA, Trepanier LL, Kumar R, et al. Neuropsychological consequences of chronic bilateral stimulation of the subthalamic nucleus in Parkinson's disease. *Brain.* 2000;123:2091-2108.

58. Leinenga G, Langton C, Nisbet R, et al. Ultrasound treatment of neurological diseases—current and emerging applications. *Nat Rev Neurol.* 2016;12(3):161-174.

59. Elias WJ, Huss D, Voss T, et al. A pilot study of focused ultrasound thalamotomy for essential tremor. *N Engl J Med.* 2013;369(7):640-648.

60. Fomenko A, Neudorfer C, Dallapiazza RF, et al. Low-intensity ultrasound neuromodulation: an overview of mechanisms and emerging human applications. *Brain Stimul.* 2018;11(6):1209-1217.

61. Poon C, McMahon D, Hynynen K, et al. Non-invasive targeted delivery of therapeutics to the brain using focused ultrasound. *Neuropsychopharmacology.* 2017;120:20-37.

62. Bowary P, Greenberg BD. Noninvasive focused ultrasound for neuromodulation: a review. *Psychiatr Clin N Am.* 2018;41(3):505-514.

63. Brinker ST, Preiswerk F, McDannold NJ, et al. Virtual brain projection for evaluating trans-skull beam behavior of transcranial ultrasound devices. *Ultrasound Med Biol.* 2019;45(7):1850-1856.

64. Zhang J, Laiwalla F, Kim JA, et al. Integrated device for optical stimulation and spatiotemporal electrical recording of neural activity in light-sensitized brain tissue. *J Neural Eng.* 2009;6(5):055007.

65. Rost BR, Schneider-Warme F, Schmitz D, et al. Optogenetic tools for subcellular applications in neuroscience. *Neuron.* 2017;96(3):572-603.

66. O'Reardon JP, Solvason HB, Janicak PG, et al. Efficacy and safety of transcranial magnetic stimulation in the acute treatment of major depression: a multisite randomized controlled trial. *Biol Psychiatry.* 2007;62(11):1208-1216.

67. Levkovitz Y, Isserles M, Padberg F, et al. Efficacy and safety of deep transcranial magnetic stimulation for major depression: a prospective multicenter randomized controlled trial. *World Psychiatry.* 2015;14(1):64-73.

68. Perera T, George MS, Grammer G, et al. The clinical TMS safety consensus review and treatment recommendations for TMS therapy in major depressive disorder. *Brain Stimul.* 2016;9(3):336-346.

69. Blumberger DM, Vila-Rodriguez F, Thorpe KE, et al. Effectiveness of theta burst versus high-frequency repetitive transcranial magnetic stimulation in patients with depression (THREE-D): a randomised non-inferiority trial. *Lancet.* 2018;391(10131):1683-1692.

70. Oberman L, Edwards D, Eldaief M, et al. Safety of theta burst transcranial magnetic stimulation: a systematic review of the literature. *J Clin Neurophysiol.* 2011;28(1):67-74.

71. Fox MD, Buckner RL, White MP, et al. Efficacy of transcranial magnetic stimulation targets for depression is related to intrinsic functional connectivity with the subgenual cingulate. *Biol Psychiatry.* 2012;72(7):595-603.

72. Weigand A, Horn A, Caballero R, et al. Prospective validation that subgenual connectivity predicts antidepressant efficacy of transcranial magnetic stimulation sites. *Biol Psychiatry.* 2018;84(1):28-37.

73. Carmi L, al Yagon U, Dar R, et al. Deep transcranial magnetic stimulation (TMS) in obsessive compulsive disorder (OCD) patients. *Eur Psychiatry.* 2015;30(Suppl 1):794.

74. Lusicic A, Schruers KR, Pallanti S, et al. Transcranial magnetic stimulation in the treatment of obsessive-compulsive disorder: current perspectives. *Neuropsychiatr Dis Treat.* 2018;14:1721-1736.

75. Palm U, Reisinger E, Keeser D, et al. Evaluation of sham transcranial direct current stimulation for randomized, placebo-controlled clinical trials. *Brain Stimul.* 2013;6(4):690-695.

76. Loo CK, Husain MM, McDonald WM, et al. International randomized-controlled trial of transcranial direct current stimulation in depression. *Brain Stimul.* 2018;11(1):125-133.

77. Loo CK, Alonzo A, Martin D, et al. Transcranial direct current stimulation for depression: 3-week, randomised, sham-controlled trial. *Br J Psychiatry.* 2012;200(1):52-59.

78. Kalu UG, Sexton CE, Loo CK. Transcranial direct current stimulation in the treatment of major depression: a meta-analysis. *Psychol Med.* 2012;42(9):1791-1800.

79. Meron D, Hedger N, Garner M, et al. Transcranial direct current stimulation (tDCS) in the treatment of depression: systematic review and meta-analysis of efficacy and tolerability. *Neurosci Biobehav Rev.* 2015;57:46-62.

80. Senço NM, Huang Y, D'Urso G, et al. Transcranial direct current stimulation in obsessive–compulsive disorder: emerging clinical evidence and considerations for optimal montage of electrodes. *Expert Rev Med Devices.* 2015;12(4):381-391.

81. Shiozawa P, Leiva APG, Castro CDC, et al. Transcranial direct current stimulation for generalized anxiety disorder: a case study. *Biol Psychiatry.* 2014;75(11):e17-e18.

82. Heeren A, Billieux J, Philippot P, et al. Impact of transcranial direct current stimulation on attentional bias for threat: a proof-of-concept study among individuals with social anxiety disorder. *Soc Cogn Affect Neurosci.* 2017;12(2):251-260.

83. Hampstead BM, Briceño EM, Mascaro N. Current status of transcranial direct current stimulation in posttraumatic stress and other anxiety disorders. *Curr Behav Neurosci Rep.* 2016;3(2):95-101.

84. van't Wout-Frank M, Shea MT, Larson VC. Combined transcranial direct current stimulation with virtual reality exposure for posttraumatic stress disorder: feasibility and pilot results. *Brain Stimul.* 2019;12(1):41-43.

85. van't Wout M, Longo SM, Reddy MK, et al. Transcranial direct current stimulation may modulate extinction memory in posttraumatic stress disorder. *Brain Behav.* 2017;7(5):e00681.

86. Asthana M, Nueckel K, Mühlberger A, et al. Effects of transcranial direct current stimulation on consolidation of fear memory. *Front Psychiatry.* 2013;4:107.

87. van't Wout M, Mariano TY, Garnaat SL, et al. Can transcranial direct current stimulation augment extinction of conditioned fear? *Brain Stimul.* 2016;9(4):529-536.

88. Mungee A, Kazzer P, Feeser M, et al. Transcranial direct current stimulation of the prefrontal cortex: a means to modulate fear memories. *NeuroReport.* 2014;25(7):480-484.

89. Abend R, Jalon I, Gurevitch G, et al. Modulation of fear extinction processes using transcranial electrical stimulation. *Transl Psychiatry.* 2016;6(10):e913.

90. Dittert N, Hüttner S, Polak T, et al. Augmentation of fear extinction by transcranial direct current stimulation (tDCS). *Front Behav Neurosci.* 2018;12:76.

91. van't Wout-Frank M, Shea MT, et al. Combined transcranial direct current stimulation with virtual reality exposure for posttraumatic stress disorder: feasibility and pilot results. *Brain Stimul.* 2019;12(1):41-43.

92. International Association for the Study of Pain (IASP). IASP terminology (updated December 14, 2017). Available at https://www.iasp-pain.org/Education/Content.aspx?ItemNumber=1698#Pain. Accessed February 16, 2020.

93. Valle A, Roizenblatt S, Botte S, et al. Efficacy of anodal transcranial direct current stimulation (tDCS) for the treatment of fibromyalgia: results of a randomized, sham-controlled longitudinal clinical trial. *J Pain Manag.* 2009;2(3):353-361.

94. Khedr EM, Omran EAH, Ismail NM, et al. Effects of transcranial direct current stimulation on pain, mood and serum endorphin level in the treatment of fibromyalgia: a double blinded, randomized clinical trial. *Brain Stimul.* 2017;10(5):893-901.

95. Fregni F, Boggio PS, Lima MC, et al. A sham-controlled, phase II trial of transcranial direct current stimulation for the treatment of central pain in traumatic spinal cord injury. *Pain.* 2006;122(1-2):197-209.

96. Antal A, Terney D, Kühnl S, et al. Anodal transcranial direct current stimulation of the motor cortex ameliorates chronic pain and reduces short intracortical inhibition. *J Pain Symptom Manag.* 2010;39(5):890-903.

97. Ahn H, Woods AJ, Kunik ME, et al. Efficacy of transcranial direct current stimulation over primary motor cortex (anode) and contralateral supraorbital area (cathode) on clinical pain severity and mobility performance in persons with knee osteoarthritis: an experimenter- and participant-blinded, randomized, sham-controlled pilot clinical study. *Brain Stimul.* 2017;10(5):902-909.

98. O'Connell NE, Marston L, Spencer S, et al. Non-invasive brain stimulation techniques for chronic pain. *Cochrane Database Syst Rev.* 2018;3:CD008208.

99. Crombez G, Eccleston C, Van Damme S, et al. Fear-avoidance model of chronic pain: the next generation. *Clin J Pain.* 2012;28(6):475-483.

100. Tang NK, Crane C. Suicidality in chronic pain: a review of the prevalence, risk factors and psychological links. *Psychol Med.* 2006;36(5):575-586.

101. Mariano TY, van't Wout M, Jacobson BL, et al. Effects of transcranial direct current stimulation (tDCS) on pain distress tolerance: a preliminary study. *Pain Med.* 2015;16(8):1580-1588.

102. Elsner B, Kugler J, Pohl M, et al. Transcranial direct current stimulation (tDCS) for idiopathic Parkinson's disease. *Cochrane Database Syst Rev.* 2016;7:CD010916.

103. Mariano TY, Burgess FW, Bowker M, et al. Transcranial direct current stimulation for affective symptoms and functioning in chronic low back pain: a pilot double-blinded, randomized, placebo-controlled trial. *Pain Med.* 2019;20(6):1166-1177. doi: 10.1093/pm/pny188.

104. Kellner CH, Knapp R, Husain MM, et al. Bifrontal, bitemporal and right unilateral electrode placement in ECT: randomised trial. *Br J Psychiatry.* 2010;196(3):226-234.

105. Husain MM, Rush AJ, Fink M, et al. Speed of response and remission in major depressive disorder with acute electroconvulsive therapy (ECT): a Consortium for Research in ECT (CORE) report. *J Clin Psychiatry.* 2004;65(4):485-491.

106. Perugi G, Medda P, Toni C, et al. The role of electroconvulsive therapy (ECT) in bipolar disorder: effectiveness in 522 patients with bipolar depression, mixed-state, mania and catatonic features. *Curr Neuropharmacol.* 2017;15(3):359-371.

107. Prudic J, Haskett RF, McCall WV, et al. Pharmacological strategies in the prevention of relapse after electroconvulsive therapy. *J ECT.* 2013;29(1):3-12.

108. Holtzheimer P, Husain M, Lisanby S, et al. Subcallosal cingulate deep brain stimulation for treatment-resistant depression: a multisite, randomized, sham-controlled trial. *Lancet Psychiatry.* 2017;4(11):839-849.

109. Dougherty D, Rezai A, Carpenter L, et al. A randomized sham-controlled trial of deep brain stimulation of the ventral capsule/ventral striatum for chronic treatment-resistant depression. *Biol Psychiatry.* 2015;78(4):240-248.

110. Bergfeld I, Mantione M, Hoogendoorn M, et al. Deep brain stimulation of the ventral anterior limb of the internal capsule for treatment-resistant depression: a randomized clinical trial. *JAMA Psychiatry.* 2016;73(5):456.

111. Schlaepfer T, Bewernick B, Kayser S, et al. Deep brain stimulation of the human reward system for major depression—rationale, outcomes and outlook. *Neuropsychopharmacology.* 2014;39(6):1303-1314.

112. Drysdale AT, Grosenick L, Downar J, et al. Resting-state connectivity biomarkers define neurophysiological subtypes of depression. *Nat Med.* 2017;23(1):28-38.

113. Goodman WK, Foote KD, Greenberg BD, et al. Deep brain stimulation for intractable obsessive compulsive disorder: pilot study using a blinded, staggered-onset design. *Biol Psychiatry.* 2010;67(6):535-542.

114. Greenberg BD, Gabriels LA, Malone DA, et al. Deep brain stimulation of the ventral internal capsule/ventral striatum for obsessive-compulsive disorder: worldwide experience. *Mol Psychiatry.* 2010;15(1):64.

115. Mallet L, Polosan M, Jaafari N, et al. Subthalamic nucleus stimulation in severe obsessive-compulsive disorder. *N Engl J Med.* 2008;359(20):2121-2134.

Psychosocial Interventions in Neuropsychiatry

Kim Willment · Abby Altman · Laura Morrissey · Meghan Searl · Lorna Campbell · Laura T. Safar

INTRODUCTION

In this chapter, we discuss general aspects of the psychosocial dimension in the assessment and care of neuropsychiatric patients, and specific interventions including case management, various psychotherapies—with emphasis on cognitive-behavioral therapy (CBT) and mindfulness training, and cognitive rehabilitation.

Why are psychosocial interventions important in neuropsychiatry? Across disorders such as dementia, epilepsy, multiple sclerosis, Parkinson's disease, and stroke, neuropsychiatric patients experience significant impact of illness on multiple domains of life[1] including:

- Emotional functioning
- Carrying out a daily routine
- Working and interpersonal relationships
- Reduced participation in the community
- Needing support from others, and limitations on independent living

Within the context of interdisciplinary care, psychosocial interventions can assist neuropsychiatric patients with all these difficulties. Research on psychosocial experiences and interventions in neuropsychiatry tends to focus on distinct neurological illnesses. There is the risk of losing specificity of experiences when generalizing across different illnesses, but there may also be some value in recognizing common experiences and needs.

THE IMPORTANCE OF CAREGIVERS

A unique aspect of psychosocial interventions in neuropsychiatry is the involvement of caregivers—they play a role in the different psychosocial interventions discussed in this chapter. Caregivers can be family members or friends, or professionals without a personal relationship with the designated patient. Caregivers facilitate and amplify the effect of psychosocial interventions. In addition, it is known that caregivers of patients with neuropsychiatric and behavioral symptoms may experience even a greater burden than caregivers of patients with motor symptoms and direct needs for physical care. Neuropsychiatric and behavioral symptoms are associated with increased burden for caregivers in all neurological illnesses. Some examples are: ALS[2]; multiple sclerosis[3]; Parkinson's disease[4,5]; post-stroke[5]; dementia.[6] In dementia, neuropsychiatric and behavioral symptoms are associated with earlier placement in skilled nursing facilities.[7,8] Some of the most challenging symptoms for caregivers include agitation, aggression, accusatory delusions, and disrupted sleep-wake cycle. It is especially hard when these symptoms are combined with constant need for supervision, as caregivers just don't get a break. All of this is magnified by the poignant fact that patients often do not seem like the persons they once were. Caregivers themselves are at significant risk for psychiatric morbidity, especially depression. The majority of people with dementia live with family caregivers who themselves are at risk for morbidity and mortality. Later in this chapter we discuss interventions that target caregiver coping style; this is a modifiable factor that mediates caregiver's experience of burden.[6]

CASE MANAGEMENT IN NEUROPSYCHIATRY

Case management in neuropsychiatry can be essential in caring for the overall health of a patient and the patient's caregivers. The National Association of Social Workers defines case management as "a process to plan, seek, advocate for and monitor services from different social services or healthcare organizations and staff on behalf of a client." Case management is ubiquitous in health care today; the term is often used to refer to brokerage of services with limited face-to-face contact with patients. The term "case management" is often used interchangeably with "care management." The case manager most typically operates in the context of a larger system. In hospitals and other health systems, the implementation of collaborative care models that include case management strategies can reduce behavioral symptoms associated with neuropsychiatric conditions, lessen caregiver burden, and reduce health care costs and

> **BOX 10-1** Principles of Clinical Case Management (Kanter[12])
>
> 1. Continuity of care
> 2. Use of the case management relationship
> 3. Titrating support and structure in response to client need
> 4. Flexibility of intervention strategies
> 5. Facilitating client resourcefulness or strengths

> **BOX 10-2** Clinical Case Management Components (Kanter[12])
>
> **Initial phase**
> 1. Engagement
> 2. Assessment
> 3. Planning
>
> **Environmental focus**
> 4. Linking with community resources
> 5. Consulting with families and caregivers
> 6. Maintaining and expanding social networks
> 7. Collaborating with physicians, social agencies, mental health, and health care facilities
> 8. Advocacy
>
> **Client focus**
> 9. Intermittent individual psychotherapy
> 10. Teaching independent living skills
> 11. Psychoeducation about psychiatric and medical disorders
>
> **Client-environmental focus**
> 12. Crisis intervention
> 13. Monitoring

utilization.[9,10] Please see Chapter 36 for further discussion about collaborative models of health care delivery.

As distinct from case management generally, **clinical** case management is a modality of practice for social workers and other mental health professionals. Clinical case management is a holistic and broad ranging approach that takes into account the interactions between patients and the systems around them including family, institutions of medical care, and the community.

Kanter[11] (see Box 10-1) defined clinical case management as "a modality of social work practice that, acknowledging the importance of biological and psychological factors, addresses the overall function and maintenance of the person's physical and social environment toward the goals of facilitating physical survival, health and mental health, personal growth, and community functioning."

Since the start of case management during deinstitutionalization in the 1970s, disagreements about combining or separating out the role of primary psychotherapist and the role of clinical case manager have persisted. In practice, resources often don't support two separate clinicians.

One key difference is that clinical case management allows for more flexible contact with patients, the systems they interact with, and their caregivers, whereas psychotherapy is more highly structured. While both psychotherapy and case management highlight the importance of the therapeutic alliance between clinician and patient, clinical case management allows the clinician to utilize a variety of approaches to meet the needs of the patient within his or her environment, from facilitating communication with medical and community providers to providing emotional support around adjustment to illness.

Box 10-2 shows the components of clinical case management. In the complex reality of the interface of patients and their environment, several of these components overlap and a clinician may be intervening at several levels simultaneously. The analogy of fitting a square peg into a round hole applies as, more often than not, work is needed for the environment and the patient to better accommodate one another.

The reasons for referral to clinical case management in neuropsychiatry are varied and ideally would support patients and their caregivers across the progression of the illness (see Box 10-3). The period around the time of a neurological diagnosis is a vulnerable one for patients and families when they may require support, as well as specific guidance around managing symptoms and adjusting to the new needs. Many neurodegenerative conditions impair cognition, insight, and judgment.

It's important for patients to complete a health care proxy and power of attorney when they still have decision-making capacity. Completing advanced planning early on can save families from having to pursue guardianship or conservatorship in the future.

Fundamental to meeting the ongoing needs of a patient is the assessment of the patient's available physical, financial, and social supports which may change over time as the disease progresses. Case managers work to link patients to available services in the community as well as helping family decision-making around transitions of care. Caregivers benefit from encouragement to use resources like respite and homecare, prioritizing their self-care, and development of adaptive coping skills. When patients have problems with non-adherence to medications, appointments, and recommendations, case managers problem-solve with them and caregivers, engage other informal supports, and refer as necessary for services like transportation or a visiting nurse.

Working to support the patient's caregiver is a pillar of clinical case management with neuropsychiatric populations. The majority of persons with dementia receive care at home from informal caregivers. According to the Alzheimer's Association, in 2017, "caregivers of people with Alzheimer's or other dementias provided an estimated 18.4 billion hours of informal (i.e., unpaid) assistance, a contribution to the nation valued at $232.1 billion." Families pay 70% of the total lifetime costs of caring for a patient with dementia.[13]

In addition to cognitive and functional decline, many patients with neurodegenerative diseases present with preexisting psychiatric conditions or an increase in behavioral or psychological disturbances. For example, the noncognitive neuropsychiatric

---

BOX 10-3 Reasons for Referral to Clinical Case Management and Possible Interventions

New diagnosis of neurological illness

- Advance directives: Health Care Proxy, Durable Power of Attorney
- Education about the condition, guided by patient and family preferences for information[19]
- Engagement of patient and family in care and treatment planning

Life-stage or care transition (patient or caregiver)

- Assessment of new needs and care planning
- Ability of environment/support network to meet patient's needs
- Patient's ability to meet role responsibilities (work; parenting)

Safety risks

- Falls
- Suicidal or homicidal risk
- Self-harming behaviors
- Neglect/abuse of elderly or disabled
- Interventions include: Safety assessment and plan, crisis intervention, mandated reporting

Caregiver burden

- Interventions: Case management (use of resources) and psychotherapy (coping skills) to offset burden

Treatment adherence problems (medication, appointments, recommendations)

- Interventions: Problem solving, engagement of informal supports, referrals to community resources

Need for increased activity, socialization, daily structure

- A clinical understanding of the individual's needs and obstacles results in a referral that is a better fit for the patient's needs

---

symptoms (NPS) of dementia are "associated with poor patient and caregiver outcomes, including excess morbidity and mortality, increased health care utilization, and earlier nursing home placement, as well as caregiver stress, depression and reduced employment."[14] The psychiatric symptoms associated with neurodegenerative diseases are believed to cause more caregiver burden than the cognitive and functional changes.[15,16] Caregiver burnout manifests in multiple ways, including tearfulness, anger, and high level of contact with providers. Clinical case managers act as the lead in helping the care team support caregivers as they adjust to the changing needs of the patient. They can assist in reducing caregiver burden and improve outcomes for patients.[17,18]

Another major function of clinical case managers is to evaluate and attempt to mitigate safety risks for neuropsychiatry patients, including suicidality, homicidality, and self-injurious behaviors. In addition, neuropsychiatric case managers are highly trained to assess for neglect or abuse of elderly and

disabled patients, given the high rates of caregiver burnout in this population and the potential vulnerability of patients due to their cognitive and physical impairments. Case management targeting caregivers can reduce depression and distress in both patient and caregivers—this has been demonstrated in different settings, including with caregivers of recently hospitalized patients with severe mental illness and neurodegenerative disease.[16]

There are various situations in which concerns may arise about caregiving arrangements, such as:

- Impairment of caregivers (e.g., aging parents caring for adults with developmental disorders)
- Patients with neuropsychiatric disorders caring for children
- Absence of identified caregivers

In these instances, clinical case managers assess needs of different family members, explore possible expanded networks of support, and develop a plan accordingly.

To meet patients' need for meaningful activity and socialization, clinical case managers differentially refer to vocational rehabilitation agencies, adult day health programs, club houses, day treatment centers, and independent living centers. A clinical case manager typically has a better understanding of the individual's needs, which results in a more relevant referral. In addition, the clinician can assist in overcoming obstacles such as avoidance, or apathy, to foster the individual's engagement in those settings.

A small sample of studies supporting the effectiveness of case management has been included. See Table 10-1 for examples of case management interventions for people with dementia living in the community with a family caregiver. These interventions are effective in delaying time to placement and reducing behavioral symptoms. Somme et al.,[20] Hickam et al.,[21] and Reilly et al.[10] present systematic reviews of trials utilizing case management for people with dementia. The most effective case management interventions include a high intensity of contact with caregivers and high levels of integration of the case manager into the treating medical team.[20] According to the 2016 World Alzheimer's Report, studies have demonstrated effectiveness when there is "a manageable caseload for delivering interventions with the required intensity; a clear role definition with adequate preparation and training; and empowerment of the case manager to access and coordinate care across providers and sectors."[22]

PSYCHOTHERAPY IN NEUROPSYCHIATRY

Psychotherapy is the primary treatment of adjustment disorder in neurological illness and functional neurological symptoms (e.g., non-epileptic seizures). It is also an adjunctive treatment of emotional and behavioral disturbances that occur both as part of a primary psychiatric illness and in the context of neurological illness. Psychotherapy can assist in the treatment of a variety of neuropsychiatric/behavioral symptoms and syndromes including mood, anxiety, and psychotic presentations, disruption of sleep-wake cycle, impulsivity, and apathy.

Psychotherapy requires some adaptation when working with neuropsychiatric patients (see Table 10-2). For patients with memory loss, this may involve the use of external aids

TABLE 10-1 • Case Management with Patients with Dementia and Their Caregivers.

Study	N	Intervention	Outcome
Mittlelman et al.[23]	406	• Individual and family counseling sessions with caregiver • Encouragement of support group • Ad hoc telephone counseling, information, and referral	• Reduced rate of placement (p=0.025), • Median delayed placement of 1.5 years • Reduction in caregiver burden and depression
Callahan et al.[9]	153	• Bimonthly to monthly sessions over 1 year with caregiver • Standardized protocols to treat behavioral and psychological symptoms of dementia	• Reduction in behavioral and neuropsychiatric symptoms (p=0.01) • Reduced caregiver burden and depression
Samus et al.[24]	303	• Individualized care planning • Referral to services • Education around disease and coping skills • Care monitoring by interdisciplinary team	• Significant delay in placement • Significantly greater reduction in proportion of unmet needs related to Safety and Advanced Care Planning • Improvement of self-reported quality of life
Thryian et al.[17]	407	• In home care management with nurse case manager	• Significantly decreased behavioral and psychological symptoms • Reduced caregiver burden

TABLE 10-2 • Psychotherapy Adaption when Working with Neuropsychiatric Patients.

Area of Deficit	Psychotherapy Adaptation
Memory	Repetition, external memory aids (written instructions, programmed reminders)
Executive dysfunction	Breaking tasks into component parts
Attention	Active focusing by therapist
Mobility impairment	Telephone and Internet technology (e.g., telehealth)
Communication impairment (e.g., hypophonia; dysarthria)	Writing and electronic devices

by writing summaries and instructions at each session and helping patients use calendars or program reminders in their electronic devices. When patients have executive dysfunction, clinicians help them break overwhelming projects into more manageable parts and set realistic schedules for completion.

Patients with attentional problems require active focusing to stay on topic. Adaptations to mobility and communication impairment are often needed, and this is even more challenging when these problems are combined (as can be the case with Parkinson's disease, multiple system atrophy, and post-stroke). When it is difficult to understand the patient and the patient doesn't have the motor skills to write or type, referral to speech and occupational therapy should be considered. An important cognitive deficit to be aware of is anosognosia. It represents impairment in the neurocognitive processes that support insight, typically due to lesion of the relevant neurocircuits. Anosognosia may be irreversible, although in certain neurological conditions (e.g., post-stroke) the individual may experience recovery. It is important to distinguish anosognosia from "denial," a lack of insight due to a psychological process.[25]

Caregivers may be included in the psychotherapy process in a variety of ways, tailored to the patient's need and illness stage. They provide important collateral observations on the patient's behavior and help the patient with psychotherapy homework or implementing strategies in between sessions. Couple and family therapy focuses on the dynamic between patients and caregivers, addressing caregiver's frustration and burden, emotional abuse, and feelings of dependency in the designated patient. When the patient has severe cognitive impairment, the interventions often primarily involve the caregiver and strategies to reduce caregiver burnout.

A comprehensive description of the various psychotherapy modalities exceeds the scope of this chapter. Please see Table 10-3 for a summary of some important psychotherapy modalities.

There is ample evidence supporting the efficacy of various psychotherapies in neuropsychiatry. A systematic review of CBT for depression in chronic neurological conditions (Parkinson's disease, dementia, multiple sclerosis, epilepsy) found cognitive and/or behavioral interventions beneficial, with largest effect sizes comparing CBT to passive control (rather than another psychotherapy).[33] Psychosocial interventions in dementia have effect sizes on behavioral and psychological symptoms at least equal to the effects of psychopharmacology. Not only do they not cause side effects, they have the added benefit of improving caregiver wellness. We review here a few studies (see Table 10-4) demonstrating the efficacy of psychotherapy for the treatment of depression in mild cognitive impairment (MCI) and dementia. This is a prevalent patient presentation and a well-researched topic, and the findings can illuminate the possibilities of psychotherapy in other neuropsychiatric disorders. Although the loss of language, memory, and insight are obstacles to the use of traditional psychotherapy, research shows that psychotherapy

TABLE 10-3 • Summary of Psychotherapy Modalities.

Cognitive-behavioral therapy (CBT)	Based in integration of classical and operant conditioning (Pavlov; Skinner) with social learning theory (Albert Bandura). Principle: cognitions, behaviors, and emotions continually reinforce one another. Includes broad range of focused short-term interventions.[26]
Behavioral management therapy/ Strategies	Behavioral therapy, adapted for individuals with cognitive impairment, trains the caregiver on behavioral strategies to alter the contingencies that relate to behavior problems. Strategies include distraction, communication, increasing pleasant events, behavioral activation, and environmental modifications.
Third wave behavioral therapies	Integrate Buddhist principles and meditation practice. Includes acceptance and commitment therapy (ACT), dialectical behavior therapy (DBT) (Marsha Linehan), and mindfulness-based cognitive therapy (MBCT).
Mind-body therapies	Intervenes with physiological state. Includes: Relaxation response (Herbert Benson) and mindfulness-based stress reduction (Jon Kabbat-Zin).
Motivation interviewing	Not a modality of psychotherapy. Techniques to facilitate and engage intrinsic motivation for change and resolving ambivalence.
Group psychotherapy	Universalizes and validates experience and provides opportunities for competence through helping others. Cost-effective delivery of skills-building treatment.[27]
Family psychotherapy	Relationship-focused interventions improve family functioning by enhancing communication, conflict resolution, problem-solving, and cohesiveness.[28]
Supportive psychotherapy	Based in ego psychology. Bolsters coping mechanisms, focuses on present, and promotes situational adaptation. Active role of therapist including reassurance and suggestion.[29] Others (e.g., Alexopoulos et al.[30]; Arean et al.[31]) describe this approach as nondirective.
Psychoanalysis, psychodynamic/ Introspective psychotherapy	Based on psychoanalytic drive theory, object relations, and self-psychology. Uses exploration and interpretation to develop insight into unconscious conflicts and influence of early relational experiences. Traditionally long-term and frequent; newer short-term models.[29,32]
Problem-solving therapy (PST)	Skills for improving patient's ability to deal with everyday life problems. Teaches a five-stage process: (1) problem orientation, (2) definition, (3) generation of solutions, (4) decision making, and (5) solution implementations and verification.

TABLE 10-4 • Studies Supporting Psychotherapy for Depression in MCI and Dementia.

Intervention (Author, Year)	Target Population	Outcome
PST vs. ST (Alexopoulos et al., 2003)[30]	Older adults with depression and cognitive deficits	Significant reduction in depression ($p=0.01$) and disability ($p=0.001$) in the PST vs. ST group
PST vs. ST (Alexopoulos et al., 2011)[36]	Older adults with depression and cognitive impairment	Positive difference in benefit for PST vs. ST higher among patients with greater cognitive impairment and more mood episodes
BT-pleasant events and problem-solving components vs. typical care and wait list control (Teri et al., 1997)[37]	Patients and caregivers	Significant reduction in depression symptoms for patients ($p<0.001$) and *caregivers* ($p<0.01$) in the BT groups; results maintained at 6 months
Cognitive-behavioral family intervention. Assessment of caregiver and patient behavior. Caregiver education, coping skills, stress management training (Marriott et al., 2000)[38]	Caregivers of individuals with dementia	Significant reductions in distress and depression in caregivers; reductions in patient behavioral disturbance; increase in patient activities at 3 months

BT, behavior therapy; PST, problem-solving therapy; ST, supportive therapy.

can be modified to effectively treat depression in the setting of cognitive dysfunction. Systematic reviews find a positive effect of psychotherapy in treatment of depression in MCI and dementia[34] with strongest evidence for problem-solving therapy (PST) and modified cognitive behavioral treatment.[35] We invite the reader to find further psychotherapy examples in the chapters for specific neuropsychiatric disorders.

COGNITIVE-BEHAVIORAL THERAPY IN NEUROPSYCHIATRY

In this section, we briefly discuss CBT and then review its use within neuropsychiatry. Lastly, we present a clinical case demonstrating the use of CBT with an individual with MCI.

Introduction to CBT

CBT is an evidence-based, goal-focused, short-term psychotherapy treatment. It considers the interrelationships between thoughts, feelings, and behaviors. This includes how cognitions or interpretations influence emotions and behaviors,[39] and how behaviors affect thought patterns and emotions.[40] Within a CBT framework, distress and psychiatric concerns may be created, exacerbated, and maintained by unhelpful patterns within an individual's way of thinking and acting. Changing or altering one or more of these patterns creates ripple effects that can alleviate distress and decrease the severity of psychiatric concerns.

In sessions with patients, CBT clinicians often draw the CBT model (see Figure 10-1) to use as a visual aid during discussions. The CBT process can be highly interactive, and illustrations can assist patients in understanding cycles and the interrelationships between factors. This model shows how individuals' thinking influences the feeling(s) experienced, and vice versa. A behavior or a series of behaviors can also impact the cycle. Utilizing this model in the session encourages patients to be scientists in their lives—to try to collect data, make hypotheses, and aim to understand what may be happening. CBT empowers patients to analyze their patterns and realize that they are changeable.

To help recognize patterns in thinking, CBT clinicians encourage patients to look for regular patterns in their thinking styles or, more specifically, cognitive distortions (see Figure 10-2). Cognitive distortions are exaggerated thought patterns believed to be involved in the onset and perpetuation of psychological distress. Cognitive distortions can cause individuals to perceive reality inaccurately.[39] In CBT, clinicians work with patients to examine how regularly they may be engaging in unhelpful cognitive distortions. They then train patients in cognitive restructuring skills, such as creating a more neutral way of speaking. Another example is to have patients engage in *Socratic questioning,* to be a scientist in their own lives. Examples may include, "Is there anything that contradicts that way of thinking?," "Is there evidence supporting that belief?," "What is the utility of thinking that statement?" Through systematic exploration and challenging of negative cognitive distortions, patients increase awareness and become open to thoughts that create a more neutral or positive emotion. They learn to create more accurate portrayals of reality.

There are three main components of CBT treatment: cognitive, behavioral, and physiologic interventions. Every CBT

Checklist of Cognitive Distortions*

1. **All-or-nothing thinking:** You look at things in absolute, black-and white categories.

2. **Over generalization:** You look a negative event as a never-ending pattern of defeat.

3. **Mental filter:** You dwell on the negatives.

4. **Discounting the positives:** You insist that your accomplishments or positive qualities don't count.

5. **Jumping to conclusions:**
   (A) **Mind-reading**—You assume that people are reacting negatively to you when there's no definite evidence;
   (B) **Fortune Telling**—You arbitrarily predict that things will turn out badly.

6. **Magnification or minimization:** You blow things way out of proportion or you shrink their importance.

7. **Emotional reasoning:** You reason from how you feel: "I feel like an idiot, so I really must be one."

8. **"Should statements":** You criticize yourself (or other people) with "shoulds," "oughts," "musts," and "have tos."

9. **Labeling:** Instead of saying "I made a mistake," you tell yourself, "I'm a jerk," or "a fool," or a "loser."

10. **Personalization and blame:** You blame yourself for something you weren't entirely responsible for, or you blame other people and deny your role in the problem.

*Copyright © 1991 by David D. Burns, MD. Revised, 1992.

FIGURE 10-2. Cognitive distortions ("Checklist of Cognitive Distortions" from *Feeling Good* by David D. Burns. Copyright © 1980 by David D. Burns, M.D. Used by permission of HarperCollins Publishers.[41]).

session may not address all three, but a course of CBT likely addresses each component at some point. As discussed above, cognitive interventions aim at modifying the individual's relationship to unhelpful cognitions, self-statements, or beliefs. The CBT clinician engages the patient in cognitive restructuring or guided discovery to help modify some of these ways of thinking by examining facts versus thoughts, with the goal of symptom relief.[42] Ultimately, if patients don't think as negatively about themselves or their symptoms, they will likely not feel as bad.

Behaviorally, a CBT clinician's goal is to decrease maladaptive behaviors and increase a patient's engagement in behaviors that increase quality of life and decrease psychiatric distress. Considering depression, an example of maladaptive behavior may be avoidance. Patients may feel low energy, sad, or disengaged, and decide to take a nap with the hope that this will bring relief. However, that nap may turn into staying in bed for the entire afternoon and missing opportunities for engagement in value-based activities, worsening rather than elevating their mood. This is an example of negative reinforcement. In addition, distress levels are usually higher since there is less engagement in what is valued by the individual. In CBT, clinicians work with patients to access positive reinforcement more regularly through engagement in nondepressed, value-based behaviors. A clinician may also target avoidance through engaging patients in exposure-based strategies to face a fear or perceived negative

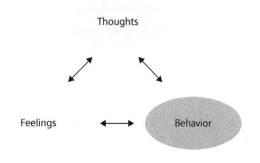

FIGURE 10-1. Cognitive model/cognitive triangle.

outcome, and to see if a new appraisal of themselves or of the situation can be learned.

Rumination can also be classified as a behavior. Often perceived as not in one's conscious awareness, rumination serves as a way a patient's mind tries to control uncertainty, solve perceived predicaments (usually feared outcomes), or avoid uncomfortable emotions. Bringing patients minds out of auto-pilot can be useful and help them evaluate if the rumination negatively influences mood and/or has less impact on outcomes than anticipated. Mindfulness is another behavioral strategy for patients to gain awareness of their thought process and potentially change the relationship they have with their thoughts.

There are also physiologic interventions. If patients are thinking negative thoughts all day, their body will likely feel tense and uncomfortable. In instances like this, CBT clinicians teach and encourage diaphragmatic breathing to help with relaxation and to correct over breathing or chest breathing. Progressive muscle relaxation may also reduce bodily tension. Clinicians notice and point out physiologic signs of depression in patients, like slouching over or turning inward (to hide or take up less space). Physiologic interventions also include suggesting better posture or encouraging patients to shift the ways they physically present themselves in the world.

CBT within Neuropsychiatry

CBT can be very effective to address multiple neuropsychiatric symptoms and disorders, including depression, anxiety, mood fluctuations, disinhibition, and impulsivity. CBT can assist patients with strategies to address these emotional states and decrease emotional distress. In addition, CBT can help patients understand the behavioral and cognitive influences that might trigger mood problems, and the reciprocal relationships between their thinking, mood, and behavior. Other manifestations of neuropsychiatric disturbances include apathy, agitation, wandering and aggressiveness, and sleep or appetite changes. CBT, especially its behavioral components, is efficacious for addressing these symptoms. For instance, clinicians can encourage patients to consider the patterns specific to *who, what, where,* and *when* the behavior is happening. In patients with limited insight due to cognitive changes, direct work with the patient to shift behavior may be difficult. With these cases, CBT clinicians may focus on changing the environment. For instance, to prevent wandering in a patient with dementia, a clinician might put a stop sign at an exit door to help cue the individual to "stop" at a door. This visual cue can be more effective than a verbal cue, given that the visual and procedural memory-based elements of the cue prompts a more reliable long-term, memory-based understanding of what an individual should do at a stop sign.

Neuropsychiatric patients may experience thoughts related to the cognitive decline they experience. They often have fears related to illness trajectory, outcomes, and what the future holds. Cognitions might be focused on worries related to their brain changes. Given this, they may be more preoccupied with the future rather than the present moment. In addition, thoughts in these patients can be more rigid and concrete given the potential impact of neuropsychiatric conditions on insight and brain functions. CBT protocols may need to be modified to account for these cognitive changes, as shown later in this chapter.

In this work, a clinician's consideration of multimodal learning strategies within a CBT session is useful. It may be valuable to have patients take notes during a session, or provide them with notes they can take home. A binder, with tabs or colors referencing a mutually decided upon organizational system, can help patients with prompting and recall. Sections reference topics from each CBT session and can be dated or organized by content. Visual aids and diagrams like the diagram of the CBT model (Figure 10-1) assist patients rehearse what they have learned. Caregivers or "coaches" may also use it to bring the CBT work into day-to-day life. The psychotherapy session can be recorded for patients to take home. Patients set a goal to listen to each session, facilitating the encoding of session information. Also, clinicians and patients can more specifically record the cognitive reframes or alternative ways of thinking created in session, so that patients can review and play these therapeutic interventions between sessions. It can be a very powerful change tool for patients to hear their own voice utilizing the CBT skills. In one recent case, a patient recorded the reframe and made it his phone's ringtone. The patient initiated this idea, with the aim of having it played/noticed over and over. As in this example, it is especially beneficial when patients creatively apply the skills learned in session in ways that may work best for them. There are a number of ways technology can also be implemented effectively through smartphone applications.[43]

Patients and their caregivers or "coaches" should create a cueing system to aid in keeping the patient oriented and help them apply and practice session information between sessions. Patients can benefit from reminders, even when not struggling with cognitive limitations. Alarms and prompts can be very effective in breaking habituated patterns and/or increase the chance information may be remembered and reviewed. Signage around patients' homes with skill reminders or other information that can be depicted visually may be beneficial. These signs or prompts help patients break patterns instead of deferring to automatic routines.

As discussed in the case management section, caregiver involvement can also be very instrumental in CBT work. Caregivers are encouraged to join for parts of sessions or be involved in phone check-ins during CBT sessions. The caregiver may take on a coaching role and help emphasize regularly the skills learned in session. Practice between sessions with support or cues from a caregiver often result in greater therapeutic benefits and provide patients with extra encouragement and accountability.

Evidence suggests that CBT is associated with brain changes detectable with current imaging techniques. For example, CBT for depression and anxiety may result in increased efficiency of the frontal-parietal executive control network, important in the regulation of emotion. An increased capacity for "top-down" emotion regulation is employed when skills taught in CBT are engaged. Functional brain imaging studies showing changes in activity of the dorsal anterior cingulate cortex could be seen as in keeping with this model.[44,45]

CBT with MCI and Dementia

Anxiety and depressive disorders frequently coexist with MCI, and untreated mood disorders can worsen cognitive concerns.[46,47] Anxiety severity may increase the rate of conversion from MCI to Alzheimer's dementia.[48] Psychosocial and behavioral approaches are the preferred initial interventions to address emotional syndromes comorbid with cognitive impairment, given the multiple drug interactions and medical comorbidities present in an aging or neuropsychiatric population.[49,50] Research[51-54] supports the efficacy of behavioral and cognitive interventions for individuals with MCI, as well as for those with mild and even moderate stages of dementia. Techniques, however, may need to be modified for these populations. Improvements can be seen in anxiety, depression, and obsessions, and decreases in caregiver distress can also be shown with the use of CBT-based protocols.[37,52,54,55]

Peaceful mind[52,56] is a CBT-based intervention for anxiety in individuals with mild or moderate dementia living in the community. Caregivers are included in the intervention, which includes in-home sessions for 3 months, and up to 8 brief telephone sessions during months 3–6. The sessions involve CBT skills such as self-monitoring for anxiety, deep breathing, coping self-statements, behavioral activation, and sleep management. The treatment is particularly suited to meet the needs of individuals with dementia through its emphasis on behavioral rather than cognitive interventions, its slower pace, limited learned material, repetition and cueing, inclusion of a "coach," and home-based sessions. This intervention can be efficacious to reduce individuals' anxiety, increase their quality of life, and decrease caregivers' distress. For the full manual and general suggestions for treatment delivery, see Paukert et al.[56] Charlesworth et al.[53] developed a 10-session CBT protocol for use in a randomized controlled trial with people with anxiety and mild-to-moderate dementia. This protocol was unique in its inclusion of person-centered approaches to CBT, with individualized tailoring to accommodate for cognitive deficits and other challenges. Within the approach, the person with dementia worked directly with clinicians and involved a "supportive other" when available and/or necessary. Spector et al.[54] developed a CBT manual for anxiety and depression in dementia. There were improvements in depression, which remained significant at 6 months.

CASE VIGNETTE 10.1

A 62-year-old, married male, who retired earlier than planned from work as a small business owner, was seen for CBT in the Geriatric Clinic at BWH. This patient was recently diagnosed with MCI, with a 2-year history of progressive short-term memory problems.

Case Interventions

During the first session, the patient was given a binder to hold session notes. The sessions were split, with half of the session with the patient alone and the other half with the patient and his wife, who acted as the treatment "coach." Color-coded tabs were used to break down items by topic and to visually cue the patient and caregiver to reference and practice the items noted

under a particular color or topic between sessions. The wife also attended a caregiver group, an evidence-based intervention that offers monthly psychoeducation and CBT strategies to support caregivers of those with neuropsychiatric and cognitive concerns.

The clinician started by providing simplified psychoeducation on the lethargy/apathy cycle. This cycle illustrates how individuals experience stress and negative life events and then experience associated reactions of negative thinking and negative self. Negative thinking can often be amplified when individuals are also engaging in depressed behaviors (e.g., staying in bed longer, avoidance, disengagement in activities). Depressed behavior can be amplified due to perceptions of needing to conserve energy or "hibernate" when managing low energy or motivation. Patients often hope that when they "recharge," they will then engage in the intended activity and/or shift their behavior. Unfortunately, that desired motivation does not surface immediately (or ever with these behavioral patterns) and individuals get stuck in this cycle. This patient also experienced negative thoughts about needing to retire earlier than planned and about his MCI diagnosis, which caused heightened negative self-talk focused on being a failure and on perceptions of not being able to remember anything. This then led the patient to take less action and to engage in less "doing" due to thoughts of wanting to decrease the possibility of not doing something "right." He stayed home and in bed more, which in the short term made him feel better. However, the longer he disengaged, the worse he felt and the more stress he experienced. For this patient and his wife, it was helpful to draw out a personalized version of the lethargy/apathy cycle in session, to help highlight the negative reinforcement patterns that were contributing to lower mood. This drawing and session notes were added to his binder under a specific color and topic heading. Buy-in around this theory and resonation with the approach lead to collaborative discussions regarding how best to intervene and what goals to set.

With patients displaying more prominent apathy and cognitive difficulties it can be helpful to begin with behavioral strategies (the "B" in CBT). The gold standard in behavioral treatments is behavioral activation.[57,58] Within behavioral activation, a clinician first asks patients to take an inventory, hour by hour, of what they do each day and to assess how enjoyable and important these activities are to them. Our patient was encouraged to set some alarms to prompt him to fill out the daily forms. The caregiver/"coach" also helped to place the forms in places to visually cue the patient to complete them. After completing the forms for about a week, the patient found that he spent about 50% of his waking hours ruminating. He was engaging in much "what if" worrying and thinking that people did not want to be in his life anymore. Ultimately, this ruminative behavior caused him to feel sadness. Engaging in the self-monitoring assessment helped him realize that he didn't value his time ruminating. As a result, the clinician targeted this ruminative behavior by asking the patient to consider, "what could I do instead?." In behavioral activation, patients learn to reflect on what their values are, versus what they are doing out of habit or due to mood state or fears.

The patient spoke about what he valued, and he noted a desire to be more engaged in his life. This included appreciating time with his grandchildren and watching college sports. He was helped to consider ways he could engage in activities reflective of these values during the time he typically spent ruminating. The goal was not to eliminate rumination, since this did not seem realistic, but to schedule more valued and enjoyable activities during the times he was ruminating. When applying his behavioral activation insights, the patient engaged in phone calls with his grandchildren and attended some college sports games at times that he normally would be ruminating. His wife acted in the "coach" role and would offer reminders and show him the hour-by-hour forms noted above, to cue him to consider engaging in the value-based activity. The patient enjoyed these activities and he noted his mood as more elevated during those times. He and his wife shared perceptions of improvement in depressed mood over the course of the day.

The clinician also provided psychoeducation and training on physiological interventions to help with relaxation, including deep, square, and diaphragmatic breathing. Square or box breathing is a technique used to facilitate slow breathing. The patient is invited to visualize a square, and to break down his or her breathing into four movements, each lasting 4 seconds, corresponding to one side of the square (*inhale, hold, exhale, hold*). The drawing of an actual square, with each of those words written on each side, can be provided to the patient. It was helpful to pair the recognition of a mood state with these physiological interventions, through a process called spaced retrieval.[59] Spaced retrieval involves practicing recalling information with a patient over progressively longer intervals of time, using retained procedural (implicit) memory. A clinician first works with a patient to identify a goal (e.g., to improve my depressed mood, to decrease my tension) and then the clinician and patient work together to pair a prompt and/or response to that goal (e.g., "when I am tense, I can breathe"). If during the session the clinician notices that the patient appears tense, or if the patient states that he/she feels tense, the clinician may ask, "what do you do if you are tense?" If the patient answers with "I can breathe," intervals between prompts may be longer. If he/she fails to correctly answer the prompt, the clinician offers a reminder and asks the question again sooner. This technique may be effective for individuals with various dementia diagnoses, by enabling them to remember information for longer periods and to better achieve long-term treatment goals.[60,61]

Cognitive interventions were also utilized. Although some cognitive approaches may need to be adapted and simplified, individuals with MCI or dementia can still benefit from identifying patterns in their thinking or shifting thoughts to more positive or neutral statements. This patient frequently found himself saying, "I forget everything" or "I have lost control." The clinician and the patient reviewed in session what thinking styles and/or cognitive distortions were present and then worked together to create more neutral statements, such as, "There are many things I can still remember" and "I do have control." The patient wrote these statements in his CBT notebook with a color-coded tab labeled "reframes" and would review these reframes when he caught himself engaging in negative thinking and in general, when he regularly looked at this notebook. His wife also cued him to look at the notebook, particularly this tabbed section, if she noticed this type of thinking.

Another approach used to target his rumination was to consider the value behind the activity in which he was engaging, not just the content on which he was ruminating. For instance, he had negative and catastrophic ruminations when he was a passenger on longer car trips. On the other hand, travel and driving were things he used to value and enjoy a great deal. As a result, in his CBT binder he wrote, "I may be feeling nervous and I also do really enjoy travel. Going somewhere new is important to me." On car trips, then, he would to turn to the "driving" tab section of his binder to read these created reframes. In one session, we also created an audio recording of his voice that stated "I enjoy driving. This is important to me" and he was prompted to listen to this voice message when applicable.

MINDFULNESS-BASED THERAPIES IN NEUROPSYCHIATRY

Introduction

One of the most commonly used definitions of mindfulness comes from Jon Kabat-Zinn, who developed one of the earliest codified, secular mindfulness training programs in the United States. He said that "mindfulness means paying attention in a particular way; on purpose, in the present moment, and non-judgmentally."[62] Mindfulness is a particular attitude toward one's own experience. It can be practiced informally by bringing the qualities of presence attention, openness, curiosity, and warmth to the experiences of day-to-day life. This attitude can be practiced in an intentional way in the context of activities such as walking, eating, running, and even washing the dishes or sweeping. It can also be practiced formally, through meditation. The type of formal mindfulness practice that has been most widely studied involves combining focused attention with an attitude of openness, interest, and nonreactivity to inner experience, including sensations, emotions, and thoughts.

In the last 5–10 years, mindfulness has increasingly emerged as a topic of interest. This may be in part because of the rapidly growing base of research demonstrating effects on health and well-being. The first publication about mindfulness and health came out in 1982.[62] Before 2002 there were 10 publications or less per year. In 2009 there were over 100 and in 2015 there were over 500.[63]

Early studies in healthy adults suggested that mindfulness training and regular practice of mindfulness could increase positive affect and decrease negative affect,[64,65] improve emotion regulation,[66,67] boost immune function,[68,69] sharpen focus,[70–72] and strengthen coping effectiveness.[73,74] Some studies even demonstrated that mindfulness training could lead to changes in gene expression.[75,76]

Mindfulness and the Brain

There is a rapidly growing literature investigating changes in brain structure and function following mindfulness training and CBT. The following summary includes findings that have particular relevance to the field of neuropsychiatry.

A number of studies of mindfulness training have demonstrated changes in the structure or function of the insula. The insula is understood to be important for interoceptive awareness, or the awareness of one's own internal experiences. A systematic review of functional imaging studies of brain activity following mindfulness-based interventions reported that one of the most consistent findings was of increased insular cortex activity.[77] Other studies have reported greater activation in the insula and anterior cingulate following mindfulness training, coupled with decreased activation in primary sensory cortex.[78] One hypothesis is that mindfulness training strengthens networks that are important for moment-to-moment awareness of experience while downregulating regions that may be active regardless of awareness, such as primary sensory cortex.

Other studies have reported changes in prefrontal-limbic connections following mindfulness training. Decreased activation in the amygdala and increased activation in prefrontal regions following mindfulness training have been reported across multiple studies. One hypothesis is that the development of mindful emotion regulation is mediated by stronger prefrontal cognitive control, which then downregulates activity in limbic areas important for affect processing, such as the amygdala. There have been some functional connectivity studies looking at changes in prefrontal and limbic regions. One such investigation[79] found that individuals with generalized anxiety showed stronger connections between the prefrontal cortex and amygdala after mindfulness training, which correlated with improvement in anxiety symptoms.

Mindfulness training has been associated with changes in the default mode network (DMN), a region of medial cortical structures thought to be important for self-referential processing and mind wandering. Brewer and colleagues were the first to demonstrate a change in the DMN associated with mindfulness training. They found that, when compared to controls, a group of expert meditators showed less activity in the DMN as well as stronger functional connectivity between DMN regions and anterior cingulate and dorsolateral prefrontal cortex. They interpreted the greater functional connectivity as indicating increased cognitive control over the function of the DMN. Changes in the DMN following mindfulness training have potential implications for therapeutic interventions in clinical populations where aberrant DMN activity has been shown. Such populations might include those with major depressive disorder, posttraumatic stress disorder, and Alzheimer's disease.[80]

Mindfulness Training

The most widely taught mindfulness training program in the United States currently is mindfulness-based stress reduction (MBSR), developed by Jon Kabat-Zinn and colleagues in the late 1970s. MBSR is an 8-week program that teaches basic mindfulness skills in a group format. It combines a set of formal mindfulness practices, such as sitting meditation and a body scan, with gentle yoga and education about the nature of stress reactivity and the potentially mitigating role of mindful awareness. Participants are expected to attend a two-and-a-half-hour class each week as well as one 6-hour partially silent retreat that takes place, typically, on a weekend day. Participants are expected to do approximately 45 minutes of daily home practice, involving a combination of audio-guided meditation or yoga and some form of informal mindfulness and self-observation. Since its development in the early 1980s, it has grown into a program

that is taught worldwide in several different languages, as well as more recently, online.

There are a number of condition-specific programs that have grown out of the MBSR model. One of the most widely known is mindfulness-based cognitive therapy (MBCT). Like MBSR, MBCT is an 8-week group program that teaches mindfulness meditation. However, unlike MBSR, MBCT integrates mindfulness training with elements of CBT. MBCT was originally developed for individuals who were in remission from major depression but at risk for future episodes of depression. It has been demonstrated to be quite effective in reducing relapse rates for this population. In recent years, it has also been adopted for use with other clinical populations, including depression not yet in remission as well as chronic pain, psychosis, and bipolar disorder. Like MBSR, there is a significant time commitment, including weekly meetings, a weekend retreat, and daily home practice. It is also taught worldwide, but tends to be less-readily available likely because it is newer than MBSR.

A number of other programs have grown out of the MBSR model. Some examples include Mindfulness Based Relapse Prevention for addiction, Mindful Self-Compassion (for adults and for teens), and Mindfulness-Based Childbirth and Parenting. Acceptance and commitment therapy and dialectical behavior therapy have not grown out of the MBSR model, but are both psychological therapies that incorporate mindfulness as one of the central tenets of the treatment. There are many other ways in which the application of mindfulness has been described in various clinical conditions, such as ADHD and anxiety, as well as in different developmental stages, such as children and older adults.

Mindfulness and Neuropsychiatry

In the past few years, a number of studies have reported looking at mindfulness training in neuropsychiatric populations. Most of these studies have been feasibility and preliminary efficacy studies.

In a study looking at mindfulness training for depression in the context of traumatic brain injury (TBI), Bédard and colleagues[81] randomly assigned patients with documented TBI to either an experimental group, which received a modified mindfulness-based cognitive therapy intervention, or a wait-list control group. The MBCT intervention was adapted to be more accessible to TBI patients in that it was broken up into more sessions (10, instead of 8) of shorter duration (90 minutes, instead of 2–2.5 hours) than the standard MBCT group. Home practices were shorter (20–30 minutes, instead of 45 minutes) and it also used simplified language and repetition to reinforce learning to accommodate problems with memory, fatigue, and concentration often experienced by people with TBI. Participants were encouraged to record their observations and questions on "new learning" forms, to facilitate deeper reflection on usual modes of behavior and habits of mind in day-to-day activities. At the end of the study, the authors found that the MBCT group showed a significantly greater reduction in total depression scores and neurovegetative symptoms compared with the control group. Increases in mindfulness were associated with improvements in depression symptoms. Importantly, the reduction in depression symptoms in the adapted-MBCT group was significant not only following the intervention delivery, but also at 3 months out.

In 2015, Tang and colleagues[82] published a study of mindfulness training in a group of individuals with drug-resistant epilepsy. The study aimed to examine effects of mindfulness training on depression, anxiety, social isolation, and overall quality of life in this population as related to having treatment refractory seizures, particularly seizures that occur in public. All of the study participants were encouraged to take care of themselves by adhering to their medication regimen, getting good sleep, and exercising. All patients were offered social support as part of their study participation, but only half were also provided with mindfulness training. The mindfulness group received training in standard mindfulness techniques in a group format and were encouraged to practice these techniques daily on their own. They also received instruction on using an active acceptance approach in coping with their seizures. Patients in the control group participated in a support group where they could reflect on their illness experience. At the end of the study, seizure frequency was significantly reduced in both groups. Both groups showed improvements in anxiety, quality of life, and subjective well-being, but patients in the mindfulness group improved to a much greater degree in these categories than the control group, particularly with regard to seizure worry and energy levels. In addition, only the mindfulness patients achieved statistically significant improvements in memory.[82]

Finally, a meta-analysis of mindfulness training for fatigue in stroke, TBI, and multiple sclerosis looked specifically at randomized and quasi-randomized controlled trials of mindfulness training for fatigue. Based on the four studies included in the final analysis, they estimated a moderate effect size of mindfulness-based interventions on fatigue in these conditions, compared to no treatment or control treatments.[83]

COGNITIVE REHABILITATION THERAPY

Cognitive rehabilitation therapy (CRT) is the treatment of cognitive limitations or deficits that result from brain disease or injury. There are many different models of CRT. This section will focus on the **comprehensive or holistic CRT model**, which is built on the premise that healthy adaptation to brain disease or injury is facilitated by attending to cognitive difficulties in combination with emotional and behavioral symptoms.[84-86] Many of the methods and the interventions within the holistic CRT model initially developed for TBI and stroke[87-89] were translated and shown to be effective in other neurologic and psychiatric conditions as well. The treatments tend to be goal oriented and highly individualized to a patient's specific cognitive profile and functional difficulties; the generalization or the transfer of skills to everyday life is one of the main treatment goals.[90,91] CRT research is still in its early stages, but there have been many research studies, including clinical trials. (See Table 10-5 for references to recent studies and review articles.) These studies have shown evidence for improvement benefits on targeted cognitive tasks, but often these changes fall short of what is deemed clinically meaningful in drug trials. They are also inconsistently associated with changes in behavioral disturbances, mood, and quality of life.

Choi and Twamley[127] defined a clinical reasoning model that outlines **neuropsychological, psychological,** and **awareness factors** to facilitate case conceptualization and treatment planning in CRT.

TABLE 10-5 • Summary of Research References in CRT.	
Disorder/Disease Population	**CRT Research References**
TBI	Bogdanova et al.[92]; Powell et al.[93]; Virk et al.[94]; Tate et al.[95]; Togher et al.[96]
MCI and Dementia	Belleville et al.[97]; Chandler et al.[98]; Clare et al.[99,100]; Cotelli et al.[101]; Hampstead, Gillis, and Stringer[102]; Huckans et al.[103]; Jean et al.[104]; Reijnders, van Heugten, and van Boxtel[105]; Simon, Yokomizo, and Bottino[106]; Stott and Spector[107]
Stroke	Chung et al.[108]; Gillespie et al.[109]; Lockwood[110]
Multiple sclerosis	Ernst et al.[111]; Goverover et al.[112]; Mitolo et al.[113]
Parkinson's disease	Alzahrani and Venneri[114]; Cerasa et al.[115]; Hindle et al.[116]; Strouwen et al.[117]
Epilepsy	Del Felice et al.[118]; Farina et al.[119]; Geraldi et al.[120]; Koorenhof et al.[121]; Maschio et al.[122]
Schizophrenia	Murthy et al.[123]; Paquin et al.[124]
Mood disorders	Kluwe-schiavon et al.[125]; Priyamvada et al.[126]

- *Neuropsychological or cognitive factors* focus on a patient's cognitive profile and history, including a patient's pattern of cognitive strengths and deficits, level of cognitive reserve, and disease specific considerations, such as whether the patient is presenting with a progressive or a static brain injury.
- *Psychological factors* largely focus on what symptoms the patient is presenting with, but also account for the patient's psychiatric history. For example, is the patient presenting with active symptoms of depression and anxiety that are resulting in negative thoughts, impacting self-efficacy, and/or perhaps leading to defeatist beliefs?
- *Awareness factors* describe the patient's understanding of their cognitive difficulties, as well as their disease or illness. If patients have limited awareness or insight about their symptoms and the source of those symptoms, then it is often quite difficult to engage them in treatment.

A comprehensive or holistic CRT is a multistage treatment approach that addresses awareness/insight factors through education and insight-oriented work, neuropsychological factors through cognitive interventions, and psychological factors through psychosocial interventions, such as CBT (Table 10-6). The progression through treatment stages is typically determined by patient and caregiver goals. Early stages of treatment tend to be focused on providing disease-specific education and reviewing details of a patient's cognitive profile. This forms the basis of treatment engagement and collaborative goal setting. Explicitly defining outcomes is necessary for setting patient and caregiver expectations and keeping treatment time-limited. Recent cognitive rehabilitation research has argued against using neuropsychological test performance as outcome measures because of the lack of ecological validity of these tests.[128] Instead functional outcomes, such as meeting stated goals, improving self-efficacy, and reducing patient and caregiver level of distress, have been shown to be more useful patient-oriented outcome measures.

Cognitive interventions are the heart of CRT and can be categorized in two ways: **compensatory and restorative** (Table 10-7). **Compensatory** approaches teach patients strategies to work around cognitive deficits that are negatively impacting their everyday life. Compensatory strategies are top-down approaches that build a scaffold, structure, and organization to support daily tasks and activities. External strategies, such as using a notebook or making lists, and internal or meta-cognitive strategies are the framework of these approaches.

TABLE 10-6 • Comprehensive or Holistic CRT.

Holistic CRT Focus	Example Treatments
Awareness/Insight building	Psychoeducation about injury, prognosis/disease course Insight-oriented focus to improve awareness of symptoms Motivational interviewing to facilitate active participation
Cognitive/ Neuropsychological	Cognitive interventions
Psychological/ Emotional adjustment	Cognitive-behavioral therapy, grief counseling, trauma therapy

TABLE 10-7 • Compensatory and Restorative Interventions in CRT.

Approach	Compensatory	Restorative
Goal	Develop and train patient on strategies to work-around or compensate for cognitive deficits	Return patient to baseline level of functioning through intensive, repetitive practice on tasks of increasing difficulty
Method	External and internal strategy training	Computerized or instructional training
Examples	CBT for ADHD, goal management training, memory support system, mnemonic training	BrainHQ, attention processing training, Lumosity, Cogmed, brain fitness

Examples of evidenced-based protocols for attention and executive functioning include CBT for ADHD,[129] goal management training,[130] and PST.[131] CBT for ADHD focuses on both external organization and internal strategies, such as a planner/calendar system, building awareness of attention span, and teaching patients how to overcome distractibility and procrastination. These strategies are helpful for anyone who has attention and executive functioning difficulties, not just individuals with developmental ADHD. Other treatments for executive dysfunction include goal management training, which places a large focus on strategies for improving performance monitoring and attentional awareness and control. A very basic form of mindfulness attention training is part of this protocol.[130] PST combines a focus on frustration tolerance with systematic steps for breaking larger goals down into smaller, more manageable steps.[131] In terms of memory, the memory support system is a framework for training people how to use a combined calendar/journal system.[132] The Ecologically Oriented Neurorehabilitation of Memory protocol focuses on mnemonic and internal memory support techniques, such as association, elaboration, and visualization.[133] O'Neil-Pirozzi, Kennedy, and Sohlberg[134] conducted a useful review of internal memory strategies in brain injury which details other protocols.

Based on learning theory, Sohlberg and Mateer[90] outline three phases of learning compensatory strategies to promote effective translation to daily life. During the acquisition phase, the components of the strategy and its intended use are taught. Next, the goal of the application phase is to apply the techniques or strategy to a patient's life. This step often involves in-session exercises to demonstrate to the patient how to use the strategy at home. The final, adaptation phase, focuses on adapting the technique or strategy into a daily routine, with the goal of making it a habit. Homework assignments are essential during this stage.

Technology now plays a very important role in supporting compensatory and behaviorally oriented treatment approaches. Smartwatches and smartphones have made it easier to deliver alerts and prompts to support attention regulation and prospective memory. Table 10-8 lists several applications and electronic devices that can be integrated to support a comprehensive CRT.

TABLE 10-8 • Applications and Electronic Devices in CRT.

App/Software	Category/Description
PaceMyDay	Planning to optimize energy
ReachMyGoals	Implement and monitor SMART goals
Evernote	Task management, note-taking
Selfcontrol	Program periods of time, disabling certain applications on your smartphone or computer to help with focus
Focus booster	Monitors usage of computer programs and applications. Sessions are automatically recorded and there is a reporting tool to help with visualizing progress.
Calendar applications	Google and other calendar programs interact directly with smartphones. Program calendar reminders and facilitate more intensive cueing interventions.
Wearable cameras	Lifelogging technologies are still in development, but some Microsoft research studies have shown them to be very powerful for patients with significant memory impairment.
RFID devices	Remote monitoring systems allow caregivers to monitor behaviors from afar.
Smart speakers	Voice-activated and can make it possible to take notes and create reminders without too much training (e.g., Amazon Echo, Google Home).

CASE VIGNETTE 10.2

This is a 50-year-old woman with recent onset seizures, depression, and anxiety. She is experiencing forgetfulness, word-finding difficulty, and reduced attention and concentration. She decided to stop working in retail because she was concerned about mistakes she was making handling money. She has felt socially isolated since she has stopped working. An example treatment plan for this patient is presented below:

Psychoeducation/Awareness-building
- Review of neuropsychological profile
- Understanding neuropsychological profile in context of patient's epilepsy, depression, and anxiety
- Monitoring of cognitive slips and errors to learn about specific functional limitations and correct any misconceptions regarding memory versus attentional errors. For example, patient was labeling her difficulty with task focus and distraction as a memory problem ("I forget what I am doing in the middle of doing it.")

Goal-setting
- Improve task focus and attentional control, and increase rate of task completion
- Improve memory for appointments and everyday activities
- Create a more regular daily schedule

Interventions
- Improving metacognitive awareness and control (adapted from goal management training[130])
  - The primary educational component of the intervention is learning about the *automatic pilot*. Many routine tasks can be completed without thinking about them, like showering or dressing. With practice, one develops a habit or automatic program to take care of routine tasks. It may be the case that individuals get used to having their attention divided across several tasks and an automatic pilot state develops, which may make it difficult to fully sustain attention on one task. This may allow individuals to get more things done, but it can also lead to cognitive slips and memory errors.
  - *STOP! State* strategy training: Periodic alerting of the sustained attention system
    - The STOP! State strategy is introduced as a way to monitor whether the use of the automatic pilot is appropriate, and break out of it if necessary. To exercise the STOP! State strategy, patients are asked to work in 30-minute intervals at the beginning of which an intention or goal is set. They then practice stopping the automatic pilot about every 5 minutes to check in whether they are still working on the goal that was set. Patients are encouraged to not set alarms to know when 5 minutes have passed, with the goal of determining if setting the intention to check in more regularly helps drive their internal monitoring. Some people may find the act of checking in every 5 minutes or so disruptive initially, but it should be highlighted that this is because they are building a new skill or habit. Over time they will develop a new "automatic pilot" habit of checking in with their attention and it will eventually be done with relatively little cognitive effort.
- Planner/Memory support system (adapted from Greenaway et al.[132])
  - The planner should have three sections, a daily calendar organized by hourly appointment slots, as section for journaling, and a place to create a daily to-do list.
  - The behavioral targets would be that the patient starts to track her appointments and activities in the paper planner (as opposed to electronic calendar on phone). She will write down notes from conversations, which can be done in the journal section. She will define one activity/appointment to do outside of the home every day.
  - The general rules for suggested usage are reviewed.
    - Patient is to review planner twice per day in the AM and PM (can be linked to meals because these are usually already part of daily routine). Reviews are a good time to look back on what took place on previous days and what is coming up in the days to come.
    - The AM review is a good time to create a daily to-do list.
    - The notebook stays in the same spot in a highly trafficked area at home to visually cue the patient to refer to it and take notes.
    - When the patient leaves the home, the planner should go with her, just like her keys and wallet.
    - If it is challenging for a patient to initially remember to take notes on their day or record conversations, an alarm or timer can be set to go off at 11 am and 3 pm to prompt them to take notes.

As mentioned above, CRT approaches can be compensatory or restorative. **Restorative** approaches are based on the theory that structure and repetitive practice of increasing demands facilitates neuroplasticity.[135] Restorative training attempts to help patients return to their baseline level of functioning through intensive, repetitive practice that gets increasing challenging or more difficult. Many of these "brain exercise" programs are implemented through computerized approaches. Some are available directly to the public, like Lumosity and BrainHQ, while others require that a trained clinician issues licenses and oversees the training process, like Cogmed. The research support for use of these programs is still unclear, particularly as it relates to generalization to real life. A multisite study consisting of 10 group-training sessions (and up to 4 boost-training sessions) focused on memory, reasoning, and processing speed resulted in less decline in instrumental activities of daily living compared with the control group, and improved reasoning and processing speed cognitive abilities for 10 years.[136] Edwards and colleagues[137] added to these findings by reporting that at 10-year follow-up, participation in the processing speed intervention (offered as part of BrainHQ) also resulted in a reduction in incident dementia. There was a significant effect of number of training sessions, such that greater risk reduction was associated with more training sessions. Cognitive training focused on memory and reasoning was not associated with decreased risk for dementia.

Summary and Key Points

- Psychosocial interventions are essential, as part of a multidisciplinary approach in neuropsychiatry, to address the multidimensional impact of neuropsychiatric illnesses in individuals' lives—including behavioral, social, vocational, and relational adjustments.
- Psychosocial interventions include case management, psychotherapy, and cognitive rehabilitation.
- Caregivers may play a key role in facilitating the execution of psychosocial interventions.
- Case management functions include to assess the individual's needs, develop a plan, seek appropriate services, connect the individual with them, and monitor the results of such connection.
- Clinical case management is a holistic approach that may assist patients across the illness continuum including initial adjustment and planning, environmental focus, psychoeducation and psychotherapy, and crisis intervention.
- There is ample evidence supporting the efficacy of various psychotherapies in neuropsychiatry, including cognitive-behavioral therapy, problem-solving therapy, mindfulness-based interventions, and others.

- Psychotherapy delivery requires adaptation when working with neuropsychiatric patients, due to their cognitive difficulties.
- Cognitive-behavioral therapy is an evidence-based, goal-focused, short-term approach. It examines and works on the interrelations between thoughts, feelings, and behaviors. Interventions may be classified as cognitive, behavioral, and physiologic. There is wide evidence supporting its use in neuropsychiatric conditions.
- Mindfulness training, particularly when appropriately adapted for specific clinical populations, is not only feasible but also effective in targeting specific symptoms, including depression, anxiety, and fatigue. Initial research demonstrates the potential impact of mindfulness training in brain structures, including increased activation of the insula, anterior cingulate, and prefrontal cortex, and decreased activation of the amygdala.
- Cognitive rehabilitation therapy may follow a holistic model that considers, in addition to cognitive dysfunction, the individual's psychological and awareness factors. It uses compensatory and restorative interventions. Treatment is most useful when individualized, and when the newly learned or improved skills can be transferable to everyday life. Nowadays, technology plays a crucial role in supporting cognitive rehabilitation strategies.

Multiple Choice Questions

1. Clinical case management may include the following interventions:
   a. Encourage patients to complete advance directives
   b. Psychotherapy
   c. Assessment of environmental needs, referring patients to the appropriate systems, and monitoring the fit between patient and systems
   d. a and c
   e. All of the above

2. In addition to standard techniques, which additional components may be included in CBT treatment of someone with MCI or dementia?.
   a. Caregiver/Coach involvement
   b. Use of a notebook with tabbed sections
   c. Use of audio-recordings of sessions or skills used
   d. Environmental modifications such as signage around the house and alarms
   e. All of the above

3. Research on the impact of mindfulness training on brain structure and function shows that:
   a. Mindfulness training may increase activity in the insular cortex.
   b. Mindfulness training may decrease activation in the amygdala and increase activation in prefrontal cortex.
   c. Expert meditators show decreased activity in the default mode network (DMN).
   d. All the above.
   e. Only a and b are correct.

4. Select the correct statement, regarding cognitive rehabilitation therapy (CRT):
   a. Having a clear understanding of a patient's cognitive strengths and deficits and customizing the appropriate, evidence-based CRT interventions to match that cognitive profile, are typically enough to maximize the chances of success of the CRT intervention.
   b. A solid improvement in neuropsychological test performance is the best indicator of CRT success.
   c. Having ecological validity, or in other terms, their applicability to everyday life, is a potential strength of compensatory CRT strategies.
   d. The goal of CBT for ADHD is to change the cognitive distortions present in ADHD.
   e. "Brain exercise" programs via widely available apps offer the same benefits of clinicians-monitored CRT, at a fraction of the cost.

Multiple Choice Answers

1. **Answer: e**
   Clinical case management may include the functions traditionally thought to belong to case management, as well as psychotherapeutic interventions.

2. **Answer: d**
   To enhance psychotherapy's efficacy and the carry-through of interventions discussed in sessions, CBT techniques may need to be modified when working with individuals with MCI or dementia.

3. **Answer: d**
   Increased insular cortex activity appears as one of the most consistent findings following mindfulness interventions, possibly related to the strengthening of networks that are important for moment-to-moment awareness of experience. Mindfulness training also seems to increase prefrontal control over emotional experiences. Lastly, expert meditators are likely to show decreased activity in the DMN, and increased functional connectivity between DMN and anterior cingulate and dorsolateral prefrontal cortex, suggesting an increased cognitive control over the function of the DMN.

4. **Answer: c**
   In addition to the cognitive profile, psychological and awareness factors play a role in the success of CRT interventions. Many researches argue that the success of CRT should be measured by functional outcomes, not just improvement in test performance. Compensatory CRT strategies aim to have ecological validity—helping individuals function better in their everyday life. CBT for ADHD addresses both, cognitive and behavioral challenges in ADHD. The research support for computerized and publicly available cognitive restorative programs is limited, particularly regarding their applicability to everyday functioning.

References

1. Coenen M, Cabello M, Umlauf S, et al. Psychosocial difficulties from the perspective of persons with neuropsychiatric disorders. *Disabil Rehabil.* 2015;18:1-12.
2. Lillo P, Mioshi E, Hodges JR. Caregiver burden in amyotrophic lateral sclerosis is more dependent on patients' behavioral changes than physical disability: a comparative study. *BMC Neurol.* 2012;12:156-162.
3. Figved N, Myhr KM, Larsen JP, Aarsland D. Caregiver burden in multiple sclerosis: the impact of neuropsychiatric symptoms. *J Neurol Neurosurg Psychiatry.* 2007;78(10):1097-1102.
4. D'Amelio M, Terruso V, Palmeri B, et al. Predictors of caregiver burden in partners of patients with Parkinson's disease. *Neurol Sci.* 2009;30(2):171-174.
5. Thommesen B, Aarsland D, Braekhus A, Oksengaard AR, Engedal K, Laake K. The psychosocial burden on spouses of the elderly with stroke, dementia and Parkinson's disease. *Int J Geriatr Psychiatry.* 2002;17(1):78-84.
6. Raggi A, Tasca D, Panerai S, Neri W, Ferri R. The burden of distress and related coping processes in family caregivers of patients with Alzheimer's disease living in the community. *J Neurol Sci.* 2015;358(1-2):77-81.
7. Steele C, Rovner B, Chase GA, Folstein M. Psychiatric symptoms and nursing home placement of patients with Alzheimer's disease. *Am J Psychiatry.* 1990;147(8):1049-1051.
8. Kopetz S, Steele CD, Brandt J, et al. Characteristics and outcomes of dementia residents in an assisted living facility. *Int J Geriatr Psychiatry.* 2000;15(7):586-593.
9. Callahan CM, Boustani MA, Unverzagt FW, et al. Effectiveness of collaborative care for older adults with Alzheimer disease in primary care: a randomized controlled trial. *JAMA.* 2006;295(18):2148-2157.
10. Reilly S, Miranda-Castillo C, Malouf R, et al. Case management approaches to home support for people with dementia. *Cochrane*

Database Syst Rev. 2015;1:CD008345. doi:10.1002/14651858. CD008345.pub2.

11. Kanter J. Clinical case management: definition, principles, components. *Hosp Community Psychiatry.* 1989;40(4):361-368.

12. Kanter J. Clinical case management. In: Brandell J, ed. *Theory and Practice of Clinical Social Work.* New York, NY: Columbia University Press; 2010:chap 20.

13. Alzheimer's Association: 2018 Alzheimer's Disease Facts and Figures. *Alzheimers Dement.* 2018;14(3):367-429. Available at https://www.alz.org/documents_custom/2018-facts-and-figures. pdf.

14. Kales HC, Gitlin LN, Lyketsos CG. Management of neuropsychiatric symptoms of dementia in clinical settings: recommendations from a multidisciplinary expert panel. *J Am Geriatr Soc.* 2014;62(4):762-769.

15. Pollock BG, Mulsant BH, Rosen J, et al. A double-blind comparison of citalopram and risperidone for the treatment of behavioral and psychotic symptoms associated with dementia. *Am J Geriatr Psychiatry.* 2007;15:942-942.

16. Johnson DK, Niedens M, Wilson JR, Swartzendruber L, Yeager A, Jones K. Treatment outcomes of a crisis intervention program for dementia with severe psychiatric complications: the Kansas bridge project. *Gerontologist.* 2013;53(1):102-112.

17. Thyrian JR, Hertel J, Wucherer D, et al. Effectiveness and safety of dementia care management in primary care: a randomized clinical trial. *JAMA Psychiatry.* 2017;74(10):996-1004.

18. Corvol A, Dreier A, Prudhomm J, Thyrian JR, Hoffmann W, Somme D. Consequences of clinical case management for caregivers: a systematic review. *Int J Geriatr Psychiatry.* 2017;32(5):473-483.

19. Werner P, Karnieli-Miller O, Eidelman S. Current knowledge and future directions about the disclosure of dementia: a systematic review of the first decade of the 21st century. *Alzheimers Dement.* 2013;9(2):74-88.

20. Somme D, Trouve H, Dramé M, Gagnon D, Couturier Y, Saint-Jean O. Analysis of case management programs for patients with dementia: a systematic review. *Alzheimers Dement.* 2012;8(5):426-436.

21. Hickam DH, Weiss JW, Guise J-M, et al. Outpatient Case management for adults with medical illness and complex care needs. *Comparative Effectiveness Review.* No. 99. (Prepared by the Oregon Evidence-based Practice Center under Contract No. 290-2007-10057-I.) AHRQ Publication No.13-EHC031-EF. Rockville, MD: Agency for Healthcare Research and Quality; January 2013. Available at www.effectivehealthcare.ahrq.gov/reports/final.cfm.

22. Prince M, Comas-Herrera A, Knapp M, Guerchet M, Karagiannidou M. *World Alzheimer Report 2016: Improving Healthcare for People Living with Dementia: Coverage, Quality and Costs Now and in the Future.* London, UK: Alzheimer's Disease International (ADI). Available at https://www.alz.co.uk/research/WorldAlzheimerReport2016.pdf 2007.

23. Mittelman MS, Haley WE, Clay OJ, Roth DL. Improving caregiver well-being delays nursing home placement of patients with Alzheimer disease. *Neurology.* 2006;67(9):1592-1599.

24. Samus Q, Johnston D, Black B, et al. A multidimensional home-based care coordination intervention for elders with memory disorders: the Maximizing Independence at Home (MIND) Pilot Randomized Trial. *Am J Geriatr Psychiatry.* 2014;22(4):398-414.

25. Ecklund-Johnson E, Torres I. Unawareness of deficits in Alzheimer's disease and other dementias: operational definitions and empirical findings. *Neuropsychol Rev.* 2005;15(3):147-166.

26. Traeger LN, Greer JA. Cognitive behavioral therapies. In: Fogel BS, Greenberg DB, eds. *Psychiatric Care of the Medical Patient.* Oxford, UK: Oxford University Press; 2015:chap 14.

27. Gore-Felton C, Spiegel D. Group psychotherapy for medically ill populations. In: Fogel BS, Greenberg DB, eds. *Psychiatric Care of the Medical Patient.* Oxford, UK: Oxford University Press; 2015:chap 13.

28. Keitner GI. Family therapy in chronic medical illness. In: Fogel BS, Greenberg DB, eds. *Psychiatric Care of the Medical Patient.* Oxford, UK: Oxford University Press; 2015:chap 11.

29. Green SA. Psychotherapeutic principles and techniques. In: Fogel BS, Greenberg DB, eds. *Psychiatric Care of the Medical Patient.* Oxford, UK: Oxford University Press; 2015:chap 10.

30. Alexopoulos GS, Raue P, Areán P. Problem-solving therapy versus supportive therapy in geriatric major depression with executive dysfunction. *Am J Geriatr Psychiatry.* 2003;11:46-52.

31. Areán PA, Raue P, Mackin RS, Kanellopoulos D, McCulloch C, Alexopoulos GS. Problem-solving therapy and supportive therapy in older adults with major depression and executive dysfunction. *Am J Psychiatry.* 2010;167:1391-1398.

32. Lynch TR, Smoski MJ. Individual and group psychotherapy. In: Blazer DG, Steffens DC, eds. *The American Psychiatric Publishing Textbook of Geriatric Psychiatry.* Arlington, VA: American Psychiatric Publishing; 2009:chap 29.

33. Fernie BA, Kollmann J, Brown RG. Cognitive behavioral interventions for depression in chronic neurological conditions: a systemic review. *J Psychosom Res.* 2015;78:411-419.

34. Orgeta V, Qazi A, Spector AE, Orrell M. Psychological treatments for depression and anxiety in dementia and mild cognitive impairment. *Cochrane Database Syst Rev.* 2014;1:1-59.

35. Regan B, Varanelli L. Adjustment, depression, and anxiety in mild cognitive impairment and early dementia: a systematic review of psychological intervention studies. *Int Psychogeriatr.* 2013;25(12):1963-1984.

36. Alexopoulos GS, Raue PJ, Kiosses DN, et al. Problem-solving therapy and supportive therapy in older adults with major depression and executive dysfunction: effect on disability. *Arch Gen Psychiatry.* 2011;68:33-41.

37. Teri L, Logsdon RG, Uomoto J, McCurry SM. Behavioral treatment of depression in dementia patients: a controlled clinical trial. *J Gerontol B Psychol Sci Soc Sci.* 1997;52:159-166.

38. Marriott A, Donaldson C, Tarrier N, Burns A. Effectiveness of cognitive-behavioural family intervention in reducing the burden of care in carers of patients with Alzheimer's disease. *Br J Psychiatry.* 2000;176:557-562.

39. Beck AT, Ruch AJ, Shaw BF, et al. *Cognitive Therapy of Depression.* New York, NY: The Guilford Press; 1979.

40. Skinner BF. *About Behaviorism.* New York, NY: Vintage; 1974.

41. Burns DD. *Feeling Good: The New Mood Therapy.* New York, NY: Penguin Books; 1991.

42. Beck JS. *Cognitive Behavior Therapy: Basics and Beyond.* 2nd ed. New York, NY: Guilford Press; 2011.

43. Wang K, Varma DS, Prosperi M. A systematic review of the effectiveness of mobile apps for monitoring and management of mental health symptoms or disorders. *J Psychiatr Res.* 2018;107:73-78.

44. Franklin G, Carson AJ, Welch KA. Cognitive behavioural therapy for depression: systematic review of imaging studies. *Acta Neuropsychiatr.* 2016;28(2):61-74.

45. Yang Y, Kircher T, Straube B. The neural correlates of cognitive behavioral therapy: recent progress in the investigation of patients with panic disorder. *Behav Res Ther.* 2014;62:88-96.

46. Hort J, O'Brien JT, Gainotti G, et al. EFNS guidelines for the diagnosis and management of Alzheimer's disease. *Eur J Neurol.* 2010;17(10):1236-1248.

47. Potter GG, Steffens DC. Contribution of depression to cognitive impairment and dementia in older adults. *Neurologist.* 2007;13(3):105-117.

48. Mah L, Binns MA, Steffens DC; the Alzheimer's Disease Neuroimaging Initiative. Anxiety symptoms in amnestic mild cognitive impairment are associated with medial temporal atrophy and predict conversion to Alzheimer's disease. *Am J Geriatr Psychiatry.* 2015;23(5):466-476.

49. Buchanan TA, Christenson A, Houlihan D, et al. The role of behavior analysis in rehabilitation of persons with dementia. *Behav Ther.* 2011;42:9-21.

50. Salzman C, Jeste D, Meyer R. Elderly patients with dementia-related symptoms of severe agitation and aggression: consensus statement on treatment options, clinical trials methodology, and policy. *J Clin Psychiatry.* 2008;9(6):889-898.

51. James IA. *Cognitive Behavioural Therapy with Older People: Interventions for Those With and Without Dementia.* London, UK: Jessica Kingsley Publishers; 2010.

52. Stanley MA, Calleo J, Bush AK, et al. The peaceful mind program: a pilot test of a cognitive-behavioral therapy-based intervention for anxious patients with dementia. *Am J Geriatr Psychiatry.* 2013;21:696-708.

53. Charlesworth G, Sadek S, Schepers A, et al. Cognitive behavior therapy for anxiety in people with dementia: a clinician guideline for a person-centered approach. *Behav Modif.* 2015;39(3):390-412.

54. Spector A, Charlesworth G, King M, et al. Cognitive behaviour therapy (CBT) for anxiety in people with dementia: a pilot randomised controlled trial. *Br J Psychiatry.* 2015;206(6):509-516.

55. Mohlman J, Gorenstein EE, Kleber M, et al. Standard and enhanced cognitive–behavioral therapy for late-life generalized anxiety disorder. *Am J Geriatr Psychiatry.* 2003;11:24-32.

56. Paukert AL, Kraus-Schuman C, Wilson N, et al. The Peaceful Mind manual: a protocol for treating anxiety in person with dementia. *Behav Modif.* 2013;37:631-664.

57. Lewinsohn PM. A behavioral approach to depression. In: Friedman RJ, Katz MM, eds. *Psychology of Depression: Contemporary Theory and Research.* Oxford, England: Wiley; 1974:157-178.

58. Martell CR, Addis ME, Jacobson NS. *Depression in Context: Strategies for Guided Action.* New York, NY: Norton; 2001.

59. Camp CJ, Stevens AB. Spaced-retrieval: a memory intervention for dementia of the Alzheimer's type (DAT). *Clin Gerontol.* 1990;10:658-661.

60. Bourgeois MS, Hickey EM. *Dementia: From Diagnosis to Management: A Functional Approach.* New York, NY: Psychology Press; 2009.

61. Hopper T, Mahendra N, Kim E, et al. Evidence-based practice recommendations for working with individuals with dementia: spaced-retrieval training. *J Med Speech Lang Pathol.* 2005;13(4).

62. Kabat-Zinn J. An outpatient program in behavioral medicine for chronic pain patients based on the practice of mindfulness meditation: theoretical considerations and preliminary results. *Gen Hosp Psychiatry.* 1982;4(1):33-47.

63. American Mindfulness Research Association. Available at http://www.goAMRA.org. 2017.

64. Jha A, Stanley EA, Kiyonaga A, et al. Examining the protective effects of mindfulness training on working memory capacity and affective experience. *Emotion.* 2010;10(1):54-64.

65. Garland E, et al. Mindfulness training promotes upward spirals of positive affect and cognition: multilevel and autoregressive latent trajectory modeling analyses. *Front Psychol.* 2015;6:15.

66. Chambers R, et al. Mindful emotion regulation: an integrative review. *Clin Psychol Rev.* 2009;29(6):560-572.

67. Chiesa A, et al. Mindfulness: top-down or bottom-up emotion regulation strategy? *Clin Psychol Rev.* 2013;33(1):82-96.

68. Pace T, et al. Effect of compassion meditation on neuroendocrine, innate immune and behavioral responses to psychosocial stress. *Psychoneuroendocrinology.* 2009;34(1):87-98.

69. Black, et al. Mindfulness meditation and the immune system: a systematic review of randomized controlled trials. *Ann N Y Acad Sci.* 2016;1373(1):13-24.

70. Tang, et al. Short-term meditation training improves attention and self-regulation. *Proc Natl Acad Sci U S A.* 2007;104(43):17152-17156.

71. Jha A, et al. Mindfulness training modifies subsystems of attention. *Cogn Affect Behav Neurosci.* 2007;7(2):109-119.

72. Mrazek M, et al. Mindfulness training improves working memory capacity and GRE performance while reducing mind wandering. *Psychol Sci.* 2013;24(5):776-781.

73. Kabat-Zinn J, et al. The clinical use of mindfulness meditation for the self-regulation of chronic pain. *J Behav Med.* 1985;8(2):163-190.

74. Grossman P, et al. Mindfulness-based stress reduction and health benefits. A meta-analysis. *J Psychosom Res.* 2004;57(1):35-43.

75. Epel E, et al. Can meditation slow rate of cellular aging? Cognitive stress, mindfulness, and telomeres. *Ann N Y Acad Sci.* 2009;1172:34-53.

76. Creswell J, et al. Mindfulness-based stress reduction training reduces loneliness and pro-inflammatory gene expression in older adults: a small randomized controlled trial. *Brain Behav Immun.* 2012;26(7):1095-1101.

77. Young KS, et al. The impact of mindfulness-based interventions on brain activity: a systematic review of functional magnetic resonance imaging studies. *Neurosci Biobehav Rev.* 2018;84:424-433.

78. Lazar SW, et al. Meditation experience is associated with increased cortical thickness. *NeuroReport.* 2005;16:1893-1897.

79. Hölzel BK, et al. Neural mechanisms of symptom improvements in generalized anxiety disorder following mindfulness training. *Neuroimage Clin.* 2013;2:448-458.

80. Brewer JA, et al. Meditation experience is associated with differences in default mode network activity and connectivity. *Proc Natl Acad Sci U S A.* 2011;108(50):20254-20259.

81. Bédard M, et al. Mindfulness-based cognitive therapy reduces symptoms of depression in people with a traumatic brain injury: results from a randomized controlled trial. *J Head Trauma Rehabil.* 2013;29(4):E13-E22.

82. Tang V, Poon WS, Kwan P. Mindfulness-based therapy for drug-resistant epilepsy: an assessor-blinded randomized trial. *Neurology.* 2015;85:1100-1107.

83. Ulrichsen K, et al. Clinical utility of mindfulness training in the treatment of fatigue after stroke, TBI, and MS: a systematic literature review and meta-analysis. *Front Psychol.* 2016;7:9-12.

84. Diller L. A model for cognitive retraining in rehabilitation. *Clinical Psychologist.* 1976;29(2):13-15.

85. Ben-Yishay Y. *Working Approaches to Remediation of Cognitive Deficits in Brain Damaged Persons.* New York, NY: New York University Medical Center; 1978.

86. Prigatano GP. *Neuropsychological Rehabilitation After Brain Injury.* Baltimore, MD: Johns Hopkins University Press; 1986.

87. Cicerone KD, Langenbahn DM, Braden C, et al. Evidence-based cognitive rehabilitation: updated review of the literature from 2003 through 2008. *Arch Phys Med Rehabil.* 2011;92(4):519-530.

88. Cappa SF, Benke T, Clarke S, et al. EFNS guidelines on cognitive rehabilitation: report of an EFNS task force. *Eur J Neurol.* 2003;10(1):11-23.

89. Cappa SF, Benke T, Clarke S, et al. EFNS guidelines on cognitive rehabilitation: report of an EFNS task force. *Eur J Neurol.* 2005;12(9):665-680.

90. Sohlberg MM, Mateer CA. *Cognitive Rehabilitation: An Integrated Neuropsychological Approach.* New York, NY: Guilford Publication; 2001.

91. Wilson B. *Memory Rehabilitation Integrating Theory and Practice.* New York, NY: Guilford Press; 2009.

92. Bogdanova Y, et al. Computerized cognitive rehabilitation of attention and executive function in acquired brain injury: a systematic review. *J Head Trauma Rehabil.* 2016;31(6):419-433.

93. Powell LE, Wild MR, Glang A, et al. The development and evaluation of a web-based programme to support problem-solving skills following brain injury. *Disabil Rehabil Assist Technol.* 2019;14(1):21-32.

94. Virk S, Williams T, Brunsdon R, Suh F, Morrow A. Cognitive remediation of attention deficits following acquired brain injury: a systematic review and meta-analysis. *NeuroRehabilitation.* 2015;36(3):367-377.

95. Tate R, Kennedy M, Ponsford J, et al. INCOG recommendations for management of cognition following traumatic brain injury, part III: executive function and self-awareness. *J Head Trauma Rehabil.* 2014;29(4):338-352.

96. Togher L, Wiseman-hakes C, Douglas J, et al. INCOG recommendations for management of cognition following traumatic brain injury, part IV: cognitive communication. *J Head Trauma Rehabil.* 2014;29(4):353-368.

97. Belleville S, Hudon C, Bier N, et al. MEMO+: efficacy, durability and effect of cognitive training and psychosocial intervention in individuals with mild cognitive impairment. *J Am Geriatr Soc.* 2018;66(4):655-663.

98. Chandler MJ, Parks AC, Marsiske M, Rotblatt LJ, Smith GE. Everyday impact of cognitive interventions in mild cognitive impairment: a systematic review and meta-analysis. *Neuropsychol Rev.* 2016;26(3):225-251.

99. Clare L, Linden DE, Woods RT, et al. Goal-oriented cognitive rehabilitation for people with early-stage Alzheimer disease: a single-blind randomized controlled trial of clinical efficacy. *Am J Geriatr Psychiatry.* 2010;18(10):928-939.

100. Clare L, Bayer A, Burns A, et al. Goal-oriented cognitive rehabilitation in early-stage dementia: study protocol for a multi-centre single-blind randomised controlled trial (GREAT). *Trials.* 2013;14:152.

101. Cotelli M, Manenti R, Zanetti O, Miniussi C. Non-pharmacological intervention for memory decline. *Front Hum Neurosci.* 2012;6:46.

102. Hampstead BM, Gillis MM, Stringer AY. Cognitive rehabilitation of memory for mild cognitive impairment: a methodological review and model for future research. *J Int Neuropsychol Soc.* 2014;20(2):135-151.

103. Huckans M, Hutson L, Twamley E, Jak A, Kaye J, Storzbach D. Efficacy of cognitive rehabilitation therapies for mild cognitive impairment (MCI) in older adults: working toward a theoretical model and evidence-based interventions. *Neuropsychol Rev.* 2013;23(1):63-80.

104. Jean L, Bergeron ME, Thivierge S, Simard M. Cognitive intervention programs for individuals with mild cognitive impairment: systematic review of the literature. *Am J Geriatr Psychiatry.* 2010;18(4):281-296.

105. Reijnders J, Van Heugten C, Van Boxtel M. Cognitive interventions in healthy older adults and people with mild cognitive impairment: a systematic review. *Ageing Res Rev.* 2013;12(1):263-275.

106. Simon SS, Yokomizo JE, Bottino CM. Cognitive intervention in amnestic Mild Cognitive Impairment: a systematic review. *Neurosci Biobehav Rev.* 2012;36(4):1163-1178.

107. Stott J, Spector A. A review of the effectiveness of memory interventions in mild cognitive impairment (MCI). *Int Psychogeriatr.* 2011;23(4):526-538.

108. Chung CS, Pollock A, Campbell T, Durward BR, Hagen S. Cognitive rehabilitation for executive dysfunction in adults with stroke or other adult non-progressive acquired brain damage. *Cochrane Database Syst Rev.* 2013;(4):CD008391.

109. Gillespie DC, Bowen A, Chung CS, Cockburn J, Knapp P, Pollock A. Rehabilitation for post-stroke cognitive impairment: an overview of recommendations arising from systematic reviews of current evidence. *Clin Rehabil.* 2015;29(2):120-128.

110. Lockwood C. Cognitive rehabilitation for memory deficits after stroke: a Cochrane review summary. *Int J Nurs Stud.* 2017;76:131-132.

111. Ernst A, Blanc F, De seze J, Manning L. Using mental visual imagery to improve autobiographical memory and episodic future thinking in relapsing-remitting multiple sclerosis patients: a randomized-controlled trial study. *Restor Neurol Neurosci.* 2015;33(5):621-638.

112. Goverover Y, Chiaravalloti ND, O'brien AR, Deluca J. Evidenced-based cognitive rehabilitation for persons with multiple sclerosis: an updated review of the literature from 2007 to 2016. *Arch Phys Med Rehabil.* 2018;99(2):390-407.

113. Mitolo M, Venneri A, Wilkinson ID, Sharrack B. Cognitive rehabilitation in multiple sclerosis: a systematic review. *J Neurol Sci.* 2015;354(1-2):1-9.

114. Alzahrani H, Venneri A. Cognitive rehabilitation in Parkinson's disease: a systematic review. *J Parkinsons Dis.* 2018;8(2):233-245.

115. Cerasa A, Quattrone A. The effectiveness of cognitive treatment in patients with Parkinson's disease: a new phase for the neuropsychological rehabilitation. *Parkinsonism Relat Disord.* 2015;21(2):165.

116. Hindle JV, Petrelli A, Clare L, Kalbe E. Nonpharmacological enhancement of cognitive function in Parkinson's disease: a systematic review. *Mov Disord.* 2013;28(8):1034-1049.

117. Strouwen C, Molenaar EA, Keus SH, et al. Protocol for a randomized comparison of integrated versus consecutive dual task practice in Parkinson's disease: the DUALITY trial. *BMC Neurol.* 2014;14:61.

118. Del Felice A, Alderighi M, Martinato M, et al. Memory rehabilitation strategies in nonsurgical temporal lobe epilepsy: a review. *Am J Phys Med Rehabil.* 2017;96(7):506-514.

119. Farina E, Raglio A, Giovagnoli AR. Cognitive rehabilitation in epilepsy: an evidence-based review. *Epilepsy Res.* 2015;109:210-218.

120. Geraldi CV, Escorsi-Rosset S, Thompson P, Silva ACG, Sakamoto AC. Potential role of a cognitive rehabilitation program following left temporal lobe epilepsy surgery. *Arq Neuropsiquiatr.* 2017;75(6):359-365.

121. Koorenhof L, Baxendale S, Smith N, Thompson P. Memory rehabilitation and brain training for surgical temporal lobe epilepsy patients: a preliminary report. *Seizure.* 2012;21(3):178-182.

122. Maschio M, Dinapoli L, Fabi A, Giannarelli D, Cantelmi T. Cognitive rehabilitation training in patients with brain

tumor-related epilepsy and cognitive deficits: a pilot study. *J Neurooncol.* 2015;125(2):419-426.

123. Murthy NV, Mahncke H, Wexler BE, et al. Computerized cognitive remediation training for schizophrenia: an open label, multi-site, multinational methodology study. *Schizophr Res.* 2012;139(1-3):87-91.

124. Paquin K, Wilson AL, Cellard C, Lecomte T, Potvin S. A systematic review on improving cognition in schizophrenia: which is the more commonly used type of training, practice or strategy learning? *BMC Psychiatry.* 2014;14:139.

125. Kluwe-schiavon B, Viola TW, Levandowski ML, et al. A systematic review of cognitive rehabilitation for bipolar disorder. *Trends Psychiatry Psychother.* 2015;37(4):194-201.

126. Priyamvada R, Ranjan R, Chaudhury S. Cognitive rehabilitation of attention and memory in depression. *Ind Psychiatry J.* 2015;24(1):48-53.

127. Choi J, Twamley EW. Cognitive rehabilitation therapies for Alzheimer's disease: a review of methods to improve treatment engagement and self-efficacy. *Neuropsychol Rev.* 2013;23(1):48-62.

128. Cicerone KD, Azulay J, Trott C. Methodological quality of research on cognitive rehabilitation after traumatic brain injury. *Arch Phys Med Rehabil.* 2009;90(11 suppl):S52-S59.

129. Safren SA, Sprich S, Perlman C, Otto M. *Mastering Your Adult ADHD: A Cognitive-Behavioral Treatment Program (Client Workbook).* New York, NY: Oxford University Press; 2005.

130. Levine B, Schweizer TA, O'connor C, et al. Rehabilitation of executive functioning in patients with frontal lobe brain damage with goal management training. *Front Hum Neurosci.* 2011;5:9.

131. Eskin M. *Problem Solving Therapy in Clinical Practice.* London/Waltham, MA: Elsevier; 2012.

132. Greenaway MC, Duncan NL, Smith GE. The memory support system for mild cognitive impairment: randomized trial of a cognitive rehabilitation intervention. *Int J Geriatr Psychiatry.* 2013;28(4):402-409.

133. Stringer AY. *Ecologically Oriented Neurorehabilitation of Memory (EON-MEM).* Los Angeles, CA: Western Psychological Services; 2007.

134. O'Neil-Pirozzi TM, Kennedy MR, Sohlberg MM. Evidence-based practice for the use of internal strategies as a memory compensation technique after brain injury: a systematic review. *J Head Trauma Rehabil.* 2016;31(4):E1-E11.

135. Mahncke HW, Bronstone A, Merzenich MM. Brain plasticity and functional losses in the aged: scientific bases for a novel intervention. *Prog Brain Res.* 2006;157:81-109.

136. Rebok GW, Ball K, Guey LT, et al. Ten-year effects of the advanced cognitive training for independent and vital elderly cognitive training trial on cognition and everyday functioning in older adults. *J Am Geriatr Soc.* 2014;62(1):16-24.

137. Edwards JD, Xu H, Clark DO, et al. Speed of processing training results in lower risk of dementia. *Alzheimers Dement.* 2017;3(4):603-611.

Neuropsychiatric Syndromes and Disorders

IV

Part A. Neurobehavioral and Neuropsychiatric Syndromes and Disorders

Mood, Psychotic, Anxiety, and Obsessive-Compulsive Disorders: A Neuropsychiatric Foundation

11

Renana Eitan · David A. Silbersweig

INTRODUCTION

Contemporary neuropsychiatry conceptualizes mental illnesses as brain disorders. In contrast to neurological disorders with identifiable lesions, mental disorders can be addressed as disorders of brain circuits. The view of mental disorders as brain circuit disorders has been further consolidated by reports on successful treatment of mental disorders with focal brain interventions. However, mental illnesses not only originate from dysfunction of different brain areas but also represent a much more complex multidimensional organization of information in the brain. The basic biological science behind some of the fundamental elements of mental illness, such as cognition, emotion, behavior, and social processes, has been advancing rapidly in the past 20 years. New scientific methods for studying the brain include structural and functional imaging of distinct neural circuit elements and connections. Genetic techniques have identified risk factors for mental illness. Novel analytic techniques such as neural networks, a biologically inspired programming paradigm which enables learning from observational data, have partially revealed the basic neural mechanisms underlying mental illness.[1] However, clinical research supporting the classification system in psychiatry has not kept up with these scientific advances.[2,3] Psychiatric diagnoses are currently distinguished based on sets of specific symptoms as detailed in the *Diagnostic and Statistical Manual of Mental Disorders*, 5th edition (*DSM-5*), released in 2013.[4] In 2009, the National Institute of Mental Health (NIMH) launched the research domain criteria (RDoC) project to develop, for research purposes, new ways of classifying mental disorders based on dimensions of observable behavior and neurobiological measures.[5] Integration of clinical experience with the rapid advancing neurobiological knowledge is essential for every treatment provider in the field of psychiatry and neuropsychiatry.[6]

Genetic, neuroimaging, and clinical analyses find overlap across a wide variety of psychiatric diagnoses, suggesting common neurobiological substrates for mental illness. For example, a morphometry meta-analysis ($n=15,892$ individuals) across six diverse diagnostic groups (schizophrenia, bipolar disorder [BPD], depression, addiction, obsessive-compulsive disorder [OCD], and anxiety) found that gray matter loss converged across diagnoses in three regions: the dorsal anterior cingulate and right and left insula.[7] Interestingly, the common neuroimaging findings in mental illness are related to cognitive functions. For example, abnormal activations in the left prefrontal cortex (PFC) and anterior insula, and the right ventrolateral PFC and intraparietal sulcus, demonstrate a common cognitive pattern of inflexibility across major psychiatric disorders.[8] In most mental illnesses, cognitive impairment has a critical role in determining the total function and quality of life. Therefore, accurate assessment and treatment of the cognitive aspects of mental illness, not just emotional or behavioral symptoms, are an integral and important part of psychiatry.

While most psychiatrists are familiar with the dimensions related to mood, psychosis, or anxiety, it is important that they also know about other dimensions related to cognitive-behavioral and social neuroscience. The role of neuropsychiatry is expanding the field of psychiatry into these new dimensions and can provide advanced approaches to diagnosis, formulation, and treatment.[9] The unique neuropsychiatric clinical skills might help in refining the diagnostic criteria of mental illnesses. Understanding neuroscience can enhance psychiatric approaches to patients and suggest new treatment targets. This chapter describes the neuropsychiatric approach to mood disorders (major depressive disorder [MDD], BPD, and mood disturbances associated with other neurological and medical disorders), psychotic disorders (schizophrenia, and psychotic disorders due to other medical/neurological conditions), anxiety disorders (idiopathic anxiety disorders, and those associated with other medical/neurological conditions), and obsessive-compulsive disorder. The discussion is focused on methods for integration of neuroscientific knowledge and neuropsychiatric skills into psychiatry. Relevant disorders are presented with a special consideration of cognitive aspects of mental illness, highlighting the most recent neurobiological findings related to these disorders and describing other brain disorders that manifest with symptoms of mental illness.

MOOD DISORDERS

Major Depressive Disorder

MDD is a mood disorder typically characterized by low mood, a feeling of sadness, and a general loss of enjoyment and interest in things. It is a debilitating medical illness that affects a person's physical and mental state, and level of functioning.

Epidemiology

The average 12-month and lifetime estimated prevalence of depression is 6% and 20%, respectively. The prevalence and most demographic characteristics of MDD are similar in many counties and cultures, although in high-income countries more patients are diagnosed and treated.[10] The World Health Organization (2018) states that depression is the leading cause of ill health and disability worldwide and estimates that more than 300 million people are now living with MDD, an increase of more than 18% between 2005 and 2015.[11] The burden of depression is further increased by its association with an increased risk of developing conditions such as diabetes mellitus, heart disease, hypertension, stroke, obesity, cancer, cognitive impairment, and Alzheimer's disease (AD).[12,13] Depressed patients are almost 20-fold more likely to die by suicide than the general population.[14]

MDD is an episodic disorder and the mean episode duration varies between 3 and 8 months. Most MDD patients recover over time: 50%, 65%, and 75% of patients recover within 3, 6, and 12 months, respectively.[15] However, among treated and non-treated MDD patients nearly 20% do not recover at 24 months.[15] In more severe and treatment-resistant MDD population, treated in outpatient care settings, the recovery rate is lower. Only 25% of these patients recover within 6 months and more than 50% of patients do not recover at 24 months. About 80% of treated and non-treated MDD patients experience at least one recurrence.

While MDD can develop at any age, the average age of onset is the mid-20s. Increasing age predicts less favorable disease course. Rates of major depression are two-fold higher for women than men, whereas for bipolar depression the sex ratios are nearly equal.[16,17] The causes of the gender difference in the prevalence of major depression include psychological or social factors, such as gender differences regarding occupation, negative life events, and role expectations.[18] Some data suggest that matching social role variables such as marital status, children, and occupational status between women and men, reduces the female excess by about 50%. Nevertheless, biological differences may be crucial. For example, hormonal etiologies of depression may be associated with the luteal phase of the menstrual cycle, the postpartum period, menopause, and oral contraceptives.

Environmental and social factors are associated with risk of depression. These factors are called the "social determinants" of depression and include socioeconomic status or events (e.g., poverty, unemployment, war, migration, discrimination, negative life events), ethnicity (even when controlling for other demographic characteristics[19]), lifestyle factors (such as diet, exercise, and sleep[20]), and substance use (alcohol use, drug abuse, etc.). In addition, chronic depression can cause a "social drift" (movement down the social scale) including interpersonal dysfunction and work and family problems. Some of the discussed social factors and depression could be related to a third risk factor such as genetic vulnerability or brain function. However, in a recent large study, the association between lower educational attainment and risk for depression was not found to reflect a measurable genetic effect but was mostly related to socioeconomic status.[21]

Pathophysiology of Depression

Despite major advances in research of the pathophysiology of depression, no single model can explain the mechanism of depression. The heterogeneity of major depression as presented by variable symptoms, course of illness, and treatment response is a major obstacle to understanding the pathophysiology of depression. Here we summarize our current understanding of the neurobiology of MDD. Figure 11-1 summarizes the pathophysiology of depression.

Environmental Factors and Stress

The risk for major depression increases with stress exposure, but stressful life events are probably not necessary or sufficient to cause major depression.[22] The brain has a major role in regulation of stress by perceiving the threats, evaluating threatening situations, and activating behavioral and physiological responses. Stress is mediated by cortisol, epinephrine, the sympathetic nervous system, pro- and anti-inflammatory cytokines, and other metabolic hormones. While in most individuals acute or chronic stress is adaptive and promotes resilience, in susceptible individuals stress-related responses might become maladaptive and cause depression. Major depression can be divided into reactive depression (i.e., a stress-responsive subtype) and endogenous depression (i.e., no apparent environmental precipitants), and it can present as a combination of the two. Not only adult stressful life events increase the risk for depression but also childhood events such as physical and sexual abuse, psychological abuse and neglect, exposure to domestic violence, or early separation from parents. In utero stress has also been shown to increase the risk of MDD later in life.[23] Adulthood and childhood stressful life events account for 10–12% of the phenotypic variance in major depression.[24] The genetic basis for major depression is different in stress exposed and unexposed groups.[24] Recent evidence suggests that childhood maltreatment changes trajectories of brain development to affect sensory systems, network architecture and circuits involved in threat detection, cortisol stress reactivity, emotional regulation, and reward anticipation.[25]

Neuroendocrinology

The hypothalamic-pituitary-adrenal (HPA) axis that regulates the secretion of corticotropin-releasing factor (CRF) and glucocorticoids is central to the stress response and is found to be disrupted in depression.[26] Steroid and other metabolic hormone receptors are expressed in most brain regions, mediate the communication between the brain and body via hormonal

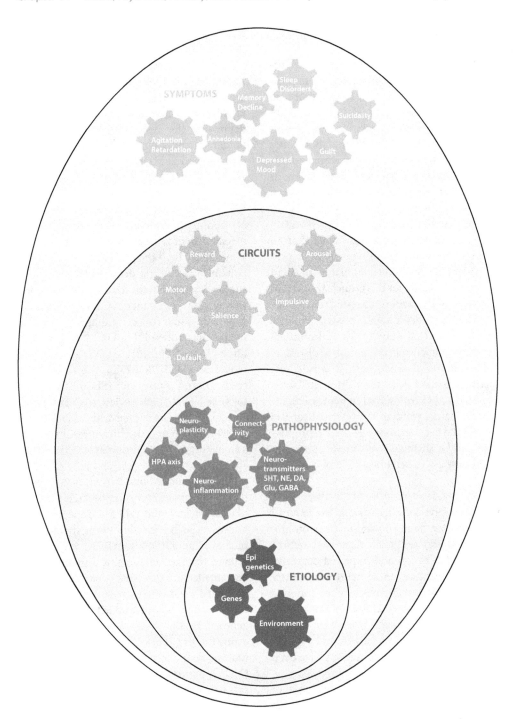

FIGURE 11-1. From etiology to pathophysiology, neuronal circuits, and symptoms of mood disorders.

and neural pathways, and activate cellular and molecular mechanisms for brain plasticity.[27] Changes in the HPA axis in depressed patients are correlated with more severe symptoms, melancholic and psychotic features, older age, higher recurrent risk, as well as with cognitive deficits in depression. Cognitive deficits, especially those closely related to hippocampus function, were found to be related to cortisol secretion in depressed patients.[28] The association between cortisol measures and cognitive performance (such as visual memory, processing speed, and executive function) exists also in MDD patients in

remission.[29] The gene encoding for corticotropin-releasing factor receptor type 1 (CRHR1) has been associated with cognitive features of depression including difficulty with decision making, higher rumination, and poorer learning and memory.[30] Similarly, the corticotropin-releasing hormone binding protein (CRHBP) gene has a role in predicting which patients will improve with antidepressants and which type of antidepressant may be most effective.[31] Neuroendocrine-based interventions to treat depression, such as anti-glucocorticoids, have yielded mixed results.[32] Stimulation of the mineralocorticoid receptors can decrease cortisol secretion and improve memory performance in depressed patients.[33]

Other neuropeptides such as the thyroid hormones and prolactin[34] are also closely related to the pathophysiology of depression (for review, see Kormos and Gaszner[35]). Hypothyroidism increases the risk for depression and thyroid hormones can augment antidepressants effects and cognitive functions.[36] Enhancement of antidepressant action by thyroid hormones may be related to their effect of increasing hippocampal neurogenesis.[37] Genetic variants of thyroid hormone transporters or of deiodinases I and II (i.e., enzymes involved in the activation or deactivation of thyroid hormones) may increase the risk to depression and influence the effectiveness of antidepressants.[38] The incidence of depression in women is much higher than in men. The excess of depression is greater during women's reproductive lives and the incident of depression is similar in men and women after menopause.[39] The reason for this is unclear, and is as likely to be social as biological. It has been suggested that female susceptibility may be linked to surges in reproductive hormones (estrogen and progesterone) during puberty. These hormonal changes might explain other women-related depressive disorders such as premenstrual dysphoric disorder, postpartum depression disorder, and perimenopausal depression disorder. Levels of estrogen have been reported to be lowered in depressed premenopausal and perimenopausal women. Depressive disorders in women emerge largely during transitions in their reproductive aging cycle, which can be attributed to internal endocrine possesses that affect emotion-associated brain circuits.

Monoamines and Other Neurotransmitter Systems

The monoamine theory of depression suggests that the reduced availability of the monoamine neurotransmitters (serotonin, norepinephrine, and dopamine) results in decreased neurotransmission that leads to depression and impaired cognitive performance.[40] Figure 11-2 illustrates these neurotramsmitter projections. Monoaminergic systems, in particular serotonergic neurotransmission, have been recognized as an important factor in many behavioral symptoms of depression, such as low mood, anhedonia, vigilance, reduced motivation, fatigue, and psychomotor agitation or retardation. Serotonin brain levels have been linked to changes in behavioral and somatic functions (appetite, sleep, sex, and circadian rhythm) with low serotonin levels in post-mortem brains of depressed patients compared to normal population. Dopamine brain levels have been linked to motivation, concentration, decision making, reward, and aggression. Norepinephrine brain levels are also linked to depressive symptoms including reduced libido, appetite, concentration, interest and motivation, as well as increased aggression.

The deficiency of monoamines in the synaptic cleft could occur through the degrading effects of the monoamine oxidases. This is supported by the increased monoamine oxidase enzyme activity in depressed patients and using monoamine oxidase inhibitors (MAOIs) as antidepressants. The serotonin transporter (SERT) is the primary regulator of serotonin levels in the brain and a key target for widely used antidepressant drugs such as selective serotonin reuptake inhibitors (SSRIs). PET studies have revealed that individuals with current MDD have altered level of serotonin receptors 5-HT1A and 5-HT1A

binding potential, especially in the anterior cingulate cortex, the PFC, and in the hippocampus.[41]

Other neurons, such as excitatory glutamate neurons, and inhibitory gamma-aminobutyric acid (GABA) interneurons, are related to atrophy of neurons in cortical and limbic brain regions and changes in connectivity and network function in depression (for review, see Duman et al.[42]). The endogenous opioid system is also involved in the regulation of mood and is dysregulated in MDD (for review, see Pecina et al.[43]).

Genetics

Many researchers have explored the nature of genetic versus environmental influences on depression and the biological mechanism of genes involved in depression. MDD is considered as modestly heritable (30–40%).[44] The odds ratio for increased risk for MDD in first-degree relatives of MDD is of 2.84.[45] Twin studies suggest that the heritability of major depression is 42% in women and 29% in men.[46] Candidate gene studies of MDD have generated some robust findings. Some of these genes include the apolipoprotein E (APOE ε2 and APOE ε4), guanine nucleotide-binding protein (GND3), methylenetetrahydrofolate reductase (MTHFR 677T), dopamine transporter (SLC6A3), the serotonin transporter (SLC6A4), and the dopamine receptor gene (DRD 4) (for review, see Flint and Kendler[47]). Although many large-scale genome-wide association studies (GWAS) for MDD failed to find significant results for genes,[48] most recently a study organized by the genetic testing company, 23andMe, has shown significant findings.[49] Many of the genetic loci found in MDD are enriched for CNS expression and important for CNS development or neurogenesis. Such genes in the European population include the OLFM4 gene (encoding olfactomedin-4, known to be expressed in brain, including in the amygdala and medial temporal lobe), MEF2C (myocyte enhancer factor 2C, known to regulate synaptic function and related to epilepsy and intellectual disability), TMEM161B (transmembrane protein 161B, related to the response to social isolation in a mouse model of depression), and MEIS2 (regulates pathways in neurogenesis). Further analysis of this set of data revealed some interesting findings. For example, a specific variant on chromosome 4 that was found in norepinephrine-dopamine reuptake inhibitor (NDRI, bupropion) responders was also associated with gene sets related to long-term depression, circadian rhythm, and vascular endothelial growth factor (VEGF) pathway.[50] An alternative approach for GWAS is to focus on a more homogeneous genetic background. The CONVERGE study, which focuses on Han Chinese females, has found unique genetic loci in MDD in this specific ethnic population: two loci contributing to the risk of MDD were found on chromosome 10, near the SIRT1 gene and an intron of the LHPP gene.[51,52]

The genetics of depression is probably polygenic and involves many genes with small effects. MDD heterogeneity may imply involvement of different gene clusters in the pathophysiology of specific depression phenotypes. Furthermore, relevant genetic variants may cause an increased risk only in the presence of exposure to stressors and other adverse environmental circumstances ("gene-environment interaction"). Epigenetic mechanisms are associated with the response to stress and trauma exposure and the development of stress-related depression (for

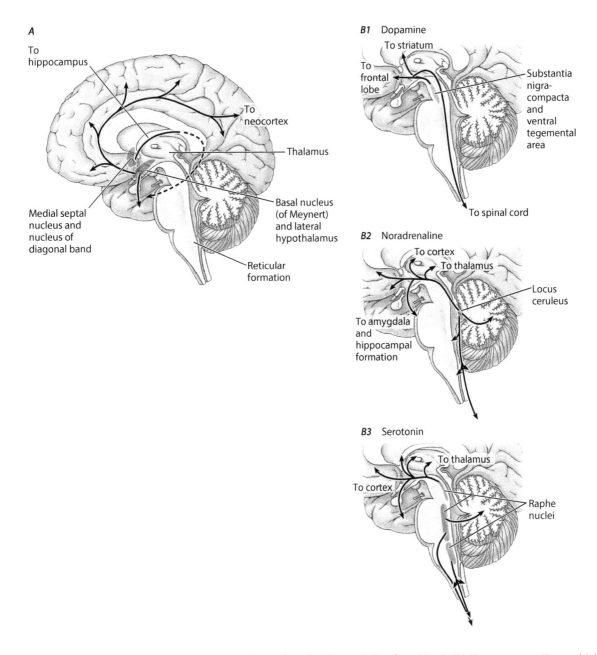

FIGURE 11-2. Illustration of neurotransmitter projections. (Reproduced with permission from Martin JH: *Neuroanatomy Text and Atlas.* 4th ed. http://neurology.mhmedical.com. Copyright © McGraw Hill LLC. All rights reserved.)

review, see Klengel and Binder[53]). In addition to postnatal epigenetic effects of stress, maternal stress during pregnancy can lead to early epigenetic programming of the fetus. For example, prenatal maternal cortisol levels reveal gender-dependent influences. Girls exhibit an adaptive response probably by increasing the neural network connectivity necessary for maintaining homeostasis and efficient brain function across the lifespan.[54] Similarly, an association of preconception parental trauma with epigenetic alterations was found in both exposed parent and offspring, providing potential insight into how a severe psychophysiological trauma can have intergenerational effects.[55]

Neuroimmunology

The neuroinflammatory hypothesis of MDD is supported by animal and human findings. Activation of the immune system causes sickness behaviors such as depressed mood, anhedonia, and weight loss. Inflammatory changes in MDD include peripheral monocyte activation, increased cytokine levels (TNF, IL-1β, and IL-6), reduced NK cell cytotoxicity, and reduced T cell proliferation (for review, see Hodes et al.[56]). The immune system mediates stress events that impact the brain. Peripheral immune functions can influence the CNS by cytokines, infiltration by peripheral immune cells or signaling via the vagus nerve. The immune signals in depression probably affect brain receptor expression in astrocytes, microglia and neurons, as well as brain neurogenesis and plasticity. Most interestingly, direct changes in microglia activity in depression were found using novel PET techniques.[57] Anti-inflammatory treatments, such as nonsteroidal anti-inflammatory drugs (NSAIDs) and cytokine inhibitors, decrease depressive symptoms.[58]

Neuroplasticity

Adult neurogenesis, the lifelong addition of new neurons, occurs in several different species including humans. The newly generated cells can mature into functional neurons. Upregulation of neurogenesis occurs in response to enriched environment, exercise, and learning, while downregulation occurs in response to aging and stress. Neurogenesis occurs mainly in the subgranular zone of the dentate gyrus of the hippocampus, from which the cells migrate to the granular zone. Reduction in hippocampal neurogenesis is hypothesized to contribute to the development of depression. It is well established that the volume of the hippocampus is decreased in patients suffering from depression. This reduction in hippocampal volume observed in depression might be related to hippocampal cell loss. In depressed patients, lower levels of factors that modulate neurogenesis, such as brain-derived neurotrophic factor (BDNF), can be found.

Neurocircuits in Depression

Depression is not a pathology in a single brain region or cell type but disrupted cortico-limbic circuits in the forebrain. See Figure 11-3 for an illustration of the limbic association areas. The PFC has been extensively studied in depression patients. Most studies show a reduction in cortical volume in the medial PFC (mPFC) and orbitofrontal cortex (OFC) in depressed individuals.[59,60] Other key network nodes for depression include the subcortical areas connected to the PFC, such as the hippocampus, nucleus accumbens (NAc), and amygdala nuclei. These brain regions are changed by depression and stress at the

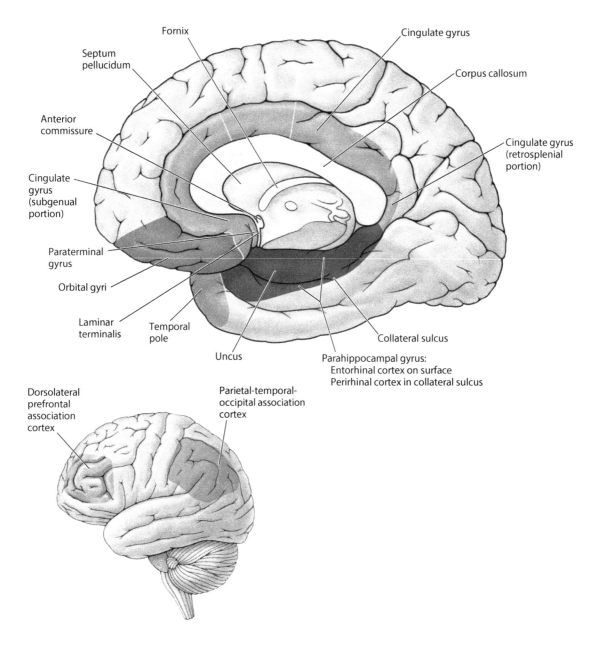

FIGURE 11-3. Illustration of the limbic association areas. (Reproduced with permission from Martin JH: *Neuroanatomy Text and Atlas.* 4th ed. http://neurology.mhmedical.com. Copyright © McGraw Hill LLC. All rights reserved.)

molecular (gene expression), cytoarchitectural (morphological changes to neurons and glia cells), anatomical (morphological changes in tissue volume), and functional levels (blood flow or metabolism). The morphometric cellular changes in specific brain areas in depression include mainly cell loss (hippocampus, subgenual PFC), cell atrophy (dorsolateral PFC and OFC), but also increased numbers of cells in other brain areas (hypothalamus, dorsal raphe nucleus).[61] The underlying mechanism of cellular changes in depression is probably related to neuroplasticity and cellular resilience.[62]

Many studies comparing depression patients to healthy individuals report atrophy of the hippocampus as well as hypoactivity of the dorsolateral PFC and hyperactivity of the subcallosal cingulate cortex, amygdala, and insula.[63] However, these imaging findings are not used as diagnostic biomarkers for depression since they have failed to differentiate between depressed and healthy subjects. Influence on these brain regions by antidepressants, behavioral treatments, or neuromodulation can change the emotion-related behaviors. Depression and its treatments not only change each brain region but also the reciprocal communication, connectivity, within the neural networks. Most recently, imaging genetics consortia such as the ENIGMA project allow researchers to study the association between specific genetic variants and magnetic resonance imaging (MRI)-based measures of brain structure. For example, specific genetic architecture in a subgroup of depression patients is correlated to both changes in hippocampal volume and clinical depressive symptoms.[64]

Animal and human studies suggest that depression is associated with disruption of specific neural circuitry: reward circuit, salience circuit, default mode network and frontoparietal cognitive control circuit.

The reward system normally aims at achieving the maximal reward that ensures our survival with optimization of independent gain and cost functions.[65] The reward circuitry makes rapid optimal tradeoffs between exploratory and definitive behaviors as well as long-term learning of optimal behavioral policy. The most characterized reward circuit is part of the ventral striatum (VS) and basal ganglia, where several cortical and subcortical loop projections interact with internal reentry loops. This complex network is ideally designed for selecting and inhibiting simultaneously occurring events of cognitive and emotional signals.[66] For example, the ventral tegmental area (VTA) dopaminergic neurons innervate the NAc as well as the PFC, amygdala, and hippocampus. The reward circuitry probably contributes to depressive symptoms by reducing responses to rewarding experiences and exaggerating responses to aversive experiences. Combined with maladaptive cognitive style, these changes can change the perception and interpretation of reward valence, the motivation for reward, and the decision-making process.[67] Anhedonia might be caused by the loss of sensitivity to reward stimuli.[68]

The salience circuit is related to the reward circuit. The salience system aims at guiding motivated behavior that is related to emotional or cognitive stimuli. This circuit detects salient changes in the environment and signals the need for additional processing and initiation of appropriate emotional or cognitive control. This network includes projections between the dorsal cingulate cortex, anterior insula, VS, and amygdala. One of the most frequent abnormalities in MDD is increased connectivity and heightened activation of the amygdala.[69] The negative affective and salience circuit contributes to depression symptoms by creating a mood-congruent negative bias and an increased maladaptive reaction to threat.

The default mode network is characterized by greater activity during "resting" states, that is, when a person is not focused on the outside world and the brain is at wakeful rest. This network is defined by the connectivity between the anterior medial PFC, posterior cingulate cortex, and angular gyrus observed under task-free conditions. In MDD patients the default network is hyperactivated and hyperconnected.[70,71] This may explain the patients' excessive self-focus, rumination, and cognitive dysfunctions.[72]

The frontoparietal cognitive control circuit is involved in many cognitive processes. MDD is characterized by hypoconnectivity within the frontoparietal network (cognitive control of attention and emotion regulation) and between frontoparietal systems and parietal regions of the dorsal attention network (attending to the external environment).[73]

Clinical Presentation

According to the *DSM-5*,[4] MDD is diagnosed by at least five of the following symptoms: depressed mood (subjective report or observation made by others); diminished interest or pleasure in activities (anhedonia); weight loss or gain; sleep disturbances (insomnia or hypersomnia); psychomotor agitation or retardation; fatigue or lack of energy; feelings of worthlessness or guilt; diminished ability to think or concentrate; recurrent thoughts of death, suicidal ideation, a specific plan for committing suicide or a suicide attempt. Depressive symptoms cause clinically significant distress or impairment in social, occupational, or other important areas of functioning. The impaired functional and symptomatic state lasts for at least 2 weeks and usually a major depressive episode (MDE) lasts for weeks, months, or even years.

Cognitive impairment is one of the diagnostic criteria for depression. Depressed patients describe cognitive deficit as impaired ability to think, remember, concentrate, or make even minor decisions. Objective measures demonstrate moderate cognitive deficits in executive function, memory, and attention as well as a biased attention to negative information in current depressed patients.[74,75] The cognitive deficit usually presents with the first episode of MDD[76] and persists beyond the acute phase of depression. Patients in remission also show moderate deficits in executive function, response inhibition, and attention but only a tendency toward minor deficits in memory.[77] Therefore, cognitive deficits probably represent a core feature of depression that cannot be considered an epiphenomenon that is entirely secondary to symptoms of low mood or lack of motivation. Persisting cognitive impairments are clinically relevant and can contribute to poor quality of life and psychosocial functioning in remitted depressed patients.[78] It is worth noting that although cognitive impairment is not present in every MDD patient, the population attributable prevalence is very high.[79]

Psychotic depression is characterized by delusions and/or hallucinations and is associated with poorer cognitive performance in some specific cognitive domains, such as visual and verbal learning and executive functions.[80] In most patients, the content of delusions and hallucinations is consistent with the typical depressive themes of personal inadequacy, guilt, disease, death, nihilism, or deserved punishment ("mood-congruent psychotic features"). Psychotic features of depression tend to reoccur in subsequent depressive episodes. The risk ratio for a prior or subsequent psychotic episode in patients whose index depressive episode was psychotic compared with those whose index episode was nonpsychotic is 7–10.[81]

Treatment

There are three main treatment options in depression: psychotherapy, pharmacotherapy, and brain stimulation. Mild MDD is usually treated with psychotherapy while moderate-to-severe MDD is treated with a combination of pharmacotherapy and psychotherapy. Brain stimulation techniques are usually reserved to more treatment-resistant MDD patients. Principles of treatment selection for MDD include measurement-based care, priority to both psychiatric and medical comorbidity, identification of depression specifiers (such as melancholy or psychosis), suicide risk assessment, and evaluation of cognitive symptoms.[82]

Psychotherapy and Physical Therapy

The most studied psychotherapy method in MDD is cognitive-behavioral therapy (CBT). MDD patients learn to identify negative, distorted thinking patterns and replace them with more accurate positive thoughts. Other psychotherapy methods include behavioral activation therapy that increases the patient's positive activities and provides a sense of pleasure; psychodynamic therapy that explores emotions, thoughts, and earlier life experiences to challenge pathological patterns; interpersonal therapy that helps patients identify difficulties in relationships and interpersonal conflicts; mindfulness-based therapy that involves regular meditative practice in which the patients learn to accept their challenges. New distance (non-face-to-face) therapy methods include computer-based and telephone-delivered psychotherapy. Patient preference in combination with evidence-based treatments and clinician or system capacity can optimize psychotherapy strategies for improving individual outcomes in MDD.[83]

Physical exercise has a moderate effect on depression compared to control conditions but no effect at follow-up.[84] The effects of exercise when compared to psychological treatments or antidepressant medication are small and not significant. However, exercise as an adjunct to antidepressant medication yields moderate effects.[85]

Pharmacotherapy

Antidepressant medications are widely used and mostly influence the functioning of certain neurotransmitters in the brain, primarily serotonin and norepinephrine. Older medications such as tricyclic antidepressants (TCAs) and MAOIs can be difficult to tolerate due to side effects or, in the case of MAOIs, dietary and medication restrictions. Medications such as the SSRIs, selective serotonin/norepinephrine reuptake inhibitors (SNRIs), and norepinephrine and dopamine reuptake inhibitors

(NDRIs), appear to have fewer side effects than the older drugs, making it easier for patients to adhere to treatment. No single medication is effective for all depressed patients, as various groups of patients will respond to one drug while other patients will require different agents. A recent meta-analysis of 21 antidepressants and over 100,000 MDD patients revealed that all antidepressants are more efficacious than placebo, but effect sizes are mostly modest (odds ratios of 1.37–2.13).[86] A large "real world" study of treatment-resistant depression (sequenced treatment alternatives to relieve depression—STAR*D) suggested that a patient with persistent depression can get well after trying multiple treatment strategies, but his or her odds of "beating" depression lessen as additional strategies are needed.[87] Persistent depression is usually treated with combination of different antidepressants or augmentation with non-antidepressant drugs such as lithium, l-triiodothyronine (T3), or atypical antipsychotics. Cognitive symptoms such as difficulty in concentrating and indecisiveness in MDD patients may limit functional recovery. Resolution of cognitive symptoms of depression could lag behind recovery from mood symptoms in many patients.[88] Several clinical trials have noted a pro-cognitive effect of antidepressants in MDD, especially in the domains of psychomotor speed and delayed recall.[89]

Novel medications for depression include glutamatergic system modulators (such as ketamine[90]), anti-inflammatory medications,[91] and opioid tone modulators and opioid-κ antagonists.[92] For a detailed review of principles of pharmacological management of depression see the Canadian Network for Mood and Anxiety Treatments (CANMAT) 2016 clinical guidelines.[93]

Brain Stimulation

Despite its high prevalence, social impact, and variety of therapeutic options for depression many patients remain treatment resistant.[94,95] For these severely ill patients who do not respond to psychotherapy and medication, electroconvulsive therapy (ECT) is often prescribed. For more than 50 years, ECT has been the only nonpharmacological, somatic treatment of psychiatric disorders in widespread clinical use. This situation is now changing with brain stimulation techniques that are rapidly becoming a highly promising novel avenue for treatment of depression.[96] These new techniques include transcranial magnetic stimulation (TMS), magnetic seizure therapy (MST), transcranial direct current stimulation (tDCS), vagus nerve stimulation (VNS), and deep brain stimulation (DBS).

ECT produces epileptiform convulsions as a treatment for depression. It is considered effective and safe but continues to be regarded with suspicion by much of the public and the medical profession.[97] Hollywood films such as The Snake Pit (1948) and One Flew Over the Cuckoo's Nest (1975) set an antipsychiatry and anti-ECT tone that has never completely abated. The epileptiform seizure may seem to be an all-or-none event but not every generalized seizure has antidepressant properties. Stimulus intensity relative to threshold and location of the electrodes (bilateral or unilateral electrode placement) are major factors in the efficacy of the therapy. To minimize short- and longer-term memory deficits associated with ECT, major research efforts have been invested in trying to limit the stimulus path and to adapt the stimulus characteristics (stimulus pulse duration) and stimulus intensity to the seizure threshold of the individual patient.[98]

TMS uses figure eight-shaped coils to create magnetic fields and to modulate neuronal activity to a maximum depth of 1.5–2.5 cm from the scalp. Many studies support the safety and efficacy of repetitive TMS (rTMS) antidepressant therapy.[99,100] A recent meta-analysis (4233 MDD patients) revealed that bilateral, low-frequency or high-frequency and θ-burst rTMS interventions are more effective than sham treatments (OR, 4.66–2.37).[101] Deep TMS (dTMS) uses H-shaped coils and can modulate neuronal activity in deeper regions of the brain. The dTMS treatment over the PFC was found to have antidepressant as well as positive cognitive effects.[102,103] Although TMS is inferior to ECT with regard to efficacy, especially in treatment-resistant MDD patients, it seems more acceptable and well tolerated by the patients.[104]

MST uses a magnetic field to induce a seizure. An rTMS device is used to induce a seizure and the procedure is carried out as is ECT using general anesthetics and muscle relaxants. Although MST is not often used, preliminary results show efficacy for MDD patients with no significant cognitive adverse effects.[105]

tDCS applies a weak direct current via scalp electrodes overlying targeted cortical areas. As a relatively new treatment, it is not clear if tDCS treatment may be efficacious for treatment of depression.[106,107] Active tDCS treatment for depression did not show cognitive benefits independent of mood effects. Rather, tDCS treatment relative to sham stimulation for major depression may instead be associated with a reduced practice effect for processing speed.[108]

VNS is carried by bipolar electrodes on the left cervical vagus nerve, which are attached to an implanted stimulator generator. Most of the vagus fibers terminate in the medulla from which there are projections to many brain regions, including the limbic circuitry. VNS has been approved for treatment-resistant MDD patients in 2005 by the Food and Drugs Administration (FDA). It seems that 3–12 months of VNS are needed for the antidepressant effect of this treatment[109] and long-term treatment can prevent reoccurrence of depression.[110] A similar method, transcutaneous auricular vagus nerve stimulation (taVNS), has been recently introduced with some reported positive effects in MDD patients.[111] See Chapter 9 for a more detailed review of neurostimulation treatments in neuropsychiatry.

For the most severely, treatment-resistant patients, several invasive ablative neurosurgical procedures have also been available (for review, see Abosch and Cosgrove[112]). Anterior capsulotomy involves a lesion in fronto-thalamic fibers that pass through the anterior limb of the internal capsule.[113] Cingulotomy involves the generation of bilateral lesions in the ACC as well as the fibers of the cingulum.[114] Subcaudate tractotomy involves the generation of bilateral lesions in the substantia innominata of the basal forebrain immediately ventral to the head of the caudate. Limbic leukotomy combines lesion formation in the ACC with subcaudate tractotomy. These ablative procedures had been associated with a high success rate in severe and treatment-resistant MDD patients, although they are now infrequently used due to potential side effects and the irreversibility of the treatment.[115] Alternative methods for noninvasive

thermal brain ablation such as the focused ultrasound ablation therapy have been explored, with no published results yet.

In the past 25 years, destructive procedures to treat Parkinson's disease (PD) and essential tremor, such a thalamotomy and pallidotomy, have been replaced by applying high-frequency electrical stimulation to these targets. A quadripolar electrode is implanted into the selected brain targets, which is connected to the pacemaker-like device (pulse generator) that is mounted under the skin of the chest. DBS has been found to have distinct advantages over ablation with the major advantage being its reversibility, as well as the option to modify specific stimulation parameters when necessary. DBS can be a potentially safe, effective, flexible, and reversible alternative to ablative surgery for treatment-resistant depression, if the optimal target can be defined and evaluated. Six DBS targets have been studied in treatment-resistant MDD patients: subcallosal cingulate gyrus (SCG), NAc, ventral capsule/VS or anterior limb of internal capsule (ALIC), medial forebrain bundle (MFB), lateral habenula (LHb), and inferior thalamic peduncle.[116] Preliminary open-label results of DBS for depression showed promising results in approximately 50% of patients suffering from severe treatment-resistant MDD. However, controlled or blinded clinical trials produced inconsistent results both in the SCG,[117,118] the VS,[119] and the ALIC.[120]

Bipolar Disorder

Bipolar disorders, formerly called manic-depressive disorder or affective psychosis, are characterized by biphasic mood episodes of depression and mania or hypomania.

Epidemiology

The lifetime and 12-month prevalence of BPD are 0.6% and 0.4% for BP-I and 0.4% and 0.3% for BP-II, respectively.[121] BPD's mean age of onset is around 20 years. BPD in individuals aged ≥60 years represent as much as 25% of the population with BPD, including those with early-onset as well as late-onset BPD.[122] As a lifelong and recurrent illness, BPD often lead to functional impairment and reduced quality of life. Early diagnosis and treatment improves prognosis and decreases number of suicide attempts.[123] Low quality of life in BPD patients is mainly associated with the length of illness (or early onset), the presence of depressive symptoms, nicotine dependence, and the lack of social support.[124] The prevalence of BP-I is similar in men and women, but BP-II is more common in women. Women with BPD are more likely than men to show a predominance of depressive polarity as well as a depressive onset while men with BPD are more likely to suffer from comorbid substance use disorders.[125] Cannabis use is associated with early age of onset of BPD and subsequent increases in manic and depressive symptoms.[126–128]

Pathophysiology

The environmental factors, neuroendocrine systems, and monoamines dysregulation present in BPD are similar to that of MDD. Some environmental factors have been shown to modify the onset and course of BPD. Perinatal risk factors such as caesarean section delivery, maternal influenza infection, maternal smoking during pregnancy, high paternal age, and childhood adverse events can increase the risk of BP disorders. Known triggers of BP disorders are change of season, increased light exposure, and sleep deprivation. The monoamines dysregulation in BPD is more focused on the dopaminergic system. Elevation in striatal D2/3 receptor availability leads to increased dopaminergic neurotransmission and mania, while increased striatal dopamine transporter (DAT) levels leads to reduced dopaminergic function and depression.[129] The genetics and brain circuits of BPD are more related to psychotic disorders than to MDD.

Genetics

BPD have high heritability rate. Patients with a BP-I and BP-II report a 41.2% and 36.3% prevalence of family history of BPD and a 18.5% prevalence of family history of MDD.[130] As with other psychiatric disorders, GWAS indicate that the heritability of BPD is attributable largely to multiple loci of small effects.[131] Analysis of genetic overlap between BPD and other psychiatric disorders has shown a substantial sharing of risk loci between BPD and schizophrenia,[132] significant commonalities with MDD, but little with autism or attention-deficit hyperactivity disorder (for review, see Harrison[133]).

In a meta-analysis of large GWAS data sets ($n = 12{,}127$), 966 genes that contained 2 or more variants associated with BPD were identified. Among these 966 genes, 226 were empirically significant and related to relevant brain pathways: corticotropin-releasing hormone signaling, phospholipase C signaling, glutamate receptor signaling, and endothelin 1 signaling.[134] Future meta-analysis might identify genetic variants in BPD that could be used to predict individual risk, the course of the disorders, or the effects of medication.[135] For example, the International Consortium on Lithium Genetics identified two genetic regions that may be useful as biomarkers for lithium response in a sample of 2563 patients.[136] Mitochondrial DNA mutations have also been reported to be associated with BPD.[137]

Neurocircuits of BPD

Neuroimaging studies of BPD demonstrate abnormalities in neural circuits of emotion processing, emotion regulation, and reward processing (for review, see Phillips and Swartz[138]). Most recently, the BPD working group within the ENIGMA Consortium examined structural brain MRI and clinical data from 6503 individuals, 2447 of which were BPD patients. They report thinner cortical gray matter in frontal, temporal, and parietal regions of both brain hemispheres in BPD patients with strongest effects in left pars opercularis, fusiform gyrus, and rostral middle frontal cortex. This reduced cortical surface area was associated with a history of psychosis and longer duration of illness.[139] Diffusion tensor imaging (DTI) is uniquely sensitive to white matter microstructure analysis including axonal coherence, fiber density, and myelin integrity. Several DTI studies indicate that white matter hyperintensities, especially in the prefrontal and frontal white matter, are associated with BPD compared with healthy controls.[140] The disruption of neural connectivity due to myelin degradation is hypothesized to play a role in the pathophysiology of BPD. Many MRI studies have reported distinct functional and structural alterations in emotion or reward processing neural circuits between MDD and BPD. Several studies performed pattern classification

analysis using structural and functional MRI data to distinguish between MDD and BPD using machine learning approaches, which yielded a moderate level of accuracy in classification.[141,142]

Clinical Presentation

According to the *DSM-5*, bipolar I disorder (BP-I) is diagnosed by a manic episode that may be preceded by and may be followed by hypomanic or MDEs.[4] Most of the patients who meet the criteria for a manic episode also experience MDEs during their lives. A manic episode is diagnosed by persistently elevated, expansive, or irritable mood, activity, or energy, lasting at least 1 week. During this time, three (or more) of the following symptoms are present: inflated self-esteem or grandiosity, decreased need for sleep, talkativeness or pressure to keep talking, flight of ideas or racing thoughts, distractibility, increased goal-directed activity or psychomotor agitation, excessive involvement in activities that have a high potential for adverse consequences. The mood disturbance is sufficiently severe to cause marked impairment in social or occupational functioning or to necessitate hospitalization to prevent harm to self or others, or there are psychotic features. Depressive episodes characteristics are similar to the criteria of MDD (as described above). Acute episodes of mood alterations in BPD can include symptoms at both poles (mixed symptoms).

Bipolar II disorder (BP-II) is diagnosed by the lifetime experience of at least one episode of major depression and at least one hypomanic episode. A hypomanic episode is shorter and associated with a milder change in functioning than a manic episode. Symptom severity as reported by the patients is greater for depressive episodes than for manic episodes. However, BP-II is not considered a milder condition than BP-I disorder, mainly because of the amount of time individuals with this condition spend in depression and because of the mood instability experienced by individuals with BP-II disorder that is typically accompanied by serious impairment in work and social functioning.

The longitudinal course of BPD is highly variable. Patients with BPD can achieve full remissions. During the symptom-free periods the disorder is considered latent ("euthymic episodes"). Unfortunately, many BPD patients have residual and subthreshold symptoms persist in a pervasive way that lower functional level. The trajectory of the residual symptoms is thought to be dependent on the clinical course, with full recovery difficult to achieve especially after a third and subsequent episodes. A subset of patients seems to present a progressive course associated with brain changes and functional impairment.[143] Risk factors associated with these unfavorable outcomes are number of mood episodes, early trauma, and psychiatric and medical comorbidity.[144] For a review of classification of staging in BPD, see Berk et al.[145]

Cognitive impairment is an important factor in the total functional impairment of BPD patients. Cognitive deficits in BPD patients are not mood-state dependent and can be detected both during depression or manic/hypomanic episodes and during remission or euthymic episodes. Cognitive impairment during affective episodes includes significant deficits in psychomotor speed, attention, working memory, and cognitive flexibility and milder deficits in verbal learning, memory, attentional switching, and verbal fluency. Cognitive impairment during euthymic episodes includes difficulties in attention, processing speed, episodic memory, executive functions (such as cognitive flexibility, response inhibition, and planning). There is no change in theory of mind.[146,147] Cognitive impairment can be detected as soon as the first BPD episode. More severe or longstanding illness and antipsychotic medication are associated with greater cognitive impairment.[148] The cognitive profile of BPD patients was thought to be of a progressive nature and associated with the number of episodes and number of hospitalizations.[149] However, a recent meta-analysis shows that BPD patients' performance on cognitive measures remain stable over time (mean follow-up period of 4–5 years).[150–152] Individuals at risk for BPD exhibit deficits in global measures of neurocognition and deficits in specific neurocognitive domains, including verbal memory and executive function. These cognitive deficits might represent potential predictors of BPD.[153]

Treatment

BPD episodes are frequent, and effective treatment includes treatment of acute depressive, hypomanic, or manic symptoms as well as the prevention of relapses. Psychotherapy and most of the brain stimulation techniques in BPD are similar to those of MDD, especially when treating the MDEs of BPD. However, pharmacotherapy in BPD is based on mood stabilizers (lithium, anticonvulsant, and antipsychotic medications).[154] Most recently, the CANMAT and the International Society for BPD (ISBD) have published recommendations for the treatment of BPD.[155] Briefly, first-line treatment for acute manic episode includes lithium, divalproex, and many antipsychotics (quetiapine, asenapine, aripiprazole, paliperidone, risperidone, and cariprazine). First-line treatment for acute BPD depression include quetiapine, lurasidone plus lithium or divalproex, lithium, lamotrigine, lurasidone, or adjunctive lamotrigine. For maintenance phase treatment, the medications that have been shown to be effective for the acute phase can be continued or lithium, quetiapine, divalproex, lamotrigine, asenapine, and aripiprazole monotherapy or combination treatments could be considered.

Individual patients may benefit from antidepressants but there is major concern about the risk of a mood switch to hypomania, mania, and mixed states. Bupropion and possibly SSRIs may have lower rates of manic switch than tricyclic and tetracyclic antidepressants and SNRIs.[156] Acute and long-term treatment of mixed states in BPD is a clinical challenge.[157] Manic symptoms in BPD mixed states are responsive to treatment with several atypical antipsychotics, with the best evidence for olanzapine. For depressive symptoms in BPD mixed states, addition of ziprasidone to treatment as usual may be beneficial.[157] Recurrence prevention can be achieved with olanzapine, quetiapine, valproate, and lithium. BPD patients have a relatively low adherence to pharmacotherapy. Some patients report that they feel depressed when they become euthymic. These patients may tend to reduce or stop the mood stabilizer medications in order to feel hypomanic.

Most mood stabilizer medications have neurologic and neurocognitive side effects.[158] The most frequent neurological side effect of mood stabilizers is tremor that occurs in 65% of patients using lithium and 1–5% of patients using valproate and

lamotrigine. Carbamazepine's side effects include ataxia, nausea, dizziness, drowsiness, vomiting, blurred vision, and diplopia. Lamotrigine can cause headache and nausea and valproate can cause sedation. Although many BPD patients report cognitive side effects when taking mood stabilizers, it is usually difficult to determine whether any cognitive changes reflect mood stabilizers itself, the serum level, residual mood symptoms, or another medical state such as hypothyroidism.[159] Many BPD patients show some impairment of executive functions and emotion recognition, regardless of their pharmacological treatment.[160] However, memory, attention, and most of the executive functions are impaired in patients who take anticonvulsants as mood stabilizers. Lamotrigine appears to have a safer neurocognitive profile than other anticonvulsants. Lithium has an impact on psychomotor speed, processing speed, intellectual abilities, and executive functioning but no impact on attention.[161] Interestingly, excellent lithium responders, having no affective recurrences during lithium therapy, perform on cognitive functions tests similar to those of age-matched, healthy control subjects.[162] Some studies also report that lithium reduces risk of dementia in BPD patients. Another important cause for neurocognitive side effects in medicated BPD patients is anticholinergic medications that are prescribed to treat extrapyramidal side effects associated with antipsychotics.[163]

Cognitive impairment can be distressing and decrease patients' compliance with treatment. Medications that have been examined as potential treatment for cognitive impairment in BPD include mifepristone (corticosteroid receptor antagonist), galantamine or donepezil (cholinesterase inhibitors), pramipexole, and modafinil.[164] However, the findings regarding efficacy of medications on cognition are overall minimal or preliminary.[164] Neurocognitive evaluation should be considered in all medicated BPD patients to better evaluate the treatment impact on neurocognition. A cognitive psychotherapy treatment such as CBT should be considered in patients with significant or treatment-related cognitive impairment. In recent years, functional remediation was studied in BPD patients and shown to be effective in improving functional outcome.[165,166] This neurocognitive intervention involves neurocognitive techniques, training, psychoeducation on cognition-related issues, and problem-solving within an ecological framework.

Mood Disturbances Associated with Other Neuropsychiatric and Medical Disorders

Depression is prevalent in many chronic general medical and neurological illnesses. The neurochemical, structural, and functional neuroanatomy pathophysiology of MDD is similar to the pathophysiology of depression in these disorders. Therefore, in patients with neuropsychiatry and medical illness, depression might be caused by the underlying neuropsychiatry or medical illness, the treatment, the emotional stress of having a chronic disease, recurrence of a comorbid mood disorder, or a combination of these factors. For example, neuroinflammatory illnesses, such as multiple sclerosis (MS), are associated with high rates of depression, probably due to shared immune system mechanism for depression. Neurodegenerative basal ganglia illnesses, such as PD, Huntington's disease, or Wilson's disease, are also associated with high rates of depression, probably due to shared pathways and monoamines in the pathogenesis of depression. Post-stroke depression involves combination of various ischemia-induced neurobiological dysfunctions, such as damage to the left frontal-basal ganglia pathways,[167] alterations of monoaminergic neurotransmitter systems, stress activation of the HPA axis, impairment of neurogenesis and mitochondrial dysfunction, in the context of psychosocial distress.[168] Psychological stress in epileptic patients explains depression in many patients but acute and temporary seizure-related states of depression or suicidality have also been reported.[169] Pharmacological or iatrogenic causes of depression include corticosteroids, alpha-interferon, or thyroid ablation. Depression is also caused by specific vitamin deficiencies, such as vitamin B12 and folic acid deficiency.[170,171]

A two-way association between depression and many neurology illnesses has been established. For example, stroke increases the risk of post-stroke depression, and depression is an independent risk factor for stroke.[171A,B] Sometimes, depression precedes the neurologic symptoms in neuropsychiatric disorders. For example, the presenting symptom of PD might be depression, anxiety, or obsessive symptoms. Depressive symptoms are prevalent, worsen the prognosis, and severely interfere with the rehabilitation process of the underlying neuropsychiatry illness. For example, post-stroke depression has been shown to inhibit physical and cognitive recovery.[172] About one in three patients with epilepsy will have experienced a psychiatric disorder in the course of their life, with mood and anxiety disorders being the most frequent, and these psychiatric symptoms are correlated with a worse quality of life and higher economic burdens of the patient and family.[173]

Memory difficulties in MDD may be the chief complaint and manifest as subcortical dementia. The memory decline in MDD may be mistaken for early signs of a dementia (which has been labelled by some as "pseudodementia").[4] It could be difficult to differentiate dementia of depression from other types of dementia until full recovery from depression is achieved. In some elderly individuals, MDE may be the initial presentation of a neurodegenerative process such as PD or AD. These depressed patients with subsequent dementia show a marked cognitive deficit.[174] Indeed, a third of patients with a neurodegenerative disease received a prior psychiatric diagnosis, most commonly depression. Frontotemporal dementia patients received a prior psychiatric diagnosis significantly more often (~50%) than patients with AD (~25%), semantic dementia (~25%), or progressive aphasia (~10%).[175] Severe cognitive impairments in elderly depressed patients should not be dismissed as dementia of depression but require clinical attention as a possible sign of incipient dementia. However, late-onset remitted depressed patients can demonstrate cognitive deficits that persist beyond the acute phase of depression such as impaired verbal memory, speed of information processing, and some executive functions. Most recently, imaging methods such as structural MRI have been suggested as a tool for the differentiation between a potential reversible dementia due to depression from dementia due to neurodegenerative disease.[176,177]

BPD has a high comorbidity rate with physical, neurological, and psychiatric diseases. BPD is associated with increased rate of dementia (hazard ratio [HR] = 2.30) which is greatest among those with late onset BPD, that is, older patients with less than 5 years of history of BPD or patients who had illness onset after 70 years of age.[178] The rate of BPD is relatively high in many primary neurologic disorders such as MS (8.5%),[179] epilepsy (12%),[180] migraine (19.2%),[181] and PD (the rate of BP is related to PINK1 mutation carriers).[182] Patients with BPD are 1.24 times more likely than normal population to have a cerebrovascular stroke.[183] The excess comorbidity in individuals with BPD is in particular caused by asthma and type-2 diabetes mellitus (T2DM).[184] BPD also has a high co-occurrence with substance use disorders.[185] Substance-induced psychosis, especially cannabis, sedatives, and alcohol, is a major risk for BP disorders.[186]

It is worth noting that neuropsychiatric patients may exhibit similar affective symptoms or a unique set of affective disorder symptoms. For example, some patients with PD complain about anhedonia while denying symptoms of depressed mood. Parkinsonian patients have a restricted range of emotional expression, often described as "poker face," that might seem similar to major depression or schizophrenia patients. An important differential diagnosis of irritable or manic affect is the pseudobulbar affect. This affect consists of uncontrollable outbursts of crying or laughter inappropriate to the external circumstances and incongruent with the internal emotional state. Pseudobulbar affect is correlated with disruption of cortico-pontine-cerebellar circuits, reducing the threshold for motor expression of emotion.[187] Anhedonia, diminished interest or pleasure in activities, is similar to another symptom, apathy, that is defined as reduced motivation for self-initiated, goal-directed behavior. Apathy is common in many neuropsychiatric disorders such as PD, AD, stroke, and other focal lesion syndromes. Indeed, apathy is related to brain circuits of depression and anhedonia such as the dorsal anterior cingulate cortex (dACC), VS, and the NAc.[188] While the relationship between sleep and mood is well documented, sleep disorders are prevalent in many neuropsychiatric disorders, in the absence of other affective symptoms.[189] Up to 90% of patients initially diagnosed with idiopathic rapid eye movement sleep behavior disorder at a sleep center later develop a defined neurodegenerative disease.[190]

PSYCHOTIC DISORDERS

The current edition of the *DSM-5* designates psychosis as a clinical syndrome that may occur in several disorders.[4] The diagnosis of psychotic disorders involves a constellation of five core symptoms: delusions, hallucinations, disorganized speech, disorganized behavior, and negative symptoms, with impaired occupational or social functioning. Delusions are fixed beliefs that would not change when provided with conflicting evidence and may include a variety of themes (e.g., persecutory, referential, somatic, religious, grandiose). Hallucinations are perception-like experiences that occur without an external stimulus that can develop in any sensory modality (auditory hallucinations are the most common in schizophrenia). Disorganized thinking (formal thought disorder) is typically inferred from the individual's speech and can include derailment or loose associations (switch from one topic to another), tangentiality (speech is obliquely related or completely unrelated), incoherence or "word salad" (speech is severely disorganized and resembles receptive aphasia). Disorganized or abnormal motor behavior may manifest itself in a variety of ways, ranging from childlike "silliness" to unpredictable agitation. Disorganized behavior includes catatonic behavior, a decreased reactivity to the environment, ranging from negativism (resistance to instructions) or mutism and stupor (lack of verbal or motor responses) to catatonic excitement (excessive motor activity).

The negative symptoms refer to lack of motivation, social withdrawal, and abnormalities in social interaction. They include: (i) diminished emotional expression or affective flattening; (ii) avolition—decreased motivated, self-initiated, purposeful activities; (iii) alogia—diminished speech output; (iv) anhedonia—decreased ability to experience or anticipate pleasure from positive stimuli; (v) asociality—lack of interest in social interaction.[191] The two factors model of negative symptoms separate them into two main groups: (1) motivation and pleasure and (2) emotional expressivity.[192]

Psychotic disorders are categorized into three pathophysiological groups:

1. Idiopathic/Primary psychoses—such as schizophrenia, schizoaffective disorder, schizophreniform disorder, brief psychotic disorder, mood disorder with psychotic features, and delusional disorder.
2. Psychoses due to medical conditions—such as Parkinson's or Huntington's disease, MS, epilepsy (ictal, postictal, and interictal psychosis), cerebrovascular disease, brain tumors, migraine, brain infections, autoimmune disorders with CNS involvement (systemic lupus erythematosus [SLE], para-neoplastic syndrome, NMDA-receptor autoimmune encephalitis), neuroendocrine disorders (hypoglycemia, thyroid, parathyroid, and adrenocortical abnormalities), neurometabolic disorders (electrolyte abnormalities, hypoxia, hypercarbia, hepatic, or renal disfunction).
3. Toxic psychoses—such as psychosis induced by recreational substances (alcohol, stimulants, hallucinogens (lysergic acid diethylamide (LSD), mescaline, and psilocybin), phencyclidine, cannabis, inhalants, sedative or hypnotic agents, etc.), psychosis induced by toxins (such as carbon mono- or dioxide, cholinesterase inhibitors, fuel or paint, organophosphates, etc.), and psychosis induced by medications (dopamimetic or anticholinergic agents, steroids or NSAIDs, anesthetic and analgesic agents, antihistamines, anticonvulsants, antidepressants, etc.).

This section is focused on the neuropsychiatric aspects of the most common idiopathic psychotic disorder, schizophrenia. Although the *DSM-5* suggests a dichotomous distinction between psychosis and health, recent data shows that psychosis is not necessarily an all-or-none phenomenon, but a continuous phenomenon across the general population, with prevalence rates of 5–8%.[193] Psychotic experiences at a subclinical level have some predictive value for psychotic disorders and for non-psychotic disorders involving functional impairment, violence, and suicide.[194] Psychosis and cognitive symptoms are more prevalent in healthy, first-degree relatives of patients with schizophrenia, suggesting that the underlying neurobiological abnormality leading to psychosis or cognitive impairment is similar in schizophrenia patients and the healthy population.[195] Therefore, understanding the spectrum of psychotic syndromes, including the negative and the cognitive symptoms, and the underlying pathophysiology and treatment strategies, is critical for a neuropsychiatric view of psychotic disorders. We then briefly discuss psychosis in other major neuropsychiatric disorders.

Schizophrenia

Epidemiology

Schizophrenia occurs with an incidence of about 0.7% of the population and is associated with a large economic burden, which is mainly driven by unemployment (38%), productivity loss due to caregiving (34%), and direct health care costs (24%).[196-198] Most patients with schizophrenia need formal or informal daily living supports.[199] The ratio of observed deaths in schizophrenia patients to expected deaths in the general population is 3.[200] In young schizophrenia patients, the main cause for this increased mortality rate is suicide, while in older schizophrenia patients it is due to neglected physical illnesses, such as cardiovascular, infectious and iatrogenic metabolic diseases.[201] Schizophrenia is slightly more frequent in men than in women, and the first episode is usually earlier in men: early to mid-20s for males and late-20s for females.[202] However, presentation of schizophrenia at different life stages varies considerably. Schizophrenia with onset prior to 40 years of age is classified as early-onset schizophrenia, schizophrenia with onset at and after 40 years of age is classified as late-onset schizophrenia, and schizophrenia with onset after 60 years of age is classified as very-late-onset schizophrenia-like psychosis. Late onset schizophrenia is relatively rare, with incidence of affective psychoses and schizophrenia of 30.9 and 7.5 per 100 000 person-years at risk, respectively, and slightly more frequent in women.[203]

Almost 100 risk factors were reported as influencing the development of schizophrenia.[204] The main factors that increase the risk of schizophrenia are cannabis use, exposure to stressful events during childhood and adulthood, history of obstetric complications, and maternal low serum folate level.[205] Other important risk factors include urban environment; birth date in late winter or spring; prenatal viral infections; older parental age; first- and second-generation immigrants; social adversity such as childhood physical abuse, sexual abuse, maltreatment, bullying as well as adulthood lack of social support or increased exposure to discrimination; and persistent abuse of amphetamine, methamphetamine, cocaine, or LSD. Direct correlation of risk factors and brain changes in schizophrenia is hard to prove. One interesting example is the finding that current (adult) city living is associated with increased amygdala activity, whereas being raised in an urban setting affects the perigenual anterior cingulate cortex.[206] Urban environment and these limbic circuits are both related to schizophrenia.

Pathophysiology

Schizophrenia is the result of complex factors related to genetics and environment and reflects abnormal brain information processing. A pathophysiologic model for schizophrenia must explain many facets of this disorder: the combination of different symptoms (positive, negative, and cognitive), periods of prominent positive symptoms as well as gradual deteriorating cognitive and social functions, and the transition from the prodromal period to the first psychotic episode. A possible model could be one of developmental anomalies secondary to variant genes, social adversity in childhood, and risks to the brain that disrupt the development and sensitize different monoamine systems in the brain.[207] In parallel, adulthood social adversity biases the cognitive schema toward psychotic interpretations. Further stress results in a chain reaction: stress causes dysregulation of monoamine release that can lead to the further biasing of cognitive schema and aberrant misinterpretation of outside or inside stimuli. In the context of biased cognitive schema, this process intensifies stress and ultimately leads to psychotic symptoms. Progressive dysregulation of the monoamine systems can lead to subsequent psychotic episodes. The critical changes in neuronal activity leading to negative symptoms are still unknown.

The original dopamine theory of schizophrenia postulated that a *hyper*dopaminergic state in the striatum was the cause of schizophrenia and the degree of blockade of dopamine D2 receptors by antipsychotic drugs correlated to their clinical antipsychotic efficacy.[208,209] Dopamimetic medications induce psychotic state (mainly paranoid delusions) and disorganized behavior and dopaminolytic medications are almost the only available antipsychotic drugs. Years later, *hypo*dopaminergic functioning in the frontal cortex was suggested as the cause of negative symptoms and cognitive deficits of schizophrenia.[210] While many studies examined dopaminergic changes in the striatum, most recently a similar deficit in the capacity for dopamine release was found in the dorsolateral PFC in schizophrenia patients in response to amphetamine challenge, and these findings were correlated to their cognitive deficit.[211] The reduced PFC dopamine release might reduce the inhibition of meso-striatal dopamine release, with a net effect of increased striatal release of dopamine. Therefore, the hyperdopaminergic state at the striatum and its cortical connections might be directly related to cognitive impairment in schizophrenia patients.[212] Molecular imaging (PET and SPECT studies) suggests presynaptic dopaminergic dysregulation as the major locus of dopamine dysfunction in schizophrenia.[213] Presynaptic dopamine dysregulation is specific to schizophrenia (and no other psychiatric disorders) and can be detected as early as the prodromal period.[214,215] Other parts of the dopaminergic system such as DAT or D2/3 receptor availabilities were not found to be impaired in drug-naïve schizophrenia patients.[216]

Other neurotransmitter systems (glutamate, GABA, acetylcholine, and serotonin) that interact with the dopaminergic system also seem to play a role in the pathogenesis of schizophrenia. Disturbances in the balance of glutamatergic-GABAergic excitation and inhibition have been suggested to cause schizophrenia.[217] Glutamate neurotransmission is important for cognition, memory, and learning. Glutamatergic models of schizophrenia are based on N-methyl-D-aspartate-type (NMDA) glutamate receptors antagonists such as ketamine and phencyclidine that can induce schizophrenia-like symptoms. NMDA receptors are important for brain plasticity (the ability to form long-term

synaptic connections) and are modulated by endogenous brain compounds such as glycine, D-serine, and glutathione.[218] NMDA antagonists have been shown to induce gamma oscillations in human EEG recordings and the cortex and striatum of rodents. Interestingly, NMDA antagonists increase gamma oscillations coherence between the cortex and basal ganglia in non-human primates. Gamma oscillation might represent the abnormal glutamate-induced connectivity of the striatum and cortex circuit in schizophrenia.[219] Reduced GABA activity can be found at the tissue and cellular level in many brain regions of schizophrenia patients, as well as in other mental illness such as depression, anxiety, and autism. The number of GABAergic neurons is not reduced in schizophrenia patients but expression of glutamate decarboxylase 1 (GAD1), the gene encoding for biosynthetic enzyme of GABA synthesis, is reduced.[220] Recent animal findings suggest that parvalbuminergic interneurons might induce, during the adolescent period, long-term plastic changes in PFC through their effect on GABAergic neurons, thereby altering perception, cognition, and behavior in the adult.[221] In contrast to dopamine and glutamate, GABA agonists only rarely induce psychosis and GABA antagonists are not used as antipsychotic.

Many genetic findings support the involvement of the monoamine systems in the pathogenesis of schizophrenia. In the most updated GWAS study, among the 108 loci that were associated with schizophrenia, one was directly related to the dopamine system (dopamine receptor 2) and others were related to dopamine synthesis, metabolism, and neurotransmission.[222] Many genes that are involved in glutamatergic neurotransmission, including NMDA and other glutamatergic receptors have also been found to be related to schizophrenia.[223] Polymorphism in the *disrupted in schizophrenia* (DISC1) gene, a protein interacting with other proteins involved in the dopamine and glutamatergic systems, is one of the most studied loci linked to an increased risk of schizophrenia.[224] Polymorphism in the catechol-O-methyl transferase (COMT) gene, a monoamine catabolic enzyme that is located within one of the strongest genetic risk factors for schizophrenia (deletion at 22q.11.2), is related to stress vulnerability and cognitive impairment in schizophrenia patients.[225] Many of the genes that have been associated with schizophrenia regulate brain development and are expressed during fetal development.[226,227] These findings are consistent with epidemiological data that correlated pre- and perinatal adverse events to the risk of schizophrenia.

A variety of infections and autoimmune conditions are associated with schizophrenia; therefore, it is possible that they share a common underlying pathway involving the inflammatory immune response.[228] The Schizophrenia Working Group of the Psychiatric Genomics Consortium have identified 128 independent associations spanning 108 loci that involve mainly the CNS and the immune systems.[222] These advances in genetics have shown that variations in the immune and complement system are associated with negative symptoms. It has been suggested that changes in the complement system cause perinatal activation of microglia and subsequent stress in adolescence triggers pathological overactivation, leading to cortical dysfunction and the development of negative symptoms in schizophrenia.[229]

Many research groups around the world aim at revealing the genetics of schizophrenia and using the data to develop new methods for early detection of the disease and new therapeutic mechanisms (for review, see the consensus paper of the World Federation of Societies of Biological Psychiatry Task Force on Genetics[230]). One example is the Genetics of Endophenotypes of Neurofunction to Understand Schizophrenia (GENUS) Consortium that aims to clarify the role of genetic variation in brain abnormalities underlying schizophrenia.[231]

Neurocircuits in Schizophrenia

Many anatomic neuroimaging studies report cortical and subcortical abnormalities in neuroleptic naïve[232-234] or chronic schizophrenia patients[235,236] and their relatives.[237] Intracranial and total brain volume are decreased by 2.0% and 2.6% respectively and lateral ventricle volumes are increased in schizophrenia patients.[238] In general, patients with schizophrenia have smaller hippocampus, amygdala, thalamus, accumbens, and anterior cingulate cortex volumes. Over time, cerebral gray matter volume, cortical volume, and thickness are decreased and correlate with cognitive impairment.[239] On the other hand, volume increases in patients with schizophrenia usually begin in the putamen and later spread to the entire striatum (larger caudate, putamen, pallidum, and a leftward asymmetry for pallidum volume).[240,241] The subcortical volume changes were found to be more highly correlated with negative symptoms than positive symptoms of schizophrenia.[242] Medications can influence brain structure volume. For example, haloperidol (typical antipsychotic drug) can decrease cortical gray matter, and whole brain and hippocampal volumes, while lithium can increase cortical gray matter volume.[243] However, the anatomical brain changes in schizophrenia patients might be of a genetic origin. For example, the volume of the pallidum is associated with the genetic risk of schizophrenia.[244] Therefore, some of the progressive loss and increase of brain tissue in schizophrenia patients might be related to genetic factors and not only to the disease process or medical treatment.

The profound anatomical changes in schizophrenia are correlated with emotional, behavioral, and cognitive findings in specific brain networks.[245] The anatomical and functional findings in schizophrenia patients are grossly correlated with the main cluster of symptoms: positive symptoms are mainly related to activity of the cortical areas (ventral medial PFC) but are also linked to the amygdala and hippocampus/parahippocampal region; negative symptoms are related to the activity of the subcortical areas (VS) but also to the ventral PFC; disorganization symptoms are related to the activity of the dorsolateral PFC.[246-248] Most recently, the structural and functional integrity of fronto-limbic brain regions was found to be related not only to specific symptoms but also to the general functional impairment in individuals with schizophrenia.[249]

The positive symptoms are mainly related to the salience network. As mentioned above (pathophysiology of MDD), this network helps control emotional or cognitive functions and depends on dopaminergic signals originating in the midbrain that project to the VS. Increased midbrain activation and dopamine uptake can be found in schizophrenia patients with both psychosis and prodromal symptoms. Although it is difficult to use brain imaging techniques while patients have active positive symptoms such as delusions, hallucinations, or disorganized behavior, a few studies have reported some interesting results.[250] Delusions are mostly correlated with abnormal anterior cingulate cortex activity.[251] Auditory hallucinations are mostly correlated with brain areas related to speech processing (the right homologue of Broca's area, bilateral insula, bilateral supra-marginal gyri, and right superior temporal gyrus) with more non-dominant lateralization during auditory hallucinations comparing to normal speech.[252] Other studies have correlated the activity of the salience network, the default mode networks, and the hippocampus in patients with visual and auditory hallucinations.[253-255] A new imaging technique, free-water corrected DTI, has recently demonstrated that delusions are associated with myelin abnormalities and possible neuroinflammation or atrophy in the cingulum bundle.[256]

Negative symptoms represent a complex aggregate of individual emotional and motivational deficits that may arise from distinct neural mechanisms.[257-259] There is still no consensus regarding brain areas and mechanisms that have causal or strong correlative relationship with negative symptoms of schizophrenia. Negative symptoms subtypes and phenotypes such as reduced reward anticipation, anhedonia, cognitive decline, and social withdrawal are correlated with specific brain areas. Similar to the positive symptoms, the negative symptoms (such as anhedonia and asociality) are also related to the salience network. Negative symptom severity is associated with decreased activity in the ventrolateral PFC (during executive functioning tasks) and the striatum (during reward conditioning tasks).[260] For example, a recent meta-analysis (over 1500 schizophrenia patients) showed bilateral VS hypoactivation during reward anticipation or feedback that was correlated to high scores of negative symptoms.[261] Another example is dysfunctional striato-cortical connectivity during a motivation challenge task that is correlated to negative symptom severity.[262] Similarly, anhedonia in schizophrenia patients with high score of negative symptoms can be manifested as reduced anterior cingulate cortex activation in response to pleasant images.[263]

Cognitive deficits in schizophrenia are mostly related to neural circuits of specific subtypes of cognitive functions. For example, working memory deficit is associated with abnormalities in the dorsolateral PFC, anterior cingulate cortex, and inferior parietal lobule, while episodic memory deficit is caused by abnormalities in the dorsolateral PFC and hippocampal formation. Abnormalities in the relationship between cortical and subcortical regions, the PFC, thalamus, basal ganglia, and cerebellum were observed in patients with schizophrenia and correlated primarily with deficits in executive functioning, processing speed, and working memory.[263-265] The cognitive symptoms of schizophrenia are also closely related to the default mode network. Many studies reported functional hyperconnectivity within the default mode network in schizophrenia patients, while some studies reported hypoconnectivity (for review, see Hu et al.[266]) (Figure 11-4).

A new imaging-genetics strategy uses imaging to evaluate genetic variation through detecting neuroimaging phenotypic differences. A recent meta-analysis has correlated the genetic load for schizophrenia with specific brain function. Task-related

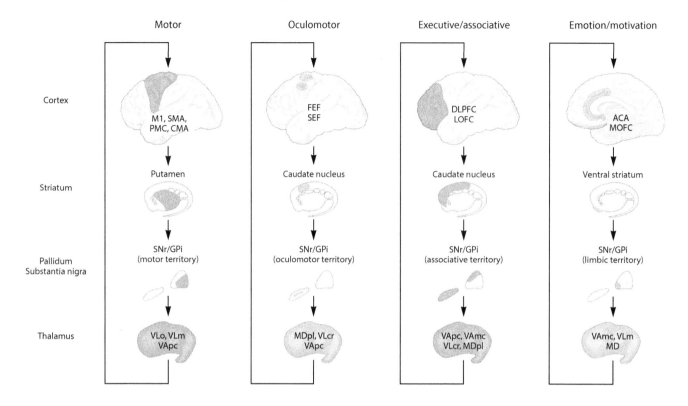

FIGURE 11-4. Anatomy of cortico-basal ganglia-thalamo-cortical circuits. (Reproduced with permission from Kandel ER, Schwartz JH, Jessell TM, et al: *Principles of Neural Science*. 5th ed. http://neurology.mhmedical.com. Copyright © McGraw Hill LLC. All rights reserved.)

recruitments of frontal areas were correlated with a few genetic variations. However, task-related recruitments of multiple brain regions were correlated with polygenic variations.[267] Future studies might provide a new insight on the correlation between genes and imaging in the pathophysiology of schizophrenia.

Clinical Presentation

Schizophrenia is a chronic and complex disorder that involves a range of emotional, behavioral, and cognitive dysfunctions. According to the *DSM-5*, the diagnosis of schizophrenia involves a constellation of five core symptoms: delusions, hallucinations, disorganized speech, disorganized behavior and negative symptoms, with impaired occupational or social functioning. The first two core symptoms, termed "positive symptoms," can more easily be controlled in most patients by antipsychotics.

Mood symptoms, mainly depressive symptoms, are common in schizophrenia and may be concurrent with active psychotic episodes. Schizoaffective disorder is characterized by a period of illness during which there is a major mood episode (major depressive or manic) concurrent with core symptoms of schizophrenia.

The cognitive symptoms of schizophrenia refer to inability to work sequentially and effectively and to organize one's life. Although cognitive symptoms are not included in the diagnostic criteria of the *DSM*, they are common in schizophrenia patients. According to the International Classification of Diseases 11th Revision (ICD-11), cognitive deficits are integral part of the symptoms of schizophrenia. Cognitive symptoms in schizophrenia include decrements in explicit (declarative) memory (especially semantic memory), working memory, language function, other executive functions, as well as slower processing speed. Although robust cognitive deficits in widespread domains may be present in schizophrenia, most cognitive deficits are separable into several neuropsychologically meaningful factors: episodic memory, working memory, perceptual vigilance, visual abstraction, and inhibitory processing.[268] Abnormalities in sensory processing and inhibitory capacity, as well as reductions in attention, are also found. Some individuals with schizophrenia show social cognition deficits, including deficits in the ability to infer the intentions of other people (theory of mind), and may attend to and then interpret irrelevant events or stimuli as meaningful, perhaps leading to the generation of explanatory delusions. Neurological signs that can be found in schizophrenia include impairments in motor coordination, sensory integration, and motor sequencing of complex movements; left-right confusion; and disinhibition of associated movements.[269] Individuals with schizophrenia may also have minor physical anomalies such as subtle morphological deviations of little functional or cosmetic consequence which may, on the other hand, represent risk markers for underlying disease susceptibility.[270]

The overt clinical features of schizophrenia typically emerge in late adolescent to young adulthood.[271] The onset may be abrupt, but most patients manifest a gradual development of positive and negative symptoms ("prodromal phase"). Once diagnosed, remission is rare, and individuals remain chronically ill. Most patients have a fluctuating course of exacerbations and remissions of positive symptoms while others have a progressive deteriorating course. Even when positive symptoms are well treated, many patients display predominantly negative symptoms from the first episode on, formerly described as the "deficit syndrome." Positive symptoms diminish over the life course, but negative symptoms tend to be persistent and disabling throughout the lifespan of schizophrenia.[272] Negative symptoms may be primary (related to the core pathophysiology of the disorder) or secondary, as a derivative of antipsychotic medication aiming at minimization of the positive symptoms.

Negative and cognitive symptoms appear to be separate domains of psychopathology that contribute to the clinical presentation and functional outcomes of schizophrenia.[273-275] Currently available antipsychotic medications predominantly treat the positive symptoms, so attention has traditionally been focused on managing them. However, negative and cognitive symptoms affect 40% and 80% of schizophrenia patients respectively, account for a considerable portion of the morbidity associated with schizophrenia, and are more related to prognosis and functioning than are positive symptoms.[276-278] Therefore, clinicians and researchers should pay special attention to these symptom domains. Classification and measurement of negative and cognitive symptoms as well as using current available treatment methods are essential to the care of schizophrenia patients.[279]

The increased interest in developing new therapies for negative and cognitive symptoms of schizophrenia has led to a reevaluation of instruments for measuring negative symptoms over the past decade. In addition to the traditional scales (the Scale for the Assessment of Negative Symptoms [SANS], the Positive and Negative Symptoms Scale [PANSS], and the Negative Symptom Assessment Scale [NSA]), two newer scales, the Brief Negative Symptom Scale (BNSS) and the Clinical Assessment Interview for Negative Symptoms (CAINS) were developed (for review, see Marder and Kirkpatrick[280]). The best-known scale to measure cognitive deficit in schizophrenia is the Measurement and Treatment Research to Improve Cognition in Schizophrenia (MATRICS) Consensus Cognitive Battery (MCCB).[281-283] Since its introduction, the MCCB has demonstrated good psychometrics and high sensitivity to improvement from interventions.[284]

Treatment

Treatment of schizophrenia includes pharmacotherapy, brain stimulation, and psychotherapy. Treatment can vary according to the symptom domain, phase, and severity of illness. In the acute psychotic episode that usually lasts weeks to months, the major treatment goals are controlling disturbed behavior and reducing the severity of psychosis and associated symptoms (such as aggression, agitation, affective symptoms, etc.). Special attention is paid to preventing harm: presence of suicidal or homicidal ideation or plans and presence of command hallucinations. In the acute psychotic stage, the treatment is based on antipsychotic medications. Antipsychotics block dopamine receptors and are classified into typical (or first-generation) and atypical (second-generation). Examples of typical antipsychotics include chlorpromazine, haloperidol, and perphenazine. Atypical antipsychotics include clozapine, olanzapine, asenapine, risperidone, quetiapine, ziprasidone, amisulpride, and aripiprazole. Atypical antipsychotics are favored over typical

antipsychotics due to the reduced risk of inducing extrapyramidal side effects (especially acute dystonic reactions, parkinsonism, and akathisia at the beginning of the treatment, and tardive dyskinesia later during the treatment).[285,286] Pharmacological treatment of extrapyramidal side effects includes benztropine, diphenhydramine, biperiden, propranolol, clonazepam or lorazepam, tetrabenazine, trihexyphenidyl, and baclofen. Metabolic parameters need to be closely controlled during treatment with antipsychotics to minimize metabolic syndrome (for review, see the World Federation of Societies of Biological Psychiatry [WFSBP] Task Force on Treatment Guidelines for Schizophrenia[287]).

In first-episode schizophrenia, early intervention is recommended.[288] Treatment strategies include antipsychotics in the lowest possible effective dose, combined with a safe and supportive environment. Benzodiazepines may be used to relieve distress, insomnia, and behavioral disturbances secondary to psychosis while antipsychotic medication takes effect. Antipsychotic treatments are introduced with great care due to the higher risk of extrapyramidal symptoms. Antipsychotics are chosen individually according to the patient's psychiatric and somatic condition with special consideration of the side-effect profile. Long-term antipsychotic medications are selected by the patient's previous experience of side effects and symptom response and preferred route of administration.[289] Symptom relapse may be the result of the natural course of the illness, despite continuing treatment. However, the most common contributors to symptoms relapse are medication non-adherence, stressful life events, and substance use. In patients with treatment-resistant schizophrenia, clozapine should be introduced because of its higher efficacy. Other treatment options include switching to another antipsychotic medication, augmentation with antidepressants or mood stabilizers, combination of antipsychotics, and ECT.[290] Other brain stimulation modalities have not been proven effective in treatment-resistant schizophrenia.[291]

Although negative and cognitive symptoms of schizophrenia determine the prognosis and functioning of patients with schizophrenia, no effective treatment for them is available. Conflicting results have been obtained with antipsychotics, anticholinergics, antidepressants, anticonvulsants, psychostimulants, glycinergic neuromodulators, modafinil, 5-HT3 receptor antagonists, and non-pharmacological therapies including psychological therapies.[292,293] Antipsychotic drugs show modest efficacy for negative symptoms, most probably through their effect on positive symptoms. Although typical antipsychotics were considered less effective than atypical antipsychotics, the CATIE study showed no significant advantages in efficacy for any of the atypical antipsychotics with regards to negative symptoms.[294] A recent meta-analysis suggested that aripiprazole might be slightly better in reducing negative symptoms than other atypical antipsychotic drugs.[295] Another recent meta-analysis that included 82 trials with 3608 study participants suggested that add-on antidepressants are efficacious for negative symptoms in patients with schizophrenia, but the effect size was small.[296] During the past decades, new therapies for negative symptoms involving the glutamatergic system were introduced, including glycine, D-cycloserine, sarcosine (N-methylglycine), glycine reuptake inhibitor (Bitopertin),[297] NMDA receptor antagonist memantine,[298–300] α7 nicotinic receptor activators,[301] and reversible acetylcholinesterase inhibitor donepezil, with no significant therapeutic effects.[302] Noninvasive brain stimulation methods such as TMS for treatment of negative symptoms are reported to have very low efficacy.[303] dTMS (deep TMS) directed at the left DLPFC did not show a difference between sham and active stimulation.[304]

Medications play a significant role in the treatment of schizophrenia. However, psychological, behavioral, psychosocial, and rehabilitation interventions have shown some efficacy when used in conjunction with antipsychotics.[305] Cognitive-behavioral therapy (CBT) is effective for the symptoms of schizophrenia but the effect is small (effect sizes are 0.33, 0.25, and 0.13 for overall symptoms, positive symptoms, and negative symptoms, respectively).[306] Cognitive remediation and training is an efficacious strategy for improving cognitive functioning, including social cognition.[307] The general treatment effect size associated with cognitive remediation therapy in schizophrenia patients is approximately 0.36–0.45.[308,309] Social cognitive training also shows small-moderate effect in schizophrenia patients.[310] Psychoeducation can improve compliance and reduce relapses and family psychoeducation programs can reduce stigma and relapse rates.[311]

Psychosis Associated with Other Neuropsychiatric and Medical Disorders

Psychotic symptoms occur in many neurodegenerative disorders including AD, dementia with Lewy bodies (DLB), PD, and frontotemporal dementia.[312] AD's psychosis is the second most prevalent psychotic disorder after schizophrenia, and it might become the first most prevalent in the coming years, as the global population ages.[313] Schizophrenia is generally regarded as an illness with onset in late adolescence or early adult life but sometimes illness onset is after 40 years of age (late-onset schizophrenia) or after 60 years (very-late-onset schizophrenia-like psychosis). Late-onset psychosis can also occur as a prodromal symptom to neurodegeneration and therefore the differential diagnosis between late-onset schizophrenia and dementia (also known as major neurocognitive disorder) is important. The phenomenology of psychosis is usually different in late-onset schizophrenia (more partition delusions [the belief that people, substances, objects, or radiation can pass through what would normally be a barrier] and auditory hallucinations of human voices) and neurodegeneration processes such as Lewy body dementia (more visual hallucinations, especially those involving animals, and less partition or paranoid delusions) or Alzheimer's dementia.[314] Cognitive deterioration in late-onset schizophrenia is characterized by deficits in (working) memory, language, psychomotor speed, and executive functioning, with the absence of neuropathological evidence for neurodegeneration.[315] It is worth noting that about 15% of middle-aged (45–65 years old) schizophrenia patients develop frontotemporal dementia, AD, or vascular dementia.[316] Schizophrenia patients, especially those younger than 65 years, have more than twofold higher risk of all-cause dementia that could not be explained by established dementia risk factors.[316A]

Psychosis due to PD is highly prevalent (50–60% of patients) and is defined as the presence of at least one of the following symptoms: illusions, false sense of presence, hallucinations, or delusions, that occur after the onset of PD and are recurrent or continuous for 1 month.[317] See Chapter 23 for discussion of the neuropsychiatry of PD and DLB. The typical clinical PD syndrome is psychosis that evolves from minor to major symptoms. In first stages of PD, symptoms include passage hallucinations (objects passing in the peripheral visual field), illusions (misinterpretation of an existing stimuli), pareidolia (the interpretation of formless visual images as real objects), and presence of hallucinations (a feeling that someone is nearby). Later in PD, symptoms include visual hallucinations, typically of animals or people, and the patient has an insight into the nature of the experience of these hallucinations. As the PD progresses, symptoms include more complex hallucinations (multimodality hallucinations) with no insight and profound delusions.[318] Psychotic symptoms in PD usually predicts cognitive decline within 2–4 years. Although PD psychosis occurs in unmedicated patients, there is a major contribution from treatment with dopamine agonists to the development of PD psychosis.[319] A few genetic mutations have been associated with PD psychosis (glucosylceramidase [GBA], microtubule-associated protein tau [MAPT], and regulator of dopamine neurotransmission [DAT1]). Treatment of PD psychosis is based on clozapine (atypical antipsychotic), pimavanserin (a 5-HT2A inverse agonist), and rivastigmine (cholinesterase inhibitor).[320]

Visual hallucinations occur in up to 80% of patients with DLB and are considered as one of the core diagnostic symptoms. These are recurrent, complex visual hallucinations, featuring people, children, or animals, sometimes accompanied by related phenomena including passage hallucinations, sense of presence, and visual illusions.[321] Severe sensitivity to antipsychotics is a supportive evidence to the diagnosis of DLB. Psychotic disorder is rare in Huntington's disease (1.2–4% of patients)[322] and is usually related to lower cognitive function and irritability.[323]

Symptoms of autoimmune encephalitis may include psychosis, other psychiatric and cognitive alterations, seizures, and movement disorders, with the most commonly affected part of the brain being the limbic system. See Chapter 26 for further review of the neuropsychiatry of neuroinflammatory and autoimmune disorders. The underlying pathophysiology of autoimmune encephalitis is critical for the diagnosis and treatment. Paraneoplastic disorders are associated with antibodies to intracellular antigens, such as anti-Hu or GAD65, and involve T-cell responses causing neuronal death. These disorders are mostly associated with cancer (the diagnosis does not require the identification of a malignancy), and the prognosis is poor. Neuronal extracellular surface antibodies, such as the N-methyl-D-aspartate receptor (NMDA-R) antibody, alpha-amino-3-hydroxy-5-methylisoxazole-4-propionic acid (AMPA) receptor antibody, and gamma-aminobutyric acid-B receptor (GABA-B) receptor antibody, usually cause a reversible effect on the neuronal function. They might be related to cancer (such as ovarian teratoma) and when treated early the prognosis is good.[324] In general, psychosis, disturbances of consciousness and orientation, catatonia, speech dysfunction, focal neurological signs, epileptic seizures/EEG abnormalities, or autonomic dysfunction have been found to be warning signs in psychiatric patients that should always lead to cerebrospinal fluid analysis with determination of antineuronal autoantibodies.[325]

Epidemiological studies have found a general association between autoimmunity and psychotic disorders. For example, 6% of schizophrenia patients have a hospital admission related to an autoimmune disease during follow-up and autoimmune disorders are associated with an increased risk of developing schizophrenia.[326] The rate of psychosis in MS is 2–4%, with over 90% of individuals having symptoms of MS prior to the onset of psychosis. The treatment of psychosis is based on anti-psychotic agents, and caution is required due to the potential for exacerbating MS symptoms, especially extrapyramidal side effects.[327] Acute disseminated encephalomyelitis (ADEM) can present as acute psychosis.[328] The rate of psychosis in SLE ranges from 2.3% to 11% in studies[329] and might be caused by the underlying disease or steroid treatment. It is worth noting that in SLE patients experiencing psychosis, this was one of the initial symptoms of SLE in up to 60% of these patients.[330] Therefore, SLE is an important differential diagnosis of an acute psychosis. Other autoimmune disorders related to psychosis are Grave's disease (hyperthyroidism with antithyroid autoantibodies), diabetes type I (with glutamic acid decarboxylase [GAD] antibodies), rheumatoid arthritis (recent studies confirm higher rate of schizophrenia in rheumatoid arthritis patients and their relatives), CNS vasculitis, psoriasis, Guillain-Barré syndrome, autoimmune hepatitis, and Crohn's disease.

Epilepsy is considered a risk factor for psychosis. Recent studies show that the prevalence of psychosis in generalized and temporal lobe epilepsy (TLE) is 5.6% and 7% respectively, and the prevalence of interictal and postictal psychosis in epilepsy is 5.2% and 2% respectively.[331] Risk factors for psychosis in TLE include early age at epilepsy onset, history of status epilepticus, hippocampal sclerosis, and left-hemisphere abnormalities.[332] Epilepsy and psychosis have a bidirectional relation, as not only are patients with epilepsy at greater risk of developing a psychotic disorder, but patients with a primary psychotic disorder are also at greater risk of developing epilepsy.[333] The treatment of most psychotic disorders in epilepsy, with the exception of ictal psychotic episodes, is low dose, preferably atypical, antipsychotic drugs. Low dosage of antipsychotic agents should be used since antipsychotics might lower the seizure threshold. See Chapter 29 for further discussion of the neuropsychiatry of epilepsy.

Post-stroke new onset psychosis is not rare and severely impacts quality of life. The prevalence of post-stroke delusions and hallucinations is 4.67% and 5.05%, respectively. Lesions in post-stroke psychosis are typically right hemisphere, particularly frontal, temporal, and parietal regions, and the right caudate nucleus.[334]

While focal lesions in the auditory and visual systems can cause hallucinations, lesions in other brain area that are connected to the primary sensory systems might also produce hallucinatory effects. Peduncular hallucinosis is a rare psychosis described as vivid, dream-like visual hallucinations that intrude on normal wakefulness. Peduncular hallucinosis appears mainly with vascular lesions or tumor compression affecting the pons, midbrain, and thalamus.[335] Charles-Bonnet syndrome is an infrequent condition of visual hallucinations occurring in patients suffering from lowered visual acuity.[336] Most recently, a pseudo-Charles-Bonnet syndrome was described with a visual loss caused by a lesion in the visual system and visual hallucinations caused by a frontal tumor.[337] Similarly, while it is well known that right frontal cortex lesions can cause a variety of delusions, lesions in other related brain areas also can lead to delusions. In a recent study, misidentification delusions were functionally connected to the left retrosplenial cortex and the right frontal cortex.[338]

ANXIETY DISORDERS

All anxiety disorders share symptoms of fear, anxiety, and behavioral and cognitive disturbances. Fear is the emotional response to real or perceived threat and is associated with autonomic arousal, fight or flight reaction, freezing, and escape behavior. A panic attack is an abrupt surge of intense fear accompanied by physical and/or cognitive symptoms. Anxiety is the anticipation of future threat and is associated with preparation for future danger and avoidant behavior.

Epidemiology

Anxiety disorders are the most prevalent mental disorders around the world (current and lifetime prevalence of 7.3% and 28.8%, respectively), and women are twice as likely as men to have an anxiety disorder.[339] Anxiety disorders are associated with significant morbidity and in 2010 they were the sixth leading cause of disability in terms of years of life lived with disability, with highest burden in women and in those aged 15–34 years.[340] Anxiety disorders are correlated with many environmental risk factors such as family history of mental disorders, low socioeconomic status, childhood maltreatment or abuse, overprotective parenting style, physical punishment in childhood, etc.

Pathophysiology

The pathophysiology of stress and the brain's role in regulation of stress are discussed above in the pathophysiology of depression section. Here we focus on the pathophysiology of fear and anxiety. The mechanism of fear involves perceiving the threats, evaluating threatening situations, and activating the behavioral and physiological response. The mechanism of anxiety involves over-generalization of conditioned fear and deficits in the extinction of conditioned fear. The mechanism of fear is relatively simple and is similar in many animals and humans. Thus, it is not surprising that the pathophysiology of fear is better understood than anxiety (for reviews, see Sylvers et al.[341]; Hofmann et al.[342]; and Tovote et al.[343]).

Many studies have used the Pavlovian fear conditioning model for studying the neurobiology of fear. In this model, a neutral stimulus (the "conditioned" stimulus, such as light or tone) evokes fear through association with a fearful stimulus (the "unconditioned" stimulus, such as foot shock or air puff). The amygdala's plasticity plays a major role in the acquisition and expression of conditioned fear. The amygdala is divided into two main structures: the basolateral amygdala has a cortex-like architecture and the central amygdala has a striatum-like architecture.[344] Fear conditioning increases the evoked responses and causes synaptic plasticity in the basolateral amygdala before the parallel changes in the cortex and the thalamus.[345] The central amygdala is also involved in fear acquisition and expression.[346] A blockade of the sensory afferents to the amygdala can inactivate conditioned fear memories.[347] The amygdala's activity is coordinated with other distributed cue- and context-specific networks for learning of fear responses that include the auditory and multimodal nuclei of the thalamus, auditory cortex, medial prefrontal cortex (mPFC), and hippocampus. Fear extinction is related to these fear conditioning brain circuits, although extinction is a new form of learning and not a simply erasing of fear memories. A specific subpopulation of cells at the basolateral amygdala, the extinction-resistant neurons, maintain the responsiveness to the conditioned stimulus, even after the extinction process.[348] The hippocampus is involved in the consolidation of contextual memories, from short-term memory to long-term memory and has a critical role in the consolidation of emotional memories such as pathological fear and traumatic events.

Although anxiety and fear are mediated by partially overlapping neuronal substrates, there are specific circuits underlying anxiety-like behavior. The bed nucleus of the stria terminalis (BNST), a target for projections from the basolateral and central amygdala, has an important role in the neural circuits of anxiety.[349] Human studies suggest that the amygdala is involved in anxiety, with mixed evidence for both enlarged and reduced amygdala volumes, that probably reflects the amygdala's role in both fear learning and extinction.[350] The ventral portion and the septum of the hippocampus mediates anxiety through pathways to the basolateral amygdala, to hypothalamic nuclei, and to the lateral septum. The mPFC modulates anxiety through pathways to the basolateral amygdala that mediate fear extinction, safety, and reduced anxiety.[351] Most recently, interconnectivity between the cerebellum and the limbic system has been shown to mediate fear and anxiety.[352,353]

Genetic and environmental factors (such as stress, early trauma, etc.) contribute to the development of anxiety disorders. Familial heritability in anxiety disorders is relatively high (30–50%), although twins, linkage, and association studies are inconclusive.[354,355] Genome-wide and gene-based association studies of anxiety disorders have revealed a few genes related to anxiety: MFAP3L (encodes a transmembrane protein, microfibrillar associated protein 3-like, that regulates metabolism, cell growth, and cell survival); NDUFAB1 (encodes a subunit of nicotinamide adenine dinucleotide hydride dehydrogenase, a nuclear encoded subunit of mitochondrial complex I, which influences fundamental cellular processes such as cellular metabolism, gene expression, and ion channel regulation); PALB2 (encodes a protein that co-localizes with BRCA2 in the cell nucleus and promotes its localization and stability in cellular structure like chromatin and nuclear matrix); CAMKMT (encodes a protein that acts in the formation of trimethyllysine in calmodulin which is involved in calcium-dependent signaling); and rs1709393 (located in an uncharacterized non-coding RNA locus on chromosomal band 3q12.3).[356,357] Some studies have identified genes for specific anxiety disorders such as GAD,[358] social anxiety,[359] or anxiety-related traits.[360] Epigenetic mechanisms are involved in anxiety disorders beginning in utero. Recent studies have shown an altered DNA methylation of the many genes related to regulation of transcription, translation, and cell division processes as well as the glucocorticoid receptor gene (NR3C1) in core blood or newborn blood of infants to mothers diagnosed with untreated anxiety disorders.[361,362]

Clinical Presentation

Normative fear and anxiety manifest in childhood as part of typical development. They are age-dependent and likely to be transient: in infancy and toddlerhood—fear of separation and stranger shyness; in early childhood—fear of darkness, thunder, nightmares, imaginary creatures or death; in childhood—fear of natural disaster, getting ill, traumatic events, school and performance anxiety; in adolescence—fear of negative evaluation and peer rejection. As the child cognitively matures, these fears begin to incorporate anticipatory events and stimuli of an imaginary or abstract nature.[363] Although anxiety disorders have distinct categorial diagnostic criteria, the distinction between developmentally normative fear or anxiety and abnormal anxiety disorders rests on clinical judgment of severity, frequency, persistency, distress, and impairment in functioning.

Anxiety disorders tend to be highly comorbid with each other and with other mental disorders such as substance use, depression, or psychosis. *DSM-5* describes seven anxiety disorders:[4]

1. *Panic disorder* consists of recurrent panic attacks, anxiety of having panic attacks, and avoidance of situations that might cause panic attacks.
2. *Generalized anxiety disorder (GAD)* consist of persistent, excessive, and uncontrollable anxiety and worry about certain domains, accompanied by physical symptoms such as restlessness, irritability, difficulty concentrating, muscle tension, fatigue, and sleep disturbance.
3. *Specific phobia* is the fear, anxiety, or avoidance of specific objects or situations such as an animal, natural environment, blood/injection/injury, etc.
4. *Social anxiety disorder* (social phobia) consists of fear, anxiety, or avoidance of social interactions and situations that involve the possibility of being scrutinized, accompanied by a cognitive ideation of being negatively evaluated, embarrassed, humiliated, rejected, etc.
5. *Agoraphobia* is the fear or anxiety about public situations such as public transportation, being in open spaces or in enclosed places, standing in line, or being in a crowd, etc.
6. *Separation anxiety disorder* consists of fear or anxiety about separation from attachment figures, usually in childhood and also throughout adulthood.
7. *Selective mutism* presents as an inability to speak in social situation.

Another anxiety-related disorder, classified by the *DSM-5* as a trauma and stressor related disorder, is *post-traumatic stress disorder (PTSD)*. PTSD develops following one or more traumatic events. The main features of PTSD are reexperiencing symptoms (such as intrusive recollections of the event, distressing dreams, or flashbacks), avoidance of stimuli associated with the trauma, arousal and reactive-externalizing symptoms, anhedonic or dysphoric mood states, negative cognitions, and dissociative symptoms (mainly depersonalization and derealization).

Substance- or medication-induced anxiety disorder may occur during intoxication or withdrawal of alcohol, caffeine, cannabis, PCP, hallucinogens, inhalants, opioids, sedatives, hypnotics, anxiolytics, stimulants (such as amphetamine), or cocaine.

Many medical conditions can cause anxiety:

▪ Endocrine diseases such as hyperthyroidism, pheochromocytoma, hypoglycemia, hyperadrenocorticism.
▪ Metabolic diseases such as porphyria, vitamin B12 deficiency.
▪ Cardiovascular disorders such as arrhythmia (especially atrial fibrillation and also increased QT interval, which may predispose to cardiac arrhythmias), pulmonary embolism, congestive heart failure.
▪ Respiratory disorders such as asthma, pneumonia, chronic obstructive pulmonary disease.

Patients with anxiety disorders present with cognitive impairments including deficits in cognitive flexibility and decision making.[364,365] Patients with anxiety disorders often make decisions that favor harm avoidance and are impaired at shifting from a previously effective strategy to a currently valid strategy. It is probably caused by their enhanced aversion to uncertainty about the decision outcome and reduced propensity to take risks rather than a stronger aversion to losses.[366] Anxiety biases attention to threat-related stimuli. Anxiety patients have a faster response detecting threat-related stimuli and therefore they are distracted by these stimuli at the expense of attention to task-relevant stimuli.[367,368] In addition to their distraction by threatening stimuli, anxiety patients are also distracted by non-threatening stimuli and display poor concentration and reduced multitasking capability.[369]

Treatment

CBT is the most common evidence-based treatment for anxiety disorders.[370] CBT focuses on challenging and changing thoughts, beliefs, attitudes, and behaviors and improving emotional regulation. CBT protocols for anxiety disorders include in vivo exposure, and the direct confrontation of feared objects, activities, or situations. Through exposure to the stimulus, the harmful conditioning can be habituated or extinguished. This treatment is short-term (usually 10–20 weeks). It reduces the cognitive biases to interpret ambiguous stimuli as threatening, replaces avoidant and safety-seeking behaviors with coping behaviors, uses relaxation and breathing training to reduce excessive autonomic arousal. The overall CBT response rates across anxiety disorders averaged 49.5% at post-treatment and 53.6% at follow-up, with an odds ratio of 2.97 compared to placebo.[371,372] Therapist-supported Internet CBT is also effective for anxiety disorders and can be used in many patients that have difficulty accessing treatment, due to a variety of obstacles.[373] Recent studies have demonstrated that anxiety patients have more negative metacognition, that is, negative beliefs about thinking such as "my worrying could make me go mad."[374,375] Negative metacognitive beliefs about the uncontrollability and

danger of worry are likely to predict anxiety and contribute to reduced investment in controlling thinking. Negative metacognition is also related to negative interpretations of internal experience, compromising choice of effective coping strategies when exposed to fear and stressful events.[376] Metacognitive training, metacognitive therapy, and metacognition reflection and insight therapy (MERIT) have been recently suggested as a treatment for anxiety disorders.[377] Other psychological treatments include psychodynamic psychotherapy, mindfulness-based, and cognitive bias modification approaches.

Evidence-based psychotherapy is usually recommended for mild-to-moderate anxiety disorders. For moderate-to-severe anxiety disorder, medications are recommended as a sole therapy or in addition to the CBT treatment (for reviews, see Stein and Sareen[377]; Craske and Stein[378]; Leichsenring and Leweke[379]; Puetz, Youngstedt, and Herring[380]). SSRIs and SNRIs are the first-line pharmacotherapy for anxiety disorders.[381] Lower starting doses and slower increasing rate are recommended in anxiety disorder patients due to higher sensitivity to drug side effects. The therapeutic dose is similar or higher than depression, and the final dosage should be maintained for a year before a trial of discontinuation can be considered. Second-line pharmacotherapies include benzodiazepines, second-generation antipsychotics, buspirone, pregabalin, and beta-blockers.[382] Although benzodiazepines are considered most effective for anxiety disorders,[383] their chronic use is controversial due to high rates of tolerance and higher risk of dementia.[384,385]

Anxiety Associated with Other Neuropsychiatric and Medical Disorders

Anxiety is highly prevalent in neuropsychiatric disorders, yet frequently underdiagnosed and undertreated, and overshadowed in research by a focus on depression.[386] Receiving a diagnosis of many neuropsychiatric disorders, such as mild cognitive impairment (MCI), dementia, PD, MS, or epilepsy, can be similar to being given a diagnosis of a terminal illness, often leading to marked anxiety.[387,388] However, in most patients with neuropsychiatric disorders the anxiety symptoms are caused by the underlying brain pathology or its treatment.

Anxiety and cognition affect each other's clinical symptoms. Anxiety symptoms have a negative impact on tests that required alternating attention, learning of new material, and abstraction abilities.[389] Anxiety is more prevalent in cognitively impaired older adults, elevated anxiety is related to poorer cognitive performance, and more severe anxiety symptoms predict future cognitive decline.[390] In people with MCI, anxiety predicts cognitive decline and the progression to dementia.[391,392] Anxiety disorders are common in people with dementia and are usually accompanied by panic attacks and agitation.[393–395]

Anxiety is related to the pathophysiology and treatment of dementia. A study in AD patients correlated higher anxiety with lower resting metabolism in bilateral entorhinal cortex, bilateral anterior parahippocampal gyrus, left anterior superior temporal gyrus, and left insula.[396] Imaging studies in PD correlated anxiety with mesolimbic changes in dopaminergic and serotonergic receptor function.[397] PD patients today are chronically treated with levodopa and develop motor fluctuations over time. Most of PD patients develop parallel non-motor fluctuations, mainly severe depression and anxiety that are mostly present in the "off" state.[398,399] Subthalamic DBS can improve these levodopa-induced emotional fluctuations in PD patients.[400]

Treatment of anxiety disorders in patients with dementia is based on CBT and pharmacotherapy.[401,402] However, CBT and other learning-based psychotherapies that are based on sound memory and executive skills might have a lower efficacy in dementia patients.[403] Other treatment options include sensory stimulation interventions such as shiatsu and acupressure, aromatherapy, massage/touch therapy, light therapy, sensory garden and horticultural activities, music/dance therapy, or multisensory stimulation therapy.[404] Please see Chapters 21 and 24, respectively, for further review of the neuropsychiatry of AD and frontotemporal dementia.

Anxiety disorders and panic attacks are also prevalent in persons with epilepsy.[405] A recent study has revealed that 40% of epileptic patients have anxiety and the most prevalent symptom of anxiety is worrying thoughts (35.6%).[406] A variety of anxiety symptoms are seen in epilepsy, including preictal (preceding a seizure), ictal (presenting as part of the seizure symptoms and signs), and postictal (occurring within 72 hours of a seizure) symptoms; symptoms resembling primary anxiety disorders (anticipatory anxiety of epileptic seizures, seizure phobia, epileptic social phobia, and epileptic panic disorder); and anxiety related to epilepsy treatment.[407] In some patients, anxiety might be a trigger for seizures. Depression, medication side effects, smoking, and illicit substance use were significantly associated with higher odds of anxiety in epileptic patients. Patients with anxiety reported more severe epilepsy, debilitating seizures, and overall lower quality of life. Focal epilepsy, especially when due to mesial temporal sclerosis, was found to be associated with high anxiety.[408] Diagnosis and treatment of anxiety disorder in epileptic patients are critical for effective treatment of epilepsy.[409]

Psychogenic non-epileptic seizures (PNES) patients present episodes resembling epileptic seizures in their semiology yet lack the underlying epileptic brain activity. Please see Chapter 13 for further review of functional neurological symptom disorder. The disorder is classified by the *DSM-5* as functional neurological symptom disorder (conversion disorder) with attacks or seizures. The classical pathophysiology of PNES has been hypothesized to be a psychodynamic mechanism where intolerable affect is converted into somatic symptoms or a dissociative process where patients utilize psychological compartmentalization to avoid traumatic memories and experiences. However, newer approaches conceptualize PNES as a panic disorder that involves cognitive and learning processes in which patients alter their attentional resources leading to dysfunctional sensory and motor networks through classical and operant conditioning mechanisms. These mechanisms are related to those of anxiety disorders, and therefore it is not surprising that the preferred treatment for PNES is an integrative psychological approach that combines CBT and rehabilitation therapy.[410]

Anxiety is a prevalent symptom in neuroinflammatory diseases. In MS, the reported prevalence of anxiety disorders is 22–40% and high anxiety scores are correlated with an increased risk of relapse.[411-413] A consistent finding in studies is that anxiety in MS is strongly associated with both high level

of disability and low quality of life.[414] This high prevalence and clinically significance of anxiety in neuroinflammatory disease is not surprising, based on the known associations between the dysregulation of the HPA axis specifically in regard to cortisol levels, as well as changes in pro- and anti-inflammatory cytokines in both anxiety and neuroinflammatory diseases.[415]

Another aspect of anxiety in neuropsychiatric syndromes is anxiety about one's health (hypochondriasis) that is a relatively common problem in neuropsychiatry settings.[416] The fear of having a serious brain disease usually leads to medical consultation and is followed by further expensive investigations being carried out unnecessarily and often worsening of anxiety when findings of marginal clinical significance are reported. The symptoms of abnormal health anxiety show little tendency to spontaneous resolution and persist for months in the absence of treatment. In many neuropsychiatric disorders, health anxiety might coexist with the primary diagnosis. These patients perceive their intact physical and cognitive performance as impaired and attribute the impairment to their illness.[417] As in other anxiety disorders, accurate diagnosis and treatment (usually CBT) could significantly improve the patients' well-being.[418]

OBSESSIVE-COMPULSIVE DISORDER

OCD is a psychiatric disorder characterized by obsessions and compulsions.

Epidemiology

OCD is among the most common, challenging, and debilitating anxiety disorders, with an estimated prevalence of 2–3%.[419] OCD usually begins in adolescence or early adulthood and the majority of individuals have a chronic waxing and waning course, with exacerbation of symptoms that may be related to stress.[420] About 15% show progressive deterioration in occupational and social functioning.[421]

Pathophysiology

Neurobiological abnormalities, such as dysregulation of neurotransmitters (mainly dopamine and serotonin) and genetic factors, may play a crucial role in the etiology and course of OCD.[422,423] The mechanisms of OCD probably involve dysfunction of cortico-striato-thalamo-cortical (CSTC) brain circuits.[424] Adult OCD patients have smaller hippocampal volumes and larger pallidum volumes while unmedicated pediatric patients have larger thalamic volumes.[425] Neuropsychological studies have demonstrated cognitive and functional abnormalities related to these structures, such as impaired executive functioning and decreased cognitive-behavioral flexibility.[426,427] Diffusion tensor imaging (DTI) and connectivity studies demonstrated abnormal and heightened connectivity of ventrolimbic corticostriatal regions in patients with OCD.[428] Functional neuroimaging studies found hyperactivity at rest in CSTC circuits in OCD that was accentuated during provocation of OCD symptoms[429,430] and was reduced after successful treatment of OCD, including pharmacological, behavioral, or neurosurgical treatments.[431]

Clinical Presentation

Obsessions are recurrent and persistent thoughts, impulses, or images that are experienced as intrusive and that cause marked anxiety and distress. The person recognizes that the obsessions are a product of his or her own mind and tries to ignore or suppress these obsessions with some other thought or actions. Compulsions are repetitive behaviors (e.g., hand washing, ordering, checking) or mental acts (e.g., praying, counting, repeating words silently) that the person feels driven to perform in response to an obsession or internal rigid rules. The compulsions are aimed at preventing or reducing distress. The person recognizes that the obsessions or compulsions are excessive or unreasonable and cause marked distress, are time-consuming, and significantly interfere with the person's normal life.

Although obsessions and compulsions can coexist in the same patient, isolated obsessions and compulsions can occur, accounting for the illness' high degree of heterogeneity. For example, some patients may have contamination obsessions and/or compulsions (i.e., "washers") while others will have compulsions to count (i.e., "checkers"). Behaviors, or compulsions, that are meant to relieve anxiety become reinforcing, leading to a vicious cycle of thoughts and actions. Heterogeneity in OCD is the rule, although it appears that activation of fear and anxiety circuitry is a common thread. OCD patients have a prominent difficulty tolerating ambiguous or uncertain situations and report heightened feeling of distress when faced with multiple possibilities.[432] They are reluctant to take risks, even in the absence of exaggerated beliefs about the probability of making a mistake.

OCD patients have a unique cognitive profile. Most OCD patients display abnormalities in cognitive flexibility, they have difficulty shifting between mental processes to generate adaptive behavioral responses, especially in the context of their symptoms.[433] OCD cognitive inflexibility is usually demonstrated by low scores in tests such as attentional set shifting, reversal and alternation, cued task-switching paradigms, cognitive control measures such as the Trail-Making, part B and Stroop tasks, and several measures of motor inhibition. Other cognitive deficits in OCD include deficits in perception, attention, memory, and executive functioning.[434]

The diagnosis of OCD was revised for the *DSM-5.*[4] OCD was separated from anxiety disorders and the OCD diagnosis contains specifiers to delineate the degree of insight.[435] As in other neuropsychiatric disorders, sleep disturbances are common among OCD patients.[436,437] The sleep pattern, as recorded in polysomnographic studies, is different in OCD compared to normal controls.[438] Sleep disturbance severity is associated with OCD severity, even when controlling for other anxiety-related or depressive disorders.[439] Specific OCD symptoms such as unacceptable thoughts, cognitive concerns, and alertness were found to be correlated with sleep disturbances.[440,441]

Treatment

Effective treatments for OCD include behavioral therapy (exposure and response/ritual prevention and CBT) and sero-tonin-reuptake inhibitors. Behavioral therapy is more effective than SSRIs and the combination of behavioral therapy plus SSRIs is most effective.[442] First-line pharmacotherapy of OCD are SSRIs such as fluoxetine, sertraline, citalopram, or TCAs such as clomipramine at the maximal tolerated dose. Second-line augmentation includes clonazepam, haloperidol, risperidone, olanzapine, or gabapentin. Preliminary data suggest efficacy and safety of other medications such as riluzole, ketamine, memantine, N-acetylcysteine, lamotrigine, celecoxib, ondansetron, either in combination with SSRIs or as monotherapy in the treatment of OCD.[443] The principal behavioral approaches in OCD are exposure and response prevention, but many patients receiving intensive CBT courses do not achieve symptomatic relief.[444,445]

The efficacy of pharmacological and non-pharmacological treatment for OCD is lower than other anxiety disorders.[446] When a new treatment is introduced, OCD patients are likely to continue engaging in some compulsions and then attribute anxiety reduction to the rituals instead of to the treatment. Although it is well known that in clinical studies for depression and anxiety, the placebo rate is high,[447] OCD patients present a lower placebo effect than other primary psychiatric disorders.[448] This relatively low placebo effect might be caused by the difficulty in shifting behaviors even when expectations are high, and anxiety is reduced. Pharmacological studies report that 50–75% of OCD patients that meet the inclusion criteria refuse to participate in blinded studies.[449] OCD patients' pervasive doubt, uncertainty, diminished feeling of confidence, and reluctance to take risks might contribute to this low recruitment rate. At least 10% of patients are refractory to the pharmacological and the behavioral treatments.[450]

The anterior limb of the internal capsule contains a rich network of fibers that connect both the PFC and anterior cingulate cortex with the hippocampus, amygdala, and the thalamus. In the past, patients with severe, refractory OCD were treated with ablative neurosurgical techniques, including anterior capsulotomy and cingulotomy.[451] Newer noninvasive approaches to anterior capsulotomy have been tried, using both gamma knife radiosurgery (GKRS) and MR-guided focused ultrasound (MRgFUS).[452–454] The anterior capsule (VS) was therefore the first target for DBS for OCD.[455] During the last decade, a few studies have suggested other DBS targets for OCD: subthalamic nucleus, NAc, and inferior thalamic peduncle. Although the overall published experience with DBS for OCD is limited, the reported results are encouraging, averaging a 50% response rate in these highly resistant OCD patients.[456–458] Current DBS studies for OCD and other psychiatric indications focus on new anatomical targets, better targeting within the above brain targets, and new physiological targets for emotional-cognitive closed-loop DBS, that is, adaptive brain stimulation based on pathologic electrophysiological activity related to emotional and cognitive symptoms.[459]

Obsessions and Compulsions Associated with Other Neuropsychiatric and Medical Disorders

OCD is related to many hyperkinetic movement disorders. *DSM-5* diagnosis of OCD includes the presence of tics as a possible specifier, based on the increasing evidence on the overlap between tic disorders and OCD. There is also a relationship between OCD and Tourette syndrome, the choreas (Huntington's disease and Sydenham's chorea), and some dystonias.[460] Among other treatments, habit reversal therapy is an effective treatment for tic disorders, Tourette syndrome, OCD, and other OC-related disorders.[461] This therapy is based on awareness training, competing response training, contingency management, relaxation training, and generalization training.[462] Obsessive-compulsive symptoms can be found in up to 50% of PD patients.[463] Parkinson's patients that are carrier of the PARKIN genotype mutation have a high rate of OC symptoms.[464]

Pediatric autoimmune neuropsychiatric disorders associated with streptococcal infections (PANDAS) and its broader iteration, pediatric acute-onset neuropsychiatric syndrome (PANS), have suggested a role for streptococcal infection in children with explosive onset OCD and tic disorders.[465] Although not included in the *DSM*, PANDAS should be suspected in abrupt OCD and other neuropsychiatric symptoms in children. Treatment of PANDAS includes antibiotics for acute and prophylactic phases, NSAIDs, SSRIs, and CBT.[466]

Epilepsy patients also have a high rate of obsessive-compulsive symptoms (up to 40%) and OCD (about 11%). TLE is associated with a higher prevalence of OCD than other forms of epilepsy.[467] High rates of OCD can also be found in MS patients (around 15%).

Summary and Key Points

- Mental disorders can be addressed as disorders of brain circuits.
- Genetic, neuroimaging, and clinical analyses find overlap across a wide variety of psychiatric diagnoses, suggesting common neurobiological substrates for mental illness.
- The role of neuropsychiatry is expanding the field of psychiatry into dimensions of cognitive-behavioral and social neuroscience and can provide advanced approaches to diagnosis, formulation, and treatment.

Multiple Choice Questions

1. The hypothalamic-pituitary-adrenal (HPA) axis is associated with the stress response. In patients suffering from depression, HPA axis alteration is associated with:
   a. Older age
   b. More severe symptoms
   c. Melancholic or psychotic depression
   d. Cognitive deficits
   e. All of the above

2. Depressed patients typically have which of the following characteristic network patterns?
   a. Hyperconnectivity within the cognitive control circuit
   b. Hyperconnectivity within the default mode network
   c. Hypoconnectivity of the amygdala with the negative affect circuitry
   d. Hypoconnectivity of the amygdala with the salience network
   e. None of the above

3. Which is the following is true regarding bipolar spectrum disorders?
   a. Bipolar II is more prevalent than bipolar I.
   b. Cognitive impairment is present in both depressive and manic episodes, but resolves during euthymic episodes.
   c. Bipolar disorder has a relatively high prevalence in multiple sclerosis and epilepsy.

   d. Bupropion may have higher risk of eliciting manic states in BPD patients compared to TCAs and SNRIs.
   e. A manic episode is not required for diagnosis of bipolar disorder if sufficient recurrent depressive episodes occur.

4. Neurobiological abnormalities in schizophrenia include:
   a. Hyperdopaminergic states in frontal cortex
   b. Hypodopaminergic states in the striatum
   c. Increased activity in striatum during reward conditioning tasks
   d. Abnormal anterior cingulate cortex activity is associated with delusions
   e. Larger hippocampus volume

5. Anxiety may be present in the following neurological disorders:
   a. As a normal reaction to the stress of receiving a neurodegenerative disorder
   b. During the "off" states of Parkinson's disease levodopa treatment
   c. In epilepsy patients, as either preictal, ictal, or postictal phenomenology
   d. Correlated to level of disability in multiple sclerosis patients
   e. All of the above

Multiple Choice Answers

1. Answer: e

Changes in the HPA axis are correlated with more severe symptoms, melancholic or psychotic features, older age, and cognitive symptoms. Unfortunately, however, neuroendocrine targeted interventions have yielded mixed results in depression treatment.

2. Answer: b

Patients with depressive symptoms typically have hyperconnectivity of the default mode network, potentially explaining ruminative self-focus. Cognitive control networks, involved in attention to external environment, tend to be hypoconnected in depressed patients, consistent with common symptoms of inattention. These examples also highlight the inverse correlation between default mode and executive control networks. Lastly, there is hyperconnectivity of the amygdala to negative affect circuitry and to the salience network.

3. Answer: c

Patients with bipolar disorder have a high relative occurrence of multiple sclerosis, epilepsy, and migraine. Bipolar II disorder has a lower lifetime prevalence (0.4%) compared to bipolar I (0.6%). Cognitive impairment is present across all affective states in bipolar disorder, with deficits spanning domains of attention, processing speed, episodic memory, and executive functioning. Though all antidepressant agents carry risk of manic conversion, bupropion is thought to have lower risk than TCAs and SNRIs. Lastly, a manic episode is a diagnostic requirement for bipolar disorder.

4. Answer: d

Delusional symptoms have been associated with anterior cingulate cortex activity abnormalities. In patients with schizophrenia, the frontal cortex generally is associated with a hypodopaminergic state, and the striatum with a hyperdopaminergic state. Individuals with schizophrenia display decreased activity in the striatum during reward conditioning tasks. The hippocampus, amygdala, thalamus, nucleus accumbens, and anterior cingulate are typically decreased in volume in schizophrenia.

5. Answer: e

All of the above are true, and are examples of the importance of screening for anxiety symptoms across varying neurological disorders.

References

1. Sullivan PF, Geschwind DH. Defining the genetic, genomic, cellular, and diagnostic architectures of psychiatric disorders. *Cell.* 2019;177(1):162-183.
2. Fung LK, Reiss AL. Moving toward integrative, multidimensional research in modern psychiatry: lessons learned from fragile x syndrome. *Biol Psychiatry.* 2016;80(2):100-111.
3. Silbersweig D, Loscalzo J. Precision psychiatry meets network medicine: network psychiatry. *JAMA Psychiatry.* 2017;74(7):665-666.
4. American Psychiatric Association. *Diagnostic and Statistical Manual of Mental Disorders.* 5th ed. Arlington, VA: American Psychiatric Association; 2013.
5. Insel T, Cuthbert B, Garvey M, et al. Research domain criteria (RDoC): toward a new classification framework for research on mental disorders. *Am J Psychiatry.* 2010;167(7):748-751.
6. Gordon JA. On being a circuit psychiatrist. *Nat Neurosci.* 2016;19(11):1385-1386.
7. Goodkind M, Eickhoff SB, Oathes DJ, et al. Identification of a common neurobiological substrate for mental illness. *JAMA Psychiatry.* 2015;72(4):305-315.
8. McTeague LM, Huemer J, Carreon DM, Jiang Y, Eickhoff SB, Etkin A. Identification of common neural circuit disruptions in cognitive control across psychiatric disorders. *Am J Psychiatry.* 2017;174(7):676-685.
9. Schildkrout B, Benjamin S, Lauterbach MD. Integrating neuroscience knowledge and neuropsychiatric skills into psychiatry: the way forward. *Acad Med.* 2016;91(5):650-656.
10. Kessler RC, Bromet EJ. The epidemiology of depression across cultures. *Annu. Rev. Public Health.* 2013;34:119-138.
11. World Health Organization: Mental Health. Available at http://www.who.int/mental_health/management/depression/en/.
12. Greenberg PE, Fournier AA, Sisitsky T, Pike CT, Kessler RC. The economic burden of adults with major depressive disorder in the United States (2005 and 2010). *J Clin Psychiatry.* 2015;76(2):155-162.
13. Walker ER, McGee RE, Druss BG. Mortality in mental disorders and global disease burden implications: a systematic review and meta-analysis. *JAMA Psychiatry.* 2015;72(4):334-341.
14. Chesney E, Goodwin GM, Fazel S. Risks of all cause and suicide mortality in mental disorders: a meta-review. *World Psychiatry.* 2014;13:153-160.
15. Spijker J, de Graaf R, Bijl RV, Beekman AT, Ormel J, Nolen WA. Duration of major depressive episodes in the general population: results from the Netherlands Mental Health Survey and Incidence Study (NEMESIS). *Br J Psychiatry.* 2002;181:208-213.
16. Seedat S, Scott KM, Angermeyer MC, et al. Cross-national associations between gender and mental disorders in the World Health Organization World Mental Health Surveys. *Arch Gen Psychiatry.* 2009;66(7):785-795.
17. Cavanagh A, Wilson CJ, Kavanagh DJ, Caputi P. Differences in the expression of symptoms in men versus women with depression: a systematic review and meta-analysis. *Harv Rev Psychiatry.* 2017;25(1):29-38.
18. Kuehner C. Why is depression more common among women than among men? *Lancet Psychiatry.* 2017;4(2):146-158.
19. Aranda MP, Chae DH, Lincoln KD, Taylor RJ, Woodward AT, Chatters LM. Demographic correlates of DSM-IV major depressive disorder among older African Americans, Black Caribbeans, and non-Hispanic Whites: results from the National Survey of American Life. *Int J Geriatr Psychiatry.* 2012;27(9):940-947.

20. Lopresti AL, Hood SD, Drummond PD. A review of lifestyle factors that contribute to important pathways associated with major depression: diet, sleep and exercise. *J Affect Disord.* 2013;148(1):12-27.

21. Peyrot WJ, Lee SH, Milaneschi Y, et al. The association between lower educational attainment and depression owing to shared genetic effects? Results in ~25,000 subjects. *Mol Psychiatry.* 2015;20(6):735-743.

22. Kendler KS, Karkowski LM, Prescott CA. Stressful life events and major depression: risk period, long-term contextual threat, and diagnostic specificity. *J Nerv Ment Dis.* 1998;186(11):661-669.

23. Entringer S, Buss C, Wadhwa PD. Prenatal stress, development, health and disease risk: a psychobiological perspective—2015 Curt Richter Award Paper. *Psychoneuroendocrinology.* 2015;62:366-375.

24. Peterson RE, Cai N, Dahl AW, et al. Molecular genetic analysis subdivided by adversity exposure suggests etiologic heterogeneity in major depression. *Am J Psychiatry.* 2018 Jun 1;175(6):545-554.

25. Teicher MH, Samson JA, Anderson CM, Ohashi K. The effects of childhood maltreatment on brain structure, function and connectivity. *Nat Rev Neurosci.* 2016;17(10):652-666.

26. Penninx BW, Milaneschi Y, Lamers F, Vogelzangs N. Understanding the somatic consequences of depression: biological mechanisms and the role of depression symptom profile. *BMC Med.* 2013;11:129.

27. McEwen BS, Bowles NP, Gray JD, et al. Mechanisms of stress in the brain. *Nat Neurosci.* 2015;18(10):1353-1363.

28. Hinkelmann K, Moritz S, Botzenhardt J, et al. Cognitive impairment in major depression: association with salivary cortisol. *Biol Psychiatry.* 2009;66(9):879-885.

29. Salvat-Pujol N, Labad J, Urretavizcaya M, et al. Hypothalamic-pituitary-adrenal axis activity and cognition in major depression: the role of remission status. *Psychoneuroendocrinology.* 2017;76:38-48.

30. Davis EG, Keller J, Hallmayer J, et al. Corticotropin-releasing factor 1 receptor haplotype and cognitive features of major depression. *Transl Psychiatry.* 2018;8(1):5.

31. O'Connell CP, Goldstein-Piekarski AN, Nemeroff CB, et al. Antidepressant outcomes predicted by genetic variation in corticotropin-releasing hormone binding protein. *Am J Psychiatry.* 2018;175(3):251-261.

32. McAllister-Williams RH, Anderson IM, Finkelmeyer A, et al. Antidepressant augmentation with metyrapone for treatment-resistant depression (the ADD study): a double-blind, randomised, placebo-controlled trial. *Lancet Psychiatry.* 2016;3(2):117-127.

33. Otte C, Wingenfeld K, Kuehl LK, et al. Mineralocorticoid receptor stimulation improves cognitive function and decreases cortisol secretion in depressed patients and healthy individuals. *Neuropsychopharmacology.* 2015;40(2):386-393.

34. Faron-Górecka A, Kuśmider M, Solich J, et al. Involvement of prolactin and somatostatin in depression and the mechanism of action of antidepressant drugs. *Pharmacol Rep.* 2013;65(6):1640-1646.

35. Kormos V, Gaszner B. Role of neuropeptides in anxiety, stress, and depression: from animals to humans. *Neuropeptides.* 2013;47(6):401-419.

36. Cooper-Kazaz R, Apter JT, Cohen R, et al. Combined treatment with sertraline and liothyronine in major depression: a randomized, double-blind, placebo-controlled trial. *Arch Gen Psychiatry.* 2007;64(6):679-688.

37. Eitan R, Landshut G, Lifschytz T, Einstein O, Ben-Hur T, Lerer B. The thyroid hormone, triiodothyronine, enhances fluoxetine-induced neurogenesis in rats: possible role in antidepressant-augmenting properties. *Int J Neuropsychopharmacol.* 2010;13(5):553-561.

38. Duntas LH, Maillis A. Hypothyroidism and depression: salient aspects of pathogenesis and management. *Minerva Endocrinol.* 2013;38(4):365-377.

39. Bebbington P, Dunn G, Jenkins R, et al. The influence of age and sex on the prevalence of depressive conditions: report from the National Survey of Psychiatric Morbidity. *Int Rev Psychiatry.* 2003;15(1-2):74-83.

40. Schildkraut JJ. The catecholamine hypothesis of affective disorders: a review of supporting evidence. *Am J Psychiatry.* 1965;122(5):509-522.

41. Jesulola E, Micalos P, Baguley IJ. Understanding the pathophysiology of depression: from monoamines to the neurogenesis hypothesis model—are we there yet? *Behav Brain Res.* 2018;341:79-90.

42. Duman RS, Sanacora G, Krystal JH. Altered connectivity in depression: GABA and glutamate neurotransmitter deficits and reversal by novel treatments. *Neuron.* 2019;102(1):75-90.

43. Peciña M, Karp JF, Mathew S, Todtenkopf MS, Ehrich EW, Zubieta JK. Endogenous opioid system dysregulation in depression: implications for new therapeutic approaches. *Mol Psychiatry.* 2019;24(4):576-587.

44. Geschwind DH, Flint J. Genetics and genomics of psychiatric disease. *Science.* 2015;349(6255):1489-1494.

45. Sullivan PF, de Geus EJ, Willemsen G, et al. Genomewide association for major depressive disorder: a possible role for the presynaptic protein piccolo. *Mol Psychiatry.* 2009;14:359-375.

46. Kendler KS, Gatz M, Gardner CO, Pedersen NL. A Swedish national twin study of lifetime major depression. *Am J Psychiatry.* 2006;163:109-114.

47. Flint J, Kendler KS. The genetics of major depression. *Neuron.* 2014;81(3):484-503.

48. Major Depressive Disorder Working Group of the Psychiatric GWAS Consortium, Ripke S, Wray NR, Lewis CM, et al. A mega-analysis of genome-wide association studies for major depressive disorder. *Mol Psychiatry.* 2013;18(4):497-511.

49. Hyde CL, Nagle MW, Tian C, et al. Identification of 15 genetic loci associated with risk of major depression in individuals of European descent. *Nat Genet.* 2016;48(9):1031-1036.

50. Li QS, Tian C, Seabrook GR, Drevets WC, Narayan VA. Analysis of 23andMe antidepressant efficacy survey data: implication of circadian rhythm and neuroplasticity in bupropion response. *Transl Psychiatry.* 2016;6(9):e889.

51. CONVERGE consortium. Sparse whole-genome sequencing identifies two loci for major depressive disorder. *Nature.* 2015;523(7562):588-591.

52. Bigdeli TB, Ripke S, Peterson RE, et al. Genetic effects influencing risk for major depressive disorder in China and Europe. *Transl Psychiatry.* 2017;7(3):e1074.

53. Klengel T, Binder EB. Epigenetics of stress-related psychiatric disorders and gene × environment interactions. *Neuron.* 2015;86(6):1343-1357.

54. Kim DJ, Davis EP, Sandman CA, et al. Prenatal maternal cortisol has sex-specific associations with child brain network properties. *Cereb Cortex.* 2017;27(11):5230-5241.

55. Yehuda R, Daskalakis NP, Bierer LM, et al. Holocaust exposure induced intergenerational effects on FKBP5 methylation. *Biol Psychiatry.* 2016;80(5):372-380.

56. Hodes GE, Kana V, Menard C, Merad M, Russo SJ. Neuroimmune mechanisms of depression. *Nat Neurosci.* 2015;18:1386-1393.

57. Setiawan E, Wilson AA, Mizrahi R, et al. Role of translocator protein density, a marker of neuroinflammation, in the brain during major depressive episodes. *JAMA Psychiatry.* 2015;72(3):268-275.

58. Köhler O, Benros ME, Nordentoft M, et al. Effect of anti-inflammatory treatment on depression, depressive symptoms, and adverse effects: a systematic review and meta-analysis of randomized clinical trials. *JAMA Psychiatry.* 2014;71(12):1381-1391.

59. Drevets WC, Price JL, Simpson JR Jr, et al. Subgenual prefrontal cortex abnormalities in mood disorders. *Nature.* 1997;386(6627):824-827.

60. Schmaal L, Hibar DP, Sämann PG, et al. Cortical abnormalities in adults and adolescents with major depression based on brain scans from 20 cohorts worldwide in the ENIGMA Major Depressive Disorder working group. *Mol Psychiatry.* 2017;22(6):900-909.

61. Rajkowska G. Postmortem studies in mood disorders indicate altered numbers of neurons and glial cells. *Biol Psychiatry.* 2000;48(8):766-777.

62. Manji HK, Moore GJ, Rajkowska G, Chen G. Neuroplasticity and cellular resilience in mood disorders. *Mol Psychiatry.* 2000;5(6):578-593.

63. Schmaal L, Veltman DJ, van Erp TG, et al. Subcortical brain alterations in major depressive disorder: findings from the ENIGMA Major Depressive Disorder working group. *Mol Psychiatry.* 2016;21(6):806-812.

64. Wigmore EM, Clarke TK, Howard DM, et al. Do regional brain volumes and major depressive disorder share genetic architecture? A study of Generation Scotland (n=19 762), UK Biobank (n=24 048) and the English Longitudinal Study of Ageing (n=5766). *Transl Psychiatry.* 2017;7(8):e1205.

65. Parush N, Tishby N, Bergman H. Dopaminergic balance between reward maximization and policy complexity. *Front Syst Neurosci.* 2011;5:22.

66. Bergman H, Katabi S, Slovik M, et al. Motor pathways, basal ganglia physiology and pathophysiology. In: Reti I, ed. *Brain Stimulation: Methodologies and Interventions.* Wiley-Blackwell; 2015.

67. Russo SJ, Nestler EJ. The brain reward circuitry in mood disorders. *Nat Rev Neurosci.* 2013;14(9):609-625.

68. Williams LM. Precision psychiatry: a neural circuit taxonomy for depression and anxiety. *Lancet Psychiatry.* 2016;3(5):472-480.

69. Hamilton JP, Chen MC, Gotlib IH. Neural systems approaches to understanding major depressive disorder: an intrinsic functional organization perspective. *Neurobiol Dis.* 2013;52:4-11.

70. Whitfield-Gabrieli S, Ford JM. Default mode network activity and connectivity in psychopathology. *Annu Rev Clin Psychol.* 2012;8:49-76.

71. Silberszweig D. Default mode subnetworks, connectivity, depression and its treatment: toward brain-based biomarker development. *Biol Psychiatry.* 2013;74(1):5-6.

72. Dutta A, McKie S, Deakin JF. Resting state networks in major depressive disorder. *Psychiatry Res.* 2014;224(3):139-151.

73. Kaiser RH, Andrews-Hanna JR, Wager TD, Pizzagalli DA. Large-scale network dysfunction in major depressive disorder: a meta-analysis of resting-state functional connectivity. *JAMA Psychiatry.* 2015;72(6):603-611.

74. Rock PL, Roiser JP, Riedel WJ, Blackwell AD. Cognitive impairment in depression: a systematic review and meta-analysis. *Psychol Med.* 2014;44(10):2029-2040.

75. Peckham AD, McHugh RK, Otto MW. A meta-analysis of the magnitude of biased attention in depression. *Depress Anxiety.* 2010;27(12):1135-1142.

76. Lee RS, Hermens DF, Porter MA, Redoblado-Hodge MA. A meta-analysis of cognitive deficits in first-episode major depressive disorder. *J Affect Disord.* 2012;140(2):113-124.

77. Bora E, Harrison BJ, Yücel M, Pantelis C. Cognitive impairment in euthymic major depressive disorder: a meta-analysis. *Psychol Med.* 2013;43(10):2017-2026.

78. Evans VC, Iverson GL, Yatham LN, Lam RW. The relationship between neurocognitive and psychosocial functioning in major depressive disorder: a systematic review. *J Clin Psychiatry.* 2014;75(12):1359-1370.

79. Cullen B, Smith DJ, Deary IJ, Evans JJ, Pell JP. The "cognitive footprint" of psychiatric and neurological conditions: cross-sectional study in the UK Biobank cohort. *Acta Psychiatr Scand.* 2017;135(6):593-605.

80. Zaninotto L, Guglielmo R, Calati R, et al. Cognitive markers of psychotic unipolar depression: a meta-analytic study. *J Affect Disord.* 2015;174:580-588.

81. Nelson JC, Bickford D, Delucchi K, Fiedorowicz JG, Coryell WH. Risk of psychosis in recurrent episodes of psychotic and nonpsychotic major depressive disorder: a systematic review and meta-analysis. *Am J Psychiatry.* 2018;175(9):897-904.

82. McIntyre RS, Suppes T, Tandon R, Ostacher M. Florida best practice psychotherapeutic medication guidelines for adults with major depressive disorder. *J Clin Psychiatry.* 2017;78(6):703-713.

83. Parikh SV, Quilty LC, Ravitz P, et al. CANMAT Depression Work Group. Canadian Network for Mood and Anxiety Treatments (CANMAT) 2016 clinical guidelines for the management of adults with major depressive disorder: section 2. Psychological treatments. *Can J Psychiatry.* 2016;61(9):524-539.

84. Krogh J, Hjorthøj C, Speyer H, Gluud C, Nordentoft M. Exercise for patients with major depression: a systematic review with meta-analysis and trial sequential analysis. *BMJ Open.* 2017;7(9):e014820.

85. Kvam S, Kleppe CL, Nordhus IH, Hovland A. Exercise as a treatment for depression: a meta-analysis. *J Affect Disord.* 2016;202:67-86.

86. Cipriani A, Furukawa TA, Salanti G, et al. Comparative efficacy and acceptability of 21 antidepressant drugs for the acute treatment of adults with major depressive disorder: a systematic review and network meta-analysis. *Lancet.* 2018;391(10128):1357-1366.

87. Rush AJ, Trivedi MH, Wisniewski SR, et al. STAR*D Study Team. Bupropion-SR, sertraline, or venlafaxine-XR after failure of SSRIs for depression. *N Engl J Med.* 2006;354(12):1231-1242.

88. Trivedi MH, Greer TL. Cognitive dysfunction in unipolar depression: implications for treatment. *J Affect Disord.* 2014;152-154:19-27.

89. Rosenblat JD, Kakar R, McIntyre RS. The cognitive effects of antidepressants in major depressive disorder: a systematic review and meta-analysis of randomized clinical trials. *Int J Neuropsychopharmacol.* 2015;19(2). pii: pyv082.

90. Molero P, Ramos-Quiroga JA, Martin-Santos R, Calvo-Sánchez E, Gutiérrez-Rojas L, Meana JJ. Antidepressant efficacy and tolerability of ketamine and esketamine: a critical review. *CNS Drugs.* 2018;32(5):411-420.

91. Noto C, Rizzo LB, Mansur RB, McIntyre RS, Maes M, Brietzke E. Targeting the inflammatory pathway as a therapeutic tool for major depression. *Neuroimmunomodulation.* 2014;21(2-3):131-139.

92. Fava M, Memisoglu A, Thase ME, et al. Opioid modulation with buprenorphine/samidorphan as adjunctive treatment for inadequate response to antidepressants: a randomized double-blind placebo-controlled trial. *Am J Psychiatry.* 2016;173(5):499-508.

93. Kennedy SH, Lam RW, McIntyre RS, et al. Canadian Network for Mood and Anxiety Treatments (CANMAT) 2016 clinical guidelines for the management of adults with major depressive disorder: section 3. Pharmacological treatments. *Can J Psychiatry.* 2016;61(9):540-560.

94. Patel V, Chisholm D, Parikh R, et al. Addressing the burden of mental, neurological, and substance use disorders: key messages from Disease Control Priorities, 3rd edition. *Lancet.* 2016;387(10028):1672-1685.

95. Akil H, Gordon J, Hen R, et al. Treatment resistant depression: a multi-scale, systems biology approach. *Neurosci Biobehav Rev.* 2018;84:272-288.

96. Eitan R, Lerer B. Nonpharmacological, somatic treatments of depression: electroconvulsive therapy and novel brain stimulation modalities. *Dialogues Clin Neurosci.* 2006;8(2):241-258.

97. Sackeim HA. Modern electroconvulsive therapy: vastly improved yet greatly underused. *JAMA Psychiatry.* 2017;74(8):779-780.

98. Sackeim HA, Prudic J, Nobler MS, et al. Effects of pulse width and electrode placement on the efficacy and cognitive effects of electroconvulsive therapy. *Brain Stimul.* 2008;1(2):71-83.

99. Gaynes BN, Lloyd SW, Lux L, et al. Repetitive transcranial magnetic stimulation for treatment-resistant depression: a systematic review and meta-analysis. *J Clin Psychiatry.* 2014;75(5):477-489; quiz 489.

100. McClintock SM, Reti IM, Carpenter LL, et al. Consensus recommendations for the clinical application of repetitive transcranial magnetic stimulation (rTMS) in the treatment of depression. *J Clin Psychiatry.* 2018;79(1). pii: 16cs10905.

101. Brunoni AR, Chaimani A, Moffa AH, et al. Repetitive transcranial magnetic stimulation for the acute treatment of major depressive episodes: a systematic review with network meta-analysis. *JAMA Psychiatry.* 2017;74(2):143-152.

102. Levkovitz Y, Isserles M, Padberg F, et al. Efficacy and safety of deep transcranial magnetic stimulation for major depression: a prospective multicenter randomized controlled trial. *World Psychiatry.* 2015;14(1):64-73.

103. Kedzior KK, Gierke L, Gellersen HM, Berlim MT. Cognitive functioning and deep transcranial magnetic stimulation (DTMS) in major psychiatric disorders: a systematic review. *J Psychiatr Res.* 2016;75:107-115.

104. Chen JJ, Zhao LB, Liu YY, Fan SH, Xie P. Comparative efficacy and acceptability of electroconvulsive therapy versus repetitive transcranial magnetic stimulation for major depression: a systematic review and multiple-treatments meta-analysis. *Behav Brain Res.* 2017;320:30-36.

105. Cretaz E, Brunoni AR, Lafer B. Magnetic seizure therapy for unipolar and bipolar depression: a systematic review. *Neural Plast.* 2015;2015:521398.

106. Meron D, Hedger N, Garner M, Baldwin DS. Transcranial direct current stimulation (tDCS) in the treatment of depression: systematic review and meta-analysis of efficacy and tolerability. *Neurosci Biobehav Rev.* 2015;57:46-62.

107. Brunoni AR, Moffa AH, Fregni F, et al. Transcranial direct current stimulation for acute major depressive episodes: meta-analysis of individual patient data. *Br J Psychiatry.* 2016;208(6):522-531.

108. Martin DM, Moffa A, Nikolin S, et al. Cognitive effects of transcranial direct current stimulation treatment in patients with major depressive disorder: an individual patient data meta-analysis of randomised, sham-controlled trials. *Neurosci Biobehav Rev.* 2018;90:137-145.

109. Carreno FR, Frazer A. Vagal nerve stimulation for treatment-resistant depression. *Neurotherapeutics.* 2017;14(3):716-727.

110. Aaronson ST, Sears P, Ruvuna F, et al. A 5-year observational study of patients with treatment-resistant depression treated with vagus nerve stimulation or treatment as usual: comparison of response, remission, and suicidality. *Am J Psychiatry.* 2017;174(7):640-648.

111. Kong J, Fang J, Park J, Li S, Rong P. Treating depression with transcutaneous auricular vagus nerve stimulation: state of the art and future perspectives. *Front Psychiatry.* 2018;9:20.

112. Abosch A, Cosgrove GR. Biological basis for the surgical treatment of depression. *Neurosurg Focus.* 2008;25(1):E2.

113. Subramanian L, Bracht T, Jenkins P, et al. Clinical improvements following bilateral anterior capsulotomy in treatment-resistant depression. *Psychol Med.* 2017;47(6):1097-1106.

114. Christmas D, Matthews K. Neurosurgical treatments for patients with chronic, treatment-refractory depression: a retrospective, consecutive, case series comparison of anterior capsulotomy, anterior cingulotomy and vagus nerve stimulation. *Stereotact Funct Neurosurg.* 2015;93(6):387-392.

115. Volpini M, Giacobbe P, Cosgrove GR, Levitt A, Lozano AM, Lipsman N. The history and future of ablative neurosurgery for major depressive disorder. *Stereotact Funct Neurosurg.* 2017;95(4):216-228.

116. Dandekar MP, Fenoy AJ, Carvalho AF, Soares JC, Quevedo J. Deep brain stimulation for treatment-resistant depression: an integrative review of preclinical and clinical findings and translational implications. *Mol Psychiatry.* 2018;23(5):1094-1112.

117. Holtzheimer PE, Husain MM, Lisanby SH, et al. Subcallosal cingulate deep brain stimulation for treatment-resistant depression: a multisite, randomised, sham-controlled trial. *Lancet Psychiatry.* 2017;4(11):839-849.

118. Eitan R, Fontaine D, Benoît M, et al. One year double blind study of high vs low frequency subcallosal cingulate stimulation for depression. *J Psychiatr Res.* 2018;96:124-134.

119. Dougherty DD, Rezai AR, Carpenter LL, et al. A randomized sham-controlled trial of deep brain stimulation of the ventral capsule/ventral striatum for chronic treatment-resistant depression. *Biol Psychiatry.* 2015;78(4):240-248.

120. Bergfeld IO, Mantione M, Hoogendoorn ML, et al. Deep brain stimulation of the ventral anterior limb of the internal capsule for treatment-resistant depression: a randomized clinical trial. *JAMA Psychiatry.* 2016;73(5):456-464.

121. Merikangas KR, Jin R, He JP, et al. Prevalence and correlates of bipolar spectrum disorder in the world mental health survey initiative. *Arch Gen Psychiatry.* 2011;68(3):241-251.

122. Sajatovic M, Strejilevich SA, Gildengers AG, et al. A report on older-age bipolar disorder from the International Society for Bipolar Disorders Task Force. *Bipolar Disord.* 2015;17(7):689-704.

123. Altamura AC, Dell'Osso B, Berlin HA, Buoli M, Bassetti R, Mundo E. Duration of untreated illness and suicide in bipolar disorder: a naturalistic study. *Eur Arch Psychiatry Clin Neurosci.* 2010;260(5):385-391.

124. Morton E, Murray G, Michalak EE, et al. Quality of life in bipolar disorder: towards a dynamic understanding. *Psychol Med.* 2018;48(7):1111-1118.

125. Nivoli AM, Pacchiarotti I, Rosa AR, et al. Gender differences in a cohort study of 604 bipolar patients: the role of predominant polarity. *J Affect Disord.* 2011;133(3):443-449.

126. Leite RT, Nogueira Sde O, do Nascimento JP, et al. The use of cannabis as a predictor of early onset of bipolar disorder and suicide attempts. *Neural Plast.* 2015;2015:434127.

127. Marwaha S, Winsper C, Bebbington P, Smith D. Cannabis use and hypomania in young people: a prospective analysis. *Schizophr Bull.* 2018;44(6):1267-1274.

128. Tyler E, Jones S, Black N, Carter LA, Barrowclough C. The relationship between bipolar disorder and cannabis use in daily life: an experience sampling study. *PLoS One*. 2015;10(3):e0118916.

129. Ashok AH, Marques TR, Jauhar S, et al. The dopamine hypothesis of bipolar affective disorder: the state of the art and implications for treatment. *Mol Psychiatry*. 2017;22(5):666-679.

130. Parker GB, Romano M, Graham RK, Ricciardi T. Comparative familial aggregation of bipolar disorder in patients with bipolar I and bipolar II disorders. *Australas Psychiatry*. 2018;26(4):414-416.

131. Mühleisen TW, Leber M, Schulze TG, et al. Genome-wide association study reveals two new risk loci for bipolar disorder. *Nat Commun*. 2014;5:3339.

132. Forstner AJ, Hecker J, Hofmann A, et al. Identification of shared risk loci and pathways for bipolar disorder and schizophrenia. *PLoS One*. 2017;12(2):e0171595.

133. Harrison PJ. Molecular neurobiological clues to the pathogenesis of bipolar disorder. *Curr Opin Neurobiol*. 2016;36:1-6.

134. Nurnberger JI Jr, Koller DL, Jung J, et al. Identification of pathways for bipolar disorder: a meta-analysis. *JAMA Psychiatry*. 2014;71(6):657-664.

135. Mistry S, Harrison JR, Smith DJ, Escott-Price V, Zammit S. The use of polygenic risk scores to identify phenotypes associated with genetic risk of bipolar disorder and depression: a systematic review. *J Affect Disord*. 2018;234:148-155.

136. Hou L, Heilbronner U, Degenhardt F, et al. Genetic variants associated with response to lithium treatment in bipolar disorder: a genome-wide association study. *Lancet*. 2016;387(10023):1085-1093.

137. Ryu E, Nassan M, Jenkins GD, et al. A genome-wide search for bipolar disorder risk loci modified by mitochondrial genome variation. *Mol Neuropsychiatry*. 2018;3(3):125-134.

138. Phillips ML, Swartz HA. A critical appraisal of neuroimaging studies of bipolar disorder: toward a new conceptualization of underlying neural circuitry and a road map for future research. *Am J Psychiatry*. 2014;171(8):829-843.

139. Hibar DP, Westlye LT, Doan NT, et al. Cortical abnormalities in bipolar disorder: an MRI analysis of 6503 individuals from the ENIGMA Bipolar Disorder working group. *Mol Psychiatry*. 2018;23(4):932-942.

140. Bellani M, Boschello F, Delvecchio G, et al. DTI and myelin plasticity in bipolar disorder: integrating neuroimaging and neuropathological findings. *Front Psychiatry*. 2016;7:21.

141. Han KM, De Berardis D, Fornaro M, Kim YK. Differentiating between bipolar and unipolar depression in functional and structural MRI studies. *Prog Neuropsychopharmacol Biol Psychiatry*. 2019;91:20-27.

142. Goya-Maldonado R, Brodmann K, Keil M, Trost S, Dechent P, Gruber O. Differentiating unipolar and bipolar depression by alterations in large-scale brain networks. *Hum Brain Mapp*. 2016;37(2):808-818.

143. Kapczinski NS, Mwangi B, Cassidy RM, et al. Neuroprogression and illness trajectories in bipolar disorder. *Expert Rev Neurother*. 2017;17(3):277-285.

144. Passos IC, Mwangi B, Vieta E, Berk M, Kapczinski F. Areas of controversy in neuroprogression in bipolar disorder. *Acta Psychiatr Scand*. 2016;134(2):91-103.

145. Berk M, Post R, Ratheesh A, et al. Staging in bipolar disorder: from theoretical framework to clinical utility. *World Psychiatry*. 2017;16(3):236-244.

146. Lee RS, Hermens DF, Scott J, et al. A meta-analysis of neuropsychological functioning in first-episode bipolar disorders. *J Psychiatr Res*. 2014;57:1-11.

147. Szmulewicz AG, Valerio MP, Smith JM, Samamé C, Martino DJ, Strejilevich SA. Neuropsychological profiles of major depressive disorder and bipolar disorder during euthymia. A systematic literature review of comparative studies. *Psychiatry Res*. 2017;248:127-133.

148. Cullen B, Ward J, Graham NA, et al. Prevalence and correlates of cognitive impairment in euthymic adults with bipolar disorder: a systematic review. *J Affect Disord*. 2016;205:165-181.

149. Cardoso T, Bauer IE, Meyer TD, Kapczinski F, Soares JC. Neuroprogression and cognitive functioning in bipolar disorder: a systematic review. *Curr Psychiatry Rep*. 2015;17(9):75.

150. Strejilevich SA, Samamé C, Martino DJ. The trajectory of neuropsychological dysfunctions in bipolar disorders: a critical examination of a hypothesis. *J Affect Disord*. 2015;175:396-402.

151. Ryan KA, Assari S, Angers K, et al. Equivalent linear change in cognition between individuals with bipolar disorder and healthy controls over 5 years. *Bipolar Disord*. 2017;19(8):689-697.

152. Martino DJ, Igoa A, Marengo E, Scápola M, Strejilevich SA. Longitudinal relationship between clinical course and neurocognitive impairments in bipolar disorder. *J Affect Disord*. 2018;225:250-255.

153. Olvet DM, Burdick KE, Cornblatt BA. Assessing the potential to use neurocognition to predict who is at risk for developing bipolar disorder: a review of the literature. *Cogn Neuropsychiatry*. 2013;18(1-2):129-145.

154. Vieta E, Berk M, Schulze TG, et al. Bipolar disorders. *Nat Rev Dis Primers*. 2018;4:18008.

155. Yatham LN, Kennedy SH, Parikh SV, et al. Canadian Network for Mood and Anxiety Treatments (CANMAT) and International Society for Bipolar Disorders (ISBD) 2018 guidelines for the management of patients with bipolar disorder. *Bipolar Disord*. 2018;20(2):97-170.

156. Pacchiarotti I, Bond DJ, Baldessarini RJ, et al. The International Society for Bipolar Disorders (ISBD) task force report on antidepressant use in bipolar disorders. *Am J Psychiatry*. 2013;170(11):1249-1262.

157. Grunze H, Vieta E, Goodwin GM, et al. The World Federation of Societies of Biological Psychiatry (WFSBP) guidelines for the biological treatment of bipolar disorders: acute and long-term treatment of mixed states in bipolar disorder. *World J Biol Psychiatry*. 2018;19(1):2-58.

158. Murru A, Popovic D, Pacchiarotti I, Hidalgo D, León-Caballero J, Vieta E. Management of adverse effects of mood stabilizers. *Curr Psychiatry Rep*. 2015 Aug;17(8):603.

159. Dols A, Sienaert P, van Gerven H, et al. The prevalence and management of side effects of lithium and anticonvulsants as mood stabilizers in bipolar disorder from a clinical perspective: a review. *Int Clin Psychopharmacol*. 2013;28(6):287-296.

160. Sabater A, García-Blanco AC, Verdet HM, et al. Comparative neurocognitive effects of lithium and anticonvulsants in long-term stable bipolar patients. *J Affect Disord*. 2016;190:34-40.

161. Paterson A, Parker G. Lithium and cognition in those with bipolar disorder. *Int Clin Psychopharmacol*. 2017;32(2):57-62.

162. Rybakowski JK. Effect of lithium on neurocognitive functioning. *Curr Alzheimer Res*. 2016;13(8):887-893.

163. Lupu AM, Clinebell K, Gannon JM, Ellison JC, Chengappa KNR. Reducing anticholinergic medication burden in patients with psychotic or bipolar disorders. *J Clin Psychiatry*. 2017;78(9):e1270-e1275.

164. Miskowiak KW, Carvalho AF, Vieta E, Kessing LV. Cognitive enhancement treatments for bipolar disorder: a systematic review and methodological recommendations. *Eur Neuropsychopharmacol*. 2016;26(10):1541-1561.

165. Torrent C, Bonnin Cdel M, Martínez-Arán A, et al. Efficacy of functional remediation in bipolar disorder: a multicenter randomized controlled study. *Am J Psychiatry*. 2013;170(8):852-859.

166. Bonnin CM, Torrent C, Arango C, et al. Functional remediation in bipolar disorder: 1-year follow-up of neurocognitive and functional outcome. *Br J Psychiatry*. 2016;208(1):87-93.

167. Grajny K, Pyata H, Spiegel K, et al. Depression symptoms in chronic left hemisphere stroke are related to dorsolateral prefrontal cortex damage. *J Neuropsychiatry Clin Neurosci*. 2016;28(4): 292-298.

168. Villa RF, Ferrari F, Moretti A. Post-stroke depression: mechanisms and pharmacological treatment. *Pharmacol Ther*. 2018;184: 131-144.

169. Elger CE, Johnston SA, Hoppe C. Diagnosing and treating depression in epilepsy. *Seizure*. 2017;44:184-193.

170. Almeida OP, Ford AH, Flicker L. Systematic review and meta-analysis of randomized placebo-controlled trials of folate and vitamin B12 for depression. *Int Psychogeriatr*. 2015;27(5):727-737.

171. Bender A, Hagan KE, Kingston N. The association of folate and depression: a meta-analysis. *J Psychiatr Res*. 2017;95:9-18.

171A. Robinson RG, Jorge RE. Post-stroke depression: a review. *Am J Psychiatry*. 2016;173(3):221-231.

171B. Pan A, Sun Q, Okereke OI, Rexrode KM, Hu FB. Depression and risk of stroke morbidity and mortality: a meta-analysis and systematic review. *JAMA*. 2011;306(11):1241-1249.

172. Chemerinski E, Levine SR. Neuropsychiatric disorders following vascular brain injury. *Mt Sinai J Med*. 2006;73(7):1006-1014.

173. Kanner AM. Psychiatric comorbidities in new onset epilepsy: should they be always investigated? *Seizure*. 2017;49:79-82.

174. Heser K, Bleckwenn M, Wiese B, et al. Late-life depressive symptoms and lifetime history of major depression: cognitive deficits are largely due to incipient dementia rather than depression. *J Alzheimers Dis*. 2016;54(1):185-199.

175. Woolley JD, Khan BK, Murthy NK, Miller BL, Rankin KP. The diagnostic challenge of psychiatric symptoms in neurodegenerative disease: rates of and risk factors for prior psychiatric diagnosis in patients with early neurodegenerative disease. *J Clin Psychiatry*. 2011;72(2):126-133.

176. Sahin S, Okluoglu-Önal T, Cinar N, Bozdemir M, Çubuk R, Karsidag S. Distinguishing depressive pseudodementia from Alzheimer disease: a comparative study of hippocampal volumetry and cognitive tests. *Dement Geriatr Cogn Dis Extra*. 2017;7(2):230-239.

177. Klöppel S, Kotschi M, Peter J, et al. Separating symptomatic Alzheimer's disease from depression based on structural MRI. *J Alzheimers Dis*. 2018;63(1):353-363.

178. Almeida OP, McCaul K, Hankey GJ, Yeap BB, Golledge J, Flicker L. Risk of dementia and death in community-dwelling older men with bipolar disorder. *Br J Psychiatry*. 2016;209(2):121-126.

179. Carta MG, Moro MF, Lorefice L, et al. The risk of bipolar disorders in multiple sclerosis. *J Affect Disord*. 2014;155:255-260.

180. Knott S, Forty L, Craddock N, Thomas RH. Epilepsy and bipolar disorder. *Epilepsy Behav*. 2015;52(pt A):267-274.

181. Kivilcim Y, Altintas M, Domac FM, Erzincan E, Gülec H. Screening for bipolar disorder among migraineurs: the impact of migraine-bipolar disorder comorbidity on disease characteristics. *Neuropsychiatr Dis Treat*. 2017;13:631-641.

182. Steinlechner S, Hagenah J, Rumpf HJ, et al. Associations of specific psychiatric disorders with isolated focal dystonia, and monogenic and idiopathic Parkinson's disease. *J Neurol*. 2017;264(6):1076-1084.

183. Wu HC, Chou FH, Tsai KY, Su CY, Shen SP, Chung TC. The incidence and relative risk of stroke among patients with

bipolar disorder: a seven-year follow-up study. *PLoS One*. 2013;8(8):e73037.

184. Schoepf D, Heun R. Bipolar disorder and comorbidity: increased prevalence and increased relevance of comorbidity for hospital-based mortality during a 12.5-year observation period in general hospital admissions. *J Affect Disord*. 2014;169:170-178.

185. Post RM, Kalivas P. Bipolar disorder and substance misuse: pathological and therapeutic implications of their comorbidity and cross-sensitisation. *Br J Psychiatry*. 2013;202(3):172-176.

186. Starzer MSK, Nordentoft M, Hjorthøj C. Rates and predictors of conversion to schizophrenia or bipolar disorder following substance-induced psychosis. *Am J Psychiatry*. 2018;175(4): 343-350.

187. Sauvé WM. Recognizing and treating pseudobulbar affect. *CNS Spectr*. 2016;21(S1):34-44.

188. Le Heron C, Apps MAJ, Husain M. The anatomy of apathy: a neurocognitive framework for amotivated behaviour. *Neuropsychologia*. 2018;118(pt B):54-67.

189. Watling J, Pawlik B, Scott K, Booth S, Short MA. Sleep loss and affective functioning: more than just mood. *Behav Sleep Med*. 2017;15(5):394-409.

190. St Louis EK, Boeve AR, Boeve BF. REM sleep behavior disorder in Parkinson's disease and other synucleinopathies. *Mov Disord*. 2017;32(5):645-658.

191. Kirkpatrick B, Fenton WS, Carpenter WT Jr, Marder SR. The NIMH-MATRICS consensus statement on negative symptoms. *Schizophr Bull*. 2006;32(2):214-219.

192. Blanchard JJ, Cohen AS. The structure of negative symptoms within schizophrenia: implications for assessment. *Schizophr Bull*. 2006;32(2):238-245.

193. van Os J, Reininghaus U. Psychosis as a transdiagnostic and extended phenotype in the general population. *World Psychiatry*. 2016;15(2):118-124.

194. Guloksuz S, van Os J. The slow death of the concept of schizophrenia and the painful birth of the psychosis spectrum. *Psychol Med*. 2018;48(2):229-244.

195. Landin-Romero R, McKenna PJ, Romaguera A, et al. Examining the continuum of psychosis: frequency and characteristics of psychotic-like symptoms in relatives and non-relatives of patients with schizophrenia. *Schizophr Res*. 2016;178(1-3):6-11.

196. Cloutier M, Aigbogun MS, Guerin A, et al. The economic burden of schizophrenia in the United States in 2013. *J Clin Psychiatry*. 2016;77(6):764-771.

197. Jin H, Mosweu I. The societal cost of schizophrenia: a systematic review. *Pharmacoeconomics*. 2017;35(1):25-42.

198. Charlson FJ, Ferrari AJ, Santomauro DF, et al. Global epidemiology and burden of schizophrenia: findings from the global burden of disease study 2016. *Schizophr Bull*. 2018;44(6): 1195-1203.

199. Harvey PD, Raykov T, Twamley EW, Vella L, Heaton RK, Patterson TL. Validating the measurement of real-world functional outcomes: phase I results of the VALERO study. *Am J Psychiatry*. 2011;168(11):1195-1201.

200. Oakley P, Kisely S, Baxter A, et al. Increased mortality among people with schizophrenia and other non-affective psychotic disorders in the community: a systematic review and meta-analysis. *J Psychiatr Res*. 2018;102:245-253.

201. Walker ER, McGee RE, Druss BG. Mortality in mental disorders and global disease burden implications: a systematic review and meta-analysis. *JAMA Psychiatry*. 2015;72(4):334-341.

202. Riecher-Rössler A, Butler S, Kulkarni J. Sex and gender differences in schizophrenic psychoses—a critical review. *Arch Womens Ment Health*. 2018;21(6):627-648.

203. Stafford J, Howard R, Kirkbride JB. The incidence of very late-onset psychotic disorders: a systematic review and meta-analysis, 1960–2016. *Psychol Med.* 2018;48(11):1775-1786.

204. Belbasis L, Köhler CA, Stefanis N, et al. Risk factors and peripheral biomarkers for schizophrenia spectrum disorders: an umbrella review of meta-analyses. *Acta Psychiatr Scand.* 2018;137(2):88-97.

205. Radua J, Ramella-Cravaro V, Ioannidis JPA, et al. What causes psychosis? An umbrella review of risk and protective factors. *World Psychiatry.* 2018;17(1):49-66.

206. Lederbogen F, Kirsch P, Haddad L, et al. City living and urban upbringing affect neural social stress processing in humans. *Nature.* 2011;474(7352):498-501.

207. Birnbaum R, Weinberger DR. Genetic insights into the neurodevelopmental origins of schizophrenia. *Nat Rev Neurosci.* 2017;18(12):727-740.

208. Carlsson A, Lindqvist M. Effect of chlorpromazine or haloperidol on formation of 3methoxytyramine and normetanephrine in mouse brain. *Acta Pharmacol Toxicol (Copenh).* 1963;20:140-144.

209. Rice MW, Roberts RC, Melendez-Ferro M, Perez-Costas E. Mapping dopaminergic deficiencies in the substantia nigra/ventral tegmental area in schizophrenia. *Brain Struct Funct.* 2016;221(1):185-201.

210. Abi-Dargham A. Do we still believe in the dopamine hypothesis? New data bring new evidence. *Int J Neuropsychopharmacol.* 2004;7(suppl 1):S1-S5.

211. Slifstein M, van de Giessen E, Van Snellenberg J, et al. Deficits in prefrontal cortical and extrastriatal dopamine release in schizophrenia: a positron emission tomographic functional magnetic resonance imaging study. *JAMA Psychiatry.* 2015;72(4):316-324.

212. Simpson EH, Kellendonk C, Kandel E. A possible role for the striatum in the pathogenesis of the cognitive symptoms of schizophrenia. *Neuron.* 2010;65(5):585-596.

213. Fusar-Poli P, Meyer-Lindenberg A. Striatal presynaptic dopamine in schizophrenia, part II: meta-analysis of [(18)F/(11)C]-DOPA PET studies. *Schizophr Bull.* 2013;39(1):33-42.

214. Egerton A, Chaddock CA, Winton-Brown TT, et al. Presynaptic striatal dopamine dysfunction in people at ultra-high risk for psychosis: findings in a second cohort. *Biol Psychiatry.* 2013;74(2):106-112.

215. Howes OD, McCutcheon R, Owen MJ, Murray RM. The role of genes, stress, and dopamine in the development of schizophrenia. *Biol Psychiatry.* 2017;81(1):9-20.

216. Howes OD, Kambeitz J, Kim E, et al. The nature of dopamine dysfunction in schizophrenia and what this means for treatment. *Arch Gen Psychiatry.* 2012;69(8):776-786.

217. Krystal JH, Anticevic A, Yang GJ, et al. Impaired tuning of neural ensembles and the pathophysiology of schizophrenia: a translational and computational neuroscience perspective. *Biol Psychiatry.* 2017;81(10):874-885.

218. Javitt DC. Current and emergent treatments for symptoms and neurocognitive impairment in schizophrenia. *Curr Treat Options Psychiatry.* 2015;1(2):107-120.

219. Slovik M, Rosin B, Moshel S, et al. Ketamine induced converged synchronous gamma oscillations in the cortico-basal ganglia network of non-human primates. *J Neurophysiol.* 2017;118:917-931.

220. Mitchell AC, Jiang Y, Peter C, Akbarian S. Transcriptional regulation of GAD1 GABA synthesis gene in the prefrontal cortex of subjects with schizophrenia. *Schizophr Res.* 2015;167(1-3):28-34.

221. Morishita H, Kundakovic M, Bicks L, Mitchell A, Akbarian S. Interneuron epigenomes during the critical period of cortical plasticity: implications for schizophrenia. *Neurobiol Learn Mem.* 2015;124:104-110.

222. Schizophrenia Working Group of the Psychiatric Genomics Consortium. Biological insights from 108 schizophrenia-associated genetic loci. *Nature.* 2014;511(7510):421-427.

223. Hall J, Trent S, Thomas KL, O'Donovan MC, Owen MJ. Genetic risk for schizophrenia: convergence on synaptic pathways involved in plasticity. *Biol Psychiatry.* 2015;77(1):52-58.

224. Dahoun T, Trossbach SV, Brandon NJ, Korth C, Howes OD. The impact of Disrupted-in-Schizophrenia 1 (DISC1) on the dopaminergic system: a systematic review. *Transl Psychiatry.* 2017;7(1):e1015.

225. Farrell MS, Werge T, Sklar P, et al. Evaluating historical candidate genes for schizophrenia. *Mol Psychiatry.* 2015;20(5):555-562.

226. Birnbaum R, Jaffe AE, Hyde TM, Kleinman JE, Weinberger DR. Prenatal expression patterns of genes associated with neuropsychiatric disorders. *Am J Psychiatry.* 2014;171(7):758-767.

227. Xia K, Zhang J, Ahn M, et al. Genome-wide association analysis identifies common variants influencing infant brain volumes. *Transl Psychiatry.* 2017;7(8):e1188.

228. Khandaker GM, Dantzer R. Is there a role for immune-to-brain communication in schizophrenia? *Psychopharmacology (Berl).* 2016;233(9):1559-1573.

229. Howes OD, McCutcheon R. Inflammation and the neural diathesis-stress hypothesis of schizophrenia: a reconceptualization. *Transl Psychiatry.* 2017;7(2):e1024.

230. Giegling I, Hosak L, Mössner R, et al. Genetics of schizophrenia: a consensus paper of the WFSBP Task Force on Genetics. *World J Biol Psychiatry.* 2017;18(7):492-505.

231. Blokland GAM, Del Re EC, Mesholam-Gately RI, et al. The Genetics of Endophenotypes of Neurofunction to Understand Schizophrenia (GENUS) consortium: a collaborative cognitive and neuroimaging genetics project. *Schizophr Res.* 2018;195:306-317.

232. Gur RE, Maany V, Mozley PD, Swanson C, Bilker W, Gur RC. Subcortical MRI volumes in neuroleptic-naive and treated patients with schizophrenia. *Am J Psychiatry.* 1998;155(12):1711-1717.

233. Spinks R, Nopoulos P, Ward J, Fuller R, Magnotta VA, Andreasen NC. Globus pallidus volume is related to symptom severity in neuroleptic naive patients with schizophrenia. *Schizophr Res.* 2005;73(2-3):229-233.

234. Glenthoj A, Glenthoj BY, Mackeprang T, et al. Basal ganglia volumes in drug-naive first-episode schizophrenia patients before and after short-term treatment with either a typical or an atypical antipsychotic drug. *Psychiatry Res.* 2007;154(3):199-208.

235. Ellison-Wright I, Glahn DC, Laird AR, Thelen SM, Bullmore E. The anatomy of first-episode and chronic schizophrenia: an anatomical likelihood estimation meta-analysis. *Am J Psychiatry.* 2008;165(8):1015-1023.

236. Goldman AL, Pezawas L, Mattay VS, et al. Heritability of brain morphology related to schizophrenia: a large-scale automated magnetic resonance imaging segmentation study. *Biol Psychiatry.* 2008;63(5):475-483.

237. Oertel-Knöchel V, Knöchel C, Matura S, et al. Cortical-basal ganglia imbalance in schizophrenia patients and unaffected first-degree relatives. *Schizophr Res.* 2012;138(2-3):120-127.

238. Haijma SV, Van Haren N, Cahn W, Koolschijn PC, Hulshoff Pol HE, Kahn RS. Brain volumes in schizophrenia: a meta-analysis in over 18 000 subjects. *Schizophr Bull.* 2013;39(5):1129-1138.

239. Kubota M, van Haren NE, Haijma SV, et al. Association of IQ changes and progressive brain changes in patients with schizophrenia. *JAMA Psychiatry.* 2015;72(8):803-812.

240. van Erp TG, Hibar DP, Rasmussen JM, et al. Subcortical brain volume abnormalities in 2028 individuals with schizophrenia and 2540 healthy controls via the ENIGMA consortium. *Mol Psychiatry.* 2016;21(4):547-553.

241. Okada N, Fukunaga M, Yamashita F, et al. Abnormal asymmetries in subcortical brain volume in schizophrenia. *Mol Psychiatry.* 2016;21(10):1460-1466.

242. Mamah D, Alpert KI, Barch DM, Csernansky JG, Wang L. Subcortical neuromorphometry in schizophrenia spectrum and bipolar disorders. *Neuroimage Clin.* 2016;11:276-286.

243. Vernon AC1, Natesan S, Crum WR, et al. Contrasting effects of haloperidol and lithium on rodent brain structure: a magnetic resonance imaging study with postmortem confirmation. *Biol Psychiatry.* 2012;71(10):855-863.

244. Caseras X, Tansey KE, Foley S, Linden D. Association between genetic risk scoring for schizophrenia and bipolar disorder with regional subcortical volumes. *Transl Psychiatry.* 2015;5:e692.

245. Li T, Wang Q, Zhang J, et al. Brain-wide analysis of functional connectivity in first-episode and chronic stages of schizophrenia. *Schizophr Bull.* 2017;43(2):436-448.

246. Kanahara N, Shimizu E, Sekine Y, et al. Does hypofrontality expand to global brain area in progression of schizophrenia?: a cross-sectional study between first-episode and chronic schizophrenia. *Prog Neuropsychopharmacol Biol Psychiatry.* 2009;33(3):410-415.

247. Gruber O, Chadha Santuccione A, Aach H. Magnetic resonance imaging in studying schizophrenia, negative symptoms, and the glutamate system. *Front Psychiatry.* 2014;5:32.

248. Moser DA, Doucet GE, Lee WH, et al. Multivariate associations among behavioral, clinical, and multimodal imaging phenotypes in patients with psychosis. *JAMA Psychiatry.* 2018;75(4):386-395.

249. Wojtalik JA, Smith MJ, Keshavan MS, Eack SM. A systematic and meta-analytic review of neural correlates of functional outcome in schizophrenia. *Schizophr Bull.* 2017;43(6):1329-1347.

250. Silbersweig DA, Stern E, Frith C, et al. A functional neuroanatomy of hallucinations in schizophrenia. *Nature.* 1995;378(6553):176-179.

251. Zhu J, Zhuo C, Liu F, Xu L, Yu C. Neural substrates underlying delusions in schizophrenia. *Sci Rep.* 2016;6:33857.

252. Sommer IE, Diederen KM, Blom JD, et al. Auditory verbal hallucinations predominantly activate the right inferior frontal area. *Brain.* 2008;131(pt 12):3169-3177.

253. Alonso-Solís A, Vives-Gilabert Y, Grasa E, et al. Resting-state functional connectivity alterations in the default network of schizophrenia patients with persistent auditory verbal hallucinations. *Schizophr Res.* 2015;161(2-3):261-268.

254. Alderson-Day B, McCarthy-Jones S, Fernyhough C. Hearing voices in the resting brain: a review of intrinsic functional connectivity research on auditory verbal hallucinations. *Neurosci Biobehav Rev.* 2015;55:78-87.

255. Hare SM, Law AS, Ford JM, et al. Disrupted network cross talk, hippocampal dysfunction and hallucinations in schizophrenia. *Schizophr Res.* 2018;199:226-234.

256. Oestreich LK, Pasternak O, Shenton ME, et al. Abnormal white matter microstructure and increased extracellular free-water in the cingulum bundle associated with delusions in chronic schizophrenia. *Neuroimage Clin.* 2016 Aug 4;12:405-414.

257. Epstein J, Silbersweig D. The neuropsychiatric spectrum of motivational disorders. *J Neuropsychiatry Clin Neurosci.* 2015;27(1):7-18.

258. Shaffer JJ, Peterson MJ, McMahon MA, et al. Neural correlates of schizophrenia negative symptoms: distinct subtypes impact dissociable brain circuits. *Mol Neuropsychiatry.* 2015;1(4):191-200.

259. Mwansisya TE, Wang Z, Tao H, et al. The diminished interhemispheric connectivity correlates with negative symptoms and cognitive impairment in first-episode schizophrenia. *Schizophr Res.* 2013;150(1):144-150.

260. Goghari VM, Sponheim SR, MacDonald AW 3rd. The functional neuroanatomy of symptom dimensions in schizophrenia: a qualitative and quantitative review of a persistent question. *Neurosci Biobehav Rev.* 2010;34(3):468-486.

261. Radua J, Schmidt A, Borgwardt S, et al. Ventral striatal activation during reward processing in psychosis: a neurofunctional meta-analysis. *JAMA Psychiatry.* 2015;72(12):1243-1251.

262. Reckless GE, Andreassen OA, Server A, Østefjells T, Jensen J. Negative symptoms in schizophrenia are associated with aberrant striato-cortical connectivity in a rewarded perceptual decision-making task. *Neuroimage Clin.* 2015;8:290-297.

263. Nelson BD, Bjorkquist OA, Olsen EK, Herbener ES. Schizophrenia symptom and functional correlates of anterior cingulate cortex activation to emotion stimuli: an fMRI investigation. *Psychiatry Res.* 2015;234(3):285-291.

264. Simpson EH, Kellendonk C, Kandel E. A possible role for the striatum in the pathogenesis of the cognitive symptoms of schizophrenia. *Neuron.* 2010;65(5):585-596.

265. Sheffield JM, Barch DM. Cognition and resting-state functional connectivity in schizophrenia. *Neurosci Biobehav Rev.* 2016;61:108-120.

266. Hu ML, Zong XF, Mann JJ, et al. A review of the functional and anatomical default mode network in schizophrenia. *Neurosci Bull.* 2017;33(1):73-84.

267. Dezhina Z, Ranlund S, Kyriakopoulos M, Williams SCR, Dima D. A systematic review of associations between functional MRI activity and polygenic risk for schizophrenia and bipolar disorder. *Brain Imaging Behav.* 2019;13(3):862-877.

268. Seidman LJ, Hellemann G, Nuechterlein KH, et al. Factor structure and heritability of endophenotypes in schizophrenia: findings from the Consortium on the Genetics of Schizophrenia (COGS-1). *Schizophr Res.* 2015;163(1-3):73-79.

269. Bachmann S, Schröder J. Neurological soft signs in schizophrenia: an update on the state- versus trait-perspective. *Front Psychiatry.* 2018 Jan 8;8:272.

270. Akabaliev VH, Sivkov ST, Mantarkov MY. Minor physical anomalies in schizophrenia and bipolar I disorder and the neurodevelopmental continuum of psychosis. *Bipolar Disord.* 2014;16(6):633-641.

271. van der Werf M, Hanssen M, Köhler S, et al. Systematic review and collaborative recalculation of 133,693 incident cases of schizophrenia. *Psychol Med.* 2014;44(1):9-16.

272. Millan MJ, Fone K, Steckler T, Horan WP. Negative symptoms of schizophrenia: clinical characteristics, pathophysiological substrates, experimental models and prospects for improved treatment. *Eur Neuropsychopharmacol.* 2014;24(5):645-692.

273. Bowie CR, Reichenberg A, Patterson TL, Heaton RK, Harvey PD. Determinants of real-world functional performance in schizophrenia subjects: correlations with cognition, functional capacity, and symptoms. *Am J Psychiatry.* 2006;163(3):418-425.

274. An der Heiden W, Häfner H. Investigating the long-term course of schizophrenia by sequence analysis. *Psychiatry Res.* 2015;228(3):551-559.

275. Mesholam-Gately RI, Giuliano AJ, Goff KP, Faraone SV, Seidman LJ. Neurocognition in first-episode schizophrenia: a meta-analytic review. *Neuropsychology.* 2009;23(3):315-336.

276. Tamminga CA, Buchanan RW, Gold JM. The role of negative symptoms and cognitive dysfunction in schizophrenia outcome. *Int Clin Psychopharmacol.* 1998;13(suppl 3):S21-S26.

277. Kotov R, Fochtmann L, Li K, et al. Declining clinical course of psychotic disorders over the two decades following first hospitalization: evidence from the Suffolk County Mental Health Project. *Am J Psychiatry.* 2017;174(11):1064-1074.

278. Chiang SK, Ni CH, Tsai CP, Lin KC. Validation of the cognitively normal range and below normal range subtypes in chronically hospitalized patients with schizophrenia. *Schizophr Res Cogn.* 2016;5:28-34.

279. Strauss GP, Cohen AS. A transdiagnostic review of negative symptom phenomenology and etiology. *Schizophr Bull.* 2017;43(4):712-719.

280. Marder SR, Kirkpatrick B. Defining and measuring negative symptoms of schizophrenia in clinical trials. *Eur Neuropsychopharmacol.* 2014;24(5):737-743.

281. Nuechterlein KH, Green MF, Kern RS, et al. The MATRICS Consensus Cognitive Battery, part 1: test selection, reliability, and validity. *Am J Psychiatry.* 2008;165:203-213.

282. Kern RS, Nuechterlein KH, Green MF, et al. The MATRICS Consensus Cognitive Battery, part 2: co-norming and standardization. *Am J Psychiatry.* 2008;165:214-220.

283. Green MF, Nuechterlein KH, Kern RS, et al. Functional co-primary measures for clinical trials in schizophrenia: results from the MATRICS Psychometric and Standardization Study. *Am J Psychiatry.* 2008;165:221-228.

284. Gray BE, McMahon RP, Green MF, et al. Detecting reliable cognitive change in individual patients with the MATRICS Consensus Cognitive Battery. *Schizophr Res.* 2014;159(1):182-187.

285. Carbon M, Hsieh CH, Kane JM, Correll CU. Tardive dyskinesia prevalence in the period of second-generation antipsychotic use: a meta-analysis. *J Clin Psychiatry.* 2017;78(3):e264-e278.

286. Mentzel CL, Bakker PR, van Os J, et al. Effect of antipsychotic type and dose changes on tardive dyskinesia and parkinsonism severity in patients with a serious mental illness: the Curaçao Extrapyramidal Syndromes Study XII. *J Clin Psychiatry.* 2017;78(3):e279-e285.

287. Hasan A, Falkai P, Wobrock T, et al. World Federation of Societies of Biological Psychiatry (WFSBP) guidelines for biological treatment of schizophrenia, part 1: update 2012 on the acute treatment of schizophrenia and the management of treatment resistance. *World J Biol Psychiatry.* 2012;13(5):318-378.

288. Correll CU, Galling B, Pawar A, et al. Comparison of early intervention services vs treatment as usual for early-phase psychosis: a systematic review, meta-analysis, and meta-regression. *JAMA Psychiatry.* 2018;75(6):555-565.

289. Takeuchi H, Kantor N, Sanches M, Fervaha G, Agid O, Remington G. One-year symptom trajectories in patients with stable schizophrenia maintained on antipsychotics versus placebo: meta-analysis. *Br J Psychiatry.* 2017;211(3):137-143.

290. Howes OD, McCutcheon R, Agid O, et al. Treatment-resistant schizophrenia: Treatment Response and Resistance in Psychosis (TRRIP) working group consensus guidelines on diagnosis and terminology. *Am J Psychiatry.* 2017;174(3):216-229.

291. Kubera KM, Barth A, Hirjak D, Thomann PA, Wolf RC. Noninvasive brain stimulation for the treatment of auditory verbal hallucinations in schizophrenia: methods, effects and challenges. *Front Syst Neurosci.* 2015;9:131.

292. Tsapakis EM, Dimopoulou T, Tarazi FI. Clinical management of negative symptoms of schizophrenia: an update. *Pharmacol Ther.* 2015;153:135-147.

293. Kishi T, Ikuta T, Oya K, Matsunaga S, Matsuda Y, Iwata N. Anti-dementia drugs for psychopathology and cognitive impairment in schizophrenia: a systematic review and meta-analysis. *Int J Neuropsychopharmacol.* 2018 May 14. doi:10.1093/ijnp/pyy045.

294. Lieberman JA, Stroup TS, McEvoy JP, et al. Effectiveness of antipsychotic drugs in patients with chronic schizophrenia. *N Engl J Med.* 2005 Sep 22;353(12):1209-1223. Epub 2005 Sep 19. Erratum in: *N Engl J Med.* 2010;363(11):1092-1093.

295. Zheng W, Zheng YJ, Li XB, et al. Efficacy and safety of adjunctive aripiprazole in schizophrenia: meta-analysis of randomized controlled trials. *J Clin Psychopharmacol.* 2016;36(6):628-636.

296. Helfer B, Samara MT, Huhn M, et al. Efficacy and safety of antidepressants added to antipsychotics for schizophrenia: a systematic review and meta-analysis. *Am J Psychiatry.* 2016;173(9):876-886.

297. Bugarski-Kirola D, Blaettler T, Arango C, et al. Bitopertin in negative symptoms of schizophrenia—results from the phase III FlashLyte and DayLyte studies. *Biol Psychiatry.* 2017;82(1):8-16.

298. Veerman SR, Schulte PF, Smith JD, de Haan L. Memantine augmentation in clozapine-refractory schizophrenia: a randomized, double-blind, placebo-controlled crossover study. *Psychol Med.* 2016;46(9):1909-1921.

299. Veerman S, Schulte P, de Haan L. Memantine add-on to clozapine treatment for residual negative symptoms of schizophrenia. *Psychopharmacology (Berl).* 2017;234(23-24):3535-3536.

300. Mazinani R, Nejati S, Khodaei M. Effects of memantine added to risperidone on the symptoms of schizophrenia: a randomized double-blind, placebo-controlled clinical trial. *Psychiatry Res.* 2017;247:291-295.

301. Wallace TL, Bertrand D. Neuronal $\alpha 7$ nicotinic receptors as a target for the treatment of schizophrenia. *Int Rev Neurobiol.* 2015;124:79-111.

302. Choi KH, Wykes T, Kurtz MM. Adjunctive pharmacotherapy for cognitive deficits in schizophrenia: meta-analytical investigation of efficacy. *Br J Psychiatry.* 2013;203(3):172-178.

303. Dougall N, Maayan N, Soares-Weiser K, McDermott LM, McIntosh A. Transcranial magnetic stimulation (TMS) for schizophrenia. *Cochrane Database Syst Rev.* 2015;(8):CD006081.

304. Rabany L, Deutsch L, Levkovitz Y. Double-blind, randomized sham controlled study of deep-TMS add-on treatment for negative symptoms and cognitive deficits in schizophrenia. *J Psychopharmacol.* 2014;28(7):686-690.

305. Morin L, Franck N. Rehabilitation interventions to promote recovery from schizophrenia: a systematic review. *Front Psychiatry.* 2017;8:100.

306. Jauhar S, McKenna PJ, Radua J, Fung E, Salvador R, Laws KR. Cognitive-behavioural therapy for the symptoms of schizophrenia: systematic review and meta-analysis with examination of potential bias. *Br J Psychiatry.* 2014;204(1):20-29.

307. Tripathi A, Kar SK, Shukla R. Cognitive deficits in schizophrenia: understanding the biological correlates and remediation strategies. *Clin Psychopharmacol Neurosci.* 2018;16(1):7-17.

308. Wykes T, Huddy V, Cellard C, McGurk SR, Czobor P. A meta-analysis of cognitive remediation for schizophrenia: methodology and effect sizes. *Am J Psychiatry.* 2011;168:472-485.

309. Keefe RS, Haig GM, Marder SR, et al. Report on ISCTM consensus meeting on clinical assessment of response to treatment of cognitive impairment in schizophrenia. *Schizophr Bull.* 2016;42(1):19-33.

310. Kurtz MM, Richardson CL. Social cognitive training for schizophrenia: a meta-analytic investigation of controlled research. *Schizophr Bull.* 2012;38(5):1092-1104.

311. Morgan AJ, Reavley NJ, Ross A, Too LS, Jorm AF. Interventions to reduce stigma towards people with severe mental illness: systematic review and meta-analysis. *J Psychiatr Res.* 2018;103:120-133.

312. Karameh WK, Murari G, Schweizer TA, Munoz DG, Fischer CE. Psychosis in neurodegenerative disorders: recent developments. *Curr Opin Psychiatry.* 2019;32(2):117-122.

313. Murray PS, Kumar S, DeMichele-Sweet MA, Sweet RA. Psychosis in Alzheimer's disease. *Biol Psychiatry.* 2014 Apr 1;75(7):542-552.

314. Van Assche L, Van Aubel E, Van de Ven L, Bouckaert F, Luyten P, Vandenbulcke M. The neuropsychological profile and

phenomenology of late onset psychosis: a cross-sectional study on the differential diagnosis of very-late-onset schizophrenia-like psychosis, dementia with Lewy bodies and Alzheimer's type dementia with psychosis. *Arch Clin Neuropsychol.* 2019;34(2): 183-199.

315. Van Assche L, Morrens M, Luyten P, Van de Ven L, Vandenbulcke M. The neuropsychology and neurobiology of late-onset schizophrenia and very-late-onset schizophrenia-like psychosis: a critical review. *Neurosci Biobehav Rev.* 2017;83:604-621.

316. Nicolas G, Beherec L, Hannequin D, et al. Dementia in middle-aged patients with schizophrenia. *J Alzheimers Dis.* 2014;39(4):809-822.

316A. Ribe AR, Laursen TM, Charles M, et al. Long-term risk of dementia in persons with schizophrenia: a Danish population-based cohort study. *JAMA Psychiatry.* 2015;72(11):1095-1101.

317. Ravina B, Marder K, Fernandez HH, et al. Diagnostic criteria for psychosis in Parkinson's disease: report of an NINDS, NIMH work group. *Mov Disord.* 2007;22(8):1061-1068.

318. Ffytche DH, Creese B, Politis M, et al. The psychosis spectrum in Parkinson disease. *Nat Rev Neurol.* 2017;13(2):81-95.

319. Morgante L, Colosimo C, Antonini A, et al. Psychosis associated to Parkinson's disease in the early stages: relevance of cognitive decline and depression. *J Neurol Neurosurg Psychiatry.* 2012;83(1):76-82.

320. Black KJ, Nasrallah H, Isaacson S, et al. Guidance for switching from off-label antipsychotics to pimavanserin for Parkinson's disease psychosis: an expert consensus. *CNS Spectr.* 2018;23(6):402-413.

321. McKeith IG, Boeve BF, Dickson DW, et al. Diagnosis and management of dementia with Lewy bodies: fourth consensus report of the DLB Consortium. *Neurology.* 2017;89(1):88-100.

322. van Duijn E, Craufurd D, Hubers AA, et al. Neuropsychiatric symptoms in a European Huntington's disease cohort (REGISTRY). *J Neurol Neurosurg Psychiatry.* 2014;85(12):1411-1418.

323. Cardoso F. Nonmotor symptoms in Huntington disease. *Int Rev Neurobiol.* 2017;134:1397-1408.

324. Lancaster E. The diagnosis and treatment of autoimmune encephalitis. *J Clin Neurol.* 2016;12(1):1-13.

325. Steiner J, Prüss H, Köhler S, Frodl T, Hasan A, Falkai P. Autoimmune encephalitis with psychosis: warning signs, step-by-step diagnostics and treatment. *World J Biol Psychiatry.* 2018:1-14.

326. Wang LY, Chen SF, Chiang JH, Hsu CY, Shen YC. Autoimmune diseases are associated with an increased risk of schizophrenia: a nationwide population-based cohort study. *Schizophr Res.* 2018;202:297-302.

327. Murphy R, O'Donoghue S, Counihan T, et al. Neuropsychiatric syndromes of multiple sclerosis. *J Neurol Neurosurg Psychiatry.* 2017;88(8):697-708.

328. Neeki MM, Au C, Richard A, Peace C, Jaques S, Johansson J. Acute disseminated encephalomyelitis in an incarcerated adolescent presents as acute psychosis: case report and literature review. *Pediatr Emerg Care.* 2019;35(2):e22-e25.

329. Jeppesen R, Benros ME. Autoimmune diseases and psychotic disorders. *Front Psychiatry.* 2019;10:131.

330. Appenzeller S, Cendes F, Costallat LT. Acute psychosis in systemic lupus erythematosus. *Rheumatol Int.* 2008;28(3):237-243.

331. Clancy MJ, Clarke MC, Connor DJ, Cannon M, Cotter DR. The prevalence of psychosis in epilepsy: a systematic review and meta-analysis. *BMC Psychiatry.* 2014;14:75.

332. Irwin LG, Fortune DG. Risk factors for psychosis secondary to temporal lobe epilepsy: a systematic review. *J Neuropsychiatry Clin Neurosci.* 2014;26(1):5-23.

333. Kanner AM, Rivas-Grajales AM. Psychosis of epilepsy: a multifaceted neuropsychiatric disorder. *CNS Spectr.* 2016;21(3):247-257.

334. Stangeland H, Orgeta V, Bell V. Poststroke psychosis: a systematic review. *J Neurol Neurosurg Psychiatry.* 2018;89(8):879-885.

335. Roser F, Ritz R, Koerbel A, Loewenheim H, Tatagiba MS. Peduncular hallucinosis: insights from a neurosurgical point of view. *Neurosurgery.* 2005;57(5):E1068; discussion E1068.

336. Boller F, Birnbaum DS, Caputi N. Charles Bonnet syndrome and other hallucinatory phenomena. *Front Neurol Neurosci.* 2018;41:117-124.

337. Kosman KA, Silbersweig DA. Pseudo-Charles Bonnet syndrome with a frontal tumor: visual hallucinations, the brain, and the two-hit hypothesis. *J Neuropsychiatry Clin Neurosci.* Winter 2018;30(1):84-86.

338. Darby RR, Laganiere S, Pascual-Leone A, Prasad S, Fox MD. Finding the imposter: brain connectivity of lesions causing delusional misidentifications. *Brain.* 2017;140(2):497-507.

339. Stein DJ, Scott KM, de Jonge P, Kessler RC. Epidemiology of anxiety disorders: from surveys to nosology and back. *Dialogues Clin Neurosci.* 2017;19(2):127-136.

340. Baxter AJ, Vos T, Scott KM, Ferrari AJ, Whiteford HA. The global burden of anxiety disorders in 2010. *Psychol Med.* 2014;44(11):2363-2374.

341. Sylvers P, Lilienfeld SO, LaPrairie JL. Differences between trait fear and trait anxiety: implications for psychopathology. *Clin Psychol Rev.* 2011;31(1):122-137.

342. Hofmann SG, Ellard KK, Siegle GJ. Neurobiological correlates of cognitions in fear and anxiety: a cognitive-neurobiological information processing model. *Cogn Emot.* 2012;26(2):282-299.

343. Tovote P, Fadok JP, Lüthi A. Neuronal circuits for fear and anxiety. *Nat Rev Neurosci.* 2015;16(6):317-331.

344. Quirk GJ, Armony JL, LeDoux JE. Fear conditioning enhances different temporal components of tone-evoked spike trains in auditory cortex and lateral amygdala. *Neuron.* 1997;19(3):613-624.

345. Johansen JP, Hamanaka H, Monfils MH, et al. Optical activation of lateral amygdala pyramidal cells instructs associative fear learning. *Proc Natl Acad Sci U S A.* 2010;107(28): 12692-12697.

346. Ciocchi S, Herry C, Grenier F, et al. Encoding of conditioned fear in central amygdala inhibitory circuits. *Nature.* 2010;468(7321):277-282.

347. Nabavi S, Fox R, Proulx CD, Lin JY, Tsien RY, Malinow R. Engineering a memory with LTD and LTP. *Nature.* 2014;511(7509):348-352.

348. Herry C, Ciocchi S, Senn V, Demmou L, Müller C, Lüthi A. Switching on and off fear by distinct neuronal circuits. *Nature.* 2008;454(7204):600-606.

349. Davis M, Walker DL, Miles L, Grillon C. Phasic vs sustained fear in rats and humans: role of the extended amygdala in fear vs anxiety. *Neuropsychopharmacology.* 2010;35(1):105-135.

350. Grupe DW, Nitschke JB. Uncertainty and anticipation in anxiety: an integrated neurobiological and psychological perspective. *Nat Rev Neurosci.* 2013;14(7):488-501.

351. Motzkin JC, Philippi CL, Wolf RC, Baskaya MK, Koenigs M. Ventromedial prefrontal cortex is critical for the regulation of amygdala activity in humans. *Biol Psychiatry.* 2015;77(3): 276-284.

352. Apps R, Strata P. Neuronal circuits for fear and anxiety—the missing link. *Nat Rev Neurosci.* 2015;16(10):642.

353. Moreno-Rius J. The cerebellum in fear and anxiety-related disorders. *Prog Neuropsychopharmacol Biol Psychiatry.* 2018; 85:23-32.

354. Shimada-Sugimoto M, Otowa T, Hettema JM. Genetics of anxiety disorders: genetic epidemiological and molecular studies in humans. *Psychiatry Clin Neurosci.* 2015;69(7):388-401.

355. Taylor MJ, Martin J, Lu Y, et al. Association of genetic risk factors for psychiatric disorders and traits of these disorders in a Swedish population twin sample. *JAMA Psychiatry.* 2019;76(3):280-289.

356. Otowa T, Maher BS, Aggen SH, McClay JL, van den Oord EJ, Hettema JM. Genome-wide and gene-based association studies of anxiety disorders in European and African American samples. *PLoS One.* 2014;9(11):e112559.

357. Otowa T, Hek K, Lee M, et al. Meta-analysis of genome-wide association studies of anxiety disorders. *Mol Psychiatry.* 2016;21(10):1391-1399.

358. Gottschalk MG, Domschke K. Genetics of generalized anxiety disorder and related traits. *Dialogues Clin Neurosci.* 2017;19(2):159-168.

359. Stein MB, Chen CY, Jain S, et al. Genetic risk variants for social anxiety. *Am J Med Genet B Neuropsychiatr Genet.* 2017;174(2):120-131.

360. Savage JE, Sawyers C, Roberson-Nay R, Hettema JM. The genetics of anxiety-related negative valence system traits. *Am J Med Genet B Neuropsychiatr Genet.* 2017;174(2):156-177.

361. Hompes T, Izzi B, Gellens E, et al. Investigating the influence of maternal cortisol and emotional state during pregnancy on the DNA methylation status of the glucocorticoid receptor gene (NR3C1) promoter region in cord blood. *J Psychiatr Res.* 2013;47(7):880-891.

362. Non AL, Binder AM, Kubzansky LD, Michels KB. Genome-wide DNA methylation in neonates exposed to maternal depression, anxiety, or SSRI medication during pregnancy. *Epigenetics.* 2014;9(7):964-972.

363. Beesdo-Baum K, Knappe S. Developmental epidemiology of anxiety disorders. *Child Adolesc Psychiatr Clin N Am.* 2012;21(3):457-478.

364. Hartley CA, Phelps EA. Anxiety and decision-making. *Biol Psychiatry.* 2012;72(2):113-118.

365. Park J, Moghaddam B. Impact of anxiety on prefrontal cortex encoding of cognitive flexibility. *Neuroscience.* 2017;345:193-202.

366. Charpentier CJ, Aylward J, Roiser JP, Robinson OJ. Enhanced risk aversion, but not loss aversion, in unmedicated pathological anxiety. *Biol Psychiatry.* 2017;81(12):1014-1022.

367. Cisler JM, Koster EH. Mechanisms of attentional biases towards threat in anxiety disorders: an integrative review. *Clin Psychol Rev.* 2010;30(2):203-216.

368. Sagliano L, Trojano L, Amoriello K, Migliozzi M, D'Olimpio F. Attentional biases toward threat: the concomitant presence of difficulty of disengagement and attentional avoidance in low trait anxious individuals. *Front Psychol.* 2014;5:685.

369. Goodwin H, Yiend J, Hirsch CR. Generalized anxiety disorder, worry and attention to threat: a systematic review. *Clin Psychol Rev.* 2017;54:107-122.

370. Zhang A, Franklin C, Jing S, et al. The effectiveness of four empirically supported psychotherapies for primary care depression and anxiety: a systematic review and meta-analysis. *J Affect Disord.* 2019;245:1168-1186.

371 Loerinc AG, Meuret AE, Twohig MP, Rosenfield D, Bluett EJ, Craske MG. Response rates for CBT for anxiety disorders: need for standardized criteria. *Clin Psychol Rev.* 2015;42:72-82.

372. Carpenter JK, Andrews LA, Witcraft SM, Powers MB, Smits JAJ, Hofmann SG. Cognitive behavioral therapy for anxiety and related disorders: a meta-analysis of randomized placebo-controlled trials. *Depress Anxiety.* 2018;35(6):502-514.

373. Olthuis JV, Watt MC, Bailey K, Hayden JA, Stewart SH. Therapist-supported Internet cognitive behavioural therapy for anxiety disorders in adults. *Cochrane Database Syst Rev.* 2016;3: CD011565.

374. Sun X, Zhu C, So SHW. Dysfunctional metacognition across psychopathologies: a meta-analytic review. *Eur Psychiatry.* 2017;45:139-153.

375. Gkika S, Wittkowski A, Wells A. Social cognition and metacognition in social anxiety: a systematic review. *Clin Psychol Psychother.* 2018;25(1):10-30.

376. Nordahl H, Hjemdal O, Hagen R, Nordahl HM, Wells A. What lies beneath trait-anxiety? Testing the self-regulatory executive function model of vulnerability. *Front Psychol.* 2019;10:122.

377. Philipp R, Kriston L, Lanio J, et al. Effectiveness of metacognitive interventions for mental disorders in adults—a systematic review and meta-analysis (METACOG). *Clin Psychol Psychother.* 2019;26(2):227-240.

378. Stein MB, Sareen J. Clinical practice. Generalized anxiety disorder. *N Engl J Med.* 2015;373(21):2059-2068.

379. Craske MG, Stein MB. Anxiety. *Lancet.* 2016;388:3048-3059.

380. Leichsenring F, Leweke F. Social anxiety disorder. *N Engl J Med.* 2017;376(23):2255-2264.

381. Puetz TW, Youngstedt SD, Herring MP. Effects of pharmacotherapy on combat-related PTSD, anxiety, and depression: a systematic review and meta-regression analysis. *PLoS One.* 2015;10(5):e0126529.

382. Strawn JR, Geracioti L, Rajdev N, Clemenza K, Levine A. Pharmacotherapy for generalized anxiety disorder in adult and pediatric patients: an evidence-based treatment review. *Expert Opin Pharmacother.* 2018;19(10):1057-1070.

383. Gomez AF, Barthel AL, Hofmann SG. Comparing the efficacy of benzodiazepines and serotonergic anti-depressants for adults with generalized anxiety disorder: a meta-analytic review. *Expert Opin Pharmacother.* 2018;19(8):883-894.

384. He Q, Chen X, Wu T, Li L, Fei X. Risk of dementia in long-term benzodiazepine users: evidence from a meta-analysis of observational studies. *J Clin Neurol.* 2019;15(1):9-19.

385. Olfson M, King M, Schoenbaum M. Benzodiazepine use in the United States. *JAMA Psychiatry.* 2015;72(2):136-142.

386. Stephens EJ, Dysch L, Gregory J. Diagnostic overshadowing of anxiety in Parkinson disease: psychosocial factors and a cognitive-behavioral model. *Cogn Behav Neurol.* 2018;31(3):123-132.

387. Hsu D, Marshall GA. Primary and secondary prevention trials in Alzheimer disease: looking back, moving forward. *Curr Alzheimer Res.* 2017;14(4):426-440.

388. Butler E, Thomas R, Carolan A, Silber E, Chalder T. 'It's the unknown'—understanding anxiety: from the perspective of people with multiple sclerosis. *Psychol Health.* 2019;34(3):368-383.

389. Yochim BP, Mueller AE, Segal DL. Late life anxiety is associated with decreased memory and executive functioning in community dwelling older adults. *J Anxiety Disord.* 2013;27(6):567-575.

390. Beaudreau SA, O'Hara R. Late-life anxiety and cognitive impairment: a review. *Am J Geriatr Psychiatry.* 2008;16(10):790-803.

391. Gulpers B, Ramakers I, Hamel R, Köhler S, Oude Voshaar R, Verhey F. Anxiety as a predictor for cognitive decline and dementia: a systematic review and meta-analysis. *Am J Geriatr Psychiatry.* 2016;24(10):823-842.

392. Li XX, Li Z. The impact of anxiety on the progression of mild cognitive impairment to dementia in Chinese and English data bases: a systematic review and meta-analysis. *Int J Geriatr Psychiatry.* 2018;33(1):131-140.

393. Van der Mussele S, Mariën P, Saerens J, Somers N, Goeman J, De Deyn PP, Engelborghs S. Behavioral syndromes in mild

cognitive impairment and Alzheimer's disease. *J Alzheimers Dis.* 2014;38(2):319-329.

394. van der Linde RM, Dening T, Stephan BC, Prina AM, Evans E, Brayne C. Longitudinal course of behavioural and psychological symptoms of dementia: systematic review. *Br J Psychiatry.* 2016;209(5):366-377.

395. Lutz SG, Holmes JD, Ready EA, Jenkins ME, Johnson AM. Clinical presentation of anxiety in Parkinson's disease: a scoping review. *OTJR (Thorofare N J).* 2016;36(3):134-147.

396. Hashimoto H, Monserratt L, Nguyen P, et al. Anxiety and regional cortical glucose metabolism in patients with Alzheimer's disease. *J Neuropsychiatry Clin Neurosci.* 2006;18(4):521-528.

397. Thobois S, Prange S, Sgambato-Faure V, Tremblay L, Broussolle E. Imaging the etiology of apathy, anxiety, and depression in Parkinson's disease: implication for treatment. *Curr Neurol Neurosci Rep.* 2017;17(10):76.

398. Martínez-Fernández R, Schmitt E, Martinez-Martin P, Krack P. The hidden sister of motor fluctuations in Parkinson's disease: a review on nonmotor fluctuations. *Mov Disord.* 2016;31(8):1080-1094.

399. van der Velden RMJ, Broen MPG, Kuijf ML, Leentjens AFG. Frequency of mood and anxiety fluctuations in Parkinson's disease patients with motor fluctuations: a systematic review. *Mov Disord.* 2018;33(10):1521-1527.

400. Abbes M, Lhommée E, Thobois S, et al. Subthalamic stimulation and neuropsychiatric symptoms in Parkinson's disease: results from a long-term follow-up cohort study. *J Neurol Neurosurg Psychiatry.* 2018;89(8):836-843.

401. Troeung L, Egan SJ, Gasson N. A waitlist-controlled trial of group cognitive behavioural therapy for depression and anxiety in Parkinson's disease. *BMC Psychiatry.* 2014;14:19.

402. Seppi K, Ray Chaudhuri K, Coelho M, et al. Update on treatments for nonmotor symptoms of Parkinson's disease—an evidence-based medicine review. *Mov Disord.* 2019;34(2):180-198.

403. Orgeta V, Qazi A, Spector A, Orrell M. Psychological treatments for depression and anxiety in dementia and mild cognitive impairment: systematic review and meta-analysis. *Br J Psychiatry.* 2015;207(4):293-298.

404. Abraha I, Rimland JM, Trotta FM, et al. Systematic review of systematic reviews of non-pharmacological interventions to treat behavioural disturbances in older patients with dementia. The SENATOR-OnTop series. *BMJ Open.* 2017;7(3):e012759.

405. Carrozzino D, Marchetti D, Laino D, et al. Anxiety in adolescent epilepsy. A clinimetric analysis. *Nord J Psychiatry.* 2016;70(6):424-429.

406. Pham T, Sauro KM, Patten SB, et al. The prevalence of anxiety and associated factors in persons with epilepsy. *Epilepsia.* 2017;58(8):e107-e110.

407. Munger Clary HM. Anxiety and epilepsy: what neurologists and epileptologists should know. *Curr Neurol Neurosci Rep.* 2014;14(5):445.

408. Munger Clary HM, Snively BM, Hamberger MJ. Anxiety is common and independently associated with clinical features of epilepsy. *Epilepsy Behav.* 2018;85:64-71.

409. Hingray C, McGonigal A, Kotwas I, Micoulaud-Franchi JA. The relationship between epilepsy and anxiety disorders. *Curr Psychiatry Rep.* 2019;21(6):40.

410. O'Neal MA, Baslet G. Treatment for patients with a functional neurological disorder (conversion disorder): an integrated approach. *Am J Psychiatry.* 2018;175(4):307-314.

411. Boeschoten RE, Braamse AMJ, Beekman ATF, et al. Prevalence of depression and anxiety in multiple sclerosis: a systematic review and meta-analysis. *J Neurol Sci.* 2017;372:331-341.

412. Rossi S, Studer V, Motta C, et al. Neuroinflammation drives anxiety and depression in relapsing-remitting multiple sclerosis. *Neurology.* 2017;89(13):1338-1347.

413. Kowalec K, McKay KA, Patten SB, et al. Comorbidity increases the risk of relapse in multiple sclerosis: a prospective study. *Neurology.* 2017;89(24):2455-2461.

414. Butler E, Matcham F, Chalder T. A systematic review of anxiety amongst people with multiple sclerosis. *Mult Scler Relat Disord.* 2016;10:145-168.

415. Furtado M, Katzman MA. Neuroinflammatory pathways in anxiety, posttraumatic stress, and obsessive compulsive disorders. *Psychiatry Res.* 2015;229(1-2):37-48.

416. Hilty DM, Bourgeois JA, Chang CH. Diagnostic and treatment interventions for hypochondriasis in the neurology setting. *Curr Treat Options Neurol.* 2006;8(5):401-409.

417. Carrigan N, Dysch L, Salkovskis PM. The impact of health anxiety in multiple sclerosis: a replication and treatment case series. *Behav Cogn Psychother.* 2018;46(2):148-167.

418. Tyrer P, Salkovskis P, Tyrer H, et al. Cognitive-behaviour therapy for health anxiety in medical patients (CHAMP): a randomised controlled trial with outcomes to 5 years. *Health Technol Assess.* 2017;21(50):1-58.

419. Lipsman N, Neimat JS, Lozano AM. Deep brain stimulation for treatment-refractory obsessive-compulsive disorder: the search for a valid target. *Neurosurgery.* 2007;61(1):1-11; discussion 3.

420. Eisen JL, Pinto A, Mancebo MC, Dyck IR, Orlando ME, Rasmussen SA. A 2-year prospective follow-up study of the course of obsessive-compulsive disorder. *J Clin Psychiatry.* 2010;71(8):1033-1039.

421. Eisen JL, Mancebo MA, Pinto A, et al. Impact of obsessive-compulsive disorder on quality of life. *Compr Psychiatry.* 2006;47(4):270-275.

422. Ozaki N, Goldman D, Kaye WH, et al. Serotonin transporter missense mutation associated with a complex neuropsychiatric phenotype. *Mol Psychiatry.* 2003;8(11):933-936.

423. Pauls DL. The genetics of obsessive-compulsive disorder: a review. *Dialogues Clin Neurosci.* 2010;12(2):149-163.

424. Ahmari SE, Dougherty DD. Dissecting OCD circuits: from animal models to targeted treatments. *Depress Anxiety.* 2015;32(8):550-562.

425. Boedhoe PS, Schmaal L, Abe Y, et al. Distinct subcortical volume alterations in pediatric and adult OCD: a worldwide meta- and mega-analysis. *Am J Psychiatry.* 2017;174(1):60-69.

426. Cavedini P, Gorini A, Bellodi L. Understanding obsessive-compulsive disorder: focus on decision making. *Neuropsychol Rev.* 2006;16(1):3-15.

427. Vaghi MM, Vértes PE, Kitzbichler MG, et al. Specific fronto-striatal circuits for impaired cognitive flexibility and goal-directed planning in obsessive-compulsive disorder: evidence from resting-state functional connectivity. *Biol Psychiatry.* 2017;81(8):708-717.

428. Reggente N, Moody TD, Morfini F, et al. Multivariate resting-state functional connectivity predicts response to cognitive behavioral therapy in obsessive-compulsive disorder. *Proc Natl Acad Sci U S A.* 2018;115(9):2222-2227.

429. Saxena S, Rauch SL. Functional neuroimaging and the neuroanatomy of obsessive-compulsive disorder. *Psychiatr Clin North Am.* 2000;23(3):563-586.

430. Simon D, Kaufmann C, Müsch K, Kischkel E, Kathmann N. Fronto-striato-limbic hyperactivation in obsessive-compulsive disorder during individually tailored symptom provocation. *Psychophysiology*. 2010;47(4):728-738.

431. Greenberg BD, Rauch SL, Haber SN. Invasive circuitry-based neurotherapeutics: stereotactic ablation and deep brain stimulation for OCD. *Neuropsychopharmacology*. 2010;35(1): 317-336.

432. Tolin DF, Abramowitz JS, Brigidi BD, Foa EB. Intolerance of uncertainty in obsessive-compulsive disorder. *J Anxiety Disord*. 2003;17(2):233-242.

433. Gruner P, Pittenger C. Cognitive inflexibility in obsessive-compulsive disorder. *Neuroscience*. 2017;345:243-255.

434. Ouimet AJ, Ashbaugh AR, Radomsky AS. Hoping for more: how cognitive science has and hasn't been helpful to the OCD clinician. *Clin Psychol Rev*. 2019;69:14-29.

435. de Avila RCS, do Nascimento LG, Porto RLM, et al. Level of insight in patients with obsessive-compulsive disorder: an exploratory comparative study between patients with "good insight" and "poor insight". *Front Psychiatry*. 2019 Jul 3;10:413.

436. Paterson JL, Reynolds AC, Ferguson SA, Dawson D. Sleep and obsessive-compulsive disorder (OCD). *Sleep Med Rev*. 2013;17(6):465-474.

437. Nordahl H, Havnen A, Hansen B, Öst LG, Kvale G. Sleep disturbances in treatment-seeking OCD-patients: changes after concentrated exposure treatment. *Scand J Psychol*. 2018 Apr;59(2):186-191.

438. Díaz-Román A, Perestelo-Pérez L, Buela-Casal G. Sleep in obsessive-compulsive disorder: a systematic review and meta-analysis. *Sleep Med*. 2015;16(9):1049-1055.

439. Cox RC, Olatunji BO. Sleep disturbance and obsessive-compulsive symptoms: results from the national comorbidity survey replication. *J Psychiatr Res*. 2016;75:41-45.

440. Raines AM, Short NA, Sutton CA, Oglesby ME, Allan NP, Schmidt NB. Obsessive-compulsive symptom dimensions and insomnia: the mediating role of anxiety sensitivity cognitive concerns. *Psychiatry Res*. 2015;228(3):368-372.

441. Kalanthroff E, Linkovski O, Weinbach N, Pascucci O, Anholt GE, Simpson HB. What underlies the effect of sleep disruption? The role of alertness in obsessive-compulsive disorder (OCD). *J Behav Ther Exp Psychiatry*. 2017;57:212-213.

442. Romanelli RJ, Wu FM, Gamba R, Mojtabai R, Segal JB. Behavioral therapy and serotonin reuptake inhibitor pharmacotherapy in the treatment of obsessive-compulsive disorder: a systematic review and meta-analysis of head-to-head randomized controlled trials. *Depress Anxiety*. 2014;31(8):641-652.

443. Hirschtritt ME, Bloch MH, Mathews CA. Obsessive-compulsive disorder: advances in diagnosis and treatment. *JAMA*. 2017 Apr 4;317(13):1358-1367.

444. Boschen MJ, Drummond LM, Pillay A. Treatment of severe, treatment-refractory obsessive-compulsive disorder: a study of inpatient and community treatment. *CNS Spectr*. 2008;13(12): 1056-1065.

445. Carpenter JK, Andrews LA, Witcraft SM, Powers MB, Smits JAJ, Hofmann SG. Cognitive behavioral therapy for anxiety and related disorders: a meta-analysis of randomized placebo-controlled trials. *Depress Anxiety*. 2018;35(6):502-514.

446. Sugarman MA, Kirsch I, Huppert JD. Obsessive-compulsive disorder has a reduced placebo (and antidepressant) response compared to other anxiety disorders: a meta-analysis. *J Affect Disord*. 2017 Aug 15;218:217-226.

447. Jakovljević M. The placebo-nocebo response in patients with depression: do we need to reconsider our treatment approach and clinical trial designs? *Psychiatr Danub*. 2014;26(2):92-95.

448. Khan A, Kolts RL, Rapaport MH, Krishnan KR, Brodhead AE, Browns WA. Magnitude of placebo response and drug-placebo differences across psychiatric disorders. *Psychol. Med*. 2005;35:743-749.

449. Foa EB, Liebowitz MR, Kozak MJ, et al. Randomized, placebo-controlled trial of exposure and ritual prevention, clomipramine, and their combination in the treatment of obsessive-compulsive disorder. *Am J Psychiatry*. 2005;162(1):151-161.

450. Attiullah N, Eisen JL, Rasmussen SA. Clinical features of obsessive-compulsive disorder. *Psychiatr Clin North Am*. 2000;23(3):469-491.

451. Brown LT, Mikell CB, Youngerman BE, Zhang Y, McKhann GM2nd, Sheth SA. Dorsal anterior cingulotomy and anterior capsulotomy for severe, refractory obsessive-compulsive disorder: a systematic review of observational studies. *J Neurosurg*. 2016 Jan;124(1):77-89.

452. Lopes AC, Greenberg BD, Canteras MM, et al. Gamma ventral capsulotomy for obsessive-compulsive disorder: a randomized clinical trial. *JAMA Psychiatry*. 2014;71(9):1066-1076.

453. Jung HH, Kim SJ, Roh D, et al. Bilateral thermal capsulotomy with MR-guided focused ultrasound for patients with treatment-refractory obsessive-compulsive disorder: a proof-of-concept study. *Mol Psychiatry*. 2015;20(10):1205-1211.

454. Kim SJ, Roh D, Jung HH, et al. A study of novel bilateral thermal capsulotomy with focused ultrasound for treatment-refractory obsessive-compulsive disorder: 2-year follow-up. *J Psychiatry Neurosci*. 2018;43(4):170188.

455. Nuttin B, Cosyns P, Demeulemeester H, Gybels J, Meyerson B. Electrical stimulation in anterior limbs of internal capsules in patients with obsessive-compulsive disorder. *Lancet*. 1999;354(9189):1526.

456. Greenberg BD, Malone DA, Friehs GM, et al. Three-year outcomes in deep brain stimulation for highly resistant obsessive-compulsive disorder. *Neuropsychopharmacology*. 2006;31(11):2384-2393.

457. Alonso P, Cuadras D, Gabriëls L, et al. Deep brain stimulation for obsessive-compulsive disorder: a meta-analysis of treatment outcome and predictors of response. *PLoS One*. 2015;10(7): e0133591.

458. de Koning PP, Figee M, van den Munckhof P, Schuurman PR, Denys D. Current status of deep brain stimulation for obsessive-compulsive disorder: a clinical review of different targets. *Curr Psychiatry Rep*. 2011;13(4):274-282.

459. Rappel P, Marmor O, Bick A, et al. Subthalamic theta activity: a novel human subcortical biomarker for obsessive compulsive disorder. *Transl Psychiatry*. 2018;8(1):118.

460. Fibbe LA, Cath DC, van den Heuvel OA, Veltman DJ, Tijssen MA, van Balkom AJ. Relationship between movement disorders and obsessive-compulsive disorder: beyond the obsessive-compulsive-tic phenotype. A systematic review. *J Neurol Neurosurg Psychiatry*. 2012;83(6):646-654.

461. Lee MT, Mpavaenda DN, Fineberg NA. Habit reversal therapy in obsessive compulsive related disorders: a systematic review of the evidence and CONSORT evaluation of randomized controlled trials. *Front Behav Neurosci*. 2019;13:79.

462. Essoe JK, Grados MA, Singer HS, Myers NS, McGuire JF. Evidence-based treatment of Tourette's disorder and chronic tic disorders. *Expert Rev Neurother*. 2019:1-13.

463. Bugalho P, da Silva JA, Cargaleiro I, Serra M, Neto B. Psychiatric symptoms screening in the early stages of Parkinson's disease. *J Neurol*. 2012;259(1):124-131.

464. Sharp ME, Caccappolo E, Mejia-Santana H, et al. The relationship between obsessive-compulsive symptoms and PARKIN genotype: the CORE-PD study. *Mov Disord*. 2015;30(2):278-283.

465. Wilbur C, Bitnun A, Kronenberg S, et al. PANDAS/PANS in childhood: controversies and evidence. *Paediatr Child Health*. 2019;24(2):85-91.

466. Chiarello F, Spitoni S, Hollander E, Matucci Cerinic M, Pallanti S. An expert opinion on PANDAS/PANS: highlights and controversies. *Int J Psychiatry Clin Pract*. 2017 Jun;21(2):91-98.

467. Bird JS, Shah E, Shotbolt P. Epilepsy and concomitant obsessive-compulsive disorder. *Epilepsy Behav Case Rep*. 2018 Jul 20;10:106-110.

12

Focal Neurobehavioral Syndromes

Michael Erkkinen · Deepti Putcha · Kirk R. Daffner

INTRODUCTION

One of the fundamental working hypotheses of modern neuroscience is that the functioning of the brain permits and shapes the expression of the mind. Cognitive, perceptual, affective, and behavioral capacities and limits are determined by neural structures and the dynamic flow of information within them. The shifting contents of momentary experience are the product of precisely coordinated, ever-changing combinations of electrical activity within richly connected neural networks. Put another way, neural states encode mental experiences. These complex neurobiological processes are scaffolded by evolution via inherited factors, animated by environmental inputs, and chiseled by experience and learning. The system learns about itself and the workings of its environment through continuous prediction and feedback, self-generated actions and environmental inputs shape this dynamic neural circuitry. Brain-behavior relationships are complex but patterned: specific neural activities support specific mental states and localized brain dysfunction leads to focal neurobehavioral changes. This schematic framework relating brain and mind is embedded in the clinical fields of behavioral neurology and neuropsychiatry and serves as this chapter's main axiom.

There are many schemas for how to understand the brain's role in supporting mental functioning. Highlighted below are several working hypotheses about brain organization that help to frame and add explanatory depth to the discussion of focal neurobehavioral syndromes. These ideas are introduced to stimulate the creative clinician to connect bedside observations not only to neuroanatomy, but to more foundational principles of cognitive neuroscience. Clinicians have a frontline opportunity to test, challenge, and improve these models to better understand and care for our patients. If past is prologue, clinician-driven ideas about brain-behavior relationships also promise to change our basic understanding of human cognition, affect, and behavior.

The brain is composed of specialized neurocomputational units whose activity is determined by local neurobiological factors

The brain is a collection of modular, often anatomically localized, units each designed to perform a specialized type of neural computation. The coordinated activity of these neural transformations form networks that encode the complex neural representations supporting cognition, affect, and behavior. Individual units receive information, perform a specific transformation, and share the result with other units. The dynamic integration of information flowing across multiple neurocomputational units supports the incredible diversity of cognitive functions. The particular transform performed by an individual unit is determined primarily by the neurobiological properties of its local brain tissue (e.g., cytoarchitecture, cell types, etc.).[1] A given unit is capable of receiving, transforming, and transmitting information from many different units/areas[2] via white matter pathways. It can contribute to a wide variety of functions depending on its connections with other units, enhancing efficiency. In contrast, a single function may be accomplished by different combinations of parts/units, which provides redundancy in case of injury. The redundancy idea—that there are multiple ways to perform a task—makes it difficult to precisely pinpoint the disrupted units/parts for any observed change in behavior. The flexible employment of these units and their networks supports mental functioning.

The pattern and strength of connectivity between units varies, and is determined by structural factors (e.g., presence/density of white matter tracts, synaptic density, etc.) and functional considerations (e.g., dynamic engagement of intact pathways in real time). Multiple units sharing and transforming information is referred to as a neural "network." Networks generate complex combinations of transformed information and support higher-order representations. Dynamic shifts in network activity support the diversity of neural processes that underlie cognition, affect, and behavior. These shifts are mediated by neurochemical and neurophysiological processes.

This organizational structure supports the capacity for single units (e.g., nodes) to participate in multiple different networks, enhancing the system's efficiency. Color combinations provide a simple illustration of this efficiency. Weighted combinations of red, yellow, and blue (i.e., a 3-unit color network, each a single computational unit) can represent a nearly infinite set of colors, which is much more efficient than representing each possible color combination as its own unique entity. Spatial coordinates are similar: an infinite possibility of three-dimensional locations can be represented as weighted values along just three axes (e.g., a 3-unit spatial network). Combining the information within these two 3-unit networks—color and space—allows any color to associate with any location, producing a nearly infinite set of color-location combinations. Because the information from each network is represented simultaneously (e.g., in parallel), an entirely new, synergistic entity is created ("color-location"), much like "green" is not just yellow-blue. For non-synergistic color-location combinations (e.g., a specific color at a specific location), a single 3-unit network can be utilized in series, with a fourth node serving to hold/store the first representation (e.g., color) while the second is being processed (e.g., location).

These same phenomena occur on larger scales in the brain and offer a conceptual mechanism by which complex states are generated via dynamic combinations of individual computational units participating in networks. Representations generated by one network (e.g., visual) can be combined with other networks (e.g., language) to form more complex representations (e.g., letters), which in turn can be combined yet again (e.g., written words). The iterative nature of the system allows a single neurocomputational unit to participate in many networks and support a wide array of mental functions.

Specific cognitive, affective, and behavioral expressions do not emerge from activity contained within single, specific, anatomically localized regions (e.g., as posited by phrenology). Precise, dynamic combinations of multiple, often anatomically disparate, interacting neurocomputational units are responsible for their genesis. Some suggest that these interactions have synergistic or emergent properties that cannot be explained by studying the individual components in isolation.

Sensory inputs are the building blocks of perception, which is also shaped by genetics, prior experience, and context

The brain uses sensory inputs to create perceptual content. Perturbations in the physical properties of the world—both the external environment and internal bodily states—are detected by biological receptors and translated into codes stored in the activity of neurons. These environmentally proximate codes/units are the raw data from which the brain models the world. These basic codes are combined, filtered, and layered together to form higher-order assemblies that constitute the architecture of perception. The assembly process is designed to detect and highlight potential salience in the data and is shaped by evolution/genetics (e.g., hard-wired recognition of salient patterns), prior experience (e.g., associative learning of stimuli with salient outcomes), and the behavioral context. Once these perceptual models have been sufficiently grounded and informed

by incoming sensory information, they can be dynamically untethered from sensory systems and repurposed for other cognitive operations such as imagination.[3]

Experience Is Animated within the Brain's Perceptual Machinery

The brain relies on its perceptual machinery to ground and express its knowledge and models of the world. These perceptual processes can be guided and manipulated by many different types of stimuli, and the nature of this influence encodes meaningful distinctions between different aspects of mentation. Perception that is constructed directly from incoming sensory streams (e.g., vision, audition), for example, supports the perception of the external world; guidance by internally generated motor plans supports perception of prepared/imagined actions; guidance by internally generated cognitive processes supports perception of thoughts, imagined scenes, or abstractions. The functioning of these different perceptual modes is shaped by one's genetic milieu, prior experiences, and the behavioral context, all of which serve to filter and inform one's perceptual expectations (see below). Perception and action are intimately connected; *action*—in its most broad sense—is that in the body or mind which disturbs perception.

The Brain Detects Patterns in Multiple Levels of Perception and Generates Predictive Models

Continuous streams of incoming sensory information are not random; they contain patterns in their sensory features and temporal flow. The brain discerns and stores these featural-temporal patterns and uses them as predictions about the state of the world. These serve to "fill in the gaps" later when incoming information is incomplete, ambiguous, or noisy. Repeated exposure to specific sensory inputs that are reliably followed by other sensory changes in close temporal proximity underlies rudimentary predictive models of *causality*. Stable sensory features across multiple temporal contexts support basic models of *form*, defined broadly as the configuration of objects and other perceptual phenomena. The information from these basic models is combined and integrated into higher-order featural-temporal assemblies, whose patterns are themselves detected, stored, and used to generate new predictions about the world. This process is iterative and expansive with each round of successive integration. The higher-level predictions feed back upon lower levels, too, creating both top-down and bottom-up influences. In totality, these dynamic multilayered prediction models constitute the large-scale, personal schematic frameworks about how the world works. They are the substrate for *expectation*, originally built into the neural structures from basic sensory building blocks. Cognitive processes combine and repurpose these working models of causality, form, and expectation to ground imaginations or abstract reasoning in conceptual schemas.

The brain constantly generates and updates predictive models about the self, the world, and their salient interactions. Data that are not consistent with expectations (i.e., a prediction error) are used to update the model's predictive settings. The ability to represent self (as distinct from nonself) and generate schemas about the world—and one's causal relationship to it—are supported by predictive processing. The predictions themselves are often used by the brain to guide decision making, judgements, and behavior, which highlights the importance of the model's accuracy and tuning. The ability to adapt one's predictive schemas based on new information varies across individuals, as does the ability to filter out data that do not fit the prediction.

The Brain's Ability to Adapt to Its Environment Depends on the Behavioral Function and Developmental Stage

The brain's different individual structures vary in their ability to adapt to changes in the environment. Many systems—often located in the brainstem—are inflexible and optimized to efficiently perform a stereotyped response whenever they become activated. These processes are often inborn and automatic, much like a motor reflex (although often more complex). Other parts of the central nervous system—particularly the cerebral cortex—are heavily dependent on environmental inputs (i.e., experience) to shape their particular expression. While certain areas are evolutionarily primed to support a particular function (e.g., inferior frontal gyrus [IFG] for speech output), their precise tuning and behavioral expressions are individualized based on one's experience (e.g., individual accents). The ability of neural tissue to adapt and reorganize itself (i.e., neuroplasticity) based on changing environmental inputs varies over the course of the lifespan. There are often critical periods of high plasticity during development, when experiences have a marked impact on neural organization and subsequent behavioral expression.

Sensory and Motor Processes Represent Two Sides of the Same Coin

Just as sensory information shapes action, actions have sensory consequences. A simple movement of the arm leads to changes in the external environment which can be detected by visual and/or somatosensory systems, and also causes changes in the internal environment which can be detected by proprioceptive and visceromotor mechanisms. *Specific* actions lead to *specific* sensory consequences, and these relationships are stored as integrated sensorimotor associations that serve as predictive models coupling actions with perceptions. The codes can be accessed in a bidirectional manner: merely *perceiving* specific actions performed by others activates the motor programs required to perform the action. This is the so-called "mirror neuron" system.[4] This perception-action coupling is what is known as the common coding hypothesis: the idea that action and perception are tightly linked[5] as two aspects of an overlapping process. The brain utilizes these common codes to plan actions based on the anticipated sensory consequences, and specific actions can be induced by perceptual inputs.

Action-perception coupling may have broad implications for understanding behavior and cognition when considered as a general principle that extends beyond simple skeletal movements and their tactile/proprioceptive consequences. Perceiving the social behavior and/or affection of others may activate similar internal self-representations ("affect sharing"),[6,7] including

visceromotor programs; specific cognitive "actions" can specifically alter the contents of one's working memory stores or imagination for problem solving. The tight linkages between different forms of action and perception offer a potential mechanism for many aspects of behavior, including reduced empathy in autism.[8]

The Brain Is Composed of Several Large-Scale, Often Anti-Correlated, Networks that Support Different Processing "Modes"

The brain tends to utilize several large-scale (e.g., multiple, anatomically distant) networks that support specialized "modes" of cognition. A mode is a wide set of preferential engagements with attentional, cognitive, perceptual, emotional, and action-generating machinery that represent restricted ways of interacting with and manipulating the mental and physical environment. These processing modes support different functions, such as tasks that require goal-driven externally directed attention or those supporting focus upon one's own internal mentalizations such as thought, imagination, recollection of prior memories, and others. The coordinated activity of these large-scale networks amplifies and dampens certain cognitive processes by facilitating different connectivity patterns between brain regions, producing a broad set of specialized and highly efficient interactions at the expense of others. The activity of one mode is often most effective when the activity in others is suppressed. The brain switches between modes depending on the needs of the individual, and certain functions necessitate multiple modes acting in concert.

Many Aspects of Neural Processing Occur Outside of Conscious Experience

Most of the brain's processing is hidden from consciousness. This is true for perception, action, cognition, and behavior. Incoming sensory stimuli, for example, are highly processed before entering one's conscious awareness and are often perceived as a cohesive whole without perception of its deconstructed low-level components. In terms of action, a high-order behavioral plan may be conceived and directed within one's consciousness while the complex series of smaller microactions needed to enact the plan within motor-effector systems are performed outside one's conscious control. Conscious ("explicit") processing is usually reserved for the highest-order functions, with most of the brain devoted to activity outside of consciousness ("implicit" processing). The reach of consciousness into lower levels may vary based on the ongoing needs of the individual.

Patients with deficient explicit processing may lack insight and have difficulty relaying the nature of their symptoms; their declared beliefs may not align with their outward behaviors. Excessive explicit processing can be disruptive, bringing into consciousness functions or stimuli that are best handled implicitly.

A Brief Note on the Problem of Consciousness

Despite the seemingly irreducible quality of one's *own* conscious awareness, direct observation and detection of *other* minds poses philosophical difficulties. Generally accepted methods of scientific inquiry measure phenomena that are accessible via a third-person perspective (e.g., physical world and its forces); the qualitative experience of consciousness is accessible only through first-person introspection. As such, mental states may only be inferred based on indirect measurements such as behavior and neurophysiological data. The tension of not being able to directly measure the object of highest interest—the mind—permeates cognitive neuroscience and its clinical companions, behavioral neurology and neuropsychiatry. Discussions of "mental" states are often avoided and are replaced by alternative terms such as "representation," which refers to neurologic states whose biological composition/readouts correlate with reported first-person experiences of specific mental states. This chapter continues in the tradition of avoiding this central philosophical mind-body problem, preferring to use "representation" when referring to psychological states.

Philosophical conceptions aside, consciousness is often divided into different components, including arousal/wakefulness and awareness. Deficits in these systems are termed disorders of consciousness. Reduced *arousal*, which is described by the amount of stimulation needed to generate the appearance of wakefulness, can manifest as total unresponsiveness, known as **coma**, or reduced responsiveness, known as **stupor** or **lethargy**. Excessive arousal may be seen in states of mania or agitation. *Awareness* is the conscious perception of specific mental representations or processes (e.g., the contents of consciousness). Many cognitive, perceptual, affective, and behavioral processes normally unfold outside of one's awareness, often in a graded manner, suggesting a physiologic role for regulating the content of one's consciousness awareness. When the control of awareness is dysfunctional, it can produce symptoms or reduced insight, known as **anosognosia**, which can be global or focal, but often involve the nondominant hemisphere.

The rest of the chapter is focused on the specific anatomical networks and organizational structures whose disruption or injury leads to common neurobehavioral syndromes. The basic principles reviewed provide a schematic context for the remainder of the chapter and serve as a foundation for the discussions about brain-behavior relationships. For a more detailed presentation of the functional neuroanatomy of cognitive processing, please see the authors' related work, Chapter 3, of this volume.

SENSORY-PERCEPTUAL PROCESSING

The brain's models about the world are informed by and grounded in its connections with the physical environment, both external and internal/body. Sensory-perceptual systems receive input from the external world in the form of light, pressure waves, chemical compounds, tactile displacement, and others, representing the basic inputs for vision, sound, olfaction and taste, and touch, respectively. They receive inputs from the body that relay information about the body's physical position in space, markers of tissue damage, and internal homeostatic functions (e.g., chemical states of the body, autonomic states, visceral organ sensation, metabolic demands, etc.), and others. These basic sensory inputs are the building blocks of perception that underlie many aspects of cognition and behavior.

Disruptions of these distal sensory systems can produce neurologic symptoms affecting aspects of cognition and behavior.

Some are intuitive: hearing loss due to inner ear damage can affect speech perception and blindness caused by ocular problems can affect reading, writing, and drawing. Others are less obvious: peripheral sensory damage can produce **"release" hallucinations** of simple or well-formed unimodal hallucinations after acquired visual or hearing loss (NB: **Charles Bonnet syndrome** refers to well-formed visual hallucinations after acquired vision loss), or the **"phantom limb" phenomenon** after limb amputations and its accompanying loss of body state inputs. Similar symptoms may also affect the olfactory system, a condition known as **phantosmia**.[9] Despite the reduced peripheral input, central perceptual representations remain intact and can become activated in the absence of sensory inputs. Activation of higher-order perceptual representations without direct stimulation from sensory inputs supports normal cognitive functions, such as imagination and language. When dysregulated, however, it can lead to experiences of excessive or inappropriate mentalization, such as hallucinations.

A sudden change in peripheral sensory functioning leads to prediction errors about the sensory consequences of one's actions. This can result in a retuning of the action-perception machinery and consequent changes in behavior. Hearing loss, for example, may cause a compensatory increase in the volume of one's speaking voice; a reduction in autonomic inputs from the body lead to compensatory tachycardia upon standing as is reported in some cases of the postural orthostatic tachycardia syndrome (POTS). Altered sensory inputs can also lead to imprecise afferent predictions, leading to incorrect central activations and misperceptions and experience of **illusions**, especially in patients with cognitive impairment. These kinds of changes are sometimes misdiagnosed as occurring secondary to central nervous system damage or primary psychiatric conditions. Screening for peripheral sensory changes is an important component of the cognitive and behavioral evaluation.

Sensory perception—the awareness of incoming sensory information—is a higher-order process that depends on the cerebral cortex. The primary sensory cortices support basic perceptual processing of unimodal sensory inputs. Damage to these primary sensory cortices can produce clinical syndromes that illustrate the distinction between sensation and perception. Bilateral damage to the primary visual cortex, for example, can produce **"blindsight,"** where patients qualitatively experience total blindness yet respond to some visual stimuli with better-than-chance success rates. Despite their insistence on being blind, affected individuals duck when an object is thrown toward them, actively avoid tripping on obstacles placed in their line of gait, and make accurate guesses about information presented in their affected visual fields. They are unable to provide an account of their vision and are often bewildered by their unexpectedly effectual behaviors. Similar syndromes are reported with other sensory modalities, including cortical deafness after bilateral superior temporal damage, and cortical somatosensory loss after lesions to the post-central gyrus. Blindsight illustrates the important role of the cortex in explicit perceptual processing and forces the realization that conscious perception—despite its subjective quality as offering an immediate, foundational, unfiltered window onto the world—is an "active" process that requires specialized cortical neural machinery to compute.

Sensory perception is a multilayered process whereby successive rounds of neural processing encode increasingly complex perceptual representations. Informational flow through these systems often occurs via distinct pathways that support different types of perceptual processing. The visual system, for example, has dedicated areas for the processing of color, depth, motion, and object forms; the auditory system has specialized pathways representing sound as language (e.g., phonology). Other sensory modalities have a similar organization with specialized unimodal features. Damage to these higher-order, "secondary" sensory processing streams can produce modality-specific focal perceptual symptoms. Damage to phonological processing areas in the bilateral posterior superior temporal lobe, for example, may cause "**pure word deafness**," whereby one cannot comprehend the meaning of spoken words but can read and understand the same words without difficulty. Disruption of the motion-sensitive areas in the visual cortex, area MT (or V5), produces symptoms of **akinetopsia** ("motion blindness").

Adjacent to the secondary sensory cortices are *multimodal* sensory areas, where information from multiple sensory modalities is integrated into high-order perceptual representations. These areas support diverse functions such as the ability to perceive the world as a multidimensional, multimodal scene (like in a movie) or conceptual schemas of objects, abstract concepts, and other types of semantic knowledge. These multimodal areas are richly connected with other neurologic systems (e.g., "hubs"), which support their role in cognition and behavior.

COGNITIVE PROCESSING

The cognitive systems are traditionally organized into domains of mental processing (e.g., attention, executive functioning, visuospatial skills, language, praxis, calculations, etc.). This scheme did not originate from an understanding of functional neuroanatomy but rather neuropsychological models of cognition. Mapping these psychologically organized functions onto neuroanatomical networks is complex. Different cognitive functions may recruit similar or overlapping networks, and similar cognitive functions may be mediated by different neural pathways. For example, both recalling past memories and imaging future scenarios are different cognitive functions that utilize similar functional neuroanatomy. Alternatively, copying a four-sided figure with equal-length lines and right angles can be achieved by simply seeing and reproducing the lines on the page without knowledge of its identity as a square; alternatively, one can recognize the figure as a square and call upon one's concept of squares to reproduce the figure. The same cognitive function—copying a figure—is potentially accomplished through multiple pathways. "Focal" neurobehavioral syndromes do not necessarily imply a specific focal anatomical lesion, but often point to disruption somewhere within a complex neural network. "Localization" of function is often characterized in terms of network failure, even when there is a solitary focal lesion. Despite the complex alignment of psychology and neuroanatomy, general principles of cognitive localization nevertheless emerge. The chapter continues the convention of organizing the cognitive system by its neuropsychological domains.

It is important to keep in mind that neuropsychological functions are hierarchical and interdependent, as the successful expression of some mental faculties requires that other functions to be at least partially intact. An obvious example is that of arousal (i.e., wakefulness): a stuporous patient will perform poorly on cognitive tests across multiple domains (e.g., attention, language, memory), even if the domain-specific neuroanatomical systems underlying these functions are themselves not damaged. Disturbances in this arousal-wakefulness system can yield a false sense of localization when not considered as part of a hierarchical organization. This is also true for motivation, as an unmotivated or unengaged participant is apt to perform poorly on many cognitive tests, which can lead to incorrect conclusions as to the localization of disrupted networks. Attention, concentration, executive functions, language, and visuospatial skills, as well as elemental neurologic functions (e.g., motor, coordination, sensation) all influence a patient's performance on testing—including on measures designed to isolate specific cognitive domains—and it is important to understand and consider the cognitive operations required to carry out each test to avoid drawing improper conclusions. It is the interdependency of these functions that makes localization so challenging … and rewarding.

The neurobiological substrates supporting language processing provide an elegant demonstration of structure-function relationships in behavioral neurology and neuropsychiatry. The chapter's early emphasis on language disorders serves to highlight general principles that apply to other neural/cognitive systems. Below, a detailed discussion of the language system is followed by briefer descriptions of the other systems.

CHARACTERIZING DEFICITS AFFECTING THE LANGUAGE SYSTEM

The faculty of communication through language is remarkable. The presence of sounds in the air, scribbles on a page, raised dots on a paper, and others, efficiently transforms the state of our brain into one of shared representations with their author, albeit filtered through our social lenses. These sensory symbols co-opt our perceptual machinery and effortlessly generate and proliferate concepts and mental imagery that spread through the nervous system to impact behavior. Human brains are uniquely designed to efficiently transmit their brain states—and receive those of others—via the coded mechanisms of language. Our facility in using these codes separates us from other animals; it allows us to communicate across time and space about specific entities that are not within our immediate perceptual environment. Language enables us to have connected brains, to be less alone, to become less isolated.

Communicating with language fundamentally requires one decode sensory inputs into language symbols, link these symbols with properly formed concepts, and produce sensory language symbols that others can interpret. These faculties comprise the core "language" system. In the real world, however, language is employed for social purposes: to share desires, concerns, and ideas, acquire knowledge from others' experiences, and develop schemas about other minds. These real-life language functions extend far beyond that of symbol-semantic relationships and depend on cognitive, motivational, and perceptual skills. Paralinguistic expressions such as affective prosody (e.g., the emotional "tones" of speech), metaphor, sarcasm, body language, and conversational turn-taking connect language skills with complex limbic, social, and perceptual networks. Storytelling engages executive control and memory systems. Listening and reading requires attention and concentration. Lesions anywhere along this extended multidomain network can manifest as difficulty communicating with language, even when the fundamental language operations are spared.

Comprehending language depends on perceiving sensory phenomena as symbolically representative of semantic concepts. Each language's sensory code is composed of a small set of learned elements (known as "features") that serve as building blocks for higher-order linguistic structures. Specific combinations of these features make up the sensory word forms that connect to specific semantic concepts. Concepts that are paired with specific word forms are referred to as lexical concepts, or lemma (colloquially, "words"). Communicating requires that speakers and listeners have a common set of word forms and shared word-concept relationships. A language's set of unique lexical concepts is known as the lexicon. The specific sensory elements utilized by language users are surprisingly arbitrary and vary across cultures. Sound and visual symbols are the most commonly used. A language's auditory and written sensory elements are termed phonemes and graphemes, respectively, and their methods for combining them into words are similarly termed phonology and orthography.

Expressing language requires a communicator to generate an idea they wish to convey (e.g., conceptual preparation), retrieve the lexical concepts that align with the intended content, represent the message as a sensory (e.g., phonological) target, and select the appropriate motor (e.g., articulatory) plan to produce external sensory perturbations that allow a listener to comprehend the utterance.[10] Producing language requires some form of motor output—most commonly speaking, writing/typing, or signing—but other methods can be utilized in situations of motor compromise.

Focal nervous system damage can disrupt language functioning in specific sensory and motor modalities while leaving others intact (e.g., pure word deafness, alexia, etc.). In people with language symptoms, it is important to determine if the deficit is modality-dependent (e.g., auditory verbal comprehension vs. reading; speaking vs. writing) or independent (e.g., poor comprehension regardless of sensory input). Modality-specific deficits suggest the potential use of alternative pathways to access—and unlock—hidden linguistic capacities.

Language deficits can disrupt affective and social functioning, often causing frustration, anxiety, withdrawal, and isolation. These reactions are often an appropriate grief response to the acquired reduced ability to communicate specific intentions, desires, and beliefs, and to understand those of other people. While an important means of social engagement, symbolic language is only one of many methods of communication between individuals and may only represent a small portion of the transmitted information between individuals. In addition, the selective loss of language functions may, in some cases, potentiate other nonlinguistic capacities.[11,12]

In classic aphasiology, the language system is lateralized to the left hemisphere in most people, and grossly divided into a posterior, sensory, receptive region (i.e., Wernicke's area) in the temporal and parietal lobes, and an anterior, motor-grammatical, expressive area (i.e., Broca's area) in the frontal lobe, which are connected by the arcuate fasciculus, a white matter tract. Damage to the posterior areas produces poor comprehension of language with spared expressive fluency (Wernicke aphasia), and anterior damage produces poor fluency with spared comprehension (Broca's aphasia). The ability to repeat is affected in both conditions. This framework serves as a foundation for the remainder of this section (please see Figure 12-1).

Basic Language Comprehension

Because so many of the formal cognitive tests across multiple domains rely on verbal comprehension, it is important to test the basic integrity of this system. The simplest way is to ask the patient to follow commands. For efficiency, it is sometimes best to begin with longer, more difficult requests (e.g., for those in

Classical Aphasiology Syndromes			
Aphasia Label	**Comprehension**	**Repetition**	**Fluency**
Normal	+	+	+
Wernicke	−	−	+
Transcortical sensory	−	+	+
Broca	+	−	−
Transcortical motor	+	+	−
Conduction	+	−	+
Global	−	−	−

FIGURE 12-1. Classical aphasiology syndromes. NB: Wernicke and transcortical sensory aphasias are also categorized as a "receptive" and Broca and transcortical motor as "expressive." + signifies intact; − signifies impaired.

Boston: "indicate with the fingers of your left hand the number that corresponds to the first letter of the name of the city we are in…"). If the patient manages this challenging task, this faculty is likely intact. If not, the examiner can pursue more elementary components of language processing. Simple, short requests are often useful as they reduce the attentional and working memory demands, a potential confounder. Successful execution of these tasks implies that basic verbal comprehension is intact.

Basic verbal comprehension requires several steps, including specialized sensory processing to decode sensory inputs into language symbols, linking the symbols with the appropriate semantic concepts, and using this integrated information to select an action that communicates understanding. Deficits in any of these steps produce different patterns of impaired language comprehension.

The ability to decode sensory inputs into language symbols is a modality-specific process accomplished within primary and secondary sensory areas (discussed below). The linkage of symbols to meaning is likely a domain-general process occurring within a multimodal convergence zone within posterior parts of temporal lobe (see Chapter 3 in this volume),[13] adjacent to high-order auditory and visual processing areas. Injury to this lexical-semantic interface is associated with **Wernicke aphasia**, which is characterized by reduced comprehension of spoken and written language with fluent verbal output that lacks meaningful content. The patients often demonstrate a striking lack of insight into their own deficits.

The ability to decode sensory inputs into language symbols occurs in secondary unimodal sensory cortices (e.g., audition, vision). Selective disruptions in this process cause comprehension deficits isolated to the affected sensory modality, even when primary sensory perceptions for that mode are intact. **Pure word deafness (or auditory verbal agnosia)**, for example, is characterized by poor comprehension of verbally presented words with preserved reading comprehension and hearing. The patient may even be able to identify and discriminate between basic phonological elements of speech. Speech may be perceived as sounding like a foreign language. This is often caused by damage to phonological processing areas within the bilateral (occasionally unilateral left-sided) superior temporal gyri. **Pure alexia (or pure word blindness)** is the parallel syndrome within the visual modality where previously-literate individuals can comprehend words presented verbally but not textually, even when the primary elements of vision are normal. They have difficulty with writing. This occurs with damage to orthographic (i.e., visual letter and word representations) processing areas located within parts of the left fusiform gyrus, which is part of the ventral visual processing stream (see below). These conditions suggest a disturbance not in the lexical-semantic interface but instead a selective problem with representing phonological and visual word forms.

Deficits in sensory decoding into language elements can be strikingly focal. The left fusiform gyrus processes increasingly complex forms of visual orthographic representations along a posterior-to-anterior gradient. The mid-anterior fusiform is appropriately known as the "visual word form area" (VWFA), as lesions cause pure alexia. If the posterior fusiform is undamaged in these cases, letter comprehension is spared, yielding the syndrome of **letter-by-letter dyslexia**.[14] This syndrome is characterized by a unique reading deficit whereby affected individuals perceive individual letters but not whole words. To overcome this, individuals read a word's letters out loud one at a time in sequence until the previously imperceptible word and its meaning are suddenly identified, presumably by utilizing an alternate phonological pathway to access the lexical-semantic interface. Patients with deficits in the visual language pathways important for decoding letter and words have concomitant difficulties spelling words that relay on phonic rules (e.g., reasoning via visual symbol-to-sound relationships).

A nearly identical pure alexia syndrome known as **alexia without agraphia** can emerge from focal damage to a different set of adjacent regions, namely the left primary visual areas in the occipital cortex and nearby posterior part of the corpus callosum (i.e., splenium). Affected individuals have a right-sided visual field deficit due to the left occipital damage; vision is intact in the left hemifield because the right occipital/visual areas are spared. Because visual information is decoded into language symbols in the left fusiform gyrus, the right occipital cortex sends its visual information across the hemispheres via the splenium of the corpus callosum to be processed for reading. Because the splenium is damaged, the left fusiform does not receive the visual inputs, causing alexia despite intact primary vision within the left hemifield. Because the language network and auditory inputs are spared, verbal comprehension, speech, and writing are intact. A striking and memorable phenomenon occurs whereby the patient writes a sentence but is unable to read what he has written only a few moments later. Neurobehavioral deficits that emerge due to poor information flow between processing areas is known as a **disconnection syndrome**.[15]

Because many components of language comprehension are modality-specific, when a deficit is identified it is important to test this system using different sensory inputs (e.g., verbal and written). Difficulties should, of course, prompt an assessment of elemental sensory and motor functions, including testing of basic hearing, vision, and the motor system.

Lexical Retrieval Deficits and Anomia

Highly effective communication depends on the ability to rapidly access specific lexical-semantic concepts and their associated sensory word forms in real time. Once a concept has been selected for expression, the appropriate lexical label (e.g., sensory word form) must be retrieved before it can be expressed as a communicative action. This lexical retrieval process is often guided by top-down (e.g., internally generated) mechanisms, but may be facilitated by exposure to sensory-perceptual features related to the word form or concept (e.g., stimulus-driven). The functional networks supporting this process are complex, and involve regions involved in perception, semantic processing, and directed search capabilities. Please see Figure 12-2, to illustrate this.

Lexical retrieval deficits commonly present as **anomic aphasia** characterized by word retrieval deficits in spontaneous speech and difficulty naming objects on confrontational testing (e.g., Boston Naming Test). In spontaneous speech, affected individuals

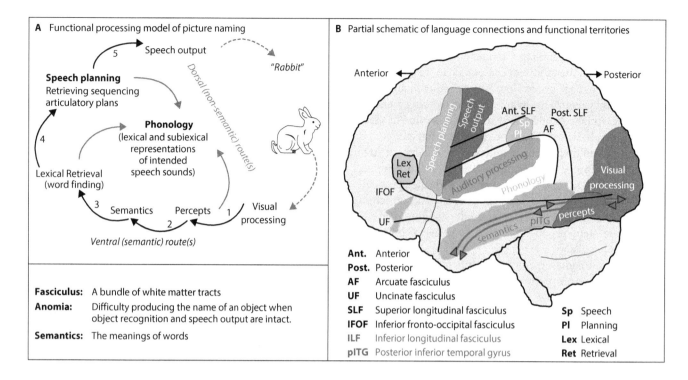

FIGURE 12-2. Networks involved in naming and lexical retrieval. (Reproduced with permission from Hope TM, Price CJ. Why the left posterior inferior temporal lobe is needed for word finding. *Brain.* 2016;139(11):2823-2826. Published by Oxford University Press on behalf of the Guarantors of Brain. All rights reserved.)

may experience a frustrating "tip of the tongue" state where they can describe the concept they wish to express without being able to recall the sensory (e.g., phonological) word form. They are often able to provide detailed descriptions of ideas they wish to express, or pantomime the use of objects, despite being unable to conjure up the appropriate and specific lexical label. Frequent use of synonyms and other circumlocutionary phrases leads to imprecise and vague-sounding content. Speaking may be interrupted by hesitations or pauses to allow time for word searching. The retrieval difficulties are most apt to occur for low-frequency words. On tests of confrontational naming, providing the first letter or sound of the elusive word often aids its retrieval. The individual is virtually always able to recognize the word from a list of multiple choices. The elusive word may spontaneously come to the speaker after a few moments. Some speakers consciously use methods to aid their word search by providing their own internal phonemic cues by silently imagining each letter of the alphabet. Slips of the tongue can occur, particularly **semantic paraphasias,** where incorrect but semantically related words are expressed (e.g., "guitar" instead of "banjo").

In anomic aphasia due to a lexical selection deficit, both the bank of semantic concepts and lexical labels (e.g., the lexicon) are intact, but their connections are disrupted. The ability of concepts to activate their lexical labels becomes less efficient, and requires top-down, frontally mediated search mechanisms or bottom-up perceptual stimulation (e.g., phonemic cues, multiple choices) to facilitate the connection. The strength of concept-label connections varies across concepts; the activation of semantically related concepts with more readily accessible lexical labels leads to semantic paraphasias. In anomic aphasia, the disruption of the lexical-semantic interface is largely unidirectional; perception of

sensory word forms (e.g., phonological word forms) efficiently activates the appropriate concepts.

Anomia symptoms are most severe when concept-to-label connections and the compensatory systems become dysfunctional. Problems with decoding language (e.g., phonological processing), semantic knowledge (e.g., reduced number and nuance of conceptual stores), and top-down directed search mechanisms can exacerbate symptoms. These functionally disparate processes seem to converge within the left temporal lobe. Deficits in lexical retrieval in anomic aphasia localize to left lateral temporal regions, including most notably the mid-to-posterior middle temporal gyrus (MTG),[17,18] mid-to-posterior inferior gyrus, superior temporal gyrus, and the associated subcortical white matter.[19] Semantic paraphasic errors, similarly, occur most commonly with damage to the posterior inferior temporal cortex.[20]

The MTG is a heteromodal region that processes highly integrated information from multiple sensory processing streams The MTG is situated adjacent to areas known to process semantic/object information, the inferior temporal cortex, and phonological information, the superior temporal cortex. Confrontation naming deficits may be category-specific based on the involved anatomy: objects/noun and action/verb impairments associate with temporal and frontal dysfunction, respectively. The precise mechanisms for this observation are debated, but may relate to category-specific differences in semantic storage, lexical access, or syntactic handling.[21]

Semantic Deficits

A critical aspect of language processing is the ability to represent and flexibly access semantic knowledge. Semantic concepts are specific, clustered combinations of sensory, motor, visceral, cognitive, affective, and linguistic information that are bound together. A simple concept would be a square, which has specific perceptual quality and a geometrically based definition. The "square" concept is likely to be similar across individuals. An individual's concept of "baseball," however, may be more complex. To some, "baseball" encompasses the sensory smell of fresh cut grass and the sound of a fastball "popping" the mitt, motor plans for swinging a bat and throwing a pitch, visceral responses watching ninth inning of the World Series, cognitive rules and strategies, affective elation of winning, and the linguistic knowledge of one's favorite players, among many others. While there are core conceptual features likely to be shared across individuals, the concept is ultimately individualized. The ability to bind complex, multimodal representations together (such as baseball) and associate them with specific lexical labels allows for efficient communication of complex ideas.

The binding process is conceived like the hub and spokes of wheel. A concept's hub has specific, weighted connections with many types of information (e.g., cognitive, visceral, perceptual, motor, limbic, etc.), the spokes, that in aggregate comprise the concept. Hubs are located in heteromodal areas, whereas the spokes are located diffusely in multiple locations depending on the representational content. Losing one or two spokes (e.g., visuospatial, lexical representations) does not lead to a complete loss of the concept, although it may be less detailed, as other features may be maintained. Damaging the hub, however, prevents the binding of features into a unified construct, causing a loss of conceptual representations.[22]

Patients with **semantic aphasia** have difficulty describing objects in precise terms and tend to offer only vague, tangential replies. Phonemic cues or multiple choices do not improve performance. Their spontaneous speech may be difficult to follow due to its lack of detail, although patients are often not bothered by their diminished verbal precision. These deficits may occur in neurodegenerative disease such as the syndrome of **semantic variant primary progressive aphasia (svPPA)**. Affected individuals usually maintain exemplar representations of categories longer and lose the fine-grained details that are constructed around these prototypes. For instance, when asked to draw pictures of a variety of animals, patients may sketch a series of basic, dog-like animals that lack distinct features central to each animal.[23] Patients speak in a similar manner, often using generic, categorical terms in place of more nuanced expressions (e.g., "my wife Anna" becomes "the woman," "my home in Cambridge" becomes "the place"). Some of these symptoms can also occur in degenerative conditions beyond that of svPPA, including Alzheimer's disease.

The bedside evaluation for semantic knowledge includes asking patients to name objects, to draw or describe objects in as much detail as possible, or to associate objects with overlapping semantic features. Testing confrontational spelling and oral reading of words can also be informative. Disproportionate errors handling words that do not follow phonetic rules (e.g., irregular words), such as "yacht," "gnome," or "choir," is called "**surface" dyslexia and dysgraphia**. Knowledge of the linguistic quirks of these words is part of their semantic representation, and when this information is compromised, a common strategy is to rely on phonetic spellings to arrive at the answer.

svPPA is associated with striking atrophy of the left > right anterior temporal lobes. The ventrolateral anterior temporal lobe is widely considered to be the site of the so-called semantic "hub." However, cases of acute, unilateral anterior temporal damage, or surgical removal of the anterior temporal lobe due to focal epilepsy, are rarely associated with major semantic loss. The functional neuroanatomical mechanisms for this finding are unclear and are vigorously debated. Damage to the "spokes" cause more restricted forms of semantic loss. Parietal lobe damage, for example, can affect one's previously acquired conceptual and procedural knowledge of how objects work and how they interface with the body, leading to the inability to pantomime learned motor acts (i.e., apraxia).

Deficits in Verbal Working Memory and the Sensory Guidance of Speech

Communicating with language expressions requires individuals to "hold in mind" what they wish to say while simultaneously formulating and executing the appropriate motor expression. This online maintenance of linguistic intention (i.e., the "phonological content buffer") is critical for continuous, smooth language output. This can be examined by asking patients to repeat phrases of increasing length. It is best to uses phrases that are semantically impoverished or unpredictable (e.g., "Arthur was an oozy, oily sneak") to prevent one from accurately reconstructing the sentence word-for-word from its semantic content alone. A common type of error is an inaccurate reproduction of phrases that nevertheless communicate the original semantic gist (e.g., "It is a rainy afternoon in Boston" becomes "It is pouring rain today in Massachusetts"). Length-dependent repetition errors often suggest a deficit in verbal working memory or a problem with the linguistic computations occurring within this buffer.

The syndrome of **conduction aphasia** is characterized by poor verbal repetition accompanied by slips of the tongue (i.e., paraphasic speech errors) despite intact comprehension and fluency. The patient may be unable to maintain longer spoken phrases online. **Paraphasic errors** are usually phonologically based, including syllable or sound substitutions, deletions, insertions, or transpositions (e.g., shortstop becomes "port-stop"), which can sometimes produce neologisms or quirky spoonerisms. These disordered phonemes are produced without articulatory distortions, suggesting intact motor-speech effector functioning. Speech errors are more apt to occur on longer, novel, and phonologically complex phrases, particularly those lacking in semantic content. The **logopenic variant of PPA** is a degenerative aphasia with many overlapping features with conduction aphasia, including paraphasias during repetition and prominent word-retrieval deficits. Note that successful repetition does not require comprehension to be intact, as one can repeat words without understanding their meaning.

Verbal working memory (the so-called "phonological loop") is supported by a network that includes the posterior superior temporal cortex and left IFG.[24] Immediate "echoic" auditory working memory (lasting a few seconds) occurs in the temporal lobe, and does not require frontal systems.[25] Active, online maintenance of verbal information beyond this short timeframe, however, recruits inferior frontal systems important for motor-speech planning. This phonological loop is often conceived as a network supporting "silent rehearsal" of motor speech acts, which sustains specific phonological contents within the verbal working memory store. Damage anywhere along this phonological loop circuit can produce length-dependent repetition errors.

More recent conceptions of the regions involved in verbal repetition have begun to shed light on the computations occurring within verbal working memory stores (see Chapter 3 in this textbook; see also Hickok and Poeppel[26] and Leonard et al.[27]). Based on incoming sensory information received by the listener, primary and secondary auditory processing areas within the superolateral temporal lobes construct phonological representations of word forms (e.g., auditory/sound "images"). During repetition tasks, these auditory images are held in a phonological working memory storage buffer and serve as the "sensory target" for the motor system, whose goal it is to reproduce that sound target as accurately as possible through the appropriate sequencing and execution of motor-articulatory actions. The selection and sequencing of articulatory gestures is performed by motor-speech areas within the left inferior frontal and ventral premotor areas, and ultimately fed forward to primary motor areas located on the precentral gyrus that interface with the articulators via corticobulbar and corticospinal projections.

This process of sensory-to-motor translation, whereby auditory images represented in superior temporal areas are mapped onto appropriate motor-articulatory templates in the left inferior frontal areas, is thought to be mediated by cortical areas within the left temporoparietal junction (TPJ, adjacent to the supramarginal gyrus and superior temporal cortex). Damage to this area causes errors in verbatim repetition and paraphasic errors,[28] possibly due to incorrect mapping of phonological targets to the appropriate motor program.

Characterizing aphasia syndromes by repetition skills aids in their categorization and localization. Intact repetition implies intact functioning of the dorsal language stream, which includes phonological encoding (e.g., bilateral superior temporal), sensorimotor translation (e.g., TPJ), and motor planning and execution (e.g., left IFG). The syndrome of poor comprehension with normal fluency and repetition suggests impairment in the ventral language stream, where sensory language symbols are mapped onto semantic networks. If semantic knowledge is intact (i.e., the patient can demonstrate knowledge of concepts that do not rely on verbal information), the problem likely is one affecting the lexical-semantic interface, putatively centered within the MTG and its connections.[26,29] This syndrome is termed **transcortical sensory aphasia** and has traditionally been conceived of as a disconnection syndrome[30] caused by white matter tract disruption between Wernicke area and semantic centers, although cortical disruption alone can reproduce the syndrome.[29]

Motor Speech Deficits and Agrammatism

Expressive linguistic communication requires motoric actions that produce interpretable sensory language symbols. For speech production, this involves central motor-articulatory processes important for planning, initiating, sequencing, and executing phonetic/articulatory actions. Downstream motor effector pathways are responsible for enacting muscle movement plans involved in speech production, and include the upper motor neurons, cranial and peripheral nerves, neuromuscular junction, and muscles themselves. When these distal effector pathways are damaged, they cause **dysarthria**, which is characterized by articulation errors due to weakness, ataxia, and/or sensory loss.

Commonly reported symptoms of central motor-speech dysfunction include reduced overall verbal output with slow, effortful speech, mispronunciations, dysarthria, apraxia of speech, and stuttering, among others. Mutism can occur in severe cases. The precise pattern of symptomatology depends on the affected neurologic territory. Speech deficits are often readily detected while observing spontaneous speech, although these systems can be taxed by asking the patient to repeat complex, multisyllabic words or phrases (e.g., tongue twisters like "Methodist Episcopalian").

Successful production of fluent language output requires that an appropriately sequenced, exquisitely coordinated series of complex movements (i.e., articulatory for speech, manual for writing, gestural with signing) unfold with precise timing. Disturbances in any of these elements—sequencing, timing, coordination—or in the processes that regulate them will lead to speech errors. The neural network underlying these processes involve both cortical-subcortical areas, including primary, premotor, and supplementary motor cortices, the basal ganglia, and the cerebellum, as well as their connections with other functional networks (e.g., cognitive, sensory, limbic, etc.). Selective damage to components of these networks tends to yield distinct patterns of aphasia. Similar to language comprehension, expressive-motor deficits can be modality-specific, with speech, writing, and signing differentially affected.

Damage to the bilateral primary motor cortex or its efferent pathway, the pyramidal tract (i.e., upper motor neuron), is associated with the pure speech disorder known as **spastic dysarthria**. The speech is slow, with a strained, "tight" quality (e.g., as though the throat is being squeezed) due to increased laryngeal muscle tone, and the articulatory movements of the lips and tongue are slow but coordinated. An exaggerated jaw jerk reflex may be elicited, reflecting loss of descending motor control and inhibition of the lower cranial nerve pathways from the cortex. Occasionally there may be **pseudobulbar affect** (i.e., "emotional incontinence"), the dysregulated and uncontrolled expression of emotion that often does not reflect the patient's internal state, also presumably is due in part to loss of corticobulbar innervation of emotion-organizing centers in the brainstem. See Chapter 8 in this textbook for further discussion of pseudobulbar affect and its treatment.[31,32] Because most of the lower cranial nerve nuclei that control guttural movements receive bilateral innervation from the primary motor cortices, unilateral lesions are unlikely to cause a severe spastic dysarthria with a strained quality. Asymmetry in tongue protrusion[33] or facial muscles can occur with unilateral damage, however, which can cause a selective and often mild lingual or buccal dysarthria. The time course of onset for spastic dysarthria varies and can develop acutely due to bilateral opercular strokes (e.g., Foix-Chavany-Marie syndrome[34]), chronically in neurodegenerative disease (e.g., amyotrophic lateral sclerosis, primary lateral sclerosis, progressive supranuclear palsy), and others in between.

Damage to the motor planning areas causes **apraxia of speech**, a condition characterized by effortful speech, inconsistent articulation errors, poor initiation, unanticipated speech errors with attempts at self-correction, stopping and starting "trial and error" corrections (aka "groping" speech), and abnormal prosody, among others.[35] Apraxia of speech occurs with disruption of motor-speech planning networks: the lateral premotor areas (e.g., ventral and dorsal) are important for sequencing, and medial premotor areas (e.g., supplementary motor area) for timing and initiation. Ventral premotor areas within the posterior aspects of the left inferior frontal cortex (i.e., posterior IFG, rostral precentral gyrus, anterior insula) contain developmentally acquired sensorimotor articulatory-motor programs that encode specific movement sequences for specific syllables or words.[36] Lesions here produce articulatory distortions and other speech apraxia symptoms in cases of acute stroke[37] or the degenerative syndrome of primary progressive apraxia of speech.[38,39] Other studies place the lesion critical for the development of primary progressive apraxia of speech more superiorly in the dorsal premotor areas and supplementary motor area.[40] In severe cases, there may be a total inability to speak despite intact writing and oropharyngeal functioning, which some have labelled **aphemia**, although there is no consensus on how this term should be used.[41]

The canonical expressive aphasia that affects all expressive modalities (i.e., speaking, writing, signing) is **Broca's aphasia**, which is characterized by reduced language output (i.e., nonfluent) and poor repetition with relatively preserved comprehension and other aspects of cognition.[42,43] The reduced expressive output is not explained by weakness. This impairment is often accompanied by **agrammatism**, in which patients do not produce nor comprehend sentences that rely on syntactic structures to convey their meaning (e.g., "The lion was eaten by the tiger—which animal is alive?").[44] Speech may be "telegraphic," where only content words (e.g., nouns, verbs, adjectives) are used, and function words such as articles and prepositions are omitted (e.g., "I want a Skittle" becomes "I want Skittle"). Apraxia of speech may also be present. Many of these symptoms are most pronounced during spontaneous, propositional speech, and fluency may improve during overlearned, automatic speech tasks such as singing, counting, and reciting the days of the week. Not surprisingly, patients with Broca's aphasia often appear frustrated and exasperated while speaking. Many of their language faculties are spared, such as single-word comprehension, intention, semantic processing, and lexical retrieval. Patients may report a normal-sounding internal monologue, suggesting spared phonological encoding (i.e., sensory targets). The deficit lies in the normally effortless translation of their linguistic intent into grammatically appropriate expressions within the motor-articulatory system.

Broca's aphasia is seen with disruption of the left IFG and several of its surrounding structures. This connected set of regions is known as "Broca's complex."[45] Broadly speaking, Broca's complex is critical for shaping language ideas into hierarchically organized grammatical structures and preparing them for motor expression. Multiple functions support this process, including accessing and holding online phonological and other sensory language representations (e.g., lexical retrieval, verbal working memory), grammatical processing, and translating these structures into exquisitely timed and sequenced motor plans for overt expression (i.e., articulatory planning). The posterior inferior frontal gyrus and surrounding areas play a critical role in packaging of verbal output in accordance with appropriate word order (syntax), phrase structure, and use of grammatical morphemes (such as word endings that modify tense or number). Disruptions of these processes will lead to focal deficits.

Verbal working memory and directed lexical retrieval (e.g., word generation), for example, are supported by the left IFG and its connections with the parieto-temporal areas. Deficits in this network will produce symptoms of losing one's train of thought and difficulty generating words without bottom-up supports. Grammatical processing similarly is mediated by the left IFG and disruption leads to difficulty producing and comprehending sentences, with symptoms of telegraphic speech. Motor-articulatory planning relies on premotor systems, with ventral areas biased toward sequencing and dorsal medial areas (SMA) for timing and initiation. Deficits in these systems lead to speech apraxia, stuttering, and in severe cases, speech arrest, sometimes known as **aphemia**.[46] These functions are supported by subcortical connections, including parts of the basal ganglia, thalamus, and cerebellum. This language production network connects more broadly to cognitive, limbic, and other areas. In this light, Broca's complex is best conceived of as an integrative hub for expressive language that facilitates the flow of information across multiple language subsystems[47,48] and its interface with other broad systems (e.g., cognitive, limbic, etc.).

Damage to Broca's area "proper," a more restricted cortical location within the posterior IFG corresponding to Brodmann area 44/45, is associated with relatively mild deficits in fluency (speaking in short sentences), agrammatism, and occasionally, a **foreign accent syndrome**. The foreign accent syndrome is a motor speech disorder where one's speech changes from their normal dialect and takes on a "foreign" sound quality, often occurring after neurologic injury. The etiologies are can be divided into functional (i.e., psychogenic) and structural. Structural etiologies (strokes, tumors, TBI, multiple sclerosis, etc.) tend to occur in the frontal lobes (or other perisylvian language/motor/sensory areas; the cerebellum may also be involved), often including different aspects of Broca's complex that is important in fluency, grammar, articulatory planning (e.g., timing, sequencing), and prosody (e.g., stressed/unstressed syllables).

A Brief Note on Prosody

Language expressions contain much more than symbolic references to semantic concepts and their hierarchical relationships. Speech is infused with emotionality, social nuance, metaphor, inference, and connation. These aspects are critical for effective social communication through language, known as pragmatics. The addition of stressed and unstressed sounds, melodic contours, intonation, variation in volume, rhythm, and others to convey additional social communicative meaning is known as prosody. Diminished or inappropriate prosody is known as **aprosodia**, or **dysprosody**. Dysprosody can present as comprehension or expressive deficit. This syndrome may develop after damage to the nondominant hemisphere, often within the perisylvian areas, although this localization is controversial.

The Language System's Interaction with Intention

A different type of motor-speech disorder, **dynamic aphasia (i.e., transcortical motor aphasia)**, is characterized by a marked reduction in spontaneous propositional speech.[49] These individuals have difficulty initiating and maintaining self-generated speech, have difficulty engaging in conversation, and appear to lack the impulse to speak. They may be misdiagnosed with depression despite insisting on a normal internal mood state. Formal language testing usually reveals intact comprehension, confrontational naming, repetition (including lengthy utterances), and grammatical processing. Different clinical subtypes of the dynamic aphasia syndrome have been described, including those with language-specific deficits (e.g., verbal planning) or domain-general processes (e.g., conceptual preparation).[50] The deficit can occur as part of a mixed aphasia syndromes. The symptoms often reflect disrupted connections of language system with other cognitive (e.g., executive skills) and affective systems (e.g., motivation).

Dynamic aphasia emerges with disruption of a network involving dorsal medial prefrontal areas,[51,52] the left IFG, their subcortical connections, and their interconnected white matter tracts.[53] The dorsal medial wall of the posterior frontal cortex houses two anatomically adjacent areas, the supplementary motor area (SMA) and pre-SMA. These areas have important connections with cognitive and motor systems and play an important role in self-initiation and energization of thought and action.[54,55] SMA connections with the left IFG play a critical role in speech timing, initiation, and monitoring[56]; pre-SMA-IFG connections provide a link between intention/motivation and language expression.[53] The pre-SMA may contribute to spontaneity in verbal expression. The white matter pathway connecting dorsomedial prefrontal cortices and the IFG is known as the frontal aslant track.[57] Reduced integrity of these fibers is associated with deficits in spontaneous propositional speech[58] in individuals with the **nonfluent variant of PPA**, a dementia syndrome associated with phenotypic features similar to Broca's aphasia.

The Language System Is an Example of the Broader Concept of Praxis

The motor-articulatory system represents a specialized example of a broader skill set: the execution of complex, learned motor actions (i.e., praxis). **Apraxia** is the "inability to correctly carry out purposeful, skilled movements when this deficit is not caused by elemental motor or sensory deficits, abnormal involuntary movements, or cognitive disorders."[59] Skilled motor performance requires knowledge about how self-generated actions impact the body and the environment, which is learned

iteratively through repeated actions, error detection, and feedback. Through experience, specific actions become associated with predictable sensory consequences, forming stored sensory-motor representations. Selection and activation of these sensorimotor programs in appropriate context supports the unfolding of complex, learned, purposeful actions. Examples include swinging a baseball bat, hammering a nail, playing the guitar, and others. These sensorimotor associations are stored as connected networks between posterior parietal and premotor cortices, often supported by subcortical network connections, with posterior areas encoding sensory-perceptual representations and frontal areas specific motor programs. These programs are subject to bottom-up, more "automatic" activation and top-down, "goal-directed" activation.[60] Apraxia occurs when these sensorimotor programs are damaged or are not accessed properly.

Acquiring these complex, specific sensorimotor representations requires a more immediate mechanism for perception-acting coupling. The so-called "mirror neuron" system matches combinations of perceptual inputs with the specific frontal motor systems most likely to accurately reproduce those inputs[61]; these relationships may be formed by experience during developmental sensorimotor learning.[62] Examples of this sensory-to-motor integration include verbal speech perception connecting with motor articulatory areas to guide speech mimicry, or visual perception of another's limb movements connecting to motor limb-kinesthetic areas to support action mimicry, or seeing a picture and drawing it. Enacting these perceptually driven action representations leads to overt sensory consequences (e.g., visual, proprioceptive, somatosensory, etc.) that are fed back into the action-perception model, setting the iterative learning process into motion.

Activation of these sensorimotor pathways is subject to top-down and bottom-up regulation. Loss of top-down regulation of these systems can produce disinhibition of the mirror neuron system,[63] leading to **echophenomena,** including the automatic mimicry of sounds, known as **echolalia**, or movement, **echopraxia**. Loss of bottom-up activation may lead to reduced mimicry and reduced imitative learning, as is seen in individuals with autism.[64]

The neural correlates of certain types of apraxia mirror those of aphasia. In both cases, perceptual inputs facilitate the selection and execution of specialized motor sequences, although in one the target is primarily auditory (i.e., spoken language), and in the other is visual-kinesthetic (i.e., limb movement). In limb praxis, three-dimensional visual-kinesthetic sensory targets are learned and stored as sensory programs and are used to guide the selection of actions to be planned and executed by the frontal lobe. These stored sensory targets, known as engrams, are stored in parieto-temporal regions and are connected to modality-specific (e.g., limb, oro-buccal) premotor areas in the frontal lobes involved in motor planning. An individual's learned set of engrams is known as the "praxicon" (similar to "lexicon" in the language system). These parieto-frontal connections support the appropriate selection of specific motor programs that enact the visual-kinesthetic engram. This parieto-premotor learned action sensorimotor network is also connected with medial prefrontal areas (e.g., SMA) important for initiation and timing of the

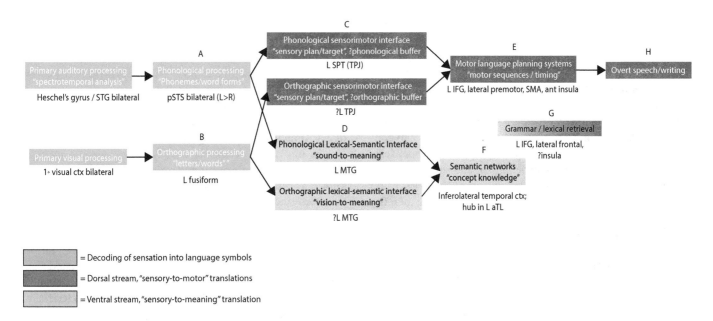

FIGURE 12-3. Summary of cortical language processing.

Expected Speech/Language Syndromes

A—Pure word deafness with phonological paraphasias; spared oral reading and reading comprehension

B—Pure alexia, malformed letters/words (?orthographic paraphasia); spared verbal comprehension

C—Repetition errors (length-dependent), phonological paraphasias (worse on long/complex words), naming errors, neologisms; intact comprehension of single words

D—Poor word deafness (i.e., verbal comprehension deficit) without phonological paraphasias; intact repetition and semantic concepts

E—Apraxia of speech (variable misarticulations, groping speech, stuttering; ?also writing), poor initiation/spontaneity, agrammatism, aphemia (when only affecting speech programs), pure agraphia (when only affecting writing programs)

F—Semantic loss, surface dyslexia

G—Agrammatism, telegraphic speech, loss of functor words

H—Dysarthria (type depends on lesion location)

—

A−D = "Wernicke"; E+G = "Broca"; C = "conduction"

? = putative role or anatomical location

movements. Dr. Kenneth Heilman has offered an apt metaphor of playing the piano: the parietal cortex contains the sheet music that provides the sensory codes, the frontal cortex represents the piano player that executes the content of the sheet music, and the primary motor effectors represent the piano itself (Dr. Kenneth Heilman, 2017, Harvard-Longwood Grand Rounds). Damage to the engram-containing regions in the parietal lobe leads to **ideomotor apraxia**, whereby individuals have difficulty knowing how to posture their limbs when executing a previously learned action generating the sensory images of the action they have previously learned.[59] **Limb-kinetic apraxia**, whereby the precise sequencing and timing of limb actions is poor, occurs with damage to frontal structures.[59] Other types of apraxias are described, including ideational, constructional, and others.

This entire process is strikingly similar to the sensory guidance of speech. Given the overlapping peripheral anatomy required for speech articulation and other oro-buccal actions (like sniffing a flower or blowing a kiss), and the somatotopic cortical representations of these areas within the primary and premotor cortex, it is not surprising that lesions within the inferior frontal areas that cause expressive aphasia also tend to cause oro-buccal, and sometimes limb-kinetic, apraxia. In these frontal lesions, the more posteriorly located sensory targets (e.g.,

engrams) are spared, and accordingly, patients are usually able to identify the correct learned motor movement, even if they are unable to execute them properly.[59]

Figure 12-3 provides a schematic summary of cortical language processing and the clinical syndromes that may result from disruption of its different components.

CHARACTERIZING DEFICITS AFFECTING EPISODIC MEMORY

One of the most common presenting symptoms in clinical settings is "memory loss." When this is the chief complaint, one must keep an open mind about the potential cognitive systems involved, as patients and families often use the term "memory" colloquially when referring to other aspects of cognition, including lexical retrieval, visuospatial dysfunction, apraxia/agnosia, and attention problems, among others. Even when formal "memory" testing is abnormal (e.g., the ability to recall a recently learned word list), the differential diagnosis includes both executive/attentional and memory processes, each of which is supported by distinct functional neuroanatomy and has its own list of potential etiologies. The precise characterization of memory deficits can determine its underlying localization and uncover consequential diagnostic, prognostic, and sometimes therapeutic information.

Memory is a broad term describing many different cognitive processes that share the property of retaining or recreating information to which the person was previously exposed. The ability to store aspects of experience allows one to adapt to a changing environment. This broad concept encompasses both explicit/declarative processes that are directly accessible to consciousness, such as episodic and autobiographical memory (e.g., replaying the content of prior experiences) and semantic memory (e.g., factual and conceptual knowledge of the world), and implicit/non-declarative process such as procedural memory (i.e., the execution of learned, complex motor actions; "tying shoes"), associative learning through operant conditioning (i.e., emotional reactions such as fear with exposure a triggering stimulus), or the effects of priming (e.g., recent exposure to a stimulus influences the response to a subsequent, related stimulus, a process not dependent on conscious intention or guidance). Brain dysfunction can impact all of these processes, although the circuits underlying each vary.

Memory may be broadly conceived of as a modulator of neural predictions, by which prior inputs exert influence over how ongoing inputs are processed, including perception.[65] Memory stores are strengthened by the salience of the inputs and their behavioral consequences.

Mechanistically, the neurotransmitter dopamine is an important modulator of neuroplasticity and learning. Its presence within synapses facilitates long-term potentiation (LTP), an important cellular mechanism for stabilizing and strengthening specific neuron-to-neuron connections.[66] Many of the brain's dopamine-releasing neurons originate in the ventral tegmental area (VTA) of the midbrain, an area activated by different types of detected environmental salience.[67] Widespread areas of the brain receive dopaminergic projections, including the prefrontal cortex, the hippocampus, and striatum. The salience-triggered release of dopamine may help to guide the brain to store inputs that are most behaviorally relevant. The neuroanatomical location of the dopamine release may support different types of memory, including the motor striatum for procedural motor learning, the ventral striatum and amygdala for emotional learning (e.g., desire/anticipation, fear), and the hippocampus for episodic memory.[68] Non-dopamine neurotransmitter systems also impact memory storage mechanisms, including acetylcholine, norepinephrine, and others.

Episodic Memory

Episodic memory refers to information acquired at a specific time, place, and circumstance (e.g., what one had for lunch yesterday), and includes the sensory, motor, cognitive, emotional aspects of experience. Some examples include remembering and reliving the memory of watching the Red Sox win the 2004 World Series, what was ordered for lunch at the hospital cafeteria yesterday, or the details of a recent conversation with my mother.

Patients with episodic memory deficits—commonly referred to as **amnesia**—have difficulty recalling information about prior experiences, or even that particular events occurred at all. In severe instances, such as reported in the famous case of H.M.,[69]

patients are completely unable to consciously recall information obtained even a few minutes earlier. When repeatedly exposed to similar circumstances, patients behave as though the experience is novel, reacting to others with surprise and treating the situation as unfamiliar. The ability to update longitudinal self-schemas and personal narratives is disrupted, as is the passage of time, yielding the phenotype of being "stuck" in a particular time period and way of relating to the world. Personal insight into these deficits is usually poor. Episodic memory may be lost for events occurring *prior* to a single point in time, known as **retrograde amnesia**, and/or *after* a point in time, as in **anterograde amnesia**.

Complete, permanent episodic memory loss is relatively rare, but can occur in conditions that cause damage to the temporal lobes bilaterally, such as limbic encephalitis (e.g., herpes simplex virus, autoimmune conditions, many others) and traumatic brain injury. **Transient global amnesia**, a fascinating and somewhat enigmatic clinical syndrome, is characterized by acute-onset complete episodic memory loss that usually resolves within several hours. The pathophysiologic mechanisms underlying the disorder are debated, but MRI often demonstrates transient signal abnormalities within hippocampus[70] or perihippocampal structures.

Symptoms of partial amnesia are common but may be subtle, often manifesting repetitive behaviors such as retelling stories and asking the same questions, forgetting details of prior conversations or story plots, misplacing items, increased reliance on lists to keep track of information, among others. **Prospective memory**, the ability to remember the timing and nature of future engagements, may also be affected.[71] Time sense can be altered, including when an event took place, how long it lasted, the sequential order of happenings, or its temporal sequence in relation to other events. Place information is often affected, including where an event took place, or what the scene looked like. The ability to remember when and where information was obtained is known as **source memory**.[72] Insight into one's own amnestic symptoms may be preserved in mild cases.

There are several ways to quantitatively test episodic memory function and learning. Tasks that rely on short-term processes (e.g., minutes) can be administered in a single office visit, allowing for a rapid assessment of these functions. Most learning protocols follow a similar series of steps: (1) exposure to new information/stimuli, (2) immediate confirmation that the information was absorbed (i.e., encoding), (3) distraction and the passage of time, (4) testing spontaneous recollection of the presented information (e.g., retrieval), and (5) assessing recognition of the information when provided clues/hints (e.g., storage). The stimuli that are used vary across tasks and may include word lists, stories, pictures/figures, word and shape associations, or the physical locations of objects hidden in a room.

Episodic memory is often conceptualized as a three-stage process: (1) encoding, (2) storage, and (3) retrieval. The 5-step bedside memory testing protocol described above allows one to isolate—at least operationally—the processing stages supporting memory formation (see Figure 12-4). The neuroscientific accounts of the stages supporting memory formation are more nuanced, detailed, and complex than what is discussed below.

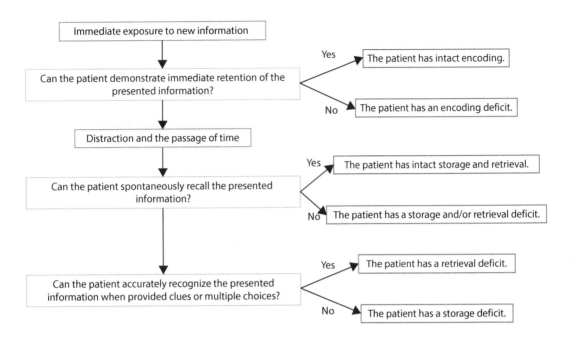

FIGURE 12-4. Schematized 5-step protocol to test memory functions. Schematized 5-step protocol to operationally isolate the memory stages of encoding, storage, and retrieval. The conclusions drawn assume that other cognitive functions known to affect memory performance (e.g., language comprehension to understand the instructions, sustained attention, effort, etc.) are controlled or otherwise accounted for.

The discussion provides a starting point for more comprehensive assessment.

An individual with difficulty demonstrating immediate retention of recently presented information is said to have deficits in encoding. If, after a period of distraction, they are unable to spontaneously recall the previously presented information, they have either a deficit in storage or retrieval. If the individual can recall the information with cues or recognize the information when presented multiple choices, the deficit is considered one of retrieval. If the individual does not improve with cues or choices, the deficit is one of storage. While this oversimplifies a complex process, it nevertheless provides a conceptual schema to frame memory processing.

Encoding is the process whereby experiential information (e.g., sensory, cognitive, emotional, etc.) is engaged by attentional and working memory systems and prepared for short-term storage. Patients unable to demonstrate their retention of newly presented information moments after the instruction is provided (and comprehended) are said to have encoding deficits. This may occur with dysfunction in attentional and working memory systems and their connections with mesial temporal and hippocampal areas. Experiential information (i.e., a multisensory perceptual traces) needs to be perceived and transformed into a format that can be stored, accessed, and re-instantiated later. This process depends on perception and attentional processing mediated by fronto-parieto-subcortical areas[73] and the memory areas subserving data preparation for storage in the mesial temporal/hippocampal areas.[74-77]

Storage deficits prevent the formation and retention of new episodic memories. Providing contextual cues does not readily facilitate the recall of information, which is unlike retrieval deficits. Storage deficits result from damage to the hippocampus, its local inputs (e.g., parahippocampal gyrus), or its connections along a larger limbic network (i.e., the Papez circuit—see Figure 3-8, Chapter 3) including the cingulate cortex, fornix, mammillary bodies, subiculum, and anterior thalamus.[78] These temporolimbic structures index experiences for later recollection and support encoding and storage. Streams of highly integrated information from sensory, cognitive, affective, and other systems—the online contents of experience—are filtered, stored, and indexed by these structures, including their occurrence at a particular time and place. Content to be remembered is selected based on its degree of salience. People tend to remember important life experiences in rich detail such as their wedding day, the birth of their children, the death of loved ones, personal traumatic experiences, or major cultural events. **Flashbulb memory** is a term used to describe the detailed memory of where a person was and what he was doing when he learned about a major event,[79] such as the 9/11 attacks, JFK's assassination, or the OJ Simpson verdict.

Recalling these stored streams of highly integrated information lets one replay and reexperience them by recapitulating their expression within perceptual areas, and their spatiotemporal markings allow one to order past events in the proper sequence at the appropriate locations.[80] Minor deficits in the storage system may limit the vividness of the recollection or cause uncertainty about when and where an episode occurred; major deficits cause a complete absence of recall. **Wernicke-Korsakoff syndrome**, characterized by profound amnesia with confabulation and poor insight, is associated with injury to parts of the temporolimbic system (e.g., mammillary bodies, anterior thalamus), and is caused by thiamine deficiency, often in people with alcohol dependence[81] or prior bariatric surgery.[82] Patients with Wernicke-Korsakoff syndrome may unintentionally produce false statements or engage in false behaviors that are reflective of inaccurate memory or belief, a symptom known as **confabulation**.

Episodic memory loss due to temporolimbic dysfunction tends to spare memory for remote events that occurred months and years ago. Remote memories often take on the character of semantic memory, becoming grounded more by their factual content and less by their experiential vividness. These remote events become stored as semantic knowledge in cortical networks outside the hippocampus. This observation was made famous in the case of H.M., who was able to recall autobiographical events from his early childhood despite a total loss of more recent events. A similar dissociation with sparing of memory for remote events occurs in the early stages of typical **Alzheimer's disease**, a degenerative condition affecting mesial temporal structures and associated with short-term episodic memory storage loss.

Access to episodic memory stores can occur via top-down, goal-directed directed retrieval (e.g., during formal memory testing) or through bottom-up, stimulus-driven mechanisms triggered by ongoing perceptual experiences (e.g., hearing a song on the radio triggers the memory of one's first kiss).[83] Goal-directed, top-down retrieval of recently presented information is supported by fronto-parietal-subcortical structures and their connections with mesial temporal memory areas.[83,84] Deficiencies in these active retrieval processes can be overcome with cues and multiple choices, which provide a robust bottom-up stimulus as alternative pathway to activate the prior memory stream. If the patient cannot give the correct answer in this aided setting, despite having successfully encoded the information earlier, the problem is believed to reflect deficient storage mechanisms.

The consequences of poor retrieval are significant. Memory traces inaccessible by top-down processes cannot be used to guide explicit, goal-directed behaviors, and leads to ill-informed decision making. Retrieval is essential for everyday functions such as remembering internet passwords, the car's location in the parking lot, or the events that occurred at a meeting. As part of the default mode internet linking motivationally relevant, internally generated, top-down processing areas in the medial prefrontal cortex with the mesial temporal episodic memory areas,[85] this retrieval system allows us to reexperience past events flexibly and on demand (see Chapter 3 of this volume).

CASE VIGNETTE 12.1

Mr. L is a 73-year-old right-handed man with past medical history of hypertension, hyperlipidemia, and sleep apnea, who initially presented with 2—3 years of progressive word-finding difficulties. His difficulty finding words is associated with circumlocutions, word substitutions, paraphasic errors, vague speech, and mild comprehension difficulties in which he asks others to clarify their utterances immediately after they speak. Other, non-language symptoms include reduced concentration and mild memory deficits. He is functionally independent.

His elemental neurologic examination is notable for mild paratonia and awkward rapid alternating movements on the right side. Neuropsychological testing demonstrates multidomain cognitive impairment, including language, executive functions, and verbal memory. His language deficits include poor confrontational naming, reduced generative fluency (semantic > phonemic), length-dependent repetition errors, and phonological paraphasias. His auditory verbal memory is much worse than his visual verbal memory, and was impaired at all levels (encoding, storage, and retrieval). His brain MRI reveals global atrophy, left more than right, with disproportionate involvement of the temporal, parietal, and dorsal parieto-frontal areas. There is a mild burden of microvascular disease as evidence by FLAIR hyperintensities. Cerebrospinal fluid analysis shows no clear evidence of inflammation. He has reduced beta-amyloid and elevated total and phosphorylated tau levels.

Mr. L has a mild neurocognitive disorder, and his symptoms localize best to dysfunction within the phonological loop (left posterior superior temporal sulcus, temporoparietal junction, left inferior frontal gyrus, arcuate fasciculus) and, to a lesser extent, dorsal frontoparietal attentional and executive control networks, and temporolimbic memory storage areas. His clinical diagnosis is mild cognitive impairment with logopenic language features. The most likely underlying etiology is neuropathological Alzheimer's disease.

CHARACTERIZING DEFICITS AFFECTING ATTENTION

The particular thoughts, feelings, or sensations that illuminate one's momentary subjective experience seem to reflect the internal gaze of one's attention. The seemingly limitless possibilities of conscious experience momentarily collapse into rather constrained chunks of subjectivity. The processes that engage, disengage, filter, select, switch, inhibit, and maintain the elements of experience comprise the mechanisms of attention.[86]

The brain's perceptual neural machinery is frequently repurposed in the name of efficiency. The same areas that represent incoming sensory information as perceptions of external reality (e.g., the tree in front of me *right now*) are also used to imagine past perceptual experiences (e.g., the tree I walked past *last week*) or to mentally simulate (i.e., "embody") semantic concepts (e.g., the concept of a tree). The mode of engagement may shift based on the behavioral context and the priorities of the individual. Detected environmental salience may redirect resources toward specific sources of incoming sensory information; a quiescent environment may shift toward internally generated stimulations for learning or preparation; other times, it is useful to explore the external environment for potential resources or threats. Flexible shifting between modes of attentional engagement optimizes the brain's limited resources.

Modes of Attention: Stimulus-Driven ("Bottom-Up"), Goal-Directed ("Top-Down"), and Stimulus-Independent ("Default Mode")

The detection of salient stimuli in the environment causes a rapid reallocation of attentional resources directed toward the stimulus. This "bottom-up," involuntarily, stimulus-driven system alerts and reorients perceptual systems to help assess the relevance, value, or meaning of a stimulus or event. If one is reading a book, for example, and is suddenly bit by a mosquito on the arm, attention may immediately shift from the story plot to the arm and an accompanying interest in the precise location of the bite, the identification of the bug, and a seemingly involuntarily quick slap. According to some models of attention, this rapid reallocation of neural resources is correlated with activity in a cortical network known as the ventral attention network (VAN), which includes ventral frontal and parietal regions, namely the IFG and the TPJ, and tends to be lateralized to the right hemisphere (see Figure 3-2B, Chapter 3).[87] The VAN is strongly connected with cortical and subcortical areas important for decoding salience from incoming sensory inputs. Activity in the VAN may encode subjective awareness of attentional shifts and/or provide signals that alter activity in other attentional networks. When a salient, bottom-up signal activates the VAN, attentional resources are shifted toward the incoming stimulus.

Attention may also be directed by top-down, goal-directed processes. Consider the example of looking for a lost set of keys. When searching, one maintains the goal of finding the keys while directing attention and eye movements to various spatial locations within the space, biasing each upcoming location to recognize the visual pattern suggestive of keys. Directed spatial exploration, where attention is directed to information at specific locations, is supported by activity in the dorsal attention network (DAN), with hubs located in the dorsal and lateral parts of the parietal (e.g., the intraparietal sulcus, IPS) and the frontal (e.g., frontal eye fields, FEF) lobes bilaterally.[87] Some investigators also include parts of the MTG in the DAN. Both the IPS and FEF contain egocentric (i.e., self at the center) spatial maps of the external environment.[88] The DAN supports shifts in spatial attention involved in the visual exploration of the environment and generating expectations about incoming information for a particular location.[89]

When unexpected or potentially relevant behavioral information is detected outside the DAN-prioritized spatial locations, the right TPJ becomes active as part of the VAN. TPJ activation marks the occurrence of bottom-up, stimulus-driven changes in attention, and supports an orienting response; right TPJ strokes impair the spatial orienting.[90] The VAN may be important for switching between other large-scale networks (e.g., default mode, central executive) when unanticipated salient changes are detected,[91] although this may also be supported directly by the broader salience network (see Chapter 3). Violations in the expected sensory consequences of actions, uncued changes in context, and the perceived beginnings and ends of behavioral events[92] are known to activate the right TPJ, all of which may provide an impetus to initiate changes in top-down attention and goal-directed behaviors.

The DAN and VAN have important interactions and they share a hub in the right middle frontal gyrus. The set-point for VAN-associated attentional shifts can be downregulated by tasks requiring a high degree of top-down attention. Professional basketball players shooting free throws, for example, are able to suppress opposing fans attempts at distraction (e.g., fans yelling their name and waving signs behind the hoop), likely reflecting suppression of the VAN. VAN activity also temporarily changes activity in the DAN.

During periods of environmental quiescence, attention can be directed away from immediate external environmental salience and toward internally generated mental states. Processes such as mental simulation and rehearsal, imagination, episodic memory recall, self-talk, and others may help prepare one for future situations, learn through analyzing prior experiences, and develop mental models to understand the world. These processes may be goal-directed or triggered by spontaneously generated internal stimuli. These internal triggers may be salient to the individual. This attentional state is supported by the so-called "default mode" network (DMN), with anatomical hubs in the medial and lateral parietal, medial prefrontal, and middle temporal cortices (see Figure 3-4 in Chapter 3).[93] The DAN and its companion, the central executive network, may coactivate with the DMN to support purposeful recollection or directed mental simulation.

Focal behavioral symptoms occur when these networks are damaged or dysregulated. Disruption of the DAN is associated with reduced top-down, goal-directed processing, and produces symptoms distractibility, loss of intention, and excessive environmental reactivity. Disruption of the VAN leads to reduced adaptability to salient changes in one's situation.

Hemispatial Neglect

Dysfunction of the DAN and VAN has important clinical consequences. **Hemispatial neglect** is characterized by a lack of awareness and inability to attend to egocentric space to the left or right of the vertical meridian. This occurs with acute damage to the nondominant (usually right-sided) hemisphere, often involving the parietal lobes, but also frontal or subcortical areas. When severe, neglect symptoms extend beyond the visual sensory modality, impacting somatosensory and auditory processing, motor intentions, and cognition, including exploratory behaviors and mental simulations. Broadly speaking, these patients lose awareness of the existence of a world beyond the left side of their egocentric vertical meridian. They may not eat food on the left side of their plate, not move their right hand beyond midline when asked to reach for their hemiparetic left hand, and be unable to generate a mental map of the United States west of Chicago. They may not acknowledge hemiparesis affecting the left side of their body (i.e., **anosognosia**), deny ownership of their own left-sided body parts (i.e., **asomatognosia**), or harbor the delusion that the left side of their body must be someone else's (i.e., **somatoparaphrenia**).

Hemispatial neglect may also be subtle, and when incomplete, may only become apparent with the introduction of competing stimuli on the non-neglected side, typically the right. This can be tested by providing double simultaneous stimulation on both sides of the patient's hemispace. If patients perceive the stimuli when tested individually on each side, but report only right-sided events with simultaneous stimulation, they are said to have extinction, a sign of unilateral neglect. Other methods include asking patients to copy figures or draw a clock, bisect a horizontal line, cross out with a pen all instances of a symbol (such as a line) on a page, or describe a map of their state or county. When severe, hemispatial neglect can be easily mistaken for a hemianopia (i.e., unilateral visual field deficit, most often due to primary visual cortex damage) and may be indistinguishable at the bedside.

Neglect associated with damage to the right parietal areas often affects both DAN and VAN machinery, although the TPJ and its white matter connections with the frontal lobes may be most critical.[94] This typically occurs with right-sided lesions and not with damage to the left. This supports the notion that the right hemisphere is important for bilateral spatial attention and the left hemisphere only for right-sided attention; damage to the right hemisphere, it follows, results in an unopposed attentional bias toward the right side of the egocentric world by the left parietal lobe.

CHARACTERIZING DEFICITS AFFECTING EXECUTIVE FUNCTIONING

Executive functioning is critical to organizing and sustaining goal-directed behaviors. These skills facilitate appropriate decision making in response to changing environmental demands. The ability to select and shift the contents of one's top-down attention (i.e., attention control) and ignore others (i.e., inhibitory control), to set and sustain behavior goals/targets, provide a cognitive platform for planning and manipulating complex mental actions (i.e., working memory), select among competing actions (i.e., conflict resolution), and monitor their outcome are some of the important operations of executive functioning.

Patients with executive dysfunction present in myriad ways, and the condition is often labeled simply as the **dysexecutive syndrome**. Symptoms of losing one's train of thought or purpose for engaging in a task may reflect poor working memory; difficulty with planning or staying organized may suggest reduced cognitive flexibility; distractibility, impulsivity, and difficulty finishing tasks may reflect poor vigilance or inhibitory control; errors in judgement or reduced insight may suggest poor conflict and internal monitoring, respectively.

The executive functions, like other aspects of the cognitive state examination, are hierarchical; it is important to test working memory early as impairments in this capacity may markedly impact the performance of other skills. Simple tests of working memory include a digit or spatial span. Processing speed can be assessed with a Stroop color naming task or Trail Making Test Part A (TMT-A). Cognitive flexibility and task switching can be examined with the Trail Making Test Part B (TMT-B) or the Wisconsin Card Sorting Testing. Response inhibition can be assessed with anti-saccades, Stroop color-word interference task, or a go/no-go task. Generative fluency may be used to assess energization and initiation. Please see Chapter 5 (Neuropsychiatric Assessment) and Chapter 7 (Neuropsychological Evaluation in Neuropsychiatry) for further discussion about testing of executive functions.

Executive functioning has traditionally been considered to be primarily supported by the prefrontal cortex, although more recent conceptions extend the neural regions involved to include the parietal cortex and subcortical network encompassing the basal ganglia, thalamus, and cerebellum. The "central executive network" (CEN) includes regions of the prefrontal cortex, including the dorsolateral prefrontal cortex (DLPFC), frontopolar cortex, orbitofrontal cortex, dorsal anterior cingulate cortex (ACC), as well as the superior and inferior parietal, temporal, and subcortical areas.[95] Damage anywhere along this network can impair functions associated with executive control.

A complete discussion of the particular contributions from each node of the network, or of each of the executive skills individually, is beyond the scope of the chapter. A few examples of executive functions are highlighted below.

Working Memory

Working memory is what allows us to hold a thought, an image, or sound—or any conscious perception—in the mind actively and continuously. It permits one to hear a phone number and keep it "online" for a few moments before dialing it, or to retain the image of one's surrounding visual environment immediately after closing the eyes. This active maintenance process has a limited storage capacity; for example, most individuals cannot immediately recall word-for-word the script of a 2-minute television ad after watching it once, or the step-for-step choreography of a dance performance. Some suggest working memory capacity to be limited to four bits of information; others suggest seven plus or minus two. How the basic perceptual content is "chunked" and held online is critical for how they are utilized by the brain for other purposes. Working memory is an essential building block for so-called "higher-order" cognitive skills, including many aspects of executive functioning important for analytical reasoning and multistep processing (see below), real-life aspects of language such as engaging in conversation and reading, and long-term memory storage, among other skills. It is thus critical for goal-directed behavior, including the skill of maintaining a goal online.

Other conceptions of working memory extend its meaning to include both the temporary storage capacity and a superimposed central executive component. Information held online is transformed through cognitive operations, and this entire process is termed working memory. This conception of working memory can be tested using tasks that require maintenance and manipulation, such as spelling words backwards or performing serial calculations.

Working memory deficits manifest symptomatically as difficulty retaining information immediately after it is presented,[96] and occur when the systems important for holding information online are dysfunctional. With disruption of auditory or verbal working memory systems (i.e., the "phonological loop"), patients cannot hold verbal information in mind, and may report that they forget what they had planned to say, that information "goes in one ear and out the other," or that they have difficulty comprehending long phrases. They may need to write things down to recall the information later. When the deficits affect visuospatial information (i.e., the "visual sketchpad"), patients cannot actively maintain recently presented visual information online. Working memory deficits associated with impairments of executive control may present as difficulty managing complex multistep tasks, deficits in problem solving, and difficulty with mental math.

The neurological systems that underlie working memory systems are discussed elsewhere in this textbook (see Chapter 3). In general, working memory requires the online maintenance of neural representations, which include both a mental "image" to be sustained (e.g., a recently presented sound, image, touch, etc.) and a mechanism for sustaining it. The mental images are sensory representations supported by visual, auditory, somatosensory, and multimodal cortices within the parietal, temporal, and occipital cortices. Active maintenance of these sensory images and its resistance to interference is subserved by dorsolateral prefrontal areas. Any pathological process affecting these fronto-parietal-subcortical networks can cause the syndrome of working memory impairment.

Working memory capacity can be tested by asking patients to hold increasingly lengthy bits of information. For auditory systems, a forward digit span or repetition of sentences are easily quantifiable methods. The visual systems can be probed using a "spatial span" test where the examiner points to different spatial locations sequentially and the patient is asked to repeat the same sequence. The number of locations to sequence becomes larger with each successive trial.

Sustained Attention and Impulsivity

The reduced ability to voluntarily sustain one's attention on a goal-directed task is referred to as **poor vigilance**. Common symptoms include difficulty concentrating and maintaining focus, distractibility, not completing tasks, and excessive mind-wandering. Vigilance testing employs tasks that require prolonged engagement without taxing other higher-order executive functions, to isolate the skill of interest. A prolonged "go/no-go" test, such as Connor's Continuous Performance Task, in which the patient responds to a target stimulus and withholds a response to foils, is a standard approach. A bedside testing example includes counting backwards from 100 to 0 by threes. The functional neuroanatomy of vigilance is complex[97] and likely represent the dynamic interplay between top-down and bottom-up attentional control systems.[98] Vigilance deficits can emerge with dysfunction of frontal and/or parietal areas that often involve the right hemisphere and/or ascending neurotransmitter systems (e.g., acetylcholine, norepinephrine, others). These systems are often disrupted in states of toxic-metabolic encephalopathy or delirium.

Response Inhibition

The ability to inhibit one's prepotent, automatic responses to stimuli is an important aspect of executive functioning. This braking function affords the opportunity to consider the consequences of impending actions and decisions. **Reduced inhibitory control** is a common symptom in attention-deficit hyperactivity disorder, which may be associated with impulsivity (e.g., blurting, talking out of turn, impatience, overeating, risky behavior) and hyperactivity (e.g., fidgety, "can't sit still"). The mechanisms underlying these symptoms are complex and generally felt to result from dysfunction within cortical-subcortical network involving the orbitofrontal cortex, right lateral inferior frontal cortex, striatum, and thalamus.

The **environmental dependency syndrome** is a behavioral syndrome characterized by excessive utilization and interaction with the contents of one's immediate environment.[99] This can manifest with **echophenomenon**, the tendency to involuntarily mimic observed behaviors, including speech ("echolalia"), gesture ("echopraxia"), and facial expressions ("echomimia"). The neural underpinnings are likely complex and potentially multifactorial; they can develop in states of reduced inhibitory control or reduced self-monitoring as can occur with disruption of bilateral frontal circuitry in conditions such as degenerative disease, catatonia, Tourette syndrome, and others.

Other Executive Functions

The DLPFC may also may be involved in holding evaluative "rules" or goals on-line,[100] and selecting among potential competing behavioral responses. Deficits in inductive, rule-based cognition can occur with DLPFC damage.[101]

The dorsal ACC contributes to cognitive control by detecting conflict. This can be examined at the bedside with a Stroop interference task, where individuals are presented written words of colors that are printed in different ink colors and asked to name the ink color instead of reading the word. The ACC receives widespread input from multiple networks, including the salience network, DMN, and others. The ACC's detection of conflict applies to a wide range of representations, including between competing motor programs, the outcome versus the expectations of actions, or even between a task-demand and one's sense of capacity to carry it out.

CHARACTERIZING DEFICITS AFFECTING VISUOSPATIAL FUNCTIONS

The cortical visual system is anchored by the occipital cortex, with primary visual areas surrounding the calcarine fissure at the occipital pole, and higher-order aspects of visual processing (e.g., color, depth, motion, object/pattern representations, etc.) supported by adjacent sites within the occipital, parietal, and temporal areas. The visual system is broadly conceptualized as being composed of two "streams" of information processing (see Chapter 3). The ventral "what" pathway, which includes the fusiform gyrus inferiorly and the occipito-temporal cortices laterally, is important for representing and identifying visual patterns important for object recognition, face recognition, reading of text, and other functions. It serves as the visual system's most direct pathway to semantic networks. The dorsal "how" (or "where") pathway, located within the superior occipital, lateral parietal, and lateral frontal cortices, uses visual information to create spatial representations that guide attentional resources and motor actions. The ventral and dorsal pathways are connected at various points along their streams, which may allow for the integration of different representations. Similar to other sensory systems, as visual information moves away from the primary visual cortex through the stream, information becomes more highly processed and is integrated with information from areas outside the visual system.

Visuospatial deficits can produce a large variety of symptoms—ranging from cortical blindness to writing deficits to clumsiness when reaching—depending on which aspect of the visual system is affected.

Not being able to see represents the most basic, and profound complaint about visual processing. Blindness can occur with lesions anywhere within the afferent visual system, including the eye and its related structures (e.g., cornea, lens, vitreous, retina), optic nerve, thalamus, subcortical white matter (e.g., "optic radiations"), and primary visual cortex. When there is concern for blindness, a clinical evaluation for lesions in these precortical areas is required, including a detailed ophthalmologic examination (e.g., visualization of the retina, optic disc, and other ocular structures) and a detailed elemental neurologic examination that specifically measures acuity, confrontational visual fields, pupillary responses, and extraocular movements. For a discussion of **cortical blindness** and **blindsight**, please see the section on sensory perception.

Some patients who experience sudden bilateral occipital lobe dysfunction will present with what is easily mistaken for an acute confusional episode. Patients may have difficulty navigating and may walk into walls or closed doors, or they may make references to seeing objects in front of them that are not actually there. The examination, however, is not suggestive of global encephalopathy (e.g., reduced arousal or hyperarousal, poor attention) or receptive aphasia (e.g., inability to follow verbal commands), but unexpectedly reveals cortical blindness. This condition goes by the eponym **Anton-Babinski syndrome**, and is characterized by cortical blindness accompanied by a lack of awareness of visual deficits (e.g., anosognosia), confabulations of visual content, and the delusional belief of intact vision despite contrary evidence.

The Dorsal Visual Stream: The Visual System's Contribution to Spatial Aspects of Cognition and Action

The dorsal stream of the visual system—the superolateral extension of the visual system into the parietal and frontal lobes—is fundamentally responsible for representing the world as a three-dimensional, extrapersonal space with the self existing at the center. The dorsal stream is where the brain computes representations of depth and distance, left and right, and relational concepts such as "in front of," "behind," "above," and "below." These spatial representations are utilized by other systems to guide movements, direct attention, and enrich or support aspects of cognition.

The elemental aspects of dorsal stream processing—depth, orientation, spatial relationships, locations—can be examined at the bedside. A basic screening test for these functions is to copy or mimic visually presented information with limited semantic content, a skill referred to as **constructional praxis**. Successful performance implies intact perceptual and constructive functions, which are supported by posterior aspects of the dorsal stream (e.g., perception) and their connections with frontal-premotor cortices, important for motor planning (e.g., construction).[102] The Rey-Osterrieth Complex Figure Test requires individuals to copy as accurately as possible a complex, multifeatured line drawing[103]; many other figures exist, including intersecting pentagons and a Benson figure.[102] See Chapters 5 and 7 for further discussion of testing of visual function. Mimicry of complex bimanual hand shapes (e.g., interlocking "A-OK" signs) can also be used.[104] Other tests of dorsal stream functions include the number location subtest of the Visual Object Spatial Perception (VOSP) battery, where one is asked to determine which number in an upper square corresponds to the same location of a dot in a lower square, the Judgement of Line Orientation test, and the Hooper Visual Organization Test. Of note, poor performance on these tests can result from non-visuospatial processes, including attention/concentration, planning/organization, and motor skills.

The ability of sensory systems to guide action selection is a recurring theme in behavioral neurology and has broad implications for how experience-driven predictive models influence action, thought, and behavior, as discussed below.

Understanding Sensory-Guided Movements

One of the central functions of the dorsal visual stream is to make visuospatial information *useful* to cognitive and motor systems. It serves as the blueprint for transforming visual sensory information into specific actions performed by frontal systems. Take the example of seeing and reaching out to pick up an apple. The frontal cortex has access to a large number of motor programs, many of which are learned and stored as an array of prepotent programs. Picking up the apple requires that a highly specific series of movements be selected (termed "action selection") that achieve a specific spatiotemporal outcome (termed "action specification"), as determined by the behavioral context.

All movements generate sensory feedback, and through repetition and experience, the brain learns to associate specific movements with specific sensory consequences. These learned sensorimotor associations become bidirectional: internally generated actions generate sensory expectations (e.g., feedforward control) and bottom-up perception of specific sensory patterns automatically activate the motor plans associated with those sensory percepts, as occurs in the so-called "mirror" system.[105] Top-down mechanisms can activate the same sensorimotor system: goal-driven selection of specific sensory outcomes (e.g., action specifications) activates the specific action plan predicted to produce the target sensory outcome.[5,106] In the case of picking up the apple, the action specification target is the specific visual and tactile sensation associated with reaching and grasping, which is then used to select the appropriate reaching and grasping movements associated with those sensory consequences.[107]

In a given context, there are likely many possible action specifications and overt actions that are possible. Inputs from cognitive (e.g., the apple is soft) and evaluative (e.g., the apple is ripe and delicious) systems may influence the action specifications and selections, ultimately yielding a decision about the motor plan to be executed.

This sensorimotor system is subject to feedback control. Actions selected based on their expected sensory consequences may not yield the expected results, possibly due to poorly tuned sensorimotor associations or errors in motor execution. The mismatch between the expected and overt sensory consequences produces an error signal which is used to select corrective actions.

The intended sensory targets, the overt feedback, and error calculation all occur in the dorsal stream via connections between parietal and prefrontal cortices. In the case of picking up an apple, when the selected action yields erroneous consequences (e.g., the arm reaches to an incorrect location), the mismatch error is detected in the sensory systems and a new, updated sensorimotor action plan is engaged to correct it (e.g., adjust the reach).

Disturbances in these visuomotor circuits produce **visually guided motor deficits**. When affecting limb movements, these errors manifest clinically as clumsiness in reaching, causing symptoms such as knocking things over or mispouring glasses of water, among others. The reaching functions can be assessed at the bedside by having the patient make a pointer with his index finger and reach out and touch the end of the examiner's similarly extended finger, preferably near the extent of the patient's reach. Deficits will manifest as slow but smooth, imprecise reaching movements to the target, often reaching beyond the target; this is a finding known as **optic ataxia**.[108] The mechanisms for this are likely myriad, including the poor spatial mapping of actions, altered depth perception, or an overreliance overt visual feedback (as opposed to feedforward) for motor control.

Deficits in visually guided eye movements can also occur, manifesting as difficulty surveying or scanning the visual environment with ease and difficulty bringing into focus objects in the visual periphery, among others. On exam, patients have difficulty moving their eyes rapidly toward a visual target (i.e., saccades) or pursuing a moving target across their visual field. They may only be able to volitionally move their eyes slowly and with great effort, or may need to close their eyes before initiating the movement, or they may turn their head without moving their eyes within the orbit. This cluster of signs is known as **oculomotor apraxia** (historically labeled "psychic paralysis of gaze"). This may be due to problems generating an egocentric spatial grid of the world, a function supported by the lateral parietal lobes, resulting in difficulty computing where objects are located in space. The lack of spatial coordinates results in poor visual sensory targets, thereby affecting the eye movement plans via abnormal signaling through the parieto-prefrontal pathway.[109]

The sensory-to-motor guidance of action is not isolated to the visual modality. Broadly speaking, there are multiple sensory areas within the lateral temporal-parietal areas (i.e., auditory, visual, somatosensory; often heteromodal) that are richly connected with effector-specific (e.g., articulators, limb, eyes) motor planning areas in the frontal lobe that together form a circuit supporting sensory-guided action. These circuits carry specific names: the "phonological loop" for phonological guidance of speech; the frontal and parietal eye fields for sensory guidance of eye movements; the "praxicon" or visuo-kinesthetic engrams for praxis-related movements. For speech processing, see Hickok et al.[110]

These strong, bidirectional sensorimotor, perception-action pathways offer a potential mechanism to explain a diverse set of mental phenomena beyond the guidance of overt skeletal muscle movement. The abstract notion of tightly coupled action-perception associations whose activity is driven by context via top-down or bottom-up mechanisms can extend to internal mental phenomena. Activating these frontal/action and parietal/perceptual networks offer a mechanism for representing simulation of episodic memories (i.e., prefrontal-hippocampal-parietal circuits), imagination, mental rotation, scene construction, and aspects of working memory.

It is possible that activation of these sensorimotor associations is important for tagging experiences as belonging to "self." When actions are selected by central processes, they contain both a movement and sensory expectation. If these connections become disturbed, selected actions become unyoked from their sensory associations and the action-driven incoming sensory information is falsely (but understandably) interpreted as coming from the external world as opposed to the action. When dovetailed with faulty belief evaluation systems, this mismatch persists and leads to reduced feelings of agency or ownership over movement. While the neural construction of these complex self-related phenomena is likely more complex than what is presented here, these principles of sensorimotor integration are important.[111] This model has broad implications for disease states, including **alien limb phenomena** where affected individuals report a reduced sense of agency over their limb movements, and elements of psychosis, including delusions of self (e.g., **somatoparaphrenia**) and hallucinations. Alien phenomenon is often reported with parietal and frontal lesions.[112,113]

Other Dorsal Stream Functions

The inability to integrate the individual elements of a visual scene into a bound-together, coherent whole is known as **simultanagnosia**. In this condition, patients are unable to integrate visual elements at different levels of their attentional zoom, possessing an inability to "see the forest for the trees." This skill requires integration of multiple stimuli occurring at different spatial locations and depends on the ability to shift attention/gaze and to hold perceptual content in working memory while it is bound together. The disrupted neuropsychological mechanisms are debated but may entail a "restricted spatial window of attention," somewhat akin to how a spotlight can produce an intense effect on a small spatial area or weak effect across a broad area, but not both simultaneously, deficits in object perception, or the interaction between both of these systems (i.e., object perception guiding spatial attention).[114] Others have suggested a combination of deficits in visual exploration and shifting of spatial attention, visual short-term memory, and visual speed of processing.[115]

Performance of this cognitive skill can be assessed in several ways. Asking the individual to describe the elements of a scene containing multiple, related simultaneous "happenings" at different spatial locations requires them to shift their attention to integrate the components into a broader whole. The Cookie Theft picture from the Boston Diagnostic Aphasia Examination or the Picnic Scene picture from the Western Aphasia Battery are two commonly used stimuli. Patients with simultanagnosia may fixate on a single aspect of the picture or be unable to combine the components into a larger narrative. Another test involves identifying all instances of a single letter that are presented in different sizes among alternative letter choices. Affected individuals are apt to perceive only the smallest letters that can be processed by focused attention and single fixations, but miss the largest letters, whose perception requires widening the attentional window and/or attentional shifts. This pattern of deficit is the opposite as one might expect from reduced visual acuity. This form of visual processing can also be tested using Navon figures, where a larger, recognizable shape (such as a letter) is composed of smaller copies of a different shape (a different letter, or number). Patients with simultanagnosia are unable to perceive the larger shape despite intact recognition of the smaller component. Simultanagnosia is associated with lesions in the bilateral parietal and occipital areas.

The Italian Renaissance-era painter, Giuseppe Arcimboldo, is well-known for his art that portrays tactfully arranged fruits and plants that create hierarchical images of expressive human faces (see Figure 12-5). Perception of these faces requires the ability to perceive larger visual structures composed of smaller individual elements. Deficits in this processing ability lead to simultanagnosia and can develop with bilateral occipito-parietal lobe injury or dysfunction. In viewing Arcimboldo's paintings, patients with simultanagnosia may not perceive the face despite seeing the individual fruits.

When optic ataxia, oculomotor apraxia, and simultanagnosia occur together, it is labeled **Balint syndrome**. Patients suffering from this condition may report not seeing things located directly in front of them ("I couldn't find the doorknob," "I missed the giant TV in the house"). Balint syndrome can occur with bilateral parieto-occipital damage due to any number of etiologies, including stroke, anoxic brain injury, traumatic brain injury, and neurodegenerative disease.

Other testable functions of the parietal lobes include skills in number processing[116] and the ability to perform mathematical calculations,[117] finger gnosis (e.g., perception of the positioning of one's finger in space),[118] distinctions between left and right, and writing skills. When these functions are disturbed concomitantly, the constellation of symptoms is referred to as **Gerstmann syndrome**, which is characterized by **dyscalculia**, **finger agnosia**, **left-right confusion**, and **dysgraphia**.[119] Gerstmann syndrome is traditionally associated with lesions of the left inferior parietal lobule (typically the angular gyrus), although the unifying neuropsychological function relating

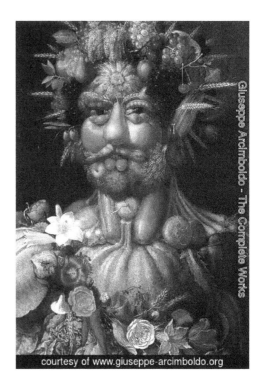

FIGURE 12-5. Examples of hierarchical visuospatial forms. The Italian Renaissance-era painter, Giuseppe Arcimboldo, is well-known for his art that portrays tactfully arranged fruits and plants that create hierarchical images of expressive human faces. Perception of these faces requires the ability to perceive larger visual structures composed of smaller individual elements. Deficits in this processing ability lead to simultanagnosia and can develop with bilateral occipito-parietal lobe injury or dysfunction. In viewing Arcimboldo's paintings, patients with simultanagnosia may not perceive the face despite seeing the individual fruits.

these skills is not entirely clear. It has also been reconsidered as a disconnection syndrome.[120] When all of these symptoms are observed along with alexia, anomia, and constructional disturbances, the pattern of deficits has been labeled the **angular gyrus syndrome**.

There are also dorsal stream connections with memory areas within the mesial temporal lobe and hippocampus via the posterior cingulate and retrosplenial cortices (PCC/Rsp), as part of the so-called parietal-mesial temporal pathway.[109] Deficits in this pathway can produce deficits in visuospatial navigation—particularly the type that relies on using landmarks for guidance—known as **topographic disorientation**. The hippocampus plays a critical role in indexing spatial locations for later recall and recognition. Damage to the hippocampus (and adjacent parahippocampal areas) is associated with poor learning and recognition of spatial landmarks, but a preserved ability to produce mental maps based on self-referential, "egocentric" coordinates (e.g., left-right, forward-back, etc.).[121] Damage to the PCC/Rsp, however, leads to a different type of topographic disorientation where patients can recognize landmarks but cannot use this knowledge to inform egocentric navigational decisions.[122] This may be due to the PCC/Rsp's role in linking externally referenced, "allocentric" locations to egocentric spatial representations, as the former is primarily supported by the mesial temporal lobe and the latter by lateral parietal cortices.

A person's ability to construct a mental map can be tested at the bedside. Asking patients to explain how to navigate from their house to a well-known location in their city, or to draw a map of their home, for example, may offer a window into the cognitive processes at play. Interpreting these narratives is limited; an accurate report does not exclude the possibility that the patient is describing routes from rote memory, and an inaccurate report may be due to deficits in other cognitive domains (e.g., expressive language, memory, etc.). Firm conclusions as to the underlying processing are problematic based on these bedside tests (see Aguirre and D'Esposito[123]). Reduced navigational skills are a common early symptom of Alzheimer's disease, which often affects both the mesial temporal, PCC/Rsp, and lateral parietal areas.

The Ventral Visual Stream: Generating Form Based on Salient Visual Patterns

Patients with dysfunction of the ventral visual processing stream present with symptoms and signs that are quite different from those of the dorsal stream. The ventral stream, which extends from the primary visual cortex anteriorly along the inferior occipito-temporal cortices, is where visual information is extracted and decoded into patterns with particular significance or meaning. The computational processing of this pathway allows for the specialized perception of faces, written text, objects, mathematical symbols, and others, and links these perceptions with semantic representations.

An important symptom of ventral stream dysfunction is **alexia** (i.e., inability to read) or **dyslexia** (e.g., difficulty with aspects of reading). As mentioned in prior sections, the processes of decoding visual information into orthographic language symbols (e.g., letters, words) occurs primarily within the fusiform gyrus. The fusiform subregion important for the decoding of whole words is known as the "visual word form area." Damage anywhere along this pathway can cause symptoms of dyslexia.

Dyslexia can result from abnormal visual processing of letters or an inability to link visual language symbols (e.g., orthography) with the appropriate vocal sounds ("decoding"), regardless of the ability to link written words with semantic networks. Errors in these processes are referred to as "**deep**" **dyslexia**. Affected individuals may be unable to read non-words or functor words, both of which are semantically empty. When asked to read the word "glove," they may read it as the semantically related word "mitten." When asked to spell, individuals with deep dyslexia may be able recall and generate written words based on previously learned semantic-symbol relationships but not use letter-sound relationships as guidance (i.e., phonics), and write "mitten" for "glove." "**Surface**" **dyslexia**, in contrast, is characterized by difficulty reading despite intact symbol-sound relationships. Correct reading of irregularly spelled words (e.g., YACHT, PINT) requires access to these words' semantic nodes, where information about their linguistic irregularities is stored. When access to semantic information is disrupted, as can occur with left anterior temporal lobe damage, patients rely on phonics as a strategy to read, which leads to errors.

Spelling deficits, a reduced ability to generate written words composed of learned collections of written symbols (e.g., letters), may co-occur with dyslexia. **Surface dysgraphia**, which occurs with reduced access to a word's semantic network, is characterized by spelling deficits occurring on irregularly spelled words (e.g., CHOIR, ALIGN), as patients rely on phonetic rules as strategy to spell (e.g., "QUIER" or "ALINE").

Prosopagnosia, the inability to perceive and recognize individual faces, is associated with focal damage within the right fusiform gyrus in a region appropriately referred to as the "fusiform face area." This capacity can be tested at the bedside in several ways, including showing pictures of famous faces (and non-famous control faces) and asking individuals to identify them (e.g., by name, stating facts about them, etc.). Human face perception requires the ability to rapidly decode many features simultaneously to produce the feeling of recognition. In prosopagnosia, semantic knowledge of the person whose face is not visually recognized is often intact and can be accessed via other modalities (e.g., gait, gesture, voice, etc.).

Ventral stream dysfunction can cause deficits in the visual perception and recognition of objects. This can be tested by asking patients to name visually presented objects (e.g., using line drawings from the Boston Naming Test). This can be confounded by deficits in lexical retrieval, which can be circumvented by providing cues or multiples choices, or asking the patient to describe the object or to pantomime its use.

The ventral stream has important interactions with attentional and limbic systems. The ability to recognize facial expressions and interpret emotional content in body language, and to detect biological motion (e.g., movements produced by animate organisms) are all supported by ventral stream processing. Attentional and affective regulation can influence the content of the ventral stream perceptions. **Conceptual priming**, where exposure to specific semantic information unconsciously lowers the activation thresholds for activating other related semantic concepts, alters the perception of incoming visual information, biasing it toward the primed concept. This is distinct from **perceptual priming**, whereby exposure to certain perceptual forms biases incoming information to more rapidly perceive those and related forms. These inputs can modulate the processing of information within the ventral stream and can generate expectations about the content—and meaning—of incoming percepts.

An interesting example of how top-down regulation of the ventral stream signaling influences the content of visual perception is **face pareidolia**. Pareidolia is finding meaning in otherwise innocuous, noisy incoming visual signals; it is the idea behind, for example, seeing the face of Jesus in a pancake. There is evidence that the top-down influence of the orbitofrontal cortex on the fusiform gyrus may underlie the phenomenon in some cases.[124]

Interactions between Visual and Memory Systems

The notion of two separate streams—the dorsal and ventral streams—is likely overly simplified, as there is cross-talk between the two systems at different levels. There are many tasks that activate both pathways simultaneously. For example, when a frisbee is tossed toward a person, he/she needs to produce a visually guided movement plan to catch or avoid it (dorsal stream) as well as identify the object accurately (ventral stream), which informs the best movement selection (dorsal stream). Misperceiving the frisbee's spatial location or speed, or its identity (e.g., as a porcelain plate), will produce an inappropriate response. Communication between the two streams can be assessed clinically. Individuals administered the Hooper Visual Organization Test, for example, are asked to identify and name objects that are presented as line drawings cut into multiple pieces whose components are displayed at different orientations. This task activates both dorsal (mental rotation) and ventral (object perception) stream visual processing areas simultaneously.[125]

Humans are able to replay prior experiences in their mind's eye, which reflects our capacity for episodic memory. Stored episodic memory traces are reconstructed within widely distributed perceptual networks to reproduce a rendition of the prior experience. This is supported by connections between mesial temporal episodic memory centers and perceptual areas. The medial parietal lobe (e.g., the posterior cingulate cortex and retrosplenial cortex), as part of the default mode network, may help mediate this process. Damage to the posterior cingulate cortex leads to deficits in episodic memory and the ability to describe imagined scenes.[126]

The medial parietal region also supports representations of familiarity, in which patients report a feeling of having previously interacted with a stimulus, even if the precise details of the prior interactions cannot be recollected. Deficits in familiarity are an important component of the **delusional misidentification syndromes**. The **Capgras syndrome**, for example, is characterized by the delusional belief that a loved one has been replaced by an identical-appearing imposter, may be driven by reduced familiarity signals associated with the loved one's face accompanied by an impaired ability to judge the plausibility of one's conception. Recent evidence suggests disruption in a network that includes the left medial parietal cortex and right inferior frontal lobe.[127]

Visual Systems and Representations of Self

Dorsal stream machinery, with the support of vestibular, proprioceptive, somatic, and auditory information, acts to situate individuals at the subjective center of their personal visuospatial universe, and represents one's conscious stream of imagery as unfolding from a single vantage point—the location of "I"—at any given moment. These hardwired, egocentric perspectives are critical in the formation of self-representations. Abnormalities within the dorsal stream, particularly within the right parietal lobe, can disrupt the feeling of automatic self-positioning, leading to symptoms such as out of body experiences,[128] autoscopy

(perception of the environment from a non-egocentric perspective),[129] and a loss of depth perception.

A BRIEF NOTE ON THE LOCALIZATION OF EMOTIONAL, SOCIAL, AND BEHAVIORAL SYMPTOMATOLOGY

This chapter's primary focus has been on the traditionally classified elements of cognition (e.g., language, praxis, memory, attention, executive functions, visuospatial skills) and not on feeling states, social behavior, personality, and motivation. This asymmetric emphasis in content risks perpetuating the great schism between cognition and affect, thinking and feeling, and neurology and psychiatry, which is the product of long-standing sociocultural influences dating back to the early 20th century.[130] While the subjective experiences of emotion and thought are often starkly different, their fundamental neuroscientific underpinnings are similarly reliant on the cellular biological properties of interacting neurons and glia that act in concert across distances to form network-based representational architectures. The anatomy supporting both phenomena are deeply interconnected in the brain at many levels. Even a superficial understanding of human behavior necessitates the integration of cognition and affect; a distinction between the two is artificial.

On a practical level, negative affective symptoms are common, distressing, and often the most proximate reason why people visit the doctor. In patients with memory loss, for example, it is often the *feelings* of worry that motivates the patient (or family) to seek medical attention. Many patients will only seek help for their limping gait when their knees start to cause *pain*, or when they become *frustrated* by their reduced walking speed or other functional limitations. It is critical to recognize the importance of emotional processing in guiding behaviors.

How the nervous system detects, evaluates, and responds to salience in the environment offers the potential to meaningfully integrate perceptual, motor, cognitive, social, and affective processing under a unified framework. These different aspects of human mental functioning are highlighted in Chapter 2 and discussed throughout this textbook.

CONCLUSION

The phenomena that comprise human experience and behavior are intimately connected to the structure and functioning of the brain. The notion that intricately timed electrical impulses traveling across complex networks of neurobiological circuitry represent and construct the incredible diversity of mental states is the great axiom of cognitive neuroscience and lies at the foundation of neuropsychiatry and behavioral neurology. The organization of this hierarchical biological system supports the many different aspects of human cognitive functioning. Focal neurobehavioral syndromes emerge when these systems are disrupted. This chapter has reviewed some of these basic structures and the symptoms that develop when damage is incurred.

Summary and Key Points

■ *Background/Fundamentals*
- Underlying the enterprise of cognitive neuroscience and clinical neuropsychiatry is the hypothesis that contents and expression of the mind (e.g., cognition, emotion, and behavior) are functions supported by the dynamic flow of electrical activity through interacting neural structures. There are several common assumptions about the underlying workings of neural systems, including (1) the brain is composed of specialized neurocomputational units, (2) sensory inputs form the building blocks of experience, (3) experience is animated within complex, multilevel perceptual machinery, (4) the brain generates and stores predictive models about the world, (5) the brain can update its models throughout the lifespan, particularly during development, (6) self-generated sensory and motor processes become tightly linked, (7) the brain operates several large-scale processing modes that support different ways of engaging with the environment, and (8) many aspects of neural processing occur outside of consciousness.
- Basic sensory-perceptual processing serves as the brain's primary interface with the environment, and these inputs provide the fundamental building blocks for higher-order predictive models about the world. Abnormal sensory-perceptual processing impacts aspects of cognition and behavior, including release phenomenon (e.g., Charles-Bonnet, phantom limb) and highlights the dissociation between explicit and implicit processing modes (e.g., blindsight). Deficits to components of the hierarchical, modular structures of the sensory-perceptual systems produce focal, higher-order clinical syndromes (e.g., pure word deafness, akinetopsia).
- Cognitive skills are traditionally grouped by the neuropsychological function, including attention, executive functioning, memory, language, visuospatial skills, praxis, and others. The mapping of these neuropsychological functions onto neuroanatomical networks is complex, hierarchical, and interdependent. Basic wakefulness, motivation, and attention are necessary for testing the contents of higher-order cognitive faculties. Deficits in perception, action, affect, and cognition are likely to impact the performance on cognitive tests designed to "isolate" a specific function.

■ *Language*
- The language system provides a unique opportunity to illustrate principles of structure-function relationships relevant to neuropsychiatry. The fundamental skill of language is the ability to link combinations of sensory symbols with semantic knowledge, and to use these relationships to communicate. Language elements are combined into larger grammatical structures (e.g., syntax, morphology) that enable the expression of hierarchical, agential relationships between the semantic elements. The core language system can be accessed via several perceptual inputs (e.g., auditory/speech, visual/writing, visual/signing) and expressed through multiple motoric means.

Language deficits may be domain-general (e.g., global comprehension or expression) or modality-specific (e.g., pure word deafness, aphemia).
- The language system is broadly divided into two processing streams: (1) a ventral stream within the temporal lobe that links sensory language symbols with semantic knowledge, and (2) a dorsal stream within the temporoparietal areas critical for using sensory language symbols for motor expression. Disruption of ventral stream processing leads to deficits in comprehension (e.g., Wernicke aphasia, pure word deafness, pure alexia, semantic aphasia, transcortical sensory aphasia). Dorsal stream disruption produces deficits in the sensory guidance of production (e.g., conduction aphasia, verbal working memory deficits). The organization of speech into hierarchical grammatical structures primarily occurs within the dominant inferior frontal gyrus, with deficits associated with agrammatism.
- The transition from language intention to motor expression (e.g., speech, writing) requires precise planning of carefully timed, appropriately sequenced actions by frontal premotor areas, and overt expression within the peripheral motor effector system. Deficits in motor-speech planning yield production deficits in the form of an apraxia of speech whereas the motor effector system disruption causes dysarthria.
- Broca's aphasia, a nonfluent, usually agrammatic aphasia with poor repetition but intact single-word comprehension, is associated with damage to the dominant inferior frontal gyrus. Wernicke aphasia, a fluent aphasia with poor comprehension, poor repetition, but intact fluency occurs with disruption of the posterior superior temporal areas.
- Symptoms impacting the successful deployment of language skills can emerge with disrupted connections to other networks. Transcortical motor aphasia, for example, occurs when the language system is disconnected from areas important for motivation and intention.

■ *Memory*
- Memory is the capacity for the brain to store aspects of experience to guide future behavior. There are many types of memory, including procedural, semantic, stimulus-reinforcement conditioning, and episodic (and many others), each supported by its own functional neuroanatomy.
- Episodic memory refers to information acquired in the context of a specific time, place, and circumstance. This type of memory can be recalled and replayed within the mind's eye. Amnesia refers to acquired episodic memory loss and is characterized by whether the memory loss affects information acquired before (i.e., retrograde amnesia) or after (i.e., anterograde amnesia) the onset of the injury. Common symptoms include repeating oneself without realizing it, an altered sense of the passage of time, misplacing items, needing to write things down to recall information later, and not being able to retrieve information about recent personal events.

- Acquisition and storage of episodic and autobiographical memories are enhanced when the events are associated with a high degree of salience (e.g., flashbulb memory).
- Episodic memory is operationally conceptualized as a three-stage process: (1) encoding, in which information is introduced and prepared for storage, (2) storage, and (3) retrieval, in which stored memories are accessed. Broadly speaking, encoding is supported by frontoparietal and temporolimbic structures, storage is supported by temporolimbic structures, and retrieval by frontoparietal structures.
- Episodic memory deficits are seen in myriad neurobehavioral syndromes, including Alzheimer's disease, transient global amnesia, Wernicke-Korsakoff syndrome, and others.

▪ *Attention and Executive Functions*
- The processes that engage, filter, select, and maintain the elements of experience comprise the mechanisms of attention. These functions support the allocation of scarce neural resources to the most relevant components of the environment to support the long-term and immediate needs of the person. Attentional resources are supported by stimulus-driven ("bottom up"), goal-directed ("top down"), and stimulus-independent, non-goal-directed processing modes. These modes are mediated by different neural networks, the ventral attention, dorsal attention, and default mode networks, respectively. Each of these circuits include distinct, circumscribed nodes within the parietal and frontal areas, with the dorsal attention network located more superiorly along the lateral surface, the ventral attention network more inferiorly along the lateral surface, with a right hemisphere dominance, and the default mode network along the medial wall.
- Improper balance between these attentional processing modes can produce focal neurobehavioral symptoms, including the environmental dependency syndrome.
- Hemispatial neglect is a disorder of spatial attention that occurs with disruption of the nondominant hemisphere and is characterized by reduced awareness of egocentric space on one half of one's vertical meridian (typically the left).
- Executive functioning is a broad term denoting a number of cognitive processes, including top-down mechanisms for shifting attention, inhibitory control, planning, organization, working memory, conflict monitoring, and self-monitoring. Because these skills are broadly supported by functional networks with hubs within the prefrontal and lateral parietal cortices, dysexecutive symptoms tend to occur together.
- Working memory deficits manifest as difficulty retaining information immediately after it is presented, and can be domain-specific (e.g., verbal, visuospatial, episodic). Other conceptions extend this idea to include both the active maintenance of and the cognitive, executive operations performed on the held information. Reduced concentration, distractibility, impulsivity, poor decision making, and impaired problem solving are common manifestations of the dysexecutive syndrome.

▪ *Visuospatial Functions*
- Visuospatial information guides our attentional gaze, helps plan and select actions, and contributes to semantic knowledge via the detection of visual patterns, among many other roles. The visuospatial system is broadly divided into a dorsal processing stream important for spatially guided actions (the "where" or "how" pathway) and a ventral stream supporting pattern recognition and semantic processing (the "what" pathway).
- Cortical visual loss from disruption of primary visual areas can manifest as cortical blindness with blindsight. Cortical blindness accompanied by a lack of insight with confabulation is referred to as the Anton-Babinski syndrome.
- Deficits in dorsal stream functioning include constructional apraxia, optic ataxia, oculomotor apraxia, and simultanagnosia. These can present separately, or together, as part of the Balint syndrome with bilateral parieto-occipital dysfunction. The Gerstmann syndrome, characterized by dyscalculia, finger agnosia, dysgraphia, and left-right confusion, is also seen with dorsal stream disruption, classically described in left parietal lobe lesions.
- Deficits in ventral stream functioning include alexia, prosopagnosia, and pareidolia. Dyslexia may manifest from disrupted relationships between visual language symbols and the appropriate sound/phonology (e.g., "deep" dyslexia), or from poor semantic representations (e.g., "surface" dyslexia).
- Reduced navigational skills can result from topographic disorientation, which is characterized by disrupted connections between parietal and temporolimbic structures important for recognizing landmarks and generating egocentric navigational relationships.
- The dorsal and ventral streams communicate, and the integration of these two types of information supports aspects of cognition and behavior.

Multiple Choice Questions

1. Which of the following is true regarding language dysfunction?
    a. Production deficits can only be caused by disruption of frontal lobe areas.
    b. Comprehension deficits can only be caused by disruption of temporal and/or parietal areas.
    c. A deficit in speech comprehension is always accompanied by a similar deficit in reading comprehension.
    d. Spastic dysarthria is caused by deficits in motor speech planning areas.
    e. Damage to the fusiform gyrus can produce letter-by-letter alexia.

2. Which of the following is false regarding episodic memory?
   a. Amnesia can occur with herpes encephalitis.
   b. Episodic memory is an important component of one's autobiographical memory.
   c. Difficulty spontaneously (i.e., without cues or multiple choices) recalling a recently learned word list only occurs with temporolimbic dysfunction.
   d. Memory encoding and storage are supported by temporolimbic structures.
   e. Not all patients with Alzheimer's disease have memory loss.

3. Which of the following symptoms is not considered part of the dysexecutive syndrome?
   a. Hemispatial neglect
   b. Distractibility
   c. Impulsivity
   d. Losing one's train of thought
   e. Poor decision making

4. Which of the following is not a function supported by the ventral visual processing stream?
   a. Reading
   b. Face recognition
   c. Object recognition
   d. Smooth reaching movements to a target

Multiple Choice Answers

1. **Answer: e**
   Within the fusiform gyrus is the so-called visual word form area (VWFA), where orthographic representations of whole words are represented. Damage to this region cause pure word blindness, a form of pure alexia with spared verbal comprehension. Some patients overcome this by spelling the words one letter at a time to presumably access the word form via an alternative, possibly auditory pathway. (a) Production deficits can occur with damage to the dominant (usually left) temporoparietal junction, as can occur in a conduction aphasia. Affected individuals have difficulty repeating complex phrases and make a high number of paraphasic errors. (b) While single-word comprehension is predominantly subserved by temporal > parietal structures, sentence and grammar comprehension uses inferior frontal systems. (c) Comprehension deficits can be domain-general (e.g., affecting both spoken and written inputs), as in the case of Wernicke and transcortical sensory aphasia, or domain-specific (e.g., affecting one modality but sparing others), as occurs in pure word deafness or pure alexia. Spastic dysarthria is caused by disruption of the bilateral corticobulbar tracts involved in the peripheral motor effector pathways.

2. **Answer: c**
   Assuming the patient was able to encode properly, poor spontaneous recall recently learned information can result from a deficit in either storage or retrieval. A storage deficit implies temporolimbic dysfunction, whereas retrieval deficits more commonly occur with frontoparietal networks disruption. (a) Herpes simplex encephalitis often affects temporolimbic structures in the mesial temporal lobe, and significant amnesia is common. (b) Autobiographical memory refers to memories related to one's personal narrative, including prior experiences stored as episodic memories. Semantic self-knowledge (i.e., one's birthday, or first word) may be autobiographical but not episodic. (d) This is true. (e) While episodic memory loss is a common symptom of typical Alzheimer's disease, in atypical cases the pathology affects other networks (e.g., visuospatial areas) while sparing the temporolimbic structures, preserving memory function.

3. **Answer: a**
   Hemispatial neglect usually occurs with disruption of neural areas important for mapping the world onto egocentric spatial coordinates, usually within the nondominant hemisphere. It does not typically cluster with the dysexecutive syndrome. (b–e) These symptoms are all part of the dysexecutive syndrome, which occurs with disruption of the executive control networks.

4. **Answer: d**
   The use of visual information to guide reaching movements to a target is a canonical function of the dorsal stream. (a–c) The use of visual information to identify patterns that can be linked to semantic networks is the primary function of the ventral stream. These functions include reading, face recognition, and object recognition, among others.

References

1. Schmahmann JD, Pandya DN. Disconnection syndromes of basal ganglia, thalamus, and cerebrocerebellar systems. *Cortex*. 2008;44(8):1037-1066.
2. Petersen SE, Sporns O. Brain networks and cognitive architectures. *Neuron*. 2015;88(1):207-219.
3. Lee S-H, Kravitz DJ, Baker CI. Disentangling visual imagery and perception of real-world objects. *NeuroImage*. 2012;59(4):4064-4073.
4. Kilner JM, Friston KJ, Frith CD. Predictive coding: an account of the mirror neuron system. *Cogn Process*. 2007;8(3):159-166.
5. Prinz W. Perception and action planning. *Eur J Cogn Psychol*. 1997;9(2):129-154.
6. Shdo SM, et al. Deconstructing empathy: neuroanatomical dissociations between affect sharing and prosocial motivation using a patient lesion model. *Neuropsychologia*. 2018;116(pt A): 126-135.
7. Keysers C, Gazzola V. Expanding the mirror: vicarious activity for actions, emotions, and sensations. *Curr Opin Neurobiol*. 2009;19(6):666-671.
8. Hadjikhani N, et al. Anatomical differences in the mirror neuron system and social cognition network in autism. *Cereb Cortex*. 2005;16(9):1276-1282.
9. Frasnelli J, et al. Clinical presentation of qualitative olfactory dysfunction. *Eur Arch Otorhinolaryngol*. 2004;261(7):411-415.
10. Levelt WJM, Roelofs A, Meyer AS. A theory of lexical access in speech production. *Behav Brain Sci*. 1999;22(1):1-38.
11. Seeley WW, et al. Unravelling Bolero: progressive aphasia, transmodal creativity and the right posterior neocortex. *Brain*. 2008;131(pt 1):39-49.
12. Erkkinen MG, et al. Artistic renaissance in frontotemporal dementia. *JAMA*. 2018;319(13):1304-1306.
13. Hickok G, Poeppel D. The cortical organization of speech processing. *Nat Rev Neurosci*. 2007;8(5):393-402.
14. Fiset D, et al. How to make the word-length effect disappear in letter-by-letter dyslexia: implications for an account of the disorder. *Psychol Sci*. 2005;16(7):535-541.
15. Geschwind N. Disconnexion syndromes in animals and man. I. *Brain*. 1965;88(2):237-294.
16. Hope TM, Price CJ. Why the left posterior inferior temporal lobe is needed for word finding. *Brain*. 2016;139(11):2823-2826.
17. Baldo JV, et al. Grey and white matter correlates of picture naming: evidence from a voxel-based lesion analysis of the Boston Naming Test. *Cortex*. 2013;49(3):658-667.
18. Win KT, et al. Neural correlates of verbal episodic memory and lexical retrieval in logopenic variant primary progressive aphasia. *Front Neurosci*. 2017;11:330.
19. Herbet G, et al. Converging evidence for a cortico-subcortical network mediating lexical retrieval. *Brain*. 2016;139(11):3007-3021.
20. Cloutman L, et al. Where (in the brain) do semantic errors come from? *Cortex*. 2009;45(5):641-649.
21. Benetello A, et al. The dissociability of lexical retrieval and morphosyntactic processes for nouns and verbs: a functional and anatomoclinical study. *Brain Lang*. 2016;159:11-22.
22. Ralph MAL, et al. The neural and computational bases of semantic cognition. *Nat Rev Neurosci*. 2016;18:42.
23. Rascovsky K, et al. 'The quicksand of forgetfulness': semantic dementia in *One Hundred Years of Solitude*. *Brain*. 2009;132(9):2609-2616.
24. Papagno C, et al. Mapping the brain network of the phonological loop. *Hum Brain Mapp*. 2017;38(6):3011-3024.
25. Buchsbaum BR, et al. Human dorsal and ventral auditory streams subserve rehearsal-based and echoic processes during verbal working memory. *Neuron*. 2005;48(4):687-697.
26. Hickok G, Poeppel D. The cortical organization of speech processing. *Nat Rev Neurosci*. 2007;8(5):393.
27. Leonard MK, et al. The peri-Sylvian cortical networks underlying single word repetition revealed by electrocortical stimulation and direct neural recordings. *Brain Lang*. 2019;193:58-72.
28. Pilkington E, et al. Sources of phoneme errors in repetition: perseverative, neologistic, and lesion patterns in jargon aphasia. *Front Hum Neurosci*. 2017;11:225.
29. Boatman D, et al. Transcortical sensory aphasia: revisited and revised. *Brain*. 2000;123(8):1634-1642.
30. Catani M, Mesulam M. The arcuate fasciculus and the disconnection theme in language and aphasia: history and current state. *Cortex*. 2008;44(8):953-961.
31. Lauterbach EC, Cummings JL, Kuppuswamy PS. Toward a more precise, clinically-informed pathophysiology of pathological laughing and crying. *Neurosci Biobehav Rev*. 2013;37(8):1893-1916.
32. Miller A, Pratt H, Schiffer RB. Pseudobulbar affect: the spectrum of clinical presentations, etiologies and treatments. *Expert Rev Neurother*. 2011;11(7):1077-1088.
33. Umapathi T, et al. Tongue deviation in acute ischaemic stroke: a study of supranuclear twelfth cranial nerve palsy in 300 stroke patients. *Cerebrovasc Dis*. 2000;10(6):462-465.
34. Weller M. Anterior opercular cortex lesions cause dissociated lower cranial nerve palsies and anarthria but no aphasia: Foix-Chavany-Marie syndrome and "automatic voluntary dissociation" revisited. *J Neurol*. 1993;240(4):199-208.
35. Ogar J, et al. Apraxia of speech: an overview. *Neurocase*. 2005;11(6):427-432.
36. Guenther FH. *Neural Control of Speech*. Cambridge, MA: MIT Press; 2016.
37. Graff-Radford J, et al. The neuroanatomy of pure apraxia of speech in stroke. *Brain Lang*. 2014;129:43-46.
38. Josephs KA, et al. Syndromes dominated by apraxia of speech show distinct characteristics from agrammatic PPA. *Neurology*. 2013;81(4):337-345.
39. Utianski RL, et al. Tau-PET imaging with [18F] AV-1451 in primary progressive apraxia of speech. *Cortex*. 2018;99:358-374.
40. Botha H, et al. Classification and clinicoradiologic features of primary progressive aphasia (PPA) and apraxia of speech. *Cortex*. 2015;69:220-236.
41. Schiff HB, et al. Aphemia. Clinical-anatomic correlations. *Arch Neurol*. 1983;40(12):720-727.
42. Broca P. Remarques sur le siège de la faculté du langage articulé, suivies d'une observation d'aphémie (perte de la parole). *Bulletin de la Société Anatomique*. 1861;6:330-357.
43. Pearce JMS. Broca's aphasias. *Eur Neurol*. 2009;61(3):183-189.
44. Friederici AD. The neural basis for human syntax: Broca's area and beyond. *Curr Opin Behav Sci*. 2018;21:88-92.
45. Ardila A, Bernal B, Rosselli M. How localized are language brain areas? A review of Brodmann areas involvement in oral language. *Arch Clin Neuropsychol*. 2016;31(1):112-122.
46. Ottomeyer C, et al. Aphemia: an isolated disorder of speech associated with an ischemic lesion of the left precentral gyrus. *J Neurol*. 2009;256(7):1166-1168.
47. Flinker A, et al. Redefining the role of Broca's area in speech. *Proc Natl Acad Sci U S A*. 2015;112(9):2871-2875.
48. Ardila A, Bernal B, Rosselli M. Why Broca's area damage does not result in classical Broca's aphasia. *Front Hum Neurosci*. 2016;10:249.

49. Robinson G, Shallice T, Cipolotti L. Dynamic aphasia in progressive supranuclear palsy: a deficit in generating a fluent sequence of novel thought. *Neuropsychologia*. 2006;44(8):1344-1360.

50. Robinson GA, Spooner D, Harrison WJ. Frontal dynamic aphasia in progressive supranuclear palsy: distinguishing between generation and fluent sequencing of novel thoughts. *Neuropsychologia*. 2015;77:62-75.

51. Ardila A, Lopez MV. Transcortical motor aphasia: one or two aphasias? *Brain Lang*. 1984;22(2):350-353.

52. Pai M-C. Supplementary motor area aphasia: a case report. *Clin Neurol Neurosurg*. 1999;101(1):29-32.

53. Crosson BA, Bohsali A, and Raymer AM. *10 Transcortical Motor Aphasia*, in *The Oxford Handbook of Aphasia and Language Disorders*. New York, NY: Oxford University Press; 2017:171.

54. Kim J-H, et al. Defining functional SMA and pre-SMA subregions in human MFC using resting state fMRI: functional connectivity-based parcellation method. *NeuroImage*. 2010;49(3):2375.

55. Zhang S, Ide JS, Li CS. Resting-state functional connectivity of the medial superior frontal cortex. *Cereb Cortex*. 2012;22(1):99-111.

56. Hertrich I, et al. The role of the supplementary motor area for speech and language processing. *Neurosci Biobehav Rev*. 2016; 68:602-610.

57. Dick AS, et al. The frontal aslant tract (FAT) and its role in speech, language and executive function. *Cortex*. 2019;111:148-163.

58. Catani M, et al. A novel frontal pathway underlies verbal fluency in primary progressive aphasia. *Brain*. 2013;136(8):2619-2628.

59. Heilman KM. Apraxia. *Continuum (Minneap Minn)*. 2010;16 (4, Behavioral Neurology):86-108.

60. Campbell MEJ, Cunnington R. More than an imitation game: top-down modulation of the human mirror system. *Neurosci Biobehav Rev*. 2017;75:195-202.

61. Iacoboni M, et al. Cortical mechanisms of human imitation. *Science*. 1999;286(5449):2526-2528.

62. Catmur C. Sensorimotor learning and the ontogeny of the mirror neuron system. *Neurosci Lett*. 2013;540:21-27.

63. Mehta UM, Basavaraju R, Thirthalli J. Mirror neuron disinhibition may be linked with catatonic echo-phenomena: a single case TMS study. *Brain Stimul*. 2013;6(4):705-707.

64. Williams JHG, Whiten A, Singh T. A systematic review of action imitation in autistic spectrum disorder. *J Autism Dev Disord*. 2004;34(3):285-299.

65. Stokes MG, et al. Long-term memory prepares neural activity for perception. *Proc Natl Acad Sci U S A*. 2012;109(6):E360-E367.

66. Frey U, Schroeder H. Dopaminergic antagonists prevent long-term maintenance of posttetanic LTP in the CA1 region of rat hippocampal slices. *Brain Res*. 1990;522(1):69-75.

67. Winton-Brown TT, et al. Dopaminergic basis of salience dysregulation in psychosis. *Trends Neurosci*. 2014;37(2):85-94.

68. Shohamy D, Adcock RA. Dopamine and adaptive memory. *Trends Cogn Sci*. 2010;14(10):464-472.

69. Scoville WB, Milner B. Loss of recent memory after bilateral hippocampal lesions. *J Neurol Neurosurg Psychiatry*. 1957;20(1):11-21.

70. Li J, Hu WL. Bilateral hippocampal abnormalities in magnetic resonance imaging in transient global amnesia. *Am J Emerg Med*. 2013;31(4):755.e1-3.

71. Gordon BA, et al. Structural correlates of prospective memory. *Neuropsychologia*. 2011;49(14):3795-3800.

72. Johnson MK, Hashtroudi S, Lindsay DS. Source monitoring. *Psychol Bull*. 1993;114(1):3.

73. Cabeza R, Nyberg L. Imaging cognition II: an empirical review of 275 PET and fMRI studies. *J Cogn Neurosci*. 2000;12(1):1-47.

74. Axmacher N, et al. Interaction of working memory and long-term memory in the medial temporal lobe. *Cereb Cortex*. 2008;18(12):2868-2878.

75. Berlingeri M, et al. Anatomy of the episodic buffer: a voxel-based morphometry study in patients with dementia. *Behav Neurol*. 2008;19(1-2):29-34.

76. Leube DT, et al. Neural correlates of verbal episodic memory in patients with MCI and Alzheimer's disease—a VBM study. *Int J Geriatr Psychiatry*. 2008;23(11):1114-1118.

77. Schmidt-Wilcke T, et al. Memory performance correlates with gray matter density in the ento-/perirhinal cortex and posterior hippocampus in patients with mild cognitive impairment and healthy controls—a voxel based morphometry study. *NeuroImage*. 2009;47(4):1914-1920.

78. Aggleton JP, et al. Thalamic pathology and memory loss in early Alzheimer's disease: moving the focus from the medial temporal lobe to Papez circuit. *Brain*. 2016;139(7):1877-1890.

79. Brown R, Kulik J. Flashbulb memories. *Cognition*. 1977;5(1):73-99.

80. Eichenbaum H. On the integration of space, time, and memory. *Neuron*. 2017;95(5):1007-1018.

81. Kopelman MD, et al. The Korsakoff syndrome: clinical aspects, psychology and treatment. *Alcohol Alcohol*. 2009;44(2):148-154.

82. Chaves LCL, et al. A cluster of polyneuropathy and Wernicke-Korsakoff syndrome in a bariatric unit. *Obes Surg*. 2002;12(3):328-334.

83. Eichenbaum H. Prefrontal–hippocampal interactions in episodic memory. *Nat Rev Neurosci*. 2017;18:547.

84. Sestieri C, Shulman GL, Corbetta M. The contribution of the human posterior parietal cortex to episodic memory. *Nat Rev Neurosci*. 2017;18(3):183-192.

85. Buckner RL, Andrews-Hanna JR, Schacter DL. The brain's default network. *Ann N Y Acad Sci*. 2008;1124:1-38.

86. Knudsen EI. Fundamental components of attention. *Annu Rev Neurosci*. 2007;30:57-78.

87. Vossel S, Geng JJ, Fink GR. Dorsal and ventral attention systems: distinct neural circuits but collaborative roles. *Neuroscientist*. 2014;20(2):150-159.

88. Jerde TA, Curtis CE. Maps of space in human frontoparietal cortex. *J Physiol Paris*. 2013;107(6):510-516.

89. Shulman GL, et al. Quantitative analysis of attention and detection signals during visual search. *J Neurophysiol*. 2003;90(5):3384-3397.

90. Rinne P, et al. Triple dissociation of attention networks in stroke according to lesion location. *Neurology*. 2013;81(9):812-820.

91. Corbetta M, Patel G, Shulman GL. The reorienting system of the human brain: from environment to theory of mind. *Neuron*. 2008;58(3):306-324.

92. Zacks JM, et al. Event perception: a mind-brain perspective. *Psychol Bull*. 2007;133(2):273-293.

93. Raichle ME. The brain's default mode network. *Ann Rev Neurosci*. 2015;38(1):433-447.

94. Toba MN, et al. Common brain networks for distinct deficits in visual neglect. A combined structural and tractography MRI approach. *Neuropsychologia*. 2018;115:167-178.

95. Niendam TA, et al. Meta-analytic evidence for a superordinate cognitive control network subserving diverse executive functions. *Cogn Affect Behav Neurosci*. 2012;12(2):241-268.

96. Baddeley A. Working memory: looking back and looking forward. *Nat Rev Neurosci*. 2003;4(10):829-839.

97. Rosenberg MD, et al. A neuromarker of sustained attention from whole-brain functional connectivity. *Nat Neurosci*. 2016;19(1):165-171.

98. Langner R, Eickhoff SB. Sustaining attention to simple tasks: a meta-analytic review of the neural mechanisms of vigilant attention. *Psychol Bull*. 2013;139(4):870-900.

99. Lhermitte F. Human autonomy and the frontal lobes. Part II: patient behavior in complex and social situations: the "environmental dependency syndrome". *Ann Neurol*. 1986;19(4):335-343.

100. Asaad WF, Rainer G, Miller EK. Task-specific neural activity in the primate prefrontal cortex. *J Neurophysiol*. 2000;84(1):451-459.

101. Reverberi C, et al. Specific impairments of rule induction in different frontal lobe subgroups. *Neuropsychologia*. 2005;43(3):460-472.

102. Possin KL, et al. Distinct neuroanatomical substrates and cognitive mechanisms of figure copy performance in Alzheimer's disease and behavioral variant frontotemporal dementia. *Neuropsychologia*. 2011;49(1):43-48.

103. Shin MS, et al. Clinical and empirical applications of the Rey–Osterrieth complex figure test. *Nat Protoc*. 2006;1(2):892-899.

104. Moo LR, et al. Interlocking finger test: a bedside screen for parietal lobe dysfunction. *J Neurol Neurosurg Psychiatry*. 2003;74(4):530-532.

105. Molenberghs P, Cunnington R, Mattingley JB. Is the mirror neuron system involved in imitation? A short review and meta-analysis. *Neurosci Biobehav Rev*. 2009;33(7):975-980.

106. Herwig A, Prinz W, Waszak F. Two modes of sensorimotor integration in intention-based and stimulus-based actions. *Q J Exp Psychol*. 2007;60(11):1540-1554.

107. Cisek P, Kalaska JF. Neural mechanisms for interacting with a world full of action choices. *Annu Rev Neurosci*. 2010;33:269-298.

108. Karnath HO, Perenin MT. Cortical control of visually guided reaching: evidence from patients with optic ataxia. *Cereb Cortex*. 2005;15(10):1561-1569.

109. Kravitz DJ, et al. A new neural framework for visuospatial processing. *Nat Rev Neurosci*. 2011;12(4):217-230.

110. Hickok G, Houde J, Rong F. Sensorimotor integration in speech processing: computational basis and neural organization. *Neuron*. 2011;69(3):407-422.

111. Synofzik M, Vosgerau G, Newen A. Beyond the comparator model: a multifactorial two-step account of agency. *Conscious Cogn*. 2008;17(1):219-239.

112. Graff-Radford J, et al. The alien limb phenomenon. *J Neurol*. 2013;260(7):1880-1888.

113. Albrecht F, et al. Unraveling corticobasal syndrome and alien limb syndrome with structural brain imaging. *Cortex*. 2019; 117:33-40.

114. Dalrymple KA, Barton JJ, Kingstone A. A world unglued: simultanagnosia as a spatial restriction of attention. *Front Hum Neurosci*. 2013;7:145.

115. Neitzel J, et al. Neuro-cognitive mechanisms of simultanagnosia in patients with posterior cortical atrophy. *Brain*. 2016;139(12):3267-3280.

116. Eger E. Neuronal foundations of human numerical representations. In: *Progress in Brain Research*. Amsterdam, NL: Elsevier; 2016:1-27.

117. Kadosh RC, Dowker A, Cappelletti M. *The Neuropsychology of Acquired Number and Calculation Disorders*. Oxford, UK: Oxford University Press; 2015.

118. Rusconi E, et al. Neural correlates of finger gnosis. *J Neurosci*. 2014;34(27):9012-9023.

119. Gerstmann J. Syndrome of finger agnosia, disorientation for right and left, agraphia and acalculia: local diagnostic value. *Arch NeurPsych*. 1940;44(2):398-408.

120. Rusconi E, et al. A disconnection account of Gerstmann syndrome: functional neuroanatomy evidence. *Ann Neurol*. 2009;66(5):654-662.

121. Herdman KA, et al. Impoverished descriptions of familiar routes in three cases of hippocampal/medial temporal lobe amnesia. *Cortex*. 2015;71:248-263.

122. Epstein RA. Parahippocampal and retrosplenial contributions to human spatial navigation. *Trends Cogn Sci*. 2008;12(10):388-396.

123. Aguirre GK, D'Esposito M. Topographical disorientation: a synthesis and taxonomy. *Brain*. 1999;122(pt 9):1613-1628.

124. Bar M, et al. Top-down facilitation of visual recognition. *Proc Natl Acad Sci U S A*. 2006;103(2):449-454.

125. Moritz CH, et al. Functional MRI neuroanatomic correlates of the Hooper Visual Organization Test. *J Int Neuropsychol Soc*. 2004;10(7):939-947.

126. Irish M, et al. Scene construction impairments in Alzheimer's disease—a unique role for the posterior cingulate cortex. *Cortex*. 2015;73:10-23.

127. Darby RR, et al. Finding the imposter: brain connectivity of lesions causing delusional misidentifications. *Brain*. 2016; 140(2):497-507.

128. De Ridder D, et al. Visualizing out-of-body experience in the brain. 2007;357(18):1829-1833.

129. Blanke O, et al. Out-of-body experience and autoscopy of neurological origin. *Brain*. 2004;127(2):243-258.

130. Baker MG, Kale R, Menken M. The wall between neurology and psychiatry. *BMJ*. 2002;324(7352):1468-1469.

13

Functional Neurological Symptom Disorder

Gaston Baslet · Mary A. O'Neal · Barbara A. Dworetzky

INTRODUCTION AND DEFINITIONS

Patients with medically unexplained symptoms (MUS) are commonly seen in all medical practices, especially in neurology and psychiatry. MUS comprise up to one-third of new referrals to an ambulatory neurology clinic.[1] Many of these patients suffer from a functional neurological symptom disorder (FNSD), a type of somatic symptom disorder also called conversion disorder or functional neurological disorder (FND). MUS is a term that implies physical complaints without a clear physiological explanation. However, in its diagnostic criteria, the *DSM-5* de-emphasizes the issue of pathogenesis to avoid grounding the diagnosis in the absence of such explanation.

Per *DSM-5* criteria, somatic symptom disorder is diagnosed when a physical symptom is the primary complaint and there is accompanying psychobehavioral criteria (excessive thinking, behaviors, and/or emotional responses) related to the primary somatic symptom. To meet *DSM-5* diagnostic criteria, patients need to have one or more somatic symptoms for a duration of at least 6 months. There may or may not be a medically diagnosed condition to explain the somatic symptoms.[2] Further, these symptoms are distressing and result in significant impairment.[3] It has been estimated that somatic symptom disorders account for an estimated 256 billion dollars/year in medical expenditures in the United States.[4]

FNSD is a disorder in which the somatic complaint consists of neurologic symptoms. Per *DSM-5* diagnostic criteria, FNSD symptoms involve altered voluntary motor or sensory function. Cognitive complaints of a functional nature (also called "cogniform" symptoms) are not included in the *DSM-5* diagnostic criteria for FNSD, although they are frequently encountered in clinical practice and have been described in the neuropsychology literature.[5] The diagnosis of FNSD is based on demonstrating that the neurologic symptom is not consistent with an alteration in the normal physiology of the nervous system, and not better explained by another medical or mental disorder. Presence of a psychological stressor or psychobehavioral criteria is not required for a diagnosis of FNSD.[2]

In this chapter, we will discuss the epidemiology, pathophysiology, clinical presentation as well as the appropriate assessment, differential diagnosis, and treatment for patients with FNSD. The discussion will include FNSDs that present with continuous symptoms, such as functional movement disorder or functional weakness, and paroxysmal "spells" known as psychogenic non-epileptic seizures (PNES), the most common subset of FNSD. Although patients with FNSD with episodic neurologic complaints share significant disability and features with those who suffer from constant symptoms, they present differently to a unique set of clinicians requiring evaluations and treatments that are distinct. There is no evidence that patients with FNSD are feigning their symptoms and there is increasingly convincing evidence that FNSD is a disorder that arises from changes in the normal function of the brain.

EPIDEMIOLOGY

Incidence and Prevalence

It is difficult to obtain accurate incidence rates due to the varied definitions for FNSD and the differences in the populations studied. In addition, estimates are likely low given the stigma and misunderstanding associated with the disorder as well as lack of knowledge and reluctance on the part of clinicians to make a definitive diagnosis and convey it with confidence to the patient. Despite these limitations, a review of studies provides an overall incidence rate of 4–12/100,000 per year.[6] In a study of 3781 ambulatory referrals to a neurology clinic in the United Kingdom, 16% were diagnosed during the initial neurology visit with FNSD, becoming the second most common diagnosis of newly referred patients after headache.[7] The incidence rate for PNES in the general U.S. population has been reported as 1.4–4.9 per 100,000.[8,9] PNES accounts for 7.4% of new neurology visits to a large ambulatory practice.[10] The prevalence in the U.S. population of FNSD is approximately 50 per 100,000[6] and for PNES it is 2–33 per 100,000.[11] For those presenting to epilepsy monitoring units (EMUs) with drug-resistant seizures, approximately 20–40% of adults[12,13] and 10–23% of children are ultimately diagnosed with PNES,[14] with the majority at some point reporting a markedly prolonged seizure-like episode.[15]

Risk Factors

Women outnumber men diagnosed with FNSD in a ratio of 2–3:1. When comparing different subtypes of FNSD, PNES usually presents with a higher female-to-male ratio (3:1) than functional movement disorder (1.5–3:1).[16] Late-onset PNES (defined as having onset after age 55) is seen more evenly distributed between the sexes.[17] Although FNSD can occur at any age, onset most commonly occurs between 35 and 50 years of age,[18] with PNES presenting earlier (mid-20s) than other subtypes of FNSD.[16] PNES rarely occurs below the age of 6 years.[19] In one study of patients presenting to an Australian outpatient neurologic clinic, FNSD patients were significantly younger with an average age of 45 compared to those presenting for other neurologic diagnoses, who had an average age of 56.[20] Another study comparing patients with a motor manifestation of FNSD to those who had a structural neurological disorder causing weakness, showed no difference in age of onset, marital status, or socioeconomic background between the two groups.[21]

Having a neurologic diagnosis is a risk factor for FNSD. There is no single category of neurologic disease which is more likely to have an associated FNSD. Stone and colleagues[22] found that 12% of patients with an established neurologic diagnosis (excluding headache) had neurologic symptoms somewhat or not at all explained by that disease. Thus, patients may present with a combination of neurologic symptoms (both organic/structural and functional).[23] In the subset of patients diagnosed with PNES, more than 40% have comorbid neurologic conditions,[24] with 10–20% having comorbid epilepsy.[25,26] In those patients with PNES and comorbid epilepsy, the epilepsy diagnosis is usually established more than a decade earlier than the PNES diagnosis.[13] Other common medical risk factors in PNES are mild traumatic brain injury, prior neurosurgery,[27] intellectual/learning disability,[28] substance use disorders, headache, chronic pain syndromes, and other MUS.[29]

Psychiatric comorbidities, including depression, anxiety, post-traumatic stress disorder (PTSD), personality disorders, and dissociative disorders are common.[30] Prior traumatic experiences are common in patients with FNSD. Rates of traumatic experiences in FNSD are significantly higher than in the general population, and most studies indicate that at least a third of FNSD patients report such histories.[31] Physical and sexual abuse are the most commonly reported type of trauma[31] with women having higher rates than men.[32–34] Stressful life events (including trauma, emotional neglect, and other stressful experiences) are highly associated with FNSD, at a frequency significantly higher than in healthy, neurological, and psychiatric control groups.[35] PNES may be associated with a higher rate of sexual abuse compared to other subtypes of FNSD.[36] Personality characteristics (such as ineffective emotion processing and interpersonal styles, alexithymia, avoidance tendencies, illness, and health misperceptions) and environmental factors (such as family discord, losses, work-related stressors) are commonly present in FNSD patients, as long-standing predisposing vulnerabilities and/or as singular precipitating factors.[37] School problems and being victims of bullying are commonly reported in children with PNES.[38–40]

Risk factors have been found to vary by age in PNES. In one study, patients with juvenile onset PNES were found to have suffered from a greater degree of abuse during childhood (but not specifically greater degree of physical or sexual abuse), school failure or bullying, and family or personal history of epilepsy, whereas in those with adult onset PNES medical comorbidities were more common.[41] Some studies on pediatric PNES have shown that the rates of physical and sexual abuse did not differ from controls,[42] pointing to a contrast with adults with PNES.

PATHOPHYSIOLOGY

Figure 13-1 summarizes a biopsychosocial model with the many predisposing, precipitating, and perpetuating factors that contribute to the development of FNSD.[37] There is no one single factor that explains the development of FNSD but rather an interaction of several factors over time. Case Vignette 13.1 illustrates an initial precipitating event of a traumatic experience leading to onset of chronic pain symptoms and recurrent PNES, in the context of avoidance strategies to cope with the initial insult.

CASE VIGNETTE 13.1

A 28-year-old woman presents to a neurologist with complaints of seizure-like episodes that have been present for 6 months. This is the third recurrence of such episodes (which previously occurred for a period of 6 months, at age 18 and at age 22). At those times, the episodes resolved on their own and the patient sought no care. The seizure-like episodes consist of a feeling of lightheadedness followed by a sense of distancing from the environment, inability to talk coherently, side-to-side head shaking, and eye fluttering. The duration is about 2–3 minutes, after which the patient is exhausted but aware of what happened. Current frequency is on average every other day. Physical pain tends to be a trigger for the episodes.

Past medical history includes a diagnosis of fibromyalgia since age 18, chronic generalized anxiety, past episodes of major depression (denies current symptoms). At age 18, the patient was in a physically abusive relationship, but she denies PTSD symptoms from it. She dedicated her life to advocate for women with trauma based on this experience. During the initial evaluation the patient said "I never had to go to therapy; helping others in a similar situation was my way of coping and forgetting about what had happened to me."

Medication: Duloxetine for fibromyalgia and anxiety.

Neurological exam and brain imaging are unremarkable. The patient underwent a long-term video-EEG monitoring and on day #2 of her monitoring, she experienced a typical episode which shows an identical semiology as described above, with no electrographic correlate.

A diagnosis of PNES was made based on the captured typical episode on video-EEG with semiology of PNES and lack of electrographic change from a normal awake rhythm.

The diagnosis was explained to the patient. The predisposing, precipitating, and perpetuating factors identified in her history were highlighted as facilitating the expression

of her functional neurological episodes. She expressed relief that she did not have epilepsy and without prompting, she was able to connect her traumatic past to the onset of her episodes and asked if her chronic pain could also be a "psychosomatic" reaction to what had happened to her.

She started cognitive-behavioral therapy for PNES. After 10 sessions, she reported cessation of her PNES events and marked reduction of her pain and anxiety symptoms.

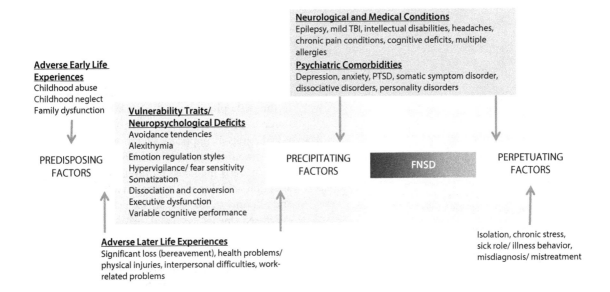

FIGURE 13-1. Risk factors in FNSD. Multiple factors are associated to FNSD including vulnerability traits/neuropsychological deficits, adverse life experiences, and psychiatric comorbidities and neurological and medical conditions. These factors interact at different time points as predisposing, precipitating, and/or perpetuating. (Reproduced with permission from Baslet G, Seshadri A, Bermeo-Ovalle A, et al. Psychogenic non-epileptic seizures: an updated primer. *Psychosomatics.* 2016;57(1):1–17. Copyright © 2016. Elsevier. https://www.sciencedirect.com/journal/psychosomatics.)

Different psychological and cognitive theories offer hypothetical mechanisms for FNSD. The classical Freudian hypothesis is based on the presumption that intolerable affect or intrapsychic conflict is "converted" into neurological symptoms (therefore the name "conversion disorder"). A dissociative hypothesis, originally postulated by Pierre Janet, conceptualizes FNSD as a disorder where dissociative mechanisms, such as compartmentalization and detachment, are originally adaptive, usually in the face of traumatic experiences. These mechanisms, however, become dysfunctional over time. According to the dissociative hypothesis, FNSD is an "autosuggestive disorder," with symptoms akin to those seen in hypnotic states.

A modern cognitive model hypothesis explains FNSD as resulting from an alteration in the allocation of attentional resources to certain sensory states (self-focus), and the activation of a dysfunctional expectation about sensory and motor function. The increased attention to the body and maladaptive expectation about neurological function lead to the development of functional neurological symptoms. The symptoms themselves lead to avoidance and other behavioral changes that reinforce and perpetuate symptoms and may lead to disability. This cascade of cognitive and behavioral processes is postulated to be precipitated by a triggering event and possibly facilitated by preexisting factors

such as prior experiences, maladaptive cognitive interpretations, learning models, or hardwired tendencies.[43,44] Figure 13-2 illustrates the cognitive hypothesis of FNSD.[45]

Electromyography studies show normal function of the primary pathways (motor efferent and sensory afferent pathways). Cortical inhibitory processes (or their impairment) are presumed to alter motor and sensory functions in FNSD. For instance, smaller motor evoked potentials were detected in patients with functional paresis compared to healthy controls during motor imagery tasks,[46] possibly indicating inhibition of corticospinal excitability during the task.

Alterations in the autonomic nervous system in PNES include lower heart rate variability, which signals lower parasympathetic activity at baseline, compared to healthy controls,[47] and variable sympathetic hyperarousal compared to epilepsy controls.[48] The lower baseline parasympathetic activity at baseline signals stress vulnerability and indicates restoration of the organism is less likely to occur during periods of reduced stress.[48]

Structural and functional imaging provide insight into the brain changes associated to FNSD. Volumetric magnetic resonance imaging (MRI) studies show evidence of differences in the anatomy of both cortical and subcortical brain regions in patients with FNSD compared to healthy controls; however,

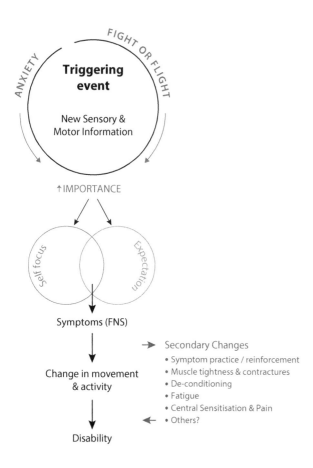

FIGURE 13-2. Cognitive model hypothesis of FNSD. (FNS, functional neurological symptoms.) (Reproduced with permission from Nielsen G, Ricciardi L, Demartini B, et al. Outcomes of a 5-day physiotherapy programme for functional (psychogenic) motor disorder. *J Neurol*. 2015; 262(3):674–681. Copyright © 2015. Springer Nature. https://www.springer.com/journal/415)

studies are limited, have varied methodologies and need replication. Some of the observed morphological changes include increased thickness in premotor cortex and decreased volumes in subcortical nuclei in functional motor disorders,[49–51] and cortical atrophy in the right motor and premotor regions and bilateral cerebellar atrophy in PNES.[52]

Functional neuroimaging, such as functional MRI, reveals differences in activity and connectivity between brain regions compared to healthy controls. Such functional alterations are reported in FNSD within (activity) and between (functional connectivity) brain areas involved in body awareness and emotion processing (insula, amygdala), self-monitoring (ventromedial prefrontal cortex [VMPFC]), cognitive control (dorsolateral prefrontal cortex [DLPFC], dorsal anterior cingulate cortex [dACC], inferior frontal gyrus), self-referential processing (temporoparietal junction [TPJ]/supramarginal gyrus) and motor intention, initiation, and inhibition (supplemental motor area [SMA]).[53]

Increased functional connectivity has been demonstrated between emotional and premotor regions (specifically amygdala and SMA) during emotion-laden tasks, and between VMPFC and motor cortex. Increased activity in the amygdala and insula at different stages of motor planning have also been documented in motor FNSD. These findings suggest a role for arousal, subjective interoception and self-monitoring processes in the pathophysiology of FNSD. Lower TPJ activity in functional tremor and lower supramarginal gyrus activity in functional paralysis implicate alterations at the level of agency and sensorimotor integration in FNSD. Other higher-order cognitive processes mediated by the DLPFC (such as intention and attention) and dACC (involved in inhibition, action monitoring, and response to conflict) are likely implicated in motor FNSD as decreased (for DLPFC) and increased activity (for dACC) have been demonstrated in functional paralysis, along with variable findings regarding connectivity between DLPFC and SMA.[54]

The neurobiology of FNSD is in the early stages of being understood. Alterations at the levels of sensory, cognitive, emotional, and motor complex processing are implicated in the disorder. Figure 13-3 offers a hypothetical pathophysiological model based on the most commonly replicated findings from functional neuroimaging studies.

CLINICAL PRESENTATION AND ASSESSMENT

The phenomenology of FNSD varies widely. Patients may present with continuous neurologic symptoms or paroxysmal episodes mimicking seizures. Symptoms of weakness, pain, paresthesia, dizziness, tremor, dystonia, visual loss, double vision and cognitive complaints are common. In each case, the diagnosis is made by demonstrating the symptom as physiologically incompatible with neurological function (or dysfunction). Table 13-1 lists neurological examination findings that can help confirm a diagnosis of FNSD, many of which were present in Case Vignette 13.2.[16,55,56]

CASE VIGNETTE 13.2

A 31-year-old woman presented to the emergency department after she awoke with right eye pain, visual blurring, right-sided weakness, and numbness one day after running a road race. She also endorsed numbness in her hands and feet, balance difficulty, and falling. She was admitted to the neurology inpatient unit.

Past medical history included a history of joint pain for which she was taking colchicine and acetaminophen. She had no prior psychiatric history.

Medications: Acetaminophen, colchicine, oral contraceptive pill

On examination: She was alert and cooperative. Her optic disks were sharp. Her cranial nerves were intact II–XII, no difficulty with visual acuity, no afferent pupillary defect. On strength testing, she had diffuse give-away weakness on the right side. Her reflexes were 2+ and symmetric without a Babinski response. When asked to lift her right leg, there was no activation of the left hamstring muscles (a positive

Hoover's sign). Sensory exam was intact to all modalities. Her coordination was normal. On gait testing, she had difficulty initiating movement and veered to either side. Her walking ability improved when she walked faster or was asked to pretend to ice-skate.

Brain magnetic resonance imaging (MRI) with gadolinium showed minimal nonspecific white matter abnormalities without enhancement. Cervical MRI with and without contrast was normal. MRI of her thoracic spine showed a small syrinx from thoracic levels 4–11.

A diagnosis of FNSD was made based on the positive findings on the neurologic exam including the give-away weakness, positive Hoover's sign, and the abnormal gait which improved with distraction and more difficult tasks of ambulation. These signs were all explained to the patient as supporting the diagnosis of FNSD.

Both the white matter abnormalities and the small thoracic syrinx were felt to be incidental and did not explain her symptoms.

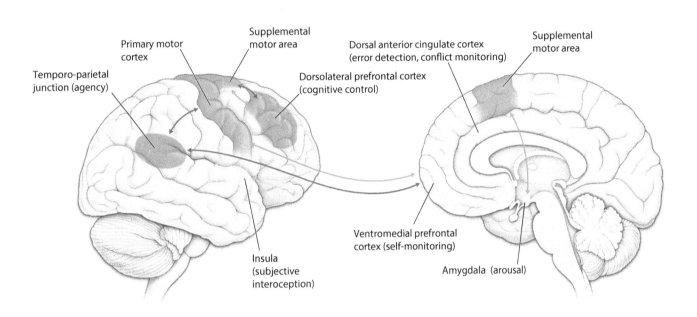

FIGURE 13-3. Pathophysiological model of FNSD based on functional neuroimaging studies. Green areas: brain regions with increased activity; red areas: brain regions with decreased activity; green arrows: connection between two areas that have increased functional connectivity; red arrows: connection between two areas that have decreased functional connectivity. The increased/decreased activity or functional connectivity is observed in FNSD subjects in relation to control subjects or control conditions and based on various functional neuroimaging studies.

In the case of seizure complaints, the neurological exam may be entirely normal. PNES should be suspected in patients with drug-resistant seizures in which multiple electroencephalographic (EEGs) examinations have been normal. The most typical presentation for PNES is loss of consciousness without motor findings,[57] but also common are out-of-phase, side-to-side prolonged shaking episodes with closed eyes, or unexplained sudden drop attacks.[58] The patient in Case Vignette 13.1 presents with a semiology very suggestive of PNES. There are proposed levels of diagnostic certainty for PNES, supported by the International League Against Epilepsy (ILAE), that take into account history, phenomenology, and electrophysiological findings (Table 13-2).[59] When episodes are frequent and resources are available, the "gold standard" for establishing the diagnosis of PNES is to record events typical for the patient on video with synchronous EEG monitoring demonstrating no epileptic correlate and that the events are atypical for any type of epileptic seizure. Prolactin levels drawn within 20 minutes of an episode

have been used to help assess whether an event is epileptic or not, however, this test has a low negative predictive value and a high false positive rate.[60,61]

In addition to a careful neurological examination, the initial evaluation should include a screening for psychiatric comorbidities and other psychosocial risk factors, as enumerated in the previous section. The patients' descriptions of their neurological symptoms may uncover panic/anxiety or dissociative symptoms as part of their experience with neurological symptoms.[62] In Case Vignette 13.1, the patient reports an experience of distancing that indicates the presence of dissociation in the context of other seizure-like symptoms. Patients with PNES have a difficult time providing details of their seizure-like episodes, offering more information on the place or state they were in rather than specific symptoms of the seizure-like episode, a linguistic characteristic termed "focusing resistance."[63]

It is common for FNSD symptoms to have an abrupt onset as demonstrated in Case Vignette 13.2. The varied

TABLE 13-1 • Neurological Examination Findings That Help Confirm the Diagnosis of FNSD

Sign	Sensitivity and Specificity	Definition	Example/Comments
Motor			
Variable strength (collapsing/give-away weakness)	Sensitivity: 63% Specificity: 97%	As the examiner applies different levels of force, the patient varies their resistance.	Limb collapses from a normal position with a light touch or normal strength is developed and then suddenly collapses (or gives way).
Hoover sign	Sensitivity: 94% Specificity: 99%	Hip extension weakness returns to normal with contralateral hip flexion against resistance.	Examiner compares felt pressure in his/her hand under weak leg's heel when weak leg pushes downward versus when normal leg pushes upward. Positive sign: less strength when weak leg pushing downward.
Motor inconsistency	Sensitivity: 13% Specificity: 98%	Inability to perform a certain movement, while performing a different movement using the same muscle is possible.	For example, weakness of ankle plantar flexion on bed, but patient able to walk on tiptoes; patient can rise from chair but unable to lift either leg off the exam table.
Co-contraction	Sensitivity: 17% Specificity: 100%	Simultaneous contraction of agonist and antagonist muscles resulting in no/little movement.	For example, when asked to flex the elbow, both biceps and triceps are activated (note: excessive antagonist activation also observed in spastic patients).
Hemiparesis in a non-cortical spinal pattern	Not validated	Weakness is equally distributed in all muscle groups (compared to upper motor neuron weakness pattern, where weakness is seen in flexors>extensors in leg and extensor>flexors in arm).	All muscles are weak, without specific pattern.
Babinski trunk-thigh test	Not validated	Lack of asymmetry between weak and normal side when attempting to sit up (compared to physiologic weakness where paretic leg will elevate and contralateral shoulder moves forward).	Patient is in supine position, with arms across chest and is asked to sit up.
Tremor			
Entrainment	Sensitivity: 91% Specificity: 91%	The tremor frequency switches to match the frequency of a voluntary rhythmical movement performed by the unaffected limb.	Patient with a unilateral tremor is asked to copy a rhythmic movement with the unaffected limb. The tremor in the affected hand either "entrains" to the rhythm of the unaffected hand, stops completely, or the patient is unable to copy the simple rhythmic movement.
Distraction	Sensitivity: 92% Specificity: 94%	The tremor changes when the examiner has the patient engage in cognitively distracting tasks.	For example, patient is asked to count backward and examiner observes change in frequency, amplitude, or rhythm of the tremor.
Variability	Sensitivity: 22% Specificity: 92%	The characteristics of the tremor (e.g., amplitude) vary during the exam.	
Sensory			
Non-anatomical sensory loss	Sensitivity: 74% Specificity: 100%	Diminished sensation that fits a non-dermatomal pattern.	For example, sensation normalizes at hip or shoulder, unilateral glove, or sock distribution.
Midline splitting	Sensitivity: 20% Specificity: 93%	Exact splitting of sensation in the midline.	The sensory nerves do not end exactly at the midline.
Splitting of vibration	Sensitivity: 95% Specificity: 14%	Difference in the sensation of a tuning fork placed over the left compared to the right side of the sternum or frontal bone.	The frontalis is a single bone, so vibration sense should be the same bilaterally.
Gait			
Dragging leg	Sensitivity: 8.4% Specificity: 100%	The leg is dragged at the hip behind the body.	In patient with cortical-spinal weakness, patients perform a circumduction of the leg.

(continued)

TABLE 13-1 • Neurological Examination Findings That Help Confirm the Diagnosis of FNSD (Continued)

Sign	Sensitivity and Specificity	Definition	Example/Comments
Excessively slow gait	Not validated	Slowness is observed in all aspects of gait.	Patients with bradykinesia display the most prominent slowness with gait initiation.
			Orthopedic patients can walk slowly to avoid pain.
Psychogenic Romberg	Not validated	Consistently falls toward or away from the examiner when performing Romberg test. Large amplitude body sway after a silent latency of a few seconds and improvement of balance with distraction.	
Non-economic posture (sometimes labelled astasia-abasia)	Not validated	A walking pattern that requires considerable effort as well as balance to maintain the posture (e.g., walking with knees flexed).	For example, knee buckling without a fall requires more strength at knee flexors.

TABLE 13-2 • Diagnostic Levels of Certainty for Psychogenic Non-epileptic Seizures (PNES)

Diagnostic Level	History	Witnessed Event	EEG
Possible	+	By witness or self-report/description	No epileptiform activity in routine or sleep-deprived interictal EEG
Probable	+	By clinician who reviewed video recording or in person, showing semiology typical of PNES	No epileptiform activity in routine or sleep-deprived interictal EEG
Clinically established	+	By clinician experienced in diagnosis of seizure disorders (on video or in person), showing semiology typical of PNES, while not on EEG	No epileptiform activity in routine or ambulatory ictal EEG during a typical ictus/event in which the semiology would make ictal epileptiform EEG activity expected during equivalent epileptic seizures
Documented	+	By clinician experienced in diagnosis of seizure disorders, showing semiology typical of PNES, while on video EEG	No epileptiform activity immediately before, during, or after ictus captured on ictal video EEG with typical PNES semiology

Source: LaFrance WC, Baker GA, Duncan R, Goldstein LH and Reuber M. Minimum requirements for the diagnosis of psychogenic nonepileptic seizures: A staged approach: A report from the International League Against Epilepsy Nonepileptic Seizures Task Force. Epilepsia. 2013;54(11):2005–2018. Reprinted with permission. Copyright © 2013. Wiley Periodicals, International League Against Epilepsy.

clinical presentations of the disorder and the number of different involved clinicians make the diagnosis of FNSD challenging. However, the diagnosis can be made accurately with low error rates.[64] Common mistakes can occur when clinicians do not consider the diagnosis in patients without significant psychiatric comorbidities (false negatives). Other common errors (false positives) include erroneously diagnosing FNSD in psychiatric patients or missing an underlying neurologic problem—including epilepsy—in someone with comorbid FNSD.

Assessment and Differential Diagnosis

The assessment of a patient with FNSD will vary depending on the presentation. For example, functional motor weakness would need to be distinguished from other causes of weakness including disorders involving the corticospinal tract, anterior horn cell, radiculopathies, plexopathies, peripheral nerve, neuromuscular junction, and muscle disorders. The initial evaluation should be thorough and tailored to exclude the likeliest possibilities. Experts in FNSD advocate that demonstrating to the patient how you know that their nervous system is intact is extremely helpful.[65] In Case Vignette 13.2, the positive Hoover's sign was demonstrated to the patient and she was educated on its meaning. The fact that her gait improved with more complex tasks such as skating and walking fast was inconsistent with a structural neurologic disorder. Referring patients to verified online resources (such as www.neurosymptoms.org, www.fndhope.org, and www.nonepilepticseizures.com) and providing educational materials can help reinforce the diagnosis and further limit skepticism.

In the case of PNES, observing an episode with typical semiology of PNES can provide a high level of certainty without capturing an event on video synchronized with EEG.[59] However, removing anticonvulsants and providing a careful team evaluation in the EMU allows for greater certainty and better outcomes[66] for those with frequent drug-resistant seizures. There

TABLE 13-3 • Comparison of Findings Between PNES and Epileptic Seizures

	PNES	Epileptic Seizures
Occurs out of sleep	No (pseudo-sleep)	Can occur
Sensation of dizziness, olfactory sensation, or numbness	Can be seen	Can be seen
Eyes	More commonly closed	More commonly opened
Significant bodily injury (broken bones, burns, etc.)	Not common	Relatively more common
Tongue biting	Anterior tip of the tongue	Lateral aspect of the tongue
Pelvic thrusting	Can be seen	Can be seen (frontal lobe seizures)
Duration	Can be prolonged	Short if frontal lobe
Ictal weeping	Yes	Unlikely
Urinary incontinence	Can be seen	Can be seen

Source: Rathod J, Benbadis S. Diagnostic challenges for the neurologist. In: Dworetzky B, Baslet G, eds. Psychogenic Nonepileptic Seizures: Towards the Integration of Care. New York, NY: Oxford University Press; 2017:123–138. Reprinted with permission of Oxford Publishing Limited through PLSclear.

are challenges associated with solely relying on a video-EEG captured event to confirm the diagnosis of PNES, such as the inability to capture a typical episode during the monitoring period and a normal EEG during an event without altered consciousness, which may occur with some focal seizures. Communicating the diagnosis of PNES can also prove challenging especially to those with definite comorbid epilepsy, alternate views of cause of the seizures, and those with intellectual disability. The most common differential diagnoses of PNES are convulsive syncope and epilepsy, especially of frontal lobe origin. Semiological features that can help distinguish PNES from epileptic seizures and PNES specifically from frontal lobe seizures are listed in Tables 13-3 and 13-4 respectively.[67] Signs with the greatest specificity in favor of PNES include long duration, fluctuating course, asynchronous movements, pelvic thrusting, side-to-side head or body movements, closed eyes, and ictal crying, whereas stertorous breathing, events occurring during EEG confirmed sleep and postictal confusion are highly specific for epileptic seizures.[68] In addition, evidence suggests that preserved memory for items presented during the event may assist in distinguishing PNES from epileptic seizures.[68] Many of the semiological signs discussed here are also described in Case Vignette 13.1.

Neuropsychological evaluation can be helpful in those patients with associated cognitive complaints. The patient's effort during neurocognitive testing can be determined by assessing performance validity, which reveals greater variability in PNES compared to epilepsy controls. Neuropsychological evaluation may also help identify some of the risk factors previously enumerated as well as personality profiles highly suggestive of FNSD.[69]

In addition to screening for well-known predisposing, precipitating, and perpetuating biopsychosocial risk factors,[37] the mental status exam of patients with FNSD may show some distinguishing features. For instance, using certain linguistic

TABLE 13-4 • Comparison of Findings Between PNES and Frontal Lobe Seizures

	PNES	Frontal Lobe Seizures
Seizure duration	Tend to be prolonged (>5 minutes)	Short (<30 seconds)
Events out of EEG-verified sleep	Never	Common
Flipping (supine to prone or prone to supine)	Can be seen	Almost never
Eyes	Closed	Open
Eye deviation	Geotropic*	Versive**
Pelvic thrusting	Can be seen	Very rare
Opisthotonic posturing	Common	Never
Bicycling/kicking	Can be seen	Very rare
Side-to-side head shaking	Common	Almost never
Tonic posturing	Not seen	Common
Clonic movements	Not seen	Common
Ictal grasping	Rare	May be seen
Intact awareness with bilateral motor activity	Common	Rare

*Geotropic eye movements occur when eyes deviate downward toward the side that the head is turned.

**Versive movement refers to the typically sustained and involuntary lateral head and eye deviation due to tonic contraction of head and eye muscles during a seizure.

Source: Rathod J, Benbadis S. Diagnostic challenges for the Neurologist. In: Dworetzky B, Baslet G, eds. Psychogenic Nonepileptic Seizures: Towards the integration of care. New York, NY: Oxford University Press; 2017:123–138. Reprinted with permission of Oxford Publishing Limited through PLSclear.

characteristics to describe symptoms (in PNES, patients provide less detail about the seizure experience itself and more about the circumstances and context surrounding the episodes), avoiding emotion-laden discussions, and having multiple other somatic complaints should alert clinicians on the possibility of FNSD as it pertains to the primary neurological complaint. None of these clinical observations, however, should be used as grounds to confirm the diagnosis, which should follow *DSM-5* criteria.

Course and Natural History

There is little information on the course and natural history of FNSD, but what is known suggests that the outcomes, including quality of life and return to gainful employment, are poor. This paucity of data is due to the relative lack of large-scale prospective trials, the poor adherence to psychiatric treatment,[70] and the frequent movement of patients from clinician to clinician in search of another explanation for their symptoms. In addition, there is some evidence that medical utilization may decrease for patients with PNES after video-EEG established diagnosis, but other somatic symptoms may continue or appear, and patients remain economically dependent.[71] For PNES, poor outcomes are correlated with comorbid epilepsy and psychiatric illness, more dramatic seizure semiology, and younger age of onset, while better outcomes have been correlated with accepting the diagnosis, higher education, shorter duration of illness, employment, and good social supports. Participation in psychotherapy treatment is associated to improved PNES frequency 1–2 years after diagnosis.[72] Seizure complaints continued in more than 70% of patients and more than 56% remained disabled after diagnosis was confirmed a mean of 4 years prior. In a long-term study of patients with FNSD, 83% of patients with either motor or sensory FNSD reported persistent symptoms a median of 12 years after initial diagnosis.[64] Other studies following patients with PNES show continued high rates of disability.[71] FNSD patients' degree of disability has been linked to continuing symptoms[73] and has been compared to that of patients with multiple sclerosis.[2] Most outcome studies in FNSD have not considered the use of evidence-based treatments. Once such treatments become commonplace in medical practice, it is hoped that outcome rates may improve.

TREATMENT

Communication of the Diagnosis and Engagement in Treatment

When FNSD is highly suspected and definitely once the diagnosis is confirmed, patients should be openly informed about FNSD. Communication of the diagnosis can lead to improvement in symptom severity[74] and medical utilization[75,76] for a subset of patients. It remains unclear for how long this initial improvement after diagnosis can be sustained without further intervention, or whether other functional symptoms may replace the original symptom over time.

Many communication strategies have been described on how to inform patients of their diagnosis.[77] Some of the most frequently emphasized elements during these communication strategies include: (1) reassure patients that the symptoms are genuine and not considered fake; (2) provide a name for the disorder and explain how the diagnosis was (or would be) confirmed; (3) highlight predisposing, precipitating, and perpetuating factors, and a mechanism for the disease; (4) state that there are treatments that work. The explanation about the disease mechanism typically consists of providing a model where the predisposing, precipitating, and perpetuating factors affect the brain, thus producing the symptoms. For instance, clinicians may say that the brain becomes overloaded and shuts down, causing the symptoms.[77] Acceptance of the diagnosis and subsequent engagement in treatment are important goals of the diagnosis communication strategy. The patient in Case Vignette 13.1 accepted the diagnosis of PNES and understood the interaction of the different factors that led to her symptoms.

Many patients with FNSD have a difficult time adhering to treatment recommendations, as shown by a longitudinal study of adherence rates to psychiatric treatment in PNES.[70] Multidisciplinary collaboration is essential during the treatment planning phase and necessary throughout treatment. The diagnosing neurologist should remain available after the diagnosis is established, ensuring that patients follow through with the recommended treatment. Specific tasks for the neurologist include management of comorbid neurologic conditions (such as headaches or epileptic seizures), management or taper of medications (for instance, removing AEDs in patients with lone PNES), and providing recommendations related to work and driving restrictions.[78]

Motivational interviewing (MI) is an intervention designed to engage patient's intrinsic motivation to generate change; it may help improve adherence to psychotherapy post PNES diagnosis.[79]

Evidence-Based Treatment

Psychotherapy

Compared to other neuropsychiatric disorders, evidence-based treatments for FNSD remain limited. The most robust evidence comes from psychotherapy interventions.

Cognitive-behavioral therapy (CBT) is usually superior to standard medical care (SMC) in somatoform disorders (the former nomenclature for what is now called somatic symptom and related disorders),[80,81] with benefits that are of small effect size and most noticeable over time.[81] When applied specifically to FNSD, most CBT programs consist of the following elements: (1) education about the disorder and the stress response cycle, (2) training on stress management techniques, (3) incorporation of new behaviors that address avoidance patterns, and (4) identification and change of unhelpful thought patterns that reinforce symptoms. Randomized trials show efficacy of CBT in PNES treatment.[82-84] The CODES trial is a multicenter randomized controlled trial (RCT) that showed significant sustained reduction (at 12 months) in a number of secondary outcome measures with CBT (12 sessions) compared to standard medical care (SMC). It did not show PNES frequency difference at 12 months.[84] CBT can also help with reduction of associated comorbidities, as illustrated in Case Vignette 13.1. The use of a self-guided CBT booklet showed significant reduction in functional neurological symptom burden at 3 and 6 months when compared to SMC.[85] CBT treatment workbooks that have been validated in randomized clinical trials in FNSD can be recommended to patients and mental health providers.[86,87]

Other psychotherapeutic interventions studied in RCTs include a brief psychoeducational intervention for PNES,[88] manualized hypnosis for motor FNSD,[89,90] a multidisciplinary psychotherapy approach,[91] CBT plus physical exercise,[92] and other behavioral interventions for PNES that focused on

paradoxical intention (using imagery exposure to induce PNES)[93] and operant conditioning (positive reinforcement and punishment through withdrawal of privileges).[94] The latter two behavioral interventions proved superior to the control intervention despite limited sample sizes and some methodological variabilities.[93,94]

The details and outcomes of these RCTs for psychotherapeutic interventions are summarized in Table 13-5. Uncontrolled studies evaluated other types of psychotherapies with promising

TABLE 13-5 • Randomized and/or Controlled Trials in FNSD

Author, Year (Country)	N (Final Analysis); Clinical Population	Intervention/s	Design	Outcome
Ataoglu et al. (2003) (Turkey)	30; PNES	Paradoxical intention 2/day (inpatient, 3 weeks) vs. diazepam (outpatient, 6 weeks)	RCT	• Significantly better response rate in paradoxical intention group in terms of PNES remission and anxiety symptoms.
Moene et al. (2002) (Netherlands)	45; Motor FNSD	Inpatient manualized hypnosis (8 weekly sessions) vs. inpatient admission without hypnosis (8 weekly nonspecific sessions)—all received other similar inpatient treatments.	RCT	• Hypnosis did not provide additional benefit. • Both groups showed improvement in functional neurological symptoms at treatment end and at 6-month follow-up. • Improvement in psychopathology not specific to intervention group.
Moene et al. (2003) (Netherlands)	44; Motor FNSD	Weekly manualized hypnosis sessions (10 weeks) vs. wait list (3 months)	RCT	• Significant improvement in functional neurological symptoms and level of impairment in the hypnosis arm at treatment end and at 6-month follow-up. • No improvement in psychopathology.
Goldstein et al. (2010) (UK)	66; PNES	CBT (12 sessions) + standard medical care (SMC) vs. SMC alone	RCT	• Significant lower PNES frequency in CBT group at treatment end; trend toward significance at 6-month follow-up. • Mood and employment status showed no change. • Both groups with decrease in medical utilization.
LaFrance et al. (2010) (US)	33; PNES	Sertraline 25–200 mg daily vs. placebo for 12 weeks	Double-blind, placebo-controlled RCT	• No difference in PNES frequency between groups. • No difference in secondary measures. • Relative change in within-group event frequency (45% decline in event frequency in sertraline group vs. 8% increase in placebo group).
Sharpe et al. (2011) (UK)	125; Various FNSD	CBT Guided Self Help (plus maximum four 30-min guidance sessions) + SMC vs. SMC	RCT	• Overall health, functional neurological symptoms, and symptom burden improved further in intervention group at 3 months. • Functional neurological symptoms improvement maintained at 6 months, plus anxiety and physical function improvement at 6 months.
Aamir et al. (2011) (Pakistan)	15; PNES	Behavior therapy (15 sessions over 2 months) vs. routine outpatient treatment; both groups with 1 initial week of inpatient treatment	RCT	• Significant reduction in PNES frequency, depression, and anxiety scores in the behavior therapy group at last follow-up. • Behavior therapy group already had significantly lower PNES frequency after 1 week of same inpatient treatment.

TABLE 13-5 • Randomized and/or Controlled Trials in FNSD (Continued)				
Author, Year (Country)	N (Final Analysis); Clinical Population	Intervention/s	Design	Outcome
Czarnecki et al. (2012) (US)	120; Psychogenic motor disorder	Intensive outpatient rehabilitation program (PT and OT) 2/day for 5 days vs. historical controls not receiving treatment	Historical cohort controlled, non-randomized	• Patient and clinician with similar ratings of improvement in intervention (PT) group upon treatment completion. • Long-term outcome (2–3 years after diagnosis) was significantly better in intervention group in terms of symptom improvement and disability.
LaFrance et al. (2014) (US)	34; PNES	CBT-informed psychotherapy (CBT-ip, 12 sessions) vs. sertraline vs. CBT-ip+sertraline vs. treatment-as-usual	RCT	• Within-group analysis showed significant decline in PNES frequency in CBT-ip and CBT-ip + sertraline groups, but not in the other groups. • Improvement in many secondary measures in both CBT-ip arms. • No comparison between groups.
Chen et al. (2014) (US)	43; PNES	Psychoeducational meetings (1.5-hour long, monthly, 3 times) vs. routine seizure clinic	RCT	• No significant differences in PNES frequency between groups at treatment end or at 3-month follow-up. • Significant improvement in work and social adjustment scale in intervention (psychoeducation) group. • Trend toward decreased medical utilization in intervention group.
Jordbru et al. (2014) (Norway)	60; Psychogenic gait disorder	Inpatient PT (multidisciplinary approach) for 3 weeks immediately vs. 4 weeks after randomization	RCT, cross-over design	• Significant difference between treatment and no treatment in functional independence and mobility. • Improvements sustained at 1 month and 1 year after intervention for all participants.
Hubschmid et al. (2015) (Switzerland)	21; Psychogenic motor disorder and PNES	Interdisciplinary group psychotherapy (4–6 sessions) including 2 consultations with neurologist and psychiatrist vs. SMC	RCT	• Significant difference in improvement in the active arm for somatic dissociation, clinical improvement, overall psychopathology, and depression scores at 12-month follow-up. • Active arm did not show greater improvement in quality of life, and no difference between the groups regarding likelihood to accept psychiatric referral. • Subjects in active arm spent fewer days in hospital after intervention.
Dallochio et al. (2014) (Italy)	37; Psychogenic motor disorder	CBT + physical activity vs. CBT alone vs. SMC	RCT	• Improvement based on psychogenic movement rating scale in both active arms, with no difference between them. • No improvement in SMC arm.
Nielsen et al. (2017) (UK)	57; Psychogenic motor disorder	Outpatient specialized PT (over a 5-day program) vs. referral to local PT with letter	RCT	• Significant difference at 6 months in ratings of physical function and percentage of self-rated improvement. Differences between groups also noted in other mobility measures. • Control intervention not standardized.
Goldstein et al. (2020)	368; PNES	CBT + SMC vs. SMC	RCT	• Reduction in 2dary outcomes, CBT, 12 mo.

PNES, Psychogenic non-epileptic seizures; CBT, cognitive-behavioral therapy; CBT-ip, CBT-informed psychotherapy; SMC, standard medical care.

results. These include long-term interpersonal psychodynamic psychotherapy for PNES,[95] short-term psychodynamic psychotherapy for psychogenic movement disorders,[96] group psychotherapy for PNES,[97] prolonged exposure for PNES with comorbid PTSD,[98] mindfulness-based psychotherapy for PNES,[99] and inpatient programs.[100]

Physical Therapy

Physical therapy (PT) was proven effective in the treatment of motor and gait manifestations of FNSD.[101] PT educates patients about their condition, emphasizes their capacity for normal movement, and limits maladaptive motor responses. PT protocols for FNSD work under the premise that self-focused attention and illness expectation create and reinforce abnormal movements, therefore education, movement re-training, and emphasis on self-management are the basic principles of treatment.[45] A randomized cross-over controlled study of 3-week inpatient PT for psychogenic gait disorder showed sustained benefit 1 year after the program was completed.[102] An intensive outpatient PT program for psychogenic motor disorder (gait, movement disorder, and weakness) also demonstrated durable improvements when compared to historical or control interventions.[103,104] These interventions are further described in Table 13-5.

Pharmacological Treatment

The positive evidence for pharmacological treatment in FNSD comes from very few uncontrolled studies that evaluated the efficacy of antidepressants in psychogenic movement disorder and PNES, respectively.[105,106] The only double-blind, placebo-controlled RCT in PNES did not demonstrate sertraline to be superior to placebo (although the study may have been under-powered).[107] The addition of sertraline to CBT did not seem to confer further benefit in the treatment of PNES in a four-arm trial for PNES, also described in Table 13-5.[83] A few studies have demonstrated efficacy of newer-generation antidepressants compared to placebo in patients with a variety of somatic symptoms.[108] Choosing which antidepressant or anxiolytic medication is most appropriate when treating FNSD should be based on treatment of the identified psychiatric comorbidities, and not the FNSD itself. Clinical judgment should be used as to when it is appropriate to initiate medications to treat psychiatric comorbidities.

Noninvasive Stimulation Therapies

Evidence of effectiveness of noninvasive stimulation therapies in functional weakness consists primarily of case series or case reports that show benefit of electroconvulsive therapy (ECT) or repetitive transcranial magnetic stimulation (rTMS),[109] with the exception of two studies. One of them is an uncontrolled retrospective study of rTMS over the contralateral motor cortex in 70 subjects with functional paralysis, which showed immediate and sustained improvement in most subjects.[110] The other study included 11 subjects with functional paresis in a single-blinded placebo controlled cross-over proof-of-principle study of rTMS over the contralateral motor cortex. The study showed immediate significant improvement in objective muscle strength for those receiving the intervention.[111] A case series of seven subjects with PNES showed improvement in event frequency with rTMS over the right TPJ.[112]

In summary, the treatment toolbox for FNSD remains limited. Some interventions are effective, although this information is based on a few RCTs. Evidence also comes from low powered and uncontrolled studies. Unless psychiatric comorbidity is a concern, functional motor disorders that present with gait, weakness, or abnormal movements should be first treated with PT. Supplementation with CBT should be considered. In the specific case of PNES, CBT has the most robust evidence and should be considered a first-line treatment. Other forms of psychotherapy lack the evidence that CBT has, but may be considered on an individual basis. Psychopharmacological interventions should be limited to the treatment of comorbid psychiatric conditions. Stimulation therapies lack sufficient evidence for the treatment of FNSD at this point, but they are promising interventions that require future investigation.

FUTURE DIRECTIONS

There is much about FNSD that is not yet known. Certain life events, particularly traumatic ones, can make patients more vulnerable to develop FNSD. Functional MRI and volumetric studies are beginning to uncover the neurobiology of FNSD and the biology of stress has been implicated. However, it is not clear as to why a particular life event precipitates FNSD (vs. another neuropsychiatric symptom) or what determines the specific phenotype of FNSD. In addition, many of the factors that predict treatment responsiveness and effectiveness are unknown.

As more is understood in terms of the pathophysiology of FNSD, more targeted treatments will be developed and offered. At a practical level, integrated care can help facilitate early engagement in treatment and possibly limit the long-term functional impact of the disease. An essential aspect of integrated care is the involvement of patients, health care providers, family members, and other social supports working toward a common goal of recovery with increased engagement in meaningful life activities.

Summary and Key Points

- The diagnosis of FNSD is made on the basis of the neurological exam, with assistance of ancillary testing if needed, showing evidence of preserved neurological function that is physiologically inconsistent with the presenting symptom.
- FNSD is commonly seen in neurologic practice. Most patients are women. History of trauma/PTSD, depression, and anxiety are among the most common psychiatric comorbidities. Neurologic diagnoses can co-occur with FNSD.
- The pathophysiology of FNSD is incompletely understood, but available studies suggest that the disorder is due to alterations in the integration of sensory, motor, cognitive, and emotional functions.
- The evaluation of FNSD should include exclusion of the likeliest differential diagnoses. However, FNSD is not a diagnosis of exclusion and is based on positive signs. Therefore, the diagnosis should be made confidently.
- Once established, the diagnosis of FNSD should be clearly communicated to the patient. The discussion should include

a name for the disorder, a mechanism for the disease, and information about resources and treatment.

■ Physical therapy has been shown to be an effective treatment for patients with motor, gait, and tremor manifestations of FNSD, whereas CBT is the best first-line treatment for patients with PNES.

■ Psychopharmacological therapy can be used to treat comorbid psychiatric conditions.

■ Many patients with FNSD remain symptomatic and disabled years after the diagnosis. However, the impact of evidence-based treatments on long-term outcomes is unknown.

Multiple Choice Questions

1. Which of the following statements about FNSD is incorrect?
   a. The majority of FNSD patients are women.
   b. Depression and post-traumatic stress disorder are common comorbidities.
   c. The diagnosis requires that the onset is associated with a psychological stressor.
   d. Many patients with FNSD are disabled.
   e. Patients are not feigning their neurological symptoms.

2. Clinical assessment and initial treatment of a patient with FNSD should include the following except:
   a. Assessment of potential psychiatric comorbidities
   b. Evaluation for coexisting neurological conditions
   c. Educating the patient about their diagnosis
   d. Exhaustive testing to exclude any other possible diagnosis, even if unlikely
   e. Demonstrating to the patient how you made the diagnosis on the basis of their neurological exam

3. Semiologic findings favoring a diagnosis of epilepsy over PNES include all except:
   a. Eyes open
   b. Postictal confusion
   c. Ictal crying
   d. Tongue bite
   e. Stertorous breathing

4. A 28-year-old woman is diagnosed with PNES through video-EEG capture of a typical PNES event. A previously started anti-epileptic drug (lamotrigine) is discontinued immediately when video-EEG shows no evidence of epilepsy. She had a past history of sexual abuse but denies active PTSD symptoms. She otherwise denies any other psychiatric symptoms, currently or in the past. There is no evidence of neurological disease. What evidence-based treatment is recommended in this case to address PNES?
   a. CBT
   b. Restart lamotrigine at mood stabilizing doses
   c. Sertraline
   d. rTMS
   e. Physical therapy

5. A patient was diagnosed with PNES. Her episodes primarily consisted of loss of consciousness and she had stopped working 6 months prior to the diagnosis. She also suffers from chronic headaches. The diagnosing neurologist sees her 6 months after the diagnosis of PNES. The following are encouraging signs of her recovery except:
   a. No recurrence of PNES (with loss of consciousness) since diagnosis
   b. Less frequent use of analgesic medication for comorbid headaches
   c. Still not working
   d. No emergency room visits in the last 6 months
   e. Actively participating in psychotherapy for PNES

Multiple Choice Answers

1. **Answer: c**
   DSM-5 no longer requires that there be any temporal relationship between psychological factors and the onset or worsening of the functional neurological symptoms. In addition, the criterion that patients are not intentionally producing their symptoms has been abandoned, as volitional control over the symptoms is extremely difficult to establish. Despite elimination of the criterion, FNSD patients are not considered to be fabricating their symptoms.

2. **Answer: d**
   Testing should be directed to exclude the likeliest diagnoses, but should be limited and completed soon after the initial visit. Extensive testing sends the message to the patient that the clinician is uncertain about the diagnosis of FNSD and will often unearth incidental findings that can unnecessarily prolong confirmation of the diagnosis and initiation of treatment.

3. **Answer: c**
   Ictal crying, pelvic thrusting, side-to-side head/body movements, prolonged episode, and eyes closed favor PNES over epilepsy.

4. **Answer: a**
   CBT has the strongest evidence in the treatment of PNES. In patients with active PTSD (not the case here), prolonged exposure could be beneficial. There is no reason to restart

lamotrigine in a patient without epilepsy or a mood disorder. Evidence for the use of antidepressants or rTMS in PNES is very limited. Physical therapy is used in motor FNSD with weakness, gait, or tremor presentations.

5. Answer: c
Participation in treatment, decreased medical utilization, decrease in other functional symptoms (such as headaches),

and PNES resolution are all encouraging signs of recovery. Inability to work remains a concern, as many patients with FNSD remain disabled many years after the diagnosis. Disability is associated with poor symptom resolution.

References

1. Carson AJ, Ringbauer B, Stone J, et al. Do medically unexplained symptoms matter? A prospective cohort study of 300 new referrals to neurology outpatient clinics. *J Neurol Neurosurg Psychiatry*. 2000;68(2):207-210.
2. American Psychiatric Association. *Diagnostic and Statistical Manual of Mental Disorders*. 5th ed. Arlington, VA: American Psychiatric Press; 2013.
3. Stone J, Sharpe M, Rothwell PM, Warlow CP. The 12 year prognosis of unilateral functional weakness and sensory disturbance. *J Neurol Neurosurg Psychiatry*. 2003;74(5):591-596.
4. Barsky AJ, Orav EJ, Bates DW. Somatization increases medical utilization and costs independent of psychiatric and medical comorbidity. *Arch Gen Psychiatry*. 2005;62(8):903-910.
5. Delis DC, Wetter SR. Cogniform disorder and cogniform condition: proposed diagnoses for excessive cognitive symptoms. *Arch Clin Neuropsychol*. 2007;22(5):589-604.
6. Akagi H, House A. The clinical epidemiology of hysteria: vanishingly rare, or just vanishing? *Psychol Med*. 2002;32(2):191-194.
7. Stone J, Carson A, Duncan R, et al. Who is referred to neurology clinics?—the diagnoses made in 3781 new patients. *Clin Neurol Neurosurg*. 2010;112(9):747-751.
8. Sigurdardottir KR, Olafsson E. Incidence of psychogenic seizures in adults: a population-based study in Iceland. *Epilepsia*. 1998;39(7):749-752.
9. Szaflarski J, Ficker D, Cahill W, Privitera M. Four-year incidence of psychogenic nonepileptic seizures in adults in Hamilton County, OH. *Neurology*. 2000;55(10):1561-1563.
10. Stone J, Carson A, Duncan R, et al. Symptoms 'unexplained by organic disease' in 1144 new neurology out-patients: how often does the diagnosis change at follow-up? *Brain*. 2009;132(pt 10):2878-2888.
11. Benbadis SR, Allen Hauser W. An estimate of the prevalence of psychogenic non-epileptic seizures. *Seizure*. 2000;9(4):280-281.
12. Martin R, Burneo JG, Prasad A, et al. Frequency of epilepsy in patients with psychogenic seizures monitored by video-EEG. *Neurology*. 2003;61(12):1791-1792.
13. Reuber M, Fernandez G, Bauer J, Helmstaedter C, Elger CE. Diagnostic delay in psychogenic nonepileptic seizures. *Neurology*. 2002;58(3):493-495.
14. Kotagal P, Costa M, Wyllie E, Wolgamuth B. Paroxysmal nonepileptic events in children and adolescents. *Pediatrics*. 2002;110(4):e46.
15. Dworetzky BA, Bubrick EJ, Szaflarski JP. Nonepileptic psychogenic status: markedly prolonged psychogenic nonepileptic seizures. *Epilepsy Behav*. 2010;19(1):65-68.
16. Stone J, Carson A. An integrated approach to other functional neurological symptoms and related disorders. In: Dworetzky B, Baslet G, eds. *Psychogenic Nonepileptic Seizures: Toward the Integration of Care*. New York, NY: Oxford University Press; 2017:290-307.
17. Duncan R, Oto M, Martin E, Pelosi A. Late onset psychogenic nonepileptic attacks. *Neurology*. 2006;66(11):1644-1647.
18. Carson A, Lehn A. Epidemiology. *Handb Clin Neurol*. 2016;139:47-60.
19. Park EG, Lee J, Lee BL, Lee M, Lee J. Paroxysmal nonepileptic events in pediatric patients. *Epilepsy Behav*. 2015;48:83-87.
20. Ahmad O, Ahmad KE. Functional neurological disorders in outpatient practice: an Australian cohort. *J Clin Neurosci*. 2016;28:93-96.
21. Stone J, Warlow C, Sharpe M. The symptom of functional weakness: a controlled study of 107 patients. *Brain*. 2010;133(pt 5):1537-1551.
22. Stone J, Carson A, Duncan R, et al. Which neurological diseases are most likely to be associated with "symptoms unexplained by organic disease". *J Neurol*. 2012;259(1):33-38.
23. Stone J, Reuber M, Carson A. Functional symptoms in neurology: mimics and chameleons. *Pract Neurol*. 2013;13(2):104-113.
24. Krumholz A, Niedermeyer E. Psychogenic seizures: a clinical study with follow-up data. *Neurology*. 1983;33(4):498-502.
25. Lesser R. Psychogenic seizures. *Neurology*. 1996;46(6):1499-1507.
26. Benbadis S, Agrawal V, Tatum W. How many patients with psychogenic nonepileptic seizures also have epilepsy? *Neurology*. 2001;57(5):915-917.
27. Reuber M, Kral T, Kurthen M, Elger CE. New-onset psychogenic seizures after intracranial neurosurgery. *Acta Neurochir (Wien)*. 2002;144(9):901-907.
28. Duncan R, Oto M. Psychogenic nonepileptic seizures in patients with learning disability: comparison with patients with no learning disability. *Epilepsy Behav*. 2008;12(1):183-186.
29. Wong V, Salinsky M. Neurological and medical factors. In: Dworetzky B, Baslet G, eds. *Psychogenic Nonepileptic Seizures: Toward the Integration of Care*. New York, NY: Oxford University Press; 2017:67-80.
30. Sar V, Akyuz G, Kundakci T, Kiziltan E, Dogan O. Childhood trauma, dissociation, and psychiatric comorbidity in patients with conversion disorder. *Am J Psychiatry*. 2004;161(12):2271-2276.
31. Roelofs K, Pasman J. Stress, childhood trauma, and cognitive functions in functional neurologic disorders. *Handb Clin Neurol*. 2016;139:139-155.
32. Oto M, Conway P, Mcgonigal A, Russell AJ, Duncan R. Gender differences in psychogenic non-epileptic seizures. *Seizure*. 2005;14(1):33-39.
33. Thomas AA, Preston J, Scott RC, Bujarski KA. Diagnosis of probable psychogenic nonepileptic seizures in the outpatient clinic: does gender matter? *Epilepsy Behav*. 2013;29(2):295-297.
34. Matin N, Young SS, Williams B, et al. Neuropsychiatric associations with gender, illness duration, work disability, and motor

subtype in a U.S. functional neurological disorders clinic population. *J Neuropsychiatry Clin Neurosci*. 2017;29(4):375-382.

35. Ludwig L, Pasman JA, Nicholson T, et al. Stressful life events and maltreatment in conversion (functional neurological) disorder: systematic review and meta-analysis of case-control studies. *Lancet Psychiatry*. 2018;5(4):307-320.

36. Driver-Dunckley E, Stonnington CM, Locke DE, Noe K. Comparison of psychogenic movement disorders and psychogenic nonepileptic seizures: is phenotype clinically important? *Psychosomatics*. 2011;52(4):337-345.

37. Baslet G, Seshadri A, Bermeo-Ovalle A, Willment K, Myers L. Psychogenic non-epileptic seizures: an updated primer. *Psychosomatics*. 2016;57(1):1-17.

38. Singh SP, Lee AS. Conversion disorders in Nottingham: alive, but not kicking. *J Psychosom Res*. 1997;43(4):425-430.

39. Carson AJ, Ringbauer B, Mackenzie L, Warlow C, Sharpe M. Neurological disease, emotional disorder, and disability: they are related: a study of 300 consecutive new referrals to a neurology outpatient department. *J Neurol Neurosurg Psychiatry*. 2000;68(2):202-206.

40. Roelofs K, Keijsers GP, Hoogduin KA, Naring GW, Moene FC. Childhood abuse in patients with conversion disorder. *Am J Psychiatry*. 2002;159(11):1908-1913.

41. Asadi-Pooya AA, Emami M. Juvenile and adult-onset psychogenic non-epileptic seizures. *Clin Neurol Neurosurg*. 2013;115(9):1697-1700.

42. Plioplys S, Doss J, Siddarth P, et al. A multisite controlled study of risk factors in pediatric psychogenic nonepileptic seizures. *Epilepsia*. 2014;55(11):1739-1747.

43. Reuber M, Brown RJ. Understanding psychogenic nonepileptic seizures—phenomenology, semiology and the Integrative Cognitive Model. *Seizure*. 2017;44:199-205.

44. Edwards MJ. Neurobiologic theories of functional neurologic disorders. *Handb Clin Neurol*. 2017;139:131-137.

45. Nielsen G, Ricciardi L, Demartini B, et al. Outcomes of a 5-day physiotherapy programme for functional (psychogenic) motor disorders. *J Neurol*. 2015;262(3):674-681.

46. Liepert J, Hassa T, Tuscher O, Schmidt R. Electrophysiological correlates of motor conversion disorder. *Mov Disord*. 2008;23(15):2171-2176.

47. Bakvis P, Roelofs K, Kuyk J, et al. Trauma, stress, and preconscious threat processing in patients with psychogenic nonepileptic seizures. *Epilepsia*. 2009;50(5):1001-1011.

48. Reinsberger C, Sarkis R, Papadelis C, et al. Autonomic changes in psychogenic nonepileptic seizures: toward a potential diagnostic biomarker? *Clin EEG Neurosci*. 2015;46(1):16-25.

49. Atmaca M, Aydin A, Tezcan E, Poyraz AK, Kara B. Volumetric investigation of brain regions in patients with conversion disorder. *Prog Neuropsychopharmacol Biol Psychiatry*. 2006;30(4):708-713.

50. Nicholson TR, Aybek S, Kempton MJ, et al. A structural MRI study of motor conversion disorder: evidence of reduction in thalamic volume. *J Neurol Neurosurg Psychiatry*. 2014;85(2):227-229.

51. Aybek S, Nicholson TR, Draganski B, et al. Grey matter changes in motor conversion disorder. *J Neurol Neurosurg Psychiatry*. 2014;85(2):236-238.

52. Labate A, Cerasa A, Mula M, et al. Neuroanatomic correlates of psychogenic nonepileptic seizures: a cortical thickness and VBM study. *Epilepsia*. 2012;53(2):377-385.

53. Perez DL, Dworetzky BA, Dickerson BC, et al. An integrative neurocircuit perspective on psychogenic nonepileptic seizures and functional movement disorders: neural functional unawareness. *Clin EEG Neurosci*. 2015;46(1):4-15.

54. Voon V, Cavanna AE, Coburn K, et al. Functional neuroanatomy and neurophysiology of functional neurological disorders (conversion disorder). *J Neuropsychiatry Clin Neurosci*. 2016;28(3):168-190.

55. Daum C, Hubschmid M, Aybek S. The value of "positive" clinical signs for weakness, sensory and gait disorders in conversion disorder: a systematic and narrative review. *J Neurol Neurosurg Psychiatry*. 2014;85(2):180-190.

56. Van Der Stouwe AM, Elting JW, Van Der Hoeven JH, et al. How typical are "typical" tremor characteristics? Sensitivity and specificity of five tremor phenomena. *Parkinsonism Relat Disord*. 2016;30:23-28.

57. Leis A, Ross M, Summers A. Psychogenic seizures: ictal characteristics and diagnostic pitfalls. *Neurology*. 1992;42(1):95-99.

58. O'neal M, Caplan R. Ambulatory presentations in adults and children. In: Dworetzky B, Baslet G, eds. *Psychogenic Nonepileptic Seizures: Toward the Integration of Care*. New York, NY: Oxford University Press; 2017:3-13.

59. Lafrance WC Jr, Baker GA, Duncan R, Goldstein LH, Reuber M. Minimum requirements for the diagnosis of psychogenic nonepileptic seizures: a staged approach: a report from the International League Against Epilepsy Nonepileptic Seizures Task Force. *Epilepsia*. 2013;54(11):2005-2018.

60. Alving J. Serum prolactin levels are elevated also after pseudo-epileptic seizures. *Seizure*. 1998;7(2):85-89.

61. Chen DK, So YT, Fisher RS. Use of serum prolactin in diagnosing epileptic seizures: report of the Therapeutics and Technology Assessment Subcommittee of the American Academy of Neurology. *Neurology*. 2005;65(5):668-675.

62. Reuber M, Chen M, Jamnadas-Khoda J, et al. Value of patient-reported symptoms in the diagnosis of transient loss of consciousness. *Neurology*. 2016;87(6):625-633.

63. Plug L, Sharrack B, Reuber M. Seizure metaphors differ in patients' accounts of epileptic and psychogenic nonepileptic seizures. *Epilepsia*. 2009;50(5):994-1000.

64. Stone J, Smyth R, Carson A, et al. Systematic review of misdiagnosis of conversion symptoms and "hysteria." *BMJ*. 2005;331(7523):989.

65. Stone J, Edwards M. Trick or treat? Showing patients with functional (psychogenic) motor symptoms their physical signs. *Neurology*. 2012;79(3):282-284.

66. Reuber M, Pukrop R, Bauer J, et al. Outcome in psychogenic nonepileptic seizures: 1 to 10-year follow-up in 164 patients. *Ann Neurol*. 2003;53(3):305-311.

67. Rathod J, Benbadis SR. Diagnostic challenges for the neurologist. In: Dworetzky B, Baslet G, eds. *Psychogenic Nonepileptic Seizures: Toward the Integration of Care*. New York, NY: Oxford University Press; 2017:123-138.

68. Avbersek A, Sisodiya S. Does the primary literature provide support for clinical signs used to distinguish psychogenic nonepileptic seizures from epileptic seizures? *J Neurol Neurosurg Psychiatry*. 2010;81(7):719-725.

69. Willment K, Loring D. Practical and diagnostic challenges for the neuropsychologist. In: Dworetzky B, Baslet G, eds. *Psychogenic Nonepileptic Seizures: Toward the Integration of Care*. New York, NY: Oxford University Press; 2017:153-178.

70. Tolchin B, Dworetzky BA, Baslet G. Long-term adherence with psychiatric treatment among patients with psychogenic nonepileptic seizures. *Epilepsia*. 2018;59(1):e18-e22.

71. Duncan R. Long-term outcomes. In: Dworetzky B, Baslet G, eds. *Psychogenic Nonepileptic Seizures: Toward the Integration of Care*. New York, NY: Oxford University Press; 2017:279-289.

72. Tolchin B, Dworetzky BA, Martino S, et al. Adherence with psychotherapy and treatment outcomes for psychogenic nonepileptic seizures. *Neurology.* 2019;92(7):e675-e679.

73. Binzer M, Kullgren G. Motor conversion disorder. A prospective 2- to 5-year follow-up study. *Psychosomatics.* 1998;39(6):519-527.

74. Hall-Patch L, Brown R, House A, et al. Acceptability and effectiveness of a strategy for the communication of the diagnosis of psychogenic nonepileptic seizures. *Epilepsia.* 2010;51(1):70-78.

75. Razvi S, Mulhern S, Duncan R. Newly diagnosed psychogenic nonepileptic seizures: health care demand prior to and following diagnosis at a first seizure clinic. *Epilepsy Behav.* 2012;23(1):7-9.

76. Jirsch JD, Ahmed SN, Maximova K, Gross DW. Recognition of psychogenic nonepileptic seizures diminishes acute care utilization. *Epilepsy Behav.* 2011;22(2):304-307.

77. Lafrance WC Jr, Reuber M, Goldstein LH. Management of psychogenic nonepileptic seizures. *Epilepsia.* 2013;54(suppl 1):53-67.

78. Berneo-Ovalle A, Kanner AM. The role of the neurologist after diagnosis. In: Dworetzky B, Baslet G, eds. *Psychogenic Nonepileptic Seizures: Toward the Integration of Care.* New York, NY: Oxford University Press; 2017:253-265.

79. Tolchin B, Baslet G, Suzuki J, et al. Randomized controlled trial of motivational interviewing for psychogenic nonepileptic seizures. *Epilepsia.* 2019;60(5):986-995.

80. Kroenke K. Efficacy of treatment for somatoform disorders: a review of randomized controlled trials. *Psychosom Med.* 2007;69(9):881-888.

81. Van Dessel N, Den Boeft M, Van Der Wouden JC, et al. Non-pharmacological interventions for somatoform disorders and medically unexplained physical symptoms (MUPS) in adults. *Cochrane Database Syst Rev.* 2014(11): CD011142.

82. Goldstein LH, Chalder T, Chigwedere C, et al. Cognitive-behavioral therapy for psychogenic nonepileptic seizures: a pilot RCT. *Neurology.* 2010;74(24):1986-1994.

83. Lafrance WC Jr, Baird GL, Barry JJ, et al. Multicenter pilot treatment trial for psychogenic nonepileptic seizures: a randomized clinical trial. *JAMA Psychiatry.* 2014;71(9):997-1005.

84. Goldstein LH, Robinson EJ, et al. CODES study group. Cognitive behavioural therapy for adults with dissociative seizures (CODES): a pragmatic, multicentre, randomised controlled trial. *Lancet Psychiatry.* 2020;7(6):491-505.

85. Sharpe M, Walker J, Williams C, et al. Guided self-help for functional (psychogenic) symptoms: a randomized controlled efficacy trial. *Neurology.* 2011;77(6):564-572.

86. Williams C, Kent C, Smith S, et al. *Overcoming Functional Neurological Symptoms: A Five Areas Approach.* London: Hodder Arnold; 2011.

87. Reiter J, Andrews D, Reiter C, Lafrance W. *Taking Control of Your Seizures Workbook.* New York, NY: Oxford University Press; 2015.

88. Chen DK, Maheshwari A, Franks R, et al. Brief group psychoeducation for psychogenic nonepileptic seizures: a neurologist-initiated program in an epilepsy center. *Epilepsia.* 2014;55(1):156-166.

89. Moene FC, Spinhoven P, Hoogduin KA, Van Dyck R. A randomised controlled clinical trial on the additional effect of hypnosis in a comprehensive treatment programme for in-patients with conversion disorder of the motor type. *Psychother Psychosom.* 2002;71(2):66-76.

90. Moene FC, Spinhoven P, Hoogduin KA, Van Dyck R. A randomized controlled clinical trial of a hypnosis-based treatment for patients with conversion disorder, motor type. *Int J Clin Exp Hypn.* 2003;51(1):29-50.

91. Hubschmid M, Aybek S, Maccaferri GE, et al. Efficacy of brief interdisciplinary psychotherapeutic intervention for motor conversion disorder and nonepileptic attacks. *Gen Hosp Psychiatry.* 2015;37(5):448-455.

92. Dallocchio C, Tinazzi M, Bombieri F, Arnó N, Erro R. Cognitive behavioural therapy and adjunctive physical activity for functional movement disorders (conversion disorder): a pilot, single-blinded, randomized study. *Psychother Psychosom.* 2016;85(6):381-383.

93. Ataoglu A, Ozcetin A, Icmeli C, Ozbulut O. Paradoxical therapy in conversion reaction. *J Korean Med Sci.* 2003;18(4):581-584.

94. Aamir S, Hamayon S, Sultan S. Behavior therapy in dissociative convulsion disorder. *J Depress Anxiety.* 2011;1(1):1-4.

95. Mayor R, Howlett S, Grunewald R, Reuber M. Long-term outcome of brief augmented psychodynamic interpersonal therapy for psychogenic nonepileptic seizures: seizure control and health care utilization. *Epilepsia.* 2010;51(7):1169-1176.

96. Kompoliti K, Wilson B, Stebbins G, Bernard B, Hinson V. Immediate vs. delayed treatment of psychogenic movement disorders with short term psychodynamic psychotherapy: randomized clinical trial. *Parkinsonism Relat Disord.* 2014;20(1):60-63.

97. Barry JJ, Wittenberg D, Bullock KD, et al. Group therapy for patients with psychogenic nonepileptic seizures: a pilot study. *Epilepsy Behav.* 2008;13(4):624-629.

98. Myers L, Vaidya-Mathur U, Lancman M. Prolonged exposure therapy for the treatment of patients diagnosed with psychogenic non-epileptic seizures (PNES) and post-traumatic stress disorder (PTSD). *Epilepsy Behav.* 2017;66:86-92.

99. Baslet G, Ehlert A, Oser M, Dworetzky BA. Mindfulness-based therapy for psychogenic nonepileptic seizures. *Epilepsy Behav.* 2020;103(Pt A):106534.

100. Kuyk J, Siffels MC, Bakvis P, Swinkels WA. Psychological treatment of patients with psychogenic non-epileptic seizures: an outcome study. *Seizure.* 2008;17(7):595-603.

101. Nielsen G, Stone J, Edwards MJ. Physiotherapy for functional (psychogenic) motor symptoms: a systematic review. *J Psychosom Res.* 2013;75(2):93-102.

102. Jordbru AA, Smedstad LM, Klungsoyr O, Martinsen EW. Psychogenic gait disorder: a randomized controlled trial of physical rehabilitation with one-year follow-up. *J Rehabil Med.* 2014;46(2):181-187.

103. Czarnecki K, Thompson JM, Seime R, et al. Functional movement disorders: successful treatment with a physical therapy rehabilitation protocol. *Parkinsonism Relat Disord.* 2012;18(3):247-251.

104. Nielsen G, Buszewicz M, Stevenson F, et al. Randomised feasibility study of physiotherapy for patients with functional motor symptoms. *J Neurol Neurosurg Psychiatry.* 2017;88(6):484-490.

105. Voon V, Lang AE. Antidepressant treatment outcomes of psychogenic movement disorder. *J Clin Psychiatry.* 2005;66(12):1529-1534.

106. Pintor L, Bailles E, Matrai S, et al. Efficiency of venlafaxine in patients with psychogenic nonepileptic seizures and anxiety and/or depressive disorders. *J Neuropsychiatry Clin Neurosci.* 2010;22(4):401-408.

107. Lafrance WC Jr, Keitner GI, Papandonatos GD, et al. Pilot pharmacologic randomized controlled trial for psychogenic nonepileptic seizures. *Neurology.* 2010;75(13):1166-1173.

108. Kleinstauber M, Witthoft M, Steffanowski A, et al. Pharmacological interventions for somatoform disorders in adults. *Cochrane Database Syst Rev.* 2014;(11): CD010628.

109. Schonfeldt-Lecuona C, Lefaucheur JP, Lepping P, et al. Non-invasive brain stimulation in conversion (functional) weakness

and paralysis: a systematic review and future perspectives. *Front Neurosci*. 2016;10:140.

110. Chastan N, Parain D. Psychogenic paralysis and recovery after motor cortex transcranial magnetic stimulation. *Mov Disord*. 2010;25(10):1501-1504.

111. Broersma M, Koops EA, Vroomen PC, et al. Can repetitive transcranial magnetic stimulation increase muscle strength in functional neurological paresis? A proof-of-principle study. *Eur J Neurol*. 2015;22(5):866-873.

112. Peterson KT, Kosior R, Meek BP, et al. Right temporoparietal junction transcranial magnetic stimulation in the treatment of psychogenic nonepileptic seizures: a case series. *Psychosomatics*. 2018;59(6):601-606.

Addiction as a Neuropsychiatric Disease

14

Claudia P. Rodriguez · Joji Suzuki

INTRODUCTION

Drug addiction is a chronic disease that is characterized by loss of control, cravings, and compulsive use despite negative consequences. As a neuropsychiatric disease, addiction is conceptualized as a cycle of binge/intoxication, withdrawal/negative affect, and preoccupation/anticipation. The stages of the cycle are directed by activity and neuroadaptations that occur at different regions of the brain with repeated drug use. As reviewed in this chapter, key structures involved in each of these stages include the ventral tegmental area (VTA) in binge/intoxication, extended amygdala (including the bed of stria terminalis, nucleus accumbens, and amygdala) in withdrawal/negative affect and craving, and orbitofrontal cortex, basolateral amygdala, and hippocampus in preoccupation/anticipation.[1]

The transition to addiction involves changes in the mesolimbic dopamine system, hypothalamic pituitary axis (HPA), and other stress systems (corticotropin-releasing factor, norepinephrine, vasopressin, dynorphin), as well as dysregulation of anti-stress systems (neuropeptide Y, nociceptin), prefrontal cortex (PFC), and the extended amygdala. These changes contribute to an increase in reward threshold, heightened sensitivity to drug rewards versus nondrug rewards, decreased ability to feel pleasure in everyday activities, increased stress reactivity, and a decreased capacity for decision making and self-regulation associated with the compulsive nature of use in addiction.[2]

Treatment of drug addiction involves using evidence-based medications to help restore healthy brain function, while utilizing behavioral therapies to improve distress intolerance, coping skills, self-compassion, and enrichment of social relationships.

EPIDEMIOLOGY

Genetic, social, and environmental factors contribute to an individual's susceptibility to addiction. Family history, presence of comorbid mental illness, history of trauma, and early exposure to drug use are factors that increase the risk for development of substance use disorders (SUD). Individuals who have a mental illness, such as major depressive disorder, are more likely to have comorbid SUD, and vice versa. Studies have shown that the co-occurring SUD and psychiatric disorders can worsen the prognosis for each disorder.[3]

There are several resources that evaluate the impact of SUD on individuals and their communities. Nationally, the annual cost of substance use related to crime, lost work, and health care exceeds $740 billion.[4] The National Epidemiologic Survey on Alcohol and Related Conditions (NESARC) is a cross-sectional study based on a nationally representative sample of the civilian noninstitutionalized population in the United States aged 18 and older sponsored by the National Institute on Alcohol Abuse and Alcoholism (NIAAA). This study is meant to assess the prevalence of alcohol use disorder (AUD) and associated disease in the surveyed population. The results of 2016 showed a prevalence of 12 month and lifetime drug use disorders of 3.9% and 9.9%, respectively.[5]

Started in 1975, the Monitoring the Future (MTF) study is a survey study that explores attitudes (perceived risk, disapproval, and availability of drugs) and drug use among 8th, 10th, and 12th graders in over 380 public and private schools in the United States.[6]

In 1975 over one-third (36%) of 12th graders had tried some illicit drug other than marijuana. By 1981, the percentage rose to 43% and declined until another increase in the 1990s when use of several drugs rose steadily but remained at values lower than in the early 1980s (Figure 14-1).

Cannabis has remained the most widely used illicit drug throughout MTF study. In 2017, the study began to include questions about vaping cannabis. In each grade, more than 25% of students who had used cannabis had experienced vaping it.[6] Like other drugs, increase in use of cannabis over time has been coupled with a decrease in the perception of harm and disapproval of cannabis use, consistent with legal and social changes related to cannabis over time (Figure 14-2). Lifetime and daily use of cigarettes declined significantly amongst all groups since its peak in the mid-1990s, with a concomitant increase in perceived risk and disapproval, and a decrease in the perception

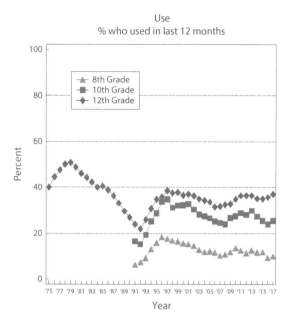

Use
% who used in last 12 months

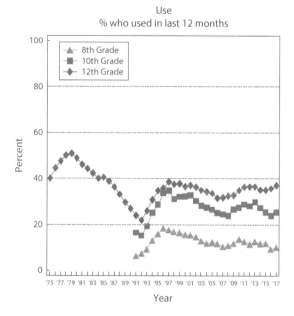

Use
% who used in last 12 months

FIGURE 14-1. Use of any illicit drug other than cannabis in the previous 12 months per year, results from Monitoring the Future study 2017. (Source: Johnston LD, Miech RA, O'Malley OM, et al. Monitoring the future national survey results on drug use: 1975-2017: Overview, key findings on adolescent drug use. Ann Arbor, MI: Institute for Social Research, The University of Michigan. 2018.)

of availability of cigarettes. Use of narcotics other than heroin, reported only for 12th graders, has shown a gradual decline since 2009 (Figure 14-3). Other prescription opioids, such as hydrocodone (Vicodin) and oxycodone hydrochloride (OxyContin), have shown a drop in use among all grades since 2010.[6]

The MTF study has allowed for observations about the dynamic relationship between specific drugs and factors that influence use.[6] One of the observations reflects a "honeymoon period" for drugs, in which perceived benefits outweigh risks and knowledge of the positive effects of specific drugs reach mainstream culture faster than the negative effects of each drug. In addition, while specific drugs may fall out of popularity at one time, they can later regain popularity through a process known as "generational forgetting," where adverse consequences of a drug may be forgotten as new generations replace the older ones.[6] This can be seen with a variety of drugs, including lysergic acid diethylamide (LSD) and methamphetamines, where perceived risk decreased as risk of use in the following generation increased. Thus, education about drug use should be drug specific, as individuals may not recognize all drugs as being equally harmful.

The National Survey on Drug Use and Health (NSDUH) provides information on the prevalence, patterns, and consequences of drug use and other mental health disorders in individuals in the United States aged 12 or older.[7] This survey includes information on use of tobacco, cannabis, alcohol, opioids, and illicit drugs (Figure 14-4), as well as patterns of alcohol use, including current, binge, and heavy alcohol use (Figure 14-5). In addition, the NSDUH explores need and receipt of treatment, highlighting the need for greater access to substance use treatment as noted in Figure 14-6. Other available resources include the National Drug Early Warning System, which monitors drug use trends in 12 sentinel communities

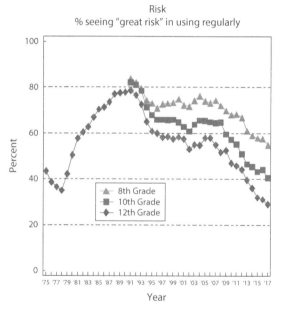

Risk
% seeing "great risk" in using regularly

FIGURE 14-2. Use of cannabis and perceived risk of regular use of cannabis per year, results from Monitoring the Future study 2017. (Source: Johnston LD, Miech RA, O'Malley OM, et al. Monitoring the future national survey results on drug use: 1975-2017: Overview, key findings on adolescent drug use. Ann Arbor, MI: Institute for Social Research, The University of Michigan. 2018.)

(Texas, Denver, San Francisco, Los Angeles, Atlanta metro, Chicago metro, Detroit/Wayne county, King County (Seattle), Maine, New York City, Philadelphia, and Southeastern Florida (Miami)) across the United States (https://ndews.umd.edu/). Finally, the Centers for Disease Control and Prevention and the National Institute of Drug Addiction provide information regarding a wide range of drug use measures and overdose deaths. Figure 14-7 shows the three waves of the rise in opioid-related overdose deaths: prescription opioids in the late-1990s, followed by heroin-related overdoses starting in 2010, and finally, as of 2013, overdose deaths driven primarily by synthetic opioids, specifically, fentanyl.[8]

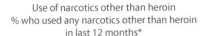

Use of narcotics other than heroin
% who used any narcotics other than heroin
in last 12 months*

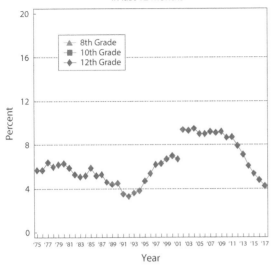

Availability of narcotics other than heroin**
% saying "fairly easy" or "very easy" to get

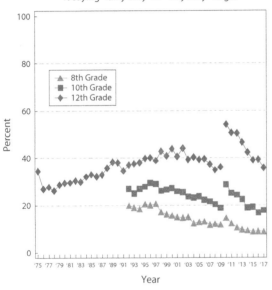

*Beginning in 2002, a revised set of questions on other narcotics use was introduced in which Talwin, laudanum, and paregoric were replaced as examples given with Vicodin, OxyContin, and Percocet.
**In 2010 the list of examples was changed from methadone, opium to Vicodin, OxyContin, Percocet, etc.

FIGURE 14-3. Use and availability of narcotics other than heroin in previous 12 months per year, results from Monitoring the Future study 2017. (Source: Johnston LD, Miech RA, O'Malley OM, et al. Monitoring the future national survey results on drug use: 1975-2017: Overview, key findings on adolescent drug use. Ann Arbor, MI: Institute for Social Research, The University of Michigan. 2018.)

PATHOPHYSIOLOGY

Several models have been proposed to understand SUD.[1,2] The 4 C's of addiction, proposed by the American Society of Addiction Medicine, can be used to screen individuals for the diagnosis of SUD, and nicely superimpose onto the *DSM-5*

criteria for SUD (Table 14-1). The brain disease model of addiction describes drug addiction as a process that involves several areas of the brain including the PFC, the mesolimbic dopaminergic system, HPA, and more. As an individual moves from a cycle of impulsivity to compulsivity, there are several neurobiological changes that occur which contribute to the loss of control and negative affect associated with SUD. Each stage of drug use, from binge/intoxication to withdrawal/negative affect and preoccupation/anticipation, is directed by neurobiological mechanisms (Figure 14-8).[2]

The mesolimbic dopaminergic system involves the primary structures of the primitive reward system. This system is activated not only by drugs of misuse, but also by other rewards that are crucial to the preservation of our species, including food, water, and sex. The system learns, through conditioning and reinforcement learning, to recognize environmental cues associated with rewards to increase the likelihood of the reward being experienced again.

At a biological level, drugs trigger release of extracellular dopamine (DA) in areas of the reward system.[1] The pharmacokinetic properties of drugs are important characteristics that affect their addiction potential based on the how quickly the drug use leads to release of DA. These factors may dictate the route of administration and frequency of drug use. Over time, repeated exposure to the reward, in conjunction with environmental cues such as drug paraphernalia, people, or specific emotional states, result in conditioning which lead to a rapid firing of DA cells in anticipation of the reward.[1,2] Cue-induced cravings involve amygdala activation that contributes to this conditioned response to the stimuli. In relapse prevention treatment, individuals are often taught to recognize and attempt to avoid "people, places, and things" that may lead to this anticipatory brain response and represent a high risk for relapse. An individual with AUD will experience an intense reaction to the site or smell of alcohol. These conditioned experiences are fixed and difficult to alter even after a prolonged period of time without drug use. Furthermore, studies have shown that the expectation of a drug's rewarding effects influences the rewarding response to the drugs. This aspect of drug use and response involves glutamate's activity which modulates the extent of release of DA in the nucleus accumbens, and therefore, the experience of reward.

Unlike nondrug rewards, which have a cessation of DA firing after repeated consumption, ongoing use of drugs continues to directly increase DA levels.[2] Also, over time, nondrug rewards decrease in value relative to drug rewards, losing some of their "motivational power," and individuals who struggle with addiction forego things like food and companionship/sex for drugs. In that way, drug seeking and taking occurs at the expense of natural rewards, affecting individuals' motivation for rewards.[2]

In addition, as individuals continue to use drugs, the DA release and activation response is altered, so that pleasure from both drug and nondrug rewards are experienced as less intense. The brain reward system is reset in a way that individuals do not get the same level of DA stimulation, or euphoria, from using a drug compared to the first time it was used. In other words, the initial motivation for substance use is positive reinforcement, or use of a substance to experience euphoria. As individuals develop an addiction, ongoing substance use is motivated

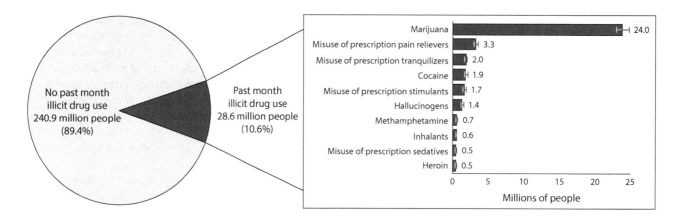

FIGURE 14-4. Past month illicit drug use among individuals 12 and older in 2016 according to the National Survey of Drug Use and Health.[7] Note: Estimated numbers of people refer to people aged 12 or older in the civilian, noninstitutionalized population in the United States. The numbers do not sum to the total population of the United States because the population for NSDUH does not include people aged 11 years old or younger, people with no fixed household address (e.g., homeless or transient people not in shelters), active-duty military personnel, and residents of institutional group quarters, such as correctional facilities, nursing homes, mental institutions, and long-term care hospitals. Note: The estimated numbers of current users of different illicit drugs are not mutually exclusive because people could have used more than one type of illicit drug in the past month. (Source: Center for Behavioral Health Statistics and Quality, Substance Abuse and Mental Health Services Administration. https://www.samhsa.gov/data/.)

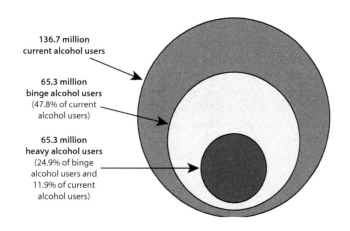

FIGURE 14-5. Current, binge, heavy alcohol use among individuals 12 and older in 2016 according to the National Survey of Drug Use and Health. (Source: Center for Behavioral Health Statistics and Quality, Substance Abuse and Mental Health Services Administration. https://www.samhsa.gov/data/.)

by negative reinforcement, or the use of substance to avoid the unpleasant feeling that arises in the absence of the drug.[2] Because our reward system is tenacious, persistent, and has a great capacity for storing ingrained memories, this process does not reverse quickly after termination of exposure to the drug.

At a biological level, the stage of withdrawal/negative affect involves the HPA, adaptations of the circuitry of the extended amygdala, and decreases in reward neurochemicals—all of which contribute to the emotional dysregulation, heightened stress sensitivity, increased brain reward threshold, and the negative motivational state of withdrawal. Neurochemical changes during this stage of withdrawal and negative affect include decreased basal DA activity, decreased D2 receptors in the PFC and ventral striatum, decreased serotonin (5HT) transmission, activation of neuropeptide Y and dynorphin, and involvement of corticotrophin-releasing factor. These changes contribute further to the

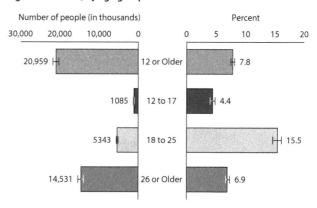

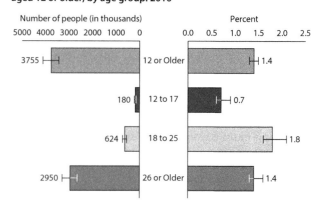

FIGURE 14-6. Comparison of need versus receipt of substance use treatment in the past year in the United States among people aged 12 or older, by age group in 2016 according to the National Survey of Drug Use and Health. (Source: Center for Behavioral Health Statistics and Quality, Substance Abuse and Mental Health Services Administration. https://www.samhsa.gov/data/.)

Drugs involved in U.S. overdose deaths, 2000 to 2016 (8)

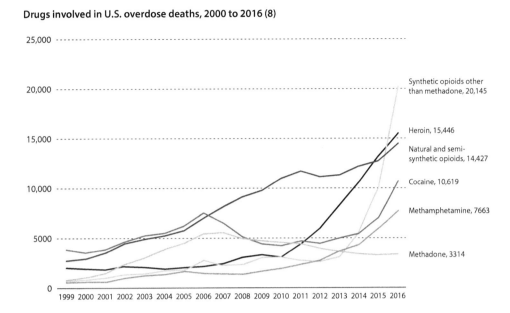

FIGURE 14-7. Drugs involved in U.S. overdose deaths, 2000–2016. (Data from National Institutes of Health: U.S. Department of Health and Human Services, National Center for Health Statistics. CDC Wonder. https://www.cdc.gov/nchs/index.htm.)

TABLE 14-1 • *DSM-5* Diagnosis of Substance Use Disorder (SUD).	
4 C's of Addiction	**DSM-5 Criteria**
	Mild: 2–3, Moderate: 4–5, Severe: 6 or more
Control	Use of substance in larger amounts or over a longer period than was intended
	A great deal of time spent on activities necessary to obtain, use, or recover from the effects of the drug
	A persistent desire or unsuccessful effort to cut down on or control use
Cravings	Craving for or a strong desire or urge to use
Consequences	Recurrent use, resulting in a failure to fulfill major obligations at work, school, or home
	Continued use despite persistent or recurrent social or interpersonal problems caused or exacerbated by the effects of substance
	Reduced participation in or avoidance of important social, occupational, or interpersonal activities
	Recurrent use in situations in which it is physically hazardous
	Continued use despite knowledge of having a persistent or recurrent physical or psychological problem that is likely to have been caused or exacerbated by the substance
Compulsive Use	Withdrawal
	Tolerance

discomfort experienced when a drug is removed, or the effect of the drug wears off.[1,2] These changes are reflected in individuals' ongoing compulsive use of drugs in the absence of positive reinforcement with drug use. Specific withdrawal syndromes vary from drug to drug and depend on molecular changes associated with each drug of abuse, duration of use, and frequency of use. Nonetheless, the above-stated changes in neurochemistry are shared among drugs of abuse, resulting in irritability, sleeplessness, and anhedonia experienced after drug use cessation.

Finally, the stage of preoccupation and anticipation involves the PFC and several deleterious changes that affect executive processes including impulse control, decision making, the capacity to distinguish between immediate and delayed rewards, and the ability to stop an action based on higher-order reasoning. This affects a person's capacity to engage in short-term versus long-term goals. The imbalance created by changes in glutamatergic connections from PFC to VTA, downregulation of DA activity in the reward system, and hyperactivity of stress systems (including the HPA axis), affect a person's ability to abstain from drug use despite intention and strong desire to do so.[2] Furthermore, drug use leads to further weakening of the PFC's ability to intervene, so that people's ability to stop taking the drug once they have used is significantly compromised. All of these stages put together serve the foundation for many of our psychotherapeutic and pharmacologic treatments for addiction.

Finally, the physical and social environment of the individual may be a significant contributor to the pathogenesis of SUD. While the classical paradigm of SUD posits that an individual becomes addicted with the repeated exposure to the substance, studies have shown that environmental factors also play a powerful role. In animal models, rats isolated in cages will compulsively consume large amounts of morphine to which it has free access. However, in a series of experiments investigators took the same rats and placed them in a much larger enclosure that

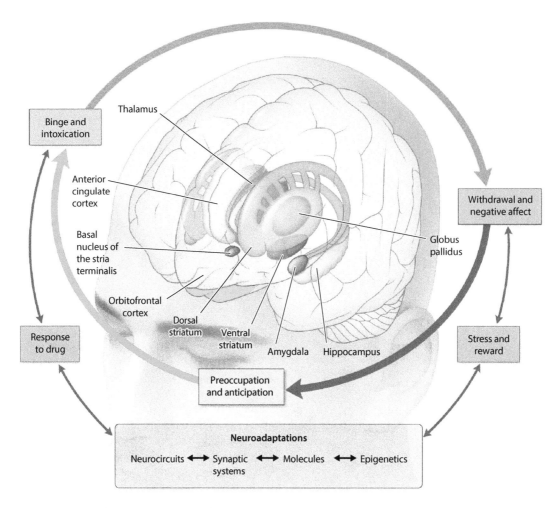

FIGURE 14-8. Neuropsychiatry of addiction. The ventral tegmental area (VTA), not identified in this figure, is a group of primarily dopaminergic neurons in the midbrain, near the substantia nigra. The VTA uses mesocortical (involved in emotion, motivation, and executive function) and mesolimbic (involved in reward processing) pathways to receive information from various regions and forward the information the nucleus accumbens that is processed in reinforcement learning and plays a role in addiction.

mimicked the rats' natural social and physical environment (i.e., presence of other rats and structured to play with, soft bedding). When such other competing rewards were present, the rats consumed far less of the morphine, even though they had free access to it. As such, the pathogenesis of SUD is likely to be a biopsychosocial process that includes the complex interplay of biology and the individuals' environment.[9]

CLINICAL PRESENTATION

This section of the chapter will focus specifically on various neuropsychiatric complications related to substance use. Topics covered will include Wernicke's encephalopathy (thiamine deficiency), alcohol-related dementia, alcohol withdrawal, opioid withdrawal, post-hypoxic and toxic leukoencephalopathies, specific intoxications related to common drugs of abuse, and cannabis use disorder.

Wernicke's Encephalopathy

Individuals with AUD exhibit varying levels of cognitive and motor impairment. Cognitive impairment can range from mild to severe, and includes Wernicke's encephalopathy (WE), associated with thiamine deficiency.

Generally, thiamine levels are maintained by a combination of oral intake through diet, active absorption in the gut, reabsorption in the kidneys, and storage in the liver.[10] Neuropsychiatric symptoms of thiamine deficiency arise when thiamine levels have fallen to 20% below normal. It can take 2–3 weeks for thiamine stores to become depleted without supplementation. In addition to poor nutrition, there are several reasons why individuals with AUD may develop WE. As mentioned earlier, a primary storage site for thiamine is the liver and chronic alcohol use affects the liver's capacity for storage.[10] Hypomagnesemia is common in individuals with AUD, and magnesium is required for utilization of thiamine. Active absorption across the gut is affected during acute alcohol intoxication and by alcohol-related gastritis. There is an increase in loss of thiamine from the kidneys due to alcohol's effects on the renal epithelial cells.[10] Finally, alcohol reduces the enzymatic activity of thiamine pyrophosphokinase, which is required for the formation of thiamine pyrophosphate, the major active form of thiamine in the central nervous system (CNS).[10] Within 10 days of thiamine depletion in the brain, cytotoxic edema, astrocyte volume increase,

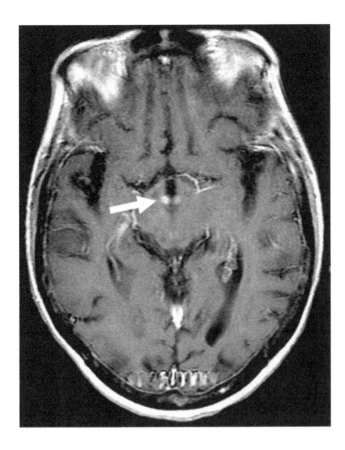

FIGURE 14-9. Wernicke's encephalopathy findings on brain magnetic resonance imaging (MRI) (mammillary bodies highlighted). (Reproduced with permission from Ropper AH, Samuels MA, Klein JP. *Adams and Victor's Principles of Neurology*. 10th ed. https://accessmedicine.mhmedical.com. Copyright © McGraw Hill LLC. All rights reserved.)

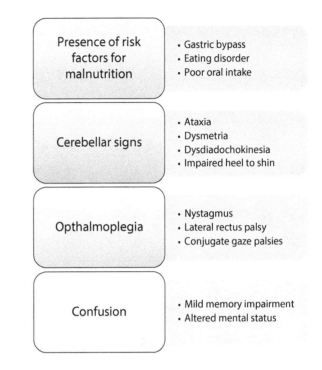

FIGURE 14-10. Caine criteria for thiamine deficiency.

endothelial cell dysfunction, nitrous oxide production, and release of intracellular glutamate into the extracellular space occur.[10] With acute alcohol withdrawal, there is additional neurotoxicity from NMDA receptor hypersensitivity. Gliosis and microhemorrhages in mammillary bodies and the periaqueductal gray can be seen on MRI imaging (Figure 14-9),[12] although imaging is not required to make the diagnosis of WE.[10]

In clinical practice, signs and symptoms of WE are identified using the Caine criteria (provided below) to determine need for treatment.[11] Serum levels are not consistent with thiamine levels in the CNS and are therefore not used in practice to determine the diagnosis or need for treatment. Thiamine deficiency should be treated with high-dose intravenous thiamine (200–500 mg three times daily) when an individual at risk (AUD, history of gastric bypass or other GI pathology that may affect absorption) presents with two of four Caine criteria: signs of malnutrition, ophthalmoplegia, cerebellar dysfunction, and confusion (Figure 14-10).[11] Cerebellar signs of ataxia may be associated with deficits in attention/working memory and upper limb motor function.[13] In addition, the most pronounced memory impairment may be seen in individuals with both cerebellar dysfunction and dietary deficiencies.[13] Treatment with high-dose thiamine allows for simple diffusion into the CNS by generating high serum concentrations, a process that cannot be saturated. Without treatment, long-term outcomes of WE can include development of Korsakoff syndrome, a disorder associated with profound anterograde amnesia and impaired recall of past events, confabulation, and deficits in executive function in an otherwise alert and responsive individual.[14]

Alcohol-Related Dementia

There have been several proposed underlying factors that may contribute to alcohol-related dementia (ARD) including neurotoxic effects of chronic exposure to alcohol (neuronal loss through glutamate excitotoxicity, oxidative stress, and disruption of neurogenesis), thiamine deficiency, and other nutritional deficiencies.[14] Frontal lobes are particularly susceptible to long-standing alcohol use with evidence showing volume shrinkage, decreased neuron density, and altered glucose metabolism.[14] Neuroimaging studies show white matter loss, primarily in the PFC, corpus callosum, and cerebellum, and neuronal loss in the superior frontal association cortex, hypothalamus, and cerebellum.[14] Patients with ARD show deficits in visuospatial tasks, working memory, motor speed, and executive function.[14] Assessment involves taking a nutritional and drinking history, treating underlying contributing factors that may contribute to cognitive changes, and assessment of cognitive status on an ongoing basis. Diagnosis of ARD consists of, in part, identifying cognitive and functional decline following a history of AUD and excluding other causes of dementia. Partial recovery of white matter disturbances can occur with abstinence and can be accompanied by clinical improvements in cognitive and motor abilities.[14] However, the pattern and rate of cognitive recovery is not fully understood.

Glu = glutamate; GABA = gamma-amino butyric acid

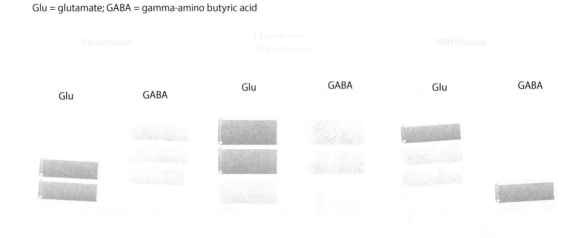

FIGURE 14-11. Changes with alcohol intoxication, chronic use, and withdrawal. Glu, glutamate; GABA, gamma-amino butyric acid.

Alcohol Withdrawal

Chronic alcohol use is associated with changes in the functioning of several neurotransmitters including DA, gamma-amino butyric acid (GABA), and glutamate. As alcohol use results in increased GABA activity, there is an associated decrease in the levels of GABA and decreased GABA receptor sensitivity. Also, with chronic alcohol use, there is an upregulation of glutamatergic activity that occurs to maintain CNS homeostasis. Upon abrupt alcohol cessation, unopposed glutamatergic activity, nervous system hyperactivity, and hyperadrenergic drive result in the clinical picture of alcohol withdrawal (Figure 14-11). DA also contributes to hallucinations, decreased seizure threshold, and autonomic hyperactivity during alcohol use and upon cessation.[15] Alcohol withdrawal symptoms typically arise within 6 hours after abrupt alcohol cessation, and range from mild to severe, including delirium tremens (DTs) (Table 14-2). Risk factors for complicated alcohol withdrawal include a history of structural brain lesions (e.g., traumatic brain injury, stroke), history of complicated withdrawal (seizures, DTs), number of past admissions for medically monitored withdrawal (>4 in past year poses greater risk), and current metabolic derangements, deranged liver enzymes, medical illness, older age, and severe withdrawal symptoms at initial assessment.[16] Assessment involves evaluation for the presence of risk factors, and use of scales, such as the Clinical Institute Withdrawal Assessment for Alcohol Scale-Alcohol Revised (CIWA-Ar), to determine severity of alcohol withdrawal and need for intervention. Treatment of alcohol withdrawal generally involves GABAergic agents to aid in reestablishing CNS homeostasis. Symptom-triggered treatment is the most common approach to treat alcohol withdrawal, with benzodiazepines being the standard medication used.

There are several models of treatment that have been studied, including symptom based, fixed tapering dose, and loading dose regimen. Current evidence supports symptom-triggered regimen (STR) in individuals who are not critically ill or showing signs of severe withdrawal (i.e., DTs or seizures). The CIWA-Ar is a 10-item scale used to classify severity of withdrawal and

TABLE 14-2 • Timeline of Onset of Symptoms in Alcohol Withdrawal.

Time of Appearance After Cessation	Symptoms
6–12 hours	Minor withdrawal symptoms: Insomnia, tremulousness, mild anxiety, GI upset, headache, diaphoresis, palpitations, anorexia
12–24 hours	Alcoholic hallucinosis: Visual, tactile, auditory hallucinations without confusion or delirium
24–48 hours	Withdrawal seizures: Generalized tonic clonic
48–72 hours	Delirium tremens: Autonomic dysfunction, alcohol withdrawal symptoms, delirium, hallucinations (mostly visual)

determine how much benzodiazepine to administer. Most studies have suggested that symptom-triggered therapy can reduce overall benzodiazepine dose, adverse drug events, and length of stay.[16] Still, other studies have not noted significant differences in length of stay with STR. Fixed tapering dose regimen is ideal for individuals who are not appropriate for CIWA, such as individuals who are delirious, unable to cooperate with assessment (e.g., postoperative), or acutely psychotic. This regimen consists of providing fixed doses at scheduled intervals and tapering over the course of several days. It is also used for individuals who are appropriate for treatment of alcohol withdrawal in the outpatient setting. Outpatient treatment may require daily assessments which can occur in a partial day treatment program setting and would be appropriate for individuals who are medically and psychiatrically stable, have mild-to-moderate withdrawal symptoms without any history of DTs or seizures, easy access to the clinic, and a non-drinking support at home.[16] The initial dose may be determined based on the severity of symptoms of withdrawal upon initial

CASE VIGNETTE 14.1

CC: "I had a bad fall"

A 49-year-old man with a past medical history of hypertension, hyperlipidemia, and psychiatric history of major depressive disorder, moderate, and alcohol use disorder who is admitted after a mechanical fall down a flight of stairs with imaging notable for C1 subluxation, right occipital condyle fracture, and right wrist pain. He denies any seizure, loss of consciousness, or chest pain related to the incident.

He is admitted to neurosurgery for additional imaging and observation.

- Onset of drinking: 20 years old, daily drinking starting at age 30
- One pint of Vodka daily—last drink 6 hours prior to admission
- History of one seizure when attempting to self-detox
- No history of DTs or ICU admissions related to alcohol withdrawal
- Five past admissions for medically monitored alcohol withdrawal—no history of complicated withdrawal in these settings
- Head injuries, one with loss of consciousness, in setting of intoxication
- Denies any other drug use

Extensive maternal family history of AUD, brother with opioid use disorder (OUD)

Medications: Citalopram 20 mg daily, ASA 81 mg daily, and Metoprolol 50 mg bid

ROS tremulousness, headache, right shoulder pain, nausea, poor appetite

Exam notable for pulse of 94, tanned complexion, tremors, dysmetria, cognitively intact

Labs notable for MCV 101, AST/ALT 82/43, Mg 1.5. BAL at presentation 106

Urine toxicology screen: Negative for THC, opiates, cocaine, benzodiazepines, PCP

VS 100.4, 140/92, 80, 17, 95% on RA

Labs (CBC, CMP) unremarkable with improved Mg after supplementation

On day 2 of hospitalization, he becomes increasingly agitated, disoriented, and impulsive requiring haloperidol 1 mg IV. Review of records indicates that he has received 6 mg of lorazepam since his admission.

Differential Diagnoses:

Delirium tremens

Thiamine deficiency (Wernicke's encephalopathy)

Benzodiazepine intoxication

Toxic encephalopathy (delirium due to other causes)

Given time frame from last drink, delirium tremens is not likely to be the diagnosis associated with the patient's presentation. He has only received 6 mg of lorazepam, so benzodiazepine intoxication is also unlikely. Although he may have thiamine deficiency in association with chronic alcohol use, acute worsening of mental status is more likely consistent with delirium rather than WE. His initial presentation was not associated with confusion. Nonetheless, he does have dysmetria on exam consistent with cerebellar dysfunction and chronic alcohol use so that treating with high-dose thiamine is warranted. Given acute change in mental status, however, it would be important to consider workup for medical causes of delirium. Given his current state of confusion and agitation, he is no longer appropriate for symptom-triggered regimen (as described in treatment section of this chapter) and should be transitioned to a fixed tapering dose regimen.

TABLE 14-3 • Benzodiazepines Commonly Used in the Treatment of Alcohol Withdrawal.

	Lorazepam	Oxazepam	Chlordiazepoxide	Diazepam
Equivalent doses	1 mg	15 mg	25 mg	5 mg
Half life	10–20 h	5–20 h	5–15 h	30–60 h
Active metabolites	None	None	Yes, t½ >100 h	Yes, t½ >100 h
Hepatic disease	↑ t½ with cirrhosis	↑ t½ with cirrhosis	↑ t½ with cirrhosis	↑ t½ with cirrhosis, acute or chronic hepatic disease
Renal disease	Impaired elimination	No effect	No effect	Decreased protein binding
Older age	No effect on t½	No effect	Slower absorption, ↑ t½	↑ t½

t½, half-life; h, hours.

assessment, known history of benzodiazepine requirements, or risk factors for complicated withdrawal. Finally, loading dose regimen consists of using a long-acting benzodiazepine, such as diazepam or chlordiazepoxide. A preestablished dose is provided every 2 hours until the patient is calm but not oversedated. Long-acting active metabolites allow these medications to self-taper. The

benzodiazepines most commonly studied for alcohol withdrawal are lorazepam, diazepam, oxazepam, and chlordiazepoxide (Table 14-3).[16] While there is no standard benzodiazepine to use for management of withdrawal, factors such as medication half-life and comorbid diseases (i.e., liver dysfunction) should be taken into account. Lorazepam and oxazepam are metabolized through glucuronidation, and thus are preferred in individuals with liver dysfunction. A few studies have shown benefits of using barbiturates for management of alcohol withdrawal, which have cross tolerance with alcohol and long-acting effects. Nonetheless, benzodiazepines remain the most commonly used medication due barbiturates' narrow therapeutic index.[16] There are several agents that can be used in conjunction with benzodiazepines that have shown to decrease symptoms of alcohol withdrawal and decrease the dose requirements of benzodiazepines (Table 14-4).[16]

Clinical Pearl

Avoid use of excess benzodiazepines in individuals with traumatic brain injuries as these may cause paradoxical agitation and impair cognition. It is preferable to avoid use of benzodiazepines if possible or use short-acting agents and titrate slowly to adequate response.

TABLE 14-4 • Adjunctive Medications Used in Alcohol Withdrawal.

Adjunctive Medications	
Carbamazepine	Effective alternative to benzodiazepine in treatment of mild-to-moderate withdrawal Superior in preventing rebound withdrawal symptoms Reduced posttreatment alcohol consumption Limited in use due to interactions with other medications NOT to be used alone in severe alcohol withdrawal
Clonidine dexmedetomidine (typically limited to ICU patients)	Both agents are alpha agonists As adjuncts, reduce sympathetic overdrive and autonomic symptoms Moderate effect in ameliorating symptoms Decrease in total amount of benzodiazepine required
Valproic acid	Consider use in individuals at risk for seizures (history of past seizures, head injury, intracranial abnormality) When used in conjunction with benzodiazepine, can reduce benzodiazepine dose requirements
Baclofen	Reduced cravings Improved CIWA-Ar scores
Gabapentin	Mixed results May reduce risk of drinking Dose ranges variable, unclear if effective in severe alcohol withdrawal

Data from CIWA-Ar, Clinical Institute Withdrawal Assessment for Alcohol Scale-Alcohol Revised.

Opioid Withdrawal

Chronic prescription or illicit opioid use results in symptoms of withdrawal that can be measured using the Clinical Opiate/Opioid Withdrawal Scale (COWS) (Table 14-5). Assessment of opioid withdrawal involves evaluation of type of drug used (e.g., heroin, fentanyl, prescription opioids), last time of use, mode of administration (i.e., insufflation, intravenous, oral), history of overdoses, access to nasal naloxone, and past history of successful attempts at recovery and/or past use of medications for opioid use disorder (OUD). Management of opioid withdrawal involves use of medications to target specific symptoms of opioid withdrawal (Figure 14-12). Medications such as methadone and buprenorphine are helpful in providing rapid and effective relief from symptoms and are also FDA-approved treatments for OUD, as discussed later in this chapter. Buprenorphine is a partial agonist of the mu opioid receptor and decreases symptoms of opioid withdrawal within 30–60 minutes following the first dose. Dose titration occurs on day 1 until resolution of withdrawal symptoms is obtained. Methadone is a full agonist at the mu opioid receptor, with more sedating properties compared to buprenorphine and more drug-drug interactions. Federal legislation allows for use of methadone in the hospital if the patient is admitted for a medical issue other than opioid withdrawal (not admitted specifically for detoxification from opioids). Under these circumstances, the patient can be provided with 30–40 mg of methadone on day 1 of their hospitalization to manage withdrawal symptoms and cravings, followed by a daily dose taper and discontinuation prior to discharge unless a direct admission to a methadone clinic is established. Federal regulations do not allow physicians to prescribe methadone for OUD treatment in the regular outpatient setting. Methadone can only be continued without taper if the patient has a methadone clinic identified that will continue their dose the day after discharge. This may happen with patients who are on chronic methadone treatment prior to their admission (as illustrated in the respective case vignettes). Both methadone and buprenorphine can be provided in the hospital setting for management of opioid withdrawal in patients admitted for reasons other than opioid withdrawal without any additional requirements from the provider. It is only in the outpatient setting that management of OUD requires engagement in a federally regulated program for methadone, and a Drug Enforcement Administration (DEA) waiver for buprenorphine prescribing. The waiver can be obtained by physicians by completing an 8-hour training, and by nurse practitioners and physician assistants after 24 hours of training. Free online waiver trainings and modules are available through https://pcssnow.org/.

The COWS is especially applicable to starting buprenorphine treatment. Buprenorphine is different from other opioids, not only due to partial agonism at the mu opioid receptor (decreased risk of overdose), but also due to its higher binding affinity and slow dissociation from the opioid receptor. Due to these properties, if an individual takes buprenorphine after recently using a full agonist opioid, buprenorphine can displace the full agonist, and lead to immediate partial agonist activity, which the patient will experience as acute withdrawal. On the other hand, if the patient is in mild-to-moderate withdrawal (COWS greater than or equal to 8), partial agonist activity will

TABLE 14-5 • Clinical Opiate Withdrawal Scale.

Clinical Opiate Withdrawal Scale (COWS)

Buprenorphine induction COWS score

Document COWS at initiation, 2 hours after first dose, and then PRN every 4 hours

Patient Name	Date:

Times of Observation

Resting pulse rate: *Measured after patient is sitting or lying for 1 minute*

0 = pulse 80 or below	2 = pulse rate 101–120
1 = pulse rate 81–100	4 = pulse rate greater than 120

Sweating: *Over past 1/2 hour not accounted by room temperature or patient activity*

0 = no report of chills or flushing	3 = beads of sweat on brow or face
1 = subjective report of chills or flushing	4 = sweat streaming off face
2 = flushed or observable moistness on face	

Restlessness: *Observation during assessment*

0 = able to sit still	3 = frequent shifting or extraneous movements of legs or arms
1 = reports difficulty sitting still but is able to	4 = unable to sit still for more than a few seconds

Pupil size

0 = pupils pinned or normal size for room light	2 = pupils moderately dilated
1 = pupils possibly larger than normal for room light	4 = pupils so dilated that only the rim of the iris is visible

Bone or joint aches: *If patient was having pain previously, only the additional component attributed to opiate withdrawal is scored*

0 = not present	2 = patient reports severe diffuse aching of joints/muscles
1 = mild diffuse discomfort	4 = patient is rubbing joints or muscles and is unable to sit because of discomfort

Runny nose or tearing: *Not accounted for by cold symptoms or allergies*

0 = not present	2 = nose running or tearing
1 = nasal stuffiness or unusually moist eyes	4 = nose constantly running or tears streaming down cheeks

GI upset: *Over last 1/2 hour*

0 = no GI symptoms	3 = vomiting or diarrhea
1 = stomach cramps	4 = multiple episodes of diarrhea or vomiting
2 = nausea or loose stool	

Tremor: *Observation of outstretched hands*

0 = no tremor	2 = slight tremor observable
1 = tremor can be felt, but not observed	4 = gross tremor or muscle twitching

Yawning: *Observation during assessment*

0 = no yawning	2 = yawning three or more times during assessment
1 = yawning once or twice during assessment	4 = yawning several times per minute

Anxiety or irritability

0 = none	2 = patient obviously irritable or anxious
1 = patient reports increasing irritability or anxiousness	4 = patient so irritable or anxious that participation in the assessment is difficult

Gooseflesh skin

0 = skin is smooth	5 = prominent piloerection
3 = piloerection of skin can be felt or hairs standing up on arm	

Reproduced with permission from Wesson DR, Ling, W. The Clinical Opiate Withdrawal Scale (COWS). *J Psychoactive Drugs*. 2003. Taylor & Francis Ltd, http://tandfonline.com.

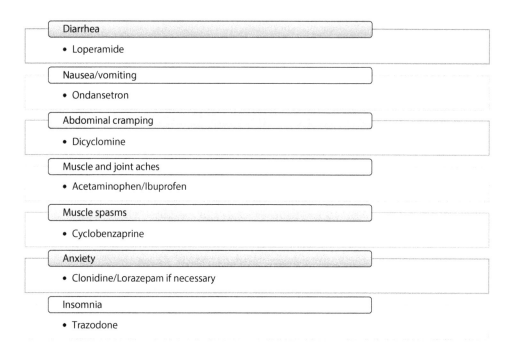

Diarrhea
- Loperamide

Nausea/vomiting
- Ondansetron

Abdominal cramping
- Dicyclomine

Muscle and joint aches
- Acetaminophen/Ibuprofen

Muscle spasms
- Cyclobenzaprine

Anxiety
- Clonidine/Lorazepam if necessary

Insomnia
- Trazodone

FIGURE 14-12. Symptomatic regimen for management of opioid withdrawal.

CASE VIGNETTE 14.2

A 43-year-old woman with a history of hepatitis C and OUD, with intravenous drug use (IVDU), is admitted after a motor vehicle accident. She is not currently in treatment for OUD. She is not interested in buprenorphine treatment. She is administered 30 mg of methadone orally. By day 5 of hospitalization, she is tapered to 0 mg of methadone and discharged with referral to an outpatient addiction recovery program.

Key points:

1. Under federal regulations, methadone cannot be prescribed for treatment of OUD in the outpatient setting outside of a federally regulated methadone treatment program.
2. Methadone can be used while patients are admitted for non-opioid withdrawal reasons to manage symptoms of opioid withdrawal.

result in relief of withdrawal symptoms without euphoria. This is beneficial in both management of withdrawal and treatment of OUD, in which patients experience decreased cravings and an increased capacity to avoid opioid use while on buprenorphine maintenance.

Clinical Pearl

Patients who suffer with chronic pain and have been prescribed opioids for a prolonged period of time will exhibit tolerance and withdrawal due to chronic prescription medication use. In these patients, if doses of opioids are escalating, providers must consider several differential diagnoses including addiction, such as recurrence of underlying disease, acute exacerbation of pain, development of tolerance, diversion, and opioid hyperalgesia. One must also consider the exacerbation of the subjective experience of pain with associated psychiatric comorbidities and target these as appropriate to aid in pain management.

Leukoencephalopathies in the Context of SUD[17]

Delayed post-hypoxic leukoencephalopathy (DPHL) is a rare demyelinating disease that can occur after a period of mild-to-moderate hypoxia. Whereas acute hypoxia generally affects gray matter, DPHL involves white matter tracts. Computed tomography (CT) scans can show diffuse hypodensities in white matter, and magnetic resonance imaging (MRI) reveals typically non-enhancing T2-sequence hyperintense lesions in the periventricular white matter of the cerebral hemispheres (Figure 14-13).[12,17] These lesions do not usually extend into the cortex and spare the cerebellum and brainstem. The onset of symptoms is days to weeks after seemingly full recovery from an acute anoxic injury, such as following an opioid overdose, with neuropsychiatric symptoms varying from agitation, confusion, and akinetic mutism to parkinsonian symptom. Treatment involves aggressive supportive care. Most patients experience recovery with varying degrees of motor and cognitive impairments.

Heroin-associated toxic leukoencephalopathy was initially described in cases of inhaled heroin vapor, a process known as "Chasing the Dragon," but can now be seen in cases of insufflated (snorted) heroin use as well. The mechanism of damage in heroin-induced leukoencephalopathy remains unclear. Given that most cases occur in temporal clusters or with

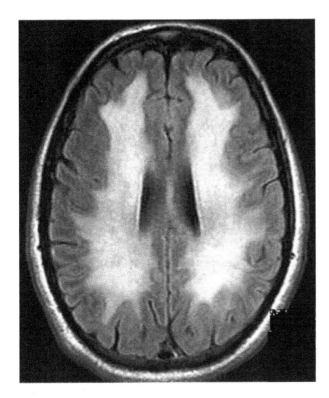

inhaled heroin, it may be associated with additives or contaminants present in heroin or the method of preparation.[16,17]

Symptoms of heroin inhalation leukoencephalopathy may arise during acute intoxication or withdrawal and are not associated with overdose from heroin.[17] The presentation is characterized by three stages, initially with cerebellar signs. Progression through stages may occur over a period of weeks to months (Figure 14-14).[17] The diagnosis requires the history of heroin inhalation, clinical presentation (which may include one or all stages), and findings on imaging that include symmetric white matter lesions of the cerebellum and posterior cerebrum, including posterior limbs of internal capsule (Figure 14-15).[17,18] Cases have been reported with cerebellar sparing that have been associated with intravenous or insufflated heroin use.[17] Treatment is primarily supportive, with some studies suggesting benefits in symptom improvement by providing antioxidant therapy (vitamin E, vitamin C, and ubiquinone).[17]

Drug Intoxication

The clinical features of drug intoxication are variable and are based on the specific drug used, including its pharmacokinetic and pharmacodynamics properties. The route of administration and speed of substance effect can affect the intensity of intoxication and likelihood of experiencing acute withdrawal. Intoxication can also be dose-dependent, as with alcohol, where blood alcohol levels (BALs) correlate with symptoms of intoxication (Table 14-6).[15] Clinical features of intoxication based on *DSM-5* criteria of common drugs of abuse are outlined in Table 14-7.[19]

Cannabis Use Disorder

Over the past decade, changes in the acceptance of cannabis use range from medical marijuana to legal recreational use of cannabis. Over the past decades, the composition of cannabis has changed, with an increase in psychoactive compound

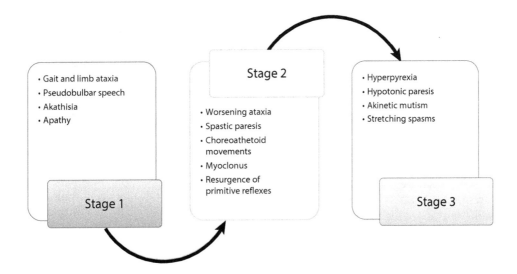

FIGURE 14-14. Progression of heroin-induced leukoencephalopathy.

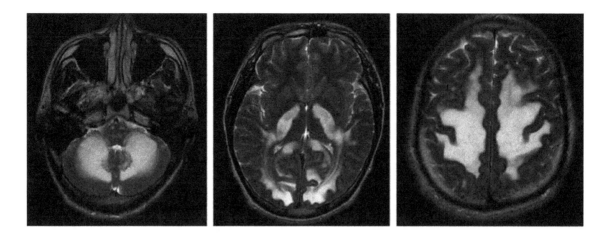

FIGURE 14-15. Brain MRI of heroin-induced leukoencephalopathy. (Reproduced with permission from Tormoehlen LM. Toxic Leukoencephalopathies. *Psychiatr Clin North Am*. 2013;36(2):277-92. https://www.sciencedirect.com/journal/neurologic-clinics.)

TABLE 14-6 • Clinical Picture of Alcohol Intoxication Based on Blood Alcohol Level.	
Blood Alcohol Level	**Clinical Picture**
20–100 mg percent	Mood and behavioral changes Reduced coordination impairment of ability to drive a car or operate machinery
101–200 mg percent	Reduced coordination of most activities Speech impairment Trouble walking General impairment of thinking and judgment
201–300 mg percent	Marked impairment of thinking, memory, and coordination Marked reduction in level of alertness Memory blackouts Nausea and vomiting
301–400 mg percent	Worsening of above symptoms with reduction in body temperature and blood pressure Excessive sleepiness Amnesia
401–800 mg percent	Difficulty walking (coma) Serious decreases in pulse, temperature, blood pressure, and rate of breathing Urinary and bowel incontinence Death

tetrahydrocannabinol and a decrease of the potentially therapeutic compound cannabidiol (CBD).[20] Increased availability of cannabis varieties that are high in THC have been associated with accelerated onset of psychosis, increased cannabis-related hospital admissions, and increased anxiety and psychotic like experiences.[20]

Studies show that with chronic cannabis exposure, neuroanatomic alterations can be seen across regions that are high in cannabinoid receptors (i.e., hippocampus, PFC, amygdala, cerebellum). These changes are thought to be mostly secondary to the neurotoxic THC component of cannabis. On the other hand, CBD has been found to have anxiolytic, antipsychotic, and therapeutic properties, and may attenuate the harmful properties of THC.[20] Research is limited by heterogeneity among studies due to variable doses, frequency, potency of cannabis used, mode of administration, age of onset of use, etc. Most measures are based on self-report, and there are no standards for quantifying exposure levels. Nonetheless, studies indicate that a greater dose of cannabis and earlier age of onset of cannabis use are risk factors associated with neurobiological changes, increased risk of psychotic illness,[20] and increased effects on cognition.[21] Also, cannabis use has been associated with worsening prognosis for individuals with schizophrenia and bipolar disorder.

Both acute and chronic cannabis use are associated with impairments in verbal learning and memory and attention.[21] Acute cannabis use is associated with deficits in psychomotor function and inhibition.[21] Evidence of recovery of cognitive dysfunction after abstinence from use is limited and mixed, though indicate some persistence in the negative effects on memory.[21] There is no FDA-approved treatment for cannabis withdrawal or cannabis use disorder, as studies with a variety of pharmacological options have mixed results.

ASSESSMENT AND DIFFERENTIAL DIAGNOSIS

Assessment of alcohol or drug intoxication, withdrawal, and associated neuropsychiatric issues involves obtaining a clinical history and reviewing laboratory tests to evaluate recent use or examine indicators of chronic use. An important part of the assessment involves obtaining a medical history, including a comprehensive substance use history (Figure 14-16). If the patient is unable to provide a history, it is important to obtain collateral information as acute intoxication may appear as delirium or a primary psychotic illness, and knowledge of drug use may affect treatment. Physical exam should

TABLE 14-7 • Signs and Symptoms of Intoxication with Common Substances Based on *DSM-5* Criteria.

Substance	Eyes	GI	Speech	Autonomic Heart Rate (HR)	Blood Pressure (BP)	Motor	Behavioral	Other	Severe
Opioid	Pupil constriction	Constipation	Slurred			Drowsiness	Euphoria Apathy Dysphoria Impairment in attention/memory		Overdose with respiratory suppression Coma
Stimulant	Pupil dilation	Nausea or Vomiting Weight loss with ongoing use		↑ or ↓ HR ↑ or ↓ BP Perspiration Chills		Psychomotor agitation/slowing Muscle weakness Dyskinesia Dystonia	Confusion Hypersexuality Hypervigilance Hyperawareness		Seizures Coma
Benzodiazepine	Nystagmus		Slurred			Incoordination Unsteady gait	Impaired cognition Mood lability Sexual or aggressive behavior		Stupor Coma
Cannabis	Conjunctival injection	↑ appetite		↑ HR		Incoordination	Euphoria/Anxiety Sensation of slowed time	Dry mouth	
Phencyclidine	Vertical or horizontal nystagmus			↑ HR ↑ BP		Ataxia Psychomotor agitation Dysarthria Muscle rigidity	Impulsiveness Assaultiveness	↓ Pain response Hyperacusis	Seizures Coma
Other hallucinogens: D-lysergic acid diethylamide (LSD), Peyote (Mescaline)	Pupil dilation Blurred vision			↑ HR Palpitations Sweating		Tremors Incoordination	Impulsiveness Assaultiveness Paranoia		
Inhalant	Nystagmus Blurred vision Diplopia		Slurred			Incoordination Unsteady gait Lethargy Depressed reflexes Tremor Muscle weakness	Euphoria Belligerence Assaultiveness Apathy	Dizziness	Stupor Coma

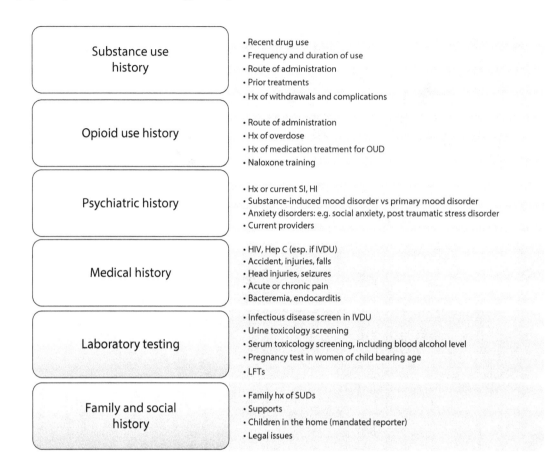

Substance use history
- Recent drug use
- Frequency and duration of use
- Route of administration
- Prior treatments
- Hx of withdrawals and complications

Opioid use history
- Route of administration
- Hx of overdose
- Hx of medication treatment for OUD
- Naloxone training

Psychiatric history
- Hx or current SI, HI
- Substance-induced mood disorder vs primary mood disorder
- Anxiety disorders: e.g. social anxiety, post traumatic stress disorder
- Current providers

Medical history
- HIV, Hep C (esp. if IVDU)
- Accident, injuries, falls
- Head injuries, seizures
- Acute or chronic pain
- Bacteremia, endocarditis

Laboratory testing
- Infectious disease screen in IVDU
- Urine toxicology screening
- Serum toxicology screening, including blood alcohol level
- Pregnancy test in women of child bearing age
- LFTs

Family and social history
- Family hx of SUDs
- Supports
- Children in the home (mandated reporter)
- Legal issues

FIGURE 14-16. Clinical assessment of substance use.

evaluate for objective signs of withdrawal and intoxication from alcohol (Tables 14-2 and 14-6) other substances (Tables 14-7 and 14-8).

It is not uncommon for individuals who are using illicit drugs to use more than one drug at a time, further complicating the clinical presentation of both intoxication and withdrawal. Urine toxicology screening becomes an essential part of the assessment of drug intoxication. Most urine drug screens include immunoassay screening for cannabis (THC), benzodiazepines, cocaine, opiates, and phencyclidine. For assessment of use of other drugs, including opioids (synthetic and semi-synthetic) such as oxycodone, methadone, fentanyl, or buprenorphine, additional testing is typically required. Finally, urine toxicology screens have limitations in their capacity to detect use of drugs such as synthetic cannabinoids, hallucinogens, and certain fentanyl analogues.

Recent alcohol use can be identified by obtaining a BAL or through use of a breathalyzer. When considering BALs, it should be noted that alcohol is metabolized by zero order kinetics, so that one drink is metabolized per hour (10–15 mg/dL/h). However, chronic drinkers metabolize alcohol at faster rates of 20–25 mg/dL/h. In addition, women metabolize alcohol differently so that higher BALs (and intoxication) will show despite drinking the same amount as their male counterparts.[15] There are several reasons for higher BALs in women including lower total body water and a lower activity of alcohol dehydrogenase

in the stomach. This contributes to a greater risk of alcohol-related illness such as liver disease and may contribute to the "telescoping" effect seen in women in which the progression from onset of drinking to AUD diagnosis and need for treatment occurs faster than in men.[15] Urine alcohol can also be obtained through immunoassay screening, which can detect alcohol 6–12 hours after the last drink. However, the urine alcohol screen carries a high risk of false positive results. Urine ethyl glucuronide and ethyl sulfate can be detected in the urine 3–5 days following the last drink depending on amount consumed and are used primarily in medical and criminal justice programs where complete abstinence is expected.[15] There are also indirect biomarkers that are associated with chronic alcohol use. These include livers transaminases, gamma glutamyl transferase (GGT), carbohydrate-deficient transferrin (CDT), and mean corpuscular volume (MCV). In alcoholic hepatitis, an elevated ratio of aspartate transaminase (AST) to alanine transaminase (ALT) of 2:1 is typically seen (normal is closer to 1). While above markers can be elevated in a variety of diseases that are not alcohol-specific, GGT and CDT, when combined, have a sensitivity and specificity for chronic alcohol use of over 90%.

Mood disorders often coexist with SUD, and current guidelines warrant treatment of both concurrently. It is helpful, if possible, to distinguish between a substance-induced mood disorder and a primary mood disorder, where a substance-induced

TABLE 14-8 • Withdrawal Signs and Symptoms from Common Substances.					
Caffeine	Cannabis	Opioids	Sedative, Hypnotics, Anxiolytics	Stimulants	Tobacco
Headache Drowsiness Dysphoric, depressed irritable mood Difficulty concentrating Flu-like symptoms	Irritability, anger, aggression Anxiety Sleep difficulty (insomnia, disturbing dreams) Decreased appetite Restlessness Depressed mood At least one of the following: Abdominal pain Shakiness/Tremor Sweating Fever Chills Headache	Dysphoric mood Nausea/vomiting Muscle aches Lacrimation/ rhinorrhea Pupil dilation Piloerection Diaphoresis Diarrhea Yawning Fever Insomnia	Autonomic hyperactivity Tremor Insomnia Nausea/Vomiting Transient visual or tactile hallucinations Psychomotor agitation Anxiety Grand mal seizures	Fatigue Vivid, unpleasant dreams Insomnia or hypersomnia Increased appetite Psychomotor retardation or agitation	Irritability Anxiety Difficulty concentrating Increased appetite Restlessness Depressed mood Insomnia

mood disorder occurs when criteria for the disorder is met during or within 1 month of intoxication with or withdrawal from a substance that is capable of causing the mental disorder.[3] If the mental disorder preceded the onset of intoxication or withdrawal or persisted for at least 1 month after the intoxication or withdrawal from the substance ended, it is more likely a primary mood disorder.

Differential diagnoses for acute intoxication and withdrawal may range from primary mood or psychotic illness to delirium (toxic metabolic encephalopathy). Review of medical comorbidities and laboratory testing will help clarify recent drug use.

TREATMENT

This section will focus on FDA-approved, evidence-based treatments for alcohol, opioid, and tobacco use disorders. Treatments for acute intoxication of substances will be explored as well. Treatment of addiction to other drugs, including stimulants and cannabis, is limited and research findings are mixed, and therefore will not be discussed in this chapter. Finally, nonpharmacologic, behavioral treatments will be discussed. Behavioral interventions play an important role in the management of addiction and help restore balance in the brain circuitry affected by drug use.[2] These treatments are geared toward improving stress reactivity, enhancing salience of natural nondrug rewards, and improving executive function and self-regulation.

Alcohol Use Disorder Treatment

The three FDA-approved medications for treatment of AUD are naltrexone, acamprosate, and disulfiram. Naltrexone is an opioid receptor blocker that works by decreasing reward following alcohol use. For all patients, an opioid-free period of at least 7–10 days is required as administration of naltrexone while on opioid medications or illicit opioid use results in abrupt, severe symptoms of opioid withdrawal. Studies

related to naltrexone in the treatment of AUD have shown that naltrexone reduces the risk of relapse, and if relapse happens, it reduces number of drinks per drinking day and the number of heavy drinking days. Sufficient blockade of opioid receptors requires 80% adherence to treatment with oral naltrexone. An injectable, extended release version of naltrexone is available, which is administered as a monthly intramuscular gluteal injection and bypasses first pass metabolism, with less associated side effects. Alternatively, disulfiram irreversibly binds to aldehyde dehydrogenase, an enzyme involved in the metabolism of alcohol (Figure 14-17). If alcohol is ingested while on the medication, dose-dependent symptoms arise, ranging from nausea and flushing to seizures and cardiovascular collapse. Consent is an important part of prescribing disulfiram as patients need to be aware of the dangers of drinking while on the medication. Additionally, because disulfiram is irreversible bound to the enzyme, it may take up to 2 weeks for the body to create enough unbound enzyme to metabolize alcohol appropriately. Finally, acamprosate is a medication, dosed three times daily, that may be used in individuals with severe liver dysfunction as it is primarily metabolized by the kidneys. Acamprosate is a glutamate/GABA system modulator and stabilizes this system, which,

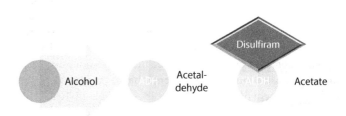

FIGURE 14-17. Mechanism of action of disulfiram activity. ADH, alcohol dehydrogenase; ALDH, aldehyde dehydrogenase.

CASE VIGNETTE 14.3

A 37-year-old man with a history of OUD, on methadone 75 mg daily, is admitted for acute onset shortness of breath. You contact his methadone clinic and obtain a "last dose letter" confirming his enrollment in the clinic and daily dose. He receives his daily 75 mg oral dose while in the hospital and is discharged with plans to obtain his daily dose at the methadone clinic the following morning. He is provided with a last dose letter to provide to his methadone clinic prior to discharge from the hospital.

Key points:

Patients who are enrolled in a methadone clinic and are admitted to the hospital should be continued on their treatment. Steps to take in the inpatient setting include:

1. Confirming last dose date and amount with methadone clinic.
2. Continue methadone at dose confirmed. If unable to confirm dose (e.g., on weekends) can provide 30–40 mg daily until able to confirm dose.
3. Provide patient with last dose letter to indicate date and dose last received in the hospital prior to discharge.

TABLE 14-9 • Medications for Management of Alcohol Use Disorder.

Drug	Dosing	Mechanism	Effects	Adverse Effects
Naltrexone	50–100 mg PO daily	Opioid antagonist	↓ cravings	Liver monitoring with oral
XR-NTX	380 mg IM		↓ heavy drinking	
			↓ EtOH effects	Opioids (at typical doses) not effective for pain while on naltrexone
Disulfiram	250 mg PO Daily	ALDH inhibitor	Supervision helps	Disulfiram reaction, dose-dependent (severity of reaction may vary depending on amount of alcohol consumed) Liver monitoring
Acamprosate	333–666 mg PO tid	Glutamate modulation	↑ abstinence Improved neurovegetative symptoms	Diarrhea, contraindicated in renal failure

ALDH, aldehyde dehydrogenase; EtOH, alcohol; IM, intramuscular; PO, oral; XR-NTX, extended release naltrexone.

as discussed earlier in the chapter in section for alcohol withdrawal, is affected by chronic alcohol use. Both acamprosate and oral naltrexone are associated with reduction in return to drinking.[22] See Table 14-9 for a summary of medications used in the treatment of AUD.

Opioid Use Disorder Treatment

The three FDA-approved medications for treatment of OUD are buprenorphine, methadone, and naltrexone (specifically extended-release injectable naltrexone). Treatment of OUD with methadone requires dosing through a federally regulated methadone clinic. Buprenorphine treatment requires physicians to obtain a waiver to prescribe this medication for treatment of OUD and allows for patients to obtain treatment in the outpatient setting. By blocking the opioid receptor, naltrexone blocks opioid activity if a patient uses an opioid while on the medication. Choosing the right medication for each patient is based on several factors, including patient preference (Figure 14-18). Table 14-10 reviews the three medications used for OUD treatment.

Nicotine Use Disorder Treatment

Nicotine replacement therapy (NRT), bupropion, and varenicline are the three FDA-approved medications to treat nicotine

use disorder. Nicotine replacement allows for a slow taper off of nicotine using a variety of modes of administration, including patches, gum, lozenges, sublingual tablets, sprays, and inhalers. Bupropion acts primarily on the DA and norepinephrine system and is also used as an antidepressant. It can be used alone or in combination with NRT to treat nicotine use disorder. Varenicline is a selective nicotine receptor partial agonist. All treatments are superior over placebo in achieving abstinence from tobacco use.[23] A recent large randomized, double blind, placebo-controlled trial comparing medications used in treatment of nicotine use disorder did not show a significant increase in neuropsychiatric adverse events attributable to varenicline or bupropion compared to nicotine patch or placebo.[23]

Drug and Alcohol Intoxication

Management of acute intoxication entails determining the degree of intoxication (e.g., BAL), and managing presenting symptoms, while ensuring safety and monitoring for onset of withdrawal. Agitation is common to most drugs of abuse, and benzodiazepines are often used as treatment to ensure patient and staff safety. Treatment may entail observation until the patient can engage in a formal assessment if unable to attend to the medical examination. Table 14-11 reviews treatment of acute intoxication with common substances.[15,24]

TABLE 14-10 • Comparison of Medications Used to Treat Opioid Use Disorder.			
Medication	**Dosing**	**Treatment**	**Adverse Effects**
Methadone	• Optimal dosing is influenced by factors including metabolism, body weight, and comorbid medical illnesses • Effective average dose range 60–120, varies per individual • Liquid formulation • Once daily dosing	• Only available at licensed opioid treatment programs • Daily attendance to obtain medication during the early phases of treatment • Gold standard in pregnancy • Risk of neonatal abstinence syndrome in infants	• QTc prolongation • Medication interactions (cytochrome P metabolism: increased levels of methadone when combined with CYP inducers) • Respiratory depression • Constipation • Sedation • Nausea • Diaphoresis
Bup/Nal **Buprenorphine monoproduct primarily used in pregnancy**	• Typical maintenance dose is 8–16 (max. typically 24 mg) • <8 mg for individuals with known OUD and who have been off opioids • Dosed daily, bid, or tid • Tid dosing for pain • Sublingual tablet or film, or buccal film formulation	• Available from physician's office • Buprenorphine prescribers must obtain a specific DEA waiver by completing an 8-hour training (MDs) or 24 hours of training (NPs and PAs) • Initiation requires the individual to be abstinent or withdrawing from opioids (avoid use of short acting opioids for at least 8–12 hours prior to induction, longer time if long-acting opioid)	• Precipitated withdrawal • Respiratory depression: especially if concurrent use of alcohol or sedatives • Constipation • Headache • Sweating
Extended release injectable naltrexone	• 380 mg • Dosed monthly • Intramuscular	• Available from physician's office—no specific training required • Initiation requires opioid free for 7–10 days	• Injection site reactions • Nausea, dizziness • Predicted need for opioids within the next month • Joint pain • Headaches

Bup/nal, buprenorphine/naloxone; DEA, Drug Enforcement Administration; NP, nurse practitioners; OUD, opioid use disorder; PA, physician assistant.

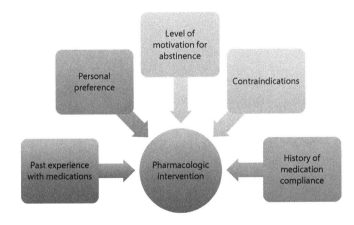

FIGURE 14-18. Choosing medication for treatment of opioid use disorder.

Nonpharmacologic Interventions

Motivational interviewing (MI) is a technique used in the treatment of SUD, which highlights individuals' autonomy in the process of recovery. It is a process that includes engagement, focusing, evoking "change talk," and planning for change that occurs dynamically over time. It is based on principles of

TABLE 14-11 • Management of Acute Intoxication with Common Drugs.	
Intoxication	**Treatment**
Alcohol	Supportive: IVFs, IV antiemetics prn, thiamine supplementation, management of alcohol withdrawal
Stimulants	Benzodiazepines for agitation Cautious use of antipsychotics (can worsen hyperthermia)
Hallucinogens	Rarely require medical treatment "Bad trip" (anxiety/panic): Benzodiazepines Cautious use of antipsychotics (can cause dysphoria and possible worsening of hallucinations with haloperidol) Hypertensive crisis: IV labetalol Serotonin syndrome: Cyproheptadine
Opioids	No treatment required, though monitoring for opioid overdose if under supervision If overdose: Naloxone (IN, IM, IV) to reverse overdose

IM, intramuscular; IN, intranasal; IV, intravenous; prn, as needed; IVFs, intravenous fluids.

collaboration, acceptance, evocation, and compassion, with a primary focus on individuals' values to identify goals.[25] Cognitive behavioral therapy (CBT) is often used in relapse prevention treatment and is helpful in assisting individuals find healthier ways to cope with their emotions, navigate their world despite stressors, and identify long-term goals.[26] Studies have also examined the role of cognitive and motivational therapies in normalizing aberrant activity of the brain's reward circuitry and recruitment of the brain's inhibitory/executive control network indicating not only behavioral changes with treatment but also neurobiological benefits.[26] Neuroimaging studies have shown that nonpharmacologic interventions, such as CBT and MI, are associated with a normalization of aberrant activity in the brain's

reward circuitry and the recruitment and strengthening of the brain's inhibitory control network.[26] Finally, peer-based support is important and is utilized in 12-step and Self-Management and Recovery Training (SMART) meetings, as well as the incorporation of recovery coaches in early recovery.

Understanding the neurobiological changes that occur with persistent exposure to substances of abuse allows providers to appreciate the pharmacologic and therapeutic interventions used, as well as their potential impact in activating hypoactive regions of the reward system, allowing for recovery and healing to occur over time, increasing an individuals' potential to remain free from drugs and alcohol.

Summary and Key Points

- The brain's reward system is affected by all drugs of abuse leading to changes in incentive salience of drug versus nondrug rewards and an increase in reward threshold. Dopamine, GABA, and endogenous opioids play a key role in the reinforcing effects of drugs.
- Recruitment of stress systems and dysregulation of neurochemicals with repeated drug use contributes to negative reinforcement of drug use, driving the compulsive nature of addiction.
- Different drugs of abuse have specific objective signs and symptoms associated with intoxication and withdrawal that can help differentiate them from other neuropsychiatric

diseases. Laboratory testing and a comprehensive substance use history are important components of the assessment for drug use.

- Current treatments are founded on the neurobiology of addiction. Evidence-based treatments exist for management of alcohol withdrawal, AUD, OUD, and tobacco use disorder.
- Further research is needed to identify treatments for management of addiction to other drugs, such as stimulants and cannabis, both of which are commonly used drugs.
- As social and legal acceptance of cannabis continues to change, further research is needed to understand long-term effects of cannabis use and to develop treatments for acute intoxication, cannabis use disorder, and acute cannabis withdrawal.

Multiple Choice Questions

1. The three stages of addiction:
   a. Include intoxication, generational forgetting, and withdrawal
   b. Involve only behavioral changes that occur as an individual moves from first use to addiction
   c. Consist of binge/intoxication, withdrawal, and preoccupation/anticipation
   d. All stages are dictated by the rewarding effects (i.e., positive reinforcement) obtained from ongoing drug use
   e. Are used to support criminalization as it emphasizes logic as the driving force in addiction

2. A 48-year-old woman with a past medical history of chronic pain from a past motor vehicle accident with lumbar radiculopathy and a psychiatric history of post-traumatic stress disorder and OUD, with a recent relapse in the setting of

divorce, is admitted to the hospital after being found down and unresponsive, requiring nasal naloxone. She is admitted for ongoing monitoring and aspiration pneumonia. She begins to experience symptoms of opioid withdrawal and asks to leave against medical advice. In an effort to ensure she remains in the hospital for additional testing and treatment, you offer the following:
   a. Unfortunately, you can only offer clonidine as you are not allowed to prescribe methadone for opioid addiction outside of a federally regulated methadone clinic
   b. High-dose benzodiazepines to manage her opioid withdrawal
   c. A psychiatry consultation as she needs additional support
   d. Methadone only as buprenorphine requires a special waiver for prescribing in the hospital
   e. Methadone or buprenorphine for management of opioid withdrawal while in the hospital

3. A 52-year-old man with a past medical history of hemochromatosis and AUD is admitted for management of alcohol withdrawal. In assessing his treatment, which of the following is true:
   a. There is no advantage of using symptom-triggered therapy over fixed dose regimen.
   b. Delirium tremens can be seen as early as 12 hours after the last drink.
   c. Visual hallucinations without delirium may indicate alcohol hallucinosis.
   d. If delirious, CIWA-Ar should be more closely monitored and additional benzodiazepines given.
   e. Diazepam is the most ideal benzodiazepine to use due to its extrahepatic metabolism via glucuronidation.

4. A 21-year-old man presents to the emergency department after developing panic symptoms at a party. He endorses use of alcohol. On exam, you notice tachycardia, rapid speech, dilated pupils, and hyperactivity. He is worried about providing laboratory tests as his parents are with him and he does not "want to get in trouble." You suspect, based on his signs and symptoms, that his urine will likely test positive for recent use of:
   a. Cannabis
   b. Cocaine
   c. Opioids
   d. Benzodiazepines
   e. Caffeine

Multiple Choice Answers

1. **Answer: c**
   Generational forgetting is a concept that involves patterns of drug use and perceived risks of harm as shown by the Monitoring the Future study in which the associated harms of specific drugs are forgotten as generational replacement takes place. Transition from one stage to another does not only reflect changes in behavior, but also neurobiological changes that affect motivational factors associated with the development of addiction. The binge/intoxication stage involves primarily the reward system, but other stages, including withdrawal/negative affect involves stress systems, and changes in our anti-reward systems, including neurochemicals such as neuropeptide Y. Neurobiological changes show that ongoing drug use is driven by changes in the emotional and reward systems rather than by logic or higher-level reasoning.

2. **Answer: e**
   Management of opioid withdrawal can involve the use of clonidine to help with hyperadrenergic drive and anxiety related to the syndrome. However, use of agonists, like methadone or buprenorphine, provide faster and more effective relief of symptoms of withdrawal. While benzodiazepines may also help with anxiety in opioid withdrawal, benzodiazepines alone are not first-line agents in management of opioid withdrawal but are the gold standard for management of alcohol withdrawal. A psychiatry consultation may be helpful to assess for capacity to leave against medical advice but will not resolve the issue of opioid withdrawal. BOTH methadone and buprenorphine can be prescribed by any physician in the hospital. Special regulations for methadone and buprenorphine prescribing apply to outpatient treatment of OUD.

3. **Answer: c**
   Alcohol hallucinosis typically resolves spontaneously within 48 hours of alcohol cessation and is not associated with confusion. It can occur in about 25% of individuals with AUD and does not require additional pharmacologic interventions. Research suggests an advantage in using symptom-triggered alcohol withdrawal treatment, such that it may lead to shorter length of hospitalization and lower benzodiazepine dose administration, without obvious differences in adverse events. DTs typically presents 48–72 hours after alcohol cessation. If a patient who is undergoing alcohol withdrawal becomes delirious, it would be best to discontinue symptom-triggered therapy, as ongoing confusion and agitation would lead to increased benzodiazepine doses and can lead to iatrogenic benzodiazepine intoxication. Delirious patients should be placed on standing taper of benzodiazepines for alcohol withdrawal management, and medical workup for alternate causes of delirium should be explored. Finally, diazepam undergoes intrahepatic metabolism and should be avoided in individuals with liver dysfunction as they are at risk of accumulating active metabolites and thus, at risk of sedation and iatrogenic benzodiazepine intoxication.

4. **Answer: b**
   Symptoms of cannabis intoxication do not include dilated pupils, but rather conjunctival injection. Anxiety and tachycardia may be presenting symptoms of cannabis intoxication, but other signs such as rapid speech are not associated with cannabis use. Opioid intoxication would be more consistent with miosis and sedation rather than hyperactivity. Benzodiazepines are typically associated with slurred speech, nystagmus, and drowsiness/sedation. While caffeine intoxication can lead to hyperactivity and tachycardia, dilated pupils are not specific to caffeine use and does not fit the clinical picture. Also, there is not a urine toxicology screen for caffeine use.

References

1. Koob GF, Volkow ND. Neurocircuitry of addiction. *Neuro-psychopharmacology*. 2010;35(1):217-238.
2. Volkow N, Koob GF, McLellan AT. Neurobiological advances from the brain disease model of addiction. *N Engl J Med*. 2016;374:363-371.
3. Teeson M, Mewton L. Epidemiology of addiction. In: Galanter M, Kleber HD, Brady KT, eds. *Textbook of Substance Abuse Treatment*. Washington, DC: American Psychiatric Publishing; 2015:P47.
4. National Institute on Drug Abuse. *Trends & Statistics*. 2017. Available at https://www.drugabuse.gov/related-topics/trends-statistics. Accessed July 12, 2019.
5. Grant BF, Saha TD, Ruan WJ, et al. Epidemiology of DSM-5 drug use disorder: results from the national epidemiologic survey on alcohol and related conditions-III. *JAMA Psychiatry*. 2016;73(1):39-47.
6. Johnston LD, Miech RA, O'Malley OM, et al. *Monitoring the Future National Survey Results on Drug Use: 1975–2017: Overview, Key Findings on Adolescent Drug Use*. Ann Arbor, MI: Institute for Social Research, The University of Michigan; 2018.
7. Substance Abuse and Mental Health Services Administration. *Key Substance Use and Mental Health Indicators in the United States: Results from the 2016 National Survey on Drug Use and Health*. HHS Publication No. SMA 17-5044, NSDUH Series H-52. Rockville, MD: Center for Behavioral Health Statistics and Quality, Substance Abuse and Mental Health Services Administration; 2017. Available at https://www.samhsa.gov/data/. Accessed July 12, 2019.
8. National Institutes of Health: U.S. Department of Health and Human Services, National Center for Health Statistics. CDC Wonder. Available at https://www.cdc.gov/nchs/index.htm. Accessed July 12, 2019.
9. Gage SH, Sumnall HR. Rat Park: how the rat paradise changed the narrative of addiction. *Addiction*. 2018;14(5):917-922.
10. Isenberg-Grzeda E, Kutner HE, Nicolson SE. Wernicke-Korsakoff-syndrome: under-recognized and under-treated. *Psychosomatics*. 2012;53:507-516.
11. Caine D, Halliday GM, Kril JJ, Harper CG. Operational criteria for the classification of chronic alcoholics: identification of Wernicke's encephalopathy. *J Neurol Neurosurg Psychiatry*. 1997;62:51-60.
12. Ropper AH, Samuels MA, Klein JP. Diseases of the nervous system caused by nutritional deficiency. In: *Adams & Victor's Principles of Neurology*. 10th ed. New York, NY: McGraw-Hill; 2014.
13. Fama R, Le Berre AP, Hardcastle C, et al. Neurological, nutritional, and alcohol consumption factors underlie cognitive and motor deficits in chronic alcoholism. *Addict Biol*. 2019;24(2):290-302.
14. Ridley NJ, Draper B, Withall A. Alcohol-related dementia: an update of the evidence. *Alzheimers Res Ther*. 2013;5(1):3.
15. Myrick H. Treatment of alcohol intoxication and alcohol withdrawal. In: *Textbook of Substance Abuse Treatment*. Washington, DC: American Psychiatric Publishing; 2015:159.
16. Sachdeva A, Choudhary M, Chandra M. Alcohol withdrawal syndrome: benzodiazepines and beyond. *J Clin Diagn Res*. 2015;9(9):VE01-VE07.
17. Tormoehlen LM. Toxic leukoencephalopathies. *Psychiatr Clin North Am*. 2013;36(2):277-292.
18. Offiah C, Hall E. Heroin-induced leukoencephalopathy: characterization using MRI, diffusion-weighted imaging, and MR spectroscopy. *Clin Radiol*. 2008;63(2):146-152.
19. Galanter M, Kleber HD, Brady KT. Appendix: DSM-5 substance related and addictive disorders. In: *American Psychiatric Association: Diagnostic and Statistical Manual of Mental Disorders*. 5th ed. Arlington, VA: American Psychiatric Association; 2013.
20. Lorenzetti V, Solowij N, Yucel M. The role of cannabinoids in neuroanatomic alterations in cannabis users. *Biol Psychiatry*. 2016;79(7):17-21.
21. Broyd S, Van Hell H, Beale C, Yucel M, Solowij N. Acute and chronic effects of cannabinoids on human cognition—a systematic review. *Biol Psychiatry*. 2016;70(7):557-567.
22. Jonas DE, Amick HR, Feltner C, et al. Pharmacotherapy for adults with alcohol use disorders in outpatient settings: a systematic review and meta-analysis. *JAMA*. 2014;311(18):1889-1900.
23. Anthenelli RM, Benowitz NL, West R, et al. Neuropsychiatric safety and efficacy of varenicline, bupropion, and nicotine patch in smokers with and without psychiatric disorder (EAGLES): a double-blind, randomised, placebo-controlled trial. *Lancet*. 2016;387(10037):2507-2520.
24. MacLean KA, Johnson MW, Griffiths RR. Hallucinogens and club drugs. In: Galanter M, Kleber HD, Brady KT, eds. *Textbook of Substance Abuse Treatment*. Washington, DC: American Psychiatric Publishing; 2015:209.
25. DiClemente CC, Greene P, Petersen AA, Thrash ST, Crouch TB. Motivational enhancement. In: Galanter M, Kleber HD, Brady KT, eds. *Textbook of Substance Abuse Treatment*. Washington, DC: American Psychiatric Publishing; 2015:397.
26. Zilverstand A, Parvaz MA, Moeller SJ, Goldstein RZ. Cognitive interventions for addiction medicine: understanding the underlying neurological mechanisms. *Prog Brain Res*. 2016;224:285-304.

15

Neuropsychiatry of Sleep and Sleep Disorders

Rebecca M. Allen · Milena Pavlova

Sleep comprises roughly one-third of an adult's life. It is an active physiological process with wide effects on health. Poor/insufficient sleep has the potential to aggravate any disease and many diseases impact sleep. Therefore, an understanding of sleep and sleep disorders is essential for the practice of neuropsychiatry. Sleep disorders epitomize neuropsychiatry, capturing the overlap between altered brain networks, behavior, and cognition. Sleep deprivation impairs almost all cognitive functions, and evidence has rapidly accumulated implicating amount and quality of sleep in disturbances of memory processing and consolidation. Furthermore, sleep disorders contribute to the morbidity of both psychiatric and neurological disease. The likelihood of having sleep problems increases with the number of psychiatric diagnoses,[1] and parasomnias are more common in psychiatric populations.[2] Sleep disturbance is now a well-recognized common consequence of traumatic brain injury (TBI) across all levels of TBI severity,[3] and sleep disruption is also prevalent in neurodegenerative disorders.[4] Sleep disorders (e.g., obstructive sleep apnea [OSA], REM behavior disorder [RBD], other parasomnias) should be carefully considered in patients with a variety of cognitive and behavioral presenting complaints. This chapter will review the basics of sleep physiology, our present understanding of the purpose of sleep, and briefly review sleep disorders.

BASICS OF HUMAN SLEEP PHYSIOLOGY

In humans, sleep typically occurs during the biological night—a phase regulated by the circadian cycle. Sleep is characterized by relative physical inactivity and unawareness of the surrounding environment, higher melatonin levels, lower cortisol levels, lower urine volume, and lower body temperature.

The most frequently used technique for studying sleep in humans is polysomnography (PSG), which records simultaneously electroencephalography (EEG), eye movements (EOG), and muscular activity (EMG). PSG data help distinguish non-rapid eye movement (NREM) sleep from rapid eye movement (REM) sleep. Physiologically, normal NREM sleep starts with a gradual change in consciousness, loss of memory for the immediately preceding interval, and overall slower activity, with a decreased heart rate (40–90 BPM), regular, slower respirations, and a mild decrease in oxygen saturation (about 2%), reflecting a lower brain metabolic activity and decreased demand. Electrographically, NREM sleep is associated with synchronous neuronal activity, represented on the EEG by high-amplitude, low-frequency rhythms. NREM sleep can be further subdivided into three distinct stages. Stage N1 represents the transition from wakefulness to sleep and is usually of short duration. It is characterized by slow roving eye movements, disappearance of the alpha activity on EEG, and appearance of slower theta rhythms. Stage N2 is the stage occupying the most time during the night, and is characterized by K complexes (biphasic negative-positive waveforms of high amplitude, 0.5 seconds in duration) and sleep spindles (brief sigma frequency activity of 15 Hz for less than a second). Progressively, the appearance of slow delta waves will delineate the transition of stage N2 to stage N3. After about 90 minutes of sleep, the first REM period is seen, characterized by eye movements, often visible through closed eyelids. Electrographically, REM sleep is distinguished from NREM sleep by three core signs: (1) a low voltage EEG activity, mainly theta and alpha rhythms; (2) characteristic REMs; and (3) muscle atonia, measured on a chin EMG channel. During REM sleep, respiration and heart rate are irregular, and cerebral metabolic rate and oxygen demand are both increased. The human brain cycles through lighter and deeper sleep, with approximately four to five cycles per night (see Figure 15-1).

The regulation of sleep is complex (see Figure 15-2 for a diagram of brainstem circuits relevant to sleep regulation). The ventrolateral preoptic nucleus (VLPO), located in the anterior hypothalamus, is a sleep promoter and is generally considered to be the "off" button of the sleep-wake switch; it regulates the wake-to-sleep transition by reducing activity of the ascending arousal systems, using GABA and galanin. The tuberomammillary nucleus in the posterior hypothalamus is the "on" button of the sleep-to-wake switch, and wakefulness is stabilized by the orexin/hypocretin system in the lateral hypothalamus. Unlike

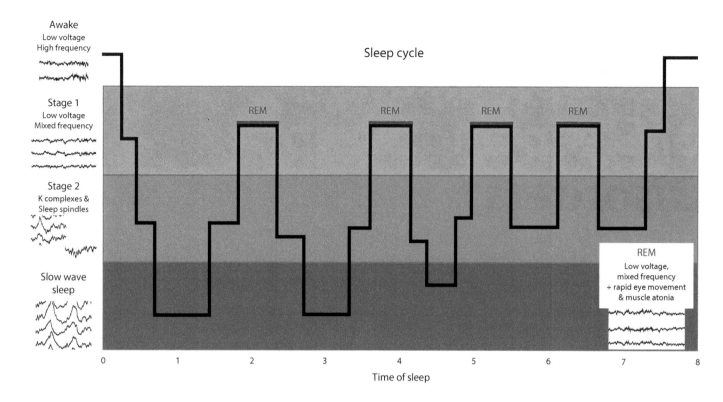

FIGURE 15-1. Sleep cycle. Throughout a typical nights' sleep, the human brain cycles through lighter and deeper sleep, with approximately four to five cycles per night. In the first half of the night, more time is spent in deep sleep (slow-wave sleep) and in the second half of the night, more time is spent in light sleep (stages 1 and 2) and REM sleep.

the sleep-wake switch, the ascending reticular activating system is more like a dimmer switch, using five key neurotransmitters (histamine, dopamine, norepinephrine, serotonin and acetylcholine) from the brainstem to the cortical arousal system to promote wakefulness.[5]

According to a model described by Borbély and Achermann,[6] sleep initiation is regulated by two independent processes. The first is the effect of the duration of wakefulness: the longer the individual is awake, the stronger the homeostatic pressure to sleep. The second process is the effect of the circadian rhythms, which control a variety of different functions and allow sustained wakefulness during the "biological day" of the individual and sleep at night. The circadian rhythm, or internal clock, is constantly reset based upon activity and light exposure. The effect of light depends on timing of exposure as well as the intensity spectrum/wavelength, with the blue spectrum of light having a stronger influence.[7] Melatonin is a key part of the circadian rhythm, and its secretion is influenced by light. Melatonin is secreted during the dark hours, even in nocturnal animals. In humans, the onset of melatonin secretion usually occurs about 2 hours prior to the usual sleep time and continues until the end of the biological night.

SLEEP, HEALTH, AND MORTALITY

Sleep deprivation has historically been linked to fatalities. In 1849, Dr. Luther Bell at the McLean Asylum for the Insane in Massachusetts described nine cases of acute exhaustive mania

characterized by delusions, hallucinations, hyperactivity, frequent fevers, and nearly no sleep, several of which ended in fatality. In retrospect it is difficult to determine if these patients had other conditions, such as an infectious disease or familial fatal insomnia, and nearly all were treated with "opening of the temporal artery," "emetic-cathartics," salts, and leeches, but at least one of Bell's cases seemed to be mania as we would diagnose it today, followed by hyperactive and then hypoactive delirium and death after about 6 weeks of very little sleep.[8]

The connection between sleep deprivation and mortality has been confirmed repeatedly in modern animal and human studies. Interestingly, in animal models the lethality of sleep deprivation varies depending on what part of sleep is lost. Rapid-eye movement deprived rats live 4–6 weeks, while total sleep deprived rats live 2–3 weeks[9]; healthy rats generally live several years.

Sleep loss is associated with many adverse health outcomes contributing to morbidity and mortality. For instance, sleep loss is associated with impaired immune function. The immune system forms "immunological memories" of antigens during sleep. One night of sleep deprivation after receiving the hepatitis A vaccine lowers the antibody titer by nearly 50% one month later, and sleep debt impairs the immune response to the influenza vaccine.[10,11] Immunological response to antigens is associated with the amount of slow-wave sleep.[12] Sleep loss is also associated with disturbances of the thyroid axis, and abnormalities in stress hormone regulation. The latter may include a failure to suppress cortisol levels at night, and acute release of cortisol after morning awakening.[10,13,14] Short sleep duration (less than

A NonREM sleep

B REM sleep

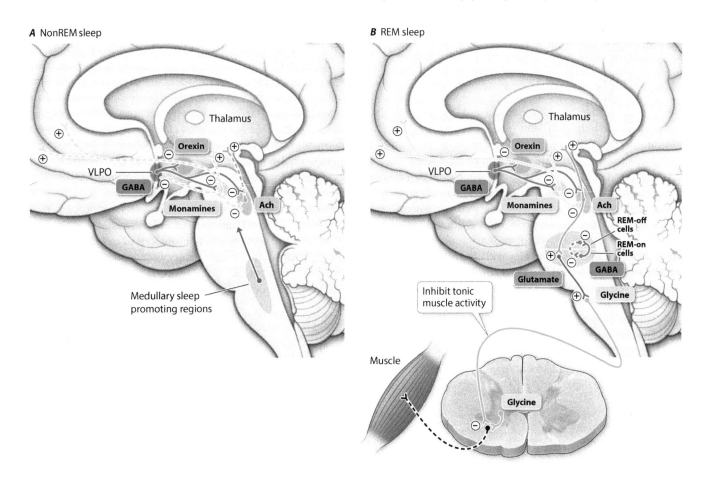

FIGURE 15-2. Brainstem circuits important for sleep regulation. **(A)** During non-REM sleep, GABAergic (and galanin) neurons in the ventral lateral preoptic area of the anterior hypothalamus inhibit neurons in the ascending activating systems, including posterior hypothalamic orexin neurons, monoamines such as histamine (in the tuberomammillary nucleus, not shown), serotonin, noradrenaline, and dopamine, as well as brainstem cholinergics (Ach). Certain regions of the medulla may also play a role in promoting non-REM sleep. **(B)** During REM sleep, monoamine transmitters, particularly noradrenaline and serotonin, are further reduced. This contributes to increased cholinergic inputs to the thalamus and EEG appearance of arousal. Pontine circuits include mutually inhibitory REM-on and REM-off cells, as well as neurons that inhibit tonic muscle activity during REM dream states. (From Blumenfeld H. *Neuroanatomy through Clinical Cases.* 2nd ed. Sunderland, MA: Sinauer Associates, an imprint of Oxford University Press; 2010. Reproduced with permission of Oxford Publishing Limited through PLSclear.)

7 hours) is also associated with coronary artery calcification,[15] increased proinflammatory biomarkers,[16] metabolic disruption (reduced leptin and elevated ghrelin),[17] higher total energy intake and fat intake,[18] insulin resistance,[19] and a significant increase in obesity, diabetes, cardiovascular disease, coronary heart disease, stroke, and all-cause mortality.[20,21] There have been similar findings associated with long sleep duration (over 9 hours), indicating a U-shaped relationship between mortality and sleep duration,[19,21,22] although short sleep is epidemiologically far more prevalent than long sleep and more of a public health concern.[23] The evidence is clear that impaired sleep causes physiological changes leading to lethal diseases.

Specifically relevant to the neuropsychiatrist, sleep deprivation is a significant and independent risk factor for suicide, nightmares are associated with suicidal behavior, sleep-disordered breathing is associated with suicidal ideation and planning, and nocturnal wakefulness is associated with completed suicide. The reasons for the association between sleep alteration and suicide are unclear and debated, but theories include

hypofrontality associated with wakefulness during the biological sleep period with resulting executive and affective dysfunction, and serotonin dysregulation.[24] Sleep deprivation results in affective volatility, amplification of negative emotion, and blunting of the positive benefit of rewarding activities.[25]

In sum: for health, adequate sleep is a requirement, not an option.

THEORIES OF WHY WE SLEEP

The purpose of sleep must be compelling. A sleeping creature cannot find food, cannot engage in reproduction, and cannot protect itself against predators. Sleep is tightly regulated and, unlike food intake, cannot be stocked for future use. Almost all species in the animal kingdom have some version of a circadian rhythm, though its nature varies widely, and whether we call the less active period "sleep" depends on how that term is defined. "Sleep" usually refers to a rapidly reversible state of immobility and greatly reduced sensory responsiveness, with the often-added criterion of lost sleep leading to increased sleep drive and sleep rebound (the tendency to sleep more after sleep deprivation). This definition separates sleep from rest, hibernation, and torpor (a similar state to hibernation, but for shorter periods and involuntary). Sleep can then further be characterized by the presence of EEG patterns similar to human REM or non-REM sleep.

In considering why humans sleep, and what might be unique about human sleep, examining sleep in other species can be informative. Indeed, most species have some kind of 24-hour rhythmicity to life. See Table 15-1 for highlights of sleep in animals, and for an excellent review of sleep in nonhumans, see Siegel.[26] Why is sleep such a preserved behavior across many species? One theory is that sleep's primary function is for cellular restoration, as sleep coincides with the release of growth hormone and the production of proteins in body cells, which is an energy-expensive process, and sleep is also important for immune function.[27,28] This theory does not explain why cellular restoration could not happen during wakefulness, nor does this theory fully account for the complexity of sleep, with different stages cycling throughout the night, nor does it explain why REM is such an active state, both for the heart and the brain. Another theory is that sleep's primary function is for energy conservation during times of the day or night when an animal cannot easily engage in productive activities (e.g., food gathering, reproduction). However, this theory is less compelling when considering the very low amount of energy actually saved during sleep, which is only very slightly more than resting.[29] If sleep existed merely to conserve energy and calories, there would be no need for complex changes in the firing of neural networks and changes in body metabolism and movement in a sequential manner over the course of the night. The energy-conservation theory also does not account for brain activity during REM being comparable to wakefulness, as normal REM sleep physiology involves high oxygen consumption, high cerebral blood flow, and high glucose utilization.

A current conceptualization of sleep in humans is that it is essential for cognition and memory consolidation, but this theory can only apply to species with large and complex brains. There is an enormous amount of literature supporting these functions of sleep in humans.[12,30,31] However, sleep clearly has multiple roles, and its purpose may be highly variable from species to species. If every species had memory consolidation as the primary purpose for sleep, for example, then we would expect that the "smartest" species would sleep the longest; but this is not the case, as some of the species that sleep the longest are the brown bat, giant armadillo, opossum, and python. Sleep deprivation is also not cognitively detrimental to all species in the way it is for humans. Sparrows manage to reduce their sleep by approximately two-thirds during the migratory season, with no deficit in cognition.[32] Interestingly, this resistance to cognitive deficits from sleep loss is only seen during migration; the same birds in the nonmigratory season do suffer cognitive consequences from lack of sleep.[32]

A unifying theory of sleep is that essential biological "house-keeping" processes, like cellular restoration, immune functions, hormone release, etc., are secondarily incorporated into the most suitable physiological slot in the 24-hour cycle after a species has already developed a stable rest-activity pattern.[29] For humans, a large part of that essential biological "house-keeping" allocated to sleep is cognitive processing.

Role of Sleep in Cognition

Sleep deprivation has been noted to impair almost every cognitive function, particularly psychomotor and cognitive speed, attention, working memory, and executive function.[33] Cognitive deficits from sleep deprivation accumulate to severe levels without full awareness by the affected individual.[33] Sleep deprivation with continued work after 17 hours awake has been shown to cause cognitive psychomotor impairment equivalent to a blood alcohol concentration of 0.05%[34]; this study was done in subjects age 30–49, so it is possible that older or more vulnerable brains would exhibit even greater impairment. Twenty-four hours of wakefulness is equivalent to a blood alcohol concentration of 0.10% (a blood alcohol concentration of 0.08% is considered inebriated).[35] This degree of sleep deprivation is unfortunately required by a number of professions.

While the majority of research on sleep and cognition has been in the area of memory, sleep does not just consolidate new memories and facilitate forgetting—sleep also facilitates

TABLE 15-1 • Highlights of Sleep in the Animal Kingdom.[26,32]	
Organism/Species	
Single-celled organisms	Circadian rhythms of activity
Bees	Circadian changes in sensory response thresholds have been documented.
Zebrafish	Circadian variations in activity and responsiveness, but no rebound after deprivation
Octopi and squids	Periods of rest, but do not have EEG patterns resembling sleep
Reptiles	Have NREM, but do not have rapid eye movement sleep
Birds	Very short rapid eye movement sleep with incomplete atonia, presumably to continue standing or grasping a branch
Sparrows	During migration, sparrows reduce sleep by approximately two-thirds, with no deficit in cognition (as measured by a repeated acquisition task involving learning patterns of pecking colored lights to get food). During the nonmigratory season, these same birds suffer cognitive consequences from lack of sleep.
Mammals	All have rapid eye movement sleep with atonia and non-rapid eye movement sleep stages, but high variation among the class.
Platypus	Occupies 60% of its sleep time in REM
Whales and dolphins	Unihemispheric sleep
Fur seals	Human-like bihemispheric sleep on land but whale-like unihemispheric sleep when in water

creativity and insight. Famous examples of these abound, but favorites among sleep researchers[25] include the dreams of August Kekulé leading to the conceptualization of the benzene ring, the dream of Dmitry Mendeleyev leading to the critical rule underlying the periodic table of the elements, and Otto Loewi's dream leading to the experimental demonstration of neurochemical transmission. We now have growing evidence from experimental models that sleep helps to intelligently assimilate new information, facilitating insight and novel solutions to problems.[25]

Within the realm of cognition, sleep has a particularly central role in memory processing. The first known research on sleep and memory is from 1885. The German psychologist Hermann Ebbinghaus conducted studies on memory of auditory strings of nonsense syllables at various intervals. He found that forgetting was drastically lessened when the intervals included sleep as compared to wake, a finding that was followed up and re-demonstrated in 1924 by Jenkins and Dallenbach.[30]

The nature of memory is that some events, even brief ones, are stored and kept for a lifetime if salient, while others are quickly forgotten. These salient events are recalled even if a person does not make a special effort to recall and relive the memory, indicating that there must be subconscious or offline processes involved in memory storage and in forgetting. Memory "consolidation" is a term coined in the early 1900s to explain the phenomenon of memories becoming increasingly resistant to interference—that is, better remembered, despite new and distracting information.[30] Sleep plays a key role in this process.

Sleep is thought to support the transition of memory from being temporarily processed in the hippocampus to being stored long term in the neocortex. The current theory is that this happens with the reactivation of newly encoded memory representations during sleep.[12] This process also happens during wake: when a memory is re-activated repeatedly, this leads to superior storage and a gradual transition to become independent of the hippocampus.[30] The hippocampus can be conceptualized as a relay center, binding together incoming streams of information, both external (sensory) and internal (thoughts), and then after a period of time stabilizing these memories in the neocortex.[36] The more a memory is reactivated, the better the storage and the less hippocampal-dependent the memory becomes; reorganization through repeated hippocampal-neocortical interaction produces neocortical connections that are sufficient for retrieval.[30] Problems in this process, such as with sleep deprivation or dementia, result in an impairment in subsequent hippocampal activity and associated encoding. Deficiency in non-REM slow-wave sleep has been shown to predict impaired overnight memory retention in middle-aged adults.[37] In mild-to-moderate Alzheimer's there is relative preservation of long-term memories, while short-term memory (hippocampal-based activity) is impaired earlier in the course of disease.

Different sleep stages may preferentially process different kinds of memory. Declarative memory ("knowing that") is primarily hippocampally based. Procedural memory ("knowing how") is acquired slowly and involves areas of the brain other than the hippocampus. Multiple studies and lines of research have attempted to differentiate declarative memory, procedural memory, and emotionally valenced memory in terms of which sleeps stages are most involved, and so far the evidence is mixed.[38] NREM, and particularly sleep spindles, has been strongly associated with declarative memory, and slow-wave sleep is also associated with motor skills. Striatal-dependent motor learning may require lower dopamine (slow-wave sleep).[36] Stronger evidence exists that REM sleep promotes consolidation of emotional memory.[38]

While the long-term potentiation (persistent strengthening of synapses based on recent patterns of activity) involved in memory formation can occur during wake and during sleep, sleep may be particularly involved in targeted forgetting, a process that is necessary for efficient learning.[36] While the majority of nap and overnight sleep studies have shown a benefit of sleep to the learning and retention of new information, there are informative exceptions pointing to the role of forgetting. For instance, in the case of the over-learned motor skill of riding a bike, a 2-hour nap with high sleep spindles and REM seemed to erase a newly learned incorrect way of riding a bike with the handlebars backward.[39] This lends support to the theory that targeted forgetting is a function of REM and sleep spindles. Norepinephrine, which promotes formation of memory and long-term potentiation, is notably turned "off" during REM sleep and transition to REM, which is theorized to allow targeted forgetting to occur.[36] Serotonin, likewise, is present in the hippocampus but greatly diminished during REM sleep.[36] This theory of the purpose of REM as a time of depotentiation and forgetting is supported by the correspondence of developmental periods of neural pruning with increases in REM sleep, both in animals and in humans.[36] However, the connection of sleep stage to targeted forgetting becomes complicated, as acetylcholine is also important to the induction of long-term potentiation and to learning in the hippocampus, and acetylcholine levels plummet during slow-wave sleep. Given this decrease in acetylcholine levels during slow-wave sleep, it is not clear why REM would be more associated with forgetting than slow-wave sleep. One theory is that firing of noradrenergic neurons of the locus ceruleus (a major source of norepinephrine) during slow-wave sleep could have a memory-guarding function; notably, pathology in the locus ceruleus is an early event in Alzheimer's disease.[36,40] In sum, targeted forgetting seems to be a function of sleep, but the mechanisms and timing are as yet unclear.

There are large bodies of work at several levels of analysis supporting sleep's role in memory consolidation. At the molecular level, sleep deprivation may impair memory consolidation by reducing synthesis of proteins needed to support synaptic plasticity. Sleep promotes mRNA translation, while sleep deprivation negatively impacts clusters of genes critical for translational processes known to be essential for memory encoding and consolidation.[31] The signaling pathways involved in synaptic plasticity and synaptic potentiation are impacted by sleep deprivation, and both REM and NREM sleep enhance previously induced synaptic potentiation.[31]

At the network level, there is a strong line of research findings indicating that NREM sleep serves to reactivate prior waking memory circuits to strengthen them.[38] During sleep after learning, ensembles of hippocampal and cortical cells demonstrate coordinated replay of prior learning-related firing patterns, both in animal models and in humans.[31] The coordinated replay occurs in the hippocampus, in the cortex, and between the hippocampus and cortex, commonly in association with specific NREM sleep oscillations.[31] The degree of this re-activation during sleep of physiological oscillations and firing patterns associated with initial learning has been associated with performance measures of how well learned information is retained.[31]

At the behavioral level, while early research focused on sleep's passive role in stabilizing memory and wake's promotion of forgetting through interference, more recent evidence has accumulated that sleep takes an active, dynamic role in changing memories and extracting the "gist" of information.[12] Sleep has been shown to affect nearly every type of memory, including motor sequence learning, procedural memory, visual perceptual learning, and auditory perceptual learning, as well as anagram problem solving, statistical learning, language abstraction in infants, and creative insight.[12,30]

While the area of sleep and memory is a rapidly growing field, there are many unanswered questions regarding the role of different sleep stages, and regarding processing of long-term memory.

Role of Sleep in Emotion Regulation

Sleep deprivation is clearly associated with magnification of negative reactions to aversive experiences, and blunting of positive reactions to pleasant experiences.[41,42] Sleep deprived and poor sleepers are more likely to interpret neutral stimuli as negative.[43] Emotional reactivity is increased following sleep deprivation, and can be seen in an increased pupillary response.[44] Data from functional magnetic resonance imaging suggest that lack of sleep inappropriately modulates the human emotional brain response to negative aversive stimuli; that is, the sleep-deprived brain has an amplified hyper-limbic response, with loss of top-down prefrontal regulation of the amygdala.[45]

Emotionally arousing stimuli are consistently remembered better than neutral stimuli, and this has been shown with narratives, components of scenes, and pictures.[46] The adrenergic system seems to enhance memory registration at the time of learning; interestingly, this benefit of enhanced memory for emotional stimuli is lost when propranolol is administered to block the adrenergic system.[46] The preferential remembering of emotional stimuli involves neurohormonal systems as well as the amygdala interacting with other key medial temporal lobe structures.[46] Sleep loss impairs the ability to form new memories, and this effect is most notable for positive emotional stimuli; the encoding of negative memories is more resistant to sleep loss. After the initial formation of a memory, there are also notable differences in what is remembered and forgotten. Sleep targets the consolidation of emotional memories, learned emotional associations between stimuli, and helps to actively generalize these learned associations to other contexts.[46] The extent of emotional memory is associated with quantity and quality of REM sleep, strongly suggesting that REM sleep is particularly important to emotional memory consolidation.[46] Aspects of REM sleep that have been suggested as predisposing to being uniquely amenable to emotional memory consolidation include elevated limbic and forebrain acetylcholine and theta oscillations.

In sum, sleep deprivation promotes negative interpretations of events, as well as negative memory formation and retention,

reinforcing depressive thinking patterns. Of course, psychiatric conditions such as major depression and post-traumatic stress disorder (PTSD) also negatively impact sleep and have sleep impairment as part of the diagnostic criteria,[47] thus this is a bidirectional relationship. Understanding the relationship of sleep to emotion regulation and emotional memory processing has particular clinical relevance for the psychiatrist and neurologist, and the importance of addressing patients' sleep disturbances cannot be overstated.

SLEEP DISORDERS

Sleep Evaluation

Clinical evaluation of sleep disorders should begin with a thorough sleep history. This should include information about bedtime, wake time, awakenings (number, length, difficulty reinstating sleep), daytime activity, overall activity level, exercise pattern, substance use or abuse, and sleep regularity. History should also include a detailed medication and substance review, as many drugs can affect sleep. This is a non-exhaustive list of examples: cocaine increases wakefulness and suppresses REM sleep,[48] ecstasy is arousing,[48] marijuana reduces REM sleep,[48] lipophilic beta blockers are associated with increased awakenings and REM suppression,[49] most antidepressants have been associated with restless legs syndrome (RLS) and periodic limb movements of sleep (PLMS),[50] bupropion may reduce RLS symptoms,[50] many serotonergic antidepressants suppress REM sleep,[51] antihistamines can improve sleep quality but also increase daytime sleepiness,[52] steroids induce insomnia,[53] and nicotine also causes insomnia.[54] Physical exam should include weight and height to calculate body mass index (BMI), blood pressure, examination of the face for micro- or retrognathia, neck circumference, airway, and examination of extrapyramidal symptoms like tremor, bradykinesia, and postural reflexes.

There are a handful of clinically useful sleep tests, as summarized in Table 15-2.

Insomnia

Insomnia is very common in modern life, whether it is a primary disorder or secondary to some other condition. Approximately 30% of the general population have complaints of sleep disruption, and approximately 10% have associated symptoms consistent with a diagnosis of insomnia.[55] These symptoms are long term for the majority of insomniacs.[55]

Insomnia criteria can be found both in the Diagnostic and Statistical Manual of Mental Disorders, 5th Edition (DSM-5), and in the International Classification of Sleep Disorders, Third Edition (ICSD-3). The disorder is characterized by a subjective report of a sleep complaint, either difficulty initiating or maintaining sleep. Sleep initiation dysfunction is termed "initial insomnia." Sleep maintenance difficulty can be awakenings in the middle of the night (middle insomnia) or awakening too early in the morning (terminal insomnia). The insomnia symptoms must occur at least three times per week over the course of at least 3 months, with at least one related daytime impairment such as fatigue, difficulty with attention, mood disturbance, or

TABLE 15-2 • Clinically Useful Sleep Tests.

Test	Description	Utility
Activity monitors, actigraphy	Wearable devices that sense movement and infer wake and sleep times based on activity	• Diagnosis of circadian rhythm disorders • Evaluation of response to sleep medications
Portable testing	Home sleep apnea test	• Diagnosis of sleep apnea
Polysomnogram (PSG)	Gold standard sleep test. Answers questions about overall sleep, including measurement of EEG, breathing, heart rate, and leg movements. Generates information about overall sleep architecture, and observation of sleep behaviors.	• Screening and diagnosis of a variety of sleep disorders, including obstructive sleep apnea, central sleep apnea, periodic limb movements of sleep, and REM sleep behavior disorder
Full montage video EEG-PSG	PSG with extended EEG and video recording.	• Diagnosing nocturnal seizures • Evaluating abnormal behaviors at night, suspected parasomnia
Multiple sleep latency test (MSLT)	Monitors daytime sleep in patients with daytime sleepiness. Takes place over a night of sleep and the following day. Patients are given five 20-minute opportunities to nap at 2-hour intervals.	• Diagnosing narcolepsy • Diagnosing other hypersomnias of central origin
Maintenance of wakefulness test (MWT)	Objectively confirms a patient's ability to sustain wakefulness. Consists of four 40-minute trials of quiet wakefulness.	• Evaluating the effectiveness of hypersomnia treatment • Evaluating if a worker in an alertness-sensitive profession can safely return to regular work

altered performance.[56] Recently, an eight-item questionnaire was introduced for diagnosis of insomnia, based on the DSM-5 insomnia criteria.[57]

The ICSD-3 requires one or more of the following for a diagnosis of insomnia: difficulty initiating sleep, difficulty maintaining sleep, waking up earlier than desired, resistance to going to bed on appropriate schedule, or difficulty sleeping without parent or caregiver intervention. The patient or caregiver also needs to report one or more of the following: fatigue/malaise, attention, concentration, or memory impairment, impaired social, family, occupational, or academic performance, mood disturbance/irritability, daytime sleepiness, behavioral problems (e.g., hyperactivity, impulsivity, aggression), reduced motivation/energy/initiative, proneness for errors/accidents, or concerns about or dissatisfaction with sleep. The sleep complaints cannot be explained purely by inadequate opportunity or inadequate circumstances (e.g., sleeping in strange situations or uncomfortable positions), and the sleep disturbance and associated daytime symptoms need to occur at least three times per week for at least 3 months.[58]

Traditionally, several subtypes of insomnia have been described. Although classification typically does not determine management, it is sometimes helpful in the evaluation. Idiopathic insomnia is a longstanding complaint, usually with an onset in infancy or early childhood. Idiopathic insomnia is usually without discernible cause and persists over time without remission. It is thought to arise from either genetically determined or congenital aberrations in the sleep-inducing or arousal systems in the brain.

Psychophysiological insomnia, or conditioned insomnia, results from heightened arousal and learned sleep-preventing associations. Patients with psychophysiological insomnia have an excessive focus on and worry about sleep and have physiological signs of cognitive and somatic arousal, particularly at

bedtime. They classically describe a better sleep in novel settings (while traveling for business or vacation) while they have difficulty sleeping in their usual sleep setting.

Paradoxical insomnia, which was previously called sleep state misperception, is the complaint of severe sleep disturbance without corroborative objective evidence. Patients with paradoxical insomnia have a marked propensity to underestimate the amount of sleep they experience and have generally normal polysomnograms. The prevalence of paradoxical insomnia ranges between 9.2% and 50% of patients with insomnia.[59]

There is also a subtype of insomnia in which patients have sleep problems due to inadequate sleep hygiene. Sleep hygiene refers to daily living activities that promote good-quality sleep and normal daytime alertness; see section "Treatment of Insomnia" for a more detailed discussion of sleep hygiene. Given the changes seen in the context of chronic disease, one can anticipate that inadequate sleep hygiene can lead to insomnia in many patients with neuropsychiatric disorders.

Insomnia aggregates in families but as of yet there is no specific genetically testable determinant. Neuroimaging findings in insomnia have included increased anterior cingulate cortical volume and reduced hippocampus volume, and changes in functional imaging have included increased thalamic activity during sleep, reduced recruitment of the caudate head, increased amygdala activity, and reduced frontal volume and task-related activity.[60,61] Reduced GABA activity was noted in a magnetic resonance spectroscopy study,[62] consistent with the concept of "hyperarousal."

Workup of Insomnia

More than one cause of insomnia in the same individual is the rule, not the exception. In the evaluation of insomnia, practitioners should consider the following:

- Is there enough sleep opportunity? People generally need over 7 hours of sleep with consistent timing.
- Is there a sleep fragmenting factor? Medications, environmental stimulation, and primary sleep disorders such as obstructive sleep apnea, restless legs syndrome, bladder or prostate issues, and pregnancy, and circadian rhythm disorder can all result in fragmented sleep.
- Does the insomnia recur? For a diagnosis of insomnia disorder, the sleep disturbance needs to occur over three times per week for over 3 months.[58]
- Does it cause a problem? For a diagnosis of insomnia disorder, patients must have impaired function, sleepiness, or malaise and daytime fatigue.
- Is insomnia the manifestation of another disorder?
- Do we anticipate a short-term treatment (i.e., insomnia in the setting of time-limited stress or another comorbid treatable condition), or a long-term treatment (i.e., idiopathic or psychophysiological insomnia)?
- When in the night is the most problematic time—sleep initiation or sleep maintenance?

The general consensus is that EEG does not provide diagnostically useful information to confirm or exclude insomnia. The American Academy of Sleep Medicine (AASM) does not recommend PSG for the routine assessment of insomnia. However, actigraphy as a measure of sleep duration may be clinically useful. A 2–4-week sleep log helps distinguish insomnia from circadian rhythm disorders and also may guide planning of any cognitive-behavioral therapy (CBT). Moreover, some researchers distinguish between insomnia with normal sleep duration and insomnia with short sleep duration as two separate phenotypes, with the latter being much more associated with physiological hyperarousal, impaired neurocognitive functioning, and risk of cardiometabolic morbidity and mortality,[63] which would make objective information regarding sleep duration prognostically useful. Information from sleep log or actigraphy (when available) regarding sleep duration can also help clinicians track response to treatment trials. A review of commercially available actigraphy and other home sleep measurement devices is beyond the scope of this chapter, but efforts to compare commercially available wrist devices to PSG have shown some limitations of the devices, particularly in differentiating sleep stages.[64]

Comorbid sleep disorders to consider and treat include movement disorders, parasomnias, circadian rhythm disorders, endocrine disorders (e.g., hypo- or hyperthyroidism), pain/neuropathy, psychiatric illness, and effects of medications. RLS should also be considered and treated. Insomnia is a common manifestation of sleep apnea, particularly in women.[65]

Treatment of Insomnia

Insomnia treatment should start with an explanation of good sleep hygiene and its value, and in some cases psychotherapy. Please see Table 15-3 for basic sleep hygiene recommendations. Avoidance of blue light in the evening or at night, such as the blue spectrum of light emitted by screens or bright indoor white lights, is strongly recommended, as the suprachiasmatic nucleus and pineal gland respond preferentially to blue light

TABLE 15-3 • Sleep Hygiene Tips.	
Good Sleep Hygiene Practices	**Bad Sleep Hygiene Practices**
• Use the bed only for sleep and sex • Keep bedroom at comfortable temperature • Blackout curtains, limit light exposure • Minimize anxiety and stressors before bedtime	• Reading in bed, using the phone in bed, watching television in the bedroom • Bright light in bedroom, especially blue spectrum light • Clocks in the bedroom • Large meals, stimulants, or vigorous exercise near bedtime • Daytime napping • Varying sleep schedule • Drinking alcohol near bedtime

when setting the circadian clock. The sleep hygiene recommendations for avoidance of napping and increased time out of bed and wakefulness serve to provide enhanced sleep drive and more intense subsequent sleep with increased slow-wave activity.[61] Alcohol consumption should also be a topic of discussion with sleep hygiene. While alcohol initially helps patients fall asleep, it suppresses REM, and there is REM rebound in the second half of the night with restlessness and poor-quality sleep. Early awakening after alcohol consumption is a result of both REM rebound and likely also the rebound of noradrenergic suppression.

The gold standard treatment of insomnia, which should ideally be trialed prior to starting any sleep medication, is cognitive-behavioral therapy for insomnia (CBT-I). As compared to those taking sleep medications (triazolam and zopiclone), patients have equal or better effects post-treatment with CBT-I and greater effects at follow-up.[66-68] Please see Table 15-4 for details of CBT-I.

Pharmacological treatment of insomnia generally suppresses the ascending arousal pathways or enhances the descending inhibitory pathways. There are many classes of insomnia medications, including benzodiazepines (triazolam, estazolam, temazepam, flurazepam, quazepam), nonbenzodiazepine hypnotics (zaleplon, zolpidem, zolpidem ultrashort acting, eszopiclone), the orexin receptor antagonist (suvorexant), the melatonin receptor agonist (ramelteon), antidepressants (e.g., doxepin), and off-label uses of other drugs such as other antidepressants, antihistamines, antipsychotics, and melatonin.

Melatonin is an exogenous mimic of an endogenous hormone, and its side effects are no different from placebo.[69] Endogenous melatonin is a hormone secreted by the pineal gland that signals "night" in mammals; even animals which are active at night release melatonin during dark hours. Its release is suppressed by light. For humans, melatonin production starts in the late afternoon, peaks in the middle of the night, then disappears on awakening.[69] Melatonin provides information to end organs on the phase of the circadian cycle. Exogenous melatonin has an acute inhibitory effect on neuronal firing of the suprachiasmatic nucleus, which thus promotes sleep, and also has a phase-shifting effect, which can delay or advance the sleep phase.[69] While systemic reviews of melatonin tend to conclude that evidence for its use in insomnia is fairly weak,[69] with

TABLE 15-4 • Cognitive-Behavioral Therapy for Insomnia (CBT-I)[68,138]

Cognitive control	Recognize, challenge, and change stressful, distorted sleep cognitions that exacerbate insomnia by elevating psychophysiological arousal.
Sleep hygiene training	Recommendations include: • Keep the bedroom at a comfortable temperature • Eliminate clocks from the bedroom • Avoid large evening meals • Avoid blue light in the evening • Avoid stimulants and vigorous exercise near bedtime
Sleep restriction therapy	Curtail time in bed to more closely approximate actual sleep time. Maintain consistent arising time, even after a poor night's sleep, to synchronize the endogenous circadian rhythm that regulates sleep and wakefulness.
Stimulus control	Goal is to associate the bed and bedtime with sleep as opposed to frustrating wakefulness. • Use the bedroom primarily for sleep and sex • Go to bed only when drowsy • If unable to fall asleep within 20–30 minutes, get out of bed and go to another room to engage in a quiet, relaxing activity until drowsy
Relaxation training	Muscle relaxation, breathing, and mental focusing techniques during the day and at bedtime.

a modest effect on sleep onset latency,[70] clinically meaningful effects with melatonin treatment have been demonstrated in placebo-controlled trials in humans, particularly in disorders associated with diminished or misaligned melatonin rhythms, such as circadian rhythm-related sleep disorders, insomnia in children with neurodevelopmental disorders, poor sleep quality, nocturnal hypertension, and Alzheimer's disease.[71] As human endogenous melatonin levels start to increase approximately 2 hours before natural sleep onset, the usual recommendation is to give melatonin 1–2 hours before the preferred bedtime. However, there is not enough research to establish optimal dose nor optimal timing for melatonin.[70,72] After melatonin intake, light should be kept low to avoid suppression of endogenous melatonin and phase delay.

Ramelteon is a melatonin agonist, which is FDA approved for insomnia characterized by difficulty with sleep onset. In Europe there is a prolonged-release melatonin agonist (Circadin®) which is approved by the European Medicines Agency for the short-term treatment of primary insomnia characterized by poor quality of sleep in patients 55 and older. Ramelteon and other melatonin receptor agonists tend to be useful for reducing sleep latency and regulating sleep cycles but are less useful for sleep maintenance.

Benzodiazepines bind to GABA-A receptors. When GABA is also bound, the benzodiazepine will cause the channel to open even more frequently than when GABA alone is present.[5]

Benzodiazepines strengthen the flip-flop sleep-wake switch by enhancing inhibitory outputs to all of the major cell groups in the brainstem and hypothalamus that promote arousal.[61] Benzodiazepines bind in a manner that changes the conformation of the GABA-A receptor, leading to the development of tolerance, dependence, and withdrawal.[5] They are inexpensive and ubiquitous, but problems include excessive sedation, high frequency of falls, hypotension, dependency and a loss of efficacy after longer term use, and significant short-term cognitive side effects.[60]

As compared to benzodiazepines, the nonbenzodiazepine hypnotics, nicknamed "Z drugs"—zolpidem, eszopiclone, and zaleplon—have a lower risk of tolerance, are less likely to cause rebound insomnia, and are less likely to exacerbate sleep apnea due to limited muscle relaxation effects.[73] Like benzodiazepines, the "Z drugs" also bind to the GABA-A receptor, but do so in a way that does not change its conformation. Several of the "Z drugs" are also specific for the alpha 1 subtype of the GABA-A receptor, which causes sedation, has anticonvulsant properties, and promotes amnesia, but is not anxiolytic or muscle relaxing like the alpha 2 and alpha 3 receptor subunits.[5] Unfortunately, evidence is accumulating that nonbenzodiazepine hypnotics may induce euphoria and can be abused.[74] Other problems include side effects such as parasomnias, over-sedation, and also the potential to lose efficacy with time. In the short term, cognitive changes associated with various "Z drugs" include decreased verbal memory, attention, processing speed, and working memory.[75] Zaleplon and zolpidem are short acting, which make them good medications for initial insomnia to help reduce sleep latency, but poor medications for sleep maintenance. Eszopiclone has a relatively longer half-life and is therefore more likely to improve sleep maintenance.

Both benzodiazepines and "Z drugs" have been associated with motor vehicle accidents and falls leading to fractures; other purported associations, such as with dementia, infections, respiratory disease exacerbation, pancreatitis, and cancer, cannot be conclusively validated due to insufficient and conflicting evidence.[76] Particularly, while benzodiazepine use correlates with poorer cognitive performance as compared to nonbenzodiazepine users, it does not seem to correlate with rate of cognitive decline.[77,78]

Antidepressants (low-dose doxepin, mirtazapine, trazodone) are more suitable for long-term use, and may also help other conditions such as depression, headaches, and pain. Doxepin has been shown to increase objective total sleep time by approximately half an hour, but studies are largely lacking for other antidepressants.[69] Doxepin is a sedating tricyclic antidepressant which treats depression through boosting serotonergic and noradrenergic neurotransmission, and which promotes sleep through the blocking of histaminergic neurons in the posterior hypothalamus. Mirtazapine is a presynaptic alpha-2 antagonist that has dual action by increasing noradrenergic and serotonergic neurotransmission, and its sedating effect is also attributed to antihistaminic (H1) activity at low doses. Trazodone is also thought to promote sleep through weak histaminergic antagonism. Antidepressants useful for sleep can also cause anticholinergic side effects and orthostatic hypotension. A 2018 Cochrane review on antidepressants for insomnia concluded that evidence was overall lacking; there may be a small improvement in sleep quality with short-term use of low-dose doxepin and trazodone compared with placebo.[79] There has been very little published research on the efficacy of mirtazapine in treatment of insomnia, but the scarce studies that do exist are promising.[80]

The most recent development in the pharmacologic treatment of insomnia is the development of the orexin receptor antagonist suvorexant. Orexinergic neurons in the lateral hypothalamus reinforce arousal pathways in the brainstem and direct excitatory input to the cerebral cortex and basal forebrain,[61] stabilizing the wake state. Suvorexant inhibits this wake-stimulatory pathway.

Rare Causes of Insomnia

Agrypnia refers to the syndrome of insomnia resulting from neuronal lesions or dysfunction of neural circuits involved in sleep regulation.[61] Examples of diseases that induce severe agrypnia include familial fatal insomnia, Morvan's syndrome, and TBI.

Familial fatal insomnia is a progressive neurodegenerative prion disease manifested by insomnia and dysautonomia, with a loss of circadian rhythmicity, increased autonomic output, and decreased melatonin. The onset is anywhere between age 18 and 60, with diagnosis typically around the age of 50. The presentation includes rapidly progressive memory impairment, myoclonus, hyperreflexia, excessive salivation, hypertension, and hallucinations. In the advanced stages, patients become unable to walk, talk, or swallow, and ultimately die; the mean survival time after diagnosis is 18 months. The etiology is autosomal dominant inheritance of a genetic mutation at the prion protein (PRNP) gene on chromosome 20, which leads to prion formation. On PET scan, patients will show reduced thalamic metabolism earlier in the disease followed by limbic and more widespread hypometabolism over time.[81] There is no effective treatment.

Morvan's syndrome is a very rare condition—so rare that as of 2012 only 28 case reports had been reported in the English literature.[82] Patients present with progressively worsening insomnia and varying degrees of neuromyotonia, memory loss, confusion, and autonomic features. It is considered an autoimmune disorder. Approximately 70% of Morvan's patients have anti-voltage-gated potassium channel antibodies (anti-VGKC-Ab).[82]

TBI results in insomnia for 30–70% of patients,[61] up to three times more prevalent than in the general population,[3] and this condition is most common in patients with left dorsomedial prefrontal damage.[83] Insomnia can persist for years after the injury.[3]

Circadian Rhythm Disorders

In the evaluation of sleep, special attention should be given to the function of circadian rhythms. Our current understanding of the major regulators of sleep initiation and continuity stipulates two independent processes of control: (1) homeostatic—a linear process, by which the pressure to be asleep increases with the duration of wakefulness; (2) circadian—a cyclical pressure to be awake during the "biological day" while supporting sleep during the "biological night." The circadian alerting process has a period of about 24 hours. These two processes, homeostatic

and circadian, oppose each other. During the day, homeostatic pressure progressively increases in one direction to increase sleepiness, while the circadian alerting signal also progressively increases in the other direction to promote wakefulness. While the effect of the homeostatic pressure can be altered by taking a nap (which will lower or eliminate this pressure), the circadian process is primarily driven by an endogenous pacemaker in the hypothalamus, and entrained to environmental conditions, primarily via the effect of light. A direct type of receptor in the retina, specific to the entraining effect of light, connects to the hypothalamus via the retinohypothalamic pathway and allows this entrainment. In dim light, melatonin is secreted by the pineal gland and is currently considered the most reliable marker of circadian phase. The effects of the circadian system extend to multiple physiological functions besides consciousness, including cortisol, prolactin, and melatonin secretion, thyroid-stimulating hormone, body temperature, urine volume, gastric acid secretion, and others. The minimum body temperature (the lowest body temperature in a 24-hour period) roughly corresponds to the "biological midnight."

The effect of light depends on intensity (roughly the stronger the intensity, the stronger the effect), spectrum (with the blue spectrum wavelengths inducing strongest effect), and time of administration relative to the individual's circadian phase.

The most commonly used laboratory biomarker for circadian phase is melatonin secretion. Melatonin can be measured in plasma, urine, and saliva. A number of studies have shown that the onset of melatonin secretion under dim light conditions (the dim light melatonin onset or DLMO) is the single most accurate marker for assessing the circadian pacemaker.[84] However, in the United States, use of this marker in the clinical setting is currently limited by lack of insurance coverage.

Disorders of the circadian rhythm occur when the sleep and wake phases of the individual are in conflict with the requirements of the environment. Delayed sleep wake phase disorder (DSWPD) represents later sleep phase of the circadian cycle, and advanced sleep wake phase disorder (ASWPD) represents an earlier sleep phase. When the sleep and wake phases of the circadian cycle do not follow a 24-hour rhythm, this is referred to as non-24-hour disorder (as seen in blind individuals). An irregular sleep wake phase disorder is seen when sleep occurs seemingly independently of the 24-hour time, and this is more common in individuals with central nervous system impairment, such as dementia.[58]

Circadian rhythm disorders can be treated with administration of light. Light administered prior to the midpoint of melatonin secretion (the halfway point between melatonin onset and end), which is usually in the middle of the night at the same time as the nadir of the core body temperature, leads to a delay of the sleep phase of the circadian rhythm. Light administered after that point (e.g., morning light) would lead to an advance of the phase. Since in DSWPD an advancement of sleep phase is needed, light is administered after the melatonin midpoint (typically in the morning, after the patient is awake), while in ASWPD light is administered in the evening. Care should be taken to not administer light too early (or too late in the case of ASPWD), as this would result in the opposite effect. These treatment suggestions, however, are based on a low number of relatively small studies.[85]

For DSWPD, use of melatonin may be effective on days of work or when there is a need for early awakening. A recent study by Sletten et al.[86] found melatonin 0.5 mg to be effective in alleviating DSWPD symptoms of patients with a delayed melatonin secretion. In this study, participants were instructed to take the melatonin an hour before they would need to be asleep to achieve adequate rest in the morning, and to be in dim light after taking melatonin. For example, an individual who has DSWPD, but needs to be awake at 7 am for work, and needs 8 hours of sleep to be rested, would take melatonin at 10 pm and stay in dim light afterwards.

The melatonin receptor agonist tasimelteon is approved for the treatment of non-24-hour sleep-wake disorder (in which the internal clock is not synchronized to the external), and other melatonin receptor agonists have been investigated for potential use in treatment of circadian rhythm sleep-wake disorders.[87]

It should be noted, however, that most treatment effects with melatonin, light, and melatonin agonists have been based on small studies. Furthermore, some treatments have been effective in select groups of patients and may not be generalizable. For example, the study by Sletten et al. demonstrated effectiveness of melatonin only in patients who also have a delayed dim light melatonin onset, stating that patients who do not have delayed dim light melatonin onset may be a different phenotype. However, in clinical practice, measurement of dim light melatonin onset is often very difficult to achieve, and also difficult to interpret. Thus, treatment methods are evolving.

Parasomnias

Parasomnias are disorders of altered behavior presenting during the sleep period. Parasomnias are highly relevant to clinical neuropsychiatric practice. They are more common in psychiatric populations, and they can resemble or co-occur with other neuropsychiatric conditions such as psychosis, depression, PTSD, epilepsy, substance abuse, and psychogenic behavioral disturbances. According to a 2017 review, the average prevalence for parasomnias in psychiatric disorders were: nightmare disorder (38.9%), sleep paralysis (22.3%), sleep-related eating disorder (9.9%), sleepwalking (8.5%), and REM Behavior Disorder (3.8%), all significantly higher than general population estimates, and not fully explained by medications.[2] Parasomnias are usually classified by the stage of sleep from which they arise, as seen later in this chapter. Parasomnias include sleepwalking, sleep talking, sleep terrors, sleep eating, sexsomnias, nocturnal groaning (catathrenia), sleep-related dissociative disorder, hallucinations, sleep paralysis, RBD, and confusional arousals. It is important to recognize RBD, due to its association with neurodegenerative disease. Parasomnias are not usually associated with a complaint of insomnia or sleepiness, and, with a few notable exceptions, most parasomnias are transient and do not require medical intervention.

There is little understanding of the pathophysiology of parasomnias. They are quite heterogeneous in their phenomenology, and their pathophysiological mechanisms also seem to be varied. Some, like confusional arousals, seem to be a combination

of the waking and sleeping states of consciousness. However, not all parasomnias fit neatly into the overlap theory of different sleep-wake states; for instance, RBD results from a lack of suppression of movement during REM, not from an intrusion of wake into REM sleep. The complex behaviors of sleep, like sleepwalking and sleep eating, are poorly understood. Similar to automatisms in seizures, complex behaviors occurring during the night (walking, eating, driving, talking) may be due to central pattern generators that are triggered, resulting in the behavior, but it is unknown how this occurs.

When evaluating an abnormal sleep behavior suggestive of a parasomnia, the most important disorder to rule out is frontal lobe epilepsy (in which seizures commonly occur out of sleep). Parasomnia episodes and nocturnal seizures are both present at night, both can be associated with amnesia, both impair sleep, and both can be worsened by stress/sleep fragmenting factors. Nocturnal seizures usually occur out of non-REM sleep and the seizures are characterized by violent movements or tonic-dystonic posturing. There are several clues that can help distinguish parasomnias from seizure activity. In about half of patients with non-REM parasomnias, an event is triggered by a stimulus like a noise or an apneic obstructive event. Parasomnias, unlike seizures, typically start with behaviors that look like the person is starting to arouse from sleep, such as eye opening, raising the head, rubbing the face, staring, yawning, or stretching. Non-REM parasomnias tend to have variable patterns and gradual onset and offset, but nocturnal frontal lobe seizures tend to be stereotyped motor patterns that last less than 2 minutes and start and stop suddenly. Non-REM parasomnias also tend to occur within the first 3 hours of sleep when slow-wave sleep predominates, but frontal lobe epilepsy can occur at any time during the night.[88] See Table 15-5 for a comparison of NREM parasomnias and frontal lobe seizures.

TABLE 15-5 • Distinguishing Features of Nocturnal Frontal Lobe Seizures versus NREM Parasomnias.	
Frontal Lobe Seizures	**NREM Parasomnias**
Similarities: • Present at night • Associated with amnesia • Impair sleep • Worsened by stress or sleep fragmentation Differences: • Usually occur out of NREM, but can occur at any time during the night • Start and stop suddenly • Last less than 2 minutes • Stereotyped motor patterns • Violent movements or tonic-dystonic posturing	Similarities: • Present at night • Associated with amnesia • Impair sleep • Worsened by stress or sleep fragmentation Differences: • Usually occur within the first 3 hours of sleep • Gradual onset and offset • Variable patterns • Events often triggered by stimulus like a noise or an apnea • Typically starts with behaviors that look like the person is trying to arouse from sleep (eye opening, raising head, rubbing face, staring, yawning, stretching)

TABLE 15-6 • Major Parasomnias.

Parasomnia	Definition	Classification
Sleepwalking	Episodes of leaving the bed and often performing complex behaviors, usually calmly and with no recall. Family history is common.	NREM
Sleep eating	Recurrent episodes of out-of-control eating during sleep, with a preference for high-calorie, unusual, or sometimes inedible items, and with partial or no awareness or memory of the event.	NREM
Sleep terrors	Episodes that consist of sudden screaming and demonstration of terror, usually arising from slow-wave sleep, and frequently with amnesia for the event. More common in children.	NREM
Confusional arousals	Episodes of mental confusion with abnormal behavior after partially awakening from NREM.	NREM
Sexsomnia	Individual engages in sexual activity despite being asleep. Behaviors may include sexual vocalizations, masturbation, fondling, or intercourse/attempted intercourse during sleep—followed by morning amnesia. Strong male predominance, with a mean disease onset between 26 and 33 years. Debated whether this is a separate parasomnia, or a subtype of confusional arousals or sleepwalking.[94]	NREM
Recurrent isolated sleep paralysis	Occurrence of REM-based atonia while the patient is conscious and aware, a frightening event that is often accompanied by dream activity in the form of multisensorial hallucinations, with full recall of the episode.	REM
Nightmare disorder	Extended, dysphoric, and well-recalled dreams that usually involve threats to survival, security, or physical integrity. When awakening from a nightmare, the person rapidly becomes oriented and alert.	REM
REM behavior disorder	A lack of REM atonia resulting in the acting out of dream activity, usually accompanied by vivid dream recall. Highly associated with later development of a Parkinsonian disorder.	REM

This chapter covers many of the primary sleep parasomnias (see Table 15-6 for characteristics of some of the better-known parasomnias). Not covered here are the secondary sleep phenomena that are often included under the broadest definition of parasomnias, as strange or undesirable events that happen during the night. Examples include seizures, headaches (vascular, nonvascular, hypnic, exploding head syndrome), cardiopulmonary parasomnias (arrhythmias, asthma, respiratory dyskinesias, sleep hiccup, sleep-related dyspnea and groaning), gastrointestinal parasomnias (gastroesophageal reflux, diffuse esophageal spasm, abnormal swallowing), and other secondary parasomnias (tinnitus, nocturnal panic attacks, psychogenic dissociative states).[89]

Non-REM Parasomnias

Normal NREM physiology involves a decrease in muscle tone, heart rate, overall oxygen demand, and regular respirations. Non-REM parasomnias are often collectively referred to as disorders of arousal, as behaviors usually associated with normal wake intrude into non-REM sleep. NREM parasomnias consist of a large variety of behaviors, including eating, locomotion, aggression, sex, and terrors. Several different behaviors can co-occur in the same patient and even during the same episode. During the episodes, patients are frequently unresponsive, and later amnestic for the event. Any factor that fragments sleep (e.g., periodic leg movements, OSA) or deepens sleep (e.g., drugs) can predispose to NREM parasomnia events. Events are often precipitated by sleep deprivation, stress, fever, and medications or substances. NREM parasomnias also tend to run in families.

It is crucial to distinguish NREM parasomnia episodes from seizures and postictal confusion. PSG is indicated for the workup of NREM parasomnias to evaluate for sleep fragmenting factors and, if possible, capture events for confirmation. EEG can help when seizures are suspected by evaluating for interictal epileptiform discharges, which are highly specific for epilepsy and seen in between seizures. A normal EEG does not rule out the possibility of epilepsy, and patients with frontal lobe seizures often have rare discharges that may not be captured during the EEG recording. Thus, in some situations, a more extensive evaluation is needed, such as long-term EEG monitoring.

Treatment recommendations for NREM parasomnias are scarce and generally based upon case reports and case series. If the episodes are rare and have so far not put the patient or others at harm, the most helpful intervention is education and reassurance, and instruction to family members to avoid aggressively trying to wake up the patient as this can prolong the episodes or, more rarely, provoke the patient into violence.[90,91]

If the episodes are harmful, the most important intervention is nonpharmacologic: safety measures to prevent the patient from doing harm during episodes. For example, with sleepwalking, safety measures could include ways to keep the patient confined to the bedroom, removal of sharp objects near the sleeping area, and devices to wake up the patient during episodes (such as an alarm that makes a noise when the patient tries to leave the room). The second most important intervention is prevention: elimination of drugs or other provoking factors, and implementation of good sleep hygiene. If all else fails, pharmacologic interventions can be used. Options include intermediate- or long-acting benzodiazepines, which may seem counterintuitive as similar medications, like nonbenzodiazepine receptor agonists, can provoke NREM parasomnias. The exact mechanism by which benzodiazepines seem to improve, rather than worsen, disorders of arousal is poorly understood.[90]

Serotoninergic antidepressants have been used to treat sleep terrors, and certain specific antidepressants (sertraline, clomipramine, imipramine, trazodone) have been used for sleep terrors and sleepwalking.[90] Single case reports have also been published on melatonin, hydroxytryptophan, and ramelteon.[90]

Sleepwalking

Sleepwalking is a non-REM parasomnia that can involve complex behaviors, including agitation, violence, driving, eating, and cooking. The patient may leave the bed, room, or even the building. Sleepwalking children are usually calm during episodes with no recall.[92] Sleepwalking has been associated with "sleepsex" or "sexsomnia," though this is more common with confusional arousals.[93,94] The lifetime prevalence of sleepwalking is up to 17%, with a peak at 8–12 years old,[92] decreasing to a prevalence of about 2–4% in adulthood.[95,96] A family history of sleepwalking is common and the disorder is thought to be highly genetic.[96] As the differential diagnosis includes confusional arousals, partial seizures, psychogenic dissociative states, and postictal confusion, a full polysomnogram with video and extended EEG is the recommended diagnostic test, and treatment should start with safety measures to prevent the patient from harm during sleepwalking episodes.

CASE VIGNETTE 15.1

A 55-year-old woman reports abnormal nocturnal behaviors that started many years ago but have recently intensified. She describes walking out of her bedroom and waking up in various parts of her apartment. In one situation, she woke up from a sensation of intense heat in her face. She realized she had started to cook while asleep and the heat from the gas stove woke her up.
Diagnosis: Sleepwalking.

Sleep Eating

Sleep-related eating disorder is characterized by recurrent episodes of out-of-control eating during sleep, with a preference for high-calorie, unusual, or sometimes inedible items, and with partial or no awareness or memory of the event. There is somewhat more evidence for the efficacy of SSRIs (fluoxetine, paroxetine, fluvoxamine) in sleep eating as compared to other NREM parasomnias.[90] Case reports support the use of dopamine agonists, and a few studies have shown good results with topiramate.[90]

Sleep Terrors

Sleep terrors are episodes that consist of sudden screaming and demonstration of terror, usually arising from slow-wave sleep, and frequently with amnesia for the event. The population prevalence of night terrors is approximately 2.2%, but this increases to about 30% in patients with mood disorders.[95] Sleep terrors are more common in children. Unlike with nightmares or RBD, if a person having a sleep terror is awakened, he or she will either not describe any dream content or report only a brief dream fragment.

Panic disorder has a high overlap with sleep terrors, and there are features of the two which are very similar.[2] They can be distinguished based on alertness and recall. While patients usually have no recall of a sleep terror, after a panic attack a person is fully alert, has full recall of the event, and has difficulty going back to sleep.

Treatment of sleep terrors includes reassurance, increasing total sleep, management of co-occurring sleep disorders if present (like OSA or RLS), safety measures, scheduled awakenings, and rarely medication.[92]

CASE VIGNETTE 15.2

A 5-year-old boy has episodes of sitting up in bed and screaming at night, and he does not have any memory of this in the morning. The boy's parents are frightened by these events, but the child is relatively unbothered.
Diagnosis: Sleep Terrors.

Confusional Arousals

Confusional arousals are episodes of mental confusion with abnormal behavior after partially awakening from NREM. The prevalence is about 17% in children,[58] and about 4.2% in adults.[95] A variant of confusional arousals is severe sleep inertia, in which a person has a period of impaired performance and grogginess after waking. Sleep-related sexual behaviors, or "sexsomnia," can be a form of confusional arousal (or can be sleepwalking related), with the caveat that there tends to be considerable overlap with other parasomnias (sleep driving, sleep eating) in patients with sexsomnia.[93] Patients with OSA have a tendency toward confusional arousals. Other predisposing factors include sleep deprivation and stress. Drugs and medications can also precipitate confusional arousals. Treatment involves sleep hygiene, avoiding central nervous system medications, and avoiding sleep deprivation.

REM Parasomnias

Normal REM physiology involves brain activity that is comparable to wakefulness, such as high cerebral blood flow, oxygen consumption, and glucose utilization. REM also, unlike wakefulness, involves blocked sensory input and blocked motor output through active hyperpolarization of alpha motor neurons. This motor output blockage is known as REM atonia. The most significant REM parasomnia is RBD (discussed below), which leads to sleep-related injuries of the patient or spouse in up to 65% of cases.[97,98] RBD often portends an impending neurological disorder. Other REM parasomnias include recurrent isolated sleep paralysis and nightmare disorder, which tend to be benign and self-limited conditions.

Recurrent Isolated Sleep Paralysis

Recurrent isolated sleep paralysis is the occurrence of REM-based atonia while the patient is conscious and aware, a frightening event that is often accompanied by dream activity in the form of multisensorial hallucinations, with full recall of the episode.[99] The paralysis may be accompanied by a constricting sensation of not being able to breathe due to paralysis of the voluntary muscles of respiration, although automatic involuntary breathing continues unabated. Eye movements are intact. There is often a feeling of an ominous presence in the room. Episodes are usually brief, seconds to minutes, with a mean duration of 6 minutes.[99]

Approximately 7.6% of the general population will experience at least one lifetime episode (one event) of sleep paralysis, with higher rates in females, students, and psychiatric patients[2,99]; recurrent episodes are very rare. A 2018 systematic review found that risk factors associated with sleep paralysis include substance use, stress and trauma, family history, physical illness (e.g., hypertension and chronic pain), personality ("imaginativeness" and hypnotizability), intelligence, anomalous beliefs (paranormal/spiritual), sleep problems and disorders (both in terms of subjective sleep quality and objective sleep disruption), symptoms of psychiatric illness in nonclinical samples (particularly anxiety symptoms), and psychiatric disorders (particularly PTSD and also panic disorder).[100]

"Isolated" sleep paralysis refers to the occurrence outside the context of another sleep disorder such as narcolepsy. A diagnosis of recurrent isolated sleep paralysis requires that these events must happen often enough to cause clinically significant distress, but criteria are nonspecific regarding number or frequency of events. Management focuses on reassurance, and at times therapeutic strategies such as trying to move a small muscle group (e.g., a pinky) may be helpful.

Nightmare Disorder

Dreams and nightmares may occur in all sleep stages, but prolonged story-type dreams tend to occur during REM sleep, while dream content from other states is briefer and more impressionistic. Nightmares are extended, dysphoric, and well-recalled dreams that usually involve threats to survival, security, or physical integrity. When awakening from a nightmare, the person rapidly becomes oriented and alert. Usually nightmares are rare and benign, but nightmare disorder is diagnosed when nightmares cause clinical significant distress or impairment.[58] Nightmare disorder affects approximately 4% of adults.[58] In addition to repeated occurrences of nightmares, the ICSD-3 requires at least one of the following for a diagnosis of nightmare disorder: mood disturbance, sleep resistance, cognitive impairments, negative impact on caregiver or family functioning, behavioral problems, daytime sleepiness, fatigue or low energy, impaired occupational or educational function, or impaired interpersonal/social function.[58] Nightmares can be associated with sleep or psychiatric disorders such as RBD, narcolepsy, sleep apnea, periodic limb movement disorder (PLMD), depression, and PTSD. Nightmare disorder and sleep paralysis occur in social anxiety disorder and generalized anxiety disorder at approximately three times the rate of the general population, and nightmare disorder co-occurs in 50–90% of patients with PTSD.[2] Nightmare disorder is also common in depression and correlates with an over fivefold suicide risk.[2] Nightmares can represent side effects of medications such as beta-blockers, antidepressants, nicotine, or the result of withdrawal from substances of abuse like alcohol.[101]

The AASM released a position paper on the treatment of nightmare disorder in adults in 2018. The previous recommendation for use of prazosin was downgraded from "recommended" to "may be used" due to one large (304 subjects) negative study in veterans in 2018 that contradicted the findings of at least 10 previous smaller studies (ranging in size from 44 to 100 subjects).[102] Thus, medications that may be used for PTSD-associated nightmares include olanzapine, risperidone, aripiprazole, clonidine, cyproheptadine, fluvoxamine, gabapentin, nabilone, phenelzine, prazosin, topiramate, trazodone, and tricyclic antidepressants.[102] For nightmare disorder that is not associated with PTSD, medications that may be used include nitrazepam, prazosin, and triazolam. For all forms of nightmares, the AASM recommends a variety of psychotherapies, including CBT and exposure, relaxation, and imagery re-scripting therapy.[102]

REM Behavior Disorder

RBD is characterized by abnormal behaviors emerging from REM sleep. Due to the normal increase of REM sleep over the course of a typical nights' sleep, these behaviors generally occur in the later parts of the night. Typical behaviors can include talking, screaming, punching, and kicking; more rarely, behaviors can be sexual in nature. RBD episodes are generally associated with vivid dream recall. The observed behaviors are the acting out of dream activity; for example, a patient who is punching his fists during sleep may later report he was dreaming about boxing. Patients commonly present with sleep-related injuries, altered dreams, dream-enacting behaviors, and sleep disruption. RBD is more common in men, with a typical onset in their 50s or 60s. Antidepressants such as SSRIs and monoamine oxidase inhibitors can cause RBD, but upward of 80% of patients with idiopathic RBD will develop a Parkinsonian disorder 5–29 years later.[103]

PSG is a necessary part of the evaluation and diagnosis to distinguish RBD from other parasomnias, seizures or postictal states, and psychiatric disturbances, and is likely to be of high clinical utility as the RBD episodes tend to occur nightly. For diagnosis, the ICSD-3 requires polysomnographic findings of REM sleep without atonia. Behavioral diagnostic criteria are a history of repeated episodes of sleep-related vocalization and/or complex motor behaviors presumed to occur during REM sleep.[58]

The most important treatment of RBD is the implementation of safety measures, such as padding beside the bed or movement sensors on the bed to wake the patient. Elimination of drugs that worsen episodes, such as SSRIs, should also be considered.[90] Clonazepam is widely and successfully used in RBD treatment,[90,97] with 0.5 mg generally the most suitable dosage (but the range in studies is from 0.25 to 4 mg). Evidence is growing in support of melatonin as an alternative with a more favorable safety and tolerability profile.[104]

CASE VIGNETTE 15.3

A 60-year-old man thrashes around in bed, yells aggressively, and on occasion punches his wife while sleeping. He has rolled out of bed and dislocated his shoulder and had other injuries in the past. Recently he has set up restraints to hold himself in bed and his wife has been sleeping elsewhere.

Diagnosis: REM Behavior Disorder.

Sleep-Disordered Breathing: Obstructive Sleep Apnea and Central Sleep Apnea

Sleep apnea is a primary sleep disorder characterized by pauses of breathing during sleep. In the general middle-aged population, moderate-to-severe sleep apnea can be found in about 30–50% of men and 11–23% of women.[105,106]

There are three main types of sleep apnea: OSA, central sleep apnea (CSA), and complex sleep apnea. An obstructive apnea is defined as a cessation of airflow for at least 10 seconds, and results from the collapse of the upper airway during sleep. It is associated with continued respiratory effort. By contrast, during a central apnea, the interruption of airflow occurs when there is a lack of drive to breathe—arising from the brain respiratory centers to the muscles that control breathing. Some patients present with a combination of both obstructive and central apnea, which is termed complex sleep apnea.

Clinical symptoms of sleep apnea most often include loud snoring, choking or gasping during sleep, apneas witnessed by the bed partner, excessive sleepiness and fatigue, non-restorative sleep, dryness of mouth on awakening, and morning headache. Sleep apnea has debilitating effects on the quality of life of patients and their families. When left untreated, OSA can also have major negative health consequences; it increases the risk of hypertension, type 2 diabetes, and cardiovascular diseases.[107] OSA is also a well-known risk factor for cognitive deficits[108] and for major depressive disorder.[109] The primary determinants of cognitive deficits in OSA are thought to be sleep disruption and blood gas abnormalities. Deficits in executive function, psychomotor function, and language are found in both OSA and chronic obstructive pulmonary disease and therefore more likely to be related to hypoxia/hypercarbia.[110] Deficits in attention and memory are found in both OSA and sleep deprivation studies and therefore more likely to be related to sleep disruption.[110] Importantly, the negative consequences of OSA can be, at least partially, reversed by consistent and appropriate treatment.

Workup of Sleep Apnea

Several screening scales for sleep apnea have been developed to identify at-risk patients, and the ones most frequently used in research and clinic settings are the Sleep Apnea Scale of the Sleep Disorders Questionnaire (SA-SDQ)[111] and the STOP-BANG questionnaire.[112] The SA-SDQ assesses nighttime symptoms related to sleep breathing disorders (e.g., loud snoring, witnessed apnea, awake gasping for breath, and nasal congestion) as well as sleep apnea risk factors such as age, weight, BMI, and smoking status. A cutoff of 36 for men and 32 for women was proposed to identify sleep apnea patients.[111] The STOP-BANG questionnaire (see Table 15-7) contains four yes-or-no questions that relate to clinical signs of sleep apnea (S: snoring; T: tiredness during daytime; O: observed apnea; P: high blood pressure), as well as four items related to the well-known sleep apnea risk factors (B: body mass index >35; A: age >50 years; N: neck circumference >40 cm; G: male gender). A patient is at high risk of sleep apnea if three or more of the eight questions are positively answered.[112]

Sleep apnea can be diagnosed during a polysomnogram, where the severity of sleep apnea is quantified by the number of respiratory events per hour of sleep (Apnea-Hypopnea Index,

	TABLE 15-7 • STOP-BANG Questionnaire to Screen for Obstructive Sleep Apnea.
S	Snoring? Do you Snore Loudly (loud enough to be heard through closed doors or your bed-partner elbows you for snoring at night)?
T	Tired? Do you often feel Tired, Fatigued, or Sleepy during the daytime (such as falling asleep during driving or talking to someone)?
O	Observed? Has anyone Observed you Stop Breathing or Choking/Gasping during your sleep?
P	Pressure? Do you have or are being treated for High Blood Pressure?
B	Body Mass Index more than 35 kg/m²?
A	Age older than 50?
N	Neck size large? (measured around Adams apple). For male, is your shirt collar 17 inches/43 cm or larger? For female, is your shirt collar 16 inches/41 cm or larger?
G	Gender = Male?

Low risk of OSA if yes to 0–2 questions, intermediate risk if yes to 3–4 questions, and high risk if yes to 5–8 questions. Also high risk if yes to 2 or more of the 4 STOP questions plus male, high BMI, or high neck circumference. (Reproduced with permission from Dr. Frances Chung. The STOP-Bang Questionnaire is proprietary to the University Health Network (UHN), Toronto, Canada. Copyright © 2012. www.stopbang.ca).

AHI). Along with clinical symptoms, at least five events per hour (AHI ≥5) are required for a diagnosis of sleep apnea.[113] An AHI between 5 and 14 is considered mild sleep apnea, between 15 and 29 is moderate sleep apnea, and more than 30 events per hour is considered severe sleep apnea.

Treatment of Sleep Apnea

Several therapeutic options are available for sleep apnea, including surgical and nonsurgical treatment approaches. For mild cases of OSA, behavioral interventions such as lifestyle changes (healthy diet, exercise, avoid alcohol and sedating medications, quit smoking) and avoiding supine position (for positional sleep apnea) should be tried first. Sufficient weight loss may even cure mild cases of OSA. The most widely used and preferred treatment for OSA is positive airway pressure (PAP) therapy. Depending on the type of sleep apnea, a different mask treatment will be used: for example, continuous PAP (CPAP) is generally used for treating OSA, as it sends a continuous flow of air into the nose. In some cases, bi-level therapy or auto-titrating PAP will be prescribed. Adaptive servo-ventilation, PAP ventilatory support that is adjusted based on the detection of apneas, can also be used to treat complex sleep apnea. CPAP therapy in OSA individuals has been found to reduce subjective daytime sleepiness, improve cognitive functioning, as well as mood and quality of life.[114-117] Treatment with CPAP also can improve blood pressure and glucose control.[118]

Surgical treatment methods include most commonly soft palate surgery, nasal surgery, and maxillomandibular surgery. These may help sleep apnea severity, although they generally do not cure sleep apnea.[119] Oral appliances such as mandibular advancement devices may be helpful for mild-to-moderate cases, but for moderate-to-severe OSA PAP therapy is more effective.[119] The hypoglossal nerve stimulator, an implanted device, is approved by the US Food and Drug Administration, and 5-year follow-up shows a response rate of 63%. Hypoglossal nerve stimulation is a reasonable alternative for patients who fail PAP therapy.[119,120]

CASE VIGNETTE 15.4

A 58-year-old woman presents to a clinic specializing in treatment-resistant depression to inquire about brain stimulation for low mood which has persisted for years and has not responded to medication. She emphasizes very low energy during the day, fatigue with frequent napping, and also reports spending prolonged amounts of time sleeping at night but wakes up feeling not refreshed. She complains that her thinking is not what it used to be, particularly that she has a hard time focusing. A history is also obtained of snoring, high blood pressure, and gradual weight gain over a number of years. She wakes up in the morning with mild headaches. She is referred for sleep evaluation. On polysomnography it is found that she has partial or complete cessation of breathing with preserved respiratory effort an average of six times per hour, resulting in desaturation and partial arousal. After starting continuous positive airway pressure therapy, her cognition and mood improve significantly.

Diagnosis: Obstructive Sleep Apnea.

Hypersomnia

Hypersomnia is defined as excessive daytime sleepiness despite sleep of normal or prolonged duration. Disorders causing central hypersomnia are rare. In contrast, poor sleep hygiene is common in modern life, and many patients presenting to clinic for fatigue and "excessive sleep" will not have a primary hypersomnia, but will have poor sleep hygiene and/or poor, inefficient sleep. A hypersomnia disorder should be considered in patients who have enough sleep opportunity, do not have insomnia, do not have significant environmental factors that would impair sleep quality or lead to inefficient sleep, and who have hypersomnia that recurs more than three times per week for >3 months. Hypersomnia disorders include narcolepsy types 1 and 2 (with and without cataplexy), idiopathic hypersomnia (with and without long sleep time), and recurrent hypersomnia such as Kleine-Levin syndrome. Hypersomnia can also be the result of TBI.

Narcolepsy

Narcolepsy is a disorder of REM regulation, with a prevalence falling between 25 and 50 per 100,000 people.[121] Daytime sleepiness is the most prominent and disabling symptom of narcolepsy. In addition, classic symptoms include sleep paralysis, hypnagogic (i.e., sleep onset) hallucinations, and, in narcolepsy type 1, cataplexy. Cataplexy consists of a loss of muscle tone, provoked typically by positive emotions, such as laughing or telling a joke. Occasionally, surprise or anger can be a trigger. Cataplexy attacks can be unilateral, mild and sometimes subtle, or sometimes more severe, with full collapse to the ground risking injury.

The pathophysiology of narcolepsy with cataplexy is hypothesized to be due to a lack of hypocretin, secondary to autoimmune destruction of most of the hypocretin-producing neurons in the hypothalamus.[122] Hypocretin (orexin) is low in cerebrospinal fluid in most cases of narcolepsy.[123] Almost all patients with narcolepsy type 1 (narcolepsy with cataplexy) carry the specific human leukocyte antigen (HLA) allele HLA-DQB1*06:02.[124,125] For diagnosis, HLA typing may be performed, however it is difficult to interpret and depends on the availability of genetic testing.

The diagnosis is made first clinically, and the multiple sleep latency test (MSLT) is needed to confirm the sleepiness. This test is typically performed on the day after a PSG and consists of five nap opportunities. Most narcolepsy patients fall asleep within minutes of a given nap opportunity, and thus a short sleep latency (average of less than 8 minutes over the five naps), as well as REM sleep during these naps would be supportive of narcolepsy. Current criteria require that REM sleep is present either in two or more naps or that REM is seen in one nap and a REM latency on the preceding PSG is less than 15 minutes. CSF measurement of hypocretin is performed in many European countries but is not currently commercially available in the United States.

Treatment of sleepiness usually starts with wakefulness agents, such as modafinil or armodafinil. If these are not tolerated or ineffective, stimulants (methylphenidate or amphetamine/dextroamphetamine) can be used. Cautions should include monitoring blood pressure and evaluating for arrhythmias, which can be worsened by these medications. None of these treatments have been approved for use in pregnancy. Cataplexy responds to antidepressants (typically SSRIs) or sodium oxybate.

Common comorbidities in narcolepsy include RBD as well as periodic limb movements in sleep.[126] Both of these may be worsened by SSRIs, including the ones used for cataplexy treatment.

Other Causes of Hypersomnia

Hypersomnia can be seen after head trauma, in some reports affecting as much as half of the patients with TBI,[127] and a quarter of these patients may have sleep disordered breathing. CSA, OSA, and upper airway resistance syndrome occur more commonly after TBI than in the general population. The pathophysiology of sleep disturbance after TBI may involve direct injury to sleep centers, neurohormonal responses to injury, and side effects of medications.[127] Sleep architecture may be impaired, with a reduced REM proportion.[128] Treatment of sleep disordered breathing may be helpful and use of any sedating medications should be judicious.

In rare instances, hypersomnia can be idiopathic. Idiopathic hypersomnia typically presents with long, non-refreshing naps. Two types exist: with a long sleep time, and without a long sleep time. The criteria for diagnosis include the clinical presentation, as well as supportive evidence from MSLT: a mean sleep latency of <8 minutes, and no sleep onset REMs. Treatment is often challenging. Modafinil or armodafinil at high doses can be used, and sometimes stimulants can be helpful.

In another rare condition, Kleine-Levin syndrome, hypersomnia is recurrent. Kleine-Levin syndrome has an estimated prevalence of 1–$5/10^6$ population.[129] This disorder typically presents in adolescence or early 20s and consists of periods that last for approximately 2 weeks, during which patients exhibit very long sleep (often 12–21 hours per day), and during the waking periods individuals exhibit cognitive abnormalities, such as major apathy, confusion, slowness, amnesia, or sometimes dream-like behavior. Hyperphagia or hypersexuality is common during the episodes as well, particularly in men, while depressed mood is seen more commonly in women. Déjà vu episodes are common. Between episodes, individuals have a grossly normal level of functioning; however, some research suggests that there may be enduring cognitive impairment between episodes.[129] The patients often have impaired recall of their episodes. The etiology is unknown. Exploration of proposed pathophysiological mechanisms have mostly not borne fruit, with the exception that genomic research has suggested that there is at least one genetic risk factor for bipolar disorder (loci near the TRANK1 gene) that also is associated with Kleine-Levin syndrome. Precipitating factors can include febrile illness or symptoms of infection, usually with no infectious agent identified, and for women menstruation can also be a precipitant.[129] It is generally thought to be a self-limiting syndrome, typically decreasing in frequency and intensity over the course of 8–12 years with full recovery of function by age 30. A patient may have episodes one to four times per year until the episodes gradually disappear, with no lasting psychiatric symptoms nor sleep-wake abnormalities.[130] Most textbooks and reviews state that Kleine-Levin patients have no lasting overt neurological deficits; however, a 2016 study of 122 patients showed that one-third had long-term cognitive deficits affecting retrieval and processing speed.[131] There is some suggestion that treatment with lithium may decrease the frequency of episodes, while stimulants have a marginal effect during the events[132]; however, there have been no good randomized controlled trials of any treatments.

Restless Legs Syndrome and Periodic Limb Movement Disorder

RLS and PLMD are movement disorders that interrupt sleep and cause daytime sleepiness. In this section, these two conditions are discussed together because PLMS are present in 80–90% of patients diagnosed with RLS.

RLS is characterized by uncomfortable sensations leading to an urge to move the limbs when a patient is resting or inactive, such as when sitting, lying down, or trying to fall asleep. The diagnosis of RLS is made by clinical history. The uncomfortable sensations of RLS occur or worsen while at rest, with consistent evening predominance, are associated with dysesthesia, and are partially relieved by physical activity. Patients often describe the sensation as "creeping, crawling tingling" or shock-like feelings, or simply indescribable discomfort. Over the course of the disease, the sensations can spread to the arms or trunk. One of the major characteristics of RLS is its worsening in the evening and at night, which results in difficulty initiating sleep, as patients often get up and pace around the room to relieve the discomfort. In turn, poor sleep often leads to fatigue and daytime sleepiness.

PLMS are regular, episodic stereotyped brief muscle activations occurring at regular intervals, typically in the lower limbs with bilateral repetitive brief thrusting dorsiflexion of the ankles.[130] For a diagnosis of PLMD, a person needs to have 15 or more PLMS events per hour and dysfunction or consequences associated with these movements.[58] PLMS can be diagnosed by clinical history, but a PSG may be useful to confirm the diagnosis, particularly in patients with unexplained symptoms of insomnia or hypersomnia. PLMS are defined as leg movements lasting from 0.5 to 10 seconds, recurring during intervals of 5–90 seconds, and organized in sequences of at least four leg movements in rapid succession.

RLS is one of the most common sleep-related movement disorder, affecting about 15% of adults.[133] Generally, RLS affects women more than men, and prevalence is also higher with advancing age.[133] While PLMS are common in healthy older adults, PLMD is thought to be rare and the prevalence is unknown.[58]

The cause of RLS can be idiopathic or secondary. In its idiopathic form, there is no known cause, but most patients will have a family history of RLS. Secondary RLS most often has a later onset course, and is associated with various neurological disorders (i.e., multiple sclerosis, Parkinson's disease,) iron deficiency (low ferritin level), or pregnancy. Movements of PLMD occur in close association with RLS, use of antidepressants, and the onset of anemia and uremia. Multiple studies highlight an important role of brain iron levels in the pathology of RLS and PLMS, which are lower in patients with RLS.[134] Dysfunction of the dopaminergic system has also been demonstrated as a potential pathophysiological mechanism for RLS. It is now thought that the reduced iron levels of the brain might impact the dopaminergic pathways.[134]

Some subjective scales have been developed and validated in patients with RLS, including the International Restless Legs Scale (IRLS), a 10-question instrument that assesses the severity of RLS.[135] RLS and PLMS frequently co-occur; the presence of PLMS is also supportive for the diagnosis of RLS.

Evaluation of serum ferritin level and replacement of iron if ferritin is below 50 pcg should be considered. Otherwise, pharmacological treatment of RLS may start with either dopamine agonists, gabapentin, or gabapentin enacarbil. Levodopa, ropinirole, pramipexole, cabergoline, pergolide, and gabapentin are all considered efficacious. The doses of dopamine agonists should be kept as low as possible to decrease the possibility of worsening symptoms over time, which is called augmentation. Augmentation may be prevented by using gabapentin or gabapentin enacarbil instead of dopamine agonists.[136] Other efficacious medications include pregabalin, gabapentin enacarbil, rotigotine. In more advanced disease, when other medications are no longer effective or in the setting of severe augmentation, oxycodone/naloxone, intravenous ferric carboxymaltose, and pneumatic compression devices are considered likely efficacious in idiopathic RLS. Bupropion and clonidine at this time appear to have insufficient evidence for efficacy.[137, 138]

Summary and Key Points

- Sleep is a complex, fascinating brain process, the purpose of which is incompletely understood but involves housekeeping processes in the brain and memory systems, including memory consolidation and targeted forgetting.
- Sleep is divided into stages based on polysomnography (PSG), with approximately four to five cycles of sleep per night consisting of a progression from light to deep sleep and to REM. There is more NREM in the first half of the night and increased REM in the second half of the night.
- Insomnia is common, and more than one cause in the same individual is the rule rather than the exception. First-line treatment for insomnia should be education regarding sleep hygiene.
- For insomnia, CBT-I should ideally be tried before medications.
- Parasomnias are more frequent in psychiatric populations.
- REM behavior disorder is an important parasomnia with which to be familiar due to its strong association with later development of Parkinsonian diseases (up to 80%). REM behavior disorder is the loss of normal REM atonia resulting in the acting out of dreams. It may occur in association with traumatic brain injury. Some antidepressants can cause or exacerbate REM behavior disorder.
- NREM parasomnias are "disorders of arousal," and consist of a variety of behaviors, including sleep walking, sleep eating, sleep terrors, sleep driving, and sleep sex. Confusional arousals are an NREM parasomnia in which a person partially awakens and is confused and behaves abnormally. Treatment focus should be on eliminating exacerbating factors and on safety measures.
- When evaluating abnormal sleep behavior suggestive of an NREM parasomnia, the most important disorder to rule out is frontal lobe epilepsy. Polysomnography is indicated.
- Moderate-to-severe obstructive sleep apnea is very common in the middle-aged population. When untreated, sleep apnea can increase the risk of diabetes, cardiovascular diseases, cognitive deficits, and depression. Clinical interview of patients with daytime fatigue should include screening for sleep apnea, with particular attention to witnessed cessation of breathing, snoring, dry mouth, morning headache, and hypertension.
- Diagnosis of sleep apnea requires at least five respiratory events per hour as measured by PSG. Treatment of sleep apnea with continuous positive airway pressure (CPAP) is very effective, and a variety of CPAP masks are available. Oral appliances can be helpful for mild-to-moderate cases but are not as effective as CPAP. Surgical implantation of a hypoglossal nerve stimulator can be considered for patients who fail CPAP; other surgical methods to treat sleep apnea are less effective.
- Narcolepsy's most prominent and disabling symptom is daytime sleepiness. In narcolepsy type 1, patients may also have cataplexy, which is a sudden loss of muscle tone typically provoked by positive emotions. Narcolepsy is hypothesized to be secondary to a lack of hypocretin-producing neurons in the hypothalamus. The multiple sleep latency test confirms sleepiness, and low CSF hypocretin is an optional test that can support the diagnosis. Wakefulness agents are key to treatment, and cataplexy responds to SSRIs or sodium oxybate.
- Restless legs syndrome (RLS) and periodic limb movement disorder (PLMD) are movement disorders that interrupt sleep and cause daytime sleepiness. Both are common, often multifactorial, often concurrent, and there are many well-studied treatment options.
- Given the significant emotional and cognitive consequences of sleep loss, and the comorbidity of sleep impairment with psychiatric and neurological illness, familiarity with disorders of sleep is necessary to the practice of neuropsychiatry.

Multiple Choice Questions

1. Sleep is regulated by:
   a. The homeostatic process, which is the internal clock and is reset based on activity and light exposure
   b. The circadian rhythm, which results in increased pressure to sleep the longer a person is awake
   c. The circadian rhythm, which is the internal clock and is reset based on activity and light exposure
   d. The homeostatic process, which results in increased pressure to sleep the longer a person is awake
   e. c and d

2. Which is correct regarding the sleep apnea risk factors included in the STOP-BANG questionnaire:
   a. Snoring, Timing, Obstruction, Pressure, BMI, Associated symptoms, Nighttime routine, Gender
   b. Snoring, Thickness of neck, Obstruction, Polysomnography, BMI, Age, Nightmares, Geriatric
   c. Snoring, Tiredness, Observed, Pressure, BMI, Age, Neck size, Gender
   d. Snoring, Timing, Obesity, Polysomnography, BMI, Age, Nightmares, Gender
   e. Snoring, Tired, Observed, Polysomnography, BMI, Associated symptoms, Neck size, Gender

3. A patient in clinic reports that she is having episodes of waking up screaming. These events usually happen in the second half of the night. She feels like her heart is racing, her breathing is rapid, and she is immediately alert. She can recall disturbing dreams right before waking up. The most likely diagnosis is:
   a. Nightmares
   b. Sleep terrors
   c. Confusional arousals
   d. REM behavior disorder
   e. Nocturnal seizures

4. A 62-year-old man presents to clinic reporting that his wife complains he is moving around a lot in his sleep, almost every night. Sometimes he makes movements like he is running and sometimes he cries out in his sleep. Once he kicked his wife hard enough to leave a bruise. Usually she will wake him up and he remembers that he was having a dream right before she woke him up. He is easy to awaken and is alert and oriented right after these events. After polysomnography confirms the diagnosis, the clinician could consider all except:
   a. Prescribe melatonin
   b. Prescribe clonazepam
   c. Prescribe an SSRI
   d. Discuss high association of this condition with later development of a neurodegenerative disorder
   e. Encourage basic safety measures, such as padding by the bed or movements sensors on the bed to wake the patient

5. A 25-year-old male patient has approximately four episodes a year of excessive sleeping and eating along with hypersexuality and childlike behavior. These episodes last 1–2 weeks each, and between episodes his behavior is almost back to his pre-morbid baseline. What is his diagnosis?
   a. Familial fatal insomnia
   b. Morvan's syndrome
   c. Agrypnia
   d. REM behavior disorder
   e. Kleine-Levin syndrome

Multiple Choice Answers

1. **Answer: e**
   The circadian rhythm is the internal clock and the homeostatic process is sleep pressure, and both regulate the sleep-wake cycle.

2. **Answer: c**
   The STOP-BANG questionnaire contains four yes-or-no questions that relate to clinical signs of sleep apnea (S: snoring; T: tiredness during daytime; O: observed apnea; P: high blood pressure), as well as four items related to the well-known sleep apnea risk factors (B: body mass index >35; A: age >50 years; N: neck circumference >40 cm; G: male gender).

3. **Answer: a**
   Although patients may self-diagnose as experiencing night terrors, due to the perception that nightmares are insignificant or less serious than terrors, in reality night terrors are rare in adults and usually not recalled. While sleep terrors arise out of NREM and thus happen more often early in the night, nightmares generally arise out of REM, when dreams are detailed and have plots, and the second half of the night

has a larger percentage of REM. With nocturnal seizures there would likely not be vivid dream recall, and with REM behavior disorder she would have acting out of dreams.

4. **Answer: c.**
   Antidepressants are known to precipitate REM behavior disorder (RBD). While stopping an antidepressant a patient is already taking that has good efficacy for depression would need to be carefully weighed in each case, a clinician would not want to start an antidepressant with the intent of treating REM behavior disorder. Safety is the number one priority in RBD. Melatonin and clonazepam are treatment options for RBD. The clinician will also need to discuss with the patient the association of RBD with later development of a neurodegenerative disorder.

5. **Answer: e**
   The description is consistent with Kleine-Levin syndrome. Familial fatal insomnia, Morvan's syndrome, and agrypnia are all forms of insomnia, not hypersomnia. REM behavior disorder is the acting out of dreams due to the loss of normal REM atonia.

References

1. Roth T, Jaeger S, Jin R, Kalsekar A, Stang PE, Kessler RC. Sleep Problems, Comorbid Mental Disorders, and Role Functioning in the National Comorbidity Survey Replication (NCS-R). *Biol Psychiatry*. 2006;60(12):1364-1371. doi:10.1016/j.biopsych.2006.05.039
2. Waters F, Moretto U, Dang-Vu TT. Psychiatric illness and parasomnias: a systematic review. *Current Psychiatry Rep*. 2017;19. Available at http://link.springer.com/10.1007/s11920-017-0789-3. Accessed May 17, 2018.
3. Grima NA, Ponsford JL, Pase MP. Sleep complications following traumatic brain injury. *Curr Opin Pulm Med*. 2017;23:493-499.
4. Dauvilliers Y. Insomnia in patients with neurodegenerative conditions. *Sleep Med*. 2007;8:S27-S34.
5. Stahl SM. *Stahl's Essential Psychopharmacology: Neuroscientific Basis and Practical Applications*. 4th ed. Cambridge, NY: Cambridge University Press. 2013.
6. Borbély AA, Achermann P. Sleep homeostasis and models of sleep regulation. *J Biol Rhythm*. 1999;14:559-570.
7. Duffy JF, Czeisler CA. Effect of light on human circadian physiology. *Sleep Med Clin*. 2009;4:165-177.
8. Bell L. On a form of disease resembling some advanced stages of mania and fever, but so contradistinguished from any ordinarily observed or described combination of symptoms, as to render it

probable that it may be an overlooked and hitherto unrecorded malady: by Luther V. Bell, M. D., Physician and Superintendent of the McLean Asylum for the Insane, Somerville, Mass. *AJP*. 1849;6:97–127.

9. Rechtschaffen A, Bergmann BM. Sleep deprivation in the rat: an update of the 1989 paper. *Sleep*. 2002;25:18–24.

10. Spiegel K, Sheridan JF, Cauter EV. Effect of sleep deprivation on response to immunization. [Letter]. *JAMA*. 2002;288:1471–1472.

11. Lange T, Perras B, Fehm HL, et al. Sleep enhances the human antibody response to hepatitis a vaccination. *Psychosom Med*. 2003;65:831–835.

12. Rasch B, Born J. About sleep's role in memory. *Physiol Rev*. 2013;93:681–766.

13. Van Cauter E, Spiegel K, Tasali E, et al. Metabolic consequences of sleep and sleep loss. *Sleep Med*. 2008;9:S23–S28.

14. Spiegel K, Leproult R, L'Hermite-Balériaux M, et al. Leptin levels are dependent on sleep duration: relationships with sympathovagal balance, carbohydrate regulation, cortisol, and thyrotropin. *J Clin Endocrinol Metab*. 2004;89:5762–5771.

15. King CR, Knutson KL, Rathouz PJ, et al. Short sleep duration and incident coronary artery calcification. *JAMA*. 2008;300:2859–2866.

16. Grandner MA, Sands-Lincoln MR, Pak VM, et al. Sleep duration, cardiovascular disease, and proinflammatory biomarkers. *Nat Sci Sleep*. 2013;5:93–107.

17. Taheri S, Lin L, Austin D, et al. Short sleep duration is associated with reduced leptin, elevated ghrelin, and increased body mass index. *PLoS Med*. 2004;1:e62.

18. Dashti HS, Scheer FA, Jacques PF, et al. Short sleep duration and dietary intake: epidemiologic evidence, mechanisms, and health implications. *Adv Nutr*. 2015;6:648–659.

19. Shan Z, Ma H, Xie M, et al. Sleep duration and risk of type 2 diabetes: a meta-analysis of prospective studies. *Diabetes Care*. 2015;38:529–537.

20. Itani O, Jike M, Watanabe N, et al. Short sleep duration and health outcomes: a systematic review, meta-analysis, and meta-regression. *Sleep Med*. 2017;32:246–256.

21. Yin J, Jin X, Shan Z, et al. Relationship of sleep duration with all-cause mortality and cardiovascular events: a systematic review and dose-response meta-analysis of prospective cohort studies. *J Am Heart Assoc*. 2017;6. Available at https://www.ncbi.nlm.nih.gov/pmc/articles/PMC5634263/. Accessed May 13, 2019.

22. Kripke DF, Langer RD, Elliott JA, et al. Mortality related to actigraphic long and short sleep. *Sleep Med*. 2011;12:28–33.

23. Grandner MA. Sleep, health, and society. *Sleep Med Clin*. 2017;12:1–22.

24. Tubbs AS, Perlis ML, Grandner MA. Surviving the long night: the potential of sleep health for suicide prevention. *Sleep Med Rev*. 2019;44:83–84.

25. Walker MP. The role of sleep in cognition and emotion. *Ann N Y Acad Sci*. 2009;1156:168–197.

26. Siegel JM. Do all animals sleep? *Trends Neurosci*. 2008;31:208–213.

27. Irwin MR. Why sleep is important for health: a psychoneuroimmunology perspective. *Ann Rev Psychol*. 2015;66:143–172.

28. Irwin MR, Opp MR. Sleep health: reciprocal regulation of sleep and innate immunity. *Neuropsychopharmacology*. 2017;42:129–155.

29. Lockley SW, Foster RG. Sleep: a very short introduction. 1st ed. Oxford, NY: Oxford University Press; 2012.

30. Antony JW, Paller KA. Hippocampal contributions to declarative memory consolidation during sleep. In: Hannula DE, Duff MC, eds. *The Hippocampus from Cells to Systems*. Cham, Switzerland: Springer International Publishing; 2017:245–280. Available at

http://link.springer.com/10.1007/978-3-319-50406-3_9. Accessed May 17, 2018.

31. Abel T, Havekes R, Saletin JM, et al. Sleep, plasticity and memory from molecules to whole-brain networks. *Curr Biol*. 2013;23:R774–R788.

32. Rattenborg NC, Mandt BH, Obermeyer WH, et al. Migratory sleeplessness in the white-crowned sparrow (*Zonotrichia leucophrys gambelii*). *PLoS Biol*. 2004;2:e212.

33. Goel N, Rao H, Durmer J, et al. Neurocognitive consequences of sleep deprivation. *Semin Neurol*. 2009;29:320–339.

34. Williamson A, Feyer A. Moderate sleep deprivation produces impairments in cognitive and motor performance equivalent to legally prescribed levels of alcohol intoxication. *Occup Environ Med*. 2000;57:649–655.

35. Dawson D, Reid K. Fatigue, alcohol and performance impairment. *Nature*. 1997;388:235.

36. Poe GR. Sleep is for forgetting. *J Neurosci*. 2017;37:464–473.

37. Backhaus J, Born J, Hoeckesfeld R, et al. Midlife decline in declarative memory consolidation is correlated with a decline in slow wave sleep. *Learn Mem*. 2007;14:336–341.

38. Sara SJ. Sleep to remember. *J Neurosci*. 2017;37:457–463.

39. Hoedlmoser K, Birklbauer J, Schabus M, et al. The impact of diurnal sleep on the consolidation of a complex gross motor adaptation task. *J Sleep Res*. 2015;24:100–109.

40. Grudzien A, Shaw P, Weintraub S, et al. Locus coeruleus neurofibrillary degeneration in aging, mild cognitive impairment and early Alzheimer's disease. *Neurobiol Aging*. 2007;28:327–335.

41. Tempesta D, Socci V, De Gennaro L, et al. Sleep and emotional processing. *Sleep Med Rev*. 2017. Available at http://linkinghub.elsevier.com/retrieve/pii/S1087079217301533. Accessed May 17, 2018.

42. Zohar D, Tzischinsky O, Epstein R, et al. The effects of sleep loss on medical residents' emotional reactions to work events: a cognitive-energy model. *Sleep*. 2005;28:47–54.

43. Tempesta D, Couyoumdjian A, Curcio G, et al. Lack of sleep affects the evaluation of emotional stimuli. *Brain Res Bull*. 2010;82:104–108.

44. Franzen PL, Buysse DJ, Dahl RE, et al. Sleep deprivation alters pupillary reactivity to emotional stimuli in healthy young adults. *Biol Psychol*. 2009;80:300–305.

45. Yoo S-S, Hu PT, Gujar N, et al. A deficit in the ability to form new human memories without sleep. *Nat Neurosci*. 2007;10:385–392.

46. Walker MP, van der Helm E. Overnight therapy? The role of sleep in emotional brain processing. *Psychol Bull*. 2009;135:731–748.

47. American Psychiatric Association. Diagnostic and statistical manual of mental disorders. 5th ed. Arlington, TX: American Psychiatric Association. 2013.

48. Schierenbeck T, Riemann D, Berger M, et al. Effect of illicit recreational drugs upon sleep: cocaine, ecstasy and marijuana. *Sleep Med Rev*. 2008;12:381–389.

49. Rosen RC, Kostis JB. Biobehavioral sequellae associated with adrenergic-inhibiting antihypertensive agents: a critical review. *Health Psychol*. 1985;4:579–604.

50. Kolla BP, Mansukhani MP, Bostwick JM. The influence of antidepressants on restless legs syndrome and periodic limb movements: a systematic review. *Sleep Med Rev*. 2018;38:131–140.

51. Wang Y-Q, Li R, Zhang M-Q, et al. The neurobiological mechanisms and treatments of REM sleep disturbances in depression. *Curr Neuropharmacol*. 2015;13:543–553.

52. Ozdemir PG, Karadag AS, Selvi Y, et al. Assessment of the effects of antihistamine drugs on mood, sleep quality, sleepiness, and dream anxiety. *Int J Psychiatry Clin Pract*. 2014;18:161–168.

53. Ismail MF, Lavelle C, Cassidy EM. Steroid-induced mental disorders in cancer patients: a systematic review. *Future Oncol.* 2017;13:2719–2731.

54. Liu X, Lu W, Liao S, et al. Efficiency and adverse events of electronic cigarettes: a systematic review and meta-analysis (PRISMA-compliant article). *Medicine (Baltimore).* 2018;97:e0324.

55. NIH State-of-the-Science Conference Statement on manifestations and management of chronic insomnia in adults. *NIH Consens State Sci Statements.* 2005;22:1–30.

56. American Psychiatric Association. *Diagnostic and Statistical Manual of Mental Disorders.* 5th ed. Washington, DC: American Psychiatric Association; 2013.

57. Espie CA, Farias Machado P, Carl JR, et al. The sleep condition indicator: reference values derived from a sample of 200 000 adults. *J Sleep Res.* 2018;27:e12643.

58. American Academy of Sleep Medicine. International Classification of Sleep Disorders. 3rd ed. Darien, IL: American Academy of Sleep Medicine. 2014.

59. Rezaie L, Fobian AD, McCall WV, et al. Paradoxical insomnia and subjective-objective sleep discrepancy: a review. *Sleep Med Rev.* 2018;40:196–202.

60. Winkelman JW, Plante DT, Schoerning L, et al. Increased rostral anterior cingulate cortex volume in chronic primary insomnia. *Sleep.* 2013;36:991–998.

61. Riemann D, Nissen C, Palagini L, et al. The neurobiology, investigation, and treatment of chronic insomnia. *Lancet Neurol.* 2015;14:547–558.

62. Winkelman JW, Buxton OM, Jensen JE, et al. Reduced brain GABA in primary insomnia: preliminary data from 4T proton magnetic resonance spectroscopy (1H-MRS). *Sleep.* 2008;31:1499–1506.

63. Vgontzas AN, Fernandez-Mendoza J, Liao D, et al. Insomnia with objective short sleep duration: the most biologically severe phenotype of the disorder. *Sleep Med Rev.* 2013;17:241–254.

64. Peake JM, Kerr G, Sullivan JP. A critical review of consumer wearables, mobile applications, and equipment for providing biofeedback, monitoring stress, and sleep in physically active populations. *Front Physiol.* 2018;9. Available at https://www.frontiersin.org/article/10.3389/fphys.2018.00743/full. Accessed May 24, 2019.

65. Nigro CA, Dibur E, Borsini E, et al. The influence of gender on symptoms associated with obstructive sleep apnea. *Sleep Breath.* 2018;22:683–693.

66. Morin CM, Hauri PJ, Espie CA, et al. Nonpharmacologic treatment of chronic insomnia. *Sleep.* 1999;22:1134–1156.

67. Wu R, Bao J, Zhang C, et al. Comparison of sleep condition and sleep-related psychological activity after cognitive-behavior and pharmacological therapy for chronic insomnia. *Psychother Psychosom.* 2006;75:220–228.

68. Jacobs GD, Pace-Schott EF, Stickgold R, et al. Cognitive behavior therapy and pharmacotherapy for insomnia: a randomized controlled trial and direct comparison. *Arch Intern Med.* 2004;164:1888–1896.

69. Dujardin S, Pijpers A, Pevernagie D. Prescription drugs used in insomnia. *Sleep Med Clin.* 2018;13:169–182.

70. Krystal AD, Prather AA, Ashbrook LH. The assessment and management of insomnia: an update. *World Psychiatry.* 2019;18:337–352.

71. Zisapel N. New perspectives on the role of melatonin in human sleep, circadian rhythms and their regulation: melatonin in human sleep and circadian rhythms. *Br J Pharmacol.* 2018. Available at http://doi.wiley.com/10.1111/bph.14116. Accessed June 13, 2018.

72. Auld F, Maschauer EL, Morrison I, et al. Evidence for the efficacy of melatonin in the treatment of primary adult sleep disorders. *Sleep Med Rev.* 2017;34:10–22.

73. Schatzberg AF, DeBattista C. *Manual of Clinical Psychopharmacology.* 8th revised ed. Washington, DC: American Psychiatric Publishing; 2015.

74. Victorri-Vigneau C, Dailly E, Veyrac G, et al. Evidence of zolpidem abuse and dependence: results of the French Centre for Evaluation and Information on Pharmacodependence (CEIP) network survey. *Br J Clin Pharmacol.* 2007;64:198–209.

75. Stranks EK, Crowe SF. The acute cognitive effects of zopiclone, zolpidem, zaleplon, and eszopiclone: a systematic review and meta-analysis. *J Clin Exp Neuropsychol.* 2014;36:691–700.

76. Brandt J, Leong C. Benzodiazepines and Z-drugs: an updated review of major adverse outcomes reported on in epidemiologic research. *Drugs R D.* 2017;17:493–507.

77. Zhang Y, Zhou X-H, Meranus DH, et al. Benzodiazepine use and cognitive decline in elderly with normal cognition. *Alzheimer Dis Assoc Disord.* 2016;30:113–117.

78. Picton JD, Marino AB, Nealy KL. Benzodiazepine use and cognitive decline in the elderly. *Am J Health Syst Pharm.* 2018;75:e6–e12.

79. Everitt H, Baldwin DS, Stuart B, et al. Antidepressants for insomnia in adults. *Cochrane Database Syst Rev.* 2018. Available at http://www.readcube.com/articles/10.1002/14651858.CD010753.pub2. Accessed June 6, 2018.

80. Karsten J, Hagenauw LA, Kamphuis J, et al. Low doses of mirtazapine or quetiapine for transient insomnia: a randomised, double-blind, cross-over, placebo-controlled trial. *J Psychopharmacol.* 2017;31:327–337.

81. Montagna P, Gambetti P, Cortelli P, et al. Familial and sporadic fatal insomnia. *Lancet Neurol.* 2003;2:167–176.

82. Abou-Zeid E, Boursoulian LJ, Metzer WS, et al. Morvan syndrome: a case report and review of the literature. *J Clin Neuromuscul Dis.* 2012;13:214–227.

83. Koenigs M, Holliday J, Solomon J, et al. Left dorsomedial frontal brain damage is associated with insomnia. *J Neurosci.* 2010;30:16041–16043.

84. Pandi-Perumal SR, Smits M, Spence W, et al. Dim light melatonin onset (DLMO): a tool for the analysis of circadian phase in human sleep and chronobiological disorders. *Prog Neuropsychopharmacol Biol Psychiatry.* 2007;31:1–11.

85. Auger RR, Burgess HJ, Emens JS, et al. Clinical practice guideline for the treatment of intrinsic circadian rhythm sleep-wake disorders: Advanced Sleep-Wake Phase Disorder (ASWPD), Delayed Sleep-Wake Phase Disorder (DSWPD), Non-24-Hour Sleep-Wake Rhythm Disorder (N24SWD), and Irregular Sleep-Wake Rhythm Disorder (ISWRD). An update for 2015. *J Clin Sleep Med.* 2015;11:1199–1236.

86. Sletten TL, Magee M, Murray JM, et al. Efficacy of melatonin with behavioural sleep-wake scheduling for delayed sleep-wake phase disorder: a double-blind, randomised clinical trial. *PLoS Med.* 2018;15:e1002587.

87. Williams WPT, McLin DE, Dressman MA, et al. Comparative review of approved melatonin agonists for the treatment of circadian rhythm sleep-wake disorders. *Pharmacotherapy.* 2016;36:1028–1041.

88. Maski K, Owens J. Pediatric sleep disorders. *Continuum (Minneap Minn).* 2018;24(1, Child Neurology):210-227.

89. Mahowald MW, Schenck CH. Non-rapid eye movement sleep parasomnias. *Neurol Clin.* 2005;23:1077–1106, vii.

90. Proserpio P, Terzaghi M, Manni R, et al. Drugs used in parasomnia. *Sleep Med Clin.* 2018;13:191–202.

91. Pressman MR. Disorders of arousal from sleep and violent behavior: the role of physical contact and proximity. *Sleep.* 2007;30:1039–1047.

92. Mason TBA, Pack AI. Pediatric parasomnias. *Sleep.* 2007;30: 141–151.

93. Schenck CH, Arnulf I, Mahowald MW. Sleep and sex: what can go wrong? A review of the literature on sleep related disorders and abnormal sexual behaviors and experiences. *Sleep.* 2007;30:683–702.

94. Dubessy A-L, Leu-Semenescu S, Attali V, et al. Sexsomnia: a specialized non-REM parasomnia?. *Sleep.* 2017;40. Available at https://academic.oup.com/sleep/sleep/article/2666486/Sexsomnia. Accessed January 13, 2019.

95. Ohayon MM, Guilleminault C, Priest RG. Night terrors, sleepwalking, and confusional arousals in the general population: their frequency and relationship to other sleep and mental disorders. *J Clin Psychiatry.* 1999;60(4):268–277.

96. Hublin C, Kaprio J, Partinen M, et al. Prevalence and genetics of sleepwalking: a population-based twin study. *Neurology.* 1997;48:177–181.

97. Olson EJ, Boeve BF, Silber MH. Rapid eye movement sleep behaviour disorder: demographic, clinical and laboratory findings in 93 cases. *Brain.* 2000;123(pt 2):331–339.

98. McCarter SJ, St. Louis EK, Boswell CL, et al. Factors associated with injury in REM sleep behavior disorder. *Sleep Med.* 2014;15:1332–1338.

99. Sharpless BA. A clinician's guide to recurrent isolated sleep paralysis. *Neuropsychiatr Dis Treat.* 2016;12:1761–1767.

100. Denis D, French CC, Gregory AM. A systematic review of variables associated with sleep paralysis. *Sleep Med Rev.* 2018;38:141–157.

101. Hogl B, Iranzo A. Rapid eye movement sleep behavior disorder and other rapid eye movement sleep parasomnias. *Continuum (Minneap Minn).* 2017;23:1017–1034.

102. Morgenthaler TI, Auerbach S, Casey KR, et al. Position paper for the treatment of nightmare disorder in adults: an American Academy of Sleep Medicine position paper. *J Clin Sleep Med.* 2018;14:1041–1055.

103. Schenck CH, MD: Update on REM sleep behavior disorder, its management, and its strong link with parkinsonism. *Sleep Rev.* Available at http://www.sleepreviewmag.com/2015/11/update-rem-sleep-behavior-disorder-management-strong-link-parkinsonism/. Accessed September 13, 2018.

104. McGrane IR, Leung JG, St. Louis EK, et al. Melatonin therapy for REM sleep behavior disorder: a critical review of evidence. *Sleep Med.* 2015;16:19–26.

105. Heinzer R, Vat S, Marques-Vidal P, et al. Prevalence of sleep-disordered breathing in the general population: the HypnoLaus study. *Lancet Respir Med.* 2015;3:310–318.

106. Arnardottir ES, Bjornsdottir E, Olafsdottir KA, et al. Obstructive sleep apnoea in the general population: highly prevalent but minimal symptoms. *Eur Respir J.* 2016;47:194–202.

107. Maeder MT, Schoch OD, Rickli H. A clinical approach to obstructive sleep apnea as a risk factor for cardiovascular disease. *Vasc Health Risk Manag.* 2016;12:85–103.

108. Rosenzweig I, Glasser M, Polsek D, et al. Sleep apnoea and the brain: a complex relationship. *Lancet Respir Med.* 2015;3(5):404–414.

109. Hobzova M, Prasko J, Vanek J, et al. Depression and obstructive sleep apnea. *Neuro Endocrinol Lett.* 2017;38:343–352.

110. Olaithe M, Bucks RS, Hillman DR, et al. Cognitive deficits in obstructive sleep apnea: insights from a meta-review and comparison with deficits observed in COPD, insomnia, and sleep deprivation. *Sleep Med Rev.* 2018;38:39–49.

111. Douglass AB, Bornstein R, Nino-Murcia G, et al. The Sleep Disorders Questionnaire I: creation and multivariate structure of SDQ. *Sleep.* 1994;17:160–167.

112. Chung F, Elsaid H. Screening for obstructive sleep apnea before surgery: why is it important? *Curr Opin Anaesthesiol.* 2009;22:405–411.

113. Iber C, Ancoli-Israel S, Chesson A, et al. The AASM manual for the scoring of sleep and associates events: rules, terminology and technical specifications. Westchester, IL: American Academy of Sleep Medicine. 2007.

114. Campos-Rodriguez F, Queipo-Corona C, Carmona-Bernal C, et al. Continuous positive airway pressure improves quality of life in women with OSA. A randomized-controlled trial. *Am J Respir Crit Care Med.* 2016;194:1286–1294.

115. Kushida CA, Nichols DA, Holmes TH, et al. Effects of continuous positive airway pressure on neurocognitive function in obstructive sleep apnea patients: the Apnea Positive Pressure Long-term Efficacy Study (APPLES). *Sleep.* 2012;35(12):1593–602.

116. Bucks RS, Olaithe M, Rosenzweig I, et al. Reviewing the relationship between OSA and cognition: where do we go from here? *Respirology.* 2017;22(7):1253–1261.

117. Rosenzweig I, Glasser M, Polsek D, et al. Sleep apnoea and the brain: a complex relationship. *Lancet Respir Med.* 2015;3:404–414.

118. Zhao YY, Redline S. Impact of continuous positive airway pressure on cardiovascular risk factors in high-risk patients. *Curr Atheroscler Rep.* 2015;17.

119. Waters T. Alternative interventions for obstructive sleep apnea. *Cleve Clin J Med.* 2019;86:34–41.

120. Woodson BT, Strohl KP, Soose RJ, et al. Upper airway stimulation for obstructive sleep apnea: 5-year outcomes. *Otolaryngol Head Neck Surg.* 2018;159:194–202.

121. Longstreth WT, Koepsell TD, Ton TG, et al. The epidemiology of narcolepsy. *Sleep.* 2007;30:13–26.

122. Liblau RS, Vassalli A, Seifinejad A, et al. Hypocretin (orexin) biology and the pathophysiology of narcolepsy with cataplexy. *Lancet Neurol.* 2015;14:318–328.

123. Nishino S, Ripley B, Overeem S, et al. Low cerebrospinal fluid hypocretin (Orexin) and altered energy homeostasis in human narcolepsy. *Ann Neurol.* 2001;50:381–388.

124. Miyagawa T, Tokunaga K. Genetics of narcolepsy. *Hum Genome Var.* 2019;6:4.

125. Mignot E, Hayduk R, Black J, et al. HLA DQB1*0602 is associated with cataplexy in 509 narcoleptic patients. *Sleep.* 1997;20:1012–1020.

126. Frauscher B, Ehrmann L, Mitterling T, et al. Delayed diagnosis, range of severity, and multiple sleep comorbidities: a clinical and polysomnographic analysis of 100 patients of the Innsbruck narcolepsy cohort. *J Clin Sleep Med.* 2013;9:805–812.

127. Vermaelen J, Greiffenstein P, deBoisblanc BP. Sleep in traumatic brain injury. *Crit Care Clin.* 2015;31:551–561.

128. Schreiber S, Barkai G, Gur-Hartman T, et al. Long-lasting sleep patterns of adult patients with minor traumatic brain injury (mTBI) and non-mTBI subjects. *Sleep Med.* 2008;9:481–487.

129. Gadoth N, Oksenberg A. Kleine–Levin syndrome: an update and mini-review. *Brain Dev.* 2017;39:665–671.

130. Kaufman DM. Major problems in neurology. In: *Kaufman's Clinical Neurology for Psychiatrists.* 8th ed. New York, NY: Elsevier. 2016.

131. Uguccioni G, Lavault S, Chaumereuil C, et al. Long-term cognitive impairment in Kleine-Levin syndrome. *Sleep.* 2016;39:429–438.

132. Arnulf I. Kleine-Levin syndrome. *Sleep Med Clin.* 2015;10:151–161.

133. Innes KE, Selfe TK, Agarwal P. Prevalence of restless legs syndrome in North American and Western European populations: a systematic review. *Sleep Med.* 2011;12:623–634.

134. Guo S, Huang J, Jiang H, et al. Restless legs syndrome: from pathophysiology to clinical diagnosis and management. *Front Aging Neurosci.* 2017;9:171.

135. The International Restless Legs Syndrome Study Group. validation of the International Restless Legs Syndrome Study Group rating scale for restless legs syndrome. *Sleep Med.* 2003;4:121–132.

136. Winkelman JW, Armstrong MJ, Allen RP, et al. Practice guideline summary: treatment of restless legs syndrome in adults. *Neurology.* 2016;87:2585–2593.

137. Winkelmann J, Allen RP, Högl B, et al. Treatment of restless legs syndrome: evidence-based review and implications for clinical practice (revised 2017). *Mov Disord.* 2018;33:1077–1091.

138. Anderson KN. Insomnia and cognitive behavioural therapy—how to assess your patient and why it should be a standard part of care. *J Thorac Dis.* 2018;10:S94–S102.

16

ADHD and Executive Function Disorders

Geoffrey Raynor · Seth Gale

INTRODUCTION

Attention deficit disorder (with or without hyperactivity) first appeared in the *Diagnostic and Statistical Manual of Mental Disorders* (*DSM*) III in 1980,[1] though reports of pathological inattention in children have appeared as early as the 18th century by physicians Melchior Weikard in Germany and Alexander Crichton in Scotland.[2] Sir Alexander Crichton wrote in 1798 about patients who are, from birth, "incapable of attending with constancy to any one object of education."[3] Of the disorder, he wrote: "...but, it seldom is in so great a degree as totally to impede all instruction; and what is very fortunate, it is generally diminished with age."[3] In time, the diagnosis evolved through subsequent *DSM* editions to be divided into three subtypes: predominantly inattentive, predominantly hyperactive-impulsive, and combined type. The diagnostic criterion regarding age of symptom onset was most recently expanded from 7 years to 12 years old.[4] Given the natural variability of attentional traits and abilities between individuals,[5,6] ongoing debate exists as to what severity of deficits "cross the threshold" to become a psychiatric illness.[7]

This chapter will review aspects of executive function disorders with a main focus on attention-deficit hyperactivity disorder (ADHD). Executive functioning refers to the brain processes that integrate, control, and regulate cognitive, affective, and behavioral functions. Although some models[8] consider attention to be in the domain of executive functioning, in this chapter we separate attention from executive function in a clinically meaningful way. Attention, at the basic level, starts with a modicum level of arousal that allows an individual to focus on a stimulus. Attention may be thought of as a prerequisite for most other cognitive abilities. More complex aspects of attention include where to pay attention in the visual world, what to pay attention to, the ability to divide attention, the sustaining of one's focus or attention for periods of time, and the ability to switch attention, with much overlap between these functions. Deficits in various aspects of attention are associated with ADHD, although problems with attention also commonly result from many other developmental and acquired conditions.

EPIDEMIOLOGY

The *DSM-5* reports a prevalence of ADHD in about 5% of children and 2.5% of adults based on a meta-analysis of global epidemiologic studies.[4,9,10] Prevalence rates in Europe and North America are comparable, while the Middle East and Africa share lower rates, possibly due to smaller sample sizes and/or sociocultural factors.[10] National registries and insurance provider databases tracking mental health disorders show significant increases in the number of ADHD diagnoses in the past 50 years, while epidemiologic studies remain mixed about whether prevalence, itself, has increased.[10,11] This increase in diagnoses with an unclear increase in prevalence established from epidemiologic studies suggests a trend toward overdiagnosis of ADHD in children and adolescents in developed countries, possibly explained by misinterpretation of normal developmental behavior as pathology, misleading information from caregivers' biases (i.e., parents with higher levels of education tend to report more inattentive ADHD symptoms), the ambiguity of diagnostic criteria, secondary gains from patients (i.e., response to academic or work demands), and pressure from health care systems and/or reimbursement models to make a diagnosis to justify a plan of treatment for any attention complaint.[11] Even within the United States, there are racial differences in ADHD diagnoses and treatment despite equal prevalence, with African American and Hispanic children diagnosed at significantly lower rates compared to their Caucasian peers.[12] ADHD is more prevalent in men than in women, with gender differences greater in children (2:1) than adults (1.6:1).[4] Age is negatively correlated with ADHD prevalence and symptom severity tends to improve with increasing age.[9] Rates of ADHD diagnosis are significantly higher in children with later birthdates when they are compared to older peers in the same school grade, suggesting an age-related contribution to ADHD symptoms.[13] This finding supports the concept that ADHD is often a disorder of delayed developmental maturation. Some research has raised the possibility of an adolescent- or adult-onset phenotype of the disorder, though these concepts are disputed in the field.[14]

The prevalence of ADHD varies widely across studies, mostly due to methodological differences in disease classification, involving different assessment scales, age of subjects, medication treatment status, whether additional informants were used, and criteria for the diagnosis itself. Given such variables, it is not surprising that study outcomes also vary significantly. In one study examining the impact of informant agreement (parents and teachers) on the report of ADHD symptoms, the diagnosis rate decreased significantly when a strict, "two-setting" requirement of symptoms was employed.[15]

Developmental-onset ADHD symptoms generally decline from childhood to adulthood and adults with a history of ADHD in childhood are much less likely to meet criteria for the disorder as they age.[16] In a prospective study of 135 children diagnosed with combined-type (hyperactive, inattentive) ADHD, only 22% of adults continued to meet criteria at age 41 (7% hyperactive, 7% inattentive, 8% combined).[16] Individuals diagnosed with childhood ADHD continued to have average to good occupational performance without impairment in social functioning. Controls without childhood diagnoses had superior social functioning, work performance, and salary, with fewer rates of divorce and incarceration. In that study, ongoing ADHD was weakly related to concurrent substance disorders and antisocial personality disorder, but not to mood or anxiety disorders.[16] A meta-analysis of follow-up studies of children with ADHD in fact revealed that around 15% had a persistence of symptoms that met full criteria for ADHD into adulthood. Importantly, that analysis also found that 40–60% of adults continued to have some ADHD symptoms, despite no longer meeting full criteria, perhaps constituting a cohort with "ADHD in partial remission."[17] This raises questions about whether characterizing adult ADHD as a "spectrum" disorder, with broadened criteria or different subtypes of severity, would more completely account for those affected.

A New Zealand study that followed over 1000 patients from birth to age 38 found a 6% prevalence of ADHD (*DSM-III* criteria) in childhood, with male predominance, and 3% prevalence at age 38, without clear sex differences.[18] Intriguingly, the two sets of patients did not overlap and only 5% of the originally diagnosed children continued to meet *DSM-5* diagnostic criteria at age 38. Of the adult ADHD group, 48% had substance dependence (alcohol, cannabis, or other recreational drugs) and 70% had some contact with a mental health professional in their adulthood. Forty-eight percent took prescription medication for a psychiatric disorder, including depression, anxiety, psychological trauma, substance treatment, or eating disorder. No significant impairment was captured on the adult ADHD patients' neuropsychological measures of IQ, working memory, and attentional vigilance, demonstrating poor correlation between symptoms and objective cognitive deficits.[18] These results suggest that new-onset adult ADHD symptoms are often not specific to that disorder and commonly arise from other etiologies.

Finally, a prospective study specifically sought to carefully assess ADHD symptoms that began in adolescence and adulthood.[14] Aimed at understanding the origin of late-onset adult ADHD diagnosis, 239 children and adolescents were studied over an average of 14 years with regular, comprehensive psychiatric evaluations and stepped diagnostic procedures as they entered young adulthood. Of the 96 "adolescent-onset" and 47 "adult-onset" (143 total) participants who met most ADHD criteria by retrospective rating scales completed by the subject and collateral informants, 95% were ultimately excluded from diagnosis of late-onset ADHD. Subjects either did not have functional impairment of clinical significance (64 adolescents, 7 adults), did not meet symptoms across two settings (7 adolescents, 1 adult), had symptoms better explained by co-occurring mental or substance-use disorders (8 adolescents, 21 adults), or a detailed interview concluded that symptoms began prior to the age of 12—when they would have met age-related criteria for ADHD (11 adolescents, 16 adults). Most of the "adolescent-onset" participants remitted in adulthood and upon further investigation had either subthreshold symptoms as children or had likely time-limited symptoms which could be explained by lagging brain development and the inability to accommodate to increasing environmental demands. The two "adult-onset" ADHD patients both had complex psychiatric history, making symptom etiology difficult to determine. Ultimately, these two patients were determined to meet criteria, despite confounding factors that may have better explained their symptoms.[14]

Taken together, these data support the conceptualization of two dominant groups of patients with ADHD symptoms: (1) those with childhood-onset symptoms of varying severity, who exhibit the neurodevelopmental dysfunction that typically defines the disorder, regardless of when in life the diagnosis is made, and (2) those with one or more neuropsychiatric disorders that produce cognitive and behavioral symptoms that mimic ADHD, but are better explained by these other disorders.

PATHOPHYSIOLOGY

We will first discuss the neuropsychology and neurobiology of attention, as a way to then better understand the pathophysiology of ADHD.

MODELS OF ATTENTION

Attention is the ability of the mind to orient toward, prioritize, and monitor salient stimuli in the external environment or within one's own thoughts (or "internal environment"). The expression to "*pay* attention" may best capture the intrinsic activity that is required when one marshals attention to any aspect of their environment. As a brain resource, attention is both limited and indispensable, providing the foundation for most other cognitive processes, like language, memory, and spatial cognition. Due to its levels of complexity, it is helpful to consider attention as part of a system of brain functions that can involve sequential and interrelated processes. One helpful paradigm to conceptualize attention defines three mental processes: alerting, orienting, and executive control.[19,20] Alerting refers to the act of "getting ready" for some anticipated stimulus, and is associated with quicker reaction times. Orienting is the ability to direct the focus of one's mental resources toward a determined aspect of the environment. Executive attention refers to higher-order processes, like conflict monitoring and error detection (see Table 16-1).[21]

In another helpful model, the executive control functions may be divided into the abilities of "selective" and "sustained" attention. Selective attention may be thought of as the active process of focusing mental effort toward a stimulus while filtering distractors.[22] Sustained attention refers to the ability to remain on task over a prolonged period without significant loss in performance. The term "vigilance" is sometimes used to refer to sustained attention that takes place in the setting of perceived danger or threat. The information flow of attention in the human brain involves both "top-down" or "bottom-up" processes. Top-down (endogenous) attention is motivated by a particular goal, whereas bottom-up (exogenous) attention occurs "automatically" in response to salient or novel environmental stimuli.[23,24] As an example, while listening to a lecture in a classroom, bottom-up processes of attention may automatically draw one's attention to one or many external, environmental stimuli, such as the sound of traffic outside or other students whispering, or to internal stimuli, like own's own distracting thoughts. Top-down processing consists of both intentionally selecting the lecturer's spoken words as the center of focus and filtering out and prioritizing the more automatic stimuli from bottom-up processes, in the service of unperturbed concentration on, and comprehension of, the lecture's content.

NEUROANATOMY AND NEUROPHYSIOLOGY

Neuroscience research over many decades has implicated a variety of brain regions in attention, reflecting the numerous mental processes subsumed under this domain. These studies, involving functional imaging and other modalities, have shown some convergence on the involvement of at least the frontoparietal regions and cortico-striato-thalamic circuits for many attention-related functions. One substrate that mediates attention can be divided into networks involving the dorsal and ventral frontoparietal cortices.[25] Executive functions that relate to the control of cognitive processes (cognitive control) are also likely organized into these dissociable dorsal/ventral modules.[26] In research on attention, this network division has largely been applied to the visual system but may be extended to the sensory processing of sound, touch, and other modalities. The dorsal attention network is responsible for voluntarily directing attention to a particular

location and/or feature within the sensory "stream" (e.g., the orange color of a ball you are holding; the corner of the room where a voice is heard). It is comprised of the frontal eye fields and intraparietal sulcus. The ventral attention network monitors environmentally salient and often unexpected data from the sensory "stream" and may mediate the reorienting of attention accordingly (e.g., a speeding car arising in a pedestrian's peripheral field). It comprises right-predominant temporoparietal junction and ventral frontal cortex.[25-27] Importantly, while the two systems have their specializations, they also function in dynamic interaction, depending on the task at hand.[25-27]

In addition to these anatomic considerations, neurotransmitter systems are also involved in regulating attention and executive functions. Cortical norepinephrine (NE) originates from the locus coeruleus in the brainstem. NE likely assists in the maintenance of arousal and the so-called attentional tone, a measure of the signal-to-noise ratio in the processing of sensory data, where a higher tone reflects enhancement of desired objects of attention ("signal") over those of non-salient or distracting objects ("noise").[28] Dopamine (DA), originating from the ventral tegmental area and substantia nigra in the brainstem/midbrain, is necessary for maintenance of appropriate behavioral engagement and is involved in reward pathways. Acetylcholine (ACh), from the brainstem ascending reticular activating system (ARAS) and the basal forebrain, may modulate activity in the thalamus and cortex, influencing overall information processing capacity. ACh is also critical for mediating the orienting of attention.[21,29]

PATHOPHYSIOLOGY OF DISRUPTED ATTENTION

The pathophysiology of inattention and ADHD will be reviewed using a framework of both neuropsychologically based models and associated neurobiological theory, with significant overlap between the two. ADHD likely arises from a complex interplay between genes, pre- and perinatal environment, and longer-term environmental factors, including epigenetic modification and psychological factors.[2] While we consider ADHD to be a neurodevelopmental disorder with onset in childhood, these models are relevant to understanding inattentive or hyperactive symptoms across the lifespan.

TABLE 16-1 • Neurobiological Organization of Attention Networks.				
Attention Process	**Example**	**Circuits/Nuclei Implicated**	**Neurotransmitters**	**Symptoms That Occur when Disrupted**
Alerting	"When will the target occur?"	-Locus coeruleus -RAS -Frontoparietal networks	Norepinephrine, acetylcholine	-Delayed response time
Orienting	"Where will the target occur and what will it look like?"	-Dorsal stream (FEF, IPS/SPL) -Ventral stream (TPJ, VFC)	Acetylcholine	-Distractibility
Executive control	"How can I monitor and prioritize multiple factors competing for attention?"	-DLPFC -Medial frontal, ACC	Dopamine	-Careless errors

ACC, anterior cingulate cortex; DLPFC, dorsolateral prefrontal cortex; FEF, frontal eye fields; IPS, intraparietal sulcus; RAS, reticular activating system; SPL, superior parietal lobe; TPJ, temporoparietal junction; VFC, ventral frontal cortex.

Inattention and hyperactivity of ADHD are characterized by various neuropsychological deficits and behavioral symptoms, including impairment in attention, inhibition, and motivation. The symptoms and cognitive deficits may vary along a continuum from mild to severe, with broad performance variability on neuropsychological testing. Thus, among those with ADHD who meet the same symptom-based disease criteria there can be widely different phenotypes. For example, individuals with ADHD may be quite like their neurotypical peers in behavior and cognition but have symptoms just severe enough to cause mild functional impairment. Overall, patients with ADHD do have consistently worse performance in cognitive tasks across many domains compared to age-matched, neurotypical individuals.[22] Patients with ADHD often have some impairment in the various processes of attention (i.e., alerting and executive attention; discussed above). Further deficits in response precision, cognitive flexibility, working memory, temporal information processing, and response inhibition have been described.[22]

In general, disruption anywhere along various frontal-subcortical and fronto-cortical circuits can lead to the behavioral outcomes seen in ADHD and executive function disorders. The frontal-subcortical networks are looped circuits, with flow of information from the prefrontal cortex to the striatum, striatum to thalamus (dorsal medial/ventral anterior nuclei), and then return to the frontal lobes (see Figure 16-1).[30] Dysfunction in fronto-striato-thalamic circuits plays a role in impairing inhibitory control, such as the control of immediate responses to the environment (response inhibition) and response to multiple, interfering stimuli (interference control). Alterations in the dorsal and ventral fronto-parietal circuits are also implicated in ADHD, resulting in difficulty with alerting and appropriately orienting attentional resources.[31] Structural MRI studies in ADHD have shown reduced volume in subcortical (basal ganglia), and cortical (frontal and parieto-temporal) that attenuate with age: generally, volume differences between patients with childhood ADHD and healthy controls are no longer detectable in adulthood.[32,33] Early regional brain volume differences may reflect a pattern of delay in prefrontal cortical and subcortical maturation in ADHD,[33] which also supports the notion that ADHD is a disorder of delayed neurodevelopment.

In functional imaging studies, control participants generally show an inverse correlation between the cognitive control network (dorsal anterior cingulate cortex, supplementary motor area, inferior frontal junction, anterior insula, and posterior parietal lobe) associated with goal-directed task engagement, and the default mode network (posterior cingulate, medial prefrontal, and the lateral and inferior parietal cortices), associated with internal reflection or mind wandering, which shows activity during mental rest. In ADHD patients, however, this inverse correlation is often reduced, suggesting that either a disruption in the activation of, or switching between, one or both these distributed networks may be implicated in the disorder.[31] Functional imaging studies in ADHD patients have also shown overactivation in the posterior cerebellum in conjunction with frontal lobe underactivation during attention tasks, suggesting that fronto-cerebellar connections may mediate some of the observed deficits.[34]

Interestingly, studies of twins and adopted children have shown that ADHD is a highly inheritable disorder, although robust genetic correlations remain elusive. The heterogeneity of the disorder has led the geneticists to approach a more dimensional construct of the disorder as a spectrum and begin to have more nuanced view of component subtypes of ADHD in order to improve search for genetic contributions.[35]

Cognitive and Affective Contributions

In some constructs of ADHD it is considered primarily a disorder of self-regulation, reflecting the inability to inhibit automatic responses.[36] This impaired self-regulation can involve overlapping dysfunction between cognitive and emotional processes, which can be difficult to dissociate. Executive dysfunction, for example, may sometimes contribute in a dominant way to the dysregulation of mood. Individuals with attention and executive dysfunction often have difficulties employing adaptive mechanisms to modulate stress, which leads to emotional dysregulation. Regulation of emotion is included on some ADHD symptom rating scales. The Utah Criteria for ADHD, for example, includes descriptions of "affective lability" or "hot temper"[37] and the Conners' Parent Rating Scale includes symptoms of being "down on self" or having a "short-fuse."[38] Conversely, mood lability and behavioral disinhibition themselves may lead to difficulties maintaining concentration and attention, both of which may be criteria used to diagnose other psychiatric disorders.[4] Most likely, there is dynamic and reciprocal interplay between aberrant cognitive and emotional processing in ADHD, which follows logically from our understanding of the functional connectivity between these highly interrelated networks.[39]

Given that patients with ADHD often have difficulty completing tasks, it is imperative to explore the contribution of deficits in motivation to their overall functioning. The mesocorticolimbic circuitry implicated in basic motivation includes the ventral striatum (especially the nucleus accumbens), anterior cingulate cortex, and orbitofrontal cortex, with connections to the amygdala mediating the emotional salience of the motivated behavior.[31,40] In a monetary incentive delay task, subjects with ADHD have shown decreased activation in the ventral striatum compared to controls while anticipating reward.[41] Impaired signaling in circuits that mediate the higher-order processing of motivation and reward, may lead to the inability to delay gratification and to impulsivity.[42] DA is an important neurotransmitter associated with impulsivity[40] and motivation.[43] There is evidence provided by molecular PET studies that DA reward/motivation pathways are disrupted in ADHD.[43] Children with ADHD overwhelmingly prefer immediate to delayed rewards.[44] The cause of decreased motivation is likely multidetermined. As impulsivity leads to impaired performance and punitive consequences, a person can develop greater aversion to engage in challenging tasks, which leads to further inattention or avoidance. With limited initial desire to complete a task, and an indifference to, or resentment about having to, do it at all, there is

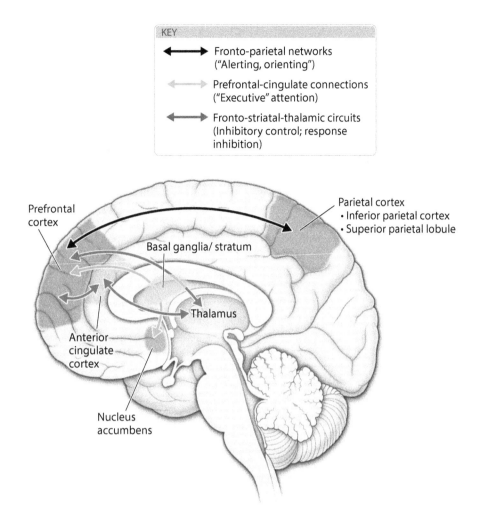

KEY

⬅➡ Fronto-parietal networks ("Alerting, orienting")

⬅➡ Prefrontal-cingulate connections ("Executive" attention)

⬅➡ Fronto-striatal-thalamic circuits (Inhibitory control; response inhibition)

Prefrontal cortex

Parietal cortex
• Inferior parietal cortex
• Superior parietal lobule

Basal ganglia/ stratum

Thalamus

Anterior cingulate cortex

Nucleus accumbens

FIGURE 16-1. Brain regions and networks involved in attention.

little incentive to engage. More concretely, if an impulsive individual is consistently having difficulty completing work and experiencing the associated, negative consequences, they may develop anxiety and low self-esteem around reengaging in any task. This lack of reengagement and positive reinforcement can then lead to a cycle of further, decreased motivation, low self-efficacy, and even worse performance.

CLINICAL PRESENTATION, DIFFERENTIAL DIAGNOSIS, AND ASSESSMENT

Clinical Presentation

The diagnosis of ADHD is based on both patients' subjective experience and observer reports of behavioral symptoms. There are no reliable biomarkers currently available in clinical care.[45] This diagnostic approach has significant limitations, particularly in the inability to correlate symptoms and behaviors with neurobiological processes. As is the case with all neuropsychiatric diagnoses, an accurate history of patients with suspected ADHD and executive disorders is the cornerstone

of the assessment. In addition to the essential interviews of patients and informants, evaluations should include a mental status examination and neuro-medical assessment. Though the *DSM-5* criteria is not without its problems, notably the overlaps in criteria, it is important to adhere to diagnostic criteria, as clinicians are known to overdiagnose ADHD based on their heuristic model and consequently overlook important exclusion criteria.[46] Our experience is that an initial, comprehensive ADHD evaluation will often take more than one appointment.

Patients with inattention or ADHD symptoms may present to their primary care physician, a psychiatrist, or a neurologist, depending on access to specialists, personal relationships to providers, and cultural practices in their community. To satisfy a diagnosis of ADHD, symptoms must not be better explained by other psychiatric disorders, such as a mood disorder, psychotic disorder, or substance use disorder. Furthermore, the manifestation of inattention and/or hyperactivity must be present across at least two settings, such as home, work, and school.[4] Vocational and social consequences of symptoms should be explored.

Patients usually seek medical attention once symptoms cause a notable interference with responsibilities at school or work. Adult patients may have recently learned about ADHD, sometimes through their own children's diagnosis or through their social milieu and may retrospectively begin to consider their own potential diagnosis. Some patients may feel a general sense of professional or social inadequacy and are searching for some medical explanation.[47] Others may seek further evaluation, after questioning whether previous diagnoses fully explain their challenges. Given the myriad of conditions that can mimic ADHD, it is imperative in all cases to take a detailed history of symptoms, hopefully augmented by collateral reports. In assessing patients' recall of their own childhood symptoms, providers must consider the normal high rates of recall bias. In one cohort study, patients above 40 years of age often falsely recalled having impairing ADHD symptoms before the age of 7, conflicting with records of parent- and self-report symptoms from childhood.[16] False negative and false positive self-reported symptoms were also fairly common in the New Zealand cohort study[18] mentioned above, substantiating a poor validity of retrospective recall of childhood symptoms. When possible, clinicians should obtain school records, report cards, and childhood neuropsychological testing results. Clinicians should also obtain a history of any other concrete measures of academic hardships, such as any need to have repeated a grade or necessity of special accommodations in school.

Symptoms of ADHD and related executive dysfunction have a wide range of clinical phenomenology. Inattention symptoms may manifest as difficulty focusing for an extended period or feeling easily distracted. Inattention may also present more covertly, with an experience of having memory problems or feeling that one's mind is "scattered." Memory complaints can be variable, and further inquiry often reveals an attention-driven memory disorder: difficulty focusing on presented information prevents its successful registration, and leads to poor, subsequent consolidation of the material into memory stores. The *DSM-5* categorizes ADHD into presentations that include predominantly inattentive, predominantly hyperactive/impulsive, or combined type. It describes inattention as difficulty remaining on task, a lack of persistence, or disorganization.[4] One consequence of inattention that patients report is a failure to pay attention to details that leads to careless mistakes at work and home. Hyperactivity is defined as "inappropriately increased motor activity" and impulsivity is referred to as engaging in hasty actions without forethought that potentially leads to adverse consequences. See Table 16-2 for other common clinical manifestations of inattention, hyperactivity, and impulsivity.[4] ADHD symptom rating scales typically have a high sensitivity but low specificity. They should be used mostly as screening measures, rather than as tools sufficient for a diagnosis.[14] For example, the commonly used Conners Adult ADHD Rating Scale has been shown to be invalid in assessing ADHD in the setting of active anxiety symptoms.[48]

In recent years an increasing number of patients in the United States have presented to providers with symptoms of inattention, and there has been a notable increase in stimulant medication prescriptions.[49] It is unclear if this trend is driven by an increased recognition by clinicians of symptoms associated with ADHD, by individuals' desire to seek cognitive enhancement to overcome social, educational, or occupational challenges, or a combination of these factors. Clinicians should be aware that some individuals do seek medical attention for the primary purpose of obtaining stimulant medications, without any desire to engage in dialogue about the comprehensive treatment of their symptoms.[50] These patients are also generally more resistant to a thorough neuropsychiatric/medical evaluation. Incentives to seek stimulant medication may include the desire to enhance academic or occupational performance, lose weight, have increased energy, decrease psychological distress, or experience stimulants' euphoric properties. Additional benefits of an ADHD diagnosis may come in the form of academic accommodations, such as extra time given on tests. ADHD symptoms can be feigned in malingering patients, especially in health systems that rely heavily on symptom checklists for diagnosis and treatment.[50] Internet forums provide detailed descriptions on how to talk about ADHD "symptoms" with providers to most effectively obtain a stimulant prescription. Both patients with ADHD and those without may misuse stimulants, highlighting the need to carefully monitor all high-risk individuals.[51] In one sample of college students at a large public university in the United States, over 60% of those prescribed a stimulant for ADHD reported having diverted their medication at least once. Patients with a history of childhood conduct disorder or illicit drug use in the past year were more likely than others to divert these controlled substances.[52]

Differential Diagnosis

As introduced above, a variety of psychiatric and medical diagnoses may also present with inattention, impulsivity, and hyperactivity. The differential diagnosis for symptoms of executive dysfunction itself is also vast. Primary psychiatric conditions, ranging from major depression to substance use disorders, have been demonstrated to be associated with cognitive dysfunction, and largely in the domains of attention and executive functioning. Inattention, for example, is one possible criterion in the *DSM-5* diagnosis of major depressive disorder and generalized anxiety disorder (GAD).[4] This is unsurprising, as the ruminative or perseverative thoughts common in these disorders detract from overall attentional resources and disrupt cognitive flexibility. Ninety percent of patients presenting to behavioral health clinics and 88% presenting to primary care clinics with depressive symptoms report difficulty with concentration[53] and up to one-half of depressed patients are thought to have continued cognitive deficits after remission.[54] Patients with bipolar disorder have shown deficits in sustained attention, planning, flexibility, and response inhibition.[55] Patients with borderline personality disorder can display impulsivity, which often leads to problems in planning and problem solving.[55] Heavy cannabis users perform consistently worse than their age-matched peers on the executive function, attention, and memory components of neuropsychological tests.[56] Mood and substance use disorders, which are commonly comorbid with ADHD, can cause similar frontal network impairment, making it difficult to dissociate ADHD from these and other conditions. Obtaining a detailed history, with a precise chronology of symptom onset and development, is paramount.

TABLE 16-2 • Symptoms/Clinical Examples of Inattention and Hyperactivity/Impulsivity.

Inattention Symptoms	Examples/Notes
Often fails to pay close attention to details or makes careless mistakes in schoolwork, at work, or during other activities	Overlooks or misses details, work is inaccurate
Often has difficulty sustaining attention during tasks or play activities	Has difficulty remaining focused during lectures, conversations, or length reading
Often does not seem to listen when spoken to directly	Mind seems elsewhere, even in the absence of obvious distraction
Often does not follow through on instructions and fails to finish schoolwork, chores, or duties in the workplace	Starts tasks but quickly loses focus and is easily sidetracked
Often has difficulty organizing tasks and activities	Difficulty managing sequential tasks; difficulty keeping materials and belongings in order; messy, disorganized work; has poor time management; fails to meet deadlines
Often avoids, dislikes, or is reluctant to engage in tasks that require sustained mental effort	Schoolwork or homework, preparing reports, completing forms, reviewing lengthy papers
Often loses things necessary for tasks or activities	May lose school materials, pencils, books, tools, wallets, keys, paperwork, eyeglasses, mobile phones
Is often easily distracted by extraneous stimuli	May include task irrelevant thoughts
Often forgetful in daily activities	Forgetful of doing chores, running errands, returning calls, paying bills, keeping appointments
Hyperactivity/Impulsivity symptoms	**Examples/Notes**
Often fidgets with or taps hands or feet or squirms in seat	Frequently bounces leg while sitting at desk
Often leaves seat in situations when remaining seated is expected	Leaves his or her place in the classroom, in the office or other workplace, or in other situations that require remaining in place
Often runs about or climbs in situations where it is inappropriate	In adults may be limited to feeling restless
Often unable to play or engage in leisure activities quietly	Feels the need to speak during a normally quiet activity, such as watching a movie.
Is often "on the go" acting as if "driven by a motor"	Is unable to be or uncomfortable being still for extended time, as in restaurants, meetings; may be experienced by others as being restless or difficult to keep up with
Often talks excessively	Others may find it exhausting to speak with the patient due to excessive talking.
Often blurts out an answer before a question has been completed	Completes other people's sentences; cannot wait in turn in conversation
Often has difficulty waiting his or her turn	Extremely impatient waiting in line
Often interrupts or intrudes on others	Butts into conversations, games, or activities; may start using other people's things without asking or receiving permission; may intrude into or take over what others are doing.

Based on DSM-5 criteria. American Psychiatric Association. Diagnostic and Statistical Manual of Mental Disorders. 5th ed. Washington, DC: American Psychiatric Association; 2013. Available at https://psychiatryon-line.org/doi/book/10.1176/appi.books.9780890425596. Accessed December 24, 2018.

In addition to mood and substance disorders, other potential sources of cognitive dysfunction that may present with impaired attention include psychotic disorders, brain injuries, other neurologic conditions, personality disorders, intellectual disability, and learning disorders (see Table 16-3). Obsessive-compulsive disorder (OCD) and tic disorders have long been associated with ADHD, however this comorbidity may be more associated within the pediatric population than in adult patients.[57] Additional culprits that can compromise attention include medications with sedating properties, such as benzodiazepines, or those with anticholinergic effects, like first-generation antihistamines or tricyclic antidepressants. A sedentary lifestyle, poor sleep routine, unhealthy diet, limited physical exercise, or non-substance addictions, like pornography or gambling, may also present with symptoms that mimic ADHD. Patients with chronic hypertension and thus often its common sequelae cerebrovascular disease, have been shown to have more attention deficits on neuropsychological evaluation than age-matched healthy controls.[58]

There is ongoing debate about whether adolescent- and adult-onset ADHD are valid disease entities.[14,59] ADHD was originally described as a neurodevelopmental disorder and consensus, generally, keeps it confined to that category. Adults presenting with new-onset ADHD symptoms are often suspected as having had ADHD from childhood but were never diagnosed. Interestingly, there is evidence that most of these patients rarely had childhood-onset symptoms.[18] Symptoms of inattention or impulsivity are present in many adolescents and adults but

TABLE 16-3 • Differential Diagnosis of ADHD.

Etiology of Inattention	Other Supporting Symptoms of This Etiology
Anxiety (GAD, social anxiety, OCD, OCPD, avoidant traits)	Frequent worries or perseveration; patterns of avoidance or procrastinating due to fear about work, failing to meet others' expectations, or other catastrophic misappraisal
Depression (MDD, PDD, dysphoria secondary to personality traits)	Depressed mood, melancholia, anhedonia, overly self-critical, feelings of worthlessness or hopelessness, or suicidality
Substance use	Heavy alcohol use, marijuana use > twice per week, use of illicit substances, positive urine toxicology
Chronic psychotic disorders (i.e., schizophrenia)	Poor reality testing, negative symptoms (blunted affect, amotivation, loss of social interest, apathy, poverty of speech and thought)
Personality disorder	Poor impulse control, emotional dysregulation, pattern of limited relationships
Sleep disorder (i.e., OSA, RLS, PLMD, narcolepsy)	Daytime fatigue, chronic insomnia, snoring, repetitive movements in sleep
Nonsubstance addictions	Difficulty with self-control and cravings of gambling, pornography, internet gaming, etc., despite negative consequences
Intellectual disability	Global impairment, including difficulties in reasoning, problem-solving, abstract thinking, and practical understanding
Learning disorder (dyslexia, specific learning disorder)	Difficulty is primarily in one domain (reading versus mathematics)
Unhealthy lifestyle	Poor diet, lack of exercise, poor sleep hygiene
Other neurologic disorder (TBI, CVD, neuroinflammatory condition)	History of moderate-to-severe head injury, neuroimaging consistent with brain pathology, focal findings on neurologic examination
Neurodegenerative disease	Progressive decline in cognitive functioning
Medication side effect	Known side effect that is temporally correlated with medication usage
Toxic-metabolic encephalopathy	Generally waxing and waning, may include disorientation, confusion, and be associated with significant medical illness
Tourette syndrome	May also include developmental pathology with attention, hyperactivity, or impulsivity. Stimulants may unmask tics

CVD, cerebrovascular disease; GAD, generalized anxiety disorder; MDD, major depressive disorder; OCD, obsessive-compulsive disorder; OCPD, obsessive-compulsive personality disorder; OSA, obstructive sleep apnea; PDD, persistent depressive disorder; PLMD, periodic limb movement disorder; RLS, restless leg syndrome; TBI, traumatic brain injury.

are either not severe enough to cause functional impairment, or, are better explained by the cognitive consequence of other disorders.

Though we do not review the differential diagnosis of ADHD symptoms in children here, it is important to be aware of potential, confounding conditions in this population, including oppositional defiant disorder, intermittent explosive disorder, reactive attachment disorder, disruptive mood dysregulation disorder, impaired hearing or vision.[4]

Assessment

As the diagnosis of ADHD is largely made by clinical interview, providers rely heavily on endorsed symptoms. Self-endorsement, sometimes problematically, depends on patients' perception of symptom severity. Self-report symptom measures may be amplified in the setting of low self-esteem, comparing one's performance to that of one's peers, and different expectations (patients, others) about what degree of inattention is acceptable. Repeated interviews in different contexts and at separated time points, along with use of informants, can help

add to the veracity and validity of symptoms. Conflict can arise when a patient of average cognitive capabilities desires to have a higher performance than may be attainable, or if anxiety over professional or academic success leads to reduced performance.[47] In other cases, when inattention is reported in the setting of low work productivity, physicians must pay careful attention to the patient's expectation of his or her performance. Extremely taxing environmental demands (e.g., high-performance expectations at work or significant responsibilities at work or home) may overwhelm one's attentional resources.[60] Some patients who present with challenges at a new job or academic program may discover that the new situation simply demands a higher degree of concentration and executive function than they can provide.

According to the *DSM-5*, a diagnosis of ADHD requires that symptoms must not be a by-product of other intentional behaviors, such as defiance, hostility, or opposition. To meet the criteria for diagnosis of the inattention or hyperactive presentation, an adult must have five of the various possible symptoms (see Table 16-2), or five symptoms from each clinical subtype, for the combined presentation. Given the neurodevelopmental origin

A 20-year-old college student without significant medical history presents for evaluation of ADHD. He has been feeling overwhelmed in his studies and has been having difficulty focusing in class. He reports becoming easily distracted when studying and often begins browsing the Internet on his phone. He remembers that he had some difficulties in elementary school with hyperactivity, fidgeting, and being a "class clown," although he progressed through high school with average grades. Transition to his college has been difficult and he has had trouble balancing his academic responsibilities with a rigorous sports training schedule and membership in a fraternity. He takes no prescription medication, though he has tried dextroamphetamine/amphetamine from a friend and found it tremendously helpful when studying for final exams. His substance history is pertinent for smoking marijuana several times per week "to relax" and otherwise drinking 4–8 beers on the weekend. On examination, his speech is loquacious, his thought pattern is somewhat circumstantial, and his affect is euthymic. He describes his mood as "okay." He asks about pharmacologic treatments for his attention.

The case described is a common presentation for symptoms of inattention and distractibility in young adults. The treating clinician must first try to differentiate between neurodevelopmental ADHD and attentional difficulties

secondary to other etiologies. This patient's history is a little ambiguous and obtaining further collateral information from his parents and school records is necessary. His substance use should be further explored and may reveal helpful avenues of treatment. His substance use may be a form of self-treatment for anxiety symptoms or may simply be for recreational purposes. In either case, he should be encouraged to reduce his marijuana and alcohol use as they certainly may be contributing to his being inattentive and easily distracted. Finally, his overall attentional capacity may be extended past its limit as he attempts to juggle the demands of multiple, time-intensive commitments. He might benefit from organizational and behavioral strategies to better manage his time and could be referred to a therapist who specializes in symptoms of inattention. The potential use of a stimulant as part of his treatment plan is complicated. Although he reported symptom improvement from stimulants, he used a medication not prescribed to him, which is a risk factor for his own misuse. He also has current substance use and his inattentive symptoms may be due to a number of factors, including mild ADHD. It would be advised to hold off on a stimulant prescription for now until further information is obtained and his adherence to other recommendations and interventions are observed over time.

of ADHD, several symptoms of attention or hyperactivity are required to be present prior to the age of 12.[4]

While assessing symptoms, it is equally important to explore their consequences. Reviewing the patients' daily activities, both on weekends and weekdays, can be helpful in elucidating the specific circumstances during which the disturbances are most prevalent. Discussing the patient's relationships amongst peers and romantic partners also provides information regarding the extent of functional impairment. Reviewing recent work performance evaluations or employer feedback can help clinicians gauge symptom impact in the occupational realm and has the added benefit of obtaining information without patients' potential biases.[61]

Attempts have been made to develop or validate more quantitative assessments for ADHD, such as the Conners' continuous performance task (CPT).[38] However, these tools have only poor-to-fair predictive power. The Conners CPT and similar instruments lack the specificity required to capture the broad heterogeneity of cognitive phenotypes that converge on the ADHD diagnosis.[62] A comprehensive neuropsychological evaluation is more likely to capture that heterogeneity, even if it may lack ecological validity, as individuals may perform differently in the controlled testing setting than in everyday circumstances. Even with this limitation, and with other barriers of cost and access to specialists in some regions, we suggest neuropsychological evaluation, when possible, as it can add significantly to ADHD evaluations and treatment planning, as well as assist with identifying comorbid learning disabilities that also may need to be addressed.

TREATMENT AND MANAGEMENT

Introduction

The treatment of adults with ADHD and attention/executive function dysfunction must be adaptable and individualized, centered on improving symptoms and daily functioning. Treatment of ADHD may include pharmacologic and non-pharmacologic interventions, with geographic variation in the sequence of treatments. In the United States, for example, the initial treatment modality is usually pharmacologic, whereas medication is often reserved for more severe cases in European countries.[2] There is a strong evidence-base for the use of psychostimulants over nonstimulants as the first line of pharmacologic treatment for ADHD in adults,[2] with support for adjunctive cognitive and behavioral strategies to improve attention and executive functioning.[63,64] As the source of cognitive dysfunction in patients with inattention often arises from various concurrent conditions, providers must have a flexible and multidimensional approach, and consider a range of treatment strategies. For example, in the setting of ADHD symptoms with concurrent psychiatric illness or substance use, it may be difficult to determine to what extent the different disorders are contributing to symptoms like concentration difficulty or decreased motivation. We recommend that physicians take a deliberate and step-wise approach in treating patients. Generally, providers should first try to target existing psychopathology, like mood disorders or anxiety, to allow for a reassessment of remaining ADHD symptoms as psychiatric symptoms improve. A step-wise treatment approach also allows for careful observation and responsive diagnostic adjustment between interventions. It can also help to disentangle symptoms and conditions from one another and shed light on any negative cycles of symptom exacerbation that occur between concurrent conditions. For example, untreated or undertreated GAD can lead to poorer concentration ability, which then worsens baseline concentration difficulties due to ADHD, which often causes worsening anxiety about one's current functioning abilities.

Addressing the contribution of depression and anxiety to attention/executive function disorders as the first step also helps to minimize associations that patients may draw between their inattention or low productivity and sense of self-worth. It is common for complaints of inattention in the depressed patient to be coupled with self-critical feelings of low self-esteem and self-worth. Patients often feel they are not "doing enough" or "being enough" to meet their own or others' expectations. If the provider's first step is to treat attention/dysexecutive symptoms with stimulants, they risk reinforcing this feeling of low self-worth by "confirming" to patients that they need better productivity to feel better. If productivity and daily functioning improve with stimulants, then a framework is established in which the patient's own accomplishments or achievements are the currency for their earning the approval and appreciation of others. Conversely, if initial treatment involves exploration to understand why they are presenting with symptoms at this point in their life and why they might feel inferior to others, then patients are more likely to achieve a healthier mindset of self-acceptance and be able to accept their limitations. Furthermore, if patients were previously functioning well, but a recent change in their work, home, or social circumstance led them to medical attention, it is beneficial for initial therapy to focus on the more recent factor causing distress. Stimulants can always be considered in a thoughtful manner for these patients, but should, ideally, be coupled with early therapy and supportive cognitive and behavioral strategies.

It is important to keep in mind that all treatments should have specific goals and there should be a plan to track potential improvement. Examples of goals include the improvement of self-reported or informant-reported symptoms, or obtaining or sustaining employment, where relevant. The alleviation of symptoms enough to improve interpersonal relationships or the ability to perform well at work can also be a critical motivator for treatment adherence. It is especially important when using cognitively enhancing medications to focus on meeting previously agreed-on goals. Patients may have positive experiences or euphoria, for example, with certain medications, and be unable to distinguish these benefits from objective improvement in cognitive or behavioral functioning.

There have been several studies on the effect of ADHD on driving, though these must be interpreted with caution. For example, some research has shown that patients with ADHD are almost four times more likely than their age-matched peers to be involved in a motor vehicle accident.[65] Importantly, the relative risk of an accident for those with ADHD decreased to

1.23, after controlling for comorbid conditions such as substance use disorder or comorbid psychiatric disorder (such as conduct disorder and oppositional defiance disorder), suggesting a significant contribution of these disorders to driving hazards.[66] The risk of a motor vehicle accident with ADHD may be equivalent to the risk with having cardiovascular disease, but lower than the risk for patients with diabetes.

Behavioral and Nonpharmacologic

In patients with ADHD and executive dysfunction, providers should be aware and encourage optimal management of any concurrent, conditions involving other systems, such as hypertension, chronic obstructive pulmonary disease, and diabetes mellitus. Untreated or undertreated systemic disease can lead to frontal-executive dysfunction and an exacerbation of ADHD symptoms. Current medication regimens should be reviewed and monitored for possible negative iatrogenic effects. Benefits of medications need to be weighed against possible neuropsychiatric side effects, including those with anticholinergic (i.e., tricyclic antidepressants),[67] sedative (i.e., benzodiazepines), or extrapyramidal/Parkinsonian (i.e., antipsychotics) properties.[68]

In addition to treating concurrent psychiatric disorders and other medical conditions, nonpharmacologic strategies and lifestyle modifications are essential in treating ADHD and executive function disorders. These can be divided into at least three categories: (a) cognitive/behavioral strategies to promote better organization and planning, (b) cognitive/behavioral strategies to decrease distractors and enhance focus, and (c) brain healthy lifestyle modifications. A meta-analysis of cognitive behavioral therapy demonstrated moderate to large effect size for the treatment of adult ADHD symptoms.[64] The *Psychosocial Interventions in Neuropsychiatry*, chapter 10 in this textbook also addresses this topic. Encouraging use of external aids to improve executive function, such as a day planner to reference regularly, alarms and notifications, and checklists are some initial steps. Organizing one's many tasks into a matrix based on urgency and importance is a helpful way to prioritize responsibilities and decrease the sense of being overwhelmed. Prioritizing tasks has the added benefit of bringing clarity to potential task-avoidance behaviors that can cause significant anxiety. It is helpful to observe for patterns of anxiety, avoidance, or poor self-esteem that emerge around task completion and daily functioning. These patterns may signal important, additional contributions to inattention and require other treatment strategies, like more psychodynamically inclined therapy.

Neuropsychiatric education about and exploration into an individual's personal attention span and executive function abilities may help patients plan more realistically and set appropriate goals. For example, patients might be attempting to work or study for long periods without breaks, which is not realistic for them and out of sync with their mental capacity. Understanding one's optimal time span for working effectively before requiring a break can improve productivity and enhance a sense of accomplishment. Even though working for short "bursts," with more frequent, time-limited breaks in between may seem counterintuitive to some, it can prove an incredibly helpful strategy for some patients. Working or studying in an environment with minimal distractors, noise cancelling headphones, or limiting e-notifications of Internet access can also be useful.

The benefits of regular exercise, sleep hygiene, a healthy diet, and mind-body practices (like mindfulness, tai chi, and yoga) have evidence-basis in the management of ADHD symptoms.[69-72] An unhealthy lifestyle has also been associated with worsened ADHD symptoms.[73] As discussed above, improvement of mood often has a clear benefit to attention. The practice of mindfulness meditation has shown benefits for different aspects of attention, including orienting, conflict monitoring, and alerting.[74] In young adult men with ADHD symptoms, 20 minutes of moderate intensity exercise led to improvement in motivation for cognitive tasks, energy, mood, and feelings of confusion.[75] Patients with impulsivity have greater risk of addiction or compulsive use of social media or gaming, and so users should be mindful of the amount of time they spend on these platforms and implications to their responsibilities or relationships.[73]

Pharmacologic

A variety of psychopharmacologic approaches allow for tailoring the treatment of patients with attention and executive function disorders. Pharmacologic treatment for ADHD is dominated by psychostimulant medications, such as methylphenidate or the amphetamines. Some medications approved in the United States for use in other disorders have been investigated for ADHD have shown additional, pro-cognitive benefits, including the antidepressants bupropion and vortioxetine.[76,77]

Psychostimulant medications act broadly in the brain and can enhance multiple cognitive domains. Amphetamine salts have been studied in ADHD and largely improve measures of selective and sustained attention, with mixed results in working memory and cognitive flexibility. Methylphenidate has a similar profile, with some demonstrated improvement in response inhibition.[22] Side effects may include exacerbation of anxiety or irritability, difficulty falling asleep, poor appetite, and exacerbation of tics. Stimulant medications, which are listed as schedule II narcotics by the FDA, have addictive properties and patients may risk development of a stimulant use disorder.[78] In higher doses and in susceptible individuals, there is a risk of psychosis. Amphetamines may carry a higher risk of precipitating a psychotic episode compared to methylphenidate.[79] Patients with heart disease may be prone to cardiovascular events with psychostimulants, including sudden death, and should either be prescribed short, low-dose trials, with cardiology consultation, or not at all.[80,81] Blood pressure should be monitored in patients on stimulants and concomitant use of monoamine oxidase inhibitors (MAOIs) should be avoided.[29] Overall, both methylphenidate and amphetamines have shown good efficacy in the treatment of ADHD, even if patients might report better tolerance and fewer side effects with amphetamines.[82]

Alternatives to stimulants include the wakefulness-promoting medications modafinil and armodafinil (the enantiopure of modafinil), which are approved in the United States for daytime sleepiness related to narcolepsy, shift work sleep disorder, and as an adjunct for obstructive sleep apnea. A meta-analysis showed that modafinil was not more efficacious than placebo in the short-term treatment of children and adults with ADHD.[83] Side effects include anxiety, insomnia, headache, nausea, decreased appetite, and hypertension. In comparison to modafinil, armodafinil reaches peak serum concentration more slowly and thus may promote a stimulating effect for longer duration.[29]

Medications such as atomoxetine, vortioxetine, bupropion, or clonidine work as catecholamine "boosters" to target symptoms of inattention. They may be appropriate for patients who have difficulty tolerating side effects of stimulants or for patients where there is a concern for the use of potentially addictive medications. Atomoxetine, for example, selectively inhibits the reuptake of NE and is approved in the United States for the treatment of ADHD.[29] It has been shown to improve cognitive flexibility and sustained attention, though appears to have minimal effect on selective attention and has mixed results with response inhibition.[22] Possible side effects include hypertension, gastrointestinal symptoms, sexual dysfunction, urinary retention, cardiac problems, and increased suicidal ideation, and should be avoided in patients with narrow-angle glaucoma or those using MAOIs. Atomoxetine has less risk of sleep disruption than psychostimulants and thus may be an appropriate alternative for patients with baseline insomnia. Bupropion is approved in the United States for major depressive disorder, seasonal affective disorder, and smoking cessation, and thus may be a good choice for inattentive patients with concurrent depressive episodes or who want to quit smoking. Bupropion's exact mechanism of action is unclear, although it likely affects NE and DA neural systems.[29] Bupropion was shown to have improvement in sustained attention and working memory without a clear effect on response inhibition.[22] Due to a side effect of lowering seizure threshold, especially by the immediate-release formulation, bupropion should be carefully considered in patients with a history of seizure disorder.

Lastly, α2-adrenergic agonists, such as clonidine or guanfacine, may improve working memory, attentional focus, and disinhibition by targeting the abundant α2 receptors in the prefrontal cortex.[29] Guanfacine has been shown to improve cognitive flexibility, but can impair selective and sustained attention and has no effect on response inhibition.[22] These α2-adrenergic agonists may be a monotherapy for ADHD or used as an adjunctive treatment to psychostimulants. Guanfacine ER is approved in the United States for the treatment of ADHD in children aged 6–12, while clonidine is only approved for hypertension. Side effects are related largely to orthostatic hypotension, including dizziness, lightheadedness, or syncope (Table 16-4).[29]

The use of psychostimulants and other cognitive enhancers raises ethical concerns that warrant discussion. The threshold for meeting criteria of functional impairment in ADHD is ill-defined, with the *DSM* advising only that symptoms must "negatively impact directly on social and academic/occupational activities."[4] This uncertainty creates a dilemma between the treating of a disorder and the neuroenhancement of individuals who have minor impairments in their functioning.

All individuals operate along a spectrum of attentional capacity and one's abilities may be overwhelmed at certain times by demanding work or school environments. Providers must guard against the medicalization of normal human experiences, emotions, and reactions to limitations in neurotypical individuals,

TABLE 16-4 • Pharmacologic Interventions.[86]

Medication	Dose Range	Comments
Dextroamphetamine/ amphetamine IR	5–40 mg divided into BID dosing	First dose upon waking, next dose 4–6 hours after (3–6-hour duration of clinical action); greater risk for misuse or diversion than extended release (ER) formulations
Dextroamphetamine/ amphetamine XL	10–30 mg once daily morning dose	Up to 8-hour duration of clinical action, can avoid need for lunchtime dosing
Lisdexamfetamine	20–70 mg once daily morning dose	10–12-hour duration of clinical action; less abusable than other stimulants; also approved for adults with binge-eating disorder
Methylphenidate IR	10–60 mg divided into BID dosing	First dose upon waking; 2–4-hour duration of clinical action; greater risk for misuse or diversion than extended-release formulations
Methylphenidate CR	18–72 mg once daily morning dose	Trilayer tablet has up to 12-hour duration of action, can avoid need for lunchtime dosing
Atomoxetine	40–100 mg daily, once in morning or divided doses	Benefit may be seen as early as first day and may continue to improve over 8–12 weeks
Clonidine	0.1–0.4 mg in divided doses	Start with bedtime dosing, when dividing doses, keep larger dose at nighttime due to sedating side effect
Guanfacine	1–2 mg daily at bedtime	Initial 1 mg nightly, then increase to 2 mg after 1 month
Bupropion XL	150–450 mg once daily morning dose	Consider using in patients with depression and cognitive side effects
Vortioxetine	5–20 mg once daily dosing	Consider using in patients with depression and cognitive side effects

who have varying life demands. The consequences of medicalization (i.e., making a diagnosis of a neuropsychiatric condition like ADHD) must be carefully weighed against the potential benefit of pharmacologic or other interventions, especially in those with mild symptomatology. Some have argued that the pharmaceutical industry, and some members of the medical community, have pathologized ordinary human experience and life events as ADHD, contributing to the compromise of individual self-esteem and self-image in some patients.[84] Stimulant medications may also lead to an advantage in competitive educational or work environments, raising ethical questions about inequality in the distribution of these neuroenhancers.[84] ADHD treatment for some individuals may be addressing inappropriate or unrealistic demands from an employer, school, or family.

Stimulant misuse among college students, defined as using medication in the absence of a prescription or using more medication than prescribed, has been a growing problem. A recent random-effects meta-analysis estimated the prevalence of stimulant misuse in college students in the United States to be about 17%.[85] Factors associated with misuse included symptoms of ADHD, concurrent substance use, membership in a college fraternity/sorority organization, and academic problems.[85] A common reason cited for misuse was to enhance academic performance, and the most common source for diverted stimulant medication was from peers in the same college community. Prescribers of controlled medications should remind patients that the diversion of these drugs is a federal offense with serious legal consequences.[84-86]

Summary and Key Points

■ Inattention, hyperactivity, or impulsivity in adult patients may represent either persistent symptoms of the neurodevelopmental disorder ADHD, or, symptoms of one or more other conditions, such as a mood or substance use disorder.

■ The available evidence, including epidemiologic and observational studies, does not seem to support the diagnosis of adult-onset ADHD. If ADHD-like symptoms have a clear onset in adulthood, they likely reflect some non-ADHD executive dysfunction, and treatment should be tailored toward the responsible condition(s).

■ Frontoparietal circuits and cortico-striato-thalamic loops are involved in various aspects of attention, and disruption anywhere along these networks potentially results in impairments.

■ For ADHD, both psychopharmacologic interventions and psychotherapy may be useful. Treatment of other underlying conditions contributing to inattention should be prioritized, including treatment of affective and substance use disorders, optimization of sleep and lifestyle, and encouraging behavioral strategies aimed at improving organization and other executive skills.

Multiple Choice Questions

1. A 25-year-old woman with history of asthma presents with complaints of difficulty focusing on her graduate studies. She explains she has been worried that her work will be not be "up to standard," which often keeps her awake at night. She has historically done well in elementary, high school, and college, achieving A's and B's. She smokes marijuana recreationally about once per month. Contributing factors to sustained inattention may include:
   a. Female gender
   b. Poor sleep
   c. Marijuana use
   d. Undiagnosed ADHD
   e. History of asthma

2. Which of the following criteria are necessary to meet *DSM-5* diagnosis of ADHD?
   a. Onset of symptoms prior to age 12
   b. Anxiety associated with symptoms
   c. Neuropsychological testing
   d. Symptoms are isolated to one setting
   e. History symptom improvement in response to stimulants

3. A 40-year-old man presents to your office as recommended by his primary care physician for evaluation of inattention. He reports he was fired from his work 2 months ago for careless mistakes and has had difficulty regaining employment. He had difficulty concentrating for extended periods of time, and would frequently procrastinate in completing his tasks or become preoccupied with other activities. He drinks two alcoholic beverages per week. He states he did "okay" in school but was held back in the second grade. He denies current significant anxiety or depressive symptoms. What is the next step during your evaluation?
   a. Prescription of bupropion to target inattention and likely underlying depression
   b. Trial of methylphenidate to assess treatment response
   c. Extended evaluation to assess symptom burden across other settings with collateral informant contribution
   d. Refer to neuropsychological testing to evaluate for ADHD
   e. Brain MRI

4. What percentage of patients presenting to mental health clinics with symptoms of depression also report concentration difficulties?
   a. 10%
   b. 40%
   c. 70%
   d. 90%
   e. 100%

Multiple Choice Answers

1. **Answer: b**
   Of the options presented, the most likely contributor to this patient's inattention is her poor sleep. Her marijuana use is relatively infrequent and unlikely to be a strong contributor to her complaints. She has history of high academic success earlier in life, which makes it less likely that her cognitive symptoms are neurodevelopmental. Asthma is not correlated with inattention. Of note, there is a gender bias in the diagnosis of ADHD, in which boys/young men are more likely to be diagnosed than girls/young women. This bias is more pronounced in early childhood and then in adolescence.

2. **Answer: a**
   Explanation: ADHD is a neurodevelopmental disorder and requires the early onset of symptoms, before age 12. Symptoms must be present across two or more settings and must cause functional impairment. The diagnosis is made by history and clinical examination rather than by neuropsychological testing. A patient's report of past improvement with a stimulant does not solidify the diagnosis, and can reflect an improvement in ADHD symptoms, or use for academic or occupational performance enhancement, weight loss, euphoric sensation, or other reasons.

3. **Answer: c**
   Explanation: The patient's clinical history should be expanded before consideration of further testing or treatment. For example, a diagnosis of ADHD requires that symptoms should occur across multiple settings. In this case, it is unclear yet if his symptoms are isolated to just his previous job. There is often pressure to prescribe medications during the first evaluation of patients presenting with ADHD symptoms. It is most important for providers to determine an accurate diagnosis and this often takes more than one appointment. As clinical history is incomplete, and he does not report depressive symptoms at this time, prescribing an antidepressant right now would not be appropriate. Similarly, prescribing a stimulant medication is likely premature as well, as the evaluation is incomplete. Neuropsychological testing might be reserved for a subsequent encounter, and is certainly a lower priority than obtaining additional history and collateral observations. A brain MRI is not indicated at this time.

4. **Answer: d**
   Explanation: The overwhelming majority of patients with depression also report concentration difficulties. This may be in part be due to the tax on attention caused by negative ruminations, feelings of guilt, and perseveration. Even after remission of a depressive episode, up to half of patients continue to have concentration difficulties.

References

1. American Psychiatric Association, Task Force on Nomenclature and Statistics, Committee on Nomenclature and Statistics. *Diagnostic and Statistical Manual of Mental Disorders*. Washington, DC: American Psychiatric Association; 1980.

2. Faraone SV, Asherson P, Banaschewski T, et al. Attention-deficit/hyperactivity disorder. *Nat Rev Dis Primers*. 2015;1:15020.

3. Lange KW, Reichl S, Lange KM, Tucha L, Tucha O. The history of attention deficit hyperactivity disorder. *Atten Deficit Hyperact Disord*. 2010;2(4):241-255.

4. American Psychiatric Association. *Diagnostic and Statistical Manual of Mental Disorders*. 5th ed. Washington, DC: American Psychiatric Association; 2013. Available at https://psychiatryonline.org/doi/book/10.1176/appi.books.9780890425596. Accessed December 24, 2018.

5. Greven CU, Merwood A, van der Meer JMJ, Haworth CMA, Rommelse N, Buitelaar JK. The opposite end of the attention deficit hyperactivity disorder continuum: genetic and environmental aetiologies of extremely low ADHD traits. *J Child Psychol Psychiatry*. 2016;57(4):523-531.

6. Martin J, Hamshere ML, Stergiakouli E, O'Donovan MC, Thapar A. Genetic risk for attention-deficit/hyperactivity disorder contributes to neurodevelopmental traits in the general population. *Biol Psychiatry*. 2014;76(8):664-671.

7. Asherson P, Trzaskowski M. Attention-deficit/hyperactivity disorder is the extreme and impairing tail of a continuum. *J Am Acad Child Adolesc Psychiatry*. 2015;54(4):249-250.

8. Baddeley A. Fractionating the central executive. In: *Principles of Frontal Lobe Function*. Stuss DT, Knight RT, eds Oxford (Oxfordshire): Oxford University Press; 2002:246-260.

9. Simon V, Czobor P, Bálint S, Mészáros Á, Bitter I. Prevalence and correlates of adult attention-deficit hyperactivity disorder: meta-analysis. *Br J Psychiatry*. 2009;194(03):204-211.

10. Polanczyk G, de Lima MS, Horta BL, Biederman J, Rohde LA. The worldwide prevalence of ADHD: a systematic review and metaregression analysis. *Am J Psychiatry*. 2007;164(6):942-948.

11. Merten EC, Cwik JC, Margraf J, Schneider S. Overdiagnosis of mental disorders in children and adolescents (in developed countries). *Child Adolesc Psychiatry Ment Health*. 2017;11(1). Available at http://capmh.biomedcentral.com/articles/10.1186/s13034-016-0140-5. Accessed March 30, 2019.

12. Alvarado C, Modesto-Lowe V. Improving treatment in minority children with attention deficit/hyperactivity disorder. *Clin Pediatr (Phila)*. 2017;56(2):171-176.

13. Layton TJ, Barnett ML, Hicks TR, Jena AB. Attention deficit–hyperactivity disorder and month of school enrollment. *N Engl J Med*. 2018;379(22):2122-2130.

14. Sibley MH, Rohde LA, Swanson JM, Hechtman LT, Molina BSG, Mitchell JT, et al. Late-onset ADHD reconsidered with comprehensive repeated assessments between ages 10 and 25. *Am J Psychiatry*. 2018;175(2):140-149.

15. Wolraich ML, Lambert EW, Bickman L, Simmons T, Doffing MA, Worley KA. Assessing the impact of parent and teacher agreement on diagnosing attention-deficit hyperactivity disorder. *J Dev Behav Pediatr*. 2004;25(1):41-47.

16. Klein RG, Mannuzza S, Olazagasti MAR, Roizen E, Hutchison JA, Lashua EC, et al. Clinical and functional outcome of childhood attention-deficit/hyperactivity disorder 33 years later. *Arch Gen Psychiatry*. 2012;69(12):1295.

17. Faraone SV, Biederman J, Mick E. The age-dependent decline of attention deficit hyperactivity disorder: a meta-analysis of follow-up studies. *Psychol Med*. 2005;36(02):159.

18. Moffitt TE, Houts R, Asherson P, Belsky DW, Corcoran DL, Hammerle M, et al. Is adult ADHD a childhood-onset neurodevelopmental disorder? Evidence from a four-decade longitudinal cohort study. *Am J Psychiatry*. 2015;172(10):967-977.

19. Posner MI, Petersen SE. The attention system of the human brain. *Annu Rev Neurosci*. 1990;13:25-42.

20. Posner MI, Petersen SE. The attention system of the human brain. *Annu Rev Neurosci*. 1990;13(1):25-42.

21. Petersen SE, Posner MI. The attention system of the human brain: 20 years after. *Annu Rev Neurosci*. 2012;35:73-89.

22. Mueller A, Hong DS, Shepard S, Moore T. Linking ADHD to the neural circuitry of attention. *Trends Cogn Sci*. 2017;21(6):474-488.

23. Posner MI. Orienting of attention. *Q J Exp Psychol*. 1980;32(1):3-25.

24. Treisman A, Geffen G. Selective attention: perception or response? *Q J Exp Psychol*. 1967;19(1):1-17.

25. Vossel S, Geng JJ, Fink GR. Dorsal and ventral attention systems. *Neuroscientist*. 2014;20(2):150-159.

26. O'Reilly RC. The what and how of prefrontal cortical organization. *Trends Neurosci*. 2010;33(8):355-361.

27. Fox MD, Corbetta M, Snyder AZ, Vincent JL, Raichle ME. Spontaneous neuronal activity distinguishes human dorsal and ventral attention systems. *Proc Natl Acad Sci U S A*. 2006;103(26):10046-10051.

28. Sara SJ. The locus coeruleus and noradrenergic modulation of cognition. *Nat Rev Neurosci*. 2009;10(3):211-223.

29. Gale S, Daffner K. Behavioral and cognitive neurology. In: *Samuel's Manual of Neurologic Therapeutics*. 9th ed. Samuels MA, Ropper AH, eds. Philadelphia, PA: Wolters Kluwer Health; 2017:492-536.

30. Alexander GE. Parallel organization of functionally segregated circuits linking basal ganglia and cortex. *Annu Rev Neurosci*. 1986;9:357-381.

31. Gallo EF, Posner J. Moving towards causality in attention-deficit hyperactivity disorder: overview of neural and genetic mechanisms. *Lancet Psychiatry*. 2016;3(6):555-567.

32. Nakao T, Radua J, Rubia K, Mataix-Cols D. Gray matter volume abnormalities in ADHD: voxel-based meta-analysis exploring the effects of age and stimulant medication. *Am J Psychiatry*. 2011;10.

33. Shaw P, Eckstrand K, Sharp W, et al. Attention-deficit/hyperactivity disorder is characterized by a delay in cortical maturation. *Proc Natl Acad Sci U S A*. 2007;104(49):19649-19654.

34. Bruchhage MMK, Bucci M-P, Becker EBE. Cerebellar involvement in autism and ADHD. In: *Handbook of Clinical Neurology*. Elsevier; 2018:61-72. Available at https://linkinghub.elsevier.com/retrieve/pii/B9780444641892000044. Accessed June 17, 2019.

35. Hawi Z, Cummins TDR, Tong J, et al. The molecular genetic architecture of attention deficit hyperactivity disorder. *Mol Psychiatry*. 2015;20(3):289-297.

36. Brown T. *ADHD Comorbidities: Handbook for ADHD Complications in Children and Adults*. Washington, DC: American Psychiatric Press; 2009.

37. Ward F. The Wender Utah Rating Scale: an aid in the retrospective diagnosis of childhood attention deficit hyperactivity disorder. *Am J Psychiatry*. 1993;150(6):885-890.

38. Conners CK, Sitarenios G, Parker JDA, Epstein JN. The Revised Conners' Parent Rating Scale (CPRS-R): factor structure, reliability, and criterion validity. *J Abnorm Child Psychol*. 1998;26(4):257-268.

39. Rubia K. Cognitive neuroscience of attention deficit hyperactivity disorder (ADHD) and its clinical translation. *Front Hum Neurosci*. 2018;12. Available at http://journal.frontiersin.org/article/10.3389/fnhum.2018.00100/full. Accessed March 2, 2019.

40. Sonuga-Barke EJS. Causal models of attention-deficit/hyperactivity disorder: from common simple deficits to multiple developmental pathways. *Biol Psychiatry*. 2005;57(11):1231-1238.

41. Plichta MM, Scheres A. Ventral–striatal responsiveness during reward anticipation in ADHD and its relation to trait impulsivity in the healthy population: a meta-analytic review of the fMRI literature. *Neurosci Biobehav Rev*. 2014;38:125-134.

42. Dalley JW, Robbins TW. Fractionating impulsivity: neuropsychiatric implications. *Nat Rev Neurosci*. 2017;18(3):158-171.

43. Volkow ND, Wang G-J, Newcorn JH, et al. Motivation deficit in ADHD is associated with dysfunction of the dopamine reward pathway. *Mol Psychiatry*. 2011;16(11):1147-1154.

44. Luman M, Oosterlaan J, Sergeant J. The impact of reinforcement contingencies on AD/HD: a review and theoretical appraisal. *Clin Psychol Rev*. 2005;25(2):183-213.

45. McGough JJ. Treatment controversies in adult ADHD. *Am J Psychiatry*. 2016;173(10):960-966.

46. Bruchmüller K, Margraf J, Schneider S. Is ADHD diagnosed in accord with diagnostic criteria? Overdiagnosis and influence of client gender on diagnosis. *J Consult Clin Psychol*. 2012;80(1):128-138.

47. Rothstein A. Neuropsychological dysfunction and psychological conflict. *Psychoanal Q*. 1998;LXVII:218-239.

48. Grogan K, Gormley CI, Rooney B, et al. Differential diagnosis and comorbidity of ADHD and anxiety in adults. *Br J Clin Psychol*. 2018;57(1):99-115.

49. Olfson M, Blanco C, Wang S, Laje G, Correll CU. National trends in the mental health care of children, adolescents, and adults by office-based physicians. *JAMA Psychiatry*. 2014;71(1):81.

50. Sansone R, Sansone L. Faking attention deficit hyperactivity disorder. *Innov Clin Neurosci*. 2011;(8):10-13.

51. Wilens TE, Adler LA, Adams J, Sgambati S, Rotrosen J, Sawtelle R, et al. Misuse and diversion of stimulants prescribed for ADHD: a systematic review of the literature. *J Am Acad Child Adolesc Psychiatry*. 2008;47(1):21-31.

52. Garnier LM, Arria AM, Caldeira KM, Vincent KB, O'Grady KE, Wish ED. Sharing and selling of prescription medications in a college student sample. *J Clin Psychiatry*. 2010;71(03):262-269.

53. Gaynes BN, Rush AJ, Trivedi M, Wisniewski SR, Balasubramani GK, Spencer DC, et al. A direct comparison of presenting characteristics of depressed outpatients from primary vs. specialty care settings: preliminary findings from the STAR*D clinical trial. *Gen Hosp Psychiatry*. 2005;27(2):87-96.

54. Rock PL, Roiser JP, Riedel WJ, Blackwell AD. Cognitive impairment in depression: a systematic review and meta-analysis. *Psychol Med*. 2014;44(10):2029-2040.

55. Gvirts HZ, Braw Y, Harari H, Lozin M, Bloch Y, Fefer K, et al. Executive dysfunction in bipolar disorder and borderline personality disorder. *Eur Psychiatry*. 2015;30(8):959-964.

56. Volkow ND, Swanson JM, Evins AE, DeLisi LE, Meier MH, Gonzalez R, et al. Effects of cannabis use on human behavior, including cognition, motivation, and psychosis: a review. *JAMA Psychiatry*. 2016;73(3):292.

57. Abramovitch A, Dar R, Mittelman A, Wilhelm S. Comorbidity between attention deficit/hyperactivity disorder and obsessive-compulsive disorder across the lifespan: a systematic and critical review. *Harv Rev Psychiatry*. 2015;23(4):245-262.

58. Ostrosky-Solis F, Mendoza VU, Ardila A. Neuropsychological profile of patients with primary systemic hypertension. *Int J Neurosci*. 2001;110:159-172.

59. Surman CBH, Goodman DW. Is ADHD a valid diagnosis in older adults? *ADHD Atten Deficit Hyperact Disord*. 2017;9(3):161-168.

60. Agnew-Blais J, Arseneault L. Late-onset ADHD: case closed or open question? *Am J Psychiatry*. 2018;175(5):481-482.

61. Gallagher R, Blader J. The diagnosis and neuropsychological assessment of adult attention deficit/hyperactivity disorder. *Ann N Y Acad Sci*. 2001;931(1):148-171.

62. Maoz H, Aviram S, Nitzan U, Segev A, Bloch Y. Association between continuous performance and response inhibition tests in adults with ADHD. *J Atten Disord*. 2018;22(3):293-299.

63. Cherkasova MV, French LR, Syer CA, et al. Efficacy of cognitive behavioral therapy with and without medication for adults with ADHD: a randomized clinical trial. *J Atten Disord*. 2016;108705471667119.

64. Knouse LE, Teller J, Brooks MA. Meta-analysis of cognitive–behavioral treatments for adult ADHD. *J Consult Clin Psychol*. 2017;85(7):737-750.

65. Barkley RA, Guevremont DC, Anastopoulos AD, Dupaul GJ, Shelton TL. Driving-related risks and outcomes of attention deficit hyperactivity disorder in adolescents and young adults: a 3- to 5-year follow-up survey. *Pediatrics*. 1993;92(2):212-218.

66. Vaa T. ADHD and relative risk of accidents in road traffic: a meta-analysis. *Accid Anal Prev*. 2014;62:415-425.

67. Bishara D, Harwood D, Sauer J, Taylor DM. Anticholinergic effect on cognition (AEC) of drugs commonly used in older people: anticholinergic effect on cognition. *Int J Geriatr Psychiatry*. 2017;32(6):650-656.

68. McIntyre RS, Lee Y, Carmona NE, Subramaniapillai M, Cha DS, Lee J, et al. Characterizing, assessing, and treating cognitive dysfunction in major depressive disorder. *Harv Rev Psychiatry*. 2018;26(5):241-249.

69. Converse AK, Ahlers EO, Travers BG, Davidson RJ. Tai chi training reduces self-report of inattention in healthy young adults. *Front Hum Neurosci*. 2014;8. Available at http://journal.frontiersin.org/article/10.3389/fnhum.2014.00013/abstract. Accessed March 3, 2019.

70. Den Heijer AE, Groen Y, Tucha L, Fuermaier ABM, Koerts J, Lange KW, et al. Sweat it out? The effects of physical exercise on cognition and behavior in children and adults with ADHD: a systematic literature review. *J Neural Transm*. 2017;124(S1):3-26.

71. Yoon SYR, Jain U, Shapiro C. Sleep in attention-deficit/hyperactivity disorder in children and adults: past, present, and future. *Sleep Med Rev*. 2012;16(4):371-388.

72. Klil-Drori S, Hechtman L. Potential social and neurocognitive benefits of aerobic exercise as adjunct treatment for patients with ADHD. *J Atten Disord*. 2016;108705471665261.

73. Weissenberger S, Ptacek R, Klicperova-Baker M, Erman A, Schonova K, Raboch J, et al. ADHD, lifestyles and comorbidities: a call for an holistic perspective—from medical to societal intervening factors. *Front Psychol*. 2017;8. Available at http://journal.frontiersin.org/article/10.3389/fpsyg.2017.00454/full. Accessed January 22, 2019.

74. Tang Y-Y, Hölzel BK, Posner MI. The neuroscience of mindfulness meditation. *Nat Rev Neurosci*. 2015;16(4):213-225.

75. Fritz KM, O'Connor PJ. Acute exercise improves mood and motivation in young men with ADHD symptoms. *Med Sci Sports Exerc*. 2016;48(6):1153-1160.

76. Frampton JE. Vortioxetine: a review in cognitive dysfunction in depression. *Drugs*. 2016;76(17):1675-1682.

77. Verbeeck W, Bekkering GE, Van den Noortgate W, Kramers C. Bupropion for attention deficit hyperactivity disorder (ADHD) in adults. Cochrane Developmental, Psychosocial and Learning Problems Group, ed. *Cochrane Database Syst Rev*. 2017. Available at http://doi.wiley.com/10.1002/14651858.CD009504.pub2. Accessed March 3, 2019.

78. Compton WM, Han B, Blanco C, Johnson K, Jones CM. Prevalence and correlates of prescription stimulant use, misuse, use disorders, and motivations for misuse among adults in the United States. *Am J Psychiatry*. 2018;175(8):741-755.

79. Moran LV, Ongur D, Hsu J, Castro VM, Perlis RH, Schneeweiss S. Psychosis with methylphenidate or amphetamine in patients with ADHD. *N Engl J Med*. 2019;380(12):1128-1138.

80. Osser D, Awidi B. Treating adults with ADHD requires special considerations. *Psychiatr News*. 2018;53(22).

81. Cooper WO, Habel LA, Sox CM, et al. ADHD drugs and serious cardiovascular events in children and young adults. *N Engl J Med*. 2011;365(20):1896-1904.

82. Cortese S, Adamo N, Del Giovane C, et al. Comparative efficacy and tolerability of medications for attention-deficit hyperactivity disorder in children, adolescents, and adults: a systematic review and network meta-analysis. *Lancet Psychiatry*. 2018;5(9):727-738.

83. Arnold VK, Feifel D, Earl CQ, Yang R, Adler LA. A 9-week, randomized, double-blind, placebo-controlled, parallel-group, dose-finding study to evaluate the efficacy and safety of modafinil as treatment for adults with ADHD. *J Atten Disord*. 2014;18(2):133-144.

84. Graf WD, Nagel SK, Epstein LG, Miller G, Nass R, Larriviere D. Pediatric neuroenhancement: ethical, legal, social and neurodevelopmental implications. *Neurology*. 2013;80(13):1251-1260.

85. Benson K, Flory K, Humphreys KL, Lee SS. Misuse of stimulant medication among college students: a comprehensive review and meta-analysis. *Clin Child Fam Psychol Rev*. 2015;18(1):50-76.

86. Stahl S. *Stahl's Essential Psychopharmacology: Prescriber's Guide*. 5th ed. New York, NY: Cambridge University Press; 2014.

Neuropsychiatry of Autism Spectrum Disorder

17

Aaron J. Hauptman · James O. Robbins · Christopher J. McDougle

INTRODUCTION

Autism spectrum disorder (ASD) is a heterogeneous developmental neuropsychiatric condition characterized by two core symptom criteria: (1) deficits in social communication and social interaction; and (2) restricted patterns of repetitive behaviors and interests or activities.[1] Previously, ASD was not a formal diagnostic term. Autistic disorder was included under the broader category of pervasive developmental disorders (PDDs) with other neurodevelopmental conditions characterized by impaired social behavior and communication along with restricted interests and repetitive behavior. Those additional conditions included Asperger's disorder, Rett's disorder, child disintegrative disorder and PDD, not otherwise specified (NOS). In *DSM-5*, autistic disorder, Asperger's disorder, and PDD NOS have been subsumed under the category of ASD while Rett's disorder and childhood disintegrative disorder have been removed and are not considered to fall within the rubric of ASD. In *DSM-5*, if ASD symptoms are clinically present in the setting of a genetic condition such as Rett's disorder, the individual is diagnosed with ASD with the specifier, "associated with a known medical or genetic condition or environmental factor."

A vast range of comorbid neuropsychiatric and medical conditions are associated with ASD. Common comorbid psychiatric conditions include anxiety, attention-deficit hyperactivity disorder (ADHD), depression, tic disorders, oppositional defiant disorder, and intellectual disability (ID).[2,3] Common medical comorbidities include gastrointestinal (GI) disturbances, sleep disorders, epilepsy, mitochondrial dysfunction, and immune system abnormalities.[4]

EPIDEMIOLOGY

Prevalence estimates for ASD have increased steadily over recent decades. For example, a 78% estimated increase in the prevalence of ASD was documented between 2002 and 2008 by the Autism and Developmental Disabilities Monitoring Network of the U.S. Centers for Disease Control and Prevention, with a rate of 1 in 88.[5] A rate of 1 in 50 was reported a few years later based on results from a 2011–2012 telephone survey study.[6] Reasons for this increase in prevalence have not been fully explained. Many factors, including changing diagnostic criteria, better identification of cases of ASD, and possibly an increase in environmental contributions may be involved. In part, increased rates in recent studies are thought to be related to improvements in identifying ASD in underserved and nonwhite populations.[7]

The gender ratio in ASD is generally reported as a 4 to 1, male to female ratio.[8] Theories to explain the reasons for the reported sex difference differ. One theory is that of "the extreme male brain." This theory posits that ASD may be mediated by abnormal prenatal sex steroids resulting in characteristics at the very far end of the normal curve of what is considered a more typical male pattern of cognitive functioning, which includes features such as higher scores in systemization tasks and a relative lack of empathic expression.[9,10] An alternative theory is "the female protective effect" model which suggests resilience to genetic insults, such as copy number variants (CNVs) and single-nucleotide variants, whereby females are protected from more severe phenotypic presentations.[11] Finally, ascertainment bias may play a role, given certain phenotypic differences, such as relatively preserved functional social abilities in females with ASD in comparison with males.[12,13]

PATHOPHYSIOLOGY

Theoretical Constructs

The cognitive profile of ASD has been described by three theories that attempt to unify conceptual and research findings: (1) Theory of Mind deficits; (2) Weak Central Coherence; and (3) Frontal-Executive Dysfunction. Theory of Mind deficits of ASD were first posited by Baron-Cohen as an explanation for the social deficits in ASD. This theory suggests the core social impairment of ASD results from an inability to "mentalize" or "mind-read," namely imagine or understand the underlying thoughts, emotions, and cognitions of others.[19] The Weak

Central Coherence theory, first posited by Frith, suggests a neurologically mediated perception of, and focus on, the parts of phenomenal experiences at the expense of the whole. This theory describes a deficit in integration of piecemeal information into more cohesive sensory or conceptual processes.[20,21] Frontal-Executive Dysfunction theory hypothesizes that impairments in frontal/executive function leading to difficulties with impulse control, attentional ability, and behavioral inhibition result in core ASD features.[22,23] Each of these theories focuses on specific aspects of the core symptom domains of ASD. Additional research will undoubtedly result in integration and expansion of these ideas as more is learned about cognitive function in ASD.

Theories meant to unify and explain the constellation of social, cognitive, behavioral, and sensory symptoms that define ASD have moved away from single brain regions or neurotransmitter systems toward network-wide, functional differences. Increasingly, ASD is approached as a developmental disconnection syndrome.[24] This shift is well-justified in the setting of consistent findings of idiosyncratically organized networks such as the frequently replicated finding of within-region enhancement of functional connectivity with decreased between-region functional connectivity as assessed via neuroimaging, particularly within the default mode network (DMN).[25–28] The DMN is a brain network of functional cortical nodes including medial prefrontal cortex, posterior cingulate cortex, precuneus, and lateral parietal cortex.[29] This network is defined by the singular characteristic of being active during rest and deactivated during cognitive tasks such as those requiring executive function.[28,30] The DMN is also noted to be involved in Theory of Mind tasks, episodic memory, and tasks involving self-reflection.[31,32] Children with ASD have been reported to have a reduction in DMN network activity and idiosyncratic organization of the network; idiosyncrasy in other large-scale networks (e.g., sensory-motor network) have been reported to correlate with ASD symptomatology as measured by the Autism Diagnostic Observation Schedule (ADOS).[33]

Genetics

Rather than being a single, phenotypically, and etiologically unified condition, ASD is increasingly appreciated as a collection of both rarer and more common underlying genetic causes that converge on specific pathways crucial for neuronal and network development. Over a dozen twin studies have been conducted to date to evaluate the interaction of genes and environment in ASD. Findings have been inconsistent, with some demonstrating a greater impact of genetic effects and others identifying the primacy of environmental influences.[14–16] There are approximately 35 neurodevelopmental syndromes with known genetic causes associated with ASD, as well as over 800 genes that have been identified with non-syndromic ASD.[17,18] Well-characterized, neurodevelopmental syndromes associated with specific, proximate genetic etiologies make up the minority of cases, but were the first genes discovered to be associated with ASD.

Recent evidence suggests there are hundreds of candidate genes with associated variants that appear to predispose to ASD.[34–38] In response to these hypotheses, murine and nonhuman primate models have been developed to investigate the genetic underpinnings of ASD-like phenotypes and their associated pathophysiology. Among genetic variations studied, synaptic genes, like those of the SHANK family, responsible for the scaffolding of postsynaptic density, are well-represented.[39] Despite the accessibility of genetically modified animal models, such as SHANK gene knock-outs, the applicability of these models for representing ASD in humans is limited. Although ASD is considered a highly heritable condition with numerous associated genetic variants, it is estimated that only 10–20% of cases of ASD have a genetic etiology involving mutations, syndromes, and de novo CNVs.[40] While individual risk genes from rare variations are observed, it is thought that the accumulation of common gene variants plays a more consequential and representative role in the etiology of ASD.[38]

In addition to polygenic variation being more etiologically representative of ASD in humans, the heterozygous genotype for a monogene mutation-of-interest in animal models often fails to produce the intended ASD phenotype. In these cases, the phenotype may only be detected in the homozygous genotype, which is rarely observed in ASD in humans. This limitation underscores the importance of polygenic variation in the etiology of ASD and the discordance between human and rodent or nonhuman primate physiology.

Environmental Factors

In addition to genetic models, a gene-by-environment interaction has also been used to explore the pathophysiology of ASD. It is suspected that, in addition to genetic abnormalities, environmental factors may contribute to the neuropathology of ASD. A genetic manipulation combined with a pre- or postnatal environmental insult may therefore act synergistically to yield a model of ASD with greater etiological validity than a genetic or environmental insult alone.

There are a multitude of environmental factors that are thought to play a role in the pathogenesis of ASD. Implication of immune system dysfunction in ASD and its study in a research setting has led to public debate over the potential harm of vaccine-use in mothers and young children. However, a large body of epidemiological literature provides no evidence in support of an association between vaccinations and the risk of developing ASD.[41] Despite the lack of association between vaccinations and ASD to date, animal models have been developed to explore the role of early-life immune insults and immune system reactivity and the ASD-like phenotypes that result. The hypotheses underlying these efforts are informed by epidemiological and experimental evidence implicating the immune system in the pathophysiology of a number of neuropsychiatric conditions, including but not limited to ASD.[42–45] Examination of more than 10,000 cases in the Danish Medical Register revealed an increased risk for ASD in the offspring of mothers who experienced viral infection during the first trimester of pregnancy and bacterial infection during the second trimester of pregnancy.[46] Additionally, proinflammatory states have been observed in multiple organ systems in patients with ASD, their siblings, and their mothers. In particular, proinflammatory biomarkers such as cytokines, activated microglia, astrocytes, and immune-related gene expression changes have been found to be increased significantly in postmortem brain tissue and cerebrospinal fluid from patients with ASD compared to controls.[47–49]

Increased exposure to synthetic and naturally occurring environmental contaminants is also thought to contribute, perhaps in isolation or with polygenic interaction, to the increasing prevalence of ASD.[50] The effects of putative developmental neurotoxicants such as heavy metals, including lead and mercury, and organohalogens, like those found in pesticides and flame retardants, and plasticizers, which have well-documented endocrine-disrupting properties, are being scrutinized in behavioral animal models of ASD, as well as in murine embryonic and neural stem cells in vitro.[51,52] Overall, these animal model data suggest a need to extend the epidemiological study of genetic, environmental, and gene-environment interactive contributions to ASD. Though achieving the statistical power to observe a gene-environment effect is a formidable challenge, prospective studies following cohorts of up to 100,000 children are underway and those data will become available for research application in the coming years.[53] These many factors combine to provide a multi-hit model to describe the complex etiopathological factors that appear to contribute to overall ASD risk (see Figure 17-1).

Inflammation and Immunity

The expression of particular cytokines, including interleukin-6 (IL-6), IL-1B, and IL-8, has been found at high concentrations in peripheral tissues in individuals with ASD compared with controls.[54] GI dysfunction is a common comorbid condition associated with ASD, and may be reflective of this proinflammatory state.[55,56] Other common comorbidities, including seizures and sleep disorders, may also be related to an inflammatory process in subtypes of ASD. Familial autoimmune disease has been observed at significantly higher rates in families of children with ASD.[57] Furthermore, higher serum antibodies specific for fetal brain proteins have been identified in a subset of mothers of children with ASD, and brain-specific plasma autoantibodies have been found at higher rates in these children as well.[58–61]

Due to the epidemiological association between gestational infection and ASD, an emergent animal model, coined maternal immune activation (MIA), involves targeting the maternal immune system during pregnancy. Herein, pregnant females are exposed to agents that share structural or compositional features with known pathogens to elicit varying responses of the maternal immune system during sensitive developmental periods of gestation. Attempts to model this phenomenon are conducted under the premise that a subtype of ASD may be caused by changes in fetal neurodevelopment due to an adverse maternal immune response. Common behavioral findings observed in pups derived from MIA models parallel the core behavioral features of ASD, including social interaction and communication deficits, along with repetitive behaviors.[62]

Immunostimulants like polyinosinic:polycytidylic acid (Poly I:C) and lipopolysaccharide (LPS), which act primarily on

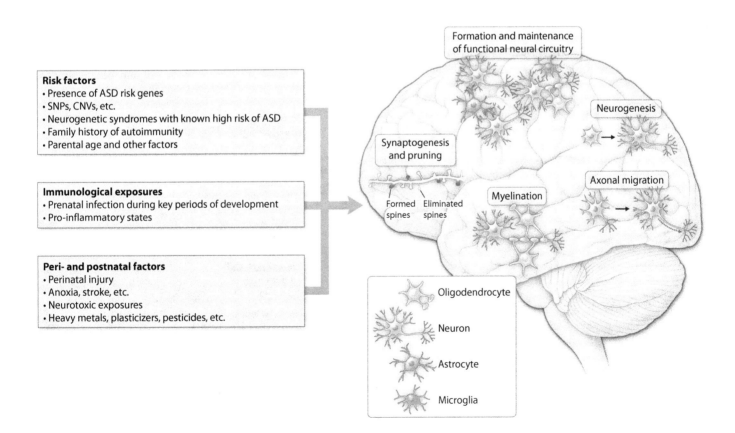

FIGURE 17-1. Multi-hit model of autism spectrum disorder.

Toll-like receptors 3 and 4, respectively, are commonly administered to pregnant females in MIA models to mimic pathogenic exposure and elicit a maternal cytokine response. Importantly, both immune agents induce a robust IL-6 response in pregnant female murine models, which has been found both responsible and critical for the ASD-like behavioral phenotype observed in the offspring.[63] In contrast, IL-10 has been deemed anti-inflammatory and protective against a gestational insult that stimulates IL-6 release.[64] However, IL-10 outside the context of MIA can itself induce behavioral changes in offspring, demonstrating the importance of balancing the contribution of proinflammatory and anti-inflammatory factors to promote healthy physiological function.[65]

Some MIA models have incorporated a "two-hit" approach wherein Poly I:C is administered to the mother during gestation and LPS is administered to the pups in the perinatal or early postnatal period.[62] "Three-hit" models have also been used, wherein a genetic manipulation is included to simulate a gene-environment interaction.[66] This approach is supported by evidence that some ASD risk-genes may not confer risk universally. That is, a particular gene variation may require a particular environmental factor to impart ASD risk.[67] This effect has been observed in animal models wherein monogenic manipulations have caused ASD-like behavior only with the addition of MIA.[68,69] Additionally, it has been observed in animal models that dysfunction of synaptic genes, which are implicated in ASD, can modulate sensitivity to environmental insults resulting in oxidative stress and hypoxia.[70,71]

Neuroanatomic Correlates

Given the complex, heterogeneous phenotypic presentation of ASD and its presumably widely variable underlying pathophysiology, it is not surprising that inconsistent findings have been reported in the neuroanatomy literature. That said, several structural and anatomical abnormalities have been consistently described in ASD, aspects of which have been utilized to explain behavioral observations (see Figure 17-2). These consist of abnormalities in overall brain volume over the course of development, microstructural anatomical abnormalities, gross neuroanatomical differences in key areas, including the prefrontal cortex, amygdala, and cerebellum, and functional connectivity findings between a number of key nodes and circuits.

Gross Anatomical Findings

Gross anatomical differences have been observed which vary in the individual over time. Enlarged brain volume is consistently found between the ages of 2 and 4 years, corresponding with increased head circumference.[72-74] A particularly consistent finding is prefrontal cortical overgrowth during early development.[75,76] The frontal lobes are involved in a vast range of functions, including higher-order neurocognitive processing, such as attention, working memory, executive function, social cognition, and others. By 5–6 years old, however, total brain volume is consistent with that of age-matched, neurotypical peers.[77] These changes are suspected to be the result of early childhood brain overgrowth with subsequent arrest in late childhood. Between this period and adulthood, overall brain volume declines, possibly as a result of decreases in cortical thickness.[78-80] Early white matter abnormalities, including increased area and thickness of the corpus callosum at 6 months, have been documented by diffusion tensor imaging in children who were eventually diagnosed with ASD compared with matched neurotypical peers.[81,82]

The cerebellum is involved in both motoric control, as well as a broad range of higher-order neurocognitive functions such as language, mood and affect regulation, and neurocognitive

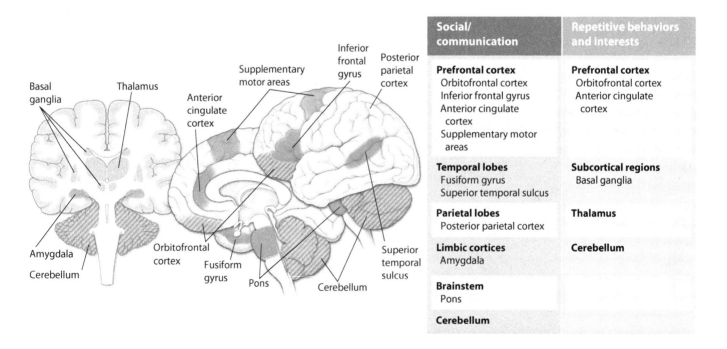

Social/communication	Repetitive behaviors and interests
Prefrontal cortex Orbitofrontal cortex Inferior frontal gyrus Anterior cingulate cortex Supplementary motor areas	**Prefrontal cortex** Orbitofrontal cortex Anterior cingulate cortex
Temporal lobes Fusiform gyrus Superior temporal sulcus	**Subcortical regions** Basal ganglia
Parietal lobes Posterior parietal cortex	**Thalamus**
Limbic cortices Amygdala	**Cerebellum**
Brainstem Pons	
Cerebellum	

FIGURE 17-2. Neuroanatomical regions implicated in autism spectrum disorder.

processing.[83] While specific neuroanatomical locations of volumetric loss are not consistent across all studies, a few findings have generally been reported. Purkinje cell hypocellularity and decreased volume of gray matter in the cerebellum have been consistently shown.[84-89] Cerebellar involvement has been hypothesized to explain aspects of sensory integration deficits, motor findings, and social pragmatic difficulties. Animal model data has been used to theorize that a range of deficits in ASD occur secondary to disrupted cerebro-cerebellar connections.[83,90-92] Correlations between specific cerebellar structural differences and patterns of behavior in ASD have been reported.[91] Additionally, the basal ganglia, a series of subcortical structures involved in motor, emotional, cognitive, habitual, and other behaviors, have also been implicated in ASD.

Morphological, neurochemical, and functional abnormalities have been described in subcortical nuclei of the basal ganglia, implicating cortico-striato-thalamo-cortical circuits.[93-95] It is speculated that basal ganglia-cerebellar connectivity findings may be mediated by abnormalities in mutual connectivity between these regions and the pons.[92]

The amygdala, a cluster of nuclei located bilaterally in the medial aspect of the temporal lobes, is linked to structures throughout the brain and is thought to play a role across a broad diversity of functions including social cognition, fear processing, and aggression, among others, and has been thought to be involved in psychiatric conditions ranging from post-traumatic stress disorder to personality disorders.[96] Atypical volumes of the amygdala have been described in ASD, albeit inconsistently, with larger volumes in early childhood that normalize over time. Amygdala abnormalities have been suggested to potentially explain the exaggerated fear conditioning and sensory reactivity seen in ASD. In addition, reports have described an association between amygdala overgrowth and the severity of clinical impairment in ASD.[97-99] In the valproic acid murine model of ASD, amygdala activation in response to a fear stimulus was double that of wild type animals and those animals demonstrated increased long-term potentiation involving the amygdala, suggestive of the possibility that amygdala hyperreactivity mediates an overgeneralized and longer-lasting fear response in individuals with ASD.[100]

Microstructure Changes

Apart from gross neuroanatomic and imaging abnormalities, microstructural changes at the level of the cortical microcolumn have been described. Studies on microstructural abnormalities in ASD are confounded by small sample sizes and methodological differences, particularly in terms of lack of genetic stratification.[76] Despite these factors, findings of focal neocortical disorganization, altered microcolumnar spacing, and abnormal cellular density have been reported.[101-104]

Functional Connectivity

Connectivity abnormalities have been described both within local microstructure, as well as between larger cortical and subcortical structures as the result of two hypothetical mechanisms: (1) imbalance between excitation and inhibition based on abnormal composition within regions; and (2) hyperconnectivity within specific regions and circuits.[76,105] Intriguingly, while

there are contradictions in the literature as to which regions experience functional enhancement and which connections are hypofunctional, it has been theorized that, perhaps, the most significant functional connectivity pattern that characterizes ASD is idiosyncratic variation of canonical functional circuitry.[106]

While abnormalities in local microcircuitry have been demonstrated, longer-range connectivity alterations have also been consistently identified. Several mechanisms have been posited to explain these abnormalities. One study identified CNVs associated with ASD and utilized gene ontology and ingenuity pathway analysis to explore common functions among the genes encoded by these regions. Many of the genes were found to have roles in axon pathfinding, among other functions.[107] Similarly, genes involved in brain patterning have been found to be down-regulated in ASD.[108] A broad range of studies have demonstrated functional and anatomic abnormalities connecting key regions in ASD, including connections between prefrontal cortex, thalamus, and cerebellum, as well as across regions involved in social processing such as the amygdala, temporo-parietal junction, and insular cortex.[109-112] Functional activity has been shown to be decreased across regions involved in language processing (temporal cortex), reward circuitry, and cognitive control (frontal-subcortical and frontal-parietal networks).[113-115]

Contextualizing Anatomical Data

Aspects of these neuroanatomic findings have been used to justify global theories of ASD, for example, arguing the "Weak Central Coherence" theory given certain findings suggestive of increased microcolumnar presence combined with enlarged prefrontal cortex.[103,116,117] This theory describes a deficit in the integration of piecemeal information into greater sensory or conceptual processes. As such, according to this interpretation of the data, excessive local connectivity with dysfunctional longer-range connectivity leads to a delay in long-range communication and transfer of information, resulting in deficits in signal-to-noise differentiation and causing large-scale circuit dysfunction.[118]

Neuroanatomically, while much of the existing data are mutually not mutually compatible, regions with known involvement can explain aspects of the reported symptomatology. For example, a frontal-subcortical connectivity disturbance within the frontal-striatal circuit may mediate repetitive and stereotypic behavior.[119] Functional lesions between key nodes required for social-emotional processing likely mediate components of the classic, core symptom deficits in social pragmatics and reciprocity.[79,89] Involvement of these brain regions does not explain the underlying disorder or the full constellation of symptoms, but does provide a neural correlate for aspects of the disorder that can be useful in conceptualizing the experience of individuals with ASD.

Associated Genetic and Neurodevelopmental Conditions

Genetic disorders with high rates of ASD, termed "syndromic autism" include Fragile X syndrome (FXS), Rett's disorder, neurocutaneous syndromes (tuberous sclerosis complex 1 and 2 [TSC 1/2] and neurofibromatosis 1 [NF1]), Prader-Willi and

Angelman syndromes, 22q11 deletion syndrome (also called velo-cardiofacial syndrome), Smith-Lemli-Opitz syndrome, Smith-Magenis syndrome, Phelan-McDermid syndrome, and others.[118]

Mendelian monogenetic syndromes associated with ASD make up the minority of cases; however, rates within these syndromes of comorbid ASD can be very high: FXS is associated with a 30% prevalence of ASD; 61% of individuals with TSC1/2 have ASD; and Rett's disorder, caused by mutations in Methyl CpG binding protein 2 (MECP2) includes autistic features as core aspects of the syndrome. Increasingly, specific CNVs are recognized for their association with ASD.[119,122] CNVs are regions of genetic duplication or deletion that occur over large expanses of genetic material and, thus, typically contain multiple genes. The result of the extensive number of genes involved contributes to uncertainty about which genes may be causally involved in the development of ASD.[123] Examples of CNVs associated with ASD include those causing Phelan-McDermid syndrome due to deletion of as many as 130 genes on Chr22q13, including certain deletions associated with ASD such as SHANK3/PROSAP2. SHANK3 is a synaptic scaffolding protein associated with language and social development impairments in ASD.[124] Other CNVs associated with ASD include deletion or duplication in chromosome regions 15q11-13 and 16p11.2 and microdeletion in 2q23.1 (see Table 17-1).[125–127]

TABLE 17-1 • Select Common Copy Number Variants (CNVs) Associated with Elevated Risk of ASD Features.

CNV	Syndrome Name	Physical Features	Neuropsychiatric Features	Core Medical Features
7q11.23[337,338]	Williams-Beuren duplication syndrome	Macrocephaly, brachycephaly, prominent forehead with deep-set eyes and straight eyebrows and high-arched palate, elfin-like facial features	Intellectual disability with visuospatial deficits and generally preserved language, anxiety spectrum disorders, attentional and behavioral problems, ASD-like features	Supravalvular aortic stenosis, hypercalcemia, hypertension
15q11-q13 (paternal)[339,340]	Prader-Willi syndrome	Characteristic body habitus with central adiposity and small limbs, thin upper lip with down-turned mouth, almond-shaped eyes	Intellectual disability, compulsive behaviors, excoriation disorder, explosive behaviors, psychosis, high rates of autistic features	Early failure to thrive followed by marked hyperphagia, decreased responsiveness to pain, self-injury
15q11-q13 (maternal)[341–343]	Angelman syndrome	Microcephaly, protruding tongue, prognathism, wide-spaced teeth, hypotonia, hyperreflexia, and characteristic gait	Motor and speech delays with greater preservation of receptive and nonverbal domains, sleep disturbance, repetitive behaviors, movement abnormalities, aggressive behaviors	Epilepsy, gastrointestinal issues, obesity, movement disorder, and ataxia
16p11.2	16p11.2 deletion syndrome	Low-set ears, webbed toes	Developmental delay, intellectual disability, high rates of ASD-like symptoms, deficits in expressive language with greater preservation of receptive language	Epilepsy
17p11.2[344]	Smith-Magenis syndrome	Square face with prominent jaw, deep-set eyes, upslanted palpebral fissures	High ASD risk and global developmental delay; behavioral problems, self-injury, sleep disturbance, and aggression	Short stature, reduced pain sensation, congenital abnormalities including heart defects and myopia
22q11.2[345,346]	Velocardiofacial syndrome/22q11 deletion syndrome	Upslanted palpebral fissures, small low-set ears, small mouth and nostrils	Increased risk for psychosis; multiple psychiatric comorbidities; lower IQ on average with nonverbal learning disorder (nonverbal learning disability)-like profile	Hypocalcemia, hypoparathyroidism, conotruncal heart defects, immune deficiencies, cleft lip and palate
22q13.3[197,347,345]	Phelan-McDermid syndrome	Dolichocephaly, ptosis, prominent ears, deep-set eyes, full brow	ASD features, global developmental delays, speech delay or absence, bipolar-like features, intellectual disability, increased risk of catatonia	Developmental regression, seizures, gastroesophageal reflux, cardiac and renal abnormalities

CLINICAL PRESENTATION, ASSESSMENT, AND DIFFERENTIAL DIAGNOSIS

In *DSM-5*, there are two core criteria necessary for a diagnosis of ASD: (1) deficits in social communication and interaction; and (2) restricted, repetitive patterns of behaviors, interests, or activities. In addition, symptoms must occur in early development, though they may only manifest later in life in the setting of certain stressors or may be masked by learned skills. Furthermore, to meet criteria for the diagnosis, symptoms must have meaningful clinical impact on current functioning and should not be the result of another underlying cause such as ID or social-pragmatic communication disorder. There are associated ASD specifiers as well, which include the presence or absence of intellectual impairment and of language impairment, the association with a known medical or genetic condition or environmental factors, the association with another neurodevelopmental or psychiatric disorder, and the presence of catatonia. Finally, the diagnosis includes three levels of severity: (1) requiring support; (2) requiring substantial support; and (3) requiring very substantial support.

There is currently no biomarker for the diagnosis of ASD; the disorder is diagnosed using criteria based on clinical presentation. Current instruments utilized for corroboration of diagnosis, primarily in research settings, include the Autism Diagnostic Interview-Revised (ADI-R) and the Autism Diagnostic Observation Schedule-Generic (ADOS-G).[128,129] The gold standard for diagnosis of ASD remains that of an experienced clinician. ASD is highly heterogeneous in its clinical presentation; some have reframed ASD as "the autisms" to emphasize the wide-ranging etiologies, pathophysiologies, and clinical presentations.[24]

Although not part of formal diagnostic criteria, behavioral symptoms are commonly associated with core features in individuals with ASD. In particular, individuals with ASD can struggle with irritability, aggression, and self-injurious behavior. This may interact with core symptoms, such as repetitive behaviors, for example in the setting of "stimming" behavior, which at times can be self-injurious. Behavioral difficulties can also be complicated by psychiatric and medical comorbidities which may contribute to or exacerbate behavioral symptoms. Challenges can occur during transition to adulthood, including loss of services, psychosocial and educational stressors, changes in levels of independence, environmental transitions, etc., which may further complicate the clinical and diagnostic picture. Such stressors may at times result in exacerbation of baseline behavioral symptoms.

Neuropsychiatric and Medical Comorbidities and Their Treatments

Comorbidities in ASD are the rule rather than the exception. Across the lifespan, a wide range of psychiatric disorders are commonly diagnosed in individuals with ASD, including mood and anxiety disorders, ADHD, and oppositional defiant disorder.[130] Obsessive-compulsive disorders and tic disorders, including Tourette syndrome and other conditions, are overrepresented in ASD.[131] These highly comorbid conditions can complicate diagnosis, treatment, and outcomes in ASD. Furthermore, behavioral changes in individuals with ASD may often occur in the setting of new-onset medical illness, such as constipation and other GI disorders, infection, and pain, among others. Onset of comorbid psychiatric conditions can also be the cause of subacute or abrupt behavioral changes and should be closely monitored for.

In addition to sequelae of core features of ASD, including associated increased risk for ID and specific neurocognitive profiles, a range of neuropsychiatric conditions are associated with ASD, as are many medical disorders which must be identified and closely monitored (see Table 17-2). Specific syndromes closely associated with ASD also carry their own unique risk factors. One example of this includes tremor ataxia syndrome which occurs in individuals with FMR1 mutation. Tremor ataxia syndrome is a neurodegenerative disorder seen in individuals with FXS, usually over the age of 50 years, and is characterized by neurocognitive decline and progressive movement abnormalities, including parkinsonism, gait ataxia, tremor, and neuropathy.[132] Other examples of elevated-risk psychiatric symptoms to be monitored for in specific genetic syndromes include severe self-injury in Lesch-Nyhan syndrome, and schizophrenia-like psychotic symptoms in velocardiofacial (22q11deletion) syndrome, which require additional specific monitoring and independent management.

Epidemiology of Psychiatric Illness in ASD

High rates of psychiatric comorbidity are present in ASD with prevalence estimates of 70% or more.[3,133] These estimates vary, with one study demonstrating comorbid social anxiety disorder in 29.2%, ADHD in 28.2%, and oppositional defiant disorder in 28.1% of patients.[3] In this study there were low comorbidity rates of major depressive disorder or dysthymia with ASD (0.9% and 0.5%, respectively), whereas other studies have demonstrated a significantly higher rate of depressive symptomatology (e.g., 49% demonstrating clinically significant depressive symptoms by PHQ-9 score).[134]

Anxiety and Mood Disorders

Rates of anxiety and depression are elevated in individuals with ASD. Epidemiological data range significantly, but pooled current prevalence in adults with ASD is estimated at 27% with lifetime prevalence of 42% for any anxiety disorder. Regarding

TABLE 17-2 • Common Neuropsychiatric and Medical Comorbidities in ASD.
Anxiety and mood disorders
Attention-deficit hyperactivity disorder
Obsessive-compulsive and related disorders
Tourette syndrome and tics
Psychotic disorders
Catatonia
Sleep disturbance
Gastrointestinal dysfunction
Epilepsy

depression, current prevalence is estimated at 23% with lifetime prevalence of 37% for depression in adults with ASD.[137] In the pediatric population, meta-analysis evaluation found 39.6% of youth with ASD have one or more comorbid anxiety disorders.[138] Heterogeneity in diagnoses, study quality, intellectual function, and other factors likely contribute to high levels of variance between studies providing epidemiological data.[137]

The presentation of anxiety and depressive disorders can be broad and may overlap with core ASD symptoms. For example, social withdrawal, ritualistic behaviors, and difficulty with novel situations, may be related to core ASD symptomatology rather than demonstrating a comorbid psychiatric diagnosis. Simultaneously, exacerbation of or change in core symptoms, such as ritualistic behaviors, obsessive interests or preoccupations, and stereotypies, may represent symptoms of a superimposed depressive episode. Notably, in individuals with communication deficits or ID, neurovegetative signs or changes in functional level, such as a decline in baseline ability to complete activities of daily living, may be the most evident signs of mood disorder.[139]

In addition to symptoms of depression, suicidality has also been reported in ASD.[135] One large-scale, health insurance-based, epidemiological study found that 3.9% of individuals with ASD attempted suicide after an average of 3.9 years following study enrollment in comparison with 0.7% of controls after an average of 6 years following study enrollment.[136] A lifetime occurrence of suicidal ideation of 72% and a history of suicide attempt in 7–47% of individuals with ASD, has been reported.[134] A lesser number of social supports, dissatisfaction with existing social supports, and higher loneliness measures were associated with a greater severity of depression and suicidal ideation while having more severe traits of ASD was associated with increased loneliness, less satisfaction with social support, and a greater severity of depression.[134]

Attention-Deficit Hyperactivity Disorder

The *DSM-IV-TR* did not allow for the codiagnosis of ADHD in patients with ASD, although *DSM-5* does. Whether they constitute separate disorders or are aspects of a common process remains to be determined. Despite this uncertainty, inattentive, hyperactive, and impulsive symptoms are common in ASD, particularly in children, with approximately 30% of individuals with ASD also meeting diagnostic criteria for ADHD.[3] As discussed above, alterations in cortical-cortical, cortical-subcortical, and long white matter tract connectivity all appear to be implicated in ASD. As a result, it is not surprising that executive dysfunction and attentional symptoms occur frequently. The primary pharmacological treatments utilized for idiopathic ADHD are psychostimulants, alpha-2 agonists, and atomoxetine (a selective norepinephrine reuptake inhibitor). Given the concerns of reduced appetite, sleep disturbance, increased irritability and agitation, and the induction or exacerbation of tics that can occur with psychostimulants, care must be taken when these medications are given to children with ASD. For example, although methylphenidate is a psychostimulant which is first line in management of idiopathic ADHD, it has been found to be less efficacious in pediatric subjects with ASD and more poorly tolerated in comparison with non-ASD

ADHD populations.[140-143] It is also notable that even greater vulnerability to side effects appears to be present in individuals with ASD that have more severe core symptomatology.[142,143] Alpha-2 agonists, including guanfacine and clonidine, may be beneficial, particularly for hyperactivity, impulsivity, and sleep disturbance and may be better tolerated than psychostimulants in patients with ASD that have comorbid tics.[144-147] Atomoxetine has shown preferential benefit for hyperactivity versus inattention in ASD as well.[148-152] There is also some evidence that the anti-glutamatergic antagonist amantadine hydrochloride may be helpful for ADHD associated with ASD, however, larger-scale studies have shown equivocal results at best.[153]

Obsessive-Compulsive and Related Disorders, Tourette Syndrome, and Tics

One of the core diagnostic criteria for ASD is the presence of repetitive and restricted behaviors.[1] A number of other conditions recognized in *DSM-5* can overlap with components of these behavioral symptoms. For example, *DSM-5* recognizes the new category of "obsessive-compulsive and related disorders" which includes conditions such as obsessive-compulsive disorder, trichotillomania, and excoriation disorder.[1] In addition, *DSM-5* defines three different tic disorders, including Tourette syndrome, persistent motor or vocal tic disorder, and provisional tic disorder.[1] As individuals with ASD can commonly experience repetitive behavioral symptoms such as repetitive ordering and touching, repeated questioning or stereotyped speech, repetitive motor stereotypies and self-injury, etc., as well as restricted interests that can appear obsessional, the potential overlap between aspects of these conditions and core ASD diagnostic criteria poses a diagnostic challenge. *DSM-5* does not disallow for comorbidity of ASD and OCD; however, it does emphasize that symptoms attributed to OCD, for example, should not be better explained by another disorder, such as repetitive patterns of behavior due to ASD.[1]

Many studies suggest significant symptom overlap and likely overrepresentation of comorbid OCD in individuals with ASD. While the rate of OCD in the general population is 1–3%, prevalence of OCD symptoms in ASD may be around 36%, with studies demonstrating a range of prevalence of OCD in ASD from 1.8% to 87%.[154-158] Overlap with core diagnostic criteria of ASD, most importantly restricted and repetitive behaviors, is a significant confounding factor as is a range of differing diagnostic criteria and patient populations. These differences become significant for many reasons, including differences in treatment. For example, classic treatment for OCD would include exposure and response prevention (ERP), where a range of behavioral and related techniques are generally utilized for management of repetitive behaviors in ASD.[159,160]

Studies have highlighted phenomenological differences between the symptoms seen in ASD versus those more typically seen in OCD. For example, repetitive ordering, hoarding, repeated questioning, tapping and touching, and self-injury are more characteristic of core repetitive behaviors in ASD, whereas OCD is better characterized by cleaning, checking, and counting behaviors.[161] Other studies demonstrate somewhat similar patterns of phenomenology in patients with ASD and a comorbid diagnosis of OCD compared to those with OCD alone. These include a decreased likelihood of checking, washing, and repetition compulsions and a greater degree of hoarding obsessions and compulsions, and repeating and ordering compulsions and less overall severity and fewer contamination and aggression obsessions.[162,163]

Tics and related disorders appear to be similarly overrepresented with ASD. As with OCD, the phenomenology of tic disorders significantly overlaps with apparent symptoms seen in ASD and must be carefully disentangled. By way of example, the rate of Tourette syndrome (characterized by two or more motor tics as well as one or more vocal tics that occur for at least a year and onset prior to age 18 without attribution to another cause such as medication) in populations with ASD varies from 2.6% to 11%.[164-166] Simultaneously, rates of ASD in populations with Tourette syndrome range from 2.9% to 20%.[167]

These elevated rates of overlap emphasize the need to differentiate between potentially similar-appearing symptoms. For example, while motor phenomena can be present in ASD, these are a result of stereotyped movements and repetitive behaviors as opposed to true tics as are present in Tourette syndrome. Additionally, while in ASD, speech symptoms may be present, these would generally be in relation to echo phenomena, which must be distinguished from true vocal tics.[165,168]

Recent data implicating abnormal frontal-striatal circuitry connectivity common between OCD and ASD implicates a shared processing alteration within the circuits that subserve motivation and reward processing as well as mediation of motor output.[169]

Psychotic Disorders

Psychosis can occur in ASD, particularly presenting with atypical psychotic symptoms. Historically, theoreticians have linked autism and psychosis, either considering autism a core feature of schizophrenia or hypothesizing the former to be the pediatric form of the latter.[170] Across a broad range of studies, among individuals with ASD, prevalence rates of schizophrenia range from 0% to 35% and rates of ASD in schizophrenia range from 3.6% to 60%.[171] Particularly high overlap has been noted in childhood-onset schizophrenia, where rates of ASD comorbidity are close to 50%.[172] There is evidence that individuals with ASD and psychosis demonstrate a particular phenotype including less stereotypy, behavioral repetitions, or restricted interests. These individuals also appear to have differences in the presentation of psychotic symptoms such that they generally meet criteria for unspecified psychosis rather than full schizophrenia criteria.[173,174]

Etiologically, it is notable that many high-risk CNVs overlap between ASD and schizophrenia, including NRXN1, CNTNAP2, 22q11.2, 1q21.1, and 15q13.3 although there is some controversy as to the significance of these associations.[175,176] Neuroanatomically, studies demonstrate a mix of structural and functional connectivity similarities and differences between ASD and schizophrenia. Similarities that have been described include patterns of right-greater-than-left gray matter volume reduction of limbic-striatal-thalamic circuits, patterns of volume reduction in middle frontal gyrus and temporo-parietal junction, corpus callosum and cingulum volume loss, medial prefrontal cortex and superior temporal sulcus hypoactivation

on tasks requiring Theory of Mind, and decreased fusiform gyrus and abnormal amygdala activation on emotion-related tasks.[177-180] These similarities, however, are offset by a broad range of dissimilar structural and functional findings, leaving more questions than answers regarding common etiopathological underpinnings.[171,178,181,182]

Distinguishing and treating comorbid psychosis in patients with ASD can be complicated and challenging. Management of schizophrenia in these instances would likely not deviate from that of standard treatment for a primary psychotic disorder. Differentiating psychotic symptoms from overvalued ideas, restricted and repetitive interests, and mental scripting (e.g., of scenes from movies) presents a difficult yet important clinical decision. This differentiation is particularly challenging if the patient is minimally or nonverbal. In this scenario, it is nearly impossible to diagnose a psychotic process with confidence. The decision of whether or not to empirically implement a trial of an antipsychotic medication is based on weighing the risks of the medication versus the severity and interference from the symptom burden.

Catatonia

Individuals with ASD are at risk for the onset of catatonia. A growing number of authors have engaged this subject recently, whether through epidemiology, exploration of theoretical underpinnings, individual and case series data, or reporting of treatment and outcomes for patients with ASD and comorbid catatonia.[183-197] Catatonia has been estimated to occur in 12–17% of individuals with ASD, with a greater risk in individuals with poor pre-morbid language development and social passivity.[183,198] Many motor signs overlap between ASD and catatonia such as stereotypy, ritualistic behavior, negativism, and echo phenomena, and individuals with a number of neurodevelopmental disorders associated with autistic features have been reported to be at risk for catatonia such as those with Down syndrome and FXS.[199-201] Catatonia has been hypothesized to occur in relation to functional connectivity abnormalities, GABAergic dysfunction, and a predisposition to mood and other psychiatric disorders.[202] Importantly, in nonverbal individuals, superimposed catatonia may be difficult to diagnose if motoric phenomena were common prior to the onset of catatonia. As a result, catatonia should be considered if there is a dramatic change in baseline motoric or echo behaviors. ASD with catatonic features is currently codified in *DSM-5* as a subtype, though without specific diagnostic guidelines.[1,183,190,192]

As with catatonia occurring in other neuropsychiatric disorders, initial management should include lorazepam challenge with an escalating dose of, ideally, intravenous or intramuscular lorazepam beginning at 1 mg and titrated to an effective dose. Maximum dosing recommendations vary, but sources site doses as high as 24 mg divided throughout day.[193,203]

Catatonia should be carefully differentiated from delirium prior to initiating treatment with lorazepam, particularly in the medically ill. The possibility of a paradoxical reaction to lorazepam, including increased agitation or dysregulated behavior, should be observed for in individuals with comorbid ASD. If treatment with lorazepam is ineffective or poorly tolerated, electroconvulsive therapy (ECT) should be considered.[190,204]

Generally, though high-dose lorazepam may be transiently effective, it may not be feasible as a long-standing treatment. ECT has been utilized safely and effectively in cases of catatonia in ASD with severe self-injurious behavior and intractable and severe behavioral dysregulation. Multiple case reports and series describing the successful use of ECT for patients with a wide range of presentations of catatonia have been published.[194,196,205]

When ECT is not available (e.g., in states where legal statute denies use for pediatric and young adolescent populations) other treatments to consider which may be more feasible for long-term use than lorazepam include other GABA-ergic and anti-glutamatergic pharmacotherapies such as zolpidem, amantadine, and memantine. To date, very little data are available for these treatments in patients with ASD and catatonia.

A possible progression of core ASD symptoms to catatonia syndrome is demonstrated in the following case vignette. Here, the evolution of symptoms and a careful ruling out of other diagnoses on the differential diagnosis in combination with a robust response to lorazepam challenge provide good evidence of the presence of catatonia. The case also demonstrates some core features commonly seen in catatonia and the need to differentiate catatonia-like features that can be present in ASD at baseline from onset of catatonia as a superimposed, secondary syndrome.

CASE VIGNETTE 17.1

Dorian is a 16-year-old, right-handed male with a long-standing diagnosis of ASD who presents to outpatient neuropsychiatry clinic with his parents due to concerns of functional decline and subacute mental status change.

At baseline, Dorian has significant communication deficits and is minimally verbal. He is able to verbally express about three words consistently and can understand only simple directions. At school and at home, he uses a pictorial representation chart on his iPad for communication with which he appears to have a vocabulary of about 25 words and, otherwise, communicates using pictures and icons. He enjoys playing simple games on his iPad or watching videos. He also enjoys movement-based therapeutic interventions such as dance therapy and yoga. When overstimulated or agitated, he will scream and pull at his ears. When younger, he would bite himself when upset or would push others if he felt that they were too close to him. In the past, he struggled with encopresis when under periods of stress which also exacerbated sleep difficulty and increased self-stimulatory behavior such as rocking. When agitated, he would hit himself but never caused serious injury. He generally could be gently redirected. He has not experienced bowel or bladder incontinence since age 8 years.

Developmentally, Dorian had no pre- or perinatal adverse events and he was typically developing until about the age of 12 months at which time he had learned three words. His parents recall behavioral and language regression soon after that time. He also had the onset of intense behavioral episodes triggered by overstimulation, transitions between activities, or other environmental triggers. He received early intervention beginning at the age of 12 months following an evaluation that was concerning for ASD in the setting of global developmental delay. He was clinically diagnosed in a specialty clinic for children with ASD and the diagnosis was corroborated with the ADOS. Genetic testing yielded no evidence of contributory, causal abnormalities. He was treated with occupational therapy, physical therapy, and speech therapy, as well as applied behavior analysis. When he entered pre-school, he received an Individualized Education Program (IEP) that provided services related to social and pragmatic communication deficits. He continued to have an IEP throughout school with periods of utilization of a one-to-one paraprofessional due to behavioral issues while in elementary school. He remained in a mainstream school in a specialized classroom for children with ASD.

Dorian takes clonidine 0.1 mg twice daily for agitation and melatonin 3 mg at night for sleep. He underwent a brief trial of risperidone 0.25 mg twice daily at age 5 years due to agitation and self-injury which was stopped after 18 months when symptoms improved with intensive behavioral management. He has also had trials of guanfacine for agitation and sertraline for presumed comorbid anxiety. These were both discontinued due to lack of benefit. Sertraline resulted in increased irritability.

Medically, Dorian is stable. He has never had a seizure or staring spell that caregivers have noted. He has a history of constipation that is intermittently treated with stool softeners. His parents attempted trials of gluten-free and ketogenic diets with the hopes of controlling his gastrointestinal symptoms that had minimal benefit. His sleep is poor historically with frequent tantrums around bedtime and both long sleep latency, as well as early morning waking. Sleep duration has improved with melatonin and clonidine, and tantrums around bedtime have lessened with carefully organized behavioral systems implemented by his family with the help of a behaviorist.

In his regular state of health, Dorian is able to feed, dress, and bathe himself with assistance. He often neglects these activities if not prompted. His day-to-day schedule is guided by a detailed picture-based calendar that is on the refrigerator of his family home. He also has a copy of the identical calendar on his iPad and another at school. Prior to any new activity, caregivers prepare Dorian for the shift in setting, activity, or transition. By doing this, they largely mitigate tantrums or dysregulated behavior that historically would occur for Dorian during these times.

He presents now along with both parents and a representative from his special education classroom due to significant recent changes in behavior and self-care. At the time of his current clinical presentation, Dorian's parents describe a gradual decline over the past 4 months. Over this period, he has ceased to use even rudimentary language and has become less responsive to verbal requests. He has become much less consistent in his use of his iPad language program, often repeatedly pressing the same icon without clear communicative intent. Whereas previously, he would respond well to a soothing voice and use of self-soothing toys such as his stuffed bear, he no longer follows basic requests. He has begun to have episodes of staring that go along with periods of decreased movement. These are punctuated by periods when he may become markedly more agitated than is consistent with his recent baseline. He is no longer able to clean himself after toileting, or shower without assistance, and he requires help with eating and dressing that he has not needed for over 5 years. His parents feel that he has lost about 10 pounds over the 4-month period.

Despite trying to correlate Dorian's change in behavior with external stressors or environmental changes, his parents and a representative from the school were unable to describe any potentially triggering events. School has noticed a similar decline in his functioning to the point where he has not been able to regularly attend for the past 2 weeks due to difficulty getting him to climb the steps onto the bus or, some days, even dressed and out of his room.

On physical examination in the office, Dorian is a slightly thin and pale-appearing boy who looks a bit younger than his 16 years. He is in a wheelchair as he was not able to respond to his parents' requests that he walk to the office from the car. His heart rate is mildly elevated at 115 beats per minute and his blood pressure is 140/80. He is not able to engage with his interviewer despite her repeated attempts to connect and he is not responsive to single, verbal commands or by means of his iPad pictorial system. His gaze is staring. He does not appear to be responding to internal stimuli. He holds his hands in a flexed posture with elbows jutting out. When the examiner lifts his right arm, it remains elevated. He is not able to engage in a general neurological or medical evaluation given his poor responsiveness. His tone is generally mildly increased. His reflexes are normal. Toes are down going bilaterally and he withdraws all limbs to a painful stimulus, although sluggishly.

His evaluator is concerned about the possibility of catatonia. She assists in arranging for an inpatient psychiatric hospitalization for intensive medical and psychiatric workup and management. She is also concerned about the possibility of behavioral decompensation secondary to an underlying medical process such as an untreated chronic medical condition or, perhaps, seizure.

Once admitted, Dorian undergoes a head CT in order to rule out an acute intracranial process which is normal. To rule out other possible contributing neurological processes, brain MRI is then completed which is also within normal limits. Blood is drawn and he undergoes a lumbar puncture. No signs of an infection or autoimmune inflammatory process are found and send-out labs for autoimmune encephalitis and paraneoplastic causes of catatonia return negative. Abdominal x-ray does not demonstrate constipation. He has no lesions or visible injuries to suggest other sources of pain or discomfort. An EEG is completed which demonstrates diffuse slowing, but no epileptiform or focal abnormalities.

Given a high index of suspicion, the treatment team initiates a trial of lorazepam 1 mg intravenously. Within 30 minutes, there is a marked change in Dorian's presentation. He shows apparent awareness of his family by his bedside. They say hello and he responds. He interacts briefly by using his iPad and pictorial system to indicate that he is hungry and would like food. After about 1 hour, he had returned to his previous state with staring gaze, minimal responsiveness, and he experienced an episode of urinary incontinence.

Over the course of the next week, escalating trials of intravenous lorazepam are given up to a dose of 10 mg divided throughout the day. With this dose, his parents describe that he has returned to his baseline. An attempt to decrease the dose the next day is met with a recrudescence of his symptoms. This is considered a positive "lorazepam challenge." Lorazepam is a benzodiazepine medication used as a "challenge" test for catatonia, whereby this medication, which normally results in mild sedation, anxiolysis, a subjective sense of relaxation and decrease in state of arousal, causes, instead, an increase in wakefulness, interactivity, arousal, and a subjective sense of cognitive and physical control. In the absence of other medical findings suggestive of an alternative cause such as encephalitis, seizure, or delirium, given this positive test, the clinical team's confidence in a diagnosis of catatonia is now high. Escalating doses of lorazepam are considered; however, the benefit of the medication continues to be transient and discharge home on high-dose lorazepam is not considered a safe and effective long-term plan.

Dorian is referred for ECT given a diagnosis of ASD with catatonia. Following successful medical clearance, he is given a course of 12 treatments over the span of 1 month with significant improvement and return to his pre-morbid level of function. The frequency of ECT is reduced over the next few weeks without symptom return. Maintenance ECT is not required. No causal etiology is found despite an extensive medical workup and his catatonia is considered to be a result of the underlying ASD. He is closely monitored, but symptoms do not recur.

Sleep Disturbance

Disordered sleep is common in ASD. Up to 50–80% of children with ASD experience a sleep disturbance, which undoubtedly contributes to behavioral problems.[206,207] Sleep problems are associated with the severity of core ASD symptoms and behavioral dysregulation.[208] Sleep disturbances may be secondary to behavioral or sleep hygiene challenges or may reflect untreated underlying comorbid psychiatric or medical conditions such as constipation, gastroesophageal reflux disease (GERD), or seizures. Significant evidence supports the use of melatonin as the first-line pharmacological agent for sleep disturbance in ASD, particularly delayed sleep-onset, with additional evidence for the alpha-2 agonist clonidine.[145,209-217] Sedative hypnotic agents are best avoided due to cognitive slowing, potential paradoxical reactions, and other risks. The antidepressant trazodone is also a generally safe alternative. Priapism (i.e., sustained penile erection) is a rare but serious potential side effect of trazodone. There is some evidence for the use of quetiapine for disturbed sleep. However, the drug should not be used solely as a sleep aide due to the risk of tardive dyskinesia and metabolic and other long-term risks.[218] Prior to consideration of pharmacotherapeutic agents, close attention to sleep hygiene, ruling out underlying medical and psychiatric conditions, and appropriate use of behavioral techniques should be utilized.

Gender Identity

Preliminary evidence indicates that the prevalence of gender dysphoria or gender variance may be increased in persons with ASD. There appears to be both notable overrepresentation of gender dysphoria or gender-variance expression in ASD and of autistic symptomatology in individuals with gender dysphoria.[219-222] This relationship is poorly understood and requires further investigation.

Gastrointestinal Dysfunction

Gastrointestinal dysfunction is a common comorbidity in patients with ASD. GI-related symptoms such as constipation, diarrhea, and GERD can contribute to behavioral changes, functional challenges, aggression, self-injury, and other symptoms. A large retrospective study, which examined the records of more than 14,000 patients with ASD across general and pediatric hospitals, found that 11.7% presented with bowel disorders (excluding inflammatory bowel disease [IBD]) compared to 1.6% of non-ASD patients.[223] Though compelling, this finding may be underrepresentative of the prevalence of GI dysfunction in ASD, reflecting confounds in the nature of its reporting. Similar studies, which have observed a prevalence of up to 70% of GI dysfunction in patients with ASD, differ greatly in their estimations.[224] Reporting challenges may contribute to the disparity in prevalence rates. Moderate-to-severe ASD-related communication deficits can limit patients' ability to express discomfort from their underlying GI pathology, which may lack typically identifiable signs during a standard physical examination.[56,225] Clinicians should pay close attention to caretaker reports of diet tolerance, stool frequency and consistency, and food preferences in these situations. The differential diagnosis should include potential medical problems, with a particular attention to constipation given its high risk, when attempting to determine the etiology of aberrant behaviors in patients with ASD.

Clinical evaluation for GI dysfunction is important not only to alleviate patient discomfort, but also because the maintenance of a healthy gut is critical for proper function of the central nervous system. The enteric nervous system (ENS), coined "the second brain," comprises approximately the same number of neurons as the spinal cord and contains roughly 95% of the serotonin in the human body. In fact, recent animal model data indicate that serotonin synthesized by the gut microbiota can regulate mood and behavior through immune cells, suggesting the convergence of two systems implicated in the pathogenesis of ASD.[226-228] The specific mechanisms linking ASD and the ENS are unclear, but the findings highlight the importance of the bidirectional communication between the gut and brain.

Though causative mechanisms remain elusive, it has been speculated that abnormalities of the GI tract in ASD may contribute to observed differences in food preference or selectivity, feeding problems, and perceived high rates of obesity.[229] Indeed, significant nutritional deficiencies have been observed in ASD populations.[230,231] However, unhealthy feeding patterns are also associated with adverse changes in gut function and microbial composition, complicating the direction of attributable causation.[232,233] This topic of ASD research has likely been superseded in the past by those of more acute medical comorbidities, such as epilepsy and catatonia. Further clinical study of nutrition in ASD is warranted, however, not only for treating unhealthy feeding behaviors but also to illuminate potential etiologic mechanisms of ASD manifestations as they relate to the gut for the development of novel treatment options.

Standard of care treatment of GI conditions for the nonpsychiatric population should be used for patients with ASD as well, to manage discomfort and improve GI function. It has been reported that treating patients with ASD with GI pathology can improve ASD-related behaviors concurrently, though it is unclear whether this effect is caused by the alleviation of GI-related discomfort or by the treatments' effects on mechanisms underlying ASD-related behavior through other mechanisms. Clinicians caring for patients with ASD must be particularly careful to note the prevalence of GI comorbidities, the potential obstacles to diagnosing GI dysfunction, and the broad scope of influence that GI dysfunction can have on all domains of the symptomatology of ASD and overall health.

Epilepsy

The estimated prevalence of epilepsy in ASD ranges from 6% to 46%, with risk factors including history of regression of social and language skills, and lower cognitive functioning.[234-241] The direction of causality between epilepsy and cognitive function is not well understood, but the association is robust: one study found that, after 10 years of age, every standard deviation decrease in IQ of patients with ASD correlated with a 47% increase in epilepsy risk.[236] Alternatively, some evidence suggests an increase in ASD-related symptoms, but not ASD, in patients with a history of the diagnosis of epilepsy leading some to speculate that the high comorbidity between ASD and epilepsy may reflect etiopathological overlap along a "spectrum of vulnerability."[242,243] A cluster analysis performed on a cohort of pediatric patients with ASD identified that the cluster with the highest rate of comorbid epilepsy exhibited the most frequent repetitive object use, motor function impairments, atypical sensory interests, and early-life ASD diagnoses.[237] The cluster analysis suggested that a particular ASD pathophysiology, with a distinct behavioral phenotype, may overlap with that of an epilepsy subtype. Though these associations may be attributable to other comorbidities shared by ASD and epilepsy, like cognitive deficits, the endophenotype described could be used as a rational framework for clinicians evaluating aberrant behaviors and individual risk of epilepsy. Onset of seizure disorder in ASD is often during late adolescence or early adulthood particularly in males who are minimally or nonverbal. This may be due to reduction in GABA-ergic function at this developmental phase that results in shifts in excitatory/inhibitory balance. A similar mechanism may be responsible for the increased prevalence of catatonia in this subgroup of individuals with ASD.

Syndromic and genetic variant subtypes of ASD also have high rates of comorbid epilepsy and thus may indicate an epileptic subtype within the autism spectrum. Because subtypes of ASD of genetic etiology are characterized by synaptic gene dysfunction, and epilepsy is characterized by intermittent dysregulation of synaptic activity on a focal or global scale, some have speculated about possible shared neurodevelopmental mechanisms.[244] Like ASD, the minority of epilepsy diagnoses are attributable to single-gene mutations or chromosomal microdeletions.[245] Also like ASD, subtypes of epilepsy with genetic etiologies, such as epileptic encephalopathies, are heterogeneous, but most reliably involve synaptic gene dysfunction.[246] Whether synaptic deficits are structural or functional, the resultant impairment in neurotransmission may lead to diverse epileptic phenotypes.

Further reinforcing the possible pathogenic overlap between ASD and epilepsy is the translational accuracy of some genetic and environmental models of ASD. Recent studies have identified epileptic phenotypes caused by monogenic mutations in both humans and rodent models of ASD. For instance, haploinsufficiency of *SYNGAP1*, an important regulator of synaptic function, is a common monogenic cause of ID in humans and has been implicated as the cause of a subtype of epileptic encephalopathy with cognitive regression.[247,248] Importantly, mutant mice heterozygous for *SYNGAP1* exhibit impaired social interaction and cognitive deficits that are causally linked to developmental dysfunction in forebrain excitatory neurons, implicating mechanisms associated with epilepsy in an ASD-like phenotype.[249]

The translational relevance of some genetic models of ASD is compelling, but the importance of environmental factors is apparent as well. Offspring in MIA models, which have an ASD-like behavioral phenotype caused by gestational or perinatal immune challenge, have exhibited patterns of spike-wave discharge, an epileptiform electroencephalogram signature, without apparent features of a generalized tonic-clonic seizure.[62] Comparable to the persistent inflammatory states of MIA offspring, some reports have found that peripheral inflammation, measured by IL-6, is predictive of interictal epileptiform activity in human patients with ASD without a history of an epilepsy diagnosis.[250] These findings suggest that the etiology of epilepsy in ASD may be as diverse and heterogeneous as the etiology of ASD itself and that further investigation of the underlying mechanisms is warranted.

There is evidence to suggest that status epilepticus contributes less to the cognitive regression characteristic of epileptic encephalopathies than do interictal EEG abnormalities.[251] These interictal spikes may occur primarily during sleep as they do in patients with continuous spike-waves during slow-wave sleep

(CSWS). Although the contribution of chronic sleep disturbance to cognitive regression has yet to be fully determined, the putative causal relationship between interictal epileptiform activity and cognitive impairment underscores the importance of evaluating sleep behaviors and biomarkers in these patients.[252] A large proportion of patients with ASD have been shown to exhibit high rates of interictal epileptiform EEG abnormalities during sleep, as well as non-seizure-related EEG abnormalities even without a history of status epilepticus.[253,254]

TREATMENTS

Pharmacological Management of Core and Associated Symptoms of ASD

There are no medications that have been consistently shown to improve the core symptoms of ASD (social-pragmatic deficits and repetitive interests and behaviors). There have been several trials of medications targeting these core symptoms, including arbaclofen (a selective GABA-B agonist), memantine (an anti-glutamatergic *N*-methyl-D-aspartate [NMDA] receptor antagonist utilized to treat memory impairment associated with Alzheimer's dementia), N-acetylcysteine (NAC; a glutamatergic modulator), oxytocin (an endogenous hormone which mediates affiliative behavior), and sulforaphane (a broadly explored, naturally occurring antioxidant found in broccoli). In general, the results of these trials have been discouraging and none of these treatments has been FDA-approved for this purpose.[255-261] Instead, the focus of psychopharmacotherapeutic management in ASD has been geared to target comorbid neuropsychiatric disorders such as anxiety disorders, ADHD, or epilepsy, or the behavioral symptoms associated with ASD, such as irritability, aggression, and self-injurious behavior. Accurately diagnosing neuropsychiatric disorders in patients with ASD is further complicated by frequent overlap between the characteristics of ASD and the comorbid conditions. This can be seen, for example, in repetitive behaviors. While behavioral repetitions are a core aspect of ASD, comorbid OCD may also occur. Careful clinical interview and behavioral observation are required to differentiate these disorders because the effective treatments are quite different.

Aggression and self-injurious behavior are common in ASD. Self-injury occurs at rates ranging from 15% to 50% in ASD, with one study reporting rates as high as 74% in an inpatient hospitalized population.[262,263] In ASD, self-injury is highly correlated with ID and generally manifests as biting, hitting, or head-banging in the context of repetitive, self-stimulatory, and sensory or emotionally overwhelming settings.[264]

Similarly, aggressive behaviors in ASD do not usually occur in the context of more typical oppositional defiant or conduct disorder symptoms, but rather when the individual is overwhelmed by sensory, emotional, or other stimuli. Aggression can also occur when the individual is frustrated, which can result from the inability to communicate thoughts, feelings, and desires adequately. Two-thirds of patients with ASD can demonstrate aggression and it is reported as one of the primary reasons for involvement of children and adolescents with

ASD in mental health services.[265,266] New-onset or exacerbation of baseline self-injury or aggression may represent an occult medical problem and should prompt careful workup.

Two medications are approved for the treatment of irritability associated with ASD, risperidone and aripiprazole. Each carries an FDA-approval for "irritability" in the context of ASD, which includes behavioral dysregulation, self-injury, and aggression. At this time, this approval pertains only to children and adolescents with ASD. Beyond these two medications, all psychopharmacological treatments in ASD are used "off-label," unless they are being utilized to target a diagnosed neuropsychiatric comorbidity. As a result of the complex comorbidities present in ASD, medication choice should be made to maximize management of the most interfering comorbid disorders while minimizing the side-effect burden.

Classes of Pharmacological Agents and Their Use in ASD

Antipsychotic Medications
The strongest evidence for treatment of behavioral dysregulation and irritability in ASD is for the atypical antipsychotics risperidone and aripiprazole.[277–280] Other second-generation antipsychotics, including olanzapine, ziprasidone, quetiapine, and clozapine, have been found to be of benefit for some patients, but in a limited number of small-scale studies.[218,277,278,281–288] The first-generation antipsychotics were initially studied as a treatment for dysregulated or aggressive behavior in ASD. Systematic trials of haloperidol demonstrated significant benefit, but equivocal and inconsistent results were obtained with the lower-potency antipsychotics such as chlorpromazine and thioridazine. Moreover, utilization of typical antipsychotics was limited by extrapyramidal symptoms and the higher risk of tardive dyskinesia.[264,289,290] Antipsychotics are also used, at times, to treat self-injurious behaviors commonly seen in ASD, though data are more limited.[264] An example of appropriately conservative and judicious use of antipsychotic medications can be seen in the case vignette, where this category of medication is used only in the absence of efficacy of behavioral therapies and medications that carry a lesser side-effect burden.

Antiepileptic and Mood-Stabilizing Medications
In addition to antipsychotics, antiepileptic medications, many of which have some mood stabilizing effects, such as divalproex sodium, lamotrigine, levetiracetam, oxcarbazepine, and topiramate, have been used to treat aggression, self-injury, and irritability.[291–297] The strongest evidence for efficacy within this category exists for divalproex sodium, although the results are mixed.[298] It should be noted that anticonvulsant medications should be specifically considered when comorbid epilepsy is present along with symptoms of aggression or self-injury. Finally, some evidence for the effectiveness of lithium exists, especially when comorbid bipolar disorder or Phelan-McDermid syndrome is present.[197,299]

Alpha-2 Agonists and Beta-Blockers
Alpha-2 agonists such as guanfacine and clonidine have been utilized for sleep, anxiety, motoric behaviors, and agitation associated with ASD, and for comorbid psychiatric disorders such as ADHD.[144–147,150,209,300–303] There are a limited number of reports of beta-blockers for management of dysregulated behaviors with mixed results.[307] Interestingly, one study demonstrated increased functional connectivity of subnetworks of the DMN in both control subjects and individuals with ASD with administration of the beta-blocker propranolol.[305] Alpha-2 agonists and beta-blockers are sometimes used early in the management of irritability due to their safer side-effect profile compared with antipsychotic medications.

Antidepressant and Related Medications
Antidepressant medications have been explored in the management of a variety of symptoms in ASD, both related to core symptomatology, as well as common comorbidities. Stereotypy or compulsive behaviors may overlap with OCD, tics, or Tourette syndrome, as well as anxiety. Selective serotonin reuptake inhibitors (SSRIs), such as fluoxetine and fluvoxamine, have shown positive benefit for adults with ASD with interfering restricted and repetitive behaviors; however, in children, SSRIs have been shown to be no more effective than placebo and with increased behavioral activating side effects.[306–309] On occasion, an SSRI may be helpful for comorbid anxiety and depression associated with ASD, but no systematic studies have demonstrated this benefit.[310–315] For self-injury, data from small-scale, open-label studies exist for paroxetine and clomipramine; side-effects of clomipramine, including onset or exacerbation of seizures, were often treatment-limiting.[306,316–318] Other medications have been explored for treating comorbid anxiety, irritability, and restricted and repetitive behaviors, including buspirone, a serotonin 1A partial agonist, which shows some promise and is generally well-tolerated.[319,320]

Behavioral Interventions for Core and Associated Symptoms of ASD

A range of nonpharmacological interventions are utilized in addressing core symptoms associated with ASD as well as comorbid conditions or ASD sequelae. These include applied behavior analysis (ABA), early intervention (specifically early intensive behavioral intervention [EIBI]), cognitive-behavioral therapy (CBT), parental training and parent-mediated therapies, music therapy, social skills training, occupational (OT), physical (PT), and speech (ST) therapies, and a range of other treatments. The data on specific interventions are often limited, but evidence does exist for utilization of these approaches.[267–273] Given the risks often associated with pharmacotherapeutic interventions, non-medication-based approaches should be strongly considered. Interventions will differ based on a broad range of factors including age, functional level, language ability, intelligence, behavioral challenges, comorbid psychiatric and medical disorders, and others. A review of the majority of these interventions is beyond the scope of this text, but a few key interventions are described.

ABA is a psychosocial intervention which targets core ASD symptoms. ABA uses principles of operant conditioning in order to facilitate learning of a new behavior and a shift away from a defined target behavior. In ABA, the antecedent events and reinforcing behavior that contribute to a target behavior are determined and positive reward for engagement in a desired alternative behavior is utilized. This is combined with interventions aimed toward extinction of problematic behavior. ABA interventions are targeted and specific and, as such, numerous specific intervention protocols are available and commonly utilized.[264]

A variety of early intervention treatments are available which can target core and ancillary ASD symptoms. A 2018 update of a 2012 Cochrane review examined the evidence for EIBI, a multiyear intervention grounded in principles of ABA that includes up to 40 hours of weekly intensive individual work.[274] EIBI targets functional skills, behavioral challenges, social skills development, and other goals in young children with the diagnosis of ASD. The review found evidence of efficacy for the intervention, but graded the evidence as weak, in large part due to small sample size and lack of high-quality, randomized-controlled trials. That said, despite the limitations of the evidence, the data suggest EIBI may contribute to gains in IQ, activities of daily living, adaptive behaviors, and social and communication skills. The greatest improvements were found within domains of IQ while the smallest were in socialization. Rigorous studies of EIBI are necessary to better evaluate outcomes, impact on families, strengths of EIBI in comparison with other interventions, and details about target populations and mitigating factors.

Interventions such as OT and ST are used for learning and facilitation of independent life skills, emotional and behavioral self-regulation, sensory integration, social comportment and language pragmatics, and other skills.[275,276] Numerous different specific treatment paradigms have been used to target age- and symptom-specific aspects of ASD. Occupational therapy and ST approaches are often highly personalized based on the needs of the individual, their family, and the relevant environment.

An example of the integration of nonpharmacological treatments and medication interventions can be seen in the case vignette. The case demonstrates the combined use of early intervention approaches with ABA, OT, PT, and ST to manage core symptoms of ASD with judicious use later on of pharmacological and medical interventions if these behavioral approaches are inadequate.

Complementary and Alternative Therapies

A broad range of complementary and alternative therapies are often utilized, frequently driven by family interest, in order to manage an array of symptoms associated with ASD. One example of such therapy is the ketogenic diet, which requires a high-fat and exceedingly low-carbohydrate intake, to induce a safe, controlled state of nutritional ketosis. The diet has been used as a treatment for refractory epilepsy since the early 20th century, and there is interest in its possible diverse application for the treatment of other neurological illnesses.[321,322] There is evidence that, in several established rodent models of ASD, restricting mice or rats to a ketogenic diet offers therapeutic potential for

treating core behavioral features of ASD and that this effect is dissociable from its antiepileptic mechanisms.[323-326] Similar improvements have been observed in humans, but further study is needed and caution should be exercised currently.[327]

The beneficial effects of the ketogenic diet are thought to be partly due to its anti-inflammatory properties, perhaps through mediation of the bioenergetic dysfunction caused by increased mitochondrial reactive oxygen species consistently observed in ASD.[328-330] Indeed, tissue-specific changes in mitochondrial dynamics have been observed in an animal model of ASD, where mice receive a ketogenic diet.[331] Though many alternative therapies are in the early stages of testing, results suggest the capacity for treatments with anti-inflammatory mechanisms, in part, to improve core behavioral symptoms of a subtype of patients with ASD.

Other diets are sometimes utilized as complementary and alternative approaches in the management of ASD symptoms. One of the more common is the gluten-free casein-free (GFCF) diet. This diet was used first based on the theory that, given evidence of increased GI permeability in ASD, an overabundance of certain peptides contained in these foods which may cross the blood-brain barrier and be centrally active, such as gluteomorphins and beta-casomorphins, may impact the endogenous opioid system causing or exacerbating core symptoms of ASD.[332,333]

Although these diets may be popular, a 2008 Cochrane review found the evidence for their efficacy to be poor and the data to be limited.[334] A 2017 review that included discussion of six small randomized trials exploring the GFCF diet concluded there to be a lack of evidence that the diet improves core ASD symptoms.[332] Both reviews cite concerns given potential physical health consequences of eliminative diets as a result of, for example, loss of the nutritional benefit of cow's milk. They also cite high financial burden of many eliminative diets and the challenge of enacting further restrictions for the child or adult with ASD given an often already significantly restricted lifestyle. Evidence also exists suggesting that utilization of the GFCF diet may substantially alter a child's eating behavior and could negatively impact social integration of a child with ASD.[335,336]

CONCLUSION

In summary, ASD is a complex, heterogeneous, developmental neuropsychiatric condition with numerous undetermined etiologies that is likely the result of a broad range of interacting genetic and environmental factors. These may include abnormalities in micro- and macro-neurocircuitry development due to polygenic variations, and aberrant inflammatory processes occurring during key developmental phases that result in deficits in the complex neural machinery responsible for social pragmatics and regulation of behavior and emotions. ASD is commonly comorbid with a range of neuropsychiatric and medical conditions including seizure disorder, mood and anxiety disorders, sleep disturbance, GI disorders, and other conditions which must be carefully attended to in clinical management.

Summary and Key Points

- Autism spectrum disorder (ASD) is a heterogeneous, developmental neuropsychiatric condition characterized by (1) deficits in social communication and interaction; and (2) restricted patterns of repetitive behaviors and interests or activities.

- Current prevalence data estimates the rate of ASD to be about 2% of the population with a 4:1 male-to-female ratio. Reasons for the increase in population prevalence of ASD over recent decades are not known but likely implicate changing diagnostic criteria, better identification of affected individuals, and possible environmental and other factors impacting underlying disease pathophysiology.

- ASD does not result from a single genetic or environmental cause. Uncommonly, ASD can occur with high likelihood in the context of specific genetic syndromes, such as Fragile X syndrome and a range of syndromes associated with specific copy number variants (CNVs). More commonly, ASD occurs in the setting of complex, polygene, and environmental interactions where, in most cases, cumulative common variation plays the most consequential and representative role in etiology.

- A number of animal models have been put forth to explore the complex, neuropsychiatric phenotypes present in ASD. To date, one of the most successful has been the maternal immune activation (MIA) model which posits an interaction between genetic predisposition and in utero exposures which, together, impact neural development via alteration of signaling pathways.

- A broad range of neuroanatomic findings are described consistently in ASD. Functional disconnection occurs between key circuits including those that subserve social cognition, frontal-executive function, and other important neurocognitive domains with possible increase in local functional connectivity. This may be governed by atypical cortical microcolumnar organization. Brain regions including the prefrontal cortex, basal ganglia, amygdala, cerebellum, and others are implicated in ASD pathophysiology. A core finding in ASD is inconsistency in patterns of functional connectivity of canonical neural circuits.

- Neuropsychiatric and medical comorbidity in ASD is the rule rather than the exception. Seizures, intellectual disability, and sleep disorders occur at high rates. Psychiatric comorbidities for which individuals with ASD are at elevated risk include ADHD, anxiety and mood disorders, catatonia, and tic and other repetitive behavior disorders among others. Individuals with ASD are at elevated risk for suicidal ideation, self-injurious behavior, and suicide attempt. Immune dysfunction and gastrointestinal disorders are common medical comorbid conditions.

- No treatments exist for the core symptoms of ASD. Risperidone and aripiprazole are the only FDA-approved treatments for ASD and are used for management of irritability and behavioral dysregulation. Otherwise, management should be geared toward identification and treatment of significantly interfering ASD comorbidities while minimizing risks of adverse effects of medications which may be more common in individuals with ASD.

- Behavioral therapies are first line for challenging behaviors, sleep disturbance, self-injury, aggression, and many other symptoms common in ASD. Applied behavior analysis and other behavioral treatments can be safely directed to target specific behavioral challenges. There is evidence for use of early intervention in ASD as demonstrating benefit across a number of domains.

- Complementary and alternative therapies are commonly utilized in the treatment of a broad range of symptoms experienced in ASD often spurred by active primary caregiver and community endorsement. Certain of these therapies, such as chelation therapy, should be universally avoided due to lack of efficacy and safety risks. Others, such as the ketogenic diet, have limited evidence, but can be carefully applied with close coordination of a clinician. Financial cost, nutritional deficiency, restrictiveness, and social isolation must all be weighed in consideration of the use of diet as a complementary and alternative therapy.

- Future directions include development of increasingly accurate and representative models for the complex gene-environment interactions believed to underlie the pathophysiology of ASD. In addition, treatment trials for core ASD symptoms are underway, although, to date, the results of these studies have been discouraging. Trials are also ongoing into complementary and alternative treatments. Much improvement continues to be made in early identification and intensive behavioral intervention in ASD.

- ASD must be approached as a complex, cross-disciplinary, neuropsychiatric condition in order to provide the most comprehensive workup and treatment plan possible. Clinicians must work closely with individuals with ASD and their families, insuring steady, ongoing communication in order to achieve the best possible outcomes.

Multiple Choice Questions

1. Which of the following is a common cause of new-onset idiopathic aberrant behavior in a nonverbal, intellectually disabled patient with ASD?
   a. Comorbid depression
   b. Tic disorder
   c. Constipation
   d. Hypoglycemia
   e. Psychosis

2. Based on the available evidence, which of the following is most likely to indicate potential immune involvement in a patient's ASD etiology?
   a. A history of HIV infection, contracted by the individual through adult sexual activity
   b. Comorbid idiopathic vocal tic
   c. Proximity of onset of ASD symptoms after receiving the measles, mumps, rubella (MMR) vaccine
   d. Family history of systemic lupus erythematosus
   e. Self-injurious behavior

3. Which of the following theoretical findings would most likely be cited as evidence to support existing theories that attempt to explain the male:female sex bias observed in ASD epidemiology?
   a. An overall decrease in expressed empathy and increase in perceived drive to systemize in the ASD population
   b. Female fetuses exhibit a greater susceptibility to miscarriage than male fetuses
   c. Fraternal siblings of female children with ASD exhibit greater ASD symptomatology than those of male children with ASD
   d. a and b
   e. a and c

4. Which of the following observations is *not* believed to be involved in the pathophysiological overlap between ASD and epilepsy?
   a. Both genetic and environmental rodent models of ASD have exhibited robust and varied epileptic phenotypes.
   b. Interictal epileptiform activity is prevalent in patients with ASD even in the absence of an epilepsy diagnosis.
   c. Both epilepsy and ASD are commonly associated with synaptic irregularities, whether structural or functional.
   d. Exposure to environmental pollutants is a primary cause of both epilepsy and ASD risk.
   e. Elevated peripheral inflammation, as measured by IL-6, has been associated with both EEG epileptiform activity and ASD.

Multiple Choice Answers

1. **Answer: c**
   Gastrointestinal conditions such as constipation may present with behavioral changes without obvious localizing symptoms. In many cases, patients who are minimally or nonverbal are unable to clearly express or demonstrate localization of discomfort and can end up with sometimes long-standing, painful medical conditions. Often, these medical comorbidities manifest with behavioral symptoms. Comorbid depression, tic disorders, low or elevated blood glucose, and psychosis are all possible causes of behavioral change; however, given the frequency of comorbid GI symptoms in ASD, including decreased gut motility, as well as the constipating, anticholinergic effects of many medications used to treat behavioral challenges in ASD, such as the antipsychotic risperidone, constipation is a particularly common cause of behavioral changes. Thus, gastrointestinal health workups should be included in the differential diagnosis in these circumstances and be included as part of an initial diagnostic workup.

2. **Answer: d**
   Family history of autoimmune disease is strongly associated with an increased risk for ASD. Although answer a involves an immune challenge, putative immune subtypes of ASD are thought to originate from the pre- and perinatal period. There is no evidence that ASD-onset is mediated by vaccines. There are many large-scale studies which refute the claim of an association between vaccination and ASD. Answers b and e do not imply an immune-mediated pathology.

3. **Answer: e**
   Answer a provides an example of the "extreme male brain" theory, wherein it is postulated that the brain of individuals with ASD exhibits what are considered to be exaggerated male characteristics, including systemization and a relative lack of empathy expression. Answer c describes potential evidence supporting the "female protective effect" theory. This theory posits that females require a greater cumulative genetic and/or environmental insult to confer risk of ASD than do males. The finding provided could support this theory because it could be inferred that siblings of females with ASD would have required greater cumulative genetic and/or environmental risk factors exposure. Despite their prominence in the field, there are ongoing debates about both theories and they require further substantiating evidence. There is no discussion in the chapter of the finding presented in answer b or of its potential relation to ASD.

4. **Answer: d**
   Answers a, b, c, and e have all been described as evidence for shared underlying pathophysiology between ASD and epilepsy. While some associations have been observed between environmental pollutant exposure and both ASD and epilepsy, environmental pollution is not considered a dominant epilepsy risk factor according to currently available evidence and is not currently believed to be a primary cause of ASD. ASD, instead, is believed to be a result of complex interplay of multi-genetic predispositions, immunological factors, and other environmental exposures of which environmental pollutants may be one.

References

1. American Psychiatric Association, DSM-5 Task Force. *Diagnostic and Statistical Manual of Mental Disorders: DSM-5*. 5th ed. Washington, DC: American Psychiatric Association; 2013.
2. Simonoff E, Jones CR, Baird G, Pickles A, Happé F, Charman T. The persistence and stability of psychiatric problems in adolescents with autism spectrum disorders. *J Child Psychol Psychiatry*. 2013;54(2):186-194.
3. Simonoff E, Pickles A, Charman T, Chandler S, Loucas T, Baird G. Psychiatric disorders in children with autism spectrum disorders: prevalence, comorbidity, and associated factors in a population-derived sample. *J Am Acad Child Adolesc Psychiatry*. 2008;47(8):921-929.

4. Bauman MD, Iosif AM, Smith SE, Bregere C, Amaral DG, Patterson PH. Activation of the maternal immune system during pregnancy alters behavioral development of rhesus monkey offspring. *Biol Psychiatry*. 2014;75(4):332-341.

5. Autism and Developmental Disabilities Monitoring Network Surveillance Year 2008 Principal Investigators; Centers for Disease Control and Prevention. Prevalence of autism spectrum disorders—Autism and Developmental Disabilities Monitoring Network, 14 sites, United States, 2008. *MMWR Surveill Summ*. 2012;61(3):1-19.

6. Blumberg SJ, Bramlett MD, Kogan MD, Schieve LA, Jones JR, Lu MC. Changes in prevalence of parent-reported autism spectrum disorder in school-aged U.S. children: 2007 to 2011-2012. *Natl Health Stat Report*. 2013(65):1-11, 1 p following 11.

7. Baio J, Wiggins L, Christensen DL, et al. Prevalence of autism spectrum disorder among children aged 8 years—Autism and Developmental Disabilities Monitoring Network, 11 sites, United States, 2014. *MMWR Surveill Summ*. 2018;67(6):1-23.

8. Werling DM, Geschwind DH. Sex differences in autism spectrum disorders. *Curr Opin Neurol*. 2013;26(2):146-153.

9. Baron-Cohen S. The extreme male brain theory of autism. *Trends Cogn Sci*. 2002;6(6):248-254.

10. Baron-Cohen S, Auyeung B, Nørgaard-Pedersen B, et al. Elevated fetal steroidogenic activity in autism. *Mol Psychiatry*. 2015;20(3):369-376.

11. Jacquemont S, Coe BP, Hersch M, et al. A higher mutational burden in females supports a "female protective model" in neurodevelopmental disorders. *Am J Hum Genet*. 2014;94(3):415-425.

12. Head AM, McGillivray JA, Stokes MA. Gender differences in emotionality and sociability in children with autism spectrum disorders. *Mol Autism*. 2014;5(1):19.

13. Halladay AK, Bishop S, Constantino JN, et al. Sex and gender differences in autism spectrum disorder: summarizing evidence gaps and identifying emerging areas of priority. *Mol Autism*. 2015;6:36.

14. Amaral DG. Examining the causes of autism. *Cerebrum*. 2017; 2017:1-17.

15. Tick B, Colvert E, McEwen F, et al. Autism spectrum disorders and other mental health problems: exploring etiological overlaps and phenotypic causal associations. *J Am Acad Child Adolesc Psychiatry*. 2016;55(2):106-113.e104.

16. Hallmayer J, Cleveland S, Torres A, et al. Genetic heritability and shared environmental factors among twin pairs with autism. *Arch Gen Psychiatry*. 2011;68(11):1095-1102.

17. Buxbaum JD, Hof PR. *The Neuroscience of Autism Spectrum Disorders*. 1st ed. Amsterdam: Elsevier/Academic Press; 2013.

18. Basu SN, Kollu R, Banerjee-Basu S. AutDB: a gene reference resource for autism research. *Nucleic Acids Res*. 2009;37(database issue):D832-D836.

19. Baron-Cohen S, Leslie AM, Frith U. Does the autistic child have a "theory of mind"? *Cognition*. 1985;21(1):37-46.

20. Frith U. *Autism: Explaining the Enigma*. Cambridge, MA: Basil Blackwell; 1989.

21. Shah A, Frith U. Why do autistic individuals show superior performance on the block design task? *J Child Psychol Psychiatry*. 1993;34(8):1351-1364.

22. Ozonoff S, Pennington BF, Rogers SJ. Executive function deficits in high-functioning autistic individuals: relationship to theory of mind. *J Child Psychol Psychiatry*. 1991;32(7):1081-1105.

23. Russell J. *Autism as an Executive Disorder*. New York, NY: Oxford University Press; 1997.

24. Geschwind DH, Levitt P. Autism spectrum disorders: developmental disconnection syndromes. *Curr Opin Neurobiol*. 2007;17(1):103-111.

25. Courchesne E, Pierce K. Why the frontal cortex in autism might be talking only to itself: local over-connectivity but long-distance disconnection. *Curr Opin Neurobiol*. 2005;15(2):225-230.

26. Happé F, Frith U. The weak coherence account: detail-focused cognitive style in autism spectrum disorders. *J Autism Dev Disord*. 2006;36(1):5-25.

27. Cherkassky VL, Kana RK, Keller TA, Just MA. Functional connectivity in a baseline resting-state network in autism. *NeuroReport*. 2006;17(16):1687-1690.

28. Washington SD, Gordon EM, Brar J, et al. Dysmaturation of the default mode network in autism. *Hum Brain Mapp*. 2014;35(4):1284-1296.

29. Raichle ME. The brain's default mode network. *Annu Rev Neurosci*. 2015;38:433-447.

30. Raichle ME, MacLeod AM, Snyder AZ, Powers WJ, Gusnard DA, Shulman GL. A default mode of brain function. *Proc Natl Acad Sci U S A*. 2001;98(2):676-682.

31. Saxe R, Kanwisher N. People thinking about thinking people. The role of the temporo-parietal junction in "theory of mind". *NeuroImage*. 2003;19(4):1835-1842.

32. Li W, Mai X, Liu C. The default mode network and social understanding of others: what do brain connectivity studies tell us. *Front Hum Neurosci*. 2014;8:74.

33. Nunes AS, Peatfield N, Vakorin V, Doesburg SM. Idiosyncratic organization of cortical networks in autism spectrum disorder. *NeuroImage*. 2019;190:182-190.

34. Neale BM, Kou Y, Liu L, et al. Patterns and rates of exonic de novo mutations in autism spectrum disorders. *Nature*. 2012;485(7397):242-245.

35. Sanders SJ, Murtha MT, Gupta AR, et al. De novo mutations revealed by whole-exome sequencing are strongly associated with autism. *Nature*. 2012;485(7397):237-241.

36. Buxbaum JD, Bolshakova N, Brownfeld JM, et al. The Autism Simplex Collection: an international, expertly phenotyped autism sample for genetic and phenotypic analyses. *Mol Autism*. 2014;5:34.

37. De Rubeis S, He X, Goldberg AP, et al. Synaptic, transcriptional and chromatin genes disrupted in autism. *Nature*. 2014;515(7526):209-215.

38. Gaugler T, Klei L, Sanders SJ, et al. Most genetic risk for autism resides with common variation. *Nat Genet*. 2014;46(8):881-885.

39. Monteiro P, Feng G. SHANK proteins: roles at the synapse and in autism spectrum disorder. *Nat Rev Neurosci*. 2017;18(3):147-157.

40. Abrahams BS, Geschwind DH. Advances in autism genetics: on the threshold of a new neurobiology. *Nat Rev Genet*. 2008;9(5):341-355.

41. Taylor LE, Swerdfeger AL, Eslick GD. Vaccines are not associated with autism: an evidence-based meta-analysis of case-control and cohort studies. *Vaccine*. 2014;32(29):3623-3629.

42. Onore C, Careaga M, Ashwood P. The role of immune dysfunction in the pathophysiology of autism. *Brain Behav Immun*. 2012;26(3):383-392.

43. McDougle CJ, Landino SM, Vahabzadeh A, et al. Toward an immune-mediated subtype of autism spectrum disorder. *Brain Res*. 2015;1617:72-92.

44. Lombardo MV, Moon HM, Su J, Palmer TD, Courchesne E, Pramparo T. Maternal immune activation dysregulation of the fetal brain transcriptome and relevance to the pathophysiology of autism spectrum disorder. *Mol Psychiatry*. 2018;23(4):1001-1013.

45. Estes ML, McAllister AK. Maternal immune activation: implications for neuropsychiatric disorders. *Science*. 2016;353(6301):772-777.

46. Atladóttir HO, Thorsen P, Schendel DE, Østergaard L, Lemcke S, Parner ET. Association of hospitalization for infection in childhood with diagnosis of autism spectrum disorders: a Danish cohort study. *Arch Pediatr Adolesc Med.* 2010;164(5):470-477.

47. Vargas DL, Nascimbene C, Krishnan C, Zimmerman AW, Pardo CA. Neuroglial activation and neuroinflammation in the brain of patients with autism. *Ann Neurol.* 2005;57(1):67-81.

48. Chez MG, Dowling T, Patel PB, Khanna P, Kominsky M. Elevation of tumor necrosis factor-alpha in cerebrospinal fluid of autistic children. *Pediatr Neurol.* 2007;36(6):361-365.

49. Morgan JT, Chana G, Pardo CA, et al. Microglial activation and increased microglial density observed in the dorsolateral prefrontal cortex in autism. *Biol Psychiatry.* 2010;68(4):368-376.

50. Ye BS, Leung AOW, Wong MH. The association of environmental toxicants and autism spectrum disorders in children. *Environ Pollut.* 2017;227:234-242.

51. Schwartzer JJ, Koenig CM, Berman RF. Using mouse models of autism spectrum disorders to study the neurotoxicology of gene-environment interactions. *Neurotoxicol Teratol.* 2013;36:17-35.

52. Kuegler PB, Zimmer B, Waldmann T, et al. Markers of murine embryonic and neural stem cells, neurons and astrocytes: reference points for developmental neurotoxicity testing. *ALTEX.* 2010;27(1):17-42.

53. Landrigan PJ, Trasande L, Thorpe LE, et al. The National Children's Study: a 21-year prospective study of 100,000 American children. *Pediatrics.* 2006;118(5):2173-2186.

54. Ashwood P, Krakowiak P, Hertz-Picciotto I, Hansen R, Pessah I, Van de Water J. Elevated plasma cytokines in autism spectrum disorders provide evidence of immune dysfunction and are associated with impaired behavioral outcome. *Brain Behav Immun.* 2011;25(1):40-45.

55. Wasilewska J, Klukowski M. Gastrointestinal symptoms and autism spectrum disorder: links and risks—a possible new overlap syndrome. *Pediatric Health Med Ther.* 2015;6:153-166.

56. Buie T, Campbell DB, Fuchs GJ, et al. Evaluation, diagnosis, and treatment of gastrointestinal disorders in individuals with ASDs: a consensus report. *Pediatrics.* 2010;125(suppl 1):S1-S18.

57. Sweeten TL, Bowyer SL, Posey DJ, Halberstadt GM, McDougle CJ. Increased prevalence of familial autoimmunity in probands with pervasive developmental disorders. *Pediatrics.* 2003;112(5):e420.

58. Wills S, Cabanlit M, Bennett J, Ashwood P, Amaral DG, Van de Water J. Detection of autoantibodies to neural cells of the cerebellum in the plasma of subjects with autism spectrum disorders. *Brain Behav Immun.* 2009;23(1):64-74.

59. Singer HS, Morris CM, Williams PN, Yoon DY, Hong JJ, Zimmerman AW. Antibrain antibodies in children with autism and their unaffected siblings. *J Neuroimmunol.* 2006;178(1-2):149-155.

60. Zimmerman AW, Connors SL, Matteson KJ, et al. Maternal antibrain antibodies in autism. *Brain Behav Immun.* 2007;21(3):351-357.

61. Croen LA, Braunschweig D, Haapanen L, et al. Maternal mid-pregnancy autoantibodies to fetal brain protein: the early markers for autism study. *Biol Psychiatry.* 2008;64(7):583-588.

62. Li Y, Missig G, Finger BC, et al. Maternal and early postnatal immune activation produce dissociable effects on neurotransmission in mPFC-amygdala circuits. *J Neurosci.* 2018;38(13):3358-3372.

63. Smith SE, Li J, Garbett K, Mirnics K, Patterson PH. Maternal immune activation alters fetal brain development through interleukin-6. *J Neurosci.* 2007;27(40):10695-10702.

64. Meyer U, Murray PJ, Urwyler A, Yee BK, Schedlowski M, Feldon J. Adult behavioral and pharmacological dysfunctions following disruption of the fetal brain balance between pro-inflammatory and IL-10-mediated anti-inflammatory signaling. *Mol Psychiatry.* 2008;13(2):208-221.

65. Mandal M, Marzouk AC, Donnelly R, Ponzio NM. Maternal immune stimulation during pregnancy affects adaptive immunity in offspring to promote development of TH17 cells. *Brain Behav Immun.* 2011;25(5):863-871.

66. Schaafsma SM, Gagnidze K, Reyes A, et al. Sex-specific gene-environment interactions underlying ASD-like behaviors. *Proc Natl Acad Sci U S A.* 2017;114(6):1383-1388.

67. D'Amelio M, Ricci I, Sacco R, et al. Paraoxonase gene variants are associated with autism in North America, but not in Italy: possible regional specificity in gene-environment interactions. *Mol Psychiatry.* 2005;10(11):1006-1016.

68. Abazyan B, Nomura J, Kannan G, et al. Prenatal interaction of mutant DISC1 and immune activation produces adult psychopathology. *Biol Psychiatry.* 2010;68(12):1172-1181.

69. Ehninger D, Sano Y, de Vries PJ, et al. Gestational immune activation and Tsc2 haploinsufficiency cooperate to disrupt fetal survival and may perturb social behavior in adult mice. *Mol Psychiatry.* 2012;17(1):62-70.

70. Hunter JW, Mullen GP, McManus JR, Heatherly JM, Duke A, Rand JB. Neuroligin-deficient mutants of *C. elegans* have sensory processing deficits and are hypersensitive to oxidative stress and mercury toxicity. *Dis Model Mech.* 2010;3(5-6):366-376.

71. Fischer M, Reuter J, Gerich FJ, et al. Enhanced hypoxia susceptibility in hippocampal slices from a mouse model of rett syndrome. *J Neurophysiol.* 2009;101(2):1016-1032.

72. Courchesne E. Abnormal early brain development in autism. *Mol Psychiatry.* 2002;7(suppl 2):S21-S23.

73. Hazlett HC, Poe M, Gerig G, et al. Magnetic resonance imaging and head circumference study of brain size in autism: birth through age 2 years. *Arch Gen Psychiatry.* 2005;62(12):1366-1376.

74. Lainhart JE, Bigler ED, Bocian M, et al. Head circumference and height in autism: a study by the Collaborative Program of Excellence in Autism. *Am J Med Genet A.* 2006;140(21):2257-2274.

75. Courchesne E, Mouton PR, Calhoun ME, et al. Neuron number and size in prefrontal cortex of children with autism. *JAMA.* 2011;306(18):2001-2010.

76. Donovan AP, Basson MA. The neuroanatomy of autism—a developmental perspective. *J Anat.* 2017;230(1):4-15.

77. Courchesne E, Karns CM, Davis HR, et al. Unusual brain growth patterns in early life in patients with autistic disorder: an MRI study. *Neurology.* 2001;57(2):245-254.

78. Lange N, Travers BG, Bigler ED, et al. Longitudinal volumetric brain changes in autism spectrum disorder ages 6-35 years. *Autism Res.* 2015;8(1):82-93.

79. Ecker C, Bookheimer SY, Murphy DG. Neuroimaging in autism spectrum disorder: brain structure and function across the lifespan. *Lancet Neurol.* 2015;14(11):1121-1134.

80. Wallace GL, Dankner N, Kenworthy L, Giedd JN, Martin A. Age-related temporal and parietal cortical thinning in autism spectrum disorders. *Brain.* 2010;133(pt 12):3745-3754.

81. Wolff JJ, Gerig G, Lewis JD, et al. Altered corpus callosum morphology associated with autism over the first 2 years of life. *Brain.* 2015;138(pt 7):2046-2058.

82. Wolff JJ, Gu H, Gerig G, et al. Differences in white matter fiber tract development present from 6 to 24 months in infants with autism. *Am J Psychiatry.* 2012;169(6):589-600.

83. Strick PL, Dum RP, Fiez JA. Cerebellum and nonmotor function. *Annu Rev Neurosci.* 2009;32:413-434.

84. Ritvo ER, Freeman BJ, Scheibel AB, et al. Lower Purkinje cell counts in the cerebella of four autistic subjects: initial findings of the UCLA-NSAC Autopsy Research Report. *Am J Psychiatry.* 1986;143(7):862-866.

85. Kemper TL, Bauman M. Neuropathology of infantile autism. *J Neuropathol Exp Neurol.* 1998;57(7):645-652.

86. Courchesne E. Brainstem, cerebellar and limbic neuroanatomical abnormalities in autism. *Curr Opin Neurobiol.* 1997;7(2):269-278.

87. Pierce K, Courchesne E. Evidence for a cerebellar role in reduced exploration and stereotyped behavior in autism. *Biol Psychiatry.* 2001;49(8):655-664.

88. Kern JK. The possible role of the cerebellum in autism/PDD: disruption of a multisensory feedback loop. *Med Hypotheses.* 2002;59(3):255-260.

89. Rojas DC, Peterson E, Winterrowd E, Reite ML, Rogers SJ, Tregellas JR. Regional gray matter volumetric changes in autism associated with social and repetitive behavior symptoms. *BMC Psychiatry.* 2006;6:56.

90. D'Mello AM, Crocetti D, Mostofsky SH, Stoodley CJ. Cerebellar gray matter and lobular volumes correlate with core autism symptoms. *Neuroimage Clin.* 2015;7:631-639.

91. D'Mello AM, Stoodley CJ. Cerebro-cerebellar circuits in autism spectrum disorder. *Front Neurosci.* 2015;9:408.

92. Subramanian K, Brandenburg C, Orsati F, Soghomonian JJ, Hussman JP, Blatt GJ. Basal ganglia and autism—a translational perspective. *Autism Res.* 2017;10(11):1751-1775.

93. Estes A, Shaw DW, Sparks BF, et al. Basal ganglia morphometry and repetitive behavior in young children with autism spectrum disorder. *Autism Res.* 2011;4(3):212-220.

94. Wegiel J, Flory M, Kuchna I, et al. Stereological study of the neuronal number and volume of 38 brain subdivisions of subjects diagnosed with autism reveals significant alterations restricted to the striatum, amygdala and cerebellum. *Acta Neuropathol Commun.* 2014;2:141.

95. Sato W, Kubota Y, Kochiyama T, et al. Increased putamen volume in adults with autism spectrum disorder. *Front Hum Neurosci.* 2014;8:957.

96. Rutishauser U, Mamelak AN, Adolphs R. The primate amygdala in social perception—insights from electrophysiological recordings and stimulation. *Trends Neurosci.* 2015;38(5):295-306.

97. Zald DH. The human amygdala and the emotional evaluation of sensory stimuli. *Brain Res Brain Res Rev.* 2003;41(1):88-123.

98. Schumann CM, Barnes CC, Lord C, Courchesne E. Amygdala enlargement in toddlers with autism related to severity of social and communication impairments. *Biol Psychiatry.* 2009;66(10):942-949.

99. Juranek J, Filipek PA, Berenji GR, Modahl C, Osann K, Spence MA. Association between amygdala volume and anxiety level: magnetic resonance imaging (MRI) study in autistic children. *J Child Neurol.* 2006;21(12):1051-1058.

100. Markram K, Rinaldi T, La Mendola D, Sandi C, Markram H. Abnormal fear conditioning and amygdala processing in an animal model of autism. *Neuropsychopharmacology.* 2008;33(4):901-912.

101. Stoner R, Chow ML, Boyle MP, et al. Patches of disorganization in the neocortex of children with autism. *N Engl J Med.* 2014;370(13):1209-1219.

102. McKavanagh R, Buckley E, Chance SA. Wider minicolumns in autism: a neural basis for altered processing? *Brain.* 2015; 138(pt 7):2034-2045.

103. Casanova MF, van Kooten IA, Switala AE, et al. Minicolumnar abnormalities in autism. *Acta Neuropathol.* 2006;112(3): 287-303.

104. Casanova MF, Buxhoeveden DP, Switala AE, Roy E. Minicolumnar pathology in autism. *Neurology.* 2002;58(3):428-432.

105. Keown CL, Shih P, Nair A, Peterson N, Mulvey ME, Müller RA. Local functional overconnectivity in posterior brain regions is associated with symptom severity in autism spectrum disorders. *Cell Rep.* 2013;5(3):567-572.

106. Hahamy A, Behrmann M, Malach R. The idiosyncratic brain: distortion of spontaneous connectivity patterns in autism spectrum disorder. *Nat Neurosci.* 2015;18(2):302-309.

107. Sbacchi S, Acquadro F, Calò I, Calì F, Romano V. Functional annotation of genes overlapping copy number variants in autistic patients: focus on axon pathfinding. *Curr Genomics.* 2010;11(2):136-145.

108. Chow ML, Pramparo T, Winn ME, et al. Age-dependent brain gene expression and copy number anomalies in autism suggest distinct pathological processes at young versus mature ages. *PLoS Genet.* 2012;8(3):e1002592.

109. Solso S, Xu R, Proudfoot J, et al. Diffusion tensor imaging provides evidence of possible axonal overconnectivity in frontal lobes in autism spectrum disorder toddlers. *Biol Psychiatry.* 2016;79(8):676-684.

110. Ashwin C, Baron-Cohen S, Wheelwright S, O'Riordan M, Bullmore ET. Differential activation of the amygdala and the 'social brain' during fearful face-processing in Asperger syndrome. *Neuropsychologia.* 2007;45(1):2-14.

111. Mason RA, Williams DL, Kana RK, Minshew N, Just MA. Theory of Mind disruption and recruitment of the right hemisphere during narrative comprehension in autism. *Neuropsychologia.* 2008;46(1):269-280.

112. Libero LE, Maximo JO, Deshpande HD, Klinger LG, Klinger MR, Kana RK. The role of mirroring and mentalizing networks in mediating action intentions in autism. *Mol Autism.* 2014; 5(1):50.

113. Eyler LT, Pierce K, Courchesne E. A failure of left temporal cortex to specialize for language is an early emerging and fundamental property of autism. *Brain.* 2012;135(pt 3):949-960.

114. Luna B, Minshew NJ, Garver KE, et al. Neocortical system abnormalities in autism: an fMRI study of spatial working memory. *Neurology.* 2002;59(6):834-840.

115. Solomon M, Ozonoff SJ, Ursu S, et al. The neural substrates of cognitive control deficits in autism spectrum disorders. *Neuropsychologia.* 2009;47(12):2515-2526.

116. Carper RA, Courchesne E. Localized enlargement of the frontal cortex in early autism. *Biol Psychiatry.* 2005;57(2): 126-133.

117. Courchesne E, Pierce K. Brain overgrowth in autism during a critical time in development: implications for frontal pyramidal neuron and interneuron development and connectivity. *Int J Dev Neurosci.* 2005;23(2-3):153-170.

118. Rudie JD, Shehzad Z, Hernandez LM, et al. Reduced functional integration and segregation of distributed neural systems underlying social and emotional information processing in autism spectrum disorders. *Cereb Cortex.* 2012;22(5):1025-1037.

119. McAlonan GM, Daly E, Kumari V, et al. Brain anatomy and sensorimotor gating in Asperger's syndrome. *Brain.* 2002;125 (pt 7):1594-1606.

120. Miles JH. Autism spectrum disorders—a genetics review. *Genet Med.* 2011;13(4):278-294.

121. Hagerman R, Hoem G, Hagerman P. Fragile X and autism: intertwined at the molecular level leading to targeted treatments. *Mol Autism.* 2010;1(1):12.

122. Percy AK. Rett syndrome: exploring the autism link. *Arch Neurol.* 2011;68(8):985-989.

123. Leppa VM, Kravitz SN, Martin CL, et al. Rare inherited and de novo CNVs reveal complex contributions to ASD risk in multiplex families. *Am J Hum Genet.* 2016;99(3):540-554.

124. Durand CM, Betancur C, Boeckers TM, et al. Mutations in the gene encoding the synaptic scaffolding protein SHANK3 are associated with autism spectrum disorders. *Nat Genet.* 2007;39(1):25-27.

125. Ornoy A, Weinstein-Fudim L, Ergaz Z. Genetic syndromes, maternal diseases and antenatal factors associated with autism spectrum disorders (ASD). *Front Neurosci.* 2016;10:316.

126. de Anda FC, Rosario AL, Durak O, et al. Autism spectrum disorder susceptibility gene TAOK2 affects basal dendrite formation in the neocortex. *Nat Neurosci.* 2012;15(7):1022-1031.

127. Talkowski ME, Mullegama SV, Rosenfeld JA, et al. Assessment of 2q23.1 microdeletion syndrome implicates MBD5 as a single causal locus of intellectual disability, epilepsy, and autism spectrum disorder. *Am J Hum Genet.* 2011;89(4):551-563.

128. Lord C, Rutter M, Le Couteur A. Autism Diagnostic Interview-Revised: a revised version of a diagnostic interview for caregivers of individuals with possible pervasive developmental disorders. *J Autism Dev Disord.* 1994;24(5):659-685.

129. Lord C, Risi S, Lambrecht L, et al. The Autism Diagnostic Observation Schedule-Generic: a standard measure of social and communication deficits associated with the spectrum of autism. *J Autism Dev Disord.* 2000;30(3):205-223.

130. Buck TR, Viskochil J, Farley M, et al. Psychiatric comorbidity and medication use in adults with autism spectrum disorder. *J Autism Dev Disord.* 2014;44(12):3063-3071.

131. Cravedi E, Deniau E, Giannitelli M, Xavier J, Hartmann A, Cohen D. Tourette syndrome and other neurodevelopmental disorders: a comprehensive review. *Child Adolesc Psychiatry Ment Health.* 2017;11:59.

132. Hall DA, Berry-Kravis E. Fragile X syndrome and fragile X-associated tremor ataxia syndrome. *Handb Clin Neurol.* 2018;147:377-391.

133. Matson JL, Williams LW. Depression and mood disorders among persons with autism spectrum disorders. *Res Dev Disabil.* 2014;35(9):2003-2007.

134. Hedley D, Uljarević M, Foley KR, Richdale A, Trollor J. Risk and protective factors underlying depression and suicidal ideation in autism spectrum disorder. *Depress Anxiety.* 2018.

135. Culpin I, Mars B, Pearson RM, et al. Autistic traits and suicidal thoughts, plans, and self-harm in late adolescence: population-based cohort study. *J Am Acad Child Adolesc Psychiatry.* 2018;57(5):313-320.e316.

136. Chen MH, Pan TL, Lan WH, et al. Risk of suicide attempts among adolescents and young adults with autism spectrum disorder: a nationwide longitudinal follow-up study. *J Clin Psychiatry.* 2017;78(9):e1174-e1179.

137. Hollocks MJ, Lerh JW, Magiati I, Meiser-Stedman R, Brugha TS. Anxiety and depression in adults with autism spectrum disorder: a systematic review and meta-analysis. *Psychol Med.* 2019;49(4):559-572.

138. van Steensel FJ, Bögels SM, Perrin S. Anxiety disorders in children and adolescents with autistic spectrum disorders: a meta-analysis. *Clin Child Fam Psychol Rev.* 2011;14(3):302-317.

139. Ghaziuddin M, Ghaziuddin N, Greden J. Depression in persons with autism: implications for research and clinical care. *J Autism Dev Disord.* 2002;32(4):299-306.

140. Birmaher B, Quintana H, Greenhill LL. Methylphenidate treatment of hyperactive autistic children. *J Am Acad Child Adolesc Psychiatry.* 1988;27(2):248-251.

141. Handen BL, Johnson CR, Lubetsky M. Efficacy of methylphenidate among children with autism and symptoms of attention-deficit hyperactivity disorder. *J Autism Dev Disord.* 2000;30(3):245-255.

142. Research Units on Pediatric Psychopharmacology Autism Network. Randomized, controlled, crossover trial of methylphenidate in pervasive developmental disorders with hyperactivity. *Arch Gen Psychiatry.* 2005;62(11):1266-1274.

143. Stigler KA, Desmond LA, Posey DJ, Wiegand RE, McDougle CJ. A naturalistic retrospective analysis of psychostimulants in pervasive developmental disorders. *J Child Adolesc Psychopharmacol.* 2004;14(1):49-56.

144. Fankhauser MP, Karumanchi VC, German ML, Yates A, Karumanchi SD. A double-blind, placebo-controlled study of the efficacy of transdermal clonidine in autism. *J Clin Psychiatry.* 1992;53(3):77-82.

145. Ming X, Gordon E, Kang N, Wagner GC. Use of clonidine in children with autism spectrum disorders. *Brain Dev.* 2008;30(7):454-460.

146. Scahill L, McCracken JT, King BH, et al. Extended-release guanfacine for hyperactivity in children with autism spectrum disorder. *Am J Psychiatry.* 2015;172(12):1197-1206.

147. Jaselskis CA, Cook EH, Fletcher KE, Leventhal BL. Clonidine treatment of hyperactive and impulsive children with autistic disorder. *J Clin Psychopharmacol.* 1992;12(5):322-327.

148. Jou RJ, Handen BL, Hardan AY. Retrospective assessment of atomoxetine in children and adolescents with pervasive developmental disorders. *J Child Adolesc Psychopharmacol.* 2005;15(2):325-330.

149. Arnold LE, Aman MG, Cook AM, et al. Atomoxetine for hyperactivity in autism spectrum disorders: placebo-controlled crossover pilot trial. *J Am Acad Child Adolesc Psychiatry.* 2006;45(10):1196-1205.

150. Posey DJ, Wiegand RE, Wilkerson J, Maynard M, Stigler KA, McDougle CJ. Open-label atomoxetine for attention-deficit/hyperactivity disorder symptoms associated with high-functioning pervasive developmental disorders. *J Child Adolesc Psychopharmacol.* 2006;16(5):599-610.

151. Troost PW, Steenhuis MP, Tuynman-Qua HG, et al. Atomoxetine for attention-deficit/hyperactivity disorder symptoms in children with pervasive developmental disorders: a pilot study. *J Child Adolesc Psychopharmacol.* 2006;16(5):611-619.

152. Harfterkamp M, van de Loo-Neus G, Minderaa RB, et al. A randomized double-blind study of atomoxetine versus placebo for attention-deficit/hyperactivity disorder symptoms in children with autism spectrum disorder. *J Am Acad Child Adolesc Psychiatry.* 2012;51(7):733-741.

153. King BH, Wright DM, Handen BL, et al. Double-blind, placebo-controlled study of amantadine hydrochloride in the treatment of children with autistic disorder. *J Am Acad Child Adolesc Psychiatry.* 2001;40(6):658-665.

154. Muris P, Steerneman P, Merckelbach H, Holdrinet I, Meesters C. Comorbid anxiety symptoms in children with pervasive developmental disorders. *J Anxiety Disord.* 1998;12(4):387-393.

155. Ghaziuddin M, Tsai L, Ghaziuddin N. Comorbidity of autistic disorder in children and adolescents. *Eur Child Adolesc Psychiatry.* 1992;1(4):209-213.

156. Le Couteur A, Rutter M, Lord C, et al. Autism diagnostic interview: a standardized investigator-based instrument. *J Autism Dev Disord.* 1989;19(3):363-387.

157. Leyfer OT, Folstein SE, Bacalman S, et al. Comorbid psychiatric disorders in children with autism: interview development and rates of disorders. *J Autism Dev Disord.* 2006;36(7):849-861.

158. Ruscio AM, Stein DJ, Chiu WT, Kessler RC. The epidemiology of obsessive-compulsive disorder in the National Comorbidity Survey Replication. *Mol Psychiatry.* 2010;15(1):53-63.

159. Watson HJ, Rees CS. Meta-analysis of randomized, controlled treatment trials for pediatric obsessive-compulsive disorder. *J Child Psychol Psychiatry.* 2008;49(5):489-498.

160. Boyd BA, McDonough SG, Bodfish JW. Evidence-based behavioral interventions for repetitive behaviors in autism. *J Autism Dev Disord.* 2012;42(6):1236-1248.

161. McDougle CJ, Kresch LE, Goodman WK, et al. A case-controlled study of repetitive thoughts and behavior in adults with autistic disorder and obsessive-compulsive disorder. *Am J Psychiatry.* 1995;152(5):772-777.

162. Lewin A, Wood J, Gunderson S, Murphy T, Storch E. Phenomenology of comorbid autism spectrum and obsessive-compulsive disorders among children. *J Dev Phys Disabil.* 2011;23:543-553.

163. Ruta L, Mugno D, D'Arrigo VG, Vitiello B, Mazzone L. Obsessive-compulsive traits in children and adolescents with Asperger syndrome. *Eur Child Adolesc Psychiatry.* 2010;19(1):17-24.

164. Kano Y, Ohta M, Nagai Y. Two case reports of autistic boys developing Tourette's disorder: indications of improvement? *J Am Acad Child Adolesc Psychiatry.* 1987;26(6):937-938.

165. Canitano R, Vivanti G. Tics and Tourette syndrome in autism spectrum disorders. *Autism.* 2007;11(1):19-28.

166. Baron-Cohen S, Scahill VL, Izaguirre J, Hornsey H, Robertson MM. The prevalence of Gilles de la Tourette syndrome in children and adolescents with autism: a large scale study. *Psychol Med.* 1999;29(5):1151-1159.

167. Huisman-van Dijk HM, Schoot R, Rijkeboer MM, Mathews CA, Cath DC. The relationship between tics, OC, ADHD and autism symptoms: a cross-disorder symptom analysis in Gilles de la Tourette syndrome patients and family-members. *Psychiatry Res.* 2016;237:138-146.

168. Mack H, Fullana MA, Russell AJ, Mataix-Cols D, Nakatani E, Heyman I. Obsessions and compulsions in children with Asperger's syndrome or high-functioning autism: a case-control study. *Aust N Z J Psychiatry.* 2010;44(12):1082-1088.

169. Akkermans SEA, Rheinheimer N, Bruchhage MMK, et al. Frontostriatal functional connectivity correlates with repetitive behaviour across autism spectrum disorder and obsessive-compulsive disorder. *Psychol Med.* 2018:1-9.

170. Shorter E, Wachtel LE. Childhood catatonia, autism and psychosis past and present: is there an 'iron triangle'? *Acta Psychiatr Scand.* 2013;128(1):21-33.

171. Chisholm K, Lin A, Abu-Akel A, Wood SJ. The association between autism and schizophrenia spectrum disorders: a review of eight alternate models of co-occurrence. *Neurosci Biobehav Rev.* 2015;55:173-183.

172. Rapoport J, Chavez A, Greenstein D, Addington A, Gogtay N. Autism spectrum disorders and childhood-onset schizophrenia: clinical and biological contributions to a relation revisited. *J Am Acad Child Adolesc Psychiatry.* 2009;48(1):10-18.

173. Selten JP, Lundberg M, Rai D, Magnusson C. Risks for nonaffective psychotic disorder and bipolar disorder in young people with autism spectrum disorder: a population-based study. *JAMA Psychiatry.* 2015;72(5):483-489.

174. Larson FV, Wagner AP, Jones PB, et al. Psychosis in autism: comparison of the features of both conditions in a dually affected cohort. *Br J Psychiatry.* 2017;210(4):269-275.

175. Carroll LS, Owen MJ. Genetic overlap between autism, schizophrenia and bipolar disorder. *Genome Med.* 2009;1(10):102.

176. Crespi B, Stead P, Elliot M. Evolution in health and medicine Sackler colloquium: comparative genomics of autism and schizophrenia. *Proc Natl Acad Sci U S A.* 2010;107(suppl 1):1736-1741.

177. Baribeau DA, Anagnostou E. A comparison of neuroimaging findings in childhood onset schizophrenia and autism spectrum disorder: a review of the literature. *Front Psychiatry.* 2013;4:175.

178. Sugranyes G, Kyriakopoulos M, Corrigall R, Taylor E, Frangou S. Autism spectrum disorders and schizophrenia: meta-analysis of the neural correlates of social cognition. *PLoS One.* 2011;6(10):e25322.

179. Abdi Z, Sharma T. Social cognition and its neural correlates in schizophrenia and autism. *CNS Spectr.* 2004;9(5):335-343.

180. Cheung C, Yu K, Fung G, et al. Autistic disorders and schizophrenia: related or remote? An anatomical likelihood estimation. *PLoS One.* 2010;5(8):e12233.

181. Shenton ME, Dickey CC, Frumin M, McCarley RW. A review of MRI findings in schizophrenia. *Schizophr Res.* 2001;49(1-2):1-52.

182. Toal F, Bloemen OJ, Deeley Q, et al. Psychosis and autism: magnetic resonance imaging study of brain anatomy. *Br J Psychiatry.* 2009;194(5):418-425.

183. Wing L, Shah A. Catatonia in autistic spectrum disorders. *Br J Psychiatry.* 2000;176:357-362.

184. Wachtel LE, Schuldt S, Ghaziuddin N, Shorter E. The potential role of electroconvulsive therapy in the 'Iron Triangle' of pediatric catatonia, autism, and psychosis. *Acta Psychiatr Scand.* 2013;128(5):408-409.

185. Ghaziuddin M, Quinlan P, Ghaziuddin N. Catatonia in autism: a distinct subtype? *J Intellect Disabil Res.* 2005;49(pt 1):102-105.

186. Dejong H, Bunton P, Hare DJ. A systematic review of interventions used to treat catatonic symptoms in people with autistic spectrum disorders. *J Autism Dev Disord.* 2014;44(9):2127-36. doi: 10.1007/s10803-014-2085-.

187. Dhossche DM, Shah A, Wing L. Blueprints for the assessment, treatment, and future study of catatonia in autism spectrum disorders. *Int Rev Neurobiol.* 2006;72:267-284.

188. Ellul P, Rotgé JY, Choucha W. Resistant catatonia in a high-functioning autism spectrum disorder patient successfully treated with amantadine. *J Child Adolesc Psychopharmacol.* 2015;25(9):726. doi: 10.1089/cap.2015.0064.

189. Faedda GL, Wachtel LE, Higgins AM, Shprintzen RJ. Catatonia in an adolescent with velo-cardio-facial syndrome. *Am J Med Genet A.* 2015;167(9):2150-2153.

190. Fink M, Taylor MA, Ghaziuddin N. Catatonia in autistic spectrum disorders: a medical treatment algorithm. *Int Rev Neurobiol.* 2006;72:233-244.

191. Haq AU, Ghaziuddin N. Maintenance electroconvulsive therapy for aggression and self-injurious behavior in two adolescents with autism and catatonia. *J Neuropsychiatry Clin Neurosci.* 2014;26(1):64-72.

192. Hare DJ, Malone C. Catatonia and autistic spectrum disorders. *Autism.* 2004;8(2):183-195.

193. Kakooza-Mwesige A, Wachtel LE, Dhossche DM. Catatonia in autism: implications across the life span. *Eur Child Adolesc Psychiatry.* 2008;17(6):327-335.

194. Mazzone L, Postorino V, Valeri G, Vicari S. Catatonia in patients with autism: prevalence and management. *CNS Drugs.* 2014;28(3):205-215.

195. Ohta M, Kano Y, Nagai Y. Catatonia in individuals with autism spectrum disorders in adolescence and early adulthood: a long-term prospective study. *Int Rev Neurobiol.* 2006;72:41-54.

196. Sajith SG, Liew SF, Tor PC. Response to electroconvulsive therapy in patients with autism spectrum disorder and intractable

challenging behaviors associated with symptoms of catatonia. *J ECT*. 2017;33(1):63-67.

197. Serret S, Thümmler S, Dor E, Vesperini S, Santos A, Askenazy F. Lithium as a rescue therapy for regression and catatonia features in two SHANK3 patients with autism spectrum disorder: case reports. *BMC Psychiatry*. 2015;15:107.

198. Dhossche DM, Wachtel LE. Catatonia is hidden in plain sight among different pediatric disorders: a review article. *Pediatr Neurol*. 2010;43(5):307-315.

199. Jacobs J, Schwartz A, McDougle CJ, Skotko BG. Rapid clinical deterioration in an individual with Down syndrome. *Am J Med Genet A*. 2016;170(7):1899-1902.

200. Kolli V, Sharma A, Amani M, Bestha D, Chaturvedi R. "Meow meow" (mephedrone) and catatonia. *Innov Clin Neurosci*. 2013;10(2):11-12.

201. Rosebush PI, Hildebrand AM, Furlong BG, Mazurek MF. Catatonic syndrome in a general psychiatric inpatient population: frequency, clinical presentation, and response to lorazepam. *J Clin Psychiatry*. 1990;51(9):357-362.

202. Hauptman AJ, Benjamin S. The differential diagnosis and treatment of catatonia in children and adolescents. *Harv Rev Psychiatry*. 2016;24(6):379-395.

203. Wachtel LE, Hermida A, Dhossche DM. Maintenance electroconvulsive therapy in autistic catatonia: a case series review. *Prog Neuropsychopharmacol Biol Psychiatry*. 2010;34(4):581-587.

204. Fink M, Taylor MA. *Catatonia: A Clinician's Guide to Diagnosis and Treatment*. Cambridge: Cambridge University Press; 2003.

205. Wachtel LE, Shorter E, Fink M. Electroconvulsive therapy for self-injurious behaviour in autism spectrum disorders: recognizing catatonia is key. *Curr Opin Psychiatry*. 2018;31(2):116-122.

206. Schreck KA, Mulick JA, Smith AF. Sleep problems as possible predictors of intensified symptoms of autism. *Res Dev Disabil*. 2004;25(1):57-66.

207. Goldman SE, Surdyka K, Cuevas R, Adkins K, Wang L, Malow BA. Defining the sleep phenotype in children with autism. *Dev Neuropsychol*. 2009;34(5):560-573.

208. Mazurek MO, Sohl K. Sleep and behavioral problems in children with autism spectrum disorder. *J Autism Dev Disord*. 2016;46(6):1906-1915.

209. Posey DJ, Puntney JI, Sasher TM, Kem DL, McDougle CJ. Guanfacine treatment of hyperactivity and inattention in pervasive developmental disorders: a retrospective analysis of 80 cases. *J Child Adolesc Psychopharmacol*. 2004;14(2):233-241.

210. Andersen IM, Kaczmarska J, McGrew SG, Malow BA. Melatonin for insomnia in children with autism spectrum disorders. *J Child Neurol*. 2008;23(5):482-485.

211. Cortesi F, Giannotti F, Sebastiani T, Panunzi S, Valente D. Controlled-release melatonin, singly and combined with cognitive behavioural therapy, for persistent insomnia in children with autism spectrum disorders: a randomized placebo-controlled trial. *J Sleep Res*. 2012;21(6):700-709.

212. Garstang J, Wallis M. Randomized controlled trial of melatonin for children with autistic spectrum disorders and sleep problems. *Child Care Health Dev*. 2006;32(5):585-589.

213. Wirojanan J, Jacquemont S, Diaz R, et al. The efficacy of melatonin for sleep problems in children with autism, fragile X syndrome, or autism and fragile X syndrome. *J Clin Sleep Med*. 2009;5(2):145-150.

214. Giannotti F, Cortesi F, Cerquiglini A, Bernabei P. An open-label study of controlled-release melatonin in treatment of sleep disorders in children with autism. *J Autism Dev Disord*. 2006;36(6):741-752.

215. Malow B, Adkins KW, McGrew SG, et al. Melatonin for sleep in children with autism: a controlled trial examining dose, tolerability, and outcomes. *J Autism Dev Disord*. 2012;42(8):1729-1737; author reply 1738.

216. Wasdell MB, Jan JE, Bomben MM, et al. A randomized, placebo-controlled trial of controlled release melatonin treatment of delayed sleep phase syndrome and impaired sleep maintenance in children with neurodevelopmental disabilities. *J Pineal Res*. 2008;44(1):57-64.

217. Wright B, Sims D, Smart S, et al. Melatonin versus placebo in children with autism spectrum conditions and severe sleep problems not amenable to behaviour management strategies: a randomised controlled crossover trial. *J Autism Dev Disord*. 2011;41(2):175-184.

218. Golubchik P, Sever J, Weizman A. Low-dose quetiapine for adolescents with autistic spectrum disorder and aggressive behavior: open-label trial. *Clin Neuropharmacol*. 2011;34(6):216-219.

219. van Schalkwyk GI, Klingensmith K, Volkmar FR. Gender identity and autism spectrum disorders. *Yale J Biol Med*. 2015;88(1):81-83.

220. Saleem F, Rizvi SW. Transgender associations and possible etiology: a literature review. *Cureus*. 2017;9(12):e1984.

221. van der Miesen AIR, de Vries ALC, Steensma TD, Hartman CA. Autistic symptoms in children and adolescents with gender dysphoria. *J Autism Dev Disord*. 2018;48(5):1537-1548.

222. Janssen A, Huang H, Duncan C. Gender variance among youth with autism spectrum disorders: a retrospective chart review. *Transgend Health*. 2016;1(1):63-68.

223. Kohane IS, McMurry A, Weber G, et al. The co-morbidity burden of children and young adults with autism spectrum disorders. *PLoS One*. 2012;7(4):e33224.

224. Chaidez V, Hansen RL, Hertz-Picciotto I. Gastrointestinal problems in children with autism, developmental delays or typical development. *J Autism Dev Disord*. 2014;44(5):1117-1127.

225. Buie T, Fuchs GJ, Furuta GT, et al. Recommendations for evaluation and treatment of common gastrointestinal problems in children with ASDs. *Pediatrics*. 2010;125(suppl 1):S19-S29.

226. Rogers GB, Keating DJ, Young RL, Wong ML, Licinio J, Wesselingh S. From gut dysbiosis to altered brain function and mental illness: mechanisms and pathways. *Mol Psychiatry*. 2016;21(6):738-748.

227. Hsiao EY, McBride SW, Hsien S, et al. Microbiota modulate behavioral and physiological abnormalities associated with neurodevelopmental disorders. *Cell*. 2013;155(7):1451-1463.

228. Yano JM, Yu K, Donaldson GP, et al. Indigenous bacteria from the gut microbiota regulate host serotonin biosynthesis. *Cell*. 2015;161(2):264-276.

229. McElhanon BO, McCracken C, Karpen S, Sharp WG. Gastrointestinal symptoms in autism spectrum disorder: a meta-analysis. *Pediatrics*. 2014;133(5):872-883.

230. Sharp WG, Berry RC, McCracken C, et al. Feeding problems and nutrient intake in children with autism spectrum disorders: a meta-analysis and comprehensive review of the literature. *J Autism Dev Disord*. 2013;43(9):2159-2173.

231. Egan AM, Dreyer ML, Odar CC, Beckwith M, Garrison CB. Obesity in young children with autism spectrum disorders: prevalence and associated factors. *Child Obes*. 2013;9(2):125-131.

232. Cox LM, Blaser MJ. Antibiotics in early life and obesity. *Nat Rev Endocrinol*. 2015;11(3):182-190.

233. Kashyap PC, Marcobal A, Ursell LK, et al. Complex interactions among diet, gastrointestinal transit, and gut microbiota in humanized mice. *Gastroenterology*. 2013;144(5):967-977.

234. Amiet C, Gourfinkel-An I, Bouzamondo A, et al. Epilepsy in autism is associated with intellectual disability and gender: evidence from a meta-analysis. *Biol Psychiatry*. 2008;64(7): 577-582.

235. Hughes JR, Melyn M. EEG and seizures in autistic children and adolescents: further findings with therapeutic implications. *Clin EEG Neurosci*. 2005;36(1):15-20.

236. Viscidi EW, Triche EW, Pescosolido MF, et al. Clinical characteristics of children with autism spectrum disorder and co-occurring epilepsy. *PLoS One*. 2013;8(7):e67797.

237. Cuccaro ML, Tuchman RF, Hamilton KL, et al. Exploring the relationship between autism spectrum disorder and epilepsy using latent class cluster analysis. *J Autism Dev Disord*. 2012;42(8):1630-1641.

238. Tuchman R, Alessandri M, Cuccaro M. Autism spectrum disorders and epilepsy: moving towards a comprehensive approach to treatment. *Brain Dev*. 2010;32(9):719-730.

239. Bolton PF, Carcani-Rathwell I, Hutton J, Goode S, Howlin P, Rutter M. Epilepsy in autism: features and correlates. *Br J Psychiatry*. 2011;198(4):289-294.

240. McDermott S, Moran R, Platt T, Wood H, Isaac T, Dasari S. Prevalence of epilepsy in adults with mental retardation and related disabilities in primary care. *Am J Ment Retard*. 2005;110(1):48-56.

241. Woolfenden S, Sarkozy V, Ridley G, Coory M, Williams K. A systematic review of two outcomes in autism spectrum disorder—epilepsy and mortality. *Dev Med Child Neurol*. 2012;54(4):306-312.

242. Gilby KL, O'Brien TJ. Epilepsy, autism, and neurodevelopment: kindling a shared vulnerability? *Epilepsy Behav*. 2013;26(3):370-374.

243. Berg AT, Plioplys S. Epilepsy and autism: is there a special relationship? *Epilepsy Behav*. 2012;23(3):193-198.

244. Lesca G, Rudolf G, Labalme A, et al. Epileptic encephalopathies of the Landau-Kleffner and continuous spike and waves during slow-wave sleep types: genomic dissection makes the link with autism. *Epilepsia*. 2012;53(9):1526-1538.

245. Steinlein OK. Genetics and epilepsy. *Dialogues Clin Neurosci*. 2008;10(1):29-38.

246. Consortium E-R, Project EPG, Consortium EK. De novo mutations in synaptic transmission genes including DNM1 cause epileptic encephalopathies. *Am J Hum Genet*. 2014;95(4):360-370.

247. Berryer MH, Hamdan FF, Klitten LL, et al. Mutations in SYNGAP1 cause intellectual disability, autism, and a specific form of epilepsy by inducing haploinsufficiency. *Hum Mutat*. 2013;34(2):385-394.

248. Carvill GL, Heavin SB, Yendle SC, et al. Targeted resequencing in epileptic encephalopathies identifies de novo mutations in CHD2 and SYNGAP1. *Nat Genet*. 2013;45(7):825-830.

249. Ozkan ED, Creson TK, Kramár EA, et al. Reduced cognition in Syngap1 mutants is caused by isolated damage within developing forebrain excitatory neurons. *Neuron*. 2014;82(6):1317-1333.

250. Inga Jácome MC, Morales Chacòn LM, Vera Cuesta H, et al. Peripheral inflammatory markers contributing to comorbidities in autism. *Behav Sci (Basel)*. 2016;6(4):29.

251. Holmes GL, Lenck-Santini PP. Role of interictal epileptiform abnormalities in cognitive impairment. *Epilepsy Behav*. 2006;8(3):504-515.

252. Singhal NS, Sullivan JE. Continuous spike-wave during slow wave sleep and related conditions. *ISRN Neurol*. 2014;2014:619079.

253. Ekinci O, Arman AR, Işik U, Bez Y, Berkem M. EEG abnormalities and epilepsy in autistic spectrum disorders: clinical and familial correlates. *Epilepsy Behav*. 2010;17(2):178-182.

254. Parmeggiani A, Barcia G, Posar A, Raimondi E, Santucci M, Scaduto MC. Epilepsy and EEG paroxysmal abnormalities in autism spectrum disorders. *Brain Dev*. 2010;32(9):783-789.

255. Ghaleiha A, Asadabadi M, Mohammadi MR, et al. Memantine as adjunctive treatment to risperidone in children with autistic disorder: a randomized, double-blind, placebo-controlled trial. *Int J Neuropsychopharmacol*. 2013;16(4):783-789.

256. Hardan AY, Fung LK, Libove RA, et al. A randomized controlled pilot trial of oral *N*-acetylcysteine in children with autism. *Biol Psychiatry*. 2012;71(11):956-961.

257. Erickson CA, Veenstra-Vanderweele JM, Melmed RD, et al. STX209 (arbaclofen) for autism spectrum disorders: an 8-week open-label study. *J Autism Dev Disord*. 2014;44(4):958-964.

258. Singh K, Connors SL, Macklin EA, et al. Sulforaphane treatment of autism spectrum disorder (ASD). *Proc Natl Acad Sci U S A*. 2014;111(43):15550-15555.

259. Singh K, Zimmerman AW. Sulforaphane treatment of young men with autism spectrum disorder. *CNS Neurol Disord Drug Targets*. 2016;15(5):597-601.

260. Lin IF, Kashino M, Ohta H, et al. The effect of intranasal oxytocin versus placebo treatment on the autonomic responses to human sounds in autism: a single-blind, randomized, placebo-controlled, crossover design study. *Mol Autism*. 2014;5(1):20.

261. Anagnostou E, Soorya L, Chaplin W, et al. Intranasal oxytocin versus placebo in the treatment of adults with autism spectrum disorders: a randomized controlled trial. *Mol Autism*. 2012;3(1):16.

262. Baghdadli A, Pascal C, Grisi S, Aussilloux C. Risk factors for self-injurious behaviours among 222 young children with autistic disorders. *J Intellect Disabil Res*. 2003;47(pt 8):622-627.

263. Handen BL, Mazefsky CA, Gabriels RL, et al. Risk factors for self-injurious behavior in an inpatient psychiatric sample of children with autism spectrum disorder: a naturalistic observation study. *J Autism Dev Disord*. 2018;48(11):3678-3688. doi:10.1007/s10803-017-3460-2.

264. Minshawi NF, Hurwitz S, Morriss D, McDougle CJ. Multidisciplinary assessment and treatment of self-injurious behavior in autism spectrum disorder and intellectual disability: integration of psychological and biological theory and approach. *J Autism Dev Disord*. 2015;45(6):1541-1568.

265. Arnold LE, Vitiello B, McDougle C, et al. Parent-defined target symptoms respond to risperidone in RUPP autism study: customer approach to clinical trials. *J Am Acad Child Adolesc Psychiatry*. 2003;42(12):1443-1450.

266. Davis NO, Carter AS. Parenting stress in mothers and fathers of toddlers with autism spectrum disorders: associations with child characteristics. *J Autism Dev Disord*. 2008;38(7):1278-1291.

267. Bearss K, Johnson C, Smith T, et al. Effect of parent training vs parent education on behavioral problems in children with autism spectrum disorder: a randomized clinical trial. *JAMA*. 2015;313(15):1524-1533.

268. Sukhodolsky DG, Bloch MH, Panza KE, Reichow B. Cognitive-behavioral therapy for anxiety in children with high-functioning autism: a meta-analysis. *Pediatrics*. 2013;132(5):e1341-e1350.

269. Ung D, Selles R, Small BJ, Storch EA. A systematic review and meta-analysis of cognitive-behavioral therapy for anxiety in youth with high-functioning autism spectrum disorders. *Child Psychiatry Hum Dev*. 2015;46(4):533-547.

270. Su Maw S, Haga C. Effectiveness of cognitive, developmental, and behavioural interventions for autism spectrum disorder in preschool-aged children: a systematic review and meta-analysis. *Heliyon*. 2018;4(9):e00763.

271. Geretsegger M, Elefant C, Mössler KA, Gold C. Music therapy for people with autism spectrum disorder. *Cochrane Database Syst Rev*. 2014(6):CD004381.

272. Oono IP, Honey EJ, McConachie H. Parent-mediated early intervention for young children with autism spectrum disorders (ASD). *Cochrane Database Syst Rev.* 2013(4):CD009774.

273. Reichow B, Steiner AM, Volkmar F. Social skills groups for people aged 6 to 21 with autism spectrum disorders (ASD). *Cochrane Database Syst Rev.* 2012(7):CD008511.

274. Reichow B, Hume K, Barton EE, Boyd BA. Early intensive behavioral intervention (EIBI) for young children with autism spectrum disorders (ASD). *Cochrane Database Syst Rev.* 2018;5:CD009260.

275. Case-Smith J, Arbesman M. Evidence-based review of interventions for autism used in or of relevance to occupational therapy. *Am J Occup Ther.* 2008;62(4):416-429.

276. Parsons L, Cordier R, Munro N, Joosten A, Speyer R. A systematic review of pragmatic language interventions for children with autism spectrum disorder. *PLoS One.* 2017;12(4):e0172242.

277. Owen R, Sikich L, Marcus RN, et al. Aripiprazole in the treatment of irritability in children and adolescents with autistic disorder. *Pediatrics.* 2009;124(6):1533-1540.

278. Marcus RN, Owen R, Manos G, et al. Safety and tolerability of aripiprazole for irritability in pediatric patients with autistic disorder: a 52-week, open-label, multicenter study. *J Clin Psychiatry.* 2011;72(9):1270-1276.

279. McDougle CJ, Scahill L, Aman MG, et al. Risperidone for the core symptom domains of autism: results from the study by the autism network of the research units on pediatric psychopharmacology. *Am J Psychiatry.* 2005;162(6):1142-1148.

280. Research Units on Pediatric Psychopharmacology Autism Network. Risperidone treatment of autistic disorder: longer-term benefits and blinded discontinuation after 6 months. *Am J Psychiatry.* 2005;162(7):1361-1369.

281. Shea S, Turgay A, Carroll A, et al. Risperidone in the treatment of disruptive behavioral symptoms in children with autistic and other pervasive developmental disorders. *Pediatrics.* 2004;114(5):e634-e641.

282. McDougle CJ, Holmes JP, Carlson DC, Pelton GH, Cohen DJ, Price LH. A double-blind, placebo-controlled study of risperidone in adults with autistic disorder and other pervasive developmental disorders. *Arch Gen Psychiatry.* 1998;55(7):633-641.

283. Malone RP, Cater J, Sheikh RM, Choudhury MS, Delaney MA. Olanzapine versus haloperidol in children with autistic disorder: an open pilot study. *J Am Acad Child Adolesc Psychiatry.* 2001;40(8):887-894.

284. Hammock R, Levine WR, Schroeder SR. Brief report: effects of clozapine on self-injurious behavior of two risperidone nonresponders with mental retardation. *J Autism Dev Disord.* 2001;31(1):109-113.

285. McDougle CJ, Kem DL, Posey DJ. Case series: use of ziprasidone for maladaptive symptoms in youths with autism. *J Am Acad Child Adolesc Psychiatry.* 2002;41(8):921-927.

286. Marcus RN, Owen R, Manos G, et al. Aripiprazole in the treatment of irritability in pediatric patients (aged 6-17 years) with autistic disorder: results from a 52-week, open-label study. *J Child Adolesc Psychopharmacol.* 2011;21(3):229-236.

287. Potenza MN, Holmes JP, Kanes SJ, McDougle CJ. Olanzapine treatment of children, adolescents, and adults with pervasive developmental disorders: an open-label pilot study. *J Clin Psychopharmacol.* 1999;19(1):37-44.

288. Duggal HS. Ziprasidone for maladaptive behavior and attention-deficit/hyperactivity disorder symptoms in autistic disorder. *J Child Adolesc Psychopharmacol.* 2007;17(2):261-263.

289. Parikh MS, Kolevzon A, Hollander E. Psychopharmacology of aggression in children and adolescents with autism: a critical review of efficacy and tolerability. *J Child Adolesc Psychopharmacol.* 2008;18(2):157-178.

290. Patel NC, Crismon ML, Hoagwood K, et al. Trends in the use of typical and atypical antipsychotics in children and adolescents. *J Am Acad Child Adolesc Psychiatry.* 2005;44(6):548-556.

291. Hellings JA, Weckbaugh M, Nickel EJ, et al. A double-blind, placebo-controlled study of valproate for aggression in youth with pervasive developmental disorders. *J Child Adolesc Psychopharmacol.* 2005;15(4):682-692.

292. Belsito KM, Law PA, Kirk KS, Landa RJ, Zimmerman AW. Lamotrigine therapy for autistic disorder: a randomized, double-blind, placebo-controlled trial. *J Autism Dev Disord.* 2001;31(2):175-181.

293. Hollander E, Chaplin W, Soorya L, et al. Divalproex sodium vs placebo for the treatment of irritability in children and adolescents with autism spectrum disorders. *Neuropsychopharmacology.* 2010;35(4):990-998.

294. Wasserman S, Iyengar R, Chaplin WF, et al. Levetiracetam versus placebo in childhood and adolescent autism: a double-blind placebo-controlled study. *Int Clin Psychopharmacol.* 2006;21(6):363-367.

295. Rugino TA, Samsock TC. Levetiracetam in autistic children: an open-label study. *J Dev Behav Pediatr.* 2002;23(4):225-230.

296. Kapetanovic S. Oxcarbazepine in youths with autistic disorder and significant disruptive behaviors. *Am J Psychiatry.* 2007;164(5):832-833.

297. Douglas JF, Sanders KB, Benneyworth MH, et al. Brief report: retrospective case series of oxcarbazepine for irritability/agitation symptoms in autism spectrum disorder. *J Autism Dev Disord.* 2013;43(5):1243-1247.

298. Accordino RE, Kidd C, Politte LC, Henry CA, McDougle CJ. Psychopharmacological interventions in autism spectrum disorder. *Expert Opin Pharmacother.* 2016;17(7):937-952.

299. Siegel M, Beresford CA, Bunker M, et al. Preliminary investigation of lithium for mood disorder symptoms in children and adolescents with autism spectrum disorder. *J Child Adolesc Psychopharmacol.* 2014;24(7):399-402.

300. Posey DJ, McDougle CJ. Guanfacine and guanfacine extended release: treatment for ADHD and related disorders. *CNS Drug Rev.* 2007;13(4):465-474.

301. Scahill L, Aman MG, McDougle CJ, et al. A prospective open trial of guanfacine in children with pervasive developmental disorders. *J Child Adolesc Psychopharmacol.* 2006;16(5):589-598.

302. Scahill L, Chappell PB, Kim YS, et al. A placebo-controlled study of guanfacine in the treatment of children with tic disorders and attention deficit hyperactivity disorder. *Am J Psychiatry.* 2001;158(7):1067-1074.

303. Handen BL, Sahl R, Hardan AY. Guanfacine in children with autism and/or intellectual disabilities. *J Dev Behav Pediatr.* 2008;29(4):303-308.

304. Sagar-Ouriaghli I, Lievesley K, Santosh PJ. Propranolol for treating emotional, behavioural, autonomic dysregulation in children and adolescents with autism spectrum disorders. *J Psychopharmacol.* 2018:269881118756245.

305. Hegarty JP, Ferguson BJ, Zamzow RM, et al. Beta-adrenergic antagonism modulates functional connectivity in the default mode network of individuals with and without autism spectrum disorder. *Brain Imaging Behav.* 2017;11(5):1278-1289.

306. McDougle CJ, Naylor ST, Cohen DJ, Volkmar FR, Heninger GR, Price LH. A double-blind, placebo-controlled study of fluvoxamine in adults with autistic disorder. *Arch Gen Psychiatry.* 1996;53(11):1001-1008.

307. Hollander E, Soorya L, Chaplin W, et al. A double-blind placebo-controlled trial of fluoxetine for repetitive behaviors and global severity in adult autism spectrum disorders. *Am J Psychiatry*. 2012;169(3):292-299.

308. McDougle CJ, Kresch LE, Posey DJ. Repetitive thoughts and behavior in pervasive developmental disorders: treatment with serotonin reuptake inhibitors. *J Autism Dev Disord*. 2000;30(5):427-435.

309. King BH, Hollander E, Sikich L, et al. Lack of efficacy of citalopram in children with autism spectrum disorders and high levels of repetitive behavior: citalopram ineffective in children with autism. *Arch Gen Psychiatry*. 2009;66(6):583-590.

310. Hellings JA, Kelley LA, Gabrielli WF, Kilgore E, Shah P. Sertraline response in adults with mental retardation and autistic disorder. *J Clin Psychiatry*. 1996;57(8):333-336.

311. DeLong GR, Teague LA, McSwain Kamran M. Effects of fluoxetine treatment in young children with idiopathic autism. *Dev Med Child Neurol*. 1998;40(8):551-562.

312. DeLong GR, Ritch CR, Burch S. Fluoxetine response in children with autistic spectrum disorders: correlation with familial major affective disorder and intellectual achievement. *Dev Med Child Neurol*. 2002;44(10):652-659.

313. McDougle CJ, Brodkin ES, Naylor ST, Carlson DC, Cohen DJ, Price LH. Sertraline in adults with pervasive developmental disorders: a prospective open-label investigation. *J Clin Psychopharmacol*. 1998;18(1):62-66.

314. Namerow L, Thomas P, Bostic JQ, Prince J, Monuteaux MC. Use of citalopram in pervasive developmental disorders. *J Dev Behav Pediatr*. 2003;24(2):104-108.

315. Owley T, Walton L, Salt J, et al. An open-label trial of escitalopram in pervasive developmental disorders. *J Am Acad Child Adolesc Psychiatry*. 2005;44(4):343-348.

316. Davanzo PA, Belin TR, Widawski MH, King BH. Paroxetine treatment of aggression and self-injury in persons with mental retardation. *Am J Ment Retard*. 1998;102(5):427-437.

317. Garber HJ, McGonigle JJ, Slomka GT, Monteverde E. Clomipramine treatment of stereotypic behaviors and self-injury in patients with developmental disabilities. *J Am Acad Child Adolesc Psychiatry*. 1992;31(6):1157-1160.

318. Lewis MH, Bodfish JW, Powell SB, Parker DE, Golden RN. Clomipramine treatment for self-injurious behavior of individuals with mental retardation: a double-blind comparison with placebo. *Am J Ment Retard*. 1996;100(6):654-665.

319. Buitelaar JK, van der Gaag RJ, van der Hoeven J. Buspirone in the management of anxiety and irritability in children with pervasive developmental disorders: results of an open-label study. *J Clin Psychiatry*. 1998;59(2):56-59.

320. Chugani DC, Chugani HT, Wiznitzer M, et al. Efficacy of low-dose buspirone for restricted and repetitive behavior in young children with autism spectrum disorder: a randomized trial. *J Pediatr*. 2016;170:45-53.e41-44.

321. Kossoff EH, Hartman AL. Ketogenic diets: new advances for metabolism-based therapies. *Curr Opin Neurol*. 2012;25(2):173-178.

322. Stafstrom CE, Rho JM. The ketogenic diet as a treatment paradigm for diverse neurological disorders. *Front Pharmacol*. 2012;3:59.

323. Ruskin DN, Svedova J, Cote JL, et al. Ketogenic diet improves core symptoms of autism in BTBR mice. *PLoS One*. 2013;8(6):e65021.

324. Mantis JG, Fritz CL, Marsh J, Heinrichs SC, Seyfried TN. Improvement in motor and exploratory behavior in Rett syndrome mice with restricted ketogenic and standard diets. *Epilepsy Behav*. 2009;15(2):133-141.

325. Nylen K, Velazquez JL, Likhodii SS, et al. A ketogenic diet rescues the murine succinic semialdehyde dehydrogenase deficient phenotype. *Exp Neurol*. 2008;210(2):449-457.

326. Ahn Y, Narous M, Tobias R, Rho JM, Mychasiuk R. The ketogenic diet modifies social and metabolic alterations identified in the prenatal valproic acid model of autism spectrum disorder. *Dev Neurosci*. 2014;36(5):371-380.

327. Evangeliou A, Vlachonikolis I, Mihailidou H, et al. Application of a ketogenic diet in children with autistic behavior: pilot study. *J Child Neurol*. 2003;18(2):113-118.

328. Kim DY, Davis LM, Sullivan PG, et al. Ketone bodies are protective against oxidative stress in neocortical neurons. *J Neurochem*. 2007;101(5):1316-1326.

329. Maalouf M, Sullivan PG, Davis L, Kim DY, Rho JM. Ketones inhibit mitochondrial production of reactive oxygen species production following glutamate excitotoxicity by increasing NADH oxidation. *Neuroscience*. 2007;145(1):256-264.

330. Sullivan PG, Rippy NA, Dorenbos K, Concepcion RC, Agarwal AK, Rho JM. The ketogenic diet increases mitochondrial uncoupling protein levels and activity. *Ann Neurol*. 2004;55(4):576-580.

331. Newell C, Shutt TE, Ahn Y, et al. Tissue specific impacts of a ketogenic diet on mitochondrial dynamics in the BTBR. *Front Physiol*. 2016;7:654.

332. Li YJ, Ou JJ, Li YM, Xiang DX. Dietary supplement for core symptoms of autism spectrum disorder: where are we now and where should we go? *Front Psychiatry*. 2017;8:155.

333. Janecka A, Staniszewska R, Gach K, Fichna J. Enzymatic degradation of endomorphins. *Peptides*. 2008;29(11):2066-2073.

334. Millward C, Ferriter M, Calver S, Connell-Jones G. Gluten- and casein-free diets for autistic spectrum disorder. *Cochrane Database Syst Rev*. 2008(2):CD003498.

335. Cornish E. Gluten and casein free diets in autism: a study of the effects on food choice and nutrition. *J Hum Nutr Diet*. 2002;15(4):261-269.

336. Francis K. Autism interventions: a critical update. *Dev Med Child Neurol*. 2005;47(7):493-499.

337. Berg JS, Brunetti-Pierri N, Peters SU, et al. Speech delay and autism spectrum behaviors are frequently associated with duplication of the 7q11.23 Williams-Beuren syndrome region. *Genet Med*. 2007;9(7):427-441.

338. Mervis CB, Klein-Tasman BP, Huffman MJ, et al. Children with 7q11.23 duplication syndrome: psychological characteristics. *Am J Med Genet A*. 2015;167(7):1436-1450.

339. Angulo MA, Butler MG, Cataletto ME. Prader-Willi syndrome: a review of clinical, genetic, and endocrine findings. *J Endocrinol Invest*. 2015;38(12):1249-1263.

340. Bennett JA, Hodgetts S, Mackenzie ML, Haqq AM, Zwaigenbaum L. Investigating autism-related symptoms in children with Prader-Willi syndrome: a case study. *Int J Mol Sci*. 2017;18(3):517.

341. Thibert RL, Larson AM, Hsieh DT, Raby AR, Thiele EA. Neurologic manifestations of Angelman syndrome. *Pediatr Neurol*. 2013;48(4):271-279.

342. Buiting K, Clayton-Smith J, Driscoll DJ, et al. Clinical utility gene card for Angelman syndrome. *Eur J Hum Genet*. 2015;23(2):e1-e3.

343. Buiting K, Williams C, Horsthemke B. Angelman syndrome—insights into a rare neurogenetic disorder. *Nat Rev Neurol*. 2016;12(10):584-593.

344. Neira-Fresneda J, Potocki L. Neurodevelopmental disorders associated with abnormal gene dosage: Smith-Magenis and Potocki-Lupski syndromes. *J Pediatr Genet*. 2015;4(3):159-167.

345. McDonald-McGinn DM, Sullivan KE. Chromosome 22q11.2 deletion syndrome (DiGeorge syndrome/velocardiofacial syndrome). *Medicine (Baltimore)*. 2011;90(1):1-18.

346. McDonald-McGinn DM, Sullivan KE, Marino B, et al. 22q11.2 deletion syndrome. *Nat Rev Dis Primers*. 2015;1:15071.

347. Egger JI, Zwanenburg RJ, van Ravenswaaij-Arts CM, Kleefstra T, Verhoeven WM. Neuropsychological phenotype and psychopathology in seven adult patients with Phelan-McDermid syndrome: implications for treatment strategy. *Genes Brain Behav*. 2016;15(4):395-404.

348. Cusmano-Ozog K, Manning MA, Hoyme HE. 22q13.3 deletion syndrome: a recognizable malformation syndrome associated with marked speech and language delay. *Am J Med Genet C Semin Med Genet*. 2007;145C(4):393-398.

Intellectual Developmental Disorders

Jung Won Kim · Christopher J. Keary · Michelle L. Palumbo · Laura C. Politte · Christopher J. McDougle · Lisa Nowinski

18

INTRODUCTION

History

A series of terms have been used over time to refer to people with varying degrees of intellectual impairment. New terms have been created to replace previous ones that were considered inappropriate or degrading, and often became viewed as derogatory themselves. For instance, the psychologist Henry Gaddard coined the term *moron* to replace the term *feeble-minded*. The term *moron*, however, became viewed as disparaging over time. In the late 19th century, the term *retarded*, which was not considered defamatory at the time, began to replace others such as *idiot*, *moron*, and *imbecile*, until it also became offensive to others by 1960.[1] On October 5, 2010, then President Barak Obama signed Rosa's law (Pub.L. 111–256), named after a girl with Down syndrome (DS), which recognized her initiatives along with those of her family in the state of Maryland, to replace *mental retardation* with *intellectual disability* and *mentally retarded individual* with *individual with intellectual disability* in federal law.[2] In 2013, the American Psychiatric Association (APA) also adopted the new term *intellectual disability* in place of *mental retardation* for the latest edition of the *Diagnostic and Statistical Manual of Mental Disorders (DSM-5)*.[3]

Terminology and Definition

Traditionally, patients younger than the age of 5 years who are not meeting their cognitive or developmental milestones, are referred to as having global developmental delay. This term is used until a comprehensive and accurate assessment of intellectual functioning can be obtained.[3] The latest version of *DSM (DSM-5)* requires "onset during the developmental period that includes both intellectual and adaptive functioning deficits in conceptual, social, and practical domains" for the diagnosis of *Intellectual Disability* (ID).[3] The *DSM-5* also included the term *Intellectual Developmental Disorder* (IDD) in parentheses next to the term *Intellectual Disability* (ID) to acknowledge changes made in the terminology in the latest version of the International Classification of Diseases (ICD-11).[3,4] Diagnostic criteria by both ICD-11 and the American Association on Intellectual and Developmental Disabilities (AAIDD) also describe ID/IDD as impairment in "intellectual functioning" and "adaptive behavior" with onset during the developmental period.[4,5] Both *DSM-5* and ICD-11 have classified ID/IDD under the parent category, *Neurodevelopmental Disorders*. The term *Intellectual Developmental Disorder* (IDD) has also been adopted by organizations including AAIDD and the U.S. Department of Education. Please see *DSM-5*, ICD-11, and AAIDD for full diagnostic criteria for ID/IDD.[3-5] *DSM-5* determines the severity of IDD as mild, moderate, severe, or profound based on the level of adaptive functioning,[3] whereas ICD-11 employs a similar classification of mild, moderate, severe, or profound (in addition to provisional or unspecified) as defined by the degree of intellectual impairment and disruption of adaptive behavior.[4]

EPIDEMIOLOGY

Prevalence

Based on a meta-analysis of 52 studies involving nearly 30 countries between 1980 and 2009, the prevalence of IDD reached about 1%, with higher estimates among low- to middle-income countries, urban locations, and child and adolescent populations.[6] Also, IDD was more prevalent in males for children, adolescents, and adults.[6] The prevalence of severe IDD is estimated to be approximately 0.3–0.5%.[7,8]

Quality of Life

Lower quality of life (QoL) is frequently reported, as measured by structured monitoring and/or survey, in patients with IDD, with risk factors such as severity of symptoms, behavioral challenges, and parental stress.[9,10] Patients with IDD also exhibit more frequent medical and psychiatric comorbidities (discussed below) and are less likely to be involved in adequate leisure activities.[11]

Mortality

Patients with IDD are reported to have a higher risk of mortality across the lifespan as compared to the general population, with an even higher risk among severely affected individuals.[12-15] The higher mortality risk in patients with IDD, however, has been found to abate over decades of one's life.[16]

Economic Cost

The total lifetime economic cost for individuals born in the year 2000 with IDD was projected to reach approximately $51.2 billion in the United States, with a per-person lifetime cost averaged at over $1 million (in equivalents of U.S. dollar values in 2003).[17]

Risk Factors

A recent systematic review and meta-analysis identified a number of risk factors associated with IDD.[18] Maternal factors include advanced age, black race, low education, third or more parity, alcohol or tobacco use, and medical illness such as diabetes, hypertension, epilepsy, or asthma. Other factors include preterm birth, male sex, and low birth weight. However, some research has suggested that there may be an overrepresentation of low-income and minority individuals identified as having an IDD.[19,20]

PATHOPHYSIOLOGY

Etiologies/Causes

Despite an immense array of possible etiologies, there is no one known causal factor. Attempts to identify causes of IDD can help with understanding the natural history, guiding the treatment, determining prognosis, and counseling for family planning. Table 18-1 summarizes the various etiologies for IDD by time and type of injury to the brain.

Pathophysiological Mechanisms

Intellectual developmental disorders can be viewed as a cluster of neurodevelopmental symptoms arising from dysfunctional neurologic system as a result of various insults to brain structure and/or neurochemistry. Although the exact pathogenesis is yet unknown, possible mechanisms include inflammatory processes, direct physical damage, neurotransmitter or network interruption, and metabolic dysfunction, among others. While some individuals with IDD show no discernable difference in brain structure, others exhibit structural malformations of the brain that may or may not be linked to an underlying genetic condition and/or epigenetic changes. Moreover, postnatal factors such as traumatic brain injury, hypoxia, infections, and exposure to toxins can result in a deterioration of intellectual functioning or development that may warrant a diagnosis of another neurocognitive disorder in addition to an IDD diagnosis (e.g., dementia in an individual with IDD).

CASE VIGNETTE 18.1

Clinical Presentation

Peter was born as the first child following a healthy and uncomplicated pregnancy. As an infant, he ate and slept well, and his parents described him as responsive and engaged. In preschool, he enjoyed playing with other children. His teachers described him as friendly, but soon started to notice differences between Peter and his peers. While the other children began to demonstrate interest in classroom learning activities like matching, sorting, and learning letters and numbers, Peter seemed drawn toward play and music. At home, Peter's parents noticed that his younger sister was quickly catching up and surpassing some of his skills. Although he spoke, Peter tended to use simple language and often preferred to watch what others were doing. He didn't seem interested in toilet training and still required full support for life skills such as dressing and brushing his teeth. In elementary school, Peter continued to require more support than the other children his age for learning. His parents and teachers ultimately developed an Individualized Education Program (IEP), and Peter began to receive modified and small group instruction for academic skills like reading, writing, and mathematics. Despite these challenges, he continued to thrive with his peers. He was friendly and playful, and his teachers called him the "mayor" of his elementary school—he seemed to know everyone. In addition, Peter developed his love for music. His favorite lesson each week was with the music teacher. His parents decided to support this interest by enrolling him in a local community choir.

As he got older, the gap between Peter and his same-age peers became increasingly noticeable. Soon, his friends began to explore the neighborhood on their own, visit each other's houses, and plan activities together. Peter was still eager to be involved, but he often required his parents' support to connect with his friends. In addition, although he had slowly developed skills for toileting and dressing independently, he required support for more complex tasks and decisions, such as determining what clothes to wear when the weather changed and finding his favorite song lyrics on the Internet. Peter's younger sister also began to help him around the house. At snack time, she would often serve his snack and remind him to wash his hands or clean up afterwards.

By the time Peter entered high school, his parents and teachers decided that he needed more intense and direct support to build his independence and functional life skills. He was enrolled in a substantially separate school program that was designed to teach individuals with intellectual and developmental disorders to be independent and successful young adults. Traditional academic instruction gave way for more functional academic applications. For example, instead of learning algebra and geometry, Peter's math lessons focused on managing a budget, making purchases, and using fractions in recipes. While his peers were learning to drive, Peter learned local bus routes and practiced walking directions to and from familiar community locations. While his peers, and even younger sister, began to apply to college and move away, Peter remained in his special education program through age 22 years. His teachers helped him build his vocational skills and explore jobs that he enjoyed. They continued to foster his love for music. Peter held an internship at a local preschool, where he helped with a daily music lesson.

As an adult, Peter continued to require support from his parents, particularly to make important life decisions around medical care, where to live, and how to manage his finances. He lived in a house with a few other young men, with some staff support to manage household tasks and maintain his schedule. He worked part-time at a local church, where he helped prepare materials for the choir. In his free time, he enjoyed taking walks in the park near his house, watching movies, and eating at his favorite local restaurant. He met a girlfriend through a local, adult activity group and they enjoyed talking to and texting each other. At the time of his 18th birthday (age of legal majority), the court determined that Peter was unable to independently make reasonably informed decisions, and his parents were granted legal guardianship to support his medical, legal, and financial decision making. Into adulthood, his parents continued to accompany him to medical visits, manage his finances, pay his rent, and they provided Peter with an allowance for spending each week. He carried a wallet with a small amount of cash and also used gift cards to make purchases from his favorite stores and download music. As Peter's parents aged, his younger sister stepped in as a new legal guardian. She continued to manage his finances and take him to medical appointments.

Phenomenology

As a lifelong developmental disability, IDD is characterized by significant deficits in intellectual capacity and concurrent impairment in adaptive functioning.[3] Figure 18-1 summarizes challenges in cognitive and adaptive skills across the lifespan. Evidence of impairment must be present before the age of 18 years and is often evident in the early developmental period. However, for individuals with milder IDD, the full extent of intellectual and adaptive skill deficits may become increasingly apparent in later childhood and adolescence when peers are generally moving away from reliance on parents or caregivers.

Early signs include delayed development of early motor milestones (i.e., rolling, sitting, crawling, or walking later than expected), delayed language development and spoken communication, and difficulty with acquisition of early adaptive skills (i.e., feeding, toileting, dressing). As children get older, they may also demonstrate difficulty reporting on and remembering events or experiences, limited ability to connect their actions with consequences, limited understanding of cause-and-effect, and impaired executive functions. In the early school-age years, this might translate to difficulty learning basic academic skills or meeting behavioral expectations in the classroom. In the later school-age years, more challenges can be noted with understanding and processing complex concepts.

Individuals with IDD can also experience wide-reaching effects on their social and vocational functioning. They will often require specialized and intensive instruction to learn new skills and may require repetition and practice over time. In addition, social relationships may be difficult to establish and maintain with typically developing peers, particularly as an individual gets older.

Common Medical and Psychiatric Symptoms and Comorbidities

Individuals with IDD are vulnerable to acquiring various medical and psychiatric comorbidities. Certainly, individuals whose IDD is related to an underlying genetic condition are at higher risk of specific medical comorbidities related to their genetic condition (e.g., cardiac problems in DS); however, there is also some research to suggest that individuals with IDD demonstrate higher rates of heart disease, diabetes, hypertension, obesity, gastrointestinal issues, and thyroid disorder, and lower rates of arthritis, migraines, back pain, and food allergies as compared to the general population,[11,21] with some of these related to underlying genetic conditions. As individuals with IDD age, issues such as "diagnostic overshadowing (the tendency to overlook symptoms of mental and physical illness as causes for decline), lack of knowledge about aging in adults with IDD, and health care disparities" may interfere with access to appropriate medical care.[22]

Beyond specific medical risk and comorbidity, it is important to note that individuals with IDD also experience psychiatric symptoms and stressors such as anxiety and depression. Although some studies have shown that the presence of an IDD does not affect the prevalence of psychiatric disorders in a subset of individuals with mild-to-moderate IDD,[23] other studies have shown that IDD is associated with higher rates of co-occurring psychopathology.[11,24] The relationship between severity of IDD

TABLE 18-1 • Etiologies/Causes of IDD by Time and Type of Injury.

Time	Type	Cause	
Prenatal	Infectious	Toxoplasmosis	
		Rubella	
		Cytomegalovirus	
		Herpes simplex virus	
	Genetic	Trisomy	Down syndrome (21)
			Edward syndrome (18)
			Patau syndrome (13)
			Triple X syndrome (X)
		Monosomy	Turner syndrome (Ring-X)
			Cri du chat syndrome (5p)
			1p36 deletion syndrome (1p36)
		Deletion	Jacobsen syndrome (11q terminal)
			Wolf-Hirschhorn syndrome (4p)
			DiGeorge syndrome (22q11.2)
		Imprinting	Prader-Willi syndrome (15)
			Angelman syndrome (15)
		Inheritable	Fragile X syndrome (X-linked)
	Teratogenic	Alcohol	
		Medications	
		Radiation	
	Hormonal	Congenital hypothyroidism	
	Treatable inborn errors of metabolism	Over 80 have been identified (e.g., phenylketonuria, coenzyme Q10 deficiency, GLUT1 deficiency syndrome, homocystinuria)	
Perinatal	Hypoxia	Maternal hypoventilation/Hypotension	
		Placental abruption	
		Umbilical cord compression	
	Prematurity	Intraventricular hemorrhage (IVH)	
		Hypoxic-ischemic encephalopathy (HIE)	
	Infection	Central nervous system (CNS) infection	
Postnatal	Traumatic	Injury/Accident	
		Neglect/Deprivation/Malnutrition	
	Toxic	Lead	
		Mercury	
	Infection	CNS infection	
	Circulatory	Stroke	
	Malignancy	Metastatic cancer	
		Brain tumor	

and psychiatric comorbidities has not been well established.[25] Rates vary dramatically with estimates ranging from 7% to 97% of adults with IDD exhibiting comorbid psychopathology or mental disorder.[26] Fletcher and colleagues estimate that 30–40% of individuals with IDD have a co-occurring mental health disorder.[27] Individuals with IDD can exhibit symptoms of anxiety, depression, other mood disorders, attention-deficit hyperactivity disorder (ADHD), stereotypic movement disorder, and impulse control disorder, among others. Some psychiatric symptoms, such as anxiety, have also been linked to challenging behaviors, such as aggression and self-injury, in individuals with IDD.[28] In addition, IDD is estimated to co-occur in more than half of all individuals with autism spectrum disorder (ASD).[29,30] Despite the clear need for psychiatric

	Cognitive challenges	Adaptive challenges
Early childhood	• Difficulty with matching, sorting, puzzles • Slow to learn • Delayed language and communication	• Delayed motor milestones • Slow feeding and toilet training • Delayed development of basic activities of daily living (e.g., dressing, self-care) • Slow to understand "stranger danger"
Adolescence	• Slow mastery of basic academic skills such as reading, writing, and arithmetic • Reduce verbal and nonverbal reasoning skills • Increased distractibility or loss of focus • Limited abstract thinking	• Continued reliance on caregiver for activities of daily living, including managing nuances of puberty • Requires more explicit instruction to learn new adaptive skills (e.g., household tasks) • Requires facilitation of recreational/leisure activities • Difficulty understanding boundaries and expectations for relationships with peers, family, and caregivers
Adulthood	• Limited ability to make informed decisions about healthcare and finances • Difficulty managing complex work tasks independently • Reduced understanding of long-term consequences of actions and behaviors	• Requires support for managing finances • May require ongoing support with daily living skills (e.g., managing medications, transportation to/from work) • Limited capacity for understanding risks in interpersonal and romantic relationships

FIGURE 18-1. Cognitive and adaptive skill challenges across the lifespan.

evaluation and care, it can be challenging to evaluate and diagnose psychiatric comorbidities in individuals with IDD, particularly those with limited language and verbal abilities, because it may be difficult to obtain an accurate report of the individuals' thoughts and feelings. In addition, it is important to note that not all atypical patterns of behavior reflect a co-occurring psychiatric condition in individuals with IDD. For example, some individuals with IDD may exhibit repetitive or peculiar vocalizations or "self-talk" that should not be considered a psychotic symptom, without further investigation.

Cognitive Dysfunction Symptoms

The cognitive profile of individuals with IDD is typically marked by global impairments in intellectual functioning, including substantially limited verbal reasoning, visual-spatial processing, and nonverbal or fluid reasoning skills. Intellectual capacity is conventionally measured with a standardized measure of general intelligence or IQ test (discussed below). Individuals with IDD demonstrate scores falling two or more standard deviations below the population mean (e.g., IQ < 70). In addition, individuals with IDD will exhibit deficits in language, learning, memory, attention, and higher-order executive functioning skills that are consistent with their impaired general intellect. Although these neurocognitive sequelae do not necessarily indicate a separate or distinct comorbid diagnosis, they can certainly exacerbate difficulties with an individual's functional skills and independence.

Although individuals with IDD are thought to have globally reduced skills, some may develop "splinter skills" that fall at or above the level expected for their age. For example, a small subset of individuals with ASD exhibit savant-like abilities in a narrow skill set.[29,30] In addition, some individuals with IDD may demonstrate some degree of variability in their core intellectual functioning, with either relative strengths or weaknesses evident in verbal or nonverbal reasoning.

Course and Natural History

IDD is a lifelong condition that is not expected to remit, even with treatment; however, with the right ongoing intervention and support, individuals with IDD have the capacity to learn and develop a number of important skills. Treatment can help an individual with IDD develop improved adaptive and self-care skills, as well as the ability to access and maintain meaningful social, vocational, and community experiences. In contrast, without ongoing intervention and support, an individual with IDD would be at substantial risk of neglect or harm, as they may struggle to meet their own basic needs independently.

Across the lifespan, an individual with IDD may require varying levels of support. For example, early on, a child with IDD may require more hands-on support for daily living skills from a parent or caregiver. Later in life, individuals with IDD may or may not require the same support for daily living skills, though they often require legal guardianship or support for higher-level tasks such as medical, legal, and financial decision making. Those with milder IDD may be successful in living independently or with minimal in-home support, whereas individuals with more severe IDD may require lifelong, intensive support for basic skills such as dressing, feeding, and bathing.

As adults with IDD enter middle age, they can be impacted by the deterioration or loss of their primary caregiver. Elderly parents may become unable to manage the demands of caregiving and individuals with significant IDD often must transition from their long-time home to residential or group home options. Other relatives may assume responsibility for caretaking or support.

Finally, as individuals with IDD enter older adulthood, there is concern for further cognitive decline or dementia in this already vulnerable population. Research has examined various factors related to the epidemiology, assessment, diagnosis, and management of dementia in IDD; however, little is known about how information regarding underlying neuropathology can be translated into more effective treatments.[31] The largest body of research is available in the DS population, with research suggesting that individuals with DS are at high risk for developing Alzheimer's disease (AD) at a relatively young age due to an overproduction of amyloid precursor protein.[32]

ASSESSMENT AND DIFFERENTIAL DIAGNOSIS

Medical, Neurological, and Psychiatric Entities That Should Be Considered

When the diagnosis of IDD is part of the differential diagnosis, a number of factors should be taken into consideration during the clinical evaluation. Genetic disorders or syndromes that are known to cause IDD should be screened or tested for (e.g., chromosomal microarray), and in particular, facial dysmorphisms, behaviors, and/or family histories that are characteristic for specific genetic disorders or syndromes warrant specific genetic testing.[33] *DSM-5* recommends that a newly identified genetic cause be added as a coexisting diagnosis to IDD.[3] While the diagnosis of IDD requires onset during the developmental period, an insult to the brain in the post-developmental period that results in impaired cognitive functions can lead to the additional diagnosis of neurocognitive disorder (e.g., various types of dementia, traumatic brain injury, Parkinson's disease, etc.).[3] Certain neurodevelopmental disorders such as ASD (refer to Chapter 17 for detailed review of ASD) and/or ADHD, can frequently coexist with IDD,[34,35] whereas others, such as specific learning disorder (SLD) may not. The diagnosis of SLD would be precluded by the diagnostic criterion that "the learning difficulties are not better accounted for by intellectual disabilities."[36] Delineating ASD in individuals with severe IDD or vice versa can be especially challenging due to potentially overlapping clinical signs and symptoms.[37,38]

Methods for Assessment and Differential Diagnosis

A comprehensive assessment and diagnosis of IDD must include two primary components. First, a complete cognitive or intellectual assessment is necessary to accurately characterize the degree of intellectual impairment. This can also provide an indication of an individual's relative strengths and challenges. There are a number of valid and reliable instruments that can be used to characterize intellectual functioning in individuals with suspected IDD. In adults, instruments such as the Stanford Binet Intelligence Scale, 5th Edition (SB-5) are particularly well suited to capture skills that may fall below the lower limits of other adult-specific assessment instruments. Figure 18-2 provides a list of commonly used cognitive and intellectual assessment instruments.

Second, a comprehensive assessment of an individual's social and adaptive functioning must also be included. Although adaptive skills have always been considered when making a diagnosis of IDD, the more recent definitions have made this even more critical. Because the newer diagnostic criteria have moved away from intellectual functioning as the primary way of determining the severity of IDD, comprehensive assessment of social and practical skills (in addition to intellectual or "conceptual" skills) is now critical. Table 18-2 provides a list of commonly used assessment instruments to capture the adaptive skills of individuals with IDD.

A comprehensive neuropsychological assessment can help to characterize the degree of cognitive impairment and subsequent impact on daily functioning. Such formal assessment may serve a range of functions including confirming diagnosis, characterizing severity of impairment, identifying additional disorders, evaluating social, emotional, or behavioral functioning, characterizing strengths and weaknesses, and measuring treatment response or progress.[39] Factors such as neglect, limited access to education, severe or untreated inattention, and social and language barriers must be considered when interpreting an individual's performance on standardized testing. Research in the field of special education has long called our attention to the problematic overrepresentation of low-income and minority students identified as having an IDD and inappropriately placed in programs designed for this population.[19,20]

TREATMENTS

Although there is currently no known cure for IDD, primary, secondary, and tertiary prevention measures can be used to both prevent the emergence of IDD and lessen its impact.[40] For example, primary efforts to prevent the development of IDD may include appropriate prenatal care and environmental health initiatives such as removing lead and other toxins from the environment. Secondary prevention may include early identification and intervention for conditions associated with IDD, and tertiary prevention includes ongoing support and accommodations such as special education programming, vocational training, and agency support. It is these tertiary prevention measures that are generally considered "treatment" for IDD. Across all levels of prevention, it is important to consider the increased risk of abuse and neglect in individuals with IDD given their intellectual and social vulnerability. Timely intervention for young patients with IDD should be considered particularly critical as evidence indicates this may result in very

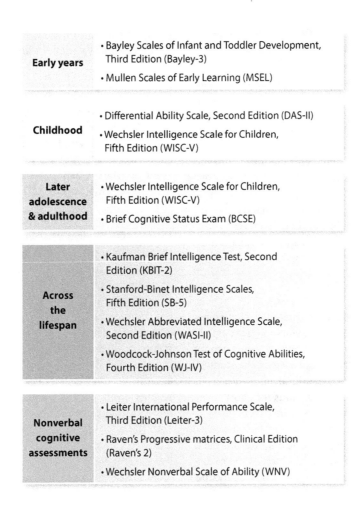

FIGURE 18-2. Commonly used cognitive and intellectual assessments/instruments.

TABLE 18-2 • Commonly Used Adaptive Skills Assessments/ Instruments.	
Early years/ Childhood	• Developmental Profile, Third Edition (DP-3)
Across the lifespan	• Adaptive Behavior Assessment System, Second Edition (ABAS-II) • Adaptive Behavior Evaluation Scale, Third Edition (ABES-3) • Scales of Independent Behavior—Revised (SIB-R) • Vineland Adaptive Behavior Scales, Third Edition (VABS-3)

significant improvement in developmental course and eventual outcome.[41]

Treatments for Reversible Causes

Identification of causes that are reversible can often translate into treatment or prevention of injury to the brain, therefore, IDD. For instance, congenital hypothyroidism is known to be one of the most frequent causes of IDD that should be screened and treated at birth.[42,43] Other examples include prevention or

timely treatment of maternal infections (e.g., rubella, cytomegalovirus, etc.) that are known to be detrimental to fetal development, avoidance of known teratogens or toxins (e.g., alcohol, drugs, radiation), and correction of treatable inborn errors of metabolism (e.g., phenylketonuria, coenzyme Q10 deficiency, GLUT1 deficiency syndrome, homocystinuria). Over 80 treatable inborn errors of metabolism have been found to be associated with IDD, the majority of which can be diagnosed with urine (organic acids, glycosaminoglycans, creatine metabolites, oligosaccharides, purines, and pyrimidines) or blood screening tests (amino acids, total homocysteine) and have available treatment options.[44] Many of these treatable causes of IDD are currently included in the newborn screening (also known as newborn blood spot), as recommended by federal and state guidelines.[45,46]

Psychotropic Medication

Many psychotropic medications can be considered as treatment options for alleviating the burden of a wide variety of comorbid psychiatric disorders and symptoms in patients with IDD. It is generally recommended that psychotropic medication options be considered after other nonpharmacologic treatments have been tried first. However, the prevalence of patients with IDD that take at least one psychotropic medication remains fairly high.[47] Prescribers should be mindful that individuals with IDD are often more sensitive to adverse effects with psychotropic medications, and lower than expected doses may be needed for tolerability. Furthermore, side effects associated with commonly used medications may exacerbate other features of the disorder, such as insomnia with stimulants, hyperactivity with SSRIs, and increased appetite with antipsychotics. It is very important that the prescribers should always start with the lowest dosage available, irrespective of age or body weight, increase the dosage at least twice as slowly as one would do for a neurotypical individual with the same target symptoms, and make only one medication change at a time. Patience should be exercised when using psychopharmacological interventions in the IDD population, despite the sense of urgency that might arise from the disturbing behavioral symptoms.

Antipsychotics

One of the most commonly encountered clinical challenges among patients with IDD is disruptive behaviors, such as aggression toward objects, self, or others.[48] Although various agents are used in clinical practice for disruptive behaviors, the atypical antipsychotics medications, *risperidone* and *aripiprazole*, have been shown to be significantly more efficacious for short-term treatment in child and adolescent patients with IDD.[49] Only a limited number of trials have evaluated the longer-term benefits of these medications. Moreover, antipsychotic medications have serious short- and long-term adverse effects, such as the metabolic syndrome, tardive dyskinesia, etc.[49] In a study analyzing 99 individuals with IDD and long-term use of antipsychotics, age and severity of IDD were positively correlated with dyskinesia and dosage with parkinsonism, while severity of IDD negatively correlated with body mass index (BMI).[50] Furthermore, evidence for the use of antipsychotics for disruptive behaviors in adult patients with IDD has not been established with larger-scale randomized controlled trials (RCTs), or the results have been inconsistent.[51] Besides antipsychotics, other agents that can be considered to treat disruptive behaviors in individuals with IDD include lithium, stimulants, and alpha-2 agonists (e.g., for symptoms associated with comorbid ADHD), whereas antiepileptics, anxiolytics, and antidepressants only have little to weak evidence.[52]

Antidepressants

Antidepressant medication—mainly selective serotonin reuptake inhibitors (SSRIs)—are one of the most commonly prescribed classes of psychotropic medication, following antipsychotics in adult patients with IDD.[47] They are often used to manage mood or anxiety symptoms and can also be considered for addressing obsessive-compulsive symptoms or intolerance to changes. However, once again, there is a lack of evidence as established with RCTs in children, adolescents, and adults with IDD, and little is known about the short- and long-term side effects in this population.[53–56]

Mood Stabilizers

Although frequently prescribed in both children and adults with IDD,[57,58] scant evidence exists for anticonvulsants, used as mood stabilizers.[59] There is more evidence in the published literature in support of lithium for alleviating challenging behavior, such as aggression, in patients with IDD.[60–62]

Stimulants and Alpha-2 Agonists

Stimulants are one of the most commonly prescribed psychotropic medications in children with IDD.[58] Methylphenidate has been established via multiple RCTs for its significant efficacy in ameliorating symptoms of ADHD in children with IDD.[63–66] Alpha-2 agonists, non-stimulant medications used for the treatment of ADHD, also have been shown to provide significant benefit for symptoms of ADHD in children with IDD.[67–69]

Benzodiazepines and Other Anxiolytics

Despite the frequent use of benzodiazepines for anxiety or agitation,[57] these drugs are known to have the risk for paradoxical worsening of maladaptive behavior in patients with IDD, a scenario that can be mistaken as lack of effectiveness rather than a worsening of challenging behaviors.[70] Other potential risks of benzodiazepines include the development of dependence, tolerance, and withdrawal, as well as worsening cognitive impairment in older patients.[71] Case reports and small case series indicate that Buspirone is effective for interfering anxiety and aggression, and well tolerated, in some individuals with IDD.[72–74] Results from open-label studies suggest that beta-blockers, like propranolol, can improve aggression in some patients with IDD.[75]

Rehabilitative Therapies

Physical Therapy

Impairment or delay in gross motor skills has been frequently reported in patients with IDD across their development and lifespan[76,77] and associated with cognitive impairment.[78] Various modalities of physical therapy, including longer-term, home-based training,[79] and body-weight-supported over-ground gait training,[80] have proven effective for improving gross motor function in patients with IDD. Although evidence for physical therapy in improving gross motor skills is currently limited,[81] most interventions are known to have very negligible risks but the practical benefit of improving QoL.[82,83]

Occupational Therapy

Occupational therapy (OT) is often considered an essential part of a special education program and for assisting with transition plans for patients with IDD.[84] Due to accompanying fine motor, sensorimotor, and/or perceptual challenges, patients with IDD frequently require or benefit from individual- or group-based OT to assist them in improving adaptability to academic and later vocational responsibilities.[84] OT can be effectively administered in the home over a longer period of time,[85] as well in school- and community-based, outpatient settings.

Psychotherapy

Psychiatric comorbidities and behavioral/developmental challenges are common in patients with IDD,[86,87] and many traditional psychotherapeutic interventions can be considered as viable treatment options. One of the most widely used treatments is cognitive-behavioral therapy (CBT). Although significant support and modification are required, patients with IDD can acquire the essential skills to participate in and benefit from CBT.[88] Despite limited evidence, appropriately modified CBT appears to be a reasonable option with potential benefits and minimal risks in alleviating depressive symptoms in patients with IDD.[89,90] Similarly, mindfulness-based cognitive therapy (MBCT) also has shown benefits in improving symptoms of depression and/or anxiety in patients with IDD.[91]

Caregiver Training and Support

High levels of stress have been observed in parents with developmentally delayed children, in particular when accompanying behavioral challenges are present.[92] Caregiver training is one of the most widely utilized approaches for improving maladaptive behavior, with fairly sustainable benefits.[93,94] Various training programs have been created and implemented in the communities with positive results. Stepping Stones Triple P (SSTP)—part of the Triple P—Positive Parenting Program in Australia—is designed as a family remedy with goals to improve behavioral, emotional, and developmental challenges in children with various neurodevelopmental conditions, by empowering parents/caregivers.[95] SSTP has shown benefits in families of patients with IDD.[96] SSTP was also effective when used with patients with various developmental disorders, including ASD, cerebral palsy, and IDD, in a group setting.[97] Parents Plus is an evidenced-based caregiver training program developed in the United Kingdom for parents with children with IDD. These are targeted programs for specific age groups—Parents Plus Early Years Program (PPEYP) for children aged 1–6 years,[98] Parents Plus Children's Program (PPCP for children aged 6–11 years,[99] and Parents Plus Adolescent Program (PPAP) for adolescents aged 11–15 years.[100] In addition to formal caregiver training curriculums, many caregivers also work with therapists and behavior specialists to address challenging behaviors and build adaptive skills. For instance, principles from applied behavior analysis (ABA) can also be effective in managing challenging behaviors in individuals with IDD.[101] ABA involves the use of highly structured principles of learning and motivation, to change or modify specific behaviors. This may include techniques such as positive reinforcement of appropriate behavior, as well as negative consequences or planned ignoring for inappropriate behaviors.

Transitional Services

Transitioning to adulthood for patients with IDD is a particularly challenging task and often a prolonged process for their families/parents. Individuals with IDD may require various aspects of support, including psychological, social, legal, financial, etc., depending on their level of functioning and adaptability. Families with young adult patients with more severe IDD are often faced with significantly more challenges yet not provided with an adequate level of resources or services within society.[102] Families need more support and assistance during transition in the areas of school, community, finances, and legal issues (e.g., guardianship).[103] Importantly, support for

parents/caregivers' well-being during the transition period should not be overlooked.[104]

Educational Services

In the United States, the Individuals with Disabilities Education Improvement Act (IDEA; 2004, P.L. 108–446) mandates individually tailored public education for students with various disabilities. Under this law, Early Intervention Programs (EIP) address special needs for infants to children up to 3 years of age, and the IEP, a special education plan available in the public education system, is used for children aged 3 years to young adults aged 21 years. Individuals are also assisted, often by their IEP teams, to begin preparing for transition to adulthood by 16 years of age, if not sooner as necessary, as mandated by IDEA.[105]

GENETIC SYNDROMES COMMONLY ASSOCIATED WITH INTELLECTUAL DEVELOPMENTAL DISORDER

The following were selected as a representation of some of the most common genetic syndromes associated with IDD—DS, Fragile X syndrome (FXS), Williams syndrome (WS), and Angelman syndrome. They reflect a range of psychiatric, neurological, and medical signs and symptoms and show differential responses to available treatment options. Understanding these hallmarks of genetic disorders most commonly associated with IDD can better inform the clinicians in identifying and treating these patients.[106]

Down Syndrome

DS is the most common known genetic cause of IDD with a birth rate at approximately 1/700.[107] Depictions of individuals with physical features of DS have been in existence since 500 BC. DS was named after John Langdon Down who described DS as a disorder in 1866. It was not until 1959 that the cause of DS was discovered by Lejeune and colleagues.[108] Ninety-five percent of cases of DS occur as a result of three copies of chromosome 21. DS resulting from a translocation or mosaicism accounts for the remaining 5% of cases. There is no single pathognomonic physical feature in DS. Commonly observed dysmorphological features include up-slanting palpebral fissures, small ears with over folded helices, epicanthal folds, a flat nasal bridge, Brushfield spots on the iris, a single palmar crease, a short fifth digit, and a wide space between the first and second toes (Figure 18-3). Common medical comorbidities include vision problems such as refractive errors, congenital heart defects such as an atrial ventricular septal defect, gastrointestinal problems such as constipation, celiac disease and Hirschsprung's disease, thyroid dysfunction such as (most commonly) hypothyroidism, short stature, and obesity. Individuals with DS are also at an increased risk of developing acute lymphocytic leukemia, atlantoaxial instability, seizures, and early-onset dementia.[109]

In terms of cognitive profile, individuals with DS have an average IQ of 50 with a range of 30–70. Cognitive development typically slows after the age of 2 years. It is not uncommon for IDD to be diagnosed later in life. There is typically a greater expressive than receptive language deficit often accompanied

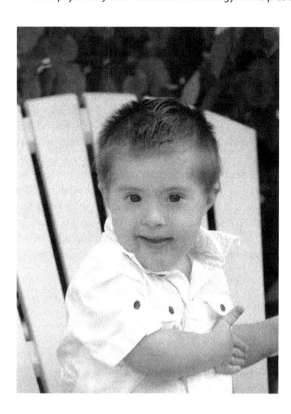

FIGURE 18-3. Commonly observed features for Down syndrome. (Reproduced with permission from Malcolm WF. Beyond the NICU: Comprehensive Care of the High-Risk Infant. https://accesspediatrics.mhmedical.com. Copyright © McGraw Hill LLC. All rights reserved.)

by significant articulation difficulties.[110] Individuals with DS are commonly characterized as being friendly, engaging, and affectionate.

Approximately one-third of individuals with DS will experience a psychiatric illness. As compared to other neurogenetic syndromes, the prevalence of psychiatric illness is lower, but it is elevated above the typical developing population. In children, externalizing disorders such as ADHD (6–34%) and oppositional defiant disorder (ODD; 10–15%) are more common than internalizing disorders (e.g., depression, anxiety). As individuals with DS age, internalizing disorders such as depression (6.1–11.4%) and anxiety (unknown prevalence) become more prevalent. ASD can also be seen in DS. There is a significant variation in the reported prevalence of ASD in DS (7–41%). Many investigators suggest that the rate of ASD is closer to 7–10%.[111–114] For depressive disorders, the available evidence for treatment is limited to case reports and small case series. In general, SSRIs are effective for depressive symptoms.[115] While not as commonly used in current practice, the tricyclic antidepressants (TCAs), such as *amitriptyline* and *imipramine*, are also effective.[115–117] For ADHD, an open-label trial of *guanfacine*, an alpha-2 adrenergic agonist, was studied for the treatment of ADHD in children with DS of ages 4–12 years by Capone and colleagues. The mean dose of *guanfacine* at the 21-week follow-up was 1.1 mg ± 0.5 mg per day or 0.07 mg/kg day ± 1.1 mg/kg with most subjects receiving *guanfacine* twice a day. Measures of irritability and hyperactivity each improved by 25%. *Guanfacine* was well tolerated. The main

side effects included nighttime sedation and asymptomatic lowering of blood pressure.[118]

Atypical antipsychotic medications have been used in DS for associated symptoms, such as aggression, irritability, and self-injurious behavior. An open-label study of *risperidone* demonstrated effectiveness for disruptive and self-injurious behaviors in patients with DS and comorbid ASD. Twenty-three subjects received *risperidone* for a mean of 95.8 ± 16.8 days with a total daily dose of 0.66 ± 0.28 mg. There was improvement in all five subscales of the Aberrant Behavior Checklist,[119] with disruptive behavior and self-injurious behavior showing the greatest magnitude of change. In addition to the target behaviors, sleep quality significantly improved in subjects with preexisting sleep problems. Side effects included increased appetite and a mean weight gain of 2.8 ± 1.5 kg. One subject had extrapyramidal symptoms (EPS) which improved with a 0.25 mg dose reduction.[120] *Aripiprazole* was effective in a 6-year-old male with DS and ASD for aggression, self-injurious behavior, and hyperactivity. *Aripiprazole* was well tolerated with some daytime sedation and mild weight gain of 0.2 kg over the course of 8 weeks.[121]

The average age at diagnosis of dementia in DS is around 55 years old.[110] In dementia without DS, the anticholinesterase inhibitors and the NMDA receptor antagonists are most commonly used in an effort to slow the progression of the disease. Randomized double-blind placebo-controlled trials of both *donepezil* (cholinesterase inhibitor) and *memantine* (NMDA receptor antagonist) found the drugs to be no better than placebo. Despite being RCTs, these studies did have their limitations including small sample size and no dementia diagnosis being required for the donepezil and memantine studies, respectively. Based upon these methodological concerns and the response data, strong conclusions about the effectiveness of these agents cannot be made. In addition to limited efficacy, interfering side effects, particularly with the cholinesterase inhibitors, including fatigue, diarrhea, insomnia, and nausea were observed.[122,123]

Clinicians providing care for individuals with DS should be aware of the common medical comorbidities that occur in DS. Obesity is very common in patients with DS. Medications with a high propensity for weight gain, such as the atypical antipsychotics, should be avoided if there are other options available. *Ziprasidone*, an atypical antipsychotic, is associated with less weight gain but needs to be used with caution in patients with congenital heart defects. An EKG as well as consultation with patient's cardiologist, if available, is advised.

Fragile X Syndrome

FXS is an X-linked neurodevelopmental disorder affecting 1 in 4000 males and 1 in 8000 females and is the most common inherited form of IDD and ASD. The syndrome results from expansion to >200 CGG trinucleotide repeats in the 5′ untranslated region of the Fragile X mental retardation-1 gene (FMR1), located at Xq27.3. The unstable expansion of CGG repeats leads to hypermethylation of the FMR1 promoter region and transcriptional silencing, resulting in insufficient or absent levels of Fragile X mental retardation protein (FMRP). FXS is diagnosed by molecular testing, including fluorescent polymerase chain reaction (PCR) to determine the number of CGG repeats and Southern blot analysis to determine methylation status.

In the absence of FMRP, an mRNA binding protein, and its mediated translational inhibition,[124] aberrant protein synthesis results in excessive activity-dependent long-term depression (LTD), synapse elimination, and loss of glutamatergic receptors (AMPAR, NMDAR) from the synaptic membrane.[125,126] The "mGluR theory" proposed by Bear and colleagues hypothesizes that the varied functional consequences of excessive mGluR-dependent protein synthesis can account for the characteristic cognitive, behavioral, and physical features.[125] FXS has similarly been described as a "synapsopathy": a disorder of synapse development and plasticity,[127] with consequential imbalance between excitatory (glutamatergic) and inhibitory (GABAergic) systems.

In males, phenotypic severity is inversely proportional to the amount of FMRP expressed. Mosaicism occurs in up to 40% of males, with the full mutation present in some cells and premutation (55–200 CGG repeats) in others. Males with FXS are typically more severely affected than females, for whom severity depends upon the degree of inactivation of the affected X chromosome. CGG amplifications between 55 and 200 repeats are termed premutation and denote FXS carrier status, which is associated with milder or absent clinical symptoms and heightened risk of expansion to the full mutation in the offspring of female carriers. Premutation amplifications do not result in the absence of FMRP, but rather increased levels of FMR1 mRNA, which may have a direct toxic effect in cells.[128,129]

Common clinical features in premutation carriers include premature ovarian failure (in women), ADHD, autistic features, learning difficulties (especially in math), and anxiety. Approximately one-third of older men (>50 years old) with premutation develop Fragile X tremor-ataxia syndrome (FXTAS), marked by intention tremor, gait ataxia, parkinsonism, autonomic dysfunction, executive function deficits, memory loss, and progression to dementia.[130] Neuroimaging typically reveals white matter lesions in the middle cerebellar peduncles, brain atrophy, and periventricular white matter disease, and postmortem findings include eosinophilic intranuclear inclusions in both neurons and astrocytes.[130,131]

Distinguishing physical features of FXS include macrocephaly, a long, narrow face, prominent forehead and chin, large ears, strabismus, high arched palate, joint hyperextensibility, and macro-orchidism in post-pubertal males (Figure 18-4). Thirteen to 20% of males and 5% of females with the full mutation develop seizures, which often resolve by adulthood. A subset of males with FXS exhibits a "Prader Willi phenotype" with obesity and hyperphagia. Hypotonia is common, and infants with FXS may present with feeding difficulties and delayed motor milestones.

The degree of neurocognitive impairment in FXS is greatest in those with the full mutation expressing minimal or no FMRP,[132] and most males with the full mutation have mild-to-moderate IDD. Among females with the full mutation, 50–71% have intellectual abilities in the borderline (IQ = 71–85) or mildly impaired (IQ = 55–70) range.[133] Affected individuals may have particular impairment in executive functioning, visuospatial skills, expressive language, and mathematics. Speech is notable

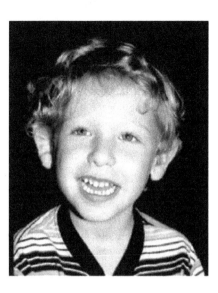

FIGURE 18-4. Commonly observed features for Fragile X syndrome. (Reproduced with permission from Carney PR, Geyer JD. *Pediatric Practice: Neurology.* https://accesspediatrics. mhmedical.com/. Copyright © McGraw Hill LLC. All rights reserved.)

for poor articulation, repetition, and short, fast utterances, and up to 10% of males with FXS are nonverbal.

Common neuropsychiatric symptoms include features of ADHD, ASD, anxiety, social phobia, insomnia, aggression, and self-injury. Symptoms of ADHD, including inattentiveness, hyperactivity, and impulsivity, are especially prominent in younger boys with FXS (approximately 75%), though hyperactivity tends to decline by young adulthood, as does agitation and aggression.[134] The prevalence of anxiety disorders in those with the full mutation exceeds 75%, with characteristic manifestations including gaze aversion, excessive shyness, and avoidance of people. Up to 25% may exhibit selective mutism, a severe expression of social anxiety.[135] On occasion, anxiety can also drive motor stereotypy (e.g., hand flapping), self-injury, and aggressive behavior. Up to one-third of individuals with FXS meet criteria for ASD, and many more have at least some features of autism, including repetitive behaviors, motor stereotypy, limited eye contact, and social communication deficits. ASD is most common in males with the full mutation and absent FMRP.

Despite greater understanding of the molecular processes owing to the development of an FXS mouse model (*Fmr1* knock-out),[136] promising preclinical results of "targeted" pharmacotherapies and repurposed older drugs have not yet demonstrated clear or consistent benefits in clinical trials (e.g., the mGluR5 antagonist mavoglurant [AFQ056]).[137–140] Other drugs of interest targeting downstream effects of mGluR5 overactivity include GABA$_A$R agonists (*acamprosate*),[141,142] glutamate modulators (*riluzole*),[143] NMDAR antagonists (*memantine*),[144] GABA$_B$R agonists (*arbaclofen*),[145,146] AMPAkines (CX516),[147] Ras-ERK1/2 inhibitors (*lovastatin*),[148] and matrix metalloproteinase-9 inhibitors (*minocycline*).[149] Studies have been hampered by small sample sizes, open-label designs, lack of

FXS-specific outcome measures, and enrolling older children and adults, perhaps missing a critical developmental window for intervention in early childhood.

In current clinical practice, interventions are typically aimed at maximizing developmental outcomes with nonpharmacological therapies, including speech and language therapy, OT, physical therapy, social skills instruction, and special education services. Psychotropic medications may be prescribed to reduce disruptive behavioral symptoms, including stimulants or alpha-2 agonists for ADHD, SSRIs for anxiety, melatonin for insomnia, and atypical antipsychotics for severe agitation, aggression, or self-injury. There is a limited body of evidence to guide treatment specifically in FXS, though following the general prescribing principles and precautions common to populations with IDD is useful, as mentioned above.

Williams Syndrome

WS is an uncommon neurodevelopmental disorder caused by a hemizygous microdeletion (only one copy present) at chromosome 7q11.23. The prevalence of WS is estimated to be between 1/7500 and 1/10,000.[150] WS is characterized by distinctive facial features. In young children, these include a flat nasal bridge, short upturned nose, periorbital puffiness, a long philtrum, and a delicate chin (Figure 18-5). Older patients have slightly coarse features with full lips, a wide smile, and a full nasal tip. Common medical comorbidities include vascular stenosis, such as supravalvular aortic stenosis, hypercalcemia and other endocrine abnormalities, sensorineural hearing loss, structural renal anomalies, and growth deficiency. The neurocognitive profile can include mild-to-moderate intellectual disability with relative strengths in language skills as compared to other cognitive domains. Individuals with WS often present with a highly social, overfriendly, and empathic personality. These personality characteristics can make these individuals vulnerable to inappropriate advances.[151]

Psychiatric comorbidities in individuals with WS include high rates of anxiety disorders (48–65%), including generalized anxiety disorder (12–25%), specific phobias (30–54%), and agoraphobia (24%), as well as ADHD (20–64.7%). Less commonly reported psychiatric disorders include depressive disorders (3–25%), obsessive-compulsive disorder (2–5%), and psychotic symptoms (5–6%).[152-154]

Only a limited number of reports of pharmacological treatment of comorbid psychiatric disorders in persons with WS exist in the medical literature. Morris et al.[155] described six children with ADHD treated with psychoactive medications. Three children were treated with *methylphenidate*, one with *pentobarbital* and *diphenhydramine*, and one with *thioridazine*, all targeting hyperactivity. The effectiveness and tolerability of these medication treatments were not reported.

A retrospective review of 18 patients with WS and comorbid ADHD treated with *methylphenidate* (mean dosage [SD] = 10.4 [5.9] mg/day) was conducted. The patients were 6.3 ± 1.4 years-old at the time of treatment initiation. Follow-up occurred 4.3 ± 3.8 years after the medication was begun. Thirteen of the 18 patients were rated as "much improved" or "very much improved" at the time of follow-up. Side effects that occurred frequently included sadness/unhappiness, poor appetite, and irritability.[156]

In the same report, the investigators described five patients with WS (12–24 years old) presenting with anxiety disorders treated with SSRIs for 1 month to 6 years. Three patients given *citalopram* (20–30 mg/day) were rated as "much improved" and one patient that received *citalopram* 20 mg/day was "minimally improved." A 12-year-old patient was treated with *fluoxetine* 20 mg/day but stopped the medication after 1 month due to headaches and abdominal pain despite showing much improvement in symptoms of anxiety. The second patient given *fluoxetine* remained unchanged after 6 months but eventually responded to *citalopram*.[156]

The atypical antipsychotic, *risperidone*, was prescribed for two young adult males with WS, one with aggression and psychotic symptoms and the other with self-injurious behavior and inappropriate sexual behavior. Improvement was seen in the presenting symptoms for both patients, but *risperidone* was stopped in both due to gastrointestinal side effects that were believed to be related to the medication.[157]

Parent surveys of the response to medication treatment of comorbid psychiatric symptoms in patients with WS have been published. One report included 513 respondents and focused on symptoms of mood, anxiety, and behavior. Twenty-four percent of subjects had been prescribed an SSRI and in 81% of cases, the response was rated "helpful" or "somewhat helpful" by parents. Twelve percent of subjects had been prescribed an antidepressant from a different class or an anxiolytic for the target symptoms. Sixty-four percent of parents reported that the medication had been "helpful" or "somewhat helpful."[158] The second parent survey asked about the effects of medication on symptoms of ADHD. The most commonly prescribed medication was a psychostimulant from the *methylphenidate* class.

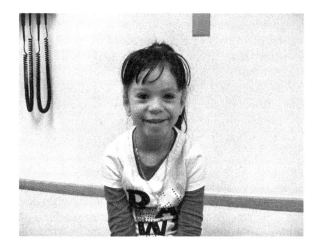

FIGURE 18-5. Commonly observed features for Williams syndrome. (Reproduced with permission from Gleason MM, Rychik J, Shaddy R. *Pediatric Practice: Cardiology.* https://accesspediatrics. mhmedical.com. Copyright © McGraw Hill LLC. All rights reserved. Image contributed by Dr. Elizabeth Goldmuntz, Children's Hospital of Philadelphia.)

Seventy-four percent of parents reported the psychostimulant to be at least "somewhat helpful."[159]

A recent report was the first to describe the co-occurrence of major depressive disorder with psychotic features in WS. Each of the three patients responded to the combination of an antidepressant and an atypical antipsychotic medication.[160]

Due to the medical comorbidities that often exist in WS, the potential benefits of psychopharmacology must be carefully weighed against the risks. Because weight gain is common in adults with WS, with two-thirds having a BMI greater than 25,[151] medications that can result in significant weight gain should be avoided whenever possible. In a meta-analysis of clinical trials of antipsychotic medications, *amisulpride, aripiprazole*, and *ziprasidone* showed the least amount of weight gain after prolonged use.[161] Weight gain is just one of the components of the metabolic syndrome that can occur with antipsychotic treatment. Dyslipidemias, increased susceptibility to diabetes, cardiac effects, and hypertension can also develop. Individuals with WS have high rates of impaired glucose tolerance,[151] and hypertension develops in approximately 50% of patients.[162] Moreover, the risk of sudden death in WS is significantly higher than in age-matched controls. In a retrospective review, 13.6% of patients with WS versus 2.0% of controls had QTc prolongation on electrocardiogram (ECG), a highly significant difference.[163] For these reasons, medications that are associated with QTc prolongation, such as *citalopram*[164] and most atypical antipsychotics,[165] should only be used in collaboration with a cardiologist, with frequent monitoring of the ECG.

Angelman Syndrome

Angelman syndrome (AS) is a neurodevelopmental disorder wherein there is impaired expression of the maternally inherited ubiquitin-protein ligase E3A gene (UBE3A) on chromosome 15.[166] AS is characterized by a host of clinical features including IDD with impaired expressive language, epilepsy, ataxia, sleep impairment, and a specific behavioral phenotype of frequent smiling and paroxysms of laughter (Figure 18-6). People with AS have significant care needs into adulthood which may include assistance with mobility and basic activities of daily living.[167] AS has an estimated incidence of 1 in 12,000–20,000 live births.[168] There are four different molecular mechanisms that result in the constellation of symptoms specific to AS. These include deletion of the maternal 15q11.2-13.1 region (about 70% of AS individuals), mutation of the maternal UBE3A gene (about 11%), paternal uniparental disomy (about 9%), and imprinting center defects (about 8%).[169] Imprinting centers are areas adjacent to genes that regulate their parental allele identity and corresponding expression. Defects in these centers can be caused by micro deletions or epimutations which lead to incorrect parent-of-origin allele identity.[170] Prader-Willi syndrome (PWS), the result of impaired expression of paternal genes from the 15q11.2-q13 region, results in a wider range of cognitive impairment than that seen in AS. Cognitive impairments in PWS may range from low-normal intelligence to moderate IDD.[171]

Problematic behavior can be common in patients with AS and can include sleep disorder,[172] hyperactivity,[173] aggressive behavior,[174] and anxiety.[175] Sleep disruption is one of the most

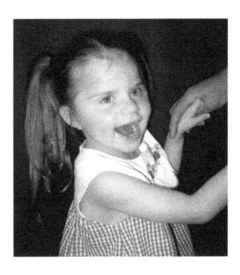

FIGURE 18-6. Commonly observed features for Angelman syndrome. (Reproduced with permission from Carney PR, Geyer JD. *Pediatric Practice: Neurology.* https://accesspediatrics.mhmedical.com/. Copyright © McGraw Hill LLC. All rights reserved.)

common behavioral challenges in children and adults with this condition. Prevalence is so high that sleep disturbance is an associated characteristic for the clinical diagnostic criteria and may affect up to 80% of individuals with the disorder.[176] Commonly reported challenges include delayed sleep initiation, frequent and prolonged nighttime awakenings, and a seemingly decreased need for total sleep. Symptoms are typically at their worst between 2 and 6 years of age[177] but may persist into adulthood.[167] Given the common co-occurrence of epilepsy and sleep disorder in AS, clinicians should be aware of the possibility that ongoing seizures may be contributing to sleep disturbance. However, many studies have found ongoing problems with sleep in participants with AS long after seizures were under control.

An agitated response to separation, particularly at bedtime, is a frequent behavioral hallmark in many patients with AS, which has led clinicians to examine behavioral strategies in improving sleep. Allen and colleagues[178] evaluated a behavioral treatment for five children with AS between the ages of 2 and 11 years who had sleep disturbance. Briefly, the behavioral treatment consisted of (1) maintaining a conducive sleep environment, (2) establishing a consistent bedtime, and (3) parent coaching to avoid responding to disruptive bedtime behaviors. Changes in the frequency of disruptive bedtime behavior and time to sleep onset were deemed statistically significant as compared to pretreatment values. Despite potential biological underpinnings of sleep disorder in AS, there is still an important role for behavioral treatments. Limited treatment trials examining the use of *melatonin* to address sleep disturbance in AS have shown promising results in decreasing sleep latency, increasing total sleep time, and reducing night awakenings.[179,180] Five milligrams were administered to participants 6 years and older and 2.5 mg to those who were younger at 7 PM.[180] Although *melatonin* usage may be ineffective or insufficient for some patients, no other medication trials have been conducted targeting sleep in this population.

Hyperactivity is a very common behavioral trait in patients with AS and may manifest in hypermotoric levels of activity.[181] Pervasive "sensory seeking" behaviors such as repetitive chewing, fidgeting, or mouthing items are common in AS and may be a reflection of this hypermotoric propensity. Hyperactivity and subsequent inattention may present challenges for patients with AS in making appropriate academic gains for their developmental level. This may slow progress in acquisition of communication strategies or lead to underestimates of cognitive abilities. One study examining the behavioral profile of 12 individuals (children and adults) with AS found elevated levels of hyperactivity as measured using the Attention Deficit Hyperactivity Disorder—Rating Scale (ADHD-RS) and Aberrant Behavioral Checklist (ABC) hyperactivity subscale.[182] Standard of care typically involves use of behavioral strategies and structure in the academic and home environment. There have been no studies of pharmacologic treatments for hyperactivity specifically for children or adults with AS.

Aggressive behavior has been consistently identified in a number of longitudinal studies as a frequent behavioral problem in AS. Two large recent studies estimated prevalence of aggressive behaviors as 73% and 72% respectively,[167,174] although other studies have found lower rates.[183] "Overactivity" was associated with physical aggression in one of these studies suggesting a possible link to hyperactivity.[174] For some patients with AS, aggression may serve a different function than the expression of explosive anger. Strachan and colleagues[184] conducted functional analyses of aggressive behaviors among 12 subjects with AS. They concluded that aggressive behaviors often served a function to maintain social attention they were receiving from adults. In support of this finding, Arron and colleagues[174] found higher levels of aggressive behavior among AS subjects with lower levels of autistic-like social interaction (i.e., intact social interest). If these behaviors reflect motivation for social interaction, families may be less likely to refer to them as "aggression" and see them as "excitability" around preferred caregivers or anxiety at the prospect of separation.

It is unclear how these factors may impact efficacy of treatment for aggressive behaviors as there have been no treatment studies. However, clinicians should consider careful assessment of precipitants for aggression in their treatment plans for patients with AS displaying aggression. Behavioral interventions that reward safe behavior with attention from preferred caregivers may be particularly effective. The association between physical aggression and "overactivity" suggests that treatments for hyperactivity may have downstream effects on reducing aggression. Finally, atypical antipsychotic medications, often used for irritability in populations with developmental disability, have particular risks in the AS population. Adults with AS have higher rates of obesity in adulthood,[167] which may be compounded from the use of atypical antipsychotic medications. Moreover, existing neurologic sequalae of AS, including tremor, may be difficult to distinguish from extrapyramidal side effects of antipsychotic medications.

Finally, anxiety has been consistently identified in population studies of adolescents and adults with AS.[175,185,186] In a study by Larson et al.,[167] 46% of caregivers identified adult study participants with AS as "showing signs of anxiety." Another study of 68 subjects found half of participants had a fear of crowds and a third had a fear of noise.[187] One cohort of 248 subjects with AS identified 45% of participants as becoming upset when routines were changed.[185] Accurate assessment of the frequency and severity of anxiety is limited by impairments in expressive language in AS.[188] Furthermore, evaluators must take into account that behaviors concerning for anxiety may instead represent pain, constipation, or unrelated sleep problems. Further research should focus on developing assessment tools specific to AS that can distinguish signs of anxiety from hyperactivity or irritability and measure improvement with treatments. While no formal treatment studies for anxiety in AS have been conducted, clinicians may opt to try *buspirone* in light of its favorable side-effect profile and levels of tolerability as drawn from neurotypical populations.[189]

Summary and Key Points

- The terminology for IDD has changed over time to avoid significant stigma associated with it.
- Understanding of IDD is advancing with accumulating knowledge of brain structure, neuro-biochemistry, genetics, etc.
- IDD is a cluster of symptoms resulting from neurologic dysfunction secondary to various forms of damage to the brain, and numerous etiologic causes for IDD have been identified.

- IDD has a huge impact on society, families, and patients' quality of life.
- Diagnosis of IDD requires deficits in intellectual and adaptive functioning with onset during the developmental period.
- Various treatment options are currently available for IDD; however, most of the current treatment options are symptomatic or rehabilitative, not curative.
- Clinicians should be well versed in multifaceted ways to support patients and families, which include not only psychological/psychiatric/neurological treatment options but also social/educational services.

Multiple Choice Questions

1. Which of the following is a possible pathophysiological mechanism for IDD?
   a. Inflammatory processes
   b. Direct physical damage
   c. Neurotransmitter or network interruption
   d. Metabolic dysfunction
   e. All of the above

2. Which of the following is mandated by the Individuals with Disabilities Education Improvement Act (IDEA; 2004, P.L. 108–446) for individually tailored public education for students with various disabilities in the United States?
   a. Early Intervention Programs (EIP)
   b. Individualized Education Program (IEP)
   c. Assistance by IEP team in preparing for transition to adulthood

   d. All of the above
   e. None of the above

3. Per the *DSM-5*, what two primary factors must be considered when determining a diagnosis of IDD during the developmental period?
   a. Academic functioning
   b. Intellectual functioning or IQ
   c. Adaptive functioning
   d. Social skills and play behaviors
   e. Both b and c are correct

4. Across the lifespan, individuals with IDD may require varying levels of support in which of the following areas?
   a. Problem-solving
   b. Academic skill acquisition and learning
   c. Basic activities of daily living
   d. Medical, legal, and financial decision making
   e. All of the above

Multiple Choice Answers

1. **Answer: e**
   IDD is believed to be a cluster of symptoms caused by failure in neurologic systems resulting from various insults to brain structure and/or neurochemistry. The exact pathogenesis is yet to be identified; possible mechanisms include inflammatory processes (e.g., prenatal infection with Rubella, CMV), direct physical damage, neurotransmitter or network interruption, and metabolic dysfunction (e.g., PKU), among many others.

2. **Answer: d**
   Currently, IDEA requires that students with various disabilities in the United States be provided with individually tailored public education. EIP addresses special needs for infants to children up to 3 years of age, while IEP provides special education plans through the public education system for children aged 3 years to young adults aged 21 years. Also,

   IEP teams often assist individuals in preparing for transition to adulthood by 16 years of age, if not sooner as necessary.

3. **Answer: e**
   The *DSM-5* currently defines IDD by deficits in intellectual function *and* deficits in adaptive functioning that result in failure to meet developmental and sociocultural standards for personal independence and responsibility. Although adaptive functioning includes conceptual, practical, and social domains, social skills and play behaviors are not included as primary diagnostic criteria.

4. **Answer: e**
   The combination of significant intellectual impairment and reduced adaptive skills often results in the need for ongoing caregiver support for the individual with IDD across the lifespan. An individual's unique profile, response to treatment, and the presence or absence of co-occurring conditions may alter the level of support required over time.

Acknowledgment

The authors thank the Nancy Lurie Marks Family Foundation for their ongoing support.

References

1. Reynolds T, Zupanick CE, Dombeck M. History of stigmatizing names for intellectual disabilities continued. MentalHelp.net. 2013.
2. 111th Congress, Public Law 111–256. 2010.
3. American Psychiatric Association. Intellectual disabilities. In: *Diagnostic and Statistical Manual of Mental Disorders (DSM-5*). Washington, DC: American Psychiatric Association Publishing; 2013:33.
4. World Health Organization. 6A00 Disorders of intellectual development. Draft ICD-11 Browser 2018. Available at https://icd.who.int/dev11/l-m/en#/http://id.who.int/icd/entity/605267007. Accessed June 19, 2018.
5. American Association on Intellectual and Developmental Disabilities. Definition of intellectual disability. 2018.

Available at http://aaidd.org/intellectual-disability/definition#.Wym5By2ZPq0. Accessed June 19, 2018.

6. Maulik PK, Mascarenhas MN, Mathers CD, Dua T, Saxena S. Prevalence of intellectual disability: a meta-analysis of population-based studies. *Res Dev Disabil*. 2011;32(2):419-436.

7. van Bakel M, et al. Monitoring the prevalence of severe intellectual disability in children across Europe: feasibility of a common database. *Dev Med Child Neurol*. 2014;56(4):361-369.

8. Roeleveld N, Zielhuis GA, Gabreels F. The prevalence of mental retardation: a critical review of recent literature. *Dev Med Child Neurol*. 1997;39(2):125-132.

9. Ncube BL, Perry A, Weiss JA. The quality of life of children with severe developmental disabilities. *J Intellect Disabil Res*. 2018;62(3):237-244.

10. Beadle-Brown J, et al. Quality of life and quality of support for people with severe intellectual disability and complex needs. *J Appl Res Intellect Disabil*. 2016;29(5):409-421.

11. Reppermund S, Trollor JN. Successful ageing for people with an intellectual disability. *Curr Opin Psychiatry*. 2016;29(2):149-154.

12. Bourke J, et al. Twenty-five year survival of children with intellectual disability in Western Australia. *J Pediatr*. 2017;188:232-239.e2.

13. Florio T, Trollor J. Mortality among a cohort of persons with an intellectual disability in New South Wales, Australia. *J Appl Res Intellect Disabil*. 2015;28(5):383-393.

14. Hosking FJ, et al. Mortality among adults with intellectual disability in England: comparisons with the general population. *Am J Pub Health*. 2016;106(8):1483-1490.

15. McCarron M, et al. Mortality rates in the general Irish population compared to those with an intellectual disability from 2003 to 2012. *J Appl Res Intellect Disabil*. 2015;28(5):406-413.

16. Landes SD. The intellectual disability mortality disadvantage: diminishing with age? *Am J Intellect Dev Disabil*. 2017;122(2):192-207.

17. Centers for Disease Control and Prevention. Economic costs associated with mental retardation, cerebral palsy, hearing loss, and vision impairment—United States, 2003. *MMWR Morb Mortal Wkly Rep*. 2004;53(3):57-59.

18. Huang J, et al. Prenatal, perinatal and neonatal risk factors for intellectual disability: a systemic review and meta-analysis. *PLoS One*. 2016;11(4):e0153655.

19. Deno E. Special education as developmental capital. *Except Child*. 1970;37(3):229-237.

20. Dunn LM. Special education for the mildly retarded—is much of it justifiable? *Except Child*. 1968;35(1):5-22.

21. Morin D, et al. A comparison of the prevalence of chronic disease among people with and without intellectual disability. *Am J Intellect Dev Disabil*. 2012;117(6):455-463.

22. Bishop KM, Robinson LM, VanLare S. Healthy aging for older adults with intellectual and development disabilities. *J Psychosoc Nurs Ment Health Serv*. 2013;51(1):15-18.

23. Turygin N, Matson JL, Adams H. Prevalence of co-occurring disorders in a sample of adults with mild and moderate intellectual disabilities who reside in a residential treatment setting. *Res Dev Disabil*. 2014;35(7):1802-1808.

24. Mohr C, Tonge BJ, Einfeld SL. The development of a new measure for the assessment of psychopathology in adults with intellectual disability. *J Intellect Disabil Res*. 2005;49 (pt 7):469-480.

25. Munir KM. The co-occurrence of mental disorders in children and adolescents with intellectual disability/intellectual developmental disorder. *Curr Opin Psychiatry*. 2016;29(2):95-102.

26. Cooper SA, et al. Psychosis and adults with intellectual disabilities. Prevalence, incidence, and related factors. *Soc Psychiatry Psychiatr Epidemiol*. 2007;42(7):530-536.

27. Fletcher RE, et al. *Diagnostic Manual—Intellectual Disability: A Textbook of Diagnosis of Mental Disorders in Persons with Intellectual Disability*. Kingston, NY: National Association for the Dually Diagnosed; 2007.

28. Pruijssers AC, et al. The relationship between challenging behaviour and anxiety in adults with intellectual disabilities: a literature review. *J Intellect Disabil Res*. 2014;58(2):162-171.

29. Charman T, et al. IQ in children with autism spectrum disorders: data from the Special Needs and Autism Project (SNAP). *Psychol Med*. 2011;41(3):619-627.

30. Fombonne E. Epidemiology of autistic disorder and other pervasive developmental disorders. *J Clin Psychiatry*. 2005;66(suppl 10):3-8.

31. Sheehan R, Ali A, Hassiotis A. Dementia in intellectual disability. *Curr Opin Psychiatry*. 2014;27(2):143-148.

32. Torr J, Strydom A, Patti P, Jokinen N. Aging in Down syndrome: morbidity and mortality. *J Policy Pract Intellect Disabil*. 2010;7(1):70-81.

33. Mefford HC, Batshaw ML, Hoffman EP. Genomics, intellectual disability, and autism. *N Engl J Med*. 2012;366(8):733-743.

34. Bourke J, et al. Population-based prevalence of intellectual disability and autism spectrum disorders in Western Australia: a comparison with previous estimates. *Medicine (Baltimore)*. 2016;95(21):e3737.

35. Memisevic H, Sinanovic O. Attention deficit hyperactivity disorder in children with intellectual disability in Bosnia and Herzegovina. *Coll Antropol*. 2015;39(1):27-31.

36. American Psychiatric Association. Specific learning disorder. In: *Diagnostic and Statistical Manual of Mental Disorders (DSM-5˚)*. Washington, DC: American Psychiatric Association Publishing; 2013:66.

37. Moss J, Howlin P. Autism spectrum disorders in genetic syndromes: implications for diagnosis, intervention and understanding the wider autism spectrum disorder population. *J Intellect Disabil Res*. 2009;53(10):852-873.

38. Matson JL, Dempsey T, Fodstad JC. The effect of autism spectrum disorders on adaptive independent living skills in adults with severe intellectual disability. *Res Dev Disabil*. 2009;30(6):1203-1211.

39. Braaten E. *The SAGE Encyclopedia of Intellectual and Developmental Disorders*. Thousand Oaks, CA: SAGE Publications; 2018.

40. Nevill RE, Havercamp SM. Intellectual disability. In: *Encyclopedia of Autism Spectrum Disorders*. Volkmar FR, eds. New York, NY: Springer; 2013:1623-1633.

41. Guralnick MJ. Early intervention for children with intellectual disabilities: an update. *J Appl Res Intellect Disabil*. 2017;30(2):211-229.

42. Rose SR, et al. Update of newborn screening and therapy for congenital hypothyroidism. *Pediatrics*. 2006;117(6):2290-2303.

43. Grosse SD, Van Vliet G. Prevention of intellectual disability through screening for congenital hypothyroidism: how much and at what level? *Arch Dis Child*. 2011;96(4):374-379.

44. van Karnebeek CD, Stockler S. Treatable inborn errors of metabolism causing intellectual disability: a systematic literature review. *Mol Genet Metab*. 2012;105(3):368-381.

45. Centers for Disease Control and Prevention. Newborn Screening Laboratory Bulletin. 2014. Available at https://www.cdc.gov/nbslabbulletin/bulletin.html. Accessed June 25, 2018.

46. Health Resources and Services Administration. Recommended Uniform Screening Panel. 2018. Available at https://www.hrsa.

gov/advisory-committees/heritable-disorders/rusp/index.html. Accessed June 25, 2018.

47. Bowring DL, et al. Prevalence of psychotropic medication use and association with challenging behaviour in adults with an intellectual disability. A total population study. *J Intellect Disabil Res.* 2017;61(6):604-617.

48. Bowring DL, et al. Challenging behaviours in adults with an intellectual disability: a total population study and exploration of risk indices. *Br J Clin Psychol.* 2017;56(1):16-32.

49. McQuire C, et al. Pharmacological interventions for challenging behaviour in children with intellectual disabilities: a systematic review and meta-analysis. *BMC Psychiatry.* 2015;15:303.

50. de Kuijper G, Mulder H, Evenhuis H, Scholte F, Visser F, Hoekstra PJ. Determinants of physical health parameters in individuals with intellectual disability who use long-term antipsychotics. *Res Dev Disabil.* 2013;34(9):2799-2809.

51. Oliver-Africano P, Murphy D, Tyrer P. Aggressive behaviour in adults with intellectual disability: defining the role of drug treatment. *CNS Drugs.* 2009;23(11):903-913.

52. Ji NY, Findling RL. Pharmacotherapy for mental health problems in people with intellectual disability. *Curr Opin Psychiatry.* 2016;29(2):103-125.

53. Aman MG, et al. Preliminary study of imipramine in profoundly retarded residents. *J Autism Dev Disord.* 1986;16(3):263-273.

54. Lewis MH, et al. Clomipramine treatment for stereotype and related repetitive movement disorders associated with mental retardation. *Am J Ment Retard.* 1995;100(3):299-312.

55. Lewis MH, et al. Clomipramine treatment for self-injurious behavior of individuals with mental retardation: a double-blind comparison with placebo. *Am J Ment Retard.* 1996;100(6):654-665.

56. Masi G, Marcheschi M, Pfanner P. Paroxetine in depressed adolescents with intellectual disability: an open label study. *J Intellect Disabil Res.* 1997;41(Pt 3):268-272.

57. Sheehan R, et al. Mental illness, challenging behaviour, and psychotropic drug prescribing in people with intellectual disability: UK population based cohort study. *BMJ.* 2015;351:h4326.

58. Doan T, et al. Psychotropic medication use in adolescents with intellectual disability living in the community. *Pharmacoepidemiol Drug Saf.* 2014;23(1):69-76.

59. Reid AH, Naylor GJ, Kay DS. A double-blind, placebo controlled, crossover trial of carbamazepine in overactive, severely mentally handicapped patients. *Psychol Med.* 1981;11(1):109-113.

60. Naylor GJ, et al. A double-blind trial of long-term lithium therapy in mental defectives. *Br J Psychiatry.* 1974;124(578):52-57.

61. Tyrer SP, et al. Factors associated with a good response to lithium in aggressive mentally handicapped subjects. *Prog Neuropsychopharmacol Biol Psychiatry.* 1984;8(4-6):751-755.

62. Craft M, et al. Lithium in the treatment of aggression in mentally handicapped patients. A double-blind trial. *Br J Psychiatry.* 1987;150:685-689.

63. Simonoff E, et al. Randomized controlled double-blind trial of optimal dose methylphenidate in children and adolescents with severe attention deficit hyperactivity disorder and intellectual disability. *J Child Psychol Psychiatry.* 2013;54(5):527-535.

64. Handen BL, et al. Efficacy of methylphenidate among preschool children with developmental disabilities and ADHD. *J Am Acad Child Adolesc Psychiatry.* 1999;38(7):805-812.

65. Pearson DA, et al. Treatment effects of methylphenidate on behavioral adjustment in children with mental retardation and ADHD. *J Am Acad Child Adolesc Psychiatry.* 2003;42(2):209-216.

66. Aman MG, Buican B, Arnold LE. Methylphenidate treatment in children with borderline IQ and mental retardation: analysis of three aggregated studies. *J Child Adolesc Psychopharmacol.* 2003;13(1):29-40.

67. Agarwal V, et al. Double-blind, placebo-controlled trial of clonidine in hyperactive children with mental retardation. *Ment Retard.* 2001;39(4):259-267.

68. Handen BL, Sahl R, Hardan AY. Guanfacine in children with autism and/or intellectual disabilities. *J Dev Behav Pediatr.* 2008;29(4):303-308.

69. Scahill L, et al. Extended-release guanfacine for hyperactivity in children with autism spectrum disorder. *Am J Psychiatry.* 2015;172(12):1197-1206.

70. Kalachnik JE, et al. Benzodiazepine behavioral side effects: review and implications for individuals with mental retardation. *Am J Ment Retard.* 2002;107(5):376-410.

71. Puustinen J, et al. CNS medications as predictors of precipitous cognitive decline in the cognitively disabled aged: a longitudinal population-based study. *Dement Geriatr Cogn Dis Extra.* 2012;2(1):57-68.

72. Balaj K, et al. Buspirone for the treatment of anxiety-related symptoms in Angelman syndrome: a case series. *Psychiatr Genet.* 2019;29(2):51-56.

73. Ratey J, Sovner R, Parks A, Rogentine K. Buspirone treatment of aggression and anxiety in mentally retarded patients: a multiple-baseline, placebo lead-in study. *J Clin Psychiatry.* 1991;52(4):159-162.

74. King BH, Davanzo P. Buspirone treatment of aggression and self-injury in autistic and nonautistic persons with severe mental retardation. *Dev Brain Dysfunct.* 1996;9:22-31.

75. Ward F, et al. Efficacy of beta blockers in the management of problem behaviours in people with intellectual disabilities: a systematic review. *Res Dev Disabil.* 2013;34(12):4293-4303.

76. Pitetti K, Miller RA, Loovis M. Balance and coordination capacities of male children and adolescents with intellectual disability. *Adapt Phys Activ Q.* 2017;34(1):1-18.

77. Carmeli E, et al. Perceptual-motor coordination in persons with mild intellectual disability. *Disabil Rehabil.* 2008;30(5):323-329.

78. Houwen S, et al. The interrelationships between motor, cognitive, and language development in children with and without intellectual and developmental disabilities. *Res Dev Disabil.* 2016;53-54:19-31.

79. Vismara L, et al. Effectiveness of a 6-month home-based training program in Prader-Willi patients. *Res Dev Disabil.* 2010;31(6):1373-1379.

80. Kurz MJ, et al. Overground body-weight-supported gait training for children and youth with neuromuscular impairments. *Phys Occup Ther Pediatr.* 2013;33(3):353-365.

81. Hocking J, McNeil J, Campbell J. Physical therapy interventions for gross motor skills in people with an intellectual disability aged 6 years and over: a systematic review. *Int J Evid Based Healthc.* 2016;14(4):166-174.

82. Shin JY, et al. The effects of a home-based intervention for young children with intellectual disabilities in Vietnam. *J Intellect Disabil Res.* 2009;53(4):339-352.

83. Ulrich DA, et al. Physical activity benefits of learning to ride a two-wheel bicycle for children with Down syndrome: a randomized trial. *Phys Ther.* 2011;91(10):1463-1477.

84. Eismann MM, et al. Characteristics of students receiving occupational therapy services in transition and factors related to postsecondary success. *Am J Occup Ther.* 2017;71(3):7103100010p1-7103100010p8.

85. Wuang YP, Ho GS, Su CY. Occupational therapy home program for children with intellectual disabilities: a randomized, controlled trial. *Res Dev Disabil.* 2013;34(1):528-537.

86. Dekker MC, Koot HM. DSM-IV disorders in children with borderline to moderate intellectual disability. I: prevalence and impact. *J Am Acad Child Adolesc Psychiatry.* 2003;42(8):915-922.

87. Dekker MC, et al. Emotional and behavioral problems in children and adolescents with and without intellectual disability. *J Child Psychol Psychiatry.* 2002;43(8):1087-1098.

88. Joyce T, Globe A, Moody C. Assessment of the component skills for cognitive therapy in adults with intellectual disability. *J Appl Res Intellect Disabil.* 2006;19(1):17-23.

89. McGillivray JA, Kershaw M. Do we need both cognitive and behavioural components in interventions for depressed mood in people with mild intellectual disability? *J Intellect Disabil Res.* 2015;59(2):105-115.

90. Unwin G, et al. Effectiveness of cognitive behavioural therapy (CBT) programmes for anxiety or depression in adults with intellectual disabilities: a review of the literature. *Res Dev Disabil.* 2016;51-52,60-75.

91. Idusohan-Moizer H, et al. Mindfulness-based cognitive therapy for adults with intellectual disabilities: an evaluation of the effectiveness of mindfulness in reducing symptoms of depression and anxiety. *J Intellect Disabil Res.* 2015;59(2):93-104.

92. Baker BL, et al. Pre-school children with and without developmental delay: behaviour problems and parenting stress over time. *J Intellect Disabil Res.* 2003;47(pt 4-5):217-230.

93. Coughlin M, et al. A controlled clinical evaluation of the Parents Plus Children's Programme: a video-based programme for parents of children aged 6 to 11 with behavioural and developmental problems. *Clin Child Psychol Psychiatry.* 2009;14(4):541-558.

94. Sanders MR, Bor W, Morawska A. Maintenance of treatment gains: a comparison of enhanced, standard, and self-directed Triple P-Positive Parenting Program. *J Abnorm Child Psychol.* 2007;35(6):983-998.

95. Sanders M, Mazzucchelli T, Studman L. *Practitioner's Manual for Standard Stepping Stones Triple P: For Families with a Child Who Has a Disability.* Brisbane, QLD: Triple P International Pty Ltd; 2012.

96. Kleefman M, et al. The effectiveness of Stepping Stones Triple P parenting support in parents of children with borderline to mild intellectual disability and psychosocial problems: a randomized controlled trial. *BMC Med.* 2014;12:191.

97. Roux G, Sofronoff K, Sanders M. A randomized controlled trial of group Stepping Stones Triple P: a mixed-disability trial. *Fam Process.* 2013;52(3):411-424.

98. Sharry J, Hampson G, Fanning M. *Parents Plus Early Years: A Practical and Positive Guide to Parenting Young Children Aged One to Six.* Manual and videos. Dublin, Ireland: Mater Hospital; 2003.

99. Sharry J, Fitzpatrick C. *Parents Plus Children's Programme: A Video-Based Parenting Guide to Managing Behaviour Problems and Promoting Learning in Children Aged Six to Eleven. Manual and videos.* Dublin: Mater Hospital; 2007.

100. Sharry J, Fitzpatrick C. *Parents Plus Adolescent Programme: A Parenting Guide to Handling Conflict and Getting on Better with Adolescents Aged Eleven to Fifteen.* Manual and videos. Dublin: Mater Hospital; 2001.

101. Smith T, Iadarola S. Evidence base update for autism spectrum disorder. *J Clin Child Adolesc Psychol.* 2015;44(6):897-922.

102. Gauthier-Boudreault C, Gallagher F, Couture M. Specific needs of families of young adults with profound intellectual disability during and after transition to adulthood: what are we missing? *Res Dev Disabil.* 2017;66:16-26.

103. Leonard H, et al. Transition to adulthood for young people with intellectual disability: the experiences of their families. *Eur Child Adolesc Psychiatry.* 2016;25(12):1369-1381.

104. Gauthier-Boudreault C, Couture M, Gallagher F. How to facilitate transition to adulthood? Innovative solutions from parents of young adults with profound intellectual disability. *J Appl Res Intellect Disabil.* 2018;31(suppl 2):215-223.

105. Jackson LL. *Occupational Therapy Services for Children and Youth Under IDEA.* Bethesda, MD: AOTA Press; 2007.

106. Van Bokhoven H. Genetic and epigenetic networks in intellectual disabilities. *Annu Rev Genet.* 2011;45:81-104.

107. Shin M, et al. Prevalence of Down syndrome among children and adolescents in 10 regions of the United States. *Pediatrics.* 2009;124(6):1565-1571.

108. Lejeune J, Gautier M, Turpin R. Study of somatic chromosomes from 9 Mongoloid children. *C R Hebd Seances Acad Sci.* 1959;248(11):1721-1722.

109. Roizen NJ, Patterson D. Down's syndrome. *Lancet.* 2003;361(9365):1281-1289.

110. Grieco J, et al. Down syndrome: cognitive and behavioral functioning across the lifespan. *Am J Med Genet C Semin Med Genet.* 2015;169(2):135-149.

111. Vicari S, Pontillo M, Armando M. Neurodevelopmental and psychiatric issues in Down's syndrome: assessment and intervention. *Psychiatr Genet.* 2013;23(3):95-107.

112. Capone G, et al. Neurobehavioral disorders in children, adolescents, and young adults with Down syndrome. *Am J Med Genet C Semin Med Genet.* 2006;142C(3):158-172.

113. Visootsak J, Sherman S. Neuropsychiatric and behavioral aspects of trisomy 21. *Curr Psychiatry Rep.* 2007;9(2):135-140.

114. Feinstein C, Chahal L. Psychiatric phenotypes associated with neurogenetic disorders. *Psychiatr Clin North Am.* 2009;32(1):15-37.

115. Myers BA, Pueschel SM. Major depression in a small group of adults with Down syndrome. *Res Dev Disabil.* 1995;16(4):285-299.

116. Szymanski LS, Biederman J. Depression and anorexia nervosa of persons with Down syndrome. *Am J Ment Defic.* 1984;89(3):246-251.

117. Storm W. Differential diagnosis and treatment of depressive features in Down's syndrome: a case illustration. *Res Dev Disabil.* 1990;11(2):131-137.

118. Capone GT, Brecher L, Bay M. Guanfacine use in children with Down syndrome and comorbid attention-deficit hyperactivity disorder (ADHD) with disruptive behaviors. *J Child Neurol.* 2016;31(8):957-964.

119. Aman MG, et al. The aberrant behavior checklist: a behavior rating scale for the assessment of treatment effects. *Am J Ment Defic.* 1985;89(5):485-491.

120. Capone GT, et al. Risperidone use in children with Down syndrome, severe intellectual disability, and comorbid autistic spectrum disorders: a naturalistic study. *J Dev Behav Pediatr.* 2008;29(2):106-116.

121. Bacanli A. Aripiprazole use in children diagnosed with Down syndrome and comorbid autism spectrum disorders. *J Child Adolesc Psychopharmacol.* 2016;26(3):306-308.

122. Prasher VP, et al. A 24-week, double-blind, placebo-controlled trial of donepezil in patients with Down syndrome and Alzheimer's disease—pilot study. *Int J Geriatr Psychiatry.* 2002;17(3):270-278.

123. Hanney M, et al. Memantine for dementia in adults older than 40 years with Down's syndrome (MEADOWS): a randomised, double-blind, placebo-controlled trial. *Lancet.* 2012;379(9815):528-536.

124. Wang H, et al. Dynamic association of the fragile X mental retardation protein as a messenger ribonucleoprotein between microtubules and polyribosomes. *Mol Biol Cell.* 2008;19(1):105-114.

125. Bear MF, Huber KM, Warren ST. The mGluR theory of fragile X mental retardation. *Trends Neurosci.* 2004;27(7):370-377.

126. Snyder EM, et al. Internalization of ionotropic glutamate receptors in response to mGluR activation. *Nat Neurosci.* 2001;4(11):1079-1085.

127. Bear MF, et al. Fragile X: translation in action. *Neuropsychopharmacology.* 2008;33(1):84-87.

128. Tassone F, et al. Elevated levels of FMR1 mRNA in carrier males: a new mechanism of involvement in the fragile-X syndrome. *Am J Hum Genet.* 2000;66(1):6-15.

129. Greco CM, et al. Neuronal intranuclear inclusions in a new cerebellar tremor/ataxia syndrome among fragile X carriers. *Brain.* 2002;125(pt 8):1760-1771.

130. Hagerman PJ, Hagerman RJ. Fragile X-associated tremor/ataxia syndrome (FXTAS). *Ment Retard Dev Disabil Res Rev.* 2004;10(1):25-30.

131. Brunberg JA, et al. Fragile X premutation carriers: characteristic MR imaging findings of adult male patients with progressive cerebellar and cognitive dysfunction. *AJNR Am J Neuroradiol.* 2002;23(10):1757-1766.

132. Loesch DZ, et al. Effect of fragile X status categories and FMRP deficits on cognitive profiles estimated by robust pedigree analysis. *Am J Med Genet A.* 2003;122a(1):13-23.

133. Tsiouris JA, Brown WT. Neuropsychiatric symptoms of fragile X syndrome: pathophysiology and pharmacotherapy. *CNS Drugs.* 2004;18(11):687-703.

134. Tranfaglia MR. The psychiatric presentation of fragile x: evolution of the diagnosis and treatment of the psychiatric comorbidities of fragile X syndrome. *Dev Neurosci.* 2011;33(5):337-348.

135. Cordeiro L, et al. Clinical assessment of DSM-IV anxiety disorders in fragile X syndrome: prevalence and characterization. *J Neurodev Disord.* 2011;3(1):57-67.

136. The Dutch-Belgian Fragile X Consortium. Fmr1 knockout mice: a model to study fragile X mental retardation. *Cell.* 1994;78(1):23-33.

137. Bailey DB Jr, et al. Mavoglurant in adolescents with fragile X syndrome: analysis of Clinical global impression-improvement source data from a double-blind therapeutic study followed by an open-label, long-term extension study. *J Neurodev Disord.* 2016;8:1.

138. Jacquemont S, et al. Epigenetic modification of the FMR1 gene in fragile X syndrome is associated with differential response to the mGluR5 antagonist AFQ056. *Sci Transl Med.* 2011;3(64):64ra1.

139. Berry-Kravis E, et al. Mavoglurant in fragile X syndrome: results of two randomized, double-blind, placebo-controlled trials. *Sci Transl Med.* 2016;8(321):321ra5.

140. Levenga J, et al. AFQ056, a new mGluR5 antagonist for treatment of fragile X syndrome. *Neurobiol Dis.* 2011;42(3):311-317.

141. Erickson CA, Mullett JE, McDougle CJ. Brief report: acamprosate in fragile X syndrome. *J Autism Dev Disord.* 2010; 40(11):1412-1416.

142. Erickson CA, et al. Impact of acamprosate on behavior and brain-derived neurotrophic factor: an open-label study in youth with fragile X syndrome. *Psychopharmacology (Berl).* 2013;228(1):75-84.

143. Erickson CA, et al. Open-label riluzole in fragile X syndrome. *Brain Res.* 2011;1380:264-270.

144. Erickson CA, Mullett JE, McDougle CJ. Open-label memantine in fragile X syndrome. *J Autism Dev Disord.* 2009;39(12):1629-1635.

145. Berry-Kravis E, et al. Arbaclofen in fragile X syndrome: results of phase 3 trials. *J Neurodev Disord.* 2017;9:3.

146. Berry-Kravis EM, et al. Effects of STX209 (arbaclofen) on neurobehavioral function in children and adults with fragile X syndrome: a randomized, controlled, phase 2 trial. *Sci Transl Med.* 2012;4(152):152ra127.

147. Berry-Kravis E, et al. Effect of CX516, an AMPA-modulating compound, on cognition and behavior in fragile X syndrome: a controlled trial. *J Child Adolesc Psychopharmacol.* 2006;16(5):525-540.

148. Caku A, et al. Effect of lovastatin on behavior in children and adults with fragile X syndrome: an open-label study. *Am J Med Genet A.* 2014;164a(11):2834-2842.

149. Leigh MJ, et al. A randomized double-blind, placebo-controlled trial of minocycline in children and adolescents with fragile x syndrome. *J Dev Behav Pediatr.* 2013;34(3):147-155.

150. Strømme P, Bjørnstad PG, Ramstad K. Prevalence estimation of Williams syndrome. *J Child Neurol.* 2002;17(4):269-271.

151. Pober BR, et al. High prevalence of diabetes and pre-diabetes in adults with Williams syndrome. *Am J Med Genet C Semin Med Genet.* 2010. Wiley Online Library. 154C(2):291-298.

152. Dodd HF, Porter MA. Psychopathology in Williams syndrome: the effect of individual differences across the life span. *J Ment Health Res Intellect Disabil.* 2009;2(2):89-109.

153. Dykens EM. Anxiety, fears, and phobias in persons with Williams syndrome. *Dev Neuropsychol.* 2003;23(1-2):291-316.

154. Leyfer OT, et al. Prevalence of psychiatric disorders in 4 to 16-year-olds with Williams syndrome. *Am J Med Genet B Neuropsychiatr Genet.* 2006;141B(6):615-622.

155. Morris CA, et al. Natural history of Williams syndrome: physical characteristics. *J Pediatr.* 1988;113(2):318-326.

156. Green T, et al. Phenotypic psychiatric characterization of children with Williams syndrome and response of those with ADHD to methylphenidate treatment. *Am J Med Genet B Neuropsychiatr Genet.* 2012;159(1):13-20.

157. Savoja V, Vicari S. Development of erosive gastrointestinal lesions during risperidone treatment in two patients with Williams syndrome. *Prog Neuropsychopharmacol Biol Psychiatry.* 2010;34(4):711-712.

158. Martens MA, et al. Parent report of antidepressant, anxiolytic, and antipsychotic medication use in individuals with Williams syndrome: effectiveness and adverse effects. *Res Dev Disabil.* 2012;33(6):2106-2121.

159. Martens MA, et al. Caregiver survey of pharmacotherapy to treat attention deficit/hyperactivity disorder in individuals with Williams syndrome. *Res Dev Disabil.* 2013;34(5):1700-1709.

160. Valdes F, et al. Brief report: major depressive disorder with psychotic features in Williams syndrome: a case series. *J Autism Dev Disord.* 2018;48(3):947-952.

161. Bak M, et al. Almost all antipsychotics result in weight gain: a meta-analysis. *PLoS One.* 2014;9(4):e94112.

162. Pober BR. Williams–Beuren syndrome. *N Engl J Med.* 2010; 362(3):239-252.

163. Collins RT 2nd, Aziz PF, Gleason MM, Kaplan PB, Shah MJ. Abnormalities of cardiac repolarization in Williams syndrome. *Am J Cardiol.* 2010;106(7):1029-1033.

164. Castro VM, et al. QT interval and antidepressant use: a cross sectional study of electronic health records. *BMJ.* 2013;346:f288.

165. Chun AK, Chua SE. Effects on prolongation of Bazett's corrected QT interval of seven second-generation antipsychotics in the treatment of schizophrenia: a meta-analysis. *J Psychopharmacol.* 2011;25(5):646-666.

166. Albrecht U, et al. Imprinted expression of the murine Angelman syndrome gene, Ube3a, in hippocampal and Purkinje neurons. *Nat Genet.* 1997;17(1):75-78.

167. Larson AM, et al. Angelman syndrome in adulthood. *Am J Med Genet A*. 2015;167A(2):331-344.

168. Williams CA, Driscoll DJ, Dagli AI. Clinical and genetic aspects of Angelman syndrome. *Genet Med*. 2010;12(7):385-395.

169. Bird LM. Angelman syndrome: review of clinical and molecular aspects. *Appl Clin Genet*. 2014;7:93-104.

170. Reik W, Walter J. Genomic imprinting: parental influence on the genome. *Nat Rev Genet*. 2001;2(1):21-32.

171. Cassidy SB, Schwartz S, Miller JL, Driscoll DJ. Prader-Willi syndrome. *Genet Med*. 2012;14(1):10-26.

172. Goldman SE, et al. Sleep in children and adolescents with Angelman syndrome: association with parent sleep and stress. *J Intellect Disabil Res*. 2012;56(6):600-608.

173. Williams CA. The behavioral phenotype of the Angelman syndrome. *Am J Med Genet C Semin Med Genet*. 2010;154C(4):432-437.

174. Arron K, et al. The prevalence and phenomenology of self-injurious and aggressive behaviour in genetic syndromes. *J Intellect Disabil Res*. 2011;55(2):109-120.

175. Smith JC. Angelman syndrome: evolution of the phenotype in adolescents and adults. *Dev Med Child Neurol*. 2001;43(7):476-480.

176. Williams CA, et al. Angelman syndrome 2005: updated consensus for diagnostic criteria. *Am J Med Genet A*. 2006;140(5):413-418.

177. Clayton-Smith J. Clinical research on Angelman syndrome in the United Kingdom: observations on 82 affected individuals. *Am J Med Genet*. 1993;46(1):12-15.

178. Allen KD, et al. Evaluation of a behavioral treatment package to reduce sleep problems in children with Angelman syndrome. *Res Dev Disabil*. 2013;34(1):676-686.

179. Zhdanova IV, Wurtman RJ, Wagstaff J. Effects of a low dose of melatonin on sleep in children with Angelman syndrome. *J Pediatr Endocrinol Metab*. 1999;12(1):57-67.

180. Braam W, et al. Melatonin for chronic insomnia in Angelman syndrome: a randomized placebo-controlled trial. *J Child Neurol*. 2008;23(6):649-654.

181. Buntinx IM, et al. Clinical profile of Angelman syndrome at different ages. *Am J Med Genet*. 1995;56(2):176-183.

182. Wink LK, et al. The neurobehavioral and molecular phenotype of Angelman syndrome. *Am J Med Genet A*. 2015;167A(11):2623-2628.

183. Summers JA, et al. Behaviour problems in Angelman syndrome. *J Intellect Disabil Res*. 1995;39(pt 2):97-106.

184. Strachan R, et al. Experimental functional analysis of aggression in children with Angelman syndrome. *Res Dev Disabil*. 2009;30(5):1095-1106.

185. Walz NC. Parent report of stereotyped behaviors, social interaction, and developmental disturbances in individuals with Angelman syndrome. *J Autism Dev Disord*. 2007;37(5):940-947.

186. Giroud M, et al. Angelman syndrome: a case series assessing neurological issues in adulthood. *Eur Neurol*. 2015;73(1-2):119-125.

187. Artigas-Pallares J, et al. Medical and behavioural aspects of Angelman syndrome. *Rev Neurol*. 2005;41(11):649-656.

188. Adams D, Oliver C. The expression and assessment of emotions and internal states in individuals with severe or profound intellectual disabilities. *Clin Psychol Rev*. 2011;31(3):293-306.

189. Riddle MA, et al. Anxiolytics, adrenergic agents, and naltrexone. *J Am Acad Child Adolesc Psychiatry*. 1999;38(5):546-556.

Tourette Syndrome and Related Neuropsychiatric Disorders

19

Erica L. Greenberg · Angela Essa · Jeremiah M. Scharf

INTRODUCTION

Tourette syndrome (TS), also known in the literature as Tourette's disorder, is a childhood-onset neuropsychiatric disorder that represents one end of a clinical spectrum of developmental tic disorders.[1] Tics are recurrent, often sudden, non-rhythmic movements or vocalizations that occur in bursts, and wax and wane over time and body location.

Currently, tic disorders are defined in *DSM-5* as distinct categorical entities, including *provisional tic disorder* (formerly transient tic disorder), *persistent (chronic) motor or vocal tic disorder*, and *Tourette's disorder*.[2] Provisional tic disorder is characterized by the presence of motor and/or vocal tics for a period of less than 1 year. Once tics have persisted for more than a year (regardless of whether some have stopped and new ones have begun), persistent (chronic) motor or vocal tic disorder is the appropriate diagnosis. If an individual has a history of *only* motor, or *only* vocal tics that have been present for more than 1 year, they would meet criteria for a persistent (chronic) motor tic disorder, or persistent (chronic) vocal tic disorder, respectively.

Based on *DSM-5* criteria, Tourette's disorder is diagnosed when an individual has had two or more motor tics, and at least one vocal tic, over the course of at least 1 year. For diagnostic purposes, it is important to note that motor and vocal tics do not both have to be present for a year, nor do they need to occur simultaneously. Furthermore, *DSM-5* criteria specifies that tics may wax and wane in frequency. Individuals may have tic-free periods of weeks to months and many individuals with mild tics do not necessarily notice their presence. Lastly, tic onset must occur prior to age 18, and must not have arisen secondary to, or solely from, an independent medical cause such as encephalitis, exposure to cocaine, or other inherited or degenerative basal ganglia disorders. Tics that onset after age 18 or that fail to meet criteria for either provisional tic disorder, persistent motor or vocal tic disorder, or Tourette's disorder, are classified as *unspecified tic disorder*.

While these diagnostic categories are still used both clinically and for research, emerging evidence from multiple types of research studies (clinical, neuroimaging, and genetic) suggest that the diagnostic boundaries between tic disorder categories are likely artificial, and that the group of developmental tic disorders may best be viewed as existing along a continuous phenotypic and developmental spectrum, akin to the unification of Autism Spectrum Disorders in *DSM-5* from the prior categories autism, Asperger's disorder, and pervasive developmental disorder not otherwise specified (PDD-NOS).[1,3]

Approximately 85% of individuals with TS presenting for clinical evaluation have one or more co-occurring psychiatric conditions.[4,5] Although obsessive-compulsive disorder (OCD) and attention-deficit hyperactivity disorder (ADHD) are the two neuropsychiatric conditions most frequently associated with TS, and are thought to have overlapping pathophysiologic mechanisms with TS and related tic disorders,[6] almost all major psychiatric disorders occur at increased rates in patients with TS compared to the prevalence of these disorders in the general population.[4] Thus, behavioral neurologists and neuropsychiatrists assessing individuals with TS need to be aware that many presenting symptoms will lie at the interface between the traditional boundaries of neurology and psychiatry and will require them to devise a formulation and treatment plan reflective of both disciplines.[7]

EPIDEMIOLOGY

In recent years, there have been multiple, large, well-designed epidemiologic studies evaluating TS prevalence worldwide.[8,9] At present, TS is thought to affect approximately 1% of school-age children. Chronic tic have not been as well studied, though may affect another 1–2%.[8] Studies have also shown that 20–25% of children will experience transient tics at some point in childhood.[10] Like most neurodevelopmental disorders, there is a male to female skew, with about a 3:1–4:1 ratio of males to females affected with TS. The mean age of onset of all tics is around ages 5–7.[11] Maximum severity is typically in early adolescence, usually between ages 10 and 13, though there is significant individual variability.[12] Fortunately, approximately two-thirds of individuals with persistent tic disorders will improve significantly over time. Conversely, approximately 10–20% of individuals with TS continue to have moderate or severely impairing tics as adults.[13] That said, those percentages are still based on limited data, and there are few predictors of adult outcomes.[14]

PATHOPHYSIOLOGY

TS and other tic disorders are developmental neuropsychiatric disorders arising from abnormalities of brain circuits involving the basal ganglia and their connections.[1] The basal ganglia consist of the striatum (including the caudate, putamen, and nucleus accumbens), the substantia nigra, the subthalamic nucleus (STN), and the globus pallidus (Figure 19-1).[6,15] The basal ganglia are subcortical nuclei that operate within the context of recurrent, parallel *cortico-basal ganglia-thalamo-cortical* (CSTC) loops, and are thought to regulate, refine, and prioritize movements, thoughts, mood, and behavior by integrating information from the external and internal environment and

providing feedback through a mechanism of reinforcement learning.[16,17]

While the basal ganglia have traditionally been viewed as the "habit system" of the brain, playing a role in motor planning and execution, they are now understood to comprise distinct associative and limbic domains, where cognition, motivation, and emotion play a driving role in movement and behavior.[18] These functional domains are thought to map onto distinct sensorimotor, associative (cognitive), and limbic (emotional) loops, with some degree of integration across circuits (Figure 19-2).[6,18] According to neuroimaging and neurophysiology studies, along with experimental results from nonhuman primates, it is likely that disruption of the orchestrated activity between the basal ganglia, cerebral cortex, thalamus, and brainstem, due to dysregulated development and/or maintenance, leads to TS and its associated co-occurring disorders (e.g., OCD, ADHD).[6,19,20] In this context, the shared familial nature of tics, OCD and ADHD appear to parallel abnormal development in motor, limbic, and associative CSTC circuits (see Genetics section below).[3,6,18,21] This parallel, yet integrated circuitry may help to explain why TS so often co-occurs with ADHD and OCD.[6]

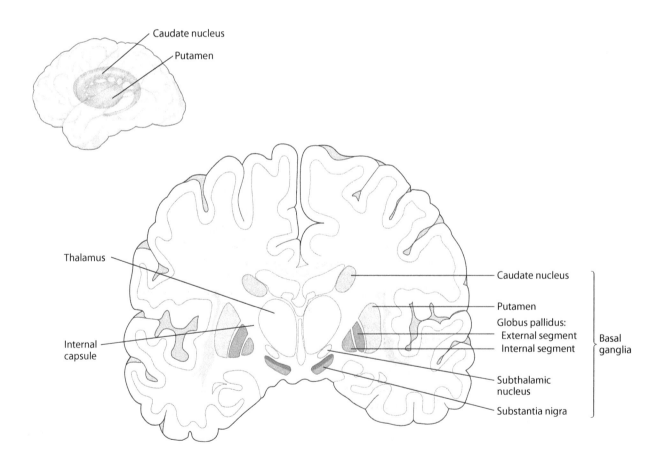

FIGURE 19-1. Nuclei of the basal ganglia. The central figures illustrates a schematic of the human brain in the coronal plane (facing head on), with the individual nuclei of the basal ganglia highlighted in blue. The smaller schematic to the upper left illustrates a view of the basal ganglia in the sagittal plane (facing the left ear) and demonstrates how the caudate nucleus extends as C-shaped subcortical structure subserving the entire cerebral cortex. (Adapted, with permission, from Nieuwenhuys R, Voogd J, van Huijzen C. *The Human Central Nervous System: A Synopsis and Atlas*. 2nd ed. Berlin: Springer; 1981 and Kandel ER, Schwartz JH, Jessell TM, Siegelbaum SA, Hudspeth AJ, Mack S. The basal ganglia. In: *Principles of Neural Science*. 5th ed. https://neurology.mhmedical.com. Copyright © 2019 McGraw Hill LLC. All rights reserved.)

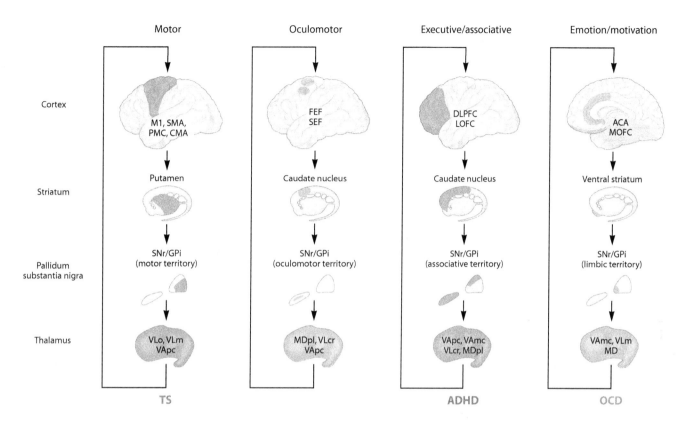

FIGURE 19-2. Cortico-striato-(pallido)-thalamo-cortical loops underlying the shared pathophysiology between Tourette syndrome, obsessive-compulsive disorder, and ADHD. ACA, anterior cingulate area; CMA, cingulate motor area; DLPFC, dorsolateral prefrontal cortex; FEF, frontal eye field; GPi, internal segment of the globus pallidus; LOFC, lateral orbitofrontal cortex; M1, primary motor cortex; MDpl, mediodorsal nucleus of thalamus, lateral part; MOFC, medial orbitofrontal cortex; PMC, premotor cortex; SEF, supplementary eye field; SMA, supplementary motor area; SNr, substantia nigra pars reticulata; VAmc, ventral anterior nucleus of thalamus, magnocellular part; VApc, ventral anterior nucleus of thalamus, parvocellular part; VLcr, ventrolateral nucleus of thalamus, caudal part, rostral division; VLm, ventrolateral nucleus of thalamus, medial part; VLo, ventrolateral nucleus of thalamus, pars oralis. (Adapted, with permission, from Wichmann T, Delong MR. Deep brain stimulation for neurologic and neuropsychiatric disorders. *Neuron.* 2006;52:197-204. https://www.sciencedirect.com/journal/neuron. Elsevier. All rights reserved, and Kandel ER, Schwartz JH, Jessell TM, Siegelbaum SA, Hudspeth AJ, Mack S. The basal ganglia. In: *Principles of Neural Science.* 5th ed. 2014. https://neurology.mhmedical.com. Copyright © McGraw Hill, LLC. All rights reserved.)

Somatotopy in the Basal Ganglia

Just as cortical mapping has demonstrated that the organization of the somatosensory and motor cerebral cortex reflects an anatomical body map, or "homunculus,"[22] stereotactic lesioning and microelectrode mapping in patients, along with high-frequency stimulation of specific areas of the putamen, STN, GPi, and motor thalamus, indicate the presence of a somatotopic organization within each nucleus of the somatosensory and motor basal ganglia.[23] Work in nonhuman primates has mapped the somatotopic organization of the putamen in finer detail, including a map for individual muscle movements of the legs, arm, and face lying anterior to an identical somatotopic map for more complex movements of adjacent muscles in each of these regions.[24] This anatomic organization also parallels the typical pattern of emergence of tics over time, in which simple tics of the eyes, nose, face, head, and shoulders often present first in patients, followed later by tics involving the arms and legs, as well as tics of increasing severity and complexity.[1,25] Therefore, the significant variability in clinical phenomenology of tics between patients with regards to body location, complexity, and severity likely correlates anatomically with more extensive involvement and dysregulation of individual CSTC circuits.

Genetics

Multiple twin and family studies have demonstrated that TS is highly heritable (~60–80%), though the disorder is not inherited in a Mendelian (single gene) fashion.[26] In addition, various studies have suggested that tics more broadly, rather than just TS alone, are increased in first-degree relatives of individuals with TS compared to rates seen in control families.[27] These findings suggest that tic disorders may represent a continuum, rather than discrete entities. More recent population-based studies using national registry data have confirmed these initial family studies, demonstrating a population-based heritability of 77%,[28,29] with a sibling recurrence risk ratio of 18.6 (95% CI, 15.3–22.6) (i.e., a child with an affected sibling has an 18.6-fold higher risk of developing TS compared to the baseline TS population prevalence) and a parent-offspring recurrent risk of 61.0 (95% CI, 44.4–83.8). Nonetheless, identification of definitive TS susceptibility genes has proved challenging, though in the last few years, significant progress has been made with identification of the first definitive, genome-wide significant TS susceptibility loci, large, rare *NRXN1* deletions and *CNTN6* duplications, as well as rare, gene-damaging de novo mutations in *CELSR3*.[30,31] Deletions in *NRXN1*, a gene encoding the presynaptic cell-adhesion molecule, Neurexin-1, that is involved in glutamatergic and GABAergic synaptogenesis, have been identified previously in other neuropsychiatric disorders including autism and schizophrenia, and therefore this mutation may confer a broader risk for neuropsychiatric disease.[32] Similarly, there has been a single case report of a child with intellectual disability and autism spectrum disorder harboring a duplication in *CNTN6*, whose protein product, Contactin-6, is also a neurodevelopmental cell-adhesion molecule.[33] To date, however, *CELSR3* mutations have only been identified in TS patients, but whether damaging alterations in this gene are specific to TS remains to be determined.

In addition to studies of single gene disruptions, a recent genome-wide association study (GWAS) of 4819 TS cases and 9488 controls demonstrated that aggregated TS-associated common risk alleles (i.e., polygenic risk scores) were most strongly enriched in DNA variants regulating gene expression in human dorsolateral prefrontal cortex.[3] While none of the other 53 human organ/tissue types were significantly enriched after correction for multiple-hypothesis testing, the 6 additional tissues nominally enriched for TS-associated gene regulatory variants came from brain structures within CSTC circuits (cortex, putamen, anterior cingulate cortex, caudate, and nucleus accumbens) as well as the cerebellum.[3] Thus, these data provide genetic support to the neuroimaging findings that CSTC dysregulation is a core feature of the disorder.

Additional analyses have leveraged TS GWAS data to examine whether the wide variation in tic severity across patients may have a genetic basis. Yu and colleagues[3] demonstrated that, in individuals with a known family history of TS or chronic tics, the relative genetic burden of TS-associated risk alleles was positively correlated with participant worst-ever tic severity, potentially reflecting more severe dysregulation within developing CSTC circuits. Similarly, the study also found that aggregated genome-wide TS common variant burden (i.e., TS polygenic risk) is present at lower levels in individuals with other tic disorders (chronic tic disorder and unspecified tic disorder), confirming that TS and other tic disorders exist along a shared gradient of genetic risk.

Finally, a few studies have examined the genetic relationship between TS, OCD, and ADHD using genome-wide association data.[34-36] These analyses indicated a significant proportion of shared polygenic risk between TS and OCD, and suggested that TS and ADHD have overlapping genetic risk as well.[36] Of note, these analyses also found evidence for genetic heterogeneity within OCD, as individuals recruited for an OCD study who either endorsed having tics, or who endorsed "symmetry," "evening up" (i.e., creating a feeling of evenness), or "just right" obsessions/compulsions without tics, had a polygenic risk profile that was more similar to TS/tic disorder than to OCD without tics.[21,35]

Nongenetic Risk Factors

A number of nongenetic risk factors have recently been identified to be increased in individuals with TS or chronic tics compared to the general population, including adverse prenatal and perinatal events, maternal smoking, and a family history of autoimmune disease.[37-41] Further work is needed to understand how these risk factors work together with genetic risk to cause disease.

CLINICAL PRESENTATION

A defining feature of tics is their partial suppressibility, which typically leads to increasing physical discomfort at the site of the tic until its release. This preceding uncomfortable physical sensation, referred to as a "premonitory urge," is often described as an "itch," "sneeze," or "tension." Most individuals with tics (especially those older than age 10) report that they perform the tic to relieve this urge.[42,43] Therefore, tics are often experienced as somewhere between "voluntary" and "involuntary" movements, as they are simultaneously experienced as being both out of one's control and requiring active participation in the movement (compared to other involuntary movement disorders, such as myoclonus or tardive dyskinesia). It is important to note that tics may continue during sleep as well.

Tics are arbitrarily divided by their complexity (simple vs. complex) and their form (motor vs. vocal) (Table 19-1).[44,45] Simple tics involve brief contractions of isolated muscle groups. Common examples of simple motor tics include eye blinking, nose twitching, head shaking, and shoulder shrugging. Phenomenologically, simple vocal tics are merely motor tics that involve contraction of the muscles in the pharynx, larynx, and/or the diaphragm. Common examples include sniffing, coughing, grunting, and throat clearing. Some experts in tic disorders prefer to use "phonic" rather than "vocal" to describe these tics, as many sound-producing tics do not engage the vocal cords and thus the term "vocal tics" may mislead clinicians and the general public that these tics require the production of words.[46]

Complex tics represent a rather broad range of repetitive movements and sounds that involve more than one muscle group and/or a temporal sequence of movements/sounds.[47] While any set of movements/sounds can comprise a complex tic, most complex motor tics often fall into one of three broad categories: (1) complex, coordinated movements or "purposeful appearing" gestures (e.g., simultaneous or sequential eye, head and shoulder jerks, skipping, jumping, deep knee bends, passing one's hands through their hair); (2) aggressive or self-injurious tics (e.g., poking, pinching, punching oneself), and (3) compulsive tics (e.g., touching, tapping, needing to repeat a tic sequence a specific number of times or to make them symmetric or even on both sides of the body). As such, it can often be quite difficult to discern where a complex tic ends and a compulsion begins; as described below, this is often a false dichotomy.[48] Complex vocal tics can include changes in intonation, syllables, words, phrases, echolalia (repeating others), palilalia (repeating oneself), and coprolalia. Of note, isolated echolalia can frequently occur in individuals with other neurodevelopmental disorders

TABLE 19-1 • Examples of Common Motor and Vocal Tics Separated by Complexity.	
Simple Tics	
Motor	Vocal
Eye blinking	Sniffing
Nose scrunching	Throat clearing
Head jerking	Coughing
Shoulder shrugging	Barking
Quick arm or hand jerks	Grunting
Abdominal muscle tensing	Squeaking
Quick arm or leg jerks	
Complex Tics	
Motor	Vocal
Eye rolling	Animal or bird noises
Touching ear to shoulder	Changes in intonation
Sequence/Chain of different tics	Sequence/Chain of vocal tics
Tapping a certain number of times	Syllables
Making tics even or symmetric	Words
Jumping	Phrases
Complex gestures or postures	Coprolalia
Echopraxia/Palipraxia	Echolalia/Palilalia
Copropraxia	

Echolalia, repeating sounds of others; palilalia, repeating oneself; echopraxia, repeating movements of others; palipraxia, repeating one's own movements.

or acquired diseases that affect frontal networks[49]; thus clinicians should be cautious about diagnosing a tic disorder when echolalia is present in the absence of other tics. Coprolalia, often thought of as swearing tics, is in fact defined as any socially inappropriate words or phrases that are stereotyped, repetitive, and occur independent of normal discourse.[47] It is important to note that coprolalia is only present in 10–20% of individuals with TS.[50] Ultimately, it may be helpful to think of tics as otherwise appropriate fragments of movements or sounds that come out at an inappropriate time.

Regarding tic phenomenology, tics most commonly involve the eyes, head, face, and neck, and typically onset in a rostral (eyes/head) to caudal (legs/feet) progression, with simple tics usually arising before complex tics, and motor before phonic tics.[1] However, by definition, tics "jump" or change over time in body location, frequency, and intensity, which is a key feature that experts use to distinguish tics from other types of repetitive movements such as complex motor stereotypies (see Differential Diagnosis section below). Additionally, baseline tic severity tends to wax and wane over periods of time, and tics themselves are known to be particularly sensitive to "modifying factors"—internal or external stimuli that serve to exacerbate or mollify tics. Common tic exacerbators include various feeling states (anxiety, tension, boredom, excitement, etc.), fatigue, and physiological stressors, such as illness. Periods of reduced stress, physiological and otherwise, and/or intense engagement/ focus (e.g., acting in a play, singing), are often associated with decreases in tics.

CO-OCCURRING NEUROPSYCHIATRIC CONDITIONS

TS rarely presents as an isolated tic disorder. About 85% of patients with TS will have at least one other neuropsychiatric condition or neurodevelopmental disorder.[4] It is important to note that, in the vast majority of those individuals, the co-occurring condition will be more impairing than the tics themselves. As such, during an initial assessment, it is imperative to screen for common associated neuropsychiatric conditions.

Obsessive-Compulsive Disorder

The most common co-occurring condition in individuals with TS or chronic tic disorder is OCD.[4,5] OCD is characterized by recurrent, bothersome, intrusive thoughts, feelings, or urges that lead to anxiety, distress, and/or disgust (obsessions), and behaviors (mental or physical) that serve to neutralize the negative feelings (compulsions). While many individuals may experience non-impairing obsessive or compulsive symptoms at some point in their lives, to meet criteria for OCD, obsessive-compulsive symptoms must be time-consuming or lead to significant distress or impairment. Between 30% and 60% of those with TS meet full criteria for OCD, with even more having subclinical obsessive-compulsive symptoms.[5] This high prevalence of co-occurring OCD in individuals with TS contrasts with the baseline OCD prevalence of 2–3% in the general adult population.[51] OCD age of onset tends to be bimodal, with one peak in the late childhood/early adolescence, and another in late teens/early 20s.[51] Of note, the early-onset subtype of OCD is more often associated with tics and TS than later onset OCD.[52] Like tics, OCD symptoms tend to wax and wane, though while tics often improve with age, OCD symptoms in those with TS have generally been thought to persist[53]; however, longitudinal outcome data has been scarce, and recent studies have found that a significant proportion of patients with TS with OCD in early adolescence experienced remission of OCD when reevaluated at age 16 or later.[13]

In general, there are many phenomenological similarities between tics and OCD. As described in the pathophysiology section (above), OCD and tics have overlapping genetic susceptibility and dysfunctional neurocircuitry. The sensory/ somatic premonitory urge that precedes tics parallels the obsessive thoughts that precede compulsions. Certain OCD symptoms are also more frequently seen in individuals with TS compared to those without, in particular symptoms of aggressive urges, sexual and symmetry obsessions, checking, touching/tapping, and evening up compulsions.[21,54] Many patients with TS and co-occurring OCD describe experiencing feelings of "not just rightness" or incompleteness preceding their compulsions (rather than obsession-related anxiety or disgust).[54]

The experience of sensory-based feelings driving compulsions, for example, having to "tap something six times so that it feels just right," is sometimes referred to as "Tourettic

OCD."[55-58] Tourettic OCD is associated with male sex, earlier age of OCD onset, worse OCD symptoms, sensory difficulties, ADHD, impulse control disorders, and anxiety disorders. Some patients with TS and OCD also experience overlapping symptoms (described previously as "compulsive tics,"[59] or, as coined by one of our patients, "ticculsions"), where an intrusive, anxiety-provoking thought (i.e., an obsession) precedes a tic, and completion of the tic briefly relieves the anxiety. It is important to note that distinguishing between "pure" tics and/or OCD, and overlapping tic/OCD symptoms (either "Tourettic OCD" or "compulsive tics/ticculsions") has treatment implications, as OCD with tics is associated with worse treatment response to selective serotonin reuptake inhibitors (SSRIs) than OCD without tics,[60] and patients with "ticculsions" often require treatments targeting the tic and OCD components simultaneously.

Attention-Deficit Hyperactivity Disorder

Another common co-occurring neuropsychiatric disorder seen in TS is ADHD. The specific prevalence of ADHD in those with TS varies widely depending on study ascertainment, ranging between 30% and 90%.[4,5] Tic disorders with co-occurring ADHD are associated with higher levels of functional impairment, worse tic severity, and additional externalizing disorders (such as oppositional defiant disorder, ODD) often seen in children with ADHD in the absence of tics.[61] Co-occurring TS, OCD, and ADHD, known as "the triad" among TS specialists, is present in ~30% of all patients with TS.

Anger Outbursts

Anger outbursts, sometimes called "rage attacks," are another commonly co-occurring, though less recognized condition that occurs in ~15–30% of individuals with TS.[62] Individuals with anger outbursts will have severe, impulsive anger, out of proportion to the trigger, which often lasts 10–15 minutes, but can extend for 1–2 hours at a time, and is often followed by significant remorse.[62] These anger outbursts occur most commonly in patients with co-occurring ADHD, mood, or anxiety disorders.

Body-Focused Repetitive Behaviors (Hair Pulling Disorder/Skin Picking Disorder)

Hair pulling disorder (HPD) and skin picking disorder (SPD), known collectively as body-focused repetitive behaviors (BFRBs), are both classified in *DSM-5* as Obsessive-Compulsive Related Disorders. They co-occur with TS at higher rates than those in the general population.[2,63] BFRBs are quite heterogeneous, but can often be associated with a physical urge/tension similar to the premonitory urge preceding tics, and, like tics, are more frequently associated with ADHD and increased impulsivity.[64] While individuals with BFRBs have high rates of co-occurring OCD, BFRBs tend not to be responsive to SSRI therapy. Behavioral therapy, including habit-reversal training (HRT) (the same behavioral therapy approach used to treat tics), is a mainstay of BFRB treatment.[65]

Other Co-occurring Neuropsychiatric Disorders

Nearly all psychiatric disorders have been demonstrated to occur at higher rates in individuals with TS compared to that of the general population[5]; however, a large family genetic study has demonstrated that TS appears to share a direct genetic relationship only with OCD and ADHD, while all other disorders segregate in families either with OCD, ADHD, or both.[4]

Anxiety and mood disorders are two of the most common non-OCD, non-ADHD disorders found in patients with TS.[66] Of note, treatment for these conditions do not generally differ from those used in children, adolescents, or adults without tics. Patients with TS often have sleep disorders (~25%) and learning disorders (~25%), though the specific type of sleep or learning disorder varies widely.[67] Individuals with TS also frequently have heightened sensitivity or intolerance to sensory stimuli.[68,69] While this sensitivity can involve any sensory modality, patients often report, for example, being bothered by tags in shirts or seams in socks. A recently defined condition, misophonia (literally "hatred of sound"), in which intolerance of specific sounds, such as loud chewing or words containing the consonants "s" or "k," elicits a feeling of anger or disgust, is frequently associated with those who have tic-OCD spectrum disorders.[70,71]

Lastly, up to 25% of patients with TS will have symptoms consistent with an autism spectrum disorder; however, given the clinical overlap between tics and motor stereotypies as well as between obsessions and restricted repetitive behaviors, one needs to be cautious about potential misdiagnosis of this condition based only on use of common rating scales.[72,73]

Individuals with TS frequently have significant psychosocial impairment. These difficulties impact youth with TS in multiple domains, including school, social activities, and home.[74] Youth with TS often experience peer victimization, suffer from low self-esteem, and experience lower quality of life compared to their peers. As those with TS and chronic tic disorders grow up, they have a significantly greater risk of attempting (OR: 3.86; 95% CI: 3.50–4.26) and/or dying by suicide (OR: 4.39; 95% CI: 2.89–6.67), even after adjusting for co-occurring psychiatric conditions.[75] TS also affects the family; parents report elevated caregiver burden and increased difficulty caring for their child compared to other children.[74] Additionally, even in the absence of a co-occurring autism spectrum disorder diagnosis, studies have identified an association between TS and social deficits.[73] It is important to note that TS-associated disability and impairment is more frequently associated with co-occurring psychiatric conditions than with the tics themselves.[76]

ASSESSMENT AND DIFFERENTIAL DIAGNOSIS

When motor and/or vocal tics are observed and the presence of the other diagnostic criteria are met, a diagnosis of a developmental tic disorder (e.g., provisional tic disorder, persistent (chronic) motor or vocal tic disorder, or TS) can be established. The most important component of the assessment is conducting a thorough history, including approximate age of onset, any precipitating factors, a list of past and current motor and/or vocal tics, confirmation of a waxing and waning pattern of symptoms with different tics appearing and disappearing over time, and the presence of a premonitory urge and brief tic suppressibility, often with subsequent rebound effects. Of note, young children often do not experience a premonitory urge, but should be able to suppress tics briefly if they are aware of them.[45] The presence of a family history of tic disorders and/or OCD can support the diagnosis, but is not always present given the non-Mendelian inheritance of the disorder.[26] Exposures to medications or recreational drugs that can exacerbate tics, such as stimulants, carbamazepine, and lamotrigine, may in some situations account for recent tic emergence or tic worsening, but are no longer thought to "cause" tics, and are not contraindicated in patients with tics.[77] Lastly, questions about any significant developmental delay, congenital anomalies, or other major neurological symptoms help to identify co-occurring conditions or rare alternative causes of tics discussed below.

In the context of a typical history and presentation, a normal neurological exam, and the absence of other systemic symptoms and/or other abnormal movements, neuroimaging or electro-encephalography is typically non-informative.[78] While the diagnosis is made clinically, the Yale Global Tic Severity Scale (YGTSS) is commonly used to assess and track severity of tic symptoms over time.[44] In the YGTSS, motor and vocal tics are assessed independently, and are scored (each 0–5) based on elements including number, frequency, intensity, complexity, and interference which are added together to form the YGTSS Total Tic Score (range 0–50). An additional YGTSS Impairment Scale (range 0–50) assesses the psychosocial consequences of the disorder and is similar to the DSM Global Assessment of Function, although higher scores represent higher levels of impairment.[44]

Tics can be present in other inherited or degenerative disorders of the basal ganglia, such as myoclonus-dystonia, acanthocytosis, or Wilson's disease, but patients with these disorders should also have other movement disorders (e.g., tremor, chorea, dystonia) in addition to tics. Tics can rarely occur following a vascular or traumatic injury, or encephalitis involving the basal ganglia. In these cases, mental status and/or the elemental neurological exam is typically abnormal, indicating the need for a more extensive workup. Anterior cingulate seizures can produce complex repetitive movements that may look like tics, though should be distinguishable from a developmental tic disorder by the absence of previous or other co-occurring tics and lack of suppressibility. Endocrine disturbances (primarily thyroid abnormalities) or medications/drugs, such as cocaine, stimulants, carbamazepine, and lamotrigine, can exacerbate existing tics or cause tics to emerge for the first time, though this is now viewed as triggering tics in individuals with a familial predisposition for a developmental tic disorder, as opposed to a primary cause.

When evaluating tics/TS, it is vital to screen for co-occurring psychiatric conditions given their high prevalence in TS patients

CASE VIGNETTE 19.1

Part I: Sam, an 11-year-old boy with no formal neurological or psychiatric diagnoses, presents with his parents for evaluation of sudden onset "movements" and "noises" over the past few months that he can't control. He is particularly bothered by a sequenced movement where he jerks his head back and grunts, as well as a need to "slap his desk" whenever he sits down in school. When asked directly, Sam reports having a "weird feeling" right before needing to make these movements/sounds, and after completing them he experiences brief relief of that feeling. He states that sometimes the movements happen without him realizing, while other times he tries to control them, but if he doesn't do them, he "will explode." In response to a screen for other movements, he reports that a few weeks ago he had to lift his shoulders up repeatedly, but these symptoms went away last week.

Sam's parents report that he has always been a very active child, and although his teachers often comment on how bright he is, they report that he has difficulty remaining in his seat, often appears to be "day-dreaming," and often gets in trouble for talking with peers during lessons or speaking without raising his hand. They note Sam seemed to "blink a lot" during his kindergarten year, and would often continue to cough or sniff long after a simple cold or allergy season had passed. He has a history of seasonal allergies and asthma, and will occasionally use an albuterol inhaler but takes no daily medications. Sam's mother experienced prolonged labor with a forceps-assisted delivery. He had a typical development, and met all milestones on time. He is very outgoing, and is well-related to his peers. Sam's parents note that he has always had trouble sleeping, and will often lie awake in bed for a few hours every night.

Regarding family history, dad reports that he "probably has ADHD," and mom denies any psychiatric family history. They note that Sam's 13-year-old sister was recently diagnosed with OCD and is currently receiving behavioral therapy. Sam lives at home with both parents and his older sister, and recently started 6th grade at the local middle school, which has been a challenging adjustment. He reports that while he had very good friends in elementary school, some of the students are now teasing him when he grunts or smacks his desk. His parents have recently found him crying at night about not wanting to go to school.

A brief neurological exam shows no focal findings, and there is no history of any other medical or neurological conditions. In meeting with Sam alone, he cautiously reveals that recently he has been getting thoughts "stuck in his head" that really scare him, specifically intrusive thoughts that he will "stab his mother." While he knows he would never do this, the more he tries to stop the thoughts, the more intense they get, and they are currently present for at least 2 hours a day and "really upset him." He also discloses that whenever he sees a hot stove top, he feels the need to touch it. Finally, he is upset because his parents are always yelling at him for not wearing a seatbelt, which he states that he can't wear, because "it's not symmetrical."

In meeting with Sam's parents separately, they state that they are concerned because "the littlest things will set Sam off." With very small provocations, he will "go from 0 to 100" and can occasionally punch holes in their walls.

In discussing Sam's diagnosis of Tourette syndrome (as he has had at least one motor tic and a phonic tic for at least a year), the physician also describes that Sam meets criteria for obsessive-compulsive disorder, and likely ADHD, though confirmation of impairment at school is necessary to make this diagnosis. His parents find it helpful to hear that, although tics, OCD, and ADHD require different treatments, they are not really three separate disorders and commonly co-occur due to their sharing of overlapping brain circuitry. In addition, the physician mentions that Sam's "rage episodes" are also related to TS, OCD, and ADHD, and that treatment of anger outbursts involves not only direct behavioral and pharmacological management of impulse control, but also targeting the tic, OCD, and ADHD symptoms that are causing impairment and lowering his tolerance threshold.

Regarding treatment, the physician describes the gold standard behavioral therapy for tics, CBIT and mentions that Sam would benefit from ERP, a type of behavioral therapy aimed at targeting OCD thoughts. Given Sam's current degree of distress secondary to tics, difficulty sleeping, impulsivity/rage and likely ADHD symptoms, alpha-agonists are discussed, and with his parents' consent, a 0.1 mg/day clonidine (patch) is started. Neuropsychological testing is also arranged given the increased rate of learning disorders seen in those with TS.

Three months later, Sam returns with his parents. He states that while the clonidine helped somewhat, he needed sequentially increases in dosing which ultimately were too sedating. He found a therapist who specialized in ERP, but wasn't able to find a CBIT provider. As such, his intrusive thoughts are improved, but he continues to have severe complex tics, and has developed new tics, including punching himself hard in the chest, and cracking his jaw until it feels painful. He also continues to have anger episodes at home, which on one occasion his parents had to call the police. Given his symptom progression, the physician discusses the risks, benefits, and potential side effects of starting aripiprazole, an atypical antipsychotic that targets tics but can also help with mood and behavioral regulation. This medication is started at 2 mg nightly, and increased to 5 mg nightly with significant tic reduction. However, Sam continues to have compulsive tics that must be done symmetrically. Escitalopram is added and titrated over the course of 6–8 weeks to 20 mg daily, with effective symptom reduction.

Part II: Two years later, Sam is doing very well. His tics, OCD symptoms, and anger outbursts are all under good control. However, now that he is in high school, he is struggling to pay attention and keep track of homework assignments. He is also distracted on the baseball field, where he is being considered for the varsity team. He has been working with an executive function coach, but, despite his best effort, he is not making progress. He and his parents ask about ADHD medications, but worry about worsening tics. The physician discusses with them that while stimulants used to be considered to be contraindicated in individuals with tics, studies have subsequently shown that stimulants are safe, well-tolerated, and quite effective in treating those with ADHD and tics, especially when combined with an alpha-agonist. Sam decides to try low-dose methylphenidate, and although he does have some increased simple motor tics, they decrease after the first week. After slow uptitration to an effective dose, he finds the medication extremely helpful for his focus.

Part III: Three more years pass, and Sam has had significant success on a regimen of escitalopram 20 mg daily, aripiprazole 5 mg nightly, and extended release methylphenidate 20 mg daily. He thinks he is ready to start weaning off his medications, as he has not had any tics in the last 2 years. He is gradually weaned off the aripiprazole over 2–3 months without recurrent tics. He initially has difficulty when tapering Escitalopram below 5 mg daily, as some of his intrusive thoughts return. However, he engages in a few "booster sessions" of ERP with his CBT therapist, and the symptoms improve. He opts to continue on methylphenidate, and has a successful senior year. He decides to go to college to study biomedical engineering in order to create devices for children with disabilities.

and their associated disability and functional impairment.[1] As outlined in the 2019 American Academy of Neurology (AAN) guidelines, these should include ADHD, OCD, anxiety, mood disorders, disruptive behaviors, and suicidality.[79] Referral for formal neuropsychological testing is recommended, given the high rate of co-occurring learning disorders as well as executive dysfunction and graphomotor impairment.

DIFFERENTIAL DIAGNOSIS

The differential diagnosis for tics includes allergies, stereotypies, dystonia, myoclonus, akathisia, tardive dyskinesia, and other inherited/acquired disorders of the basal ganglia.

Allergies can usually be easily distinguished from tics, as allergies are associated with local irritation or inflammation such as eye redness or mucus production, while tics are not. Furthermore, simple vocal tics such as sniffing or throat clearing often have an underlying, stereotyped pattern that differs from the more varied sounds associated with an allergic response. Lastly, sniffing, throat clearing, or coughing due to allergies or an upper respiratory infection (URI) should be time-limited. Of note, a common condition seen by pediatric pulmonary and otorhinolaryngology specialists is "habit cough," in which children develop persistent throat clearing or coughing following a URI.[80,81] While no longitudinal or family studies have been conducted on this entity, habit cough has the same characteristics as transient/provisional tic disorder, and the primary treatment is behavior therapy that is quite similar to habit reversal training (HRT), the established behavioral therapy used for tic disorders.[80]

Stereotypies, formally known as complex motor stereotypies (CMS), are frequently observed in individuals with an autism spectrum disorder, but can also occur in typically developing children[82,83] and have multiple features to distinguish them from tics. While tics tend to onset after age 5, motor stereotypies typically onset early in life and almost always before age 3. Tics typically start in the eyes, face, head, or shoulders, and, by definition, change in location over time (e.g., first blinking, then head shaking, then shoulder shrugs, etc.). In contrast, CMS are fixed, intermittent, repeated bilateral arm and hand movements, usually with flexion/extension and pronation/supination of the arms, though other common variations involve bringing both hands to the midline and/or up to the face. Unlike tics, CMS do not "move," that is, do not change in body location over time, and instead continue to consist of bilateral upper extremity movements. Some patients with stereotypies can have simultaneous mouth opening, humming, and/or standing on tiptoes occurring along with their bilateral arm/hand movements, but the entire set of movements remains part of a single, recurrent, stereotyped sequence. Third, all intended actions generally cease while individuals engage in stereotypies, while tics will occur in the background of ongoing speech and movement. Lastly, stereotypies are not associated with a premonitory tension/urge compared to the sensory symptoms that precede tics, though as noted above, younger children with tics do not always experience this premonitory urge. Of note, stereotypies typically do not respond to medications, but, if impairing, can be reduced through behavioral therapy.[84]

Myoclonus is defined by sudden, rapid, "shock-like," muscle jerks that, unlike tics, are not suppressible and not associated with a premonitory urge. **Dystonia** is characterized by simultaneous contractions of agonist/antagonist muscles resulting in spasms that are distinct from most tics. While some complex tics can have dystonic features, these are unlikely to occur without a prior or concurrent history of simple tics. **Akathisia** consists of non-stereotyped, non-repetitive movements and thus should be easily distinguishable from tics. Like tics, akathisia arises from an uncomfortable internal feeling, though this differs from the premonitory urge of tics by a feeling of inner restlessness that is typically relieved by moving one's legs. Lastly, the oro-buccal, lingual, or facial movements associated with **tardive dyskinesia** can overlap in appearance with facial tics. However, tics can be voluntarily suppressed for brief periods of time and can often disappear for minutes, hours, or days, while tardive dyskinesia is not suppressible and is typically continuous.

PANDAS (pediatric autoimmune neuropsychiatric disorder associated with streptococcal infections), hypothesized to be a postinfectious autoimmune disorder akin to Sydenham Chorea, is characterized by an abrupt, "explosive" onset and dramatic symptom exacerbation of OCD and/or tics, along with hyperactivity and other "neurological abnormalities" (e.g., unusual/jerky movements), with a temporal relationship to group A beta-hemolytic streptococcal infection.[85] It has since been associated with other acute neuropsychiatric changes,

including separation anxiety, mood lability, anger outbursts, anorexia, sleep changes, increased urinary frequency, handwriting changes, and joint pain, and has been expanded to capture a wider range of potential infectious triggers (pediatric acute neuropsychiatric syndrome, PANS).[86] The diagnosis continues to be controversial, and, in the absence of definitive biomarkers, it is still unclear whether those with PANDAS/PANS have a distinct neuroimmune condition or whether they have OCD and/or tics as well as an independent susceptibility to recurrent infections.[87] Recent research has demonstrated an elevated risk of autoimmune disorders in relatives of individuals with OCD and/or tic disorders compared with population controls.[88] However, a double-blind, randomized controlled trial of intravenous immunoglobulin (IVIG) for treatment of PANDAS did not identify a significant benefit between the active and control groups, although all patients subsequently improved in the open-label phase of the study.[89] Thus, further research is needed before formal diagnostic and treatment guidelines can be established.

TREATMENT

Tics in and of themselves do not necessarily require treatment; treatment is recommended only if the tics cause difficulties in self-esteem, academic progress, or physical pain. If tics are upsetting to parents and/or school teachers, but not the child, treatment is not typically recommended, though psychoeducation for both family and educators is crucial.

In 2019, AAN published the first national guidelines for evaluation and treatment of individuals with TS and chronic tic disorders.[79] These guidelines recommend that clinicians provide psychoeducation about the natural course of tic disorders, common co-occurring conditions and their treatments, and that they consider the degree of functional impairment secondary to tics when recommending treatment. As previously noted, watchful waiting is an acceptable treatment approach if the tics themselves are not causing functional impairment. Clinicians should also counsel patients that, even with treatment, complete tic cessation is unlikely.

Treatments for tics can be divided into two subcategories: behavioral and pharmacological. Behavioral therapy for tics, known as Comprehensive Behavioral Intervention for Tics (CBIT), has been demonstrated to be effective in two randomized, controlled multicenter clinical trials, one in children and one in adults, with effect sizes favoring CBIT compared to supportive therapy at the same magnitude as those observed in RCTs of atypical neuroleptics versus placebo.[90,91] Based on these findings, the recent AAN treatment guidelines recommend that CBIT should be considered first-line treatment where available.[79]

Behavioral Therapy for Tics (CBIT)

Multiple studies have shown efficacy of CBIT in both children and adults.[79,90,91] CBIT typically consists of three components, functional-based assessment/intervention, habit reversal training, and relaxation training. The functional-based evaluation/intervention and HRT are believed to be most important in treatment success. During the function-based evaluation/

intervention component, the treater works with the patient to identify the contextual factors that support, maintain, or dampen expression of tics. It is also well known that tics worsen during times of stress, anxiety, overexcitement, boredom, tiredness, etc., and reduce during periods of intense concentration or relaxation. Part of the function-based evaluation/intervention is to reduce unnecessary tic-exacerbating periods, and increase times associated with decreased tics. The most common and helpful response to tics is often benign ignoring. It is important to note that although these symptoms are being treated with behavioral interventions, it does not mean that the tics themselves are therefore "behavioral" in origin, or that the individual is performing them intentionally. It should be noted that this first component of CBIT is completed for each tic individually, as some tics may improve with certain environmental/behavioral interventions whereas others may not.

The second part of CBIT is HRT, which itself consists of three components: awareness training, competing response, and social support. In awareness training, the individual works with the therapist to be able to identify the sensations/feelings that just precede the tic (premonitory urges). Once the individual is successfully "aware" of the tic, they develop a "competing response" which is a movement that is physically incompatible with the tic and less noticeable than the tic. When the individual senses the premonitory urge, they engage in the competing response, and hold it for either 1 minute or until the premonitory urge passes (whichever is longer). Of note, there is some recent research showing that the competing response does not have to be physically incompatible with the tic, and as such, may be more due to directed attention. Finally, social support involves one or more individuals close to the patient helping them to achieve their goal of tic reduction. The "social support" learns to help prompt the patient to do the competing response, and to praise them when they engage in it. A 2010 study demonstrated that CBIT was more effective than psychoeducation and supportive therapy, reduced total tic severity in children (52.5% vs. 18.5%), and improved psychological, social, and school functioning—all factors associated with TS in youth.[90]

Pharmacological Treatments for Tics

Pharmacological treatments are considered in three tiers, stratified based on therapeutic and side-effect profiles.[45] In current practice, first-generation antipsychotics, such as haloperidol and pimozide, are saved for the last resort (third tier). The first tier includes alpha-2 agonists, such as clonidine and guanfacine. These medications can be very helpful for tics, especially (and possibly specifically) when there is a co-occurring ADHD diagnosis.[79] The clonidine patch can be particularly helpful when oral clonidine is too sedating, though up to 25% of users develop a focal contact rash that limits use due to irritation and pruritus. The predominant side effects that can limit use of alpha-2 agonists are sedation, dry mouth, and occasionally orthostasis and new-onset bad dreams.[78]

Tier 2 agents include atypical neuroleptics, with efficacy proportional to the D2 receptor binding affinity of the drug.[78] Thus, risperidone and aripiprazole are effective tic suppressants,

while olanzapine and quetiapine are not particularly effective. Currently, aripiprazole is the only FDA-approved atypical neuroleptic for treatment of tics; however, risperidone is widely used based on results from randomized, placebo-controlled clinical trials.[79] Ziprasidone, which also has high D2 receptor binding, can also be effective, but often to a lesser degree than risperidone or aripiprazole, though has the benefit of being more weight-neutral. Unfortunately, there is a large gap between the tolerability and effectiveness of Tier 1 and Tier 2 treatments, due to the high rates of sedation, weight gain with associated hyperlipidemia, and potential risk of tardive dyskinesia associated with atypical neuroleptics.[79]

The third tier treatments for tics are the first-generation antipsychotics, and specifically the three agents with the highest D2 receptor binding potential: haloperidol, pimozide, and fluphenazine. These medications are quite efficacious in reducing tics, but also are associated with significant side effects that limit their effectiveness, including the highest risk of extrapyramidal symptoms, such as parkinsonism, oculogyric crisis, and tardive dyskinesia.[79] That said, much lower doses of these medications (typical range 0.5–5 mg) are often used to treat tics compared to the doses used for psychotic disorders.[78] Of the three high-potency neuroleptics, haloperidol and pimozide are FDA approved for the treatment of tics, but pimozide is associated with significant QTc prolongation and has multiple drug-drug interactions that tend to limit its use compared to haloperidol and fluphenazine.[79] As when using neuroleptic medications for other disorders, physicians should monitor weight, fasting glucose, and fasting lipids at baseline and intermittently thereafter as per APA Guidelines.[92] Intermittent exams for drug-induced movement disorders are also warranted.

There are a number of other off-label medications that have some evidence in reducing tics, but in general have not been shown to have significant efficacy in double-blind, randomized placebo-controlled trials. Some of those medications include clonazepam, topiramate, and baclofen.[79] Tetrabenazine has been shown to be effective in treating tics, but it can cause significant weight gain and parkinsonism, and can lead to depression in ~15% of patients.[93]

Other Biological Treatments for Tics

Botulinum toxin injections have some evidence base for treating focal simple motor tics of the eyes, face, and neck, as well as for vocal tics, in adolescents and adults where the benefits outweigh the risks.[94,95] In addition, based on state legislation, physicians may consider treatment with cannabis-based medication in adults who are otherwise treatment resistant, though evidence from randomized controlled clinical trials is lacking.[96]

Deep brain stimulation can be considered in treatment-refractory patients with severe TS after undergoing a multidisciplinary evaluation and failing multiple classes of medication and behavioral therapy.[97] However, there is still a lack of consensus as to the optimal placement of DBS leads, and there are little long-term data from randomized, placebo-controlled trials.[79]

The AAN guidelines also recommend that clinicians assess for and appropriately treat the frequent co-occurring psychiatric conditions seen in patients with TS.[79] It is also important to take these co-occurring disorders into account when deciding which medication(s) to prescribe. While stimulants are no longer contraindicated in those with tics and ADHD,[79] one might consider using an alpha-agonist as a first-line medication if the child is experiencing a combination of tics and ADHD symptoms. It should also be noted that using a combination of alpha-agonists and stimulants has been shown in a randomized, double-blind, placebo-controlled trial to be synergistic in patients with tics and ADHD, improving both the tics and the ADHD symptoms better than either treatment type individually.[98] Given that OCD so commonly co-occurs with TS, individuals with tics and OCD often require augmentation with SSRIs, particularly when tics have an additional compulsive component.[59]

OCD Treatments

Serotonin reuptake inhibitors (including SSRIs and clomipramine [CMI], a highly serotonergic tricyclic antidepressant) and cognitive behavioral therapy (CBT) have both been shown to be effective in treating OCD.[99,100] Exposure response prevention (ERP), a type of CBT, is considered first-line treatment. A seminal randomized, blinded placebo-controlled trial comparing CMI, ERP, combination treatment, and placebo in adults with OCD demonstrated that all active treatments (CMI, ERP, CMI+ERP) were superior to placebo.[101] ERP alone and combined treatment did not differ significantly from one another, and both were superior to CMI alone. In children and adolescents with OCD, a similar randomized, placebo-controlled trial comparing CBT, SSRIs (sertraline), combined treatment, and placebo demonstrated that CBT, sertraline, and combined treatment were all statistically superior to placebo.[102]

Based on clinical trials and the favorable side-effect profile of SSRIs relative to CMI, the first-line pharmacological treatment for OCD is SSRIs. Studies in adults have shown that OCD requires higher doses of SSRIs compared to depression and/or anxiety.[60,103] While fluvoxamine is often mentioned as a preferred agent, multiple meta-analyses have demonstrated that all SSRIs have equal efficacy in treating OCD.[100,104] When combined with ERP, up to 75% of individuals will experience some symptom relief.[51] CMI, a tricyclic antidepressant, with potent serotonergic properties, is the gold standard pharmacological OCD treatment, but is often not used first due to increased side effects (dry mouth, constipation, sedation, etc.).[51] It is important to note that having OCD and tics is associated with worse treatment response to SSRIs than OCD without tics.[60] Not infrequently, those patients will require augmenting agents in addition to the SSRI, namely neuroleptic medications.[60] As such, patients with "ticculsions" may often require treatments targeting the tic and OCD components simultaneously.

ADHD Treatments

While the use of stimulants in individuals with tics was long thought to be contraindicated, as these medications had been observed to produce and/or worsen tics, convergent evidence in recent years has demonstrated that stimulants do not *cause* tics.[98,105] Rather, stimulants may unmask tics in an individual with a strong biological predisposition for tics, as children with TS and ADHD generally experience ADHD onset a year or two prior to tic onset, even in the absence of exposure to stimulants.[4,77] Furthermore, a large-scale meta-analysis of pediatric clinical trials of stimulants did not identify a significant excess of emergent tics in children receiving stimulants compared to placebo,[105] and a seminal randomized double-blind, controlled trial by the Tourette Syndrome Study Group demonstrated that combined use of low-dose stimulants and an alpha-2 agonist significantly reduced both ADHD and tic symptoms in children with ADHD and persistent tic disorders.[98] Thus, as noted above, the AAN treatment guidelines recommend that stimulants are appropriate to prescribe in this patient population.[79]

While the gold standard treatment for ADHD in children and adolescents are stimulants, due to their larger effect size compared to other treatments and high efficacy rates,[106] if stimulants are not tolerated in any particular patient, alpha-2 agonists have also shown to be effective in treating ADHD symptoms, though tend to be less potent.[107]

Summary and Key Points

- Tourette syndrome (TS) is a neuropsychiatric disorder that represents one end of a continuous spectrum of developmental tic disorders.
- TS is more common than previously recognized, with an estimated prevalence of ~1% of school-aged children.
- The vast majority of individuals with TS have one or more co-occurring psychiatric disorders that often cause more impairment than the tics themselves.
- Tourette and other tic disorders are thought to arise from dysregulated cortico-striato-thalamo-cortical circuits that overlap with similar circuitry underlying OCD and ADHD pathophysiology.

- Comprehensive Behavioral Intervention for Tics (CBIT) is an effective treatment for tics both in children and adults and should be considered first-line treatment when tics cause impairment.
- Individuals with TS and OCD can often have symptoms that lie at the interface between the two disorders, which may require treatments targeting both tic and OCD components.
- The use of psychostimulants to treat ADHD in individuals with tics are no longer thought to be contraindicated and can often be tolerated with slow uptitration and/or co-treatment with an alpha-2 agonist.

Multiple Choice Questions

1. The dysregulation of which neural circuits are most commonly associated with Tourette syndrome?
   a. Cortico-hippocampal-mammillo-thalamo-cortical
   b. Lateral lemniscus
   c. Spino-reticulo-thalamic
   d. Cortico-striatal-thalamo-cortical
   e. Inferior longitudinal fasciculus

2. Which disorders most frequently co-occur in individuals with Tourette syndrome?
   a. Obsessive-compulsive disorder (OCD) and attention-deficit/hyperactivity disorder (ADHD)
   b. ADHD and conduct disorder
   c. Bipolar disorder and generalized anxiety disorder
   d. OCD and major depressive disorder
   e. Major depressive disorder and generalized anxiety disorder

3. What medication combination might be necessary for an individual with "Tourettic OCD" where there is overlap between tics and compulsions (also known as "ticculsions" or "compulsive tics")?
   a. Alpha-2 agonist and atypical neuroleptic
   b. Atypical neuroleptic and serotonin reuptake inhibitor (SRI)
   c. Serotonin reuptake inhibitor and benzodiazepine
   d. Alpha-2 agonist and benzodiazepine
   e. Mood stabilizer and atypical neuroleptic

4. The gold standard pharmacological treatment for which condition that commonly co-occurs with Tourette syndrome was previously prohibited for fear it would cause/exacerbate tics?
   a. ADHD
   b. OCD
   c. Rage attacks
   d. Body-focused repetitive disorders
   e. Autism spectrum disorder

Multiple Choice Answers

1. **Answer: d**
   Abnormal development and/or regulation of cortico-striatal-thalamo-cortical circuits are thought to underlie the pathophysiology of Tourette syndrome and other tic disorders.

2. **Answer: a**
   OCD and ADHD. In individuals with TS, 30–60% meet criteria for OCD, and 30–90% meet criteria for ADHD, with about 30% meeting criteria for tics, OCD, and ADHD together. These three conditions are all associated with dysregulation of cortico-striatal-thalamo-cortical circuits, with tics, OCD, and ADHD symptoms appearing to have parallel developmental abnormalities in motor, limbic, and associative CSTC circuits, respectively.

3. **Answer: b**
   Atypical neuroleptic and serotonin reuptake inhibitor (SRI). OCD with co-occurring tics is less responsive to SRI monotherapy compared to OCD without tics. Similarly, individuals with tics that have a compulsive component to their tics often fail to respond to monotherapy with either an alpha-2 agonist or neuroleptic medication. Evidence from the OCD literature supports addition of an atypical neuroleptic to augment SRIs in individuals with tics. In those already taking an atypical neuroleptic for tics who continue to have compulsive tics, targeting the OCD component with an SRI can be helpful.

4. **Answer: a**
   ADHD. Until recently, there was widespread belief that stimulants could cause tics in patients without tic disorders and could not be used in individuals with TS without making tics worse. However, a seminal randomized, double-blind, placebo-controlled trial by the Tourette Syndrome Study Group demonstrated that the combined use of low-dose stimulants and an alpha-2 agonist significantly reduced both tics and ADHD symptoms in children with ADHD and persistent tic disorders compared to placebo or either medication alone. In addition, a large meta-analysis of pediatric clinical trials of stimulants did not identify a significant excess of emergent tics in children receiving stimulants compared to placebo.[98,105] As such, the American Academy of Neurology treatment guidelines recommend that stimulants are appropriate to prescribe in this patient population.

References

1. Robertson MM, Eapen V, Singer HS, et al. Gilles de la Tourette syndrome. *Na Rev Dis Primers*. 2017;3:16097.
2. American Psychiatric Association. *Diagnostic and Statistical Manual of Mental Disorders*. 5th ed. Washington, DC: American Psychiatric Association; 2013.
3. Yu D, Sul JH, Tsetsos F, et al. Interrogating the genetic determinants of Tourette's syndrome and other tic disorders through genome-wide association studies. *Am J Psychiatry*. 2019;176:217.
4. Hirschtritt ME, Lee PC, Pauls DL, et al. Lifetime prevalence, age of risk, and genetic relationships of comorbid psychiatric disorders in Tourette syndrome. *JAMA Psychiatry*. 2015;72:325.
5. Freeman RD, Fast DK, Burd L, Kerbeshian J, Robertson MM, Sandor P. An international perspective on Tourette syndrome: selected findings from 3,500 individuals in 22 countries. *Dev Med Child Neurol*. 2000;42:436.
6. Jahanshahi M, Obeso I, Rothwell JC, Obeso JA. A fronto-striato-subthalamic-pallidal network for goal-directed and habitual inhibition. *Nat Rev Neurosci*. 2015;16:719.

7. Perez DL, Keshavan MS, Scharf JM, Boes AD, Price BH. Bridging the great divide: what can neurology learn from psychiatry? *J Neuropsychiatry Clin Neurosci.* 2018;30:271.

8. Knight T, Steeves T, Day L, Lowerison M, Jette N, Pringsheim T. Prevalence of tic disorders: a systematic review and meta-analysis. *Pediatr Neurol.* 2012;47:77.

9. Scharf JM, Miller LL, Gauvin CA, Alabiso J, Mathews CA, Ben-Shlomo Y. Population prevalence of Tourette syndrome: a systematic review and meta-analysis. *Mov Disord.* 2015; 30:221.

10. Snider LA, Seligman LD, Ketchen BR, et al. Tics and problem behaviors in schoolchildren: prevalence, characterization, and associations. *Pediatrics.* 2002;110:331.

11. Leckman JF, Zhang H, Vitale A, et al. Course of tic severity in Tourette syndrome: the first two decades. *Pediatrics.* 1998;102:14.

12. Bloch MH, Peterson BS, Scahill L, et al. Adulthood outcome of tic and obsessive-compulsive symptom severity in children with Tourette syndrome. *Arch Pediatr Adolesc Med.* 2006;160:65.

13. Groth C, Mol Debes N, Rask CU, Lange T, Skov L. Course of Tourette syndrome and comorbidities in a large prospective clinical study. *J Am Acad Child Adolesc Psychiatry.* 2017;56:304.

14. Bloch MH, Sukhodolsky DG, Dombrowski PA, et al. Poor fine-motor and visuospatial skills predict persistence of pediatric-onset obsessive-compulsive disorder into adulthood. *J Child Psychol Psychiatry.* 2011;52:974.

15. Lanciego JL, Luquin N, Obeso JA. Functional neuroanatomy of the basal ganglia. *Cold Spring Harb Perspect Med.* 2012;2:a009621.

16. Doya K. Complementary roles of basal ganglia and cerebellum in learning and motor control. *Curr Opin Neurobiol.* 2000;10:732.

17. Ito M, Doya K. Multiple representations and algorithms for reinforcement learning in the cortico-basal ganglia circuit. *Curr Opin Neurobiol.* 2011;21:368.

18. Haber SN, Knutson B. The reward circuit: linking primate anatomy and human imaging. *Neuropsychopharmacology.* 2010;35:4.

19. Worbe Y, Marrakchi-Kacem L, Lecomte S, et al. Altered structural connectivity of cortico-striato-pallido-thalamic networks in Gilles de la Tourette syndrome. *Brain.* 2015;138:472.

20. Worbe Y, Gerardin E, Hartmann A, et al. Distinct structural changes underpin clinical phenotypes in patients with Gilles de la Tourette syndrome. *Brain.* 2010;133:3649.

21. Darrow SM, Hirschtritt ME, Davis LK, et al. Identification of two heritable cross-disorder endophenotypes for Tourette syndrome. *Am J Psychiatry.* 2017;174:387.

22. Penfield W. Functional localization in temporal and deep sylvian areas. *Res Publ Assoc Res Nerv Ment Dis.* 1958;36:210.

23. Maillard L, Ishii K, Bushara K, Waldvogel D, Schulman AE, Hallett M. Mapping the basal ganglia: fMRI evidence for somatotopic representation of face, hand, and foot. *Neurology.* 2000;55:377.

24. Romanelli P, Esposito V, Schaal DW, Heit G. Somatotopy in the basal ganglia: experimental and clinical evidence for segregated sensorimotor channels. *Brain Res Brain Res Rev.* 2005;48:112.

25. Hirschtritt ME, Darrow SM, Illmann C, et al. Social disinhibition is a heritable subphenotype of tics in Tourette syndrome. *Neurology.* 2016;87(5):497-504.

26. Pauls D, Fernandez T, Mathews CA, State M, Scharf JM. The inheritance of Tourette disorder: a review. *J Obsess Compuls Relat Disord.* 2014;3:380.

27. O'Rourke JA, Scharf JM, Yu D, Pauls DL. The genetics of Tourette syndrome: a review. *J Psychosom Res.* 2009;67:533.

28. Browne HA, Hansen SN, Buxbaum JD, et al. Familial clustering of tic disorders and obsessive-compulsive disorder. *JAMA Psychiatry.* 2015;72:359.

29. Mataix-Cols D, Isomura K, Perez-Vigil A, et al. Familial risks of Tourette syndrome and chronic tic disorders. A population-based cohort study. *JAMA Psychiatry.* 2015;72:787.

30. Huang AY, Yu D, Davis LK, et al. Rare copy number variants in NRXN1 and CNTN6 increase risk for Tourette syndrome. *Neuron.* 2017;94:1101.

31. Wang S, Mandell JD, Kumar Y, et al. De novo sequence and copy number variants are strongly associated with Tourette disorder and implicate cell polarity in pathogenesis. *Cell Reports.* 2018;24:3441.

32. Castronovo P, Baccarin M, Ricciardello A, et al. Phenotypic spectrum of NRXN1 mono- and bi-allelic deficiency: a systematic review. *Clin Genet.* 2020;97(1):125-137.

33. Tassano E, Uccella S, Giacomini T, et al. Clinical and molecular characterization of two patients with CNTN6 copy number variations. *Cytogenet Genome Res.* 2018;156:144.

34. Davis LK, Yu D, Keenan CL, et al. Partitioning the heritability of Tourette syndrome and obsessive compulsive disorder reveals differences in genetic architecture. *PLoS Genet.* 2013;9:e1003864.

35. Yu D, Mathews CA, Scharf JM, et al. Cross-disorder genome-wide analyses suggest a complex genetic relationship between Tourette's syndrome and OCD. *Am J Psychiatry.* 2015;172(1):82-93.

36. Anttila V, Bulik-Sullivan B, Finucane HK, et al. Analysis of shared heritability in common disorders of the brain. *bioRxiv.* 2016. doi:https://doi.org/10.1101/048991

37. Mathews CA, Bimson B, Lowe TL, et al. Association between maternal smoking and increased symptom severity in Tourette's syndrome. *Am J Psychiatry.* 2006;163:1066.

38. Mathews CA, Scharf JM, Miller LL, Macdonald-Wallis C, Lawlor DA, Ben-Shlomo Y. Association between pre- and perinatal exposures and Tourette syndrome or chronic tic disorder in the ALSPAC cohort. *Br J Psychiatry.* 2014;204:40.

39. Dalsgaard S, Waltoft BL, Leckman JF, Mortensen PB. Maternal history of autoimmune disease and later development of Tourette syndrome in offspring. *J Am Acad Child Adolesc Psychiatry.* 2015;54:495.

40. Browne HA, Modabbernia A, Buxbaum JD, et al. Prenatal maternal smoking and increased risk for Tourette syndrome and chronic tic disorders. *J Am Acad Child Adolesc Psychiatry.* 2016;55:784.

41. Brander G, Rydell M, Kuja-Halkola R, et al. Perinatal risk factors in Tourette's and chronic tic disorders: a total population sibling comparison study. *Mol Psychiatry.* 2018;23:1189.

42. Leckman JF, Bloch MH, Scahill L, King RA. Tourette syndrome: the self under siege. *J Child Neurol.* 2006;21:642.

43. Bliss J. Sensory experiences of Gilles de la Tourette syndrome. *Arch Gen Psychiatry.* 1980;37:1343.

44. Leckman JF, Riddle MA, Hardin MT, et al. The Yale Global Tic Severity Scale: initial testing of a clinician-rated scale of tic severity. *J Am Acad Child Adolesc Psychiatry.* 1989;28:566.

45. McNaught KS, Mink JW. Advances in understanding and treatment of Tourette syndrome. *Nat Rev Neurol.* 2011;7:667.

46. Jankovic J, Kurlan R. Tourette syndrome: evolving concepts. *Mov Disord.* 2011;26:1149.

47. Kurlan R, Daragjati C, Como PG, et al. Non-obscene complex socially inappropriate behavior in Tourette's syndrome. *J Neuropsychiatry Clin Neurosci.* 1996;8:311.

48. Worbe Y, Mallet L, Golmard JL, et al. Repetitive behaviours in patients with Gilles de la Tourette syndrome: tics, compulsions, or both? *PLoS One.* 2010;5:e12959.

49. Ganos C, Ogrzal T, Schnitzler A, Munchau A. The pathophysiology of echopraxia/echolalia: relevance to Gilles de la Tourette syndrome. *Mov Disord.* 2012;27:1222.

50. Freeman RD, Zinner SH, Muller-Vahl KR, et al. Coprophenomena in Tourette syndrome. *Dev Med Child Neurol.* 2009;51:218.

51. Hirschtritt ME, Bloch MH, Mathews CA. Obsessive-compulsive disorder: advances in diagnosis and treatment. *JAMA.* 2017; 317:1358.

52. Geller DA. Obsessive-compulsive and spectrum disorders in children and adolescents. *Psychiatr Clin N Am.* 2006;29:353.

53. Bloch MH, Leckman JF. Clinical course of Tourette syndrome. *J Psychosom Res.* 2009;67:497.

54. Leckman JF, Grice DE, Barr LC, et al. Tic-related vs. non-tic-related obsessive compulsive disorder. *Anxiety.* 1994;1:208.

55. Conelea CA, Walther MR, Freeman JB, et al. Tic-related obsessive-compulsive disorder (OCD): phenomenology and treatment outcome in the Pediatric OCD Treatment Study II. *J Am Acad Child Adolesc Psychiatry.* 2014;53:1308.

56. Leckman JF, Walker DE, Goodman WK, Pauls DL, Cohen DJ. "Just right" perceptions associated with compulsive behavior in Tourette's syndrome. *Am J Psychiatry.* 1994;151:675.

57. Mansueto CS, Keuler DJ. Tic or compulsion? It's Tourettic OCD. *Behav Modif.* 2005;29:784.

58. Cath DC, Spinhoven P, Hoogduin CA, et al. Repetitive behaviors in Tourette's syndrome and OCD with and without tics: what are the differences? *Psychiatry Res.* 2001;101:171.

59. Palumbo D, Kurlan R. Complex obsessive compulsive and impulsive symptoms in Tourette's syndrome. *Neuropsychiatr Dis Treat.* 2007;3:687.

60. Bloch MH, Landeros-Weisenberger A, Kelmendi B, Coric V, Bracken MB, Leckman JF. A systematic review: antipsychotic augmentation with treatment refractory obsessive-compulsive disorder. *Mol Psychiatry.* 2006;11:622.

61. Debes NM, Hjalgrim H, Skov L. The presence of comorbidity in Tourette syndrome increases the need for pharmacological treatment. *J Child Neurol.* 2009;24:1504.

62. Budman CL, Bruun RD, Park KS, Lesser M, Olson M. Explosive outbursts in children with Tourette's disorder. *J Am Acad Child Adolesc Psychiatry.* 2000;39:1270.

63. Greenberg E, Tung ES, Gauvin C, et al. Prevalence and predictors of hair pulling disorder and excoriation disorder in Tourette syndrome. *Eur Child Adolesc Psychiatry.* 2018;27:569.

64. Woods DW, Houghton DC. Diagnosis, evaluation, and management of trichotillomania. *Psychiatr Clin N Am.* 2014;37:301.

65. Grant JE, Chamberlain SR. Trichotillomania. *Am J Psychiatry.* 2016;173:868.

66. Coffey BJ, Biederman J, Smoller JW, et al. Anxiety disorders and tic severity in juveniles with Tourette's disorder. *J Am Acad Child Adolesc Psychiatry.* 2000;39:562.

67. Glaze DG, Frost JD Jr, Jankovic J. Sleep in Gilles de la Tourette's syndrome: disorder of arousal. *Neurology.* 1983;33:586.

68. Cohen AJ, Leckman JF. Sensory phenomena associated with Gilles de la Tourette's syndrome. *J Clin Psychiatry.* 1992;53:319.

69. Soler N, Hardwick C, Perkes IE, et al. Sensory dysregulation in tic disorders is associated with executive dysfunction and comorbidities. *Mov Disord.* 2019;34:1901.

70. Schroder A, Vulink N, Denys D. Misophonia: diagnostic criteria for a new psychiatric disorder. *PLoS One.* 2013;8:e54706.

71. Taylor S, Conelea CA, McKay D, Crowe KB, Abramowitz JS. Sensory intolerance: latent structure and psychopathologic correlates. *Compr Psychiatry.* 2014;55:1279.

72. Huisman-van Dijk HM, Schoot R, Rijkeboer MM, Mathews CA, Cath DC. The relationship between tics, OC, ADHD and autism symptoms: a cross-disorder symptom analysis in Gilles de la Tourette syndrome patients and family-members. *Psychiatry Res.* 2016;237:138.

73. Darrow SM, Grados M, Sandor P, et al. Autism spectrum symptoms in a Tourette's disorder sample. *J Am Acad Child Adolesc Psychiatry.* 2017;56:610.

74. Eapen V, Cavanna AE, Robertson MM. Comorbidities, social impact, and quality of life in Tourette syndrome. *Front Psychiatry.* 2016;7:97.

75. Fernandez de la Cruz L, Rydell M, Runeson B, et al. Suicide in Tourette's and chronic tic disorders. *Biol Psychiatry.* 2017;82:111.

76. Pringsheim T, Lang A, Kurlan R, Pearce M, Sandor P. Understanding disability in Tourette syndrome. *Dev Med Child Neurol.* 2009;51:468.

77. Hirschtritt ME, Dy ME, Yang KG, Scharf JM. Child neurology: diagnosis and treatment of Tourette syndrome. *Neurology.* 2016;87:e65.

78. Scahill L, Erenberg G, Berlin CM Jr, et al. Contemporary assessment and pharmacotherapy of Tourette syndrome. *NeuroRx.* 2006;3:192.

79. Pringsheim T, Okun MS, Muller-Vahl K, et al. Practice guideline recommendations summary: treatment of tics in people with Tourette syndrome and chronic tic disorders. *Neurology.* 2019;92:896.

80. Weinberger M. The habit cough: diagnosis and treatment. *Pediatr Pulmonol.* 2018;53:535.

81. Irwin RS, Glomb WB, Chang AB. Habit cough, tic cough, and psychogenic cough in adult and pediatric populations: ACCP evidence-based clinical practice guidelines. *Chest.* 2006;129: 174S.

82. Mahone EM, Bridges D, Prahme C, Singer HS. Repetitive arm and hand movements (complex motor stereotypies) in children. *J Pediatr.* 2004;145:391.

83. Harris KM, Mahone EM, Singer HS. Nonautistic motor stereotypies: clinical features and longitudinal follow-up. *Pediatr Neurol.* 2008;38:267.

84. Specht MW, Mahone EM, Kline T, et al. Efficacy of parent-delivered behavioral therapy for primary complex motor stereotypies. *Dev Med Child Neurol.* 2017;59:168.

85. Swedo SE, Leonard HL, Mittleman BB, et al. Identification of children with pediatric autoimmune neuropsychiatric disorders associated with streptococcal infections by a marker associated with rheumatic fever. *Am J Psychiatry.* 1997;154:110.

86. Chang K, Frankovich J, Cooperstock M, et al. Clinical evaluation of youth with pediatric acute-onset neuropsychiatric syndrome (PANS): recommendations from the 2013 PANS Consensus Conference. *J Child Adolesc Psychopharmacol.* 2015;25:3.

87. Singer HS, Gilbert DL, Wolf DS, Mink JW, Kurlan R. Moving from PANDAS to CANS. *J Pediatr.* 2012;160:725.

88. Mataix-Cols D, Frans E, Perez-Vigil A, et al. A total-population multigenerational family clustering study of autoimmune diseases in obsessive-compulsive disorder and Tourette's/chronic tic disorders. *Mol Psychiatry.* 2018;23:1652.

89. Williams KA, Swedo SE, Farmer CA, et al. Randomized, controlled trial of intravenous immunoglobulin for pediatric autoimmune neuropsychiatric disorders associated with streptococcal infections. *J Am Acad Child Adolesc Psychiatry.* 2016; 55:860.

90. Piacentini J, Woods DW, Scahill L, et al. Behavior therapy for children with Tourette disorder: a randomized controlled trial. *JAMA.* 2010;303:1929.

91. Wilhelm S, Peterson AL, Piacentini J, et al. Randomized trial of behavior therapy for adults with Tourette syndrome. *Arch Gen Psychiatry.* 2012;69:795.

92. American Diabetes Association, American Psychiatric Association, American Association of Clinical Endocrinologists,

North American Association for the Study of Obesity. Consensus development conference on antipsychotic drugs and obesity and diabetes. *Diabetes Care*. 2004;27:596.

93. Kenney C, Hunter C, Mejia N, Jankovic J. Is history of depression a contraindication to treatment with tetrabenazine? *Clin Neuropharmacol*. 2006;29:259.

94. Marras C, Andrews D, Sime E, Lang AE. Botulinum toxin for simple motor tics: a randomized, double-blind, controlled clinical trial. *Neurology*. 2001;56:605.

95. Trimble MR, Whurr R, Brookes G, Robertson MM. Vocal tics in Gilles de la Tourette syndrome treated with botulinum toxin injections. *Mov Disord*. 1998;13:617.

96. Muller-Vahl KR. Treatment of Tourette syndrome with cannabinoids. *Behav Neurol*. 2013;27:119.

97. Martinez-Ramirez D, Jimenez-Shahed J, Leckman JF, et al. Efficacy and safety of deep brain stimulation in Tourette syndrome: The International Tourette Syndrome Deep Brain Stimulation Public Database and Registry. *JAMA Neurol*. 2018;75:353.

98. Tourette Syndrome Study Group. Treatment of ADHD in children with tics: a randomized controlled trial. *Neurology*. 2002;58:527.

99. McGuire JF, Piacentini J, Lewin AB, Brennan EA, Murphy TK, Storch EA. A meta-analysis of cognitive behavior therapy and medication for child obsessive-compulsive disorder: moderators of treatment efficacy, response, and remission. *Depress Anxiety*. 2015;32:580.

100. Soomro GM, Altman D, Rajagopal S, Oakley-Browne M. Selective serotonin re-uptake inhibitors (SSRIs) versus placebo for obsessive compulsive disorder (OCD). *Cochrane Database Syst Rev*. 2008;CD001765.

101. Foa EB, Liebowitz MR, Kozak MJ, et al. Randomized, placebo-controlled trial of exposure and ritual prevention, clomipramine, and their combination in the treatment of obsessive-compulsive disorder. *Am J Psychiatry*. 2005; 162:151.

102. Pediatric OCD Treatment Study Group. Cognitive-behavior therapy, sertraline, and their combination for children and adolescents with obsessive-compulsive disorder: the Pediatric OCD Treatment Study (POTS) randomized controlled trial. *JAMA*. 2004;292:1969.

103. Bloch MH, Storch EA. Assessment and management of treatment-refractory obsessive-compulsive disorder in children. *J Am Acad Child Adolesc Psychiatry*. 2015;54:251.

104. Geller DA, Biederman J, Stewart SE, et al. Which SSRI? A meta-analysis of pharmacotherapy trials in pediatric obsessive-compulsive disorder. *Am J Psychiatry*. 2003;160:1919.

105. Cohen SC, Mulqueen JM, Ferracioli-Oda E, et al. Meta-analysis: risk of tics associated with psychostimulant use in randomized, placebo-controlled trials. *J Am Acad Child Adolesc Psychiatry*. 2015;54:728.

106. Cortese S, Adamo N, Del Giovane C, et al. Comparative efficacy and tolerability of medications for attention-deficit hyperactivity disorder in children, adolescents, and adults: a systematic review and network meta-analysis. *Lancet Psychiatry*. 2018;5:727.

107. Ruggiero S, Clavenna A, Reale L, Capuano A, Rossi F, Bonati M. Guanfacine for attention deficit and hyperactivity disorder in pediatrics: a systematic review and meta-analysis. *Eur Neuropsychopharmacol*. 2014;24(10):1578-1590.

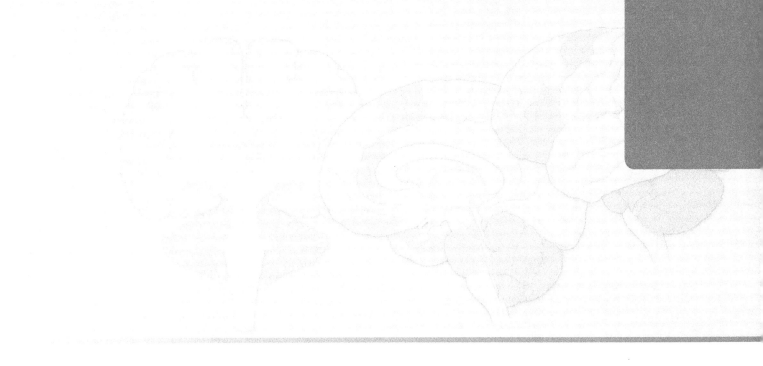

Part B. Neuropsychiatry of Neurological and Medical Disorders

Approach to Neurocognitive Disorders

Scott M. McGinnis

20

INTRODUCTION

The purpose of this chapter is to provide a framework for approaching cognitive disorders based on anatomical localization and time course. In so doing we will review key clinical considerations in the diagnosis and management of conditions with acute/subacute onset versus those with insidious onset (Figure 20-1). In each case, it is important to know the cardinal features of the more common conditions as well as atypical features that should prompt consideration of alternative, less common conditions. For conditions with acute/subacute onset this involves understanding core aspects of delirium (exceedingly common) and features that might alternatively suggest conditions in the differential diagnosis of rapidly progressive dementia (RPD; relatively less common). For conditions with insidious onset, the chapter reviews a basic workup and considers a high-level distinction between two categories of presentations: nonprogressive disorders, and gradually progressive neurodegenerative (±vascular) diseases. Within the category of neurodegenerative disorders, we will explore the utility of a comprehensive diagnostic formulation encompassing syndrome, severity, and suspected underlying neuropathology. The chapter concludes by examining key elements of relatively more common conditions—late-onset, amnesic, and dysexecutive syndromes associated with underlying Alzheimer's disease (AD) and Lewy body disease (LBD) neuropathology—and atypical features that might suggest relatively less common conditions such as non-amnesic presentations of AD and syndromes within the spectrum of frontotemporal lobar degeneration (FTLD) neuropathology.

ACUTE AND SUBACUTE ONSET PRESENTATIONS

Cognitive disorders with acute and subacute manifestations evolving over hours, days, or weeks are frequently encountered in the inpatient setting due to their dramatic impact and requirement for urgent diagnosis and management. Distinguishing between delirium[1] and RPD represents a key first step in determining the cause of cognitive dysfunction presenting acutely over days or weeks. The hallmarks of delirium include a primary disturbance in attention (including directing, focusing, sustaining, and shifting attention) representing a change from baseline and tending to fluctuate over the course of the day.[1] Table 20-1 lists features used to distinguish delirium from RPD. Notably, delirium occurs most frequently from the indirect impact of underlying general medical conditions, medications, or drug intoxication or withdrawal on the brain as opposed to a primary neurological condition. It is critical to establish the presence of inattention via mental status examination and to assess for localizing signs via a targeted, efficient screening elemental neurological examination (see Chapter 5).

Given the possibility that, in selected circumstances primary neurological conditions might present with delirium, studies such as MRI brain, electroencephalogram (EEG), and lumbar puncture for analysis of cerebrospinal fluid (CSF) are indicated when a preliminary workup for metabolic, toxic, and infectious causes fails to reveal evidence of a general medical etiology, additional elements of the presentation point toward a neurological condition such as stroke, seizure, or central nervous system (CNS) infection, or a patient demonstrates persistent delirium despite appropriate medical care for an initial suspected cause. These same studies prove very useful when it

---

[1] In some contexts, "delirium" is considered a subtype of "acute confusional state" characterized by hypervigilance, psychomotor agitation, and autonomic hyperactivity. Here, the term encompasses the spectrum of acute confusional states with and without these characteristics.

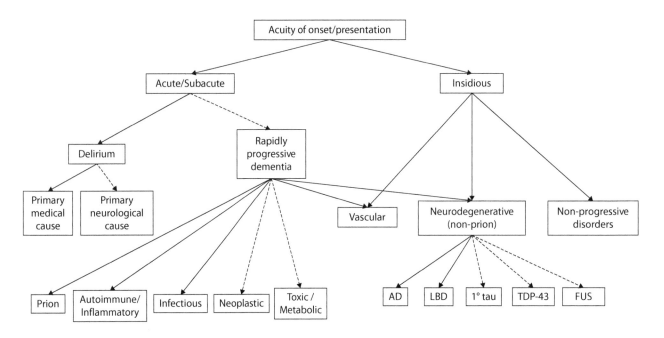

FIGURE 20-1. Flowchart depicting major etiologic categories for cognitive disorders with acute/subacute onset or insidious onset. Specific conditions within these etiologic categories are reviewed in the text. Solid lines depict relatively more prevalent conditions, dashed lines less prevalent conditions. 1° tau, primary tauopathy; AD, Alzheimer's disease; FUS, fused in sarcoma neuropathology; LBD, Lewy body disease; TDP-43, TDP-43 proteinopathy.

TABLE 20-1 • Features Distinguishing Delirium from Rapidly Progressive Dementia.		
	Delirium	**Rapidly Progressive Dementia**
Time course	Fluctuating	Rapidly progressive over days/weeks
Level of consciousness	More likely fluctuating, with disrupted circadian rhythm	Less likely fluctuating
Principal cognitive domain(s) affected	Attention	Variable
"Cortical" signs*	Present less frequently	Present more frequently
Motor signs	Isolated asterixis and/or myoclonus possible	Extrapyramidal, pyramidal, cerebellar signs more likely; myoclonus likely
Etiology	Usually general medical condition, medication side effect, drug intoxication/withdrawal	Usually primarily neurological

*"Cortical" signs include aphasia, apraxia, alexia, agraphia, acalculia, agnosia, cortical sensory signs, and neglect.

comes to establishing the etiology of a RPD, as reviewed below. Chapter 25 covers delirium in detail.

RPDs involve progression of cognitive symptoms over a time course of weeks to months to a point of dementia—defined by a loss of functional independence due to cognitive impairment.[2] While prion diseases have been considered the "prototypical" RPDs—accounting for roughly 68% of cases in published series—the relative frequency of prion versus non-prion conditions in published retrospective RPD cohorts depends highly on the geographic location and clinical setting of the site reporting the cases. Large samples from prion specialty centers have reported confirmed or likely prion diseases in 56–92% of cases,[2–6] whereas samples from tertiary care hospitals in various locations around the world have reported prion diseases in 7–31% of RPD cases.[7–10] Analysis of the non-prion cases from both prion specialty centers and tertiary care hospitals reveals atypically rapid presentations of other neurodegenerative diseases (e.g., AD, LBD, FTLD), autoimmune/inflammatory disorders, infections, and vascular disorders of the CNS to be the most common causative categories, followed by neoplasms, toxic or metabolic conditions, and miscellaneous other causes (Figure 20-2).

Considering the broad differential diagnosis of RPD it is advantageous to take a structured approach to diagnosis, thinking systematically across etiological categories. Achieving a specific diagnosis hinges upon identifying key disease-associated signs and features and narrowing the differential following an initial screening evaluation including selected high-yield blood tests, MRI brain, CSF analysis, and EEG. Tables 20-2 through 20-5 display conditions, associated features, initial studies, and secondary studies across selected etiological categories of RPD.

Prion Diseases

Prion diseases are neurodegenerative illnesses involving the conversion of a normal host cell prion protein (PrP^C) into an

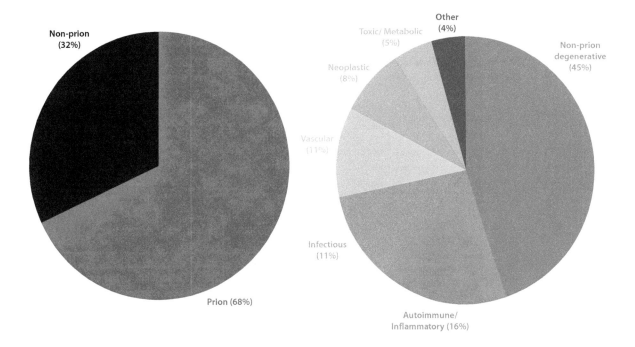

FIGURE 20-2. Proportions of prion and non-prion causes of rapidly progressive dementia, and etiological categories in the subset of non-prion cases pooled from multiple retrospective cohorts).[2-10]

TABLE 20-2 • Neurodegenerative Causes of Rapidly Progressive Dementia.		
	Prion	**Non-Prion Neurodegenerative**
Conditions	*Sporadic*: **Sporadic Jakob-Creutzfeldt disease** Genetic: Genetic Jakob-Creutzfeldt disease; fatal familial insomnia; Gerstmann-Straüssler-Scheinker syndrome *Acquired*: Variant Jakob-Creutzfeldt disease; iatrogenic Jakob-Creutzfeldt disease	Alzheimer's disease Lewy body disease FTLD: Primary tauopathy (Pick disease, CBD, PSP, others); TDP-43 proteinopathy (including FTLD with MND)
Associated features	Myoclonus, extrapyramidal, pyramidal, cerebellar, cortical signs	Extrapyramidal signs, pyramidal signs, cortical signs
Tests and studies	*CSF*: **RT-QuIC, 14-3-3, t-tau** *MRI*: **DWI/ADC**, T2/FLAIR *EEG*: Synchronous bi- or triphasic periodic sharp wave complexes *Other*: PRNP gene sequencing; brain biopsy	*CSF*: Aβ42, t-tau, p-tau (AD) *MRI*: **High-resolution T1**, T2/FLAIR, GRE/SWI *EEG*: Focal or diffuse slowing *Other*: FDG-PET; DaT imaging; EMG/NCV; brain biopsy

Aβ42, beta-amyloid (1, 42); CBD, corticobasal degeneration; DaT, dopamine transporter; DWI/ADC, diffusion-weighted/apparent diffusion coefficient imaging; EMG/ NCV, electromyography/nerve conduction velocities; FDG-PET, fluorodeoxyglucose positron emission tomography; GRE, T2* gradient echo; MND, motor neuron disease; PSP, progressive supranuclear palsy; p-tau, phosphorylated tau; RT-QuIC, real-time quaking-induced prion conversion; SWI, susceptibility-weighted imaging; t-tau, total tau. Conditions and studies with high clinical relevance are depicted in bold.

abnormal, pathological scrapie isoform (PrP^Sc), which subsequently spreads inexorably through the brain by further inducing the pathogenic conformational change in previously healthy cells. Resulting histopathological changes also include spongiform change due to vacuolization within neurons, and neuronal loss without inflammation. Prion disease occurs 80–95% of the time spontaneously as sporadic Jakob-Creutzfeldt disease (JCD), 10–15% of the time in genetic forms including genetic JCD, Gerstmann-Straüssler-Scheinker (GSS) syndrome, and fatal familial insomnia (FFI), and less than 1% of the time in acquired infectious/transmitted form (Table 20-2).[11] Genetic prion diseases are invariably caused by mutations in the human

prion protein gene, *PRNP*, the relatively rare syndromes of GSS and FFI usually being characterized by progressive ataxia and progressive insomnia and dysautonomia, respectively. Rare to begin with, the incidence of acquired prion diseases has decreased with (1) the implementation of modified surgical procedures to prevent transmission via corneal transplants, EEG depth electrodes, and dura mater graft transplants; (2) the use of recombinant pituitary hormones as opposed to cadaveric hormone extracts; (3) the cessation of ritual cannibalism in Papua New Guinea to prevent kuru; and (4) efforts to eradicate bovine spongiform encephalopathy to prevent variant JCD via ingestion of contaminated meat products.

TABLE 20-3 • Autoimmune/Inflammatory and Infectious Causes of Rapidly Progressive Dementia.

	Autoimmune/Inflammatory	Infections
Conditions	*Antibody-mediated*: **Paraneoplastic encephalitis/ degeneration; non-paraneoplastic Ab-mediated encephalitis** *Demyelinating*: ADEM; multiple sclerosis; systemic autoimmune disorders[a] *Vasculitis*: Primary CNS angiitis; secondary CNS vasculitides[b] *Steroid-responsive*: Hashimoto encephalopathy; steroid-responsive encephalopathy associated with systemic autoimmune disorders[a] *CNS involvement of systemic disorders*: Neurosarcoidosis; CNS lupus; Behçet syndrome	*Viral and virus-related*: **HSV; HIV**; PML; SSPE; **other viral encephalitides** *Bacterial*: **Neurosyphilis**, CNS tuberculosis, atypical mycobacteria; other atypical bacteria (e.g., *Bartonella*, *Mycloplasma*, *Brucella*, CNS Whipple) rarely *Fungal*: *Cryptococcus*, *Coccidiodes*, *Aspergillus*, *Toxoplasma*, others *Parasitic*: *Balamuthia*, *Baylisascaris*, others
Associated features	Cancer-related signs; systemic autoimmune-related symptoms/ signs	Headache, fever, meningeal signs
Tests and studies	*Blood*: **ESR, CRP, ANA; paraneoplastic, autoimmune Abs**; ANCA, dsDNA, anti-Sm, anti-RNP, SCL-70, SSA/SSB, RF, C3, C4, CH50, anti-Jo, anti-centromere; anti-thyroglobulin, anti-thyroid peroxidase *CSF*: **Protein, glucose, cell count/diff; IgG index, oligoclonal bands; paraneoplastic, autoimmune Abs** *MRI*: **T2/FLAIR**, contrast *Other*: Brain biopsy	*Blood*: **CBC/diff, RPR/TA-IgG, HIV** *Urine*: **Urinalysis, urine culture** *CSF*: **Protein, glucose, cell count/diff; VDRL**; Cryptococcal Ag, viral PCRs, Abs, cultures; bacterial, fungal, AFB stains, cultures; Whipple PCR *MRI*: Contrast

[a]*Examples include Sjögren syndrome and systemic lupus erythematosus.*
[b]*Examples include Behçet syndrome, polyarteritis nodosa, ANCA-associated, and cryoglobulinemic vasculitis.*
Ab, antibody; ADEM, acute disseminated encephalomyelitis; AFB, acid fast bacilli; Ag, antigen; ANA, antinuclear antibody; ANCA, antineutrophil cytoplasmic antibody; anti-RNP, anti-ribonucleoprotein; anti-Sm, anti-Smith; CBC/diff, complete blood count with differential; CH50, total complement activity; CRP, c-reactive protein; dsDNA, anti-double stranded DNA; ESR, erythrocyte sedimentation rate; PCR, polymerase chain reaction; PML, progressive multifocal leukoencephalopathy; RF, rheumatoid factor; RPR, rapid plasma reagin; SCL-70, anti-topoisomerase I; SSA/SSB, anti-Sjögren's syndrome related A and B; SSPE, subacute sclerosing panencephalitis; TA-IgG, Treponema pallidum antibody IgG; VDRL, Venereal Disease Research Laboratory test. Conditions and studies with high clinical relevance are depicted in bold.

TABLE 20-4 • Vascular and Neoplastic Causes of Rapidly Progressive Dementia.

	Vascular	Neoplastic
	Ischemic: **Strategic infarcts**, diffuse embolic infarcts, diffuse subcortical leukoencephalopathy *Hemorrhagic*: Intraparenchymal hemorrhage, bilateral subdural hematoma *Other*: Cerebral amyloid angiopathy, superficial siderosis, venous sinus thrombosis, dural arteriovenous fistula	*Lymphoma/Lymphoproliferative*: **Primary CNS lymphoma**, intravascular lymphoma, leptomeningeal lymphoma, lymphomatosis cerebri, lymphomatoid granulomatosis *Glioma*: Glioblastoma, gliomatosis cerebri *Metastatic*: Leptomeningeal carcinomatosis, parenchymal metastases
Associated features	Colocalizing focal signs; headache	Colocalizing focal signs; cranial nerve signs; blurred vision; headache; seizures
Tests and Studies	*Blood*: Coagulation profile; hypercoagulability testing *MRI*: **DWI/ADC, T2/FLAIR, GRE/SWI**, T1, **MRA**, MRV *Other*: CTA, CTV; carotid ultrasound; TTE, TEE; conventional angiography	*Blood*: SPEP, immunoelectrophoresis, CA-125 *CSF*: **Cytology, flow cytometry**; β_2-microglobulin, EBV PCR *MRI*: MR spectroscopy *Other*: **CT chest, abdomen pelvis with and without contrast**; FDG-PET/CT; testicular or pelvic ultrasound; mammogram; ophthalmologic examination, vitreous sampling

CTA/V, computed tomography angiography/venography; MRA/MRV, magnetic resonance angiography/venography; SPEP, serum protein electrophoresis; TEE, transesophageal echocardiography; TTE, transthoracic echocardiography. Conditions and studies with high clinical relevance are depicted in bold.

Sporadic JCD has an incidence of approximately one case per million per year worldwide.[12] Early symptoms are most commonly cognitive, though might also be cerebellar (e.g., ataxic gait), behavioral (e.g., agitation, depression, apathy, personality change), constitutional (e.g., dizziness, fatigue, sleep disturbance, weight loss), motor, sensory, or visual.[11] Even if absent initially, myoclonus is present in over 90% of cases at some point in the illness, cerebellar signs are present in over 50% of cases, and extrapyramidal or pyramidal motor signs are likewise present in over 50% of cases.[13-15] Consensus clinical diagnostic criteria for sporadic JCD from UCSF and from the World Health Organization (WHO)/European MRI-CJD Consortium require

TABLE 20-5 • Toxic and Metabolic Causes of Rapidly Progressive Dementia.		
	Toxic	**Metabolic**
	Medications: Lithium, methotrexate *Recreational drugs:* Alcohol, cocaine, heroin *Environmental/ Occupational:* Bismuth, mercury	*Vitamin deficiencies:* **Thiamine (B1)**, niacin (B3), cyanocobalamin (B12) *End-organ disease:* Portosystemic shunt, hepatic encephalopathy, hepatorenal syndrome, hypoxemia/hypercarbia *Electrolyte-related:* Extrapontine myelinolysis *Endocrine:* Hypothyroidism, hyperparathyroidism, hypoglycemia, hyperosmolar hyperglycemia *Genetic:* Adult-onset leukodystrophies; glycogen storage diseases; liposomal storage diseases; MELAS; Wilson disease
Associated features	Signs vary according to condition	
Tests and studies	*Blood:* Medication levels, toxicology screen *Urine:* Toxicology screen; heavy metal screen (24 hour)	*Blood:* **CMP, Ca, P, Mg**; **TFTs, vitamin B12**, homocysteine, MMA; copper, ceruloplasmin; ammonia; thiamine *Urine:* Copper (24 hour); porphobilinogen/delta-aminolevulinic acid

CMP, comprehensive metabolic profile; MELAS, mitochondrial encephalomyopathy, lactic acidosis, and stroke-like episodes; MMA, methylmalonic acid; P, phosphate; TFTs, thyroid function tests. Conditions and studies with high clinical relevance are depicted in bold.

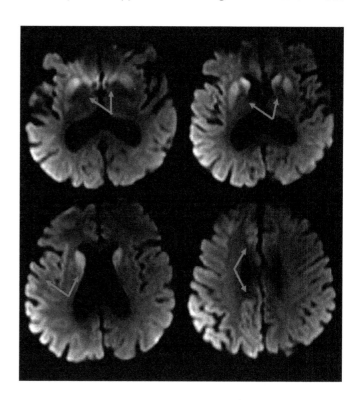

FIGURE 20-3. Diffusion-weighted MRI sequence from a patient with Jakob-Creutzfeldt disease demonstrating restricted diffusion in the striatum and along the cortical ribbon.

(1) rapidly progressive cognitive decline/dementia; (2) at least two of the following signs: myoclonus, pyramidal/extrapyramidal dysfunction, cerebellar dysfunction, visual dysfunction, or akinetic mutism in addition to suggestive EEG and/or MRI. The UCSF criteria also include focal cortical signs and the WHO criteria includes elevated CSF 14-3-3 protein.[15,16] Clinical features in JCD are influenced by molecular subtype, itself determined by two factors: the methionine (M) versus valine (V) polymorphism at codon 129 of *PRNP*, and the size of PrP^Sc following partial digestion with protease K (type 1 vs. type 2). Because MM1 and MV1 are considered nearly identical, and MM2 has both "cortical" and "thalamic" forms, the six recognized subtypes include MM1/MV1, VV1, VV2, MV2, MM2-cortical, and MM2-thalamic.[17]

The finding of restricted diffusion along the cortical ribbon and/or within deep gray matter nuclei (caudate, putamen, or thalamus)—visualized on diffusion weighted and apparent diffusion coefficient (DWI/ADC) sequences (Figure 20-3)—has higher than 90% sensitivity and specificity regardless of molecular subtype.[18,19] Molecular subtypes influence the results

of diagnostic studies in JCD with some subtypes (VV1, MM2-cortical) more likely to demonstrate a cortical pattern and others (VV2, MV2, MM2-thalamic) more likely to demonstrate a subcortical pattern.[20] The classic EEG finding of periodic synchronous bi- or triphasic sharp wave complexes (PSWCs) is often not present until middle and late stages of illness and more likely to be seen in the MM1/MV1 subtype (~70–80% sensitive) than in all other subtypes.[13,14,17,21] CSF 14-3-3 protein similarly appears more sensitive in MM1/MV1 JCD than other subtypes,[13,22] with overall (pooled) sensitivity ~90% or higher.[23] Owing to much lower specificity, elevated CSF 14-3-3 and total tau levels are best considered as nonspecific markers of neuronal injury, neither to be used as a screening test when the pretest probability of JCD is low nor as confirmation of the diagnosis when there are nonsuggestive features and other causes of RPD remain in the differential diagnosis. Recently available real-time quaking-induced conversion (RT-QuIC) assays that amplify detection of PrP^Sc in CSF or olfactory mucosa brushings have thus far demonstrated excellent specificity (>95%), thus showing promise as a confirmatory test.[24] Brain biopsy continues to represent the gold standard for confirming the diagnosis of JCD, though if clinical features, CSF, and MRI are all suggestive and treatment-responsive mimics such as inflammatory encephalitides have been effectively ruled out, then diagnostic confirmation via brain biopsy may not provide additive value.

Management of prion diseases is strictly supportive, as there are no treatments to alter the disease course. Death occurs within 1 year of symptom onset in most cases, with median survival around 6 months.[25]

Neurodegenerative Diseases (Non-Prion)

Neurodegenerative diseases that are usually insidious in onset and slowly progressive may, at times, present with a more rapid onset and progression of symptoms so as to be considered RPDs. Neurodegenerative diseases represent the most common non-prion etiology of RPD in multiple retrospective cohort studies.[2,3,6,8,9] Within the differential diagnosis of non-prion neurodegenerative diseases, FTLD with motor neuron disease, 4-repeat tauopathies (progressive supranuclear palsy and corticobasal degeneration), and diffuse LBD may be disproportionately more commonly represented and AD less commonly represented in subsets of patients with rapidly progressive versus slowly progressive time courses (Table 20-2).[26] Rapid progression in AD has been associated with early appearance of motor symptoms, concomitant presence of additional neuropathologies (e.g., LBD and/or vascular disease), and high levels of CSF total tau or phosphorylated tau.[5,27]

Non-prion neurodegenerative diseases are reviewed in greater detail below, and in Chapters 21, 23, and 24.

Autoimmune/Inflammatory Diseases

Consideration and recognition of autoimmune and inflammatory causes of RPD are critical because they tend to be more responsive to treatment than many other etiologies and because they can mimic less treatment-responsive conditions such as prion disease.[28,29] The spectrum of autoimmune/inflammatory diseases (Table 20-3) consists of conditions with different pathophysiological mechanisms, including antibodies against specific neural antigens, demyelination, vasculitis, perivascular inflammation, meningoencephalitis, and mechanisms that remain unclear to date (Hashimoto encephalopathy, others).

Antibody-mediated encephalitides are noteworthy given an ever-growing number of antibodies directed against specific anti-neural antigens identified in recent years, frequent limbic/paralimbic localization producing prominent temporolimbic amnesia and neuropsychiatric symptoms—including but not limited to psychosis, mania, and obsessive-compulsive symptoms—and possible presentation with restricted diffusion along the cortical ribbon resembling that occurring in JCD (Figure 20-4).[28] Among paraneoplastic conditions, some of the more frequent antibodies associated with encephalitis include anti-Hu (ANNA-1), anti-CRMP5, and anti-Ma2.[30] Encephalitis associated with antibodies against neuronal cell surface/synaptic proteins may occur in the presence or absence of underlying cancer, the classic exemplar being anti-NMDA receptor encephalitis (sometimes associated with ovarian teratoma). In addition to amnesia and psychiatric symptoms, characteristics of anti-NMDA receptor encephalitis include prodromal symptoms (headache, fever), language-output related changes (e.g., mutism, echolalia), dyskinesias, seizures, diminished level of consciousness, and autonomic instability.[31]

Workup of autoimmune/inflammatory conditions can yield results with variable specificity. Nonspecific findings include abnormalities in the CSF (elevated protein, lymphocytic pleiocytosis, elevated IgG index, oligoclonal bands), EEG (focal or generalized slowing, periodic lateralized epileptiform discharges, epileptiform activity), and/or MRI (T2/FLAIR

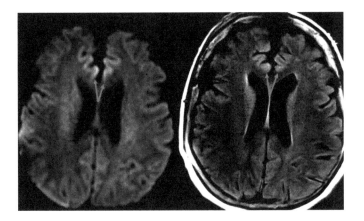

FIGURE 20-4. Diffusion-weighted and fluid-attenuated inversion recovery sequences from a patient with antibodies against leucine-rich, glioma inactivated 1 (LG1) protein subunit of the voltage-gated potassium channel complex. Images demonstrate restricted diffusion and increased T2 signal in the anterior cingulate cortex. The patient improved clinically, and radiographic findings resolved following treatment with high-dose corticosteroids and rituximab.

hyperintensities). Detection of antibodies in the blood and/or CSF has greater specificity, though not 100%.[32] As diagnosis can sometimes be challenging and it is imperative to avoid missing treatable causes, standard management algorithms for RPD suggest treatment with high-dose corticosteroids (e.g., IV methylprednisolone 1 g daily for 5 days) if CSF and brain and body imaging findings are not diagnostic and infection and lymphoma have been effectively ruled out.[2]

Autoimmune/inflammatory conditions and paraneoplastic antibody-mediated encephalitis are reviewed in greater detail in Chapters 26 and 28, respectively.

Infections

Another potentially treatable category, CNS infections, are a proportionally more common cause of RPD in developing countries and in immunocompromised individuals in developed countries.[7,10,33] The presence of headache, fever, meningeal signs, or inflammatory CSF should prompt consideration of infectious etiologies, possibilities including viruses, bacteria, fungi, and parasites (Table 20-3). Less common in the era of antiretroviral therapy (ART) than previously, HIV-associated dementia should be considered, particularly when a presentation suggests a "subcortical" process involving psychomotor slowing, attention and executive dysfunction, depression, and/or apathy. HSV encephalitis is the most common form of sporadic encephalitis, characteristically affecting the temporal lobes to produce cognitive manifestations such as impairments in episodic memory and/or semantic processing and behavioral changes that might include hypomania, psychosis, or Klüver-Bucy syndrome.[34] Neurosyphilis can cause cognitive impairment and dementia both in its early forms—for example, as an encephalitis occurring more frequently in immunocompromised individuals[35]—and more classically in the late form of general paresis, frequently associated with neuropsychiatric signs such as depression, mania, and psychosis.

Blood and CSF tests are particularly useful to establish a diagnosis in many cases of RPD due to a CNS infection. The neuropsychiatry of infectious disorders is covered in detail in Chapter 26.

Vascular Conditions

As cognitive changes can follow a wide variety of vascular lesions, vascular dementia diagnosed clinically is a heterogeneous construct that requires one's best effort to correlate cognitive changes with lesions, temporally, spatially (based on known principles of localization), or both. Multiple mechanisms of ischemic stroke may apply (Table 20-4), including intrinsic small, medium, or large vessel vasculopathies, atheroembolism, cardioembolism, central venous thrombosis, hypoperfusion, hyperviscosity, and others. Similarly, multiple types or categories of hemorrhage can impair cognition, including intraparenchymal hemorrhage, cerebral amyloid angiopathy (CAA) with numerous lobar microhemorrhages and/or extensive superficial siderosis (superficial hemorrhage into the cortical sulci), and bilateral subdural hematomas. Dementia and RPD may result from a limited number of focal (i.e., "strategic") lesions or from the cumulative effects of more widespread lesions, as occurs with extensive subcortical small vessel ischemic disease or diffuse cortical emboli. Importantly, in many older individuals establishing the presence of vascular disease does not rule out concomitant neurodegenerative neuropathology.[36]

Neuroimaging studies, particularly the diffusion, T2/FLAIR, and susceptibility sequences of MRI and vascular imaging with CT and/or MR angiography and venography are very useful in the diagnosis of vascular causes of RPD. Conventional angiography is typically required to diagnose selected causes including dural arteriovenous fistulae. In some cases of subacute, multifocal infarcts, brain biopsy may be required to identify a condition such as intravascular lymphoma or CNS vasculitis.

Chapter 22 covers the neuropsychiatry of stroke and cerebrovascular diseases.

Neoplasms

Neoplasms uncommonly present with progressive cognitive impairment as the most prominent feature. Possibilities within this category include various presentations of lymphoma, glioma, and metastatic disease (Table 20-4). While the finding of an enhancing lesion or lesions on contrast MRI can be a helpful clue in some scenarios, in other cases changes might be more diffuse/infiltrating (e.g., as with lymphomatosis or gliomatosis cerebri), suggestive of multifocal infarction (e.g., as with intravascular lymphoma) or limited to subtle leptomeningeal findings. Patients with CNS neoplasms may demonstrate signs of elevated intracranial pressure. Those with leptomeningeal involvement may have signs referable to single or multiple cranial nerves.

Multiple large volume lumbar punctures for CSF cytology and flow cytometry are indicated for evaluation of potential CNS lymphoma. Other studies of potential value include testicular ultrasound in men and slit lamp examination of the eyes for evaluation of possible ocular disease and consideration of intraocular biopsy. When negative, stereotactic brain biopsy is frequently required. Corticosteroids are contraindicated prior to biopsy because they cause necrosis of lymphoma cells which can render the biopsy non-diagnostic.

Chapter 28 covers the neuropsychiatry of cancer and its treatment.

Toxic/Metabolic Conditions

The toxic/metabolic category comprises causes of RPD with varying responsiveness to treatment depending upon the specific etiology. Major subcategories within the "toxic" group include iatrogenic toxins (i.e., medications, chemotherapy), recreational drugs, environmental or occupational exposures. Subcategories within the "metabolic" group include vitamin deficiencies, sequelae of end-organ dysfunction (liver, kidneys, heart, lung), endocrine conditions, electrolyte-related conditions, and genetic metabolic disorders (Table 20-5). A thorough history is particularly important when evaluating for potential toxic exposures and risk factors for metabolic disease, for example, conditions predisposing one to malnutrition. Knowledge of associated general medical and neurological signs is likewise useful here, since toxic and metabolic conditions often affect more than just the CNS. For example, niacin (vitamin B3) deficiency is associated with a photosensitive pigmented dermatitis and diarrhea in addition to dementia (pellagra), and cyanocobalamin (vitamin B12) deficiency is associated with macrocytic anemia, glossitis, symmetrical numbness/paresthesias, and gait changes.[37]

Thiamine (vitamin B1) deficiency or Wernicke encephalopathy accounts for a relatively high proportion of toxic/metabolic RPDs[3,7] and can present with features similar to JCD, that is, ataxia and restricted diffusion in the diencephalon on MRI DWI.[38] A majority of patients with neuropathological evidence of thiamine deficiency do not demonstrate the full classic triad of cognitive changes, oculomotor dysfunction, and gait ataxia.[39] All patients in whom the diagnosis is being considered should be treated urgently with intravenous thiamine.

Other Conditions

Additional causes of RPD include primary psychiatric disorders, hydrocephalus, seizures (particularly focal status epilepticus), and mesial temporal sclerosis. Causative primary psychiatric disorders include melancholic depression, psychotic disorders, bipolar-spectrum disorders, and catatonia. The neuropsychiatry of catatonia is reviewed in Chapter 25.

INSIDIOUS ONSET PRESENTATIONS

"Memory loss" in an older patient represents the most common chief complaint/reason for referral to an outpatient subspecialty cognitive/behavioral neurology clinic. Used colloquially, it can refer to problems in any number of areas (cognitive domains), including but not limited to difficulty recalling recent events and information (episodic memory); losing track of one's train of thought and/or action or difficulties holding information in mind (attention and working memory), problems with the acquisition and retrieval of information that one can still store well, difficulties completing complex tasks, and changes in problem solving, reasoning, and judgment (executive functions); difficulty

TABLE 20-6 • Major Diagnostic Considerations in Cognitive Presentations with Insidious Onset and/or Chronic Time Course.

	Attention/Executive	Episodic Memory	Other Domains
Relatively static (nondegenerative)	**Dysexecutive syndrome due to aging + superimposed factors ± developmental weakness** Developmental disorders Prior monophasic frontal-associated network injury[*]	Prior monophasic temporolimbic network injury	Prior monophasic injury to language, visual/spatial, cortical sensory/motor, social cognitive networks Developmental disorders
Gradually progressive (neurodegenerative ± vascular)	**Lewy body syndromes/diseases** Progressive dysexecutive syndrome due to AD or FTLD Progressive dysexecutive syndrome due to vascular disease Normal pressure hydrocephalus	**Progressive amnesic syndrome due to AD** Progressive amnesic syndrome due to FTLD	Progressive aphasia due to FTLD or AD Progressive visuospatial syndrome (PCA) due to AD or LBD Corticobasal syndrome due to FTLD or AD bvFTD due to FTLD

[*]Monophasic neurologic injuries include (but are not limited to) vascular, infectious, toxic/metabolic, autoimmune/inflammatory events, resected neoplasm, and traumatic brain injury.
AD, Alzheimer's disease; bvFTD, behavioral variant frontotemporal dementia; FTLD, frontotemporal lobar degeneration; PCA, posterior cortical atrophy. Conditions with high clinical relevance are depicted in bold.

retrieving words in order to convey intended meaning (language); and/or difficulty recalling a route one navigates (visuospatial functions). Subjective observations about the time course of symptoms do not always reflect the objective time course. Given the critical importance of localization and time course in diagnosing cognitive disorders with insidious onset, much of the art of diagnosis reduces to the clinician's ability to determine these elements by history and examination (Table 20-6). Once accomplished, the remainder of the evaluation—that is, laboratory and neuroimaging studies—serves to assess for potentially modifiable contributing factors to cognitive dysfunction and to test one's already-formulated hypothesis about the most likely etiology underlying the cognitive dysfunction. This section starts with a description of the general approach to the evaluation of neurocognitive disorders of insidious presentation, including history, examination, laboratory, and neuroimaging workup. It then reviews the main disorders included in this category.

History and Examination

Chapter 3 of this textbook reviews concepts of localization of cognitive processes to large-scale brain networks, and Chapters 4–7 review methodologic considerations in neuropsychiatric workups in detail. Here, we briefly review a reasonable standard of care in the outpatient workup of a patient being evaluated for potential cognitive impairment of insidious onset. In most cases, history should be obtained both from the patient and from a reliable informant who knows the patient well because cognitive disorders by their nature frequently affect an individual's ability to accurately self-report. It is useful to begin with open-ended questions about observations and concerns, and with a request for examples, a goal being to determine whether there are symptoms referable to key cognitive domains affected by the more common etiologic considerations and incorporated in consensus diagnostic criteria for dementia.[1,40] If open-ended questioning does not cover all key domains, targeted questioning to assess for characteristic symptoms helps to fill in the gaps (Table 20-7). A detailed history further provides the first opportunity to

examine important areas including social/comportmental cognition, attention, language, and episodic memory.

Structured questionnaires such as scales to assess level of functioning in activities of daily living (ADLs)[41,42] and neuropsychiatric symptoms[43,44] can be useful to obtain needed information about the impact of cognitive difficulties on the patient's functioning in usual activities and a relevant survey of mood, anxiety, psychosis, and additional neuropsychiatric elements. Reviewing elements pertaining to sleep (initiation, maintenance, snoring/breathing, restless legs symptoms, dream enactment), daytime energy and alertness (including dozing, napping, fluctuations), basic sensory and motor functions (walking, balance, tremor, fine manual dexterity, vision, hearing, smell), autonomic symptoms (orthostatic lightheadedness, constipation, loose stools, urinary frequency/urgency/incontinence, erectile dysfunction, changes in sweating or salivation), and pain allows for a comprehensive consideration of additional potential etiologic and/or contributing factors.

Pertinent goals of the initial cognitive examination are to supplement the history in establishing and localizing cognitive dysfunction and to establish a baseline for potential future comparison toward the aim of determining time course. A key question is whether the patient has objective evidence of cognitive changes above and beyond what might be attributed to normal aging, where possible factoring in what is known about the patient's educational history and/or premorbid level of intelligence. An examination should therefore provide a reasonable survey of the core cognitive domains noted above. Embedding an established, validated cognitive assessment tool such as the Montreal Cognitive Assessment[45] or the Addenbrooke's Cognitive Examination-Revised[46] into one's examination can provide a solid foundation on which to add selected supplemental measures and yield a global score that can aid in longitudinal tracking. However, as these tools may not prove sufficient to survey all domains, supplementation with additional high-yield single-domain cognitive tests is recommended (Table 20-7).[47] Referral to a neuropsychologist or cognitive disorders specialist is indicated if time does not permit a comprehensive initial

TABLE 20-7 • Relevance of Commonly Reported Symptoms and Cognitive Tests to Cognitive Domains in Patients Evaluated for Cognitive Impairment with Insidious Onset.

Domain	Symptoms	Examples of Tests
Episodic memory	Rapidly forgetting recent information or events Repeating questions or statements without awareness Producing fabricated, distorted, or misinterpreted memories without intention to deceive (confabulation)	Supra-span word list tests (e.g., CERAD word list, Hopkins Verbal Learning Test, Rey Auditory Verbal Learning Test) MoCA: Five item word list
Attention/Working memory	Losing train of thought in the middle of a sentence or task Difficulty holding information "in mind" (e.g., forgetting reason for walking into a room) Difficulty multitasking	Trail Making Test, A and B Digit Span Forward and Backward Sequential Operation Series (e.g., months of the year backward) Stroop test MoCA: Trail making; digit span; vigilance; serial 7 subtractions
Executive functioning	Difficulty completing complex, multistep tasks Difficulties planning, organizing, or problem-solving Difficulty retrieving information that comes back later and/or with cues[a] Changes in reasoning and judgment	Antisaccade test Frontal assessment battery Clock-drawing test Controlled Oral Word Association[b] MoCA: Clock drawing (interpreted); abstraction
Language	Difficulty retrieving words leading to hesitancy, pauses, using more words to convey meaning, or using incorrect words Mispronouncing words (phonological errors)	Boston naming test-15 item Semantic category fluency MoCA: Naming; sentence repetition[c]
Visual/Spatial	Difficulties navigating and/or orienting in space Difficulty locating items in one's field of view, especially when other items are present	Cube copying test Cancellation test Line bisection test MoCA: Cube; clock drawing
Higher sensory/Motor	Difficulty using tools	Limb apraxia testing Graphesthesia testing In-between test (finger agnosia) Interlocking finger test

[a]Associated with executive dysfunction and possible early temporolimbic amnesia.
[b]Tests executive functioning and language.
[c]Tests language and verbal working memory.
CERAD, Consortium to Establish a Registry for Alzheimer's Disease; MoCA, Montreal Cognitive Assessment.

history and cognitive examination, or if one's own initial assessment fails to achieve the key goals of establishing neuroanatomic localization and time course.

An initial elemental neurological examination serves to screen for neurological signs including but not limited to signs potentially associated with neurodegenerative conditions (parkinsonism, upper motor neuron signs,[2] "primitive" reflexes[3]),

prior stroke or other focal brain injury, or other neurological conditions with potential to impact the patient's functional status (e.g., vision loss, hearing loss, peripheral neuropathy). It can be useful to embed tests for hemineglect, simultanagnosia, limb apraxia, and cortical sensory signs into one's screening examination.

Laboratory and Neuroimaging Workup

The goal of core basic laboratory studies in patients with insidious onset cognitive impairment is more frequently to identify potentially modifiable factors contributing to cognitive symptoms and/or risk than it is to identify fully reversible etiologies. Experts typically recommend that most or all patients have the following checked: comprehensive metabolic profile (including electrolytes, renal function tests, fasting glucose level, and liver function tests), thyroid-stimulating hormone (with additional T4 if high or low), vitamin B12 (with reflex homocysteine and methylmalonic acid if low or borderline-low), and complete blood counts.[48] Additional testing (e.g., for infectious, autoimmune/inflammatory, or other nondegenerative conditions) is

---

[2] Signs of upper motor neuron lesions include spasticity (velocity-dependent resistance to passive movement of a limb), hyperreflexia, extensor plantar response, and pattern of weakness more prominently affecting shoulder abduction (vs. adduction), elbow extension (vs. flexion), wrist extension (vs. flexion), hip abduction (vs. adduction), knee flexion (vs. extension), and ankle extension (vs. flexion).

[3] "Primitive" reflexes are present in infancy and disappear as brain development leads to their inhibition. Reappearance usually suggests dysfunction in the frontal lobes and/or diffuse cerebral dysfunction. Examples include the palmar grasp, palmomental, rooting, sucking, and snout reflexes. The glabellar reflex is also frequently present in the context of extrapyramidal dysfunction.

determined by clinical circumstances and the anticipated utility/value of the test being considered.

Structural neuroimaging—preferably with MRI—is recommended for purposes of assessing: (1) the burden of suspected vascular disease in forms of leukoariosis, chronic infarcts, and/or microhemorrhages or superficial siderosis; (2) for focal patterns of atrophy as may occur in AD or FTLD; (3) additional (relatively rare) lesions or structural changes potentially associated with cognitive dysfunction (e.g., hydrocephalus, neoplasm, infectious/inflammatory diseases, etc.). In most cases, when structural neuroimaging results corroborate one's diagnostic impression no further workup is indicated or necessary.

In special circumstances additional workup for biomarkers of neurodegeneration or molecular neuropathology can provide value, particularly if results would affect the plan of care and/or if establishing a diagnosis with greater confidence would be useful to the patient and/or those close to her or him. Analysis of CSF beta-amyloid (1,42), total tau, and phosphorylated tau levels can yield information regarding the likelihood of underlying AD neuropathology, most commonly useful when a patient has one of the following: persistent, unexplained mild cognitive impairment (MCI)—defined by subjective concerns about changes in memory or thinking, corroborated by cognitive testing, but not at a severity precluding independence in usual activities[49]; MCI or dementia with onset at an early age (<65); or MCI or dementia that is atypical for AD on the basis of cognitive profile, dominant behavioral symptoms at presentation, or additional evidence of vascular disease, LBD, FTLD, or other cognitively impairing conditions.[50] Though not-specific for molecular neuropathology, ^{18}F-fluorodeoxyglucose (FDG) positron emission tomography (PET) can be similarly helpful to distinguish AD from frontotemporal dementias (FTDs) and/or dementia with Lewy bodies (DLB), and, in some cases to determine the likelihood of a neurodegenerative cause of persistent, unexplained cognitive impairment at a level of MCI or dementia.[51,52] Also not specific for molecular neuropathology, dopamine transporter imaging with ^{18}F-flourodopa PET or ^{123}I-ioflupane single photon emission computed tomography is useful to distinguish degenerative from nondegenerative causes of parkinsonism.[53] Amyloid PET imaging provides information generally comparable to that provided by CSF AD biomarkers but is obtained less frequently in clinical practice because it has not been routinely covered by health insurance.[54]

Genetic testing for mutations associated with familial AD—mutations in the genes encoding amyloid precursor protein (APP), presenilin-1 (PSEN1), and presenilin-2 (PSEN2)—is recommended only in select circumstances, for example, when a patient has AD dementia with early-onset (defined arbitrarily as onset of symptoms before age 65) and family history of dementia, family history suggestive of autosomal dominant dementia and at least one case of early-onset AD, and in individuals with a relative who has a known gene mutation.[55] Similar principles apply when considering testing for mutations in genes associated with familial FTLD—chromosome 9 open reading frame-72 (C9orf72), microtubule-associated protein tau (MAPT), and granulin (GRN)—though one should also consider family history of amyotrophic lateral sclerosis

(ALS) and Parkinson's disease (PD) diagnosed clinically to be relevant, especially with onset at 65-years-old or younger.[56] Genetic testing is usually best carried out by genetics counselors, who offer detailed education and recommendations prior to tests being completed.

Nonprogressive Disorders of Attention and Executive Functioning

"Normal cognitive aging," a challenging concept for many reasons, has been defined operationally as performance within 1.5–2 standard deviations of the mean for age on neuropsychological testing.[57] Aging frequently brings cognitive changes in processing speed and aspects of attention, working memory, and executive functioning.[58–60] Superimposed factors that affect the brain diffusely or frontal-associated brain networks specifically cause attention and/or executive deficits at a level beyond those changes attributable to normal aging, that nonetheless do not progress to dementia as would neurodegenerative conditions at a comparable level of impairment.[61] A variety of superimposed factors have been implicated, categories including primary psychiatric conditions, sleep disorders (including but not limited to obstructive sleep apnea), chronic general medical illness, chronic pain, and medications with the potential to adversely affect cognition.[62–64] It is also possible for normal aging (plus or minus a superimposed acquired factor) to unmask preexisting developmental weaknesses that were previously compensated and not active or bothersome throughout adulthood, leading up to the onset of presenting symptoms.[65]

The standard workup outlined above may provide information to indicate a dysexecutive syndrome due to suspected nondegenerative factors, suggestive elements being a cognitive profile limited to attention and/or executive dysfunction (i.e., without compelling evidence of temporolimbic amnesia or cortical language, visual/spatial or sensory/motor signs), the identification of potentially causative superimposed factors in reasonable temporal proximity to the onset of cognitive symptoms, establishing a nonprogressive time course, and neuroimaging without evidence of significant cerebral atrophy. However, distinguishing nondegenerative etiologies from neurodegenerative etiologies early in their time course is not always straightforward. AD or LBD may present with a predominantly dysexecutive cognitive profile,[66–68] the former more frequently in individuals with sporadic early-onset presentations (with onset of symptoms in their 50s or early 60s) and frequent comorbid depression and/or anxiety that might be mistaken as a cause of the cognitive dysfunction. In other situations, nondegenerative dysexecutive disorder might be misdiagnosed as MCI or dementia due to a suspected neurodegenerative disease when a patient and/or someone who knows them well reports a clearly progressive time course, when comorbid superimposed contributing factors are not readily identified, or when structural neuroimaging results are ambiguous with respect to evidence of focal atrophy suggestive of neurodegeneration. Depending on the specifics of the situation, additional workup with biomarkers of neurodegeneration or molecular neuropathology might provide value.

Progressive Neurodegenerative ± Vascular Disorders

While a detailed, mechanistic understanding of the pathophysiology of neurodegenerative diseases remains elusive, important insights have been gained in recent decades. Some of the more important insights are as follows: (1) pathophysiological disease processes as reflected by their characteristic microscopic misfolded protein inclusions—which constitute the diagnostic gold standard—start years in advance of the first symptoms noted[69]; (2) neurodegenerative diseases target large-scale brain networks (defined by structural and functional connectivity), starting focally and propagating along the connected nodes of the networks[70,71]; and (3) different neurodegenerative pathologies frequently co-occur in the same individual, and also frequently co-occur with vascular pathology.[72] These insights have ramifications for how we think about an appropriate diagnostic framework for neurodegenerative cognitive disorders in addition to their implications for developing disease-modifying therapeutics.

Comprehensive Diagnostic Formulation

It is advantageous to consider a comprehensive diagnostic formulation including the *primary neurodegenerative cognitive syndrome*, the *stage* of illness, and the *suspected underlying neuropathology*. Features of a *secondary syndrome*, if present, should be noted and additional factors with potential to negatively impact cognition should be identified. This scheme represents a departure from historical concepts of conditions such as clinically diagnosed AD being interwoven with "dementia" and often considered synonymously with neuropathological AD (defined by intermediate-to-high levels of beta-amyloid plaques and tau neurofibrillary tangles). The previously widely used National Institute of Neurological and Communicative Disorders and Stroke-Alzheimer's Disease and Related Disorders (NINCDS-ADRDA) consensus clinical diagnostic criteria for AD indicated a requirement for dementia in all patients for whom a diagnosis of possible AD or probable AD might be considered.[73] Accommodating evidence that accumulation of beta-amyloid plaques starts before changes in memory and thinking becoming apparent,[74,75] the 2011 National Institute on Aging-Alzheimer's Association workgroups on diagnostic guidelines for AD offered revised criteria for a diagnosis of AD at different levels of clinical severity by incorporating biomarker data: normal cognition (preclinical AD), MCI due to AD, and dementia due to AD.[40,69,76] Similar principles of neuropathological changes starting before symptoms likely apply in Lewy body disorders and FTLD.[77,78] While the pathophysiological significance of preclinical neuropathological protein inclusions remains unclear and the utility of preclinical disease as a construct has yet to be firmly established in clinical practice, understanding MCI and dementia as *stages* of illness rather than diagnostic endpoints in and of themselves has great value. Used accordingly, these terms can be applied across the spectrum of neurodegenerative syndromes and neuropathologies in a staging scheme based on the degree to which cognitive changes impact a patient's level of functioning in ADLs (Table 20-8).

TABLE 20-8 • Staging in Neurodegenerative Cognitive Disorders.

Stage	Cognition	Functioning
Early preclinical	No symptoms, normal testing	Normal
Late preclinical (SCD)	Subjective concerns, normal testing	
Mild cognitive impairment	Impairment in one or more cognitive domains	Usual activities but not at usual level (independent in iADLs[a])
Mild dementia		Dependent in one or more complex iADLs
Moderate dementia	Impairment in two or more cognitive domains	Widespread dependence in iADLs and some aspects of basic ADLs (e.g., personal hygiene)[b]
Severe dementia	Global cognitive impairment	Widespread dependence in basic ADLs
End-stage dementia	Global cognitive impairment and basic motor dysfunction	Complete dependence in basic ADLs

[a]*Instrumental activities of daily include driving (and other forms of transportation within the community), taking prescribed medications, managing finances, shopping for groceries and necessities, preparing meals, and using the telephone and other forms of communication (e.g., email).*
[b]*Basic activities of daily living include bathing/showering, tending to personal hygiene/grooming, dressing, toileting, functional mobility, and self-feeding. SCD, Subjective cognitive decline.*

As prior diagnostic constructs linked a diagnosis of AD with dementia, so did they link AD with the syndrome of progressive declining episodic memory. The NINCDS-ADRDA and *Diagnostic and Statistical Manual of Mental Disorders, Fourth Edition (DSM-IV)* criteria for AD required impairment in episodic memory and at least one other cognitive domain.[73,79] In the years since these criteria were proposed, two significant limitations have become apparent based on clinical-neuropathological correlation studies. First, patients with neuropathological AD may present with primary impairment in a cognitive domain other than episodic memory.[4,80–82] Second, patients presenting with amnesic dementia satisfying the NINCDS-ADRDA or DSM-IV criteria turn out to have a primary neuropathological diagnosis other than AD about 15% of the time, even when the diagnosis is made by experts in AD research centers.[83] Both limitations highlight important diagnostic principles, also apparent when one examines clinical-neuropathological correlation studies in other conditions such as FTLD: clinical syndromes are determined by the brain networks that degenerate, and the correspondence between specific patterns of network degeneration

---

[4] This is particularly relevant in sporadic early-onset AD, in which approximately one-third of patients present atypically with primary cognitive dysfunction in a domain other than episodic memory.

TABLE 20-9 • Major Features and Clinical-Neuropathological Correlations in Neurodegenerative Cognitive Disorders.

Syndrome		Major Features	Most Common 1° Pathologies	Less Common 1° Pathologies
Amnesic		**Progressive amnesia**; variable early executive dysfunction, word-retrieval difficulties, visual/spatial dysfunction	**AD** (± LBD, VaD, TDP)	1° tau[a], TDP, VaD, LBD, HS
Dysexecutive	DLB syndrome	**Parkinsonism, visual hallucinations, dream enactment**, fluctuations; dysautonomia, hyposmia, neuroleptic-sensitivity, delusions, apathy, anxiety, depression	**LBD** (± AD, VaD)	VaD, AD
	Other dysexecutive	**Prominent executive dysfunction**; variable early amnesia, word-retrieval difficulties, visual/spatial dysfunction, social/comportmental changes	**AD** (± LBD, VaD)	VaD, 1° tau, TDP
Aphasic (PPA)	Logopenic	**Word-retrieval difficulties, poor sentence repetition**; phonological errors	**AD** (± LBD, VaD)	TDP, 1° tau, LBD
	Nonfluent/ agrammatic	**Impaired syntax and grammar**; possible apraxia of speech; impaired comprehension of complex sentences	**1° tau**	TDP, AD, LBD
	Semantic	**Impaired single word comprehension, confrontation naming**; impaired object knowledge, surface dyslexia or dysgraphia	**TDP**	AD, 1° tau
Visuospatial (PCA)		**Visual attention and perceptual deficits[b], constructional dyspraxia**; oculomotor, dressing, and/or limb apraxia; optic ataxia, acalculia, agraphia, left/right disorientation, finger agnosia	**AD** (± LBD, VaD)	1° tau, LBD, TDP
Social/Comportmental (bvFTD)		**Behavioral disinhibition, apathy, obsessive-compulsive/perseverative behaviors, loss of sympathy/empathy, hyperorality/changes in food preference, executive dysfunction**	**TDP, 1° tau**	AD, FUS
Sensory/Motor (CBS)		**Asymmetrical cortical (orobuccal or limb apraxia, cortical sensory deficit, alien limb) and motor (limb rigidity or akinesia, limb dystonia, myoclonus)**	**1° tau**	AD, TDP

[a]*Primary tauopathies include corticobasal degeneration, progressive supranuclear palsy, Pick disease, argyrophilic grain disease, and primary age-related tauopathy.*
[b]*Include space and/or object perception deficits, simultanagnosia, apperceptive prosopagnosia, environmental agnosia, alexia, and homonomous visual field defect.*
1°, Primary; AD, Alzheimer's disease; bvFTD, behavioral variant frontotemporal dementia; CBS, corticobasal syndrome; FUS, fused in sarcoma; HS, hippocampal sclerosis; LBD, Lewy body disease; PCA, posterior cortical atrophy; PPA, primary progressive aphasia; TDP, TDP-43 proteinopathy; VaD, vascular disease.

and neuropathologies is not one-to-one. Table 20-9 lists key features and most frequent clinical-neuropathological associations of major neurodegenerative cognitive syndromes.

Given the lack of clarity that inevitably arises from conflating syndromic and neuropathological diagnoses, it is useful to consider these as separate elements in the diagnostic formulation.[84] In most cases neuropathology is not known but rather suspected based on established clinical-neuropathological associations, and where available, information from biomarkers and/or secondary syndromic features.[5] In rare instances

underlying neuropathology might be effectively known, as in the case of a familial autosomal dominant condition with confirmed neuropathology.

Common versus Less Common Neurodegenerative Cognitive Syndromes

One should have a high index of suspicion for syndromes associated with AD neuropathology or LBD neuropathology due to their relatively high prevalence in older adults presenting for evaluation of cognitive impairment.[85,86] AD presents most frequently as a progressive amnesic syndrome characterized by difficulty retaining recent information, examples including not remembering important details from recent life events (and conversations) and repeating the same questions or statements without awareness of doing so. Milder impairments in executive functions, language (word retrieval), and visuospatial functions are present relatively early in many cases,[87] though a proportion

---

[5] As an example, a patient presenting with a progressive decline in memory for recent events and information, might have CSF evidence of underlying AD neuropathology yet also evolve to develop elements potentially suggestive of LBD (e.g., formed visual hallucinations, dream enactment, mild parkinsonism). In this case, it would be reasonable to suspect mixed AD and LBD underlying neuropathology.

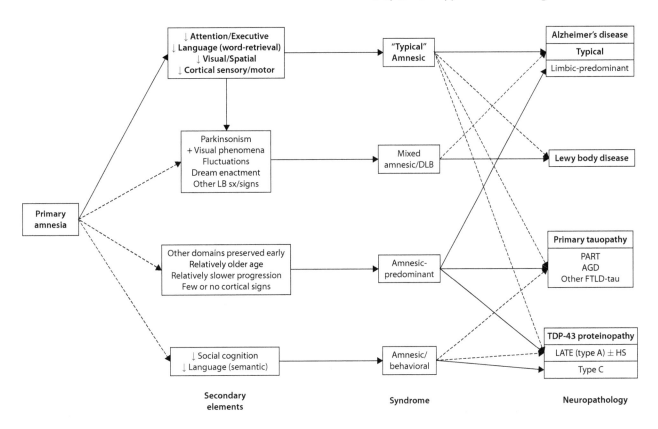

FIGURE 20-5. Syndrome-neuropathological associations in patients presenting with progressive amnesia as the most prominent early feature. Bold arrows and text depict the most common secondary elements, syndromic diagnosis, and primary underlying neuropathologies. Dashed lines depict relatively less common primary neuropathologies and/or secondary neuropathologies. AGD, argyrophilic grain disease; CBD, corticobasal degeneration; HS, hippocampal sclerosis; JCD, Jakob-Creutzfeldt disease; LATE, limbic-predominant age-related TDP-43 encephalopathy; PART, primary age-related tauopathy; PD, Parkinson's disease; PSP, progressive supranuclear palsy; VCI, vascular cognitive impairment. Please refer to Table 20-9 for key to additional abbreviations.

has markedly progressive amnesia with relative sparing of non-memory functions, possibly due to a "limbic-predominant" pattern of tau neurofibrillary tangle pathology.[88] Figure 20-5 illustrates syndrome-neuropathological associations in patients presenting with progressive amnesia as the most prominent early feature. Chapter 21 reviews AD and its associated neuropsychiatric features in detail.

LBD occurs on a phenotypic spectrum from predominant early motor symptoms (PD syndrome) to predominant early cognitive and neuropsychiatric symptoms (DLB syndrome). Patients with PD and no cognitive dysfunction at presentation may develop cognitive impairment and dementia at a later point in time. The cognitive profiles of both PD dementia and DLB tend to involve impaired attention and executive functioning. DLB is more frequently associated with additional impairments in tasks involving visuospatial functions than is PDD.[89,90] The "typical" parkinsonism seen in PD syndrome involves relatively prominent early asymmetrical resting tremor, bradykinesia, limb rigidity, less prominent early postural instability, and symptomatic responsiveness to levodopa, whereas toward the DLB end of the spectrum there is frequently greater symmetry of motor symptoms, more prominent early postural instability, and less responsiveness to levodopa.[91] A nontrivial proportion of individuals with diffuse neocortical LBD neuropathology lack parkinsonian symptoms and signs

well into their symptomatic disease course.[92] Both PD and DLB are associated with sensitivity to dopamine-blocking medications (including antipsychotics) such that treatment frequently exacerbates (or, in some cases of DLB, precipitates) motor symptoms.

Recent clinical diagnostic criteria for a diagnosis of "probable DLB" indicate a requirement for dementia with at least two of four "core" clinical features: fluctuating cognition with pronounced variations in attention and alertness; recurrent visual hallucinations that are typically well formed and detailed; REM sleep behavior disorder, which may precede cognitive decline; one or more spontaneous cardinal features of parkinsonism (bradykinesia, rest tremor, or rigidity).[86] While formed visual hallucinations are required to meet the core criterion, a patient might have "minor hallucinations/illusions" including vividly sensing the presence of someone else in the room when no one was there, experiencing a brief vision of movement in the room, or looking at something and perceiving it as something else.[93] Chapter 23 reviews Lewy body disorders and their associated neuropsychiatry features in detail.

FTD syndromes—including, but not limited, to the behavioral variant of FTD (bvFTD) and the semantic and nonfluent/agrammatic variants of primary progressive aphasia (PPA)—represent, along with AD, the most frequently encountered early-onset neurodegenerative dementias.[94,95] Table 20-9 contains

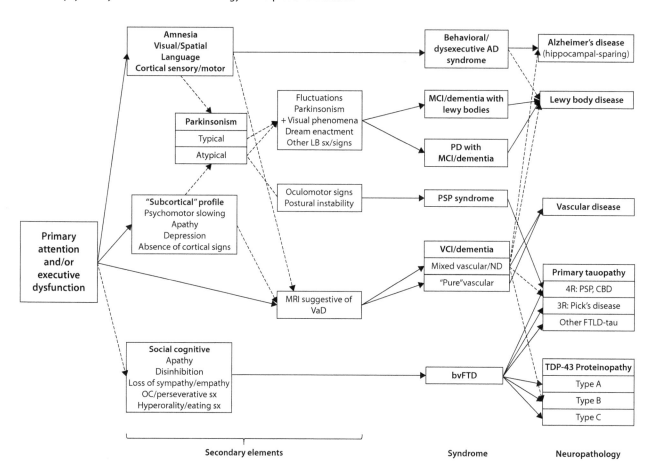

FIGURE 20-6. Syndrome-neuropathological associations in patients presenting with attention/executive dysfunction as the most prominent early feature. Bold arrows and text depict the most common secondary elements, syndromic diagnosis, and primary underlying neuropathologies. Dashed lines depict relatively less common primary neuropathologies and/or secondary neuropathologies. AGD, argyrophilic grain disease; CBD, corticobasal degeneration; HS, hippocampal sclerosis; JCD, Jakob-Creutzfeldt disease; LATE, limbic-predominant age-related TDP-43 encephalopathy; PART, primary age-related tauopathy; PD, Parkinson's disease; PSP, progressive supranuclear palsy; VCI, vascular cognitive impairment. Please refer to Table 20-9 for key to additional abbreviations.

key elements of these and selected other neurodegenerative cognitive syndromes, Figures 20-6 through 20-8 review syndrome-neuropathological correlations, and Chapter 24 reviews FTD in detail.

Pathophysiological Considerations

Important questions pertaining to disease mechanisms in neurodegenerative cognitive disorders remain unanswered or incompletely answered. One major question involves the relative importance of the disease-defining misfolded proteins in the disease process.[96] To date, efforts to target beta-amyloid in clinical therapeutic studies in AD have not yielded favorable results.[97,98] Whether these treatment failures are due to intervening too late in the disease process to be of benefit, failure of drugs to target the most important forms of beta-amyloid, or because the strategy of targeting beta-amyloid itself is not likely to yield benefit is unclear.

The pathophysiological basis of network-based neurodegeneration likewise remains unclear. Proposed mechanisms include metabolic stress (to key network nodes), trophic failure,

transneuronal spread of pathological proteins (prion-like mechanisms), and shared vulnerability of network regions based on developmental factors.[99] In view of the variable correspondence between networks and neuropathologies, neurodegeneration might arise as a "final common pathway" response to more than one type of physiological stressor across the lifespan. The spectrum of gene variants that increase risk of neurodegeneration is broad, implicating intracellular mechanisms (mitochondrial function, oxidative damage/repair, ubiquitin/proteasomal system functioning, apoptosis, autophagy), local tissue environment factors (cell adhesion, endocytosis, neurotransmission, other transmissible factors), systemic factors (immunological, inflammatory, metabolic, endocrine, vascular), and factors pertaining to development and aging (neurotrophic factors, epigenetics, telomeres).[100] There are likewise numerous epidemiological risk factors for late-life dementia with relatively small effect sizes, including but not limited to developmental learning disorders,[101–103] mid-life medical conditions (hypertension, high cholesterol, diabetes mellitus, obesity, vascular disease, sleep disorders),[104] psychiatric conditions (depression, PTSD, schizophrenia),[105–107] habits (physical activity, mental inactivity), toxin

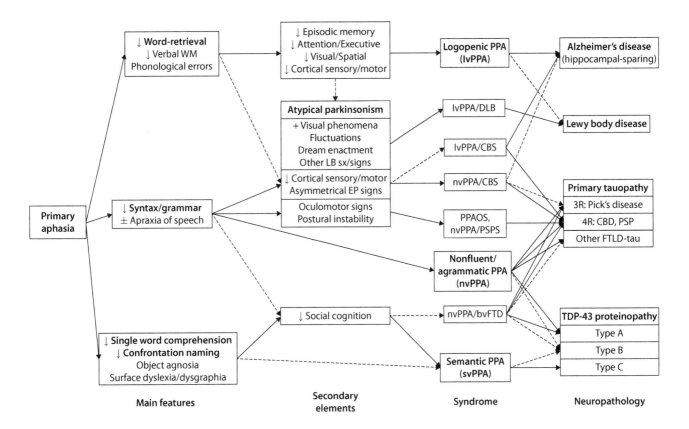

FIGURE 20-7. Syndrome-neuropathological associations in patients presenting with aphasia as the most prominent early feature. Bold arrows and text depict the most common secondary elements, syndromic diagnosis, and primary underlying neuropathologies. Dashed lines depict relatively less common primary neuropathologies and/or secondary neuropathologies. AGD, argyrophilic grain disease; CBD, corticobasal degeneration; HS, hippocampal sclerosis; JCD, Jakob-Creutzfeldt disease; LATE, limbic-predominant age-related TDP-43 encephalopathy; PART, primary age-related tauopathy; PD, Parkinson's disease; PSP, progressive supranuclear palsy; VCI, vascular cognitive impairment. Please refer to Table 20-9 for key to additional abbreviations.

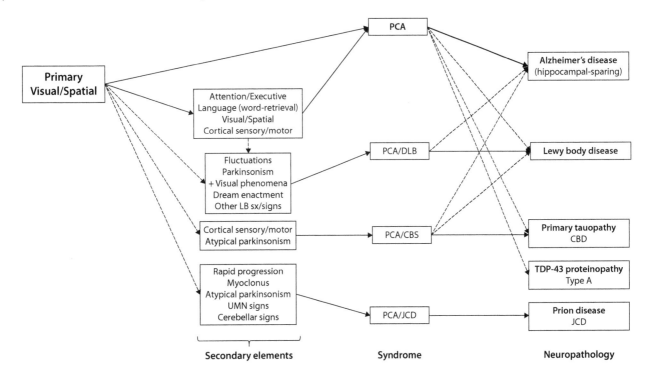

FIGURE 20-8. Syndrome-neuropathological associations in patients presenting with visual/spatial dysfunction as the most prominent early feature. Bold arrows and text depict the most common secondary elements, syndromic diagnosis, and primary underlying neuropathologies. Dashed lines depict relatively less common primary neuropathologies and/or secondary neuropathologies. AGD, argyrophilic grain disease; CBD, corticobasal degeneration; HS, hippocampal sclerosis; JCD, Jakob-Creutzfeldt disease; LATE, limbic-predominant age-related TDP-43 encephalopathy; PART, primary age-related tauopathy; PD, Parkinson's disease; PSP, progressive supranuclear palsy; VCI, vascular cognitive impairment. Please refer to Table 20-9 for key to additional abbreviations.

exposures (smoking, pesticides, environmental toxins),[108] and head trauma.[109] Heterogeneity and multiplicity of disease risk factors and mechanisms across individuals sharing the same syndromic and primary neuropathological diagnosis represent a possible reason for the presence and heterogeneity of secondary neuropathologies, for example, cerebrovascular, Lewy body, and TDP-43 pathologies in subsets of individuals with a primary neuropathological diagnosis of AD.[36,110,111]

If network degeneration occurs as a "final common pathway" phenomenon, an approach to identifying the genetic and acquired risk factors and associated disease mechanisms in subgroups within the various syndromic/neuropathological populations might be indicated to achieve the most effective disease-modifying treatments. This idea has precedent in other areas of "personalized medicine" such as cancer treatment.

Summary and Key Points

- Localizing cognitive symptoms and establishing the time course form a foundation for diagnosis in both acute/subacute onset, rapidly progressive and insidious onset, gradually progressive scenarios.
- The differential diagnosis of RPD is broad, with JCD, autoimmune/inflammatory, infections, and vascular diseases occurring relatively more frequently than conditions in other etiological categories.

- Non-prion neurodegenerative disorders are optimally characterized considering syndromic presentation, severity, and suspected underlying neuropathology, with amnesic and/or dysexecutive syndromes in the context of AD and/or LBD ± vascular disease, encountered more frequently than primary aphasic, visuospatial, or social/comportmental syndromes associated with AD or FTLD.
- Biomarkers of molecular neuropathology and/or neurodegeneration are increasingly available and useful for diagnosis in appropriate contexts.

Multiple Choice Questions

1. Which of the following diagnostic tests has the greatest specificity for Jakob-Creutzfeldt disease?
   a. Periodic sharp wave complexes on EEG
   b. CSF real-time quaking-induced conversion (RT-QuIC) test for protein seeding activity
   c. Diffusion restriction in the basal ganglia and/or two or more cortical regions on MRI
   d. Elevated CSF 14-3-3 protein
   e. *PRNP* gene sequencing

2. Which of the following conditions is a relatively common cause of cognitive dysfunction in individuals over the age of 65?
   a. Alzheimer's disease (AD)
   b. Primary medical illness, psychiatric illness, or other factors (e.g., suboptimal sleep, pain, medication side effects) superimposed on normal aging
   c. Lewy body disease (LBD)
   d. Frontotemporal lobar degeneration (FTLD)
   e. a, b, and c

3. Which of the following is *not* a component of a standard workup for cognitive impairment with insidious onset?
   a. Detailed history from the patient and an informant who knows the patient well
   b. Mental status examination to survey all major cognitive domains and general neurological examination for localizing signs (including but not limited to parkinsonism, upper motor neuron signs, and primitive reflexes)

   c. Laboratory workup for potentially modifiable factors causing or contributing to cognitive dysfunction
   d. Functional brain imaging (with FDG-PET, amyloid PET, or dopamine transporter imaging) or lumbar puncture (to rule out normal pressure hydrocephalus and to assess CSF biomarkers of Alzheimer's disease neuropathology)
   e. Structural neuroimaging with MRI (or, if not possible CT) to evaluate for focal atrophy, findings suggestive of vascular disease, and other lesions potentially associated with cognitive dysfunction

4. Which of the following statements is *not* true?
   a. Dementia and Major Neurocognitive Disorder are synonymous terms.
   b. Alzheimer's disease is most commonly associated with a decline in memory for recent events and information as a relatively prominent early symptom.
   c. Alzheimer's disease, Lewy body disease, and vascular dementia are mutually exclusive and should not be diagnosed in the same patient.
   d. Subjective cognitive dysfunction (without objective evidence of cognitive impairment on testing) might be related to nondegenerative factors (e.g., medical, psychiatric conditions), neurogenerative disease, or both.
   e. A comprehensive diagnostic formulation for patients with suspected neurodegenerative cognitive disorders requires identification of the primary neurodegenerative cognitive syndrome, the stage of illness, and suspected underlying neuropathology.

Multiple Choice Answers

1. Answer: b
Real-time quaking-induced conversion (RT-QuIC)—an in vitro assay specifically targeting the pathological prion protein (PrP^{Sc})—has diagnostic sensitivity over 80% and specificity over 95%. This specificity is superior to that of periodic sharp wave complexes on EEG (~85–90% specific), DWI restriction in the basal ganglia and/or two or more locations along the cortical ribbon (~90–95% specific), and elevated CSF 14-3-3 protein (~60–70% specific). *PRNP* gene sequencing is useful to identify cases of genetic, but not sporadic JCD.

2. Answer: e
Alzheimer's disease and Lewy body disease are both relatively common causes of progressive cognitive dysfunction in older individuals. Primary medical illness, psychiatric illness, and/or additional "non-neurological" factors commonly present as nonprogressive disorders of attention and executive functioning in older individuals. FTLD is proportionally a more common cause of early-onset dementia, with incidence and prevalence figures comparable to AD, in individuals under the age of 65.

3. Answer: d
Functional brain imaging techniques and/or lumbar puncture are not routinely required in a workup for cognitive dysfunction. Their use should be reserved for special circumstances in which a diagnosis is ambiguous, and the information to-be-provided has anticipated value. All other components listed (a, b, c, and e) represent important components of a standard workup for cognitive dysfunction.

4. Answer: c
Clinical/pathological correlation studies have consistently demonstrated that multiple/mixed neuropathological diagnoses are the "rule" rather than the "exception." All other statements (a, b, d, and e) are true. "Major Neurocognitive Disorder" is a DSM-5 construct with a comparable definition to that for "dementia." Alzheimer's disease neuropathology is most commonly associated with a clinical syndrome involving early impairment in episodic memory, though less commonly can present with impairments in executive, language, visuospatial, or higher sensory/motor functioning. Neurodegenerative conditions start years prior to onset of symptoms and progress through stages of normal cognition, subjective cognitive decline, mild cognitive impairment, and dementia. A comprehensive diagnostic formulation implicitly recognizes the distinction between neurodegenerative syndromes, terms denoting severity (e.g., MCI or mild/moderate/severe dementia), and underlying neuropathological changes.

REFERENCES

1. American Psychiatric Association. *DSM-5 Task Force. Diagnostic and Statistical Manual of Mental Disorders: DSM-5*. 5th ed. Washington, DC: American Psychiatric Association; 2013.
2. Geschwind MD. Rapidly progressive dementia. *Continuum (Minneap Minn)*. 2016;22(2 Dementia):510-537.
3. Chitravas N, Jung RS, Kofskey DM, et al. Treatable neurological disorders misdiagnosed as Creutzfeldt-Jakob disease. *Ann Neurol*. 2011;70(3):437-444.
4. Begue C, Martinetto H, Schultz M, et al. Creutzfeldt-Jakob disease surveillance in Argentina, 1997-2008. *Neuroepidemiology*. 2011;37(3-4):193-202.
5. Grau-Rivera O, Gelpi E, Nos C, et al. Clinicopathological correlations and concomitant pathologies in rapidly progressive dementia: a brain bank series. *Neurodegener Dis*. 2015;15(6):350-360.
6. Heinemann U, Krasnianski A, Meissner B, et al. Creutzfeldt-Jakob disease in Germany: a prospective 12-year surveillance. *Brain*. 2007;130(pt 5):1350-1359.
7. Anuja P, Venugopalan V, Darakhshan N, et al. Rapidly progressive dementia: an eight year (2008-2016) retrospective study. *PLoS One*. 2018;13(1):e0189832.
8. Papageorgiou SG, Kontaxis T, Bonakis A, Karahalios G, Kalfakis N, Vassilopoulos D. Rapidly progressive dementia: causes found in a Greek tertiary referral center in Athens. *Alzheimer Dis Assoc Disord*. 2009;23(4):337-346.
9. Sala I, Marquie M, Sanchez-Saudinos MB, et al. Rapidly progressive dementia: experience in a tertiary care medical center. *Alzheimer Dis Assoc Disord*. 2012;26(3):267-271.
10. Studart Neto A, Soares Neto HR, Simabukuro MM, et al. Rapidly progressive dementia: prevalence and causes in a neurologic unit of a tertiary hospital in Brazil. *Alzheimer Dis Assoc Disord*. 2017;31(3):239-243.
11. Geschwind MD. Prion diseases. *Continuum (Minneap Minn)*. 2015;21(6 Neuroinfectious Disease):1612-1638.
12. Ladogana A, Puopolo M, Croes EA, et al. Mortality from Creutzfeldt-Jakob disease and related disorders in Europe, Australia, and Canada. *Neurology*. 2005;64(9):1586-1591.
13. Collins SJ, Sanchez-Juan P, Masters CL, et al. Determinants of diagnostic investigation sensitivities across the clinical spectrum of sporadic Creutzfeldt-Jakob disease. *Brain*. 2006;129(pt 9):2278-2287.
14. Parchi P, Giese A, Capellari S, et al. Classification of sporadic Creutzfeldt-Jakob disease based on molecular and phenotypic analysis of 300 subjects. *Ann Neurol*. 1999;46(2):224-233.
15. Zerr I, Kallenberg K, Summers DM, et al. Updated clinical diagnostic criteria for sporadic Creutzfeldt-Jakob disease. *Brain*. 2009;132(pt 10):2659-2668.
16. Vitali P, Maccagnano E, Caverzasi E, et al. Diffusion-weighted MRI hyperintensity patterns differentiate CJD from other rapid dementias. *Neurology*. 2011;76(20):1711-1719.
17. Puoti G, Bizzi A, Forloni G, Safar JG, Tagliavini F, Gambetti P. Sporadic human prion diseases: molecular insights and diagnosis. *Lancet Neurol*. 2012;11(7):618-628.
18. Shiga Y, Miyazawa K, Sato S, et al. Diffusion-weighted MRI abnormalities as an early diagnostic marker for Creutzfeldt-Jakob disease. *Neurology*. 2004;63(3):443-449.
19. Young GS, Geschwind MD, Fischbein NJ, et al. Diffusion-weighted and fluid-attenuated inversion recovery imaging in

Creutzfeldt-Jakob disease: high sensitivity and specificity for diagnosis. *AJNR Am J Neuroradiol.* 2005;26(6):1551-1562.

20. Meissner B, Kallenberg K, Sanchez-Juan P, et al. MRI lesion profiles in sporadic Creutzfeldt-Jakob disease. *Neurology.* 2009;72(23):1994-2001.

21. Hamaguchi T, Kitamoto T, Sato T, et al. Clinical diagnosis of MM2-type sporadic Creutzfeldt-Jakob disease. *Neurology.* 2005;64(4):643-648.

22. Sanchez-Juan P, Green A, Ladogana A, et al. CSF tests in the differential diagnosis of Creutzfeldt-Jakob disease. *Neurology.* 2006;67(4):637-643.

23. Muayqil T, Gronseth G, Camicioli R. Evidence-based guideline: diagnostic accuracy of CSF 14-3-3 protein in sporadic Creutzfeldt-Jakob disease: report of the guideline development subcommittee of the American Academy of Neurology. *Neurology.* 2012;79(14):1499-1506.

24. Lattanzio F, Abu-Rumeileh S, Franceschini A, et al. Prion-specific and surrogate CSF biomarkers in Creutzfeldt-Jakob disease: diagnostic accuracy in relation to molecular subtypes and analysis of neuropathological correlates of p-tau and Abeta42 levels. *Acta Neuropathol.* 2017;133(4):559-578.

25. Pocchiari M, Puopolo M, Croes EA, et al. Predictors of survival in sporadic Creutzfeldt-Jakob disease and other human transmissible spongiform encephalopathies. *Brain.* 2004;127(pt 10):2348-2359.

26. Josephs KA, Ahlskog JE, Parisi JE, et al. Rapidly progressive neurodegenerative dementias. *Arch Neurol.* 2009;66(2):201-207.

27. Schmidt C, Wolff M, Weitz M, Bartlau T, Korth C, Zerr I. Rapidly progressive Alzheimer disease. *Arch Neurol.* 2011;68(9):1124-1130.

28. Geschwind MD, Tan KM, Lennon VA, et al. Voltage-gated potassium channel autoimmunity mimicking Creutzfeldt-Jakob disease. *Arch Neurol.* 2008;65(10):1341-1346.

29. Seipelt M, Zerr I, Nau R, et al. Hashimoto's encephalitis as a differential diagnosis of Creutzfeldt-Jakob disease. *J Neurol Neurosurg Psychiatry.* 1999;66(2):172-176.

30. Gultekin SH, Rosenfeld MR, Voltz R, Eichen J, Posner JB, Dalmau J. Paraneoplastic limbic encephalitis: neurological symptoms, immunological findings and tumour association in 50 patients. *Brain.* 2000;123(pt 7):1481-1494.

31. Dalmau J, Lancaster E, Martinez-Hernandez E, Rosenfeld MR, Balice-Gordon R. Clinical experience and laboratory investigations in patients with anti-NMDAR encephalitis. *Lancet Neurol.* 2011;10(1):63-74.

32. Angus-Leppan H, Rudge P, Mead S, Collinge J, Vincent A. Autoantibodies in sporadic Creutzfeldt-Jakob disease. *JAMA Neurol.* 2013;70(7):919-922.

33. McGinnis SM. Infectious causes of rapidly progressive dementia. *Semin Neurol.* 2011;31(3):266-285.

34. Fisher CM. Hypomanic symptoms caused by herpes simplex encephalitis. *Neurology.* 1996;47(6):1374-1378.

35. Johns DR, Tierney M, Felsenstein D. Alteration in the natural history of neurosyphilis by concurrent infection with the human immunodeficiency virus. *N Engl J Med.* 1987;316(25):1569-1572.

36. Custodio N, Montesinos R, Lira D, Herrera-Perez E, Bardales Y, Valeriano-Lorenzo L. Mixed dementia: a review of the evidence. *Dement Neuropsychol.* 2017;11(4):364-370.

37. Stabler SP. Clinical practice. Vitamin B12 deficiency. *N Engl J Med.* 2013;368(2):149-160.

38. Halavaara J, Brander A, Lyytinen J, Setala K, Kallela M. Wernicke's encephalopathy: is diffusion-weighted MRI useful? *Neuroradiology.* 2003;45(8):519-523.

39. Torvik A, Lindboe CF, Rogde S. Brain lesions in alcoholics. A neuropathological study with clinical correlations. *J Neurol Sci.* 1982;56(2-3):233-248.

40. McKhann GM, Knopman DS, Chertkow H, et al. The diagnosis of dementia due to Alzheimer's disease: recommendations from the National Institute on Aging-Alzheimer's Association workgroups on diagnostic guidelines for Alzheimer's disease. *Alzheimer Dement.* 2011;7(3):263-269.

41. Galasko D, Bennett D, Sano M, et al. An inventory to assess activities of daily living for clinical trials in Alzheimer's disease. The Alzheimer's Disease Cooperative Study. *Alzheimer Dis Assoc Disord.* 1997;11(suppl 2):S33-S39.

42. Johnson N, Barion A, Rademaker A, Rehkemper G, Weintraub S. The Activities of Daily Living Questionnaire: a validation study in patients with dementia. *Alzheimer Dis Assoc Disord.* 2004;18(4):223-230.

43. Cummings JL, Mega M, Gray K, Rosenberg-Thompson S, Carusi DA, Gornbein J. The Neuropsychiatric Inventory: comprehensive assessment of psychopathology in dementia. *Neurology.* 1994;44(12):2308-2314.

44. Kaufer DI, Cummings JL, Ketchel P, et al. Validation of the NPI-Q, a brief clinical form of the Neuropsychiatric Inventory. *J Neuropsychiatry Clin Neurosci.* 2000;12(2):233-239.

45. Nasreddine ZS, Phillips NA, Bedirian V, et al. The Montreal Cognitive Assessment, MoCA: a brief screening tool for mild cognitive impairment. *J Am Geriatr Soc.* 2005;53(4):695-699.

46. Mioshi E, Dawson K, Mitchell J, Arnold R, Hodges JR. The Addenbrooke's Cognitive Examination Revised (ACE-R): a brief cognitive test battery for dementia screening. *Int J Geriatr Psychiatry.* 2006;21(11):1078-1085.

47. Daffner KR, Gale SA, Barrett AM, et al. Improving clinical cognitive testing: report of the AAN Behavioral Neurology Section Workgroup. *Neurology.* 2015;85(10):910-918.

48. Knopman DS, DeKosky ST, Cummings JL, et al. Practice parameter: diagnosis of dementia (an evidence-based review). Report of the Quality Standards Subcommittee of the American Academy of Neurology. *Neurology.* 2001;56(9):1143-1153.

49. Petersen RC, Smith GE, Waring SC, Ivnik RJ, Tangalos EG, Kokmen E. Mild cognitive impairment: clinical characterization and outcome. *Arch Neurology.* 1999;56(3):303-308.

50. Shaw LM, Arias J, Blennow K, et al. Appropriate use criteria for lumbar puncture and cerebrospinal fluid testing in the diagnosis of Alzheimer's disease. *Alzheimers Dement.* 2018;14(11):1505-1521.

51. Frey KA, Lodge MA, Meltzer CC, et al. ACR-ASNR practice parameter for brain PET/CT imaging dementia. *Clin Nucl Med.* 2016;41(2):118-125.

52. Nobili F, Arbizu J, Bouwman F, et al. European Association of Nuclear Medicine and European Academy of Neurology recommendations for the use of brain (18) F-fluorodeoxyglucose positron emission tomography in neurodegenerative cognitive impairment and dementia: Delphi consensus. *Eur J Neurol.* 2018;25(10):1201-1217.

53. Marshall VL, Patterson J, Hadley DM, Grosset KA, Grosset DG. Two-year follow-up in 150 consecutive cases with normal dopamine transporter imaging. *Nucl Med Commun.* 2006;27(12):933-937.

54. Landau SM, Lu M, Joshi AD, et al. Comparing positron emission tomography imaging and cerebrospinal fluid measurements of beta-amyloid. *Ann Neurol.* 2013;74(6):826-836.

55. Goldman JS, Hahn SE, Catania JW, et al. Genetic counseling and testing for Alzheimer disease: joint practice guidelines of the American College of Medical Genetics and the National Society of Genetic Counselors. *Genet Med.* 2011;13(6):597-605.

56. Wood EM, Falcone D, Suh E, et al. Development and validation of pedigree classification criteria for frontotemporal lobar degeneration. *JAMA Neurol*. 2013;70(11):1411-1417.

57. Daffner KR. Promoting successful cognitive aging: a comprehensive review. *J Alzheimers Dis*. 2010;19(4):1101-1122.

58. Charlton RA, Barrick TR, McIntyre DJ, et al. White matter damage on diffusion tensor imaging correlates with age-related cognitive decline. *Neurology*. 2006;66(2):217-222.

59. Van Petten C, Plante E, Davidson PS, Kuo TY, Bajuscak L, Glisky EL. Memory and executive function in older adults: relationships with temporal and prefrontal gray matter volumes and white matter hyperintensities. *Neuropsychologia*. 2004;42(10): 1313-1335.

60. Salthouse TA. The processing-speed theory of adult age differences in cognition. *Psychol Rev*. 1996;103(3):403-428.

61. Ganguli M, Jia Y, Hughes TF, et al. Mild cognitive impairment that does not progress to dementia: a population-based study. *J Am Geriatr Soc*. 2019;67(2):232-238.

62. Colenda CC, Legault C, Rapp SR, et al. Psychiatric disorders and cognitive dysfunction among older, postmenopausal women: results from the Women's Health Initiative Memory Study. *Am J Geriatr Psychiatry*. 2010;18(2):177-186.

63. Moore AR, O'Keeffe ST. Drug-induced cognitive impairment in the elderly. *Drugs Aging*. 1999;15(1):15-28.

64. Morley JE. Cognition and chronic disease. *J Am Med Dir Assoc*. 2017;18(5):369-371.

65. Ivanchak N, Fletcher K, Jicha GA. Attention-deficit/hyperactivity disorder in older adults: prevalence and possible connections to mild cognitive impairment. *Curr Psychiatry Rep*. 2012;14(5):552-560.

66. Emre M, Aarsland D, Brown R, et al. Clinical diagnostic criteria for dementia associated with Parkinson's disease. *Mov Disord*. 2007;22(12):1689-1707; quiz 1837.

67. Ossenkoppele R, Pijnenburg YA, Perry DC, et al. The behavioural/dysexecutive variant of Alzheimer's disease: clinical, neuroimaging and pathological features. *Brain*. 2015;138(pt 9): 2732-2749.

68. Salmon DP, Galasko D, Hansen LA, et al. Neuropsychological deficits associated with diffuse Lewy body disease. *Brain Cogn*. 1996;31(2):148-165.

69. Sperling RA, Aisen PS, Beckett LA, et al. Toward defining the preclinical stages of Alzheimer's disease: recommendations from the National Institute on Aging-Alzheimer's Association workgroups on diagnostic guidelines for Alzheimer's disease. *Alzheimers Dement*. 2011;7(3):280-292.

70. Pievani M, de Haan W, Wu T, Seeley WW, Frisoni GB. Functional network disruption in the degenerative dementias. *Lancet Neurol*. 2011;10(9):829-843.

71. Seeley WW, Crawford RK, Zhou J, Miller BL, Greicius MD. Neurodegenerative diseases target large-scale human brain networks. *Neuron*. 2009;62(1):42-52.

72. Bennett DA, Wilson RS, Arvanitakis Z, Boyle PA, de Toledo-Morrell L, Schneider JA. Selected findings from the Religious Orders Study and Rush Memory and Aging Project. *J Alzheimers Dis*. 2013;33(suppl 1):S397-S403.

73. McKhann G, Drachman D, Folstein M, Katzman R, Price D, Stadlan EM. Clinical diagnosis of Alzheimer's disease: report of the NINCDS-ADRDA Work Group under the auspices of Department of Health and Human Services Task Force on Alzheimer's Disease. *Neurology*. 1984;34(7):939-944.

74. Price JL, Morris JC. Tangles and plaques in nondemented aging and "preclinical" Alzheimer's disease. *Ann Neurol*. 1999;45(3): 358-368.

75. Bateman RJ, Xiong C, Benzinger TL, et al. Clinical and biomarker changes in dominantly inherited Alzheimer's disease. *N Engl J Med*. 2012;367(9):795-804.

76. Albert MS, DeKosky ST, Dickson D, et al. The diagnosis of mild cognitive impairment due to Alzheimer's disease: recommendations from the National Institute on Aging-Alzheimer's Association workgroups on diagnostic guidelines for Alzheimer's disease. *Alzheimers Dement*. 2011;7(3):270-279.

77. Frigerio R, Fujishiro H, Ahn TB, et al. Incidental Lewy body disease: do some cases represent a preclinical stage of dementia with Lewy bodies? *Neurobiol Aging*. 2011;32(5):857-863.

78. Rohrer JD, Nicholas JM, Cash DM, et al. Presymptomatic cognitive and neuroanatomical changes in genetic frontotemporal dementia in the Genetic Frontotemporal dementia Initiative (GENFI) study: a cross-sectional analysis. *Lancet Neurol*. 2015;14(3):253-262.

79. American Psychiatric Association. *Task Force on DSM-IV. Diagnostic and Statistical Manual of Mental Disorders: DSM-IV-TR*. 4th ed. Washington, DC: American Psychiatric Association; 2000.

80. Alladi S, Xuereb J, Bak T, et al. Focal cortical presentations of Alzheimer's disease. *Brain*. 2007;130(pt 10):2636-2645.

81. Balasa M, Gelpi E, Antonell A, et al. Clinical features and APOE genotype of pathologically proven early-onset Alzheimer disease. *Neurology*. 2011;76(20):1720-1725.

82. Koedam EL, Lauffer V, van der Vlies AE, van der Flier WM, Scheltens P, Pijnenburg YA. Early-versus late-onset Alzheimer's disease: more than age alone. *J Alzheimers Dis*. 2010;19(4):1401-1408.

83. Beach TG, Monsell SE, Phillips LE, Kukull W. Accuracy of the clinical diagnosis of Alzheimer disease at National Institute on Aging Alzheimer Disease Centers, 2005-2010. *J Neuropathol Exp Neurol*. 2012;71(4):266-273.

84. Dickerson BC, McGinnis SM, Xia C, et al. Approach to atypical Alzheimer's disease and case studies of the major subtypes. *CNS Spectr*. 2017;22(6):439-449.

85. Ballard C, Gauthier S, Corbett A, Brayne C, Aarsland D, Jones E. Alzheimer's disease. *Lancet*. 2011;377(9770):1019-1031.

86. McKeith IG, Boeve BF, Dickson DW, et al. Diagnosis and management of dementia with Lewy bodies: fourth consensus report of the DLB Consortium. *Neurology*. 2017;89(1):88-100.

87. Gurnani AS, Gavett BE. The differential effects of Alzheimer's disease and Lewy body pathology on cognitive performance: a meta-analysis. *Neuropsychol Rev*. 2017;27(1):1-17.

88. Murray ME, Graff-Radford NR, Ross OA, Petersen RC, Duara R, Dickson DW. Neuropathologically defined subtypes of Alzheimer's disease with distinct clinical characteristics: a retrospective study. *Lancet Neurol*. 2011;10(9):785-796.

89. Calderon J, Perry RJ, Erzinclioglu SW, Berrios GE, Dening TR, Hodges JR. Perception, attention, and working memory are disproportionately impaired in dementia with Lewy bodies compared with Alzheimer's disease. *J Neurol Neurosurg Psychiatry*. 2001;70(2):157-164.

90. Mondon K, Gochard A, Marque A, et al. Visual recognition memory differentiates dementia with Lewy bodies and Parkinson's disease dementia. *J Neurol Neurosurg Psychiatry*. 2007;78(7):738-741.

91. Aarsland D, Ballard C, McKeith I, Perry RH, Larsen JP. Comparison of extrapyramidal signs in dementia with Lewy bodies and Parkinson's disease. *J Neuropsychiatry Clin Neurosci*. 2001;13(3):374-379.

92. Irwin DJ, Grossman M, Weintraub D, et al. Neuropathological and genetic correlates of survival and dementia onset in

synucleinopathies: a retrospective analysis. *Lancet Neurol.* 2017;16(1):55-65.

93. Williams DR, Warren JD, Lees AJ. Using the presence of visual hallucinations to differentiate Parkinson's disease from atypical parkinsonism. *J Neurol Neurosurg Psychiatry.* 2008;79(6):652-655.

94. Mercy L, Hodges JR, Dawson K, Barker RA, Brayne C. Incidence of early-onset dementias in Cambridgeshire, United Kingdom. *Neurology.* 2008;71(19):1496-1499.

95. Ratnavalli E, Brayne C, Dawson K, Hodges JR. The prevalence of frontotemporal dementia. *Neurology.* 2002;58(11):1615-1621.

96. Jack CRJr, Bennett DA, Blennow K, et al. A/T/N: an unbiased descriptive classification scheme for Alzheimer disease biomarkers. *Neurology.* 2016;87(5):539-547.

97. Egan MF, Kost J, Voss T, et al. Randomized Trial of verubecestat for prodromal Alzheimer's disease. *N Engl J Med.* 2019;380(15):1408-1420.

98. Salloway S, Sperling R, Fox NC, et al. Two phase 3 trials of bapineuzumab in mild-to-moderate Alzheimer's disease. *N Engl J Med.* 2014;370(4):322-333.

99. Zhou J, Gennatas ED, Kramer JH, Miller BL, Seeley WW. Predicting regional neurodegeneration from the healthy brain functional connectome. *Neuron.* 2012;73(6):1216-1227.

100. Ramanan VK, Saykin AJ. Pathways to neurodegeneration: mechanistic insights from GWAS in Alzheimer's disease, Parkinson's disease, and related disorders. *Am J Neurodegener Dis.* 2013;2(3):145-175.

101. Curtin K, Fleckenstein AE, Keeshin BR, et al. Increased risk of diseases of the basal ganglia and cerebellum in patients with a history of attention-deficit/hyperactivity disorder. *Neuropsychopharmacology.* 2018;43(13):2548-2555.

102. Miller ZA, Rosenberg L, Santos-Santos MA, et al. Prevalence of mathematical and visuospatial learning disabilities in patients with posterior cortical atrophy. *JAMA Neurol.* 2018;75(6):728-737.

103. Rogalski E, Johnson N, Weintraub S, Mesulam M. Increased frequency of learning disability in patients with primary progressive aphasia and their first-degree relatives. *Arch Neurol.* 2008;65(2):244-248.

104. Ritchie K, Carriere I, Ritchie CW, Berr C, Artero S, Ancelin ML. Designing prevention programmes to reduce incidence of dementia: prospective cohort study of modifiable risk factors. *BMJ.* 2010;341:c3885.

105. Katon W, Pedersen HS, Ribe AR, et al. Effect of depression and diabetes mellitus on the risk for dementia: a national population-based cohort study. *JAMA Psychiatry.* 2015;72(6):612-619.

106. Ribe AR, Laursen TM, Charles M, et al. Long-term risk of dementia in persons with schizophrenia: A Danish population-based cohort study. *JAMA Psychiatry.* 2015;72(11):1095-1101.

107. Yaffe K, Vittinghoff E, Lindquist K, et al. Posttraumatic stress disorder and risk of dementia among US veterans. *Arch Gen Psychiatry.* 2010;67(6):608-613.

108. Lee PC, Bordelon Y, Bronstein J, Ritz B. Traumatic brain injury, paraquat exposure, and their relationship to Parkinson disease. *Neurology.* 2012;79(20):2061-2066.

109. Johnson VE, Stewart W, Smith DH. Widespread tau and amyloid-beta pathology many years after a single traumatic brain injury in humans. *Brain Pathol.* 2012;22(2):142-149.

110. James BD, Wilson RS, Boyle PA, Trojanowski JQ, Bennett DA, Schneider JA. TDP-43 stage, mixed pathologies, and clinical Alzheimer's-type dementia. *Brain.* 2016;139(11):2983-2993.

111. Walker L, McAleese KE, Thomas AJ, et al. Neuropathologically mixed Alzheimer's and Lewy body disease: burden of pathological protein aggregates differs between clinical phenotypes. *Acta Neuropathol.* 2015;129(5):729-748.

21

The Neuropsychiatry of Alzheimer's Disease

Hema Kher · Kelsey D. Biddle · Nancy J. Donovan

EPIDEMIOLOGY

Prevalence/Incidence

More than 5.7 million Americans are currently living with Alzheimer's disease (AD) dementia, a condition that affects 1 in 10 U.S. adults over the age of 65.[1] AD is the primary etiology for the majority of dementia cases, accounting for 60–80% of dementia cases worldwide.[1] The prevalence of AD dementia increases with age, from 3% of people age 65–74, to 17% of people age 75–84, to 32% of people age 85 years and older.[2] As the U.S. population ages, the number of Americans with AD dementia is projected to expand more than twofold to 13.8 million by 2050 (Figure 21-1).[2] It is now recognized that AD begins with a long silent interval prior to the onset of symptoms. Therefore, current prevalence data for AD underestimate the true number of Americans affected across the disease spectrum—individuals who are impaired as well as those with presymptomatic disease who are at high risk of progression to impairment.[3–5]

Risk Factors

The strongest known risk factors for sporadic or late-onset AD are older age,[6] family history of dementia,[7] and the apolipoprotein E ε4 (APOE4) allele.[8] Clinically diagnosed probable AD dementia is more common in women compared to men, with women accounting for nearly two-thirds of affected individuals.[2] This gender discrepancy is commonly attributed to women having a longer life expectancy than men,[9] however, other sex-specific factors have been reported.[10–13] AD prevalence rates also differ across racial and ethnic groups. Compared to Caucasian Americans, Hispanics are one and one-half times more likely to develop AD dementia.[14] African Americans are twice as likely to have AD dementia than older white Americans.[14–16] Lower educational attainment and socioeconomic status are independent risk factors for AD that contribute to differences in AD risk by race.[17–20] Significant traumatic brain injury has been associated in some studies with increased risk of developing AD dementia later in life.[21,22] Accumulating evidence suggests

that neuropsychiatric symptoms, such as depression, anxiety, and apathy, may be initial manifestations of neurodegenerative brain changes and, when present, these symptoms increase both the risk and rate of progression to dementia.[23] Risk of cognitive impairment due to AD may be mitigated by lifestyle factors, particularly when addressed or implemented in young adulthood or middle age. Regular physical exercise,[24] a healthy diet,[25] management of cardiovascular risk factors including hypertension, dyslipidemia, and diabetes mellitus,[26] and lifelong social[27] and cognitive engagement[28,29] may be protective factors that lower an individual's risk of AD onset.[30]

Genetics in AD

AD can be classified as familial or sporadic based on the presence or absence of a history of AD in second-, third-degree, or closer, affected family members.[31] It is further classified as early-onset or late-onset based on symptom onset before or after age 65.[31] An estimated 15–25% of late-onset AD cases are familial, in comparison to close to half of early-onset cases.[32] Fewer than 5% of AD cases demonstrate an autosomal dominant pattern of inheritance. Although approximately 95% of AD cases are late-onset, AD is among the most common causes of early-onset dementia, with incidence figures comparable to frontotemporal lobar degeneration (FTLD).

The apolipoprotein E ε4 (APOE4) allele is the strongest genetic risk factor for sporadic AD and familial AD that is not due to an autosomal dominant gene mutation. APOE4 is a susceptibility gene that elevates risk of developing AD and lowers age of onset of cognitive impairment in a dose-dependent fashion.[33] The APOE gene has three isoforms—APOE2, E3, and E4. Individuals with one APOE4 allele (heterozygotes) have a 25–30% risk of developing mild cognitive impairment (MCI) or dementia due to AD by age 85, the risk increasing to 50–60% in those with two copies of the allele (homozygotes).[34]

Familial autosomal dominant AD usually leads to early-onset AD, at times with onset of symptoms in the fourth or fifth decade of life.[35] Nearly all cases of familial autosomal dominant AD

Projected number of people age 65 and older (total and by age)
in the U.S. population with Alzheimer's Dementia, 2010 to 2050

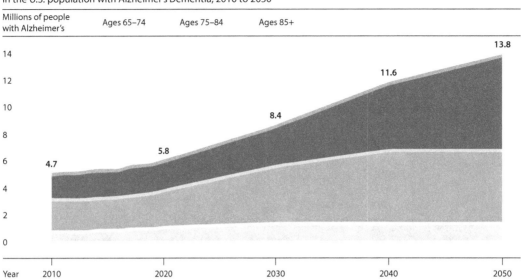

FIGURE 21-1. Alzheimer's disease is a growing public health problem. As the population ages, Alzheimer's disease is expected to become increasingly prevalent (prevalence is measured in millions). (Created with data from Hebert et al. (2013). Reproduced with permission from the Alzheimer's Association, 2020 Alzheimer's Disease Facts and Figures.)

with early onset are linked to three hallmark genes involved in beta-amyloid (Aβ) generation: amyloid precursor protein (*APP*), presenilin-1 (*PSEN1*), and presenilin-2 (*PSEN2*), with causative mutations leading to overproduction of Aβ (reviewed below).[36]

PATHOPHYSIOLOGY

Beta-Amyloid and Tau

AD is a pathobiologic process defined by the deposition of protein aggregates in the form of Aβ containing plaques and tau-containing neurofibrillary tangles (NFTs) which accumulate in characteristic brain regions over a period of decades (Figure 21-2).[37] Multiple brain changes associated with these pathological aggregates include synaptic dysfunction, aberrant neuronal network activity, neuronal toxicity, and ultimately neuronal death and neurodegeneration.[38] These accumulating pathologies and ensuing brain changes are associated with progressive cognitive, neuropsychiatric and functional impairment, and early mortality.

Aβ plaque accumulation is among the first identifiable brain changes associated with AD, predating the development of clinical signs and symptoms of AD by at least a decade.[39] Plaques are mostly comprised of Aβ protein, formed by the proteolytic cleavage of APP by beta- and gamma secretases.[40] Aβ monomers vary in length between 36 and 43 amino acids. These peptides may assume a variety of conformations, from dimers (two monomers) and soluble oligomers (a molecular complex composed of a few monomers) to larger polymers arranged into insoluble fibrils.[38] Monomeric Aβ-40 is the most prevalent Aβ peptide in the brain and is produced by initial gamma-secretase cleavage of APP. Alternate proteolytic processing of APP initiated by the beta-secretase enzyme produces the soluble Aβ-42

peptide which forms neurotoxic oligomers and other intermediate assemblies that are prone to aggregate into plaques. APP is encoded by the gene *APP*. Gamma secretases comprise multiple proteins, including presenilins encoded by genes *PSEN1* and *PSEN2*.[41] In familial autosomal dominant AD, mutations in *APP*, *PSEN1*, and *PSEN2* can lead to the increased formation of toxic Aβ-42 and increase the ratio of Aβ-42 to Aβ-40. A similar phenomenon occurs in Down's syndrome, as individuals have three copies of the *APP* gene (located on chromosome 21).

The pathophysiological mechanisms and significance of Aβ accumulation in sporadic AD and non-autosomal dominant familial AD are topics being actively researched and debated. Aβ accumulation may occur from overproduction of aggregation-prone Aβ species or from decreased degradation or clearance of Aβ across the blood-brain barrier. *APOE4* has been associated with decreased efficiency of Aβ clearance (compared to *APOE2* and *APOE3*) owing to a role of apolipoprotein E in this process. Other *APOE4* non-amyloid-dependent disease mechanisms have been proposed, including impaired synaptogenesis and hippocampal neurogenesis, effects on mitochondrial function, and maladaptive response to neuronal stress and injury.[42] Additional hypothesized factors associated with Aβ accumulation include cumulative metabolic stress in highly active brain regions over the lifespan[43] and formation of Aβ as a physiological response to microbial infection.[44] Once present, soluble and insoluble forms of Aβ have been linked with activation of microglia involved in their clearance, resulting in the release of neurotoxic fragments and proinflammatory mediators, oxidative stress, and damage to mitochondria.[45] Soluble Aβ oligomers may impair synaptic function and thereby promote aberrant neuronal network activity.[46]

NFTs are dense, intracellular protein aggregates containing abnormal configurations of the protein tau (Figure 21-2). In

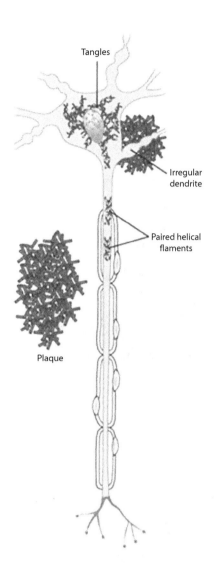

FIGURE 21-2. Abnormalities in a neuron are associated with Alzheimer's disease. The cytopathologic hallmarks are intracellular neurofibrillary tangles and extracellular amyloid plaques that have a core of β-amyloid peptides surrounded by altered nerve fibers and reactive glial cells. (Reproduced with permission from Kandel ER, Schwartz JH, Jessell TM, et al: Principles of Neural Science. 5th ed. https://neurology.mhmedical.com. Copyright © McGraw Hill LLC. All rights reserved.)

its normal form, tau protein is present in axons and is involved in microtubule assembly and organization.[47] When phosphorylated, tau is more likely to aggregate into NFTs,[48] which accumulate in neuronal cell bodies and dendrites and impair neurotransmission and neuronal function.[49] The localization and quantity of NFTs correlates with other markers of neurodegeneration such as cortical atrophy and also strongly correlates with type and progression of clinical signs and symptoms of AD (Figure 21-3).[50,51]

The mechanisms by which Aβ and tau pathologies interact with each other and co-pathogenic factors to produce clinical signs and symptoms and neurodegeneration are incompletely understood. While pathologic tau may develop independently from Aβ,[52] its accumulation appears to be potentiated by high Aβ.[53,54] NFT-mediated disruption of cytoskeletal integrity and

neurotransmission represents a plausible mechanism leading to synaptic loss and cell death. Recent studies suggest that pathological tau may be transmitted transynaptically to downstream neurons within networks, representing a potential mechanism contributing to progressive neurodegeneration.[55] Additional potential disease-modifying factors include genetic variations, comorbidities such as inflammatory, endocrine, or vascular disease, and shared or contributing factors underlying the development of other pathologic proteinopathies (e.g., synucleinopathies, FTLD).

Biomarkers of AD Pathophysiology

Recent research utilizing in vivo neuroimaging and cerebrospinal fluid (CSF) AD biomarkers has provided important insights into the time course of AD pathological changes across presymptomatic and symptomatic stages of the disease.[56] Biomarkers of Aβ deposition include low levels of soluble Aβ-42 in the CSF, as well as increased uptake of Aβ PET tracer ligands that correlate with greater plaque burden (see Chapter XX for a review of neuroimaging biomarkers in AD) (Figure 21-4). Biomarkers of pathological tau include elevated levels of total and phosphorylated tau in the CSF, and regional brain uptake of PET ligands specific for paired helical filament tau. Characteristic neuroimaging markers of neurodegeneration occurring early in AD include hypometabolism in vulnerable regions such as the lateral temporalparietal cortices and posterior cingulate cortex/precuneus measured with FDG PET[57] and atrophy in medial temporal and basal-lateral temporal regions captured on MRI.[37] These findings may all be present prior to the development of cognitive symptoms and clinical diagnosis of AD and become more pronounced with disease progression.[37]

In 2018, the National Institute on Aging—Alzheimer's Association (NIA-AA) published new research guidelines which established a biological definition of AD based strictly on biomarker criteria,[56] notable because prior consensus diagnostic criteria for AD required the presence of suggestive clinical symptoms and signs.[58,59] Within this "AT(N)" framework individuals are classified into pathological categories based on the presence or absence of biomarkers of Aβ ("A"), tau ("T"), or neurodegeneration [("N")]. Biomarker evidence of both abnormal amyloid and tau ("A+T+") is necessary to meet criteria for AD. Individuals with biomarker evidence of abnormal amyloid (PET ligand binding or low CSF Aβ-42) in the absence of CSF or PET markers of tau or neurodegeneration ("A+T-N-") are classified into an alternate category designated as "Alzheimer's pathologic change." Those who have biomarker evidence of tau pathology and/or neurodegeneration in the absence of Aβ are classified as having "Non-AD pathologic change."

This framework offers several advantages to promote ongoing research into the pathophysiology of AD. Separating clinical symptoms and signs from molecular and neurodegenerative biomarkers accommodates a current conceptualization of AD as a disease process that starts well in advance of symptoms and progresses through stages of subjective cognitive decline (SCD), mild cognitive impairment (MCI), and mild, moderate, and severe stages of dementia. This biological definition avoids the imperfect correlation between clinical signs and symptoms

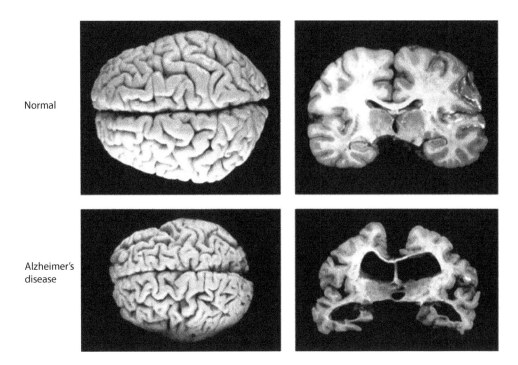

FIGURE 21-3. Normal brain viewed from above and in coronal section, compared with brain from a patient with Alzheimer's disease, showing cortical atrophy (widened sulci) and ex vacuo hydrocephalus (enlarged ventricles due to cerebral atrophy). (Whole brain photos reproduced with permission from the University of Alabama at Birmingham Department of Pathology PEIR Digital Library© (http://peir.net). Brain slice photos used with permission from A. C. McKee.)

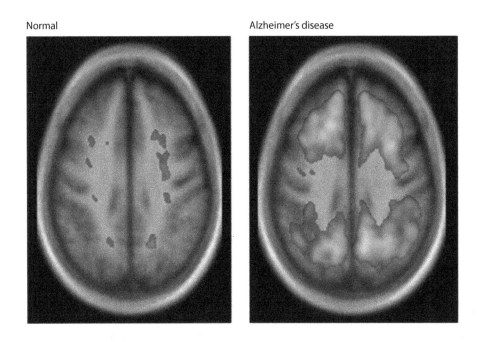

FIGURE 21-4. Visualizing Alzheimer's disease in the living brain. The density of β-amyloid plaques is indicated by the red regions in these images made after administration of Pittsburgh compound B, a fluorescent analog of thioflavin T. (Reproduced with permission from Buckner RL, Snyder AZ, Shannon BJ, et al: Molecular, structural, and functional characterization of Alzheimer's disease: Evidence for a relationship between default activity, amyloid, and memory. JNeurosci. 2005; 25:7709-7717. https://doi.org/10.1523/JNEUROSCI.2177-05.2005)

suggestive of AD and neuropathologically confirmed AD, and it accommodates individuals with AD pathologic markers who present atypically with prominent early impairment in non-memory cognitive domains. Further, it offers a framework into which biomarkers of other pathophysiological processes (e.g., synucleinopathies, FTLD, cerebrovascular pathology) might be incorporated when available. In so doing, the hope will be to obtain a better understanding of relationships between Aβ, tau, additional pathophysiological processes, neurodegeneration, and clinical symptoms and signs.

CLINICAL PRESENTATION

Cognitive Symptoms in AD

Older adults often experience changes in cognitive function that do not interfere with everyday function, do not manifest as deficits on formal neuropsychological testing, and may be ascribed to normal cognitive aging. Individuals with these mild subjective changes were previously described as "worried well." However, recent Aβ and/or tau biomarker studies suggest that a subset of individuals with SCD may be more accurately considered to be in the earliest symptomatic stages of AD.[60] Research criteria have described these early cognitive changes in biomarker-positive older adults as "transitional" AD-related symptoms.[61]

MCI (also known by the *DSM-5* designation as mild neurocognitive disorder)[62] refers to individuals with cognitive symptoms corroborated by objective performance deficits on cognitive testing greater than expected for age and educational background but not associated with loss of independence in basic or instrumental activities of daily living (IADLs). MCI may be characterized according to whether deficits occur within a single cognitive domain or multiple domains, with standard domains comprising episodic memory, attention, language, executive functions, visuospatial functions, and social cognition. Of these domains, clinically significant impairments in episodic memory are most characteristic of MCI due to underlying AD, particularly when occurring with an insidious onset and gradually progressive time course. In these cases, there is a high probability of progression to dementia (also known as major neurocognitive disorder in the *DSM-5* nomenclature) likely due to AD. In addition to a prominent early impairment in episodic memory, dementia due to AD is frequently characterized by additional, less prominent impairments in language (e.g., word retrieval), executive functions, and visuospatial functions. In sporadic early-onset cases, AD may present with primary early impairment in language, visuospatial functions, or executive functions. However, these patterns of early deficits are generally less common in AD.

Dementia, or major neurocognitive disorder, is diagnosed when a patient loses independence in IADLs such as driving, managing finances, taking medications, shopping, preparing meals, completing household chores, and using the telephone or other forms of communication.[59] Please refer to Chapter 20, Approach to Neurocognitive Disorders, for a more detailed description of the clinical features of this entity.

Assessment and Differential Diagnosis

For both MCI and dementia due to AD, diagnosis requires that other systemic and neurological causes of cognitive impairment be ruled out.[59] For example, evidence of significant cerebrovascular disease or prior stroke may indicate vascular cognitive

impairment as a primary etiology rather than AD. Visual hallucinations, parkinsonian motor changes, dream enactment behaviors, and profound fluctuations in attention or alertness may suggest an underlying Lewy body disorder (reviewed in Chapter XX). Prominent social cognitive changes (i.e., frank disinhibition, severe apathy, loss of sympathy and/or empathy, obsessive-compulsive and/or perseverative behaviors, hyperorality and/or changes in food preference) may suggest underlying FTLD (reviewed in Chapter 24). However, many patients exhibit a mixed presentation of symptoms, such as a typical AD presentation with concurrent presence of cerebrovascular disease or features of another type of dementia.[63] Indeed, neuropathological data suggest that most dementia cases among community-dwelling older adults are associated with mixed brain pathologies.[64]

In addition to detailed history, physical and neurological examinations, the recommended standard workup for patients with memory loss potentially due to AD includes detailed cognitive testing sufficient to assess performance in all major cognitive domains relative to expectations for age and education, laboratory workup for potentially modifiable factors associated with cognitive impairment, and structural neuroimaging to assess for evidence of vascular disease and/or focal atrophy. Clinical use of in vivo molecular biomarker studies of Aβ and/or tau is reserved for select diagnostic circumstances other than AD dementia with a typical amnesic presentation. The clinical assessment of AD includes the review of the individual's level of independence with IADLs and basic ADLs such as bathing, eating, and toileting. Safety issues to be assessed include medication compliance, home safety (cooking, firearms, ability to be alone), and community safety (driving, wandering). The status of legal issues (power of attorney, health care proxy, advance directives) should be evaluated as well. See Chapter 20 for a review of diagnostic approach to MCI and Major Neurocognitive Disorder.

NEUROPSYCHIATRIC SYMPTOMS IN AD

Epidemiology and Clinical Presentation

Neuropsychiatric symptoms (NPS) are increasingly recognized as core features of AD that occur early in the disease process and become more prevalent across later disease stages.[65] NPS in AD are associated with decreased patient quality of life,[66] increased caregiver burden and depression,[67] higher health care utilization and cost,[68] increased institutionalization,[69] more rapid disease progression, and earlier mortality.[70] Thus, appropriate identification and management of NPS may lead to more favorable outcomes for patients with AD and their caregivers.

Commonly recognized NPS in clinically diagnosed AD include apathy, depression, agitation/aggression, anxiety, sleep disturbances, irritability, appetite disturbances, aberrant motor behaviors, delusions, disinhibition, hallucinations, and euphoria (in order of decreasing frequency) (Figure 21-5).[71-73] At the MCI stage, approximately 50% of individuals experience one or more NPS. At the dementia stage, the prevalence of NPS increases: an estimated 75% of individuals with dementia experience at least one NPS in a given month, and nearly all individuals will experience NPS during the course of their disease.[65,74]

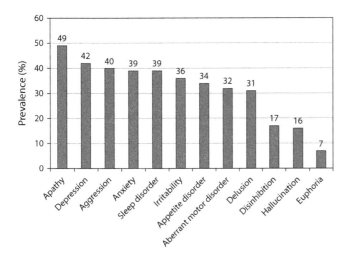

FIGURE 21-5. The prevalence of neuropsychiatric symptoms in Alzheimer's disease dementia. (Reproduced with permission from Zhao QF, Tan L, Wang HF, et al. The prevalence of neuropsychiatric symptoms in Alzheimer's disease: Systematic review and meta-analysis. *J Affect Disord.* 2016;190:264–271. Elsevier. https://www.sciencedirect.com/journal/journal-of-affective-disorders.)

The profile of NPS also varies with disease progression. Irritability, depression, apathy, and sleep disturbances are frequently reported at the stage of MCI and may emerge even earlier in the disease process when individuals are cognitively unimpaired.[75,76]

Prevalence of anxiety, appetite changes, and agitation increases across MCI and ensuing dementia stages. Apathy, the most common NPS, is substantially associated with degree of cognitive impairment and becomes more severe with disease progression.[77,78] Other NPS, including motor disturbances, hallucinations, delusions, and disinhibition are more likely to develop at advanced stages of dementia.[23,76,78] Agitation and aggression are more prevalent at the moderate and severe stages of dementia, and are among the most common NPS in late dementia.[65,79]

NPS in AD may differ from the classic presentation of psychiatric symptoms observed in younger and older patients with depression who are cognitively unimpaired. Depression in AD, for example, may present with subsyndromal symptoms or short-lived, recurrent disturbances in mood. Sadness may be less common than irritability, fear, or anxiety. Apathy, characterized by lack of motivation, emotional indifference, and social withdrawal, is often a symptom of depression, but can also present as a distinct symptom in AD.[80] Depressed patients with AD may experience greater difficulty with ADLs, difficulty falling or staying asleep, decreased appetite, and weight loss. Guilt and suicidal ideation are not common, but clinicians should elicit input from patient and caregiver to screen thoroughly for these symptoms.[81] Older adults with dementia have been found to have a higher risk of a suicide compared to those without dementia, particularly in the first 6 months after diagnosis.[82]

Psychosis in AD also differs from psychosis of schizophrenia and other primary psychotic disorders. In AD dementia, the most common psychotic symptoms are hallucinations and delusions. Visual hallucinations are more common than auditory, in contrast to schizophrenia. Delusions are typically paranoid and often pertain to thoughts of persecution, abandonment, infidelity, or misidentification.[83] Delusions of misidentification include thoughts that a family member is another person or an imposter (Capgras syndrome), the belief that a stranger is a familiar person (Fregoli syndrome), the belief that a deceased family member is still alive, the belief that a new place is home or a familiar location (reduplicative paramnesia), or the idea that one's home is not one's home (foreign reduplicative paramnesia).[83] Distorted thinking in AD may also be confabulatory or an elaboration of cognitive dysfunction rather than a fixed delusional belief. Patients with psychosis in dementia are unlikely to have a history of psychotic episodes prior to development of dementia.[84]

Pathophysiology of NPS in AD

Theoretical models have been proposed to describe the relationship of NPS to biological and clinical features of AD. According to the *symptom hypothesis*, NPS are understood to be manifestations of AD linked to disease-specific pathology.[85] Others have proposed that NPS may occur as a reaction or response to the development of cognitive or other clinical symptoms in AD, a form of *reverse causality*.[86] Alternately, the *risk factor hypothesis* considers that NPS and AD share common risk factors or a common etiology, and thus they co-occur but progress along distinct pathways.[85] The *unmet needs hypothesis* describes NPS as symptoms arising from unrecognized deficits in function or well-being that affected individuals are unable to fulfill on their own or express to others.[85] Other models suggest that NPS may be an independent cause of neurodegeneration that worsens AD-related clinical decline or NPS may be a disease-modifying factor which interacts with other environmental and genetic risk factors.[86]

Emerging neurobiological models propose that NPS develop in AD due to multileveled disruptions of neural circuits, networks, and neurotransmitter systems regulating cognition and emotion.[86] See Table 21-1 for a summary of this topic. For example, neuroimaging studies have found associations of apathy in AD dementia with decreased perfusion, hypometabolism, and volume loss in the anterior cingulate[87–90] and orbitofrontal[87–89,91,92] cortices, brain regions involved in the integration of emotional, motor, and cognitive information necessary for decision making and initiation of motivated behavioral responses.[93–95] Consistent with these in vivo findings, neurofibrillary tau tangle burden in the anterior cingulate cortex at autopsy has been correlated with higher apathy ratings in patients with AD, directly linking apathy with regional AD pathology.[96] Apathy has also been positively associated with neocortical Aβ deposition measured by PET.[97] More recent studies in unimpaired older adults and those with MCI point to associations of greater apathy with cortical thinning and hypometabolism in inferior temporal and posterior cingulate cortices, posterior cortical regions which undergo neurodegeneration in early AD.[98–100] Abnormalities in cholinergic and dopaminergic function have also been associated with apathy in AD and provide the rationale for the success of certain trials of cholinergic[101] and dopaminergic agents[102] for the treatment of apathy.

Agitation in AD has been associated with atrophy and/or changes in network connectivity in frontal, anterior cingulate, posterior cingulate, and orbitofrontal cortices and in the

TABLE 21-1 • Summary of Neurobiological Correlates of Neuropsychiatric Symptoms of Alzheimer's Disease and Their Potential Treatments.

Neuropsychiatric Symptoms of Alzheimer's Disease	Neurotransmitter Mechanisms	Neuroimaging Correlates	Treatments: Evidence-Based or Used by Practitioners
Depression	Monoaminergic, noradrenergic, gamma amino butyric acid (GABA) neurotransmission dysfunction	Reduced entorhinal cortex thickness; accelerated atrophy in anterior cingulate cortex; decreased cerebral glucose in frontal and parietal cortices	Nonpharmacological treatments; selective serotonin reuptake inhibitors, dual serotonin-norepinephrine reuptake inhibitors
Apathy	Lower dopamine transporter binding; lower cholinergic receptor binding	Decreased metabolic activity in anterior cingulate cortex and orbitofrontal cortex; functional deficits in several medial and inferior frontal cortical regions	Nonpharmacological treatments; methylphenidate, amantadine, D-amphetamine, modafinil
Agitation and aggression	Cholinergic neurotransmission deficits; increased D2/D3 receptor availability; monoaminergic (5-HT2A) transmission defects	Atrophy of cingulate and frontal cortices; insula, amygdala, and hippocampal atrophy; lower metabolic activity in temporal, frontal, and cingulate cortices; anterior salience network connectivity changes	Nonpharmacological treatments; citalopram, atypical antipsychotic medications, anti-epileptic mood stabilizers
Psychosis	D2/D3 receptor availability, monoaminergic, cholinergic	Lower regional cerebral blood flow in angular gyrus and occipital lobe; increased atrophy in frontal, parietal, and cingulate cortices	Nonpharmacological treatments; atypical antipsychotic medications

Adapted with permission from Nowrangi MA, Lyketsos CG, Rosenberg PB. Principles and management of neuropsychiatric symptoms in Alzheimer's dementia. Alzheimers Res Ther. 2015;7:12. Springer Nature. https://alzres.biomedcentral.com.

amygdala, insula, and hippocampus.[103] It is hypothesized that neurodegeneration in these regions involved in the assessment of salience and in emotional regulation may predispose to both an overestimation of threat and maladaptive emotional and behavioral responses.[23] Greater measures of disinhibition have similarly been associated with atrophy in bilateral anterior cingulate and right medial frontal regions.[104] Neuropathological studies have correlated agitation or aggression with reduced markers of cholinergic, dopaminergic, or serotonergic function[105,106] as well as CSF markers of tau and phospho-tau[107] in patients with AD. These widespread pathological changes and broad neurochemical deficits are consistent with agitation as a symptom of advanced disease and late rather than early clinical stage.

Psychotic symptoms (hallucinations and delusions) often co-occur with agitation and they are commonly studied together. Structural and functional deficits most often associated with delusions have been localized to the anterior cingulate cortex and orbitofrontal, dorsolateral frontal, and inferior frontal regions (as reviewed by Rosenberg).[90] In other work, psychotic symptoms (hallucinations, delusions, and night time agitation) were associated with reduced cerebral blood flow in the right angular gyrus and right occipital lobe.[108] Psychotic symptoms in AD have been correlated with increased neocortical NFTs[109] but not neocortical plaque density.[110] Psychotic symptoms in AD have also been associated with increased nucleus accumbens dopamine D3 receptor density independent of neuroleptic exposure or Lewy body pathology,[111] lower cell counts in the dorsal raphe nucleus,[112] increased ratio of acetylcholinesterase/5-HT levels, and increased synaptic loss.[83] Notably, cohort studies have demonstrated familial aggregation of psychosis in AD suggesting that genetic variants modify the

pathology and accelerate the course of disease in affected individuals with psychosis.[83]

Other NPS such as depression have also been associated with neurodegenerative changes in various brain regions including depression-related neuronal loss in the locus coeruleus, the raphe nucleus,[113] the entorhinal cortex,[114] and frontoparietal hypometabolism,[115,116] though these studies are less numerous and findings less consistent.

Assessment and Differential Diagnosis of NPS

Regular screening for NPS in AD and offering recommendations for managing these symptoms are key practices for improving the quality of life of dementia patients and caregivers, as published in the joint statement from the American Psychiatric Association and American Association of Neurology multidisciplinary work group.[117,118] Recent American Psychiatric Association practice guidelines also recommend that patients with dementia be regularly assessed for the type, frequency, severity, pattern, and timing of behavioral and psychological symptoms.[118]

Assessment and management of NPS comprise an iterative process which requires understanding of patient, caregiver, and environmental factors that may be contributing to symptoms.[119] Patients with AD may not be able to voice their needs in the face of physical or emotional distress. Reversible conditions contributing to NPS in AD may include medical illness, pain, side effects of medications, and interactions between medications. Preexisting primary psychiatric or personality disorders should also be considered when evaluating NPS. Caregivers are the primary sources of information regarding AD patients' behavioral and psychological symptoms. Many factors specific to caregivers themselves, such as stress, depression, and level of knowledge about dementia, may affect their assessment of patients' symptoms. Finally, environmental factors contributing to NPS should be identified, such as over- and under-stimulation, changes to routine, and overwhelming social situations,[120] which, of note, may include abuse by caregivers. Concerns for home and personal safety (self-neglect, access to firearms) may be heightened in individuals with both cognitive impairment and NPS.

Several scales have been developed and validated to assess depression and other NPS in older adult patients with and without dementia. The Neuropsychiatric Inventory (NPI), possibly the most widely used instrument, is completed as an interview of caregivers, or other knowledgeable informants, of patients. The NPI assesses the presence, severity, and level of caregiver distress associated with 12 common behavioral disturbances including delusions, hallucinations, agitation/aggression, depression/dysphoria, anxiety, elation/euphoria, disinhibition, irritability/lability, apathy/indifference, aberrant motor activity, sleep, and appetite/eating disorders.[71] The NPI Questionnaire (NPI-Q) was developed as a more abbreviated form of the NPI which can be self-administered by a caregiver or other informant.[121] The NPI scales screen for numerous possible symptoms, whereas other instruments focus specifically on one NPS. The Geriatric Depression Scale, Cornell Scale for Depression in Dementia, and Cohen-Mansfield Agitation Inventory assess more specific neuropsychiatric dimensions in greater depth than the NPI alone. These scales are commonly used in research settings. However, some of these instruments, such as the NPI-Q and Geriatric Depression Scale, are also used in clinical settings.

International consensus criteria for apathy[122] and agitation[123] in AD and other neurodegenerative disorders have been developed to facilitate research and regulatory applications for drug development programs. The Mild Behavioral Impairment Checklist is a novel research instrument developed by expert consensus to advance the detection and classification of NPS in pre-dementia stages of neurodegenerative disorders such as AD.[124]

Treatment of NPS in AD

Annual, or more frequent, screening for NPS with validated instruments such as the NPI is recommended to allow for early detection of symptoms, education and counseling for caregivers, and timely intervention.[125]

Nonpharmacologic Therapy

Nonpharmacologic approaches are recommended as first-line therapy for NPS in AD in non-emergent situations and should be incorporated into comprehensive care of dementia patients. Compared to pharmacologic therapies, nonpharmacologic strategies may better address underlying causes of NPS such as environmental stressors and unmet needs, may promote caregiver education, and may minimize potential adverse effects.[125]

Interventions aimed at modifying the environment of AD patients have been shown to prevent and reduce behavioral symptoms. Such interventions include optimizing structured routines, reducing overstimulation (e.g., excess noise, clutter), and eliminating environmental safety concerns such as access

to sharp objects.[120] Creating visual cues or reminders to reduce confusion may also reduce NPS.[125] Exercise training has been found to improve depressive symptoms[126] and disordered sleep.[125] Music therapy has been shown to improve anxiety, depression, agitation, and aggression.[127,128] Cognitive stimulation therapy is an intervention aimed at stabilizing and improving cognitive impairment. This intervention was also found to reduce apathy, depression, and overall severity of NPS.[129] Cognitive-behavioral therapy has also been found to be effective for the treatment of depression for individuals with MCI as well as for those with mild-to-moderate dementia (reviewed in Chapter 10 "Psychosocial Interventions in Neuropsychiatry"). Strongest evidence supports problem solving and modified cognitive behavioral treatment approaches.[130]

Interventions that are patient-centered and caregiver-directed aim to improve the identification of precipitating causes as well as strategies to modify these triggers.[120] These interventions have shown to not only reduce behavioral and psychiatric symptoms in patients but also decrease caregiver distress, improve caregiver confidence, and enhance caregiver communication with AD patients.[120] Ultimately, they help integrate nonpharmacologic, medical, and psychopharmacologic treatments.

Pharmacologic Therapy

There are currently no FDA-approved medications for the management of psychiatric and behavioral symptoms in AD. However, risperidone is approved in Europe and Canada for the treatment of persistent agitation in moderate and severe AD dementia. Certain pharmacologic therapies have been shown to benefit specific NPS and are often prescribed off-label to target these symptoms.

Depression

To date, antidepressants have shown minimal benefit when used to treat depression in AD dementia. The DIADS-2 randomized control trial (RCT) assessed the efficacy of sertraline for the treatment of depressive symptoms and showed no significant improvement in depression compared to placebo.[131] Another RCT examining the effects of sertraline and mirtazapine on depressive symptoms showed no significant improvement from either antidepressant compared to placebo or compared to each other.[132] Notably, in both studies, depression scores declined in both active treatment and placebo groups which may point to treatment effects from clinical management alone. A meta-analysis of RCTs similarly showed no significant benefit of sertraline, mirtazapine, fluoxetine, and tricyclic antidepressants imipramine and clomipramine compared to placebo.[133] Despite this lack of supportive evidence specific to older adults with dementia, antidepressants are still often prescribed for depression of AD based on their established efficacy for the treatment of depression more broadly. SSRIs are commonly prescribed, possibly due to their perceived low side-effect profile. However, the DIADS study found sertraline was associated with significantly higher rates of side effects, including diarrhea, indigestion, dry mouth, and dizziness, compared to placebo.[131] Preliminary evidence points to possible protective effects of SSRIs in reducing risk of progression from MCI to AD dementia.[134]

Apathy

The ADMET trial compared the effects of methylphenidate to placebo on apathy in AD dementia. This trial showed an improvement in two out of three outcome measures, including apathy severity scores. A nonsignificant improvement in cognition measured by the Mini Mental State Exam was also observed in patients receiving methylphenidate compared to placebo. Methylphenidate was not associated with significantly elevated risk of adverse effects.[102] Additional studies have also compared methylphenidate, acetylcholinesterase inhibitors (including donepezil and galantamine), memantine, and modafinil to placebo for treatment of apathy with mixed results. A meta-analysis of these pharmacologic treatments found no significant effect on apathy.[135]

Agitation and Psychosis

Antipsychotic medications are often prescribed for treatment of agitation, aggression, and psychosis in AD. Some typical and atypical antipsychotics have been shown to be more efficacious than others. However, they are also associated with significant adverse effects. In 2008, the FDA instituted a black-box warning for all antipsychotic medications, advising that elderly patients with dementia-related psychosis who are treated with antipsychotics have a 1.6 to 1.7 times greater risk of death compared to those without antipsychotic exposure. Because of the significant risk associated with these medications, their use is most appropriate in patients whose symptoms are severe, dangerous, and/or cause significant distress to the patient and is ill-advised for non-approved indications such as insomnia.[136]

Atypical, or second-generation, antipsychotics are prescribed for the treatment of psychosis and agitation in AD dementia. The CATIE-AD trial was an effectiveness study in which olanzapine, risperidone, and quetiapine were compared to one another and to placebo for the treatment of agitation, aggression, and psychosis in AD dementia. Compared to placebo, olanzapine and risperidone were significantly more effective, indicated in this study by significantly delayed discontinuation of those medications due to inefficacy.[137] Patients randomized to olanzapine and risperidone also demonstrated significant reduction in other outcomes, including the overall NPI score and the hostile suspiciousness subcategory of the Brief Psychiatric Rating Scale (BPRS).[138] Risperidone was also associated with decreased psychosis.[138]

Meta-analysis has shown risperidone is superior to placebo in treatment of psychosis of dementia, particularly in patients with severe symptoms and aggression.[139] The overall effect size is weak, but given the large number of studies with adequate sample sizes and study designs, risperidone was judged to have moderate evidence of efficacy by an expert panel.[118]

Aripiprazole also has moderate evidence to support its use in treatment of psychosis and agitation in dementia.[118] In a meta-analysis of three placebo-controlled RCTs, aripiprazole was associated with significant reduction in total NPI and BPRS scores. Two of these studies examined efficacy in nursing home patients, and these studies also demonstrated significant reduction in Cohen-Mansfield Agitation Inventory (CMAI) scores. There was no significant improvement in psychosis.[140] The magnitude of the effects of aripiprazole is weak, indicated by relatively small effect sizes.[118]

Olanzapine and quetiapine have less evidence supporting their efficacy for the treatment of NPS in dementia, compared to risperidone and aripiprazole.[118] Meta-analysis examining olanzapine in nursing home patients did not demonstrate efficacy as there was no significant improvement in NPI and BPRS scores or psychosis subscales.[140]

Quetiapine likewise has not demonstrated significant effect on NPS in meta-analysis including three studies of nursing home patients with AD and behavioral symptoms. However, this analysis was limited by differences in outcome measures.[140] The CATIE-AD trial also did not demonstrate effectiveness of quetiapine in outpatients, though this was likely limited by inadequate dosing.[137] Thus, the evidence for quetiapine use in treatment of NPS is weak.

Atypical antipsychotics are associated with significant adverse effects that should be weighed against the potential benefits in treating NPS. Risperidone is associated with increased risk of sedation, extrapyramidal symptoms,[139] confusion,[137] and cerebrovascular events.[140] Adverse effects associated with olanzapine include somnolence, edema,[140] extrapyramidal symptoms, confusion, and cognitive disturbance.[137] Quetiapine is associated with increased risk of sedation and cognitive impairment.[137]

Haloperidol is a typical, or first-generation, antipsychotic available in oral, intramuscular, and intravenous formulations which is sometimes prescribed for agitation and psychosis in patients with AD dementia. Compared to placebo, haloperidol is associated with significant decrease in aggression in

---

CASE VIGNETTE 21.1

A 77-year-old man presented for evaluation with a 2-year history of progressive difficulty retrieving words and the names of friends, poor recall of information while reading, problems locating common kitchen items, and an impaired ability to use the computer. There was a 6-month history of anxiety, irritability, and decreased sense of humor. A former chief financial officer, he was unable to prepare his personal taxes. A basic metabolic panel, complete blood count, thyroid function tests, and levels of B12 and folate were normal. Brain imaging showed mild bilateral frontal, parietal, and anterior temporal atrophy and an absence of subcortical white matter changes. He was diagnosed with Alzheimer's disease dementia and was prescribed donepezil and citalopram.

patients with dementia, but otherwise has limited efficacy for other measures of agitation.[141] This medication is also associated with increased risk of extrapyramidal symptoms.[141] A study examining the mortality risk with individual antipsychotics among patients with dementia found haloperidol to be associated with the highest relative risk of mortality.[142] The use of haloperidol in nonemergency settings and in the absence of delirium is therefore not recommended as a first-line agent.[136]

First- and second-generation antipsychotics are associated with an increased mortality risk, evidenced by retrospective cohort data and black-box warning stating their use for treatment of dementia-related psychosis carries an increased risk of death compared to placebo. Within the first 6 months of treatment initiation, haloperidol is associated with the greatest mortality risk, followed by olanzapine and risperidone. Quetiapine is associated with the lowest mortality risk. The mortality risk associated with haloperidol is highest in the first 30 days of treatment, whereas the risk attributed to olanzapine and risperidone is highest in the first 120 days.[142]

Strong evidence suggests that citalopram may be used as an alternative to antipsychotics for treatment of agitation in AD dementia. The CitAD study was a double-blind, placebo-controlled RCT which examined the effects of citalopram on agitation in a predominantly outpatient, noninstitutionalized population. Compared to placebo, citalopram showed superiority in reduction of agitation, global clinical improvement, reduction in total NPI score, and reduction in caregiver distress.[143] In secondary analyses, citalopram was also associated with significant improvement in delusions, anxiety, irritability,

and lability.[144] There were small but measurable adverse effects of citalopram on cognition and QTc prolongation.[143] Although the CitAD trial evaluated citalopram 30 mg daily as the target dose, current practice standards recommend a maximum dose of citalopram 20 mg daily for adults age 60 and older to minimize the risk of QTc prolongation.

Anticonvulsants such as divalproex sodium, gabapentin, lamotrigine, and oxcarbamezapine have been studied for the treatment of agitation in AD dementia without clear evidence of efficacy to date.[145-148]

Other NPS

There have been no RCTs evaluating psychotropic medications for anxiety or irritability in AD, although SSRIs or SNRIs are commonly used for these symptoms and for anxiety disorders in older individuals with and without AD. Paroxetine and tricyclic antidepressants are not recommended in these older adults due to anticholinergic effects, including adverse effects on cognition.[149] Benzodiazepines are also generally avoided because of their association with cognitive impairment, delirium, falls, fractures, and motor vehicle accidents in older adults.[149] There is limited evidence to support the use of trazodone for sleep disturbance in AD dementia and it is commonly used for this purpose in clinical practice.[150] A systematic review found no evidence of benefit or harm in the use of either melatonin or ramelteon in the treatment of sleep disturbances in AD.[151] A small placebo-controlled RCT examining the use of mirtazapine in AD-related sleep disturbances found no significant improvement in nocturnal sleep but did find a significant increase in daytime sleepiness.[152]

Summary and Key Points

- AD is a common cause of neuropsychiatric, cognitive, and functional morbidity and mortality in older adults, affecting more than 1 in 10 Americans age 65 and older. The prevalence of AD dementia expected to more than double by 2050 as the U.S. population ages.
- AD is now defined as a biologic construct characterized by in vivo or neuropathological evidence of beta-amyloid plaques and neurofibrillary tau tangles, pathologies which are present at presymptomatic and symptomatic disease stages.
- Nearly all patients with AD will experience at least one neuropsychiatric symptom during the course of their illness. Apathy, anxiety, and depression often emerge early in the disease process of AD, while psychosis and agitation are more typical of later disease stages.

- Neuropsychiatric symptoms are associated with increased caregiver burden and distress, increased costs of care, risk of hospitalization and long-term care placement, more rapid disease progression, and early death.
- Nonpharmacologic interventions are recommended as first-line treatments in non-emergent settings.
- Evidence supporting the pharmacologic treatment for depression is limited. However, the antidepressant citalopram has been shown to be effective for reducing agitation and other neuropsychiatric symptoms in AD dementia.
- Antipsychotics are used for treatment of severe agitation and psychosis in AD, although evidence supporting their efficacy is mixed. Antipsychotics carry an increased risk of mortality in patients with dementia, and their risks and benefits should be weighed before initiation.

Multiple Choice Questions

1. Which of the following is not a recognized risk factor for the development of Alzheimer's disease dementia?
   a. Advanced age
   b. Apolipoprotein E ε2 allele
   c. Female sex
   d. Family history of dementia
   e. Lower educational attainment

2. Which of the following is true regarding amyloid plaques in Alzheimer's disease?
   a. Amyloid plaques are dense, intracellular protein aggregates.
   b. Gene mutations associated with familial (or early-onset) AD contribute to AD pathology primarily through decreased clearance of beta amyloid.
   c. Elevated Aβ-42 in cerebrospinal fluid is a biomarker of AD pathology.
   d. Aβ oligomers contribute to AD pathophysiology through impairment of synaptic functions and signaling pathways.
   e. All individuals with biomarker evidence of amyloid plaque accumulation will go on to develop cognitive impairment.

3. Which neuropsychiatric symptom is most prevalent in AD?
   a. Apathy
   b. Anxiety
   c. Depression
   d. Euphoria
   e. Agitation

4. Which of the following is true regarding the use of citalopram in treatment of neuropsychiatric symptoms of Alzheimer's disease dementia?
   a. It is FDA-approved for the treatment of agitation in AD.
   b. There is strong evidence for the use of citalopram in the treatment of depression in AD.
   c. Citalopram carries a black-box warning due to increased risk of death in patients with dementia compared to placebo.
   d. Use of citalopram in dementia is associated with improvements in agitation, caregiver distress, and overall NPI scores.
   e. Treatment with citalopram improves cognition in patients with AD.

Multiple Choice Answers

1. **Answer: b**
   Advanced age, female sex, family history of dementia, and low educational attainment are all independent risk factors for AD dementia. The Apolipoprotein E ε4 allele (APOE4) is a recognized risk factor for sporadic, or late-onset, Alzheimer's disease. The APOE4 allele is associated with less efficient clearance of Aβ from the central nervous system compared to APOE3 or APOE2 alleles. APOE4 genotypes have also been implicated in non-amyloid-dependent disease mechanisms such as impaired synaptogenesis and hippocampal neurogenesis.

2. **Answer: d**
   Neurofibrillary tangles are dense, intracellular protein aggregates containing pathological tau. Amyloid plaques are extracellular protein aggregates containing fibrils of beta-amyloid dimers, oligomers, and polymers. Gene mutations associated with early-onset AD include APP, PSE1, and PSE2, all of which are associated with increased production of Aβ, rather than decreased clearance. Monomeric Aβ-40 is the most prevalent Aβ peptide, but Aβ-42 is the peptide most prone to aggregation and formation of amyloid plaques. Low levels of Aβ-42 in cerebrospinal fluid and high levels of brain amyloid plaques detected by positron emission tomography are in vivo biomarkers of AD. Soluble Aβ oligomers are associated with impaired synaptic functions and aberrant neuronal activity. Although abnormal amyloid pathology is necessary for pathogenesis of AD, many individuals with evidence of amyloid plaque accumulation remain cognitively intact.

3. **Answer: a**
   Apathy is the most common neuropsychiatric symptom in Alzheimer's disease and typically becomes more prevalent and severe with advanced disease. The overall prevalence of apathy in individuals with probable AD dementia was 49% in pooled meta-analytic data. Prevalence for depression was 42%, aggression/agitation 40%, and anxiety 39%. The prevalence of elation/euphoria was 7%, the lowest of the commonly measured neuropsychiatric symptoms.

4. **Answer: d**
   There are currently no FDA-approved pharmacologic treatments for neuropsychiatric symptoms in Alzheimer's disease dementia. However, there have been studies supporting off-label use for some psychotropic medications. The CitAD trial was a randomized control trial which examined the effects of citalopram on agitation in a predominantly outpatient population with Alzheimer's disease dementia. Citalopram was shown to have a significant effect on decreasing agitation, as well as improvements in overall scores on the Neuropsychiatric Index (NPI) and caregiver distress. Secondary analyses also demonstrated improvements in delusions, anxiety, irritability, and lability. There have been no studies of citalopram for the treatment of depression in AD, and evidence for effective treatments for depression in AD is lacking overall. Citalopram does carry a risk of side effects such as prolonged QT interval and possible worsening cognitive symptoms in AD dementia patients. However, unlike antipsychotics, citalopram is not associated with higher mortality and does not carry a black-box warning.

References

1. Alzheimer's Association 2018 Alzheimer's disease facts and figures. *Alzheimers Dement*. 2018;14(3):367-429.
2. Hebert LE, Weuve J, Scherr PA, Evans DA. Alzheimer disease in the United States (2010-2050) estimated using the 2010 census. *Neurology*. 2013;80(19):1778-1783.
3. Bradford A, Kunik ME, Schulz P, Williams SP, Singh H. Missed and delayed diagnosis of dementia in primary care: prevalence and contributing factors. *Alzheimer Dis Assoc Disord*. 2009;23(4):306-314.
4. Kotagal V, Langa KM, Plassman BL, et al. Factors associated with cognitive evaluations in the United States. *Neurology*. 2015;84(1):64-71.
5. Taylor DH Jr, Ostbye T, Langa KM, Weir D, Plassman BL. The accuracy of Medicare claims as an epidemiological tool: the case of dementia revisited. *J Alzheimers Dis*. 2009;17(4):807-815.
6. Hebert LE, Bienias JL, Aggarwal NT, et al. Change in risk of Alzheimer disease over time. *Neurology*. 2010;75(9):786-791.
7. Mayeux R, Sano M, Chen J, Tatemichi T, Stern Y. Risk of dementia in first-degree relatives of patients with Alzheimer's disease and related disorders. *Arch Neurol*. 1991;48(3):269-273.
8. Saunders AM, Strittmatter WJ, Schmechel D, et al. Association of apolipoprotein E allele epsilon 4 with late-onset familial and sporadic Alzheimer's disease. *Neurology*. 1993;43(8):1467-1472.
9. Hebert LE, Scherr PA, McCann JJ, Beckett LA, Evans DA. Is the risk of developing Alzheimer's disease greater for women than for men? *Am J Epidemiol*. 2001;153(2):132-136.
10. Chene G, Beiser A, Au R, et al. Gender and incidence of dementia in the Framingham Heart Study from mid-adult life. *Alzheimers Dement*. 2015;11(3):310-320.
11. Carter CL, Resnick EM, Mallampalli M, Kalbarczyk A. Sex and gender differences in Alzheimer's disease: recommendations for future research. *J Womens Health (Larchmt)*. 2012;21(10): 1018-1023.
12. Altmann A, Tian L, Henderson VW, Greicius MD, Alzheimer's Disease Neuroimaging Initiative I. Sex modifies the APOE-related risk of developing Alzheimer disease. *Ann Neurol*. 2014;75(4):563-573.
13. Ungar L, Altmann A, Greicius MD. Apolipoprotein E, gender, and Alzheimer's disease: an overlooked, but potent and promising interaction. *Brain Imaging Behav*. 2014;8(2):262-273.
14. Gurland BJ, Wilder DE, Lantigua R, et al. Rates of dementia in three ethnoracial groups. *Int J Geriatr Psychiatry*. 1999;14(6): 481-493.
15. Green RC, Cupples LA, Go R, et al. Risk of dementia among white and African American relatives of patients with Alzheimer disease. *JAMA*. 2002;287(3):329-336.
16. Demirovic J, Prineas R, Loewenstein D, et al. Prevalence of dementia in three ethnic groups: the South Florida program on aging and health. *Ann Epidemiol*. 2003;13(6):472-478.
17. Yaffe K, Falvey C, Harris TB, et al. Effect of socioeconomic disparities on incidence of dementia among biracial older adults: prospective study. *BMJ*. 2013;347:f7051.
18. Glymour MM, Manly JJ. Lifecourse social conditions and racial and ethnic patterns of cognitive aging. *Neuropsychol Rev*. 2008;18(3):223-254.
19. Fitzpatrick AL, Kuller LH, Ives DG, et al. Incidence and prevalence of dementia in the Cardiovascular Health Study. *J Am Geriatr Soc*. 2004;52(2):195-204.
20. McDowell I, Xi G, Lindsay J, Tierney M. Mapping the connections between education and dementia. *J Clin Exp Neuropsychol*. 2007;29(2):127-141.
21. Barnes DE, Kaup A, Kirby KA, et al. Traumatic brain injury and risk of dementia in older veterans. *Neurology*. 2014;83(4): 312-319.
22. Yaffe K, Lwi SJ, Hoang TD, et al. Military-related risk factors in female veterans and risk of dementia. *Neurology*. 2019;92(3): e205-e211.
23. Lanctot KL, Amatniek J, Ancoli-Israel S, et al. Neuropsychiatric signs and symptoms of Alzheimer's disease: new treatment paradigms. *Alzheimers Dement (NY)*. 2017;3(3):440-449.
24. Stephen R, Hongisto K, Solomon A, Lonnroos E. Physical activity and Alzheimer's disease: a systematic review. *J Gerontol A Biol Sci Med Sci*. 2017;72(6):733-739.
25. Barberger-Gateau P, Raffaitin C, Letenneur L, et al. Dietary patterns and risk of dementia: the Three-City cohort study. *Neurology*. 2007;69(20):1921-1930.
26. Baumgart M, Snyder HM, Carrillo MC, et al. Summary of the evidence on modifiable risk factors for cognitive decline and dementia: a population-based perspective. *Alzheimers Dement*. 2015;11(6):718-726.
27. Krueger KR, Wilson RS, Kamenetsky JM, et al. Social engagement and cognitive function in old age. *Exp Aging Res*. 2009;35(1): 45-60.
28. Karp A, Paillard-Borg S, Wang HX, et al. Mental, physical and social components in leisure activities equally contribute to decrease dementia risk. *Dement Geriatr Cogn Disord*. 2006;21(2):65-73.
29. Sajeev G, Weuve J, Jackson JW, et al. Late-life cognitive activity and dementia: a systematic review and bias analysis. *Epidemiology*. 2016;27(5):732-742.
30. Livingston G, Sommerlad A, Orgeta V, et al. Dementia prevention, intervention, and care. *Lancet*. 2017;390(10113):2673-2734.
31. Goldman JS, Hahn SE, Catania JW, et al. Genetic counseling and testing for Alzheimer disease: joint practice guidelines of the American College of Medical Genetics and the National Society of Genetic Counselors. *Genet Med*. 2011;13(6):597-605.
32. Brickell KL, Steinbart EJ, Rumbaugh M, et al. Early-onset Alzheimer disease in families with late-onset Alzheimer disease: a potential important subtype of familial Alzheimer disease. *Arch Neurol*. 2006;63(9):1307-1311.
33. Bonham LW, Geier EG, Fan CC, et al. Age-dependent effects of APOE epsilon4 in preclinical Alzheimer's disease. *Ann Clin Transl Neurol*. 2016;3(9):668-677.
34. Genin E, Hannequin D, Wallon D, et al. APOE and Alzheimer disease: a major gene with semi-dominant inheritance. *Mol Psychiatry*. 2011;16(9):903-907.
35. Joshi A, Ringman JM, Lee AS, Juarez KO, Mendez MF. Comparison of clinical characteristics between familial and non-familial early onset Alzheimer's disease. *J Neurol*. 2012;259(10):2182-2188.
36. Lanoiselee Y, Grebenkov DS. Unraveling intermittent features in single-particle trajectories by a local convex hull method. *Phys Rev E*. 2017;96(2-1):022144.
37. Jack CR Jr, Knopman DS, Jagust WJ, et al. Tracking pathophysiological processes in Alzheimer's disease: an updated hypothetical model of dynamic biomarkers. *Lancet Neurol*. 2013;12(2):207-216.
38. Huang Y, Mucke L. Alzheimer mechanisms and therapeutic strategies. *Cell*. 2012;148(6):1204-1222.
39. Mintun MA, Larossa GN, Sheline YI, et al. [11C]PIB in a nondemented population: potential antecedent marker of Alzheimer disease. *Neurology*. 2006;67(3):446-452.
40. Citron M. Alzheimer's disease: strategies for disease modification. *Nat Rev Drug Discov*. 2010;9(5):387-398.

41. Rosenberg RN, Lambracht-Washington D, Yu G, Xia W. Genomics of Alzheimer disease: a review. *JAMA Neurol.* 2016;73(7):867-874.

42. Kim J, Basak JM, Holtzman DM. The role of apolipoprotein E in Alzheimer's disease. *Neuron.* 2009;63(3):287-303.

43. Vlassenko AG, Vaishnavi SN, Couture L, et al. Spatial correlation between brain aerobic glycolysis and amyloid-beta (Abeta) deposition. *Proc Natl Acad Sci U S A.* 2010;107(41):17763-17767.

44. Moir RD, Lathe R, Tanzi RE. The antimicrobial protection hypothesis of Alzheimer's disease. *Alzheimers Dement.* 2018;14(12):1602-1614.

45. Cummings JL. Alzheimer's disease. *N Engl J Med.* 2004;351(1):56-67.

46. Palop JJ, Mucke L. Amyloid-beta-induced neuronal dysfunction in Alzheimer's disease: from synapses toward neural networks. *Nat Neurosci.* 2010;13(7):812-818.

47. Mietelska-Porowska A, Wasik U, Goras M, Filipek A, Niewiadomska G. Tau protein modifications and interactions: their role in function and dysfunction. *Int J Mol Sci.* 2014;15(3):4671-4713.

48. Alonso AD, Grundke-Iqbal I, Barra HS, Iqbal K. Abnormal phosphorylation of tau and the mechanism of Alzheimer neurofibrillary degeneration: sequestration of microtubule-associated proteins 1 and 2 and the disassembly of microtubules by the abnormal tau. *Proc Natl Acad Sci U S A.* 1997;94(1):298-303.

49. Mattson MP. Pathways towards and away from Alzheimer's disease. *Nature.* 2004;430(7000):631-639.

50. Arriagada PV, Growdon JH, Hedley-Whyte ET, Hyman BT. Neurofibrillary tangles but not senile plaques parallel duration and severity of Alzheimer's disease. *Neurology.* 1992;42(3 pt 1):631-639.

51. Xia C, Makaretz SJ, Caso C, et al. Association of in vivo [18F] AV-1451 tau PET imaging results with cortical atrophy and symptoms in typical and atypical Alzheimer disease. *JAMA Neurol.* 2017;74(4):427-436.

52. Braak H, Del Tredici K. The pathological process underlying Alzheimer's disease in individuals under thirty. *Acta Neuropathol.* 2011;121(2):171-181.

53. Rapoport M, Dawson HN, Binder LI, Vitek MP, Ferreira A. Tau is essential to beta-amyloid-induced neurotoxicity. *Proc Natl Acad Sci U S A.* 2002;99(9):6364-6369.

54. Garcia ML, Cleveland DW. Going new places using an old MAP: tau, microtubules and human neurodegenerative disease. *Curr Opin Cell Biol.* 2001;13(1):41-48.

55. de Calignon A, Polydoro M, Suarez-Calvet M, et al. Propagation of tau pathology in a model of early Alzheimer's disease. *Neuron.* 2012;73(4):685-697.

56. Jack CR Jr, Lowe VJ, Weigand SD, et al. Serial PIB and MRI in normal, mild cognitive impairment and Alzheimer's disease: implications for sequence of pathological events in Alzheimer's disease. *Brain.* 2009;132(pt 5):1355-1365.

57. Jack CR Jr, Bennett DA, Blennow K, et al. A/T/N: an unbiased descriptive classification scheme for Alzheimer disease biomarkers. *Neurology.* 2016;87(5):539-547.

58. McKhann G, Drachman D, Folstein M, et al. Clinical diagnosis of Alzheimer's disease: report of the NINCDS-ADRDA Work Group under the auspices of Department of Health and Human Services Task Force on Alzheimer's disease. *Neurology.* 1984;34(7):939-944.

59. Albert MS, DeKosky ST, Dickson D, et al. The diagnosis of mild cognitive impairment due to Alzheimer's disease: recommendations from the National Institute on Aging-Alzheimer's Association workgroups on diagnostic guidelines for Alzheimer's disease. *Alzheimers Dement.* 2011;7(3):270-279.

60. Jessen F, Amariglio RE, van Boxtel M, et al. A conceptual framework for research on subjective cognitive decline in preclinical Alzheimer's disease. *Alzheimers Dement.* 2014;10(6):844-852.

61. Jack CR Jr, Bennett DA, Blennow K, et al. NIA-AA research framework: toward a biological definition of Alzheimer's disease. *Alzheimers Dement.* 2018;14(4):535-562.

62. *Diagnostic and Statistical Manual of Mental Disorders: DSM-5.* 5th ed. Arlington, VA: American Psychiatric Association; 2013.

63. McKhann GM, Knopman DS, Chertkow H, et al. The diagnosis of dementia due to Alzheimer's disease: recommendations from the National Institute on Aging-Alzheimer's Association workgroups on diagnostic guidelines for Alzheimer's disease. *Alzheimers Dement.* 2011;7(3):263-269.

64. Schneider JA, Arvanitakis Z, Bang W, Bennett DA. Mixed brain pathologies account for most dementia cases in community-dwelling older persons. *Neurology.* 2007;69(24):2197-2204.

65. Lyketsos CG, Lopez O, Jones B, et al. Prevalence of neuropsychiatric symptoms in dementia and mild cognitive impairment: results from the cardiovascular health study. *JAMA.* 2002;288(12):1475-1483.

66. Gonzalez-Salvador T, Lyketsos CG, Baker A, et al. Quality of life in dementia patients in long-term care. *Int J Geriatr Psychiatry.* 2000;15(2):181-189.

67. Mohamed S, Rosenheck R, Lyketsos CG, Schneider LS. Caregiver burden in Alzheimer disease: cross-sectional and longitudinal patient correlates. *Am J Geriatr Psychiatry.* 2010;18(10):917-927.

68. Murman DL, Chen Q, Powell MC, et al. The incremental direct costs associated with behavioral symptoms in AD. *Neurology.* 2002;59(11):1721-1729.

69. Yaffe K, Fox P, Newcomer R, et al. Patient and caregiver characteristics and nursing home placement in patients with dementia. *JAMA.* 2002;287(16):2090-2097.

70. Peters ME, Schwartz S, Han D, et al. Neuropsychiatric symptoms as predictors of progression to severe Alzheimer's dementia and death: the Cache County Dementia Progression Study. *Am J Psychiatry.* 2015;172(5):460-465.

71. Cummings JL, Mega M, Gray K, et al. The Neuropsychiatric Inventory: comprehensive assessment of psychopathology in dementia. *Neurology.* 1994;44(12):2308-2314.

72. Lyketsos CG, Carrillo MC, Ryan JM, et al. Neuropsychiatric symptoms in Alzheimer's disease. *Alzheimers Dement.* 2011;7(5):532-539.

73. Zhao H, Tang W, Xu X, Zhao Z, Huang L. Functional magnetic resonance imaging study of apathy in Alzheimer's disease. *J Neuropsychiatry Clin Neurosci.* 2014;26(4):134-141.

74. Steinberg M, Shao H, Zandi P, et al. Point and 5-year period prevalence of neuropsychiatric symptoms in dementia: the Cache County Study. *Int J Geriatr Psychiatry.* 2008;23(2):170-177.

75. Geda YE, Roberts RO, Mielke MM, et al. Baseline neuropsychiatric symptoms and the risk of incident mild cognitive impairment: a population-based study. *Am J Psychiatry.* 2014;171(5):572-581.

76. Masters MC, Morris JC, Roe CM. "Noncognitive" symptoms of early Alzheimer disease: a longitudinal analysis. *Neurology.* 2015;84(6):617-622.

77. Panza F, Frisardi V, Capurso C, et al. Effect of donepezil on the continuum of depressive symptoms, mild cognitive impairment, and progression to dementia. *J Am Geriatr Soc.* 2010;58(2):389-390.

78. Zhao QF, Tan L, Wang HF, et al. The prevalence of neuropsychiatric symptoms in Alzheimer's disease: systematic review and meta-analysis. *J Affect Disord.* 2016;190:264-271.

79. Sadak TI, Katon J, Beck C, Cochrane BB, Borson S. Key neuropsychiatric symptoms in common dementias: prevalence and implications for caregivers, clinicians, and health systems. *Res Gerontol Nurs.* 2014;7(1):44-52.

80. Benoit M, Berrut G, Doussaint J, et al. Apathy and depression in mild Alzheimer's disease: a cross-sectional study using diagnostic criteria. *J Alzheimers Dis.* 2012;31(2):325-334.

81. Lyketsos CG, Lee HB. Diagnosis and treatment of depression in Alzheimer's disease. A practical update for the clinician. *Dement Geriatr Cogn Disord.* 2004;17(1-2):55-64.

82. Erlangsen A, Zarit SH, Conwell Y. Hospital-diagnosed dementia and suicide: a longitudinal study using prospective, nationwide register data. *Am J Geriatr Psychiatry.* 2008;16(3):220-228.

83. Murray PS, Kumar S, Demichele-Sweet MA, Sweet RA. Psychosis in Alzheimer's disease. *Biol Psychiatry.* 2014;75(7):542-552.

84. Jeste DV, Finkel SI. Psychosis of Alzheimer's disease and related dementias. Diagnostic criteria for a distinct syndrome. *Am J Geriatr Psychiatry.* 2000;8(1):29-34.

85. Peters ME, Lyketsos CG. Beyond memory: a focus on the other neuropsychiatric symptoms of dementia. *Am J Geriatr Psychiatry.* 2015;23(2):115-118.

86. Geda YE, Schneider LS, Gitlin LN, et al. Neuropsychiatric symptoms in Alzheimer's disease: past progress and anticipation of the future. *Alzheimers Dement.* 2013;9(5):602-608.

87. Benoit M, Clairet S, Koulibaly PM, Darcourt J, Robert PH. Brain perfusion correlates of the apathy inventory dimensions of Alzheimer's disease. *Int J Geriatr Psychiatry.* 2004;19(9):864-869.

88. Lanctot KL, Moosa S, Herrmann N, et al. A SPECT study of apathy in Alzheimer's disease. *Dement Geriatr Cogn Disord.* 2007;24(1):65-72.

89. Robert PH, Darcourt G, Koulibaly MP, et al. Lack of initiative and interest in Alzheimer's disease: a single photon emission computed tomography study. *Eur J Neurol.* 2006;13(7):729-735.

90. Rosenberg PB, Nowrangi MA, Lyketsos CG. Neuropsychiatric symptoms in Alzheimer's disease: what might be associated brain circuits? *Mol Aspects Med.* 2015;43-44:25-37.

91. Marshall GA, Monserratt L, Harwood D, et al. Positron emission tomography metabolic correlates of apathy in Alzheimer disease. *Arch Neurol.* 2007;64(7):1015-1020.

92. Tunnard C, Whitehead D, Hurt C, et al. Apathy and cortical atrophy in Alzheimer's disease. *Int J Geriatr Psychiatry.* 2011;26(7):741-748.

93. MacDonald AW 3rd, Cohen JD, Stenger VA, Carter CS. Dissociating the role of the dorsolateral prefrontal and anterior cingulate cortex in cognitive control. *Science.* 2000;288(5472):1835-1838.

94. Paus T. Primate anterior cingulate cortex: where motor control, drive and cognition interface. *Nat Rev Neurosci.* 2001;2(6):417-424.

95. Zhou J, Seeley WW. Network dysfunction in Alzheimer's disease and frontotemporal dementia: implications for psychiatry. *Biol Psychiatry.* 2014;75(7):565-573.

96. Marshall GA, Fairbanks LA, Tekin S, Vinters HV, Cummings JL. Neuropathologic correlates of apathy in Alzheimer's disease. *Dement Geriatr Cogn Disord.* 2006;21(3):144-147.

97. Marshall GA, Donovan NJ, Lorius N, et al. Apathy is associated with increased amyloid burden in mild cognitive impairment. *J Neuropsychiatry Clin Neurosci.* 2013;25(4):302-307.

98. Donovan NJ, Wadsworth LP, Lorius N, et al. Regional cortical thinning predicts worsening apathy and hallucinations across the Alzheimer disease spectrum. *Am J Geriatr Psychiatry.* 2014;22(11):1168-1179.

99. Delrieu J, Desmidt T, Camus V, et al. Apathy as a feature of prodromal Alzheimer's disease: an FDG-PET ADNI study. *Int J Geriatr Psychiatry.* 2015;30(5):470-477.

100. Gatchel JR, Donovan NJ, Locascio JJ, et al. Regional 18F-fluorodeoxyglucose hypometabolism is associated with higher apathy scores over time in early Alzheimer disease. *Am J Geriatr Psychiatry.* 2017;25(7):683-693.

101. Feldman H, Gauthier S, Hecker J, et al. A 24-week, randomized, double-blind study of donepezil in moderate to severe Alzheimer's disease. *Neurology.* 2001;57(4):613-620.

102. Rosenberg PB, Lanctot KL, Drye LT, et al. Safety and efficacy of methylphenidate for apathy in Alzheimer's disease: a randomized, placebo-controlled trial. *J Clin Psychiatry.* 2013;74(8):810-816.

103. van den Elsen GA, Ahmed AI, Verkes RJ, et al. Tetrahydrocannabinol for neuropsychiatric symptoms in dementia: a randomized controlled trial. *Neurology.* 2015;84(23):2338-2346.

104. Serra L, Perri R, Cercignani M, et al. Are the behavioral symptoms of Alzheimer's disease directly associated with neurodegeneration? *J Alzheimers Dis.* 2010;21(2):627-639.

105. Minger SL, Esiri MM, McDonald B, et al. Cholinergic deficits contribute to behavioral disturbance in patients with dementia. *Neurology.* 2000;55(10):1460-1467.

106. Garcia-Alloza M, Gil-Bea FJ, Diez-Ariza M, et al. Cholinergic-serotonergic imbalance contributes to cognitive and behavioral symptoms in Alzheimer's disease. *Neuropsychologia.* 2005;43(3):442-449.

107. Bloniecki V, Aarsland D, Cummings J, Blennow K, Freund-Levi Y. Agitation in dementia: relation to core cerebrospinal fluid biomarker levels. *Dement Geriatr Cogn Dis Extra.* 2014;4(2):335-343.

108. Banno K, Nakaaki S, Sato J, et al. Neural basis of three dimensions of agitated behaviors in patients with Alzheimer disease. *Neuropsychiatr Dis Treat.* 2014;10:339-348.

109. Farber NB, Rubin EH, Newcomer JW, et al. Increased neocortical neurofibrillary tangle density in subjects with Alzheimer disease and psychosis. *Arch Gen Psychiatry.* 2000;57(12):1165-1173.

110. Sweet RA, Hamilton RL, Lopez OL, et al. Psychotic symptoms in Alzheimer's disease are not associated with more severe neuropathologic features. *Int Psychogeriatr.* 2000;12(4):547-558.

111. Sweet RA, Hamilton RL, Healy MT, et al. Alterations of striatal dopamine receptor binding in Alzheimer disease are associated with Lewy body pathology and antemortem psychosis. *Arch Neurol.* 2001;58(3):466-472.

112. Forstl H, Burns A, Levy R, Cairns N. Neuropathological correlates of psychotic phenomena in confirmed Alzheimer's disease. *Br J Psychiatry.* 1994;165(1):53-59.

113. Lyness SA, Zarow C, Chui HC. Neuron loss in key cholinergic and aminergic nuclei in Alzheimer disease: a meta-analysis. *Neurobiol Aging.* 2003;24(1):1-23.

114. Zahodne LB, Gongvatana A, Cohen RA, et al. Are apathy and depression independently associated with longitudinal trajectories of cortical atrophy in mild cognitive impairment? *Am J Geriatr Psychiatry.* 2013;21(11):1098-1106.

115. Lee DY, Choo IH, Jhoo JH, et al. Frontal dysfunction underlies depressive syndrome in Alzheimer disease: a FDG-PET study. *Am J Geriatr Psychiatry.* 2006;14(7):625-628.

116. Sultzer DL, Mahler ME, Mandelkern MA, et al. The relationship between psychiatric symptoms and regional cortical metabolism in Alzheimer's disease. *J Neuropsychiatry Clin Neurosci.* 1995;7(4):476-484.

117. Sanders AE, Nininger J, Absher J, et al. Quality improvement in neurology: dementia management quality measurement set update. *Am J Psychiatry*. 2017;174(5):493-498.

118. Association AP. *The American Psychiatric Association Practice Guideline on the Use of Antipsychotics to Treat Agitation or Psychosis in Patients with Dementia*. Washington, DC: American Psychiatric Association Publishing; 2016:218.

119. Kales HC, Gitlin LN, Lyketsos CG; Detroit Expert Panel on Assessment and Management of Neuropsychiatric Symptoms of Dementia. Management of neuropsychiatric symptoms of dementia in clinical settings: recommendations from a multidisciplinary expert panel. *J Am Geriatr Soc*. 2014;62(4):762-769.

120. Kales HC, Gitlin LN, Lyketsos CG. Assessment and management of behavioral and psychological symptoms of dementia. *BMJ*. 2015;350:h369.

121. Kaufer DI, Cummings JL, Ketchel P, et al. Validation of the NPI-Q, a brief clinical form of the Neuropsychiatric Inventory. *J Neuropsychiatry Clin Neurosci*. 2000;12(2):233-239.

122. Robert P, Onyike CU, Leentjens AF, et al. Proposed diagnostic criteria for apathy in Alzheimer's disease and other neuropsychiatric disorders. *Eur Psychiatry*. 2009;24(2):98-104.

123. Cummings J, Mintzer J, Brodaty H, et al. Agitation in cognitive disorders: International Psychogeriatric Association provisional consensus clinical and research definition. *Int Psychogeriatr*. 2015;27(1):7-17.

124. Ismail Z, Smith EE, Geda Y, et al. Neuropsychiatric symptoms as early manifestations of emergent dementia: provisional diagnostic criteria for mild behavioral impairment. *Alzheimers Dement*. 2016;12(2):195-202.

125. Gitlin LN, Kales HC, Lyketsos CG. Nonpharmacologic management of behavioral symptoms in dementia. *JAMA*. 2012;308(19):2020-2029.

126. Williams CL, Tappen RM. Exercise training for depressed older adults with Alzheimer's disease. *Aging Ment Health*. 2008;12(1):72-80.

127. Guetin S, Portet F, Picot MC, et al. Effect of music therapy on anxiety and depression in patients with Alzheimer's type dementia: randomised, controlled study. *Dement Geriatr Cogn Disord*. 2009;28(1):36-46.

128. Abraha I, Rimland JM, Trotta FM, et al. Systematic review of systematic reviews of non-pharmacological interventions to treat behavioural disturbances in older patients with dementia. The SENATOR-OnTop series. *BMJ Open*. 2017;7(3):e012759.

129. Niu YX, Tan JP, Guan JQ, Zhang ZQ, Wang LN. Cognitive stimulation therapy in the treatment of neuropsychiatric symptoms in Alzheimer's disease: a randomized controlled trial. *Clin Rehabil*. 2010;24(12):1102-1111.

130. Regan B, Varanelli L. Adjustment, depression, and anxiety in mild cognitive impairment and early dementia: a systematic review of psychological intervention studies. *Int Psychogeriatr*. 2013;25(12):1963-1984.

131. Rosenberg PB, Drye LT, Martin BK, et al. Sertraline for the treatment of depression in Alzheimer disease. *Am J Geriatr Psychiatry*. 2010;18(2):136-145.

132. Banerjee S, Hellier J, Dewey M, et al. Sertraline or mirtazapine for depression in dementia (HTA-SADD): a randomised, multicentre, double-blind, placebo-controlled trial. *Lancet*. 2011;378(9789):403-411.

133. Orgeta V, Tabet N, Nilforooshan R, Howard R. Efficacy of antidepressants for depression in Alzheimer's disease: systematic review and meta-analysis. *J Alzheimers Dis*. 2017;58(3):725-733.

134. Bartels C, Wagner M, Wolfsgruber S, et al. Impact of SSRI therapy on risk of conversion from mild cognitive impairment to Alzheimer's dementia in individuals with previous depression. *Am J Psychiatry*. 2018;175(3):232-241.

135. Ruthirakuhan MT, Herrmann N, Abraham EH, Chan S, Lanctot KL. Pharmacological interventions for apathy in Alzheimer's disease. *Cochrane Database Syst Rev*. 2018;5:CD012197.

136. Reus VI, Fochtmann LJ, Eyler AE, et al. The American Psychiatric Association practice guideline on the use of antipsychotics to treat agitation or psychosis in patients with dementia. *Am J Psychiatry*. 2016;173(5):543-546.

137. Schneider LS, Tariot PN, Dagerman KS, et al. Effectiveness of atypical antipsychotic drugs in patients with Alzheimer's disease. *N Engl J Med*. 2006;355(15):1525-1538.

138. Sultzer DL, Davis SM, Tariot PN, et al. Clinical symptom responses to atypical antipsychotic medications in Alzheimer's disease: phase 1 outcomes from the CATIE-AD effectiveness trial. *Am J Psychiatry*. 2008;165(7):844-854.

139. Katz I, de Deyn PP, Mintzer J, et al. The efficacy and safety of risperidone in the treatment of psychosis of Alzheimer's disease and mixed dementia: a meta-analysis of 4 placebo-controlled clinical trials. *Int J Geriatr Psychiatry*. 2007;22(5):475-484.

140. Schneider LS, Dagerman K, Insel PS. Efficacy and adverse effects of atypical antipsychotics for dementia: meta-analysis of randomized, placebo-controlled trials. *Am J Geriatr Psychiatry*. 2006;14(3):191-210.

141. Lonergan E, Luxenberg J, Colford J. Haloperidol for agitation in dementia. *Cochrane Database Syst Rev*. 2002(2):CD002852.

142. Kales HC, Kim HM, Zivin K, et al. Risk of mortality among individual antipsychotics in patients with dementia. *Am J Psychiatry*. 2012;169(1):71-79.

143. Porsteinsson AP, Drye LT, Pollock BG, et al. Effect of citalopram on agitation in Alzheimer disease: the CitAD randomized clinical trial. *JAMA*. 2014;311(7):682-691.

144. Leonpacher AK, Peters ME, Drye LT, et al. Effects of citalopram on neuropsychiatric symptoms in Alzheimer's dementia: evidence from the CitAD study. *Am J Psychiatry*. 2016;173(5):473-480.

145. Tariot PN, Schneider LS, Cummings J, et al. Chronic divalproex sodium to attenuate agitation and clinical progression of Alzheimer disease. *Arch Gen Psychiatry*. 2011;68(8):853-861.

146. Cooney C, Murphy S, Tessema H, Freyne A. Use of low-dose gabapentin for aggressive behavior in vascular and mixed vascular/Alzheimer dementia. *J Neuropsychiatry Clin Neurosci*. 2013;25(2):120-125.

147. Suzuki H, Gen K. Clinical efficacy of lamotrigine and changes in the dosages of concomitantly used psychotropic drugs in Alzheimer's disease with behavioural and psychological symptoms of dementia: a preliminary open-label trial. *Psychogeriatrics*. 2015;15(1):32-37.

148. Sommer OH, Aga O, Cvancarova M, et al. Effect of oxcarbazepine in the treatment of agitation and aggression in severe dementia. *Dement Geriatr Cogn Disord*. 2009;27(2):155-163.

149. American Geriatrics Society Beers Criteria® Update Expert Panel. American Geriatrics Society 2019 Updated AGS Beers Criteria(R) for Potentially Inappropriate Medication Use in Older Adults. *J Am Geriatr Soc*. 2019;67(4):674-694.

150. Camargos EF, Louzada LL, Quintas JL, et al. Trazodone improves sleep parameters in Alzheimer disease patients: a randomized, double-blind, and placebo-controlled study. *Am J Geriatr Psychiatry*. 2014;22(12):1565-1574.

151. McCleery J, Cohen DA, Sharpley AL. Pharmacotherapies for sleep disturbances in dementia. *Cochrane Database Syst Rev*. 2016;11:CD009178.

152. Scoralick FM, Louzada LL, Quintas JL, et al. Mirtazapine does not improve sleep disorders in Alzheimer's disease: results from a double-blind, placebo-controlled pilot study. *Psychogeriatrics*. 2017;17(2):89-96.

The Neuropsychiatry of Stroke

Hope Schwartz · John Sullivan · Daniel Talmasov · Laura T. Safar

INTRODUCTION

Stroke is the fifth leading cause of death in the United States and an important cause of disability. Every year, about 795,000 people in the United States have a stroke. About 610,000 of these are first or new strokes; 185,000 are recurrent strokes.[1] Stroke is characterized by the sudden occurrence of a neurologic deficit or syndrome. Typically, especially as it pertains to physical symptoms, the resultant neurologic syndrome corresponds to the portion of the brain supplied by the respective cerebral vessels affected by the stroke (see Figures 22-1 and 22-2). Strokes are broadly categorized as ischemic or hemorrhagic.[2] The underlying cause of the vascular occlusion in ischemic strokes may be: (i) atherosclerosis with superimposed thrombosis, affecting large cerebral or extracerebral blood vessels (Figure 22-3), (ii) cerebral embolism, and (iii) occlusion of small cerebral vessels within the parenchyma of the brain. Alternative pathologic processes that may result in ischemic brain damage include arterial dissection, inflammatory conditions such as vasculitis, thrombosis of cerebral veins, and dural sinuses, thrombosis of cerebral vessels due to hypercoagulable conditions, vasospasm, and other mechanisms. Hemorrhagic strokes (Figure 22-4) are caused by the rupture of blood vessels and subsequent bleeding into the brain parenchyma (intracerebral hemorrhage) or the subarachnoid space (Figure 22-5). Contributing factors to hemorrhagic strokes are weakened blood vessels, for instance due to aneurysms or arteriovenous malformations, and hypertension. Hemorrhagic strokes typically do not respect vascular territories and thus may result in more complex syndromes.

The focus of this chapter is the neuropsychiatric disorders and symptoms that may occur as a consequence of stroke. This includes the discussion of post-stroke depression (PSD), anxiety, mania, and psychosis, apathy, emotional aprosodia, and pathological laughing and crying. In addition, this chapter reviews the topic of vascular depression, a disorder characterized by depression, executive dysfunction, and subcortical microvascular disease.

POST-STROKE DEPRESSION

PSD is diagnosed based on the temporal relationship between a clinically apparent stroke and the onset of depression. Unlike idiopathic major depressive disorder, PSD primarily has onset late in life. It has modifiable risk factors, which coincide with the risk factors for cerebrovascular disease itself. Anticipation, recognition, and treatment of depression associated with cerebrovascular disease can reduce its morbidity, and improve outcomes related to vascular disease itself.[3]

Epidemiology

It is estimated that 6.8 million Americans over the age of 20 have suffered a stroke, with an annual incidence of approximately 795,000.[4] Among the approximately 75% who survive a stroke, one-third will experience PSD, significantly higher than the incidence in the general population, which ranges from 5% to 13%.[5] A study of 4022 patients followed for 15 years in the South London Stroke Register estimated a cumulative incidence of PSD of 55%, with greatest risk in the first year after stroke and 33% of cases occurring in the first 3 months.[6-8] The most consistent predictors of PSD include physical disability, stroke severity, and cognitive impairment.[5] Two large systematic reviews identified lack of family and social support, history of depression, and post-stroke anxiety as additional risk factors for PSD.[7-9] Confounding the relationship between post-stroke impairment and PSD, however, is the observation that the presence of PSD worsens outcomes and increases the degree of residual disability after stroke.[10]

Pathophysiology

Several factors may mediate the development of depression in neurological illnesses, including both psychosocial and biological etiologies. Psychologically, the experience of stroke as a sudden loss of physical, verbal, or cognitive function, and the immediate onset of significant disability is a traumatic

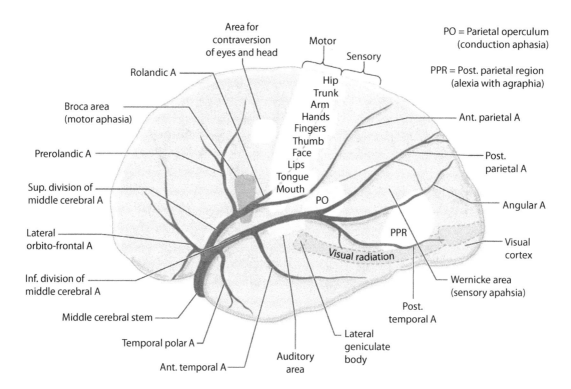

FIGURE 22-1. Diagram of the left cerebral hemisphere, lateral aspect, showing the courses of the middle cerebral artery and its branches and the principal regions of cerebral localization. Below are the lists of the clinical manifestations of infarction in the territory of this artery and the corresponding regions of cerebral damage. (Reproduced with permission from Ropper AH, Samuels MA, Klein JP, Prasad S. Stroke and cerebrovascular diseases. In: *Adams and Victor's Principles of Neurology.* 11th ed. https://accessmedicine.mhmedical.com. Copyright © McGraw Hill LLC. All rights reserved.)

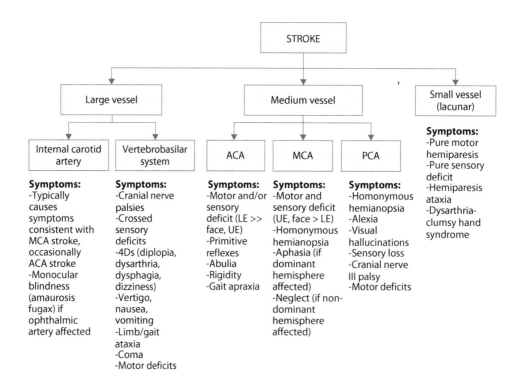

FIGURE 22-2. Clinical characteristics of stroke dependent on vascular territory affected. ACA, anterior cerebral artery; LE, lower extremity; MCA, middle cerebral artery; PCA, posterior cerebral artery; UE, upper extremity. (Reproduced with permission from Mitra R. Stroke rehabilitation. In: *Principles of Rehabilitation Medicine.* https://accessmedicine.mhmedical.com. Copyright © McGraw Hill LLC. All rights reserved.)

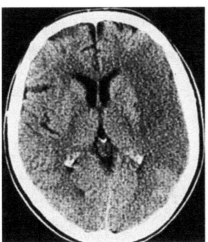 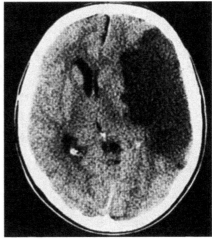

FIGURE 22-3. Large ischemic infarction of the left cerebral hemisphere mainly in the distribution of the superior division of the middle cerebral artery. CT at 24 hours (left) and 72 hours (right) following the onset of stroke symptoms. The second scan (right) demonstrates marked swelling of the infarcted tissue and rightward displacement of central structures. (Reproduced with permission from Ropper AH, Samuels MA, Klein JP, Prasad S. Stroke and cerebrovascular diseases. In: *Adams and Victor's Principles of Neurology*. 11th ed. https://accessmedicine.mhmedical.com. Copyright © McGraw Hill LLC. All rights reserved.)

experience, and PSD shares some of its origins in the reactive nature of depression that emerges in the wake of any significant medical diagnosis or illness. The relationship between severity of post-stroke physical and cognitive impairment and development of PSD symptoms supports the theory that PSD may arise in part from challenges of coping with medical sequelae of the injury itself.[11,12] However, larger physical and cognitive impairments may imply a larger stroke. In addition, the stroke location can contribute directly, by affecting the neurocircuitry mediating mood, to more severe depression. Although there is ongoing debate about whether lesion location increases the likelihood of developing PSD, evidence suggests that infarcts in the left frontal lobe and basal ganglia are more likely to precipitate depression. Although not consistently observed, PSD seems to correlate with the proximity of the infarct to the anterior pole of the left frontal lobe.[13,14] This correlation was not observed among patients with right-hemisphere stroke.[13] A prospective study of 68 first-time ischemic stroke patients demonstrated a relationship between lesions disrupting the left limbic-cortical-striatal-palladial-thalamic circuit and PSD onset. PSD was specifically associated with lesions of the ventral ACC, dorsal ACC, subgenual cortex, amygdala, and subiculum.[15]

Changes in monoamine neurotransmitters may also be involved in the development of PSD, with serotonergic system disruption specifically implicated in PSD.[16,17] Rodent models of stroke have shown ipsilateral depletion of serotonin, norepinephrine, and dopamine after stroke, and reduction of monoamine metabolites has been demonstrated in the CSF of human patients with PSD, suggesting alterations of the monoaminergic circuits as a consequence of the stroke. PET imaging of 5-HT2 receptors shows evidence of greater upregulation of serotonin receptors in the right hemisphere compared to the left in patients with depression after a right-hemisphere stroke. This finding supports the hypothesis of monoamine alterations

leading to PSD.[18] Proinflammatory cytokines resulting from the underlying cerebrovascular injury may play a role in disrupting serotonin synthesis and disrupting the HPA axis, further contributing to depressive symptoms.[19] Small studies of the role of genetic factors in PSD risk have indicated that higher serotonin transporter gene (SLC6A4) methylation in the presence of the s/s (short/short alleles) 5-HTTLPR genotype, as well as higher BDNF gene methylation and BDNF polymorphism val66met, were independently associated with incident PSD.[20,21]

Clinical Presentation

Symptoms of PSD do not significantly differ from those of idiopathic major depressive disorder. Because of overlapping symptoms of stroke and depression (e.g., changes in energy, sleep, appetite, libido, and cognition), several studies have examined the validity of DSM criteria for major depression in the setting of stroke. Adjusting diagnostic criteria, however, to account for the origin of neurovegetative symptoms (i.e., attempts to exclude symptoms judged to be direct sequelae of the stroke) does not improve the sensitivity or specificity of DSM criteria for major depressive disorder in the setting of stroke.[22] In sum, DSM criteria for major depressive disorder are sensitive and apply to PSD as well. Several screening measures may aid in the diagnosis of PSD, displaying high sensitivity in the post-stoke setting. These include the Center of Epidemiological Studies-Depression Scale (CES-D), Hamilton Depression Rating Scale (HDRS), and Patient Health Questionnaire (PHQ-9).[5] The symptoms of PSD do not differentiate it from other forms of late-life depression. The particular presentation of individual cases likely depends on the lesion location and the extent of disability, combined with the individual's reaction to the stroke due to the new and potentially traumatic onset of functional impairment.

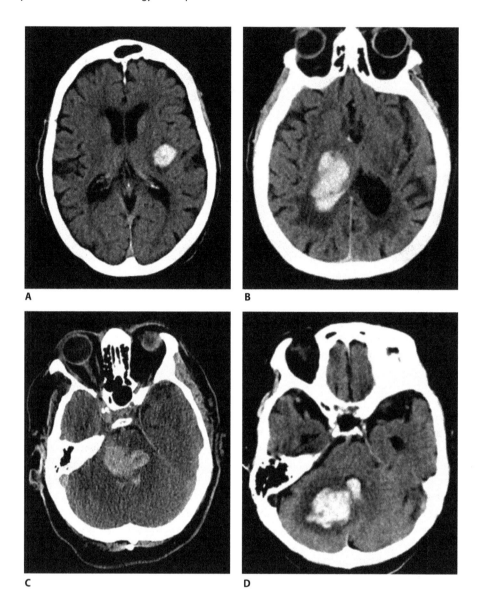

FIGURE 22-4. Unenhanced CT showing hypertensive hemorrhages in the putamen **(A)**, thalamus **(B)**, pons **(C)**, and cerebellum **(D)**. The thalamic hemorrhage (B) has extended into the posterior horn of the right lateral ventricle and the cerebellar hemorrhage (D) has extended into the fourth ventricle. (Reproduced with permission from Ropper AH, Samuels MA, Klein JP, Prasad S. Stroke and cerebrovascular diseases. In: *Adams and Victor's Principles of Neurology.* 11th ed. https://accessmedicine.mhmedical.com. Copyright © 2019 McGraw Hill LLC. All rights reserved.)

Course and Natural History

The course of PSD has been examined in several longitudinal studies, but the conclusions have been inconsistent and the degree of treatment in most case series has not been clearly delineated. There is some consensus, however, that depressive symptoms that emerge rapidly, within hours to days of stroke, tend to peak within 3–6 months of onset and approximately 50% experience remission by 1 year. Patients who develop the onset of depression 2 months after stroke or later, however, typically have a more protracted course, and up to 50% remain depressed 2 years after their stroke. One confounding factor is the degree of physical disability, which correlates with risk of depression; patients with greater disability tend to be overrepresented in the hospital and rehabilitation settings where patients have been

recruited for many of these studies.[23] The early identification and treatment of PSD has important implications for both medical and psychiatric outcomes from stroke. Patients with PSD are more likely to have worse functional outcomes with lower participation in rehabilitation, lower QOL, and higher mortality (especially in patients under 65).[5]

Assessment and Differential Diagnosis

Lack of awareness of the high prevalence of PSD, misattribution of depressive symptoms to physical consequences of the stroke, and perception that the patient's distress may be an "appropriate" reaction to stroke all likely lead to the underdiagnosis of PSD. Recognition of this entity, however, is important, because appropriate treatment of depression can alleviate the

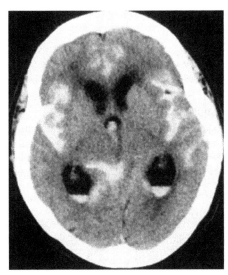
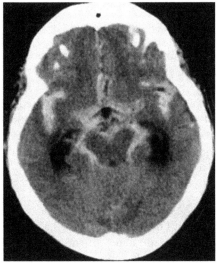

FIGURE 22-5. Subarachnoid hemorrhage as a result of rupture of a basilar artery aneurysm. **Left**: Axial CT at the level of the lateral ventricles showing widespread hyperdense blood in the subarachnoid spaces and layering within the ventricles with resultant hydrocephalus. There is a blood-CSF level in the posterior horns of the lateral ventricles, typical of recent bleeding. **Right**: At the level of the basal cisterns, blood can be seen surrounding the brainstem, in the anterior sylvian fissures, and the anterior interhemispheric fissure. The temporal horns of the lateral ventricles are enlarged, reflecting acute hydrocephalus. (Reproduced with permission from Ropper AH, Samuels MA, Klein JP, Prasad S. Stroke and cerebrovascular diseases. In: *Adams and Victor's Principles of Neurology.* 11th ed. https://accessmedicine.mhmedical.com. Copyright © 2019 McGraw Hill LLC. All rights reserved.)

suffering of the depressed patient as well as improve rehabilitation outcomes. As discussed, DSM criteria for major depressive disorder are sensitive and specific for PSD. The defining characteristic of this entity is onset after a clinically apparent stroke. Other symptoms can emerge after stroke, however, that can complicate or confound the diagnosis of depression. The most common post-stroke symptom that mimics depression is apathy. Apathy is a reduction of motivation not attributable to emotional distress, cognitive impairment, or level of consciousness.[24] Apathy is also a common feature of depression and is included on the Hamilton Depression Rating Scale. However, several studies and reviews demonstrate that apathy and depression are not always correlated and can be differentiated.[25] A case series[26] compared apathy and depression levels across stroke, Alzheimer's disease, and idiopathic major depression. While the relationship between apathy and depression varied among the groups, patients with major depression or left-hemisphere stroke tended to have higher depression scores and lower apathy scores. Patients with right-hemisphere stroke had high levels of both apathy and depression, although these symptoms did not correlate with each other in this group. A longitudinal study of patients with PSD found that within 3 months of a stroke, levels of apathy and depression did not correlate, but that a correlation emerged over time and was significant at 1 year. Both apathy and depression were predicted by the presence of dementia, but depression was independently predicted by psychosocial factors, such as not living with a family member. Although the correlation increased, there were a significant number of patients at 1 year who demonstrated apathy or depression, but not both.[27]

Although apathy and depression are likely related to the disruption of frontal-subcortical networks, distinguishing the two phenomena has treatment implications: apathy is less likely to be responsive to antidepressants[28] than PSD. When apathy occurs after stroke, careful assessment for other symptoms of depression is required to differentiate the two syndromes. If apathy coexists with depression, the treatment of both syndromes may be indicated.

Treatment

Treatment of PSD is important, as degree of depressive symptoms negatively correlates with rehabilitation potential[3] and post-stroke outcomes.

Psychopharmacological Treatment

Numerous studies comparing antidepressants against alternate agents or placebo have demonstrated widely varying efficacy in antidepressant treatment for PSD. The range of study types, enrollment criteria, and means of assessment make it difficult to draw firm conclusions, but several studies have demonstrated efficacy of antidepressant agents in this population. The most commonly studied agents are selective serotonin reuptake inhibitors (SSRIs) and tricyclic antidepressants (TCAs). In general, antidepressants from either class outperform placebo, although placebo response is high, which is typical for antidepressant trials. Nortriptyline has been shown to significantly outperform both fluoxetine and placebo.[23] Tricyclic agents may be effective, but their use is limited by their adverse effects. Patients with PSD tend to be elderly and are more likely to have vascular disease. Anticholinergic effects and risk of cardiac arrhythmias may lead most clinicians to reject these agents in favor of SSRI antidepressants. SSRIs, particularly fluoxetine, may have the added benefit of improving motor recovery—in the FLAME trial, a double-blind, placebo-controlled study of 231 ischemic stroke patients showed that 20 mg fluoxetine plus physiotherapy outperformed physiotherapy alone in motor recovery outcomes at 3 months.[29]

Several case series and chart reviews have demonstrated the safety and tolerability of psychostimulants in PSD, but data on effectiveness are limited. One placebo-controlled trial of 21 patients in the rehabilitation setting showed that methylphenidate (30 mg/day) improved depressive symptoms and motor recovery.[30] Stimulants may be used an adjunct therapy with SSRIs, especially with comorbid cognitive impairment or fatigue, but cardiovascular side effects should be carefully considered and monitored.[5]

Brain Stimulation Therapies

Two retrospective chart reviews have demonstrated the safety and efficacy of ECT for PSD, with some patients receiving treatment within 1 month of stroke.[31] Repetitive transcranial magnetic stimulation (rTMS) has growing evidence for use in recovery of motor and cognitive stroke symptoms, as well as management of post-stroke central pain, but evidence for its efficacy in PSD is limited.[32,33]

Psychosocial Treatment

Post-stroke patients struggle with issues of loss of function and many times loss of independence. They may depend on caregivers and the inclusion of caregivers in treatment may increase effectiveness of the interventions. The potential for rehabilitation may change the dynamics of the relationship with caregivers over time. Different approaches including cognitive behavioral therapy (CBT), mindfulness-based interventions, and acceptance and commitment therapy have been used. While the evidence of benefit of psychotherapy in this population has been limited,[34] small trials of brief psychosocial interventions (6–20 sessions) have shown some benefit in treating PSD.[5]

POST-STROKE ANXIETY

Epidemiology

Anxiety disorders are among the most prevalent psychiatric disorders, with up to 33.7% lifetime prevalence in the general population. They include general anxiety disorder (GAD), panic disorder, social anxiety disorder (SAD), obsessive-compulsive disorder (OCD), and post-traumatic stress disorder (PTSD).[35] While all anxiety disorders described in the DSM have been reported after stroke, GAD is the most commonly described.[36] A meta-analysis of 44 observational studies reported the prevalence of anxiety as 20% in the first month after stroke, 23% in months 2 through 5, and 24% after 6 months.[37] Additional studies report post-stroke anxiety prevalence of 3–30%, with over half of patients experiencing anxiety in the 10 years after injury.[38–40]

Several factors increase risk for post-stroke anxiety, including young age (below 65 years old), female gender, inability to work, premorbid anxiety or depression, and smoking or alcohol abuse, with stroke severity contributing additional risk.[40,41] A longitudinal study of 101 acute stroke patients found that anxiety prevalence remained constant over a 3-year period (even as depression prevalence declined) and was most affected by female gender and previous anxiety diagnoses.[42] Premorbid

cognitive function, particularly cognitive speed, has been associated with the development of anxiety 3 months post-stroke.[43]

Limited research examines the effect of premorbid anxiety on risk of stroke. A prospective study of 2625 community-dwelling individuals found no association between HADS-A score and stroke, with no differences reported between anxiety disorder subtypes.[44] Anxiety post-stroke is associated with decreased quality of life and functional outcomes, including dependence and social network size.[45,46] Ample literature supports a relationship between post-stroke anxiety and depression, with co-occurrence rates between 17% and 80% reported.[37,47]

Pathophysiology

The relationship between lesion location and neuropsychiatric outcomes is difficult to assess due to small sample sizes and suboptimal imaging data, with studies relying on CT rather than MRI.[48] In a cross-sectional study of 693 acute stroke admissions with MRI, right frontal infarcts were associated with an increased rate of post-stroke anxiety.[48] This research supports previous findings in TBI patients linking right orbitofrontal lesions to development of anxiety symptoms.[49] Neurocircuitry models of anxiety describe the interaction between the amygdala and cortices, implicating the amygdala in the generation of fear responses and the medial and ventromedial prefrontal cortex in fear extinction.[50] Research in rodent and primate models suggest that frontal lesions may lead to dysregulated top-down control of negative emotion, which contributes to anxiety disorders.[51–53] In human subjects, medial orbitofrontal cortex abnormalities are associated with trait anxiety,[54] and functional imaging studies reveal decreased connectivity between the amygdala and medial prefrontal cortex in several anxiety disorders including SAD, PTSD, and GAD.[55] However, the effect of lesion location in post-stroke anxiety remains poorly understood. A meta-analysis of 5760 stroke patients found no statistically significant relationship between lesion location and development of post-stroke anxiety.[37] Comorbid anxiety and depression seem to be more likely associated with lesions in the left hemisphere; however, anxiety without depression seems to be more likely associated with lesions in the right hemisphere.[46] Cerebral atrophy is associated with development of chronic depression and anxiety but is not associated with psychiatric symptoms in the acute stage.[46]

The development of post-stroke anxiety disorders may be mediated by the trauma of the cerebrovascular event itself and the psychological distress of extended hospitalization and rehabilitation. Iatrogenic PTSD is well-described in acute medical illness, including asthma, myocardial infarction, and physical trauma.[56,57] A review of 1138 stroke and TIA survivors found that up to one-fourth of hospitalized patients may develop significant PTSD symptoms related to the cerebrovascular event.[58] Negative cognitive appraisal,[56] poor coping strategies, and an unfavorable psychosocial environment contribute to the severity of neuropsychiatric outcomes post-stroke.[41] In a 2-year longitudinal study of 142 stroke patients, anxiety was associated with greater functional impairment and depression scores in the 2 years after stroke.[59] Increased comorbidities, disability, and recurrent stroke or TIA have also been implicated in post-stroke anxiety disorders.[60]

The relationship between stroke and anxiety also may be influenced by genetics. One study associates tryptophan hydroxylase 2 (TPH2) polymorphisms with development of post-stroke anxiety in a Han Chinese sample.[61] This research supports previous reports linking TPH2 variants with anxiety-related disorders.[62,63] TPH is the rate-limiting step in serotonin synthesis, and dysregulated TPH2 expression in rodent models is associated with alterations in serotonergic pathways that cause increased anxiety-related behavior.[64]

Clinical Presentation

The phenomenology of post-stroke anxiety disorders is diverse, and may include GAD, panic disorder, SAD, OCD, and PTSD. The DSM describes GAD as excessive anxiety and worry that is difficult to control and occurs more often than not, for a period of at least 6 months, with a negative impact on daily functioning and well-being.[65] Criteria require at least three additional symptoms, including restlessness, decreased energy, poor concentration, irritability nervous tension, or insomnia.[65] While GAD is the most commonly described subtype of anxiety in the post-stroke population, phobic disorders, especially agoraphobia, may also be a frequent presentation of post-stroke anxiety.[66] In a prospective study of 175 stroke patients 3 months post-injury, 10% displayed phobic disorders, while 7% displayed both phobic disorders and GAD, and 4% displayed GAD only.[45] Phobic disorders included agoraphobia, social phobia, and specific injury-related fears such as recurrence, headache, physical exertion, and falls.[45] Even in the absence of a formal diagnosis of an anxiety disorder, subthreshold fears specific to functional status or stroke recurrence may significantly impact quality of life.[67,68] Anxiety is commonly comorbid with PSD and may worsen the prognosis of depressive disorders.[37,69] Given the substantial co-occurrence of depression and anxiety in post-stroke patients, it is important to consider and treat anxiety in patients diagnosed with PSD.[47] Patients with comorbid depression are at greater risk of developing chronic or long-standing anxiety.[42]

Ample research suggests that post-stroke anxiety negatively impacts the course of recovery from stroke. Patients with anxiety had greater functional and social limitations and lower quality of life 3 months post-stroke.[40,45,69] However, a study of global cognitive performance (measured by MMSE) showed no relationship between post-stroke anxiety and cognitive impairment in the acute phase or long-term follow-up in 142 patients.[69] The limited studies on the time course and natural history of post-stroke anxiety show that patients who develop anxiety in the acute phase tend to remain anxious in medium and long-term follow-up. In a 6-month, prospective study of 532 consecutive stroke survivors, 40% of patients with initial anxiety continued to experience anxiety at 6 months, while 7% of initially non-anxious patients developed new-onset anxiety at 6 months.[70] In additional longitudinal studies, rates of post-stroke anxiety remain high at 3 and 10 years after diagnosis, and patients who had not recovered by 1 year were at significant risk for developing chronic anxiety.[40,46] A longitudinal study of 220 patients found that prevalence of anxiety 5 years after stroke was 29%, significantly higher than at 6 months after stroke, indicating that new-onset anxiety may develop even after the acute recovery phase.[71]

Assessment and Differential Diagnosis

Psychiatric needs often go unaddressed in the acute hospitalization post-stroke. In a survey of 1251 post-stroke patients in the United Kingdom, dissatisfaction with the psychological services was widespread.[72] Anxiety in the post-stoke population remains less recognized or studied than PSD.[37] Several factors contribute to underdiagnosis of anxiety in post-stroke patients. There is substantial overlap between symptoms of anxiety and sequalae of the cerebrovascular event itself, including fatigue and sleep disturbance.[37] Characteristics of the patient population represented in acute stroke survivors, such as advanced age and limited verbal ability, are associated with difficultly diagnosing anxiety.[73]

The hallmark of post-stroke anxiety is onset after an acute stroke. Clinical characteristics include worry, restlessness, decreased energy, poor concentration, irritation, nervous tension, and insomnia.[41] The differential diagnosis includes medical conditions that may present with similar symptoms, including endocrine (hyperthyroidism, pheochromocytoma, or hyperparathyroidism), cardiopulmonary (arrhythmia or obstructive pulmonary diseases), sequelae of the stroke itself, or comorbid neurological illnesses.[74] Given detailed medication monitoring in the hospital setting, substance use or withdrawal are less likely but should be ruled out.[74] Complicating the differential diagnosis is the increased likelihood of comorbidity with another psychiatric condition. Patients with generalized anxiety often meet criteria for major depressive disorder, and anxiety commonly co-occurs with other mood disorders.[75] As discussed above, it is important to consider and address anxiety in patients diagnosed with PSD.

Validated, patient-reported scales can be used to supplement clinical interview and patient history. The Hospital Anxiety and Depression Scale (HADS) is a 14-item self-assessment questionnaire that measures depression and anxiety and was developed for use in nonpsychiatric hospital settings.[76] In a review of eight screening tools for anxiety, HADS was the only tool with adequate sensitivity and specificity in the post-stroke population.[37] The HADS-Anxiety subscale is the most commonly used in post-stroke anxiety research, though several studies using the HADS-A suggest that lower cutoff scores in post-stroke patients versus the general population should be considered for greater clinical validity.[77-82] In patients who are unable to self-report symptoms of anxiety, the Behavioral Outcomes of Anxiety (BOA) scale reported by the caregiver has shown adequate sensitivity and specificity in a small sample of post-stroke survivors but has yet to be validated on a large scale.[83] The Beck Anxiety Inventory, Hamilton Anxiety and Depression Scale, and General Health Questionnaire-30 have also been used in studies of post-stroke patients.[59,84] Given the correlation between early-onset post-stoke anxiety and previous psychiatric disorders, attention should be given to assessing premorbid psychiatric state.[59]

Treatment

Studies of optimal treatment for anxiety in the post-stroke patient population are limited. Guidance can be taken from the treatment of idiopathic anxiety, with additional consideration for patient-specific risk factors including age, cardio/cerebrovascular disease, and interactions with other medications. The timely diagnosis and treatment of anxiety post-stroke has important implications for medical and psychological outcomes. Treatment for anxiety is likely to be multimodal and include pharmacotherapy and psychosocial interventions such as patient education and lifestyle modification.[41]

Pharmacological

Pharmacological treatment for anxiety disorders may include SSRI/serotonin and norepinephrine reuptake inhibitors (SNRIs), TCAs, benzodiazepines, buspirone, and pregabalin, among others. SSRIs increase available serotonin in the brain by inhibiting serotonin reuptake by presynaptic nerve terminals and are typically prescribed for a wide variety of anxiety disorders including panic disorders, OCD, and PTSD.[85,86] Considering the frequency of comorbid depression in this population, SSRIs[47] and SNRIs may be useful in improving psychiatric outcomes by targeting symptoms of both anxiety and depression. Paroxetine with or without psychotherapy reduced symptoms of anxiety compared to standard care in patients with comorbid anxiety and depression post-stroke but is not well-studied in patients with anxiety alone.[86] In a post-stroke GAD prevention study, participants treated prophylactically with 5 mg/day or 10 mg/day of escitalopram had significantly reduced risk of developing post-stroke anxiety.[87] There is some clinical evidence that SSRIs in post-stroke patients may improve motor recovery and reduce dependence, disability, and neurological impairment, though most studies are small and heterogenous and the mechanism is poorly understood.[88-90] One large RCT of physical therapy plus fluoxetine (20 mg/day) or placebo showed enhanced motor recovery at 3 months in the fluoxetine arm.[91] SSRIs are generally well-tolerated in elderly populations, with lower anticholinergic effects than TCAs.[92] However, the known side effects of SSRIs merit additional caution in post-stroke patients. SSRIs increase bleeding risk, which should be considered in patients with risk factors for hemorrhagic stroke.[93] Patients with acute cerebrovascular events are at greater risk for cardiac arrhythmias,[94] which may be exacerbated by the risk of QTc prolongation with SSRI use.[95] SNRIs may cause hypertension, which is itself an independent risk factor for stroke.[96]

Nortriptyline has the strongest evidence base of the TCAs for anxiety after stroke. In a study of 104 post-stroke patients, nortriptyline treatment (100 mg/day) over 12 weeks significantly reduced anxiety and depression symptoms versus SSRI fluoxetine (40 mg/day) and placebo.[97] In a merged analysis, nortriptyline outperformed placebo in improving anxiety and depression symptoms in patients with comorbid PSD and GAD.[98] In elderly patients with or at-risk for cognitive impairment, and/or patients with vascular disease, the anticholinergic effects of TCAs should be avoided where possible.[99] Risk of falls due to postural hypotension should also be considered.[100] Of the TCAs, nortriptyline and desipramine have the smallest anticholinergic effect.[100]

Benzodiazepines are GABA-enhancing anxiolytics that reduce somatic symptoms of anxiety disorders including insomnia and muscle tension.[86] Benzodiazepines should generally be avoided in the elderly, and usually are not considered the first line of treatment for post-stroke anxiety, as their complications may include increased fall risk and cognitive decline, in addition to rebound insomnia and anxiety with withdrawal.[101] There is limited evidence for buspirone, a partial serotonin agonist, with one RCT of 72 subjects reporting reduction in anxiety symptoms in patients with comorbid anxiety and depression.[102] However, the quality of evidence in this study was low, with reported doses in the first week (20–30 mg/day) and second week (40–60 mg/day) but no information about weeks 3 and 4 and a high dropout rate of 22.6%.[86] Pregabalin, approved for treatment of epilepsy, fibromyalgia, and neuropathic pain, may have some clinical utility in treating both post-stroke anxiety disorders and central post-stroke pain.[103]

Psychosocial and Behavioral Interventions

There are few large-scale studies of behavioral and psychosocial interventions in post-stroke anxiety. Psychotherapy, particularly CBT with cognitive rehabilitation strategies, may be useful for improving mood and reducing symptoms of anxiety.[104-106] Studies of CBT in acquired brain injury provide strong evidence that therapeutic delivery modified for cognitive deficits increases efficacy in treating anxiety and depression.[107-109] Relaxation therapy teaches coping strategies for decreasing arousal and has shown promise in the post-stroke population. A 1-month, home-based intervention delivered by CD reduced anxiety symptoms on the HADS at 3 months, and treatment effects remained robust after 1 year.[110,111] Multimodal psychosocial interventions focusing on building patient self-efficacy and acceptance, motivational interviewing for mood, at home leisure activity, and vascular risk management have shown promise in small pilot studios and are a topic for continuing research.[112-116] Lifestyle education and modification, including efforts to improve sleep hygiene and exercise as tolerated, may help address somatic symptoms of anxiety including fatigue and restlessness.

POST-STROKE MANIA

Epidemiology

Secondary mania is a rare but potentially debilitating consequence of stroke. Quality data regarding the incidence of post-stroke mania is sparse, and to date there has been no large prospective study on the sequelae of stroke wherein patients were systemically examined for signs of mania. Retrospective case reviews report a low incidence—Starkstein et al.[117] reported only three cases of post-stroke mania in a series of 700 stroke patients (0.4%), and a smaller series reported three cases of mania in 188 stroke patients (1.6%).[118,119]

Pathophysiology

The pathophysiology of stroke-induced mania is incompletely understood. Lesions leading to the emergence of secondary mania have been hypothesized to disrupt neuroanatomic networks important in the regulation of mood, emotional modulation, reward processing, and behavior,[117,119-121] but lesion locations contributing to onset of secondary mania are anatomically heterogeneous, and it does not appear that direct damage to any single structure can be considered necessary for the emergence of secondary mania.[122] Among these heterogeneous lesion locations, stroke locations reported in association with mania have been hypothesized to be part of a ventral limbic circuit, including the right orbitofrontal and basotemporal cortices, caudate, and thalamus.[119] A recent systematic review broadens this scope, identifying associations between secondary mania and lesions in the superior frontal gyrus, medial orbitofrontal cortex, hippocampus and parahippocampal gyrus, superior and middle temporal poles, middle and inferior temporal gyrus, fusiform gyrus, anterior cingulate gyrus (ACG), and thalamus.[119,122]

Some authors, after observing that a family history of affective disorder appeared more common in patients who developed secondary mania, hypothesized that genetic loading may also play a role[123]; though sample sizes are too limited to be definitive. It has been suggested that right-hemispheric lesions are more likely to lead to secondary mania than left-sided lesions—this was supported by a recent systematic review of lesion imaging associated with secondary mania.[117,120–122] However, left-sided lesions have also been reported in association with mania.[117,119,124] A study employing network analysis using human connectome data demonstrated that diverse lesions leading to secondary mania shared common patterns of functional connectivity to orbitofrontal and temporal cortices.[125]

Clinical Presentation

The clinical manifestations of post-stroke mania are similar to those in primary mania, with characteristic symptoms including elevated or irritable mood, pressured speech, flight of ideas, grandiosity, psychomotor agitation, and insomnia/decreased subjective need for sleep.[119] The frequency of these symptoms does not appear to differ significantly between primary and secondary mania.[121] In addition to the symptoms of mania, patients affected by post-stroke mania may experience periods of depression,[126] and may exhibit cognitive dysfunction including memory disturbances for events that occur during the manic period.[127] Patients may also exhibit a wide range of additional neurologic symptoms including motor deficits, hemineglect, focal sensory deficits, and others, based on lesion location. Importantly, other neurologic deficits in post-stroke mania may go underreported, either due to a general lack of insight or anosognosia due to stroke or due to an exaggerated sense of well-being associated with the manic episode.[127]

Assessment and Differential Diagnosis

The differential diagnosis for post-stroke mania includes a primary psychiatric disorder (bipolar affective disorder, or a primary psychotic disorder), other causes of secondary mania (including mania due to a mass lesion, drug toxicity [e.g., antidepressants, corticosteroids], or metabolic effects), substance use, delirium, and mania due to other medical condition (such has hyperthyroidism, hypothyroidism, or Cushing's disease).[128] Clinicians should consider post-stroke mania in a patient with vascular risk factors who presents with mania atypical for classic bipolar disorder (e.g., first manic episode after the age of 40 years, no prior history of depression or affective disorder, no family history of bipolar illness, presence of neurologic deficits).[120]

Evaluation for post-stroke mania should begin with a thorough history, including the timing and onset of manic symptoms, the concurrence of and temporal relationship to any new neurologic deficits, screening for vascular risk factors, and screening for personal and family history of affective or psychotic disorders. Patients in whom there is ample suspicion for a secondary cause of mania should undergo further workup with neuroimaging. A brain MRI with evidence of stroke in a patient with new-onset mania and no prior history of bipolar affective disorder can be suggestive of secondary mania if there is a temporal relationship between the occurrence of a new lesion and the onset of manic symptoms.

Treatment

Treatment of patients with post-stroke mania should emphasize both the management of vascular risk factors to prevent development of an additional stroke[128] as well as treatment of the manic episode. The range of psychopharmacologic treatments employed in post-stroke mania is wide and reflects those drugs used in primary mania, but the vast majority of treatment data is on a case report level and it is difficult to draw comparisons between the relative effectiveness of different anti-manic therapies at this time.[119] Pharmacologic treatments can include lithium or valproate monotherapy,[119,127,128] other mood stabilizers (carbamazepine), and first- (haloperidol) or second-generation antipsychotics (olanzapine, risperidone, and others).[119] Clinicians should remain mindful of the potential risks and side effects when selecting an agent for treating secondary mania, especially in the stoke population (e.g., metabolic syndrome associated with some second-generation antipsychotics may worsen neurovascular risk, drug-induced parkinsonism may exacerbate gait difficulties in patients with post-stroke paresis).

POST-STROKE PSYCHOSIS

Epidemiology

Post-stroke psychosis is a relatively rare phenomenon, defined by the presence of hallucinations and/or delusions after stroke. In the post-acute phase (0–6 months), a meta-analysis of 2234 post-stroke patients estimated the 12-year incidence of psychosis at 6.7%, with 4.67% of patients experiencing delusions and 5.05% of patients experiencing hallucinations.[129] In a comprehensive, retrospective study of 1129 stroke patients in Western Australia, 6.7% developed a psychotic disorder over the 12-year follow-up period, with mean onset at 6 months following stroke.[130] In the acute setting, psychosis may be over-diagnosed due to similarities in clinical presentation to delirium, a reversible syndrome presenting with acute confusion and cognitive impairment caused by altered brain function.[65]

Reported risk factors for post-stroke psychosis include previous psychiatric history, with depression and alcohol use disorder most commonly reported in the literature.[129,131–133] Imaging studies comparing patients who developed post-stroke psychosis to lesion-matched controls suggest that preexisting subcortical atrophy and right-hemisphere lesion location may also confer increased risk.[134]

Pathophysiology

Studies looking at the neuropathological basis of delusions suggest that disrupted functional connectivity of the right frontal cortex impairs belief evaluation, prediction error signaling, internal monitoring, attentional surveillance, pragmatic communication, and perceptual integration.[131,135–137] A case series of 15 patients showing an association between right posterior temporoparietal lesions and development of delusional ideations within 24 hours of stroke onset[138] lends support to this right-hemisphere disconnection hypothesis. A small study of eight patients with right caudate strokes and age-matched controls implicates frontal-subcortical circuits connecting the frontal lobe to the basal ganglia in the formation of content-specific delusions.[132]

Clinical Presentation

Post-stroke psychosis most commonly presents as delusional disorder, including persecutory delusions, Othello syndrome, reduplicative paramnesia, and somatic delusions.[129] Schizophrenia-like psychosis with hallucinations (auditory more common than visual) and mood disorder with psychotic features have also been described.[131,134] Unlike post-stoke delirium, post-stroke psychosis is more likely to have a delayed onset similar to post-TBI psychosis, appearing several months after the cerebrovascular accident.[139] A multicenter study of 145 patients in skilled nursing facilities found that psychosis was significantly higher in patients who were not successfully discharged after 1 year; optimal management of post-stroke psychosis may improve rehabilitation outcomes.[140] Post-stroke psychosis has been associated with higher mortality rates at 10-year follow-up.[130]

Assessment and Differential Diagnosis

The delayed onset and poor prognosis of post-stroke psychosis elucidate the importance of screening, monitoring, and early intervention, including eliciting caregiver-reported symptoms during rehabilitation. The literature estimates that 14–56% of hospitalized patients over the age of 65 experience delirium.[141] While post-stroke delirium most typically occurs in the acute phase and post-stroke psychosis has a delayed onset, it is important to consider delirium in the differential diagnosis because patients with history of stroke remain at high risk for developing delirium due to their brain injury.

Treatment

Psychopharmacological treatment for post-stoke psychosis typically consists of antipsychotics. Typical or atypical antipsychotics may be used, with haloperidol and risperidone reported most frequently in the literature.[129] The side effects of antipsychotics in the post-stroke population should be carefully considered. While atypical antipsychotics are less likely to cause extrapyramidal symptoms or tardive dyskinesia, they may confer increased risk of weight gain, diabetes mellitus, and other metabolic side effects that are independent risk factors for stroke.[142,143] Antipsychotics should be avoided, if possible, in elderly patients with dementia due to increased risk of stroke and sudden death.[144]

POST-STROKE APATHY

Epidemiology

A systematic review of 19 studies found that apathy was present in 36.6% of stroke survivors, with similar rates in acute (<15 days post-injury) and post-acute phases of recovery, and was associated with greater depression and cognitive impairment.[145] One study of 76 stroke patients showed that apathy was present in 17 patients in the acute phase, and 7 of the acute apathetic patients remained apathetic at 1 year. In addition, 11 new cases of post-stroke apathy were detected at 1 year, suggesting that apathy should be assessed in both phases.[146] Post-stroke apathy is associated with poorer functional recovery, physical health, and social participation.[147–149]

Pathophysiology

The literature lacks consensus on the relationship between lesion location and post-stroke apathy risk. A recent review found an association between subcortical infarcts, specifically those involving the basal ganglia, and post-stroke apathy.[150] This finding is supported by the high prevalence of apathy in neurological conditions affecting the basal ganglia such as PSP, Parkinson's disease (PD), and Huntington's disease.[151,152] Dysfunction in frontal-subcortical circuits may result in reduced motivation mediated by the anterior cingulate.[150,153–155] Most large reviews have not found an association between apathy and laterality or anatomical location. One meta-analysis of 149 studies showed that lesion type may play a role, with hemorrhagic lesions presenting higher apathy risk in the acute phase and ischemic strokes presenting with increased apathy risk in the post-acute phase.[156]

Clinical Presentation and Diagnosis

Post-stroke apathy is marked by low motivation and presents with decreased motor, verbal, and behavioral output, often accompanied by lack of interest in activities and hobbies. While patients with PSD express low mood and sadness regarding decreased activity, patients with isolated symptoms of apathy often deny low mood and may present with emotional indifference.[157] Despite these differences, it is important to remember that besides being an independent entity, apathy can also be one of the symptoms of depression. In addition, apathetic and depressive syndromes can coexist. Though post-stroke apathy is a clinical diagnosis, validated scales may be helpful in establishing this diagnosis and differentiating the presentation from depression. For example, the Apathy Evaluation Scale is commonly used in research and validated in elderly populations and patients with neurological injury.[158–161]

Treatment

Psychopharmacological treatment of post-stroke apathy may include dopaminergic agents, including amantadine, methylphenidate-levodopa, and rotigotine, as well as stimulants to increase motivation and activation. A review of 227 patients in trials of dopamine agonists has shown promise in reducing symptoms of apathy following stroke.[162] There is some evidence for the use of stimulants for apathy, including methylphenidate and modafinil.[163,164] However, cardiovascular side effects, including heart rate and blood pressure elevation, should be carefully monitored in a post-stroke population with underlying cardiovascular risk factors.[165] Cholinergic agents such as donepezil may also be used to increase activation.[166] In a double-blind, randomized, controlled trial of 70 patients with post-stroke apathy, the nootropic nefiracetam (targeting choline, monoamine, and GABA pathways) showed that 900 mg/day significantly reduced apathy scores compared to a lower dose or placebo.[167] In the setting of comorbid depression, antidepressants with dopaminergic or noradrenergic activity may be particularly useful, including bupropion[157] or SNRIs such as levomilnacepram, milnacipram, duloxetine, and venlafaxine. A study of problem-solving therapy versus escitalopram (5–10 mg/day depending on age) found that both interventions were more effective in preventing apathy 1-year post-stroke than placebo.[168]

POST-STROKE EMOTIONAL APROSODIA

Post-stroke emotional aprosodia presents with deficits in the expression or comprehension of the emotional and social components of language—the changes in pitch, loudness, rate, or rhythm that convey a speaker's emotional intent (linguistic prosody).[169] Receptive (or sensory) aprosodia is characterized by difficulty interpreting other's emotions and decreased empathy, while expressive (or motor) aprosodia is characterized by difficulty inserting emotion into speech through prosody.[170,171] Patients may present a combination of both expressive and receptive aprosodia. Estimates of prevalence in the literature vary, ranging from 30% to 49% in the acute setting with relatively few well-characterized cohorts.[172,173]

While expression and interpretation of emotion are governed by a bilaterally distributed network, right prefrontal and temporal regions play a particularly important role

---

CASE VIGNETTE 22.1

Ms. M was a 56-year-old right-handed woman who presented to the ED with new-onset left facial weakness and numbness, and drooling. On exam, she was found to have left facial weakness sparing the forehead and left V2-V3 sensory loss. Her brain MRI showed small scattered foci of acute infarction in the right insula and right frontal lobe (MCA territory). MR angiogram showed mild atherosclerotic changes of the origin of the right ICA and left ECA without significant stenosis.

Transthoracic echocardiogram showed LVEF of 60% with diastolic dysfunction. There were no regional wall motion abnormalities. Agitated saline bubble study showed no evidence of right-to-left shunting. Left and right atrial sizes were normal. EKGs showed sinus rhythm. After discharge she had a 30-day cardiac monitor study which showed no significant arrhythmia.

Lipid profile showed markedly elevated LDL and triglycerides. HbA1C was 5.8. ESR was normal.

She had a history of obesity, HTN, hyperlipidemia, and a psychiatric history of generalized anxiety disorder (GAD) and major depressive disorder (MDD), recurrent, moderate, both in full remission by the time of the stroke. She did not smoke and had no history of alcohol or drug abuse. Her medications were HCTZ, venlafaxine XR 150 mg QAM, clonazepam 1 mg QHS.

Her father had type II DM and HTN. Her brother died at 56 of an MI and stroke; he was a smoker with DM, HTN, and hyperlipidemia. She was married and had two children.

She worked as a bank teller for 30 years and retired a short time before her stroke.

She was started on aspirin 325 mg daily, atorvastatin 80 mg daily before discharge from the hospital. On follow-up exam 2 weeks post-stroke, there was very subtle residual weakness of the left lower face, with a tendency to drool from the left side of the mouth. The rest of the exam was normal. The summary assessment was that she had a small ischemic stroke in the right MCA territory. The mechanism was likely embolic, and no cardiac source was found. She had multiple vascular risk factors and mild carotid atherosclerosis. Her stroke was likely due to artery-to-artery embolism from her carotid disease. The recommendations from neurology included secondary stroke prevention with low-dose aspirin and optimal control of her multiple risk factors (HTN, hyperlipidemia, and obesity), including a high-intensity statin agent, a low-calorie and low-fat diet, and regular aerobic exercise. She was encouraged to see her psychiatrist for exacerbation of her anxiety and mood difficulties.

At a visit with her psychiatrist 1-month post-stroke, she presented with fears about her health and about stroke recurrence. She had a feeling of impending doom. She was sleeping well at night but felt anxious throughout the day. She denied depression. She had reduced her psychiatric medications on her own because of fear of taking medications that could sedate her—she was afraid of dying during her sleep. She was now taking Clonazepam 0.5 mg QHS, and had fully stopped her venlafaxine. On mental status exam, her mood and affect were anxious. She also appeared as mildly disinhibited and labile—she was more talkative than at her baseline, and teared up easily. Her MMSE was 30/30; she drew an accurate clock and line bisection was within normal limits. She was attentive through the visit, provided a good history of recent events, and her receptive and expressive language appeared within normal limits.

The impression was that her anxiety and affect changes were likely of multifactorial origin, with contributions from her baseline psychiatric illness, psychological adjustment difficulties to stroke, discontinuation syndrome from her stopping venlafaxine, and effects of the stroke on mood and affect regulation.

Eight months after her initial presentation, she had a second stroke. Her left-sided weakness worsened and included weakness of her left arm. Brain MRI showed an acute ischemic stroke in the right basal ganglia, and MR angiogram showed no flow in the right superior division of the MCA. There was a large flow defect consistent with a large atheroma in the right carotid bulb. This did not cause significant ICA stenosis. Evaluation included telemetry showing no significant arrhythmia, transthoracic echocardiogram showing no significant lesion, no embolic source, LVEF 60%, normal RA and LA sizes, lipid profile with total cholesterol 247, triglycerides 135, HDL 57, LDL elevated to 162. An EEG which showed no epileptiform features.

She acknowledged that she was not taking her medications regularly, including the atorvastatin, before this most recent stroke. She was restarted on aspirin, atorvastatin, and venlafaxine XR 37.5 mg/day before discharge.

A 30-day cardiac rhythm monitoring study post-discharge showed no significant arrhythmia.

On neurological exam 1 month after her second stroke, she presented subtle residual weakness of the left lower face, with a trace of drooping of the left corner of the mouth. There was very mild weakness of the left arm, seen as orbiting on examination. The rest of the exam was normal. She was assessed as having a second ischemic stroke in the right MCA territory, likely embolic, due to artery-to-artery embolism.

On psychiatric examination, also 1 month after her second stroke, she again reported concerns about her health, but appeared much less anxious than previously. However, she cried very intensely during the appointment and was described by her daughter as being "very sensitive about nothing." Her daughter provided numerous examples of emotionally neutral situations (such as watching TV or having a trivial conversation) where Ms. M had crying spells that she could not explain. These crying outbursts were taking place at least once a day, most days of the week. She denied depression. She had normal levels of energy, activity, appetite, and sleep. She was enthusiastic about her participation in physical rehabilitation and was proud about her recovery. She was assessed—in addition to her baseline GAD and MDD—to present with a syndrome of pathological laughter and crying (PLC), in this case without the laughter component. Her venlafaxine XR was increased to 75 mg/day, and at follow-up 1 month later her crying spells were much diminished.

in production and perception of emotion through prosody, based on ERP, fMRI, and lesion studies.[172,174,175] Affective aprosodia is most commonly associated with lesions in the right hemisphere, and most typically occurs in right cortical versus subcortical lesions.[176-178] Emotional aprosodia following acute cerebrovascular injury is a strong indicator of right-hemisphere dysfunction—in a study of 28 hospitalized patients and age-matched controls, impairment in receptive prosody outperformed unilateral spatial neglect as a reliable measure of right-hemisphere injury.[179] Lesions in the right posterior-inferior frontal region are typically associated with motor aprosodia, while lesions in the right posterior-superior temporal region are typically associated with sensory aprosodia.[172,177,180] Patients with impaired expressive and receptive prosody are more likely to have lesions in the right anterior temporal pole, suggesting that this region may play a role in a presumed common component underlying both motor and sensory aspects of prosody.[177]

Motor aprosodia may present with flattened speech and affect, often co-occurring with difficulty expressing or interpreting facial expressions, while sensory aprosodia manifests as a lack of empathy or appropriate emotional response to others.[171,181] There may be significant variation in deficits, with some patients experiencing motor aprosodia with no sensory aprosodia, or vice versa.[171] Formal bedside testing with the Aprosodia Battery may be helpful in distinguishing flat affect due to impaired prosody from depressive or dysarthric symptoms.[171,182] The Aprosodia Battery tests spontaneous production, repetition, and comprehension of affective prosody and has been validated in a number of neurologic conditions.[176]

Early identification and treatment of emotional aprosodia have important implications for rehabilitation. Prosody impairments may significantly affect quality of life in post-stroke patients, including decreased psychological well-being, difficulties in interpersonal relationships, increased burden of care, and marital dissatisfaction.[169,183,184] In a survey of 28 caregivers, the most commonly reported sequela of right-hemisphere stroke was loss of emotional empathy.[185] A study of 49 post-stroke patients showed that affective motor aprosodia was strongly predictive of subsequent PSD 3 months post-injury.[186] Emotional aprosodia may be especially difficult to identify and treat because right-hemisphere lesions are often associated with anosognosia, in which patients fail to identify or acknowledge impairment, and/or executive/attentional deficits that may impair performance on formal testing.[169,171]

Treatment approaches for emotional aprosodia typically consist of speech therapy and cognitive rehabilitation services.[187] A limited body of literature supports the hypothesis that prosody can be improved with behavioral treatment in patients with impaired communication.[171,188,189] Cognitive-linguistic and motor-imitative therapies have shown promise in small studies, with one small study reporting that 12 of 14 subjects with acquired brain injury responded to one or both treatments.[190]

POST-STROKE PATHOLOGICAL LAUGHING AND CRYING

Pathological laughing and crying (PLC) is a syndrome characterized by frequent, brief, and intense bouts of uncontrollable crying and/or laughing, due to a neurological disorder.[191] In addition to post-stroke, PLC may be commonly associated with several other neurological conditions: Alzheimer's disease, amyotrophic lateral sclerosis, multiple sclerosis, PD, and traumatic brain injury. Other names used for this syndrome include pseudobulbar affect, emotional lability, and emotional incontinence.

Epidemiology

The prevalence of post-stroke PLC is estimated to be about 11%. This value may vary widely across studies due to the different groups evaluated (e.g., clinic-based or population-based), the definition of PLC considered, and the sensitivity/specificity of the instruments used for identifying this syndrome.[191,192]

Pathophysiology

PLC may result from lesions that disrupt the neurocircuitry involved in emotional regulation and expression.[192] Lesions of heterogeneous localization may precipitate PLC (frontal and parietal lobes, descending pathways to the brain stem, subcortical tracts involving the cerebellum),[193,194] in line with a model of an extended emotion and affect regulation neural network that can be affected at different points. A traditional view posits that the cerebral cortex is crucial for the appraisal of the contextual information of an emotional stimulus, and the modulation of the intensity, frequency, and duration of the emotional response. This top-down model proposes that emotional modulation is facilitated by cortico-bulbar pathways, and that PLC may occur due to lesions in cortex, or in these descending tracts.

A more specific description of this model proposes a volitional system, involving frontoparietal (primary motor, premotor, supplementary motor, posterior insular, dorsal ACG, primary sensory, and related parietal) corticopontine projections, and an emotional pathway, involving projections from orbitofrontal cortex, ventral ACG, anterior insular, inferior temporal, and parahippocampal areas, that regulate the amygdala. The amygdala and hypothalamus, in turn, activate the periaqueductal gray (PAG)-dorsal tegmentum (dTg) complex, which activates the displays of laughing and crying. The volitional system inhibits the emotional pathway at multiple levels. Lesions of the volitional corticopontine projections (or of their feedback or processing circuits) can produce PLC.[195]

An alternative model considers that the cerebellum plays a significant role in modulating emotional expression, and thus lesions that impact the cerebro-ponto-cerebellar pathways responsible for adjusting the automatic execution of laughter or crying can provoke PLC.[193]

Monoaminergic neurotransmitter systems and specific receptors that may be implicated in PLC include glutamatergic NMDA, muscarinic M1-3, GABA-A, dopamine D2, norepinephrine alpha-1,2, serotonin 5HT1a, 5HT1b/d, and sigma-1 receptors. This explains the efficacy of diverse pharmacological agents active in these systems in patients with PLC.[191,195,196]

Clinical Presentation

The individual with PLC presents uncontrollable episodes of crying and/or laughing that are mood-incongruent, thus not related to feelings of sadness or joy. In some individuals, there may be an underlying emotional state present (e.g., sad mood), but the affect displayed is clearly excessive with respect to the mood. Similarly, the intense affective display is incongruent with the context surrounding the individual, or a clearly exaggerated response. For instance, a sad commercial may trigger profuse, disproportionate tearfulness. PLC may present as comorbid with other neuropsychiatric disorders, including mood and cognitive disorders.[197]

Assessment and Differential Diagnosis

Obtaining a very detailed history may be sufficient to assess the presence of this syndrome. On the other hand, because of its overlap with other psychiatric disorders, the use of specific rating scales may be helpful with screening and diagnosis. The Center for Neurologic Study—Lability Scale (CNS-LS, range 7–35) is a self-report measure initially developed to assess affective lability in individuals with ALS,[198] later validated for other disorders. It includes an auxiliary subscale for episodes of anger/frustration. The presence of a mood disorder such as major depression may result in a confoundedly high score, potentially producing a false positive for PLC.[197] Similarly, a proposed cutoff score of 13 is highly sensitive but not specific. A more conservative cutoff score of 21 appears to be more accurate.[192] The Pathological Laughter and Crying Scale (PLACS, range 0–54) is a clinician-administered instrument that measures the severity of PLC symptoms. It was developed for PLC in stroke patients.[199] A proposed cutoff of >13 renders a similar PLC prevalence as the CNS-LS cutoff of >21.[192]

In terms of differential diagnoses, it is important to assess the presence of PLC or a mood disorder such as depression or bipolar disorder and its spectrum. In these mood disorders, mood and affect are congruent. However, PLC may coexist with any of these mood disorders—in this clinical situation it is advised to treat the mood disorder first, as many times this also results in resolution of the PLC manifestations. In rare cases where the bouts of laugher or crying are very stereotyped and present with alteration of consciousness, they may represent seizure activity (gelastic or dacrystic, respectively). Regular EEG, and in some cases video-monitoring EEG, may be indicated.[191]

Treatment

PLC should be treated when this syndrome is bothersome to the individual or results in social or occupational dysfunction.[191] Multiple pharmacological agents have been shown to be effective.[191,200] Tricyclic antidepressants (nortriptyline, amitriptyline, imipramine) have demonstrated to be effective for PLC[200] and nortriptyline showed efficacy specifically for post-stroke PLC in a double-blind trial.[199]

Among the SSRIs, fluoxetine, sertraline, and citalopram showed efficacy for post-stroke PLC in double-blind trials.[200] Importantly, SSRIs tend to be used at low therapeutic doses, and the therapeutic response may be evident within the first few weeks, typically sooner than in depression. The combination dextromethorphan/quinidine has proven useful for treatment of PLC in stroke.[201] Quinidine prolongs the QT interval, although at the dose used in the dextromethorphan/quinidine combination the risk is considered minor.

Lamotrigine showed effectiveness for post-stroke PLC in a case report.[202] Agents that have demonstrated effectiveness in addressing PLC in other neurological illnesses, as indicated in case reports include venlafaxine, duloxetine, reboxetine, mirtazapine,[191,203] and valproic acid.[204] They should be reserved for cases in which more established agents fail, or added therapeutic benefits (dual action on mood and pain; mood stabilizing properties) are important. Levodopa and amantadine also showed some benefit for post-stroke PLC[205] but given the limited evidence for their efficacy, these agents should be considered only when other options have failed.

VASCULAR DEPRESSION

Vascular depression is an evolving concept that arose from the observation of the correlation between depression and subcortical microvascular disease. This condition has become more widely appreciated in the age of increasingly available MRI. Although cases of depressed elderly patients with atherosclerosis have long been described, "vascular depression" was first hypothesized as a distinct syndrome when Alexopoulos et al.[206] described an association of late-life depression with impaired executive function and white matter hyperintensities on T2-weighted MRI. This suggested areas for further investigation, including involvement of frontal-subcortical circuits in idiopathic depression, and also evolved into a recognizable subtype of depression. However, there is not yet a consensus for criteria defining vascular depression, and it is not included in the *DSM-5*, which complicates attempts to investigate the syndrome. Some investigators prefer the term "subcortical ischemic depression," and others refer to "depression executive dysfunction," which describes the syndrome symptomatically, while allowing for other causes. Despite terminology differences, most investigators agree that the triad of depression onset after sixth decade, white matter hyperintensities found on MRI, and executive dysfunction comprise the core features of vascular depression. Additional features may include lack of personal or family history, persistent symptoms without discrete episodes, and lack of insight of patients into their affective symptoms.[207]

Epidemiology

Estimating the prevalence of vascular depression is complicated by the general under-recognition of late-life depression and the requirement of imaging and cognitive assessment for diagnosis. In a large cross-sectional study of 16,423 older adults, vascular depression prevalence was estimated at 3.4% of Americans aged 50 and older, approximately 2.64 million people.[208] Vascular depression was defined in terms of meeting *DSM-4* criteria for major depression within the last year, in a person with cardiovascular or cerebrovascular disease or risk factors. However, the criteria in this study do not include imaging findings or measures of cognitive impairment, and included patients with PSD,

which is a separate diagnostic entity. These factors may have led to an overestimate of prevalence. A smaller study of 783 older adults in Korea that used an imaging-based definition of vascular depression estimated the prevalence at 2.4%.[209]

Pathophysiology

Studies on the mechanism of vascular depression have centered on the MRI white matter hyperintensities which represent microvascular disease. The amount of white matter hyperintensities correlates with age, regardless of the presence of depression. There is a correlation between the white matter disease burden in the frontal lobes and the incidence of depression. Periventricular hyperintensities appear equally prevalent in depressed and nondepressed subjects. Deep white matter hyperintensities, however, have consistently been found to be more prevalent in depressed subjects, and in those with late-onset depression in particular.[210] These deep white matter lesions are thought to be disruptive to frontal-subcortical-limbic networks crucial to mood regulation, and may also disrupt temporal lobe function to a lesser extent.[211]

The correlation of executive dysfunction with white matter disease and depression suggests disruption of dorsolateral-prefrontal-striatal circuits. Post-mortem tissue analysis demonstrates that subcortical ischemia disproportionately affects the dorsolateral prefrontal cortex in patients with late-life depression,[212] and that white matter hyperintensities in vascular depression are ischemic, rather than inflammatory.[213]

Clinical Presentation

Vascular depression differs from other forms of depression in several ways, although there is significant overlap.[214] Emerging criteria for vascular depression include low energy, reduced insight, anhedonia, deficits in initiation, and slowed processing speed.[211] Executive dysfunction, commonly seen in dysfunction of the dorsolateral prefrontal cortex or its connections, is a defining characteristic of vascular depression. Vascular depression shares characteristics with frontal lobe syndromes, particularly those arising from dysfunction of medial or dorsolateral prefrontal cortices. On neuropsychological testing, patients with vascular depression may demonstrate difficulty with task completion, decision making, processing speed, concentration, and attention.[207] These cognitive deficits are often paired with irritability and social withdrawal, although cognitive symptoms may be more pronounced and troubling to the patient than mood symptoms.[207] Anhedonia as a major symptom is more common in vascular depression than subjectively depressed or low mood. Family history of mood disorder is less common in vascular depression than in idiopathic depression.

Course and Natural History

The clinical course of vascular depression is similar to that of refractory major depression in that it generally becomes a chronic condition and tends not to respond to antidepressant treatment. Progression of white matter disease is a risk factor for the onset of vascular depression,[215] but it is not known whether progression of subcortical vascular disease in an individual patient correlates with worsened depression. Patients with diagnosed vascular depression are at increased risk for dementia, as microvascular disease causes subcortical vascular depression and also exacerbates dementia from other etiologies, such as Alzheimer's disease. A meta-analysis of 23 studies found that late-life depression, including vascular depression, increased the risk of Alzheimer's disease dementia and vascular dementia.[216] An MRI-based study of 161 older depressed subjects showed that both white matter hyperintensity volume and subcortical gray matter hyperintensity volume were associated with incident dementia.[217] Vascular depression tends to decrease ability to manage medical comorbidities, and is associated with increased impairments in daily functioning, frailty, and shortened life span.[218,219] Even if mood symptoms do not meet DSM criteria for major depression, subthreshold depressive disorders are associated with increased mortality, and decreased functional status and quality of life.[220]

Assessment and Differential Diagnosis

The presence of executive dysfunction in vascular depression may lead to some confusion over whether a given patient's symptoms represent depression or dementia. The syndrome of "reversible dementia of depression," also known as "pseudodementia," has long been described, with deficits not only of memory but also of executive function. Concern over this syndrome has been that clinicians often overlook depressive symptoms in the presence of cognitive impairment in elderly patients. Awareness of the entity of vascular depression, however, introduces a third consideration in addition to the possible diagnoses of idiopathic depression and dementia due to neurodegenerative process. Vascular depression comprises symptoms of both depression and executive dysfunction and shares features with depression and dementia of other etiologies. Diagnosis of vascular depression, however, implies the presence of microvascular disease, demonstrated by subcortical white matter hyperintensities on T2-weighted MRI. Brain imaging in this setting may help distinguish among idiopathic depression and vascular depression in elderly patients or patients with significant vascular risk factors. Given the high prevalence of white matter hyperintensities in older patients, MRI findings may be read as normal or unremarkable for age. However, in the context of clinical depressive and cognitive symptoms, the presence of imaging-defined cerebrovascular disease, indicated by deep white matter and periventricular hyperintensities as well as subcortical gray matter lesions, may be an important diagnostic clue.[207]

The syndrome of apathy can also present a diagnostic challenge. Apathy and executive dysfunction may present as features of vascular depression, but also can signify the emergence of a neurodegenerative disorder or the sequelae of a stroke or other structural lesion. Differentiation of apathy from depression has been previously covered in the discussion of PSD, and similar considerations apply with vascular depression.

Treatment

Psychopharmacological Treatment

Given its likely distinct psychopathology, it seems intuitive that the treatment profile of vascular depression would differ at least partially from idiopathic depression. Several studies have demonstrated variable response to SSRIs in these patients. Response to these medications seems to correlate with the degree of neuropsychological impairment and inversely correlate with the progression of white matter hyperintensities.[215] In a nonrandomized trial, 33% of patients achieved remission over 12 weeks with SSRI treatment. The likelihood of remission, assessed by MADRS score, diminished with increasing deficits in overall executive function, language processing, episodic memory, and processing speed.[221] In general, vascular depression confers an increased risk of nonresponse to treatment with antidepressant medications, with a low expected remission rate of 33%.[221] A placebo-controlled trial of sertraline in elderly patients with depression (but not specifically with vascular depression) found that sertraline performed worse than placebo in patients with impaired executive function, as measured by response inhibition.[222] This suggests that elderly patients with executive dysfunction and depression, including those with vascular depression, may be subject to the side effects of antidepressants but not their therapeutic effects on mood symptoms. Emerging research suggests that SSRIs may improve neural plasticity[223,224] and decrease amyloid-beta production[225]—however, especially in the absence of measurable affective benefits, the clinical value of this information remains uncertain.

Brain Stimulation Therapies

A study comparing rTMS of the left dorsolateral prefrontal cortex to sham rTMS for patients with vascular depression found a response rate of 39% and a remission rate of 27%,[226] including in patients previously unresponsive to treatment with antidepressants. Unlike antidepressants, response to treatment did not correlate with degree of cognitive impairment or executive dysfunction. There was a decreasing response to rTMS with increasing age and also with decreased volume of frontal gray matter. There is limited evidence regarding use of electroconvulsive therapy (ECT) in vascular depression, but one small series and several case reports suggest it is effective and generally well-tolerated, although perhaps with increased risk of delirium compared to ECT in idiopathic depression.[227] In elderly patients, cognitive side effects tend to be transient, regardless of underlying cognitive impairment.[228] In a study of 81 elderly inpatients with major depression, investigators found a 58% remission rate for a subgroup with more than one cardiovascular risk factor, and the response to ECT was independent of cardiovascular risk.[229]

Psychosocial Treatment

Given the usual age of onset of vascular depression, psychotherapy with these patients shares characteristics with psychotherapy with other ill, elderly patients. CBT for insomnia may be useful in addressing sleep disturbances contributing to cognitive deficits. Executive dysfunction may be targeted through problem-solving therapy or problem-adaptation therapy, and cognitive rehabilitation therapy may play a role in helping develop behavioral strategies to circumvent cognitive deficits.[207] An important role of psychotherapy with this population is to support the work patients need to do in sustaining positive health behaviors, to help decrease their vascular risk factors. Managing sleep, exercise, diet, medication adherence, hypercholesterolemia, hypertension, and other metabolic disorders is an important component of therapy for vascular depression. Several aspects of psychotherapy in the context of cognitive impairment, including supportive therapy and behavioral activation, apply to this population as well; importantly, the inclusion of caregivers in the plan of care may augment treatment results. See Chapter 10 for further discussion about the adaptation of psychosocial approaches when treating individuals with cognitive impairment.

Summary and Key Points

- In addition to significant physical disability, stroke can also have neuropsychiatric sequelae, which can be an independent cause of disability and exacerbate the residual physical symptoms of a stroke.
- In general, neuropsychiatric disorders after stroke lead to poorer functional outcomes in rehabilitation. Their treatment may include medication, psychosocial interventions, and brain stimulation with rTMS or ECT.
- Pharmacological treatment generally follows the guidelines of the treatment of primary psychiatric disorders, with additional considerations for increased adverse effects due to age, poor balance/fall-risk, cognition (anticholinergic effects), and cardiovascular risk factors in stroke patients.
- Depression can emerge after an infarct to many different neuroanatomic locations (especially left frontal lobe), with up to one-third of post-stroke patients experiencing PSD. Patients with personal and family histories of depression are at higher risk. TCAs and SSRIs have demonstrated efficacy, and ECT has been successfully used in severe and refractory depression.
- The prevalence of anxiety after stroke has been reported from 3% to 30%, commonly presenting as GAD or phobic disorders, with substantial overlap between anxiety and PSD.

Risk factors include young age, premorbid psychiatric history, and substance dependence.
- Apathy is reported in 36.6% of stroke survivors and is often associated with subcortical infarcts, especially in the basal ganglia. Apathy may be a symptom of PSD or a distinct clinical diagnosis in the absence of low mood.
- Mania and psychosis are rare but debilitating and may lead to underreporting of cognitive and functional limitations. Stroke locations reported in association with mania have included a right ventral limbic circuit, including the right orbitofrontal and basotemporal cortices, caudate, and thalamus.
- The estimated prevalence of emotional aprosodia ranges from 30% to 49%. It may present with expressive or receptive deficits in emotional expression through language. Treatment typically consists of speech and cognitive rehabilitation therapy.
- Pathological laughing and crying is prevalent in approximately 11% of stroke patients and is associated with disruption of circuits mediating emotional and affect regulation.
- Vascular depression often presents with cognitive symptoms characteristic of subcortical dementia and is associated with subcortical microvascular disease. Response to antidepressants appears to be poor in vascular depression; prevention of cerebral microvascular disease through managing CVD risk factors may offer protection.

Multiple Choice Questions

1. Which of the following is incorrect regarding PSD and vascular depression?
   a. Vascular depression is associated with white matter hyperintensities on MRI.
   b. Vascular depression presents with cognitive deficits including executive dysfunction and slowed processing speed, while the presentation of cognitive deficits in PSD is variable.
   c. Vascular depression is generally more responsive to SSRIs than PSD.
   d. Age is a risk factor for vascular depression, but not clearly so for PSD.
   e. Family history of psychiatric disorders is less common in vascular depression than PSD.

2. Which of the following pharmacological agents—side effects matches is correct, and an important consideration when treating patients with cerebrovascular injury?
   a. SSRIs—anticholinergic effects
   b. Atypical antipsychotics—weight loss
   c. Benzodiazepines—bleeding risk
   d. Mirtazapine—QTc prolongation
   e. SNRIs—increased blood pressure

3. Which of the following statements about post-stroke anxiety is false?
   a. Rates of post-stroke anxiety are high in the weeks following stroke, and a large proportion of patients continue to report symptoms of anxiety 6 months later.
   b. Nortriptyline has the strongest evidence base, among the tricyclic antidepressants, for the treatment of post-stroke anxiety.
   c. Cognitive limitations after a cerebrovascular injury can interfere with the timely diagnosis of anxiety.
   d. Benzodiazepines are the first line of treatment for post-stroke anxiety.
   e. Post-stoke anxiety is likely to present with symptoms of GAD and/or phobic disorders.

4. Which of the following is not associated with increased risk of post-stroke depression?
   a. Infarcts in the right frontal lobe or basal ganglia
   b. Post-stroke anxiety
   c. Lack of family and social support
   d. Severity of functional impairment and physical disability
   e. History of premorbid depression

Multiple Choice Answers

1. Answer: c
While SSRIs have been effective in treating post-stroke mood symptoms and enhancing motor recovery, their efficacy is limited in vascular depression. SSRIs are more effective in vascular depression patients with less white matter burden and executive dysfunction. PSD primarily onsets in later life because the risk of stroke is higher; however, age is not a known independent risk factor for the development of depression given a cerebrovascular injury.

2. Answer: e
SNRIs are associated with increased risk of hypertension, which is an important consideration in the post-stroke population to manage risk of recurrence. SSRIs are associated with increased bleeding risk and QTc prolongation.

Atypical antipsychotics and mirtazapine are associated with weight gain.

3. Answer: d
Benzodiazepines are not a preferred treatment option as they carry a risk of worsening cognition, cause balance problems, and other side effects.

4. Answer: a
The risk of post-stroke depression is increased in the presence of post-stroke anxiety, physical/functional limitations, or lack of social support structures. History of premorbid depression also increases risk. While depression can emerge after an infarct in any location, evidence suggests that post-stroke depression is more likely to be associated with lesions in the left frontal lobe or basal ganglia.

References

1. Benjamin EJ, Blaha MJ, Chiuve SE, et al. Heart disease and stroke statistics—2017 update: a report from the American Heart Association. *Circulation.* 2017;135:e229-e445.

2. Cerebrovascular diseases. Ropper AH, Samuels MA, Klein JP, eds. *Adams & Victor's Principles of Neurology.* 10th ed. New York, NY: McGraw-Hill; 2014:chap 34. http://neurology.mhmedical.com/content.aspx?bookid=690&sectionid=50910885. Accessed March 10, 2019.

3. Gillen R, Tennen H, McKee TE, Gernert-Dott P, Affleck G. Depressive symptoms and history of depression predict rehabilitation efficiency in stroke patients. *Arch Phys Med Rehabil.* 2001;82(12):1645-1649.

4. Go AS, Mozaffarian D, Roger VL, et al. Heart disease and stroke statistics—2013 update: a report from the American Heart Association. *Circulation.* 2013;127(1):e6-e245.

5. Towfighi A, Ovbiagele B, El Husseini N, et al. Poststroke depression: a scientific statement for healthcare professionals from the American Heart Association/American Stroke Association. *Stroke.* 2017;48(2):e30-e43.

6. Hackett ML, Yapa C, Parag V, Anderson CS. Frequency of depression after stroke: a systematic review of observational studies. *Stroke.* 2005;36(6):1330-1340.

7. Ayerbe L, Ayis S, Crichton S, Wolfe CDA, Rudd AG. The natural history of depression up to 15 years after stroke: the South London Stroke Register. *Stroke.* 2013;44(4):1105-1110.

8. Ayerbe L, Ayis S, Wolfe CDA, Rudd AG. Natural history, predictors and outcomes of depression after stroke: systematic review and meta-analysis. *Br J Psychiatry.* 2013;202(1):14-21.

9. De Ryck A, Brouns R, Geurden M, Elseviers M, De Deyn PP, Engelborghs S. Risk factors for poststroke depression: identification of inconsistencies based on a systematic review. *J Geriatr Psychiatry Neurol.* 2014;27(3):147-158.

10. Sinyor D, Amato P, Kaloupek DG, Becker R, Goldenberg M, Coopersmith H. Post-stroke depression: relationships to functional impairment, coping strategies, and rehabilitation outcome. *Stroke.* 1986;17(6):1102-1107.

11. Nys GMS, van Zandvoort MJE, van der Worp HB, de Haan EHF, de Kort PLM, Kappelle LJ. Early depressive symptoms after stroke: neuropsychological correlates and lesion characteristics. *J Neurol Sci.* 2005;228(1):27-33.

12. Ng KC, Chan KL, Straughan PT. A study of post-stroke depression in a rehabilitative center. *Acta Psychiatr Scand.* 1995;92(1):75-79.

13. Narushima K, Kosier JT, Robinson RG. A reappraisal of post-stroke depression, intra- and inter-hemispheric lesion location using meta-analysis. *J Neuropsychiatry Clin Neurosci.* 2003;15(4):422-430.

14. Robinson RG, Szetela B. Mood change following left hemispheric brain injury. *Ann Neurol.* 1981;9(5):447-453.

15. Terroni L, Amaro E, Iosifescu DV, et al. Stroke lesion in cortical neural circuits and post-stroke incidence of major depressive episode: a 4-month prospective study. *World J Biol Psychiatry.* 2011;12(7):539-548.

16. Newberg AR, Davydow DS, Lee HB. Cerebrovascular disease basis of depression: post-stroke depression and vascular depression. *Int Rev Psychiatry.* 2006;18(5):433-441.

17. Rocco A, Afra J, Toscano M, et al. Acute subcortical stroke and early serotonergic modification: a IDAP study. *Eur J Neurol.* 2007;14(12):1378-1382.

18. Mayberg HS, Robinson RG, Wong DF, et al. PET imaging of cortical S2 serotonin receptors after stroke: lateralized changes and relationship to depression. *Am J Psychiatry.* 1988;145(8):937-943.

19. Spalletta G, Bossù P, Ciaramella A, Bria P, Caltagirone C, Robinson RG. The etiology of poststroke depression: a review of the literature and a new hypothesis involving inflammatory cytokines. *Mol Psychiatry.* 2006;11(11):984-991.

20. Kim J-M, Stewart R, Kang H-J, et al. A longitudinal study of SLC6A4 DNA promoter methylation and poststroke depression. *J Psychiatr Res.* 2013;47(9):1222-1227.

21. Kim J-M, Stewart R, Kang H-J, et al. A longitudinal study of BDNF promoter methylation and genotype with poststroke depression. *J Affect Disord.* 2013;149(1–3):93-99.

22. Spalletta G, Ripa A, Caltagirone C. Symptom profile of DSM-IV major and minor depressive disorders in first-ever stroke patients. *Am J Geriatr Psychiatry.* 2005;13(2):108-115.

23. Whyte EM, Mulsant BH. Post stroke depression: epidemiology, pathophysiology, and biological treatment. *Biol Psychiatry.* 2002;52(3):253-264.

24. Marin RS. Differential diagnosis and classification of apathy. *Am J Psychiatry.* 1990;147(1):22-30.

25. Levy ML, Cummings JL, Fairbanks LA, et al. Apathy is not depression. *J Neuropsychiatry Clin Neurosci*. 1998;10(3):314-319.

26. Marin RS, Firinciogullari S, Biedrzycki RC. Group differences in the relationship between apathy and depression. *J Nerv Ment Dis*. 1994;182(4):235-239.

27. Withall A, Brodaty H, Altendorf A, Sachdev PS. A longitudinal study examining the independence of apathy and depression after stroke: the Sydney Stroke Study. *Int Psychogeriatr*. 2011;23(2):264-273.

28. Berman K, Brodaty H, Withall A, Seeher K. Pharmacologic treatment of apathy in dementia. *Am J Geriatr Psychiatry*. 2012;20(2):104-122.

29. Chollet F, Tardy J, Albucher J-F, et al. Fluoxetine for motor recovery after acute ischaemic stroke (Flame): a randomised placebo-controlled trial. *Lancet Neurol*. 2011;10(2):123-130.

30. Grade C, Redford B, Chrostowski J, Toussaint L, Blackwell B. Methylphenidate in early poststroke recovery: a double-blind, placebo-controlled study. *Arch Phys Med Rehabil*. 1998;79(9):1047-1050.

31. Currier MB, Murray GB, Welch CC. Electroconvulsive therapy for post-stroke depressed geriatric patients. *J Neuropsychiatry Clin Neurosci*. 1992;4(2):140-144.

32. Klein MM, Treister R, Raij T, et al. Transcranial magnetic stimulation of the brain: guidelines for pain treatment research. *Pain*. 2015;156(9):1601-1614.

33. Hackett ML, Anderson CS, House A, Xia J. Interventions for treating depression after stroke. *Cochrane Database Syst Rev*. 2008;(4):CD003437.

34. Duan X, Yao G, Liu Z, Cui R, Yang W. Mechanisms of transcranial magnetic stimulation treating on post-stroke depression. *Front Hum Neurosci*. 2018;12:215.

35. Bandelow B, Michaelis S. Epidemiology of anxiety disorders in the 21st century. *Dialogues Clin Neurosci*. 2015;17(3):327-335.

36. Ferro JM, ed. *Neuropsychiatric Symptoms of Cerebrovascular Diseases*. London: Springer; 2013.

37. Burton CAC, Murray J, Holmes J, et al. Frequency of anxiety after stroke: a systematic review and meta-analysis of observational studies. *Int J Stroke*. 2013;8(7):545-559.

38. Robinson RG. Neuropsychiatric consequences of stroke. *Ann Rev Med*. 1997;48(1):217-229.

39. Rafsten L, Danielsson A, Sunnerhagen KS. Anxiety after stroke: a systematic review and meta-analysis. *J Rehabil Med*. 2018;50(9):769-778.

40. Ayerbe L, Ayis SA, Crichton S, et al. Natural history, predictors and associated outcomes of anxiety up to 10 years after stroke: the South London Stroke Register. *Age Ageing*. 2014;43(4):542-547.

41. Ferro JM, Caeiro L, Figueira ML. Neuropsychiatric sequelae of stroke. *Nat Rev Neurol*. 2016;12(5):269-280.

42. Morrison V, Pollard B, Johnston M, et al. Anxiety and depression 3 years following stroke: demographic, clinical, and psychological predictors. *J Psychosom Res*. 2005;59(4):209-213.

43. Barker-Collo SL. Depression and anxiety 3 months post stroke: prevalence and correlates. *Arch Clin Neuropsychol*. 2007;22(4):519-531.

44. Portegies MLP, Bos MJ, Koudstaal PJ, et al. Anxiety and the risk of stroke: the Rotterdam Study. *Stroke*. 2016;47(4):1120-1123.

45. Chun HY, Whiteley WN, Dennis MS, et al. Anxiety after stroke: the importance of subtyping. *Stroke*. 2018;49(3):556-564.

46. Aström M. Generalized anxiety disorder in stroke patients. A 3-year longitudinal study. *Stroke*. 1996; 27(2):270-275.

47. Wright F, Wu S, Chun HY, et al. Factors associated with post-stroke anxiety: a systematic review and meta-analysis. *Stroke Res Treat*. 2017;2017:2124743.

48. Tang WK, Chen Y, Lu J, et al. Frontal infarcts and anxiety in stroke. *Stroke*. 2012;43(5):1426-1428.

49. Grafman J, Vance SC, Weingartner H, et al. The effects of lateralized frontal lesions on mood regulation. *Brain*. 1986;109 (pt 6):1127-1148.

50. Milad MR, Rauch SL. The role of the orbitofrontal cortex in anxiety disorders. *Ann N Y Acad Sci*. 2007;1121(1):546-561.

51. Agustín-Pavón C, Braesicke K, Shiba Y, et al. Lesions of ventrolateral prefrontal or anterior orbitofrontal cortex in primates heighten negative emotion. *Biol Psychiatry*. 2012;72(4):266-272.

52. Kuniishi H, Ichisaka S, Matsuda S, et al. Chronic inactivation of the orbitofrontal cortex increases anxiety-like behavior and impulsive aggression, but decreases depression-like behavior in rats. *Front Behav Neurosci*. 2016;10:250.

53. Shiba Y, Kim C, Santangelo AM, et al. Lesions of either anterior orbitofrontal cortex or ventrolateral prefrontal cortex in marmoset monkeys heighten innate fear and attenuate active coping behaviors to predator threat. *Front Syst Neurosci*. 2014;8:250.

54. Xue SW, Lee TW, Guo YH. Spontaneous activity in medial orbitofrontal cortex correlates with trait anxiety in healthy male adults. *J Zhejiang Univ Sci B*. 2018;19(8):643-653.

55. Duval ER, Javanbakht A, Liberzon I. Neural circuits in anxiety and stress disorders: a focused review. *Ther Clin Risk Manag*. 2015;11:115-126.

56. Garton ALA, Sisti JA, Gupta VP, et al. Poststroke post-traumatic stress disorder: a review. *Stroke*. 2017;48(2):507-512.

57. Zatzick D, Jurkovich GJ, Rivara FP, et al. A national US study of posttraumatic stress disorder, depression, and work and functional outcomes after hospitalization for traumatic injury. *Transac Meet Am Surg Assoc*. 2008;126:79-87.

58. Edmondson D, Richardson S, Fausett JK, et al. Prevalence of PTSD in survivors of stroke and transient ischemic attack: a meta-analytic review. *PLoS One*. 2013;8(6):e66435.

59. Schultz SK, Castillo CS, Kosier JT, et al. Generalized anxiety and depression. Assessment over 2 years after stroke. *Am J Geriatr Psychiatry*. 1997;5(3):229-237.

60. Goldfinger JZ, Edmondson D, Kronish IM, et al. Correlates of post-traumatic stress disorder in stroke survivors. *J Stroke Cerebrovasc Dis*. 2014;23(5):1099-1105.

61. Chi S, Teng L, Song J-H, et al. Tryptophan hydroxylase 2 gene polymorphisms and poststroke anxiety disorders. *J Affect Disord*. 2013;144(1–2):179-182.

62. Serretti A, Liappas I, Mandelli L, et al. TPH2 gene variants and anxiety during alcohol detoxification outcome. *Psychiatry Res*. 2009;167(1–2):106-114.

63. Laas K, Kiive E, Mäestu J, et al. Nice guys: homozygocity for the TPH2-703G/T (rs4570625) minor allele promotes low aggressiveness and low anxiety. *J Affect Disord*. 2017;215:230-236.

64. Donner NC, Johnson PL, Fitz SD, et al. Elevated tph2 mRNA expression in a rat model of chronic anxiety. *Depress Anxiety*. 2012;29(4):307-319.

65. American Psychiatric Association. *Diagnostic and Statistical Manual of Mental Disorders*: DSM-5. 5th ed. Washington, DC: American Psychiatric Association; 2013.

66. Burvill PW, Johnson GA, Jamrozik KD, et al. Anxiety disorders after stroke: results from the Perth Community Stroke Study. *Br J Psychiatry*. 1995;166(3):328-332.

67. Townend E, Tinson D, Kwan J, et al. Fear of recurrence and beliefs about preventing recurrence in persons who have suffered a stroke. *J Psychosom Res.* 2006;61(6):747-755.

68. Watanabe Y. Fear of falling among stroke survivors after discharge from inpatient rehabilitation. *Int J Rehabil Res.* 2005;28(2):149-152.

69. Shimoda K, Robinson RG. Effect of anxiety disorder on impairment and recovery from stroke. *J Neuropsychiatry Clin Neurosci.* 1998;10(1):34-40.

70. De Wit L, Putman K, Baert I, et al. Anxiety and depression in the first six months after stroke. A longitudinal multicentre study. *Disabil Rehabil.* 2008;30(24):1858-1866.

71. Lincoln NB, Brinkmann N, Cunningham S, et al. Anxiety and depression after stroke: a 5 year follow-up. *Disabil Rehabil.* 2013;35(2):140-145.

72. McKevitt C, Fudge N, Redfern J, et al. Self-reported long-term needs after stroke. *Stroke.* 2011;42(5):1398-1403.

73. van Rijswijk E, van Hout H, van de Lisdonk E, et al. Barriers in recognising, diagnosing and managing depressive and anxiety disorders as experienced by Family Physicians: a focus group study. *BMC Fam Pract.* 2009;10:52.

74. Locke AB, Kirst N, Shultz CG. Diagnosis and management of generalized anxiety disorder and panic disorder in adults. *Am Family Physician.* 2015;91(9):617-624.

75. Zimmerman M, McGlinchey JB, Chelminski I, et al. Diagnostic co-morbidity in 2300 psychiatric out-patients presenting for treatment evaluated with a semi-structured diagnostic interview. *Psychol Med.* 2008;38(2):199-210.

76. Zigmond AS, Snaith RP. The Hospital Anxiety and Depression Scale. *Acta Psychiatr Scand.* 1983;67(6):361–370.

77. Burton L-J, Tyson S. Screening for mood disorders after stroke: a systematic review of psychometric properties and clinical utility. *Psychol Med.* 2015;45(1):29-49.

78. Sagen U, Vik TG, Moum T, et al. Screening for anxiety and depression after stroke: comparison of the Hospital Anxiety and Depression Scale and the Montgomery and Asberg Depression Rating Scale. *J Psychosom Res.* 2009;67(4):325-332.

79. O'Rourke S, MacHale S, Signorini D, et al. Detecting psychiatric morbidity after stroke: comparison of the GHQ and the HAD scale. *Stroke.* 1998;29(5):980-985.

80. Aben I, Verhey F, Lousberg R, et al. Validity of the beck depression inventory, hospital anxiety and depression scale, SCL-90, and Hamilton depression rating scale as screening instruments for depression in stroke patients. *Psychosomatics.* 2002;43(5):386-393.

81. Bjelland I, Dahl AA, Haug TT, et al. The validity of the hospital anxiety and depression scale. *J Psychosom Res.* 2002;52(2):69-77.

82. Johnson G, Burvill PW, Anderson CS, et al. Screening instruments for depression and anxiety following stroke: experience in the Perth community stroke study. *Acta Psychiatr Scand.* 1995;91(4):252-257.

83. Linley-Adams B, Morris R, Kneebone I. The Behavioural Outcomes of Anxiety scale (BOA): a preliminary validation in stroke survivors. *Br J Clin Psychol.* 2014;53(4):451-467.

84. Castillo CS, Schultz SK, Robinson RG. Clinical correlates of early-onset and late-onset poststroke generalized anxiety. *Am J Psychiatry.* 1995;152(8):1174-1179.

85. Craig CR, Stitzel RE, eds. *Modern Pharmacology with Clinical Applications.* 6th ed. Philadelphia, PA: Lippincott Williams & Wilkins; 2004.

86. Knapp P, Campbell Burton CA, Holmes J, et al. Interventions for treating anxiety after stroke. *Cochrane Database Syst Rev.* 2017;5:1-39.

87. Mikami K, Jorge RE, Moser DJ, et al. Prevention of post-stroke generalized anxiety disorder, using escitalopram or problem-solving therapy. *J Neuropsychiatry Clin Neurosci.* 2014;26(4):323-328.

88. Siepmann T, Penzlin AI, Kepplinger J, et al. Selective serotonin reuptake inhibitors to improve outcome in acute ischemic stroke: possible mechanisms and clinical evidence. *Brain Behav.* 2015;5(10).

89. Pinto CB, Saleh Velez FG, Lopes F, et al. SSRI and motor recovery in stroke: reestablishment of inhibitory neural network tonus. *Front Neurosci.* 2017;11:637.

90. Mead GE, Hsieh C-F, Lee R, et al. Selective serotonin reuptake inhibitors (SSRIs) for stroke recovery. *Cochrane Database Syst Rev.* 2012;11:CD009286.

91. Chollet F, Tardy J, Albucher J-F, et al. Fluoxetine for motor recovery after acute ischaemic stroke (Flame): a randomised placebo-controlled trial. *Lancet Neurol.* 2011;10(2):123-130.

92. Wiese B. Geriatric depression: the use of antidepressants in the elderly. *B C Med J.* 2011;53(47):341-347.

93. Laporte S, Chapelle C, Caillet P, et al. Bleeding risk under selective serotonin reuptake inhibitor (SSRI) antidepressants: a meta-analysis of observational studies. *Pharmacol Res.* 2017;118:19-32.

94. Kallmünzer B, Breuer L, Kahl N, et al. Serious cardiac arrhythmias after stroke. *Stroke.* 2012;43(11):2892-2897.

95. Funk KA, Bostwick JR. A comparison of the risk of QT prolongation among SSRIs. *Ann Pharmacother.* 2013;47(10):1330-1341.

96. Zhong Z, Wang L, Wen X, et al. A meta-analysis of effects of selective serotonin reuptake inhibitors on blood pressure in depression treatment: outcomes from placebo and serotonin and noradrenaline reuptake inhibitor controlled trials. *Neuropsychiatr Dis Treat.* 2017;13:2781-2796.

97. Robinson RG, Schultz SK, Castillo C, et al. Nortriptyline versus fluoxetine in the treatment of depression and in short-term recovery after stroke: a placebo-controlled, double-blind study. *Am J Psychiatry.* 2000;157(3):351-359.

98. Kimura M, Tateno A, Robinson RG. Treatment of poststroke generalized anxiety disorder comorbid with poststroke depression: merged analysis of nortriptyline trials. *Am J Geriatr Psychiatry.* 2003;11(3):320-327.

99. Khalid MM, Waseem M. Tricyclic antidepressant toxicity. In: *StatPearls.* Treasure Island, FL: StatPearls Publishing; 2018. Available at http://www.ncbi.nlm.nih.gov/books/NBK430931/.

100. Frank C. Pharmacologic treatment of depression in the elderly. *Can Fam Physician.* 2014;60(2):121-126.

101. Markota M, Rummans TA, Bostwick JM, et al. Benzodiazepine use in older adults: dangers, management, and alternative therapies. *Mayo Clin Proc.* 2016;91(11):1632-1639.

102. Zhang Y, Zhang H, Wang H. Effects of buspirone hydrochloride on post-stroke affective disorder and neural function. *Chinese J Clin Rehabil.* 2005;9(12):8-9.

103. Kim JS, Bashford G, Murphy TK, et al. Safety and efficacy of pregabalin in patients with central post-stroke pain. *Pain.* 2011;152(5):1018-1023.

104. Kneebone II, Jeffries FW. Treating anxiety after stroke using cognitive-behaviour therapy: two cases. *Neuropsychol Rehabil.* 2013;23(6):798-810.

105. Thomas SA, Walker MF, Macniven JA, et al. Communication and Low Mood (CALM): a randomized controlled trial of behavioural therapy for stroke patients with aphasia. *Clin Rehabil.* 2013;27(5):398-408.

106. Broomfield NM, Laidlaw K, Hickabottom E, et al. Post-stroke depression: the case for augmented, individually tailored cognitive behavioural therapy. *Clin Psychol Psychother.* 2011;18(3):202-217.

107. Bradbury CL, Christensen BK, Lau MA, et al. The efficacy of cognitive behavior therapy in the treatment of emotional distress after acquired brain injury. *Arch Phys Med Rehabil.* 2008;89(12 suppl):S61-S68.

108. Arundine A, Bradbury CL, Dupuis K, et al. Cognitive behavior therapy after acquired brain injury: maintenance of therapeutic benefits at 6 months posttreatment. *J Head Trauma Rehabil.* 2012;27(2):104-112.

109. Waldron B, Casserly LM, O'Sullivan C. Cognitive behavioural therapy for depression and anxiety in adults with acquired brain injury: what works for whom? *Neuropsychol Rehabil.* 2013;23(1):64-101.

110. Golding K, Kneebone I, Fife-Schaw C. Self-help relaxation for post-stroke anxiety: a randomised, controlled pilot study. *Clin Rehabil.* 2016;30(2):174-180.

111. Golding K, Fife-Schaw C, Kneebone I. Twelve month follow-up on a randomised controlled trial of relaxation training for post-stroke anxiety. *Clin Rehabil.* 2017;31(9):1164-1167.

112. Fang Y, Mpofu E, Athanasou J. Reducing depressive or anxiety symptoms in post-stroke patients: pilot trial of a constructive integrative psychosocial intervention. *Int J Health Sci.* 2017;11(4): 53-58.

113. Watkins CL, Auton MF, Deans CF, et al. Motivational interviewing early after acute stroke: a randomized, controlled trial. *Stroke.* 2007;38(3):1004-1009.

114. Desrosiers J, Noreau L, Rochette A, et al. Effect of a home leisure education program after stroke: a randomized controlled trial. *Arch Phys Med Rehabil.* 2007;88(9):1095-1100.

115. Graham CD, Gillanders D, Stuart S, et al. An Acceptance and Commitment Therapy (ACT)–based intervention for an adult experiencing post-stroke anxiety and medically unexplained symptoms. *Clin Case Stud.* 2015;14(2):83-97.

116. Ihle-Hansen H, Thommessen B, Fagerland MW, et al. Effect on anxiety and depression of a multifactorial risk factor intervention program after stroke and TIA: a randomized controlled trial. *Aging Ment Health.* 2014;18(5):540-546.

117. Starkstein SE, Boston JD, Robinson RG. Mechanisms of mania after brain injury. 12 case reports and review of the literature. *J Nerv Ment Dis.* 1988;176(2):87-100.

118. Caeiro L, Ferro JM, Albuquerque R, Figueira ML. Mania no AVC agudo. *Sinapse.* 2002;(2):90.

119. Santos CO, Caeiro L, Ferro JM, Figueira ML. Mania and stroke: a systematic review. *Cerebrovasc Dis.* 2011;32(1):11-21.

120. Satzer D, Bond DJ. Mania secondary to focal brain lesions: implications for understanding the functional neuroanatomy of bipolar disorder. *Bipolar Disord.* 2016;18(3):205-220.

121. Starkstein SE, Pearlson GD, Boston J, Robinson RG. Mania after brain injury. A controlled study of causative factors. *Arch Neurol.* 1987;44(10):1069-1073.

122. Barahona-Correa JB, Cotovio G, Costa RM, et al. Right-sided brain lesions predominate among patients with lesional mania: evidence from a systematic review and pooled lesion analysis. *bioRxiv.* 2018:1-25. doi: https://doi.org/10.1101/433292. If you need to add when it was accessed: Accessed June 15 2019.

123. Robinson RG, Boston JD, Starkstein SE, Price TR. Comparison of mania and depression after brain injury: causal factors. *Am J Psychiatry.* 1988;145(2):172-178.

124. Liu CY, Wang SJ, Fuh JL, Yang YY, Liu HC. Bipolar disorder following a stroke involving the left hemisphere. *Aust N Z J Psychiatry.* 1996;30(5):688-691.

125. Lee I, Nielsen K, Nawaz U, et al. Diverse pathophysiological processes converge on network disruption in mania. *J Affect Disord.* 2019;244:115-123.

126. Starkstein SE, Fedoroff P, Berthier ML, Robinson RG. Manic-depressive and pure manic states after brain lesions. *Biol Psychiatry.* 1991;29(2):149-158.

127. Cummings JL, Mendez MF. Secondary mania with focal cerebrovascular lesions. *Am J Psychiatry.* 1984;141(9):1084-1087.

128. Taylor JB, Prager LM, Quijije NV, Schaefer PW. Case 21-2018: A 61-year-old man with grandiosity, impulsivity, and decreased sleep. *N Engl J Med.* 2018;379(2):182-189.

129. Stangeland H, Orgeta V, Bell V. Poststroke psychosis: a systematic review. *J Neurol Neurosurg Psychiatry.* 2018;89(8):879-885.

130. Almeida OP, Xiao J. Mortality associated with incident mental health disorders after stroke. *Aust N Z J Psychiatry.* 2007;41(3):274-281.

131. Devine MJ, Bentley P, Jones B, et al. The role of the right inferior frontal gyrus in the pathogenesis of post-stroke psychosis. *J Neurol.* 2014;261(3):600-603.

132. McMurtray AM, Sultzer DL, Monserratt L, et al. Content-specific delusions from right caudate lacunar stroke: association with prefrontal hypometabolism. *J Neuropsychiatry Clin Neurosci.* 2008;20(1):62-67.

133. van Almenkerk S, Depla MFIA, Smalbrugge M, et al. Institutionalized stroke patients: status of functioning of an under researched population. *J Am Med Dir Assoc.* 2012;13(7):634-639.

134. Rabins PV, Starkstein SE, Robinson RG. Risk factors for developing atypical (schizophreniform) psychosis following stroke. *J Neuropsychiatry Clin Neurosci.* 1991;3(1):6-9.

135. Darby RR, Laganiere S, Pascual-Leone A, et al. Finding the imposter: brain connectivity of lesions causing delusional misidentifications. *Brain.* 2017;140(2):497-507.

136. Gurin L, Blum S. Delusions and the right hemisphere: a review of the case for the right hemisphere as a mediator of reality-based belief. *J Neuropsychiatry Clin Neurosci.* 2017;29(3):225-235.

137. Corlett PR, Murray GK, Honey GD, et al. Disrupted prediction-error signal in psychosis: evidence for an associative account of delusions. *Brain.* 2007;130(pt 9):2387-2400.

138. Kumral E, Oztürk O. Delusional state following acute stroke. *Neurology.* 2004;62(1):110-113.

139. Stéfan A, Mathé J-F. What are the disruptive symptoms of behavioral disorders after traumatic brain injury? A systematic review leading to recommendations for good practices. *Ann Phys Rehabil Med.* 2016;59(1):5-17.

140. Buijck BI, Zuidema SU, Spruit-van Eijk M, et al. Neuropsychiatric symptoms in geriatric patients admitted to skilled nursing facilities in nursing homes for rehabilitation after stroke: a longitudinal multicenter study. *Int J Geriatr Psychiatry.* 2012;27(7): 734-741.

141. Fong TG, Tulebaev SR, Inouye SK. Delirium in elderly adults: diagnosis, prevention and treatment. *Nat Rev Neurol.* 2009;5(4):210-220.

142. Hirsch L, Yang J, Bresee L, et al. Second-generation antipsychotics and metabolic side effects: a systematic review of population-based studies. *Drug Saf.* 2017;40(9):771-781.

143. Uçok A, Gaebel W. Side effects of atypical antipsychotics: a brief overview. *World Psychiatry.* 2008;7(1):58-62.

144. Gareri P, Segura-García C, Manfredi VGL, et al. Use of atypical antipsychotics in the elderly: a clinical review. *Clin Interven Aging.* 2014;9:1363-1373.

145. Caeiro L, Ferro JM, Costa J. Apathy secondary to stroke: a systematic review and meta-analysis. *Cerebrovasc Dis.* 2013;35(1):23-39.

146. Caeiro L, Ferro JM, Pinho E Melo T, Canhão P, Figueira ML. Post-stroke apathy: an exploratory longitudinal study. *Cerebrovasc Dis.* 2013;35(6):507-513.

147. Mayo NE, Fellows LK, Scott SC, et al. A longitudinal view of apathy and its impact after stroke. *Stroke.* 2009;40(10):3299-3307.

148. Hama S, Yamashita H, Shigenobu M, et al. Depression or apathy and functional recovery after stroke. *Int J Geriatr Psychiatry.* 2007;22(10):1046-1051.

149. Harris AL, Elder J, Schiff ND, et al. Post-stroke apathy and hypersomnia lead to worse outcomes from acute rehabilitation. *Transl Stroke Res.* 2014;5(2):292-300.

150. van Dalen JW, Moll van Charante EP, Nederkoorn PJ, et al. Poststroke apathy. *Stroke.* 2013;44(3):851-860.

151. Bogart KR. Is apathy a valid and meaningful symptom or syndrome in Parkinson's disease? A critical review. *Health Psychol.* 2011;30(4):386-400.

152. Chase TN. (2011). Apathy in neuropsychiatric disease: diagnosis, pathophysiology, and treatment. *Neurotox Res.* 2011;19(2):266-278.

153. Levy R, Dubois B. Apathy and the functional anatomy of the prefrontal cortex-basal ganglia circuits. *Cereb Cortex.* 2006;16(7):916-928.

154. Le Heron C, Apps MAJ, Husain M. The anatomy of apathy: a neurocognitive framework for amotivated behaviour. *Neuropsychologia.* 2018;118(pt B):54-67.

155. Tekin S, Cummings JL. Frontal-subcortical neuronal circuits and clinical neuropsychiatry: an update. *J Psychosom Res.* 2002;53(2):647-654.

156. Douven E, Köhler S, Rodriguez MMF, et al. Imaging markers of post-stroke depression and apathy: a systematic review and meta-analysis. *Neuropsychol Rev.* 2017;27(3):202-219.

157. Ferro JM, Caeiro L, Figueira ML. Neuropsychiatric sequelae of stroke. *Nat Rev Neurol.* 2016;12(5):269-280.

158. Marin RS, Biedrzycki RC, Firinciogullari S. Reliability and validity of the Apathy Evaluation Scale. *Psychiatry Res.* 1991;38(2):143-162.

159. Lane-Brown AT, Tate RL. Measuring apathy after traumatic brain injury: psychometric properties of the Apathy Evaluation Scale and the Frontal Systems Behavior Scale. *Brain Injury.* 2009;23(13–14):999-1007.

160. Resnick B, Zimmerman SI, Magaziner J, et al. Use of the Apathy Evaluation Scale as a measure of motivation in elderly people. *Rehabil Nurs.* 1998;23(3):141-147.

161. Brodaty H, Sachdev PS, Withall A, et al. Frequency and clinical, neuropsychological and neuroimaging correlates of apathy following stroke—the Sydney Stroke Study. *Psychol Med.* 2005;35(12):1707-1716.

162. Sami MB, Faruqui R. The effectiveness of dopamine agonists for treatment of neuropsychiatric symptoms post brain injury and stroke. *Acta Neuropsychiatrica.* 2015;27(6):317-326.

163. Rosenberg PB, Lanctôt KL, Drye LT, et al. Safety and efficacy of methylphenidate for apathy in Alzheimer's disease: a randomized, placebo-controlled trial. *J Clin Psychiatry.* 2013;74(8):810-816.

164. Frakey LL, Salloway S, Buelow M, et al. A randomized, double-blind, placebo-controlled trial of modafinil for the treatment of apathy in individuals with mild-to-moderate Alzheimer's disease. *J Clin Psychiatry.* 2012;73(6):796-801.

165. Sinha A, Lewis O, Kumar R, et al. Adult ADHD medications and their cardiovascular implications. *Case Rep Cardiol.* 2016:2343691.

166. Waldemar G, Gauthier S, Jones R, et al. Effect of donepezil on emergence of apathy in mild to moderate Alzheimer's disease. *Int J Geriatr Psychiatry.* 2011;26(2):150-157.

167. Robinson RG, Jorge RE, Clarence-Smith K, et al. Double-blind treatment of apathy in patients with poststroke depression using nefiracetam. *J Neuropsychiatry Clin Neurosci.* 2009;21(2):144-151.

168. Mikami K, Jorge RE, Moser DJ, et al. Prevention of poststroke apathy using escitalopram or problem-solving therapy. *Am J Geriatr Psychiatry.* 2013;21(9):855-862.

169. Leon SA, Rodriguez AD. Aprosodia and its treatment. *Perspect Neurophysiol Neurogen Speech Lang Disord.* 2008;18(2):66.

170. Ross ED, Shayya L, Rousseau JF. Prosodic stress: acoustic, aphasic, aprosodic and neuroanatomic interactions. *J Neurolinguist.* 2013;26(5):526-551.

171. Leon SA, Rosenbek JC, Crucian GP, et al. Active treatments for aprosodia secondary to right hemisphere stroke. *J Rehabil Res Dev.* 2005;42(1):93-101.

172. Wright AE, Davis C, Gomez Y, et al. Acute ischemic lesions associated with impairments in expression and recognition of affective prosody. *Perspect ASHA Spec Interest Groups.* 2016;1(2):82-95.

173. Starkstein SE, Federoff JP, Price TR, et al. Neuropsychological and neuroradiologic correlates of emotional prosody comprehension. *Neurology.* 1994;44(3 pt 1):515-522.

174. Dara C, Kirsch-Darrow L, Ochfeld E, et al. Impaired emotion processing from vocal and facial cues in frontotemporal dementia compared to right hemisphere stroke. *Neurocase.* 2013;19(6):521-529.

175. Blonder LX, Pettigrew LC, Kryscio RJ. Emotion recognition and marital satisfaction in stroke. *J Clin Exp Neuropsychol.* 2012;34(6):634-642.

176. Ross ED, Thompson RD, Yenkosky J. Lateralization of affective prosody in brain and the callosal integration of hemispheric language functions. *Brain Lang.* 1997;56(1):27-54.

177. Ross ED, Monnot M. Neurology of affective prosody and its functional-anatomic organization in right hemisphere. *Brain Lang.* 2008;104(1):51-74.

178. Guranski K, Podemski R. Emotional prosody expression in acoustic analysis in patients with right hemisphere ischemic stroke. *Neurol Neurochir Pol.* 2015;49(2):113-120.

179. Dara C, Bang J, Gottesman RF, et al. Right hemisphere dysfunction is better predicted by emotional prosody impairments as compared to neglect. *J Neurol Transl Neurosci.* 2014;2(1):1037.

180. Heilman KM, Leon SA, Rosenbek JC. Affective aprosodia from a medial frontal stroke. *Brain Lang.* 2004;89(3):411-416.

181. Shatzman S, Mahajan S, Sundararajan S. Often overlooked but critical: poststroke cognitive impairment in right hemispheric ischemic stroke. *Stroke.* 2016;47(9):e221-e223.

182. House A, Rowe D, Standen PJ. Affective prosody in the reading voice of stroke patients. *J Neurol Neurosurg Psychiatry.* 1987;50(7):910-912.

183. Blonder LX, Bowers D, Heilman KM. The role of the right hemisphere in emotional communication. *Brain.* 1991;114(3):1115-1127.

184. Eslinger PJ, Parkinson K, Shamay SG. Empathy and social-emotional factors in recovery from stroke. *Curr Opin Neurol.* 2002;15(1):91-97.

185. Hillis AE, Tippett DC. Stroke recovery: surprising influences and residual consequences. *Adv Med.* 2014.

186. Villain M, Cosin C, Glize B, et al. Affective prosody and depression after stroke: a pilot study. *Stroke.* 2016;47(9):2397-2400.

187. Lehman Blake M, Duffy J, Tompkins C, et al. Right hemisphere syndrome is in the eye of the beholder. *Aphasiology.* 2003;17(5):423-432.

188. Hargrove P, Anderson A, Jones J. A critical review of interventions targeting prosody. *Int J Speech Lang Pathol.* 2009;11(4):298-304.

189. Tompkins CA. Rehabilitation for cognitive-communication disorders in right hemisphere brain damage. *Arch Phys Med Rehabil.* 2012;93(1):S61-S69.

190. Rosenbek JC, Rodriguez AD, Hieber B, et al. Effects of two treatments for aprosodia secondary to acquired brain injury. *J Rehabil Res Dev.* 2006;43(3):379.

191. Wortzel HS, Oster TJ, Anderson CA, Arciniegas DB. Pathological laughing and crying—epidemiology, pathophysiology and treatment. *CNS Drugs.* 2008;22:531-545.

192. Work SS, Colamonico JA, Bradley DG, Kaye RE. Pseudobulbar affect: an under-recognized and under-treated neurological disorder. *Adv Ther.* 2011;28:586-601.

193. Parvizi J, Coburn KL, Shillcutt SD, et al. Neuroanatomy of pathological laughing and crying: a report of the American Neuropsychiatric Association Committee on Research. *J. Neuropsychiatry Clin Neurosci.* 2009;21:75-87.

194. Ghaffar O, Chamelian L. Feinstein A. Neuroanatomy of pseudobulbar affect: a quantitative MRI study in multiple sclerosis. *J Neurol.* 2008;406-412.

195. Lauterbach EC, Cummings JL, Kuppuswamy PS. Toward a more precise, clinically-informed pathophysiology of pathological laughing and crying. *Neurosci Biobehav Rev.* 2013;37:1893-1916.

196. Stahl SM. Dextromethorphan-quinidine-responsive pseudobulbar affect (PLC): psychopharmacological model for wide-ranging disorders of emotional expression? *CNS Spectr.* 2016;21 (6):419-423.

197. Hanna J, Feinstein A, Morrow SA. The association of pathological laughing and crying and cognitive impairment in multiple sclerosis. *J Neurol Sci.* 2016;361:200-203.

198. Moore SR, Gresham LS, Bromberg MB, et al. A self report measure of affective lability. *J Neurol Neurosurg Psychiatry.* 1997;63:89-93.

199. Robinson RG, Parikh RM, Lipsey JR, et al. Pathological laughing and crying following stroke: validation of a measurement scale and a double-blind treatment study. *Am J Psychiatry.* 1993;150:286-293.

200. Pioro EP. Current concepts in the pharmacotherapy of pseudobulbar affect. *Drugs.* 2011;71:1193-1207.

201. Hammond FM, Alexander DN, Cutler AJ, et al. PRISM II: an open-label study to assess effectiveness of dextromethorphan/quinidine for pseudobulbar affect in patients with dementia, stroke or traumatic brain injury. *BMC Neurol.* 2016;16:160.

202. Ramasubbu R. Lamotrigine treatment for post-stroke pathological laughing and crying. *Clin Neuropharmacol.* 2003;26(5):233-235.

203. Ferentinos P, Paparrigopoulos T, Rentzos M, Evdokimidis I. Duloxetine for pathological laughing and crying. *Int J Neuropsychopharmacol.* 2009;12:1429-1430.

204. Johnson B, Nichols S. Crying and suicidal, but not depressed. Pseudobulbar affect in multiple sclerosis successfully treated with valproic acid: case report and literature review. *Palliat Support Care.* 2015;13:1797-1801.

205. Udaka F, Yamao S, Nagata H, et al. Pathologic laughing and crying treated with levodopa. *Arch Neurol.* 1984;41:1095-1097.

206. Alexopoulos GS, Meyers BS, Young RC, Campbell S, Silbersweig D, Charlson M. "Vascular depression" hypothesis. *Arch Gen Psychiatry.* 1997;54(10):915-922.

207. Taylor WD, Schultz SK, Panaite V, Steffens DC. Perspectives on the management of vascular depression. *Am J Psychiatry.* 2018;175(12):1169-1175.

208. González HM, Tarraf W, Whitfield K, Gallo JJ. Vascular depression prevalence and epidemiology in the United States. *J Psychiatr Res.* 2012;46(4):456-461.

209. Park JH, Lee SB, Lee JJ, et al. Epidemiology of MRI-defined vascular depression: a longitudinal, community-based study in Korean elders. *J Affect Disord.* 2015;180:200-206.

210. O'Brien J, Desmond P, Ames D, Schweitzer I, Harrigan S, Tress B. A magnetic resonance imaging study of white matter lesions in depression and Alzheimer's disease. *Br J Psychiatry.* 1996;168(4):477-485.

211. Aizenstein HJ, Baskys A, Boldrini M, et al. Vascular depression consensus report—a critical update. *BMC Med.* 2016a;14(1):161. Available at https://doi.org/10.1186/s12916-016-0720-5. Accessed June 15, 2019.

212. Thomas AJ, Perry R, Kalaria RN, Oakley A, McMeekin W, O'Brien JT. Neuropathological evidence for ischemia in the white matter of the dorsolateral prefrontal cortex in late-life depression. *Int J Geriatr Psychiatry.* 2003;18(1):7-13. Available at https://doi.org/10.1002/gps.720. Accessed June 15, 2019.

213. Thomas AJ, O'Brien JT, Davis S, et al. Ischemic basis for deep white matter hyperintensities in major depression: a neuropathological study. *Arch Gen Psychiatry.* 2002;59(9):785-792.

214. Pimontel MA, Reinlieb ME, Johnert LC, Garcon E, Sneed JR, Roose SP. The external validity of MRI-defined vascular depression. *Int J Geriatr Psychiatry.* 2013;28(11):1189-1196.

215. Taylor WD, Steffens DC, MacFall JR, et al. White matter hyperintensity progression and late-life depression outcomes. *Arch General Psychiatry.* 2003;60(11):1090-1096.

216. Diniz BS, Butters MA, Albert SM, Dew MA, Reynolds CF. Late-life depression and risk of vascular dementia and Alzheimer's disease: systematic review and meta-analysis of community-based cohort studies. *Br J Psychiatry.* 2013;202(5):329-335.

217. Steffens DC, Potter GG, McQuoid DR, et al. Longitudinal magnetic resonance imaging vascular changes, apolipoprotein E genotype, and development of dementia in the neurocognitive outcomes of depression in the elderly study. *Am J Geriatr Psychiatry.* 2007;15(10):839-849.

218. Almeida OP, Hankey GJ, Yeap BB, Golledge J, Norman PE, Flicker L. Depression, frailty, and all-cause mortality: a cohort study of men older than 75 years. *J Am Med Dir Assoc.* 2015;16(4):296-300.

219. Paulson D, Lichtenberg PA. Vascular depression and frailty: a compound threat to longevity among older-old women. *Aging Ment Health.* 2013;17(7):901-910.

220. Ho CS, Jin A, Nyunt MSZ, Feng L, Ng TP. Mortality rates in major and subthreshold depression: 10-year follow-up of a Singaporean population cohort of older adults. *Postgrad Med.* 2016;128(7):642-647.

221. Sheline YI, Barch DM, Garcia K, et al. Cognitive function in late life depression: relationships to depression severity, cerebrovascular risk factors and processing speed. *Biol Psychiatry.* 2006;60(1):58-65.

222. Sneed JR, Culang ME, Keilp JG, Rutherford BR, Devanand DP, Roose SP. Antidepressant medication and executive dysfunction: a deleterious interaction in late-life depression. *Am J Geriatr Psychiatry.* 2010;18(2):128-135.

223. Taler M, Miron O, Gil-Ad I, Weizman A. Neuroprotective and procognitive effects of sertraline: in vitro and in vivo studies. *Neurosci Lett.* 2013;550:93-97.

224. Boldrini M, Santiago AN, Hen R, et al. Hippocampal granule neuron number and dentate gyrus volume in antidepressant-treated and untreated major depression. *Neuropsychopharmacology.* 2013;38(6):1068-1077.

225. Sheline YI, West T, Yarasheski K, et al. An antidepressant decreases CSF Aβ production in healthy individuals and in transgenic AD mice. *Sci Transl Med.* 2014;6(236):236re4.

226. Jorge RE, Moser DJ, Acion L, Robinson RG. Treatment of vascular depression using repetitive transcranial magnetic stimulation. *Arch General Psychiatry.* 2008;65(3):268-276.

227. Coffey CE, Hinkle PE, Weiner RD, et al. Electroconvulsive therapy of depression in patients with white matter hyperintensity. *Biol Psychiatry.* 1987;22(5):629-636.

228. Meyer JP, Swetter SK, Kellner CH. Electroconvulsive therapy in geriatric psychiatry: a selective review. *Psychiatric Clin N Am.* 2018;41(1):79-93.

229. Spaans HP, Kok RM, Bouckaert F, et al. Vascular risk factors in older patients with depression: outcome of electroconvulsive therapy versus medication. *Int J Geriatr Psychiatry.* 2018;33(2):371-378.

The Neuropsychiatry of Parkinson's Disease and Dementia with Lewy Bodies

Irina A. Skylar-Scott · Adrienne D. Taylor · Katiuska J. Ramirez · John Sullivan

INTRODUCTION

The focus of the first section of this chapter is the epidemiology and pathophysiology of non-motor features of Parkinson's disease (PD), as well as the clinical presentation and approaches to diagnosis and treatment of PD. The second section emphasizes parallel features of dementia with Lewy bodies (DLB).

Parkinson's disease (also called Parkinson's disease) is a progressive, neurodegenerative disorder attributable to dopaminergic neuronal deterioration and loss in the substantia nigra pars compacta (SNc) and ventral tegmental area (VTA) of the midbrain. Although James Parkinson, a physician working in London in 1817, described "the absence of any injury to the senses and to the intellect," in An Essay on the Shaking Palsy, the core clinical attributes of PD are now widely acknowledged to include both motor and non-motor signs and symptoms.[1] Motor clinical features—asymmetric resting tremor, rigidity, akinesia or bradykinesia, and later, postural instability—result largely from disruption of nigrostriatal pathways, which extend from the midbrain's pigmented SNc to the dorsal "motor" striatum (caudate and putamen; see Figure 23-1). The term *striatum* refers to the striped appearance of gray and white matter. These motor features manifest due to decreased dopaminergic input to the basal ganglia and resultant thalamic inhibition and reduced excitatory input to the motor cortex. The role of direct and indirect striatal output circuitry on promoting and inhibiting movement, respectively, are outside the scope of this chapter; for details, please see a review by Calabresi and colleagues.[2]

The non-motor features of PD include mood dysregulation, anxiety, psychosis, sleep disturbances, personality changes, and cognitive impairment, among others. Other non-motor manifestations of PD, including olfactory, autonomic, and gastrointestinal dysfunction, are not reviewed here. Cognitive impairment and neuropsychiatric manifestations result, at least partially, from the respective disruption of the dopaminergic mesocortical and mesolimbic pathways—this disruption is mediated by deterioration of dopaminergic neurons

in the VTA. Although SNc neurons are the most susceptible dopaminergic neurons to degeneration in PD (with average degeneration in PD of approximately 80% of SNc neurons), about 50% of dopaminergic neurons within the VTA deteriorate as well.[3] Mesocortical pathways, implicated in cognitive impairment in PD, extend from the VTA to the prefrontal cortex. Emotional dysregulation in PD occurs due to disruption of mesolimbic "reward" pathways, which project from the VTA to the ventral striatum (primarily to the nucleus accumbens, or NAc) in the basal forebrain anterior to the hypothalamus (Figure 23-2).

In parallel to these neurochemical changes, α-synuclein protein cytoplasmic inclusions in neurons and neuron projections (Lewy bodies and Lewy neurites) are distributed across the central and peripheral nervous system over time (Figure 23-3). Neuropathologist Heiko Braak proposed a six-stage progression in 2003 ("Braak staging," which was expanded upon in 2009) wherein in presymptomatic stages 1 and 2, Lewy body pathology arises in the olfactory bulb, medulla, and pons; in stages 3 and 4, pathologic changes occur in the SNc as well as the amygdala and then the temporal lobes; and in stages 5 and 6, pathology develops in the neocortex. Prior to stage 1, α-synuclein may form in the enteric nervous system, which connects to the medulla via the vagus nerve, and the peripheral nervous system. Synuclein aggregates in limbic and cortical areas are thought to coincide with neuropsychiatric and cognitive sequelae, respectively (Figures 23-4 and 23-5).[4,5] However, researchers have increasingly questioned the predictive utility and accuracy of this model.[6] For an excellent review of the neuropathologic discoveries in PD over the last century, please see Goedert et al.[7]

Overall, PD is the second most common neurodegenerative disease after Alzheimer's disease (AD). Nearly 1 million Americans have PD, and the global prevalence is over 6 million.[8,9] For individuals aged 40 years in the United States, the lifetime risk of PD is 2% for men and 1.3% for women.[10] PD is thought to be the fastest growing source of patient disability among all neurologic disorders.[11] Neuropsychiatric and

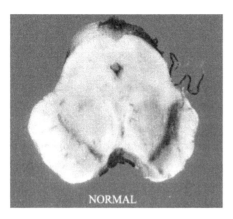
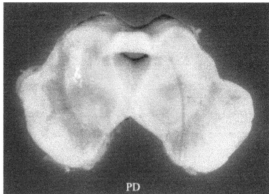

FIGURE 23-1. Macroscopic view of the normal pigmentation pattern of the substantia nigra in a gross specimen slice through the midbrain (left) and the depigmentation in the Parkinson's disease patient (right) due to dopaminergic cell loss. (Reproduced with permission from Watts RL, Standaert DG, Obeso JA. Parkinson's disease: neuropathology. In: *Movement Disorders.* 3rd ed. https://neurology.mhmedical.com/content. Copyright © McGraw Hill LLC. All rights reserved.)

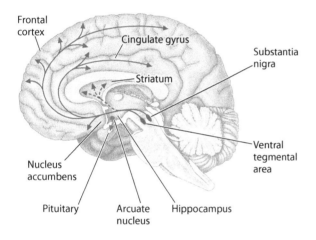

FIGURE 23-2. The major dopaminergic projections in the central nervous system include the nigrostriatal (dashed blue arrows), mesocorticolimbic (solid blue arrows), and tuberoinfundibular (red arrows) pathways. Disruption of the dopaminergic mesocortical and mesolimbic pathways plays a critical role in cognitive impairment and neuropsychiatric manifestations, respectively, in Parkinson's disease. (Reproduced with permission from Brunton LL, Hilal-Dandan R, Knollmann BC. 5-Hydroxytryptamine (serotonin) and dopamine. In: *Goodman & Gilman's: The Pharmacological Basis of Therapeutics.* 13th ed. https://accessmedicine.mhmedical.com/content. Copyright © McGraw Hill LLC. All rights reserved)

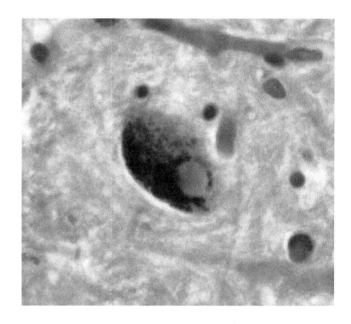

FIGURE 23-3. A round, eosinophilic Lewy body inclusion within the cytoplasm of a neuron in the substantia nigra. (Reproduced with permission from Frosch MP, Anthony DC, De Girolami U. The central nervous system. In *Robbins and Cotran Pathologic Basis of Disease.* 8th ed. © Saunders/Elsevier. All rights reserved.)

cognitive non-motor features of PD contribute substantially to this disability; in a cross-sectional study, non-motor symptoms (primarily depression and cognitive impairment) accounted for 37–54% of the total variance in disability among subjects.[12] Thus, it remains essential to identify and treat non-motor manifestations in PD patients. A schematic illustrating the natural history of both motor and non-motor clinical features of PD is shown in Figure 23-6.

DEPRESSION

Epidemiology

Psychiatric symptoms are common in PD, and depression is the most frequent among these. Estimates of depression rates in PD vary widely, but it is estimated that 17% of patients with PD meet *Diagnostic and Statistical Manual of Mental Disorders, Fifth Edition* (*DSM-5*) criteria for major depressive disorder. An additional 35% of PD patients meet criteria for dysthymia or subsyndromal depression.[13] Thus, over half of patients with PD suffer from depressed mood.

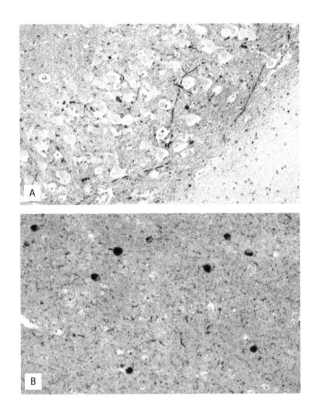

FIGURE 23-4. Lewy pathology develops characteristic regional differences. This is an alpha-synuclein staining in the hippocampus showing a network of Lewy neuritis **(A)** and in the limbic cortex showing cortical Lewy bodies in pyramidal cells as well as Lewy neurites **(B)** in a patient with Lewy pathology. (Reproduced with permission from Watts RL, Standaert DG, Obeso JA. Parkinson's disease: neuropathology. In: *Movement Disorders*. 3rd ed. https:// neurology.mhmedical.com. Copyright © McGraw Hill LLC. All rights reserved.)

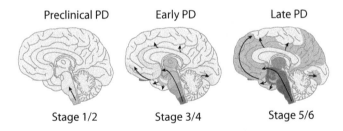

FIGURE 23-5. Classically, Lewy body pathology is thought to begin in the autonomic nervous system and then extends from the medulla up to the midbrain. It then ascends into the limbic system, and finally, the neocortex, and this can contribute to emotional and cognitive disturbances, respectively ("Braak staging"). Researchers have recently questioned this model, however. (Reproduced with permission from Watts RL, Standaert DG, Obeso JA. Parkinson's disease: neuropathology. In: *Movement Disorders*. 3rd ed. https://neurology.mhmedical.com. Copyright © McGraw Hill LLC. All rights reserved.)

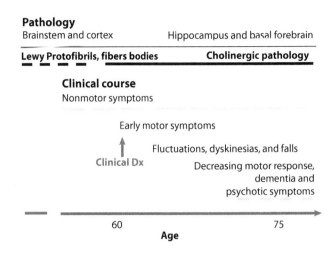

FIGURE 23-6. Natural history of Parkinson's disease, including motor and non-motor features. (Reproduced with permission from Fauci AS, Braunwald E, Kasper DL, et al. *Harrison's Principles of Internal Medicine*, 17th ed. https://accessmedicine.mhmedical.com. Copyright © McGraw Hill LLC. All rights reserved.)

more depression compared with healthy controls at baseline and at 2 years of follow-up. Mood symptoms can precede clinical motor parkinsonism by up to 20 years, but peak onset is 3–6 years prior to onset of motor symptoms and PD diagnosis.[17,18] It should be noted that most reports of depression onset rely in part upon patients' recall and are thus subject to some degree of reporting bias. However, support for an association between depression and PD was corroborated by a retrospective cohort study of patients with depression in which the date of depression diagnosis was logged by general practitioners at the time of diagnosis. The study identified a hazard ratio for developing PD of 3.13 among patients diagnosed with depression using International Classification of Primary Care (ICPC) criteria.[19]

Pathophysiology

While psychological reactions to the diagnosis and long-term prognosis of PD as well as the degree of PD-related disability have a role in the development of depression in PD, studies suggest that the neurobiological pathophysiology underlying PD also contributes to the development of depressive symptoms.[20] The correlation between depressive and certain motor symptoms supports the idea of a common pathophysiologic pathway. For example, there is a higher prevalence of depression in patients with predominantly akinetic-rigid motor symptoms versus tremor-rigid-bradykinetic symptoms.[21] Overall, the basal ganglia have a significant role in emotional processing as part of the prefrontal-striatal-thalamic circuits; the ventral striatum is particularly implicated in these emotional processing circuits.

Specialized positron emission tomography (PET) imaging called [11C]RTI-32 PET serves as an in vivo marker of neurotransmitter transporter binding. PET imaging of dopamine (DA) and norepinephrine (NE) transport receptors in patients with PD with and without depression shows that decreased DA and NE receptor binding correlates with depression symptom severity, as measured by the Beck Depression Inventory (BDI), in the left ventral striatum (NB: "receptor binding" refers

On the whole, rates of depression in patients who are ultimately diagnosed with PD are about double that of the general population.[14,15] De la Riva and colleagues[16] studied de novo PD patients and found that this population experienced significantly

to binding of ligands DA or NE to their respective receptors; this term does not refer to embedding of receptors within cell membranes). In general, patients with PD and depression have reduced receptor binding in the locus coeruleus (blue-pigmented nucleus in the pons and primary site of NE production), mediodorsal and inferior thalamus, left ventral striatum, and right amygdala when compared to patients with PD without depression. However, all PD patients had decreased binding in the left ventral striatum compared to healthy controls.[22] This suggests that depression in PD may be a consequence of a subset of the pathological processes of PD itself, although the authors did not compare nondepressed PD patients to controls (and, therefore, neurochemical changes in the depressed PD subgroup may be driving this difference between PD subjects and controls). It remains unclear whether development of depression in PD is related to underlying, individual vulnerabilities to disease progression.

Structural and functional imaging studies further highlight the involvement of the mediodorsal thalamus or "limbic thalamus" in depression associated with PD, in addition the neurochemical changes discussed above. In a study comparing patients with PD with and without depression, Cardoso and colleagues[23] identified increased volume in bilateral mediodorsal thalami in the PD depressed group based on voxel-based morphometry. There is convergent data that depressed patients, in general, have increased numbers of neurons in the mediodorsal thalamus, but it is unclear whether these are excitatory projection neurons or inhibitory interneurons.[24] In the PD subjects with increased mediodorsal thalamic volume, there was also reduced activation in the left mediodorsal thalamus and in the left dorsomedial prefrontal cortex on task-based functional magnetic resonance imaging (fMRI) scans of depressed participants compared with those without depression.[23] Potential effects of the loss of dopaminergic projections to the mediodorsal thalami, and how this might affect the above results, need to be further elucidated.

Notably, hypodopaminergic states can be particularly associated with anhedonia (diminished interest in previously enjoyed activities), a key feature of MDD. This is due to resultant hypoactive mesocorticolimbic reward circuitry[25] to which patients with PD are particularly vulnerable. Indeed, several studies of dopamine receptor agonist (DA) pramipexole, which has a preferential binding profile for D3 receptors in the limbic striatum, have demonstrated positive effects on anhedonia.[26–28]

Clinical Presentation

Depression often emerges before PD diagnosis, but it may also occur in the early or late stages of disease. Depression and anxiety are often comorbid.[18] Somatic symptoms of depression may be masked or confounded by parkinsonian motor manifestations such as bradykinesia and hypomimia. Additionally, hypomimia can affect patients' social and emotional lives and relationships. Many patients with PD who do not have depression experience early waking, decreased energy, and psychomotor retardation. Other symptoms, however, such as decreased appetite and libido, increased sleep latency (time to fall asleep) and overnight awakening, and non-somatic depressive symptoms—such

as low mood, anhedonia, feelings of guilt, and preoccupation with death—are generally attributable to depression.[29]

PD patients on levodopa may experience dysphoria and/or anxiety, combined with their motor fluctuations, as part of the "on/off" cycle. In most cases, the effect of levodopa gradually wears off a few hours after each dose. Additionally, after long-term use, levodopa may not work optimally. During these "off" periods, PD patients experience exacerbation of the PD motor symptoms and may also become more depressed and anxious. During the "on" periods after levodopa doses, PD patients' mobility increases (possibly with added dyskinesias), and mood improves. Thus, patients with PD may present with a uniquely cyclical form of depressed mood.[30]

Course and Natural History

Evolution of depressive symptoms in PD tends to mirror evolution of the motor symptoms. A longitudinal study of non-motor symptoms[31] showed that depressive symptoms decrease over the first 2 years after PD diagnosis as dopaminergic therapy is initiated and titrated. As neurodegeneration progresses, however, depressive symptoms return and become more refractory, similar to the motor and autonomic symptoms.

Depression can exacerbate the disability produced by motor symptoms and can be considered a marker of disease severity. In fact, depression is independently correlated with degree of disability in PD.[11] Patients with PD recognize the morbidity associated with depression. In a patient survey,[32] patients with early (<6 years) PD rate "mood" as the sixth most bothersome symptom. Patients with more advanced illness (>6 years) however, rate "mood" as the second most bothersome symptom behind medication-related symptom fluctuations.

Assessment and Differential Diagnosis

There are no specific criteria for diagnosis of depression in PD, and DSM criteria are generally used. Marsh and colleagues[29] recommend an "inclusive" approach to diagnosis that considers all pertinent symptoms that relate to depression, regardless of their overlap with symptoms of PD or other medical conditions, thus considering symptoms based on observation rather than presumed etiology. They also recommend a careful assessment of anhedonia to distinguish it from apathy, the latter of which may appear in patients with PD who are not depressed. Lastly, they encourage the identification and diagnosis of minor depression or dysthymia in PD, as these symptoms can cause significant distress and functional impairment in PD without rising to the level of major depression.[29]

Depression scales may be useful in PD to screen for unreported or difficult-to-detect depression and to monitor the progression of symptoms. The BDI,[33] Hamilton Rating Scale for Depression (HAM-17),[34] and Montgomery-Asberg Depression Rating Scale (MADRS),[34] are validated instruments for diagnosing and assessing severity of depression in PD, although the cutoffs for clinical significance tend to slightly overdiagnose depression because of the confounding effect of motor symptoms (please see the Clinical Presentation section above for discussion of overlapping motor and depressive symptoms).

Because of its inherent morbidity and association with greater functional impairment, diagnosis of depression in PD is as important as it can be difficult due to this confounding effect. In one prospective study, diagnostic accuracy of the treating neurologist during routine visits was only 35% when compared with a BDI cutoff score of 10, an accepted threshold.[35] Routine screening of PD patients for depression and other non-motor symptoms should be commonplace and can be effectively accomplished using self-report checklists such as the BDI.

Treatment

Psychopharmacologic Treatment

Although controlled trial data are limited, clinicians have used antidepressants to treat depression in patients with PD with encouraging results. It is reasonable to start with selective serotonin reuptake inhibitors (SSRIs) given their preferred side-effect profile compared with that of tricyclic antidepressants (TCAs).[36] One controlled trial in 2009 comparing TCA nortriptyline and SSRI paroxetine for depression in PD showed significant advantages of nortriptyline,[37] although this study had several limitations including its brief duration, relatively small size, and high dropout rate.[38] This study notwithstanding, TCAs and paroxetine are often avoided in elderly patients with PD who may be at risk for anticholinergic side effects, including cognitive dysfunction.[39]

A randomized, double blind, placebo-controlled study established that both venlafaxine, a serotonin-norepinephrine reuptake inhibitor (SNRI), and paroxetine may improve depression in subjects with PD.[40] A small series demonstrated a beneficial effect with the use of duloxetine, another SNRI.[41] Of note, some researchers have raised concern over the potential exacerbation of extrapyramidal side effects by serotonergic agents; however, the evidence remains inconclusive.[42,43] Proposed mechanisms for worsening motor symptoms due to SSRIs include inhibition by serotonin of nigrostriatal DA release, effects of SSRIs on sigma 2 receptors, and increased raphe nuclei projection activity on nigral cells resulting in decreased DA turnover.[44] Bupropion, an antidepressant which inhibits reuptake of norepinephrine and dopamine (NDRI), should theoretically be of benefit in PD, given its dopaminergic mechanism of action. It has been reported as effective anecdotally in a case report, and further study is recommended because of its low likelihood of worsening—and, in fact, potential for ameliorating—motor symptoms.[45,46]

Monoamine oxidase inhibitors (MAOIs) can provide benefits in reducing "on/off" motor fluctuations in addition to treating depression. MAO-B inhibitors selegiline and rasagiline are most commonly used. One trial comparing two doses of rasagiline in 22 patients with comorbid PD and depression showed improvement in motor symptoms without significant differences in motor symptoms between patients receiving 1 or 2 mg/d. All patients also showed improvement in depressive symptoms, but patients receiving the higher dose showed greater improvement compared with those receiving the lower dose.[47] This suggests that the antidepressant benefits of rasagiline are independent of its motor benefits and that this medication may be particularly useful in patients with PD who are depressed. Selegiline

or rasagiline should be used with caution in combination with SSRIs and TCAs due to the risk of serotonin syndrome. Notably, a trial of 1174 subjects with PD randomized to rasagiline versus placebo included 191 subjects on rasagiline and concurrent SSRI or TCA medication. Of these 191 individuals, none experienced serotonin syndrome.[48] Patients on MAOIs should be counseled to limit or avoid tyramine-containing foods such as animal liver, alcoholic beverages, and aged cheeses given the risk that tyramine can increase NE release, without the counteracting effects of MAO to metabolize the excess NE, and lead to hypertensive crisis.

Treatment of PD itself, with dopaminergic medications such as levodopa and DAs, can also treat concomitant depression. In contrast, other non-motor manifestations of PD such as cognitive impairment benefit minimally from dopaminergic medications, and moreover, hallucinations and delusions can be exacerbated by dopaminergic medications.[49] DAs such as pramipexole are commonly used to treat PD motor symptoms, and they may also benefit PD depression. However, the evidence from controlled studies is still insufficient to recommend DAs as a first line of treatment for depression. Of note, potential side effects of the addition or uptitration of dopaminergic medications include nausea, orthostasis, confusion, hallucinations, and impulse control disorders (ICDs are discussed later in this chapter). Long-term dopaminergic therapy can also result in motor fluctuations, failed doses, involuntary movements known as dyskinesias, and abnormal cramps and postures of the trunk and postures known as dystonias.[50]

Brain Stimulation Therapies

While there has not been a randomized controlled trial (RCT) of electroconvulsive therapy (ECT) for depression in PD, there are numerous uncontrolled studies reporting efficacy and tolerability. It has been hypothesized to enhance DA neurotransmission and increase sensitivity of DA receptors. ECT should certainly be considered as a treatment for medication-refractory or severe depression in patients with PD.[43] Repetitive transcranial magnetic stimulation (rTMS) has shown promising results in patients with PD and depression. Beneficial effects on motor and cognitive symptoms have also been reported.[36,51]

Deep brain stimulation (DBS) has emerged as an important treatment option for motor symptoms of PD, particularly in patients with advanced disease or with side effects that limit the usefulness of dopaminergic medications. The most common sites for stimulator placement in PD are the subthalamic nucleus (STN) and the globus pallidus internus (GPi, medial "pale globe" in Latin) of the basal ganglia. The effects of DBS for PD are most clearly seen in the improvement of motor symptoms, but changes in mood have been observed as well. The evidence has been mixed, with some early reports of increased incidence of depression following DBS surgery and subsequent larger randomized trials showing little difference in mood outcomes of DBS versus medical management of PD.[52] Although some reports have suggested greater risk of depression following DBS placement in the STN as compared with the GPi, a study designed to compare these sites using mood and cognitive measures as primary endpoints failed to find a significant difference.[53]

Furthermore, stimulation of STN often allows for reduction of dopaminergic medication due to less prominent motor symptoms, but dose reduction of levodopa or DAs may exacerbate underlying depressive symptoms, which these medications had been treating as well. Although premorbid, well-controlled depression is not a contraindication to DBS, surgery can be associated with a depression relapse.[54]

There has been concern that DBS targeting of the STN may increase suicide risk, in particular, but this link has not been firmly established.[55] In one international survey of 55 centers with over 5000 patients with DBS in the STN, the suicide rate in the first year after surgery was 0.26% per year, which was 13 times higher than the suicide rate of age, gender, and country-matched general population controls.[56] It is therefore reasonable to screen DBS candidates for suicide risk and to carefully monitor for symptoms of depression and suicidal ideation postoperatively. Please see the section on neuropsychiatric effects of DBS later in this chapter for more details.

Psychosocial Treatment

Psychosocial treatments appear useful for depression in PD as well. An RCT of cognitive behavioral therapy (CBT) for depression in PD included exercise, behavioral activation, thought monitoring and restructuring, sleep hygiene, worry control, and relaxation training. It was supplemented with individual sessions with caregivers designed to equip them with the skills necessary to facilitate the practice of CBT at home.[57] In comparison with the control group, which received clinical monitoring alone, the treatment group showed significant improvement in measures of depression. Furthermore, this study revealed that caregiver participation, rather than patient factors (motor disability, psychiatric comorbidity, and executive function), predicted treatment response.[57,58] Patient Education Program Parkinson (PEPP), a standardized program using CBT techniques administered to small groups of patients and their caregivers, also showed mood improvement in the treatment group.[59,60] There is some evidence for group therapy in the treatment of depression in PD. A small, waitlist-controlled RCT of group therapy demonstrated a significant reduction in depression in group participants; the group therapy used psychodrama methods (e.g., role play and emotional expression with sessions focused on disease education, discussing emotions, and providing tools to adapt to circumstances) in 12 sessions, provided education on PD, and information on coping skills and adaptive resources.[61]

Interventions that primarily target motor symptoms of PD can also have secondary benefits on mood.[61] There is evidence to suggest that Tai Chi is one such intervention; there is also preliminary evidence in favor of yoga and music therapy, but further study is needed.[62] Also, a study of multidisciplinary rehabilitation including individually administered physical, occupational, and speech therapies, group relaxation exercises, expert lectures, and caregiver groups showed significant improvement in mood, although the benefits were not sustained 6 months after termination.[63,64] This result suggests the need for longer-term interventions or maintenance sessions to address the continuing needs of patients and the progressive nature of PD itself.

ANXIETY

Epidemiology

Up to 40% of PD patients meet criteria for one of several anxiety disorders, as defined by the DSM. An additional 15% may experience significant anxiety symptoms without meeting DSM criteria.[65] The prevalence rates of anxiety in PD vary widely in the literature. A 2016 systematic review by Broen et al. found that the average prevalence of an anxiety disorder in PD patients was 31%. The most frequent diagnosis was generalized anxiety disorder (GAD) with a prevalence of 14.2%. Other diagnoses included social phobia (prevalence of 13.9%), anxiety disorder not otherwise specified (13.3%), and specific phobia (13.9%). One-third of PD patients diagnosed with anxiety had two or more anxiety disorders.[66] Additionally, in a prospective study of 89 subjects with mild PD evaluated for depression and anxiety (using the Geriatric Depression Scale and Hospital Anxiety and Depression Scale—"Anxiety" subscale, respectively) every 6 months for 18 months, depression and anxiety were comorbid in 13.5% of the sample.[67]

Demographic factors associated with anxiety in PD include younger age, female gender, and younger age of PD onset.[68] In terms of PD clinical characteristics, associations between anxiety and disease duration and severity have been found in some, but not all, studies. A prior history of anxiety and anxiety-related personality traits (neuroticism, harm avoidance) have also been associated with anxiety in PD patients.[69]

Pathophysiology

There is ongoing research into the neurobiological alterations that contribute to anxiety in PD. Implicated pathways and structures include (1) neurodegeneration of mesolimbic and mesocortical dopaminergic projections, (2) dysfunction of the amygdala, and (3) degeneration of brainstem nuclei responsible for NE and serotonin synthesis.[69,70]

Dopaminergic alterations can be directly related to anxiety symptoms in PD. The positive relationship between anxiety and "on/off" motor fluctuations, as well as that of anxiety and withdrawal of dopaminergic medication, provides clinical evidence to support dopaminergic involvement in PD-associated anxiety. The dopaminergic theory suggests that the neurodegeneration of mesolimbic and mesocortical dopaminergic projections, which is observed as a primary neuroanatomical alteration in PD, is strongly associated with anxiety in PD. The mesolimbic dopaminergic pathway has projections to the amygdala, which is a key structure implicated in the production and regulation of anxiety. More directly, functional alterations and neurodegeneration in the amygdala have been implicated in the emotional dysfunction and anxiety symptoms in PD.[69]

Degeneration of brainstem structures such as the raphe nuclei (in the midbrain, pons, and medulla) and the blue-pigmented pontine locus coeruleus—both structures important in the regulation of anxiety in general—may be implicated in PD-related anxiety, as well. The raphe nuclei are abundant in serotonin while the locus coeruleus is rich in NE, and the depletion of these neurotransmitters is thought to result in enhanced anxiety in PD. The association between premorbid anxious personality and PD as well as the high prevalence of anxiety disorders among family members of patients with PD suggest a genetic predisposition to PD-related anxiety. However, studies corroborating this, such as investigations of genetic polymorphisms directly associated with neurotransmitter systems implicated in PD and in anxiety, are limited.[69,70] From the psychosocial perspective, anxiety is often a part of the psychological response to a chronic and progressive neurological diagnosis.[69]

Clinical Presentation

Anxiety in PD commonly includes symptoms of inability to relax, restlessness, tension, and worrying thoughts. It also encompasses sleep disturbances and fatigue. PD patients also experience a range of anxiety symptoms specific to PD, or that are particularly prominent in PD, such as worsening of parkinsonian resting tremor as well as embarrassment or self-consciousness over parkinsonian symptoms. Additionally, PD patients have increased anxiety in the context of needing more assistance due to disability and due to fear of falling. The onset of anxiety symptoms in PD can take place before or after the diagnosis of PD. Anxiety in PD that precedes motor symptoms may be a premotor manifestation of the illness, resulting from early neurobiological changes related to the disease, which suggests a common pathological mechanism underlying anxiety and the motor symptoms of PD.[69]

Anxiety in PD can co-occur with and be exacerbated by disease-related motor signs and symptoms (e.g., postural instability, freezing of gait, gait impairment, bradykinesia, resting tremor, muscle cramps, dystonia, and overall freezing). Patients with PD are particularly vulnerable during the nadir of dopaminergic stimulation ("off" periods) and in the context of treatment-related complications (e.g., dyskinesias).[68] Studies that have tried to elucidate the association between anxiety and extrapyramidal clinical features have identified that patients with PD may suffer from excessive, recurrent, and anticipatory anxiety in relation to "off" periods.[69] Panic attacks have been called an "abstinence syndrome" because they occurred 90.3% of the time during "off" periods in patients on levodopa or dopaminergic agonists.[71] Research on whether the prevalence of obsessive-compulsive disorder is higher in PD compared with the general population have been mixed[72]; for details of possible fastidious and obsessive personality traits in PD, please see the Parkinsonian Personality section. For details on impulsive-compulsive behaviors, please see the Impulse Control Disorders section.

Assessment and Differential Diagnosis

The diagnosis of anxiety disorders in PD is typically made based on anxiety symptoms and following classic DSM criteria. Rating scales, such as the Beck Anxiety Inventory (BAI) and the Hamilton Anxiety Rating Scale (HARS), can be helpful in identifying the presence of anxiety. They can also be useful in monitoring patients' clinical course over time and responses to treatment. The BAI has a predominant focus on physical anxiety symptoms (such as those presenting in panic attacks), and the HARS focuses on assessing symptoms of generalized anxiety.[66]

Recognizing and treating anxiety in PD patients is imperative because anxiety can have a substantial impact on quality of life and functioning. Clinicians fail to recognize more than half of cases with clinically significant anxiety symptoms (as determined by cutoff score thresholds on anxiety rating scales), suggesting that anxiety in PD is underrecognized and undertreated.[69] Both when assessing anxiety via a clinical evaluation of symptoms, or with the use of rating scales, it is important to be aware of the possible fluctuations of anxiety correlating with the fluctuations of the effect of dopaminergic medication and motor symptoms.

There are limitations to the use of anxiety rating scales among PD patients, compared to the general population, because these scales may not be sensitive to lower, but bothersome, levels of anxiety or to anxiety in the context of motor fluctuations. They may not adequately differentiate between PD symptoms, physical or neurovegetative symptoms of anxiety (e.g., fatigue, muscle tension, insomnia, and agitation), or a combination thereof.[69,70] There are also limitations with the clinical diagnosis of anxiety disorders in PD via the *DSM-5*, as patients with PD may present with anxiety symptoms that do not correspond clearly to the different DSM anxiety disorders. Reciprocally, the DSM group of anxiety disorders may not capture the subtypes of anxiety present in PD described above, including anxiety related to motor symptoms and anxiety related to DA fluctuations.[69]

Treatment

There is limited research dedicated to the treatment of anxiety in PD. Most drug trials have primarily targeted depression and motor symptoms in PD. SSRIs are used to treat depression in PD and are also utilized to reduce comorbid anxiety symptoms. The SSRI citalopram can help achieve longer remission rates in cases of anxious depression. However, in a double-blind, placebo-controlled RCT, citalopram did not cause a significant decline in anxiety symptoms. Paroxetine also failed to show a reliable effect in decreasing depressive or anxiety symptoms when compared to the placebo group in another double-blind, placebo-controlled RCT.[70] Uncontrolled studies have shown efficacy of SSRIs in treating PD-related anxiety, however.[73-75] SNRI data is limited; one 12-week RCT of 115 subjects in the SAD-PD group did not find a significant difference in treatment effect between placebo, venlafaxine, and paroxetine groups; however, these results should be interpreted cautiously because anxiety was only a secondary outcome.[76]

TCAs are both noradrenaline and serotonin reuptake inhibitors and may have advantages to treating anxiety in PD due to their action on two neurotransmitter systems. Although a double-blind, placebo-controlled RCT showed that desipramine significantly impacted depressive symptoms and was quicker to act compared to citalopram, it did not significantly decrease anxiety symptoms when compared to the placebo group. However, amitriptyline significantly decreased anxiety symptoms when compared to placebo and paroxetine. SSRIs such as citalopram frequently lead to fewer side effects compared to TCAs, and this often guides clinical practice.[70]

Mirtazapine is an agent that acts via noradrenaline and serotonin reuptake and has been shown to decrease depressive and anxiety symptoms in PD, in addition to tremor and dyskinesias related to levodopa therapy. Buspirone, a specific serotonin receptor agonist, has also been helpful in the treatment of anxiety in PD and in addressing levodopa-related dyskinesias. Benzodiazepines are not generally recommended because of potential adverse reactions like increased risk of falling and cognitive dysfunction.[70]

CBT offers a nonpharmacological approach to the treatment of anxiety in PD that has been most effective when tailored to PD patients and when taking into account their motor symptoms. A blinded RCT showed that CBT for depression in PD led to significant improvements in depression, anxiety, motor decline, and quality of life. Further research is needed to compare CBT to pharmacological options and to determine when CBT should be administered in conjunction with pharmacological options.[70]

PSYCHOSIS

Epidemiology

More than 50% of all PD patients experience psychotic symptoms, and up to 75% of patients with PD dementia experience psychotic symptoms.[77] Patients with Parkinson's disease psychosis (PDP) are more likely to experience a poorer quality of life, increased disability, and increased caregiver burden compared with their PD counterparts without psychosis. PDP also increases the risk of nursing home placement and mortality. Risk factors for PDP include longer disease duration, more advanced disease, cognitive impairment, rapid eye movement (REM) behavior sleep disorder, and depression.[78,79] The prevalence of specific psychotic symptoms in PD is discussed below (please see the Clinical Presentation section).

Pathophysiology

Dopaminergic medications may contribute to or exacerbate psychotic symptoms, but psychotic symptoms in PD can arise in medication-naïve patients; overall, the pathology of PDP is complex and not solely medication-related.[78,79] There is ongoing research into the pathogenesis of PDP—to date, studies have identified disruption of visual processing and executive function pathways, and temporo-limbic structures and neocortical gray matter have also been implicated.[79]

Stebbins and colleagues[80] found that PD subjects who were hallucinating had increased fMRI activation of frontal (Brodmann areas 44 and 46) and subcortical (caudate) areas and less visual cortex activation compared with PD subjects who were not hallucinating; the authors proposed that disinhibition of "top-down" processing resulted in release of internally generated images into areas that process externally generated ones. Additionally, when pathologic specimens were compared in 10 PD patients with hallucinations and 10 PD without them, the former group had significantly greater amygdalar and cortical Lewy bodies.[81] With regard to neurotransmitter systems, research to date has implicated DA dysregulation most consistently in PD-related psychosis, but serotonin and acetylcholine have also been implicated.[82]

Clinical Presentation

The spectrum of characteristic symptoms in PDP includes minor phenomena, visual and nonvisual hallucinations, and delusions. Minor phenomena include presence hallucinations (experiencing the sense that another is present), passage hallucinations (experiencing imagery, such as animals, in one's periphery), and illusions (external stimuli that are misperceived or misinterpreted).[78,79] The most common symptoms in PDP include mild visual distortions and more complex visual hallucinations, including images of animals or people.[77-79] The prevalence of minor phenomena in PD patients is 20–45%; 13–27% of these patients have co-occurring hallucinations.[79] Less common psychotic symptoms include delusions, which affect 5–30% of PD patients, and auditory hallucinations, which affect 8% of PD patients.[77] Delusions, or fixed false beliefs, tend to be of a paranoid nature and usually relate to infidelity. Less commonly, persecutory, religious, or grandiose delusions can occur.[78,79]

Assessment and Differential Diagnosis

The National Institute of Neurological Disorders and Stroke (NINDS) and the National Institute of Mental Health (NIMH) set forth the following diagnostic criteria for PDP in 2007: characteristic symptoms (e.g., illusions, presence hallucinations, hallucinations, and/or delusions) that are recurrent or persistent for ≥1 month, a PD diagnosis via the UK Brain Bank criteria,[83] onset of characteristic symptoms after the PD diagnosis, and the exclusion of other probable diagnoses (e.g., DLB, psychiatric disorder, and delirium) (Table 23-1).[79,84]

An American Academy of Neurology review in 2006 was unable to recommend any psychosis rating scale for use in PD. Although a 2008 Movement Disorder Society Rating Scale Task Force recommended 4 of 12 psychosis rating scales for use in PD, it also cautioned that these scales were still limited with regards to capturing the full spectrum of PDP symptoms. The recommended scales included the Neuropsychiatric Inventory (NPI), Brief Psychiatric Rating Scale (BPRS), Positive

TABLE 23-1 · NINDS/NIMH Criteria for the Diagnosis of Parkinson's Disease Psychosis.	
Criteria	**Details**
Characteristic symptoms that are recurrent or persistent for ≥1 month	Illusions Presence hallucinations Hallucinations Delusions
PD diagnosis	UK Brain Bank criteria[22]
Onset of characteristic symptoms after the PD diagnosis	
Exclusion of other probable diagnoses	Dementia with Lewy bodies Psychiatric disorder Delirium

NINDS/NIMH, National Institute of Neurological Disorders and Stroke/National Institute of Mental Health; PD, Parkinson's disease.
Adapted from Ravina B, Marder K, Fernandez HH, et al. Diagnostic criteria for psychosis in Parkinson's disease: Report of an NINDS, NIMH Work Group. Mov Disord. 2007;22(8):1061-1068. https://doi.org/10.1002/mds.21382.

and Negative Syndrome Scale (PANSS), and Schedule for Assessment of Positive Symptoms for Parkinson's Disease Psychosis (SAPS-PD). Further investigation is necessary to assess the utility of newer scales like the SAPS-PD.[79,84,85] A discussion of potential medical contributors to psychosis is detailed below (please see the Treatment section).

Treatment

Management of PDP first involves assessment of the nature and severity of the characteristic symptoms since not all psychotic symptoms are distressing or disabling to patients, and, consequently, may not need further intervention. If intervention is deferred, patients should be monitored for progression of psychotic symptoms, especially in the context of new medical or pharmacological triggers or stressors. It is imperative to evaluate for any possible medical contributors to psychosis, such as febrile illness, infections, or structural brain lesions. PD is an independent risk factor for delirium, and PD patients are vulnerable to adverse medication events, syncope, falls, pneumonia, genitourinary infections, trauma, and mobility complications.

A careful evaluation of PD and non-PD medications should also be undertaken, since these may be causal or exacerbating factors.[78,79] Careful consideration into the timing of starting or adjusting medications and the onset of psychotic symptoms may be helpful. Nonessential non-PD medications, which can be contributing to psychotic symptoms, such as benzodiazepines, anticholinergics, bladder antispasmodics, muscle relaxants, and opioids, should be discontinued.

Dopamine replacement therapy (DRT) can exacerbate delusions and hallucinations; PD medications may need to be adjusted with the goal of ameliorating/resolving psychotic symptoms while maintaining motor function. PD medications should be removed gradually in the following order, in an attempt to reduce psychotic symptoms: anticholinergics (including benztropine and trihexyphenidyl, which are sometimes used for tremor reduction in PD patients), MAO-B inhibitors, amantadine, DAs, and catechol-O-methyltransferase (COMT) inhibitors (e.g., entacapone). Any levodopa adjustments should be made last. It is worth noting that, in the process of discontinuing other PD medications, levodopa may need to be increased to preserve motor function.[78,79]

When the above interventions are insufficient to ameliorate or resolve disabling or distressing psychotic symptoms, antipsychotic medications should be considered. All typical antipsychotics and most atypical antipsychotics are not recommended in this patient population due to their negative impact on motor function, mostly via significant D2 receptor antagonism. The exceptions are clozapine and quetiapine. Clozapine, a weak D2 antagonist and more significant 5HT2A and D4 antagonist, seems to be the most efficacious, but its clinical use has been limited due to the risk of agranulocytosis and the need for regular laboratory monitoring.[79,80] In two randomized control trials of clozapine in PD psychosis, both studies showed significant improvement (using the Clinical Global Improvement Scale or CGIS) when clozapine was compared to placebo. Additionally, motor function did not worsen (as measured by the motor Unified Parkinson's Disease Rating Scale or UPDRS) following

clozapine use for 4 weeks.[85] Common side effects of clozapine are sedation and postural hypotension, but the low effective doses (up to 50 mg daily) of clozapine in PDP do not seem to be associated with metabolic syndrome as seen with the long-term use of clozapine at 300–900 mg per day for psychosis in schizophrenia.

Quetiapine, a weak D2 antagonist and more significant 5HT2A antagonist, is used more routinely in clinical practice since it does not require the same regular laboratory monitoring as clozapine and causes very limited motor impairment. Clinical trials have provided mixed results with regards to its efficacy. Two clinical trials compared quetiapine to clozapine in the treatment of psychosis in PD, and while one of these showed them to be equally efficacious, the other showed clozapine to be superior.[78,79]

In 2016, pimavanserin became the first medication to receive FDA approval for the treatment of psychosis in PD. It is a 5HT2A selective inverse agonist with negligible binding to dopaminergic, adrenergic, histaminergic, and muscarinic receptors. A phase III randomized, double-blind, placebo-controlled study showed that pimavanserin had significant antipsychotic efficacy with improvements on the SAPS-PD, improved caregiver burden, and no motor impairment.[78,79]

Other potential non-antipsychotic pharmacological interventions include cholinesterase inhibitors (CHEIs). Although no double-blind, placebo-controlled trials have been conducted to determine the efficacy of CHEIs in psychosis, smaller studies, case series, and open label trials have found these agents (rivastigmine has been more studied than donepezil) to positively impact cognitive impairment and have more subtle positive treatment effects on visual hallucinations. Delusions did not improve in these studies. Memantine, an NDMA receptor antagonist, has been found to worsen psychosis in patients with PD and DLB.[78,79,86]

Overall, further investigation will be necessary to determine the longer-term efficacy and safety of pimavanserin and the utility of other pharmacological agents in the treatment of PDP.

APATHY

Epidemiology

Reported frequencies of apathy in PD range from 15% to 70%, and this variability is likely due to the differences in diagnostic approaches when assessing for PD-related apathy. Apathy may occur in up to 25% of PD patients during early stages of the disease. In the absence of dementia, its prevalence increases to 40% after 5–10 years of disease. The prevalence further increases to 60% when dementia is present.[87,88]

Pathophysiology

In a PET functional neuroimaging study, PD individuals with apathy demonstrated a blunted response to a spatial search task for reward money compared with PD participants without apathy in the areas implicated in representations of reward values, including ventromedial prefrontal cortex, left amygdala, left striatum, and VTA.[89] In another PET study examining DA radioligand binding in PD subjects with and without apathy following STN-DBS, there was increased binding in the orbitofrontal cortex, dorsolateral PFC, cingulate cortex, left ventral striatum, and right amygdala in the apathetic subjects; this may be interpreted as either an increased DA receptor density or a reduction of endogenous DA levels.[90] In non-demented patients, disruptions in activation in the lateral (dorsolateral and ventrolateral) PFC and caudate are implicated in cognitive apathy (please see the Clinical Presentation section).[87,88] These studies underscore the role of the hypodopaminergic state in the mesocorticolimbic system in emotional and cognitive dysregulation in PD.

Clinical Presentation

Apathy is a behavioral syndrome that results in a state of reduced motivation and a decrease in goal-directed behavior, with associated emotional and cognitive features.[87,88,91] Apathy in PD can manifest predominantly within one domain or with a combination of characteristics from four different domains: decreased emotional valence (reward deficiency syndrome), depression, decreased cognitive interest (executive dysfunction), and an absence of spontaneous activation of mental processes (auto-activation deficit).[87,88,92,93]

Apathy, independent of cognitive impairment or depression, can present throughout the disease course of PD. It can also manifest after DBS, especially in the context of a reduction or withdrawal of dopaminergic medications.[87,88] Although there can be overlap between apathy and depression in PD, depression can be distinguished by the presence of comparatively more negative emotions, thoughts, and beliefs (Table 23-2).[88]

In contrast to PD without apathy, PD with apathy can herald decreased functioning in activities of daily living and is associated with more severe motor impairment, worse executive dysfunction, decreased treatment response, poor outcome, diminished quality of life, significant caregiver distress, and a higher risk of developing dementia.[87,88]

This section discusses apathy in the context of PD. For a more general discussion of the syndrome of apathy in different neuropsychiatric disorders and its treatment, please see the chapter 8 *Psychopharmacology in Neuropsychiatric Syndromes*, in this textbook.

Assessment and Differential Diagnosis

There is a lack of widely accepted diagnostic criteria for apathy in PD. There are ongoing efforts to improve the standardization and generalizability of tools and criteria that can be used among physicians and research groups. To date, only two studies have published clinical criteria for apathy in PD and apathy in AD and other neuropsychiatric disorders.[87,88]

A 2008 task force commissioned by the Movement Disorders Society, which assessed the clinical validity properties of apathy and anhedonia scales in PD patients, only recommended the Apathy Scale (AS) to assess for apathy in PD. Although item 4 (motivation/initiative) of the UPDRS also met criteria for recommendation, the task force suggested it only be used for the screening of apathy in PD, given its limitation as a single item construct. The task force "suggested" (a step below

TABLE 23-2 • Symptoms of Apathy, Symptoms of Depression, and Overlapping Symptoms of Apathy and Depression in Parkinson's Disease.		
Apathetic Symptoms	**Overlapping Symptoms**	**Emotional Symptoms of Depression**
• Reduced initiative • Loss of interest in social events or everyday activities • Willing to participate only if another person is engaging her/him • Decreased interest in starting new activities • Decreased interest in the world around him/her • Emotional indifference • Diminished emotional reactivity • Less affectionate • Lack of concern	• Psychomotor retardation • Anhedonia • Anergia • Less active than usual • Less enthusiastic about his/her usual interests	• Sadness • Feelings of guilt • Negative thoughts and feelings • Helplessness • Hopelessness • Pessimism • Self-criticism • Anxiety • Suicidal ideation

"recommended") the following scales for the screening of apathy in PD: the Apathy Evaluation Scale (AES), the Lille Apathy Rating Scale (LARS), or item 7 (apathy) of the NPI. Of note, the LARS would now meet "recommended" criteria given its use outside the scope of its original development.[87,88,94]

Treatment

Studies have investigated CHEIs, dopaminergic agents, and antidepressants for the treatment of apathy in PD. A double-blind, placebo-controlled study of PD patients without dementia and depression showed improvement of apathy (assessed using the LARS) after 6 months on rivastigmine 9.5 mg/d. Furthermore, in a 12-week prospective, placebo-controlled, randomized, double-blind trial, the D2/D3 dopamine agonist piribedil significantly improved apathy (assessed using the AS) that had arisen following STN-DBS. The D2/D3 dopamine agonist ropinirole also significantly improved apathy (assessed using the AS) that had arisen following STN-DBS in an open-label study of 8 PD patients. Methylphenidate was helpful for apathy in PD in a case report, but evidence remains limited. Bupropion, a norepinephrine-dopamine reuptake inhibitor, may improve motivation.[87,88]

The use of SSRIs for the treatment of apathy in PD is controversial; in some studies, SSRIs have been associated with increased apathy among elderly depressed patients and in PD patients. Case reports of patients with apathy following subthalamic nucleus DBS indicate that the apathy was resistant to SSRI treatment but responded to dopaminergic treatment.[87,88]

IMPULSE CONTROL DISORDERS

Impulsive-compulsive behaviors (ICBs) in PD include impulse control disorders (ICDs), punding, and DA dysregulation syndrome. ICDs are non-motor complications of PD in which a person fails to resist the drive to engage in repetitive, excessive, and compulsive behaviors (please see the Clinical Presentation section below for additional details). This condition can be triggered by DRT, especially with DA treatment.[95]

Epidemiology

DRT appears to be the main risk factor for occurrence of ICDs. At least one ICD has been reported in 7.2% for those patients treated with levodopa only, 14% of patients on DAs only, 17.7% of PD patients treated with both levodopa and DAs, and 1.7% in PD patients not prescribed either levodopa or DA.[95] Many studies have shown that the strongest association is reported with DAs (vs. levodopa); there is inconsistent evidence regarding a dose-response relationship between DRT and ICDs and related behaviors, however.[96,97] Evidence suggests that PD in the absence of treatment does not result in increased risk for development of ICDs or related behaviors, reinforcing the association between DRT and ICDs. Nonpharmacological risk factors include early age of disease onset, male gender, personal or family history of alcohol abuse or pathological gambling, novelty-seeking personality traits, cognitive or psychiatric disorders, and sleep disorders.[98-101]

Pathophysiology

Experimental research on the pathophysiology of ICDs in PD patients remains an emerging field. D1 and D2 receptors are found predominately in the dorsal striatum, while D3 receptors localize to the ventral striatum. While DA in the dorsal striatum may improve motor symptoms, activation of D3 receptors in the ventral striatum may induce impulsive behaviors. Thus, DAs such as pramipexole, which have been shown to be relatively selective to D3 receptors, result in increased risk of ICDs.[102]

Imaging and clinical studies have demonstrated that nigrostriatal degeneration and overactivity of structures within and interacting with the mesocorticolimbic pathway (orbitofrontal cortex or OFC, amygdala, hippocampus, and insula) could play a role in some behavioral processes relevant to pathophysiology of ICD including several features of impulsivity and inability to learn from negative outcomes without affecting behavior on probabilistic/gambling-like schedules of reinforcement.[103,104]

Clinical Presentation

ICDs are non-motor complications of PD in which a person fails to resist the drive to engage in repetitive, excessive, and compulsive behaviors that can be dangerous for themselves or other people and/or interfere in major areas of life functioning. ICDs can be defined as "behavioral" addictions and include compulsive eating, gambling, buying, and sexual behavior.[100,101] ICDs fall under the umbrella of ICBs, which also include punding (stereotyped, repetitive, and purposeless behaviors such as rearranging papers), hobbyism (excessive or compulsive Internet use, reading, art work, and work on projects), aimless wandering, hoarding, and dopamine dysregulation syndrome (DDS, characterized by compulsive overuse of DRT particularly with L-dopa and short-acting DAs).[104-108] Punding and DDS will be discussed in more detail later in this chapter. These behaviors vary in severity and excessive nature but may lead to major functional decline or impairment in quality of life, both for the individual with PD and family members. Generally speaking, these behaviors become a disorder when they become harmful for patients, become harmful for their relatives, or interfere with social relationships.[104]

Assessment and Differential Diagnosis

Patients often do not report ICBs to their providers due to lack of awareness of the association with their behaviors and antiparkinsonian medications or due to embarrassment. Therefore, vigilant, ongoing screening and the use of rating instruments are important to diagnose these disorders, monitor changes in symptoms over time, and assess response to treatment.[105]

The modified version of the Minnesota Impulsive Disorders Interview (MIDI) is a semi-structured interview used to assess the degree of impulsivity related to compulsive behavior, including compulsive buying, pathological gambling, hypersexuality, compulsive eating, as well as other impulsive disorders not commonly reported in PD (e.g., pyromania, kleptomania, trichotillomania, and pathological skin picking). Although the MIDI is a widely used clinical and research tool, neither the internal consistency of the items nor the inter-rater reliability of the diagnoses has been demonstrated in PD patients. In addition, the MIDI does not feature punding, DDS, or hobbyism.[109]

The screening Questionnaire for Impulsive-Compulsive disorders in Parkinson's disease (QUIP) and Rating Scale version (QUIP-RS) are validated tools to assess ICDs and related disorders. While the first of these questionnaires, QUIP, is valid as a screening instrument for ICDs, it does not allow for the assessment of the severity of these disorders—an assessment that is necessary to establish diagnosis cutoff points and for follow-up of these behaviors. The QUIP-RS, conversely, has cutoff points for the diagnosis of ICDs with >80% sensitivity and specificity. Both of these instruments can be self- or rater-administered and have been translated and validated in numerous languages. The interrater reliability between trained rater and self-rater assessments was 0.95 for the total ICD score and 0.93 for the total QUIP-RS score.[110,111]

The Scales for Outcomes in Parkinson's disease-Psychiatric Complications (SCOPA-PC)[112] is another validated screening instrument for psychiatric complications in PD including hallucinations, illusions, paranoid ideation, altered dream phenomena, and confusion with one question about sexual preoccupation and one question about compulsive shopping or gambling. A new instrument, the Ardouin Scale of Behavior in Parkinson's disease (ASBPD), consists of a semi-structured standardized interview designed to assess neuropsychiatric features in PD using three domains: (1) hypodopaminergic disorders, (2) non-motor fluctuations, and (3) hyperdopaminergic behaviors.[113] This scale allows for a quantitative measurement and is therefore a valuable tool for long-term follow-up.

Treatment

Management of ICDs consists of patient and caregiver education with active screening and clinical understanding of the risks and benefits of alternative drug treatment. Caregivers should be actively involved in ensuring medication compliance and in monitoring of behaviors, including hoarding and medication overuse. ICDs and related behaviors often improve or resolve with dose reduction of DRT, switching to a different agonist, or withdrawal of DRT entirely. In a recent observational study, patients who discontinued or significantly decreased DAs experienced remission or significant reduction of ICD behaviors.[114] Therefore, when tolerated, the initial step to address ICDs would be to decrease DRT to the lowest effective daily dose.

When changes in DRT are ineffective or not tolerated, psychotropic medications and psychotherapy provide a secondary treatment course. Atypical neuroleptics, particularly clozapine, risperidone, and quetiapine, have been reported to control ICDs.[115,116] Mood stabilizers, such as valproate and lithium, have also been reported to help in individual patients with ICDs.[117] SSRIs have not been shown to have a positive effect, despite well-documented benefit in obsessive-compulsive disorders.[118,119] Caregivers are integral to implementing environmental modifications such as limiting patient's access to financial resources or the Internet. Counseling and CBT can also be useful as an adjunctive approach although several reports show disappointing results.[116]

DOPAMINE DYSREGULATION SYNDROME AND PUNDING

Dopamine dysregulation syndrome (DDS) and punding are relatively recently described iatrogenic disturbances that may complicate long-term symptomatic therapy of PD. DDS was originally described as "hedonistic homeostatic dysregulation" by Giovannoni et al.[120]—it is characterized by patients requesting early and increased doses of dopaminergic drugs or self-escalation of these medications without physicians' approval in excess of those required to control their motor symptoms.[121-123] Punding, as described in the ICD section above, refers to stereotyped, repetitive, and purposeless behaviors, such as rearranging papers.

Epidemiology

The prevalence of DDS in the general population of patients with PD is often difficult to ascertain as current studies are from specialist referral centers with inherent biases.[121] Within those limitations, it appears to range between 3% and 4%. Current data on punding are equally limited with prevalence ranging from 1% to 14%. Punding has been observed in PD patients exhibiting ICDs without DDS, emphasizing the degree of overlap between the ICD and punding behaviors.[121,124] Patients with PD who later develop DDS tend to have PD diagnoses at younger ages, premorbid histories of alcohol or substance abuse, impulsive and novelty-seeking personality traits, and histories of depressive disorders (Table 23-3).[121]

TABLE 23-3 • Risk Factors and Probable Contributors to the Development of Dopamine Dysregulation Syndrome in Parkinson's Disease Patients.
Strong risk factors
Young onset of Parkinson's disease (<45 years of age)
Previous history of alcohol or illicit drug abuse
Impulsive sensation-seeking personality traits, previous "risk-taking" activities
Probable contributors
History of depressive symptoms
Use of large amounts of rapidly acting dopamine replacement therapies (rapid-release levodopa formulations, bolus apomorphine injections)
Various candidate genes (e.g., DRD2) that are linked to addiction and high novelty-seeking personalities
Impaired decision making in PD due to disruption in reciprocal loops between striatum and structures in the prefrontal cortex following dopamine depletion

Pathophysiology

Because of the occurrence of punding in cocaine and amphetamine users, DDS and punding have been proposed to relate to DA excess.[125] Various candidate genes have been linked to addiction, impulsivity, and sensation seeking, particularly variants of the D_2 receptor gene (DRD2). These variants have been associated with comorbid antisocial personality disorder symptoms, high novelty-seeking behaviors, and various ICDs.[126] The TaqI A1 allele is one example. The A1 allele is a genetic polymorphism in the D2 receptor gene that results in a reduction in D2 receptor density by up to 30%, and it may play a role in less efficient learning, particularly as it relates to learning to avoid negative consequences of actions and reward-based decision making.[127,128] D2 receptor agonist cabergoline has been shown to increase positive-feedback related activity in individuals with the allele compared with those without it, and thus, the additional D2 stimulation may drive increased reward responses and addictive behaviors such as those seen in ICBs. Cohen and colleagues[128] refer to a "Goldilocks zone of dopamine stimulation" and speculate that cabergoline overstimulates D2 receptors in those without the allele, and therefore, this group is less likely to engage in excess reward-seeking behaviors. The disruption of reciprocal loops between the striatum and the prefrontal cortex in PD can lead to impaired decision making in PD and subsequent addictive behaviors. Some studies have shown that medicated PD patients displayed enhanced positive-feedback learning, adaptation of behavior according to changes in stimulus-reward contingencies, and other frontally predominant functions.[129,130] These findings may support an "overdose hypothesis" wherein DRT causes overstimulation of the ventral striatum, which is relatively spared from DA depletion in early-stage PD and is therefore vulnerable to excess DA.[131]

Levodopa is considered the most potent trigger of DDS in PD patients. Some cases have been reported in patients using subcutaneous apomorphine and oral DAs.[131,132] The potency and rapid action of levodopa and apomorphine may be more likely to give the patient a subjective "high" and therefore increase the risk of excessive use. Punding is most commonly seen in patients prescribed both levodopa and DAs but has also been shown to occur in patients taking levodopa alone.[125]

The development of physiological tolerance to levodopa is mediated by central pharmacokinetic and pharmacodynamic changes related to progressive dopaminergic denervation.[121] DA projections to the nucleus accumbens are implicated in behaviors such as the acquisition and consumption of food, sexual intercourse, and other rewards, and these projections are thought to play a role in addiction. DRT-induced neuroplasticity within the ventral and dorsal striatal systems and subsequent long-term disruptions of signaling in the basal ganglia have been proposed to cause the development of behavioral and motor complications of compulsive medication use in PD.[133,134] Indeed, molecular imaging studies have shown that PD patients with DDS exhibited enhanced ventral striatal DA release that was induced by levodopa compared to PD patients without DDS.[135] Overall, sensitization of ventral striatal networks to DRT resulting in appetitive behaviors may be analogous to the neuroplastic changes in the dorsal striatum thought to contribute to the motor complications of DRT such as dyskinesias and repetitive motor acts.[136]

Clinical Presentation

DDS can result from an addictive pattern of DRT use that is seen in association with distressing psychomotor "off period" DA withdrawal states; as a result, patients request increased doses of DRT or self-escalate these medications without physicians' approval. The dose escalation is typically in excess of that required to control motor symptoms.[121-123] A minority of patients may also describe a subjective "kick," "rush," "high," or mood benefit after taking short-acting dopaminergic medications.[120]

As treatment continues, drug-induced dyskinesias often emerge, along with socially harmful behaviors reminiscent of those seen in stimulant substance users. The psychological effects of "weaning off" often precede any discernable physical changes, and severe dysphoria often dominates the clinical picture. Craving, euphoria/hypomania, appetitive behaviors, aggression, psychosis, and motor stereotypies (compulsive behaviors) are also commonly seen.[136] Patient often report avoidance and anxiety related to periods of "off" non-motor symptoms as reasons for taking more medications. Patients with DDS will devote significant amount of time to complex and frequent drug administration regimens, hoarding of medication, and purchases of additional dopaminergic treatment. Often, any attempt to reduce the medication dose by the physician is met with strong resistance.

Like DDS, punding was first described in amphetamine and cocaine users.[137,138] Punding is a complex, stereotyped behavior in PD patients on DRT characterized by one or more of the following: (1) an intense fascination with repetitive manipulations of technical equipment; (2) the continual handling, collecting, examining, and sorting of common objects; (3) grooming; (4) hoarding; (5) pointless driving or walkabouts; and (6) engagement in extended monologues devoid of content.[136]

There is a compulsive nature to the behavior in that the person is often distracted but becomes irritable and anxious if prevented from resuming the behavior. They are often able to acknowledge the futile and self-destructive nature of the behaviors but find it difficult to prevent themselves from doing them. The activity chosen by a punder often relates to a previous occupation or interest; however, the patient often has an inability to complete the task efficiently or leaves a chaotic or untidy mess. Punding often leads to social avoidance, severe sleep deprivation, and alienation of family members.

Assessment and Differential Diagnosis

Despite recent increasing awareness, DDS (along with other ICBs) remains frequently unrecognized. Patients are often reluctant to divulge details regarding symptoms because the behaviors are often perceived as embarrassing. Therefore, collateral information from family members is essential. Severe, continuous dyskinesias should alert the physician to the possibility of DDS, particularly when associated with complaints that the medication is not working. Diagnosis is based on clinical presentation. Providers can also utilize diagnostic criteria proposed by Giovannoni et al.[120] to assist with diagnosis (Table 23-4).

Patients with DDS often have higher scores on ISS ratings with a wide range of responses on novel stimuli and cues predictive of reward, including positive affect (elation and expectation), increased energy, and enhanced psychomotor activity that are thought to be mediated by the mesolimbic dopaminergic systems.[139,140]

DDS is not always easily distinguished from maladaptive dependence or addiction. Patients with PD require dopaminergic medication to control motor symptoms, which when taken correctly, may represent an "adaptive dependence."[141] In contrast to stimulant users, patients with PD rarely describe punding behaviors as pleasurable.[142]

TABLE 23-4 • Diagnostic Criteria of Dopamine Dysregulation Syndrome.

Parkinson's disease with documented levodopa responsiveness

Need for increasing doses of DRT in excess of those normally required to relieve parkinsonian symptoms and signs

Pattern of pathological use; expressed need for increased DRT in the presence of excessive and significant dyskinesias despite being "on," drug hoarding or drug-seeking behavior, unwillingness to reduce DRT, absence of painful dystonias

Impairment in social or occupational functioning: fights, violent behavior, loss of friends, absence from work, loss of job, legal difficulties, arguments or difficulties with family

Development of hypomanic, manic, or cyclothymic affective syndrome in relation to DRT

Development of a withdrawal state characterized by dysphoria, depression, irritability, and anxiety on reducing level of DRT

Duration of disturbance of at least 6 months

DRT, dopamine replacement therapy.
Source: Giovannoni G, O'Sullivan JD, Turner K, et al. *Hedonistic homeostatic dysregulation in patients with Parkinson's disease on dopamine replacement therapies.* J Neurol Neurosurg Psychiatry. 2000;68(4):423-428, Reproduced with permission from BMY Publishing Group Ltd.

Treatment

The patient's family, caregivers, physicians, and pharmacist may all need to be involved in gradual decreasing dopaminergic doses and instituting a fixed and rigid rationing program.[119] "Booster" medications such as subcutaneous bolus doses of apomorphine and rapid-acting levodopa formulations should be stopped immediately. Hypomanic and psychotic symptoms associated with DDS are best managed in the hospital setting. If dose reductions are not effective, antipsychotic medications such as quetiapine should be considered. Aripiprazole is used in severe cases[121]; please see the Psychosis section, earlier in this chapter, for considerations surrounding antipsychotic use in PD patients. Dopaminergic drug dosage reduction may occasionally precipitate a more severe depression or anxiety state, which requires intensive inpatient treatment with antidepressant and behavioral therapy. Valproic acid can be an effective tool in treating DDS.[143,144]

Psychosocial treatments, including contingency management, relapse prevention, family-based approaches, and general CBT, have been shown to be beneficial in treatment of substance use disorders, but there is currently no clear evidence of its usefulness in DDS.[121] There is some evidence of symptom remission in patients who underwent DBS surgery.[145] However, further research is required to identify factors that can predict patient with DDS or ICDs who would most benefit from DBS.

PSYCHIATRIC EFFECTS OF DBS FOR PARKINSON'S DISEASE

DBS is a successful treatment of motor symptoms in PD with common therapeutic targets including the STN, GPi, and ventral intermediate nucleus (VIM) of the thalamus. The STN and globus pallidus are shown in Figure 23-7; Figure 23-8 shows an MRI brain following DBS implantation.

DBS surgery may markedly improve "off"-medication motor symptoms, and STN-DBS has the potential to allow significant reductions in drug dose (on average by about 50%).[146] However, there are frequent related psychiatric and cognitive symptoms, many reproducible with stimulation. These symptoms can often fluctuate after DBS placement due to changes in dopaminergic medications and stimulation parameters. Therefore, patients should undergo individualized evaluation, and a risk/benefit discussion should be part of their pre-DBS evaluation.

The psychiatric effects of GPi-DBS for PD have been much less examined to date compared to those associated with STN-DBS. Many of the general points and treatment principles discussed below on STN-DBS also apply to GPi-DBS for PD unless otherwise stated. Patients with depression and apathy have been hypothesized to have a lower density of presynaptic dopaminergic terminals predominantly in the mesocorticolimbic system and CNS monoamine cell dysfunction in the SNc prior to onset of PD.[147-149] Long-term treatment with dopaminergic agents leads to alterations in DA receptor potentiation along the nigrostriatal pathway, possible causing apathy. Dopaminergic medications are often decreased in the postoperative period, which can result in mood changes as well as decreased motivation or apathy despite good motor outcomes.[150] Postoperative depression may occur in about 8% of patients who undergo STN-DBS,[151] although evidence is mixed. A recent meta-analysis showed that the incidence of suicide post-DBS is quite rare and appears to be related to rapid reductions in dopaminergic medications rather than direct stimulation effects.[152] However, monitoring for suicidal risk post-DBS remains important. Preoperative depression is predictive of postoperative depression and overall decrease in quality of life, regardless of target.[153] Development or worsening of apathy in the postsurgical period has been observed most in patients with STN lead placement. In the short term, STN-DBS generally has a positive effect on anxiety while some

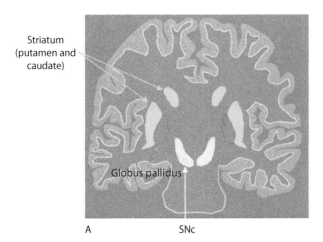
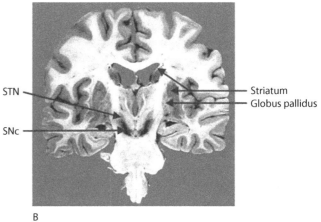

FIGURE 23-7. There is a schematic **(A)** and a post-mortem coronal section **(B)** demonstrating the dorsal striatum (caudate and putamen), subthalamic nucleus (STN), globus pallidus (GP), and substantia nigra pars compacta (SNc). The most common sites for the deep brain stimulation (DBS) placement are the STN and the globus pallidus interna (GPi, medial aspect of the GP). (Reproduced with permission from Jameson J, Fauci AS, Kasper DL, et al. Parkinson's disease. In: *Harrison's Principles of Internal Medicine.* 20th ed. https://accessmedicine. mhmedical.com. Copyright © McGraw Hill LLC. All rights reserved.)

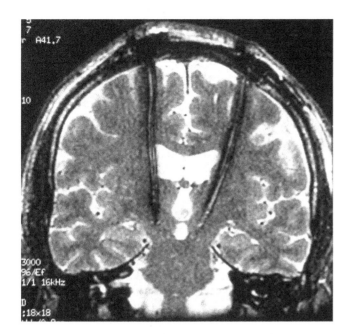

FIGURE 23-8. This fat spin echo coronal magnetic resonance imaging demonstrates the positions of the deep brain stimulator leads in the subthalamic nuclei bilaterally. (Reproduced with permission from Brunicardi F, Andersen DK, Billiar TR, et al. In: *Schwartz's Principles of Surgery.* 11th ed. https://accessmedicine. mhmedical.com. Copyright © McGraw Hill LLC. All rights reserved.)

reports have shown worsening in anxiety with GPi-DBS.[154,155] About 4% of STN-DBS patients can develop postsurgical mania or hypomania with resolution of mania by changing stimulation settings.[151,156]

Due to the ability to decrease dopaminergic medications dosages after surgery, STN-DBS is potentially a treatment option for patients with dopaminergic drug-related behaviors. For patients with DDS, ICDs, or punding, STN-DBS may appear to be a better placement option, given its greater effects on parkinsonism. This may enable drug reductions in contrast to GPi DBS where drug therapy usually remains unchanged.[157] After DBS placement, preexisting ICDs can continue, worsen, or develop de novo after STN-DBS implementation with punding, hypersexuality, pathological gambling, binge eating, and compulsive shopping most commonly reported.[158] However, STN-DBS appears to convey an overall benefit.

The development of cognitive impairment with DBS is less understood given that cognitive changes following surgery are often heterogeneous and can be related to disease progression, medication side effects, and microlesional changes.[159,160] Including all therapeutic DBS targets and reasons for treatment, cognition post-DBS improved in 31% of PD patients, deteriorated in 12%, and remained unchanged in 13%.[161] Executive function was shown to decline in 36% of patients 1 year after surgery[162] with predictive factors of cognitive decline including preoperative executive dysfunction, advanced age, and poor L-dopa response.[163] Effects of STN-DBS on verbal fluency can be attributed to stimulation effects (results in the "on" versus "off" stimulation condition literature are variable; see Schroeder et

al.[164] vs. Morrison et al.[165]), disease progression, or microlesional effects.[166–168] In the COMPARE trial, Okun and colleagues[169] suggested verbal fluency loss was the consequence of surgery and microlesional effects, rather than stimulation, given that the post-DBS STN group demonstrated verbal fluency deterioration compared with the pre-DBS group, especially when off DBS. Some studies have demonstrated phonemic fluency deficits alone,[170] while others have identified deleterious effects on both semantic and phonemic fluency.[171]

SLEEP DISORDERS IN PARKINSON'S DISEASE

The majority of patients with PD suffer from some form of sleep disruption, and studies show that this usually starts early in the disease course.[172,173] The causes of these sleep disturbances are multifactorial. Neurodegeneration of central sleep regulation centers in the brainstem and dysfunction of thalamocortical pathways are likely involved. Along with abnormalities in sleep architecture, PD-related symptoms such as nocturia may have a secondary effect on the quality of sleep.

Excessive Daytime Sleepiness

Excessive daytime sleepiness and involuntary dozing affect up to 50% of patients with PD and could be a preclinical marker.[174] This is an important symptom to identify early in the disease course since it can substantially affect quality of life. A combination of the disease course itself, the effect of nocturnal sleep disruption, and antiparkinsonian drugs probably contribute to the development of excessive daytime sleepiness. In some patients, it has been linked to the development of sudden-onset sleep and an abnormal period of sleep latency (<5 min) in 30% of patients with PD.[175,176]

REM Sleep Behavior Disorder

REM sleep behavior disorder (RBD) occurs in about a third of patients with PD.[177] This disorder is characterized by loss of normal skeletal muscle atonia during REM sleep, thus allowing affected patients to physically act out their dreams, which are often vivid or unpleasant. Vocalizations (talking, shouting, and verbal threats) and abnormal movements (arm or leg jerks, falling out of bed, and violent assaults) are commonly reported by bed partners. RBD is found to precede the onset of motor symptoms in PD patients in up to 40% of patients. It is theorized that RBD occurs due to the degeneration of lower brainstem nuclei, including the pedunculopontine and subcoeruleal nucleus.[178,179]

COGNITIVE DYSFUNCTION AND DEMENTIA IN PD

Mild cognitive impairment in PD (PD-MCI) is defined as cognitive decline attributable to PD that is excessive for age but associated with preserved functional abilities for daily activities.[180] Mild neurocognitive disorder (mild NCD) is the *DSM-5* nomenclature for MCI. Clinical diagnostic criteria for Parkinson's disease dementia (PDD), as defined by a task force of the Movement Disorder Society (MDS), distinguished *probable* from *possible* PDD. Both require two core features: (1) PD diagnosis based on the Queen Square Brain Bank Criteria[83] and (2) a dementia with insidious onset and slow progression with impairment in more than one cognitive domain, a decline from premorbid level, and deficits severe enough to impair daily life. Probable PDD requires a typical cognitive profile in at least two cognitive domains and at least one behavioral symptom, while possible PDD is characterized by an atypical cognitive profile with one or more impaired domains; additionally, behavioral symptoms are optional in possible PD. Another disorder, such as vascular disease, may coexist with PD in possible PDD but judged not to be the cause of dementia. In possible PDD, there may be an unknown time interval between motor and cognitive symptom onset. Finally, in both cases, there cannot be features that suggest other conditions as the cause of mental impairment.[181]

Major neurocognitive disorder (major NCD) is the *DSM-5* nomenclature for dementia. A diagnosis of major NCD or dementia implies, in addition to cognitive decline, a substantial functional impairment. The criteria for a *DSM-5* diagnosis of NCD due to PD has many overlapping features with the MDS criteria; the following features are required: (1) mild or major NCD criteria met, (2) cognitive decline after PD diagnosis, (3) insidious onset and gradual progression, and (4) no other medical cause. However, the *DSM-5* definitions of Possible and Probable NCD due to PD differ from the MDS criteria; Possible and Probable NCD due to PD require one or two features, respectively, of the following: (1) no mixed etiology and/or (2) PD diagnosis before NCD diagnosis. Please see chapter 20 in this textbook for further information on this topic.

Epidemiology

Approximately 26.7% of patients with PD and without dementia have PD-MCI.[180] Furthermore, in a systematic review of PDD, the proportion of PD subjects with PDD was 24–31%. Additionally, 3–4% of subjects with dementia had PDD. In the general population over the age of 65, the prevalence of PDD is 0.2–0.5%.[182] In a UK cohort of 86 PD subjects without dementia followed for 4 years, risk factors for development of dementia included older age, later age of onset of PD, hallucinations, and impairment in memory and language function at baseline. Dementia is a predictor for institutional placement in PD.[183]

Pathophysiology

There is an association between cortical Lewy body pathology (Lewy bodies and Lewy neurites) and PDD; nonetheless, not all patients with PD and dementia have cortical Lewy bodies.[184] Lewy bodies are characterized by abnormal neuronal cytoplasmic inclusions with alpha-synuclein protein aggregates (see Figure 23-3). In PD, Lewy body pathology is initially most prominent in the olfactory system and lower brainstem; this progresses to involve the midbrain. Subsequently, other brain structures including the cortex become involved (see Figure 23-5). In a study of 22 individuals with PD who were followed until their autopsy—18 of whom had dementia—all subjects had limbic or neocortical Lewy body disease. The Lewy body score was associated with the rate of cognitive decline.[185] In a separate study of 22 subjects with PD, clinical dementia rating (CDR) scores

correlated with Lewy body scores in the entorhinal cortex and Brodmann area 24 (anterior cingulate). Lewy body density in the entorhinal cortex accounted for 36% of the variability in CDR scores; senile plaques accounted for 19%. Lewy body density in the anterior cingulate explained 25% of the CDR variability. Neurofibrillary tangle density did not predict CDR scores.[186]

Although dopaminergic loss predicts motor symptoms in PD, it does not consistently predict cognitive impairment.[187] Of note, AD amyloid and tau pathology is often comorbid with cortical Lewy body and neurite pathology; in one study of 140 subjects with PD—in whom 92 developed dementia—approximately one-quarter had sufficient pathology for comorbid AD.[188]

Clinical Presentation

In PDD, motor symptoms (e.g., tremor, rigidity, akinesia or bradykinesia, and postural instability) usually precede the onset of dementia. The typical profile of cognitive deficits in PDD includes impaired attention which may fluctuate, impaired executive function, impaired visuospatial function, and impaired free memory recall that improves with cueing. Visuospatial and verbal memory tasks decline more rapidly in PDD patients followed longitudinally compared with their AD counterparts, even after controlling for motor slowing.[189] In fact, deterioration of visuospatial abilities may predict cognitive impairment and dementia. Language impairment, including sentence comprehension and production, may precede progression to dementia.[190]

Although a lack of behavioral symptoms does not exclude a diagnosis of PDD, the presence of one or more behavioral symptoms supports the diagnosis; as mentioned above, according to MDS diagnostic criteria, behavioral symptoms are optional in possible PDD and required for probable PD.[181] Behavioral symptoms in PDD patients include depressed or anxious mood, apathy, hallucinations, delusions, and excessive daytime sleepiness. Although these behavioral symptoms can occur in PD patients with or without dementia, daytime sleepiness and visual hallucinations are both predictors for dementia.[180]

Among patients with PD-MCI, single domain cognitive impairment is most common. Additionally, non-amnestic presentations are more common than amnestic ones.[180] In terms of clinical course, Hu and colleagues[191] reported on 486 subjects with PD who had been diagnosed with PD within the previous 3.5 years; 41% had MCI at study onset, 21% developed MCI after 18 months of follow-up, and 5% progressed from MCI to dementia over those 18 months.

Assessment and Differential Diagnosis

The diagnostic criteria and clinical features of PDD are described above. When considering PDD, the differential diagnosis includes other synucleinopathies such as DLB, which is discussed in more detail in the section below (see Table 23-5 for comparison of cognitive and behavioral features of PDD and DLB). In a Mayo Clinic Study comparing cohorts of PDD and DLB subjects (46 and 64 subjects, respectively), there was a statistically significant difference in DLB versus PDD in terms of both the frequency of hallucinations (40% in DLB vs. 9% in PDD) and cognitive

TABLE 23-5 • Early Cognitive, Psychomotor, and Behavioral Symptoms Associated with Parkinson's Disease Dementia (PDD) and Dementia with Lewy Bodies.

Disorder	Symptom Onset, Progression Rate	Memory	Attention	Executive Functions	Language	Visuospatial Function	Psychomotor Function	Behavior
PDD	Insidious, varied	Recent: possible deficits Recognition: variable Remote: intact Procedural: possible impairments	Intact primary attention span, impaired selective/ divided attention; fluctuations	Difficulty planning/ shifting set	Verbal fluency, mechanical aspects of speech impaired	May be impaired	Resting tremor, bradykinesia, rigidity, postural instability, shuffling gait	Depression common, may exhibit hallucinations/ delusions (less common than DLB)
DLB	Insidious, varied	Recent: usually less than AD Recognition: variable Remote: intact Procedural: intact	Significant fluctuations in attention	Variable	Variable; fluency may be impaired	Impaired construction, copy, visuospatial planning, and problem solving	May exhibit a range of parkinsonian symptoms	Hallucinations, delusions, depression

Adapted with permission from Halter JB, Ouslander JG, Tinetti ME, et al. Hazzard's Geriatric Medicine and Gerontology, 6th ed. http://accessmedicine.mhmedical.com. Copyright © McGraw Hill LLC. All rights reserved.

fluctuations (16% in DLB vs. 4% in PDD); a comparison of the incidence of myoclonus (8% in DLB, 2% in PDD) in both groups did not result in a statistically significant difference.[192] The differential diagnosis also includes other synucleinopathies like multiple systems atrophy (MSA) and tauopathies like progressive supranuclear palsy (PSP) and corticobasal syndrome (CBS), in addition to AD and frontotemporal lobar degeneration. Please see Table 23-6 for a brief review of parkinsonian syndromes.

TABLE 23-6 • Clinical Features of the Parkinsonian Syndromes Which Are Included in the Differential Diagnosis for Parkinson's Disease Dementia.

	Parkinson's Disease[a]	Dementia with Lewy Bodies[a]	Multiple Systems Atrophy	Progressive Supranuclear Palsy	Corticobasal Syndrome
Distinguishing features	Parkinsonism (begins unilaterally, may become bilateral) Dyskinesias with DRT Depression Anxiety Apathy Psychosis Impulsive-compulsive behaviors RBD	Parkinsonism (bilateral) Dementia Hallucinations (minor phenomena, well-formed) Fluctuations Depression RBD	Parkinsonism (bilateral) Autonomic dysfunction Cerebellar signs Depression RBD	Parkinsonism (bilateral) Early falls Vertical gaze dysfunction Axial rigidity Apathy Pathologic emotionality Mild depression Mild anxiety	Parkinsonism (unilateral) Alien limb Apraxia Myoclonus (often unilateral) Personality changes Depression
Dementia	Late	Early (visuospatial dysfunction prominent)	Present in some patients	Early (executive dysfunction prominent)	Late
Average age of onset	60s	50s–80s	50s	60s	60s
Neuroimaging	No pathognomonic findings	Temporo-occipital hypometabolism on PET	Hot cross buns sign in pons	Humming bird and Mickey Mouse signs due to midbrain atrophy	Asymmetric parietal/basal ganglia atrophy and hypometabolism
Pathology	Synuclein	Synuclein	Synuclein	Tau	Tau, amyloid

[a]See chapter text for detailed review of neuropsychiatric features.
DRT, dopamine replacement therapy; PET, positron emission tomography; RBD, rapid eye movement (REM) behavior disorder.
Adapted from Craft et al.[218] and Lauterbach.[219]

CASE VIGNETTE 23.1

A 64-year-old man developed bradykinesia, rigidity, and postural instability, and he was subsequently diagnosed with Parkinson's disease (PD). He was initially treated with rasagiline, and levodopa-carbidopa was added 2 years later. He also developed dysautonomia with hypotension, which was treated with midodrine. Eight years after initial diagnosis, he was referred to a neuropsychiatry clinic with depression, anxiety, and poor sleep in the setting of functional limitations due to PD. He was started on escitalopram 5 mg daily and mirtazapine 15 mg daily with good response. However, his mood later worsened, and he developed anhedonia due to multiple stressors including dismantling his business; at this time the escitalopram was increased to 10 mg daily, and he was referred to psychotherapy. A while after his depression remitted, he developed worsening neurovegetative symptoms, which were attributed to PD progression rather than depression. The day prior to hospitalization for a fall, he had hallucinations of cabinets opening and closing. He subsequently became disoriented. He underwent a workup for delirium, and he was found to have a urinary tract infection. He received antibiotics, and the hallucinations resolved. Antipsychotics were avoided due to the risk of worsening his parkinsonism.

At the time of initial presentation to neuropsychiatry clinic, he underwent neuropsychological testing that suggested PD-MCI. His testing demonstrated evidence of cognitive and motor slowing, executive dysfunction, and visuospatial dysfunction. He was inattentive, and he would lose track of task demands. Memory performance was slightly below expected values with primary difficulties at the level of encoding. Although his wife helped him with instrumental activities of daily living (iADLs) at that time, this was largely due to his motor functional limitations rather than cognitive limitations. Over the course of treatment, his cognition continued to decline, and he was diagnosed with Parkinson's disease dementia 3 years later after his performance on the above measures declined. He increasingly relied on his wife for iADLs due to both cognitive and functional impairment. An MRI of his brain demonstrated moderate parietal and mild frontal volume loss. He was started on a cholinesterase inhibitor and was referred to cognitive rehabilitation.

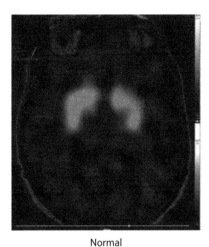
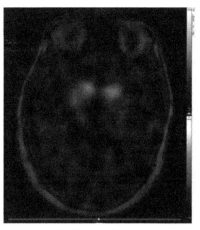

Normal   Parkinson's disease

FIGURE 23-9. Dopamine transporter scan (DaTscan) of a healthy individual (left) and an individual with Parkinson's disease and decreased striatal radiotracer (Iofluplane) uptake (right). (From Biller J, Gruener G, Brazis PW. Ancillary neurodiagnostic procedures—lumbar puncture and neuroimaging. In: *DeMyer's The Neurologic Examination: A Programmed Text.* 7th ed. https://neurology.mhmedical.com. Copyright © McGraw Hill LLC. All rights reserved. Reproduced with permission from Robert Wagner, M.D.)

Dopamine transporter imaging (DaTscans) in PD typically demonstrate decreased dopaminergic activity in the striatum, but this is nonspecific and can be seen with other disorders that affect dopaminergic pathways, such as MSA or LBD. However, it can be helpful in distinguishing PDD from AD or FTLD in clinically ambiguous situations (Figure 23-9).

Treatment

There have been several large RCTs evaluating treatment of cognitive impairment in PD-MCI and PDD. A double-blind RCT study of rasagiline, an MAO-B inhibitor, in PD-MCI over 12 weeks demonstrated an improvement in compositional z-attention score in rasagiline versus placebo arms, but other cognitive domains tested did not significantly improve.[193] Patients on rasagiline should be counseled about dietary restrictions, as detailed in the Depression section above.

CHEIs donepezil and rivastigmine have been studied in PDD individuals using RCT paradigms. A 24-week study of donepezil did not demonstrate a significant difference in cognitive subscale of the Alzheimer's Disease Assessment Scale (ADAS-cog) scores, but using a treatment-by-country interaction analysis, both 5 mg and 10 mg daily were significant compared with placebo. Additionally, based on Clinicians Interview Based Impression of Change with Caregiver input (CIBIC+) scores, the 10 mg arm was significantly different from placebo. There was no difference between the 5 mg and placebo arms on the CIBIC+. Similarly, rivastigmine was tested using a 24-week protocol, and both the ADAS-Cog and Alzheimer's Disease Co-operative Study Clinicians Global Impression of Change (ADCS-CGIC) endpoints were significantly different when compared with placebo.[193]

In one meta-analysis of 10 studies, both CHEIs and memantine resulted in a small improvement in clinicians' global impression of change. Additionally, CHEIs but not memantine improved Mini-Mental State Examination (MMSE) scores.

These drugs also had good safety profiles, although rivastigmine demonstrated an increased risk of mild or moderate adverse events compared with placebo. There was no difference in risk of serious adverse events when rivastigmine was compared with placebo.[194] Notably, it is important to counsel patients with PDD that CHEIs can worsen tremor, and memantine can worsen extrapyramidal symptoms.[193]

PARKINSONIAN PERSONALITY

Personality differences have long been reported in PD patients before the onset of motor symptoms and during early stages of the disease. Indeed, James Parkinson noted that his first case "had industriously followed the business of a gardener, leading a life of remarkable temperance and sobriety."[195] PD patients are often described as being fastidious, industrious, anhedonic, obsessive, cautious, and inflexible.[196,197] They have less novelty-seeking and more harm avoidance traits compared with control populations.[198] One study showed that changes in novelty seeking and harm reduction were related to the asymmetric pattern of motor symptom onset[199]—patients whose illness developed initially on the right side of the body showed reduced novelty seeking when compared with matched healthy controls. In contrast, patients whose illness began on the left side of the body reported increased levels of harm avoidance.

Of note, most studies that have looked at distinctive prodromal or preclinical personality profiles before the onset of motor symptoms in PD have been limited by personality inventories that were not developed for retrospective use and have been based on retrospective case-control studies prone to recall bias.[200] In a prospective study, the Mayo Clinic Study of Personality and Aging, researchers followed 6822 subjects over four decades; the Minnesota Multiphasic Personality Inventory (MMPI) was completed between 1962 and 1965 and was used to obtain measures of extraversion, introversion, and neuroticism personality traits. In this study, neuroticism, which included psychoasthenia, pessimism, and depression subscales, showed a significant association with later development of PD, largely due to an anxious personality (psychoasthenia) subscale. The pessimism subscale showed a week association, and the depression subscale did not demonstrate any association. In this study, the sensation seeking and constraint subscales of the extraversion and introversion personality trait scales, respectively, did not show an association with development of PD.[198]

DEMENTIA WITH LEWY BODIES

Dementia with Lewy bodies (DLB), which is also known as Lewy body dementia, is the second most common form of dementia after AD. Because PD and DLB both involve Lewy body pathology, they are often thought of as two ends of a disease continuum wherein the clinical hallmark of DLB is the onset of cognitive impairment prior to motor impairment whereas the hallmark of PD is motor impairment on presentation. The psychiatric hallmarks of DLB are discussed below (please see the Clinical Presentation section).

Epidemiology

DLB in the Population

In one study of more than 5000 subjects over age 65, the incidence of dementia was 3.6% a year, and the incidence of DLB was 0.1% a year.[201] The range of DLB prevalence in the 65 and older general population is 0.1–2%.[202]

DLB Among Dementia Patients

The incidence of DLB is 3.2–4.5% annually among individuals with dementia in population-based studies. The average prevalence of DLB in clinic-based studies of dementia is approximately 7.5% (or 1 in every 13 dementia subjects), but variance is high, and these numbers approach 25% of dementia subjects in some clinic studies.[203]

Age and Sex in DLB

The mean age of onset of DLB is 75. Unlike studies of AD that demonstrate a female predominance, the literature about gender differences in DLB is mixed; in one systematic review of eight studies, five described a female predominance while three described a male predominance.[203]

Pathophysiology

As mentioned in the discussion of PDD pathology, Lewy bodies are round, eosinophilic cytoplasmic inclusions, and Lewy neurites are fibrils made of insoluble polymers deposited in neuronal projections (see Figure 23-3). They are strongly immunoreactive for the protein alpha-synuclein. Although the function of alpha-synuclein is poorly understood, it may be a lipid-binding protein. In both PDD and LBD, alpha-synuclein accumulates in the presynapses resulting in interference in axonal transport and in neurotransmitter depletion.[204,205]

In addition to Lewy body pathology in the substantia nigra, one of the defining neuropathologic characteristics of DLB is the presence of Lewy bodies in the cortex, particularly in the temporal (including hippocampal regions) and parietal lobes (see Figure 23-4). Within the hippocampus, alpha-synuclein load is most pronounced in the CA1 and CA2 areas. There is also a higher alpha-synuclein load in the amygdala of DLB patients compared with their PD counterparts (92% vs. 30%, respectively).[204,205] In fact, in a study of 12 neocortical, limbic, and brainstem sites in 10 patients with a pathologic diagnosis of DLB, the mean density of Lewy bodies in limbic areas was significantly higher than in neocortical areas; in this study, the highest density of Lewy bodies was found in the amygdala, and the lowest density was found in the occipital lobes. In limbic areas, Lewy body formation positively correlated with neuritic plaque but not neurofibrillary tangle deposition.[206]

Amyloid beta load, if present, is more severe and extended in the cortex and striatum in LBD compared with PDD; AD pathology is often comorbid with DLB, which often results in a mixed dementia presentation (see Figure 23-10). In a

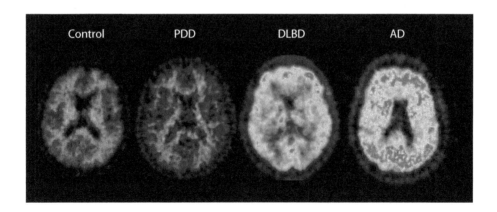

FIGURE 23-10. 11C-PiB uptake, indicating amyloid deposition, in positron emission tomography (PET) scans. Left to right: The brains of a control subject, a patient with Parkinson's disease dementia (PDD), a patient with diffuse Lewy body disease (DLBD), and a patient with Alzheimer's disease (AD). Increased PiB uptake is visible in the AD and DLBD patients. (Reproduced with permission from Watts RL, Standaert DG, Obeso JA. Neuroimaging of movement disorders. In: *Movement Disorders*. 3rd ed. https://neurology.mhmedical.com. Copyright © McGraw Hill LLC. All rights reserved.)

TABLE 23-7 • Diagnostic Criteria for Dementia with Lewy Bodies (DLB).

Essential
   Dementia, defined as progressive cognitive decline that interferes with social or occupational functions or with usual daily activities
Probable DLB
   Two or more core clinical features, with or without biomarkers, or one core clinical feature with one or more biomarkers
Possible DLB
   One core clinical feature with no biomarker evidence
   One or more biomarkers but no core clinical features
Core clinical features
   Fluctuating cognition with pronounced variations in attention and alertness
   Recurrent visual hallucinations that are typically well formed and detailed
   REM sleep behavior disorder, which may precede cognitive decline
   One or more spontaneous cardinal features of parkinsonism: bradykinesia, rest tremor, or rigidity
Supportive clinical features
   Severe sensitivity to antipsychotic agents
   Postural instability
   Repeated falls
   Syncope or other transient episodes of unresponsiveness
   Severe autonomic dysfunction (e.g., constipation, orthostatic hypotension, urinary incontinence)
   Hypersomnia
   Hyposmia
   Hallucinations in other modalities
   Systematized delusions
   Apathy
   Anxiety
   Depression
Indicative biomarkers
   Reduced dopamine transporter uptake in basal ganglia as demonstrated by SPECT or PET
   Abnormal (low uptake) ^{123}iodine-MIBG myocardial scintigraphy
   Polysomnographic confirmation of REM sleep without atonia
Supportive biomarkers
   Relative preservation of medial temporal lobe structures on CT/MRI scan
   Generalized low uptake on SPECT/PET perfusion/metabolism scan with reduced occipital activity ± the cingulate island sign on FDG-PET imaging
   Prominent posterior slow-wave activity on EEG with periodic fluctuations in the pre-alpha/theta range

Source: McKeith IG, Boeve BF, Dickson DW, et al. Diagnosis and management of dementia with Lewy bodies: Fourth consensus report of the DLB Consortium. Neurology. 2017;89(1):88-100. https://n.neurology.org/content/89/1/88.

neuropathology study by Irwin and colleagues evaluating AD co-pathology with DLB, 69 of 98 (70%) of individuals with a clinical diagnosis of DLB had intermediate or high level AD pathology. About 60% of patients with a clinical diagnosis of DLB or PDD as well as diffuse neocortical LBD neuropathology had intermediate or high level AD pathology; two-thirds of these patients with neocortical LBD pathology had a clinical diagnosis of DLB.[207] Tau load is typically most prominent in the mesial temporal lobes in DLB. Substantia nigra neuron loss involves the dorsolateral SNc preferentially, but pedunculopontine cholinergic cell loss is not common; the latter is common in PPD patients with hallucinations, however, which may indicate a different pattern of degeneration in DLB compared with PDD. Of interest, patients with DLB have high serotonin receptor binding density in the cortex.[204]

Clinical Presentation

DLB is diagnosed when cognitive dysfunction precedes motor parkinsonism or when cognitive dysfunction begins within 1 year of onset of motor features of PD. Dementia, defined as progressive cognitive decline resulting in interference of function, is essential for a DLB diagnosis (Table 23-7). Early cognitive deficits include difficulties with attention, executive function, and visuospatial abilities; memory impairment is typically present after disease progression.[208] In a study of 111 patients with probable DLB, 42 of whom had a CSF profile consistent with AD, individuals with comorbid DLB and AD had significantly worse memory profiles (as measured by the Visual Association Test and Rey Auditory Verbal Learning Test) compared with those with DLB alone. There were no differences between the groups based on performance on tests of executive function, attention, language, or visuospatial function.[209]

Core Clinical Features

Fluctuating cognition with changes in attention and level of alertness, recurrent visual hallucinations, and REM sleep behavior disorder typically occur early in the disease. The visual hallucinations are classically detailed and fully formed. Cardinal features of parkinsonism, including bradykinesia, resting tremor, or rigidity, are also considered core clinical features of DLB; one or more must be present.[208]

Supportive Clinical Features

It is important to obtain information about potentially supportive clinical features, including sensitivity to antipsychotic medications, postural instability, repeated falls, syncope, autonomic dysfunction (including constipation, orthostasis, urinary incontinence, hypersomnia, and hyposmia), hallucinations in other sensory modalities, and minor hallucinations. As mentioned in the PDD section above, minor hallucinations include presence hallucinations (experiencing the sense that another is present), passage hallucinations (experiencing imagery in one's periphery), and illusions (external stimuli that are misperceived or misinterpreted). It is also helpful to determine the presence of comorbid psychiatric symptoms, including depression, anxiety, apathy, and delusions which commonly occur in DLB.[208]

Assessment and Differential Diagnosis

Differential Diagnosis

PDD is on the differential when considering DLB. The two dementias have a great deal of clinical overlap including motor symptoms (rigidity, akinesia) and cognitive impairments (including frontal executive and visual-construction impairment as well as mild language impairment). Additionally, both are frequently characterized by comorbid mood disturbances, REM sleep behavior disorder, and neuroleptic sensitivity.[204]

However, attentional and episodic verbal memory impairments tend to be more prominent in DLB. Tremor occurs less frequently in DLB. Conversely, DLB is associated with slower walk time, more impaired balance, and more frequent orthostasis compared with PDD. Visual hallucinations, delusions, and fluctuations in attention are more common in DLB. Furthermore, visual hallucinations occur spontaneously in DLB whereas they occur most commonly after L-dopa therapy in PDD (although DA therapy-naïve patients with PDD can suffer from spontaneous hallucinations, as well). Finally, while PDD dementia age of onset is often earlier than that of DLB, cognitive decline is often faster in DLB.[204]

The differential diagnosis also includes AD, MSA, PSP, and frontotemporal lobar degeneration, among others. As mentioned above, AD pathology is often comorbid with DLB, frequently resulting in a mixed dementia presentation. However, when DLB presents in isolation, verbal memory (including storage and retrieval) is relatively preserved until late stages compared with that of typical AD patients. Additionally, DLB patients will have relative preservation of hippocampal volumes on MRI. On single-photon emission computed tomography (SPECT) scans, there is robust uptake in the caudate and putamen in AD and normal controls ("comma appearance") in contrast to uptake restricted to the caudate in DLB ("period" or "full stop" appearance). Temporoparietal hypoperfusion on SPECT is seen in both AD and DLB, but occipital hypoperfusion is more commonly seen in DLB (Figure 23-11). Indeed, fluorodeoxyglucose (FDG) PET may demonstrate widespread metabolic reduction in DLB, but reduction in visual association cortex is often particularly more pronounced in DLB groups compared to AD groups; also, reduced uptake in the posterior cingulate is seen in AD but not DLB.[205,209–211]

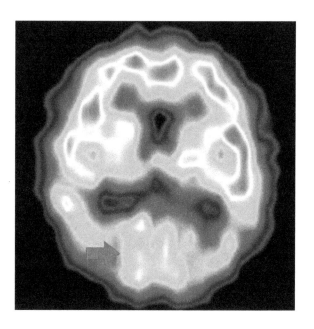

FIGURE 23-11. Dementia with Lewy bodies (DLB) is characterized by fluorodeoxyglucose positron emission tomography (FDG PET) hypometabolism (green color) throughout the entire cerebral cortex, including occipital lobe involvement (red arrow), unlike Alzheimer's disease. The preservation of posterior cingulate metabolism, which is often seen in DLB, is not shown in this slice. (From Usatine RP, Smith MA, Mayeaux, Jr. EJ, Chumley HS. Dementia. In: *The Color Atlas and Synopsis of Family Medicine*. 3rd ed. https://accessmedicine.mhmedical.com. Copyright © McGrraw Hill LLC. All rights reserved. Reproduced with permission from Bundhit Tantiwongkosi, M.D.)

Assessment

Please see the Clinical Presentation section above for clinical aspects of assessment. Although DLB patients have been found to have more atrophy overall than PDD patients in one study, these subtle differences are unlikely to aid in the diagnosis of one syndrome or the other.[208] SPECT scans show decreased occipital perfusion, and PET scans show decreased occipital metabolism as mentioned above[209,210]—these findings can be used to distinguish between AD and DLB when clinical features are equivocal. Additionally, as mentioned, patients with DLB may have a "cingulate island sign" on PET scans wherein posterior cingulate metabolism is preserved with surrounding occipital hypometabolism.[210-212]

DaTscans in DLB typically demonstrate decreased dopaminergic activity in the striatum, but this is nonspecific and can be seen with other hypodopaminergic states, such as PD and MSA (see Figure 23-9). However, it can be helpful in distinguishing DLB from AD.[208,213] Finally, alpha-synuclein deposition is being explored as a biomarker, but further research is needed.[214]

Treatment

Treatment for DLB is often based on expert consensus opinion rather than clinical trials. Preliminary data supports exercise for motor and cognitive benefits, cognitive training, and caregiver-oriented education to manage psychiatric symptoms. Additionally, clinical trials support the use of CHEIs donepezil and rivastigmine to improve cognition and function as well as treat apathy, visual hallucinations, and delusions.[208]

Dopaminergic agents should be used with caution in DLB patients due to the risk of worsening psychosis. In one study of 19 subjects meeting criteria for probable DLB, one-third demonstrated a motor benefit on the UPDRS, and one-third developed exacerbation of hallucinations or psychosis. Only 4 of 19 (22%) experienced motor benefit without worsening psychosis.[214]

Antipsychotics for the management of behavioral disturbances, hallucinations, and delusions carry the risk of increased mortality risk in patients with dementia as well the risk of a sensitivity reaction in DLB patients. Drugs used in PD, including quetiapine and clozapine, are used widely with limited evidence in DLB; a small placebo-controlled trial of quetiapine in 23 subjects with DLB was negative, although the drug was well-tolerated. The trial was confounded by a design change, incomplete recruitment, a large placebo effect, inadequate dosage (mean 120 mg daily), and inadequate power.[215,220] There is currently no controlled clinical trial data on the role of pimavanserin, a 5-HT$_{2A}$ inverse agonist that was FDA approved in April 2016 for the treatment of PD psychosis, in DLB; a retrospective case series revealed clinical improvement in four of four DLB patients started on pimavanserin, but the benefit for one of these individuals waned after 5 months.[208,216] Finally, although evidence is scant, depression is DLB is often treated similarly to depression in other dementias with SSRIs, SNRIs, or mirtazapine.

Summary and Key Points

- Parkinson's disease (PD) is a neurodegenerative illness wherein the core pathology is characterized by loss of dopaminergic neurons in the nigrostriatal pathway, which results in extrapyramidal signs and symptoms; dopaminergic disruption in mesolimbic and mesocortical pathways result in neuropsychiatric manifestations and cognitive impairment, respectively.
- **Depression in PD:** The reduction in dopaminergic tone in the ventral striatum is associated with emergence of depression in patients with PD. The disruption of mesolimbic pathways, decreased receptor binding in the ventral striatum, and structural changes in the mediodorsal thalamus have been implicated. The diagnosis of, and the disability from, a neurodegenerative process can be psychologically destabilizing and also trigger depression in PD. Depression is highly prevalent among patients with PD and can lead to significant additional morbidity. Recognition of depression in PD can be challenging, due to the overlap between neurovegetative symptoms of depression and motor symptoms of PD. Multiple treatment modalities are beneficial, including SSRIs, SNRIs, TCAs, and bupropion. Treatment of PD with levodopa and DAs can also ameliorate depression. MAO-B inhibitors, such as rasagiline, can be used to treat PD motor symptoms and comorbid depression. ECT should be considered for severe or medication-refractory depression. There is mixed evidence regarding the role of DBS in exacerbating depression and suicide risk. Psychosocial treatments such as individual and group cognitive behavioral therapy for both patients and caregivers can provide benefit.
- **Anxiety in PD:** Recognizing and treating anxiety in PD patients is imperative because anxiety can have a significant impact on quality of life and functioning. There are limitations when using anxiety rating scales and *DSM-5* criteria for the assessment and diagnosis of anxiety among PD patients, since they may not pick up on subthreshold but significant anxiety, anxiety related to PD manifestations, and anxiety related to motor fluctuations. Treatment options include certain antidepressants with favorable side-effect profiles and nonpharmacological approaches like CBT.
- **Psychosis in PD:** More than 50% of all PD patients experience psychotic symptoms, and up to 75% of patients with PD dementia experience psychotic symptoms. Management of Parkinson's disease psychosis (PDP) involves assessment of the nature and severity of the characteristic symptoms since not all psychotic symptoms are distressing or disabling to patients. Then, the next step is to evaluate for any possible medical contributors of psychosis. Subsequently, adjustment of PD medications is considered with the goal of ameliorating or resolving psychotic symptoms while maintaining motor function. If psychotic symptoms persist after these steps, antipsychotic medication use in this population is then carefully considered; quetiapine and clozapine are most frequently utilized.
- **Apathy in PD:** Apathy, independent of cognitive impairment or depression, has been described throughout the disease course of PD and can also manifest after deep brain stimulation (DBS), especially in the context of a reduction or withdrawal of dopaminergic medications. Reported frequencies in the literature range from 15% to 70%, and this variability is likely due to the differences in diagnostic approaches. Studies have investigated cholinesterase inhibitors, dopaminergic agents, and SSRIs for the treatment of apathy in PD. While the first two medication classes have been found to be helpful, SSRIs may worsen apathy in PD patients.
- **Impulse control disorders (ICDs):** Current estimates suggest that ICDs are a common side effect of DRT in PD patients. ICDs typically identified in PD fall into several domains, including compulsive eating, gambling, buying, and sexual behavior. Excessive engagement in these behaviors might be associated with guilt or embarrassment. Risk factors for ICDs in PD include young age, impulsive or novelty-seeking personality, personal or family history of psychiatric illness or substance abuse, prior history of ICDs, and dopamine receptor agonist therapy. ICDs after DRT might be considered a behavioral addiction due to a dysfunction in the ventral striatum and mesocorticolimbic pathway. Treatments can involve dose reduction or complete withdrawal of DRT, switching dopaminergic therapies, selected psychotropics, behavioral treatments, and engaging spouses or other family members to assist in implementing environmental modifications.
- **Dopamine dysregulation syndrome (DDS) and punding:** DDS is an iatrogenic disturbance where patients develop an additive pattern of DRT use, administering doses in excess of those required to control their motor symptoms. This syndrome may complicate long-term symptomatic therapy of PD. Punding refers to stereotyped, repetitive, and purposeless behaviors such as rearranging papers. Antipsychotics, mood stabilizers, and DBS have been shown to be effective in treatment.

- **Deep brain stimulation (DBS):** Along with motor improvement, DBS therapies may result in unanticipated non-motor symptoms after implantation; these risks underscore the importance of neuropsychiatric screening prior to intervention. Unanticipated non-motor symptoms post-DBS include depression, apathy, and mania. STN-DBS may convey a benefit in DDS, punding, and ICDs, although the results are mixed. Risk of development of neuropsychiatric and cognitive deficits are worth discussing with any prospective DBS candidates, as these factors can greatly undermine quality of life.
- **Sleep disorders in PD:** Excessive daytime sleepiness and REM sleep behavior disorder are common symptoms of PD which often precede motor or other observable symptoms of PD.
- **Cognitive dysfunction in PD:** Mild cognitive impairment in PD (PD-MCI) is characterized by cognitive decline that is not normal for age but with normal functional activities. Parkinson's disease dementia (PDD) involves both cognitive and functional decline. About 27% of PD patients have PD-MCI, and 24–31% have PDD. PDD is often associated with limbic and neocortical Lewy body disease. Cholinesterase inhibitors donepezil and rivastigmine have been shown to improve clinicians' global impression of change (and rivastigmine improved MMSE scores), but the effects are modest.
- **Parkinsonian personality:** Historically, there has been a description in the literature of a distinct premorbid parkinsonian personality profile, which includes traits such as diligence at work and aversion to risk, but there has not been consistent evidence for this in the literature.
- **Dementia with Lewy bodies:** Dementia with Lewy bodies (DLB) is the second most common form of dementia after Alzheimer's disease. Fluctuating cognition with changes in attention and level of alertness, recurrent visual hallucinations, and REM sleep behavior disorder typically occur early in the disease. PD and DLB are thought to lie on the same clinical spectrum. Clinically, they have overlapping parkinsonian features, including bradykinesia, limb rigidity, and gait disorder. Although parkinsonism in DLB is often more symmetric and less severe than PD, there is no feature of motor parkinsonism that can reliably distinguish one from another. Additionally, with regard to PDD versus DLB, a somewhat arbitrary classification has been defined wherein parkinsonism must be present for 1 year or more before dementia onset in order for the clinical presentation to be classified as PDD; in contrast, in DLB, dementia occurs prior to or at the same time as parkinsonism. In both, the substantia nigra and locus coeruleus may show pallor on neuropathological evaluation. Similarly, both may result in Lewy bodies in cortical, limbic, and brainstem areas. Data on effective symptomatic management remain limited. Dopaminergic agents and antipsychotics should be used with caution in DLB.

Multiple Choice Questions

1. A 65-year-old man with Parkinson's disease (PD) presents to clinic with a new onset of visual hallucinations and paranoid thought content, both of which are distressing to him. Which of the following statements is true?
   a. It would be appropriate to immediately start an atypical antipsychotic, like quetiapine or clozapine, to address his psychotic symptoms.
   b. It is imperative to first evaluate for any possible medical or pharmacological contributors of psychosis.
   c. It may be helpful to adjust his PD medications, especially decreasing levodopa right away.
   d. If he also has memory impairment, it may be beneficial to start a cholinesterase inhibitor to address his memory issues and psychotic symptoms.
   e. If starting an atypical antipsychotic, the best option would be risperidone.

2. A 70-year-old man with Parkinson's disease (PD) presents to clinic with his wife. She reports that her husband has been progressively less energetic, affectionate, and engaged in social activities and in his usual hobbies over the past several months. Of note, he recently had STN-DBS. Which of the following statements is **false**?
   a. The patient seems to have some characteristics of apathy, which is a behavioral syndrome that results in a state of reduced motivation and a decrease in goal-directed behavior with emotional and cognitive features.
   b. Although there is a lack of widely accepted diagnostic criteria for apathy in PD, there are helpful scales for the assessment of apathy in PD.
   c. Apathy in PD can manifest after DBS, especially in the context of a reduction or withdrawal of dopaminergic medications.
   d. SSRIs are first-line agents for the treatment of apathy in PD.
   e. Although there can be overlap between apathy and depression in PD, depression can be distinguished by the presence of more negative emotions, thoughts, and beliefs.

3. Which of the following refers to a behavior characterized by stereotyped, repetitive, and purposeless behaviors such as rearranging papers, which can be seen in patients with Parkinson's disease?
   a. Punding
   b. Dopamine dysregulation syndrome
   c. Impulse control disorders
   d. Hobbyism

4. All of the following have been associated with parkinsonian personality except:
   a. Industrious
   b. Anhedonic
   c. Thrill-seeking
   d. Cautious
   e. Inflexible

Multiple Choice Answers

1. Answer: b

When a PD patient has a new onset of psychotic symptoms, it is imperative to first evaluate for any possible medical or pharmacological contributors of psychosis, such as febrile illness, infections, structural brain lesions, or recent medication changes. PD is an independent risk factor for delirium, and PD patients are vulnerable to adverse medication events, syncope, falls, pneumonia, genitourinary infections, trauma, and mobility complications.

Dopamine replacement therapy (DRT) can exacerbate delusions and hallucinations; PD medications may thus need to be adjusted with the goal of ameliorating or resolving psychotic symptoms while maintaining motor function. However, when PD medications are adjusted, any levodopa adjustments should be made last. Other pharmacological interventions for the treatment of Parkinson's disease psychosis (PDP) include specific atypical antipsychotic agents (i.e., quetiapine, clozapine, and pimavanserin), which have different side-effect profiles and monitoring parameters. Further investigation into the efficacy of cholinesterase inhibitors for the treatment of PDP is needed.

2. Answer: d

Studies have investigated cholinesterase inhibitors, dopaminergic agents, and antidepressants for the treatment of apathy in PD. Some studies have shown rivastigmine to be helpful for apathy in PD, and the D2/D3 dopamine agonists piribedil and ropinirole improved apathy that had arisen after STN-DBS. While bupropion, a norepinephrine-dopamine reuptake inhibitor, may improve motivation, SSRIs have been associated with increased apathy among elderly depressed patients and in PD patients in some studies. Methylphenidate was helpful for apathy in PD in a case report, but more evidence is needed regarding its efficacy for apathy in AD.

3. Answer: a

Punding refers to stereotyped, repetitive, and purposeless behaviors such as rearranging papers. Punding often leads to social avoidance, severe sleep deprivation, and alienation of family members. Because patients don't often mention these behaviors, it is important to ask screening questions of patients and caregivers. Dopamine dysregulation syndrome refers to compulsive overuse of dopamine replacement therapy, particularly with L-dopa and short-acting dopamine agonists. Impulse control disorders (ICDs) are non-motor complications of PD in which a person fails to resist the drive to engage in repetitive, excessive behaviors such as shopping, gambling, or sexual activities. Hobbyism refers to excessive or compulsive Internet use, reading, art work, and work on projects. All of the answer choices fall under the umbrella of impulsive-compulsive behaviors (ICBs).

4. Answer: c

Patients with Parkinson's disease have been associated with industrious, anhedonic, cautious, and inflexible personality features. However, the description of these characteristics in individuals with Parkinson's disease is mostly based on retrospective case-control studies, which are prone to recall bias. These features may instead represent changes in behavioral style of individuals secondary to PD itself.

References

1. Parkinson J. An essay on the shaking palsy. *J Neuropsychiatry Clin Neurosci*. 2002;14(2):223-236.
2. Calabresi P, Picconi B, Tozzi A, Ghiglieri V, Di Filippo M. Direct and indirect pathways of basal ganglia: a critical reappraisal. *Nat Neurosci*. 2014;17(8):1022.
3. Brichta L, Greengard P. Molecular determinants of selective dopaminergic vulnerability in Parkinson's disease: an update. *Front Neuroanat*. 2014;8:152.
4. Braak H, Del Tredici K, Rüb U, De Vos RA, Steur EN, Braak E. Staging of brain pathology related to sporadic Parkinson's disease. *Neurobiol Aging*. 2003;24(2):197-211.
5. Braak de H DT. Neuroanatomy and pathology of sporadic Parkinson's disease. *Adv Anat Embryol Cell Biol*. 2009;201:1-19.
6. Burke RE, Dauer WT, Vonsattel JP. A critical evaluation of the Braak staging scheme for Parkinson's disease. *Ann Neurol*. 2008;64(5):485-491.
7. Goedert M, Spillantini MG, Del Tredici K, Braak H. 100 years of Lewy pathology. *Nat Rev Neurol*. 2013;9(1):13.
8. Alves G, Forsaa EB, Pedersen KF, Dreetz Gjerstad M, Larsen JP. Epidemiology of Parkinson's disease. *J Neurol*. 2008;255(S5):18-32.
9. Pringsheim T, Jette N, Frolkis A, Steeves TD. The prevalence of Parkinson's disease: a systematic review and meta-analysis. *Mov Disord*. 2014;29(13):1583-1590.
10. Ascherio A, Schwarzschild MA. The epidemiology of Parkinson's disease: risk factors and prevention. *Lancet Neurol*. 2016;15(12):1257-1272.
11. Dorsey ER, Elbaz A, Nichols E, et al. Global, regional, and national burden of Parkinson's disease, 1990–2016: a systematic analysis for the global burden of disease study 2016. *Lancet Neurol*. 2018;17(11):939-953.
12. Weintraub D, Moberg PJ, Duda JE, Katz IR, Stern MB. Effect of psychiatric and other non-motor symptoms on disability in Parkinson's disease. *J Am Geriatr Soc*. 2004;52(5):784-788.
13. Reijnders JSAM, Ehrt U, Weber WEJ, Aarsland D, Leentjens AFG. A systematic review of prevalence studies of depression in Parkinson's disease. *Mov Disord*. 2008;23(2):183-189. doi:10.1002/mds.21803.
14. Ishihara L, Brayne C. A systematic review of depression and mental illness preceding Parkinson's disease. *Acta Neurol Scand*. 2006;113(4):211-220.
15. Noyce AJ, Bestwick JP, Silveira-Moriyama L, et al. Meta-analysis of early non-motor features and risk factors for Parkinson disease. *Ann Neurol*. 2012;72(6):893-901.
16. de la Riva P, Smith K, Xie SX, Weintraub D. Course of psychiatric symptoms and global cognition in early Parkinson disease. *Neurology*. 2014;83(12):1096-1103.
17. Tolosa E, Compta Y, Gaig C. The premotor phase of Parkinson's disease. *Parkinsonism Relat Disord*. 2007;13:S2-S7.

18. Schapira AH, Chaudhuri KR, Jenner P. Non-motor features of Parkinson disease. *Nat Rev Neurosci.* 2017;18(7):435.

19. Schuurman AG, van den Akker M, Ensinck KTJL, et al. Increased risk of Parkinson's disease after depression: a retrospective cohort study. *Neurology.* 2002;58(10):1501-1504.

20. Menza MA, Mark MH. Parkinson's disease and depression: the relationship to disability and personality. *J Neuropsychiatry.* 1994;6(2):165-169.

21. Starkstein SE, Petracca G, Chemerinski E, et al. Depression in classic versus akinetic-rigid Parkinson's disease. *Mov Disord.* 1998;13(1):29-33.

22. Remy P, Doder M, Lees AJ, Turjanski N, Brooks DJ. Depression in Parkinson's disease: loss of dopamine and noradrenaline innervation in the limbic system. *Brain.* 2005;128(6):1314-1322.

23. Cardoso EF, Maia FM, Fregni F, et al. Depression in Parkinson's disease: convergence from voxel-based morphometry and functional magnetic resonance imaging in the limbic thalamus. *NeuroImage.* 2009;47(2):467-472.

24. Young KA, Holcomb LA, Yazdani U, Hicks PB, German DC. Elevated neuron number in the limbic thalamus in major depression. *Am J Psychiatry.* 2004;161(7):1270-1277.

25. Heinz A, Schmidt LG, Reischies FM. Anhedonia in schizophrenic, depressed, or alcohol-dependent patients: neurobiological correlates. *Pharmacopsychiatry.* 1994;27(S 1):7-10.

26. Lemke MR, Brecht HM, Koester J, Kraus PH, Reichmann H. Anhedonia, depression, and motor functioning in Parkinson's disease during treatment with pramipexole. *J Neuropsychiatry Clin Neurosci.* 2005;17(2):214-220.

27. Fujiwara S, Kimura F, Hosokawa T, Ishida S, Sugino M, Hanafusa T. Anhedonia in Japanese patients with Parkinson's disease. *Geriatr Gerontol Int.* 2011;11(3):275-281.

28. Miura S, Kida H, Nakajima J, et al. Anhedonia in Japanese patients with Parkinson's disease: analysis using the Snaith–Hamilton Pleasure Scale. *Clin Neurol Neurosurg.* 2012;114(4):352-355.

29. Marsh L, McDonald WM, Cummings J, Ravina B, NINDS/NIMH Work Group on Depression and Parkinson's Disease. Provisional diagnostic criteria for depression in Parkinson's disease: report of an NINDS/NIMH Work Group. *Mov Disord.* 2006;21(2):148-158.

30. Storch A, Schneider CB, Wolz M, et al. Nonmotor fluctuations in Parkinson disease: severity and correlation with motor complications. *Neurology.* 2013;80(9):800-809.

31. Erro R, Picillo M, Vitale C, et al. Non-motor symptoms in early Parkinson's disease: a 2-year follow-up study on previously untreated patients. *J Neurol Neurosurg Psychiatry.* 2013;84(1):14-17.

32. Politis M, Wu K, Molloy S, G Bain P, Chaudhuri KR, Piccini P. Parkinson's disease symptoms: the patient's perspective. *Mov Disord.* 2010;25(11):1646-1651.

33. Leentjens AFG, Verhey FRJ, Luijckx G-J, Troost J. The validity of the Beck Depression Inventory as a screening and diagnostic instrument for depression in patients with Parkinson's disease. *Mov Disord.* 2001;15(6):1221-1224.

34. Leentjens AFG, Verhey FRJ, Lousberg R, Spitsbergen H, Wilmink FW. The validity of the Hamilton and Montgomery-Asberg depression rating scales as screening and diagnostic tools for depression in Parkinson's disease. *Int J Geriatr Psychiatry.* 2000;15(7):644-649.

35. Shulman LM, Taback RL, Rabinstein AA, Weiner WJ. Non-recognition of depression and other non-motor symptoms in Parkinson's disease. *Parkinsonism Relat Disord.* 2002;8(3):193-197.

36. Seppi K, Ray Chaudhuri K, Coelho M, et al. Update on treatments for non-motor symptoms of Parkinson's disease—an evidence-based medicine review. *Mov Disord.* 2019;34(2):180-198.

37. Menza M, Dobkin RD, Marin H, et al. A controlled trial of antidepressants in patients with Parkinson disease and depression. *Neurology.* 2009;72(10):886-892.

38. Okun MS, Fernandez HH. Will tricyclic antidepressants make a comeback for depressed Parkinson disease patients? *Neurology.* 2009;72(10):868-869.

39. Connolly B, Fox SH. Treatment of cognitive, psychiatric, and affective disorders associated with Parkinson's disease. *Neurotherapeutics.* 2014;11(1):78-91.

40. Richard IH, McDermott MP, Kurlan R, et al. A randomized, double-blind, placebo-controlled trial of antidepressants in Parkinson disease. *Neurology.* 2012;78(16):1229-1236.

41. Bonuccelli U, Meco G, Fabbrini G, et al. A non-comparative assessment of tolerability and efficacy of duloxetine in the treatment of depressed patients with Parkinson's disease. *Expert Opin Pharmacother.* 2012;13(16):2269-2280.

42. Simons JA. Fluoxetine in Parkinson's disease. *Mov Disord.* 1996;11(5):581-582.

43. Kulisevsky J, Pagonabarraga J, Pascual-Sedano B, Gironell A, García-Sánchez C, Martínez-Corral M. Motor changes during sertraline treatment in depressed patients with Parkinson's disease. *Eur J Neurol.* 2008;15(9):953-959.

44. Dell'Agnello G, Ceravolo R, Nuti A, et al. SSRIs do not worsen Parkinson's disease: evidence from an open-label, prospective study. *Clin Neuropharmacol.* 2001;24(4):221-227.

45. Raskin S, Durst R. Bupropion as the treatment of choice in depression associated with Parkinson's disease and its various treatments. *Med Hypotheses.* 2010;75(6):544-546.

46. Zaluska M, Dyduch A. Bupropion in the treatment of depression in Parkinson's disease. *Int Psychogeriatr.* 2011;(23):325-327.

47. Korchounov A, Winter Y, Rossy W. Combined beneficial effect of rasagiline on motor function and depression in de novo PD. *Clin Neuropharmacol.* 2012;35:121-124.

48. Smith KM, Eyal E, Weintraub D. Combined rasagiline and antidepressant use in Parkinson disease in the ADAGIO study: effects on non-motor symptoms and tolerability. *JAMA Neurol.* 2015;72(1):88-95.

49. Chaudhuri KR, Schapira AH. Non-motor symptoms of Parkinson's disease: dopaminergic pathophysiology and treatment. *Lancet Neurol.* 2009;8(5):464-474.

50. Aquino CC, Fox SH. Clinical spectrum of levodopa-induced complications. *Mov Disord.* 2015;30(1):80-89.

51. Aarsland D, Pahlhagen S, Ballard C, et al. Depression in Parkinson disease—epidemiology, mechanisms and management. *Nat Rev.* 2012;8:35-47.

52. Schuepbach WM, Rau J, Knudsen K, et al. EARLYSTIM Study Group. Neurostimulation for Parkinson's disease with early motor complications. *N Engl J Med.* 2013;368:610-622.

53. Okun MS, Fernandez HH, Wu SS, et al. Cognition and mood in Parkinson's disease in subthalamic nucleus versus globus pallidus interna deep brain stimulation: the COMPARE trial. *Ann Neurol.* 2009;65:586-595.

54. Okun MS, Wu SS, Foote KD, et al. Do stable patients with a premorbid depression history have a worse outcome after deep brain stimulation for Parkinson disease? *Neurosurgery.* 2011;69:357-360.

55. Doshi PK, Chhaya N, Bhatt MH. Depression leading to attempted suicide after bilateral subthalamic nucleus stimulation for Parkinson's disease. *Mov Disord.* 2002;17(5):1084-1085.

56. Voon V, Krack P, Lang AE, et al. A multicentre study on suicide outcomes following subthalamic stimulation for Parkinson's disease. *Brain.* 2008;131(10):2720-2728.

57. Dobkin RD, Menza M, Allen LA, et al. Cognitive-behavioral therapy for depression in Parkinson's disease: a randomized, controlled trial. *Am J Psychiatry*. 2011;168(10):1066-1074.

58. Dobkin RD, Rubino JT, Allen LA, et al. Predictors of treatment response to cognitive-behavioral therapy for depression in Parkinson's disease. *J Consult Clin Psychol*. 2012;80(4):694-699.

59. A'Campco LE, Wekking EM, Slpithoff-Kamminga NG, et al. The benefits of a standardized patient education program for patients with Parkinson's disease and their caregivers. *Parkinsonism Relat Disord*. 2010;16(2):89-95.

60. Sproeseer E, Viana MA, Quagliato EM, et al. The effect of psychotherapy in patients with PD: a controlled study. *Parkinsonism Relat Disord*. 2010;16(4):89-95.

61. Yang S, Sajatovic M, Walter B. Psychosocial interventions for depression and anxiety in Parkinson's disease. *J Geriatr Psychiatry Neurol*. 2012;25(2):113-121.

62. Bega D, Zadikoff C. Complementary and alternative management of Parkinson's disease: an evidence-based review of eastern influenced practices. *J Mov Disord*. 2014;7(2):57.

63. Trend P, Kaye J, Gage H, Owen C, Wade D. Short-term effectiveness of intensive multidisciplinary rehabilitation therapy for people with Parkinson's disease and their carers. *Clin Rehabil*. 2002;16(7):717-725.

64. Wade DT, Gage H, Owen C, Wade D. Multidisciplinary rehabilitation for people with Parkinson's disease: a randomized controlled study. *J Neurol Neurosurg Psychiatry*. 2003;74(2):158-162.

65. Pontone GM, Williams JR, Anderson KE, et al. Anxiety and self-perceived health status in Parkinson's disease. *Parkinsonism Relat Disord*. 2011;17(4):249-254.

66. Broen MP, Narayen NE, Kuijf ML, Dissanayaka NN, et al Prevalence of anxiety in Parkinson's disease: a systematic review and meta-analysis. *Mov Disord*. 2016;31:1125-1133.

67. Wee N, Kandiah N, Acharyya S, et al. Depression and anxiety are co-morbid but dissociable in mild Parkinson's disease: a prospective longitudinal study of patterns and predictors. *Parkinsonism Relat Disord*. 2016;23:50-56.

68. Lutz SG, Holmes JD, Ready EA, et al. Clinical presentation of anxiety in Parkinson's disease: a scoping review. *OTJR*. 2016;36(3):134-147.

69. Dissanayaka NN, White E, O'Sullivan JD, et al. The clinical spectrum of anxiety in Parkinson's disease. *Mov Disord*. 2014;29:967-975.

70. Coakeley S, Martens KE, Almeida QJ. Management of anxiety and motor symptoms in Parkinson's disease. *Exp Rev Neurotherapeut*. 2014;14(8):937-946.

71. Vázquez A, Jimenez-Jimenez FJ, Garcia-Ruiz P, Garcia-Urra D. "Panic attacks" in Parkinson's disease: a long-term complication of levodopa therapy. *Acta Neurol Scand*. 1993;87(1):14-18.

72. Alegret M, Junque C, Valldeoriola F, Vendrell P, Marti MJ, Tolosa E. Obsessive-compulsive symptoms in Parkinson's disease. *J Neurol Neurosurg Psychiatry*. 2001;70(3):394-396.

73. Menza M, Marin H, Kaufman K, Mark M, Lauritano M. Citalopram treatment of depression in Parkinson's disease: the impact on anxiety, disability, and cognition. *J Neuropsychiatry Clin Neurosci*. 2004;16(3):315-319.

74. Tarczy MI, Szombathelyi E. Depression in Parkinson's disease with special regard to anxiety: experiences with paroxetine treatment. *Mov Disord*. 1998;13(suppl 2):275.

75. Shulman LM, Singer C, Liefert R, Mellman T, Weiner W. Therapeutic effects of sertraline in patients with Parkinson's disease. *Mov Disord*. 1996;11:603.

76. Richard IH, McDermott MP, Kurlan R, et al. A randomized, double-blind, placebo-controlled trial of antidepressants in Parkinson disease. *Neurology*. 2012;78(16):1229-1236.

77. Cooney JW, Stacy M. Neuropsychiatric issues in Parkinson's disease. *Curr Neurol Neurosci Rep*. 2016;16(5):49.

78. Chang A, Fox SH. Psychosis in Parkinson's disease: epidemiology, pathophysiology, and management. *Drugs*. 2016;76(11):1093-1118.

79. Schneider RB, Iourinets J, Richard IH. Parkinson's disease psychosis: presentation, diagnosis and management. *Neurodegener Dis Manag*. 2017;7(6):365-376.

80. Stebbins GT, Goetz CG, Carrillo MC, et al. Altered cortical visual processing in PD with hallucinations: an fMRI study. *Neurology*. 2004;63(8):1409-1416.

81. Papapetropoulos S, McCorquodale DS, Gonzalez J, Jean-Gilles L, Mash DC. Cortical and amygdalar Lewy body burden in Parkinson's disease patients with visual hallucinations. *Parkinsonism Relat Disord*. 2006;12(4):253-256.

82. Zahodne LB, Fernandez HH. Pathophysiology and treatment of psychosis in Parkinson's disease. *Drugs Aging*. 2008;25(8):665-682.

83. Hughes AJ, Daniel SE, Kilford L, Lees AJ. Accuracy of clinical diagnosis of idiopathic Parkinson's disease: a clinico-pathological study of 100 cases. *J Neurol Neurosurg Psychiatry*. 1992;55(3):181-184.

84. Ravina B, Marder K, Fernandez HH, et al. Diagnostic criteria for psychosis in Parkinson's disease: report of an NINDS, NIMH Work Group. *Mov Disord*. 2007;22(8):1061-1068.

85. Fernandez HH, Aarsland D, Fénelon G, et al. Scales to assess psychosis in Parkinson's disease: critique and recommendations. *Mov Disord*. 2008;23(3):484-500.

86. Connolly B, Fox SH. Treatment of cognitive, psychiatric, and affective disorders associated with Parkinson's disease. *Neurotherapeutics*. 2014;11(1):78-91.

87. Pagonabarraga J, Kulisevsky J. Apathy in Parkinson's disease. *Int Rev Neurobiol*. 2017;133:657-678.

88. Pagonabarraga J, Kulisevsky J, Strafella AP, Krack P. Apathy in Parkinson's disease: clinical features, neural substrates, diagnosis, and treatment. *Lancet Neurol*. 2015;14(5):518-531.

89. Lawrence AD, Goerendt IK, Brooks DJ. Apathy blunts neural response to money in Parkinson's disease. *Soc Neurosci*. 2011;6(5-6):653-662.

90. Thobois S, Ardouin C, Lhommée E, et al. Non-motor dopamine withdrawal syndrome after surgery for Parkinson's disease: predictors and underlying mesolimbic denervation. *Brain*. 2010;133(4):1111-1127.

91. Marin RS. Apathy: a neuropsychiatric syndrome. *J Neuropsychiatry Clin Neurosci*. 1991;3(3):243-254.

92. Marin RS. Apathy: concept, syndrome, neural mechanisms, and treatment. *Semin Clin Neuropsychiatry*. 1996;1(4):304-314.

93. Starkstein SE. Apathy in Parkinson's disease: diagnostic and etiological dilemmas. *Mov Disord*. 2012;27(2):174-178.

94. Leentjens AF, Dujardin K, Marsh L, et al. Apathy and anhedonia rating scales in Parkinson's disease: critique and recommendations. *Mov Disord*. 2008;23(14):2004-2014.

95. Weintraub D, Koester J, Potenza MN, et al. Impulse control disorders in Parkinson disease: a cross-sectional study of 3090 patients. *Arch Neurol*. 2010;67(5):589-595.

96. Weintraub D, Siderowf AD, Potenza MN, et al. Association of dopamine agonist use with impulse control disorders in Parkinson's disease. *Arch Neurol*. 2006;63(7):969-973.

97. Lee JY, Kim JM, Kim JW, et al. Association between the dose of dopaminergic medication and the behavioral

disturbances in Parkinson disease. *Parkinsonism Relat Disord.* 2010;16(3):202-207.

98. Fantini ML, Macedo L, Zibetti M, et al. Increased risk of impulse control symptoms in Parkinson's disease with REM sleep behavior disorder. *J Neurol Neurosurg Psychiatry.* 2015;86(2):174-179.

99. Vitale C, Santangelo G, Trojano L, et al. Comparative neuropsychological profile of pathological gambling, hypersexuality, and competitive eating in Parkinson's disease. *Mov Disord.* 2011;26(5):830-836.

100. Voon V, Fox SH. Medication-related impulse control and repetitive behaviors in Parkinson disease. *Arch Neurol.* 2007; 64(8):1089-1096.

101. Voon V, Sohr M, Lang AE, et al. Impulse control disorders in Parkinson disease: a multicenter case-control study. *Ann Neurol.* 2011;69(6):986-996.

102. Balarajah S, Cavanna AE. The pathophysiology of impulse control disorders in Parkinson disease. *Behav Neurol.* 2013; 26(4):237-244.

103. Marques A, Durif F, Fernagut PO. Impulse control disorder in Parkinson's disease. *J Neural Transmission.* 2018;125:1299-1312.

104. Weintraub D, David AS, Evans AH, et al. Clinical spectrum of impulse control disorders in Parkinson's disease. *Mov Disord.* 2015;30(2):121-127.

105. Evans AH, Katzenschlager R, Paviour D, et al. Punding in Parkinson's disease: its relation to the dopamine dysregulation syndrome. *Mov Disord.* 2004;19(4):397-405.

106. Weintraub D, Papay K, Siderowf A; Parkinson's Progression Markers Initiative. Screening for impulse control symptoms in patients with de novo Parkinson disease: a case-control study. *Neurology.* 2013;80(2):176-180.

107. Giovannoni G, O'Sullivan J, Turner K, et al. Hedonistic homeostatic dysregulation in patients with Parkinson's disease on dopamine replacement therapies. *J Neurol Neurosurg Psychiatry.* 2000;68(4):423-428.

108. O'Sullivan SS, Djamshidian A, Evans AH, et al. Excessive hoarding in Parkinson's disease. *Mov Disord.* 2010;25(8):1026-1033.

109. Christenson GA, Faber RJ, De Zwaan M, et al. Compulsive buying: descriptive characteristics and psychiatric comorbidity. *J Clin Psychiatry.* 1994;55(1):5-11.

110. Weintraub D, Hoops S, Shea JA, et al. Validation of the questionnaire for impulsive-compulsive disorders in Parkinson's disease. *Mov Disord.* 2009;24(10):1461-1467.

111. Weintraub D, Mamikonyan E, Papay K, et al. Questionnaire for impulsive-compulsive in Parkinson's disease—rating scale. *Mov Disord.* 2012;27(2):242-247.

112. Visser M, Verbaan D, van Rooden SM, et al. Assessment of psychiatric complications in Parkinson's disease: the SCOPA-PA. *Mov Disord.* 2007;22(15):2221-2228.

113. Rieu I, Martinez-Martin P, Pereira B, et al. International validation of behavioral scale in Parkinson's disease without dementia. *Mov Disord.* 2015;30(5):705-713.

114. Mamikonyan E, Siderowf AD, Duda JE, et al. Long-term follow-up of impulse control disorders in Parkinson's disease. *Mov Disord.* 2008;23(1):75-80.

115. Giovannoni G, O'Sullivan JD, Turner K, et al. Hedonistic homeostatic dysregulation in patients with Parkinson's disease on dopamine replacement therapy. *J Neurol Neurosurg Psychiatry.* 2000;68:423-428.

116. Ceravolo R, Frosini D, Rossi C, et al. Impulse control disorders in Parkinson's disease: definition, epidemiology, risk factors, neurobiology and management. *Parkinsonism Relat Disord.* 2009;15(S4): S111-S115.

117. Klos KJ, Bower JH, Josephs KA, et al. Pathological hypersexuality predominately linked to adjuvant dopamine agonist therapy in Parkinson's disease and multiple system atrophy. *Parkinsonism Relat Disord.* 2005;11(6):381-386.

118. Kurlan R. Disabling repetitive behaviors in Parkinson's disease. *Mov Disord.* 2004;19(4):433-437.

119. Courty E, Durif F, Zenut M, et al. Psychiatric and sexual disorders inducted by apomorphine in Parkinson's disease. *Clin Neuropharmacol.* 1997;20(2):140-147.

120. Giovannoni G, O'Sullivan JD, Turner K, et al. Hedonistic homeostatic dysregulation in patients with Parkinson's disease on dopamine replacement therapies. *J Neurol Neurosurg Psychiatry.* 2000;68(4):423-428.

121. O'Sullivan SS, Evans AH, Lees AJ. Dopamine dysregulation syndrome: an overview of its epidemiology, mechanisms and management. *CNS Drugs.* 2009;23(2):157-170.

122. Lawrence AD, Evans AH, Lees AJ. Compulsive use of dopamine replacement therapy in Parkinson's disease: reward systems gone awry? *Lancet Neurol.* 2003;2(10):595-604.

123. Evans AH, Katzenschlager R, Paviour D, et al. Punding in Parkinson's disease: its relation to the dopamine dysregulation syndrome. *Mov Disord.* 2004;19(4):397-405.

124. Evans AH, Lees AJ. Dopamine dysregulation syndrome in Parkinson's disease. *Curr Opin Neurol.* 2004;17(4):393-398.

125. Voon V. Repetition, repetition, repetition: compulsive and punding behaviors in Parkinson's disease. *Mov Disord.* 2004; 19(4):367-370.

126. Blum K, Noble EP, Sheridan PJ, et al. Allelic association of human dopamine D2 receptor gene in alcoholism. *JAMA.* 1990;263(15):2055-2060.

127. Klein TA, Neumann J, Reuter M, et al. Genetically determined differences in learning from errors. *Science.* 2007; 318(5856):1642-1645.

128. Cohen MX, Krohn-Grimberghe A, Elger CE, Weber B. Dopamine gene predicts the brain's response to dopaminergic drug. *Eur J Neurosci.* 2007;26(12):3652-3660.

129. Frank MJ, Seeberger LC, O'Reilly RC. By carrot or by stick: cognitive reinforcement learning in parkinsonism. *Science.* 2004;306(5703):1940-1943.

130. Swainson R, Rogers RD, Sahakian BJ, et al. Probabilistic learning and reversal deficits in patients with Parkinson's disease or frontal or temporal lobe lesions: possible adverse effects of dopaminergic medication. *Neuropsychologia.* 2000;38(5):596-612.

131. Cools R, Barker RA, Sahakian BJ, Robbins T. Enhanced or impaired cognitive function in Parkinson's disease as a function of dopaminergic medication and task demands. *Cereb Cortex.* 2001;11(12):1136-1143.

132. Spigset O, von Schelle C. Levodopa dependence and abuse in Parkinson's disease. *Pharmacotherapy.* 1997;17(5):1027-1030.

133. Pezzella FR, Colosimo C, Vanacore N, et al. Prevalence and clinical features of hedonistic homeostatic dysregulation in Parkinson's disease. *Mov Disord.* 2005;20(1):77-81.

134. Pavese N, Evan AH, Tai YF, et al. Compulsive use of dopamine replacement therapy in Parkinson's disease: in vivo evidence of dopaminergic reward system dysregulation with PET. *Neurology.* 2004;62(suppl):A431.

135. Evan AH, Pavese N, Lawrence AD, et al. Compulsive drug use linked to sensitized ventral striatal dopamine transmission. *Ann Neurol.* 2006;59(5):852-858.

136. Nocjar C, Panksepp J. Chronic intermittent amphetamine pretreatment enhances future appetive behavior for drug- and natural-reward: interaction with environmental variables. *Behav Brain Res.* 2002;128:189-203.

137. Rylander G. Pyschoses and the punding and choreiform syndromes in addiction to central stimulant drugs. *Psychiatr Neurol Neurochir.* 1972;75(3):203-212.

138. Schiorring E. Psychopathology induced by "speed drugs." *Pharmacol Biochem Behav* 1981;14(suppl 1):109-122.

139. Cloninger CR. A systematic method for clinical description and classification of personality variants: a proposal. *Arch Gen Psychiatry.* 1987;44(6):573-588.

140. Leyton M, Boileau I, Benkelfat C, et al. Amphetamine-induced increases in extracellular dopamine, drug wanting, and novelty seeking: a PET/[11C]raclopride study in healthy men. *Neuropsychopharmacology.* 2002;27(6):1027-1035.

141. Bearn J, Evans AH, Kelleher M, Turner K, Lees AJ. Recognition of a dopamine replacement therapy dependence syndrome in Parkinson's disease: a pilot study. *Drug Alchol Depend.* 2004;76(3):305-310.

142. Fernandez HH, Friedman JH. Punding on L-dopa. *Mov Disord.* 1999;14(5):836-838.

143. Epstein J, Madiedo CJ, Lai L, Hayes MT. Successful treatment of dopamine dysregulation syndrome with valproic acid. *J Neuropsychiatry Clin Neurosci.* 2014;26(3):E3-E3.

144. Sriram A, Ward HE, Hassan A, et al. Valproate as a treatment for dopamine dysregulation syndrome (DDS) in Parkinson's disease. *J Neurol.* 2013;260(2):521-527.

145. Cilia R, Siri C, Canesi M, et al. Dopamine dysregulation syndrome in Parkinson's disease: from clinical and neuropsychological characterization to management and long-term outcome. *J Neurol Neurosurg Psychiatry.* 2013;85(3):311-318.

146. Limousin P, Krack P, Pollak P, et al. Electrical stimulation of the subthalamic nucleus in advanced Parkinson's disease. *N Engl J Med.* 1998;339(16):1105-1111.

147. Eskow Jaunarajs KL, Angoa-Perez M, Kuhn DM, Bishop C. Potential mechanisms underlying anxiety and depression in Parkinson's disease: consequences of L-DOPA treatment. *Neurosci Biobehav Rev.* 2001;35(3):556-564.

148. Braak H, Ghebremedhin E, Rüb U, et al. Stages in the development of Parkinson's disease-related pathology. *Cell Tissue Res.* 2004;318(1):121-134.

149. Thobois S, Ardouin C, Lhommée E, et al. Non-motor dopamine withdrawal syndrome after surgery for Parkinson's disease: predictors and underlying mesolimbic denervation. *Brain.* 2010;133(pt 4):1111-1127.

150. Nassery A, Palmese CA, Sarva H, et al. Psychiatric and cognitive effects of deep brain stimulation for Parkinson's disease. *Curr Neurol Neurosci Rep.* 2016;16(10):87.

151. Temel Y, Kessels A, Tan S, et al. Behavioural changes after bilateral subthalamic stimulation in advanced Parkinson disease: a systemic review. *Parkinsonism Relat Disord.* 2006;12(5):265-272.

152. Weintraub D, Duda JE, Carlson K, et al. Suicide ideation and behaviours after STN and GPi DBS surgery for Parkinson's disease: results from a randomised, controlled trial. *J Neurol Neurosurg Psychiatry.* 2013;84:1113-1118.

153. Pinsker M, Amtage F, Berger M, Nikkhah G, van Elst LT. Psychiatric side-effects of bilateral deep brain stimulation for movement disorders. *Acta Neurochir Suppl.* 2013;117:47-51.

154. Couto MI, Monteiro A, Olivera A, Lunet N, Massano J. Depression and anxiety following deep brain stimulation in Parkinson's disease: systematic review and meta-analysis. *Acta Medica Port.* 2014;27(3):372-382.

155. Okun MS, Wu SS, Fayad S, Ward H, Bowers D. Acute and chronic mood and apathy outcomes from a randomized study of unilateral STN and GPi DBS. *PLoS One.* 2014;9(12):e114140.

156. Raucher-Chene D, Charrel CL, de Maindreville AD, Limosin F. Manic episode with psychotic symptoms in a patient with Parkinson's disease treated by subthalamic nucleus stimulation: improvement on switching targets. *J Neurol Sci.* 2008;273(1-2):116-117.

157. Volkmann J, Allert N, Voges J, et al. Long-term results of bilateral pallidal stimulation in Parkinson's disease. *Ann Neurol.* 2004;55(6):871-875.

158. Lim SY, O'Sullivan SS, Kotschet K, Gallagher DA, Lacey C. Dopamine dysregulation syndrome, impulse control disorders and punding after deep brain stimulation surgery for Parkinson's disease. *J Clin Neurosci.* 2009;16:1148-1152.

159. Aybek S, Gronchi-Perrin A, Berney A, et al. Long-term cognitive profile and incidence of dementia after STN-DBS in Parkinson's disease. *Mov Disord.* 2007;22(7):974-981.

160. Witt K, Granert O, Daniels C, et al. Relation of lead trajectory and electrode position to neuropsychological outcomes of subthalamic neurostimulation in Parkinson's disease: results from a randomized trial. *Brain.* 2013;136(pt 7):2109-2119.

161. Appleby BS, Duggan PS, Regenberg A, Rabins PV. Psychiatric and neuropsychiatric adverse events associated with deep brain stimulation: a meta-analysis of 10 years' experience. *Mov Disord.* 2007;22(12):1722-1728.

162. Fasano A, Romito LM, Daniele A, et al. Motor and cognitive outcome in patients with Parkinson's disease 8 years after subthalamic implants. *Brain.* 2010;133(9):2664-2676.

163. Smeding HM, Speelman JD, Huizenga HM, Schuurman PR, Schmand B. Predictors of cognitive and psychosocial outcome after STN DBS in Parkinson's disease. *J Neurol Neurosurg Psychiatry.* 2011;82(7):754-760.

164. Schroeder U, Kuehler A, Lange KW, et al. Subthalamic nucleus stimulation affects a frontotemporal network: a PET study. *Ann Neurol.* 2003;54(4):445-450.

165. Morrison CE, Borod JC, Perrine K, et al. Neuropsychological functioning following bilateral subthalamic nucleus stimulation in Parkinson's disease. *Arch Clin Neuropsychol.* 2004;19(2):165-181.

166. Ehlen F, Krugel LK, Vonberg I, et al. Intact lexicon running slowly—prolonged response latencies in patients with subthalamic DBS and verbal fluency deficits. *PLoS One.* 2013;8(11):e79247.

167. Williams AE, Arzola GM, Strutt AM, et al. Cognitive outcome and reliable change indices 2 years following bilateral subthalamic nucleus deep brain stimulation. *Parkinsonism Relat Disord.* 2011;17(5):321-327.

168. Castelli L, Rizz L, Zibetti M, et al. Neuropsychological changes 1-year after subthalamic DBS in PD patients: a prospective controlled study. *Parkinsonism Relat Disord.* 2010;16(2):115-118.

169. Okun MS, Fernandez HH, Wu SS, et al. Cognition and mood in Parkinson's disease in subthalamic nucleus versus globus pallidus interna deep brain stimulation: the COMPARE trial. *Ann Neurol.* 2009;65(5):586-595.

170. Mikos A, Bowers D, Noecker AM, et al. Patient-specific analysis of the relationship between the volume of tissue activated during DBS and verbal fluency. *NeuroImage.* 2011;54:S238-S246.

171. De Gaspari D, Siri C, Di Gioia M, et al. Clinical correlates and cognitive underpinnings of verbal fluency impairment after chronic subthalamic stimulation in Parkinson's disease. *Parkinsonism Relat Disord.* 2006;12(5):289-295.

172. Chaudhuri KR. Nocturnal symptom complex in PD and its management. *Neurology.* 2003;61(6 suppl 3):S17-S23.

173. Garcia-Borreguero D, Larosa O, Bravo M. Parkinson's disease and sleep. *Sleep Med Rev.* 2003;7(2):115-119.

174. Abbott RD, Ross GW, White LR, et al. Excessive daytime sleepiness and subsequent development of Parkinson disease. *Neurology.* 2005;65(9):1442-1446.

175. Tracik F, Ebersbach G. Sudden daytime sleep onset in Parkinson's disease: polysomnographic readings. *Mov Disord*. 2001;16(3):500-506.

176. Ulivelli M, Rossi S, Lombardi C, et al. Polysomnographic characterization of pergolide-induced sleep attacks in idiopathic PD. *Neurology*. 2002;58(3):462-465.

177. Olson EJ, Boeve BF, Silber MH. Rapid eye movement sleep behaviour disorder: demographic, clinical and laboratory findings in 93 cases. *Brain*. 2000;123(pt 2):331-339.

178. Fantini ML, Ferini-Strambi L, Montplaisir J. Idiopathic REM sleep behavior disorder: toward a better nosologic definition. *Neurology*. 2005;64(5):780-786.

179. Chaudhuri KR, Healy DG, Schapira AHV. Non-motor symptoms of Parkinson's disease: diagnosis and management. *Lancet Neurol*. 2006;5(3):235-245.

180. Litvan I, Aarsland D, Adler CH, et al. MDS Task Force on mild cognitive impairment in Parkinson's disease: critical review of PD-MCI. *Mov Disord*. 2011;26(10):1814.

181. Emre M, Aarsland D, Brown R, et al. Clinical diagnostic criteria for dementia associated with Parkinson's disease. *Mov Disord*. 2007;22(12):1689-1707.

182. Aarsland D, Zaccai J, Brayne C. A systematic review of prevalence studies of dementia in Parkinson's disease. *Mov Disord*. 2005;20(10):1255-1263.

183. Hobson P, Meara J. Risk and incidence of dementia in a cohort of older subjects with Parkinson's disease in the United Kingdom. *Mov Disord*. 2004;19(9):1043-1049.

184. Fields JA. Cognitive and neuropsychiatric features in Parkinson's and Lewy body dementias. *Arch Clin Neuropsychol*. 2017;32(7):786-801.

185. Aarsland D, Perry R, Brown A, Larsen JP, Ballard C. Neuropathology of dementia in Parkinson's disease: a prospective, community-based study. *Ann Neurol*. 2005;58(5):773-776.

186. Kövari E, Gold G, Herrmann FR, et al. Lewy body densities in the entorhinal and anterior cingulate cortex predict cognitive deficits in Parkinson's disease. *Acta Neuropathol*. 2003;106(1):83-88.

187. Press DZ, Mechanic DJ, Tarsy D, Manoach DS. Cognitive slowing in Parkinson's disease resolves after practice. *J Neurol Neurosurg Psychiatry*. 2002;73(5):524-528.

188. Irwin DJ, White MT, Toledo JB, et al. Neuropathologic substrates of Parkinson disease dementia. *Ann Neurol*. 2012;72(4):587-598.

189. Johnson DK, Galvin JE. Longitudinal changes in cognition in Parkinson's disease with and without dementia. *Dement Geriatr Cogn Disord*. 2011;31(2):98-108.

190. Roheger M, Kalbe E, Liepelt-Scarfone I. Progression of cognitive decline in Parkinson's disease. *J Parkinsons Dis*. 2018;8(2):183-193.

191. Hu MT, Szewczyk-Królikowski K, Tomlinson P, et al. Predictors of cognitive impairment in an early stage Parkinson's disease cohort. *Mov Disord*. 2014;29(3):351-359.

192. Savica R, Grossardt BR, Bower JH, Boeve BF, Ahlskog JE, Rocca WA. Incidence of dementia with Lewy bodies and Parkinson disease dementia. *JAMA Neurol*. 2013;70(11):1396-1402.

193. Connolly B, Fox SH. Treatment of cognitive, psychiatric, and affective disorders associated with Parkinson's disease. *Neurotherapeutics*. 2014;11(1):78-91.

194. Wang HF, Yu JT, Tang SW, et al. Efficacy and safety of cholinesterase inhibitors and memantine in cognitive impairment in Parkinson's disease, Parkinson's disease dementia, and dementia with Lewy bodies: systematic review with meta-analysis and trial sequential analysis. *J Neurol Neurosurg Psychiatry*. 2015;86(2):135-143.

195. Martyn C, Gale C. Tobacco, coffee and Parkinson's disease. *BMJ*. 2003;326(7389):561-562.

196. Todes CJ, Lees AJ. The pre-morbid personality of patients with Parkinson's disease. *J Neurol Neurosurg Psychiatry*. 1985;48(2):97-100.

197. Menza MA, Golbe LI, Cody RA, et al. Dopamine-related personality traits in Parkinson's disease. *Neurology*. 1993;43(3 pt 1):505-508.

198. Poletti M, Bonuccelli U. Personality traits in patients with Parkinson's disease: assessment and clinical implications. *J Neurol*. 2012;259(6):1029-1038.

199. Tomer R, Aharon-Peretz J. Novelty seeking and harm avoidance in Parkinson's disease: effects of asymmetric dopamine deficiency. *J Neurol Neurosurg Psychiatry*. 2004;75(7):972-975.

200. Ishihara L, Bryane C. What is the evidence for a premorbid parkinsonian personality: a systematic review. *Mov Disord*. 2006;21(8):1066-1072.

201. Miech RA, Breitner JC, Zandi PP, et al. Incidence of AD may decline in the early 90s for men, later for women: the Cache County study. *Neurology*. 2002;58:209-218.

202. Zaccai J, McCracken C, Brayne C. A systematic review of prevalence and incidence studies of dementia with Lewy bodies. *Age Ageing*. 2005;34(6):561-566.

203. Jones SV, O'Brien JT. The prevalence and incidence of dementia with Lewy bodies: a systematic review of population and clinical studies. *Psychol Med*. 2014;44(4):673-683.

204. Jellinger KA, Korczyn AD. Are dementia with Lewy bodies and Parkinson's disease dementia the same disease? *BMC Med*. 2018;16(1):34.

205. Goedert M. Alpha-synuclein and neurodegenerative diseases. *Nat Rev Neurosci*. 2001;2(7):492.

206. Rezaie P, Cairns NJ, Chadwick A, Lantos PL. Lewy bodies are located preferentially in limbic areas in diffuse Lewy body disease. *Neurosci Lett*. 1996;212(2):111-114.

207. Irwin DJ, Grossman M, Weintraub D, et al. Neuropathological and genetic correlates of survival and dementia onset in synucleinopathies: a retrospective analysis. *Lancet Neurol*. 2017;16(1):55-65.

208. McKeith IG, Boeve BF, Dickson DW, et al. Diagnosis and management of dementia with Lewy bodies: fourth consensus report of the DLB Consortium. *Neurology*. 2017;89(1):88-100.

209. Lemstra AW, De Beer MH, Teunissen CE, et al. Concomitant AD pathology affects clinical manifestation and survival in dementia with Lewy bodies. *J Neurol Neurosurg Psychiatry*. 2017;88(2):113-118.

210. Beyer MK, Larsen JP, Aarsland D. Gray matter atrophy in Parkinson disease with dementia and dementia with Lewy bodies. *Neurology*. 2007;69(8):747-754.

211. Lobotesis K, Fenwick JD, Phipps A, et al. Occipital hypoperfusion on SPECT in dementia with Lewy bodies but not AD. *Neurology*. 2001;56(5):643-649.

212. Okamura N, Arai H, Higuchi M, et al. [18F] FDG-PET study in dementia with Lewy bodies and Alzheimer's disease. *Prog Neuropsychopharmacol Biol Psychiatry*. 2001;25(2):447-456.

213. Ceravolo R, Volterrani D, Gambaccini G, et al. Presynaptic nigro-striatal function in a group of Alzheimer's disease patients with parkinsonism: evidence from a dopamine transporter imaging study. *J Neural Transm*. 2004;111(8):1065-1073.

214. Beach TG, Adler CH, Sue LI, et al. Multi-organ distribution of phosphorylated α-synuclein histopathology in subjects with Lewy body disorders. *Acta Neuropathol*. 2010;119(6):689-702.

215. Goldman JG, Goetz CG, Brandabur M, Sanfilippo M, Stebbins GT. Effects of dopaminergic medications on psychosis and motor function in dementia with Lewy bodies. *Mov Disord.* 2008;23(15):2248-2250.

216. Friedman JH. A retrospective study of pimavanserin use in a movement disorders clinic. *Clin Neuropharmacol.* 2017;40(4):157-159.

217. Berkowitz A. *Lange Clinical Neurology and Neuroanatomy: A Localization-Based Approach.* New York, NY: McGraw-Hill Education; 2016.

218. Craft S, Cholerton B, Reger M. Cognitive changes associated with normal and pathological aging. In: *Hazzard's Geriatric Medicine and Gerontology.* Halter JB, Ouslander JG, Tinettie ME, Studenski S, High KP, Asthana S, eds. New York: NYMcGraw Hill Medical.

219. Lauterbach EC. The neuropsychiatry of Parkinson's disease and related disorders. *Psychiatr Clin.* 2004;27(4):801-825.

220. Kurlan R, Cummings J, Raman R, Thal L. Quetiapine for agitation or psychosis in patients with dementia and parkinsonism. *Neurology.* 2007;68(17):1356-1363.

24

Frontotemporal Dementia

Bradford C. Dickerson · Megan Quimby · Katherine Brandt · Diane E. Lucente · Bonnie Wong

INTRODUCTION

Professor Arnold Pick first reported, in 1892, a 71-year-old patient with progressive language and cognitive decline, and grossly visible anterior temporal lobe atrophy post-mortem.[1] This is thought to be the first report of a patient with what was later called semantic dementia by Professors John Hodges and Julie Snowden. Professor Alois Alzheimer subsequently described the microscopic histologic abnormalities that were later called "Pick's disease" by Drs. Onari and Spatz. Professor Schneider published a detailed report on clinical course of the disease, highlighting the insidious early changes in behavior and personality and—in contrast with Alzheimer's disease (AD)—the typical relative preservation of memory and orientation.[2] Through most of the rest of the century, patients with behavioral-comportmental dementias were usually diagnosed as having "Pick's disease." In the 1980s and 1990s, Professors Marsel Mesulam, Sandra Weintraub, John Hodges, Julie Snowden, Andrew Kertesz, and others reignited the interest of the behavioral neurology and neuropsychiatry field in progressive aphasias.[3-5] In the 1980s, the Lund[6] and Manchester[7] groups reported important early studies generating renewed interest in the behavioral phenotype of frontotemporal dementia (FTD), soon thereafter proposing clinical and pathological diagnostic criteria.[8] In the late 1990s, formal international consensus diagnostic criteria[9] were developed for three major clinical phenotypes: "frontotemporal dementia," "progressive nonfluent aphasia," and "semantic dementia." In the early 2000s, interest in the syndromes we now call FTDs surged, leading to the development and evolution of clinical and pathological criteria for the diagnosis and, more recently, an explosion in scientific understanding of this family of diseases, as well as a robust international clinical-scientific organization devoted to the diseases (http://www.isftd.org) with biannual international conferences sparking tremendous collaborative energy.[10] Important advances were formalized in 2011 when new consensus diagnostic criteria were published for primary progressive aphasia (PPA)[11] and the behavioral variant of FTD (bvFTD).[12] These criteria were then largely incorporated with some simplification into the fifth edition of the American Psychiatric Association Diagnostic and Statistical Manual in 2013.

Although terminology remains confusing in this family of diseases, we continue to recognize the syndromes of bvFTD, semantic variant PPA (svPPA), and nonfluent or agrammatic variant PPA (nfvPPA) to present in the context of a neuropathological family of diseases termed frontotemporal lobar degeneration (FTLD). The third major subtype of PPA, the "logopenic" variant, is usually associated with AD pathology. FTLD is a loosely knit group of neurodegenerative diseases that preferentially affect the frontal and anterior temporal lobes, with relative sparing of other cortical regions in many cases, and often affecting basal ganglia and in some cases basal forebrain and brainstem nuclei. Largely for reasons of pathological overlap, several other diseases have also now been included in this clinical and pathological spectrum, including progressive supranuclear palsy (PSP), corticobasal degeneration (CBD), and FTD with motor neuron disease or amyotrophic lateral sclerosis (FTD-MND or FTD-ALS).

EPIDEMIOLOGY

FTLD is thought to be the third most common degenerative cause of dementia, after AD and Lewy body disease (LBD), accounting for 5–15% of dementias. FTLD often causes early-onset dementia, typically affecting people in their mid-40s to mid-60s. In people younger than 65 years old, it is thought to be the second most common cause of dementia. Nevertheless, pathologically confirmed cases have been reported with age of clinical symptom onset as young as age 21[13] and as old as age 85.[14] Some epidemiologic studies raise the question of whether it is being substantially underreported,[15] suggesting that it may be more common than previously thought, including in the elderly.[16,17]

The incidence and prevalence rates of FTD have received little study with widely ranging results, from a prevalence of ~1.1 per 100,000 cases in a study from the Netherlands[18] to 15–17 per 100,000 cases in two studies from the United Kingdom[19,20] and one from Northern Italy[16] to 35 per 100,000 cases from a door-to-door investigation in Southern Italy.[21] With regard to incidence, an American study reported incidence rates in Rochester, Minnesota of 2.2 per 100,000 between ages 40 and 49, 3.3 per 100,000 between ages 50 and 59, and 8.9 per 100,000 between ages 60 and 69.[17]

NEUROPATHOLOGY OF FTLD

The hallmark of the neuropathology of FTLD is its topographic distribution—which in some cases is strikingly focal—in the frontal and anterior temporal lobes, as well as often involving the hippocampus, amygdala, basal ganglia, diencephalon, brainstem nuclei, and sometimes cerebellum.

Dr. Pick described the focal "knife-like" atrophy of anterior temporal and frontal cortex that later came to be called FTLD.[22,23] Using silver staining histopathologic techniques, Dr. Alzheimer reported two important microscopic lesions[24]: intraneuronal argyrophilic inclusion bodies which were later called the "Pick body" and achromatic neuronal balloon cells which were called "Pick cells."[25] During the mid-20th century, detailed reports of such cases provided further insights,[26–28] describing the major features of what came to be known as "Pick's disease," including atrophy, neurodegeneration, and tau pathology in prefrontal cortex, frontoinsula, anterior cingulate, and anterior temporal cortex, with relative sparing of the posterior third of the superior temporal gyrus and primary visual cortex.[29,30] It has since become clear that there is often prominent white matter tau pathology as well,[31] including near the cortical gray matter-white matter junction.[32] The basal ganglia, basal forebrain, and brainstem structures are prominently affected in some patients and minimally affected in others.[32] Drs. Kertesz and Munoz conceptualized Pick's disease as one of a spectrum of tauopathies that can present as PPA or bvFTD, including the tauopathies PSP and CBD.[33–36]

In the 1970s and 1980s, observations were made that some patients with what otherwise appeared clinically to be a frontal lobe-type dementia did not exhibit classical Pick's disease neuropathology. Constantinidis and colleagues[37] developed a classification system that recognized three major types of so-called "Pick's disease," the first of which is classical Pick's pathology, the second is CBD, and the third lacked specific histological characteristics. Brun and Gustafson recognized a "frontal lobe degeneration of non-Alzheimer type" that was neither AD nor Pick's disease, and other investigators also reported on this mysterious disease,[7,38] with one particularly memorable moniker being "dementia lacking distinctive histology (DLDH)."[39]

In the early 2000s, it became clear that most DLDH cases were immunoreactive to ubiquitin (FTLD-U). The breakthrough came in 2006, with the demonstration that the majority of cases showed intraneuronal inclusions of transactive DNA binding protein, molecular weight 43 kilodalton (TDP-43).[40] Professor Ian Mackenzie and others[41] described distinct subtypes (A, B, C, and D) based on the intracellular localization and morphology of the inclusions. This proteinaceous inclusion is also found in most cases of ALS, leading these diseases to be called TDP proteinopathies.[42] Within a few years, most of the remaining ~10%

of pathologically unclassified FTLD cases were determined to be immunoreactive to the fused in sarcoma (FUS) protein.[43] Therefore, except for a very small number of cases, the majority of FTLD neuropathology is now possible to classify as (1) FTLD-tau (~40–50% of cases), (2) FTLD-TDP-43 (~40–50% of cases), or (3) FTLD-FUS (~5% of cases), and several other rare proteinopathies.

Meanwhile, Professor William Seeley identified the selective loss of the von Economo neuron (VEN), a specific cell type found in the anterior cingulate and frontoinsular cortex of evolutionarily advanced mammals.[44] This spindle-shaped neuron appears to be reduced substantially in these brain regions in patients with FTLD but not in patients with AD. Remaining VEN neurons showed pathologic features in FTLD, but appeared morphologically normal in AD. So-called fork cells are also selectively vulnerable to FTLD pathology.[45] Further research on selectively vulnerable cell types in FTLD may reveal new insights into the mechanisms of neuropathology and the predilection for certain brain regions in these diseases.

GENETICS OF FTLD

Genetic Mutations Associated with FTLD

In the mid- to late-20th century it became clear that Pick's disease could be observed in multiple generations.[27,46–48] Approximately 20–40% of cases of FTLD exhibit a family history of a similar or related condition, and 10–20% of cases have a family history consistent with an autosomal dominant inheritance pattern.[49] When linkage studies identified loci on chromosomes 3, 9, and 17, the hunt for specific genetic mutations was on.

In 1998, mutations of the microtubule-associated protein tau (*MAPT*) gene on chromosome 17q21 were reported, with many patients in the initially reported families also exhibiting parkinsonism, leading to the term FTD-parkinsonism linked to chromosome 17 (FTDP-17).[50,51] More than 44 *MAPT* mutations have been reported in over 100 families in the world.[52] MAPT mutations are toxic gain-of-function abnormalities that reduce the ability of the tau protein to bind to and stabilize microtubules. The clinical phenotypes of patients with *MAPT* mutations include bvFTD, PSP syndrome, corticobasal syndrome (CBS), or rarely PPA. A fascinating aspect of this and other forms of autosomal dominant FTD is that patients within the same family with the same genetic mutation may present with distinct clinical phenotypes, including PPA, CBS, or bvFTD.[53]

Despite these advances in understanding, it became apparent that there were a number of families with autosomal dominant FTLD with linkage to chromosome 17q21 who did not have *MAPT* gene mutations—none of the cases in these families that came to autopsy had tau pathology, but instead demonstrated what was originally described as DLDH and subsequently FTLD-U. The cause was elucidated in 2006 with reported mutations in the progranulin (*GRN*) gene,[54,55] which is also on 17q21 and very close to the *MAPT* gene. *GRN* mutations are associated with FTLD-TDP-43 pathology. More than 70 *GRN* mutations have been reported, which are thought to result in a degraded protein whose function is lost ("loss of function") due to haploinsufficiency. Mutations in *GRN* are the second most common genetic cause of familial FTLD (4–26% of familial FTLD). Age of symptom onset averages between ages 53 and 64, but varies widely, from as young as age 35 to as old as 88. The clinical phenotypes of *GRN* carriers include bvFTD (most common), PPA, CBS, and a progressive amnesic syndrome similar to that associated with AD. *GRN* mutation carriers who present with bvFTD tend to exhibit apathy, executive dysfunction, and social withdrawal rather than disinhibition or compulsive behavior. Those with PPA usually present with a nonfluent form, but may have logopenic features. Parietal degeneration is common, more prominently than in most other forms of FTLD, and frequently giving rise to limb apraxia, spatial disorientation, and related symptoms. Extrapyramidal features are also common, and psychosis is more common than in sporadic FTLD. Importantly, a common variant in the gene *TMEM106B* modifies the expression of *GRN*, delaying age of onset.[56]

Another major discovery in the genetics of FTLD was made in 2011. Families with members affected with FTD or ALS or both (FTD-ALS) had been reported with linkage to chromosome 9p, but the responsible gene remained unknown until reports of an expanded GGGGCC hexanucleotide repeat in the chromosome 9 open reading frame 72 gene (*C9orf72*).[57,58] This important finding brought the FTD and ALS research communities together to investigate common biological mechanisms. It has since become clear that *C9orf72* repeat expansions are the most common genetic cause of FTD (29% of familial FTD), ALS (38% of familial ALS), and FTD-ALS (88% of familial FTD-ALS). In patients without a family history of FTD or ALS, expansions in *C9orf72* are occasionally found, that is, patients with sporadic FTD or ALS are rarely determined to have this genetic abnormality.[59] Age of symptom onset averages between ages 50 and 64, but—like *GRN*—also varies widely, from as young as age 27 to as old as 83. As with *GRN*, variants in *TMEM106B* seem to protect against FTD due to *C9orf72* but does not influence ALS in the same way.[60] The clinical phenotypes of *C9orf72* include bvFTD, ALS, and FTD-ALS, with bulbar symptoms appearing to be more common than in sporadic ALS. Psychosis and other neuropsychiatric symptoms, including anxiety, are much more common than in sporadic FTD. Memory loss is common, as are language symptoms, although primary amnesic or aphasic phenotypes without behavioral symptoms are relatively uncommon. Extrapyramidal features are not any more common than in sporadic FTD.

Tank-binding kinase 1 (*TBK1*, located on chromosome 12) was discovered in 2015 as the third most common cause of FTLD in a large Belgian cohort, after *GRN* and *C9orf72*.[61] *TBK1*-related disease has been noted to cause bvFTD with prominent disinhibition, and, in a series of cases, with memory loss as an important associated symptom in the initial phase of the disease.[62] Some patients exhibit ALS. Neuroimaging has demonstrated widespread frontotemporal atrophy. Neuropathology in two patients demonstrated TDP-43 type B pathology.[62]

Very rarely, familial FTLD can be associated with mutations in other genes, such as *CHMP2B*[63] and valosin-containing protein (*VCP*).[64] In 2009, mutations in the *FUS* gene were discovered in association with familial ALS,[65,66] but nearly all FTLD-FUS cases examined to date do not appear to be associated with *FUS* mutations or other known genetic abnormalities (i.e., they appear to be sporadic).[67]

Detailed clinical and clinicopathologic studies of families in which FTLD is associated with particular genetic mutations have revealed important heterogeneity. Members of families with the same genetic mutation can develop pathology localized in different brain regions, and therefore present with different clinical phenotypes. This was first described clearly in families with *MAPT* mutations.[52,53,68] Although the major clinical phenotype association with *MAPT* mutations is a behavioral-dysexecutive syndrome, some patients present with extrapyramidal dysfunction, CBS, or PPA. This phenotypic heterogeneity was later also observed in families with *GRN* mutations, with some patients developing bvFTD, some PPA, and some CBS or other phenotypes.[69] Note that CBS is much more common in patients with *GRN* mutations (~4%) than it is in patients with *MAPT* mutations (~2%). A few *GRN* cases have even presented with a posterior cortical atrophy syndrome.[70,71] Families with the *C9orf72* mutation are now the prototypical example of markedly different clinical phenotypes, with some patients exhibiting bvFTD, others with ALS, and others with FTD-ALS. The bvFTD phenotype associated with *C9orf72* mutations is also unusual in that psychosis is much more prominent than in typical bvFTD; bizarre delusions are commonly a symptom very early in the course of the *C9orf72* bvFTD phenotype.[72] A growing research effort is being devoted to trying to understand this genetic-clinical heterogeneity. Families such as this imply the presence of modifying influences on the initial localization of pathology; some of these are likely genetic but it is also possible that some are developmental or environmental.

Genetic Counseling and Testing in FTD

The clinical practice of genetic counseling and testing in patients and families with FTD is complex; we and other specialty groups follow an approach similar to that summarized in several reviews.[73–75] The foundation for genetic counseling is a confident diagnosis of the likely etiology of the patient's syndrome, since the likely molecular pathology dictates genetic considerations. When we begin working with a patient and family we start by evaluating our confidence in the diagnosis. Then, we carefully obtain a family history ideally encompassing three generations, recording each blood relative's age of death, cause of death if known, and general cognitive/behavioral/neuropsychiatric status in later life (Figure 24-1). We summarize with the family that FTD and related conditions were often not diagnosed or may have been misdiagnosed in prior generations. If the family chose to have an autopsy performed, valuable information can be obtained, but in prior generations brain autopsy is relatively infrequent. If there is a potential family history of FTD or related disorders, we ask the family to try to obtain additional information or records about the affected relatives, and to consider meeting with our group's genetic counselor. If there is clearly not a family history of FTD or related disorders, and family members lived past typical age of onset, there is usually a low likelihood of the presence of a genetic mutation.[76] If family history information is unavailable or blood relatives died at a younger age, we suggest that the patient/family work with our genetic counselor to discuss the issues involved. In a patient with FTD with age of

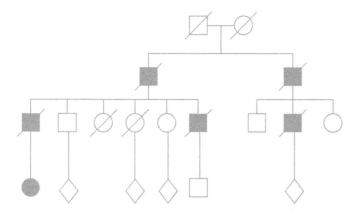

FIGURE 24-1. Pedigree of a family with familial FTD with all cases presenting with behavioral variant FTD with age of onset in the late 50s or early to mid-60s. The genetic mutation identified in this family was *MAPT* P301L. Six out of seven cases in this family were male, leading family members to believe women in the family were at lower risk. Since this genetic abnormality is inherited with an autosomal dominant pattern, it was important during genetic counseling to emphasize the fact that each offspring has a 50% likelihood of inheriting the mutation regardless of sex.

onset younger than 50 years, we and others often recommend that the patient undergo genetic testing. In patients who are older than 50, we typically do not recommend genetic testing when there is not a family history of FTD or related disorders and family members lived past age 75, since there is such a low likelihood of an abnormality.

When the patient's genetic test results are returned, there are three possible results: positive, negative, or variant of unknown significance (VUS). The interpretation of a VUS can be difficult for health professionals, and, if possible, it may be worth testing additional affected or unaffected family members if available. The identification of a positive test result for a known, pathogenic FTD gene mutation in a patient usually has a powerful impact on the family and patient. A genetic counselor can guide families in planning the disclosure of results to other family members. In some families, such results may provide relief in explaining a mysterious familial condition, while in other families this kind of result may lead to fear and stigma. Genetic counseling plays an important role in helping family members with this complex and emotionally challenging medical information. If a patient with FTD is found to have a pathogenic mutation associated with FTD, first-degree relatives have a 50% chance of inheriting it (since they are autosomal dominant). Asymptomatic blood relatives can choose to undergo presymptomatic genetic testing under the guidance of a genetic counselor. Most genetic counselors follow the so-called Huntington's disease protocol for performing this kind of counseling and testing. Individuals who test positive for a pathogenic mutation will almost certainly develop symptoms if they live long enough and each offspring has a 50% chance of inheriting the genetic abnormality. The types of symptoms and age of onset vary by gene and are best discussed with a genetic counselor experienced with FTD. If individuals test negative for the pathogenic FTD gene mutation that runs in their family, their lifetime risk

of disease drops to the general population risk, and they will not pass the genetic abnormality to offspring.

CLINICAL CHARACTERISTICS OF FTLD

It is essential to try to determine the earliest clinical symptoms that were present, which may or may not be the symptoms most troublesome to the patient and/or family at the time of evaluation. A direct history with a spouse or adult child informant in private is essential, and it is often helpful to obtain documentation through medical records or other notes of concerns at the time of symptom onset. Although time-consuming, this approach facilitates an open discussion of symptoms (informants may be uncomfortable discussing some issues in front of the patient) and enables the clinician to evaluate insight and concern in the patient separately from influence by informants. Lack of awareness or concern is often a core element of the clinical presentation in patients with bvFTD. Since many of the early symptoms are related to changes in affect or personality, it is not surprising that patients may first present to psychiatrists or other mental health professionals.

Behavioral Variant FTD

FTLD neuropathology is often associated with a clinical phenotype involving the insidious development of changes in interpersonal and emotional behavior, commonly accompanied by executive dysfunction. This clinical syndrome has historically been referred to as "Pick's disease" but is now called bvFTD. Based on a variety of concerns regarding prior criteria,[77] new international consensus diagnostic criteria were published in 2011 (Table 24-1).[12] BvFTD appears to be the most common syndrome associated with FTLD. The specific symptoms of this variant depend on the particular regions of frontotemporal cortical and frontostriatal brain systems involved and their laterality.

Disinhibition is a common early symptom, and can manifest as socially inappropriate behavior such as overly familiar interactions with strangers; loss of manners or violations of social normative behavior such as public urination or changes in behavior during social meals; or impulsive actions such as unnecessary or excessive purchasing or shoplifting.[78–80] Sometimes patients who are very active, jocular, and making rash decisions or going on spending sprees can be mistakenly diagnosed with mania or hypomania. Disinhibition appears to be related particularly to orbitofrontal and cingulo-opercular abnormalities in FTD.[81]

Another very common early symptom is apathy, including loss of interest in hobbies or leisure activities and social withdrawal[82–84]; these behavioral changes are often mistaken for depression. Yet patients with bvFTD do not usually exhibit sadness or cry, do not talk about concerns, worries, or thoughts of worthlessness or hopelessness, and do not usually exhibit the loss of appetite or sleep disturbance often seen in depression. Some investigators have suggested that bvFTD may present as a "disinhibited" or "inert" (apathetic) subtype[80] while many patients present with intermixed symptoms of both types.[85] Atrophy in the anterior cingulate cortex, dorsolateral prefrontal cortex,[84] and striatum[86] has been observed in association with apathy in bvFTD.

TABLE 24-1 • Diagnostic Criteria for bvFTD.

Evidence of neurodegenerative disease by progressive deterioration of cognition or behavior based on observation or history	
Possible bvFTD (at least 3 of the following must be present early [<3 years] in the course)	
Behavioral disinhibition	Socially inappropriate behavior; loss of manners or decorum; impulsivity
Apathy or inertia	
Loss of sympathy or empathy	Diminished response to other people's needs and feelings; diminished social interest
Perseverative, stereotyped, or compulsive behavior	Simple repetitive movements; complex compulsive or ritualistic behavior; stereotypy of speech
Hyperorality and dietary changes	Altered food preferences; binge eating or increased consumption of alcohol or cigarettes; oral exploration of inedible objects
Neuropsychological profile of executive dysfunction with relative sparing of episodic memory and visuospatial skills	
Probable bvFTD	
Meets criteria for possible bvFTD	
Exhibits functional decline	
Imaging results consistent with bvFTD	Frontal and/or anterior temporal atrophy or hypometabolism or perfusion
bvFTD with definite FTLD pathology	
Meets criteria for possible or probable bvFTD	
Histopathological evidence of FTLD on biopsy or autopsy	
Presence of a known pathogenic mutation	
Exclusionary criteria for bvFTD	
Pattern of deficits is better accounted for by another neuromedical disorder	
Behavioral disturbance is better accounted for by a psychiatric disorder	
Biomarkers strongly indicative of Alzheimer's disease or another neurodegenerative process	

Source: Rascovsky K, Hodges JR, Knopman D, et al. Sensitivity of revised diagnostic criteria for the behavioural variant of frontotemporal dementia. Brain. 2011;134(9):2456-2477. Published by Oxford University Press on behalf of the Guarantors of Brain. All rights reserved.

Loss of empathy or sympathy toward the spouse, other family members, and friends is very common and can be subtle in some cases, depending in part on premorbid personality traits.[87–89] These behavioral changes may concern family members for some time before it becomes obvious that something is wrong, which often occurs when the patient exhibits a highly unusual response to an event that almost universally provokes a vigorous, uniform emotion in most people, such as the death of a close friend or family member, or the birth of a child. Even under these circumstances, the behavior is commonly attributed to depression or another psychiatric illness or to stress or a mid-life crisis. Right anterior temporal cortex, anterior insula, and striatal abnormalities have been most consistently identified as related to loss of empathy.[90,91]

Compulsive, ritualistic, or repetitive behaviors are common in bvFTD, often early in the illness, and can be very distressing to family members.[92,93] In some cases, they may be the presenting symptom.[94] Examples of these symptoms include repetitive "projects" (e.g., stereotyped writing of greeting cards), chores (e.g., repeated emptying of trash), or playing of card or computer games or repetitive watching of a particular television show.[95] Speech patterns may be stereotyped (e.g., catch phrases, telling of stories as if by a script). Some of these symptoms appear similar to those of obsessive-compulsive disorder (OCD) but usually bvFTD patients do not describe obsessive thoughts or any relief of such thoughts by a compulsive activity, as is typically described in primary OCD. Some patients have very rigid routines that must be performed identically each day (often at a particular time, associated with "clock watching"); if these routines are disrupted, some patients become very upset. These symptoms may change as the disease progresses, in some cases becoming simpler. Simple repetitive behaviors include tapping or moving a limb, licking lips, picking skin, grunting, or moaning. These may appear similar to choreiform movements seen in dyskinetic movement disorders or tardive dyskinesia. Anatomic abnormalities associated with compulsive behaviors include striatal and anterior temporal atrophy.[96–98]

Changes in eating behavior are common and may include altered food preferences (such as an increased sweet tooth or a rigid stereotypye in the foods eaten from day to day) or gluttonous or binge-like eating.[95,99] This may—but does not always—result in substantial weight gain. Normative social eating conventions are often violated, including rapid eating or stuffing food in the mouth, taking food from others' plates, or belching. Patients may exhibit changes in the consumption of alcohol or cigarettes, sometimes resulting in extreme intoxication or vomiting. Occasionally early, but more often later, in the course of the disease patients may explore inedible objects by placing them in their mouth similar to the behavior seen in Kluver-Bucy syndrome. The neurobiological basis of changes in eating behavior in FTD appears to involve right lateralized ventral anterior insula, striatum, and orbitofrontal cortex on structural MRI voxel-based morphometry,[100,101] as well as degenerative changes in the hypothalamus.[102,103]

Executive dysfunction (problems with organization, planning, sequencing, decision making, multitasking, or monitoring performance) is very common in bvFTD.[95] Symptoms described by family members often include difficulty with financial management, poor decision making, inability to complete tasks (particularly novel tasks), or not recognizing or correcting mistakes. Despite the report of these symptoms in daily life, patients may still perform within normal limits on neuropsychological tests of executive function.[104] Progressive impairment of executive abilities may lead to job loss or disastrous mismanagement of money. In many cases, it can be difficult to determine which problems in daily life are caused by executive dysfunction as opposed to apathy. This is not surprising given that constructs of the executive functions usually include initiation or "energization" as a component process. Although executive dysfunction is typically thought of as being caused by dorsolateral prefrontal cortical involvement, it can originate in anterior cingulate, insular, parietal, or subcortical nodes of large-scale executive systems.

Another important clinical feature of bvFTD is lack of insight. This symptom was considered a core element of the Neary et al.[9] diagnostic criteria but was not included in the new international consensus diagnostic criteria because it was thought to be too difficult to ascertain consistently. Nevertheless, it is well established that many patients with bvFTD, and some patients with semantic dementia (SD), have a striking lack of insight[105-107] even when confronted with obvious impairments. Clinically, this can be particularly challenging when the patient refuses to make office follow-up visits because he or she is convinced there is not a problem. Lack of insight in FTD has been associated with right-lateralized ventromedial prefrontal atrophy.[108]

Another core feature of bvFTD is personality change. Alterations in personality can be prominent in bvFTD and also in SD.[109] Although questionnaire-based instruments to assess classical dimensional personality traits are readily available, changes in personality might be best understood clinically by considering more specific process-oriented functions contributing to personality traits. When faced with a family member who says "my spouse is not the person I married, his/her personality is completely different," it is incumbent upon the clinician to probe further to ascertain the specific changes being described. Some symptoms may include changes in the expression or comprehension of emotion, social withdrawal or disinhibition, or loss of empathy. In some cases, a previously gruff or aggressive individual becomes docile. The patient's insight into these changes is often poor. We have reported on a bvFTD patient who developed the Geschwind syndrome of hyperreligiosity, hypergraphia, irritability, and other symptoms.[110] Other symptoms that may also be described as personality changes include obsessive-compulsive behaviors, such as hoarding, and those involving changes in appetitive drives, such as sexual, eating, or drinking behaviors.

Despite the inclusion in the 2011 bvFTD diagnostic criteria of "the relative preservation of memory," memory impairment can be a prominent early feature in some cases of bvFTD,[111,112] including those that are pathologically proven.[113] In some cases, memory symptoms are reported by the patient and/or family but test performance is normal; this may reflect executive contributions to memory encoding or retrieval in daily life which may be relatively controlled in the office setting.[114] In other cases, day-to-day memory is preserved but psychometric test performance is impaired due to the magnitude of executive or semantic deficits, thereby resulting in an overestimation of memory impairment. In our clinical practice, we do not avoid the clinical diagnosis of bvFTD in a patient with well-documented amnesia if the remainder of the clinical presentation is consistent with bvFTD, especially if supported by neuroimaging test results.

Unlike the language-dominant types of FTLD, language may be relatively intact early in the course of bvFTD. This is particularly true on basic neuropsychological tests of language performance. Higher-order language abilities at the level of discourse,[115] as well as emotionally laden forms of communication including prosody, irony, sarcasm, and humor, are often abnormal early in the course of bvFTD.[91,116] As the disease progresses, semantic and other impairments often become prominent.[117]

Psychosis has been thought unusual in bvFTD, but the discovery of the *C9orf72* expansion has highlighted the common presence of psychosis in patients as well as non-demented family members with this genetic mutation.[72,118]

Progressive Aphasic Subtypes of FTLD

The other major clinical phenotype associated with FTLD involves a primary language disturbance. According to the Neary et al.[9] diagnostic criteria, such a patient would have been diagnosed as having a language-predominant form of FTD (and likely FTLD), and further subtyped into progressive nonfluent aphasia (PNFA) or SD. At present, the approach suggested by the recent international consensus diagnostic criteria for PPA[11] focuses on determining the precise clinical phenotype without reference to the presumed underlying pathology. Three canonical clinical phenotypes of PPA are currently recognized: the nonfluent/agrammatic variant (nfvPPA, which likely captures most of the patients formerly diagnosed with PNFA), the semantic variant (svPPA, which likely captures most of the patients formerly diagnosed with SD), and the logopenic variant (lvPPA). Some patients with clinical phenotype consistent with SD do not meet criteria for svPPA because they present with prosopagnosia or visual object agnosia or with relatively prominent behavioral symptoms and thus do not meet core criteria for PPA. lvPPA is most frequently associated with biomarkers of underlying AD and ultimately AD pathology, and thus would not be considered a major clinical subtype of FTLD. Nevertheless, a minority of lvPPA patients do not demonstrate biomarkers of AD pathobiology in vivo[119] and in fact have solely FTLD neuropathology post-mortem (usually FTLD-TDP-43).[120] Thus, while lvPPA is often considered nearly synonymous with an atypical language variant of AD, these recent observations support the inclusion of this clinical phenotype as a part—if small—of the FTLD spectrum.

As its name implies, PPA is a disorder that can only be diagnosed when language is the sole of major dysfunction early in the illness, usually considered to be at least 2 years (Table 24-2); when other cognitive dysfunction is clearly present, such as loss of memory for daily events, visuospatial dysfunction, or behavioral symptoms, the diagnosis of PPA cannot be made.[121-123] In some patients, language dysfunction can slowly progress and be the principal impairment for as long as a decade, but in many patients, impairments in other cognitive functions emerge after the first few years.[124]

Although patients with progressive aphasias may have personality, comportmental, and social symptoms, they are, by definition, less prominent than the language impairment early in the course of the disorder. The presence of prominent early neuropsychiatric or behavioral symptoms is generally considered exclusionary for PPA. In spite of this distinction, which is particularly important for clinical research on these disorders, some patients whose diagnosis would be best considered as PPA have prominent early neuropsychiatric or behavioral symptoms (a point discussed briefly in the 2011 diagnostic criteria). Many others have relatively mild but notable symptoms, particularly as PPA progresses to involve abilities beyond language.[125]

TABLE 24-2 • Diagnostic Criteria for PPA.
The following three conditions must all be present.
1. A new and progressive language disorder (aphasia) as documented by abnormalities in one or more of the following domains: grammaticality of sentence production, word retrieval in speech, object naming, word and sentence comprehension, spelling, reading, repetition.
2. Relative preservation of episodic memory, executive functions, visuospatial skills and comportment as documented by history, medical records, and/or neuropsychological testing.
3. Imaging and other pertinent neurodiagnostic test results that rule out causes other than neurodegeneration.
Nonfluent/Agrammatic variant (nfvPPA)
Impaired grammatical structure of spoken or written language in the absence of significant word comprehension impairments. Output is usually of low fluency.
Semantic variant (svPPA)
Impaired word comprehension in the absence of significant impairment of grammar. Object naming is severely impaired. Output is motorically fluent but often contains word-finding hesitations, semantic paraphasias, and circumlocutions.
Logopenic variant (lvPPA)
No significant grammar or word comprehension impairment. Speech contains many word-finding hesitations and phonemic paraphasias. Object naming may be impaired and may constitute the only significant finding in the examination. Current classification systems require repetition impairments for diagnosing this subtype.
Anomic subtype
All features as in lvPPA except that repetition is intact. In some cases, this subtype represents a prodromal stage of svPPA.[197]
Mixed subtype
Impaired grammatical structure and word comprehension, even at the early stages of disease.

Source: Gorno-Tempini ML, Hillis AE, Weintraub S, et al. Classification of primary progressive aphasia and its variants. Neurology. 2011;76(11): 1006-1014. https://n.neurology.org/content/76/11/1006.

Nonfluent/Agrammatic Variant PPA

The core features of nfvPPA are an impairment of grammar and, commonly, defective motor speech production. The characteristics of nonfluent speech are typically an effortful and halting speech with sound errors and distortions, with agrammatism in language production and/or comprehension.[126,127] Agrammatism is characterized by omissions of grammatical words and morphemes, reduced production of verbs,[128,129] incorrect argument structures, and decreased utterance length and complexity, often with reduced mean length of utterances and fewer embedded clauses.[115,130,131] Comprehension of simple declarative sentences is usually good, reflecting relatively intact single-word comprehension, but performance on tasks requiring the comprehension of complex syntactic structures is typically impaired.[132,133]

The disorder most often evolves to an aphasic picture similar to Broca's aphasia due to cerebrovascular disease.[130,134]

Some patients with nfvPPA present with relatively pure agrammatic language, while many present with an accompanying motor speech disorder, such as apraxia of speech (AOS) or dysarthria. Although a strict definition of PPA requires the presence of aphasia, some patients present with an isolated dysarthria and/or AOS[135,136] without obvious aphasia. NfvPPA is commonly associated with distorted sound substitutions and additions with length or complexity effects, while "pure" AOS or nfvPPA with prominent AOS are characterized by syllable segmentation and lengthened intersegment durations. Some patients also exhibit limb apraxia or other elements of an extrapyramidal (parkinsonian) syndrome.[137] Many others develop these symptoms or others consistent with a CBS or a PSP syndrome as the illness progresses.

The localization of symptoms in nfvPPA is typically linked to the prefrontal rolandic operculum, anterior insula, and possibly the opercular portion of Broca's area. The diagnosis of imaging-supported nfvPPA indeed requires focal left-sided perisylvian regions involvement, particularly of the inferior posterior frontal gyrus and insula.[11,138,139] The involvement of the "dorsal" language pathways appears to be responsible for syntactic dysfunction.[140] AOS is associated with neurodegeneration in the left posterior inferior frontal lobe or supplementary motor area, while orofacial apraxia is associated with neurodegeneration in the left middle frontal, premotor, and supplementary motor cortical; and limb apraxia is associated with left inferior parietal lobe damage.[137,141]

In nfvPPA, neuropsychiatric symptoms are less frequent initially, but as the illness progresses it becomes increasingly common to see apathy, depression, or irritability. In some cases these symptoms are present early in the illness, which may lead to misdiagnosis as a primary psychiatric disorder (often depression).

Semantic Variant PPA

Patients with svPPA develop prominent word-finding difficulty in spontaneous speech, maintaining fluency but with a tendency to rely more on high (rather than specific low) frequency nouns, and exhibiting severe anomia in confrontation naming tasks. As semantic memory loss progresses, it impairs single-word comprehension, impacting the differentiation between within-category subordinate words.[142] As the disease progresses, between-category words are affected and concepts become blurred, although speech may still be fluent. Impaired reading of words with irregular spelling is also typical of this disorder.[143] Syntactic processing is typically spared.[144] Nonverbal skills are usually minimally affected in the early stages.[142]

The dominant hemisphere anterior temporal lobe is often prominently atrophic even at initial presentation, with varying degrees of bilateral involvement.[145,146] The atrophy predominantly involves inferior and middle temporal gyri, anterior fusiform gyrus, perirhinal cortex, amygdala, and hippocampus,[147-149] but the most prominent atrophy appears to be at the tip of the left temporal pole.[150] Preserved motor speech and syntactic function reflect the integrity of the dorsal language regions and of the corresponding white matter connections.[146,151]

SvPPA patients commonly exhibit neuropsychiatric symptoms, often relatively early and in a fairly stereotypical fashion. Many of these symptoms are similar to those of bvFTD, including loss of empathy, changes in eating behavior, compulsive behavior, and disinhibition. Although these symptoms are highly consistent with FTD, depending on when they begin and how they are reported by informants, it may be difficult for the clinician to be confident in assigning a subtype diagnosis (i.e., bvFTD vs. svPPA vs. SD). The Neary et al.[9] diagnostic criteria for FTD included loss of sympathy or empathy and narrowed preoccupations (mental rigidity) as diagnostic features. Aberrant motor behavior is also reported as common in some studies; in our experience this often includes elaborate kinds of movements related to repetitive or compulsive behaviors. Depression is also reported as common in svPPA in some studies; in our experience, however, at least some patients say certain phrases repetitively (i.e., "catch phrases") that appear to express negative emotion (e.g., "I feel so stupid," "I used to know that and now I just don't know anything"), but with minimal affective behavior consistent with depression, and a structured interview with some of these patients' caregivers reveals little behavior in daily life that appears consistent with a diagnosis of depression. As the degeneration progresses, both anterior temporal lobes as well as the ventromedial and posterior orbital frontal cortices, the insula, anterior cingulate cortex, and amygdala often become involved, overlapping with the imaging features of bvFTD patients.[152]

Some patients present with semantic impairment that is more prominent for objects, people, or environmental sounds rather than words, suggesting a right-lateralized syndrome that is otherwise very similar to svPPA but likely best classified as SD.[153] SD is a broader diagnostic construct that can be considered an umbrella term for patients with svPPA and patients with agnostic and/or amnesic impairments as well as semantic memory loss.

Logopenic Variant PPA

Patients with lvPPA present with variably hesitant speech and typically without articulation deficits, but with many false starts and phonological errors, long word-finding pauses, impaired sentence comprehension and naming, with spared single-word comprehension and nonverbal semantics.[126] Patients with this syndrome typically exhibit a conduction aphasia-like deficit in repetition that is attributed to impaired phonological loop functions which is considered a core element of the syndrome.[133,154] Since all patients pause when they are attempting to retrieve low-frequency words, and many patients make speech-sound errors and have difficulty understanding of grammatically complex sentences, they may be misdiagnosed as having nfvPPA. But in fact their unconstrained, spontaneous speech is often fluent, the speech-sound errors are phonologic rather than articulatory, and grammatical production and comprehension is not impaired when sentences do not exceed their limited auditory-verbal working memory capacity (or when they are reading or writing). Thus, fluency in lvPPA has been described as "intermediate"[154]; we prefer to describe them as "variably" fluent. Note that some authors have used the term anomic aphasia to describe patients who fulfill lvPPA criteria but whose repetition is normal.

The localization of neurodegeneration in lvPPA typically involves the left posterior superior and middle temporal gyri, and inferior parietal lobule,[126,138,139,154] consistent with the hypothesis of a phonologic short-term memory impairment as the core cognitive deficit. As will be discussed below, this clinical phenotype is usually associated with underlying AD pathology rather than FTLD.

In lvPPA, neuropsychiatric symptoms are relatively infrequent early but increase as the illness progresses and include agitation, anxiety, irritability, and apathy. In many cases we have seen, the clinical phenomenology of neuropsychiatric symptoms appears similar to that seen in typical clinical forms of AD.

DIAGNOSTIC ASSESSMENT OF SUSPECTED FTLD

As with all neurodegenerative diseases, a careful clinical history taken from the patient and a knowledgeable informant is usually the single most important element of assessment. Specific FTD symptom inventories,[80,95] such as the Cambridge Behavioral Inventory,[155] the Frontal Behavioral Inventory,[156] and the Neuropsychiatric Inventory (NPI),[157] are very useful in ascertaining symptoms of FTD in a structured manner. Some of these instruments can be given to caregivers in advance as questionnaires, or used to structure an office-based interview. We have developed structured assessment scales for patients with FTD and related disorders that provide semiquantitative ratings of the types and severity of specific language impairments—the Progressive Aphasia Severity Scale (PASS)[139]—and social impairments—the Social Impairment Rating Scale.[158] As mentioned above, we believe it is essential to interview the patient separately from informants. The interview with the patient should include a psychiatric evaluation of mood and affect, thought content (e.g., is there evidence of psychosis?), and insight. Some instruments, such as the Everyday Cognition (Ecog) scale,[159] have both patient and informant forms which allows for an assessment of insight by comparing the two.

An important step in history-taking is to try to determine whether the symptoms are interfering with independent function or not (i.e., does the patient have a clinical stage of impairment consistent with dementia or mild cognitive impairment?). Some patients with PPA present with no or minimal functional impairment (problems performing activities that had previously been routine for the person, such as occupational activities or community or household activities). If function is impaired in PPA, by definition it should be attributable to compromised language and not to impairments in other domains of cognition or behavior. We have seen many patients with a progressive aphasic multidomain syndrome, with prominent aphasia but also impaired executive function, memory, or other functions. It may be possible to clearly document by history or through medical records that such a patient would have met PPA diagnostic criteria previously, but they cannot be diagnosed with PPA currently if these other domains are impaired. In other patients, it may be impossible to determine whether they ever fit into the construct of PPA, and they are best described as having a multidomain dementia with prominent aphasia (we often call this "aphasic dementia" to differentiate it from amnesic dementia).

Because the core symptoms relate to socioaffective function, many patients with bvFTD present after having lost social or occupational function, and therefore would be diagnosed with dementia even if cognitive examination and/or neuropsychological evaluation is within normal limits. Some patients have prodromal behavioral symptoms for some period of time without symptoms or signs of cognitive impairment. Some patients with so-called "mild behavioral impairment" (MBI) syndromes are in fact in the earliest stages of FTD, while other patients with MBI have etiologies other than FTD such as AD.[160,161] Since these patients do not have cognitive impairment, and it can be difficult to be sure of the etiology at this clinical stage, it is reasonable to classify such patients as having MBI, with further description of the clinical phenotype. In some cases this clinical phenotype may be consistent with bvFTD and in other cases it may be ambiguous, or consistent with late-onset bipolar illness or another kind of syndrome.

In the initial office assessment of a patient with one of the FTD clinical syndromes, a basic cognitive examination is essential. Most commonly used cognitive screening instruments, such as the Mini Mental State Examination, are insensitive to the cognitive and behavioral deficits of bvFTD. Office-based general cognitive testing instruments thought to be more sensitive to FTD include the Montreal Cognitive Assessment (MoCA)[162] and Addenbrooke's Cognitive Examination (ACE) III.[163] The Frontal Assessment Battery[164] is a brief (~10 minutes) cognitive and psychomotor assessment that has demonstrated sensitivity to FTD. Although these tests will often identify deficits in patients with FTD, some patients perform normally early in the course of the disease. In contrast, some patients with language impairments have a great deal of difficulty with tests such as the MoCA, leading to overestimation of their impairments because these tests involve many verbally mediated cognitive tests.

Finally, a neurologic examination is essential, working especially to determine whether there are abnormalities in eye movements or gait, limb or buccofacial apraxia, extrapyramidal signs, primitive reflexes, or evidence of motor neuron disease. These signs may provide important indications suggestive of possible PSP or CBD pathology, and may raise concerns regarding motor dysfunction as a contributor to functional impairment. Impersistence, perseveration, and distractibility can present challenges during the neurologic exam but are helpful signs suggestive of frontal systems dysfunction.

Neuropsychological assessment can be invaluable in patients suspected of having an FTD-spectrum disorder. Although some patients may perform adequately on brief office-based cognitive testing typically performed by a neurologist, psychiatrist, geriatrician, or other physician, the neuropsychologist may be able to detect abnormalities on extended testing using performance-based measures sensitive to functioning across cognitive domains. The use of standardized neuropsychological tests allows for comparison of the patient's cognitive abilities to that of an age- and education-matched normative sample, providing a measurement of the magnitude of departure from normal/intact performance, and serving as a valuable baseline against which future evaluations can be compared. The specific profile of spared or impaired cognitive abilities generated from neuropsychological testing also enables the clinician to identify subtypes of FTD. In at least some very mild cases of FTD, however, performance on reasonably extensive neuropsychological assessment can be normal.[165] Aiming to assemble a neuropsychological test battery tailored to bvFTD, Torralva

and colleagues[166] compiled a set of previously developed tests emphasizing "real-life" elements of executive function as well as social cognition. This test battery demonstrated higher sensitivity to mild FTD than many standard tests included in typical dementia neuropsychological batteries. Another similar approach was taken by Funkiewiez and colleagues, who assembled the Social Cognition and Emotion Assessment (SEA), and ultimately found that a subset (facial emotion recognition and faux pas identification) of the original tests were most sensitive to bvFTD, deriving the mini-SEA.[167]

The combination of findings from the assessments described above can be used to determine whether a patient fulfills current diagnostic criteria[12] for "possible" bvFTD or one of the progressive aphasias. For bvFTD, the clinician's confidence can be formally elevated to "probable" bvFTD if neuroimaging findings are present as described next. A similar approach is taken by many clinicians in diagnosing PPA, arriving at a diagnosis of imaging-supported PPA.[11]

When a patient is suspected of having PPA, or when communication or speech symptoms are present, it can be very helpful to obtain a consultation with a speech-language pathologist. An evaluation by a speech-language pathologist offers an opportunity to clarify the diagnostic formulation, may provide ideas to develop compensatory strategies, or may help identify and monitor speech or swallowing impairments. Speech pathologists offer a growing array of approaches to the development of treatment approaches for patients with PPA or other forms of FTD.[168]

Neuroimaging and Other Diagnostic Tests

Neuroimaging is an important part of the diagnostic workup of FTD, and has made valuable contributions to our understanding of the specific subtype disorders. Both structural (MRI) and functional (PET, SPECT) neuroimaging may be valuable for the investigation of anatomic, metabolic, or perfusion abnormalities in the spectrum of FTD.

MRI is critical in the diagnostic workup of suspected FTD for both the exclusion of other potential causes of slowly progressive frontal lobe syndromes, such as tumors, cerebrovascular disease, or the newly identified "sagging brain syndrome,"[169] and for the identification of abnormalities consistent with FTD neurodegenerative syndromes. Frontal and/or anterior temporal atrophy is the typical finding, and is often more prominent in the right hemisphere in bvFTD and the left hemisphere in PPA (Figure 24-2A). Metabolic or perfusion imaging can be useful in addition to MRI for the identification of abnormalities when anatomic changes are subtle or undetectable (Figure 24-2B). In some cases, both structural and functional neuroimaging may be normal early in the course of what ultimately declares itself over time as FTD.[165] Electroencephalography is not commonly recommended in the diagnostic evaluation of suspected FTD, but may demonstrate anterior or focal slowing consistent with frontal neurodegeneration.

Cerebrospinal fluid (CSF) biomarkers are being investigated in the clinical conditions thought to be due to FTLD pathology,[170] but are not yet mature enough for use in clinical practice. In some cases, the exclusion of an atypical form of AD can be

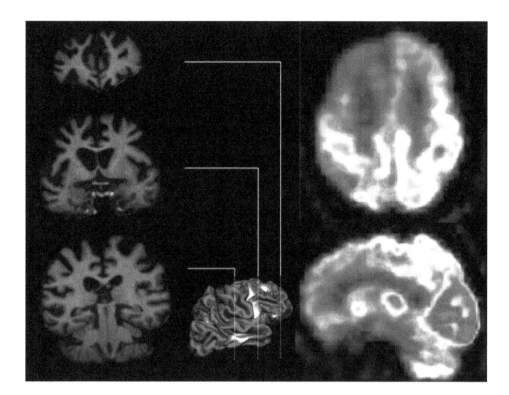

FIGURE 24-2. A 58-year-old man presented with apathy, impulsive eating, and executive dysfunction. **(A)** MRI demonstrated bilateral (right greater than left) frontal, temporal, and parietal atrophy, quantified with a map of cortical thickness compared to controls. **(B)** FDG PET showed prominent bilateral (right greater than left) frontal and temporal hypometabolism. He was found to have a Q300X (premature termination) mutation in *GRN*. His clinical syndrome lasted 5 years from first symptoms to death. Post-mortem examination revealed the expected TDP-43 Type A pathology.

helpful by analyzing CSF for amyloid-β and tau. General CSF investigation may be valuable to rule out other neurologic disorders if the patient has atypical features or a more rapid course.

If clinical evidence of motor neuron disease is present, especially if it is subtle, electromyography can provide valuable information regarding the presence of upper or lower motor neuron dysfunction, which may be critical for prognosis (Figure 24-3).

In Vivo Neuroimaging of Neuropathologic Markers

With the advent of neuroimaging tracers that bind to specific pathologic molecules, such as Pittsburgh compound B (PiB) for fibrillar beta-amyloid[171] and a growing number of putative tau-binding ligands,[172–175] it is possible to investigate clinicopathologic relationships in vivo. Extensive efforts are underway to develop tracers specific for additional pathologic markers. This will surely lead to a revolution in our understanding of the spectrum of FTD. In the first study of FTD with PiB, a comparison was made between PiB tracer uptake in 12 FTD cases, 7 AD cases, and 8 controls. The FTD cases included five patients with behavioral FTD, two with FTD/ALS, four with SD, and one with progressive aphasia. The results indicated that all AD patients had "positive" PiB PET scans, 7/8 controls had negative PiB scans, while 8 of 12 FTD cases had negative PiB PET scans.

Although this initially seemed to be a high number of amyloid-positive FTD cases, it may not be particularly surprising

in light of several autopsy studies showing the presence of AD pathology in 20–30% of FTD cases, with or without the presence of additional FTLD-type pathology.[176–179] The distribution of PiB tracer uptake in these four cases was similar to that typically seen in AD. Two of the cases carried clinical diagnoses of bvFTD, and the other two were clinically diagnosed with SD. Of note, some elements of the cognitive profiles and the FDG-PET metabolic deficits of these four cases showed features more often associated with AD than FTLD. Of the two FTD patients who have come to autopsy in this series, one had a tauopathy and one had a ubiquitinopathy: both were PiB negative.

A large multicenter study of more than 1200 patients with PPA demonstrated that more than 85% of lvPPA patients exhibited amyloid pathology, while only 20% of nfvPPA patients demonstrated amyloid pathology and 16% of svPPA patients showed amyloid pathology.[180] At least some cases of likely underlying FTLD pathology in PPA patients may exhibit dual pathology, and thus may have a positive amyloid PET scan.[181,182]

CLINICAL COURSE OF FTD

The early symptoms help determine the major subtype of FTD, but as the disease progresses, involvement of other frontotemporal and subcortical brain regions often result in the development of symptoms characteristic of the other subtypes of the diseases.[183] For example, patients with svPPA may develop disinhibition, compulsivity, and other behavioral symptoms, while

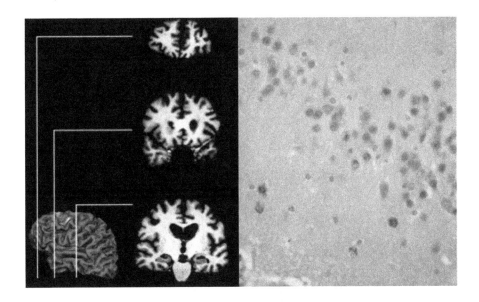

FIGURE 24-3. A 59-year-old man presented with loss of empathy, aggression, lack of insight, executive dysfunction, and word-finding difficulties. Within 1 year of symptom onset he developed dysarthria and dysphagia and was found to have clinical evidence of motor neuron disease with bulbar predominance (tongue weakness, fasciculations, lip weakness, as well as mild shoulder weakness and fasciculations with lower extremity hyperreflexia and extensor plantar responses). Electromyography showed sharp waves, fibrillation potentials, and fasciculation potentials in cervical, thoracic, and lumbar myotomes with long duration, high amplitude, polyphasic potentials with reduced recruitment and rapid firing. **(A)** MRI demonstrated bilateral (left greater than right) frontal atrophy, quantified with a map of cortical thickness compared to controls. His clinical syndrome lasted 3.5 years from first symptoms to death. **(B)** Post-mortem examination revealed the expected TDP-43 Type B pathology (TDP-43 immunohistochemistry of dentate gyrus of hippocampus).

CASE VIGNETTE 24.1

A 50-year-old man presented with depression and left-hand apraxia without rigidity, alien hand syndrome, or eye movement abnormalities, followed shortly by executive dysfunction, word-finding difficulty, and memory loss. When he was first evaluated, the neuroimaging examination revealed markedly asymmetric dominant hemisphere FDG-PET hypometabolism and atrophy extending from peri-Rolandic and dorsal parietal cortex into peri-sylvian cortex and ventral temporal cortex, with relative preservation of frontal cortex and striatum (Figure 24-4). Initial clinical syndromic diagnosis was CBS. Dopaminergic treatments did not change symptoms, as is often the case in CBS. He was treated with occupational therapy, speech-language therapy, as well as psychosocial support and multidisciplinary care planning with him and his family. Surprisingly (given his motor impairments), he was able to enjoy skiing and playing pool as well as a variety of other social and hobby-related activities for several years. His symptoms gradually progressed to include severe asymmetrical hand apraxia with rigidity (resulting in a complete loss of function of his dominant hand), and he also exhibited an increasingly prominent aphasia with dysarthria.

Symptoms progressed to include episodic and semantic memory impairment, compulsive behavior, impulsive eating, and agitation. Some of these behavioral symptoms responded to antidepressant and anticonvulsant treatments, and additional behavioral strategies and education and support helped his family develop a structured care plan with the involvement of home health aides and companions. Along with the progression of symptoms, atrophy progressed over a 4-year interval to include ventral and anterior temporal, insular, and posterior frontal cortex (Figure 24-4). Eventually the disease progressed into a terminal phase of severe rigidity with dementia lasting about a year, and he finally passed away in home hospice after an 8-year clinical course. We expected to find CBD pathology, but neuropathological examination identified Pick's disease (FTLD tau pathology, Pick's type). Given the absence of a family history and the identification of this pathology, we counseled the family that this is typically a sporadic condition for which other family members are not likely at elevated risk. To confirm this prediction, sequencing of the *MAPT* gene was performed and did not reveal any abnormalities.

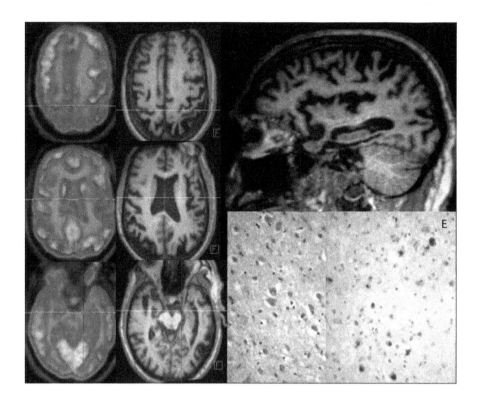

FIGURE 24-4. A 50-year-old man with a clinical syndromic diagnosis of corticobasal syndrome. The first neuroimaging examination revealed markedly asymmetric dominant hemisphere FDG-PET hypometabolism (A, B, C, left column) and atrophy (A, B, C, right column) extending from peri-Rolandic and dorsal parietal cortex (**A**) into perisylvian cortex (**B**) and ventral temporal cortex (**C**) with relative preservation of frontal cortex and striatum. Along with the progression of symptoms, atrophy progressed from parietal and posterolateral temporal over a 4-year interval to include ventral and anterior temporal, insular, and posterior frontal cortex (**D**). Although this man's clinical and imaging features pointed toward corticobasal degeneration as the likely etiology, histological examination revealed Pick bodies (**E**, left) and tau immunoreactive pathology (**E**, right) consistent with pathological Pick's disease (frontotemporal lobar degeneration tau pathology, Pick type).

bvFTD patients may develop speech, language, and/or semantic deficits.

Overall, survival after diagnosis is typically 6–10 years, with PPA-semantic variant patients having the longest survival.[184] A more recent study suggests a slightly better prognosis for bvFTD patients, with a median survival of 4.2 years from diagnosis.[185] The development of early motor symptoms or signs is a poor prognostic feature in all forms of FTD,[186] as is early language impairment in bvFTD.[185] Recent data suggest that SD patients may commonly have a very slow progression, with 50% of patients alive at 12.8 years after diagnosis in a large cohort of 100 patients.[187] The ultimate development of markers of the specific form of neuropathology may be important for prognostication, with one autopsy study of 71 patients indicating that tau pathology was associated with shorter (3 years) survival than non-tau forms of FTLD pathology (8 years).[188]

In our practice, we always discuss the value of autopsy with family members and with patients if possible (see the Case Vignette as an illustration of the value of autopsy). Despite continued improvements in the use of clinical and biomarker data for probabilistic prediction of FTLD or non-FTLD pathology, every specialized center continues to observe surprising cases. Not only is autopsy information important for providing family members with the greatest detail possible about the patient's disease, it also contributes in extremely valuable ways to ongoing research efforts.

TREATMENT OF AND CARE PLANNING FOR PATIENTS AND FAMILIES WITH FTD

Once a diagnosis of one of the forms of FTD is made, the clinician unfortunately needs to deliver the news that, at present, there are no disease-modifying therapies for FTD (as is the case for all other major neurodegenerative diseases). Nevertheless, despite the fact that we are not yet able to reverse or slow the progression of FTD and related disorders, these diseases are treatable if we approach the patient and family using a biopsychosocial model of care plan development. Treatment includes empiric pharmacologic management of symptoms, nonpharmacologic management of symptoms, management of comorbid conditions which may exacerbate cognitive-behavioral impairment, psychosocial support, and education of the family and patient.[189] A multidisciplinary team of specialists is instrumental in caring for patients and families suffering from FTD.[190] Pharmacologic and nonpharmacologic management depends on the identification and grading of severity of specific symptoms (including cognitive, behavioral, and motor symptoms), followed by their prioritization and monitoring over time. Once this is done, judicious empiric use of medications can be tackled. At present, no medications are approved for the symptomatic treatment of FTD, but many medications have demonstrated utility in small studies or case series.[191–193] For example, selective serotonin reuptake inhibitors or other antidepressants can modulate disinhibition or compulsive behavior, stimulants or pro-dopaminergic agents can sometimes reduce apathy or attentional impairment, and anticonvulsants/mood stabilizers or antipsychotic compounds can ameliorate aggression or agitation.[193,194] Side effects of these medications may in some cases outweigh benefits, and patients always need close monitoring. Cholinesterase inhibitors are generally not helpful in patients with FTD, and in some cases may exacerbate problem behaviors.

Nonpharmacologic symptom management strategies generally require the expertise of an experienced specialist clinician or team.[195,196] These include speech and language therapy for communication or swallowing issues, occupational therapy for problems with hand-eye coordination or planning that impacts instrumental or basic activities of daily living, physical therapy for gait disorders, and in some cases psychotherapy for the patient. A growing body of evidence supports the utility of speech-language therapy in PPA.[197] A driving assessment is critical, as is the evaluation of financial or health care decision-making capacity. Social work assistance with facilitating disability compensation can be very helpful. Paid or volunteer companions or home health aides to help patients remain active yet safe can be valuable. Day programs or respite residential programs may play important roles at some point in the course of the illness. Advanced care planning discussions should be considered early in the course of the illness.

Ultimately, because the myriad of resources that may be helpful to patients and family members can be difficult to identify, it is essential to dedicate time and effort toward specialized education for the patient/family through the clinician or multidisciplinary team or the Association for FTD (http://www.theaftd.org/) or Alzheimer's Association (http://www.alz.org). Psychosocial support resources can also be valuable for nearly all families and for some patients. Evidence is accruing that caregiver interventions improve quality of life in caregivers of patients with FTD.[198] The development of close links between the FTD specialty care team and the primary care physician is very important to assist in general management, including monitoring comorbid conditions and considering the role of standard prophylactic care in the context of FTD.

Finally, it is critical late in the course of the illness to assist patients and families with end of life care, facilitating access to palliative care resources and ideally obtaining nursing home and hospice care at the appropriate time. There continues to be a desperate need for residential or nursing facilities that have the capacity and skill to care for patients with FTD. And although research at present focuses largely on understanding the disease and offers little if any novel putative treatment options for patients with FTD, participation in studies can provide some meaning in an otherwise entirely tragic situation. Ultimately, the quality of the partnership between care providers experienced with FTD and patients/families with these diseases is a critical factor that influences the experience of living with FTD.

Summary and Key Points

- Frontotemporal dementia (FTD) encompasses a spectrum of clinical dementia phenotypes including behavioral variant FTD, primary progressive aphasias (PPA), corticobasal degeneration, progressive supranuclear palsy, and FTD with motor neuron disease or FTD with amyotrophic lateral sclerosis.
- The clinical syndromes of FTD arise from a diverse set of pathological diseases known as frontotemporal lobar degeneration (FTLD), with two major types: FTLD tau and FTD TDP-43, as well as several rare pathologies.
- Age of onset is usually between 45 and 65, although cases as young as 21 and as old as 85 have been reported.
- Diagnosis can be challenging, and usually requires a comprehensive multimodal assessment.
- Some cases of FTD arise as a result of an autosomal dominant genetic abnormality; the three major genes associated with FTD include *MAPT*, *GRN*, and *c9orf72*, as well as several rare genes.
- Management is at present focused on empirical treatment of symptoms and supportive multidisciplinary care.
- The pathophysiology of FTLD is only beginning to be understood, but is providing a foundation for clinical trials of potential therapeutics.

Multiple Choice Questions

1. The following points are true regarding the pathophysiology of FTLD:
   a. FTLD involves the aggregation of proteins that have important cellular functions which are then disrupted.
   b. FTLD involves tau or TDP-43 pathology and possibly interactions between them in some forms of the disease.
   c. Amyloid pathology plays a key role in FTLD.
   d. Genetic abnormalities in some cases are illuminating FTLD pathophysiologic mechanisms.
   e. a, b, and d.

2. The clinical presentation of FTD
   a. Often includes memory loss as an early feature.
   b. Typically includes prominent behavioral or language symptoms.
   c. Often includes a prominent early motor component.
   d. Is usually obvious at first evaluation and easy to diagnose.
   e. Can easily be confirmed with a blood test.

3. The assessment of patients with FTD typically includes all of the following except:
   a. Detailed history
   b. Neurologic and psychiatric exam
   c. Brain MRI
   d. FDG PET
   e. Amyloid PET

4. Evidence supports the following treatment options for some patients with FTD:
   a. Antidepressant medications
   b. Speech-language therapy
   c. Cholinesterase inhibitors
   d. Caregiver support
   e. a, b, and d

Multiple Choice Answers

1. Answer: e

As discussed in the pathophysiology section, amyloid does not play a role in FTLD. The other points are correct.

2. Answer: b

Most patients with FTD present with behavioral or language symptoms. Although many patients have memory loss as part of their clinical phenotype, it is not usually the most prominent early feature. Motor symptoms or signs often occur as FTD progresses, but only a minority of cases exhibit motor impairment as an early feature (i.e., PSP, CBS, or FTD-MND). There are no blood tests for pathologic markers of FTLD at present.

3. Answer: e

Although amyloid PET may play a role in ruling out AD in some cases of FTD, it is not part of the typical clinical evaluation at most centers in part because of availability. In many cases, the clinician will be highly confident in the diagnosis after a, b, and c.

4. Answer: e

As discussed in the section on treatment, there is evidence for the use of each of these therapies in at least some patients with FTD or their caregivers. Cholinesterase inhibitors are not effective in treating FTD.

References

1. Pick A, Girling DM, Berrios GE. On the symptomatology of left-sided temporal lobe atrophy. Classic Text No. 29. (Translated and annotated by D.M. Girling and G.E. Berrios.). *Hist Psychiatry*. 1997;8(29 pt 1):149-159.
2. Berrios GE, Girling DM. Introduction: Pick's disease and the 'frontal lobe' dementias. *Hist Psychiatry*. 1994;5(20 pt 4):539-547.
3. Mesulam MM. Slowly progressive aphasia without generalized dementia. *Ann Neurol*. 1982;11(6):592-598.
4. Goulding PJ, Northen B, Snowden JS, Macdermott N, Neary D. Progressive aphasia with right-sided extrapyramidal signs: another manifestation of localised cerebral atrophy. *J Neurol Neurosurg Psychiatry*. 1989;52(1):128-130.
5. Hodges JR, Patterson K, Oxbury S, Funnell E. Semantic dementia. Progressive fluent aphasia with temporal lobe atrophy. *Brain*. 1992;115(pt 6):1783-1806.
6. Gustafson L. Frontal lobe degeneration of non-Alzheimer type. II. Clinical picture and differential diagnosis. *Arch Gerontol Geriatr*. 1987;6(3):209-223.
7. Neary D, Snowden JS, Northen B, Goulding P. Dementia of frontal lobe type. *J Neurol Neurosurg Psychiatry*. 1988;51(3):353-361.
8. Brun A, Englund E, Gustafson L, et al. Clinical and neuropathological criteria for frontotemporal dementia. The Lund and Manchester Groups. *J Neurol Neurosurg Psychiatry*. 1994;57(4):416-418.
9. Neary D, Snowden JS, Gustafson L, et al. Frontotemporal lobar degeneration: a consensus on clinical diagnostic criteria. *Neurology*. 1998;51(6):1546-1554.
10. Dickerson BC. *Hodges' Frontotemporal Dementia*. 2nd ed. Cambridge, UK: Cambridge University Press; 2016.
11. Gorno-Tempini ML, Hillis AE, Weintraub S, et al. Classification of primary progressive aphasia and its variants. *Neurology*. 2011;76(11):1006-1014.
12. Rascovsky K, Hodges JR, Knopman D, et al. Sensitivity of revised diagnostic criteria for the behavioural variant of frontotemporal dementia. *Brain*. 2011;134(pt 9):2456-2477.
13. Snowden JS, Neary D, Mann DM. Autopsy proven sporadic frontotemporal dementia due to microvacuolar-type histology, with onset at 21 years of age. *J Neurol Neurosurg Psychiatry*. 2004;75(9):1337-1339.
14. Gislason TB, Sjogren M, Larsson L, Skoog I. The prevalence of frontal variant frontotemporal dementia and the frontal lobe syndrome in a population based sample of 85 year olds. *J Neurol Neurosurg Psychiatry*. 2003;74(7):867-871.
15. Ibach B, Koch H, Koller M, Wolfersdorf M. Hospital admission circumstances and prevalence of frontotemporal lobar degeneration: a multicenter psychiatric state hospital study in Germany. *Dement Geriatr Cogn Disord*. 2003;16(4):253-264.
16. Borroni B, Alberici A, Grassi M, et al. Is frontotemporal lobar degeneration a rare disorder? Evidence from a preliminary study in Brescia county, Italy. *J Alzheimers Dis*. 2010;19(1):111-116.
17. Knopman DS, Petersen RC, Edland SD, Cha RH, Rocca WA. The incidence of frontotemporal lobar degeneration in Rochester, Minnesota, 1990 through 1994. *Neurology*. 2004;62(3):506-508.
18. Rosso SM, Donker Kaat L, Baks T, et al. Frontotemporal dementia in The Netherlands: patient characteristics and prevalence estimates from a population-based study. *Brain*. 2003;126 (pt 9):2016-2022.
19. Harvey RJ, Skelton-Robinson M, Rossor MN. The prevalence and causes of dementia in people under the age of 65 years. *J Neurol Neurosurg Psychiatry*. 2003;74(9):1206-1209.

20. Ratnavalli E, Brayne C, Dawson K, Hodges JR. The prevalence of frontotemporal dementia. *Neurology*. 2002;58(11):1615-1621.

21. Bernardi L, Frangipane F, Smirne N, et al. Epidemiology and genetics of frontotemporal dementia: a door-to-door survey in southern Italy. *Neurobiol Aging*. 2012;33(12):2948.e1-2948.e10.

22. Pick A. Über die Beziehungen der senilen Hirnatrophie zur Aphasie. *Prager medicinische Wochenschrift*. 1892;17:165-167.

23. Munoz DG, Morris HR, Rosser M. Pick's disease. In: Dickson DW, Weller RO, eds. *Neurodegeneration: The Molecular Pathology of Dementia and Movement Disorders*. 2nd ed. Hoboken, NJ: Wiley-Blackwell; 2011.

24. Alzheimer A. Über eigenartige Krankheitsfälle der späteren Alters. *Z Gesamte Neurol Psychiatrie*. 1911;4:356-385.

25. Onari K, Spatz H. Anatomische Beiträge zur Lehre von der Pickschen umschriebenen Grosshirnrinden-Atrophie ('Picksche Krankheit'). *Z Neurol*. 1926;101:470-4511.

26. Binns JK, Robertson EE. Pick's disease in old age. *J Ment Sci*. 1962;108:804-810.

27. Schenk VW. Re-examination of a family with Pick's disease. *Ann Hum Genet*. 1959;23:325-333.

28. Neumann MA. Pick's disease. *J Neuropathol Exp Neurol*. 1949;8(3):255-282.

29. Yoshimura N. Topography of Pick body distribution in Pick's disease: a contribution to understanding the relationship between Pick's and Alzheimer's diseases. *Clin Neuropathol*. 1989; 8(1):1-6.

30. Hof PR, Bouras C, Perl DP, Morrison JH. Quantitative neuropathologic analysis of Pick's disease cases: cortical distribution of Pick bodies and coexistence with Alzheimer's disease. *Acta Neuropathol*. 1994;87(2):115-124.

31. Zhukareva V, Mann D, Pickering-Brown S, et al. Sporadic Pick's disease: a tauopathy characterized by a spectrum of pathological tau isoforms in gray and white matter. *Ann Neurol*. 2002;51(6): 730-739.

32. Dickson DW. Neuropathology of Pick's disease. *Neurology*. 2001;56(11 suppl 4):S16-S20.

33. Dickson DW, Kouri N, Murray ME, Josephs KA. Neuropathology of frontotemporal lobar degeneration-tau (FTLD-tau). *J Mol Neurosci*. 2011;45(3):384-389.

34. Kertesz A, Davidson W, Munoz DG. Clinical and pathological overlap between frontotemporal dementia, primary progressive aphasia and corticobasal degeneration: the Pick complex. *Dement Geriatr Cogn Disord*. 1999;10(suppl 1):46-49.

35. Hoglinger GU, Respondek G, Stamelou M, et al. Clinical diagnosis of progressive supranuclear palsy: the Movement Disorder Society criteria. *Mov Disord*. 2017;32(6):853-864.

36. Armstrong MJ, Litvan I, Lang AE, et al. Criteria for the diagnosis of corticobasal degeneration. *Neurology*. 2013;80(5):496-503.

37. Constantinidis J, Richard J, Tissot R. Pick's disease. Histological and clinical correlations. *Eur Neurol*. 1974;11(4):208-217.

38. Clark AW, Manz HJ, White CL3rd, Lehmann J, Miller D, Coyle JT. Cortical degeneration with swollen chromatolytic neurons: its relationship to Pick's disease. *J Neuropathol Exp Neurol*. 1986;45(3):268-284.

39. Knopman DS, Mastri AR, Frey WH2nd, Sung JH, Rustan T. Dementia lacking distinctive histologic features: a common non-Alzheimer degenerative dementia. *Neurology*. 1990; 40(2):251-256.

40. Neumann M, Sampathu DM, Kwong LK, et al. Ubiquitinated TDP-43 in frontotemporal lobar degeneration and amyotrophic lateral sclerosis. *Science*. 2006;314(5796):130-133.

41. Mackenzie IR, Rademakers R, Neumann M. TDP-43 and FUS in amyotrophic lateral sclerosis and frontotemporal dementia. *Lancet Neurol*. 2010;9(10):995-1007.

42. Tan RH, Kril JJ, Fatima M, et al. TDP-43 proteinopathies: pathological identification of brain regions differentiating clinical phenotypes. *Brain*. 2015:138(10):3110-3122.

43. Neumann M, Rademakers R, Roeber S, Baker M, Kretzschmar HA, Mackenzie IR. A new subtype of frontotemporal lobar degeneration with FUS pathology. *Brain*. 2009;132(pt 11):2922-2931.

44. Seeley WW, Carlin DA, Allman JM, et al. Early frontotemporal dementia targets neurons unique to apes and humans. *Ann Neurol*. 2006;60(6):660-667.

45. Kim EJ, Sidhu M, Gaus SE, et al. Selective frontoinsular von Economo neuron and fork cell loss in early behavioral variant frontotemporal dementia. *Cereb Cortex*. 2012;22(2):251-259.

46. Groen JJ, Endtz LJ. Hereditary Pick's disease: second re-examination of the large family and discussion of other hereditary cases, with particular reference to electroencephalography, a computerized tomography. *Brain*. 1982;105(pt 3):443-459.

47. Heston LL. The clinical genetics of Pick's disease. *Acta Psychiatr Scand*. 1978;57(3):202-206.

48. Foster NL, Wilhelmsen K, Sima AA, Jones MZ, D'Amato CJ, Gilman S. Frontotemporal dementia and parkinsonism linked to chromosome 17: a consensus conference. Conference Participants. *Ann Neurol*. 1997;41(6):706-715.

49. Goldman JS, McCarty Wood E. Genetic counseling for FTD. In: Dickerson BC, ed. *Hodges' Frontotemporal Dementia*. 2nd ed. Cambridge, UK: Cambridge University Press; 2016:153-164.

50. Hutton M, Lendon CL, Rizzu P, et al. Association of missense and 5′-splice-site mutations in tau with the inherited dementia FTDP-17. *Nature*. 1998;393(6686):702-705.

51. Poorkaj P, Bird TD, Wijsman E, et al. Tau is a candidate gene for chromosome 17 frontotemporal dementia. *Ann Neurol*. 1998;43(6):815-825.

52. Rademakers R, Cruts M, van Broeckhoven C. The role of tau (MAPT) in frontotemporal dementia and related tauopathies. *Hum Mutat*. 2004;24(4):277-295.

53. Bugiani O, Murrell JR, Giaccone G, et al. Frontotemporal dementia and corticobasal degeneration in a family with a P301S mutation in tau. *J Neuropathol Exp Neurol*. 1999;58(6):667-677.

54. Baker M, Mackenzie IR, Pickering-Brown SM, et al. Mutations in progranulin cause tau-negative frontotemporal dementia linked to chromosome 17. *Nature*. 2006;442(7105):916-919.

55. Cruts M, Gijselinck I, van der Zee J, et al. Null mutations in progranulin cause ubiquitin-positive frontotemporal dementia linked to chromosome 17q21. *Nature*. 2006;442(7105):920-924.

56. Finch N, Carrasquillo MM, Baker M, et al. TMEM106B regulates progranulin levels and the penetrance of FTLD in GRN mutation carriers. *Neurology*. 76(5):467-474.

57. Renton AE, Majounie E, Waite A, et al. A hexanucleotide repeat expansion in C9ORF72 is the cause of chromosome 9p21-linked ALS-FTD. *Neuron*. 2011;72(2):257-268.

58. DeJesus-Hernandez M, Mackenzie IR, Boeve BF, et al. Expanded GGGGCC hexanucleotide repeat in noncoding region of C9ORF72 causes chromosome 9p-linked FTD and ALS. *Neuron*. 2011;72(2):245-256.

59. Wood EM, Falcone D, Suh E, et al. Development and validation of pedigree classification criteria for frontotemporal lobar degeneration. *JAMA Neurol*. 2013;70(11):1411-1417.

60. van Blitterswijk M, Mullen B, Nicholson AM, et al. TMEM106B protects C9ORF72 expansion carriers against frontotemporal dementia. *Acta Neuropathol*. 2014;127(3):397-406.

61. Gijselinck I, Van Mossevelde S, van der Zee J, et al. Loss of TBK1 is a frequent cause of frontotemporal dementia in a Belgian cohort. *Neurology*. 2015;85(24):2116-2125.

62. Van Mossevelde S, van der Zee J, Gijselinck I, et al. Clinical features of TBK1 carriers compared with C9orf72, GRN and non-mutation carriers in a Belgian cohort. *Brain*. 2016;139(pt 2): 452-467.

63. Skibinski G, Parkinson NJ, Brown JM, et al. Mutations in the endosomal ESCRTIII-complex subunit CHMP2B in frontotemporal dementia. *Nat Genet*. 2005;37(8):806-808.

64. Cruts M, Van Broeckhoven C. Genetics of frontotemporal dementia and related disorders. In: Dickerson BC, ed. *Hodges' Frontotemporal Dementia*. 2nd ed. Cambridge, UK: Cambridge University Press; 2016.

65. Kwiatkowski TJJr, Bosco DA, Leclerc AL, et al. Mutations in the FUS/TLS gene on chromosome 16 cause familial amyotrophic lateral sclerosis. *Science*. 2009;323(5918):1205-1208.

66. Vance C, Rogelj B, Hortobagyi T, et al. Mutations in FUS, an RNA processing protein, cause familial amyotrophic lateral sclerosis type 6. *Science*. 2009;323(5918):1208-1211.

67. Huey ED, Ferrari R, Moreno JH, et al. FUS and TDP43 genetic variability in FTD and CBS. *Neurobiol Aging*. 2011;33(5): 1016.e9-1016.e17.

68. Janssen JC, Warrington EK, Morris HR, et al. Clinical features of frontotemporal dementia due to the intronic tau 10(+16) mutation. *Neurology*. 2002;58(8):1161-1168.

69. Snowden JS, Pickering-Brown SM, Mackenzie IR, et al. Progranulin gene mutations associated with frontotemporal dementia and progressive non-fluent aphasia. *Brain*. 2006;129 (pt 11):3091-3102.

70. Mitchell SB, Lucente D, Larvie M, Cobos MI, Frosch M, Dickerson BC. A 63-year-old man with progressive visual symptoms. *JAMA Neurol*. 2017;74(1):114-118.

71. Caroppo P, Belin C, Grabli D, et al. Posterior cortical atrophy as an extreme phenotype of GRN mutations. *JAMA Neurol*. 2015;72(2):224-228.

72. Boeve BF, Boylan KB, Graff-Radford NR, et al. Characterization of frontotemporal dementia and/or amyotrophic lateral sclerosis associated with the GGGGCC repeat expansion in C9ORF72. *Brain*. 2012;135(pt 3):765-783.

73. Fong JC, Karydas AM, Goldman JS. Genetic counseling for FTD/ALS caused by the C9ORF72 hexanucleotide expansion. *Alzheimers Res Ther*. 2012;4(4):27.

74. Goldman JS, Rademakers R, Huey ED, et al. An algorithm for genetic testing of frontotemporal lobar degeneration. *Neurology*. 2011;76(5):475-483.

75. Quaid KA. Genetic counseling for frontotemporal dementias. *J Mol Neurosci*. 2011;45(3):706-709.

76. Wood EM, Falcone D, Suh E, et al. Development and validation of pedigree classification criteria for frontotemporal lobar degeneration. *JAMA Neurol*. 2013;70(11):1411-1417.

77. Rascovsky K, Hodges JR, Kipps CM, et al. Diagnostic criteria for the behavioral variant of frontotemporal dementia (bvFTD): current limitations and future directions. *Alzheimer Dis Assoc Disord*. 2007;21(4):S14-S18.

78. Miller BL, Darby A, Benson DF, Cummings JL, Miller MH. Aggressive, socially disruptive and antisocial behaviour associated with fronto-temporal dementia. *Br J Psychiatry*. 1997;170:150-154.

79. Miller BL, Cummings JL, Villanueva-Meyer J, et al. Frontal lobe degeneration: clinical, neuropsychological, and SPECT characteristics. *Neurology*. 1991;41(9):1374-1382.

80. Snowden JS, Bathgate D, Varma A, Blackshaw A, Gibbons ZC, Neary D. Distinct behavioural profiles in frontotemporal dementia and semantic dementia. *J Neurol Neurosurg Psychiatry*. 2001;70(3):323-332.

81. O'Callaghan C, Hodges JR, Hornberger M. Inhibitory dysfunction in frontotemporal dementia: a review. *Alzheimer Dis Assoc Disord*. 2013;27(2):102-108.

82. Shinagawa S, Ikeda M, Fukuhara R, Tanabe H. Initial symptoms in frontotemporal dementia and semantic dementia compared with Alzheimer's disease. *Dement Geriatr Cogn Disord*. 2006;21(2):74-80.

83. Chow TW, Binns MA, Cummings JL, et al. Apathy symptom profile and behavioral associations in frontotemporal dementia vs dementia of Alzheimer type. *Arch Neurol*. 2009;66(7):888-893.

84. Massimo L, Powers C, Moore P, et al. Neuroanatomy of apathy and disinhibition in frontotemporal lobar degeneration. *Dement Geriatr Cogn Disord*. 2009;27(1):96-104.

85. Le Ber I, Guedj E, Gabelle A, et al. Demographic, neurological and behavioural characteristics and brain perfusion SPECT in frontal variant of frontotemporal dementia. *Brain*. 2006;129 (pt 11):3051-3065.

86. Rosen HJ, Allison SC, Schauer GF, Gorno-Tempini ML, Weiner MW, Miller BL. Neuroanatomical correlates of behavioural disorders in dementia. *Brain*. 2005;128(pt 11):2612-2625.

87. Mendez MF, Perryman KM. Disrupted facial empathy in drawings from artists with frontotemporal dementia. *Neurocase*. 2003;9(1):44-50.

88. Rankin KP, Kramer JH, Miller BL. Patterns of cognitive and emotional empathy in frontotemporal lobar degeneration. *Cogn Behav Neurol*. 2005;18(1):28-36.

89. Lough S, Kipps CM, Treise C, Watson P, Blair JR, Hodges JR. Social reasoning, emotion and empathy in frontotemporal dementia. *Neuropsychologia*. 2006;44(6):950-958.

90. Rankin KP, Gorno-Tempini ML, Allison SC, et al. Structural anatomy of empathy in neurodegenerative disease. *Brain*. 2006;129(pt 11):2945-2956.

91. Perry RJ, Rosen HR, Kramer JH, Beer JS, Levenson RL, Miller BL. Hemispheric dominance for emotions, empathy and social behaviour: evidence from right and left handers with frontotemporal dementia. *Neurocase*. 2001;7(2):145-160.

92. Ames D, Cummings JL, Wirshing WC, Quinn B, Mahler M. Repetitive and compulsive behavior in frontal lobe degenerations. *J Neuropsychiatry Clin Neurosci*. 1994;6(2):100-113.

93. Nyatsanza S, Shetty T, Gregory C, Lough S, Dawson K, Hodges JR. A study of stereotypic behaviours in Alzheimer's disease and frontal and temporal variant frontotemporal dementia. *J Neurol Neurosurg Psychiatry*. 2003;74(10):1398-1402.

94. Mendez MF, Perryman KM, Miller BL, Swartz JR, Cummings JL. Compulsive behaviors as presenting symptoms of frontotemporal dementia. *J Geriatr Psychiatry Neurol*. 1997;10(4):154-157.

95. Bozeat S, Gregory CA, Ralph MA, Hodges JR. Which neuropsychiatric and behavioural features distinguish frontal and temporal variants of frontotemporal dementia from Alzheimer's disease? *J Neurol Neurosurg Psychiatry*. 2000;69(2):178-186.

96. Josephs KA, Whitwell JL, Jack CR Jr. Anatomic correlates of stereotypies in frontotemporal lobar degeneration. *Neurobiol Aging*. 2008;70(11):1411-1417.

97. Rosso SM, Roks G, Stevens M, et al. Complex compulsive behaviour in the temporal variant of frontotemporal dementia. *J Neurol*. 2001;248(11):965-970.

98. Perry DC, Whitwell JL, Boeve BF, et al. Voxel-based morphometry in patients with obsessive-compulsive behaviors in behavioral variant frontotemporal dementia. *Eur J Neurol*. 2012;19(6):911-917.

99. Miller BL, Darby AL, Swartz JR, Yener GG, Mena I. Dietary changes, compulsions and sexual behavior in frontotemporal degeneration. *Dementia*. 1995;6(4):195-199.

100. Whitwell JL, Sampson EL, Loy CT, et al. VBM signatures of abnormal eating behaviours in frontotemporal lobar degeneration. *NeuroImage*. 2007;35(1):207-213.

101. Woolley JD, Gorno-Tempini ML, Seeley WW, et al. Binge eating is associated with right orbitofrontal-insular-striatal atrophy in frontotemporal dementia. *Neurology*. 2007;69(14):1424-1433.

102. Piguet O, Petersen A, Yin Ka Lam B, et al. Eating and hypothalamus changes in behavioral-variant frontotemporal dementia. *Ann Neurol*. 2011;69(2):312-319.

103. Ahmed RM, Ke YD, Vucic S, et al. Physiological changes in neurodegeneration—mechanistic insights and clinical utility. *Nat Rev Neurol*. 2018;14(5):259-271.

104. Gregory CA, Hodges JR. Clinical features of frontal lobe dementia in comparison to Alzheimer's disease. *J Neural Transm Suppl*. 1996;47:103-123.

105. Banks S, Weintraub S. Self-awareness and self-monitoring of cognitive and behavioral deficits in behavioral variant frontotemporal dementia, primary progressive aphasia and probable Alzheimer's disease. *Brain Cogn*. 2008;67(1):58-68.

106. Eslinger PJ, Dennis K, Moore P, Antani S, Hauck R, Grossman M. Metacognitive deficits in frontotemporal dementia. *J Neurol Neurosurg Psychiatry*. 2005;76(12):1630-1635.

107. Williamson C, Alcantar O, Rothlind J, Cahn-Weiner D, Miller BL, Rosen HJ. Standardised measurement of self-awareness deficits in FTD and AD. *J Neurol Neurosurg Psychiatry*. 2009;81(2):140-145.

108. Rosen HJ, Alcantar O, Rothlind J, et al. Neuroanatomical correlates of cognitive self-appraisal in neurodegenerative disease. *NeuroImage*. 2010;49(4):3358-3364.

109. Rankin KP, Baldwin E, Pace-Savitsky C, Kramer JH, Miller BL. Self awareness and personality change in dementia. *J Neurol Neurosurg Psychiatry*. 2005;76(5):632-639.

110. Veronelli L, Makaretz SJ, Quimby M, Dickerson BC, Collins JA. Geschwind syndrome in frontotemporal lobar degeneration: neuroanatomical and neuropsychological features over 9 years. *Cortex*. 2017;94:27-38.

111. Hornberger M, Piguet O, Graham AJ, Nestor PJ, Hodges JR. How preserved is episodic memory in behavioral variant frontotemporal dementia? *Neurology*. 2010;74(6):472-479.

112. Pennington C, Hodges JR, Hornberger M. Neural correlates of episodic memory in behavioral variant frontotemporal dementia. *J Alzheimers Dis*. 2011;24(2):261-268.

113. Graham A, Davies R, Xuereb J, et al. Pathologically proven frontotemporal dementia presenting with severe amnesia. *Brain*. 2005;128(pt 3):597-605.

114. Pasquier F, Grymonprez L, Lebert F, Van der Linden M. Memory impairment differs in frontotemporal dementia and Alzheimer's disease. *Neurocase*. 2001;7(2):161-171.

115. Ash S, Moore P, Antani S, McCawley G, Work M, Grossman M. Trying to tell a tale: discourse impairments in progressive aphasia and frontotemporal dementia. *Neurology*. 2006;66(9):1405-1413.

116. Kipps CM, Nestor PJ, Acosta-Cabronero J, Arnold R, Hodges JR. Understanding social dysfunction in the behavioural variant of frontotemporal dementia: the role of emotion and sarcasm processing. *Brain*. 2009;132(pt 3):592-603.

117. Hardy CJ, Buckley AH, Downey LE, et al. The language profile of behavioral variant frontotemporal dementia. *J Alzheimers Dis*. 2016;50(2):359-371.

118. Devenney EM, Ahmed RM, Halliday G, Piguet O, Kiernan MC, Hodges JR. Psychiatric disorders in *C9orf72* kindreds: study of 1,414 family members. *Neurology*. 2018;91(16):e1498-e1507.

119. Leyton CE, Villemagne VL, Savage S, et al. Subtypes of progressive aphasia: application of the International Consensus Criteria and validation using beta-amyloid imaging. *Brain*. 2011;134(pt 10):3030-3043.

120. Mesulam M, Wicklund A, Johnson N, et al. Alzheimer and frontotemporal pathology in subsets of primary progressive aphasia. *Ann Neurol*. 2008;63(6):709-719.

121. Mesulam M-M, Weintraub S. Spectrum of primary progressive aphasia. In: Rossor MN, ed. *Unusual Dementias*. London: Baillière Tindall; 1992:583-609.

122. Mesulam M-M. Primary progressive aphasia. *Ann Neurol*. 2001;49:425-432.

123. Mesulam M-M. Primary progressive aphasia: a language-based dementia. *N Engl J Med*. 2003;348:1535-1542.

124. Weintraub S, Rubin NP, Mesulam MM. Primary progressive aphasia. Longitudinal course, neuropsychological profile, and language features. *Arch Neurol*. 1990;47(12):1329-1335.

125. Modirrousta M, Price BH, Dickerson BC. Neuropsychiatric symptoms in primary progressive aphasia: phenomenology, pathophysiology, and approach to assessment and treatment. *Neurodegener Dis Manag*. 2013;3(2):133-146.

126. Gorno-Tempini ML, Dronkers NF, Rankin KP, et al. Cognition and anatomy in three variants of primary progressive aphasia. *Ann Neurol*. 2004;55:335-346.

127. Hodges JR, Patterson K. Nonfluent progressive aphasia and semantic dementia: a comparative neuropsychological study. *J Int Neuropsychol Soc*. 1996;2(6):511-524.

128. Hillis AE, Oh S, Ken L. Deterioration of naming nouns versus verbs in primary progressive aphasia. *Ann Neurol*. 2004;55(2):268-275.

129. Cotelli M, Borroni B, Manenti R, et al. Action and object naming in frontotemporal dementia, progressive supranuclear palsy, and corticobasal degeneration. *Neuropsychology*. 2006;20(5):558-565.

130. Wilson SM, Henry ML, Besbris M, et al. Connected speech production in three variants of primary progressive aphasia. *Brain*. 2010;133(pt 7):2069-2088.

131. Ash S, Evans E, O'Shea J, et al. Differentiating primary progressive aphasias in a brief sample of connected speech. *Neurology*. 2013;81(4):329-336.

132. Grossman M, Mickanin J, Onishi K, et al. Progressive nonfluent aphasia: language, cognitive, and PET measures contrasted with probable Alzheimer's disease. *J Cogn Neurosci*. 1996;8(2):135-154.

133. Charles D, Olm C, Powers J, et al. Grammatical comprehension deficits in non-fluent/agrammatic primary progressive aphasia. *J Neurol Neurosurg Psychiatry*. 2014;85(3):249-256.

134. Josephs KA, Duffy JR, Strand EA, et al. Characterizing a neurodegenerative syndrome: primary progressive apraxia of speech. *Brain*. 2012;135(pt 5):1522-1536.

135. Ogar J, Slama H, Dronkers N, Amici S, Gorno-Tempini ML. Apraxia of speech: an overview. *Neurocase*. 2005;11(6):427-432.

136. Josephs KA, Duffy JR, Strand EA, et al. Syndromes dominated by apraxia of speech show distinct characteristics from agrammatic PPA. *Neurology*. 2013;81(4):337-345.

137. Rohrer JD, Rossor MN, Warren JD. Apraxia in progressive nonfluent aphasia. *J Neurol*. 2010;257(4):569-574.

138. Rogalski E, Cobia D, Harrison TM, Wieneke C, Weintraub S, Mesulam MM. Progression of language decline and cortical atrophy in subtypes of primary progressive aphasia. *Neurology*. 2011;76(21):1804-1810.

139. Sapolsky D, Bakkour A, Negreira A, et al. Cortical neuroanatomic correlates of symptom severity in primary progressive aphasia. *Neurology*. 2010;75(4):358-366.

140. Wilson SM, Galantucci S, Tartaglia MC, et al. Syntactic processing depends on dorsal language tracts. *Neuron*. 2011;72(2):397-403.

141. Josephs KA, Duffy JR, Strand EA, et al. Clinicopathological and imaging correlates of progressive aphasia and apraxia of speech. *Brain*. 2006;129(pt 6):1385-1398.

142. Mesulam MM, Wieneke C, Hurley R, et al. Words and objects at the tip of the left temporal lobe in primary progressive aphasia. *Brain*. 2013;136(2):601-618.

143. Hodges JR, Graham N, Patterson K. Charting the progression in semantic dementia: implications for the organisation of semantic memory. *Memory*. 1995;3(3-4):463-495.

144. Meteyard L, Patterson K. The relation between content and structure in language production: an analysis of speech errors in semantic dementia. *Brain Lang*. 2009;110(3):121-134.

145. Gorno-Tempini ML, Murray RC, Rankin KP, Weiner MW, Miller BL. Clinical, cognitive and anatomical evolution from nonfluent progressive aphasia to corticobasal syndrome: a case report. *Neurocase*. 2004;10(6):426-436.

146. Wilson SM, Brambati SM, Henry RG, et al. The neural basis of surface dyslexia in semantic dementia. *Brain*. 2009;132(pt 1):71-86.

147. Mummery CJ, Patterson K, Price CJ, Ashburner J, Frackowiak RSJ, Hodges JR. A voxel-based morphometry study of semantic dementia: relationship between temporal lobe atrophy and semantic dementia. *Ann Neurol*. 2000;47:36-45.

148. Galton CJ, Patterson K, Graham K, et al. Differing patterns of temporal atrophy in Alzheimer's disease and semantic dementia. *Neurology*. 2001;57(2):216-225.

149. Chan D, Fox NC, Scahill RI, et al. Patterns of temporal lobe atrophy in semantic dementia and Alzheimer's disease. *Ann Neurol*. 2001;49(4):433-442.

150. Collins JA, Montal V, Hochberg D, et al. Focal temporal pole atrophy and network degeneration in semantic variant primary progressive aphasia. *Brain*. 2017;140(pt 2):457-471.

151. Agosta F, Henry RG, Migliaccio R, et al. Language networks in semantic dementia. *Brain*. 2010;133(pt 1):286-299.

152. Rosen HJ, Gorno-Tempini ML, Goldman WP, et al. Patterns of brain atrophy in frontotemporal dementia and semantic dementia. *Neurology*. 2002;58(2):198-208.

153. Gainotti G. Why are different the right and left hemisphere conceptual representations? *Behav Neurol*. 2014:603134.

154. Gorno-Tempini ML, Brambati SM, Ginex V, et al. The logopenic/phonological variant of primary progressive aphasia. *Neurology*. 2008;71(16):1227-1234.

155. Wear HJ, Wedderburn CJ, Mioshi E, et al. The Cambridge Behavioural Inventory revised. *Dement Neuropsychol*. 2008;2(2):102-107.

156. Kertesz A, Davidson W, Fox H. Frontal behavioral inventory: diagnostic criteria for frontal lobe dementia. *Can J Neurol Sci*. 1997;24(1):29-36.

157. Cummings JL. The Neuropsychiatric Inventory: assessing psychopathology in dementia patients. *Neurology*. 1997;48(5 suppl 6):S10-S16.

158. Bickart KC, Brickhouse M, Negreira A, Sapolsky D, Barrett LF, Dickerson BC. Atrophy in distinct corticolimbic networks in frontotemporal dementia relates to social impairments measured using the Social Impairment Rating Scale. *J Neurol Neurosurg Psychiatry*. 2014;85(4):438-448.

159. Farias ST, Mungas D, Reed BR, et al. The measurement of everyday cognition (ECog): scale development and psychometric properties. *Neuropsychology*. 2008;22(4):531-544.

160. Taragano FE, Allegri RF, Lyketsos C. Mild behavioral impairment: a prodromal stage of dementia. *Dement Neuropsychol*. 2008;2(4):256-260.

161. Ismail Z, Smith EE, Geda Y, et al. Neuropsychiatric symptoms as early manifestations of emergent dementia: provisional diagnostic criteria for mild behavioral impairment. *Alzheimers Dement*. 2016;12(2):195-202.

162. Freitas S, Simoes MR, Alves L, Duro D, Santana I. Montreal Cognitive Assessment (MoCA): validation study for frontotemporal dementia. *J Geriatr Psychiatry Neurol*. 2012;25(3):146-154.

163. Hsieh S, Schubert S, Hoon C, Mioshi E, Hodges JR. Validation of the Addenbrooke's Cognitive Examination III in frontotemporal dementia and Alzheimer's disease. *Dement Geriatr Cogn Disord*. 2013;36(3-4):242-250.

164. Dubois B, Slachevsky A, Litvan I, Pillon B. The FAB: a frontal assessment battery at bedside. *Neurology*. 2000;55(11):1621-1626.

165. Gregory CA, Serra-Mestres J, Hodges JR. Early diagnosis of the frontal variant of frontotemporal dementia: how sensitive are standard neuroimaging and neuropsychologic tests? *Neuropsychiatry Neuropsychol Behav Neurol*. 1999;12(2):128-135.

166. Torralva T, Roca M, Gleichgerrcht E, Bekinschtein T, Manes F. A neuropsychological battery to detect specific executive and social cognitive impairments in early frontotemporal dementia. *Brain*. 2009;132(pt 5):1299-1309.

167. Funkiewiez A, Bertoux M, de Souza LC, Levy R, Dubois B. The SEA (Social cognition and Emotional Assessment): a clinical neuropsychological tool for early diagnosis of frontal variant of frontotemporal lobar degeneration. *Neuropsychology*. 2012;26(1):81-90.

168. Kortte KB, Rogalski EJ. Behavioural interventions for enhancing life participation in behavioural variant frontotemporal dementia and primary progressive aphasia. *Int Rev Psychiatry*. 2013;25(2):237-245.

169. Wicklund MR, Mokri B, Drubach DA, Boeve BF, Parisi JE, Josephs KA. Frontotemporal brain sagging syndrome: an SIH-like presentation mimicking FTD. *Neurology*. 2011;76(16):1377-1382.

170. Hu WT, Chen-Plotkin A, Grossman M, et al. Novel CSF biomarkers for frontotemporal lobar degenerations. *Neurology*. 2011;75(23):2079-2086.

171. Klunk WE, Engler H, Nordberg A, et al. Imaging brain amyloid in Alzheimer's disease with Pittsburgh compound-B. *Ann Neurol*. 2004;55(3):306-319.

172. Small GW, Kepe V, Ercoli LM, et al. PET of brain amyloid and tau in mild cognitive impairment. *N Engl J Med*. 2006;355(25):2652-2663.

173. Chien DT, Bahri S, Szardenings AK, et al. Early clinical PET imaging results with the novel PHF-tau radioligand [F-18]-T807. *J Alzheimers Dis*. 2013;34(2):457-468.

174. Maruyama M, Shimada H, Suhara T, et al. Imaging of tau pathology in a tauopathy mouse model and in Alzheimer patients compared to normal controls. *Neuron*. 2013;79(6):1094-1108.

175. Fodero-Tavoletti MT, Okamura N, Furumoto S, et al. 18F-THK523: a novel in vivo tau imaging ligand for Alzheimer's disease. *Brain*. 2011;134(pt 4):1089-1100.

176. Kertesz A, McMonagle P, Blair M, Davidson W, Munoz DG. The evolution and pathology of frontotemporal dementia. *Brain*. 2005;128(pt 9):1996-2005.

177. Knibb JA, Xuereb JH, Patterson K, Hodges JR. Clinical and pathological characterization of progressive aphasia. *Ann Neurol*. 2006;59(1):156-165.

178. Davies RR, Hodges JR, Kril JJ, Patterson K, Halliday GM, Xuereb JH. The pathological basis of semantic dementia. *Brain*. 2005;128(pt 9):1984-1995.

179. Forman MS, Farmer J, Johnson JK, et al. Frontotemporal dementia: clinicopathological correlations. *Ann Neurol*. 2006;59(6):952-962.

180. Bergeron D, Gorno-Tempini ML, Rabinovici GD, et al. Prevalence of amyloid-beta pathology in distinct variants of primary progressive aphasia. *Ann Neurol.* 2018;84(5):729-740.

181. Caso F, Gesierich B, Henry M, et al. Nonfluent/agrammatic PPA with in-vivo cortical amyloidosis and Pick's disease pathology. *Behav Neurol.* 2013;26(1-2):95-106.

182. Mesulam MM, Dickerson BC, Sherman JC, et al. Case 1-2017. A 70-year-old woman with gradually progressive loss of language. *N Engl J Med.* 2017;376(2):158-167.

183. Seeley WW, Bauer AM, Miller BL, et al. The natural history of temporal variant frontotemporal dementia. *Neurology.* 2005;64(8):1384-1390.

184. Grasbeck A, Englund E, Horstmann V, Passant U, Gustafson L. Predictors of mortality in frontotemporal dementia: a retrospective study of the prognostic influence of pre-diagnostic features. *Int J Geriatr Psychiatry.* 2003;18(7):594-601.

185. Garcin B, Lillo P, Hornberger M, et al. Determinants of survival in behavioral variant frontotemporal dementia. *Neurology.* 2009;73(20):1656-1661.

186. Hu WT, Seelaar H, Josephs KA, et al. Survival profiles of patients with frontotemporal dementia and motor neuron disease. *Arch Neurol.* 2009;66(11):1359-1364.

187. Hodges JR, Mitchell J, Dawson K, et al. Semantic dementia: demography, familial factors and survival in a consecutive series of 100 cases. *Brain.* 2010;133(pt 1):300-306.

188. Xie SX, Forman MS, Farmer J, et al. Factors associated with survival probability in autopsy-proven frontotemporal lobar degeneration. *J Neurol Neurosurg Psychiatry.* 2008;79(2):126-129.

189. Cardarelli R, Kertesz A, Knebl JA. Frontotemporal dementia: a review for primary care physicians. *Am Fam Physician.* 2010;82(11):1372-1377.

190. Wylie MA, Shnall A, Onyike CU, Huey ED. Management of frontotemporal dementia in mental health and multidisciplinary settings. *Int Rev Psychiatry.* 2013;25(2):230-236.

191. Jicha GA, Nelson PT. Management of frontotemporal dementia: targeting symptom management in such a heterogeneous disease requires a wide range of therapeutic options. *Neurodegener Dis Manag.* 2011;1(2):141-156.

192. Piguet O, Hornberger M, Mioshi E, Hodges JR. Behavioural-variant frontotemporal dementia: diagnosis, clinical staging, and management. *Lancet Neurol.* 2011;10(2):162-172.

193. Manoochehri M, Huey ED. Diagnosis and management of behavioral issues in frontotemporal dementia. *Curr Neurol Neurosci Rep.* 2012;12(5):528-536.

194. O'Brien JT, Burns A, Group BAPDC. Clinical practice with anti-dementia drugs: a revised (second) consensus statement from the British Association for Psychopharmacology. *J Psychopharmacol.* 2011;25(8):997-1019.

195. Gitlin LN, Kales HC, Lyketsos CG. Nonpharmacologic management of behavioral symptoms in dementia. *JAMA.* 2012;308(19):2020-2029.

196. Shnall A, Agate A, Grinberg A, Huijbregts M, Nguyen MQ, Chow TW. Development of supportive services for frontotemporal dementias through community engagement. *Int Rev Psychiatry.* 2013;25(2):246-252.

197. Henry ML, Hubbard HI, Grasso SM, et al. Retraining speech production and fluency in non-fluent/agrammatic primary progressive aphasia. *Brain.* 2018;141(6):1799-1814.

198. Dowling GA, Merrilees J, Mastick J, Chang VY, Hubbard E, Moskowitz JT. Life enhancing activities for family caregivers of people with frontotemporal dementia. *Alzheimer Dis Assoc Disord.* 2014;28(2):175-181.

199. Mesulam M-M, Wieneke C, Thompson C, Rogalski E, Weintraub S. Quantitative classification of primary progressive aphasia at early and mild impairment stages. *Brain.* 2012;135(pt 5):1537-1553.

25

Delirium and Catatonia

Sejal B. Shah · Nomi C. Levy-Carrick · Ian Steele · Robyn Thom

INTRODUCTION

This chapter comprises the clinical entities of delirium and catatonia. These syndromes, while presenting different and specific pathophysiology and phenomenology, may share a number of characteristics, including subacute alterations in mental status, precipitation by medical comorbidities, need for inpatient level of care, and others. The differential diagnosis and institution of timely and appropriate therapeutic and supportive measures are essential for prognosis.

DELIRIUM

Epidemiology

Delirium, a constellation of symptoms sometimes described in neurologic contexts as encephalopathy, is the most common neuropsychiatric syndrome observed among medically hospitalized patients.[1] Rates of delirium vary based upon setting, with elderly and more severely ill patients at highest risk. Among general medical inpatients, the prevalence of delirium per admission is between 11% and 42%, with a prevalence rate of 10–31% at the time of admission.[2] Among critically ill, mechanically ventilated patients, the prevalence of delirium is upwards of 54%, with some studies citing rates greater than 80%.[3,4] In addition to high rates of delirium among critically ill patients, the syndrome is common among burn patients and nonelective surgical patients, with incidence rates of 39% and greater than 50% respectively.[5,6] Delirium affects up to 85% of terminally ill patients during their final few weeks of life.[7]

Significant risk factors for delirium include age, cognitive impairment including both mild cognitive disorder and dementia, high degree of illness severity, visual impairment, urinary catheterization, nutritional deficiency, and length of hospital stay.[8,9] Neither genetic factors nor family history is known to contribute to the risk of developing delirium. The relationship between sociodemographic factors (e.g., race, socioeconomic status [SES], and education) and delirium is unclear.[10]

Pathophysiology

As delirium symptoms arise secondary to underlying etiologies and are often multifactorial, the pathophysiology remains complex and variable across patient populations, as it can be for an individual patient over time. Complementary processes of inflammation, oxidative stress, hypoxia, and a variety of toxic-metabolic insults contribute to increased vulnerability of brain circuits and structures to impairment: delirium is the final common neurobehavioral pathway of these systemic disturbances.[11]

Clinical Presentation

Phenomenology

Delirium is an acute confusional state caused by an underlying physiologic disturbance. According to the Diagnostic and Statistical Manual of Mental Disorders, fifth edition (DSM-5),[12] delirium is characterized by a disturbance in consciousness (attention and awareness) accompanied by at least one other cognitive deficit, that develops over a short period of time, fluctuates, and cannot be accounted for by a preexisting cognitive disorder. The phenomenology of delirium is varied, as a range of cognitive impairments can be observed, including deficits in memory, language, and visuospatial processing. Psychotic symptoms such as hallucinations, delusions, or paranoia occur in more than 40% of delirious patients.[13] In addition to alterations in consciousness and cognition, derangements of the sleep-wake cycle, emotional instability, and psychomotor changes are often observed. There are three motor subtypes of delirium: hyperactive, hypoactive, and mixed.[14] Hyperactive delirium is characterized by hyperactivity, restlessness, and hypervigilance, while hypoactive delirium is characterized by lethargy, psychomotor slowing, and apathy. In mixed delirium, features of both hyperactive and hypoactive delirium are observed. While hyperactive delirium is most readily recognized, it accounts for only 25% of delirium cases, and hypoactive/mixed delirium is associated with poorer outcomes.[15] See Boxes 25-1 and 25-2 for key features and common etiologies of delirium.

CASE VIGNETTE 25.1

Mr. X is a 70-year-old man with a history of depression, anxiety, mild cognitive impairment, restless leg syndrome, restrictive cardiomyopathy, and end-stage renal disease who is admitted for a heart failure exacerbation with the plan to start hemodialysis. He has had difficulty tolerating dialysis. His behavioral manifestations include yelling out, restlessness, irritability, and attempts to remove lines. He complains of cramping and discomfort in his legs. The team is concerned that Mr. X's anxiety has been limiting the success of dialysis; they have been administering diphenhydramine and lorazepam several times per day to address this. Neither of these medications has achieved behavioral control so psychiatry is consulted. On assessment, Mr. X is found to be asleep during the middle of the day. According to nursing staff, his nighttime sleep has been poor. When awakened, his movements and speech are notably slowed.

He is inattentive, frequently glancing around the room, and requiring questions to be repeated. He is oriented only to self and does not recall going to dialysis earlier in the day. He denies perceptual disturbances or paranoia. Laboratory studies are notable for blood urea nitrogen (BUN) level 49, creatinine 3.8, hemoglobin 9.4, and iron 32 μg/dL. He is diagnosed with delirium of multifactorial etiology (uremia and medication effect). The recommendations to the team include reviewing his medication list and discontinuing deliriogenic medications including diphenhydramine and lorazepam. Low-dose olanzapine is started at bedtime to facilitate nighttime sleep and is also dosed prior to dialysis. Iron supplementation is administered and his restless leg symptoms improve. The following day, he is able to tolerate a full run of dialysis, which contributes to a gradual improvement of mental status over the next several days.

BOX 25-1   Key Features of Delirium

- Hallmark symptoms: impaired arousal, attention, and orientation
- Additional symptoms: cognitive impairment (language, perception, memory, spatial, orientation), emotional lability, psychotic symptoms (hallucinations, delusions, paranoia), sleep impairment, psychomotor changes (hyperactive, hypoactive, or both)
- Time course: onset occurs over hours to days, and symptom severity fluctuates throughout the day
- Mental status changes are a direct consequence of another medical condition, substance intoxication, or withdrawal

---

BOX 25-2   Common Etiologies of Delirium

- Medication effect
- Electrolyte disturbance
- Infection
- Reduced sensory input
- Intracranial disorders
- Bowel/Bladder dysfunction
- Cardiopulmonary disorders

Course and Natural History

Although delirium was previously thought to be a transient disorder with a complete return to baseline level of cognitive function once the underlying medical illness was treated, increasing evidence has demonstrated it may have serious and long-term sequelae. These include prolonged hospital length of stay, which increases the risk of medical complications,[16] as well as increased risk of death, institutionalization, and sustained cognitive impairment.[17]

While the average of length of delirium is listed as about 1 week in the *DSM-5*,[11] the symptoms can persist for much longer, and sometimes never completely resolve. A systematic review of rates of persistent delirium in hospitalized older adults (>50 years) reported recovery rates of delirium at 2 weeks, 1 month, 3 months, and 6 months to be 55.3%, 67.2%, 74.4%, and 79% respectively.[18] Thus, it is not uncommon for delirium to persist for weeks to months beyond the time of initial diagnosis. The persistence of delirium after discharge likely impacts mobility, self-care, and adherence to medical care, contributing to the observed poor outcomes associated with delirium.

Prospective epidemiologic studies have demonstrated a bidirectional relationship between delirium and dementia: dementia is an important risk factor for delirium and delirium is strongly associated with a subsequent diagnosis of dementia.[19,20] Whether there is a mechanistic relationship between the two, or whether delirium simply unmasks symptoms of a previously unrecognized dementia, remains controversial. It has been hypothesized that neurotoxic mechanisms that drive delirium (including inflammation, hypoxia, and hypoglycemia) may also directly accelerate neuropathology associated with dementia.[21] In contrast to this hypothesis, a prospective study of greater than 500 patients demonstrated that while delirium increased the risk of incident dementia by more than eightfold, delirium was not clearly associated with neuropathological correlates of dementia such as tau and amyloid burden.[22] A separate study showed that elevated levels of amyloid-β were correlated with long-term subjective cognitive impairment among patients with low levels of inflammatory markers.[23] Taken together, these results demonstrate that the interface between delirium and dementia is complex, likely multifactorial, and driven by pathophysiologic mechanisms that may be both distinct and shared.[21] In addition to cognitive impairment, delirium may be associated with post-traumatic stress disorder (PTSD) and mood disorder, along with cognitive and physical functional deficits that compromise a post-intensive care syndrome.[24]

Assessment and Differential Diagnosis

Clinical Evaluation and Assessment Tools

The gold standard for the diagnosis of delirium is a careful clinical assessment for the key features described above. A clinical assessment for delirium is focused on the review of information regarding acuity of mental status changes, previous history of delirium or cognitive impairment, and precipitating factors. A delirious patient may or may not be able to participate in the interview, depending on the severity of disturbance in attention and awareness. Patients with delirium may provide extraneous information, inadequate information, or may not speak at all. In all these cases, it is important to obtain collateral information through reviewing the record, as well as by speaking with hospital staff and family. It can be helpful to interview the patient in the presence of family, as this allows for group discussion, the opportunity to model how to interact with the delirious patient, and a chance to provide psychoeducation. As many delirious patients cannot provide a coherent narrative, observation is key in performing the mental status exam. Assessment of the patient's appearance, level of consciousness, psychomotor activity, and ability to sustain attention during the interview all provide important diagnostic information.

The diagnosis of delirium relies on a high index of suspicion, as cases frequently go undiagnosed. A study comparing clinical recognition of delirium by nursing staff to research assessments demonstrated that only 31% of delirious cases are identified.[25] Another study demonstrated that 40% of patients referred to a consultation-liaison psychiatry service for depression were found to be delirious.[26] Given the frequency of under- and misdiagnosis of delirium, standardized screening tools that are administered at regular intervals, particularly in high-risk populations, can be helpful in improving detection and prompting further consultation. Multiple screening tools, including the Confusion Assessment Method (CAM), Confusion Assessment Method for the Intensive Care Unit (CAM-ICU), Intensive Care Delirium Screening Checklist (ICDSC), and Delirium Rating Scale-Revised-98 (DRS-R-98), have been validated for use by nonpsychiatric clinicians to screen for delirium. Among the multiple screening tools available, a recent systematic review examining the accuracy of 11 such instruments demonstrated that the CAM, which takes 5 minutes to administer, had the best supportive data as a bedside screening tool (positive likelihood ratio [LR] 9.6; 95% confidence interval [CI], 5.8–16.0; negative LR 0.16; 95% CI, 0.09–0.29).[27] Although this is an ongoing area of research, there is currently no biomarker or bedside procedure with high sensitivity and specificity for delirium. Generalized slowing observed on electroencephalography (EEG) studies can support a diagnosis delirium; however, these results must be interpreted within the clinical context, as the false negative and false positive rates each approach 20%.[28] Recent research into the role of continuous EEG (cEEG) in the diagnosis of delirium in septic patients supports the association of neuronal desynchronization and loss of power in high-frequency EEG

activity with delirium. It further suggests the possibility that the beta band may be a simple indicator of non-delirium in select ICU patients with sepsis. The absence of delirium was independently associated with preserved high-frequency beta activity (>13 Hz).[29]

Differential Diagnosis

Newly diagnosed delirium should be considered a neuropsychiatric emergency, as it can signal an underlying life-threatening illness. Once the diagnosis of delirium is made—or suspected—the differential diagnoses of the underlying medical factors contributing to its onset should be undertaken. Although virtually any physiologic disturbance can result in decompensated brain function, some of the most common modifiable contributors to delirium include medication effect (intoxication or withdrawal), electrolyte disturbances, infections, reduced sensory input, intracranial disorders, bowel/bladder dysfunction, and cardiopulmonary disorders.[15] While numerous medications have been associated with delirium, commonly prescribed deliriogenic medication classes include analgesics (e.g., opioids), anticholinergics (e.g., diphenhydramine, atropine, benzotropine, tricyclics), stimulants (e.g., amphetamines, pseudoephedrine), and sedative-hypnotics (e.g., benzodiazepines, barbiturates) (Table 25-1). The need for laboratory tests and imaging should

TABLE 25-1 • Common Deliriogenic Medication Classes.		
Class	**Type**	**Examples**
Anxiolytic, sedative-hypnotic	Benzodiazepine	Midazolam Alprazolam Lorazepam
Analgesics	Narcotics	Meperidine, tramadol
	NSAIDs	Ibuprofen
Antihistamines		Diphenhydramine
		Hydroxyzine
Gastrointestinal agents	Antispasmodics	Loperamide Dicyclomine
	H2-blockers	Famotidine Cimetidine Ranitidine
Antibiotics	Fluoroquinolones	Levofloxacin Ciprofloxacin
Psychotropics	Tricyclic antidepressants	Amitriptyline Nortriptyline
		Lithium
Steroids		Prednisone Dexamethasone
Cardiovascular agents	Antiarrhythmics	Amiodarone
	Digitalis	
	Antihypertensives (i.e., beta-blockers)	Metoprolol
Anticonvulsants	Barbiturates	
Anti-parkinsonians		Benztropine Trihexyphenidyl
Antinausea meds		Scopolamine

be determined based on the clinical history and physical exam. Commonly obtained studies include a complete blood count (CBC), electrolytes, blood-urea-nitrogen and creatinine, liver enzymes, urinalysis, chest radiography, and electrocardiography. Brain imaging should be obtained if there is a history of trauma or focal neurological deficits are identified. EEG may be considered if the history is suspicious for seizures or less specific alterations in mental status with no clear etiology (which could represent non-convulsive status). Additional tests should be considered based on clinical judgment.

The neuropsychiatric differential diagnosis for etiologies contributing to delirium should include dementia, primary psychiatric illness, acute neurologic illness (e.g., stroke or seizure), and psychiatric symptoms attributable to a medical illness (e.g., neuropsychiatric systemic lupus erythematosus, previously classified as lupus cerebritis). Syndromes from these classes often co-occur.[15]

Regarding its differential diagnosis with primary psychiatric illness: Because the presentation of delirium may span multiple neuropsychiatric domains including cognitive, affective, and psychotic symptoms, delirium is frequently under- or misdiagnosed. When delirium presents with psychotic symptoms, it can be mistakenly diagnosed as a primary psychotic disorder. The psychomotor restlessness observed in hyperactive delirium can mimic mania, while the apathy, withdrawal, and psychomotor retardation of hypoactive delirium can mimic depression. Phenomenological features that are specific to delirium and not typically present in primary psychiatric illness include evolution of symptoms over a short time course (hours to days), disturbance in consciousness, waxing and waning time course (over minutes to hours), and an underlying medical illness or toxic exposure. It can also be helpful to consider the risk factors, typical presentation, and natural history of the primary psychiatric illness in question. For example, onset of a primary psychotic illness (e.g., schizophrenia) after the age of 60 is extremely rare. Finally, it should be noted that the presence of delirium and a primary psychiatric illness are not mutually exclusive. Definitively establishing the diagnosis of a comorbid psychiatric illness in the presence of active delirium is challenging due to the wide array of neuropsychiatric symptoms seen in delirium. Therefore, treatment of delirium and addressing its underlying medical illness should take precedence.

Features that would suggest primary neurologic illness include new focal neurologic findings on exam, or sustained deficits that do not wax/wane or improve as the presumed underlying etiology is addressed.

Treatment

Identification and Management of Underlying Cause(s) and Perpetuating Factors

The definitive treatment of delirium is the identification and treatment of the underlying medical illness. Often, however, the underlying etiology may not be readily apparent. Furthermore, delirium is rarely caused by a single factor; it is more often the final result of multiple insults. Thus, while addressing the underlying illness is paramount, medical treatment must also address precipitating and contributing factors, such as noxious

brain insults that occur during the hospitalization, which also serve to sustain delirium. A prospective cohort study identified five independent contributing factors for delirium including use of physical restraints (RR 4.4; 95% CI, 2.5–7.9), malnutrition (RR 4.0; 95% CI, 2.2–7.4), initiation of more than three medications during the period 48–24 hours before the onset of delirium (RR 2.9; 95% CI, 1.6–5.4), use of a bladder catheter (RR 2.4; 95% CI, 1.2–4.7), and any iatrogenic event defined as an illness or harmful occurrence that was not a consequence of the underlying illness such as a hospital-acquired infection, medication-related complication, and unintentional injury (RR 1.9; 95% CI, 1.1–3.2).[30]

Routine care of a delirious patient should deliberately target these five common precipitating factors. Behavioral interventions, such as providing a calm environment, frequent reorientation, provision of sensory aids (hearing aids and glasses), and protection of the sleep-wake cycle, should be implemented to reduce confusion and agitation, which often lead to utilization of physical restraints. Catheters and lines should be removed or replaced as soon as medically appropriate. Supportive measures, including addressing nutritional and volume status, should also be implemented. Nutritional deficiencies, particularly thiamine (vitamin B1), can lead to a myriad of mental status changes including delirium. Thiamine deficiency should be suspected not only in alcoholism, but also in any condition that results in malnutrition, including anorexia nervosa, orofacial cancers, gastric bypass surgery, and gastrointestinal cancers.[31] Early mobilization and deep vein thrombosis prophylaxis are important to reduce iatrogenic risks including deep vein thrombosis, pressure ulcers, and aspiration pneumonias. Finally, a thorough medication reconciliation should be performed, with attention to deliriogenic medication classes, potential medication interactions, and any recent changes including new medications, discontinued medications, or dose changes.

Symptomatic Treatment by Medication Class

1. Antipsychotics

Although there is no FDA-approved medication for the treatment of delirium, antipsychotics are the most commonly used class of medication to manage its symptoms while the underlying inciting and perpetuating medical etiologies are being addressed. The use of antipsychotics for the treatment of delirium remains controversial: While recent high-quality systematic reviews and meta-analyses have demonstrated that antipsychotics have not been shown to impact delirium incidence, duration, severity, or hospital length of stay,[32,33] we currently lack data on the effect of antipsychotics on patient-centered measures of delirium, including their effect on psychotic symptoms, emotional distress, and long-term functional outcomes. Clinical experience and multiple consensus statements including those by the American Psychiatric Association (APA), Canadian Coalition for Seniors' Mental Health (CCSMH), and the National Institute for Health and Care Excellence (NICE), suggest using antipsychotics to target specific symptoms of delirium when the symptoms incite patient distress, pose an immediate physical safety risk, or impeded the delivery of medical care. In these cases, it is

TABLE 25-2 • Antipsychotics Commonly Used in the Symptomatic Treatment of Delirium.[92]					
Antipsychotic	Route	Half-Life	Starting Dose	Maximum Daily Dose	Special Considerations
Haloperidol	PO, IV, IM	14–30 hours	0.5–1 mg BID	Upper limit has not been established	Minimal effect on vital signs; higher EPS risk
Quetiapine	PO	6–7 hours	12.5–25 mg BID	800 mg	Less likely to affect motor symptoms of Parkinson's; sedating
Risperidone	PO, ODT	20–30 hours	0.5 mg BID PRN	8 mg	Dose adjusted for renal dysfunction
Olanzapine	PO, ODT, IM	30 hours	2.5–5 mg BID	20 mg	Avoid in patients receiving parenteral benzodiazepines; has antiemetic properties; sedating

IM, intramuscular; IV, intravenous; ODT, oral dissolving tablets; PO, per os, oral formulation. Note that this may also be crushed and administered through percutaneous endoscopic gastrostomy (PEG).

reasonable to embark on a judicious, time-limited trial of antipsychotics to target specific symptoms such as insomnia, hallucinations, paranoia, delusions, or psychomotor agitation.

As no single antipsychotic has been demonstrated to be superior in treating delirium, selection of the antipsychotic agent should be based upon optimization of the medication's pharmacodynamics, side-effect profile, and available route of administration to the clinical situation. See Table 25-2 for a summary comparison of antipsychotics that may be used in delirium. In cases of extreme agitation, intravenous administration may be required to achieve rapid and reliable drug serum levels. Haloperidol can be administered intravenously, intramuscularly, or orally, and has been demonstrated to have minimal effects of vital signs, negligible anticholinergic activity, and minimal medication interactions; thus, it may be most appropriate for medically unstable or critically ill patients.[34] Time to onset of haloperidol is 30–60 minutes, with peak action occurring between 2 and 6 hours after administration. Risks of haloperidol include increased likelihood of extrapyramidal symptoms (EPS) as compared with lower potency or second-generation antipsychotics. For patients who have difficulty swallowing tablets, both risperidone and olanzapine are available in dissolvable tablet preparations. Patients who have insomnia may benefit from more sedating antipsychotics dosed at bedtime, such as olanzapine or quetiapine. In terms of disease-specific considerations, cancer patients receiving chemotherapy often benefit from the antiemetic properties of olanzapine.[35] Parkinson's patients are best treated with low-potency antipsychotics, such as quetiapine, as they are less likely to worsen the motor symptoms of Parkinson's (though they may be also less robust in addressing psychotic symptoms).[36]

When administering antipsychotics, it is important to monitor whether treatment targets are achieved, and to adjust the medication and dose accordingly. Additionally, patients should be carefully monitored for antipsychotic-class side effects. Three of the most serious medical risks of antipsychotic use include prolonged QTc interval, EPS, and neuroleptic malignant syndrome (NMS). QTc prolongation, particularly in patients with medical illness, has been associated with lethal ventricular arrhythmias, such as torsades de pointes (TdP). While all antipsychotics can increase the QTc interval, absolute increases

tend to be modest, ranging from a 5 to 20 ms increase, with ziprasidone being associated with the greatest QTc prolongation.[37] It is important to obtain a baseline EKG prior to administration of antipsychotics, address modifiable risk factors for prolonged QTc (e.g., replete electrolytes, minimize other medications that prolong QTc), and reassess the QTc interval after initiating an antipsychotic to ensure it has not significantly increased. Patients must also be monitored for EPS, including acute dystonia and akathisia, which can exacerbate symptoms of restlessness in delirium. Finally, all patients who are newly initiated on antipsychotic treatment must be routinely assessed for NMS, a rare but life-threatening condition, characterized by lead-pipe rigidity, fever, mental status changes, and autonomic instability.[38] If NMS is suspected, the antipsychotic medication should be immediately discontinued and aggressive supportive care should be instituted.

Finally, as the response to antipsychotics can be variable, they should be initiated at low doses and used on an as-needed basis for the minimum time required. If only partial responses are achieved, the dose may be gradually increased up to the daily maximum limits while monitoring for side effects. For cases of severe or prolonged delirium, if as-needed doses are being used regularly, it may be necessary to institute routine doses. However, in all cases, antipsychotics should be used for the minimal duration necessary and a clear plan for taper or discontinuation must be arranged prior to discharge.

2. Non-antipsychotics: Benzodiazepines, alpha agonists, and antiepileptics

Although antipsychotic medications are most commonly used for the management of delirium symptoms, other classes of medications may be helpful in certain clinical situations. Benzodiazepines are typically discontinued during acute delirium due to their propensity to perpetuate delirium, but they are the preferred agent in the treatment of delirium that is due to alcohol or benzodiazepine withdrawal. When benzodiazepines are administered, patients must be carefully monitored for signs of benzodiazepine toxicity including nystagmus, oversedation (leading to respiratory depression), slurred speech, and ataxia.

Dexmedetomidine, a parenterally administered selective alpha-2 agonist, which is used as an alternative or augmenting sedation strategy in intensive care settings, has been demonstrated in randomized controlled trials to decrease the incidence and duration of delirium when compared with benzodiazepines.[39,40] Due to the risk of bradycardia and hypotension associated with dexmedetomidine, it is used exclusively in intensive care settings. Clonidine, an oral alpha-2 agonist, has less CNS selectivity than dexmedetomidine, but can be safely administered in non-intensive care unit settings. While initial pilot data suggests that transitioning from dexmedetomidine to enteral clonidine in ICU patients is safe and feasible,[41] the role of clonidine in the treatment of non-ICU delirium has not been well studied. A randomized controlled trial comparing clonidine to placebo in elderly delirious general medical patients is currently underway.[42]

Among patients for whom antipsychotics are poorly tolerated or relatively contraindicated (e.g., history of NMS, prolonged QTc in an unstable cardiac patient), antiepileptic drugs may be considered for the management of agitation associated with delirium. A retrospective study has demonstrated that valproic acid is effective in reducing agitation and duration of delirium.[43] Valproic acid may be administered either orally or intravenously. It may be a particularly favorable choice in patients with suspected seizures or seizure risk factors, history of head injury, or comorbid mood disorder. Baseline liver enzymes and CBCs should be obtained prior to initiating it; two common side effects that warrant monitoring are hyperammonemia (19%) and thrombocytopenia (13%).[44]

Psychotherapy

As discussed above, prolonged states of delirium in critically ill patients may be associated with symptoms of PTSD, including nightmares, panic attacks, low mood, and flashbacks.[44] A cohort study demonstrated that the development of PTSD and panic symptoms post-intensive care unit stay was associated with delusional memories of the intensive care experience.[45] Although research on the effect of psychotherapy to treat longer-term psychiatric sequelae after delirium remains in its infancy, ICU diaries have emerged as one potential low-cost psychotherapeutic tool. An ICU diary is a diary written in everyday language for patients by staff and family members, describing events that occurred during an ICU stay. It is often accompanied by photographs of the patient's surroundings in the intensive care unit. The goal of the diary is to help patients reconcile frightening or delusional memories with the care and treatments they received while sedated or ventilated. The feasibility of implementing this type of intervention and its effects on mental health outcomes remain controversial, with some studies citing benefit and others demonstrating minimal effect on long-term outcomes.[46,47] A multicenter, randomized controlled trial assessing the effect of an ICU diary on patients' and families' symptoms of PTSD, anxiety, and depression symptoms is currently underway.[48]

CATATONIA

Introduction

Catatonia has been described in the literature for almost 150 years. The term was first coined by Dr. Karl Ludwig Kahlbaum

in 1874.[49] Catatonia is a syndrome comprised by a cluster of motor symptoms brought about by a wide variety of illnesses. Originally it was thought to be due to psychiatric illness, mainly schizophrenia, and for many years it was labelled as a subtype of schizophrenia (schizophrenia, catatonic type). However, over the past decades, it has become clear that catatonia can be a manifestation of a spectrum of neuropsychiatric and medical illnesses. Catatonia is currently a separate entity in the *DSM-5*. The *DSM-5* categorizes catatonia subtypes with specifiers based upon underlying etiologies. These subtypes are "Catatonia associated with another mental disorder" (e.g., depression, schizophrenia, etc.); "Catatonic disorder due to another medical condition" (e.g., hepatic encephalopathy, etc.); and "Unspecified catatonia," used when the underlying etiology is unclear, full criteria for catatonia are not met, or there is insufficient information to make a more specific diagnosis.[11] Two other types of catatonia present in the literature, idiopathic and periodic catatonia,[50,51] are much rarer and the subject of debate. Idiopathic catatonia is catatonia that has no identified medical or psychiatric cause and would be labeled "Unspecified catatonia" in the *DSM-5*.

Epidemiology

Prevalence and Incidence

The overall prevalence of catatonia is difficult to determine because it varies based upon the setting in which catatonia is studied (inpatient psychiatry units, medical units, outpatient, etc.). Furthermore, depending on the setting, the etiologies of catatonia in each can be quite different. Acknowledging this bias, we will discuss the prevalence of catatonia and the range of etiologies based on the different settings. The prevalence of catatonia in inpatient psychiatry units is roughly 10%, though studies show ranges from 4.8% to 20%.[52-57] The most common etiologies appear to be primary affective disorders followed by primary psychotic disorders, but medical/neurological etiologies are also found in these settings. The leading psychiatric illness in cases of catatonia due to psychiatric illness is bipolar disorder (20.1–46%).[57-59] The next most common one is schizophrenia (20–33%),[57,59,60] followed by schizoaffective disorder (2–6%),[57,59] and major depressive disorder (2.9–18%).[59] Other psychiatric conditions with much lower numbers include Tourette syndrome, anxiety spectrum disorders, and OCD.[61]

The recognition of nonpsychiatric causes of catatonia has led to an increase in its diagnosis in acute medical settings. When looking at patients admitted to a general medical hospital, the prevalence appears to be roughly 4–5%[62,63]; but ranges from 1.6% to 6.3%.[64] The etiologies of catatonia in patients on medical/surgical floors are more likely to be from neurological or medical problems than psychiatric illness, with a ratio up to 3:1.[52,65,66] Within this population, the most common etiologies appear to be: encephalitis (25–38.2%)[52,66–68]; central nervous system structural abnormalities (up to 30%)[64]; psychiatric disorder (17%)[52]; epilepsy (8–15%)[52,64,67]; and drug/medication-related conditions (10.29%).[52]

Risk and Associated Factors

There is currently minimal data showing any direct associations between genetic links or hereditary influence, and catatonia.

The two leading psychiatric causes of catatonia are bipolar disorder and schizophrenia, both of which have a strong hereditary component. This suggests that a related hereditary component may be present in catatonia. Periodic catatonia (defined under atypical presentations below), for instance, seems to be associated with a high familial incidence of psychoses in first-degree relatives.[51] Other factors associated with an increased risk for developing catatonia include exposure to infections during perinatal period,[61] previous episodes of catatonia,[61] a history of experiencing EPS from antipsychotics, and a recent substantial weight loss (>5% loss of body weight in 3 weeks or >20% loss of body weight in 6 months).[61]

Demographic Characteristics

There does not seem to be a gender difference in catatonia due to a psychiatric illness. Idiopathic catatonia seems to be more likely in females.[51] Patients with chronic psychotic disorders tend to have lower levels of education, income, and SES. Catatonia due to chronic psychotic disorders is likely associated with these factors as well. Among the neurological/medical population, there does not appear to be any association between demographic factors and catatonia. The one exception may be in catatonia due to anti-NMDA receptor encephalitis, since this entity is far more common in women (up to 80% of cases).[54]

Pathophysiology

Neurostructural Aspects

Several areas of the cortex have been implicated in catatonia. Involved dysfunctional areas within the frontal cortex may include the dorsolateral prefrontal cortex (PFC),[69] left lateral PFC,[70] anterior cingulate cortex,[54,71] the motor system (primary motor and supplementary motor areas),[53,71] and orbitofrontal PFC.[50,53] The parietal cortex, most commonly in the right hemisphere, has also been associated with symptoms of catatonia.[50,54]

The subcortical areas thought to be involved in the pathophysiology of catatonia include the basal ganglia,[54] the thalamus,[71] anterior cingulate cortex,[54,71] the cerebellum,[55,61] and the pons and brainstem areas.[61]

Several pathways may be implicated in the development of catatonia. They include the anterior cingulate and medial orbitofrontal circuit (limbic)[54,71]; medial orbital PFC to the amygdala[72]; the orbital PFC to the basal ganglia[69]; the orbital PFC to the parietal cortex[69]; the orbital PFC to the premotor and motor areas[61]; and the cerebellum/pons to the frontal network by way of the thalamus.[61]

Neurotransmitters

A few main neurotransmitters have been implicated in the pathophysiology of catatonia. There is evidence of major alterations and abnormal reactivity of GABA-A receptors in right orbitofrontal, motor cortex, anterior cingulate gyrus, and right parietal cortex in patients with catatonia.[50,53,69–71] There are also high densities of GABA-ergic neurons in the thalamus, basal ganglia, pons, and cerebellum that are involved in catatonic symptoms.[61] It may not be a simple deficit of GABA-A receptors, but also an imbalance of GABA-A (decreased) and GABA-B (increased) receptor activity that leads to catatonia.[61]

While dopamine has been largely implicated in catatonia, the mechanism of its involvement is not fully understood. It may be dependent upon the underlying etiology (psychiatric vs. medical), which may play a role in the alterations of dopamine activity during the catatonic state. There are high densities of dopamine receptors and neurons in the frontal circuitry and basal ganglia. Alterations in dopamine in the frontal networks can lead to dysfunction of other areas by way of the neuronal circuits, and vice versa.[61,69]

Glutamate has also been implicated in catatonia. The orbitofrontal and parietal circuitry have glutamatergic connections, and alterations in activity of glutamate lead to various symptoms of catatonia. Glutamate is also thought be involved in catatonia based on therapeutic efficacy of glutamatergic substances like amantadine in the treatment of catatonia.[70]

Symptom Neurobiology

Studies have often divided the symptoms of catatonia into three categories (motor, behavioral, and emotional) when linking them to the areas of the brain thought to be contributing.

The "motor" symptoms, including akinesia, posturing, and catalepsy, have been linked to dysfunction of the right parietal and the orbital prefrontal cortices.[50,69,72] The right parietal cortex is involved in the spatial awareness of one's body. An insult to this region can lead to anosognosia (i.e., lack of awareness of one's condition). Patients with catatonia can be viewed as having "motor anosognosia" (i.e., they remain unaware of their postures) due to right parietal dysfunction.[50,70] The orbital PFC was found to have decreased connections with the premotor and motor areas, which may lead to symptoms of akinesia.[50] The motor loop (which includes connections from motor cortex/supplemental motor area to putamen, from putamen to internal pallidum, and from there via mediodorsal thalamic nuclei back to motor cortex/supplemental motor area) was found to remain intact in patients with catatonia, but becomes downregulated by dysfunction of the orbital PFC due to transmitter alterations (i.e., GABA and DA).[50] Deficits in self-monitoring may be also associated with motor problems, linked to dysfunction in the lateral orbital PFC, the cingulate gyrus, and dorsolateral PFC.[50,61] Alterations of dopamine activity and decreased density of GABA-A receptors in the right DLPFC, the orbitofrontal cortex, and posterior parietal cortex[70,73] may be also associated with catatonia motor symptoms.

Regarding the "behavioral" symptoms of catatonia, the echophenomena (echolalia/echopraxia defined as mimicking of examiner's movements/speech) have been associated with dysfunction in the activity of motor mirror neurons.[73] Several symptoms stem from inability to inhibit behaviors, both internally motivated (i.e., perseveration, stereotypies) and externally motivated (i.e., mitmeghen, defined as exaggerated movements in response to light finger pressure despite instructions to the contrary), and this may be associated with dysfunction of the lateral orbital PFC.[50]

The "emotional" symptoms (intense anxiety, fear, euphoria, etc.) have been linked to altered functioning in the orbital PFC, right DLPFC, vmPFC, and the connections between the amygdala and orbital PFC.[50,55,73] Neurotransmitters abnormalities related to the affective symptoms seem significantly associated with decreased GABA-A receptors density in the DLPFC, which is involved during negative emotional processing.[50,53,71,73]

Clinical Presentation

Phenomenology

Currently, there are 23 symptoms that make up the syndrome of catatonia including excitement, immobility/stupor, mutism, staring, grimacing, stereotypy, mannerisms, rigidity, negativism (automatic resistance to instructions or attempts to examine the patient/does exact opposite of instruction), withdrawal, posturing/catalepsy, echopraxia/echolalia, verbigeration (i.e., repetition of phrases or sentences like a scratched record), waxy flexibility, impulsivity, automatic obedience, mitgehen, gegenhalten (resistance to passive movement, which is proportional to strength of stimulus and appears automatic rather than willful), ambitendency (the patient appears motorically "stuck" in indecisive, hesitant movements), grasp reflex, perseveration, combativeness, and autonomic abnormality.[49,69] Phenomenologically, catatonia is described as three different subtypes: stuporous, excited, or mixed (showing both stuporous and excited symptoms).[54]

The most common symptoms present in individuals with catatonia are staring (87%), immobility/stupor (90.6%), mutism (84.4%), and withdrawal (90%).[52,53,74] In addition to the physical symptoms, patients will often have concurrent psychotic symptoms (present in roughly 77% of patients with catatonia), which often go unnoticed given the mutism and stupor.[50,53] The studies did not comment on whether the high prevalence of psychotic symptoms was higher in psychiatric or medical etiologies. After their catatonia has been treated, patients have retrospectively reported that during the catatonic state, the dominating emotion was anxiety due to paranoia, hallucinations, depressive mood, or traumatic experiences. Other emotions that have been reported include extreme joy, depression, euphoria, and erotomania.[50,70]

As previously noted, the list of possible etiologies of catatonia is vast and varies according to the clinical context. There have been studies comparing the presentation of catatonia in patients with a primary psychiatric etiology and those with a primary neurologic/medical disorder. They have many overlapping symptoms, but some symptoms present more or less frequently based on the underlying etiology.

Both patients with catatonia due to primary psychiatric and medical disorders present with similarly high rates of immobility, mutism, staring, posturing, negativism, and withdrawal. Patients with psychiatric disorders may present higher rates of ambitendency, mitgehen, and automatic obedience.[52] Psychiatric patients more often present with the stuporous type, while medical patients more often exhibit a mixed type of catatonia.[52] Medical patients have higher rates of rigidity, excitement, grimacing, and echopraxia/echolalia. They also appear to have higher rates of perseveration, combativeness, grasp reflex, autonomic instability, and verbigeration (though the rates of these are low overall, 11–26%).[52]

When using the Bush-Francis Catatonia Rating Scale (BFCRS), medical patients generally present more symptoms than psychiatric patients, and greater severity. Patients who were in the medical wards (catatonia due to medical or neurological problems) had longer rates of stays and more days with catatonia versus psychiatric patients.[52] The medical patients with severe catatonia had higher levels of creatine phosphokinase (CK) and white blood cell counts than patients in whom the severe catatonia was due to a psychiatric illness.[52]

Atypical Presentations

Idiopathic catatonia is a type of catatonia that does not appear to have any identifiable underlying diagnosable psychiatric or medical condition. When compared to catatonic patients with schizophrenia or depression, idiopathic catatonic patients are more likely to be female, have shorter duration of illness, and lower psychopathology scores on the Brief Psychiatric Rating Scale (BPRS). Higher rates of catatonic symptoms of negativism, waxy flexibility, mitgehen, and ambitendency have been noted.[51]

Periodic catatonia tends to present with psychotic symptoms, though the course and symptom presentation appear distinct. Patients tend to alternate between stupor and excitement in a very rapid manner (minutes to days). They can also have symptoms of impulsivity, affective tension, parakinesis (the incorporation of a choreiform or involuntary movement into a voluntary one), stiff/choppy movements, grimaces especially in the upper face, iterative motor stereotypes, and negativism. There have been reports describing phases of catatonic symptoms that quickly alternate between periods of being asymptomatic to symptomatic and back, even appearing catatonic one day and then completely asymptomatic the next.[51,61,75]

Anti-NMDA receptor antibody encephalitis is a type of autoimmune encephalitis precipitated by anti-NMDA receptor-1 antibodies that can lead to psychiatric symptomatology like catatonia. It can often appear at first as a first break psychosis, then progress to catatonia. The time course tends to have a more rapid onset and progression. There is an association with many underlying medical conditions (e.g., most commonly ovarian teratomas), but the exact mechanism of anti-NMDA antibody encephalitis in relation to its catatonic/psychiatric symptoms remains unclear.[54]

Common Medical Comorbidities due to Catatonia

In addition to treating catatonia itself, prophylaxis and/or treatment of comorbidities associated with catatonia is vital. In patients presenting with a stuporous catatonia, the lack of eating and drinking for a prolonged period can lead to dehydration, metabolic derangements, constipation, severe weight loss, thiamine deficiency, and cardiovascular collapse. If patients are immobile for long periods of time, complications such as decubitus ulcers, contractures, and deep vein thrombosis/pulmonary emboli may occur. In patients with a more excited catatonia, excessive motor activity can lead to hyperthermia, seizures, or death. Aspiration pneumonia and other infections can be common in these patients.[54,62,69] Medical catatonic patients appear to have higher rates of concomitant complications compared to psychiatric patients.[52] Malignant catatonia, a particularly severe form, is further characterized by fever and increasing autonomic instability and is associated with mortality rates as high as 75–100% in some studies.[61,62]

Symptoms of Cognitive Dysfunction

Along with motor symptoms, there are also specific cognitive abnormalities in acute catatonia, and appear to be separate from the underlying etiology. Interestingly, in akinetic catatonia, the lack of meaningful responses to external stimuli should not be interpreted as a lack of awareness of surroundings. Many patients who have experienced catatonia and were successfully treated report that they were completely aware during their catatonic period and can retrospectively talk about their experience in great detail,[50,53] demonstrating no deficits in their general awareness or episodic memory. Neurocognitive studies of patients post treatment of akinetic catatonia found no issues with general intelligence, attention, executive function, and non-right parietal visual-spatial ability. However, catatonic patients showed significantly lower performance in visual-object space and perception tests related to the right parietal cortical area (Visual-Object-Space and Perception Test, VOSP), and problems with working memory.[76] There are also deficits with emotionally guided decisions, thought to be related to orbital PFC dysfunction.[50]

Retrospective subjective reports indicate that patients were not aware of any alterations in their movements and felt that their movements were "normal." Patients have also reported that despite long periods of posturing, there was no experience of being tired, experiencing pain, or increased sensation of effort.[50]

Course and Natural History

Untreated catatonia can last for weeks, months, and even years. More timely diagnosis and effective treatments have contributed to a shortening of its course.[61,75] When untreated, patients will often appear disheveled, cachectic (depending on duration), and incontinent.[53,75] Left untreated, it can lead to severe medical complications and death.[75]

Assessment and Differential Diagnosis

Scales

The assessment of patients for possible catatonia is largely clinical, and benefits from the utilization of rating scales. There are several rating scales for catatonia, and each has its own benefits and limits, often based on the setting or patient population.

The most commonly used scale is the BFCRS.[77] This is a 23-item scale that assesses for the symptoms of catatonia. The scale also has a screening instrument built in. The screening instrument (first 14 symptoms on the scale) are scored as either "absent or present." If two or more of these symptoms are present for 24 hours or longer, catatonia is considered a possibility. All items on the BFCRS are also rated on a scale from 0 to 3 points, with higher scores correlating with a higher severity of catatonia.[77,78] It is important to note that the scale is a screening tool and the diagnosis should also include a physical exam and review of medications and laboratory data.

Other scales were developed to help with the diagnosis of catatonia in certain conditions but are not as widely used in clinical practice. The Rogers Catatonia Scale (RCS)[79] was designed specifically to help diagnose catatonia in depressed patients. One caveat to using this scale is that it has to be done in conjunction with a standard neuromotor examination.[78] The Modified

Rogers Scale (MRS)[80,81] was found to be most useful in patients with chronic schizophrenia. This scale also requires a standard neuromotor examination. The Kanner Scale[82] was developed to help with the diagnosis of catatonia in autism and other pervasive developmental disorders. This scale does require using nursing notes as well as a neuromotor examination.[78]

Other existing scales are primarily used in research. The Braunig Catatonia Rating Scale (BCRS)[83] takes 45 minutes and needs a trained examiner.[78] The Northoff Catatonia Rating Scale (NCRS)[84] includes 40 items, which can make it less practical in clinical practice, but does have excellent specificity and sensitivity.[78]

The *DSM-5* diagnostic criteria require the patient to have three symptoms (instead of two) to make this diagnosis. This may lead to missing some patients with catatonia. Another concern is that the diagnostic criteria for catatonic disorder due to another medical condition states that the disturbance does not occur exclusively during the course of delirium, which has been proposed to be incorrect.[64,74]

Laboratory and Imaging Tests

The workup for catatonia should involve several laboratory tests including CBC, electrolytes, BUN, creatinine, hepatic enzymes, CK, serum iron levels, thyroid function tests, toxic panels, and a urinalysis.[53,64] Vital signs should also be monitored, specifically monitoring for autonomic instability.[53] Other tests that should be included in the workup are neuroimaging (MRI or CT), EEG, and lumbar puncture. In pure psychiatric illness catatonia, the EEG should be normal, however, catatonia due to medical causes (e.g., encephalitis, seizures, etc.) may have abnormal EEG findings. Over 80% of medical catatonia patients in one study exhibited abnormal EEG findings, the most common being diffuse slowing.[64,69] When performing a lumbar puncture, the sample should be tested for anti-NMDA receptor antibodies.[69]

Differential Diagnosis

There are several conditions that should be in the differential diagnosis when evaluating someone with symptoms that may represent catatonia. They include medical, psychiatric, and neurological disorders. One helpful approach was delineated by Rustad et al.,[69] dividing the differential diagnosis into two different groups: (1) patients who cannot interact with interviewer and (2) patients who refuse to interact with interviewer. Table 25-3 provides a differential diagnosis based on these two categories.

Treatment

The underlying etiology of catatonia guides its treatment. After determining that the patient has catatonia, the next step should be discontinuing any neuroleptics and other dopamine depleters and restarting any recently stopped dopamine agonists.[69,85] A variety of agents are used for the symptomatic treatment of catatonia.

Benzodiazepines

The first-line treatment for catatonia, regardless of the underlying etiology, is with benzodiazepines. The most commonly utilized and evidence-based agent is lorazepam. Benzodiazepines

TABLE 25-3 • Differential Diagnosis in Catatonia.	
(1) Those who cannot interact with interviewer	
Psychiatric	Functional neurologic disorder (conversion disorder)
	Dissociative state
	Serotonin syndrome
	Neuroleptic malignant syndrome
Neurologic	Seizure
	Locked-in-syndrome
	Coma
	Akinetic mutism
Medical	Delirium
(2) Those who refuse to interact with interviewer	
Psychiatric	Factious disorder
	Malingering

Source: Rustad JK, Landsman HS, Ivkovic A, et al. Catatonia: An Approach to Diagnosis and Treatment. Prim Care Companion CNS Disord. 2018; 20(1):17f02202.

have been the gold standard for treating catatonia since the 1980s.[56] Roughly 60–90% of patients with catatonia will respond to lorazepam.[50,53] Other benzodiazepines have been used in the treatment of catatonia such as diazepam, oxazepam, and clonazepam. They are not commonly used because they are not available in IV or IM formulations and have longer half-lives.[85-87] When treated with benzodiazepines, complete resolution of symptoms is on average 3–7 days after treatment initiation.[69,85,86]

Typical dosages of lorazepam in the treatment of catatonia range from 8 to 24 mg per day (via any route IV/IM/PO) and are usually tolerated without sedation.[85,88] Response to lorazepam is usually very quick, roughly 5–10 minutes (when given intravenously) or 20–30 minutes when given orally. However, it may take up to 24 hours.[50] The recommendation for the initial regimen is starting with lorazepam 1–2 mg Q4–12H, and adjusting the dose based on the alleviation of symptoms without sedating the patient.[85,88] If the patient becomes sedated, the dose may be too high. Gradual uptitration allows for better tolerability than a more rapid dosing strategy. Starting with lower doses in patients who are elderly, young, or medically compromised, especially in patients with obstructive sleep apnea, is recommended.[53]

The duration of treatment with benzodiazepines is usually based on the underlying etiology. Regardless, it is important to avoid discontinuing the benzodiazepine too quickly, as catatonia may reemerge.[85] When the etiology is a medical/neurological process, relapse of symptoms can occur if the benzodiazepine is stopped before the treatment of the underlying illness.[53]

Below is a commonly used algorithm[53,61,69]:

1. IV lorazepam challenge typically starts with 1–2 mg of lorazepam administered intravenously and observation for effect (usually 5–10 minutes). If there is no effect/change, a second dose is given and reassessed after another 5–10 minutes.
   - A positive response is defined as a reduction in symptoms (at least 50%) as measured on a standardized catatonia scale (e.g., BFCRS).

Note: If lorazepam is given intramuscularly or orally, the interval for the second dose should be longer: 15 minutes for intramuscularly and 30 minutes for orally.

2. If there is no effect, the same dose may be repeated in 3 hours, and it can be done again in 3 hours if necessary.
3. At least 6 mg should be given over the course of 24 hours.
4. For those patients who show partial improvement on the first day of treatment, our recommendation is to continue 2 mg of IV lorazepam every 8 hours for at least 3–4 days, and it may be continued longer to maintain improvement, particularly if catatonia has been present more than a month.

There is some evidence to guide which patients are more likely to respond to benzodiazepines. Patients who report feeling strong, intense, and uncontrollable emotions often respond well to lorazepam.[50] Patients whose catatonia displays waxy flexibility and stupor,[85,86] those for whom the primary etiology is an affective illness (depression, bipolar),[86] and those who have previously responded quickly to treatment with benzodiazepines[85] also show good response to benzodiazepine treatment.

Patients who may not respond as well to lorazepam include those with a long duration of catatonic symptoms,[50,53,85,86] higher number of episodes,[85] patients whose primary condition causing catatonia is schizophrenia (having third-person auditory hallucinations, persecutory delusions),[57,85,86] and patients who display severe mutism during a catatonia state.[85,86]

Electroconvulsive Treatment

The second line treatment of catatonia is electroconvulsive treatment (ECT). Like benzodiazepines, ECT has GABA-ergic effects that may explain its therapeutic efficacy in catatonia. The response rates for ECT in catatonic patients range from 60% to 100%.[85,87] This treatment is often initiated when there is insufficient response to benzodiazepines or in life-threatening conditions such as malignant catatonia.[53,55,85,87,91] The frequency of treatment is usually three times per week, but in more severe cases it may be given daily and then reduced to every other day once symptoms begin to improve.[85] There are cases in which maintenance ECT may be necessary.[85] In these cases, symptoms return after stopping ECT treatment, often within the first few months to a year, despite ongoing pharmacologic treatment (antipsychotics, mood stabilizers). These patients require ongoing ECT treatment to prevent return of catatonic symptoms. There is no reliable way to identify patients who will need maintenance ECT and should be evaluated on an individual basis.[85]

Patients who may be more likely to have a good response to ECT are those with a shorter duration of catatonia,[85] higher scores on BFCRS,[85] waxy flexibility,[85] gegenhaltenm,[85] younger age,[85] and those exhibiting autonomic dysregulation.[85] Patients with an affective illness appear to respond better to ECT than those with a diagnosis of schizophrenia.[85] Patients who may not respond well to ECT tend to have catatonia attributable to medical illness.[85] Common side effects from ECT include memory impairments and headache.[87]

Zolpidem

There has been some evidence (mostly case reports and case series) using non-benzodiazepine hypnotics in the treatment of catatonia, such as zolpidem. Patients who were treated with zolpidem had tried lorazepam and/or ECT without response.[85] Dose ranges were typically 7.5–40 mg per day.[85] Similar to the lorazepam challenge test, there is a zolpidem challenge test. This involves first the administration of 10 mg of zolpidem orally (no current IV/IM route) and examining the patient after 30 minutes. A positive response is a reduction of at least 50% of the BFCRS-score.[85]

TMS

Transcranial magnetic stimulation (TMS) has been employed in the treatment of catatonia. It has been used in patients with catatonia due to various etiologies (psychosis, mood, autism, and neuromedical) as a monotherapy agent. TMS has been shown to be effective when targeting the dorsolateral PFC unilaterally on either side as well as bilaterally.[56,89] However, these were only single case reports (N = 6).

Antipsychotics

The use of antipsychotics in the treatment of catatonia has been limited, especially given that antipsychotics have been implicated in causing or worsening catatonia. In addition, patients with catatonia seem to be at a higher risk of developing NMS

when treated with an antipsychotic, compared to all patients treated with antipsychotic medications—this is more likely with first-generation antipsychotics.[53]

Patients with catatonia who are usually candidates for treatment with antipsychotics are those with a primary diagnosis of schizophrenia. As mentioned above, these patients are less likely to respond to benzodiazepines or ECT.[55,56]

Catatonic patients with schizophrenia should initially be treated with a benzodiazepine or with ECT. Once the symptoms of catatonia start to improve, there may be a role for an antipsychotic to help treat residual psychotic symptoms such as delusions or hallucinations, or as a prophylactic treatment in psychotic disorders and mood disorders (bipolar patients).[85] Second-generation antipsychotics with relatively lower D2 receptor blockade (quetiapine, clozapine) or with D2 partial agonism (aripiprazole) are preferable.[85] Second-generation antipsychotics also have GABA-agonist activity and 5HT2-antagonism that could stimulate dopamine release in the PFC and thus alleviate catatonic symptoms.[85] Antipsychotics that have been used in this setting include aripiprazole (3–30 mg daily), clozapine (150–800 mg daily), olanzapine (2.5–20 mg daily), risperidone (0.5–8 mg daily), and quetiapine (300–1100 mg daily).[56,85,87,90] Some of these

CASE VIGNETTE 25.2

Mr. Random Person is a 30-year-old man with a psychiatric history of bipolar disorder, cocaine use disorder, and a TBI after a motor vehicle accident, who was brought to the emergency department by family after they had noted some changes in his behavior over past several days.

His family reports that Mr. Person was diagnosed with bipolar disorder several years ago and has been intermittently adherent to his psychiatric medications, and more recently he has not been following up with his psychiatrist. Over the past several days, Mr. Person's family members noted that he has been less interactive with them and he has not been talking or eating much. They have been finding him in various rooms of the house standing in strange postures.

The emergency department physicians did a medical workup that included a complete blood count, complete metabolic panel, creatine phosphokinase, toxicology screen (both urine and blood), urinalysis, electroencephalogram (EEG), and head imaging. They also provided him with intravenous fluids, given he was not taking in much nutrition over the past several days. All of the lab results were normal, including his toxicology screen. His EEG did not show signs of seizure activity or diffuse background slowing. His vital signs were reassuring (blood pressure of 117/79; heart rate 82; temperature 98.7°F). After the emergency room physicians ruled out any acute medical problems, the psychiatry team was consulted for evaluation of the patient's presentation, given his psychiatric history.

Upon their examination, they found Mr. Person sitting straight up in the bed staring forward. He did not seem to acknowledge that the team had entered his room. He was minimally responsive to questions, and when he did respond

it was with the same response over and over. His right arm was lifted, abducted with wrist flexed backward. He kept his arm in that position for several minutes until the physician placed it back into his lap. Mr. Person would frequently reach and pull at his left ear but there did not appear to be any reason for doing this. The psychiatry team had a high suspicion that his presentation was due to catatonia given his symptoms of staring, stupor, verbigeration, stereotypy, posturing, waxy flexibility, and withdrawal. They requested that the emergency physician order 2 mg of lorazepam to be given intravenously immediately. After roughly 10–15 minutes had past, Mr. Pearson started to interact more with the team. He was answering questions in an appropriate manner, he was no longer repeatedly touching his left ear, and he no longer demonstrated waxy flexibility. He reported that he was hearing voices and expressed paranoid delusions. About 1–2 hours later, he again started to become less responsive to questions and to demonstrate verbigeration, waxy flexibility, and stereotypy.

Mr. Pearson was started on a standing regimen of lorazepam 2 mg every 3 hours. An antipsychotic medication was not initially started for his hallucinations/delusions due to concern that this may lead to malignant catatonia. After several days, he started to show some symptoms of sedation on this regimen, and his lorazepam was then slowly titrated down over another 2 weeks. By this time his catatonia symptoms were no longer present (lorazepam was tapered off), so he was started on low-dose risperidone for his psychotic symptoms and lithium for ongoing maintenance of his bipolar disorder. He was stabilized and discharged home after a 5-week psychiatric hospitalization.

patients were using both benzodiazepine and an antipsychotic.[56] Patients with chronic catatonia seem to benefit from a combination of ECT and clozapine.[55] There is no consensus on the definition of chronic catatonia, but patients who were given the diagnosis had either a prolonged duration of catatonic symptoms (1 month–1 year), or frequent relapses of symptoms after treatment was stopped.[91]

NMDA-Antagonists

There have been case reports demonstrating successful use of NMDA receptor antagonists (such as amantadine, memantine) for the treatment of catatonia after insufficient or failed trials of a benzodiazepine. Amantadine has been successfully used as monotherapy for treatment of catatonia ($N = 18$ cases), mostly in patients with schizophrenia.[56,85,87] Dosages have been 100–600 mg daily, averaging 200 mg daily[56] but up to 100–500 mg TID.[85] Memantine has also been successfully used in the treatment of catatonia ($N = 9$ cases) in patients with a diagnosis of schizophrenia and was combined with lorazepam.[56] Dosages were from 5 to 20 mg per day.[56] The evidence for the use of these medications are currently only based on case reports and no large studies have been done comparing them to other treatments.

Mood Stabilizers

Mood stabilizers have been used in the treatment of catatonia, usually after a lack of response to benzodiazepines. Valproic acid has been shown to be useful in the treatment of catatonia ($N = 5$ cases). The studies using valproic acid have been in both schizophrenia and bipolar disorder. Valproic acid may be useful in prophylaxis of catatonia in bipolar patients.[56,85] Dosages of valproic acid ranged from 600 to 4000 mg per day.[56] Topiramate has also been found to help successfully treat catatonia in a case series of four patients with a diagnosis of schizophrenia. The dosing was 200 mg per day and was always used in conjunction with benzodiazepines. Monotherapy treatment using carbamazepine (dosing of 100–1000 mg daily) in patients with mood disorders was also found to be successful in seven cases.[56,87] Lithium was found to be helpful for prophylaxis of catatonia, but not for its treatment.[85]

Supportive Treatments

Supportive care for patients with catatonia consists of hydration, nutrition, mobilization, anticoagulation (to prevent thrombophlebitis), and aspiration precautions.[69,85,88] Vital signs should be closely monitored as well, as changes in these may be a warning of emerging malignant catatonia or NMS.[69]

Summary and Key Points

- Delirium is an acute confusional state caused by an underlying physiologic disturbance.
- Clinical assessment is the gold standard for the diagnosis of delirium and a high index of suspicion is required.
- Newly diagnosed delirium is a neuropsychiatric emergency, as it can signal an underlying life-threatening illness.
- The definitive treatment of delirium is the identification and treatment of the underlying medical illness.
- There are no FDA-approved medications for the treatment of delirium, however antipsychotics are commonly used to manage hyperactive or psychotic symptoms. Non-antipsychotic alternatives include alpha agonists and antiepileptic drugs.
- Catatonia is a syndrome of motor, behavioral, and affective symptoms that can be due to both psychiatric and medical illnesses. In inpatient psychiatric settings, the prevalence is roughly 10%. The most common psychiatric disorder associated with catatonia is bipolar disorder (46%). Within the acute medical setting, the prevalence is about 4–5%. The most common medical causes are encephalitis (35–38%) and CNS structural abnormalities (up to 30%).

- There are 23 symptoms that make up the syndrome of catatonia. The most common symptoms are staring, immobility, mutism, and withdrawal.
- Several areas of the brain have been implicated in the pathophysiology of catatonia including cortical (right dorsolateral PFC, left lateral PFC, primary and supplementary motor areas, orbitofrontal PFC, right parietal cortex) and subcortical (basal ganglia, thalamus, anterior cingulate gyrus, cerebellum, pons, and brainstems).
- The gold standard treatment for catatonia in both psychiatric and medical etiologies is lorazepam. Dosages range from 8 to 24 mg per day and symptoms usually resolve within 3–7 days. The treatment of choice for individuals who do not respond to lorazepam or develop malignant catatonia is ECT.
- After a diagnosis of catatonia, antipsychotics should be discontinued. Antipsychotics should not be started until catatonia symptoms have been adequately treated. Use of antipsychotics in acute catatonia can lead to malignant catatonia or neuroleptic malignant syndrome, which are life-threatening.
- Untreated catatonia can lead to serious medical complications including dehydration, metabolic derangements, contractures, deep vein thrombosis, cardiovascular collapse, and possibly death.

Multiple Choice Questions

1. Which of the following statements about the clinical features of delirium is true?
   a. Mental status changes develop over months to years.
   b. The symptoms are the direct consequence of another medical condition, substance intoxication, or withdrawal.
   c. Psychotic symptoms are required to make the diagnosis.
   d. Mental status changes are stable throughout the duration of delirium.

2. Which of the following symptoms is a reasonable treatment target if using antipsychotics for delirium?
   a. Disorientation
   b. Decreased level of consciousness
   c. Memory impairment
   d. Hallucinations

3. Which pair contains the most common underlying psychiatric and medical conditions that lead to catatonia?
   a. Major depressive disorder and epilepsy
   b. Stroke and bipolar disorder
   c. Schizophrenia and medication intoxication
   d. Schizoaffective disorder and multiple sclerosis
   e. Encephalitis and bipolar disorder

4. What is the gold standard in the symptomatic treatment of catatonia?
   a. Antipsychotics
   b. Antidepressants
   c. Antiepileptic drugs
   d. Benzodiazepines
   e. Electroconvulsive therapy

Multiple Choice Answers

1. Answer: b

Mental status changes occur acutely in delirium and wax and wane. Psychotic symptoms may be present but are not required to make the diagnosis. The mental status changes seen in delirium are the consequence of an underlying toxic or medical condition.

2. Answer: d

Antipsychotics have not been shown to improve disorientation, level of consciousness, or memory impairment in delirium. They may be helpful for decreasing hallucinations.

3. Answer: e

Bipolar disorder is the most common psychiatric cause of catatonia, roughly 46% of catatonic cases found in the psychiatric setting. Encephalitis is the most common cause of catatonia in the acute medical setting, not a psychiatric condition. To assume all catatonia is due to a psychiatric condition may lead the clinician to miss the presence of life-threatening medical conditions. This is important to know because the treatment of catatonia involves treating the symptoms of catatonia and the underlying cause (whether it is psychiatric or medical).

4. Answer: d

Benzodiazepines (most commonly lorazepam) are the first-line treatment for catatonia in both psychiatric and medical settings. Roughly 60–90% patients' symptoms will respond to lorazepam, often within 5–10 minutes if using IV or 20–30 minutes by PO. Patients with catatonia often require doses ranges from 8 to 24 mg per day. If the individual's symptoms do not respond within 3–7 days or he/she starts exhibiting symptoms of malignant catatonia, then ECT would be the next choice.

References

1. Maldonado JR. Acute brain failure: pathophysiology, diagnosis, management, and sequelae of delirium. *Crit Care Clin.* 2017;33:461-519.
2. Siddiqi N, House AO, Holmes JD. Occurrence and outcome of delirium in medical in-patients: a systematic literature review. *Age Ageing.* 2006;35:350-364.
3. Mehta S, Cook D, Devlin JW, et al. Prevalence, risk factors, and outcomes of delirium in mechanically ventilated adults. *Crit Care Med.* 2015;43:557-566.
4. Pisani MA, McNicoll L, Inouye SK. Cognitive impairment in the intensive care unit. *Clin Chest Med.* 2003;24:727-737.
5. Holmes EG, Jones SW, Laughon SL. A retrospective analysis of neurocognitive impairment in older patients with burn injuries. *Psychosomatics.* 2017;58:386-394.
6. Marcantonio ER. Postoperative delirium: a 76-year-old woman with delirium following surgery. *JAMA.* 2012;308:73-81.
7. Breitbart W, Strout D. Delirium in the terminally ill. *Clin Geriatr Med.* 2000;16:357-372.
8. Ahmed S, Leurent B, Sampson EL. Risk factors for incident delirium among older people in acute hospital medical units: a systematic review and meta-analysis. *Age Ageing.* 2014;43:326-333.
9. Racine AM, Fong TG, Gou Y, et al. Clinical outcomes in older surgical patients with mild cognitive impairment. *Alzheimers Dement.* 2018;14(5):590-600.
10. Khan BA, Perkins A, Hui SL, et al. Relationship between African-American race and delirium in the ICU. *Crit Care Med.* 2016;44:1727-1734.
11. Maldonado JR. Neuropathogenesis of delirium: review of current etiologic theories and common pathways. *Am J Geriatr Psychiatry.* 2013;21:12.
12. American Psychiatric Association. *Diagnostic and Statistical Manual of Mental Disorders.* 5th ed. Arlington, VA: American Psychiatric Association; 2013.
13. Webster R, Holroyd S. Prevalence of psychotic symptoms in delirium. *Psychosomatics.* 2000;41:519-522.
14. Peterson JF, Pun BT, Dittus RS, et al. Delirium and its motoric subtypes: a study of 614 critically ill patients. *J Am Geriatr Soc.* 2006;54:479-484.
15. Marcantonio ER. Delirium in hospitalized older adults. *N Engl J Med.* 2017;377:1456--1466.
16. Ely EW, Inouye SK, Bernard GR, et al. Delirium in mechanically ventilated patients: validity and reliability of the Confusion Assessment Method for the Intensive Care Unit (CAM-ICU). *JAMA.* 2001;286:2703-2710.

17. Witlox J, Eurelings LSM, de Jonghe JFM, Kalisvaart KJ, Eikelenboom P, van Gool WA. Delirium in elderly patients and the risk of postdischarge mortality, institutionalization, and dementia: a meta-analysis. *JAMA.* 2010;304:443-451.

18. Cole MG, Ciampi A, Belzile E, Zhong L. Persistent delirium in older hospital patients: a systematic review of frequency and prognosis. *Age Ageing.* 2008;38:19-26.

19. Girard TD, Jackson JC, Pandharipande PP, et al. Delirium as a predictor of long-term cognitive impairment in survivors of critical illness. *Crit Care Med.* 2010;38:1513-1520.

20. Sakuramoto H, Subrina J, Unoki T, Mizutani T, Komatsu H. Severity of delirium in the ICU is associated with short term cognitive impairment. A prospective cohort study. *Intensive Crit Care Nurs.* 2015;31:250-257.

21. Fong TG, Davis D, Growdon ME, Albuquerque A, Inouye SK. The interface between delirium and dementia in elderly adults. *Lancet Neurol.* 2015;14:823-832.

22. Davis DHJ, Muniz Terrera G, Keage H, et al. Delirium is a strong risk factor for dementia in the oldest-old: a population-based cohort study. *Brain.* 2012;135:2809-2816.

23. van den Boogaard M, Kox M, Quinn KL, et al. Biomarkers associated with delirium in critically ill patients and their relation with long-term subjective cognitive dysfunction; indications for different pathways governing delirium in inflamed and noninflamed patients. *Crit Care.* 2011;15:R297.

24. Lane-Hall MB Kuza CM, Fakhry S, Kaplan LJ. The lifetime effects of injury: postintensive care syndrome and posttraumatic stress disorder. *Anesthesiology Clin.* 2019;37(1):135-150.

25. Inouye SK, Foreman MD, Mion LC, Katz KH, Cooney LM. Nurses' recognition of delirium and its symptoms: comparison of nurse and researcher ratings. *Arch Intern Med.* 2001;161:2467-2473.

26. Farrell KR, Ganzini L. Misdiagnosing delirium as depression in medically ill elderly patients. *Arch Intern Med.* 1995;155:2459-2464.

27. Wong CL, Holroyd-Leduc J, Simel DL, Straus SE. Does this patient have delirium? *JAMA.* 2010;304:779.

28. Trzepacz PT, Brenner RP, Coffman G, van Thiel DH. Delirium in liver transplantation candidates: discriminant analysis of multiple test variables. *Biol Psychiatry.* 1988;24:3-14.

29. Nielsen RM, Urdanibia-Centelles O, Vedel-Larsen E, et al. Continuous EEG monitoring in a consecutive patient cohort with sepsis and delirium. *Neurocrit Care.* 2019. doi:10.1007/s12028-019-00703-w. [Epub ahead of print]

30. Inouye S, Charpentier P. Precipitating factors for delirium in hospitalized elderly persons: predictive model and interrelationship with baseline vulnerability. *JAMA.* 1996;20:852-857.

31. Olsen RQ, Regis JT. Delirious deficiency. *Lancet.* 2010; 376:1362.

32. Neufeld KJ, Yue J, Robinson TN, Inouye SK, Needham DM. Antipsychotic medication for prevention and treatment of delirium in hospitalized adults: a systematic review and meta-analysis. *J Am Geriatr Soc.* 2016;64:705-714.

33. Siddiqi N, Harrison JK, Clegg A, et al. Interventions for preventing delirium in hospitalised non-ICU patients. *Cochrane Database Syst Rev.* 2016;3:CD005563.

34. Hays H, Jolliff HA, Casavant MJ. The psychopharmacology of agitation: consensus statement of the American Association for Emergency Psychiatry Project BETA Psychopharmacology workgroup. *West J Emerg Med.* 2012;13:536.

35. Navari RM, Gray SE, Kerr AC. Olanzapine versus aprepitant for the prevention of chemotherapy-induced nausea and vomiting: a randomized phase III trial. *J Support Oncol.* 2011;9:188-195.

36. Desmarais P, Massoud F, Filion J, Nguyen QD, Bajsarowicz P. Quetiapine for psychosis in parkinson disease and neurodegenerative parkinsonian disorders. *J Geriatr Psychiatry Neurol.* 2016;29:227-236.

37. Harrigan EP, Miceli JJ, Anziano R, et al. A randomized evaluation of the effects of six antipsychotic agents on QTc, in the absence and presence of metabolic inhibition. *J Clin Psychopharmacol.* 2004;24:62-69.

38. Strawn JR, Keck PE, Caroff SN. Neuroleptic malignant syndrome. *Am J Psychiatry.* 2007;164:870-876.

39. Pandharipande PP, Pun BT, Herr DL, et al. Effect of sedation with dexmedetomidine vs lorazepam on acute brain dysfunction in mechanically ventilated patients: the MENDS randomized controlled trial. *JAMA.* 2007;298:2644-2653.

40. Riker RR, Shehabi Y, Bokesch PM, et al. Dexmedetomidine vs midazolam for sedation of critically ill patients: a randomized trial. *JAMA.* 2009;301:489-499.

41. Gagnon DJ, Riker RR, Glisic EK, Kelner A, Perrey HM, Fraser GL. Transition from dexmedetomidine to enteral clonidine for ICU sedation: an observational pilot study. *Pharmacotherapy.* 2015;35:251-259.

42. Neerland BE, Hov KR, Bruun Wyller V, et al. The protocol of the Oslo Study of clonidine in elderly patients with delirium; LUCID: a randomised placebo-controlled trial. *BMC Geriatr.* 2015;15:7.

43. Gagnon DJ, Fontaine G V, Smith KE, et al. Valproate for agitation in critically ill patients: a retrospective study. *J Crit Care.* 2017;37:119-125.

44. Bashar FR, Vahedian-Azimi A, Hajiesmaeili M, et al. Post-ICU psychological morbidity in very long ICU stay patients with ARDS and delirium. *J Crit Care.* 2018;43:88-94.

45. Jones C, Griffiths RD, Humphris G, Skirrow PM. Memory, delusions, and the development of acute posttraumatic stress disorder-related symptoms after intensive care. *Crit Care Med.* 2001;29:573-580.

46. Jones C, Bäckman C, Capuzzo M, et al. Intensive care diaries reduce new onset post traumatic stress disorder following critical illness: a randomised, controlled trial. *Crit Care.* 2010;14:R168.

47. Schoeman T, Sundararajan K, Micik S, et al. The impact on new-onset stress and PTSD in relatives of critically ill patients explored by diaries study (the "INSPIRED" study). *Aust Crit Care.* 2017;31:382-389.

48. Garrouste-Orgeas M, Flahault C, Fasse L, et al. The ICU-Diary study: prospective, multicenter comparative study of the impact of an ICU diary on the wellbeing of patients and families in French ICUs. *Trials.* 2017;18:542.

49. Kahlbaum K. Die katatonie oder das spannungsirresein. Klinische Abhandlugen uber psychische Kranekhieten, Berlin, Germany; 1874.

50. Northoff G. What catatonia can tell us about "top-down modulation": a neuropsychiatric hypothesis. *Behav Brain Sci.* 2002a;25:555-604.

51. Gazdag G, Takacs R, Ungvari GS. Catatonia as a putative nosological entity: a historical sketch. *World J Psychiatr.* 2017;7(3):177-183.

52. Espinola-Nadurille M, Ramirez-Bermudez J, Fricchione GL, et al. Catatonia in neurologic and psychiatric patients at a tertiary neurological center. *J Neuropsychiatry Clin Neurosci.* 2016;28(2):124-130.

53. Rasmussen SA, Mazurek MF, Rosebush PI. Catatonia: our current understanding of its diagnosis, treatment and pathophysiology. *World J Psychiatr.* 2016;6(4):391-398.

54. Brar K, Kaushik SS, Lippmann S. Catatonia update. *Prim Care Companion CNS Disord.* 2017;19(5):16br02023.

55. Walther S, Strik W. Catatonia. *CNS Spectr.* 2016;21:341-348.

56. Beach SR, Gomez-Bernal F, Huffman JC, Fricchione GL. Alternative treatment strategies for catatonia: a systematic review. *Gen Hosp Psychiatry.* 2017;48:1-19.

57. Rosenbush PI, Mazurek MF. Catatonia and its treatment. *Schizophr Bull.* 2010;36(2):239-242.

58. Solmi M, Pigato GG, Roiter B, et al. Prevalence of catatonia and its moderators in clinical samples: results from a meta-analysis and meta-regression analysis. *Schizophr Bull.* 2018;44(5):1133-1150.

59. Grover S, Chakrabarti S, Ghormode D, et al. Catatonia in inpatients with psychiatric disorders: a comparison of schizophrenia and mood disorders. *Psychiatry Res.* 2015;229:919-925.

60. Ungvari GS, Caroff SN, Gerevich J. The catatonia conundrum: evidence of psychomotor phenomena as a symptom dimension in psychotic disorders. *Schizophr Bull.* 2010;36(2):231-238.

61. Fink M, Taylor MA. *Catatonia: A Clinician's Guide to Diagnosis and Treatment.* New York, NY: Cambridge University Press; 2003.

62. Saddawi-Konefka D, Berg SM, Nejad SH, Bittner EA. Catatonia in the ICU: an important and underdiagnosed cause of altered mental status. A case series and review of the literature. *Online Case Rep.* 2013;42(3):e234-e241.

63. Jaimes-Albornoz W, Serra-Mestres J. Catatonia in a liaison psychiatry service of a general hospital: prevalence and clinical features. *Eur Psychiatry.* 2015;30(suppl 1):28-31.

64. Oldham M, Lee HB. Catatonia vis-à-vis delirium: the significance of recognizing catatonia in altered mental status. *Gen Hosp Psychiatry.* 2015;37:554-559.

65. Rizos D, Peritogiannis V, Gkogkos C. Catatonia in the intensive care unit. *Gen Hosp Psychiatry.* 2011;33(1):500-505.

66. Carroll BT, Anfinson TJ, Kennedy JC, Yendreck R, Boutros M, Bilon A. Catatonic disorder due to general medical conditions. *J Neuropsychiatry Clin Neurosci.* 1994;6:122-133.

67. De Figueiredo NS, Angst DB, Neto AM, et al. Catatonia, beyond a psychiatric syndrome. *Dement Neuropsychol.* 2017;11(2):209-212.

68. Smith JH, Smith VD, Philbrick KL, Kumar N. Catatonia disorder due to a general medical or psychiatric condition. *J Neuropsychiatry Clin Neurosci.* 2012;24:198-207.

69. Rustad JK, Landsman HS, Ivkovic A, Finn CT, Stern TA. Catatonia: an approach to diagnosis and treatment. *Prim Care Companion CNS Disord.* 2018;20(1):17f02202.

70. Northoff G. Catatonia and neuroleptic malignant syndrome: psychopathology and pathophysiology. *J Neural Transm.* 2002b;109:1453-1467.

71. Walther S. Psychomotor symptoms of schizophrenia map on the cerebral motor circuit. *Psychiatry Res.* 2015;233:293-298.

72. Northoff G. Brain imaging in catatonia: current findings and a pathophysiologic model. *CNS Spectr.* 2000;5(7): 34-46.

73. Ellul P, Choucha W. Neurobiological approach of catatonia and treatment perspectives. *Front Psychiatry.* 2015;6(182):1-4.

74. Wilson JE, Niu K, Nicolson SE, Levine SZ, Heckers S. The diagnostic criteria and structure of catatonia. *Schizophr Res.* 2015;164:256-262.

75. Wilcox JA, Duffy PR. The syndrome of catatonia. *Behav Sci.* 2015;5:576-588.

76. Northoff G, Nagel D, Danos P, Leschinger A, Lerche J, Bogerts B. Impairment in visual-spatial function in catatonia: a neuropsychological investigation. *Schizophr Res.* 1999;37(2):133-147.

77. Bush G, Fink M, Petride G, Dowling F, Francis A. Catatonia I. Rating scale and standardizing examination. *Acta Psychiatr Scand.* 1996;93:129-136.

78. Sienaert P, Rooseleer J, De Fruyt J. Measuring catatonia: a systematic review of rating scales. *J Affect Disord.* 2011;135:1-9.

79. Starkstein SE, Petracca G, Teson A, et al. Catatonia in depression: prevalence, clinical correlates, and validation of a scale. *J Neurol Neurosurg Psychiatry.* 1996;60:326-332.

80. Lund CE, Mortimer AM, Rogers D, McKenna PJ. Motor, volitional and behavioural disorders in schizophrenia. 1: assessment using the Modified Rogers Scale. *Br J Psychiatry.* 1991;158:323-327.

81. McKenna PJ, Lund CE, Mortimer AM, Biggins CA. Motor, volitional and behavioural disorders in schizophrenia. 2: the 'conflict of paradigms' hypothesis. *Br J Psychiatry.* 1991;158:328-336.

82. Carroll BT, Kirkhart R, Ahuja N, et al. Katatonia: a new conceptual understanding of catatonia and a new rating scale. *Psychiatry.* 2008;5:42-50.

83. Braunig P, Kruger S, Shugar G, Hoffler J, Borner I. The catatonia rating scale I—development, reliability, and use. *Compr Psychiatry.* 2000;41:147-158.

84. Northoff G, Koch A, Wenke J, et al. Catatonia as a psychomotor syndrome: a rating scale and extrapyramidal motor symptoms. *Mov Disord.* 1999;14:404-416.

85. Sienaert P, Dhossche DM, Vancamfort D, De Hert M, Gazdag G. A clinical review of treatment of catatonia. *Front Psychiatry.* 2014;5:181.

86. Narayanaswamy JC, Tibrewal P, Zutshi A, Srinivasaraju R, Math SB. Clinical predictors of response to treatment in catatonia. *Gen Hosp Psychiatry.* 2012;34:312-316.

87. Pelzer A, van der Heijden F, den Boer E. Systematic review of catatonia treatment. *Neuropsychiatr Dis Treat.* 2018;14:317-326.

88. Clinebell K, Azzam PN, Gopalan P, Haskett R. Guidelines for preventing common medical complications of catatonia: case report and literature review. *J Clin Psychiatry.* 2014;75(6):644-651.

89. Costanzo F, Menghini D, Casula L, et al. Transcranial direct current stimulation treatment in an adolescent with autism and drug-resistant catatonia. *Brain Stimul.* 2015;8(6):1223-1240.

90. Yoshimura B, Hirota T, Takaki M, Kishi Y. Is quetiapine suitable for treatment of acute schizophrenia with catatonic stupor? A case series of 39 patients. *Neuropsychiatric Dis Treat.* 2013;9:1565-1571.

91. De Silva V, Lakmini W, Gunawardena H, Hanwella R. Chronic catatonia treated with electroconvulsive therapy: a case report. *J Med Case Rep.* 2013;7:2019.

92. Stahl SM. *Stahl's Essential Psychopharmacology: Prescriber's Guide.* 5th ed. New York, NY: Cambridge University Press; 2014.

Neuropsychiatry of Inflammatory, Autoimmune, and Infectious Disorders

26

Jessica Harder · Tamar Katz · Irina A. Skylar-Scott

INTRODUCTION

Inflammatory, autoimmune, and infectious disorders represent some of the classic medical conditions associated with neuropsychiatric symptomatology. From systemic lupus erythematosus (SLE), the archetypal example of a rheumatologic condition that can present with prominent neuropsychiatric symptoms, to Susac's syndrome, a far less commonly known entity with documented neuropsychiatric disturbance typically limited to cognitive dysfunction, these conditions include the full range of clinical presentations, pathophysiologic mechanisms, and approaches to management. Immune-mediated processes contribute to the pathophysiology by which many inflammatory and infectious disorders cause brain damage and neuropsychiatric manifestations. To do justice to the wide range of disorders potentially included in this chapter would require a book in itself. Given the limitations of space and the desire to present a useful reference to the reader interested in the spectrum of neuroinflammatory/neuroimmunologic disease, this chapter discusses in detail some representative examples and presents summary tables about different categories of disorders. Please see Table 26-1 for key cognitive and neuropsychiatric features of selected rheumatic diseases, including SLE.[1-19]

Another rapidly developing field with critical implications for neuropsychiatry is the study of autoimmune or antibody-mediated encephalitides. Some of the best known of these, including NMDA-receptor encephalitis, are frequently paraneoplastic, and as such are treated in detail in the chapter devoted to neuropsychiatric aspects of cancer (Chapter 28). Table 26-2 outlines features of selected antibody-mediated encephalitides that may occur with or without an oncologic association.[20-39] The characteristic mesial temporal lobe changes associated with limbic encephalitis are shown in Figure 26-1.

Other important autoimmune conditions with neuropsychiatric symptoms are treated in other chapters in this book, including a chapter devoted to neuropsychiatric disorders in multiple sclerosis (Chapter 27).

Of course, neuroinflammatory and infectious processes do not always have an autoimmune pathogenic mechanism. Many neurologic infections can wreak havoc on the central nervous system both directly and through the immune processes that they trigger. Please see Table 26-3 for the main features of selected neuroinfectious diseases with neuropsychiatric manifestations.[40-69] Here, we discuss in detail HIV, herpes simplex encephalitis (as the prototypical infectious limbic encephalitis), and neurosyphilis (as a classic exemplar of neuroinfectious disease).

SYSTEMIC LUPUS ERYTHEMATOSUS

Epidemiology

SLE is a chronic inflammatory disease of unknown etiology that can have widely variable manifestations between affected individuals. The incidence and prevalence of SLE vary by geography, ethnicity, and gender and estimates of worldwide disease burden vary substantially. SLE is more common in urban than rural areas, with African Americans, Hispanics, and Asians more often affected than non-Hispanic Caucasians.[70] Women are more commonly affected than men for every age and ethnic group. Estimates of prevalence vary from 23.2/100,000 people to 241/100,000 with African American women being most highly represented.[71] Worldwide, the incidence has nearly tripled in the past 50 years due to improved detection of mild disease. Current incidence estimates range from 1 to 25 cases per 100,000 across North America, South America, Europe, and Asia.[70,71]

SLE affecting the nervous system and manifesting with either neurologic or psychiatric symptoms is termed neuropsychiatric systemic lupus erythematosus (NPSLE), previously called lupus cerebritis. The prevalence of NPSLE varies widely among different reports and across populations, with estimates ranging from 10% to 80%[72,73] in adults and 22–95% in children.[74] Interestingly, rates of NPSLE appear to differ between ethnic groups and certain ethnic groups reportedly have higher or lower rates

TABLE 26-1 • Clinical Features of Rheumatic Diseases with Cognitive and Neuropsychiatric Sequelae.

Disorder	Psychiatric Manifestations	Cognitive Manifestations	Other Distinguishing Clinical Features
Systemic lupus erythematosus	*Depression (39%),* anxiety (13%), psychosis (5–7%), mood disorder with mixed features (4%)	*Memory impairment (43%),* inattention (26%), visuospatial processing (26%), decreased psychomotor speed (26%), encephalopathy (7%)	Cutaneous manifestations (e.g., malar rash), oral ulcers, alopecia, synovitis, serositis, renal injury (e.g., proteinuria), low cell counts (anemia, leukopenia, and/or thrombocytopenia), seizures, neuropathy (cranial or peripheral), myelitis, fatigue, vision loss (e.g., due to optic neuritis, retinopathy, vitreous hemorrhage), arterial strokes
Sjögren's syndrome	*Hypochondriasis (91%), depression (48%),* behavior/personality changes (33%), somatization (33%), dissociation (23%), anxiety/panic (12.5%), hypomania followed by depression (5%), hypomania (2.5%), paranoia (2%)	*Aphasia (5%),* encephalopathy (2.4%)	Peripheral neuropathy, stroke- or multiple sclerosis-like symptoms, sicca (including dry mouth, dry eyes), enlarged parotid glands
Behçet's disease	*Behavior/personality changes (30%; of these, one-third with apathy and two-third with disinhibition),* anxiety (24%), mixed psychiatric disorder (21%), depression (21%), mania (6%), hypersomnia (3%), psychosis (3%)	*Memory impairment (88%, learning and recall more impaired than recognition, both visual and verbal impairment),* inattention 60%, executive dysfunction (52%), visuospatial dysfunction (9%), abstraction (8%), aphasia (<5% including 1% anomia)	Oral/GI and genital ulcers, erythema nodosum, arthritis/arthralgia, uveitis, venous and arterial thrombi, ophthalmoparesis, cranial neuropathy, cerebellar dysfunction, extrapyramidal dysfunction, myelopathy, hemiparesis, hemisensory loss, seizures
Susac's syndrome	*Emotional disturbance (16%),* behavior/personality changes (12–15%), apathy (12%), psychosis (10%)	*Acute encephalopathy (76%),* cognitive impairment (48%, usually loss of memory, attention, and executive function), decreased level of consciousness (9%)	Branch retinal arterial occlusion (BRAO), hearing loss
CNS vasculitis	*Behavior/personality changes (up to 95% in small vessel pediatric cohort, otherwise N/A)*	*Aphasia (28–84%, including language production and/or comprehension),* decreased level of consciousness (47%), amnestic syndrome (9%)	Prodromal period lasting months, headache, focal neurologic signs (e.g., hemiparesis or vision loss, including due to strokes or transient ischemic attacks), ataxia, seizures, papilledema, diplopia
Neurosarcoidosis	*Depression (variable cohorts, 3–66%),* irritability/agitation (up to 44%), decreased initiative/apathy (33%), euphoria (up to 22%), impaired judgment (11%), visual hallucinations (up to 11%), emotional lability (8%), behavior/personality changes (8%)	*Decreased level of consciousness (7–33%),* memory impairment (11–23%), inattention (22%), encephalopathy (3–7%), aphasia (2–8%)	Extraneurologic: malaise, fever; erythema nodosum, hepatosplenomegaly, uveitis, exophthalmos, diabetes insipidus, amenorrhea
			Neurologic: seizures, hyperreflexia, cerebellar syndrome, cranial neuropathies, peripheral neuropathies

of NPSLE than would be expected as compared to the prevalence of SLE within that demographic (see Figure 26-2A and B).[75] For example, Caucasians represent approximately 11% of all patients with SLE; however they comprise almost 40% of all patients with NPSLE". In contrast, Hispanics have lower rates of NPSLE than expected, with 33% of all patients with SLE stemming from the Hispanic communities while only 15% of NPSLE

cases fall within that demographic. The reason for the discrepancy in presentation between ethnic groups is unknown. It may represent variation in diagnosis between providers and clinical sites, given that NPSLE is currently a clinical diagnosis without consistently reliable biomarkers; perhaps with a contribution from neurophysiological differences among demographic groups. Reports vary widely as to how frequently and how

TABLE 26-2 • Clinical Features of Autoimmune Encephalitides.

Antigen	Demographic Data	Psychiatric Manifestations	Cognitive Manifestations	Other Distinguishing Features
N-methyl-D-aspartate (NMDA) receptor	Three-quarters women, one-third children and adolescents	*Initial agitation followed by catatonia (88%),* psychosis (40%, including delusions, paranoia, visual or auditory hallucinations), behavioral/personality change (20%)	*Encephalopathy or decreased level of consciousness (88%),* amnestic syndrome (23%), aphasia (including unintelligible speech, 50%)	Viral prodrome, speech changes, central hypoventilation, seizures, autonomic instability, orofacial and "piano-playing" dyskinesias and other extrapyramidal disorders; associated with ovarian teratomas (40% of patients have neoplasm)
Voltage-gated potassium channel (VGKC) complex-associated antigens (leucine-rich glioma-inactivated protein 1 [LGI1] and contactin-associated protein-like 2 [Caspr2])	More common in men than women; middle-aged or older	*Sleep disturbance (24%, including insomnia, hypersomnia, sleep reversal),* irritability/agitation (13%), psychomotor slowing (13%), visual hallucinations (13%), delusions (13%), behavioral/personality change (13%)	*Verbal memory deficits/ amnestic syndrome (80%), encephalopathy (80%), disorientation (80%),* REM sleep behavior disorder (4%), visual memory deficits (frequency not specified)	Seizures, autonomic dysfunction, neuromyotonia (peripheral hyperexcitability syndrome with cramps/ stiffness), neuropathic pain, weight loss; hyponatremia (60%); rarely associated with tumors (thymoma most common if association)
Alpha-amino-3-hydroxy-5-methyl-4-isoxazolepropionic acid (AMPA) receptor (glutamate receptors 1 and 2 subunits, [GluR1 and GluR2])	Most common in women ages 50–70	*Agitation/aggressive behavior (50%),* depression (10%), apathy (10%), perseveration (10%), insomnia (10%), hallucinations (10%)	*Amnestic syndrome (50% with limbic encephalitis in isolation, the rest have limbic encephalitis and other symptoms), encephalopathy (50%),* decreased level of consciousness (30%), disorientation (20%), confabulation (30%), reduced verbal fluency (10%)	Seizures, nystagmus; associated with breast cancer, lung cancer, and thymoma
Gamma-aminobutyric acid-A (GABA-A) receptor	Male predominance; equally likely in children and adults	*Psychosis (12%; including hallucinations),* depression (6%), disordered affect (6%); insomnia (6%), psychomotor agitation (6%)	*Rapidly progressive encephalopathy (100%),* decreased level of consciousness (17%), amnestic syndrome (12%), aphasia or decreased verbal output (12%)	Seizures and status epilepticus; most patients do not have a tumor (rare association with thymoma)
Gamma-aminobutyric acid-A (GABA-B) receptor	Males and females equally likely, middle-aged	*Agitation or behavioral disturbances (20%),* hallucinations (13%), paranoia (13%)	Amnestic syndrome (100%), encephalopathy (100%), decreased level of consciousness (13%), receptive aphasia (7%), confabulation (7%), disorientation (7%)	Seizures; associated with small-cell lung cancer
65 kDa glutamic acid decarboxylase (GAD65)	Most common in women ages 20–50	*Hallucinations (2%)*	*Amnestic syndrome (5%), encephalopathy (5%),* dysexecutive syndrome (2%, difficulties with planning, decision making), impaired attention (2%), impaired abstraction (2%)	Stiff person syndrome ("Frankenstein gait"), ataxia, brainstem encephalitis, ophthalmoplegia, parkinsonism, myelopathy, palatal tremor, nystagmus; rarely associated with tumors (thymoma, breast cancer, or neuroendocrine tumors most common if association)

(Continued)

TABLE 26-2 • Clinical Features of Autoimmune Encephalitides. (*Continued*)

Antigen	Demographic Data	Psychiatric Manifestations	Cognitive Manifestations	Other Distinguishing Features
Calcium channel (N and P/Q types)	Middle-aged	*Disordered affect and hallucinations if anti-hu co-occurring (8–12% of small cell lung cancer patients with anti-hu have calcium channel antibodies)*	*Short-term memory loss, encephalopathy, personality change, decreased level of consciousness (frequency unknown; multiple case reports)*	Sensory neuropathy, Lambert-Eaton myasthenic syndrome (P/Q type; proximal weakness and dysautonomia), subacute onset and rapidly progressive ataxia, nystagmus, diplopia, dysphagia, dysarthria, dizziness, nausea/vomiting; associated with SCLC
Ganglionic acetylcholine receptor	55% male, age most commonly mid-sixties	*10% with cognitive or psychiatric manifestations; most common psychiatric manifestations are depression and psychosis*	*Mild amnestic syndrome (among 10% with cognitive/psychiatric manifestations)*, subacute encephalopathy (8%), dysexecutive syndrome (1%)	Subacute or insidious dysautonomia including GI dysmotility, orthostasis, and sicca syndrome; tonic pupils; sensory polyneuropathy, rare association with myasthenia gravis; associated with adenocarcinoma (lung most common)

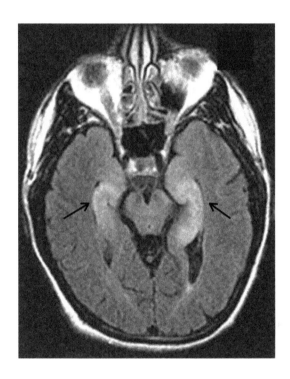

FIGURE 26-1. This FLAIR MRI image demonstrates mesial temporal hyperintensities in a patient with limbic encephalitis. (Reproduced with permission from Jameson J, Fauci AS, Kasper DL, et al. *Harrison's Principles of Internal Medicine.* 20th ed. https://accessmedicine. mhmedical.com. Copyright © McGraw Hill LLC. All rights reserved.)

accurately neuropsychiatric symptoms are diagnosed. Many studies estimate that up to 90% of patients with SLE have at least one neuropsychiatric symptom (which can be either primary or secondary) with the most common being headaches, cognitive impairment, and depression, all of which have a prevalence around 50%.[73] Approximately ¼–½ of cases of NPSLE manifest prior to or concurrent with the diagnosis of SLE, and ⅔ within

the first year of diagnosis.[76] Over the last few decades, incidence of NPSLE has increased though this is likely due to improved awareness and diagnostic capabilities including autoantibody testing and functional neuroimaging.

A complicating factor that may account for the wide variation between studies is the difficulty in determining whether neuropsychiatric symptoms are a direct effect of SLE autoantibodies on the brain or nervous system (i.e., meeting criteria for NPSLE) versus symptoms that are secondary sequelae of the illness or primary neuropsychiatric conditions that may occur around the time of diagnosis of SLE but are not necessarily related to the autoimmune activity. Some secondary sequelae of SLE include the increased incidence of thromboembolic events and stroke related to antiphospholipid syndrome, infections related to immunosuppressive therapy, or neurotoxic medication side effects.

Pathophysiology

The pathophysiology of SLE involves immunologic dysfunction characterized by the production of antinuclear antibodies that circulate systemically, deposit within tissues, and invoke an inflammatory response within the affected organ system. Injury to the CNS is thought to be mediated by specific autoantibodies generated during active stages of the illness as well as activation of complement and cytokine factors such as interleukin-1(IL-1), interleukin-6 (IL-6), tumor necrosis factor (TNF), and interferon-γ (IFN-γ) that promote inflammation and cause cytotoxic injury.[77,78] Patients with NPSLE have been found to have elevated levels of autoantibodies in their CSF, including lupus anticoagulant, antiphospholipid antibody, and antineuronal antibodies, among others,[79] as well as increased complement deposition in post-mortem studies[77] as compared to control patients with SLE who demonstrate elevated serum levels though lesser CSF involvement. The most common histopathological findings in post-mortem studies are vascular infarcts (both macro- and

TABLE 26-3 • Clinical Features of Neuroinfectious Diseases with Cognitive and Neuropsychiatric Sequelae.

Disorder	Psychiatric Manifestations	Cognitive Manifestations	Other Distinguishing Clinical Features
Herpes simplex virus (HSV) encephalitis	*Personality/behavior change (64%, including aggression and disinhibition)*, hallucinations (21%), irritability (11%), other psychosis (5%)	*Encephalopathy (91%)*, memory impairment (69%, anterograde>retrograde), decreased level of consciousness (67%, including coma), aphasia/mutism (33%, including semantic aphasia—loss of word meaning)	Prodrome (fever, headache, malaise), focal neurologic signs (e.g., aphasia, hemiparesis), seizures, anosmia, Klüver-Bucy syndrome (docility, compulsive eating, hypersexuality, hyperorality, visual agnosia)
Varicella zoster virus (VZV) encephalitis	*Personality/behavior change (70%)*, irritability (40%)	*Decreased level of consciousness (80%, including 20% with coma)*, executive dysfunction/inattention (e.g., on Stroop test as well as deficits in planning/impulse control, 36–50%), anomia (43%), amnestic syndrome (36%, immediate and delayed recall)	Seizures, rash, fever, immunocompromised/immunosuppressed patients, cranial neuropathy
Cytomegalovirus (CMV) encephalitis	*Apathy (60%)*, psychomotor retardation (57%)	*Encephalopathy (up to 90%)*, decreased level of consciousness (62%), memory impairment (60–71%); patients with CMV retinitis have difficulties with tasks of attention (73%), verbal fluency (33%), and abstraction (30%)	Disorders of retina, blood, adrenal glands, and GI tract; immunocompromised/immunosuppressed patients (e.g., HIV with CD4<50), cranial nerve palsies, fever, myelitis, polyradiculopathy
Human immunodeficiency virus (HIV)	*Depression (36%)*, dysthymia (26.5%), generalized anxiety (15.8%), drug dependence (12.5%), panic attacks (10.5%)	*Memory impairment (delayed recall, 29%)*, inattention (18%), reduced information processing speed (18%), impaired abstraction (11%), executive dysfunction (14%), verbal fluency (11%)	Fever, lymphadenopathy, sore throat, rash, myalgia/arthralgia, headache, painful mucocutaneous ulcers, opportunistic infections
Progressive multifocal leukoencephalopathy (PML, due to JC virus)	*Behavior/personality change (21%)*	*Aphasia (19%)*, reduced processing speed (4%), encephalopathy (4%)	Subacute onset hemiparesis, dysarthria, gait disturbance/ataxia, sensory deficit, visual loss (e.g., hemianopsia), seizures, immunocompromised/immunosuppressed patients (e.g., HIV with CD4<100 or natalizumab treatment)
Neurosyphilis (bacteria *Treponema pallidum*)	5–25 years after syphilis infection: *Delusions (61%)*, hallucinations (22%), depression (17%), anxiety (11%), pathological gambling (11%)	*Memory impairment (44%)*, executive dysfunction (33%), impaired judgment (28%), inattention (17%), perseveration (17%), aphasia (17%), visuospatial deficits (11%)	Primary: chancre
			Secondary: condyloma latum warts, rash on trunk/extremities including papules/nodules
			Tertiary: gummas (tumor-like balls occurring anywhere in body), neurosyphilis: seizures, meningitis, poor balance, weakness, Argyll Robertson pupils (constrict to accommodation but not light), cardiovascular syphilis (aortitis)
CNS Whipple's disease (bacteria *Tropheryma whipplei*)	*Behavior/personality change (26%, including irritability/aggression)*, hypersomnia (17–21%) or insomnia (5%), emotional lability (5%)	*Memory impairment (21–61%)*, inattention (11–61%), decreased level of consciousness (17%), executive dysfunction (17%), encephalopathy (5–17%), progressive dementia (16%), aphasia (5%)	Weight loss, steatorrhea or diarrhea, arthralgia, fever, ataxia, seizures, oculomasticatory myorhythmia (OMM, pendular nystagmus and masticatory muscle contraction, pathognomonic)

(Continued)

TABLE 26-3 • Clinical Features of Neuroinfectious Diseases with Cognitive and Neuropsychiatric Sequelae. *(Continued)*

Disorder	Psychiatric Manifestations	Cognitive Manifestations	Other Distinguishing Clinical Features
Cryptococcal meningitis (yeast *Cryptococcus neoformans*)	*Psychosis (at least 5 case reports, including hallucinations, delusions)*, insomnia (at least 4 case reports), personality/behavior changes (at least 3 case reports, including aggression/irritability, disinhibition), elated mood (at least 2 case reports), impaired reality testing (at least 1 case report)	*Changes in cognition (19%, including decreased attention/concentration, visuospatial abilities, abstraction, perceptual reasoning, working memory)*, decreased level of consciousness (7%), encephalopathy (6%)	Fever, nuchal rigidity, vomiting, increased intracranial pressure, photophobia, headaches, immunocompromised/immunosuppressed patients (e.g., HIV with CD4<100)
Toxoplasmosis (parasite *Toxoplasma gondii*)	*Psychomotor retardation (38%)*, behavior/personality changes (4%)	*Encephalopathy (52%)*, decreased level of consciousness (42%, including mild 27%, minimally responsive 11%, obtunded 3%), aphasia (8%)	Pulmonary and ocular findings; fever, seizures, headaches, immunocompromised/immunosuppressed patients (e.g., HIV with CD4<100)
Neurocysticercosis (parasite *Taenia solium*)	*Depression (78%)*, schizoaffective psychosis (13%), panic attacks (13%), phobias (13%), suicidal ideation (13%), generalized anxiety (9%), behavior/personality changes (9%), mania (4.3%), cyclothymia (4.3%), antisocial personality disorder (4.3%)	*Executive dysfunction (57.5%)*, inattention (55%), memory impairment (55%), aphasia (55%), visuospatial impairment (52.5%), apraxia (47.5%)	Seizures, focal neurologic signs, headache, altered vision, meningismus, nausea/vomiting
Creutzfeldt-Jakob disease (CJD, due to prions)	*Personality/behavior change (12%, including irritability/aggression)*, depression (4%), insomnia (2%), restlessness (2%), apathy (2%), panic attack (1%), social isolation (1%), mania (1%)	*Memory impairment (22%)*, aphasia (8%, including akinetic mutism), encephalopathy (6%), executive dysfunction (6%), decreased level of consciousness (6%), visuospatial impairment (4%), inattention (2%), apraxia (1%)	Extrapyramidal signs, ataxia, myoclonus, dysphagia, dizziness, weakness, paresthesias, diplopia
CNS tuberculosis (*Mycobacterium tuberculosis*)	*Personality/behavior change (13–39%)*, apathy (33%), depression (20%)	*Decreased level of consciousness (36%)*, chronic cognitive impairment (12–55%), including impairment in processing speed (27%), attention/working memory (27%), executive function (27%), impaired memory/learning (20%), impaired fluency (20%, categorical>phonemic), visuospatial (13%)	Pulmonary: chest pain, sputum-producing cough, hemoptysis; CNS prodrome: malaise, fever, headaches; meningitis: stiff neck, seizures, nausea/vomiting, cranial neuropathies, choroid tubercles on fundoscopy (pathognomonic); vasculopathy: strokes; tuberculoma or tuberculous brain abscess: papilledema; encephalopathy: disseminated intravascular coagulation (DIC); immunocompromised/immunosuppressed patients (e.g., HIV with CD4<500)

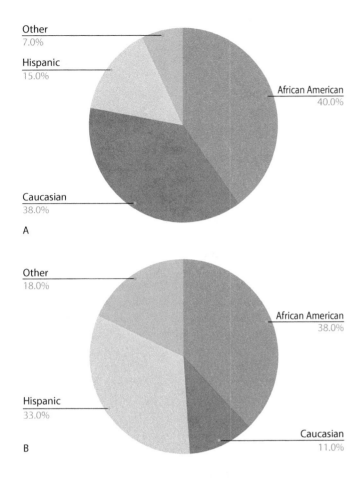

FIGURE 26-2. **A.** Estimated prevalence of patients with SLE displayed by ethnic group. **B.** Estimated prevalence of NPSLE by demographic. This pie chart represents all patients with NPSLE who fall within each of the displayed ethnic groups.

TABLE 26-4 • Neuropsychiatric Syndromes of Systemic Lupus Erythematosus per the American College of Rheumatology.
Central nervous system
Aseptic meningitis
Cerebrovascular disease
Cognitive dysfunction
Headache
Movement disorder (chorea)
Seizures
Acute confusional state
Anxiety disorder
Mood disorder
Psychosis
Demyelinating syndrome
Myelopathy (transverse myelitis)
Peripheral nervous system
Autonomic disorder
Mononeuropathy
Cranial neuropathy
Plexopathy
Polyneuropathy
Acute inflammatory demyelinating polyradiculoneuropathy (Guillain-Barré syndrome)
Myasthenia gravis

microinfarcts), hemorrhage, ischemic demyelination, patchy areas of demyelination, and cortical atrophy[77,80] and these are often visible post-mortem in patients in whom findings were not detected on MRI. Additionally, lupus vasculitis can affect cerebral blood vessels of all sizes and may or may not be visible as beading on MRI caused by asymmetric thickening of the vessel wall. Post-mortem case reports have shown vessel necrosis and inflammation on brain biopsy due primarily to lymphocyte infiltration of the vessel wall and deposition of IgG and complement in vessel walls.[81] Cerebral vasculitis or vasospasm may be a pathophysiologic cause of NPSLE symptoms. Moreover, studies are emerging that implicate blood-brain barrier dysfunction that may allow circulating antibodies to enter the brain parenchyma.[82] Taken together, vasculopathies generally are suspected to mechanistically underlie many of the symptoms of NPSLE.

Clinical Presentation

The most common manifestations of SLE involve fever, fatigue, myalgias, skin rashes, arthritis, and arthralgias, though many patients experience renal, pulmonary, gastrointestinal, or cardiac symptoms. The clinical manifestations of SLE can vary widely from patient to patient and may fluctuate over time within a particular individual. A diagnosis of NPSLE is considered for a patient with SLE manifesting at least 1 of 19 specific neuropsychiatric syndromes as outlined by the American College of Rheumatology (Table 26-4),[83,84] when the neuropsychiatric symptoms are thought to be due to cerebral involvement of SLE rather than an independent psychiatric illness. Unfortunately, many aspects of NPSLE are poorly understood and this determination can be challenging.[85]

Possible presentations of NPSLE include headaches, strokes, seizures, movement disorders, myelitis, cranial or peripheral neuropathies, or with psychiatric symptoms such as delirium, psychosis, mania, anxiety, or depression,[86] among others.

Neurologic Presentations

Stroke Syndromes

Longitudinal studies have shown that younger patients with SLE are at significantly higher risk of stroke as compared to the general population, with ischemic stroke (90%) more prevalent than hemorrhagic stroke (10%). The difference in risk is no longer clinically significant past age 60. Strokes have been reported in up to 19% of patients with SLE[87] with TIAs and small vessel infarcts being the most common. There appears to be a high correlation between antiphospholipid antibodies and the risk of stroke,[88] suggesting a primary etiology. Antiphospholipid antibodies are a heterogeneous group of antibodies that react with several phospholipid binding proteins and can cause thromboses through interactions with the antigen surface of platelets, hematopoietic serum cofactors, or endothelial cells. Secondary causes of stroke such as hypertension associated with chronic steroid therapy, infection from immunosuppression, or valvular heart disease leading to cardiac emboli all increase risk.[87,88]

Seizures

Approximately 10–20% of patients with SLE develop seizures[89] that may be of any semiology and in a minority of cases may be a presenting symptom of the illness, particularly in younger patients with a higher disease burden.[90] Focal seizures with impaired awareness are more common than generalized tonic-clonic seizures (GTCs), though GTCs in particular are more common in patients with lupus nephritis and hypertension.[91] Per some reports, seizures are correlated with psychotic symptoms and focal EEG abnormalities specifically in the temporal lobe.[91] As with strokes, seizures can also result from secondary manifestations of the SLE such as hypertension, infections, drug toxicity, or history of stroke.

Headache

Headaches are the most common neuropsychiatric symptom in patients with SLE with prevalence of up to 95% by some reports[92]—though it is unclear to what extent the prevalence of headaches in patients with SLE differs from control subjects and no specific pathological mechanism for headaches as related to SLE has been identified. Given the high prevalence it is difficult to distinguish between primary NPSLE versus secondary causes of headache, making studies variable and unreliable. Isolated headaches in patients with SLE therefore do not require any specific workup or specialized treatment recommendations, and should be managed according to standard practice.

Neuropathy

Patients with SLE are at higher risk of developing neuropathy that can be either peripheral or autonomic in nature, believed to be due to autoimmune inflammation of the small arteries that supply the nerve bed.[93] Symptoms are typically mild and asymmetric, may involve mono- or polyneuropathy, and tend to occur later in the course of the illness with decreased nerve conduction velocities noted on electromyography (EMG).[93] Cranial neuropathies have been reported though are very rare. In such cases symptoms may include optic neuritis (evident on MRI), extraocular muscle involvement, sensorineural hearing reduction, diplopia, trigeminal neuralgia, and facial weakness with dysarthria, among others.[93,94]

Other Neurological Manifestations

There are multiple uncommon neurological manifestations of SLE, including movement disorders, meningitis, and transverse myelitis. These are typically associated with active signs of brain or spinal cord involvement demonstrated on MRI and rarely occur in isolation as the primary presenting symptom of SLE. Infectious etiologies must be considered.

Ocular symptoms occur relatively commonly in patients with SLE and may involve the optic nerve, retina, uvea, conjunctiva, or eyelids.

Neuropsychiatric Presentations

Cognitive Dysfunction

Cognitive deficits occur in a majority of patients with SLE, with some studies suggesting a prevalence of over 80%.[86] Symptoms may include memory impairment, difficulties with complex attention, verbal memory and verbal reasoning, executive functioning, and personality changes, or any combination of these symptoms and may eventually progress to a diagnosis of dementia.[95] Cognitive deficits may be determined via bedside or office cognitive testing, neuropsychological testing, or by general impairments in functioning. There is no specific type of antineuronal or antiphospholipid antibody that has been consistently implicated in contributing to the cognitive deficits of NPSLE; some studies have shown an association with specific antibody subtypes though this has not been consistently validated,[96] and it remains debatable whether neuroimaging has any diagnostic value.[97,98] Cognitive dysfunction is often most acute during active stages of the disease, though may manifest even during latent periods of the illness. It remains unclear to what extent cognitive deficits associated with NPSLE are due to primary brain dysfunction arising from the direct effects of SLE on the brain, or due to the secondary effects of this chronic illness such as poor sleep, pain, anxiety, or psychological stress. Cognitive deficits tend to improve over time in patients who remain on immunosuppressant medications or antithrombotic agents, suggesting that inflammatory and thrombotic mechanisms are associated with cognitive impairment.[99] Cognitive dysfunction can be exacerbated by other symptoms of the illness such as vascular infarcts or hypertension, or by medication side effects from corticosteroids.[100]

Mood Disorders

Depression is the most common psychiatric diagnosis associated with SLE, and can be either a direct manifestation of the disease or a secondary mechanism associated with the stress of chronic illness. In the former case, multiple studies have demonstrated an association with anti-ribosomal P antibodies (in some studies up to 75–88% of patients)[101,102] and proteinuria,[103] and a few studies have found correlation with anti-NMDA antibodies, though this has not been consistently validated.[104] For a diagnosis of primary causality, depressive symptoms tend to occur acutely in the context of active disease, and a history of premorbid depression should be ruled out. Depressive illness in patients with SLE or NPSLE follows the expected course for depression, with the average depressive episode resolving within 1 year, and patients with psychosocial support faring better than those without.[105] Depression often entails a number of somatic complaints including insomnia or hypersomnia, decreased appetite, anergia, myalgias, constipation, decreased libido, and impaired concentration, all of which can be related either to depression, the primary symptoms of SLE, or both.[103,105] Other mood symptoms, such as a cyclical disturbance in mood including both manias and depressions, have also been seen in NPSLE, though are very uncommon, occurring in fewer than 1% of patients.[106] In contrast, steroid-induced mania occurs more commonly than bipolar disorder as discussed below.

Psychosis

Unlike primary psychotic disorders that often have a progressive and recurrent course, psychosis secondary to NPSLE typically occurs within the first year of diagnosis and may not recur.[39,40,93,94] Approximately 5% of patients with SLE develop associated psychosis, and up to 80% of these cases occur within

1 year of diagnosis. Unlike primary psychotic disorders that often have a progressive and recurrent course, psychosis secondary to NPSLE typically occurs within the first year of diagnosis, often as a presenting symptom of the illness, and may not recur.[107,108] Delusions of grandiosity or paranoia are the most common feature, followed by auditory hallucinations.[109] The diagnostic criteria for NPSLE-associated psychosis are similar to those for primary psychosis, including disorganized thinking, delusions, paranoia, or hallucinations among other symptoms. Unfortunately, no single imaging modality or biomarker is available to distinguish between psychosis secondary to NPSLE versus psychosis that is not, though some symptom variability may guide diagnostic impressions, for example visual or tactile hallucinations are more common in NPSLE-associated psychosis.[107,108] The ICD-10 guidelines[110] can be helpful in making the determination between NPSLE-associated psychosis versus that which is not, including (1) psychosis with a comorbid diagnosis of SLE, (2) a temporal relationship between the onset of psychiatric symptoms and the underlying disease state, (3) remission of symptoms with treatment of the underlying disease state, and (4) absence of evidence to suggest an alternative cause of a primary psychiatric condition (such as history of trauma, family history, substance use or a specific environmental trigger).

Assessment and Differential Diagnosis

The diagnosis of NPSLE requires both that a patient have an established diagnosis of SLE and that there be clinical evidence linking neurological and/or psychiatric symptoms with SLE-related disease mechanisms by time course, exam, and when applicable biomarkers. As with many psychiatric diagnoses, a diagnosis of NPSLE is considered a diagnosis of exclusion. Other etiologies including infectious, medication side effect, new onset primary psychiatric disorder, substance use, limbic seizure, stroke, and primary medical causes (primary brain tumors, electrolyte abnormalities, paraneoplastic processes for example) should be excluded. Often the timing of symptom presentation can be a helpful guideline as psychiatric manifestations of SLE tend to present within the first 2 years of diagnosis.[111] Like other manifestations of SLE, NPSLE is believed to be antibody mediated, though neuropsychiatric symptoms can be present even when other disease symptoms are stable or absent. This may occur, in part, due to variation in subtypes of antibodies leading to variable symptom pathology (see Table 26-5), such as anti-ribosomal P antibodies being more highly correlated with psychosis[101] than with peripheral complaints, for example, whereas antiphospholipid antibodies are more highly correlated with movement disorders.[112] Antineuronal and antiphospholipid antibodies are believed to increase the risk of stroke, seizure, and cortical atrophy in patients with SLE.[102,103] Several other autoantibodies subtypes including lymphocytotoxic antibodies, anti-ribosomal P antibodies, anti-endothelial cell antibodies, and cross-reacting antibodies to the NMDA receptor have been suggested to play a role in the mechanism of NPSLE, possibly through disruption of the blood-brain barrier, although this relationship remains to be confirmed.[104,115–119] Anti-ribosomal P antibodies have also been implicated in NPSLE-associated depression[120] and psychosis. Some reports suggest

that persistently elevated antiphospholipid antibodies (such as anticardiolipin antibody)[121,122] are associated with greater cognitive impairment though other studies dispute these findings.[123] Despite much research, the role of specific antibody subtypes in the pathophysiology of particular symptoms remains ambiguous, and it is difficult to distinguish causative from correlative effects. Therefore, the American College of Rheumatology does not currently recommend that clinicians pursue testing for specific autoantibodies in serum or CSF as diagnostic biomarkers for a classification of NPSLE as their association with specific symptoms remains inconclusive.

The most common MRI findings of NPSLE include cortical atrophy, micro- and macroinfarcts, hyperintense white matter lesions, and dilated ventricles,[124] with MRI findings most highly correlated with elevated CSF antibody levels rather than serum antibody levels.[125] The most commonly affected areas on MRI include the cerebral cortex, thalamus, hippocampus, pons, brainstem, and cerebellum.[126,127] However, a normal structural MRI does not exclude the diagnosis of NPSLE. PET and MR-spectroscopy may detect white matter hypometabolism in patients in whom structural MRI is unremarkable[128] though similarly a normal functional MRI does not exclude the diagnosis.[129] In addition to neuroimaging modalities, rapidly developing next generation genetic sequencing techniques are yielding new information with regard to genetic markers of SLE and potentially novel therapeutic targets. This, when taken together with the growing field of biomarkers and brain neuroimaging, may lead to novel personalized treatment.[130]

Treatment

Treatment involves administering the standard of care for SLE, then further addressing considerations specific to the presenting manifestation(s). Specific examples include the following:

Stroke(s)

Treatment via anticoagulation with aspirin or warfarin is recommended in stable patients with no evidence of hemorrhage. A target INR of 2.0–3.0 on warfarin has been shown to be as effective for reducing stroke as more intensive anticoagulation.[131] For patients with antiphospholipid syndrome the treatment is more controversial with some reports suggesting anticoagulation with warfarin (despite a lack of randomized clinical trials to support this to date) while others suggest treatment with antiplatelet therapy.[132] Adjunctive therapy with glucocorticoids to suppress production of antibodies may be utilized in patients with a concurrent lupus flare.[133]

Seizures

Treatment of seizures involves utilizing antiepileptic drugs according to routine standards of care as there are currently no randomized controlled trials specifically for the treatment of seizures in patients with SLE. One important treatment difference is that in patients with a single presenting seizure thought to represent an active inflammatory state, providers may choose to treat with pulse or IV steroids such as prednisone or methylprednisolone, or other anti-inflammatory treatments such as cyclophosphamide to reduce SLE-related inflammation rather than with antiseizure medications.[134]

TABLE 26-5 • Association of Specific Antibody Subtypes with Symptoms of NPSLE*.

Antibodies, Cytokines, and Chemokines	Associated Psychiatric Condition	Associated Neurological Conditions
Anti-NMDA • Found in CSF of 30% of patients with NPSLE	Mood disorders	Cortical atrophy Neuropathy
Anti-ribosomal P	Psychosis (strong correlation) Mood disorders (moderate correlation)	Cognitive dysfunction Seizures
Antineuronal • Antibody levels 8-fold higher in the CSF than in serum	IgG antibodies in the CSF highly correlated with NPSLE diffusely, though not with specific symptoms.	IgG antibodies in the CSF highly correlated with NPSLE diffusely, though not with specific symptoms.
Antiphospholipid (specifically, anti-β2-glycoprotein 1—IgG, IgM, and anti-cardiolipin IgG, IgM have shown the highest correlation in this class)	Dementia Mood disorders Psychosis	Cognitive dysfunction[95] Cortical atrophy[115] Seizure[114,115] Movement disorders[113,114] Stroke/Vascular/Migraine[90,134]
Anti-ganglioside antibodies	IgM-specific antibodies linked to depression[117]	IgG-specific antibodies linked to migraine, dementia, peripheral neuropathy
Complement	Increased circulating levels found in the CSF of patients with NPSLE as compared to patients with SLE without neuropsychiatric involvement, however no correlation to particular neuropsychiatric symptoms	
Anti-dsDNA • May cross react with anti-ribosomal P or anti-NMDAR antibody testing* • Several studies have shown lower antibody levels in CSF compared to serum	Depression	Cognitive dysfunction Hippocampal atrophy[127,225]

*Note: While some studies suggest a correlation between specific antibody subtypes and neuropsychiatric symptoms, study results are variable and inconsistently validated.[29]

Neuropathy

Treatment is based on severity, and may include glucocorticoids (typically prednisone 1 mg/kg), low-dose tricyclic antidepressants (TCAs), or gabapentin. In rare cases, an acute inflammatory polyradiculopathy can progress over the course of weeks to months with symptoms similar to Guillain-Barré syndrome in which case more aggressive immunosuppressant therapy such as cyclophosphamide may be indicated.[135]

Mood Disorders

Antidepressants, mood stabilizers, and antianxiety medications may be used per standard protocols, with SSRIs being first-line treatment for depression and mood stabilizers utilized for bipolar and manic disorders.[105,106] Anxiety may also manifest in patients with NPSLE, often with comorbid depression, and may also be treated with SSRIs.[136] In patients with lupus nephritis, the half-life of the medication (such as fluoxetine, which has a long half-life) should be considered and patients should be monitored closely for side effects.

Psychosis

Treatment involves immediate symptom control via administration of second-generation antipsychotics as well as treatment of the underlying SLE pathology using immunosuppressant agents such as prednisone, cyclophosphamide, or azathioprine. There

are currently no specific guidelines and no published randomized controlled trials with regard to preferential use of specific second-generation antipsychotics in the treatment of NPSLE-related psychosis. In fact, reports have been contradictory with some suggesting benefit with risperidone, olanzapine, and lurasidone,[109] while others suggest that risperidone and olanzapine are risk factors for adverse cerebrovascular events and should be avoided,[137] instead recommending use of quetiapine.[138] Long-term treatment with antipsychotics is typically not required as symptoms resolve with immunosuppressive treatment of the underlying SLE pathology.[108,109,132]

In treatment refractory cases, sequential treatment with steroids followed by immunomodulating therapy has shown good results. One open label study demonstrated that prednisolone followed by sequential oral cyclophosphamide and oral azathioprine was associated with a remission rate of over 92%.[109] Maintenance therapy with azathioprine or cyclosporin are commonly used though their efficacy has not been established by randomized controlled trials.[109]

Importantly, psychotic symptoms may also result from glucocorticoid steroid treatment used to treat SLE, in which case symptoms are most likely to occur within 6 weeks of steroid administration (often sooner), are dose dependent, and typically resolve with discontinuation of steroids.[139]

Currently, there are many experimental treatments being utilized either individually or in combination therapy for treatment refractory NPSLE. These treatments include IVIG, plasma exchange, rituximab, cyclosporins, interferon-receptor antagonists, and monoclonal antibodies, all of which have shown promise in open label studies or case reports and may provide corticosteroid sparing effects.[109] Currently these treatments await validation in randomized controlled trials. The increased application of genome wide association studies may also identify specific subtypes of antibodies or cytokines involved in the pathogenesis of NPSLE that may yield targeted biological treatment.

HUMAN IMMUNODEFICIENCY VIRUS

Epidemiology

Human immunodeficiency virus (HIV) has an estimated prevalence in the United States of 1.1 million as of 2015 (CDC, *HIV Surveillance Supplemental Report*) and an estimated annual incidence of 38,500 (CDC, *HIV Surveillance Supplemental Report*). HIV is associated with pathology of the nervous system, including direct pathologic effects of viral invasion leading to HIV-associated neurocognitive disorder (HAND) as well as the associated effects of CNS opportunistic infections and malignancies, together comprising neuroAIDS.[140] HAND can be further subdivided into asymptomatic neurocognitive impairment (ANI), mild neurocognitive disorder (MND), and HIV-associated dementia (HAD). Overall prevalence of HAND is high, with about 50% of treated patients with HIV showing cognitive impairment although prevalence of more severe forms of cognitive impairment has diminished with the availability of antiretroviral treatment.[140]

In addition, HIV is associated with a number of comorbid neuropsychiatric conditions, including depression, mania, psychosis, substance abuse, and post-traumatic stress disorder (PTSD). Depression prevalence estimates in HIV-positive patients vary widely by population and study methodology, with some as high as 60%.[141] A meta-analysis found that people with HIV had nearly twice the frequency of depression seen in the general population.[142] Recent studies after the advent of antiretroviral therapy (ART) suggest a depression prevalence in treated populations in the 20–25% range.[141] Depression in HIV-infected patients is more likely in those with symptomatic disease, those with a prior history of major depression, or those with other lifetime psychiatric comorbidities, but appears to be unaffected by life adversity or by disease progression.[143]

Patients with HIV may have mania in the context of a classic idiopathic bipolar disorder, or they may experience mania in the setting of more advanced HIV infection (lower CD4 count), which has been termed AIDS mania or secondary mania. The latter appears to be more commonly associated with cognitive impairment, and less associated with family history of bipolar disorder.[144] Prevalence of mania in one study was found to range between 1% in HIV positive individuals to nearly 5% in those with AIDS[145]; other series have found higher prevalence in the AIDS population.[146] The relationship between antiretroviral treatment and risk for mania is not entirely clear; while mania has been reported as a side effect of several antiretroviral agents,[147] a case control study of patients with HIV-associated mania actually found that any exposure to ART was protective,[148] perhaps suggesting that the neurotoxic effects of both the virus and antiretroviral treatment can be contributory.

New-onset psychosis has a prevalence of 3.7 per 100 HIV-1-infected persons in one study, and was associated with a prior psychiatric history, lower cognitive performance overall, and lack of ART.[149]

PTSD is common in persons living with HIV and AIDS. Living in poverty may represent one shared risk factor for both conditions in that poor neighborhoods see high rates of trauma exposure and inhabitants may have increased risk for substance abuse and unprotected sex.[150] Perhaps related to rates of trauma exposure, women who are HIV-positive have high rates of PTSD of around 30%, five times the rates in HIV-negative women.[150]

Substance abuse is an important comorbidity for people with HIV. Prevalences reported for these comorbidities vary widely, but ranges for alcohol abuse and dependence are 22–60% and 12–41% and one study reported comorbid IV cocaine or heroin use of 12%.[151] It is likely that comorbid opioid use in HIV patients has dramatically increased in recent years in parallel with the overall opioid epidemic.

Certain diagnoses also increase risk for acquisition of HIV; in a population-wide study in Sweden, patients with a severe mental illness such as schizophrenia, schizoaffective disorder, or bipolar disorder were significantly more likely to have HIV infection, with substance abuse contributing substantially to this increased risk.[152]

Pathophysiology

Initial HIV infection appears to be accompanied by direct viral invasion into the CNS.[153] Even in the early phases of HIV infection pathologic changes can be observed in the brain. These include diffuse myelin pallor affecting the deep white matter, thought possibly to be related to increased blood-brain barrier permeability, as well as reactive astrocytosis.[153] HAND appears to be associated with degree of host inflammatory response, although there is a limited association between viral load and severity of neurocognitive impairment.[140] Observed HIV-related pathologic changes include diffuse white matter pallor, multinucleated giant cells, reactive gliosis, and astrocytosis, affecting the putamen, globus pallidus and hippocampus primarily, but also reported in the corpus callosum and brainstem.[154] These changes may be responsible for some of the cognitive deficits and neuropsychiatric changes seen in HIV/AIDs patients. Figure 26-3 highlights the imaging features of HIV leukoencephalopathy in a patient with HIV-associated dementia (AIDS dementia).

Another pathophysiologic mechanism of neuropsychiatric disease burden in HIV is due to opportunistic infections, including cryptococcal meningitis, tubercular meningitis, *Toxoplasma* encephalitis, and JC virus (progressive multifocal leukoencephalopathy or PML). These are more common in developing countries where access to antiretroviral treatment is more limited.[140] Figures 26-4 and 26-5 highlight the characteristic imaging findings in patients with HIV and comorbid toxoplasmosis and PML, respectively.

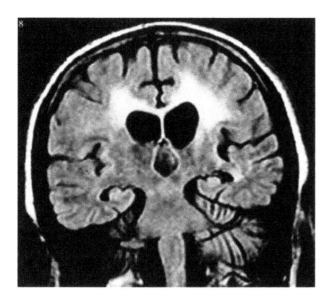

FIGURE 26-3. Coronal FLAIR MRI of HIV leukoencephalopathy in a patient with AIDS dementia. Cortical atrophy, ventricular enlargement, and large areas of white matter hyperintensities are visible. (Reproduced with permission from Ropper AH, Samuels MA, Klein JP, Prasad S. *Adams and Victor's Principles of Neurology,* 11th ed. https://accessmedicine. mhmedical.com. Copyright © McGraw Hill LLC. All rights reserved.)

Clinical Presentation

HIV presents clinically due to the reductions it effects on populations of immune cells including natural killer cells and T lymphocytes.[141] As mentioned above, the neuropsychiatric presentations associated with HIV infection are numerous. In terms of HIV-associated neurocognitive impairment, there are considered to be three stages of severity: asymptomatic, mild, and HAD, with the latter indicating associated functional impairment. HIV-associated dementia (formerly known as AIDS dementia complex or ADC and sometimes called HIV encephalitis or HIV encephalopathy) is considered to be a subcortical dementia characterized by progressive decline in attention and motor speed; it often leads to death within a year.[140] However, this clinical presentation of HAND as primarily causing motor slowing and slowed information processing was identified prior to ART. In the era of combination antiretroviral therapy (cART), HAND is associated with more learning and executive functioning deficits.[155] Before antiretroviral treatment, both HIV load and CD4 count were associated with neuropsychological impairment. However, with advances in treatment this is no longer the case, although a lower CD4 nadir remains a risk factor for HAND. Early treatment of HIV appears to be protective against neurocognitive impairment.[140]

There are also neurologic effects secondary to the presence of opportunistic infections and cancers that develop in the context of HIV infection, and that can vary in clinical presentation by type of infection or malignancy and by location (e.g., of mass effect from a primary CNS lymphoma). Common comorbid conditions that affect neurologic function include *Toxoplasma* encephalitis, primary CNS lymphoma, progressive multifocal leukoencephalopathy, cytomegalovirus encephalitis, and neurosyphilis. Syndromes such as *Toxoplasma* encephalitis may

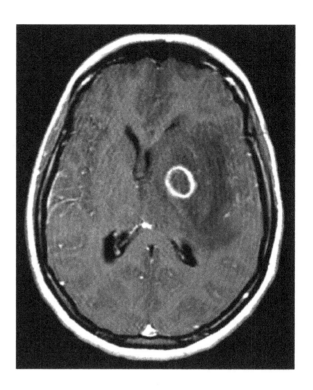

FIGURE 26-4. This MRI shows a ring-enhancing abscess due to toxoplasmosis in the deep left cerebral hemisphere in an HIV-positive patient. These lesions are sometimes accompanied by mass effect and surrounding edema, as seen here. (Reproduced with permission from Ropper AH, Samuels MA, Klein JP, Prasad S. *Adams and Victor's Principles of Neurology,* 11th ed. https://accessmedicine. mhmedical.com. Copyright © McGraw Hill LLC. All rights reserved.)

present with confusion, behavior changes, neuropsychiatric symptoms, coma, or nothing at all,[156] so diagnostic procedures including imaging, serum antibodies, and CSF testing can be helpful to identify the etiology of a change in mental status.

Depression is common in persons with HIV infection, and may be related to viral disruption of frontostriatal circuits, to psychosocial factors such as stigmatization and lack of social support, and to chronic immune activation and disruption of the HPA axis leading to increased levels of inflammatory cytokines.[141] Depression can affect the course of HIV infection. It has been associated with decreased adherence to antiretroviral treatment, with declines in several lymphocyte populations, and with disrupted HPA axis functioning that can negatively affect immune function.[141] Perhaps related to these, untreated depression is associated with a shorter time to development of AIDS and with shorter survival times.[141]

Mania secondary to HIV infection may present somewhat differently from mania due to bipolar disorder. One study found that those with mania secondary to HIV infection had more irritability (vs. elevated mood), more aggressive behavior, and more frequent paranoid delusions and hallucinations than those with mania due to bipolar disorder.[157] They were also more likely to have cognitive impairment accompanying their mania than those with a bipolar mania.[157]

Psychosis in HIV-infected populations has been reported to develop acutely or subacutely, and to include delusions, hallucinations, and bizarre behavior.[158] It has even been a presenting manifestation of HIV infection and AIDS.[158]

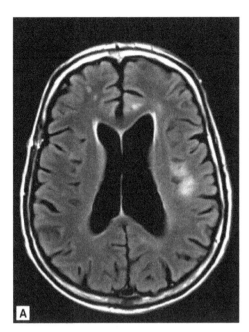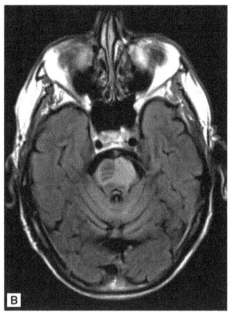

FIGURE 26-5. This is the MRI of a 31-year-old patient with HIV who developed progressive multifocal leukoencephalopathy (PML). Axial FLAIR sequences demonstrate multiple subcortical white matter lesions in **(A)** both hemispheres and in **(B)** the left pons. There was no abnormal enhancement (not shown). (Reproduced with permission from Ropper AH, Samuels MA, Klein JP, Prasad S. *Adams and Victor's Principles of Neurology,* 11th ed. https://accessmedicine.mhmedical.com. Copyright © McGraw Hill LLC. All rights reserved.)

Comorbid PTSD is associated with worse outcomes in HIV-infected individuals.[150] Possible contributors to this relationship include PTSD avoidance-related reductions in medication adherence and exaggerated immune disruption in HIV patients with PTSD.[150]

Substance abuse is also associated with poorer outcomes for HIV-infected persons, with more rapid declines in CD4 counts, increased rates of progression to AIDS, and decreased acceptance of and adherence to ART.[159] Carrying either or both a psychiatric and a substance use diagnosis also places HIV-positive individuals at increased risk for death, particularly when untreated.[160] Treating either condition helps to mitigate this risk.[160]

Assessment and Differential Diagnosis

An assessment of the HIV-positive patient with a change in cognition or behavior should begin with a thorough history, including attention to the time course of onset and symptom progression, the domains affected, and the degree of functional impairment. A clinical exam can further evaluate the presence of neuropsychiatric symptoms, degree and domains of neuropsychological deficits, and presence and type of motor disturbance, as well as help to rule out other potential contributing causes. Laboratory evaluations of the degree to which HIV is controlled (viral load and CD4 counts) can help to determine whether patient is at high risk for some HIV-associated conditions. Additional laboratory studies can help exclude other medical contributions to change in mental status, whether general medical conditions (such as metabolic disturbances) or specific comorbidities (such as syphilis). Recommended analyses include complete blood count, electrolyte panel, liver function

tests, serologies for hepatitis and syphilis, and pertinent vitamin levels (B12, folate), among others.[161]

Imaging studies can help to support or argue against a diagnosis of HAND but are not definitive. Structural imaging has demonstrated cerebral atrophy in HAD, with the bicaudate ratio (the distance between the caudate heads at their closest point divided by the width of the brain at the same line) as well as cortical thinning correlating with neurocognitive impairment.[162] Other findings in HAND include hippocampal atrophy and diffuse periventricular white matter changes, and caudate atrophy which correlates with motor dysfunction. Unfortunately, there is no pattern of changes specific enough to diagnose HAND.[162] However, imaging may also be helpful to rule out or identify space-occupying lesions such as toxoplasmosis or lymphoma that could be contributing to the presentation.

Lumbar puncture is valuable in defining the state of the central nervous system infection. Valuable CSF studies include HIV-RNA, protein levels, cell counts, oligoclonal bands, and assessments for concomitant neurosyphilis.[161]

Cognitive screening for HAND is recommended in all HIV-positive patients, at baseline (prior to initiation of combination ART), and then at least every 12–24 months (6–12 months in high-risk patients) or whenever clinically warranted.[163] A comprehensive neuropsychological assessment is optimal, but in resource-constrained settings cognitive screening tools, functional assessment, and limited neuropsychological testing can provide diagnostic information.[163] Evaluation of functional status is also recommended.[161]

The differential diagnosis for change in mental status in HIV-positive patients is broad, and includes HIV/AIDS-related conditions such as CNS lymphoma and *Toxoplasma* infection, as well as the usual range of neoplastic, infectious, endocrine, cerebrovascular, toxic, and metabolic causes.

Treatment

Treatment of the neuropsychiatric effects of HIV can be broadly divided into treatments designed to address cognitive dysfunction and those targeted at specific neuropsychiatric symptoms such as mood disturbance or psychosis. We will address these sequentially.

cART is critical for both prevention and treatment of HIV-associated neurocognitive deficits. Improved cognition has been demonstrated in HIV-positive individuals starting 4–8 months after the initiation of cART, and degree of improvement is associated with severity of initial deficit and with increase in CD4 cells.[164] In those already taking cART, adaptation of the antiretroviral regimen to one with better CNS penetration may be necessary to better control viral replication within the CNS, though the degree to which this has clinical impact on cognition has been inconsistent across studies.[164] There is also some evidence that therapies specifically targeting monocytes may improve cognitive performance in those patients with HAND.[165] Overall, optimizing neurocognitive functioning seems to depend on both successful suppression of viral activity with cART and on avoiding severe immunosuppression (no CD4 count below 200 in the patient's medical history).[155] Despite tremendous advances in ART, HIV-associated cognitive deficits persist and adjunctive treatments are often needed.

Unfortunately, psychotropic medications in general have not been demonstrated to yield significant benefit for HAND; these included cognitive-enhancing medications such as cholinesterase-inhibitors, NMDA-receptor antagonists, and stimulants.[164] There is some limited evidence that rivastigmine helps with processing speed, but it has not improved performance in other cognitive domains.[166] Memantine showed no cognitive benefit.[167] Similarly, armodafinil was not helpful.[168]

There is some evidence that cognitive rehabilitation therapies can be helpful in HAND, with benefit across a number of domains including learning and memory, abstraction, executive function, attention, and working memory.[169] Computerized cognitive stimulation may also be helpful; in an Internet-based cognitive rehabilitation program, those who used the program the most showed improvement in a global measure of cognitive impairment.[170]

With HAND persisting well into the cART era, the question of neurotoxicity associated with ART has naturally arisen. Indeed, there is some evidence for neurotoxicity at concentrations seen in the CSF, with greater toxicity associated with abacavir, efavirenz, etravirine, nevaripine, and atazanavir than for other agents.[171] As described above, effective viral suppression is considered essential for the management of HIV-associated cognitive deficits but at the same time there is evidence that certain regimens may have deleterious effects on isolated cognitive domains as shown in Kahouadji et al.[172] Additional data will clarify the optimal approach for cognitive preservation.

As with cognitive impairment, ART can be important for the prevention of neuropsychiatric symptoms like depression, mania, and psychosis. An association has been suggested

between treatment with ART and protection from developing psychosis.[149] With many of the neuropsychiatric symptoms associated with HIV, other treatment approaches also exist.

Antidepressant treatment in people with HIV tends to focus on pharmacologic therapies, and there is some data to suggest greater efficacy for antidepressant medication as compared to placebo.[173] However, a Cochrane review found that while antidepressants may be beneficial for people with HIV and depression, the overall quality of evidence was limited, which made it difficult to come to firm conclusions. That said, there was limited evidence that mirtazapine could have superiority in treating depression in this population when compared to SSRIs.[141] In this population, particular attention needs to be paid to CYP450 interactions given that antiretroviral agents can induce or inhibit cytochrome P450 enzymes which affect metabolism of a number of antidepressants.[174] Mirtazapine's minimal P450 interactions thus may make it useful in this population. Due to their minimal P450 interactions, citalopram and escitalopram are popular SSRI choices.[175] Bupropion levels may be increased when used in combination with NNRTIs and some protease inhibitors, and decreased when in combination with ritonavir, due to interactions at the 2B6 cytochrome enzyme.[175] Stimulants and modafinil have also been shown to be effective for some symptoms of depression, including low mood and energy.[175]

Psychotherapy can also be helpful; cognitive behavioral therapy has shown some benefit for management of depression in HIV-infected individuals[2] and brief interpersonal psychotherapy is another approach that demonstrated efficacy, even when administered telephonically.[176] The use of ECT to successfully treat depression in HIV-positive individuals has been described[177] and one small study supports the use of transcranial direct current stimulation to treat depression in HIV patients.[178]

The management of mania in treated patients with HIV is complicated by the risks associated with enzyme induction from ART influencing drug levels.[175] Valproic acid has therefore become a preferred agent, with lamotrigine another favored choice, although the latter may need dosing adjustments if prescribed alongside ritonavir.[175] There is some evidence supporting use of risperidone for mania and psychosis in patients with HIV.[179] However, HIV-positive patients have been reported to have increased risk for extrapyramidal side effects on high-potency D2-blocking medications, and so some treaters may prefer agents perceived as more tolerable, such as quetiapine.[175] As with other medication classes, CYP450 enzyme interactions are of concern; ritonavir in particular may affect levels of risperidone and olanzapine.[175] Clozapine should generally be avoided in the HIV-positive population due to risks of side effects and toxicity in combination with ritonavir.[175] The use of ECT to treat HIV-associated mania has been described,[180] but other forms of brain stimulation to treat mania or psychosis have not been portrayed in the literature.

Treatment of anxiety, in addition to relying on SSRI or SNRI medications, may involve use of benzodiazepines. Given the high rates of substance abuse in the HIV-positive population, attention should be paid to dependency concerns as this is a potentially serious issue.[181] As with other psychotropic drug classes, CYP enzyme interactions, especially in combination with ritonavir, could result in oversedation with alprazolam, midazolam, and triazolam.[181] Ritonavir also increases glucuronidation, which lowers the levels of oxazepam, lorazepam, and temazepam.[181] Group psychosocial interventions for individuals with comorbid HIV and anxiety have not consistently demonstrated benefit in one Cochrane review.[182] However, evaluation of a group intervention specifically to address coping with post-traumatic stress symptoms in HIV-positive people did find some benefit.[183]

Treatment for substance abuse can include opioid replacement therapy, medications to reduce cravings or substance use, psychotherapies, and group interventions. Studies of treating HIV-infected patients with comorbid substance abuse found improved treatment outcomes when the substance abuse treatment is colocated with the HIV treatment.[159] Methadone maintenance can be valuable to drug users with HIV, particularly for intravenous drug users.[184] However, buprenorphine/naloxone may be preferable to methadone for opioid maintenance therapy in HIV-positive patients as the buprenorphine combination is less dependent on CYP enzymes for clearance and may be used in conjunction with NNRTIs without the need for dose adjustments.[185] Medications such as naltrexone and disulfiram have not been well-studied in HIV-positive populations.[184] Cognitive behavioral therapy for substance abuse in conjunction with behavioral approaches like contingency management has shown variable benefit, with some of the variability being across different drugs of abuse.[184] Motivational interviewing on the other hand has benefitted outcomes for HIV-positive drug users.[184]

In addition to the necessity of treating comorbid neuropsychiatric symptoms in HIV-positive populations, there is also the issue of treating the virus itself. As noted above, antiretrovirals can have beneficial effects on neuropsychiatric symptoms, but adverse effects also occur. Many HIV drugs have known neuropsychiatric side effects, particularly non-nucleoside reverse transcriptase inhibitor (NNRTI) drugs. Some antiretroviral drugs have neuropsychiatric effects in almost 2% of those taking them, and can be a reason for discontinuation. Switching regimens can be helpful in managing such adverse effects. The NNRTI medication efavirenz in particular has been reported to be associated with mood symptoms, including depression, mania, and suicidality, and needs careful monitoring in patients with a history of depression.[175] Other symptoms reported with efavirenz include, commonly, irritability, aggression, anxiety, and insomnia, and less commonly memory loss and hallucinations.[147] Although studies have reported CNS toxicity in over 50% of those taking efavirenz, this prevalence is hard to interpret due to highly variable definitions of what qualifies as toxicity.[147] NRTI medications such as zidovudine and abacavir can cause neuropsychiatric symptoms as well, including mania and psychosis.[147] Certain alleles for cytochrome P450 2B6 may contribute to risk of neuropsychiatric side effects. Protease inhibitors (like ritonavir) are metabolized by the CYP450 system and therefore may have an indirect effect on the neural toxicity of coadministered medications.[147] Of note, newer HIV integrase inhibitors, C-C chemokine receptor type 5 (CCR5) inhibitors, and fusion inhibitors appear to be less likely to cause neuropsychiatric symptoms.[147]

HERPES VIRUS ENCEPHALITIS

Epidemiology

Viral encephalitis affects about 20,000 people per year in the Unites States.[40] Overall, herpes simplex virus (HSV) infection is quite common, with HSV type 1 (HSV-1) estimated to affect 67% of the global population aged 0–49.[186] Herpes simplex virus type 2 (HSV-2) is estimated to affect 11% of the global population aged 15–49 as of 2012.[186] There are an estimated 19.2 million new HSV-2 infections per year as of 2012 (0.5% of the global population).[186] HSV-1 typically causes peri-oral and HSV-2 genital lesions. However, HSV-2 is also a common cause of viral meningitis and HSV-1 is the most common identified cause of sporadic acute viral encephalitis.[40] HSV represented the cause for 8% of cases of encephalitis and meningitis in one large-scale study of over 26,000 patients.[187] Some estimates of the proportion of sporadic acute encephalitis cases caused by HSV are much higher, in the range of 25–50%.[40] In either case, it is certainly an important cause of acute encephalitis worldwide in the immunocompetent individual. HSV encephalitis (HSVE) occurs in all age groups.[40] Mortality rates are high in HSVE, up to 70% without treatment but remaining at 25–50% even with treatment.[40]

CASE VIGNETTE 26.1

Herpes simplex virus encephalitis (HSVE)

A 73-year-old retired heavy equipment operator presented to his PCP office with 2 weeks of memory loss and visuospatial issues as well as symptoms of decreased verbal output and withdrawal, food refusal, fatigue, and occasional anxiety. His wife noted that he had to double check to make sure he completed tasks, forgot where his tools were (even though they had been in the same place for years), did not recall a trip to his nephew's house, and took wrong turns on familiar streets. He also noted that food tasted bland, and he lost his sense of smell.

He was admitted to a local hospital. On initial exam, he demonstrated difficulties with memory encoding, storage, and retrieval. He had difficulty recalling autobiographical events, such as how he celebrated an important holiday 3 months prior to evaluation. He also made errors on testing of abstraction and orientation, and his performance on categorical and phonemic fluency tests was borderline.

An MRI brain demonstrated bilateral temporal FLAIR/T2 hyperintensities. A subsequent lumbar puncture demonstrated xanthochromia, lymphocytic pleocytosis, elevated CSF protein, and normal glucose. He was started empirically on ceftriaxone and acyclovir. His hospital course was complicated by confusion, lethargy, and visual hallucinations, which improved with IV acyclovir treatment.

His CSF workup included reassuring bacterial culture, gram stain, and cytology. His HSV PCR came back positive, alternative CSF viral studies were negative, and his ceftriaxone was discontinued.

He was subsequently discharged home with a PICC line, and he completed his treatment after a total of 21 days. In subsequent clinic visits, his wife noted that he continued to be forgetful (e.g., forgetting where the bathroom soap was located), and he was frequently tearful (e.g., when families members would leave), which was out of character. On subsequent evaluations, his orientation and fluency testing performance improved, but his memory performance remained stably impaired. He was started on sertraline for anxiety, irritability, and depressed mood, and these symptoms improved. Following neuropsychological testing, he was referred to cognitive rehabilitation. He was also referred to social work to assist with evaluation of psychosocial needs and resources for in-home support following discharge.

Neuropsychiatric symptoms are common in HSVE. They can vary from depression and anxiety to irritability, agitation, mood lability, mania, and psychosis, to amnesia, apathy, and more. Data on the frequency with which these symptoms occur in the acute stage of the illness are scant, with one study simply reporting that abnormal behavior was the presenting symptom in 24% of cases.[42] Long-term sequelae of HSVE has been better studied. One study found rates of depression in 18%, anxiety in 45%, panic attacks in 27%, irritability in 64%, and apathy in 1% of HSVE survivors studied 6 months after their encephalitis.[188] Another study found that 45% of survivors had behavioral abnormality at long-term follow-up, 69% had memory impairment, 17% had depression requiring treatment, 7% had obsessive-compulsive behavior, 3% had aggression, and 3% had hyperphagia.[42] Prevalences for anxiety, irritability, and emotional lability were reported as present in 20–35% of patients.[42] Kluver-Bucy syndrome, characterized by increased sexual behavior, hyperorality, and loss of normal fear and anger responses, is uncommon now that HSVE is treated with acyclovir.[188] Long-term functional difficulties can be more often related to persistent emotional or behavioral disturbances than to memory deficits.[188,189] The mean risk of depression in HSVE compared to other infectious diseases is summarized in Figure 26-6.

Pathophysiology

It has not been definitively established whether HSVE results from primary or latent infection, but some sources say both, with an estimated 30% of cases attributed to primary infections and the remaining 70% attributed to reactivation.[59] Evidence supporting primary infection as the source includes isolation of a different viral strain as the etiologic agent for the encephalitis from the strain causing that individual's cold sores.[59] Hypothesized routes of entry to the brain include via the olfactory nerve, via the trigeminal nerve into the frontal and temporal lobes after reactivation in the trigeminal ganglion, or direct reactivation within the brain.[59]

It is thought that the virus evades host immune response by inhibiting autophagy and by disrupting major histocompatibility complex antigen expression on infected neurons.[59] Affected regions develop edema and then evolve to hemorrhagic necrosis, with cytolysis of neurons, astrocytes, and oligodendrocytes.[59] It is unclear whether the brain regions affected are due to a particular affinity of the virus for these regions or whether it is simply due to their being closely located to the nasal cavity from which the virus is plausibly thought to enter.[59] Affected brain regions include the orbitofrontal regions, the temporal lobes including insular cortex and hippocampus, and the cingulate gyrus.[59]

A prospective study of HSVE survivors found varying patterns of temporal lobe involvement, including amygdala alone and amygdala plus hippocampus, and also left prefrontal hypoperfusion associated with long-term psychiatric sequelae, suggesting that ongoing behavioral disturbance may be related to amygdalar and frontal damage.[188] In the same study persistent memory impairment was found to be related to hippocampal and amygdalar damage, and to the overall size of the lesion.[188]

The HSV is also known to modify gene expression involving over 1300 host genes including susceptibility genes for depression, bipolar, schizophrenia, autism, neurodegeneration, and other neuropsychiatric conditions suggesting a possible genetic contribution mechanistically to behavioral change associated with herpes infections.[190] Vulnerability to developing HSVE may also be to some extent genetically determined: defects in the innate immune response, particularly mutations affecting toll-like receptors, have been shown to increase susceptibility to HSVE.[191] Mouse models have also suggested that controlling the degree of immune activation in HSVE with agents like corticosteroids or TNF alpha inhibitors may actually increase survival rates.[191]

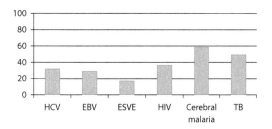

FIGURE 26-6. Mean risk of depression for infectious diseases (% prevalence). (Reproduced with permission from Barsky AJ, Silbersweig DA, Boland RJ. *Depression in Medical Illness.* https://neurology.mhmedical.com Copyright © McGraw Hill LLC. All rights reserved.)

Clinical Presentation

HSVE can present suddenly, with an acute onset, but may also be preceded by a prodrome involving fever and headache. Then alterations in consciousness, changes in personality and behavior, seizures, and motor disturbances can set in.[45] Focal neurological symptoms can include anosmia, and hallucinations can be olfactory and/or gustatory.[59] Untreated HSVE can be fatal in up to 70% of cases, with appropriate treatment reducing mortality to 25–30%.[40] Neuropsychiatric symptoms in HSVE can be complex and may not necessarily fit with conventional psychiatric disease categories, such as depression or mania. Case reports may describe elements from multiple psychiatric syndromes without the full complement of symptoms that might confirm this diagnostic category. For example, elevated mood together with confusion and disinhibition may be observed, but without all the accompanying symptoms that would merit a diagnosis of mania.[192] On the other hand, a study of the presentations of 108 acute encephalitis cases found that symptoms did tend to cluster into four categories: psychosis, catatonia, depression with psychotic features, and mania, but could have overlapping symptoms or transition from one category to another during the course of the illness.[193] This study included non-HSV causes of acute encephalitis, but the exhaustive exploration of psychiatric signs helps us to understand the range of behaviors that may be observed in acute encephalitis, including all manner of delusional thinking (paranoid, nihilistic, grandiose, religious, infestation, pseudocyesis), hallucinations (auditory, visual, olfactory, and gustatory), agitation (irritability, aggression, and violence), catatonic-like behavior (mutism, staring, food refusal, withdrawal, echolalia, excitation, and negativism), psychomotor (restlessness, hyperactivity), anxiety (fear, terror), disinhibited (sucking, biting, nudism, lewd behavior, cursing, screaming), depressed (sobbing, suicidal), manic (pressured speech, euphoria, flight of ideas), derealization, insomnia, catalepsy, perseveration, and confusion.[193] Perhaps it is unsurprising then that in the long term, encephalitis survivors can be left with significantly elevated levels of psychopathology, including increased interpersonal sensitivity, depression, phobic anxiety, and obsessive-compulsive behaviors.[194]

Memory disorders are also common in HSVE and as sequelae of the illness, and include deficits in anterograde worse than retrograde memory.[59] Other cognitive deficits observed include executive dysfunction, visuospatial deficits, and language difficulties.[59] Kluver-Bucy syndrome, which includes hypersexual behavior, hyperphagia, and atypical emotional responses, can also occur.[59] Studies of neuropsychological function after recovery from HSVE can show variable patterns and levels of impairment. One study found that encoding of new material, object naming, and semantic memory were impaired in all subjects, whereas executive function, working memory, and autobiographical memory were impaired in a smaller proportion (75%) of those studied and visuospatial function was impaired in still fewer (50%).[194]

Assessment and Differential Diagnosis

Treatment for suspected HSVE need not wait for definitive diagnosis, given the high rates of morbidity and mortality if treatment is deferred. Evaluation of suspected HSVE includes clinical history, examination, neuroimaging, lumbar puncture, and electroencephalographic (EEG) evaluation.[45] Focal neurological signs, seizures, confusion or decreased consciousness, especially if accompanied by fever, are suggestive of a possible

encephalitis.[45] Even a new-onset psychiatric disturbance without accompanying neurologic signs may raise suspicion for encephalitis, especially if there is no personal or family history of psychopathology.[193]

Elevated opening pressure on lumbar puncture, xanthrochromic CSF, and a lymphocyte-predominant elevated leukocyte count of anywhere from 10 to 2000 cells/mL are suggestive of a herpetic meningoencephalitis.[40] Typically these are accompanied by elevated CSF protein with normal glucose levels. Important CSF evaluations include a PCR analysis for HSV-1, antibody titers to rule out alternative viral agents, and Gram's stain, bacterial and fungal cultures, acid-fast preparations, and cytologic examinations, to rule out bacterial, fungal, or neoplastic causes of the encephalitis.[40] Of note, PCR is typically positive within 24 hours of symptom onset and remains so for the first week of antiviral therapy, but if a negative result is found despite a strong clinical suspicion for HSVE the CSF PCR should be repeated.[191] There are a number of other common causes of viral encephalitis, and St. Louis encephalitis virus, western and eastern equine encephalitis viruses, West Nile virus, varicella zoster virus, HIV-1, mumps, and cytomegalovirus are all on the differential.[40] A study of 432 patients with a clinical presentation suggestive of HSVE found that in addition to the viral encephalitides mentioned above and the immune-mediated limbic encephalitides, a number of other conditions can mimic HSVE, including subdural empyema, a variety of infections (e.g., tuberculosis and meningococcal meningitis), some tumors, subdural hematoma, lupus, adrenal leukodystrophy, progressive multifocal leukoencephalopathy, subacute sclerosing panencephalitis, vascular disease, and toxic encephalopathy, among others.[195]

Imaging early in the course can help to identify any alternative focal process, but imaging very early on may not yet show abnormalities associated with HSVE. With time, imaging studies will typically detect edema, signal changes, and sometimes hemorrhages in the temporal lobe, sometimes unilateral early on but becoming bilateral (see Figure 26-7).[196] Lesions can also involve inferior frontal lobes, parietal, and occipital lobes.[196] MRI is preferred over CT, which is relatively insensitive, and diffusion weighted imaging (DWI) sequences are superior to fluid attenuated inversion recovery (FLAIR) sequences early on in the clinical course.[191]

EEG findings may include nonspecific slowing, asymmetric spikes, slow waves, and intermittent periodic lateralizing epileptiform discharges (PLEDs).[196]

In the recovery phase after acute HSVE, additional evaluations may be helpful to guide neuropsychiatric management, including neuropsychological assessment, psychiatric evaluation, and repeat assessment for seizures, as postencephalitic epilepsy can develop well after the acute illness.[197] Thorough neuropsychological characterization is particularly valuable in determining the degree and type of residual cognitive impairment in order to guide rehabilitation interventions.[197]

Treatment

As mentioned previously, treatment for HSVE should begin empirically given the high morbidity and mortality associated with deferring initiation of antiviral medication. Treatment for

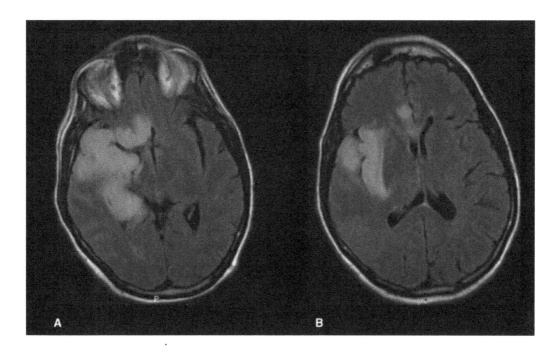

FIGURE 26-7. Axial FLAIR MRI of a patient with HSV encephalitis (HSVE) demonstrating T2/FLAIR hyperintensity in the **(A)** right medial and anterior temporal lobe and inferior frontal lobe as well as the **(B)** right insula. (Reproduced with permission from Berkowitz AL. *Clinical Neurology and Neuroanatomy: A Localization-Based Approach.* https://neurology.mhmedical.com Copyright © McGraw Hill LLC. All rights reserved.)

suspected or diagnosed HSVE is intravenous acyclovir for up to 21 days.[196] The literature available on the management of neuropsychiatric symptoms associated with both acute HSVE and its long-term sequelae is extremely limited and amounts to case reports. One report found benefit from risperidone for a woman with apathy, distractibility, and odd affect but who was not demonstrating overt psychotic symptoms.[198] Another case report found the mood stabilizers olanzapine and valproate helpful for manic-like symptoms of elevated mood, disinhibition, and hypersexuality after HSVE.[192] There are also case reports suggesting that carbamazepine can be helpful for behavioral disturbance,[199] even in the absence of EEG abnormalities.[200] Ropinirole has been reported to be helpful for postencephalitic apathy and depression.[201] While data are not available for the efficacy of antidepressant or antianxiety medications, or for most mood stabilizers and neuroleptics, common sense can still guide treatment selection, which should be symptomatically targeted. Given the high rate of seizure disorders after HSVE, bupropion may be best avoided as it can lower the seizure threshold. In post-HSVE patients with both behavioral disturbance and seizures, some anticonvulsants may provide a dual benefit. With a lack of published data to guide pharmacologic management of neuropsychiatric sequelae of HSVE, previous authors have advocated for empiric trials as necessary with medication classes including antipsychotics, anticonvulsants, antidepressants, benzodiazepines, cholinesterase inhibitors, and stimulants.[40] There is some evidence to suggest that antipsychotics carry heightened risk in the acute encephalitis patient, with reports of neuroleptic malignant syndrome, extrapyramidal side effects, and catatonia, and so use of these medications

should be undertaken at low-to-moderate doses and with close monitoring.[193]

The success of psychotherapeutic efforts may depend in part on the degree of residual cognitive dysfunction the individual is left with after recovery from the acute illness. In some cases,[202] the degree of memory or other cognitive impairment is such that it precludes the successful application of psychotherapy techniques such as cognitive behavioral therapy, which rely to some extent on memory and language functions and insight, all of which may be impacted by this illness.

Behavioral interventions, on the other hand, particularly those with simple designs, clear contingencies, and very limited cognitive/memory load for the patient, may meet with more success. This has been demonstrated to be helpful in challenging post-HSVE cases with frequent aggression that can respond well to a negative response cost design, that is, a setup in which the patient was "charged" a token for each time he engaged in an undesirable behavior; at the end of a brief set time period he could exchange remaining tokens, if enough remained, for a desired "reinforcer."[202,203]

Identifying triggers for agitation and aggression can help lay the groundwork for targeted interventions to reduce these symptoms. For example, an amnestic post-HSVE patient became agitated and aggressive over concerns about his finances and was perseverative on when his monthly social security check would arrive. Work with occupational therapy and speech and language therapy eventually enabled him to adopt a calendar system to track the days until his check, with some benefit.[202]

"Errorless learning," or being prevented from making any errors while learning new information, has been shown to help some HSVE survivors with memory deficits, particularly those with severe anterograde amnesia, although numerous learning trials are needed and heavy cuing may be needed to generalize the newly learned information to other contexts.[202] Visually presented material combined with audio (such as video footage of their early life combined with preferred music) can build upon what individuals do retain from their relatively intact retrograde memory, reinforcing correct information and building a basis on which to portray more recent, unrecalled autobiographical information.[202] A case report showed that *motor movement training* (associating a movement to a new name, for example) may be more effective than a visual imagery approach.[204]

Electroconvulsive therapy (ECT) has been reportedly used with some success in encephalitis patients with psychiatric features, especially in those with catatonia.[193] On the other hand, use of transcranial direct current stimulation to try to treat residual aphasia after HSVE was associated in one case report with recurrence of the encephalitis thought to be related to facilitated migration of activated HSV.[205]

In summary, HSV, which is highly prevalent, can sporadically develop into HSVE that can be associated with abrupt changes in mental status and persistent neuropsychiatric disturbance after recovery from the acute illness. Early treatment with acyclovir is essential. A multipronged approach to rehabilitation can help these encephalitis survivors to regain function, which is often adversely affected as much by psychiatric symptoms as by amnesia.

NEUROSYPHILIS

Epidemiology

Syphilis, a sexually transmitted infection caused by the spirochete bacterium *Treponema pallidum*, is perhaps the classic example of an infection pertinent to neuropsychiatry and historically has been a major cause of neuropsychiatric symptoms. Over the course of the second half of the last century, the prevalence of primary and secondary syphilis declined, from 71 cases per 100,000 persons in 1946 to a historic low of 2.1 cases per 100,000 persons in 2000.[206] However, over the ensuing years syphilis rates have been steadily rising again, reaching 9.5 per 100,000 persons in 2017.[207] Notably, rates of primary and secondary syphilis are particularly high among men who have sex with men (MSM), accounting for 58% of cases in 2017.[208] In addition to MSM, sex workers, transgender women, and incarcerated individuals have also been identified as at elevated risk for contracting syphilis.[209] Neurosyphilis—including syphilitic meningitis, meningovascular syphilis, tabes dorsalis, and general paresis—specifically is most often seen in individuals with HIV infection, although it remains unclear whether this is due to increased susceptibility or due to overlapping risk factors such as unprotected anal intercourse. Among HIV-negative individuals with syphilis, male gender and older age appear to be associated with increased risk for the development of neurosyphilis.[210]

Neurosyphilis can be associated with a variety of neuropsychiatric symptoms, including mood disturbance (both depressed mood and euphoria), anxiety, hallucinations, delusional thought, apathy, disinhibition, and irritability. There is very limited data published on the prevalence of neuropsychiatric symptoms. One author reports that mania accounts for less than 6% of mood disorders in neurosyphilis, with depression being much more common.[211] A case-control study of 91 neurosyphilis cases found that neuropsychiatric symptoms were more common in those at the dementia stage than in those at the mild cognitive impairment (MCI) stage, with frequency of depression ranging from 14% in the MCI cases to 27% in the dementia cases.[212] Euphoria rates here were higher than in earlier reports, with 5% of MCI stage and 26% of dementia stage experiencing euphoria.[213] Psychotic symptoms were also common, with delusions in 24–40% and hallucinations in 14–29% of MCI and dementia cases respectively.[213] Irritability, apathy, anxiety, and disinhibition were also notable in both populations, in decreasing order of frequency.[213]

Pathophysiology

Syphilitic invasion of the central nervous system often occurs during secondary syphilis; some cases are asymptomatic, while others present with aseptic meningitis including lymphocytic pleocytosis in the CSF.[206] The lack of surface-exposed proteins on the outer membrane of *T. pallidum* may help it to escape the immune system.[206] For all disease stages, the primary pathophysiologic mechanism is obliterative endarteritis.[206] Such an inflammation of the intima, the inner lining of the artery, can actually occlude the lumen of the vessel. This type of vascular involvement can lead to focal ischemia and a wide variety of focal neurologic deficits.[206] However, parenchymal damage from syphilis infection can also occur, and some of the late neurological complications of syphilis, including general paresis and tabes dorsalis, are attributed to this mechanism.[206]

Clinical Presentation

Syphilis has a number of stages and an infamously variable clinical presentation. Primary syphilis often shows up approximately 3 weeks after initial infection as the characteristic "chancre," a localized skin lesion that begins as a painless papule and ulcerates into a 1–2 cm ulcer with a raised margin, most commonly found on the genitalia. The infection quickly disseminates systemically and within a few months, approximately one-quarter of those with untreated infection develop the systemic illness of secondary syphilis. Secondary syphilis often occurs with constitutional symptoms, adenopathy, and a characteristic rash, classically maculopapular and affecting the palms and the soles, although variations in rash often occur. Condylomata lata (hypertrophic papules most commonly found on the mucous membranes) may develop in this stage as well. Syphilis can have a latent period during which the individual is asymptomatic, and can be subcategorized as early (infection within past year) or late (infection over a year ago or at an unknown time). Between 25% and 40% of those with untreated syphilis go on to develop tertiary syphilis including cardiovascular manifestations (e.g., aortitis) or gummatous syphilis (disseminated granulomatous lesions).[214]

Neurosyphilis can occur at any point in the course of infection. Involvement of the CNS can occur early in infection but may be asymptomatic. The evolution of neurosyphilis is summarized in Figure 26-8.

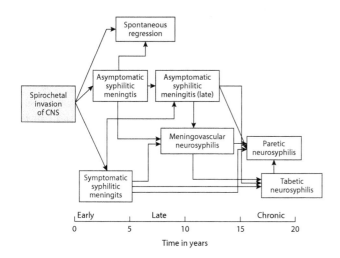

FIGURE 26-8. Diagram of the progression of neurosyphilis. (Reproduced with permission from Ropper AH, Samuels MA, Klein JP, Prasad S. *Adams and Victor's Principles of Neurology,* 11th ed. https://accessmedicine.mhmedical.com. Copyright © McGraw Hill LLC. All rights reserved.)

Clinical presentation of neurosyphilis seems to be approximately correlated with duration of infection, although this is not the case for all aspects of the presentation. Secondary syphilis may present with meningitis which can range from mild meningeal symptoms to a severe meningitis.[215] Unilateral or bilateral cranial nerve palsies can occur with syphilitic meningitis, with cranial nerves II, III, VI, VII, and VIII particularly likely to be involved.[206] Meningovascular syphilis, marked by stroke or stroke-like manifestations of small- and medium-sized CNS arteries, occurs approximately 5–10 years after infection and may present with aphasia, hemiplegia, or seizures.[215] Decades of infection may lead to two additional manifestations of neurosyphilis, general paresis of the insane and tabes dorsalis. General paresis of the insane (referred to as general paresis from this point on) presents as dementia, is progressive, and is often accompanied by a diverse array of neuropsychiatric symptoms as well as seizures.[215] Tabes dorsalis, a manifestation of involvement of the posterior columns of the spinal cord, can present with ataxia from reduced proprioception, impaired vibratory sense, diminished reflexes, severe radicular pain, and the Argyll-Robinson pupil.[215]

General paresis can present with the full spectrum of neuropsychiatric symptoms. Symptoms can include changes in motivation (apathy), mood and affect (depression, euphoria, irritability), behavior (disinhibition, agitation), and reality testing (delusions, hallucinations).[213] One retrospective study of 169 neurosyphilis cases found that 31% presented with psychiatric manifestations as a primary symptom and many patients experienced multiple psychiatric symptoms.[212] There are insufficient data available to distinguish between primary psychiatric illness and psychiatric presentations of neurosyphilis based on clinical phenomenology alone.

There is limited data on the patterns of neuropsychological impairment observed in patients with neurosyphilis and extremely limited data on changes in impairment level over time,[216] but overall, the condition is seen as one of progressive cognitive decline if left untreated. One evaluation of general paresis patients found global cognitive dysfunction, with memory impairment significantly greater than controls and comparable to the memory deficits seen in Alzheimer's disease (AD).[217] This study also found that general paresis patients performed significantly worse than controls on measures of attention, executive functioning, language, and spatial cognition.[217] Whether the course of cognitive decline is altered in neurosyphilis patients appropriately treated with antibiotics remains unclear. A systematic review found some evidence of short-term improvement on a cognitive screen in neurosyphilis patients treated with penicillin, but insufficient evidence to support a long-term improvement in cognitive function from antibiotic treatment.[218]

Assessment and Differential Diagnosis

The diagnosis of syphilis is typically made by serologic testing, with a variety of tests available that differ in sensitivity and specificity. Direct detection of the organism itself is made more difficult due to limited accessibility of the methods and expertise for these approaches.[215] A two-step process is most often used, with a positive initial test for IgG and IgM antibodies produced in response to *T. pallidum* infection (such as rapid plasma regain [RPR] or venereal disease research laboratory [VDRL] tests) typically followed up by a test for antibodies to treponemal antigens (such as fluorescent treponemal antibody adsorbed tests [FTA-ABS], *T. pallidum* particle agglutination, or enzyme immunoassays).[215] Since RPR and VDRL antibody titers can decline spontaneously and become nonreactive even without treatment,[215] it may be helpful to perform both types of testing if there is high clinical suspicion for syphilis even if initial screening is negative. Some advocate for a reverse algorithm approach, in which a treponemal antibody test is performed first and positive results are confirmed with RPR or VDRL.[219] The reverse algorithm approach appears to have higher sensitivity than the traditional strategy.[219]

For the diagnosis of neurosyphilis, CSF analysis is helpful but is only recommended currently in a limited subset of patients, including those with a suggestive clinical presentation or to evaluate for treatment failure.[215] A CSF VDRL test is typically done first, with a CSF FTA-ABS test done in those with suspected neurosyphilis and a negative CSF VDRL.[215] That said, neurologic symptoms alone are not reliable guides to the presence of syphilis in the CNS. A study of syphilis patients did not find any particular neurologic symptom to be more common in those with a reactive CSF-VDRL than those without, although in HIV-infected syphilis patients the odds of neurologic involvement were higher with moderate-to-severe photophobia, vision loss, hearing loss, or gait incoordination.[220]

Imaging unfortunately appears to add little to the diagnostic process, and indeed it would be challenging to identify neurosyphilis on the basis of MRI alone. An analysis of 35 patients with CSF-confirmed neurosyphilis found protean imaging manifestations of the disease, including diffuse cerebral atrophy, mesial temporal lobe, temporal, and frontal signal changes, infarcts, nonspecific white matter changes, sulcal exudates, progressive multifocal leukoencephalopathy, and hypothalamic enhancement, as well as some normal studies,[51] with no clear patterns identified. The findings do suggest that neurosyphilis should remain on the differential for a broad variety of MRI presentations, including mesial temporal lobe atrophy and signal change, ischemic or multifocal white matter changes, and spinal cord signal changes with or without enhancement.[51] There appears to be some association between diffuse cortical atrophy and dementia and between frontotemporal lobe predominance in those with neuropsychiatric presentations,[51] as might be expected.

Thus far, no convincing pattern of neuropsychological deficits has been established that definitively separates dementia due to neurosyphilis from dementia from other causes. Indeed, a comparison of the neuropsychological profiles among patients with general paresis of the insane (neurosyphilis), AD, and frontotemporal dementia found impairments in memory, language, and executive function that resembled those seen in the AD patients.[217]

The range of disorders that may be considered in the course of establishing a diagnosis of neurosyphilis is quite broad, in keeping with its reputation as "the great mimicker." One study of neurosyphilis patients found that the majority were initially felt to have other disorders, including AD, parkinsonism, epilepsy, hypertensive stroke, transient ischemic attack, alcoholic encephalopathy, viral encephalitis, depression, and unspecified encephalopathy.[212] Of note, the above patients had no history of major mental illness, substance abuse other than alcohol, or family history of psychiatric disturbance,[212] which suggests that a lack of personal and family psychiatric history may help point to a possible infectious cause.

HIV infection represents an important comorbidity as the rate of neurosyphilis may be higher among HIV-positive individuals who acquire syphilis.[212]

Treatment

The treatment of syphilis rests primarily on penicillin, with a single injection possible for early primary or secondary disease or three weekly injections for those with late or unknown-duration disease.[215] For neurosyphilis significantly higher doses of intravenous penicillin are recommended every 4 hours for up to 2 weeks, and managements with other antibiotics in those with a penicillin allergy or desensitization may be attempted.[215] In neurosyphilis, monitoring for response to therapy is complicated by the challenge of getting follow-up lumbar punctures, and so monitoring of changing response to the RPR test is often used as it predicts resolution of neurologic symptoms.[215]

Despite neuropsychiatric symptoms regularly occurring as part of neurosyphilis, there is little published on their management, and no consensus guidelines. One approach that has been suggested is to identify target symptoms or behavioral disturbances that are familiar from other clinical contexts, and treat these with agents that have been helpful for such target symptoms in other settings.[221] A case series found benefit for antipsychotic medications, both typical (haloperidol) and atypical (risperidone, quetiapine), for psychosis in this population.[221] They also found benefit from valproic acid derivatives for agitation

and mood stabilization.[221] Their recommended approach also includes use of the lowest effective doses and making attempts to reduce or discontinue psychotropic agents when feasible, balancing this goal against the risk associated with target symptoms should they reemerge.[221] The use of psychotherapies in the management of neurosyphilis is not described in the literature.

Case reports support the use of ECT for the treatment of depression[222] and psychosis[223] associated with neurosyphilis. There are no published data on the use of other brain stimulation therapies (such as transcranial magnetic stimulation or direct current stimulation) for the neuropsychiatric symptoms of neurosyphilis.

There is very limited evidence for an approach to the cognitive impairment of neurosyphilis, but a case report demonstrated significant improvement in score on a cognitive screen with donepezil treatment; cognition then worsened off of the cholinesterase-inhibitor and again improved back on it, suggesting some benefit.[224]

In summary, neurosyphilis can represent a complication of both early and late infection with *T. pallidum*, and is more common in the era of widespread infectious immunodeficiency syndromes. Neurosyphilis has a range of clinical presentations up to and including dementia, psychosis, and significant mood disturbance, and very limited data on symptomatic management exist.

NEUROPSYCHIATRIC MANIFESTATIONS OF COVID-19

In December 2019 a new respiratory illness was noticed to be affecting individuals in Wuhan, China. Today the disease Covid-19, now known to be caused by the severe acute respiratory syndrome (SARS)-CoV-2 coronavirus, has affected millions worldwide and is understood to have protean manifestations that extend to many organ systems, including the nervous system.

Data on prevalence of neuropsychiatric conditions associated with Covid-19 are limited not just by the newness of this disease and associated lack of follow-up, but by the limitations on testing that have challenged accurate data on disease prevalence as a whole: without an accurate denominator it is not possible to fully assess the proportion with neuropsychiatric disease. In spite of these limitations, emerging data suggest that over a third and perhaps more than half of hospitalized patients with Covid-19 have neurologic manifestations, with central nervous system (CNS) symptoms or signs occurring in ~25% of hospitalized cases.[226,227] In one case series, 45.5% of patients with severe illness and 30% of patients with non-severe illness had neurological manifestations.[226] Disease severity may thus represent one risk factor for neurologic complications. Disease severity, as well as older age, appear to be risk factors for disorders of consciousness, while milder cases were more often associated with anosmia and dysgeusia.[227]

Several pathogenic mechanisms have been proposed to explain the varied neurological/neuropsychiatric manifestations of Covid-19. There has been conflicting information about whether SARS-CoV-2 directly enters the CNS. Experimental evidence of SARS-CoV intranasal infection in rodents has shown retrograde axonal transport from the olfactory bulb,[228] however it is unclear whether this is generalizable to humans and to SARS-CoV-2. Hematogenous spread to the CNS, by viral infection of endothelial cells of the blood-brain barrier, is one plausible mechanism, and is supported by findings of viral budding across brain capillary endothelial cells.[229] However while viral particles have been found in frontal lobe neurons post-mortem[229] and SARS-CoV-2 RNA has been identified in the CSF in individual cases,[230] larger case series have failed to find the CSF positive for viral RNA in neurologically involved patients,[227] raising the possibility that indirect mechanisms are at play. Systemic inflammation can lead to blood-brain barrier breakdown through several different pathways, including its damage by circulating cytokines which can then pass into the CNS causing a neuroinflammatory reaction.[227,231] Severe hypoxemia associated with critical respiratory insufficiency can cause disorders of consciousness. In patients with severe illness, the alterations in mental status can have contributions from hypoxemia, blood-brain barrier dysfunction, cytokine release, cerebrovascular injury, and metabolic derangements (uremia, increased ammonia, electrolyte disturbances).[227] Cerebrovascular disease in Covid-19 may be caused by a combination of endothelial damage (as discussed, due to direct viral infection or by cytokines) and hypercoagulability. It has been proposed that certain neurological manifestations (e.g., acute demyelinating polyneuropathy [AIDP], optic neuritis) that have tended to occur during recovery from the acute phase of the illness may represent a parainfectious process, a dysimmune response triggered by the infection.[227] Neuropsychiatric symptoms like anxiety, mood changes, and insomnia may be linked to pathophysiologic mechanisms described above, or to psychological effects of social isolation, concern about survival/disease outcome, and stigma encountered by disease survivors.

The neurologic/neuropsychiatric clinical manifestations of Covid-19 are varied. Early in the disease course it appears that anosmia (in 5%) and dysgeusia (in 6%) are common neurologic symptoms, and may represent the first clinical sign of infection.[227] Nonspecific symptoms like headache (14%), dizziness (6%), and myalgias (17%) also tend to occur early on.[227] Other neurologic disturbances have included myopathy (3%), dysautonomia (<3%), and cerebrovascular disease (<2%).[227] In a series reported by Romero-Sánchez et al.,[227] stroke was due to ischemia in over 1% of cases and intracranial hemorrhage in <1%; over a third of the ischemic stroke cases involved the posterior artery territory and some cases involved multiple vascular territories. Arterial dissection and CNS vasculitis were also seen.[227] Other studies have found higher rates of ischemic stroke, ranging from 2.5% of all consecutive symptomatic hospitalized patients with confirmed Covid-19232 to 23% of ICU Covid-19 patients with acute respiratory distress syndrome (ARDS).233 Seizures and movement disorders occurred in less than 1% of cases, with encephalitis, Guillain-Barré syndrome, AIDP, and optic neuritis being reported even more rarely.[227]

Disorders of consciousness were among the most common neuropsychiatric presentations, occurring in almost 20% of Covid-19 patients in one large series, and were frequently associated with hypoxemia.[227] Additional data on disorders of consciousness from a systematic review of published data and preprints found prevalence rates between 2% and 22%, including a rate of 21% among patients who subsequently died.[234]

Cognitive and neuropsychiatric disturbances have been identified as well. One study found a dysexecutive syndrome in 36% and agitation in 69% of Covid-19 patients admitted to ICU, with dysexecutive symptoms persisting to hospital discharge in a third of patients.[233] It was unclear to what extent these manifestation were directly related to a Covid-19 encephalopathy, cytokines, or the effect of sedating medications and their withdrawal.

In one series, neuropsychiatric symptoms of insomnia, anxiety, depression, and psychosis occurred (in aggregate) in approximately 20% of Covid-19 hospitalized patients, and are listed here in order of frequency,[227] but other studies have found higher prevalence rates. A hospital sample from Wuhan found rates of depression and anxiety to be 29% and 35% respectively.[235] In another sample of hospitalized patients with "mild" Covid-19 disease, a high rate of depression (60%) and anxiety (55%) symptoms were reported using the PHQ-9 and GAD-7 scales. It is important to consider that physical symptoms of Covid-19 can overlap with some symptoms of depression and anxiety, which may result in an artificially high prevalence or severity of anxiety and depression, as measured by these two scales. Seventeen point five percent of those patients reported moderate-to-severe symptoms of depression and 6.8% reported moderate-to-severe anxiety. These were significantly higher than the comparable rates in healthy controls.[236] While prevalence of anxiety and depression symptoms meeting clinical cutoffs were not reported, another study of hospitalized patients with Covid-19 found significantly higher scores on anxiety and depression rating scale scores compared to those with non-Covid pneumonia.[237]

A systematic review of data from the SARS and Middle East respiratory syndrome (MERS) outbreaks indicates that in the post-acute phase rates of depression, anxiety, post-traumatic stress disorder, and fatigue were high.[234] If these findings can be extrapolated to the SARS-CoV-2 outbreak, we may anticipate increased prevalence of these conditions in survivors going forward. It should be noted, too, that even slight increases in prevalence of neuropsychiatric disorders associated with SARS-CoV-2 infection could lead to substantial worldwide increases in associated disease burden, given the unprecedented scale of this outbreak.

Assessments that may help identify neurologic manifestations of Covid-19 include the standard neurologic exam, which revealed corticospinal tract signs in 67%.[233] Brain MRI may be helpful in identifying some neurological complications of Covid-19, including strokes and limbic encephalitis. One series of 13 patients with Covid-19 and unexplained encephalopathy found frontotemporal hypoperfusion in all 11 patients who were tested, and leptomeningeal enhancement in 62% of cases.[233] Given the small sample and possible confounding factors, these findings need further evaluation.[238-240] CSF analysis in neurologically affected patients has often shown negative RT-PCR for SARS-Cov-2 RNA, as it was for 100% of cases in one series.[233]

This section has incorporated the available data on Covid-19 as this book went to press. However, information about this disease is accumulating rapidly, and we expect data on neuropsychiatric sequelae of the disease to change in the months and years to come. In particular, data on late or delayed sequelae and on therapeutic approaches are not currently available due to the virus' recent emergence.

Summary and Key Points

- The understanding of the interactions between inflammatory/neuroimmunologic disease and neuropsychiatric disturbance is increasingly a focus of inquiry. Additional research is critical to better elucidating the complexity of these relationships.
- Neuropsychiatric symptoms are common in neuroinfectious conditions and often require symptomatic treatment, with a paucity of published data to guide therapy selection.
- Diagnosis often rests on the combination of epidemiologic risk factors, clinical presentation, serum and cerebrospinal fluid testing, neuroimaging, electroencephalography, and neuropsychological assessment.
- Treatment and rehabilitation efforts including psychopharmacological interventions, psychotherapies, behavioral treatments, brain stimulation, occupational, physical, and speech and language therapies, and cognitive training all may contribute to optimize neuropsychiatric outcomes in patients affected by neuroimmune conditions.

Multiple Choice Questions

1. Which of the following statements is true regarding concomitant symptoms in systemic lupus erythematosus (SLE):
   a. Younger patients with SLE are at significantly higher risk for stroke compared to the general population but this differential risk disappears after age 60.
   b. Certain neuropsychiatric symptoms are pathognomonic for neuropsychiatric SLE (NPSLE).
   c. Anti-ribosomal P antibodies are primarily correlated with peripheral neuropathy in SLE patients.
   d. Hemorrhagic stroke is more common in SLE than ischemic stroke.
   e. Seizures are the most common neuropsychiatric symptom in SLE.

2. Which of the following patients may be at highest risk for a current diagnosis of neurosyphilis?
   a. 40-year-old female with multiple sexual partners and a history of human papilloma virus infection
   b. 15-year-old male who recently had his first sexual experience and presents with vesicular lesions on his genitals
   c. 55-year-old male who reports both male and female sexual partners and carries the human immunodeficiency virus
   d. 21-year-old female with a recent syphilitic chancre that was treated promptly with penicillin
   e. 30-year-old female with a new-onset psychosis and an unexplained rash

3. An HIV-positive patient presents to your clinic with psychotic depression. Particular attention needs to be paid to which of the following concomitant medications in selecting an agent to treat him with?
   a. Maraviroc, due to significant neuropsychiatric side effects of CCR5 inhibitors
   b. Mirtazapine, due to its effects on the CYP450 enzymes
   c. Ritonavir, due to its effects on the CYP450 enzymes
   d. Citalopram, due to the risk of serotonin syndrome
   e. Lorazepam, due to the risk of oversedation and respiratory depression

4. Rehabilitation of the patient recovering from herpes simplex virus encephalitis (HSVE) would likely be optimized by:
   a. Treating disinhibition and hypersexual behavior with carbamazepine and aphasia with transcranial direct current stimulation
   b. Treating depression symptoms with bupropion and executive dysfunction and amnesia with occupational therapy
   c. Avoiding pharmacologic interventions and focusing on insight-oriented psychotherapy for mood symptoms combined with speech and language therapy for any residual aphasia
   d. Treating disinhibition and hypersexual behavior with carbamazepine, aggressive tendencies with negative response-cost interventions, and anterograde memory impairment with visually presented material and other tools such as movement association training
   e. Treating depression symptoms with sertraline and verbal agitation with a computerized system of monthly rewards for calm behavior

Multiple Choice Answers

1. **Answer: a**

   Younger individuals with SLE are at increased risk for stroke compared to the general population, but after the age of 60 there is no longer a significant difference in risk. Neuropsychiatric SLE (NPSLE) is considered a diagnosis of exclusion, and the presentation can include a wide range of neuropsychiatric symptoms. Anti-ribosomal P antibodies are more highly correlated with psychotic symptoms than with peripheral complaints in SLE patients. Ischemic stroke (90%) is more common than hemorrhagic (10%) stroke in SLE. Headaches are the most common neuropsychiatric symptom in SLE with prevalence of up to 95%; cognitive impairment and depression are also common neuropsychiatric symptoms in SLE, with prevalences for each around 50%. Seizures have a prevalence of around 10–20% in SLE patients.

2. **Answer: c**

   While all of the described individuals may have some degree of risk for acquisition of syphilis or for its development into neurosyphilis, rates of neurosyphilis are highest among those also infected with HIV. Rates of syphilis are particularly high among men who have sex with men, and male gender and older age appear to be risk factors for the development of neurosyphilis even in HIV-negative populations.

3. Answer: c

Careful selection of psychotropic medication in HIV-positive individuals includes attention to drug-drug interactions. Ritonavir is particularly likely to interact with psychotropic medication via its effect on the CYP450 enzymes. Mirtazapine has efficacy in this population and actually has minimal P450 interactions. Citalopram is often a preferred antidepressant in this population due to limited drug-drug interactions. As a chemokine receptor type 5 inhibitor, maraviroc is actually less likely to cause neuropsychiatric symptoms than other classes of antiretroviral medications.

4. Answer: d

The limited evidence available on pharmacologic interventions after HSVE suggests that anticonvulsants, especially carbamazepine, may be helpful in controlling manic-like behavior. Amnestic post-HSVE patients respond best to behavioral interventions with simple designs, clear contingencies, and very limited memory load; rewards must be delivered quickly as the patient may not retain information for even a few minutes. Complex reward tracking involving use of a computerized device or the need to wait days or weeks for contingencies are unlikely to be as helpful given frequent postencephalitic issues with executive function and memory. Similarly, these patients are unlikely to retain the cognitive capacity sufficient to engage in insight-oriented psychotherapy. Treating depression symptoms with sertraline is a reasonable approach, but given high rates of seizure disorder in this population bupropion should be avoided. Occupational and speech and language therapy can both be helpful measures in rehabilitation. Post-HSVE patients may respond best to new information presented in a visual format or learned in association with a motor task.

References

1. Kayser MS, Dalmau J. The emerging link between autoimmune disorders and neuropsychiatric disease. *J Neuropsychiatry Clin Neurosci.* 2011;23(1):90-97.
2. Tobin WO, Pittock SJ. Autoimmune neurology of the central nervous system. *Contin Lifelong Learn Neurol.* 2017;23(3, Neurology of Systemic Disease):627-653.
3. Dimberg EL. Rheumatology and neurology. *Contin Lifelong Learn Neurol.* 2017;23(3, Neurology of Systemic Disease):691-721.
4. Borchers AT, Aoki CA, Naguwa SM, Keen CL, Shoenfeld Y, Gershwin ME. Neuropsychiatric features of systemic lupus erythematosus. *Autoimmun Rev.* 2005;4(6):329-344.
5. Ainiala H, Loukkola J, Peltola J, Korpela M, Hietaharju A. The prevalence of neuropsychiatric syndromes in systemic lupus erythematosus. *Neurology.* 2001;57(3):496-500.
6. Delalande S, De Seze J, Fauchais A-L, et al. Neurologic manifestations in primary Sjögren syndrome: a study of 82 patients. *Medicine (Baltimore).* 2004;83(5):280-291.
7. Garcia-Carrasco M, Ramos-Casals M, Rosas J, et al. Primary Sjögren syndrome: clinical and immunologic disease patterns in a cohort of 400 patients. *Medicine (Baltimore).* 2002;81(4):270-280.
8. Malinow KL, Molina R, Gordon B, Selnes OA, Provost TT, Alexander EL. Neuropsychiatric dysfunction in primary Sjögren's syndrome. *Ann Intern Med.* 1985;103(3):344-350.
9. Talarico R, d'Ascanio A, Figus M, et al. Behçet's disease: features of neurological involvement in a dedicated centre in Italy. *Clin Exp Rheumatol.* 2012;30(3):S69.
10. Abdelraheem T, Habib HM, Eissa AA, Radwan NM. Psychiatric disorders and MRI brain findings in patients with systemic lupus erythematosus and Behcet's disease: a cross sectional study. *Acta Rheumatol Port.* 2013;38:252-260.
11. Akman-Demir G, Serdaroglu P, Taşçi B, The Neuro-Behçet Study Group. Clinical patterns of neurological involvement in Behçet's disease: evaluation of 200 patients. *Brain.* 1999;122(11):2171-2182.
12. Dörr J, Krautwald S, Wildemann B, et al. Characteristics of Susac syndrome: a review of all reported cases. *Nat Rev Neurol.* 2013;9(6):307.
13. Twilt M, Benseler SM. The spectrum of CNS vasculitis in children and adults. *Nat Rev Rheumatol.* 2012;8(2):97.
14. Salvarani C, Brown RDJr, Calamia KT, et al. Primary central nervous system vasculitis: analysis of 101 patients. *Ann Neurol.* 2007;62(5):442-451.
15. Hutchinson C, Elbers J, Halliday W, et al. Treatment of small vessel primary CNS vasculitis in children: an open-label cohort study. *Lancet Neurol.* 2010;9(11):1078-1084.
16. Chapelon C, Ziza JM, Piette JC, et al. Neurosarcoidosis: signs, course and treatment in 35 confirmed cases. *Medicine (Baltimore).* 1990;69(5):261-276.
17. Joseph FG, Scolding NJ. Neurosarcoidosis: a study of 30 new cases. *J Neurol Neurosurg Psychiatry.* 2009;80(3):297-304.
18. Nozaki K, Judson MA. Neurosarcoidosis: clinical manifestations, diagnosis and treatment. *Presse Médicale.* 2012;41(6):e331-e348.
19. Höök O. Sarcoidosis with involvement of the nervous system: report of nine cases. *AMA Arch Neurol Psychiatry.* 1954;71(5):554-575.
20. Kayser MS, Kohler CG, Dalmau J. Psychiatric manifestations of paraneoplastic disorders. *Am J Psychiatry.* 2010;167(9):1039-1050.
21. Graus F, Titulaer MJ, Balu R, et al. A clinical approach to diagnosis of autoimmune encephalitis. *Lancet Neurol.* 2016;15(4):391-404.
22. McKeon A, Lennon VA, Lachance DH, Fealey RD, Pittock SJ. Ganglionic acetylcholine receptor autoantibody: oncological, neurological, and serological accompaniments. *Arch Neurol.* 2009;66(6):735-741.
23. Lancaster E, Lai M, Peng X, et al. Antibodies to the GABAB receptor in limbic encephalitis with seizures: case series and characterisation of the antigen. *Lancet Neurol.* 2010;9(1):67-76.
24. Pelosof LC, Gerber DE. Paraneoplastic syndromes: an approach to diagnosis and treatment. In: *Mayo Clinic Proceedings.* Philadelphia, PA: Elsevier; 2010:838-854.
25. Ogawa E, Sakakibara R, Kawashima K, et al. VGCC antibody-positive paraneoplastic cerebellar degeneration presenting with positioning vertigo. *Neurol Sci.* 2011;32(6):1209-1212.
26. Kaira K, Okamura T, Takahashi H, et al. Small-cell lung cancer with voltage-gated calcium channel antibody-positive paraneoplastic limbic encephalitis: a case report. *J Med Case Rep.* 2014;8(1):119.

27. Xia Z, Mehta BP, Ropper AH, Kesari S. Paraneoplastic limbic encephalitis presenting as a neurological emergency: a case report. *J Med Case Rep*. 2010;4(1):95.

28. Dalmau J, Graus F, Rosenblum MK, Posner JB. Anti-Hu–associated paraneoplastic encephalomyelitis/sensory neuronopathy. A clinical study of 71 patients. *Medicine (Baltimore)*. 1992;71(2):59-72.

29. Lancaster E, Dalmau J. Neuronal autoantigens—pathogenesis, associated disorders and antibody testing. *Nat Rev Neurol*. 2012;8(7):380.

30. Senties-Madrid H, Vega-Boada F. Paraneoplastic syndromes associated with anti-Hu antibodies. *Isr Med Assoc J*. 2001;3(2):94-103.

31. Saiz A, Blanco Y, Sabater L, et al. Spectrum of neurological syndromes associated with glutamic acid decarboxylase antibodies: diagnostic clues for this association. *Brain*. 2008;131(10):2553-2563.

32. Hernández-Echebarría L, Saiz A, Arés A, et al. Paraneoplastic encephalomyelitis associated with pancreatic tumor and anti-GAD antibodies. *Neurology*. 2006;66(3):450-451.

33. Petit-Pedrol M, Armangue T, Peng X, et al. Encephalitis with refractory seizures, status epilepticus, and antibodies to the GABAA receptor: a case series, characterisation of the antigen, and analysis of the effects of antibodies. *Lancet Neurol*. 2014;13(3):276-286.

34. Lai M, Hughes EG, Peng X, et al. AMPA receptor antibodies in limbic encephalitis alter synaptic receptor location. *Ann Neurol*. 2009;65(4):424-434.

35. Gable MS, Gavali S, Radner A, et al. Anti-NMDA receptor encephalitis: report of ten cases and comparison with viral encephalitis. *Eur J Clin Microbiol Infect Dis*. 2009;28(12):1421-1429.

36. Lancaster E, Huijbers MG, Bar V, et al. Investigations of caspr2, an autoantigen of encephalitis and neuromyotonia. *Ann Neurol*. 2011;69(2):303-311.

37. Irani SR, Alexander S, Waters P, et al. Antibodies to Kv1 potassium channel-complex proteins leucine-rich, glioma inactivated 1 protein and contactin-associated protein-2 in limbic encephalitis, Morvan's syndrome and acquired neuromyotonia. *Brain*. 2010;133(9):2734-2748.

38. Dalmau J, Gleichman AJ, Hughes EG, et al. Anti-NMDA-receptor encephalitis: case series and analysis of the effects of antibodies. *Lancet Neurol*. 2008;7(12):1091-1098.

39. Dalmau J, Lancaster E, Martinez-Hernandez E, Rosenfeld MR, Balice-Gordon R. Clinical experience and laboratory investigations in patients with anti-NMDAR encephalitis. *Lancet Neurol*. 2011;10(1):63-74.

40. Arciniegas DB, Anderson CA. Viral encephalitis: neuropsychiatric and neurobehavioral aspects. *Curr Psychiatry Rep*. 2004;6(5):372-379.

41. Munjal S, Ferrando SJ, Freyberg Z. Neuropsychiatric aspects of infectious diseases: an update. *Crit Care Clin*. 2017;33(3):681.

42. McGrath N, Anderson N, Croxson M, Powell K. Herpes simplex encephalitis treated with acyclovir: diagnosis and long term outcome. *J Neurol Neurosurg Psychiatry*. 1997;63(3):321-326.

43. Chow FC, Glaser CA, Sheriff H, et al. Use of clinical and neuroimaging characteristics to distinguish temporal lobe herpes simplex encephalitis from its mimics. *Clin Infect Dis*. 2015;60(9):1377-1383.

44. Granerod J, Ambrose HE, Davies NW, et al. Causes of encephalitis and differences in their clinical presentations in England: a multicentre, population-based prospective study. *Lancet Infect Dis*. 2010;10(12):835-844.

45. Grahn A, Nilsson S, Nordlund A, Lindén T, Studahl M. Cognitive impairment 3 years after neurological varicella-zoster virus infection: a long-term case control study. *J Neurol*. 2013;260(11):2761-2769.

46. Arribas JR, Storch GA, Clifford DB, Tselis AC. Cytomegalovirus encephalitis. *Ann Intern Med*. 1996;125(7):577-587.

47. McCutchan JA. Clinical impact of cytomegalovirus infections of the nervous system in patients with AIDS. *Clin Infect Dis*. 1995;21(suppl 2):S196-S201.

48. Justice AC, McGinnis KA, Atkinson JH, et al. Psychiatric and neurocognitive disorders among HIV-positive and negative veterans in care: Veterans Aging Cohort Five-Site Study. *AIDS*. 2004;18:49-59.

49. Bing EG, Burnam MA, Longshore D, et al. Psychiatric disorders and drug use among human immunodeficiency virus–infected adults in the United States. *Arch Gen Psychiatry*. 2001;58(8):721-728.

50. Berger JR, Pall L, Lanska D, Whiteman M. Progressive multifocal leukoencephalopathy in patients with HIV infection. *J Neurovirol*. 1998;4(1):59-68.

51. Nagappa M, Sinha S, Taly AB, et al. Neurosyphilis: MRI features and their phenotypic correlation in a cohort of 35 patients from a tertiary care university hospital. *Neuroradiology*. 2013;55(4):379-388.

52. Panegyres PK, Edis R, Beaman M, Fallon M. Primary Whipple's disease of the brain: characterization of the clinical syndrome and molecular diagnosis. *J Assoc Physicians*. 2006;99(9):609-623.

53. Prakash PY, Sugandhi RP. Neuropsychiatric manifestation of confusional psychosis due to *Cryptococcus neoformans* var. *grubii* in an apparently immunocompetent host: a case report. *Cases J*. 2009;2(1):9084.

54. French N, Gray K, Watera C, et al. Cryptococcal infection in a cohort of HIV-1-infected Ugandan adults. *Aids*. 2002;16(7):1031-1038.

55. Zuger A, Louie E, Holzman RS, Simberkoff MS, Rahal JJ. Cryptococcal disease in patients with the acquired immunodeficiency syndrome: diagnostic features and outcome of treatment. *Ann Intern Med*. 1986;104(2):234-240.

56. Porter SB, Sande MA. Toxoplasmosis of the central nervous system in the acquired immunodeficiency syndrome. *N Engl J Med*. 1992;327(23):1643-1648.

57. Rodrigues CL, De Andrade DC, Livramento JA, et al. Spectrum of cognitive impairment in neurocysticercosis: differences according to disease phase. *Neurology*. 2012. doi:10.1212/WNL.0b013e31824c46d1.

58. Rabinovici GD, Wang PN, Levin J, et al. First symptom in sporadic Creutzfeldt–Jakob disease. *Neurology*. 2006;66(2):286-287.

59. Więdłocha M, Marcinowicz P, Stańczykiewicz B. Psychiatric aspects of herpes simplex encephalitis, tick-borne encephalitis and herpes zoster encephalitis among immunocompetent patients. *Adv Clin Exp Med*. 2015;24(2):361-371.

60. Clifford DB, DeLuca A, Simpson DM, Arendt G, Giovannoni G, Nath A. Natalizumab-associated progressive multifocal leukoencephalopathy in patients with multiple sclerosis: lessons from 28 cases. *Lancet Neurol*. 2010;9(4):438-446.

61. Compain C, Sacre K, Puéchal X, et al. Central nervous system involvement in Whipple disease: clinical study of 18 patients and long-term follow-up. *Medicine (Baltimore)*. 2013;92(6):324.

62. Lu C-H, Chen H-L, Chang W-N, et al. Assessing the chronic neuropsychologic sequelae of human immunodeficiency virus–negative cryptococcal meningitis by using diffusion tensor imaging. *Am J Neuroradiol*. 2011;32(7):1333-1339.

63. Forlenza OV, Filho AH, Nobrega JP, et al. Psychiatric manifestations of neurocysticercosis: a study of 38 patients from a neurology clinic in Brazil. *J Neurol Neurosurg Psychiatry*. 1997;62(6):612.

64. Cherian A, Thomas SV. Central nervous system tuberculosis. *Afr Health Sci*. 2011;11(1):116-127.

65. Satishchandra P, Nalini A, Gourie-Devi M, et al. Profile of neurologic disorders associated with HIV/AIDS from Bangalore, South India (1989–96). *Indian J Med Res*. 2000;111:14-23.

66. Chen H-L, Lu C-H, Chang C-D, et al. Structural deficits and cognitive impairment in tuberculous meningitis. *BMC Infect Dis.* 2015;15(1):279.

67. Kalita J, Misra UK, Ranjan P. Predictors of long-term neurological sequelae of tuberculous meningitis: a multivariate analysis. *Eur J Neurol.* 2007;14(1):33-37.

68. Albertyn CH. *Cognitive Outcomes in Adults with HIV-Associated Tuberculous Meningitis* [PhD thesis]. Cape Town, ZA: University of Cape Town; 2017.

69. Sütlaş PN, Ünal A, Forta H, Şenol S, Kırbaş D. Tuberculous meningitis in adults: review of 61 cases. *Infection.* 2003;31(6):387-391.

70. Danchenko N, Satia J, Anthony M. Epidemiology of systemic lupus erythematosus: a comparison of worldwide disease burden. *Lupus.* 2006;15(5):308-318.

71. Rees F, Doherty M, Grainge MJ, Lanyon P, Zhang W. The worldwide incidence and prevalence of systemic lupus erythematosus: a systematic review of epidemiological studies. *Rheumatology.* 2017;56(11):1945-1961.

72. Muscal E, Brey R. Neurologic manifestations of systemic lupus erythematosus in children and adults. *Neurol Clin.* 2010;28(1):61-73.

73. Gulinello M, Wen J, Putterman C. Neuropsychiatric symptoms in lupus. *Psychiatr Ann.* 2012;42(9):322-328.

74. Hiraki L, Benseler S, Tyrrell P. Clinical and laboratory characteristics and long-term outcome of pediatric systemic lupus erythematosus: a longitudinal study. *J Pediatr.* 2008;152(4):550-556.

75. Gómez-Puerta JA, Barbhaiya M, Guan H, Feldman CH, Alarcón GS, Costenbader KH. Racial/ethnic variation in all-cause mortality among United States Medicaid recipients with systemic lupus erythematosus: a Hispanic and Asian paradox. *Arthritis Rheumatol.* 2015;67(3):752-760.

76. Hanly J, Urowitz M, Sanchez-Guerrero J. Neuropsychiatric events at the time of diagnosis of systemic lupus erythematosus: an international inception cohort study. *Arthritis Rheum.* 2007;56(1):265-273.

77. Cohen D, Rijnink E, Nabuurs R. Brain histopathology in patients with systemic lupus erythematosus: identification of lesions associated with clinical neuropsychiatric lupus syndromes and the role of complement. *Rheumatol Oxf.* 2017;56(1):77-86.

78. Stock A, Wen J, Putterman C. Neuropsychiatric lupus, the blood brain barrier, and the TWEAK/Fn14 pathway. *Front Immunol.* 2013;4:484.

79. Ho R, Thiaghu C, Ong H. A meta-analysis of serum and cerebrospinal fluid autoantibodies in neuropsychiatric systemic lupus erythematosus. *Autoimmun Rev.* 2016;15(2):124-138.

80. Hanly J, Walsh N, Sangalang V. Brain pathology in systemic lupus erythematosus. *J Rheumatol.* 1992;19(5):732-741.

81. Rowshani AT, Remans P, Rozemuller A, Tak PP. Cerebral vasculitis as a primary manifestation of systemic lupus erythematosus. *Ann Rheum Dis.* 2005;64(5):784-786.

82. Jafri K, Patterson SL, Lanata C. Central nervous system manifestations of systemic lupus erythematosus. *Rheum Dis Clin.* 2017;43(4):531-545.

83. Liang MH, Corzillius M, Bae S, Lew, RA, et al. The American College of Rheumatology nomenclature and case definitions for neuropsychiatric lupus syndromes. *Arthritis Rheum.* 1999;42(4):599-608.

84. Vivaldo J, de Amorim J, Julio P. Definition of NPSLE: does the ACR nomenclature still hold? *Front Med Lausanne.* 2018;5:138.

85. Sciascia S, Bertolaccini M, Baldovino S. Central nervous system involvement in systemic lupus erythematosus: overview on classification criteria. *Autoimmun Rev.* 2013;12(3):426-429.

86. Hanly J, Kozora E, Beyea S. Nervous system disease in systemic lupus erythematosus: current status and future directions. *Arthritis Rheumatol.* 2019;71(1):33-42.

87. Mikdashi J, Handwerger B, Langenberg P. Baseline disease activity, hyperlipidemia, and hypertension are predictive factors for ischemic stroke and stroke severity in systemic lupus erythematosus. *Stroke.* 2007;38(2):281-285.

88. Koskenmies S, Vaarala O, Wide E. The association of antibodies to cardiolipin, β2-glycoprotein I, prothrombin, and oxidized low-density lipoprotein with thrombosis in 292 patients with familial and sporadic systemic lupus erythematosus. *Scand J Rheumatol.* 2004;33(4):246-252.

89. González-Duarte A, Cantú-Brito C, Ruano-Calderón L. Clinical description of seizures in patients with systemic lupus erythematosus. *Eur Neurol.* 2008;59(6):320-323.

90. Joseph F, Lammie G, Scolding N. CNS lupus: a study of 41 patients. *Neurology.* 2007;69(7):644-654.

91. Andrade R, Alarcón G, González L. Seizures in patients with systemic lupus erythematosus: data from LUMINA, a multiethnic cohort (LUMINA LIV). *Ann Rheum Dis.* 2008;67(6):829-834.

92. Mayes B, Brey R. Evaluation and treatment of seizures in patients with systemic lupus erythematosus. *J Clin Rheumatol.* 1996;2(6):336-345.

93. Saigal R, Bhargav R, Goyal L. Peripheral neuropathy in systemic lupus erythematosus: clinical and electrophysiological properties and their association with disease activity parameters. *J Assoc Physicians India.* 2015;63(12):15-19.

94. Florica B, Aghdassi E, Su J. Peripheral neuropathy in patients with systemic lupus erythematosus. *Semin Arthritis Rheum.* 2011;41(2):203-211.

95. Leslie B, Crowe S. Cognitive functioning in systemic lupus erythematosus: a meta-analysis. *Lupus.* 2018;961203317751859.

96. Kozora E, Hanly J, Lapteva L. Cognitive dysfunction in systemic lupus erythematosus: past present and future. *Arthritis Rheum.* 2008;58(11):3286-3298.

97. Barraclough M, Elliott R, McKie S. Cognitive dysfunction and functional magnetic resonance imaging in systemic lupus erythematosus. *Lupus.* 2015;24(12):1239-1247.

98. Sahebari M, Rezaieyazdi Z, Khodashahi M. Brain single photon emission computed tomography scan (SPECT) and functional MRI in systemic lupus erythematosus patients with cognitive dysfunction: a systematic review. *Asia Ocean J Nucl Med Biol.* 2018;6(2):97-107.

99. Ceccarelli F, Perricone C, Pirone C. Cognitive dysfunction improves in systemic lupus erythematosus: results of a 10 years prospective study. *PLoS One.* 2018;13(5):e0196103.

100. Conti F, Alessandri C, Perricone C. Neurocognitive dysfunction in systemic lupus erythematosus: association with antiphospholipid antibodies, disease activity and chronic damage. *PLoS One.* 2012;7(3):e33824.

101. Abdel-Nasser A, Ghaleb R, Mahmoud J. Association of anti-ribosomal P protein antibodies with neuropsychiatric and other manifestations of systemic lupus erythematosus. *Clin Rheumatol.* 2008;27(11):1377-1385.

102. Karimifar M, Sharifi I, Shafiey K. Anti-ribosomal P antibodies related to depression in early clinical course of systemic lupus erythematosus. *J Res Med Sci.* 2013;18(10):860-864.

103. Zhang L, Fu T, Yin R. Prevalence of depression and anxiety in systemic lupus erythematosus: a systematic review and meta-analysis. *BMC Psychiatry.* 2017;17(1):70.

104. Lapteva L, Nowak M, Yarboro C. Anti-N-methyl-D-aspartate receptor antibodies, cognitive dysfunction, and depression in systemic lupus erythematosus. *Arthritis Rheum.* 2006; 54(8):2505-2514.

105. Jump R, Robinson M, Armstrong A. Fatigue in systemic lupus erythematosus: contributions of disease activity, pain, depression, and perceived social support. *J Rheumatol.* 2005;32(9):1699-1705.

106. Hanly J, Su L, Urowitz M. Mood disorders in systemic lupus erythematosus: results from an international inception cohort study. *Arthritis Rheumatol*. 2015;67(7):1837-1847.

107. Nayak R, Bhogale G, Patil N. Psychosis in patients with systemic lupus erythematosus. *Indian J Psychol Med*. 2012;34(1):90-93.

108. Pego-Reigosa J, Isenberg D. Psychosis due to systemic lupus erythematosus: characteristics and long-term outcome of this rare manifestation of the disease. *Rheumatol Oxf*. 2008;47(10):1498-1502.

109. Kang D, Mok CC. Management of psychosis in neuropsychiatric lupus. *J Clin Rheumatol Immunol*. 2019;19(01):9-17.

110. World Health Organization. *The ICD-10 Classification of Mental and Behavioural Disorders: Clinical Descriptions and Diagnostic Guidelines*. Geneva: World Health Organization; 1992.

111. Beltrão S, Gigante L, Zimmer D. Psychiatric symptoms in patients with systemic lupus erythematosus: frequency and association with disease activity using the Adult Psychiatric Morbidity Questionnaire. *Rev Bras Reum*. 2013;53(4):328-334.

112. Dale R, Yin K, Ding A. Antibody binding to neuronal surface in movement disorders associated with lupus and antiphospholipid antibodies. *Dev Med Child Neurol*. 2011;53(6):522-528.

113. Toubi E, Khamashta M, Panarra A. Association of antiphospholipid antibodies with central nervous system disease in systemic lupus erythematosus. *Am J Med*. 1995;99(4):397-401.

114. Wilson H, Winfield J, Lahita R. Association of IgG anti-brain antibodies with central nervous system dysfunction in systemic lupus erythematosus. *Arthritis Rheum*. 1979;22(5):458-462.

115. Borowoy A, Pope J, Silverman E. Neuropsychiatric lupus: the prevalence and autoantibody associations depend on the definition: results from the 1000 faces of lupus cohort. *Semin Arthritis Rheum*. 2012;42(2):179-185.

116. Faria R, Gonçalves J, Dias R. Neuropsychiatric systemic lupus erythematosus involvement: towards a tailored approach to our patients? *Rambam Maimonides Med J*. 2017;8(1):e00001.

117. Colasanti T, Delunardo F, Margutti P. Autoantibodies involved in neuropsychiatric manifestations associated with systemic lupus erythematosus. *J Neuroimmunol*. 2009;212(1-2):3-9.

118. Denburg S, Behmann S, Carbotte R. Lymphocyte antigens in neuropsychiatric systemic lupus erythematosus. Relationship of lymphocyte antibody specificities to clinical disease. *Arthritis Rheum*. 1994;37(3):369-375.

119. Abbott N, Mendonça L, Dolman D. The blood-brain barrier in systemic lupus erythematosus. *Lupus*. 2003;12(12):908-915.

120. Karimifar M, Sharifi I, Shafiey K. Anti-ribosomal P antibodies related to depression in early clinical course of systemic lupus erythematosus. *J Res Med Sci*. 2013;18(10):860-864.

121. Menon S, Jameson-Shortall E, Newman S. A longitudinal study of anticardiolipin antibody levels and cognitive functioning in systemic lupus erythematosus. *Arthritis Rheum*. 1999;42(4):735-741.

122. Denburg S, Denburg J. Cognitive dysfunction and antiphospholipid antibodies in systemic lupus erythematosus. *Lupus*. 2003;12(12):883-890.

123. Duarte-García A, Romero-Díaz J, Juárez S. Disease activity, autoantibodies, and inflammatory molecules in serum and cerebrospinal fluid of patients with systemic lupus erythematosus and cognitive dysfunction. *PLoS One*. 2018;13(5):e0196487.

124. Arinuma Y, Kikuchi H, Wada T. Brain MRI in patients with diffuse psychiatric/neuropsychological syndromes in systemic lupus erythematosus. *Lupus Sci Med*. 2014;1(1):e000050.

125. Tan Z, Zhou Y, Li X. Brain magnetic resonance imaging, cerebrospinal fluid, and autoantibody profile in 118 patients with neuropsychiatric lupus. *Clin Rheumatol*. 2018;37(1):227-233.

126. Zaky M, Shaat R, El-Bassiony S. Magnetic resonance imaging (MRI) brain abnormalities of neuropsychiatric systemic lupus

erythematosus patients in Mansoura city: relation to disease activity. *ScienceDirect*. 2015;37(4):S7-S11.

127. Appenzeller S, Carnevalle A, Li L. Hippocampal atrophy in systemic lupus erythematosus. *Ann Rheum Dis*. 2006;65(12):1585-1589.

128. Sarbu N, Bargalló N, Cervera R. Advanced and conventional magnetic resonance imaging in neuropsychiatric lupus. *F1000Res*. 2015;4:162.

129. Amin O, Kaul A, Smith T. Comparison of structural magnetic resonance imaging findings between neuropsychiatric systemic lupus erythematosus and systemic lupus erythematosus patients: a systematic review and meta-analysis. *Rheum Pr Res*. 2017;2:1-11.

130. Ma Y, Shi N, Li M. Applications of next-generation sequencing in systemic autoimmune diseases. *Genomics Proteom Bioinf*. 2015;13(4):242-249.

131. Crowther MA, Ginsberg JS, Julian J, Denburg J, Hirsh J, Douketis J, et al. A comparison of two intensities of warfarin for the prevention of recurrent thrombosis in patients with the antiphospholipid antibody syndrome. *N Engl J Med*. 2003;349(12):1133-1138.

132. Popescu A, Kao AH. Neuropsychiatric systemic lupus erythematosus. *Curr Neuropharmacol*. 2011;9(3):449-457.

133. Mikdashi J, Handwerger B, Langenberg P. Baseline disease activity, hyperlipidemia, and hypertension are predictive factors for ischemic stroke and stroke severity in systemic lupus erythematosus. *Stroke*. 2007;38(2):281-285.

134. Mayes B, Brey R. Evaluation and treatment of seizures in patients with systemic lupus erythematosus. *J Clin Rheumatol*. 1996;2(6):336-345.

135. Gao Z, Li X, Peng T. Systemic lupus erythematosus with Guillian-Barre syndrome: a case report and literature review. *Medicine (Baltimore)*. 2018;97(25):e11160.

136. Figueiredo-Braga M, Cornaby C, Cortez A. Depression and anxiety in systemic lupus erythematosus: the crosstalk between immunological, clinical, and psychosocial factors. *Medicine (Baltimore)*. 2018;97(28):e11376.

137. Herrmann N, Lanctot KL. Do atypical antipsychotics cause stroke? *CNS Drugs*. 2005;19(2):91-103.

138. Mak A, Ho RCM, Lau CS. Clinical implications of neuropsychiatric systemic lupus erythematosus. *Adv Psychiatr Treat*. 2009;15(6):451-458.

139. Kohen M, Asherson R, Gharavi A. Lupus psychosis: differentiation from the steroid-induced state. *Clin Exp Rheumatol*. 1993;11(3):323-326.

140. Clifford DB, Ances BM. HIV-associated neurocognitive disorder (HAND). *Lancet Infect Dis*. 2013;13(11):976-986.

141. Eshun-Wilson I, Siegfried N, Akena DH, Stein DJ, Obuku EA, Joska JA. Antidepressants for depression in adults with HIV infection. *Cochrane Database Syst Rev*. 2018;1:CD008525.

142. Ciesla JA, Roberts JE. Meta-analysis of the relationship between HIV infection and risk for depressive disorders. *Am J Psychiatry*. 2001;158(5):725-730.

143. Atkinson JH, Heaton RK, Patterson TL, et al. Two-year prospective study of major depressive disorder in HIV-infected men. *J Affect Disord*. 2008;108(3):225-234.

144. Lyketsos CG, Schwartz J, Fishman M, Treisman GJ. AIDS mania. *J Neuropsychiatry Clin Neurosci*. 1997;9(2):277-279.

145. Ellen SR, Judd FK, Mijch AM, Cockram A. Secondary mania in patients with HIV infection. *Aust N Z J Psychiatry*. 1999;33(3):353-360.

146. Lyketsos CG, Hanson AL, Fishman M, Rosenblatt A, McHugh PR, Treisman GJ. Manic syndrome early and late in the course of HIV. *Am J Psychiatry*. 1993;150(2):326-327.

147. Abers MS, Shandera WX, Kass JS. Neurological and psychiatric adverse effects of antiretroviral drugs. *CNS Drugs.* 2014;28(2):131-145.

148. Mijch AM, Judd FK, Lyketsos CG, Ellen S, Cockram A. Secondary mania in patients with HIV infection: are antiretrovirals protective? *J Neuropsychiatry Clin Neurosci.* 1999;11(4):475-480.

149. De Ronchi D, Faranca I, Forti P, et al. Development of acute psychotic disorders and HIV-1 infection. *Int J Psychiatry Med.* 2000;30(2):173-183.

150. Neigh GN, Rhodes ST, Valdez A, Jovanovic T. PTSD co-morbid with HIV: separate but equal, or two parts of a whole? *Neurobiol Dis.* 2016;92:116-123.

151. Fiellin D. Substance use disorders in HIV-infected patients: impact and new treatment strategies. *Top HIV Med.* 2004;12(3):77-82.

152. Bauer-Staeb C, Jörgensen L, Lewis G, Dalman C, Osborn DPJ, Hayes JF. Prevalence and risk factors for HIV, hepatitis B, and hepatitis C in people with severe mental illness: a total population study of Sweden. *Lancet Psychiatry.* 2017;4(9):685-693.

153. Gray F, Scaravilli F, Everall I, Chretien F, An S, Boche D, et al. Neuropathology of early HIV-1 infection. *Brain Pathol.* 1996;6(1):1-12.

154. Kopnisky KL, Bao J, Lin YW. Neurobiology of HIV, psychiatric and substance abuse comorbidity research: workshop report. *Brain Behav Immun.* 2007;21(4):428-441.

155. Heaton RK, Franklin DR, Ellis RJ, McCutchan JA, Letendre SL, LeBlanc S, et al. HIV-associated neurocognitive disorders before and during the era of combination antiretroviral therapy: differences in rates, nature, and predictors. *J Neurovirol.* 2011;17(1):3-16.

156. Ayoade F, Chandranesan J, Stevenson A. HIV-1 associated opportunistic infections, toxoplasmosis. In: StatPearls. Treasure Island, FL: StatPearls Publishing; 2018. Available at http://www.ncbi.nlm.nih.gov/books/NBK441877/. Accessed October 2, 2018.

157. Nakimuli-Mpungu E, Musisi S, Mpungu SK, Katabira E. Primary mania versus HIV-related secondary mania in Uganda. *Am J Psychiatry.* 2006;163(8):1349-1354; quiz 1480.

158. Harris MJ, Jeste DV, Gleghorn A, Sewell DD. New-onset psychosis in HIV-infected patients. *J Clin Psychiatry.* 1991;52(9):369-376.

159. Lucas GM. Substance abuse, adherence with antiretroviral therapy, and clinical outcomes among HIV-infected individuals. *Life Sci.* 2011;88(21):948-952.

160. DeLorenze GN, Satre DD, Quesenberry CP, Tsai A-L, Weisner CM. Mortality after diagnosis of psychiatric disorders and co-occurring substance use disorders among HIV-infected patients. *AIDS Patient Care STDs.* 2010;24(11):705-712.

161. Gallego L. Diagnosis and clinical features of major neuropsychiatric disorders in HIV infection. 2011;13(3):171-179.

162. Goodkin K, Alger JR, Maudsley AA, Govind V, Sheriff S, Zhang JM. Clinical utility of magnetic resonance spectroscopy to enhance diagnosis of HIV-associated mild neurocognitive disorder. *Neuropsychiatry.* 2012;2(5):379-383.

163. Antinori A, Arendt G, Grant I, et al. Assessment, diagnosis, and treatment of HIV-associated neurocognitive disorder: a consensus report of the Mind Exchange Program. *Clin Infect Dis.* 2013;56(7):1004-1017.

164. Eggers C, Arendt G, Hahn K, et al. HIV-1-associated neurocognitive disorder: epidemiology, pathogenesis, diagnosis, and treatment. *J Neurol.* 2017;264(8):1715-1727.

165. Ndhlovu LC, Umaki T, Chew GM, et al. Treatment intensification with maraviroc (CCR5 antagonist) leads to declines in CD16-expressing monocytes in cART-suppressed chronic HIV-infected subjects and is associated with improvements in neurocognitive test performance: implications for HIV-associated neurocognitive disease (HAND). *J Neurovirol.* 2014;20(6):571-582.

166. Simioni S, Cavassini M, Michel M, et al. Rivastigmine for the treatment of HIV-associated neurocognitive disorders: a randomized, double-blind, placebo-controlled, crossover pilot study. *Neurology.* 2012;78(1 suppl):S37.005.

167. Schifitto G, Navia BA, Yiannoutsos CT, et al. Memantine and HIV-associated cognitive impairment: a neuropsychological and proton magnetic resonance spectroscopy study: AIDS. 2007;21(14):1877-1886.

168. McElhiney M, Rabkin J, Van Gorp W, Rabkin R. Effect of armodafinil on cognition in patients with HIV/AIDS and fatigue. *J Clin Exp Neuropsychol.* 2013;35(7):718-727.

169. Livelli A, Orofino GC, Calcagno A, et al. Evaluation of a cognitive rehabilitation protocol in HIV patients with associated neurocognitive disorders: efficacy and stability over time. *Front Behav Neurosci.* 2015;9:306.

170. Becker JT, Dew MA, Aizenstein HJ, et al. A pilot study of the effects of internet-based cognitive stimulation on neuropsychological function in HIV disease. *Disabil Rehabil.* 2012;34(21):1848-1852.

171. Robertson K, Liner J, Meeker RB. Antiretroviral neurotoxicity. *J Neurovirol.* 2012;18(5):388-399.

172. Kahouadji Y, Dumurgier J, Sellier P, et al. Cognitive function after several years of antiretroviral therapy with stable central nervous system penetration score. *HIV Med.* 2013;14(5):311-315.

173. Iovieno N, Tedeschini E, Ameral VE, Rigatelli M, Papakostas GI. Antidepressants for major depressive disorder in patients with a co-morbid axis-III disorder: a meta-analysis of patient characteristics and placebo response rates in randomized controlled trials. *Int Clin Psychopharmacol.* 2011;26(2):69-74.

174. Eshun-Wilson I, Siegfried N, Akena DH, Stein DJ, Obuku EA, Joska JA. Antidepressants for depression in adults with HIV infection. *Cochrane Database Syst Rev.* 2018;1:CD008525.

175. Brogan K, Lux J. Management of common psychiatric conditions in the HIV-positive population. *Curr HIV/AIDS Rep.* 2009;6(2):108-115.

176. Heckman TG, Markowitz JC, Heckman BD, et al. A randomized clinical trial showing persisting reductions in depressive symptoms in HIV-infected rural adults following brief telephone-administered interpersonal psychotherapy. *Ann Behav Med.* 2018;52(4):299-308.

177. Schaerf FW, Miller RR, Lipsey JR, McPherson RW. ECT for major depression in four patients infected with human immunodeficiency virus. *Am J Psychiatry.* 1989;146(6):782-784.

178. Knotkova H, Rosedale M, Strauss SM, et al. Using transcranial direct current stimulation to treat depression in HIV-infected persons: the outcomes of a feasibility study. *Front Psychiatry.* 2012;3:59.

179. Singh AN, Golledge H, Catalan J. Treatment of HIV-related psychotic disorders with risperidone: a series of 21 cases. *J Psychosom Res.* 1997;42(5):489-493.

180. Ferrando SJ, Nims C. HIV-associated mania treated with electroconvulsive therapy and highly-active antiretroviral therapy. *Psychosomatics.* 2006;47(2):170-174.

181. Thompson A, Silverman B, Dzeng L, Treisman G. Psychotropic medications and HIV. *Clin Infect Dis.* 2006;42(9):1305-1310.

182. van der Heijden I, Abrahams N, Sinclair D. Psychosocial group interventions to improve psychological well-being in adults living with HIV. *Cochrane Database Syst Rev.* 2017;3:CD010806.

183. Sikkema KJ, Hansen NB, Kochman A, et al. Outcomes from a group intervention for coping with HIV/AIDS and childhood sexual abuse: reductions in traumatic stress. *AIDS Behav.* 2007;11(1):49-60.

184. Durvasula R, Miller TR. Substance abuse treatment in persons with HIV/AIDS: challenges in managing triple diagnosis. *Behav Med.* 2014;40(2):43-52.

185. McCance-Katz EF, Moody DE, Morse GD, et al. Interactions between buprenorphine and antiretrovirals. I. The nonnucleoside reverse-transcriptase inhibitors efavirenz and delavirdine. *Clin Infect Dis.* 2006;43(suppl 4):S224-S234.

186. Looker KJ, Magaret AS, May MT, et al. Global and regional estimates of prevalent and incident herpes simplex virus type 1 infections in 2012. *PLoS One.* 2015;10(10):e0140765.

187. Hasbun R, Rosenthal N, Balada-Llasat JM, et al. Epidemiology of meningitis and encephalitis in the United States, 2011–2014. *Clin Infect Dis.* 2017;65(3):359-363.

188. Caparros-Lefebvre D, Girard-Buttaz I, Reboul S, et al. Cognitive and psychiatric impairment in herpes simplex virus encephalitis suggest involvement of the amygdalo-frontal pathways. *J Neurol.* 1996;243(3):248-256.

189. Hokkanen L, Launes J. Cognitive recovery instead of decline after acute encephalitis: a prospective follow up study. *J Neurol Neurosurg Psychiatry.* 1997;63(2):222-227.

190. Carter CJ. Susceptibility genes are enriched in those of the herpes simplex virus 1/host interactome in psychiatric and neurological disorders. *Pathog Dis.* 2013;69(3):240-261.

191. Gnann JW, Whitley RJ. Herpes simplex encephalitis: an update. *Curr Infect Dis Rep.* 2017;19(3):13.

192. Vasconcelos-Moreno MP, Dargél AA, Goi PD, Bragatti JA, Kapczinski F, Kauer-Sant'Anna M. Improvement of behavioural and manic-like symptoms secondary to herpes simplex virus encephalitis with mood stabilizers: a case report. *Int J Neuropsychopharmacol.* 2011;14(05):718-720.

193. Caroff S, Mann S, Gliatto M, Sullivan K, Camp. Psychiatric manifestation of acute viral encephalitis. *Psychiatr Ann.* 2001;31:193-204.

194. Pewter SM, Williams WH, Haslam C, Kay JM. Neuropsychological and psychiatric profiles in acute encephalitis in adults. *Neuropsychol Rehabil.* 2007;17(4/5):478-505.

195. Whitley RJ, Cobbs CG, Alford CA, et al. Diseases that mimic herpes simplex encephalitis: diagnosis, presentation, and outcome. *JAMA.* 1989;262(2):234-239.

196. Studahl M, Lindquist L, Eriksson B-M, et al. Acute viral infections of the central nervous system in immunocompetent adults: diagnosis and management. *Drugs.* 2013;73(2):131-158.

197. Harder J, Mariano T. The importance of comprehensive neuropsychiatric care in the postencephalitic patient. *Future Neurol.* 2018;13(4):173-176.

198. Guaiana G, Markova I. Antipsychotic treatment improves outcome in herpes simplex encephalitis: a case report. *J Neuropsychiatry Clin Neurosci.* 2006;18(2):247-247.

199. Vallini AD, Burns RL. Carbamazepine as therapy for psychiatric sequelae of herpes simplex encephalitis. *South Med J.* 1987;80(12):1590-1592.

200. Gaber T, Eshiett M, Kennedy P, Chaudhuri A. Resolution of psychiatric symptoms secondary to herpes simplex encephalitis. *J Neurol Neurosurg Psychiatry.* 2003;74(8):1164.

201. Kohno N, Nabika Y, Toyoda G, Bokura H, Nagata T, Yamaguchi S. The effect of ropinirole on apathy and depression after herpes encephalitis. *Cogn Behav Neurol.* 2012;25(2):98-102.

202. Griffin S, Shannon T. Managing aggression in global amnesia following herpes simplex virus encephalitis: the case of E.B. *Brain Inj.* 2015;29(1):118-124.

203. Alderman N, Burgess P. A comparison of treatment methods for behaviour disorder following herpes simplex encephalitis. *Neuropsychol Rehabil.* 1994;4:31-48.

204. Miotto EC. Cognitive rehabilitation of amnesia after virus encephalitis: a case report. *Neuropsychol Rehabil.* 2007;17(4/5):551-566.

205. Yang Y, Xiao J, Song H, Wang R, Hussain M, Song W. Relationship of herpes simplex encephalitis and transcranial direct current stimulation—a case report. *J Clin Virol.* 2015;65:46-49.

206. Cohen SE, Klausner JD, Engelman J, Philip S. Syphilis in the modern era. *Infect Dis Clin North Am.* 2013;27(4):705-722.

207. Table 1—2017 Sexually transmitted diseases surveillance. 2018. Available at https://www.cdc.gov/std/stats17/tables/1.htm. Accessed December 4, 2018.

208. STD facts—Syphilis (detailed). 2018. Available at https://www.cdc.gov/std/syphilis/stdfact-syphilis-detailed.htm. Accessed December 4, 2018.

209. Kitayama K, Segura ER, Lake JE, et al. Syphilis in the Americas: a protocol for a systematic review of syphilis prevalence and incidence in four high-risk groups, 1980–2016. *Syst Rev.* 2017; 6(1):195.

210. Shi M, Peng R-R, Gao Z, et al. Risk profiles of neurosyphilis in HIV-negative patients with primary, secondary and latent syphilis: implications for clinical intervention. *J Eur Acad Dermatol Venereol.* 2016;30(4):659-666.

211. Barbosa IG, Vale TC, Macedo DL de, Gomez RS, Teixeira AL. Neurosyphilis presenting as mania. *Bipolar Disord.* 2012;14(3):309-312.

212. Lin L-R, Zhang H-L, Huang S-J, et al. Psychiatric manifestations as primary symptom of neurosyphilis among HIV-negative patients. *J Neuropsychiatry Clin Neurosci.* 2014;26(3):233-240.

213. Zhong X, Shi H, Hou L, et al. Neuropsychiatric features of neurosyphilis: frequency, relationship with the severity of cognitive impairment and comparison with Alzheimer disease. *Dement Geriatr Cogn Disord.* 2017;43(5-6):308-319.

214. Hicks C, Clement M. Syphilis: epidemiology, pathophysiology, and clinical manifestations in HIV-uninfected patients—UpToDate. 2018. Available at https://www.uptodate.com/contents/syphilis-epidemiology-pathophysiology-and-clinical-manifestations-in-hiv-uninfected-patients?search=syphilis&source=search_result&selectedTitle=3~150&usage_type=default&display_rank=3#H8. Accessed December 7, 2018.

215. Hook EW. Syphilis. *Lancet.* 2017;389(10078):1550-1557.

216. Beauchemin P, Laforce R. Neurocognitive changes in tertiary neurosyphilis: a retrospective chart review. *Can J Neurol Sci.* 2014;41(4):452-458.

217. Wang J, Guo Q, Zhou P, Zhang J, Zhao Q, Hong Z. Cognitive impairment in mild general paresis of the insane: AD-like pattern. *Dement Geriatr Cogn Disord.* 2011;31(4):284-290.

218. Moulton CD, Koychev I. The effect of penicillin therapy on cognitive outcomes in neurosyphilis: a systematic review of the literature. *Gen Hosp Psychiatry.* 2015;37(1):49-52.

219. Tipple C, Taylor GP. Syphilis testing, typing, and treatment follow-up: a new era for an old disease. *Curr Opin Infect Dis.* 2015;28(1):53-60.

220. Davis AP, Stern J, Tantalo L, et al. How well do neurologic symptoms identify individuals with neurosyphilis? *Clin Infect Dis.* 2017;66(3):363-367.

221. Sanchez FM, Zisselman MH. Treatment of psychiatric symptoms associated with neurosyphilis. *Psychosomatics.* 2007;48(5):440-445.

222. Weaver G, Remick R. Electroconvulsive treatment of depression associated with neurosyphilis. *J Clin Psychiatry.* 1982;43(11):468-469.

223. Pecenak J, Janik P, Vaseckova B, Trebulova K. Electroconvulsive therapy treatment in a patient with neurosyphilis and psychotic disorder: case report and literature review. *J ECT*. 2015;31(4):268-270.

224. Wu Y-S, Lane H-Y, Lin C-H. Donepezil improved cognitive deficits in a patient with neurosyphilis. *Clin Neuropharmacol*. 2015;38(4):156-157.

225. Cohen D, Rijnink E, Nabuurs R. Brain histopathology in patients with systemic lupus erythematosus: identification of lesions associated with clinical neuropsychiatric lupus syndromes and the role of complement. *Rheumatol Oxf*. 2017;56(1):77-86.

226. Mao L, Jin H, Wang M, et al. Neurologic manifestations of hospitalized patients with coronavirus disease 2019 in Wuhan, China. *JAMA Neurol*. 2020;77(6):1-9. doi:10.1001/jamaneurol.2020.1127. [Epub ahead of print, April 10, 2020]

227. Romero-Sánchez CM, Díaz-Maroto I, Fernández-Díaz E, et al. Neurologic manifestations in hospitalized patients with COVID-19: the ALBACOVID registry. *Neurology*. 2020. doi:10.1212/WNL.0000000000009937. [Epub ahead of print, June 1, 2020]

228. Desforges M, Le Coupanec A, Dubeau P, et al. Human coronaviruses and other respiratory viruses: underestimated opportunistic pathogens of the central nervous system? *Viruses*. 2019;12(1):14. doi:10.3390/v12010014.

229. Paniz-Mondolfi A, Bryce C, Grimes Z, et al. Central nervous system involvement by severe acute respiratory syndrome coronavirus-2 (SARS-CoV-2). *J Med Virol*. 2020;92(7):699-702. doi:10.1002/jmv.25915.

230. Moriguchi T, Harii N, Goto J, et al. A first case of meningitis/encephalitis associated with SARS-Coronavirus-2. *Int J Infect Dis*. 2020;94:55-58. doi:10.1016/j.ijid.2020.03.062.

231. Varatharaj A, Galea I. The blood-brain barrier in systemic inflammation. *Brain Behav Immun*. 2017;60:1-12. doi:10.1016/j.bbi.2016.03.010.

232. Lodigiani C, Iapichino G, Carenzo L, et al. Venous and arterial thromboembolic complications in COVID-19 patients admitted to an academic hospital in Milan, Italy. *Thromb Res*. 2020;191:9-14. doi:10.1016/j.thromres.2020.04.024.

233. Helms J, Kremer S, Merdji H, et al. Neurologic features in severe SARS-CoV-2 infection. *N Engl J Med*. 2020; 382(23):2268-2270. doi:10.1056/NEJMc2008597.

234. Rogers JP, Chesney E, Oliver D, et al. Psychiatric and neuropsychiatric presentations associated with severe coronavirus infections: a systematic review and meta-analysis with comparison to the COVID-19 pandemic. *Lancet Psychiatry*. 2020;7(7):611-627. doi:10.1016/S2215-0366(20)30203-0.

235. Kong X, Zheng K, Tang M, et al. Prevalence and factors associated with depression and anxiety of hospitalized patients with COVID-19. medRxiv. 2020. doi:10.1101/2020.03.24.20043075. [Epub April 5]

236. Guo Q, Zheng Y, Shi J, et al. Immediate psychological distress in quarantined patients with COVID-19 and its association with peripheral inflammation: a mixed-method study. *Brain Behav Immun*. 2020;88:17-27. doi:10.1016/j.bbi.2020.05.038.

237. Yang L, Wu D, Hou Y, et al. Analysis of psychological state and clinical psychological intervention model of patients with COVID-19. medRxiv. 2020. doi:10.1101/2020.03.22.20040899. [Epub March 24]

238. Larvie M, Lev MH, Hess CP. More on neurologic features in severe SARS-CoV-2 infection. *N Engl J Med*. 2020;382(26):e110. doi:10.1056/NEJMc2015132.

239. Sarikaya B. More on neurologic features in severe SARS-CoV-2 infection. *N Engl J Med*. 2020;382(26):e110. doi:10.1056/NEJMc2015132.

240. Helms J, Kremer S, Meziani F. More on neurologic features in severe SARS-CoV-2 infection. Reply. *N Engl J Med*. 2020;382(26):e110. doi:10.1056/NEJMc2015132.

27

Neuropsychiatry of Multiple Sclerosis

Laura T. Safar · Tarun Singhal · Nicole C. Feng · Elizabeth Misasi · Lindsay Barker

INTRODUCTION

In this chapter, we first review general concepts about multiple sclerosis (MS) and its treatment and general considerations to take into account when assessing and treating neuropsychiatric disorders in patients with MS. We then discuss specific neuropsychiatric disorders in MS.

Multiple Sclerosis: General concepts

MS is an immune-mediated demyelinating disease of the central nervous system (CNS).[1] MS is the most common cause of non-traumatic neurological disability among young adults. Its prevalence is approximately 50–300 per 100,000 population, with an estimated 2.3 million MS patients living worldwide. MS patients typically present between 20 and 40 years of age, with a female-to-male ratio of approximately 2.3:1. MS patients present with a relapsing remitting course at the time of disease onset in 85–90% of individuals, and approximately half of these patients may evolve into a secondary progressive MS phenotype with gradual accumulation of neurologic disability over years. A minority of patients may present with a progressive course at disease onset and are classified as primary progressive MS.

MS has been traditionally considered to be mediated by toxicity of autoreactive T-lymphocytes against the myelin sheath, and demyelinated plaques in white matter (WM) are pathological hallmarks of the disease. However, accumulating evidence suggests key roles of other immune cells, such as B-lymphocytes and glial cells (microglia, astrocytes, dendritic cells) in the pathogenesis of MS. Further, in addition to WM demyelination, there has been an increasing recognition of gray matter (GM) pathology, axonal injury, oligodendrocyte apoptosis, and neuronal loss in MS.

The most common presenting symptoms of MS include visual impairment due to optic neuritis, diplopia due to brainstem involvement, sensory impairment and focal weakness due to involvement of long tracts, ataxia, fatigue, sleep problems, and bladder and bowel impairment. Additionally, a significant proportion of MS patients complain of neuropsychiatric symptoms including, depression, anxiety, and cognitive disturbances, among others.

Magnetic resonance imaging (MRI) plays a key role in the diagnosis and monitoring of MS (see Figure 27-1). Table 27-1 shows a list of different MRI lesions in MS and their significance. Diagnosis of MS requires evidence of demyelinating lesions that are "disseminated in space" and "disseminated in time." Current diagnostic criteria allow for a diagnosis of MS based on a single MRI scan, in the appropriate clinical context. Simultaneous presence of a gadolinium-contrast enhancing lesion on T1-weighted MRI, along with a T2-bright lesion on T2/fluid attenuation inversion recovery (FLAIR) MRI sequence can provide evidence for dissemination in time. Similarly, presence of lesions in two of four locations (periventricular WM, juxtacortical WM, posterior fossa, or spinal cord) provides evidence for dissemination in space and helps distinguish MS lesions from vascular and nonspecific causes of WM abnormalities on MRI. MRI scanners with higher magnetic strength (e.g., 3 and 7 Tesla) enable in vivo visualization of cortical GM plaques that may play a key role in MS pathogenesis. Cortical lesions in MS may be leukocortical (involving both GM and WM, or Type I), intracortical (small lesions within the cortical GM, or Type II), subpial (Type III), or may extend throughout the cortex (Type IV). Leptomeningeal enhancement (LME) has been recently postulated as a biomarker for brain atrophy and disease progression in MS. The relationship between neuroinflammation and neurodegeneration is a key factor under active investigation for furthering the understanding of progressive MS. A possible way to conceptualize the relationship between LME and neurodegeneration is that LME may represent inflammatory follicles which secrete antibodies/cytokines/other potential toxic factors. These may directly cause neuronal injury and may also stimulate glial cells—which in turn cause neuronal injury as well, leading to neurodegeneration. Other advanced MRI techniques including magnetization transfer ratio (MTR), diffusion weighted imaging (DWI), diffusion tensor imaging (DTI), and magnetic resonance spectroscopy (MRS) have demonstrated

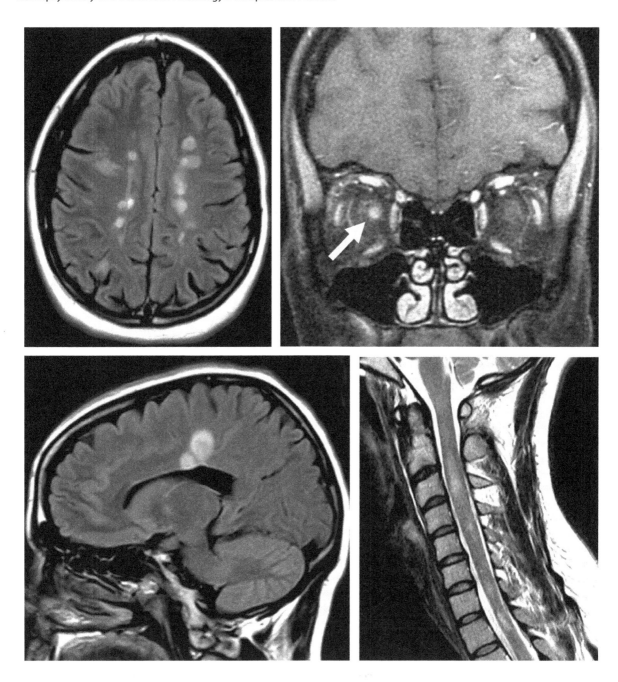

FIGURE 27-1. MRI lesions in multiple sclerosis. (Reproduced with permission from Ropper AH, Samuels MA, Klein JP. *Adams and Victor's Principles of Neurology*. 10th ed. https://accessmedicine.mhmedical.com. Copyright © McGraw Hill LLC. All rights reserved.)

CASE VIGNETTE 27.1

Ms. A is a highly accomplished professional female, with "type A" baseline personality and no previous psychiatric or neurological history. At age 40 she developed new on-set, severe agitated depression. She also had very mild hand paresthesias. Her astute primary care doctor ordered a brain MRI which showed widespread MS lesions. She required psychiatric hospitalization and parallel treatment of her severe depression and her MS. In about 4 months, she returned to her high-functioning baseline. However, in the 3 years since

MS onset, she has had three mild-to-moderate depression exacerbations. An MS exacerbation, interferon, and psycho-social stressors appear to have contributed at different times to her depression bouts. This case illustrates depression as the initial manifestation of MS. It also shows the increased vulnerability for depression relapses in MS, as well as the complex interactions between biological and psychosocial aspects: in the past, she would have likely handled the psychosocial stressors without developing depression.

TABLE 27-1 • MRI Findings in MS and Their Pathological/ Clinical Correlation.

MRI Finding	Pathological/Clinical Correlation
T2-Hyperintense lesions	Nonspecific. May represent demyelination, edema, gliosis, or tissue loss. Demonstrate weak cross-sectional correlation with disability. Appearance of new lesions reflects disease activity.
T1-Hypointense lesions or "black holes"	Axonal injury. May be transient after an acute relapse. Chronic T1-hypointensities (>6–12 months) represent persistent axonal injury and correlate better with disability.
Gadolinium-enhancing lesions	Disruption of blood-brain barrier. Incomplete or "partial" ring enhancement suggests a demyelinating etiology.
Brain atrophy	Neuronal and axonal loss affecting gray and white matter. Reflects neurodegenerative aspect of MS. Accelerated brain atrophy rates are seen in SPMS and RRMS as compared to healthy controls. "Pseudoatrophy" may be seen early after initiation of treatment due to reduction of inflammation.
Cortical lesions	Cortical demyelination which correlates with disability, cognitive symptoms
Leptomeningeal enhancement	Inflammatory follicles in the leptomeninges, comprising of B-cells, T-cells, and macrophages. Possible marker of brain atrophy and disease progression.

abnormalities in the normal appearing WM, which coincides with pathological evidence for demyelination, axonal loss, and glial activation in MS.

Cerebrospinal fluid examination may reveal presence of increased number of oligoclonal bands and elevated IgG index, which represent abnormal intrathecal production of immunoglobulins in MS. In individual cases, additional workup may be performed to rule out MS-mimics such as systemic lupus erythematosus, antiphospholipid syndrome, neurosarcoidosis, neuromyelitis optica, and vascular, metabolic, or other causes.

Management of MS patients requires a comprehensive strategy including pharmacological and nonpharmacological approaches (e.g., physical, occupational, and psychotherapeutic approaches). Pharmacological treatment includes disease-modifying therapies (DMTs) and symptomatic management, which play a key role in practical management of MS patients. There are currently over a dozen DMTs for MS that influence different aspects of MS pathogenesis and help reduce the frequency of relapses and disability progression.[2] Interferon beta-1a, interferon beta-1b, glatiramer acetate, and peginterferon beta-1a are currently approved injectable MS DMTs that are self-administered by patients intramuscularly or subcutaneously. Fingolimod, teriflunomide, and dimethyl fumarate are

currently approved oral DMTs that are taken in daily, once a day, or twice a day dosing. Natalizumab is a monoclonal antibody that prevents the entry of pathogenic lymphocytes across the blood-brain barrier and has high efficacy in MS treatment. Ocrelizumab is a monoclonal antibody directed against the CD20 marker present on B-lymphocytes and is approved for treatment of both relapsing remitting and primary progressive MS. Alemtuzumab is a lymphocyte-depleting monoclonal antibody directed against CD52 marker present on mature T- and B-lymphocytes, which has reported high efficacy in RRMS but is associated with secondary autoimmunity, particularly thyroid dysfunction in over 30% of individuals receiving this treatment. In addition to management of neuropsychiatric symptoms, pharmacological treatment of MS includes drugs to treat physical symptoms such as spasticity, reduced mobility, urinary urgency and/or retention, constipation, and tremor. These include drugs such as baclofen, tizanidine, benzodiazepines, dalfampridine, anticholinergics such as oxybutynin, solifenacin, and botulinum toxin, among others. The aim of this chapter is to focus on neuropsychiatric manifestations of MS.

Assessment and Management of Neuropsychiatric Disorders in MS: General Considerations

Neuropsychiatric disorders are highly prevalent in MS, and they severely impact quality of life, functioning, and MS prognosis. Identifying, evaluating, and treating them is extremely important. Neuropsychiatric symptoms may be the first manifestation of MS and, in a patient with an established MS diagnosis, they can signal an MS relapse. However, the diagnosis of MS is often missed when the initial manifestation consists of neuropsychiatric complaints. For example, a young woman reports: "I'm having a hard time multitasking. Things are taking me longer to do." Because the presentation is vague, her complaints may be attributed to stress, anxiety, depression, or in general, be dismissed. It is unlikely for such patients to undergo brain imaging at this stage. Typically, only when a patient develops optic neuritis or other physical symptoms will the clinician order a brain MRI, which then leads to an MS diagnosis. Interestingly, once the MS diagnosis has been made, many patients recall cognitive or mood symptoms that perhaps in retrospect could have been attributable to MS. To add to the diagnostic challenge, some physical symptoms of MS may mimic neuropsychiatric disorders. An example of this is fatigue and its functional consequences (hypoactivity, psychomotor retardation) which can be misdiagnosed as depression. While it would be uneconomical to order brain imaging for all patients with psychiatric complaints, this should be considered in certain clinical circumstances such as the presence of mild neurological symptoms (which should be screened for, as part of the psychiatric evaluation) and the lack of response to standard psychiatric treatment.

A comprehensive assessment of neuropsychiatric disorders in MS includes the understanding of both the clinical presentation and the pathophysiology: What are the symptoms and syndromes present? What are the pathogenic factors behind them? The assessment of the clinical presentation must include screening for the psychiatric disorders that are most prevalent in MS. An efficient way to do this is to have patients fill out screening instruments before the appointment which will be reviewed with the patient during the clinical encounter. Depending on the presentation, the clinician can devote more time to certain measures, as appropriate. In other words, screen widely, and then focus on the most relevant aspects. The less pressing matters may be addressed later in treatment. In our MS Neuropsychiatric Clinic at Brigham and Women's Hospital, we use the following instruments for screening:

- PHQ-9[3] for depression, GAD-7[4] for anxiety
- Center for Neurologic Study-Lability Scale (CNS-LS)[5] for pathological affect
- Mood Disorders Questionnaire (MDQ) to screen for symptoms in the bipolar disorder spectrum[6]
- Modified Fatigue Impact Scale (MFIS)[7] to understand the impact of fatigue on physical and cognitive functioning
- Audit-C[8] to screen for alcohol use disorder
- MoCA for general cognitive screening.[9] We add other tests based on the presentation and refer to neuropsychological evaluation when relevant.
- For patients with more advanced MS, we evaluate their functioning with the Lawton's Instrumental Activities of Daily Living Scale.[10]
- In addition, during the clinical meeting, we assess suicide risk and access to firearms. Compared to the general population, individuals with MS are more likely to have suicidal ideation, make suicide attempts, and complete suicide. It is important to screen and monitor these issues, to educate family members, and to document appropriately. Suicide risk factors are similar to those in primary psychiatric illnesses. Risk factors specific to MS include high level of disability and progressive illness.
- The risk assessment may also include: Risks related to errors when taking prescribed medications, fall risk, and driving risk. In patients with more advanced illness we also assess other factors, such as risk for causing fires when cooking, and risks due to abuse or exploitation by caregivers.

The causes underlying psychiatric manifestations of MS can be multifactorial. The individual with MS may present with an independent and comorbid primary psychiatric disorder, such as major depressive disorder (MDD). The neuropsychiatric manifestations may be a direct physiological consequence of MS, due to general CNS inflammation/autoimmune processes or related to the localization, type, and load of brain lesions. Psychiatric symptoms can be secondary to medications commonly prescribed to patients with MS, including the DMTs (see Table 27-2) and symptomatic treatments. Among the DMTs, interferon beta and natalizumab can cause depression as a side effect. Alternatively, if they are effective in treating MS, they may help reduce depression—since, as discussed, depression may be a direct physiological consequence of MS. Unfortunately, DMT trials have not typically included psychiatric measures among their outcomes. One exception is a trial of Fingolimod, which demonstrated benefit for patients' fatigue and depression.[11] Similarly, patients' cognition can potentially improve with successful MS treatment. The agents used for symptomatic treatments (see Table 27-3) may include commonly prescribed

TABLE 27-2 • Possible Psychiatric Side Effects of DMTs.

DMT	Possible Psychiatric Side Effects/Other Notes
Interferon beta-1a	Depression
	Psychosis
Interferon beta-1b	Depression
	Psychosis
Glatiramer	Anxiety
Natalizumab	Depression
Fingolimod	Can cause QTc prolongation and bradyarrhythmia. Avoid concurrent use of psychotropics that cause QTc prolongation.

TABLE 27-3 • Symptomatic Treatments in MS*

Spasticity	Bowel and bladder
• Baclofen	• Oxybutynin
• Diazepam	• Tolterodine
• Dantrolene	• Amitriptyline
• Tizanidine	• Darifenacin
• Intrathecal baclofen	• Trospium
• Cannabinoids	**Insomnia**
Pain treatment	• Antihistaminics
• Phenytoin	• Hypnotics
• Carbamazepine	**Fatigue**
• Amitriptyline or nortriptyline	• Amantadine
• Gabapentin	• Modafinil/Armodafinil
• Pregabalin	• Stimulants
• Duloxetine	**Dalfampridine**
• Opioids	
Corticosteroids	

Medications used for management of MS symptoms may contribute to psychiatric morbidity as a side effect.

CNS depressants such as baclofen, tizanidine, and others used to treat pain and spasticity. They may also include medications with anticholinergic effects used for urinary and bowel symptoms and for pain, such as tricyclic antidepressants. When evaluating depression and cognitive dysfunction, it is important to assess for contribution from these agents and to remove them or lower their dose if possible. Modafinil and stimulants may help fatigue and cognition, but may cause anxiety, irritability, and insomnia. Intravenous corticosteroids, used for MS relapses, may cause agitation, mania, insomnia, depression, and psychosis. Patients with a known previous psychiatric reaction to steroids can be premedicated with a mood stabilizer or an antipsychotic before the course of steroids, or be started on the psychiatric medication soon after the initial infusion. Quetiapine, for instance, can be helpful for agitation and insomnia triggered

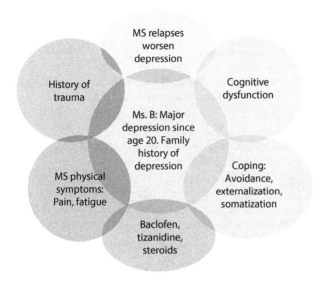

FIGURE 27-2. Multifactorial pathogenesis of psychiatric symptoms in a patient with MS.

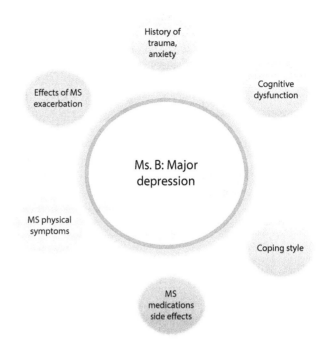

FIGURE 27-3. A simplistic assessment ignores comorbid symptoms and pathogenic factors. It is more likely to result in inadequate treatment response.

by steroids. Cannabinoids can be useful for MS spasticity, but may worsen apathy and cognitive slowing. Other contributing factors to psychiatric symptoms may be MS physical symptoms such as pain from spasticity, fatigue, and sleep disorders highly prevalent in MS such as restless legs syndrome (RLS). From the psychosocial perspective, factors such as stressful life events, social support, and the individual's coping style may influence psychiatric pathogenesis.[12] Individuals with MS who have a proactive, problem-solving coping style are less likely to develop depression than those with an emotion-focused coping style.

Most typically, patients present with a combination of these mechanisms. The case of Ms. B, as shown in Figure 27-2, illustrates the coexistence of several pathophysiological factors. She had major depression with onset at age 20. Family history of major depression, a personal history of trauma, and coping skills deficits were considered contributors to her major depression. Since her MS onset at age 30, she has noticed a worsening of depression secondary to MS flairs—her mood symptoms start concurrently or even precede physical symptoms—this suggests they are physiologically related to the MS exacerbation. Cognitively, she presents executive dysfunction—this affects her functioning and contributes to low self-esteem and depression. She is bothered by MS physical symptoms such as pain from spasticity—they add to her suffering and negative mood. Lastly, the agents to treat her physical symptoms have slowed her down even further, contributing to her hypoactivity.

Treatment follows assessment: Armed with a good understanding of the clinical presentation and pathogenic factors, the clinician uses this information to guide the selection of relevant treatments. Factors to consider in the process of treatment planning include evidence-based literature, patient's preferences, access and feasibility, cost, and benefit/risk analysis. The treatment plan is designed in partnership with the patient, caregivers, and treatment team. Continuing with the example of Ms. B, a narrow-scoped assessment would, for instance, focus on her

depression syndrome (Figure 27-3). This could lead to a diagnosis of MDD and the prescription of an SSRI. This intervention could result in a partial response to treatment, or no response at all. Understanding and addressing comorbid symptoms and biopsychosocial pathogenic factors increases the chances of therapeutic success. When treating patients with psychiatric disorders and neurological illnesses, a helpful tip may be to keep in mind the expression "the two sides of the coin." One side represents the treatment of the psychiatric syndrome in the same way one would treat a primary psychiatric disorder (e.g., an antidepressant for a depressed patient with MS). The other side represents the awareness of other pathogenic factors that may need to be addressed. In the case of MS, this may entail reviewing whether the current DMT is effective, addressing fatigue and pain, and minimizing CNS depressants to the extent possible.

Treatment must be interdisciplinary: It is very difficult to treat these patients in isolation, given the interrelationship of contributing factors. It is important to coordinate care with MS neurologists, neuropsychologists, case managers, psychotherapists, and rehabilitation therapists (e.g., cognitive, physical, occupational) to treat the primary problem(s), ameliorate symptoms, and help patients remain functional. Patients may need to see other medical specialists (e.g., pain, sleep, urology). Members of the treatment team outside of the medical center may include the patient and his/her family or support network; organizations such as the National MS Society and its resources, including online educational materials, support groups, and care managers. Patients may need to consult an attorney for situations regarding school and employment accommodations, disability, power of attorney, and so on.

Treatment along the lifespan: MS is a chronic illness, and patients' needs vary with time. Treatment must not only accompany patients at each life stage, but also educate them, anticipate their needs, and help them prepare for any upcoming challenges. MS is usually first diagnosed in young adulthood. At the time of MS onset, patients typically are in a very active stage of their lives, juggling school, work, family, and social life. Treatment must support positive adaptation and help patients sustain their engagement in things that matter to them. In patients who experience illness progression, healthy adaptation may involve sustaining an engaged lifestyle, treating the illness and its symptoms as proactively as possible, while they also learn to pace themselves and accept some of the functional changes they may experience.

Specific Neuropsychiatric Disorders in MS

Adjustment Disorder

In the period after initial MS diagnosis, patients may show symptoms of anxiety and depression, which gradually subside after a few weeks or months, in most cases. However, MS relapses may re-exacerbate anxiety and depression. A recurrent theme when working with patients with MS is uncertainty: patients do not know what course their illness will take, if it will respond to the prescribed disease-modifying drug, or their prognosis. Uncertainty plays a critical role in the onset and continued presence of anxiety. A significant role of the health care provider in this setting is to assist patients in working through important life decisions, such as motherhood, educational, and occupational plans.

While the most common reaction to an MS diagnosis is a combination of depression and anxiety, patients may react in a variety of ways. One possible response is anger or defiance/ denial, characterized by thoughts that include, "This is not happening to me" or "I don't need to take this drug (DMT) because the doctor misdiagnosed me." Some individuals exhibit catastrophic reactions and have great difficulty incorporating the MS diagnosis into their lives. A couple of patients we treated in our clinic, both young women, became more impulsive in the weeks after learning of their MS diagnosis. One of them started using cocaine, which she had never used before, and went shopping more often. She did not present hypomanic symptoms otherwise. She justified her actions by saying, "I have to live it up. I have to live my life now that I have this terminal diagnosis." Patients with MS react to their diagnosis based on their premorbid personality and tend to rely on the same coping mechanisms they have used in the past. During this early phase of treatment clinicians have an opportunity to provide education about the advances in possible treatments for MS, the importance of treatment adherence, and the impact of adherence on prognosis. While impossible to predict an individual's prognosis with certainty, education about treatment options and providing information that many patients do quite well even decades after an MS diagnosis may alleviate these early adjustment difficulties.

Depression
Epidemiology
Depression is common in patients with MS. Unfortunately, it is often unrecognized and undertreated.[13,14] Its detection and management may improve adherence to MS treatment, illness prognosis, and quality of life of patients with MS.[15] The lifetime prevalence of MDD in MS patients, based on data from population studies is 23.7% (95% CI: 17.4–30.0%).[16] Depression is more prevalent in the MS population than in comparable populations, including individuals with other chronic illnesses and the general public.[16] The point prevalence of depressive symptoms (as opposed to MDD) ranges from 31.4% to 79%.[17–20] Early MS onset,[20] greater illness severity, and level of disability[19] are associated with increased depression risk.

Patients with MS have approximately twice the rate of suicide than that of the general population.[21,22] A quarter of patients with MS may have lifetime suicidal intent.[23] Given this high risk, vigilance is warranted. Risk factors for suicide in patients with MS include depression severity, social isolation, younger age, progressive disease subtype, lower income, earlier disease course, and higher levels of physical disability.[24]

Pathophysiology
The pathophysiology of depression in MS is multifactorial. Premorbid factors, illness-related biological and clinical characteristics, treatment effects, the individual's response, and elements of the social environment may impact the development and course of depression. A family history of major depression seems to have less weight in MS patients than in patients with primary MDD,[25,26] suggesting that genetic factors play a relatively smaller role in the development of depression in MS patients, compared to individuals without MS. Several studies have evaluated the relationship between structural and functional brain changes in MS and depression. A study assessing the potential negative effect of demyelination on mood found that increased hyperintense lesion load in the left arcuate fasciculus region correlated with depressive symptoms.[27] Another study found that superior frontal and superior parietal hypointense T1 lesions predict the presence of depression, while superior frontal, superior parietal and temporal T1 lesions, third and lateral ventricles enlargement, and frontal atrophy predict the severity of depression.[28] Greater lesion volume in the left medial inferior prefrontal cortex, and anterior temporal[29] and hippocampal atrophy may also be associated with depression in MS.[30,31] The latter may be concurrent with increased cortisol levels. Right hippocampal shape changes were found in depressed patients with MS, and right hippocampal volumes were found to be smaller in those patients with higher level of depression.[32] Berg et al.[33] found that depressed MS patients had a significantly larger temporal lesion load than nondepressed MS patients, especially on the right side. Zorzon et al.[34] found that depression diagnosis and severity had a weak correlation with right frontal lesion load and right temporal brain volume. Total temporal and right hemisphere brain volume correlated significantly with depression severity. A trend of difference was detected for lesions of the right parietal and right frontal lobes, the cerebellum, and the total lesion load. In summary, studies have had heterogeneous findings. The reasons for this heterogeneity are not fully understood. Hypotheses include the limitation of the currently available neuroimaging technology; the complexity of the emotional neurocircuitry, where lesions in different localizations may result in a major depressive syndrome; the heterogeneity of the

depressive syndromes; the complex pathogenesis of depression, where in addition to lesion localization, other factors (impact of inflammation, independent from the lesions; coping style; etc.) can contribute to depression onset. Within these heterogeneous findings, however, some common themes across studies seem to be that depression in MS is associated with temporal lesions and atrophy, frontal lesions, high overall lesion load, and atrophy. It is possible that both lesions with strategic localization in the neurocircuitry mediating emotions such as hippocampal lesions, as well as more heterogeneously distributed lesions that affect the expansive network involved in emotional regulation, can cause depression. The use of DTI highlights the importance of more subtle brain connectivity changes[35] as reduced fractional anisotropy and higher mean diffusivity in left anterior temporal normal-appearing WM and GM, as well as higher mean diffusivity in right inferior frontal hyperintense lesions, correlate with depression. The contributions from functional neuroimaging techniques include an early PET study where increased perfusion in limbic areas significantly correlated with depression.[36] In a functional MRI (fMRI) study, nondepressed patients with MS showed increased activity in the ventrolateral prefrontal cortex (VLPFC) and lack of connectivity between the amygdala and PFC when processing emotional stimuli.[37] These findings may suggest that patients with MS are particularly vulnerable to developing a mood disorder and that they may be applying an ongoing compensatory mechanism to maintain euthymic mood.

Immunological and inflammatory factors and dysfunction of the hypothalamic-pituitary-adrenal (HPA) axis may have a role in MS-related depression.[38] The increase in proinflammatory cytokines, activation of the HPA, and reduction in neurotrophic factors that occur in MS may each account for the increased rate of depression in this illness.[39] Evidence supporting the role of an HPA axis dysfunction in MS-related depression includes the finding that evening cortisol concentrations do not decline in MS patients with depression.[40] Raised cortisol levels may not be suppressed by exogenous steroids administration in these patients, and this may correlate with enhanced brain lesions.[41] The corticosteroids used to treat MS may contribute to depressive symptoms; some of the immune-modulatory agents used in MS treatment may also have a role in the development of depression, such as interferon beta-1b and natalizumab.[42-44]

From a psychosocial perspective, a stress and coping strategies model is useful in understanding the pathophysiology of depression in MS. Predictors of depression may include stress, limited social support, loss of hope, uncertainty about prognosis, and use of emotion-focused coping strategies.[12,25,45] Cognitively impaired patients with MS are more likely to use high levels of avoidance as a coping strategy, which also may render them at an increased risk for depression.[46] Decreased use of active coping strategies and increased avoidance may increase depression risk; increased use of active coping strategies may result in decreased depressed mood longitudinally.[47]

Clinical Presentation

The phenomenology of major depression in patients with MS is similar to that described in the general population. There is a significant overlap between several MS symptoms such as fatigue, sleep and cognitive disturbances, and symptoms of depression. As discussed in the assessment section, different strategies can assist in diagnosing depression in this context. Fatigue may be the most frequent symptom in MS with a prevalence of up to 80% in MS patients. It has a reciprocal relationship with physical disability and depression.[48] Factors involved in its pathogenesis may include neuroconduction delay, monoamine disturbances, lesion localization, and immunomodulatory and inflammatory factors. Amantadine, modafinil and related agents, stimulants, and exercise programs are used for its treatment. Fatigue can also be secondary to sleep disturbances and to anxiety and depression, in which case addressing the primary disorder is key. Sleep disorders as a group may present in about 50% of patients with MS. These may include insomnia, nocturnal movement disorders, sleep-disordered breathing, narcolepsy, and REM sleep behavior disorder. Sleep disturbances may be secondary to other MS symptoms such as pain, spasticity, and nocturia; they may be side effects of medications or secondary to neuropsychiatric disorders such as depression and anxiety. Their management warrants a thorough clinical assessment with possible inclusion of a polysomnogram, and treatment according to the etiology.[49] Sleep disorders may worsen and contribute to depressive symptoms; thus, their treatment constitutes part of the treatment of depression. Cognitive deficits may contribute to the development of depression and in turn, depression may worsen cognition.[50-54] Other commonly comorbid symptoms include apathy and anxiety.

Patients with MS may present a wide range of mood and affect symptoms, often in combination with depression. These manifestations may include pathological or pseudobulbar affect, anger, agitation, irritability, euphoria, and disinhibition. All these may co-occur with depression at higher rates than in primary MDD, and without other associated bipolar symptoms.[17,18,55]

Patients with MS present an increased rate of suicide ideation and attempts; it is important to screen and monitor for suicidal risk in MS patients, including evaluation of the risk factors detailed above. Somatic pain is rated by as many as 32% of MS patients as one of their worst symptoms. Depression and pain may reciprocally potentiate each other and it is important to address both in treatment.

MS exacerbations and progression may contribute to the development of depression.[56-58] The Kurtzke Expanded Disability Status Scale (EDSS) quantifies MS-related disability in eight functional systems (pyramidal, cerebellar, brainstem, sensory, bowel and bladder, visual, cerebral, and other) and allows clinicians to assign a functional system score (FSS) for each of these categories. Higher levels of disability may be associated with higher levels of depression.[19,59] Untreated depression, in turn, may negatively affect the course of MS. Depression can adversely impact the physical outcome and disease exacerbations, cognitive function, adherence to treatment, suicide risk, and quality of life of patients and their caregivers.[15,60] MS can significantly impact families: children whose parents have MS may manifest greater emotional and behavioral problems than children of healthy parents.[61] As a result, this may contribute to feelings of inadequacy and guilt in depressed MS patients.

Assessment and Differential Diagnosis

Given its high prevalence and potential negative impact, clinicians should screen for depression in patients with MS. Depression as a symptom may be part of different disorders, including adjustment disorder, MDD, and bipolar disorder during a depressive or mixed episode. Several of the *DSM-5* major depression criteria may also be symptoms of MS itself: fatigue, psychomotor retardation, and problems with sleep, appetite, or concentration.

Several instruments or scales can assist in screening and diagnosing depression in MS. A self-administered scale, the Beck Depression Inventory (BDI), is validated for use in MS patients.[62] The nine-item, self-administered Patient Health Questionnaire (PHQ-9) may be useful in this population as well.[3] The SCID-IV 2-Question can be used to screen for depression, and the 28-item General Health Questionnaire may be useful to screen for depression and other emotional disturbances.[63] Clinicians should be aware that scores in items such as fatigue and concentration problems may have contributions from MS itself. The Hospital Anxiety and Depression Scale (HADS) and the Beck Fast Screen (BDI-FS) for Medically Ill Patients may be less problematic in terms of symptom overlap with the neurological illness.[64] The MS-BDI is a modified version of the BDI in which only the items known to be more related to depression in MS were retained. When comparing the performance of several measures, the BDI-FS (cutoff of 4), the BDI-II (cutoff of 14), and the Chicago Multiscale Depression Inventory (CMDI) Mood scale (cutoff of 23) appear as reliable tools to detect or screen for depression in MS. For diagnostic purposes, a cutoff of 8 on the MS-BDI, a cutoff of 22 on the CMDI Evaluative scale, and a cutoff of 19 on the BDI-II are recommended.[65] Given the burden that both MS and depression may pose on caregivers, screening and treating caregivers for depression or other emotional disturbances should be considered.

Treatment

The treatment of depression in MS patients should be interdisciplinary and use an integrated biopsychosocial approach.[66] Treating depression may bring several benefits to patients and caregivers, including enhancement of adherence to disease-modifying agents.[44] MS-related factors, such as the presence of temporal lobe lesions, may affect treatment efficacy—this is possibly due to the direct effect of structural changes in the brain.[67] For this reason, it is important to remember that effective treatment of MS itself is a fundamental part of the treatment of depression.

Psychopharmacological Treatment

There are a very limited number of studies evaluating pharmacologic options. A study comparing the antidepressant sertraline with individual cognitive-behavioral therapy (CBT) and supportive-expressive group therapy (SEG) to treat major depression found that CBT and sertraline were more effective than SEG at reducing depression.[68] A 2011 Cochrane review[69] identified only two randomized, placebo-controlled trials. Desipramine showed a trend toward efficacy in a small study.[70] Patients treated with paroxetine showed a higher response rate than those on placebo, but the difference did not reach statistical significance.[71]

Moclobemide,[72] duloxetine,[73] fluoxetine,[74] sertraline,[75] and tranylcypromine[76] may be effective per evidence from small open-label trials.

Pathologic or pseudobulbar affect may be comorbid with depression. Different antidepressants including selective serotonin reuptake inhibitors and tricyclics, as discussed later in this chapter, may be effective for treating both conditions. Small, preliminary studies looked at the potential neuroprotective or MS disease-modifying effects of SSRIs in MS,[77,78] an interesting notion that needs further exploration.

Brain Stimulation Therapies

Electroconvulsive therapy (ECT) appears to be an effective treatment for depression in MS according to the limited evidence available, which includes several case reports and small case series. Most of the 21 cases reported received ECT for severe depression; a few of those had comorbid psychotic symptoms, bipolar depression, or catatonia. Almost all the patients responded to ECT.[79] It should be reserved for patients with severe and treatment-resistant depression, and acute suicidal risk.[80,81] There has been concern, based on isolated case reports, that some patients with MS may suffer neurological deterioration after ECT. The presence of contrast-enhanced lesions may be a risk factor for disease exacerbation with ECT and the possible value of gadolinium-enhanced (Gd+) MRI pre-ECT for identifying high-risk patients has been discussed.[82] There have been four reports of neurological complications post-ECT including hemiparesis, cognitive and gait changes, delirium, and grand mal seizures.[79,83]

A small randomized, sham-controlled study of the safety and efficacy of transcranial magnetic stimulation (rTMS) on fatigue and depression in patients with MS showed potential benefits.[84] There is no conclusive information to date regarding the potential effectiveness of transcranial direct current stimulation (tDCS) for depression in MS.[85] Light therapy can be beneficial for individuals with a seasonal worsening of depression in the fall and winter. To date, there are no specific studies demonstrating its effect specifically for MS patients with depression, with or without seasonal worsening. Research studies are currently underway to evaluate the potential benefit of light therapy on MS-related fatigue.

Psychotherapy

Psychotherapy can be very effective for the treatment of depression in MS. It can be administered by itself when depression is milder, and alongside psychopharmacology in moderate and severe cases. CBT, mindfulness training, acceptance and commitment therapy, and positive psychology have shown benefits for the treatment of depression in MS patients. There is significant evidence that CBT can be effective in the reduction of depressive symptoms and improvement in quality of life.[86] CBT can be time-limited, improve awareness of maladaptive coping styles, and increase use of healthy coping skills. The MS population has many challenges with access and consistency in treatment given disease exacerbations, symptom burden, and disability factors. Flexibility in the delivery of psychotherapy may improve completion of treatment and follow-through. CBT may be effective for patients with MS and depression delivered in group[87] or individual format[68] and also when administered by phone.[88] Computerized CBT programs have also been attempted to overcome patient access challenges, however these programs have not shown the same improvements in symptoms.[89] The concept of computerized interventions is very attractive in terms of facilitating access and reducing cost, and further research is needed in this area. One benchmarking study offered home-based psychotherapy to increase engagement in treatment and proved to be effective.[90] Other modalities that may be effective for depression in MS include behavioral activation and motivational interviewing for exercise training programs.[91] A randomized trial shows that mindfulness-training is effective to reduce depression and fatigue and improve quality of life.[92]

Bipolar Disorder and other Mood Disorders
Epidemiology

Bipolar Disorder is an important contributor to worsening quality of life in MS,[93] and its prevalence in MS is about twice that of the general population.[94,95]

There is a wide range, between 0% and 16.2%, in lifetime prevalence of bipolar disorder in individuals with MS, according to different studies.[96] Reasons for this variation include differences in the questionnaires used, and population-based versus clinic-based study designs. One population-based study estimated the prevalence to be 5.83%.[95]

Pathophysiology

Bipolar symptoms may represent the influence of MS lesions in strategic locations affecting the mood regulating neurocircuitry.[97] To date, there have been limited MRI studies seeking to understand the relationship between bipolar symptoms and the characteristics of MS lesions. The symptom of elation may correlate with the presence of widespread MRI abnormalities.[98] Further, the occurrence of mania with psychotic symptoms may be more likely in the presence of MS plaques distributed predominantly in the bilateral temporal horn areas.[99]

Several studies have shown an association between WM lesions and primary bipolar disorder in the absence of MS.[100] Thus, the specific significance of WM lesions in bipolar symptoms in patients with MS requires further clarification.

Medications frequently prescribed to individuals with MS, such as steroids, baclofen, dantrolene, and tizanidine, can precipitate and contribute to a bipolar syndrome.[101] Medications to treat fatigue and cognitive disorders in MS, such as modafinil, armodafinil, and stimulants, can similarly cause bipolar symptoms.

A genetic mechanism has been presented as a possible factor,[102] but so far this hypothesis has not been validated.[103,104]

Clinical Presentation

Patients may present a full syndrome of mania or hypomania, similar to that of primary bipolar disorder. However, the most common presentation is that of one or several subsyndromal bipolar symptoms. Several symptoms classically associated with bipolar disorder are significantly more prevalent in MS than in healthy controls, including irritability, lability, euphoria, and disinhibition.[105] These symptoms may present combined with a major depressive syndrome or episode, resembling a bipolar mixed episode. In sum, mood symptoms in patients with MS appear to present in a continuum: the clinician can clearly delineate a major depressive, mixed, or manic syndrome in some cases, while others are more difficult to separate categorically.

In 1926, Cottrell and Wilson[106] found that over two-thirds of their sample of 100 cases presented "euphoria sclerotica," a state of "emotional or affective well-being," despite their illness. This high prevalence is considered an artifact of measurement[107] and a more accurate quantification of the prevalence rate may be 12%.[105]

Euphoria sclerotica may be more common in patients with greater degree of brain atrophy and cognitive impairment.[108] More specifically, GM atrophy may be associated with euphoria and disinhibition.[109] Thus, paradoxically, an individual with more advanced illness may present with expansive mood.

Assessment and Differential Diagnosis

Tools validated for the screening of bipolar disorders in the general population, such as the MDQ, can be useful to screen for the presence of bipolar symptoms in MS. For an accurate diagnosis of bipolar disorder and its further characterization (bipolar type I, II, type of episode, etc.), a careful review of past and present symptoms must be performed during the clinical encounter.

Due to the imprecision of retrospective recollection, collateral information from family members may be required. Given the discussed dimensional clinical presentation of mood symptoms in MS, it is important to establish if the individual is indeed presenting with a complete bipolar syndrome, or (simply) exhibiting isolated symptoms of the bipolar spectrum such as irritability, euphoria, impulsivity, or lability. This distinction may have treatment implications. For instance, a serotoninergic antidepressant may be indicated for a patient with major depression combined with irritability, while a mood stabilizer may be the treatment of choice if a complete hypomanic syndrome is present, to avoid precipitating mania.

Treatment

As discussed in the general guidelines, treatment should follow the "two sides of the same coin" model:

- Treat bipolar disorder with mood stabilizers and atypical antipsychotics, the same agents we would use in primary bipolar disorder, keeping both their therapeutic and side-effect profiles in mind. It has been suggested that lithium[110] as well as valproic acid and some atypical antipsychotics such as quetiapine[111] may have neuroprotective or neurotrophic properties. Further study is needed to determine the specific implications of this for MS. The potential negative side effects of lithium, carbamazepine, and valproic acid on cognitive performance need to be considered. Lamotrigine might have a less problematic impact on memory compared to other anticonvulsants.[112] Lithium can cause polyuria—a concern in patients with MS-associated bladder dysfunction. Antipsychotics should be used with caution due to their potential adverse effects on motor function including effects on balance and coordination—they may worsen MS motor symptoms and risk for falls. Those antipsychotic medications with high risk for causing metabolic syndrome should also be used with caution, as MS physical symptoms may increase a tendency to sedentarism and weight gain.

- Treat MS and remove (or taper) the medications that may be triggering bipolar symptoms. When patients with a known manic reaction require steroids, they can be premedicated with mood stabilizers such as lithium, anticonvulsants,[101] or atypical antipsychotics. Depending on the extent (severity, duration) of the reaction these medications can be used long term, or, in some cases, started right before or concurrent with the steroids.

Anxiety Disorders

In addition to their high prevalence and negative impact on quality of life, anxiety disorders may increase rates of physical symptomatology, social dysfunction, and suicidal ideation.[113] This underscores the importance of diagnosing and treating anxiety disorders in this population. Since its first description by Charcot, psychological stress has been thought to be a potential contributing factor to MS pathology. A panel of experts summarized the existing evidence in 2005,[114] concluding that data was lacking to support a strong causal relationship between stress and MS exacerbation or disease progression. Anecdotal evidence supports the association of stressful life events and exacerbation of MS, so inclusion of psychological interventions and stress management programs in MS standard of care has been encouraged. While evidence supports the use of these interventions for the treatment of psychiatric conditions and improvement of quality of life,[115] more data are needed before those interventions can be recommended as having any disease-modifying effects in MS. The researchers added that there are no data that suggest MS patients should refrain from controllable, time-limited activities associated with psychological stress (e.g., examinations) or physical activity (e.g., sports), particularly if these activities are important to the individual.

Later studies have contributed additional evidence to this possible association between stress and MS pathology. Burns et al.[116] found that patients with MS showed an increased risk of new Gd+ lesions and new or enlarging T2 lesions on MRI scans 29–62 days after a major negative life event. Positive stressful events were associated with less risk for subsequent new or enlarging T2 lesions, and with lower risk for Gd+ lesions. The results were similar when controlling for measures of perceived stress, anxiety, and depressive symptoms; thus, the relationship between stressful events and subsequent brain lesions do not seem to be driven by the psychiatric distress associated with stressful events. A stress management intervention resulted in fewer Gd+ and T2 lesions and fewer reported negative stressful events.[117]

Epidemiology

The lifetime prevalence of anxiety disorders in population-based studies using validated instruments, such as the HADS, Hamilton Anxiety Rating Scale, State-Trait Anxiety Inventory, and Beck Anxiety Inventory, is estimated to be 25.5%.[96]

Risk factors for anxiety disorders in MS include being recently diagnosed with this neurological illness; being female; experiencing pain, fatigue, or sleep disturbance; a comorbid diagnosis of depression; limited social support; and the misuse of alcohol or substances.[118,119]

Pathophysiology

From a biological perspective, there seem to be no association between symptoms of anxiety and MS MRI characteristics.[34]

Of the DMTs, glatiramer has been associated with anxiety. The reaction may also include physical symptoms: flushing, chest pain, palpitations, dyspnea, constriction of the throat, and urticaria. These symptoms are generally transient and do not require treatment.[120] Steroids can also cause anxiety as a side effect.

Psychosocially, the unpredictability of this illness—in terms of when an MS relapse may occur or what the individual's prognosis will be—is a key contributing factor to anxiety. Individuals' coping strategies may influence the development of anxiety. The use of avoidance and emotional preoccupation strategies may be associated with anxiety in people with MS.[121]

Clinical Presentation

Generalized anxiety disorder is the most common anxiety disorder reported in MS, followed by panic disorder, obsessive compulsive disorder, and social anxiety disorder.[102]

Symptoms of anxiety may present de novo after MS diagnosis, as part of an adjustment reaction. Individuals with premorbid anxiety disorders may present with an exacerbation of anxiety symptoms after MS diagnosis. MS relapses may also precipitate a new bout of more acute anxiety symptoms, given the disruptive nature of physical symptoms which remind individuals of the presence of this illness in their lives, thereby bringing back their fears. MS symptoms such as fatigue and pain, as well as severe physical disability, increase the risk of anxiety.[122]

An avoidant reaction may cause some individuals with MS to delay acceptance of the diagnosis and initiation of treatment. Patients may also present specific injection-related anxiety or phobia. This may influence their DMT choice. In cases where the avoided DMT is highly recommended by the patient's neurologist, the phobia should be addressed with treatment, preferably with CBT.[123]

Common themes of individuals' worries include concerns about their prognosis. This may take different forms, including fears about worsening physical symptoms and physical disability, and fears about inability to continue working and potential financial concerns for themselves and their family.

Anxiety may trigger an increased use of CNS depressants, such as alcohol, cannabis, and benzodiazepines. The use of these substances may worsen psychomotor retardation, fatigue, and cognitive problems, thus potentially contributing to functional problems and, paradoxically, increased anxiety.

Assessment and Differential Diagnosis

As with screening measures for depression, researchers and clinicians should exercise caution when using brief screening measures for anxiety in patients with MS.[124] Due to the physical symptoms of MS, patients may obtain an inaccurately high score on anxiety scales that take into account somatic symptoms. In addition, normal level of concern about current physical symptoms may be confused with pathological worry. Scales are very helpful in efficiently screening for anxiety symptoms, but clinical correlation is needed for an accurate diagnosis of an anxiety disorder.

A subset of patients may present somatic symptoms (e.g., paresthesias, wobbliness) that appear to be driven by anxiety[124] or "functional" factors. In these cases, the differential diagnosis between an MS flare, physical symptoms due to anxiety, and a somatic symptom disorder may be challenging. Discerning the difference is fundamental and yields important treatment implications.

Treatment
Pharmacotherapy
There are no clinical trials to guide the pharmacotherapy of anxiety disorders specifically in MS; currently, clinicians who treat this patient population follow the same guidelines as those within general psychiatry. Selective serotonin reuptake inhibitors are typically the first line of treatment. However, in the case of patients with prominent fatigue or cognitive difficulties, an agent with combined noradrenergic effects such as venlafaxine may be preferred. In patients suffering from pain or neuropathy, duloxetine may be the agent of choice. Given the increased prevalence of RLS in MS,[125] it is important to remember that serotoninergic agents[126] can worsen this problem and clinicians should monitor for this. Gabapentin and pregabalin are not typically considered first line of treatment in primary anxiety disorders. However, in MS patients with comorbid paresthesias and RLS, they may be helpful: a larger dose in the evening hours or before bedtime may be advisable to lessen the side effects of the medication, such as fatigue and cognitive slowing.

Benzodiazepines should be restricted to occasional use. Cases for which use of these medications can be considered include acute anxiety about obtaining MRI studies in patients with claustrophobia, or patients with severe anxiety who fail other psychopharmacological and psychotherapeutic measures.

Psychotherapy
Many of the same psychotherapy interventions used to treat depression have also been found to be effective for the treatment of anxiety. However, despite the high prevalence of anxiety in MS patients, research remains limited on clinical intervention specifically targeting anxiety.[127] Mindfulness-based interventions,[128] CBT,[129] and ACT have all been shown to decrease anxiety symptoms and related distress. More broadly, general stress management counseling was linked to a reduction in not only stress but also Gd+ brain lesions.[117] This finding provides evidence for the clinical benefits of psychotherapy for the management of anxiety and stress as well as its potential positive impact on the MS disease course.

Cognitive Disorders
Epidemiology
Cognitive impairment was first described as a feature of MS over a century ago.[130] However, it was initially felt to be uncommon until the 1980s, when advances in neuroimaging and the use of psychometrics enabled more quantifiable measurement.[131] Prevalence estimates of cognitive dysfunction in MS vary based on the sample studied. In 1991, Rao found 43% of individuals in a community-based sample exhibited cognitive impairment.[132] Estimates within clinic samples are as high as 60–70%.[133] Over the last 30 years, cognitive impairment in MS has been extensively studied and is now considered a core feature of the disease. It is known to have a significant impact on quality of life, social functioning,[134] and is the strongest predictor of vocational disability.[133,135]

The presence and course of cognitive impairment in MS is heterogeneous. Cognitive disorders can occur early in the disease process including in clinically isolated syndrome.[136,137] In contrast, some patients do not exhibit cognitive changes until late in the course. While cognitive impairment may occur in all disease subtypes, it is more common in progressive stages of the disease especially in secondary progressive MS, which is associated with increased brain atrophy.[138,139] Cognitive impairment may also differ qualitatively among individuals with progressive versus relapsing disease.[140] Benedict and Zivadinov[131] reported risk factors associated with cognitive impairment in MS include early age of disease onset, male sex, neurodegeneration as indicated by GM brain atrophy, and low baseline intelligence. Factors such as education and intellectual enrichment, which impact cognitive reserve, may also attenuate the development of cognitive impairment.[141]

The role of health-related factors in the development of cognitive impairment has also been examined although findings have been largely inconclusive. Smoking is a susceptibility risk factor for MS[142] and has been suggested as a risk factor for cognitive decline, although a recent meta-analysis concluded the effect on the progression of disease is less certain.[143] Cannabis is frequently used by MS patients for symptoms such as pain and spasticity and may impact the development of cognitive disorders, although the effects on cognition have not been thoroughly examined in large clinical trials. There is some preliminary evidence of detrimental effects of inhaled cannabis.[144] Inefficient patterns of cerebral activation during fMRI task performance[145] and brain volume reductions[146] have been associated with cognitive impairment in MS cannabis users compared to MS noncannabis users. Exercise may be an important modifiable factor impacting cognition. In the general population, beneficial effects of exercise training on cognition have been shown although randomized controlled trials of exercise on cognition in MS revealed mixed results on the effectiveness of physical activity to improve selected domains of cognitive function.[147]

The majority of studies on cognitive impairment in MS have been cross-sectional, thus few studies have examined cognitive decline over time. Of the few longitudinal studies conducted, the percentage of patients with cognitive impairment tended to increase over 10-year follow-up periods particularly on tests of working memory and processing speed.[148,149] However, no specific characteristics were found to be predictive of worsening cognitive function other than the presence of cognitive impairment at baseline.

Finally, it is unknown at this point whether the prevalence of cognitive impairment has changed with advances in newer DMTs. Studies with DMTs have shown weak positive effects on cognitive function in MS, but their methodological limitations reduce the strength of the results.[150]

Pathophysiology
Cognitive impairment in MS is complex and multifactorial, with both WM and GM damage implicated. Radiographic studies have provided much information regarding the neuroanatomic substrate of cognition in MS, although its pathophysiology is not fully understood. The relationship between inflammatory lesions and cognitive impairment has been well established. Early research[151] linked cognitive deficits to greater lesion load and has been replicated in many other studies.[152,153] Lesion location has also been associated with specific cognitive impairments. For example,

high lesion frequency in the corpus callosum has been associated with impairments in processing speed.[153] Demyelinating lesions also occur in the cortex and have been associated with worse performance on neuropsychological measures of memory, processing speed, and verbal fluency.[154] Using higher resolution imaging such as 7T MRI scans, it has been shown that cortical lesions are commonly associated with cognitive impairment in MS.[155]

In addition to inflammatory lesions, MS brain pathology also involves neurodegeneration. Whole brain atrophy has been strongly linked to cognitive impairment in MS and neocortical volume loss in particular.[156] In fact, measures of brain atrophy are more strongly related to cognitive impairment than conventional MRI lesion measures. In addition to cortical atrophy, cognitive deficits are tightly linked to measures of deep GM atrophy, such as the thalamus,[157] hippocampus,[158] and basal ganglia.[159] Third-ventricle width has been used as a marker of thalamic atrophy and found to be a strong predictor of impairment on tests of memory and processing speed.[160]

Notably, although correlations between MRI findings and cognitive impairment are robust, they only explain up to one-half of the variance. Thus, other factors such as brain and cognitive reserve may play a role in the negative effect of disease pathology on the expression of cognitive impairment. fMRI studies in patients with MS have shown increased cerebral activation, more widely distributed cortical recruitment, and modifications of functional connectivity relative to normal controls with similar task performance.[161] These findings implicate compensatory brain plasticity or adaptive mechanisms, which may play a role in the clinical presentation of cognitive impairment.

Finally, given the connectivity between GM and WM structures, each may contribute uniquely and additively to MS-related cognitive impairment.[162] However, additional research is needed to understand how cortical lesions, GM atrophy, and WM pathology interact in the expression of cognitive impairment.

Clinical Presentation

Classically, MS-related cognitive impairment has been characterized as a subcortical dementia, yet there is a wide variability in the clinical presentation, likely due to heterogeneity of MS cerebral pathology. Most common deficits involve speed of processing, attention, episodic memory, executive function, and verbal fluency.[163] Processing speed and episodic memory encoding and retrieval are most commonly affected. A large cross-sectional study in MS found that about 28–52% of patients were impaired on tests of speed and 30–55% on tests of memory.[164] In fact, processing speed is considered a core deficit which may be associated with other cognitive skills.[165] Clinically, slowing of information processing or bradyphrenia is sometimes observable, although other cognitive deficits may be subtle and difficult to detect without neuropsychological testing. However, it is also essential to recognize the varying clinical presentation of cognitive disorders and possible different phenotypes. For example, some patients may present solely with processing speed deficits while others present with more prominent executive compromise.

Simple attention, core language skills, and IQ are typically not affected.[163]

Overt dementia has been reported to be rare; however, the concept of dementia or "major neurocognitive disorder" by

DSM-5 classification has been largely absent from the literature and therefore the prevalence of dementia in MS is unknown. Benedict and Bobholz[166] indicate that 22% of the patients in their clinic sample study met their criteria for dementia (i.e., impairment 2 SD below the mean on at least one memory test and one neuropsychological test in another domain, combined with impairment in vocational status). They describe the cognitive deficits in these patients as virtually always including memory and processing speed. Atypical presentations have also been reported in the literature, highlighting the heterogeneity of cognitive disorders. While the majority of patients present with more subtle and specific deficits, cases have been reported of cognitive or cerebral types of MS in patients presenting with severe cognitive impairment as a primary symptom.[167–169]

The presence of comorbid psychiatric symptoms, which have been discussed previously, likely play a role in the clinical presentation of cognitive impairment in MS, although the relationship between depression and cognitive functioning is not clear due to mixed findings. Fatigue theoretically may also impact cognitive symptoms, although subjective fatigue has not correlated with objective measures of cognitive performance in the literature.[170]

Assessment and Differential Diagnosis

Despite the high prevalence of cognitive impairment in MS, it is frequently unrecognized for several of reasons. First, cognition is not routinely assessed as part of standard MS care. The gold-standard for measuring and tracking disability in MS is the EDSS, which measures physical symptoms and includes only a rough estimate of cognitive/cerebral function. In addition, subjective report of cognitive impairment is not a valid measure of objective cognitive ability, and deficits can also be subtle and easily missed in routine care. For these reasons, appropriate and reliable neuropsychological assessment is essential. Clinically, baseline cognitive assessment in newly diagnosed patients also helps to assess and monitor cognitive disability progression as well as potentially evaluating treatment efficacy.

Two main cognitive batteries that have wide acceptance for use with MS patients based their sensitivity and specificity in discriminating cognitively impaired from cognitively intact MS patients. These include the 45-minute Brief Repeatable Battery developed by Rao and colleagues[171] and 90-minute Minimal Assessment of Cognitive Function in MS,[172] which was developed by a consensus panel of MS experts in 2002. See Table 27-4 for a summary of these batteries. Both batteries include measures of processing speed and working memory, verbal and visual episodic memory, and verbal fluency. They have been found to have comparable discriminative validity, equally distinguishing MS from healthy controls, and are considered to be equally useful in the detection of the cognitive impairment commonly seen among patients with MS.[173] The MACFIMS was specifically developed in an attempt to include measures of visual processing and executive function felt to be commonly impacted in MS but not included in the earlier BRB. The Symbol Digit Modalities Test (SDMT)[174] is a component of both batteries. Many studies have shown it to be the most valid and reliable measure of neuropsychological status in MS, and it can be used for early baseline and periodic screening for cognitive

TABLE 27-4 • Comparison of Neuropsychological Batteries Established for Use in MS.

Cognitive Domain	BRB	MACFIMS	BiCAMS
Auditory processing speed and working memory	PASAT	PASAT	
Visual processing speed and working memory	SDMT	SDMT	SDMT
Verbal memory	SRT	CVLT-II	CVLT-II Immediate Recall
Visual memory	10/36 Spatial Recall Test	BVMT-R	BVMT-R Immediate Recall
Verbal fluency	COWAT	COWAT	
Visuospatial processing		JLO	
Executive function		D-KEFS Sorting	

BiCAMS, Brief International Cognitive Assessment for Multiple Sclerosis; BRB, Brief Repeatable Battery; BVMT-R, Brief Visuospatial Memory Test-Revised; COWAT, Controlled Oral Word Association Test; CVLT-II, California Verbal Learning Test-Second Edition; D-KEFS, Delis Kaplan Executive Function Scale; JLO, Judgment of Line Orientation; MACFIMS, Minimal Assessment of Cognitive Function in Multiple Sclerosis; PASAT, Paced Auditory Serial Addition Test; SDMT, Symbol Digit Modalities Test; SRT, Selective Reminding Test.

dysfunction in MS.[175] A shorter 15-minute battery based on the MACFIMS has also been proposed, the Brief International Cognitive Assessment for Multiple Sclerosis (BICAMS).[176]

While various neuropsychological batteries such as the BRB and the MACFIMS have been well established for use with MS patients, they do not fully replace the role of a clinical neuropsychological evaluation, which is comprehensive and tailored to the specific patient. In addition to specific measures found to be sensitive to MS-related cognitive impairment, clinical evaluations typically also include estimates of premorbid functioning, functional status, and assessment of other comorbidities such as fatigue and depression, which may affect cognitive skills. Collateral information from family members can be especially useful, in particular when cognition and/or insight are more severely compromised. Specific recommendations can be especially helpful to patients and families based on the neuropsychological profile including appropriateness for cognitive rehabilitation as well as vocational and academic accommodations.

Lastly, assessment is helpful in determining severity and differential diagnosis of neurocognitive disorders (minor vs. major neurocognitive disorder) and, less frequently, clarifying the differential diagnosis between an MS-related cognitive disorder and a primary neurodegenerative condition in patients with more atypical presentations.

Treatment

The treatment of cognitive dysfunction should address the continuum from mild symptomatology to major neurocognitive disorder. For instance, patients who have very mild executive dysfunction but notice its deleterious effect on their work, school, or IADLs performance, may benefit from interventions including counseling on cognitive compensatory strategies. It is important to address the different pathogenic factors that may be contributing to cognitive disorders, and this includes treating MS with DMTs. Effects of cognition have not been adequately and systematically tested in the majority of DMT trials, but a small number of studies showed that DMTs may have weak positive effects in cognition. Medications that cause cognitive slowing or have anticholinergic side effects should be lowered or discontinued if possible. Sleep disorders, pain, depression, anxiety, and any other disorders that may be contributing to the individual's cognitive impairment should be addressed.

Medications and cognitive rehabilitation therapy are indicated for minor and major neurocognitive disorder due to MS. In addition to treatment, patients may require accommodations in the academic setting or workplace.

Pharmacotherapy

Disease-Modifying Therapies A shared assumption among most MS clinicians is that the treatment of MS itself, as the primary culprit for cognitive impairment in these patients, should benefit cognition and help prevent or delay cognitive impairment. If a DMT is effective in reducing relapses and progression, it should also help mitigate and possibly reverse some of the MS cognitive symptoms. Specific scientific evidence supporting this common-sense statement, however, is somewhat limited. Importantly, this is because most DMTs trials have not commonly evaluated for cognitive effects as one of their outcomes or have done so with methodological limitations.[150,177] Interferon beta-1a showed significant benefits for processing speed and memory, compared to placebo.[178] Oral fingolimod[179,180] and interferon beta-1b[181,182] have also shown benefits. Compared with interferon beta-1a, treatment of relapsing forms of MS with ocrelizumab resulted in improved cognitive performance.[183,184]

Stimulants Methylphenidate (10 mg) improved attention and working memory of the treatment group, in a single-dose randomized, double blind, placebo-controlled trial (RCT) of 26 subjects.[185] In another single-dose RCT, l-amphetamine (45 mg) improved processing speed and working memory. There was a trend toward improved memory with the 30 and 45 mg doses.[186] A RCT of 151 subjects treated with l-amphetamine 30 mg per day during 1 month versus placebo showed statistically significant improvement in total learning and delayed recall in the active group[187] but no significant differences on the SDMT (processing speed and working memory). Patients with baseline memory impairment were more likely to experience benefit.[188] Lisdexamfetamine started at 30 mg and titrated to 70 mg showed benefits for processing speed, working memory, and learning (SDMT and CVLT2) in an 8-week RCT (n=63). There were no significant differences in side effects between the active and placebo groups.[189] When stimulants are used, their efficacy for cognition and MS fatigue should be tested periodically, for instance having the patient take a few days of "medication holidays" and monitor for differences in symptoms and functioning (Table 27-5).

TABLE 27-5 • Stimulants Trials for Cognitive Dysfunction in Patients with MS.

Medication	Study	Results	Article
Methylphenidate 10 mg	Double blind RCT (n=26)	Improved attention—1 h post-dose	Harel et al. (2009)[185]
l-amphetamine 15, 30, 45 mg	Within-subject design (n=19)	Improved processing speed, working memory (45 mg) Trend toward improved memory	Benedict et al. (2008)[186]
l-amphetamine 30 mg	Double-blind RCT (n=151); 1 month	Improved total learning and delayed recall; no processing speed difference	Morrow et al. (2009)[187]
l-amphetamine 30 mg	Double-blind RCT (n=151); 1 month	Improved memory for patients with baseline memory impairment	Sumowski et al. (2011)[188]
Lisdexamfetamine 30–70 mg	Double-blind RCT (n=63); 8 weeks	Improved processing speed, working memory, learning	Morrow et al. (2013)[189]

TABLE 27-6 • Acetylcholinesterase Inhibitors Trials for Cognitive Dysfunction in Patients with MS.

Medication	Study	Result	Article
Donepezil	RCT (n=69); 24 weeks	Improved memory	Krupp et al. (2004)[190]
Donepezil	RCT (n=120); 24 weeks	No effect of treatment	Krupp et al. (2011)[191]
Rivastigmine	RCT (n=60); 12 weeks	No effect of treatment	Shaygannejad et al. (2008)[192]
Rivastigmine	RCT (n=86); 16 weeks	Trend toward improved memory	Maurer et al. (2013)[193]

TABLE 27-7 • Other Medication Trials for Cognitive Dysfunction in Patients with MS.

Medication	Study	Result	Article
Modafinil	Double-blind RCT (n=21); 8 weeks	Improved fatigue, attention, dexterity	Lange et al. (2009)[194]
Modafinil	Double-blind RCT (n=121); 4 and 8 weeks	Primary and secondary endpoints not met; positive trend for improved fatigue; contradictory results for cognition	Moller et al. (2011)[195]
Amantadine	RCT (n=45)	No effect	Geisler et al. (1996)[197]
Amantadine	RCT (n=24)	Trend toward processing speed improvement	Sailer et al. (2000)[196]
Memantine 20 mg	RCT (n=114); 12 weeks	No effect in cognition measures; greater fatigue and side effects in active arm	Lovera et al. (2010)[198]
Memantine	RCT (n=19); 1 year	Terminated due to worsening of neurological symptoms	Villoslada et al. (2009)[199]

Acetylcholinesterase Inhibitors A handful of randomized, double-blind, placebo-controlled studies testing the effect of acetylcholinesterase inhibitors in patients with MS had mixed results. Donepezil (10 mg daily) showed benefits for memory compared to placebo in a 24 weeks' study.[190] However, this result was not replicated in a larger study of 120 subjects of the same duration, where no significant differences were observed between patients on donepezil or placebo.[191] Rivastigmine showed no statistically significant effects in two studies lasting 12 and 16 weeks each,[192,193] although the latter showed a trend toward improvement in memory in the active arm (see Table 27-6).

Several questions remain unanswered, including if these agents could be of benefit in more prolonged and larger trials, and if they may have a useful neuroprotective effect, especially for patients who are taking needed medications with anticholinergic effects, such as those for bladder dysfunction.

Wakefulness-Promoting Agents Modafinil improved attention and performance in a motor dexterity test (Nine Hole Peg Test) in a small (n=21) RCT of 8-weeks' duration.[194] However, the potential cognitive benefits of this agent were not replicated in a larger 8-week RCT of 121 subjects (Table 27-7).[195]

Other Agents Amantadine showed a trend toward processing speed improvement in patients with MS in one study,[196] but no differences with placebo in another.[197] Memantine was associated with no benefits on cognition and possible worsening of neurological symptoms in two studies.[198,199] It is not recommended to use this agent for patients with MS, given the currently available data.

Cognitive Rehabilitation

Cognitive rehabilitation is an emerging field in MS, which involves learning compensatory strategies to improve day-to-day functioning, and carrying out cognitive exercises aimed at restoring impaired cognitive functions. The efficacy for such interventions in MS is currently inconclusive, mainly due to the limited number of studies and methodological issues of the available ones, including small sample sizes, incomplete cognitive evaluations, multifaceted interventions, poorly described training interventions, and problematic or nonexistent control groups.[200,201] However, a few randomized clinical trials (RCT) of cognitive rehabilitation for MS cognitive impairment have shown benefit.[175] A home-based, remotely supervised and delivered cognitive remediation program resulted in improved performance in cognitive measures and motor tasks. Another RCT consisting of an at-home computer-based attention intervention combined with in-person counseling showed improvement in attention tasks.[175] Given the substantial variability in MS cognitive impairment, group level cognitive interventions may fail to address individual training needs unless they include modules or components that can be customized, as needed. A challenge remains to translate the gains of cognitive rehabilitation into practical applications for improved day-to-day function and specific real-world improvements.[202] Clinician- guided cognitive rehabilitation programs, customized for the individual's needs, are more likely to translate into real-life functional improvement than standard computer programs or apps. MS clinical providers often recommend individualized cognitive rehabilitation therapy for MS patients to help implement various strategies to compensate for their unique cognitive difficulties. MS patients are often in the work force, in school, or managing complex demands from family life. As such, they can often benefit from implementing strategies in their daily lives to provide additional coping mechanisms that support improved function. For example, practical strategies for coping with slowed processing speed might include being taught to slow the speed of incoming information by taking notes and asking clarifying questions in conversations or lectures. Adhering to routines and structure can be especially helpful for individuals with executive function impairments.[202]

Psychosis
Epidemiology
In a large population sample, the prevalence of psychotic disorders among people with MS was found to be approximately two to three times higher than that in the general population.[203] The lifetime prevalence of psychosis in MS is estimated to be 4.3%.[16]

Pathophysiology
The low rate of family psychiatric history in patients with psychosis and MS suggests that hereditary factors play a limited role and psychotic symptoms are related to MS rather than a separate psychotic disorder.[204] Genetic factors may, however, have a role in the increased prevalence of psychosis in MS. There seems to be a significant genetic overlap between schizophrenia and MS, driven by genes related to the major histocompatibility complex.[205] Brain inflammation or immunological processes, such as brain-reactive antibodies, may also play a role in the development of psychosis in MS.[206] Psychotic symptoms may be part of the symptomatology in patients with MS who present with delirium.[207] Psychotic symptoms appear more likely to occur in the presence of temporal,[208,209] temporoparietal,[98] and frontotemporal lesions.[18] Steroids[210,211]

and medicinal cannabis, used by MS patients to treat spasticity and other symptoms, may precipitate psychosis.[204] Agents used to treat MS fatigue and cognitive problems, such as modafinil and stimulants, can also precipitate psychosis. Psychosis has also been reported as a side effect of baclofen. Psychotic symptoms rarely occur during interferon-α and interferon-β-1a/1b therapies, but clinicians should closely monitor patients to ensure treatment is well-received and beneficial.[212]

Clinical Presentation
As discussed in the general principles section, psychiatric symptoms may be the initial manifestation of MS. This is of particular significance in the case of bipolar type I or psychotic presentations, in which patients may be hospitalized in a psychiatric ward, leaving their MS undiagnosed for months. The prevalence of MS among psychiatric inpatients may be between 0.37% and 0.83%, higher than that in the general population.[213,214] There have been numerous case reports of patients presenting with psychosis as their initial MS manifestation. In addition, psychosis may present as the only symptom of an MS flare. In both instances, psychosis can occur in the absence of accompanying focal neurological symptoms.[215]

Compared to primary psychiatric disorders such as schizophrenia, psychosis in MS may have a later onset.[99] Positive symptoms, such as hallucinations and paranoid delusions, are the most common presentation. Visual hallucinations seem to be more common than in primary psychotic illness. Auditory hallucinations are also frequently present,[204] but tactile ones are rare. Other reported psychotic manifestations include different delusional content (infidelity, grandiosity, erotomania, ideas of reference); catatonia; and Capgras, Cotard, and Klein-Levine syndromes.[215,216]

Psychotic syndromes in MS may resemble the phenomenology of any primary psychotic disorder (brief psychotic disorder, schizophrenia, schizoaffective disorder, schizophreniform disorder, delusional disorder). This happens in about 50% of cases reported in the literature, according to a comprehensive review of 91 cases.[215] Alternatively, in about 37% of cases, psychotic symptoms occur as part of a mood disorder (major depression or bipolar, with psychotic symptoms).

Psychotic symptoms may present as part of a syndrome of delirium. This may be more common in patients with MS who are taking multiple pharmacological agents that affect the CNS, and in patients with acute MS who present with widespread lesions and CNS inflammation.[217]

Assessment and Differential Diagnosis
Patients with a first psychotic episode or a first bipolar I episode should be evaluated with a brain MRI with contrast. This type of imaging can help determine the presence of MS or other neurological disorders that cause these syndromes. This is particularly important for patients with concurrent physical neurological symptoms or for those who do not respond to classic psychiatric treatments.

For a patient with known MS who presents with psychosis, it is important to assess the phenomenology and identify the syndrome present, as this has treatment implications. Do the psychotic symptoms occur in isolation, in the setting of a mood disorder, or in delirium? What is their level of severity? Is there risk of self-harm or harm to others due to distorted perception or thinking?

It is also important to try to understand the mechanism behind the onset of psychosis, as this also has treatment implications. A brain MRI will assist in elucidating which scenario is present: brain inflammation with contrast-enhancing MS lesions, or psychotic symptoms in a patient with otherwise inactive MS. Assessing the possible contribution from prescribed medications or substances of abuse is also critical.

Treatment

The most common treatment modality for psychotic symptoms in MS is antipsychotic medications.[215,218] There have been case reports utilizing each one of these agents: chlorpromazine, haloperidol, perphenazine, aripiprazole, risperidone, clozapine, quetiapine, olanzapine, and ziprasidone. Since the existing evidence is derived from case reports or small case series, choosing an antipsychotic agent should be determined in the same way clinicians do in general psychiatry: consider the desired therapeutic effect and avoid the potentially most bothersome side effects for each patient. Antipsychotics with a high rate of extrapyramidal side effects can worsen motor symptoms from MS. Those with high risk of metabolic syndrome should be avoided in MS patients with obesity and a sedentary lifestyle (e.g., patients who use wheelchairs for mobility).

Corticosteroids can cause psychosis as a side effect in some patients. On the other hand, they can be useful for treating psychosis in MS. In a review of 91 case reports of patients with MS and psychosis,[215] a total of 26 were treated with steroids, with or without concurrent antipsychotics. The amelioration of psychosis in MS after treatment with steroids—without antipsychotics—has been clearly documented.[219] The presence of Gd+ lesions coinciding with the onset of psychosis and the response to corticosteroids suggests that the psychiatric symptoms are an acute manifestation of MS.

There is little evidence regarding the efficacy of the DMTs to treat psychotic symptoms in MS. Their use is instituted to treat the baseline neurological illness.[220]

If a syndrome of delirium with psychotic symptoms is present, the standard of care is to treat the underlying cause of delirium. This syndrome may be the result of a large array of disorders that include metabolic, toxic, and infectious ones. An acute presentation of severe MS with widespread and active demyelination may present as delirium. In such a case, intravenous steroids may be the best course of action. In addition, the patient can be treated symptomatically with antipsychotics.

If there is concern that a medication or substance contributed to the onset of psychosis, it is important to remove the offending factor. Such patients may also need antipsychotic treatment.

In cases of depression with psychotic symptoms, the treatment of choice is a combination of an antidepressant and an antipsychotic. Cases that do not respond to medication treatment may be treated with ECT.[221]

In cases of bipolar disorder with psychosis, a combination of an antipsychotic and a mood stabilizer may be the treatment of choice. Lithium, valproic acid, oxcarbazepine, and lamotrigine have been used.[204] Atypical antipsychotics can be used alone, as they also have mood-stabilizing properties. Here too, if enhancing MS lesions are present and are thought to be causing the affective and psychotic syndrome, the combination of a psychotropic and a corticosteroid may be the treatment of choice.[222]

Pathological Laughing and Crying

Pathological laughing and crying (PLC) is a syndrome characterized by frequent, brief, and intense bouts of uncontrollable crying and/or laughing due to a neurological disorder.[223] Other names used for this presentation include pseudobulbar affect and emotional incontinence. For a more general discussion of this topic, including its impact in other neurological disorders, please refer to Chapter 8.

Epidemiology

The point prevalence of PLC in MS clinic and epidemiological samples is estimated to be around 10%.[224,225]

Pathophysiology

PLC may result from MS lesions that disrupt the neurocircuitry involved in emotional regulation and expression.[223] A traditional view posits that PLC results from the damage of pathways that arise in inhibitory cortical areas such as the prefrontal cortex.[226,227] Lesions "release" the emotional expression of laughter and crying, which results from activity in subcortical emotional centers. Alternatively, lesions may impact the cerebro-ponto-cerebellar pathways through which the cerebellar structures adjust the automatic execution of laughing or crying.[228]

A more specific model of the emotional neurocircuit and its disruption proposes a volitional system involving frontoparietal (primary motor, premotor, supplementary motor, posterior insular, dorsal anterior cingulate gyrus [ACG], primary sensory, and related parietal) corticopontine projections that inhibit a second network involving frontotemporal (orbitofrontal, ventral ACG, anterior insular, inferior temporal, and parahippocampal) projections. The latter, in turn, target the amygdala-hypothalamus-periaqueductal gray (PAG)-dorsal tegmentum (dTg) complex that regulates emotional displays. Lesions of the volitional corticopontine projections (or of their feedback or processing circuits) can produce PLC.[229] Lesions in the frontal lobes, parietal lobes, the descending pathways to the brainstem, and the cerebellum can correlate with PLC.[230,231] This wide variety of regions implicated is in line with the model suggesting that lesions in different locations may alter the emotion and affect regulation neurocircuitry, thus provoking PLC.

Several monoaminergic neurotransmitter systems and specific receptors may be implicated in PLC, including glutamatergic NMDA, muscarinic M1-3, GABA-A, dopamine D2, norepinephrine alpha-1,2, serotonin 5HT1a, 5HT1b/d, and sigma-1 receptors. This explains PLC response to diverse pharmacological agents active in these systems.[223,232,233]

Clinical Presentation

The individual presents with uncontrollable episodes of crying and/or laughing that are mood-incongruent, thus not related to feelings of sadness or joy. In some individuals, there may be an underlying emotional state present (e.g., sad mood), but the affect displayed is clearly excessive with respect to the mood. Similarly, the intense affective display is incongruent with the context surrounding the individual, or reflects a clearly exaggerated response. For instance, a sad commercial may trigger profuse, disproportionate tearfulness.

PLC may present more commonly in long-term and progressive MS.[224] In individuals with MS, PLC very commonly presents as comorbid with other neuropsychiatric disorders including mood disorders and cognitive deficits. As has been described with other neuropsychiatric manifestations, PLC may be the first overt manifestation of MS.[234] The comorbid cognitive difficulties may include deficits in verbal fluency, verbal learning, and executive dysfunction.[226,227] As discussed, these deficits suggest dysfunction of prefrontal cortex networks, possibly mechanistically associated with the presence of PLC.

Assessment and Differential Diagnosis

PLC is often underrecognized, or misdiagnosed. It is important to screen for it, and to educate patients, family members, and medical providers about this syndrome.[225] Clinicians may confuse it with depression or bipolar disorder. PLC can cause social distress and embarrassment, given its prominent and odd phenomenology. Family members may worry or be critical about this exaggerated affective expression.

Obtaining a very detailed history may be sufficient to assess the presence of this syndrome. On the other hand, because of its overlap with other psychiatric manifestations, the use of specific rating scales may be helpful with screening and diagnosis. The CNS-LS is a self-report measure initially developed to assess affective lability in individuals with ALS,[235] later validated for MS.[236] It includes an auxiliary subscale for episodes of anger/frustration. When administering the CNS-LS, caution should be exercised as the presence of a mood disorder such as major depression may result in a confoundedly high score, potentially producing a false positive.[227] Similarly, a proposed cutoff score of 13 is highly sensitive but not specific. A more conservative cutoff score of 21 appears to result in more accurate diagnosis.[225] The Pathological Laughter and Crying Scale (PLACS) is a clinician-administered instrument that measures the severity of PLC symptoms. It was developed for PLC in stroke patients.[237] A proposed cutoff of >13 renders a similar PLC prevalence as the CNS-LS cutoff of >21.[225]

In terms of differential diagnoses, it is important to assess if a patient's symptoms reflect PLC or a mood disorder such as depression, bipolar disorder and its spectrum, or euphoria in the absence of a full bipolar syndrome. In all the latter diagnoses, mood and affect are congruent. However, mood disorders including all those mentioned above may coexist with PLC.

In rare cases where the bouts of laugher or crying are very stereotyped and present with alteration of consciousness, they may represent an episode of epilepsy (gelastic or dacrystic, respectively). Regular EEG, and in some cases video-monitoring EEG, may be indicated.[223]

Treatment

Treatment should be instituted when PLC is bothersome to the individual or results in social or occupational dysfunction.[223] Multiple pharmacological agents have been shown to be effective for PLC in MS, as well as in other neurological illnesses.[223,238]

- **SSRIS** (fluoxetine, fluvoxamine, citalopram,[229] paroxetine, sertraline) may be effective for PLC in MS, as well as in stroke, ALS,

TBI, and other illnesses. Evidence supporting the use of SSRIs includes case series, open-label trials, and double-blind trials. These medications tend to be used at low therapeutic doses, and the therapeutic response may be evident within the first few weeks, typically sooner than typically observed in depression.
- **TCAs** (nortriptyline, amitriptyline, imipramine) have been demonstrated to be effective as well. Most studies have involved their use in PLC post-stroke, including a double-blind trial that showed effectiveness of nortriptyline for PLC post-stroke.[237] A small (n=12) double-blind crossover study showed amitriptyline's effectiveness in treating PLA in MS.[239]
- **Dextromethorphan/Quinidine** has proven useful for treatment of PLC in MS.[240,241] It can also treat symptoms of frustration and anger.[242] These clinical difficulties may represent the involvement of similar pathophysiological mechanisms, even if they do not strictly fit the clinical definition of PLC. Dextromethorphan is a weak, uncompetitive N-methyl-D-aspartate (NMDA) receptor antagonist, a sigma-1 receptor agonist, a serotonin and norepinephrine reuptake inhibitor, and an α3β4 neuronal nicotinic receptor antagonist. However, the mechanism whereby it exerts its clinical effects is not fully elucidated. Normally, dextromethorphan is rapidly metabolized through the cytochrome P450 2D6 (CYP2D6) isoenzyme, limiting its CNS bioavailability. Low-dose quinidine (10 mg) is a potent inhibitor of cytochrome P450 2D6 that substantially increases DM bioavailability.[243]

When mood or anxiety disorders are comorbid with PLC, SSRIs are the first line of treatment. TCAs should be considered especially in the presence of comorbid neuropathic symptoms and headaches. Dextromethorphan/quinidine has shown benefit in large trials and should be considered as well.

Other agents possibly efficacious for PLC in various neurological illnesses as indicated in case reports include venlafaxine, duloxetine, reboxetine, mirtazapine, lamotrigine,[223,244] and valproic acid.[245] They should be reserved to cases in which better proven agents fail, or where added therapeutic benefits (dual action on mood and pain; mood stabilizing properties) are important. Agents that enhance dopaminergic activity (levodopa, methylphenidate) and amantadine, possibly through its action as an NMDA receptor antagonist,[223] have also shown therapeutic benefits in case reports.

Alcohol and Substance Use Disorders
Introduction

There is a paucity of specific data regarding alcohol and substance use disorders in individuals with MS. However, as is the case for other neurologic disorders, abuse of alcohol and substances may contribute to the damage of the CNS and can contribute to cognitive, emotional, motor, and other disorders.[246] The abuse of alcohol and substances may interfere with the efficacy of therapeutic interventions, such as psychotherapy and antidepressant medications.[247] Alcohol and substance abuse can worsen impulsivity and suicidal risk.[248]

Individuals with MS may use alcohol and substances to help mitigate MS physical symptoms, such as chronic pain, spasticity, and fatigue. They may also abuse medications that were appropriately prescribed to alleviate those symptoms. MS physical symptoms can be exacerbated by comorbid depression and anxiety, and patients may self-medicate with alcohol or substances to alleviate these negative emotions.

For all these reasons, it is important to screen for the presence of alcohol and substance use disorders in patients with MS. Screening tools like the Audit-C and CAGE questionnaires may be helpful and should be followed by a clinical interview to assess for the presence and severity of these disorders.

Pathophysiology

There is limited data regarding the pathophysiology of alcohol or substance use disorders specifically in MS. The high prevalence of mood disorders, impulsivity, and bothersome physical symptoms such as chronic pain in MS may predispose these individuals to misuse of alcohol and substances.[8]

Alcohol Use Disorder

The lifetime prevalence of alcohol use disorders in individuals with MS is 18.8%. Several studies have shown higher rates of alcohol misuse among MS patients, compared to the general population.[16] Alcohol misuse significantly correlates with severity of depression symptoms[249] and appears to be more frequent in men[8,250] and in younger MS patients.[249]

Because rates of alcohol-related disorders are comparable to those in primary medical care settings, MS clinicians should consider routine screening for alcohol misuse as is recommended in primary care.[246]

Substance Use Disorder

The prevalence of drug abuse in individuals with MS is reported to range from 2.5% to 7.4%.[249,251] Younger MS patients may be more likely to abuse alcohol and substances.[249] They may abuse medications prescribed to help manage MS physical, psychiatric, and cognitive symptoms such as benzodiazepines, baclofen, opioids, stimulants, modafinil, and others.

Cannabis

In a 2006 survey conducted in the United Kingdom, about 43% of MS patients in clinical settings reported using cannabis at least once in their lifetime, with the first use of cannabis split evenly between before and after the MS diagnosis. Patients who begin using cannabis after the MS diagnosis typically do so to manage their MS symptoms, in particular pain and spasms. Of the MS patients who have not used cannabis, 71% expressed interest in trying the drug if it were legal or available by prescription.[252]

Several trials[253-263] have examined the effects of cannabis-based preparations on pain and spasticity among patients with MS. While some of the findings across studies are inconsistent,[264] evidence seems to support the use of cannabis for spasticity and symptoms of pain, excluding central neuropathic pain, in patients with MS.[265,266] The use of cannabis may increase the risk for the development or worsening of psychotic disorders, cognitive dysfunction, anxiety disorders, mood disorders, and addiction disorders.[264,266] Cannabis preparations may also worsen physical symptoms, such as dizziness, fatigue, somnolence, and loss of balance.[267] However, ongoing research suggests that cannabidiol (CBD) may reduce psychiatric symptoms, for instance, of anxiety disorders. Further randomized controlled studies with larger samples are needed to confirm these preliminary observations.[268]

Medical cannabinoids primarily exist in three forms: oral, oromucosal, and nasal spray. Oral versions may present a more favorable benefit to side-effects ratio.[265,269] Tetrahydrocannabinol (THC) and CBD are the two cannabinoids of most medical relevance. THC is a psychoactive compound, and CBD is largely non-psychoactive. Studies in MS have included either a combination of THC and CBD in varying ratios or stand-alone THC or CBD. The ideal ratio or doses are not yet clear.[270]

Other Neuropsychiatric Manifestations in MS: Apathy, Disinhibition, and Personality Changes

Patients with MS may present an array of neuropsychiatric symptoms, not always falling perfectly into classic nosological categories. Both apathy and disinhibition can occur in MS, either independently or in combination with other disorders, such as apathy combined with depression, or disinhibition with a bipolar-spectrum disorder. As discussed earlier in this chapter, other common neuropsychiatric manifestations include irritability, emotional lability, euphoria, and lack of insight.[105] At times, these presentations may be described as personality changes, especially if they appear to be sustained over time.[271]

The localization and type of MS lesions in individuals' brains may be among the most important factors determining these varied presentations. Lesions in the medial frontal-anterior cingulate circuit may be associated with apathy, while lesions of the orbitofrontal circuit may be associated with irritability, agitation, emotional lability, and disinhibition.[272]

The prevalence of apathy in MS clinic populations ranges from 19% to 35% in different studies,[18,273,274] and the prevalence of disinhibition ranges from 13% to 25%.[18,273,274] In the case of irritability, the range is 35–61%,[18] while the prevalence of euphoria is around 14%.[18,273]

Summary and Key Points

- Neuropsychiatric disorders are highly prevalent in multiple sclerosis. They can constitute part of the initial presentation prior to MS diagnosis, or occur later during this illness. They may significantly impact functioning, quality of life, adherence to MS treatment, and prognosis. Therefore, it is important to screen, assess, and treat them.

- The most common disorders are depression, anxiety, and cognitive dysfunction. Other phenomenology includes bipolar disorder and symptoms in the bipolar spectrum, psychosis, pathological affect, and abuse of alcohol and substances. Suicide risk is high and should be screened for.

- The pathophysiology is often complex and multifactorial. The components at play may include CNS inflammatory and autoimmune processes, MS brain lesions, DMTs and symptomatic treatments, effects of MS physical symptoms such as fatigue and pain, alcohol and substances of abuse, and individuals' coping strategies and personality traits.

- The treatment should be interdisciplinary. It typically includes routine psychiatric interventions, such as psychotropics and psychotherapy. In parallel, however, clinicians should remain vigilant about potential pathogenic contributions from active MS and other factors cited above. In certain scenarios, a DMT change and corticosteroids may bring therapeutic benefits for psychiatric symptoms.

- Future directions: Much remains to be learned about neuropsychiatric manifestations in MS. The phenomenology of the different disorders has been only partially characterized.

Biological markers to help understand the pathophysiology of psychiatric manifestations are nonexistent or inadequate. Specific therapeutic trials for mood, anxiety, psychotic, and cognitive disorders in MS are very limited. Widespread access to treatment continues to be a problem and needs creative solutions—collaborative care models and the integration of electronic tools in the continuum of treatment strategies are areas of interest. Lastly, despite the progress in the last few decades, the general split between the fields of neurology and psychiatry in the study of this illness and the care of these patients is still present. This textbook and our practice at Brigham and Women's Hospital are a part of many integrative efforts that we hope will continue to flourish.

Multiple Choice Questions

1. Which of the following statements about major depression in MS is true?
   a. The lifetime prevalence of major depression in MS is estimated to be around 15%.
   b. Bilateral parietal lesions were the most frequently ones to correlate with major depression, in studies looking at lesion localization and depression in MS.
   c. Patients with relapsing remitting MS are most likely to develop major depression because of the repeated psychological trauma involved in the flare-ups.
   d. The presence of contrast-enhanced lesions pretreatment may indicate a higher risk for worsening of neurological symptoms post-ECT.
   e. The high prevalence of cognitive dysfunction makes patients with MS nonresponsive to cognitive behavioral therapy for depression.

2. Which of the following statements about major neurocognitive disorder (MND) in MS is true?
   a. The hallmark of MND in MS is the presence of memory storage deficits.
   b. MND in MS, a classic example of subcortical dementia, occurs solely due to lesions in the cortical-subcortical tracts and thalamic atrophy.
   c. The two most common clinical complaint in patients with MND and MS are slow processing speed and spatial disorientation.
   d. Given its capacity to block NMDA receptors and decrease glutamatergic activity, memantine is the cognitive enhancer of choice in MS.
   e. The MS disease-modifying therapies (DMTs) can improve cognitive dysfunction in individuals with MS.

3. Which of the following statements is incorrect?
   a. About 85% of patients with MS have a relapsing remitting course early in their illness.
   b. Patients with *euphoria sclerotica* probably present concurrent cognitive impairment.
   c. The myth that stress may contribute to MS pathology has been fully discredited by more recent studies.
   d. Glatiramer, an injectable DMT, can cause anxiety as a side effect.
   e. Cognitive impairment is more common in progressive stages of MS.

4. A 34-year-old woman with MS is brought to the ED by her husband. For the last 2 days, she has been angry at him and convinced about his unfaithfulness. She perseverates on this same topic when interviewed by the psychiatry resident on call. She is agitated and presents a disorganized thought process. She has been taking higher doses of her prescribed baclofen and "borrowed" oxycodone pills from her sister, to alleviate her severe pain from MS spasticity. Which of the following statements about her assessment and management is incorrect?
   a. Bedside cognitive exam can assist in the differential diagnosis in her case.
   b. A brain MRI with contrast is indicated because active MS lesions may be causing her psychiatric symptoms.
   c. While useful for MS somatic exacerbations, intravenous corticosteroids are contraindicated in her case because they may exacerbate psychosis and agitation.
   d. Antipsychotics are likely to provide therapeutic benefits.
   e. Medical cannabinoids may have a role in the long-term management of her spasticity, once the current acute episode is treated and she is back to baseline.

Multiple Choice Answers

1. Answer: d

ECT can be effective in patients with MS and severe major depression and is generally considered to be safe in this population. However, isolated case reports showed worsening of neurological symptoms post-ECT. The presence of active, contrast-enhancing MS lesions may indicate a higher risk for neurological worsening post-ECT.

2. Answer: e

There is limited evidence that MS disease-modifying therapies (DMTs) can improve cognitive dysfunction in individuals with MS. Further research is needed in this important area.

3. Answer: c

While an expert panel concluded that data was lacking to support a causal relationship between stress and MS pathology in 2007, findings from subsequent studies suggest that negative stressful events may contribute to MS pathology, and stress-management interventions may be of benefit. Further research is needed to confirm these findings.

4. Answer: c

Corticosteroids may be of benefit in the treatment of acute psychotic manifestations of MS. They may have a role in the treatment of this case, if her brain MRI shows active MS lesions.

References

1. Thompson AJ, Baranzini SE, Geurts J, Hemmer B, Ciccarelli O. Multiple sclerosis. *Lancet.* 2018;391(10130):1622-1636.
2. Faissner S, Gold R. Efficacy and safety of the newer multiple sclerosis drugs approved since 2010. *CNS Drugs.* 2018;32(3):269-287.
3. Sjonnesen K, Berzins S, Fiest KM, et al. Evaluation of the 9-item Patient Health Questionnaire (PHQ-9) as an assessment instrument for symptoms of depression in patients with multiple sclerosis. *Postgrad Med.* 2012;124(5):69-77.
4. Plummer F, Manea L, Trepel D, McMillan D. Screening for anxiety disorders with the GAD-7 and GAD-2: a systematic review and diagnostic metaanalysis. *Gen Hosp Psychiatry.* 2016;39:24-31.
5. Smith RA, Berg JE, Pope LE, et al. Validation of the CNS emotional lability scale for pseudobulbar affect (pathological laughing and crying) in multiple sclerosis patients. *Mult Scler.* 2004;10(6):679-685.
6. Zimmerman M, Galione JN, Chelminski I, et al. Psychiatric diagnoses in patients who screen positive on the Mood Disorder Questionnaire: implications for using the scale as a case-finding instrument for bipolar disorder. *Psychiatry Res.* 2011;185(3):444-449.
7. Coghe G, Corona F, Marongiu E, et al. Fatigue, as measured using the Modified Fatigue Impact Scale, is a predictor of processing speed improvement induced by exercise in patients with multiple sclerosis: data from a randomized controlled trial. *J Neurol.* 2018;265(6):1328-1333.
8. Beier M, D'Orio V, Spat J, et al. Alcohol and substance use in multiple sclerosis. *J Neurol Sci.* 2014;338(1-2):122-127.
9. Freitas S, Batista S, Afonso AC, et al. The Montreal Cognitive Assessment (MoCA) as a screening test for cognitive dysfunction in multiple sclerosis. *Appl Neuropsychol Adult.* 2018;25(1):57-70.
10. Gold DA. An examination of instrumental activities of daily living assessment in older adults and mild cognitive impairment. *J Clin Exp Neuropsychol.* 2012;34(1):11-34.
11. Montalban X, Comi G, O'Connor P, et al. Oral fingolimod (FTY720) in relapsing multiple sclerosis: impact on health-related quality of life in a phase II study. *Mult Scler.* 2011;17:1341-1350.
12. Pakenham KI. Adjustment to multiple sclerosis: application of a stress and coping model. *Health Psychol.* 1999;18(4):383-392.
13. Mohr DC, Hart SL, Fonareva I, Tasch ES. Treatment of depression for patients with multiple sclerosis in neurology clinics. *Mult Scler.* 2006;12(2):204-208.
14. McGuigan C, Hutchinson M. Unrecognized symptoms of depression in a community-based population with multiple sclerosis. *J Neurol.* 2006;253(2):219-223.
15. D'Alisa S, Miscio G, Baudo S, Simone A, Tesio L, Mauro A. Depression is the main determinant of quality of life in multiple sclerosis: a classification-regression (CART) study. *Disabil Rehabil.* 2006;28(5):307-314.
16. Marrie RA, Reingold S, Cohen J, Stuve O. The incidence and prevalence of psychiatric disorders in multiple sclerosis: a systematic review. *Mult Scler.* 2015;21:305-317.
17. Figved N, Klevan G, Myhr KM, et al. Neuropsychiatric symptoms in patients with multiple sclerosis. *Acta Psychiatr Scand.* 2005;112(6):463-468.
18. Diaz-Olavarrieta C, Cummings JL, Velazquez J, Garcia de la Cadena C. Neuropsychiatric manifestations of multiple sclerosis. *J Neuropsychiatry Clin Neurosci.* 1999;11(1):51-57.
19. Chwastiak L, Ehde DM, Gibbons LE, Sullivan M, Bowen JD, Kraft GH. Depressive symptoms and severity of illness in multiple sclerosis: epidemiologic study of a large community sample. *Am J Psychiatry.* 2002;159(11):1862-1868.
20. Beiske AG, Svensson E, Sandanger I, et al. Depression and anxiety amongst multiple sclerosis patients. *Eur J Neurol.* 2008;15(3):239-245.
21. Sadovnick AD, Eisen K, Ebers GC, Paty DW. Cause of death in patients attending multiple sclerosis clinics. *Neurology.* 1991;41(8):1193-1196.
22. Stenager EN, Stenager E, Koch-Henriksen N, et al. Suicide and multiple sclerosis: an epidemiological investigation. *J Neurol Neurosurg Psychiatry.* 1992;55(7):542-545.
23. Feinstein A. An examination of suicidal intent in patients with multiple sclerosis. *Neurology.* 2002;59(5):674-678.
24. Pompili M, Forte A, Palermo M, et al. Suicide risk in multiple sclerosis: a systematic review of current literature. *J Psychosom Res.* 2012;73:411-417.
25. Patten SB, Metz LM, Reimer MA. Biopsychosocial correlates of lifetime major depression in a multiple sclerosis population. *Mult Scler.* 2000;6(2):115-120.
26. Joffe RT, Lippert GP, Gray TA, Sawa G, Horvath Z. Personal and family history of affective illness in patients with multiple sclerosis. *J Affect Disord.* 1987;12(1):63-65.
27. Pujol J, Bello J, Deus J, Marti-Vilalta JL, Capdevila A. Lesions in the left arcuate fasciculus region and depressive symptoms in multiple sclerosis. *Neurology.* 1997;49(4):1105-1110.

28. Bakshi R, Czarnecki D, Shaikh ZA, et al. Brain MRI lesions and atrophy are related to depression in multiple sclerosis. *Neuroreport.* 2000;11(6):1153-1158.

29. Feinstein A, Roy P, Lobaugh N, Feinstein K, O'Connor P, Black S. Structural brain abnormalities in multiple sclerosis patients with major depression. *Neurology.* 2004;62(4):586-590.

30. Gold SM, Kern KC, O'Connor MF, et al. Smaller cornu ammonis 2-3/dentate gyrus volumes and elevated cortisol in multiple sclerosis patients with depressive symptoms. *Biol Psychiatry.* 2010;68(6):553-559.

31. Kiy G, Lehmann P, Hahn HK, Eling P, Kastrup A, Hildebrandt H. Decreased hippocampal volume, indirectly measured, is associated with depressive symptoms and consolidation deficits in multiple sclerosis. *Mult Scler.* 2011;17(9):1088-1097.

32. Gold SM, O'Connor MF, Gill R, et al. Detection of altered hippocampal morphology in multiple sclerosis-associated depression using automated surface mesh modeling. *Hum Brain Mapp.* 2014;35:30-37.

33. Berg D, Supprian T, Thomae J, et al. Lesion pattern in patients with multiple sclerosis and depression. *Mult Scler.* 2000;6:156-162.

34. Zorzon M, deMassi R, Nasuelli D, et al. Depression and anxiety in multiple sclerosis. A clinical and MRI study in 95 subjects. *J Neurol.* 2001;248:416-421.

35. Feinstein A, O'Connor P, Akbar N, Moradzadeh L, Scott CJ, Lobaugh NJ. Diffusion tensor imaging abnormalities in depressed multiple sclerosis patients. *Mult Scler.* 2010;16(2):189-196.

36. Sabatini U, Pozzilli C, Pantano P, et al. Involvement of the limbic system in multiple sclerosis patients with depressive disorders. *Biol Psychiatry.* 1996;39(11):970-975.

37. Passamonti L, Cerasa A, Liguori M, et al. Neurobiological mechanisms underlying emotional processing in relapsing-remitting multiple sclerosis. *Brain.* 2009;132(pt 12):3380-3391.

38. Michelson D, Stone L, Galliven E, et al. Multiple sclerosis is associated with alterations in hypothalamic-pituitary-adrenal axis function. *J Clin Endocrinol Metab.* 1994;79(3):848-853.

39. Pucak ML, Carroll KA, Kerr DA, Kaplin AI. Neuropsychiatric manifestations of depression in multiple sclerosis: neuroinflammatory, neuroendocrine, and neurotrophic mechanisms in the pathogenesis of immune-mediated depression. *Dialogues Clin Neurosci.* 2007;9(2):125-139.

40. Gold SM, Kruger S, Ziegler KJ, et al. Endocrine and immune substrates of depressive symptoms and fatigue in multiple sclerosis patients with comorbid major depression. *J Neurol Neurosurg Psychiatry.* 2011;82(7):814-818.

41. Fassbender K, Schmidt R, Mossner R, et al. Mood disorders and dysfunction of the hypothalamic-pituitary-adrenal axis in multiple sclerosis: association with cerebral inflammation. *Arch Neurol.* 1998;55(1):66-72.

42. Feinstein A, O'Connor P, Feinstein K. Multiple sclerosis, interferon beta-1b and depression: a prospective investigation. *J Neurol.* 2002;249(7):815-820.

43. Mohr DC, Likosky W, Dwyer P, Van Der Wende J, Boudewyn AC, Goodkin DE. Course of depression during the initiation of interferon beta-1a treatment for multiple sclerosis. *Arch Neurol.* 1999;56(10):1263-1265.

44. Mohr DC, Goodkin DE, Likosky W, Gatto N, Baumann KA, Rudick RA. Treatment of depression improves adherence to interferon beta-1b therapy for multiple sclerosis. *Arch Neurol.* 1997;54(5):531-533.

45. Lynch SG, Kroencke DC, Denney DR. The relationship between disability and depression in multiple sclerosis: the role of uncertainty, coping and hope. *Mult Scler.* 2001;7(6):411-416.

46. Arnett PA, Higginson CI, Voss WD, Randolph JJ, Grandey AA. Relationship between coping, cognitive dysfunction and depression in multiple sclerosis. *Clin Neuropsychol.* 2002;16(3):341-355.

47. Arnett PA, Randolph JJ. Longitudinal course of depression symptoms in multiple sclerosis. *J Neurol Neurosurg Psychiatry.* 2006;77(5):606-610.

48. Bakshi R, Shaikh ZA, Miletich RS, et al. Fatigue in multiple sclerosis and its relationship to depression and neurologic disability. *Mult Scler.* 2000;6(3):181-185.

49. Lunde HMB, Bjorvatn B, Myhr K-M, Bo L. Clinical assessment and management of sleep disorders in multiple sclerosis: a literature review. *Acta Neurol Scand.* 2013;127(196):24-30.

50. Arnett PA, Higginson CI, Voss WD, Bender WI, Wurst JM, Tippin JM. Depression in multiple sclerosis: relationship to working memory capacity. *Neuropsychology.* 1999;13(4):546-556.

51. Arnett PA, Higginson CI, Voss WD, et al. Depressed mood in multiple sclerosis: relationship to capacity-demanding memory and attentional functioning. *Neuropsychology.* 1999;13(3):434-446.

52. Demaree HA, Gaudino E, DeLuca J. The relationship between depressive symptoms and cognitive dysfunction in multiple sclerosis. *Cogn Neuropsychiatry.* 2003;8(3):161-171.

53. Figved N, Benedict R, Klevan G, et al. Relationship of cognitive impairment to psychiatric symptoms in multiple sclerosis. *Mult Scler.* 2008;14(8):1084-1090.

54. Patel VP, Feinstein A. The link between depression and performance on the Symbol Digit Modalities Test: mechanisms and clinical significance. *Mult Scler.* 2019;25(1):118-121.

55. Minden SL, Orav J, Reich P. Depression in multiple sclerosis. *Gen Hosp Psychiatry.* 1987;9(6):426-434.

56. Dalos NP, Rabins PV, Brooks BR, O'Donnell P. Disease activity and emotional state in multiple sclerosis. *Ann Neurol.* 1983;13(5):573-577.

57. Zabad RK, Patten SB, Metz LM. The association of depression with disease course in multiple sclerosis. *Neurology.* 2005;64(2):359-360.

58. Lorefice L, Fenu G, Trincas G, et al. Progressive multiple sclerosis and mood disorders. *Neurol Sci.* 2015;36:1625-1631.

59. Patten SB, Lavorato DH, Metz LM. Clinical correlates of CES-D depressive symptom ratings in an MS population. *Gen Hosp Psychiatry.* 2005;27(6):439-445.

60. Figved N, Myhr KM, Larsen JP, Aarsland D. Caregiver burden in multiple sclerosis: the impact of neuropsychiatric symptoms. *J Neurol Neurosurg Psychiatry.* 2007;78(10):1097-1102.

61. Diareme S, Tsiantis J, Kolaitis G, et al. Emotional and behavioural difficulties in children of parents with multiple sclerosis: a controlled study in Greece. *Eur Child Adolesc Psychiatry.* 2006;15(6):309-318.

62. Benedict RH, Fishman I, McClellan MM, Bakshi R, Weinstock-Guttman B. Validity of the Beck Depression Inventory-Fast Screen in multiple sclerosis. *Mult Scler.* 2003;9(4):393-396.

63. Minden SL, Feinstein A, Kalb RC, et al. Evidence-based guideline: assessment and management of psychiatric disorders in individuals with MS: report of the Guideline Development Subcommittee of the American Academy of Neurology. *Neurology.* 2014;82:174-181.

64. Feinstein A, Magalhaes S, Richard JF, et al. The link between multiple sclerosis and depression. *Nat Rev Neurol.* 2014;10:507-517.

65. Strober LB, Arnett PA. Depression in multiple sclerosis: the utility of common self-report instruments and development of a disease-specific measure. *J Clin Exp Neuropsychol.* 2015;37:722-732.

66. Goldman Consensus Group. The Goldman Consensus statement of depression in multiple sclerosis. *Mult Scler.* 2005;11:328-337.

67. Mohr DC, Epstein L, Luks TL, et al. Brain lesion volume and neuropsychological function predict efficacy of treatment for depression in multiple sclerosis. *J Consult Clin Psychol.* 2003;71:1017-1024.

68. Mohr DC, Boudewyn AC, Goodkin DE, Bostrom A, Epstein L. Comparative outcomes for individual cognitive-behavior therapy, supportive-expressive group psychotherapy, and sertraline for the treatment of depression in multiple sclerosis. *J Consult Clin Psychol.* 2001;69(6):942-949.

69. Koch MW, Glazenborg A, Uyttenboogaart M, Mostert J, De Keyser J. Pharmacologic treatment of depression in multiple sclerosis. *Cochrane Database Syst Rev.* 2011;2.

70. Schiffer RB, Wineman NM. Antidepressant pharmacotherapy of depression associated with multiple sclerosis. *Am J Psychiatry.* 1990;147(11):1493-1497.

71. Ehde DM, Kraft GH, Chwastiak L, et al. Efficacy of paroxetine in treating major depressive disorder in persons with multiple sclerosis. *Gen Hosp Psychiatry.* 2008;30(1):40-48.

72. Barak Y, Ur E, Achiron A. Moclobemide treatment in multiple sclerosis patients with comorbid depression: an open-label safety trial. *J Neuropsychiatry Clin Neurosci.* 1999;11(2):271-273.

73. Solaro C, Bergamaschi R, Rezzani C, et al. Duloxetine is effective in treating depression in multiple sclerosis patients: an open label multicenter study. *Clin Neuropharmacol.* 2013;36(4):114-116.

74. Shafey H. The effect of fluoxetine in depression associated with multiple sclerosis. *Can J Psychiatry.* 1992;37:147-148.

75. Scott TF, Nussbaum P, McConnell H, Brill P. Measurement of treatment response to sertraline in depressed multiple sclerosis patients using the Carroll scale. *Neurol Res.* 1995;17:421-422.

76. Silberberg D, Armstrong R. Tranylcypromine in multiple sclerosis. *Lancet.* 1965;2:852-853.

77. Mostert JP, Sijens PE, Oudkerk M, De Keyser J. Fluoxetine increases cerebral white matter NAA/Cr ratio in patients with multiple sclerosis. *Neurosci Lett.* 2006;402:22-24.

78. Mostert JP, Admiraal-Behloul F, Hoogduin JM, Luyendijk J. Effect of fluoxetine on disease activity in relapsing multiple sclerosis: a double-blind, placebo-controlled, exploratory study. *J Neurol Neurosurg Psychiatry.* 2008;9:1027-1031.

79. Palm U, Ayache SS, Padberg F, Lefaucher JP. Non-invasive brain stimulation therapy in multiple sclerosis: a review of tDCS, rTMS and ECT results. *Brain Stimul.* 2014;7:849-854.

80. Rasmussen KG, Keegan BM. Electroconvulsive therapy in patients with multiple sclerosis. *J ECT.* 2007;23(3):179-180.

81. Pontikes TK, Dinwiddie SH. Electroconvulsive therapy in a patient with multiple sclerosis and recurrent catatonia. *J ECT.* 2010;26(4):270-271.

82. Mattingly G, Baker K, Zorumski CF, Figiel GS. Multiple sclerosis and ECT: possible value of gadolinium-enhanced magnetic resonance scans for identifying high-risk patients. *J Neuropsychiatry Clin Neurosci.* 1992;4(2):145-151.

83. Urban-Kowalczyk M, Rudecki T, Wróblewski D, et al. Electroconvulsive therapy in patient with psychotic depression and multiple sclerosis. *Neurocase.* 2014;20:452-455.

84. Schippling S, Tiede M, Lorenz I, et al. Deep transcranial magnet stimulation can improve depression and fatigue in multiple sclerosis—a clinical phase I/IIa study. *Neurology.* 2014;82:S33.007.

85. Lefaucheur JP. A comprehensive database of published tDCS clinical trials (2005-2016). *Neurophysiol Clin.* 2016;46:319-398.

86. Hind D, Cotter J, Thake A, et al. Cognitive behavioural therapy for the treatment of depression in people with multiple sclerosis: a systemic review and meta-analysis. *BMC Psychiatry.* 2014;14:5.

87. Larcombe NA, Wilson PH. An evaluation of cognitive-behaviour therapy for depression in patients with multiple sclerosis. *Br J Psychiatry.* 1984;145:366-371.

88. Mohr DC, Hart SL, Julian L, et al. Telephone-administered psychotherapy for depression. *Arch Gen Psychiatry.* 2005;62(9):1007-1014.

89. Hind D, O'Cathain A, Cooper CL, et al. The acceptability of computerised cognitive behavioural therapy for the treatment of depression in people with chronic physical disease: a qualitative study of people with multiple sclerosis. *Psychol Health.* 2010;25(6):699-712.

90. Askey-Jones S, David AS, Silber E, et al. Cognitive behaviour therapy for common mental disorders in people with multiple sclerosis: a bench marking study. *Behav Res Ther.* 2013;51:648-655.

91. Ensari I, Motl RW, Pilutti LA. Exercise training improves depressive symptoms in people with multiple sclerosis: results of a meta-analysis. *J Psychosom Res.* 2014;76:465-471.

92. Grossman P, Kappos L, Gensicke H, et al. MS quality of life, depression, and fatigue improve after mindfulness training: a randomized trial. *Neurology.* 2010;75(13):1141-1149.

93. Carta MG, Moro MF, Lorefice L, et al. Multiple sclerosis and bipolar disorders: the burden of comorbidity and its consequences on quality of life. *J Affect Disord.* 2014;167:192-197.

94. Schiffer RB, Wineman NM, Weitkamp LR. Association between bipolar affective disorder and multiple sclerosis. *Am J Psychiatry.* 1986;143(1):94-95.

95. Marrie RA, Fisk JD, Yu BN, et al. Mental comorbidity and multiple sclerosis: validating administrative data to support population-based surveillance. *BMC Neurol.* 2013;13:16.

96. Marrie RA, Reingold S, Cohen J, et al. The incidence and prevalence of psychiatric disorders in multiple sclerosis: a systematic review. *Mult Scler.* 2015;21(3):305-317.

97. Phillips LH, Henry JD, Nouzova E, Cooper C, Radklak B, Summers F. Difficulties with emotion regulation in multiple sclerosis: links to executive function, mood, and quality of life. *J Clin Exp Neuropsychol.* 2004;36:831-842.

98. Ron MA, Logsdail SJ. Psychiatric morbidity in multiple sclerosis: a clinical and MRI study. *Psychol Med.* 1989;19(4):887-895.

99. Feinstein A, du Boulay G, Ron MA. Psychotic illness in multiple sclerosis. A clinical and magnetic resonance imaging study. *Br J Psychiatry.* 1992;161:680-685.

100. Beyer J, Young R, Kuchibhatla M, Krishnan K. Hyperintense MRI lesions in bipolar disorder: a meta-analysis and review. *Int Rev Psychiatry.* 2009;21(4):394-409.

101. Jefferies K. The neuropsychiatry of multiple sclerosis. *Adv Psychiatr Treat.* 2006;12:214-220.

102. Murphy R, O'Donoghue SO, Counihan T, et al. Neuropsychiatric syndromes in multiple sclerosis. *Neurol Neurosurg Psychiatry.* 2017;88:697-708.

103. Johansson V, Lundholm C, Hillert J, et al. Multiple sclerosis and psychiatric disorders: comorbidity and sibling risk in a nationwide Swedish cohort. *Mult Scler.* 2014;20:1881-1891.

104. Marrie RA. Psychiatric comorbidity in multiple sclerosis: it's not the genes. *Mult Scler.* 2014;20:1803-1805.

105. Rosti-Otajärvi E, Hämäläinen P. Behavioural symptoms and impairments in multiple sclerosis: a systematic review and meta-analysis. *Mult Scler.* 2013;19:31-45.

106. Cottrell SS, Wilson SA. The affective symptomatology of disseminate sclerosis: a study of 100 cases. *J Neurol Psychopathol.* 1926;7(25):1-30.

107. Duncan A, Malcolm-Smith S, Ameen O, Solms M. The incidence of euphoria in multiple sclerosis: artefact of measure. *Mult Scler Int.* 2016;8:1-8.

108. Benedict RHB, Carone D, Bakshi R. Correlating brain atrophy with cognitive dysfunction, mood disturbances, and personality disorder in multiple sclerosis. *J Neuroimaging.* 2004;14:36S-46S.

109. Sanfilipo M, Benedict R, Weinstock-Guttman B, Bakshi R. Gray and white matter brain atrophy and neuropsychological impairment in multiple sclerosis. *Neurology.* 2006;685-692.

110. Chiu CT, Chuang DM. Molecular actions and therapeutic potential of lithium in preclinical and clinical studies of CNS disorders. *Pharmacol Ther.* 2010;128:281-304.

111. Hunsberger J, Austin DR, Henter ID, Chen G. The neurotrophic and neuroprotective effects of psychotropic agents. *Dialogues Clin Neurosci.* 2009;11(3):333-348.

112. Dols A, Sienaert P, van Gerven H, et al. The prevalence and management of side effects of lithium and anticonvulsants as mood stabilizers in bipolar disorder from a clinical perspective: a review. *Int Clin Psychopharmacol.* 2013;28(6):287-296.

113. Feinstein A, O'Connor P, Gray T, et al. The effects of anxiety on psychiatric morbidity in patients with multiple sclerosis. *Mult Scler.* 1999;5:323-326.

114. Heesen C, Mohr DC, Huitinga I, et al. Stress regulation in multiple sclerosis—current issues and concepts. *Mult Scler.* 2007;13:143-148.

115. Hart S, Fonareva I, Merluzzi N, et al. Treatment for depression and its relationship to improvement in quality of life and psychological well-being in multiple sclerosis patients. *Qual Life Res.* 2005;14:695-703.

116. Burns M, Nawacki E, Kwasny M, et al. Do positive or negative stressful events predict the development of new brain lesions in people with multiple sclerosis? *Psychol Med.* 2014;44(2):349-359.

117. Mohr DC, Lovera J, Brown T, et al. A randomized trial of stress management for the prevention of new brain lesions in MS. *Neurology.* 2012;79:412-419.

118. Chwastiak LA, Ehde DM. Psychiatric issues in multiple sclerosis. *Psychiatr Clin North Am.* 2007;30(4):803-817.

119. Janssens AC, Buljevac D, van Doorn PA, et al. Prediction of anxiety and distress following diagnosis of multiple sclerosis: a two-year longitudinal study. *Mult Scler.* 2006;12(6):794-801.

120. Product Information. COPAXONE(R) subcutaneous injection solution, glatiramer acetate subcutaneous injection solution. TEVA Pharmaceuticals USA, Inc. (per FDA), North Wales, PA; 2014.

121. Goretti B, Portaccio E, Zipoli V, et al. Coping strategies, psychological variables and their relationship with quality of life in multiple sclerosis. *Neurol Sci.* 2009;30(1):15-20.

122. Butler E, Matcham F, Chalder T. A systematic review of anxiety amongst people with multiple sclerosis. *Mult Scler Relat Disord.* 2016;10:145-168.

123. Mohr DC, Cox D, Epstein L, et al. Teaching patients to self-inject: pilot study of a treatment for injection anxiety and phobia in multiple sclerosis patients prescribed injectable medications. *J Behav Ther Exp Psychiatry.* 2002;33:39-47.

124. Ó Donnchadha S, Burke T, Bramham J, et al. Symptom overlap in anxiety and multiple sclerosis. *Mult Scler.* 2013;19(10):1349-1354.

125. Sieminski M, Losy J, Partinen M. Restless legs syndrome in multiple sclerosis. *Sleep Med. Rev.* 2015;22:15-22.

126. Perez-Lloret S, Rey MV, Bondon-Guitton E, et al. Associated with restless legs syndrome: a case/noncase study in the French Pharmacovigilance Database. *J Clin Psychopharmacol.* 2012;32(6):824-827.

127. Fiest KM, Walker JR, Bernstien CN, et al. Systematic review and meta-analysis of interventions for depression and anxiety in persons with multiple sclerosis. *Mult Scler Relat Disord.* 2016;5:12-26.

128. Simpson R, Booth J, Lawrence M, et al. Mindfulness based interventions in multiple sclerosis—a systemic review. *BMC Neurol.* 2014;14:15.

129. Askey-Jones S, David AS, Silber E, et al. Cognitive behavior therapy for common mental disorders in people with multiple sclerosis: a bench marking study. *Behav Res Ther.* 2013;51:648-655.

130. Charcot JM. *Lectures on the Diseases of the Nervous System.* London: New Sydenham Society; 1877.

131. Benedict RHB, Zivadinov R. Risk Factors for and management of cognitive dysfunction in multiple sclerosis. *Nature.* 2011;7:332-342.

132. Rao SM, Leo GJ, Bernardin L, et al. Cognitive dysfunction in multiple sclerosis. I. Frequency, patterns and prediction. *Neurology.* 1991;41(5):685-691.

133. Morrow SA, Drake A, Zivadinov R, Munschauer F, Weinstock-Guttman B, Benedict RH. Predicting loss of employment over three years in multiple sclerosis: clinically meaningful cognitive decline. *Clin Neuropsychol.* 2010;24:1131-1145.

134. Rao SM, Leo GJ, Ellington L, et al. Cognitive dysfunction in multiple sclerosis. II. Impact on employment and social functioning. *Neurology.* 1991;41(5):692-696.

135. Flensner G, Landtblom AM, Soderhamn O, Ek AC. Work capacity and health-related quality of life among individuals with multiple sclerosis reduced by fatigue: a cross-sectional study. *BMC Pub Health.* 2013;13:224.

136. Glanz BI, Holland CM, Gauthier SA, et al. Cognitive dysfunction in patients with clinically isolated syndromes or newly diagnosed multiple sclerosis. *Mult Scler.* 2007;13(8):1004-1010.

137. Anhoque CF, Domingues S, Teixeira AL, et al. Cognitive impairment in clinically isolated syndrome: a systematic review. *Dement Neuropsychol.* 2010;4(2):86-90.

138. Comi G, Filippi M, Martinelli V, et al. Brain MRI correlates of cognitive impairment in primary and secondary progressive multiple sclerosis. *J Neurol Sci.* 1995;132(2):222-227.

139. Fisher E, Lee J, Nakamura K, Rudick RA. Gray matter atrophy in multiple sclerosis: a longitudinal study. *Ann Neurol.* 2008;64(3):255-265.

140. Sumowski JF, Benedict R, Enzinger C, et al. Cognition in multiple sclerosis: state of the field and priorities for the future. *Neurology.* 2018;90(6):278-288.

141. Sumowski JF, Leavitt VM. Cognitive reserve in multiple sclerosis. *Mult Scler.* 2013;19(9):1122-1127.

142. Hawkes CH. Smoking is a risk factor for multiple sclerosis: a metaanalysis. *Mult Scler.* 2007;13(5):610-615.

143. Handel AE, Williamson AJ, Disanto G, Dobson R, Giovannoni G, Ramagopalan SV. Smoking and multiple sclerosis: an updated meta-analysis. *PLoS One.* 2011;6(1):e16149.

144. Corey-Bloom J, Wolfson T, Gamst A, et al. Smoked cannabis for spasticity in multiple sclerosis: a randomized, placebo-controlled trial. *CMAJ.* 2012;184:1143-1150.

145. Pavisian B, MacIntosh BJ, Szilagyi G, et al. Effects of cannabis on cognition in patients with MS: a psychometric and MRI study. *Neurology.* 2014;82:1879-1887.

146. Romero K, Pavisian B, Staines WR, Feinstein A. Multiple sclerosis, cannabis, and cognition: a structural MRI study. *NeuroImage.* 2015;8:140-147.

147. Morrison JD, Mayer L. Physical activity and cognitive function in adults with multiple sclerosis: an integrative review. *Disabil Rehabil.* 2017;39(19):1909-1920.

148. Amato MP, Ponziani G, Siracusa G, Sorbi S. Cognitive dysfunction in early-onset multiple sclerosis: a reappraisal after 10 years. *Arch Neurol.* 2001;58(10):1602-1606.

149. Schwid SR, Goodman AD, Weinstein A, McDermott MP, Johnson KP; Copaxone Study Group. Cognitive function in relapsing multiple sclerosis: minimal changes in a 10-year clinical trial. *J Neurol Sci.* 2007;255(1-2):57-63.

150. Niccolai C, Goretti B, Amato MP. Disease modifying treatments and symptomatic therapies for cognitive impairment in multiple sclerosis: where do we stand? *Mult Scler Demyelinating Disord.* 2017;2:8.

151. Rao SM, Leo GJ, Haughton VM, St Aubin-Faubert P, Bernardin L. Correlation of magnetic resonance imaging with neuropsychological testing in multiple sclerosis. *Neurology*. 1989;39(2 pt 1):161-166.

152. Patti F, Failla G, Ciancio MR, L'Episcopo MR, Reggio A. Neuropsychological, neuroradiological and clinical findings in multiple sclerosis. A 3 year follow-up study. *Eur J Neurol*. 1998;5(3):283-286.

153. Rossi F, Giorgio A, Battaglini M, et al. Relevance of brain lesion location to cognition in relapsing remitting multiple sclerosis. *PLoS One*. 2012;7:e44826.

154. Bagnato F, Salman Z, Kane R, et al. T1 cortical hypointensities and their association with cognitive disability in multiple sclerosis. *Mult Scler*. 2010;16(10):1203-1212.

155. Nielsen S, Kinkel RP, Madigan N, Tinelli E, Benner T, Mainero C. Contribution of cortical lesion subtypes at 7T MRI to physical and cognitive performance in MS. *Neurology*. 2013;81(7):641-649.

156. Portaccio E, Amato MP, Bartolozzi ML, et al. Neocortical volume decrease in relapsing-remitting multiple sclerosis with mild cognitive impairment. *J Neurol Sci*. 2006;245(1-2):195-199.

157. Houtchens MK, Benedict RHB, Killiany R, et al. Thalamic atrophy and cognition in multiple sclerosis. *Neurology*. 2007;69(12): 1213-1223.

158. Sicotte NL, Kern KC, Giesser BS, et al. Regional hippocampal atrophy in multiple sclerosis. *Brain*. 2008;131(pt 4):1134-1141.

159. Batista S, Zivadinov R, Hoogs M, et al. Basal ganglia, thalamus and neocortical atrophy predicting slowed cognitive processing in multiple sclerosis. *J Neurol*. 2012;259(1):139-146.

160. Benedict RHB, Weinstock-Guttman B, Fishman I, Sharma J, Tjoa CW, Bakshi R. Prediction of neuropsychological impairment in multiple sclerosis: comparison of conventional magnetic resonance imaging measures of atrophy and lesion burden. *Arch Neurol*. 2004;61(2):226-230.

161. Rocca MA, Amato MP, De Stefano N, et al. Clinical and imaging assessment of cognitive dysfunction in multiple sclerosis. *Lancet Neurol*. 2015;14:302-317.

162. DeLuca GC, Yates RL, Beale H, Morrow SA. Cognitive impairment in multiple sclerosis: clinical, radiologic and pathologic insights. *Brain Pathol*. 2015;25(1):79-98.

163. Chiaravalloti ND, DeLuca J. Cognitive impairment in multiple sclerosis. *Lancet Neurol*. 2008;7(12):1139-1151.

164. Benedict RHB, Cookfair D, Gavett R, et al. Validity of the minimal assessment of cognitive function in multiple sclerosis (MACFIMS). *J Int Neuropsychol Soc*. 2006;12:549-558.

165. DeLuca J, Chelune GJ, Tulsky DS, Lengenfelder J, Chiaravalloti ND. Is speed of processing or working memory the primary information processing deficit in multiple sclerosis? *J Clin Exp Neuropsychol*. 2004;26(4):550-562.

166. Benedict RHB, Bobholz JH. Multiple sclerosis. *Semin Neurol*. 2007;27(1):78-85.

167. Assouad R, Tourbah A, Papeix C. Cognitive presentation in multiple sclerosis. *Neurology*. 2008;70(5):68.

168. Staff NP, Lucchinetti CF, Keegan BM. Multiple sclerosis with predominant, severe cognitive impairment. *Arch Neurol*. 2009;66:1139-1143.

169. Zarei M. Clinical characteristics of cortical multiple sclerosis. *J Neurol Sci*. 2006;245:53-58.

170. Morrow SA, Weinstock-Guttman B, Munschauer FE, Hojnacki D. Subjective fatigue is not associated with cognitive impairment in multiple sclerosis: cross-sectional and longitudinal analysis. *J Neurol Sci*. 1995;132(2):222-227.

171. Rao SM. *Neuropsychological Screening Battery for Multiple Sclerosis*. New York, NY: National Multiple Sclerosis Society; 1991.

172. Benedict RHB, Fischer JS, Archibald CJ, et al. Minimal neuropsychological assessment of MS patients: a consensus approach. *Clin Neuropsychol*. 2002;16(3):381-397.

173. Strober L, Englert J, Munschauer F, Weinstock-Guttman B, Rao S, Benedict RHB. Sensitivity of conventional memory tests in multiple sclerosis: comparing the Rao Brief Repeatable Neuropsychological Battery and the Minimal Assessment of Cognitive Function in MS. *Mult Scler*. 2009;15(9): 1077-1084.

174. Smith A. *Symbol Digit Modalities Test: Manual*. Los Angeles, CA: Western Psychological Services; 1982.

175. Kalb R, Beier M, Benedict R, et al. Recommendations for cognitive screening and management in multiple sclerosis care. *Mult Scler*. 2018;24(13):1665-1680.

176. Langdon D, Amato M, Boringa J, et al. Recommendations for a Brief International Cognitive Assessment for Multiple Sclerosis (BICAMS). *Mult Scler*. 2012;18(6):891-898.

177. Roy S, Benedict RH, Drake AS, Weinstock-Guttman B. Impact of pharmacotherapy on cognitive dysfunction in patients with multiple sclerosis. *CNS Drugs*. 2016;30:209-225.

178. Fischer JS, Priore RL, Jacobs LD, et al. Neuropsychological effects of interferon beta-1a in relapsing multiple sclerosis. Multiple Sclerosis Collaborative Research Group. *Ann Neurol*. 2000;48:885-892.

179. Cohen JA, Barkhof F, Comi G, et al. Oral fingolimod or intramuscular interferon for relapsing multiple sclerosis. *N Engl J Med*. 2010;362:402-415.

180. Kappos L, Radue EW, O'Connor P, et al. A placebo-controlled trial of oral fingolimod in relapsing multiple sclerosis. *N Engl J Med*. 2010;362:387-401.

181. Kappos L, Polman CH, Freedman MS, et al. Treatment with interferon beta-1b delays conversion to clinically definite and McDonald MS in patients with clinically isolated syndromes. *Neurology*. 2006;67:1242-1249.

182. Penner IK, Stemper B, Calabrese P, et al. Effects of interferon beta-1b on cognitive performance in patients with a first event suggestive of multiple sclerosis. *Mult Scler*. 2012;18:1466-1471.

183. Miller AE, de Seze J, Hauser SL, et al. The effect of ocrelizumab on cognitive functioning in relapsing multiple sclerosis: analysis of the phase 3 interferon beta-1a-controlled OPERA studies. Presented at: 2017 Consortium of Multiple Sclerosis Centers Annual Meeting; 2017; New Orleans, LA. Abstract DX09.

184. Hauser SL, Bar-Or A, Comi G, et al. Ocrelizumab versus interferon beta-1a in relapsing multiple sclerosis. *N Engl J Med*. 2017;376:221-234.

185. Harel Y, Appleboim N, Lavie M, Achiron A. Single dose of methylphenidate improves cognitive performance in multiple sclerosis patients with impaired attention process. *J Neurol Sci*. 2009;276:38-40.

186. Benedict RH, Munschauer F, Zarevics P, et al. Effects of l-amphetamine sulfate on cognitive function in multiple sclerosis patients. *J Neurol*. 2008;255:848-852.

187. Morrow SA, Kaushik T, Zarevics P, et al. The effects of L-amphetamine sulfate on cognition in MS patients: results of a randomized controlled trial. *J Neurol*. 2009;256:1095-1102.

188. Sumowski JF, Chiaravalloti N, Erlanger D, et al. L-amphetamine improves memory in MS patients with objective memory impairment. *Mult Scler*. 2011;17:1141-1145.

189. Morrow SA, Smerbeck A, Patrick K, et al. Lisdexamphetamine dimesylate improves processing speed and memory in cognitively impaired MS patients: a phase II study. *J Neurol*. 2013;260:489-497.

190. Krupp LB, Christodoulou C, Melville P, et al. Donepezil improved memory in multiple sclerosis in a randomized clinical trial. *Neurology*. 2004;63:1579-1585.

191. Krupp LB, Christodoulou C, Melville P, et al. Multicenter randomized clinical trial of donepezil for memory impairment in multiple sclerosis. *Neurology.* 2011;76:1500-1507.

192. Shaygannejad V, Janghorbani M, Ashtari F, et al. Effects of rivastigmine on memory and cognition in multiple sclerosis. *Can J Neurol Sci.* 2008;35:476-481.

193. Mäurer M, Ortler S, Baier M, et al. Randomised multicentre trial on safety and efficacy of rivastigmine in cognitively impaired multiple sclerosis patients. *Mult Scler.* 2013;19:631-638.

194. Lange R, Volkmer M, Heesen C, Liepert J. Modafinil effects in multiple sclerosis patients with fatigue. *J Neurol.* 2009;256:645-650.

195. Möller F, Poettgen J, Broemel F, et al. HAGIL (Hamburg Vigil Study): a randomized placebo-controlled double-blind study with modafinil for treatment of fatigue in patients with multiple sclerosis. *Mult Scler.* 2011;17:1002-1009.

196. Sailer M, Heinze HJ, Schoenfeld MA, et al. Amantadine influences cognitive processing in patients with multiple sclerosis. *Pharmacopsychiatry.* 2000;33:28-37.

197. Geisler MW, Sliwinski M, Coyle PK, et al. The effects of amantadine and pemoline on cognitive functioning in multiple sclerosis. *Arch Neurol.* 1996;53:185-188.

198. Lovera JF, Frohman E, Brown TR, et al. Memantine for cognitive impairment in multiple sclerosis: a randomized placebo-controlled trial. *Mult Scler.* 2010;16:715-723.

199. Villoslada P, Arrondo G, Sepulcre J, et al. Memantine induces reversible neurologic impairment in patients with MS. *Neurology.* 2009;72:1630-1633.

200. Amato MP, Langdon D, Montalban X, et al. Treatment of cognitive impairment in multiple sclerosis: position paper. *J Neurol.* 2013;260(6):1452-1468.

201. Filippi M, Rocca MA. Let's rehabilitate cognitive rehabilitation in multiple sclerosis. *Neurology.* 2013;81(24):2060-2061.

202. Pepping M, Brunings J, Goldberg M. Cognition, cognitive dysfunction, and cognitive rehabilitation in multiple sclerosis. *Phys Med Rehabil Clin North Am.* 2013;24(4):663-672.

203. Patten SB, Svenson LW, Metz LM. Psychotic disorders in MS: population-based evidence of an association. *Neurology.* 2005;65(7):1123-1125.

204. Kosmidis MH, Giannakou M, Lambros M, et al. Psychotic features associated with MS. *Int Rev Psychiatry.* 2010;22:55-56.

205. Andreassen OA, Harbo HF, Wang Y, et al. Genetic pleiotropy between multiple sclerosis and schizophrenia but not bipolar disorder: differential involvement of immune-related gene loci. *Mol Psychiatry.* 2015;20:207-214.

206. Suvisaari J, Mantere O. Inflammation theories in psychotic disorders: a critical review. *Infect Disord Drug Targets.* 2013;13(1):59-70.

207. Mahboobi N, Nolden-Hoverath S, Rieker O. Multiple sclerosis presenting as a delirium: a case report. *Med Princ Pract.* 2015;24:388-390.

208. Feinstein A, du Boulay G, Ron MA. Psychotic illness in multiple sclerosis. A clinical and magnetic resonance imaging study. *Br J Psychiatry.* 1992;161:680-685.

209. Honer WG, Hurwitz T, Li DK, et al. Temporal lobe involvement in multiple sclerosis patients with psychiatric disorders. *Arch Neurol.* 1987;44:187-190.

210. Kershner P, Wang-Cheng R. Psychiatric side effects of steroid therapy. *Psychosomatics.* 1989;30:135-139.

211. Sechi GP, Piras MR, Demurtas A, et al. Dexamethasone-induced schizoaffective-like state in multiple sclerosis: prophylaxis and treatment with carbamazepine. *Clin Neuropharmacol.* 1987;10:453-457.

212. Goeb JL, Even C, Nicolas G, et al. Psychiatric side effects of interferon-beta in multiple sclerosis. *Eur Psychiatry.* 2006;21:186-193.

213. Pine DS, Douglas CJ, Charles E, et al. Patients with multiple sclerosis presenting to psychiatric hospitals. *J Clin Psych.* 1995;56:297-306.

214. Lyoo IK, Seol HY, Byun HS, et al. Unsuspected multiple sclerosis in patients with psychiatric disorders: a magnetic resonance imaging study. *J Neuropsychiatry Clin Neurosci.* 1996;8:54-59.

215. Camara-Lemarroy CR, Ibarra-Yruegas BE, Rodriguez-Gutierrez R, et al. The varieties of psychosis in multiple sclerosis: a systematic review of cases. *Mult Scler Relat Disord.* 2017;12:9-14.

216. Testa S, Opportuno A, Gallo P, et al. A case of multiple sclerosis with an onset mimicking the Kleine-Levin syndrome. *Ital J Neurol Sci.* 1987;8:151-155.

217. Felgenhauer K. Psychiatric disorders in the encephalitic form of multiple sclerosis. *J Neurol.* 1990;237:11-18.

218. Davis E, Hartwig U, Gastpar M. Antipsychotic treatment of psychosis associated with multiple sclerosis. *Prog Neuropsychopharmacol Biol Psychiatry.* 2004;28:743-744.

219. Thone J, Kessler E. Improvement of neuropsychiatric symptoms in multiple sclerosis subsequent to high-dose corticosteroid treatment. *Prim Care Companion J Clin Psychiatry.* 2008;10:163-164.

220. Asghar-Ali AA, Taber KH, Hurley RA, et al. Pure neuropsychiatric presentation of multiple sclerosis. *Am J Psychiatry.* 2004;161:226-231.

221. Corruble E, Awad H, Chouinard G, et al. ECT in delusional depression with multiple sclerosis. *Am J Psychiatry.* 2004;161:1715.

222. Hotier S, Maltete D, Bourre B, et al. A manic episode with psychotic features improved by methylprednisolone in a patient with multiple sclerosis. *Gen Hosp Psychiatry.* 2015;37:621.

223. Wortzel HS, Oster TJ, Anderson CA, Arciniegas DB. Pathological laughing and crying—epidemiology, pathophysiology and treatment. *CNS Drugs.* 2008;22:531-545.

224. Feinstein A, Feinstein K, Gray T, O'Connor P. Prevalence and neurobehavioral correlates of pathological laughing and crying in multiple sclerosis. *Arch Neurol.* 1997;54:1116-1121.

225. Work SS, Colamonico JA, Bradley DG, Kaye RE. Pseudobulbar affect: an under-recognized and under-treated neurological disorder. *Adv Ther.* 2011;28:586-601.

226. Feinstein A, O'Connor P, Gray T, Feinstein K. Pathological laughing and crying in multiple sclerosis: a preliminary report suggesting a role for the prefrontal cortex. *Mult Scler.* 1999;5:69-73.

227. Hanna J, Feinstein A, Morrow SA. The association of pathological laughing and crying and cognitive impairment in multiple sclerosis. *J Neurol Sci.* 2016;361:20-203.

228. Parvizi J, Anderson SW, Martin CO, et al. Pathological laughter and crying: a link to the cerebellum. *Brain.* 2001;124:1708-1719.

229. Andersen G, Vestergaard K, Riis JO. Citalopram for post-stroke pathological crying. *Lancet.* 1993;342:837-839.

230. Parvizi J, Coburn KL, Shillcutt SD, et al. Neuroanatomy of pathological laughing and crying: a report of the American Neuropsychiatric Association Committee on Research. *J Neuropsychiatry Clin Neurosci.* 2009;21:75-87.

231. Ghaffar O, Chamelian L, Feinstein A. Neuroanatomy of pseudobulbar affect: a quantitative MRI study in multiple sclerosis. *J Neurol.* 2008;406-412.

232. Lauterbach EC, Cummings JL, Kuppuswamy PS. Toward a more precise, clinically-informed pathophysiology of pathological laughing and crying. *Neurosci Biobehav Rev.* 2013;37:1893-1916.

233. Stahl SM. Dextromethorphan-quinidine-responsive pseudobulbar affect (PLC): psychopharmacological model for wide-ranging disorders of emotional expression? *CNS Spectr.* 2016;21(6):419-423.

234. Harel Y, Barak Y, Achiron A. Dysregulation of affect in multiple sclerosis: new phenomenological approach. *Psychiatry Clin Neurosci.* 2007;61:94-98.

235. Moore SR, Gresham LS, Bromberg MB, et al. A self report measure of affective lability. *J Neurol Neurosurg Psychiatry.* 1997;63:89-93.

236. Smith RA, Berg JE, Pope LE, et al. Validation of the CNS emotional lability scale for pseudobulbar affect (pathological laughing and crying) in multiple sclerosis patients. *Mult Scler.* 2004;10:679-685.

237. Robinson RG, Parikh RM, Lipsey JR, et al. Pathological laughing and crying following stroke: validation of a measurement scale and a double-blind treatment study. *Am J Psychiatry.* 1993;150:286-293.

238. Pioro EP. Current concepts in the pharmacotherapy of pseudobulbar affect. *Drugs.* 2011;71:1193-1207.

239. Schiffer RB, Herndon RM, Rudick RA. Treatment of pathologic laughing and weeping with amitriptyline. *N Engl J Med.* 1985;312:1480-1482.

240. Panitch H, Thisted R, Smith R, et al. Randomized, controlled trial of dextromethorphan/quinidine for pseudobulbar affect in multiple sclerosis. *Ann Neurol.* 2006;59:780-787.

241. Pioro EP, Brooks BR, Cummings J, et al. Dextromethorphan plus ultra low-dose quinidine reduces pseudobulbar affect. *Ann Neurol.* 2010;68:693-702.

242. Smith RA, Licht JM, Pope LE, et al. Combination dextromethorphan quinidine in the treatment of frustration and anger in patients with involuntary emotional expression disorder (IEED). *Ann Neurol.* 2006;60:S50.

243. Hammond FM, Alexander DN, Cutler AJ, et al. PRISM II: an open-label study to assess effectiveness of dextromethorphan/quinidine for pseudobulbar affect in patients with dementia, stroke or traumatic brain injury. *BMC Neurol.* 2016;16:89.

244. Ferentinos P, Paparrigopoulos T, Rentzos M, Evdokimidis I. Duloxetine for pathological laughing and crying. *Int J Neuropsychopharmacol.* 2009;12:1429-1430.

245. Johnson B, Nichols S. Crying and suicidal, but not depressed. Pseudobulbar affect in multiple sclerosis successfully treated with valproic acid: case report and literature review. *Palliat Support Care.* 2015;13:1797-1801.

246. Chwastiak LA, Ehde DM. Psychiatric issues in multiple sclerosis. *Psychiatr Clin North Am.* 2007;30:803-817.

247. Sullivan LE, Fiellin DA, O'Connor PG. The prevalence and impact of alcohol problems in major depression: a systematic review. *Am J Med.* 2005;118:330-341.

248. Feinstein A. Multiple sclerosis, depression, and suicide. *BMJ.* 1997;315:691-696.

249. Bombardier CH, Blake KD, Ehde DM, et al. Alcohol and drug abuse among persons with multiple sclerosis. *Mult Scler.* 2004;10:35-40.

250. Pakpoor J, Goldacre R, Disanto G, et al. Alcohol misuse disorders and multiple sclerosis risk. *JAMA Neurol.* 2014;71:1188-1189.

251. Nuyen J, Schellevis FG, Satariano WA, et al. Comorbidity was associated with neurologic and psychiatric diseases: a general practice-based controlled study. *J Clin Epidemiol.* 2006:1274-1284.

252. Chong MS, Wolff K, Wise K, et al. Cannabis use in patients with multiple sclerosis. *Mult Scler.* 2006;12:646-651.

253. Zajicek JP, Hobart JC, Slade A, et al. Multiple sclerosis and extract of cannabis: results of the MUSEC trial. *J Neurol Neurosurg Psychiatry.* 2012;83:1125-1132.

254. Rog DJ, Nurmikko TJ, Friede T, Young CA. Randomized, controlled trial of cannabis-based medicine in central pain in multiple sclerosis. *Neurology.* 2005;65:812-819.

255. Wade DT, Robson P, House H, et al. A preliminary controlled study to determine whether whole-plant cannabis extracts can improve intractable neurogenic symptoms. *Clin Rehabil.* 2003;17:21-29.

256. Collin C, Ehler E, Waberzinek G, et al. A double-blind, randomized, placebo-controlled, parallel-group study of Sativex, in subjects with symptoms of spasticity due to multiple sclerosis. *Neurol Res.* 2010;32:451-459.

257. Corey-Bloom J, Wolfson T, Gamst A, et al. Smoked cannabis for spasticity in multiple sclerosis: a randomized, placebo-controlled trial. *CMAJ.* 2012;184:1143-1145.

258. Wade DT, Makela P, Robson P, et al. Do cannabis-based medicinal extracts have general or specific effects on symptoms in multiple sclerosis? A double-blind, randomized, placebo-controlled study on 160 patients. *Mult Scler.* 2004;10:434-441.

259. Langford RM, Mares J, Novotna A, et al. A double-blind, randomized, placebo-controlled, parallel-group study of THC/CBD oromucosal spray in combination with the existing treatment regimen, in the relief of central neuropathic pain in patients with multiple sclerosis. *J Neurol.* 2013;260:984-997.

260. van Amerongen G, Kanhai K, Baakman AC, et al. Effects on spasticity and neuropathic pain of an oral formulation of Δ9-tetrahydrocannabinol in patients with progressive multiple sclerosis. *Clin Ther.* 2018;40(9):1467-1482.

261. Zajicek J, Fox P, Sanders H, et al. Cannabinoids for treatment of spasticity and other symptoms related to multiple sclerosis (CAMS study): multicentre randomised placebo-controlled trial. *Lancet.* 2003;362:1517-1526.

262. Zajicek J, Sanders HP, Wright DE, et al. Cannabinoids in MS (CAMS) study: safety and efficacy data for 12 months follow up. *J Neurol Neurosurg Psychiatry.* 2005;76:1664-1669.

263. Vaney C, Heinzel-Guttenbrenner M, Jobin P, et al. Efficacy, safety, and tolerability of an orally administered cannabis extract in the treatment of spasticity in patients with MS: a randomized, double-blind, placebo-controlled, cross-over study. *Mult Scler.* 2004;10:417424.

264. Nugent SM, Morasco BJ, O'Neil ME, et al. The effects of cannabis among adults with chronic pain and an overview of general harms: a systematic review. *Ann Intern Med.* 2017;167:319-331.

265. Yadav V, Bever C, Bowen J, et al. Summary of evidence-based guideline: complementary and alternative medicine in MS. *Neurology.* 2014;82:1083-1092.

266. Hill KP. Medical marijuana for treatment of chronic pain and other medical and psychiatric problems: a clinical review. *JAMA.* 2015;313:2474-2483.

267. Whiting PF, Wolff RF, Deshpande S, et al. Cannabinoids for medical use: a systematic review and meta-analysis. *JAMA.* 2015;313:2456-2473.

268. Mandolini GM, Lazzaretti M, Pigoni A, et al. Pharmacological properties of cannabidiol in the treatment of psychiatric disorders: a critical overview. *Epidemiol Psychiatr Sci.* 2018;27(4):327-335.

269. Fernández Ó. THC:CBD in daily practice: available data from UK, Germany and Spain. *Eur Neurol.* 2016;75:1-3.

270. Chohan H, Greenfield AL, Yadav V, Graves J. Use of cannabinoids for spasticity and pain management in MS. *Curr Treat Options Neurol.* 2016;18:1.

271. Paparrigopoulos T, Ferentinos P, Kouzoupis A, et al. The neuropsychiatry of multiple sclerosis: focus on disorders of mood, affect and behavior. *Int Rev Psychiatry.* 2010;22:14-21.

272. Cummings JL. Frontal-subcortical circuits and human behavior. *Arch Neurol.* 1993;50:873-880.

273. Fishman I, Benedict RH, Bakshi R, et al. Construct validity and frequency of euphoria sclerotica in multiple sclerosis. *J Neuropsychiatry Clin Neurosci.* 2004;16(3):350-356.

274. Chiaravalloti ND, DeLuca J. Assessing the behavioral consequences of multiple sclerosis: an application of the Frontal Systems Behavior Scale (FrSBe). *Cogn Behav Neurol.* 2003;16:54-67.

Neuropsychiatric Complications of Cancer and its Treatments

Stephanie Tung · Rahul Gupta · Halyna Vitagliano · Fremonta L. Meyer

INTRODUCTION

This chapter aims to review common neuropsychiatric manifestations seen in patients with cancer, as well as principles of assessment and management that can be used in treating these patients. It will start with a discussion of primary brain tumors and explore their epidemiology, classification, pathophysiology, and clinical presentation. It will then examine neuropsychiatric manifestations of cancers that metastasize to the brain, and rare complications including leptomeningeal carcinomatoses. Subsequently, paraneoplastic syndromes, which are infrequent but challenging causes of neuropsychiatric symptoms in cancer patients, will be discussed. This will be followed by a review of commonly encountered neuropsychiatric symptoms in cancer patients. Additionally, the neuropsychiatric side effects of cancer treatments, including radiation therapy, chemotherapy, antiepileptic drugs, and steroids will be considered. Finally, the chapter will address the treatment of neuropsychiatric symptoms in cancer patients using pharmacologic and behavioral approaches.

Cancer and its treatment may affect the brain both directly and indirectly with profound neuropsychiatric consequences. There are nearly 700,000 individuals in the United States with a brain tumor, which are categorized as primary when they originate in the brain, or metastatic when they originate from other parts of the body. Approximately 138,000 of all brain tumors are malignant, constituting brain cancer. Central and peripheral nervous system cancers represent a smaller fraction (approximately 1.4%) of all new brain cancer diagnoses. On the other hand, metastatic brain cancers are more prevalent, since approximately 20–40% of all cancers metastasize to the brain.

Neuropsychiatric and cognitive disorders are extremely common in individuals with brain tumors. More than 50% of brain tumor patients meet diagnosable criteria for a psychiatric disorder. Similarly, cognitive dysfunction is present in over 70% of patients with central nervous system (CNS) malignancies. The manifestations of these disorders are determined by two main factors: (a) the location and affected neurological circuits; and (b) the growth and infiltration pattern of the particular tumor and associated edema.[1] It is important to appreciate that manifestations of cognitive dysfunction and psychiatric disorders may vary through the cancer course, in accordance with tumor localization and specific treatments received.

PRIMARY BRAIN TUMORS

Epidemiology

Primary brain tumors are a relatively uncommon form of cancer, with high mortality rates.[2] As a group, these tumors are heterogeneous. Primary brain tumors may arise from the parenchyma or surrounding structures, such as the meninges, neuroepithelial tissues, pituitary, cranial nerves, and germ cells.

There is a 0.6% lifetime risk of being diagnosed with a brain or other nervous system cancer.[3] The overall incidence of primary brain tumors is 10.82 per 100,000 person-years.[4] In the United States, there were an estimated 23,380 new cases diagnosed in 2014 accounting for 1.4% of all new cases of cancer.[3] In the same year primary brain tumors led to 14,320 deaths, accounting for 2.4% of all cancer-related deaths.[3]

The prevalence of primary brain tumors has been increasing due to improvements in detection and treatment. In 2004, the prevalence of primary brain tumors in the United States was 209 per 100,000. By 2010 it had increased to 221 per 100,000.[5] Peak prevalence is between 55 and 64 years of age, with a slightly higher incidence in men than in women.[3] For adults with primary brain tumors, the average 5-year survival rate is 33.4%, although this rate varies widely among the specific types of tumors: 100% for pilocytic astrocytoma, 58% for low-grade astrocytoma, 11% for anaplastic astrocytoma, and 1.2% for glioblastoma.[3] From 1999 to 2007, death rates for adults with malignant brain tumors decreased at a rate of 1.2% per year, a trend being driven by more targeted radiation as well as newer and lower-dose chemotherapies.[5]

Neuropsychiatric symptoms are common in individuals with brain cancer, although exact incidence rates are poorly characterized. Compared with other cancer patient populations, the prevalence of depression is higher among patients with brain tumors.[5] Left frontal lobe tumors have been associated with depressed feelings and right frontal lobe tumors have been found to raise spirits and lead to euphoria.[6] Some initial studies suggested an independent association between depressive symptoms and frontal lobe tumors.[7] Anatomical studies reported a statistically significant association with tumors in the "ventral frontal" lobe and postoperative depression.[8] However, later studies found no association between tumors in the frontal lobe and depression.[9-13] Currently there is no consistent evidence that tumor location and depression are associated.[14] Right hemisphere lesions have been reported to present as manic symptoms.[15-17] Right frontal tumors have also been reported to be associated with patients' underestimation of the significance of their illness.[6] A large meta-analysis reported that several regions demonstrated an increased likelihood of associated symptoms when compared with other regions, but apart from a statistically significant association between anorexia symptoms and hypothalamic tumor no other definitive associations could be determined.[18]

Depressed patients do not appear to differ from nondepressed patients in terms of sociodemographic characteristics, tumor malignancy, or tumor location.[9] Not surprisingly, depression is the most independent predictor of health-related quality of life (HRQOL) in patients with brain tumors. Treatment of neuropsychiatric symptoms is critical in helping patients achieve higher levels of functioning.[5]

Classification

Primary brain tumors are classified according to World Health Organization (WHO) criteria based on their cell of origin and degree of malignancy. Higher-grade tumors confer a worse prognosis.[19]

Gliomas are the most common primary brain tumors, constituting about 15% of brain/CNS tumors.[20] Gliomas develop from glial cells (astrocytes or oligodendrocytes), which surround and support neurons in the brain.[21] They occur more frequently in men and the elderly.[20] Approximately 20% of gliomas are slow growing, low-grade tumors. They are frequently associated with epileptic seizures and have a median survival of 6–15 years, depending on the genetic profile of the tumor.[21] Poorer outcomes have been associated with older age, astrocytoma histology, tumor size >6 cm, and tumor affecting both sides of the brain.[21]

In contrast to the slow-growing gliomas, glioblastomas are associated with a higher malignancy grade and poorer prognosis.[3] Glioblastomas account for 15% of primary brain tumors.[3] Median survival time for glioblastomas can be as short as 12–15 months,[22] and largely depends on the grade. Only one-quarter of adults with the most common type of glioblastoma multiforme (GBM) survive for 2 years after diagnosis.[21]

Meningiomas are another common type of primary brain tumor. These tumors are generally slow growing and well encapsulated.[22] They develop from meningothelial cells of the arachnoid membrane covering the brain and spinal cord. They occur more frequently in women and the elderly, and

are often cured by surgery.[21] However, they can be a source of extensive morbidity including seizures and focal neurological dysfunction.[22] Seizures occur in 30% of intracranial meningiomas.[22]

Pathophysiology

This discussion focuses on the pathophysiology of brain tumors' neuropsychiatric manifestations. Brain tumors can compromise brain function via various disease mechanisms. They can infiltrate and displace brain tissue and cause symptoms according to their brain localization, as discussed below with the examples of frontal and temporal lobe tumors. Other mechanisms by which they may cause symptoms and brain dysfunction include increased intracranial pressure (ICP), seizures, and disruption of structural and functional brain connectivity.[23]

With regards to cognitive symptoms, it is traditionally believed that certain cognitive deficits may be specific for brain tumor location. For instance, left-sided tumors will cause impairment of verbal functions. However, this association between tumor localization and cognitive performance is not consistently observed. In a retrospective study, 62 patients with brain tumors were referred for neuropsychological assessment before neurosurgery, and no significant difference in cognitive performance could be linked to the brain tumor location, type, or lateralization.[11] A possible explanation for this finding is that cognitive defects may be caused by other factors, beyond the tumor's effect directly due to its localization. They may arise from mass effects imposed on the opposite hemisphere or adjacent structures, epileptic discharges, and brain compensatory mechanisms in cases of slow-growing tumors. They may also occur as a result of the cancer treatment, psychological distress, or a combination of these factors.[3]

Frontal Lobe Tumors

The frontal lobe is the most common location for brain tumors, and is associated with a great number of neuropsychiatric effects. Patients with frontal lobe tumors have been shown to have higher levels of apathy, along with disinhibition and executive dysfunction.[24]

There are three key areas of the frontal lobe that may produce distinct syndromes when affected by disease: dorsolateral, orbitofrontal, and anterior cingulate. Dorsolateral prefrontal syndrome is the most common and is typically associated with executive dysfunction. This may include difficulties with planning and goal setting, initiating or persisting in activities, and problems with sustained attention, sequencing, and perseverative behavior.

Orbitofrontal syndrome is associated with changes in personality, irritability and lability, poor judgment, and lack of insight. The development of emotional lability and mood disturbances in brain tumor patients has been linked to orbitofrontal cortex lesions. This area is known for its importance in regulating adherence to social conventions.[24] In these patients, social awareness can be affected, resulting in reduced concern about the consequences of their behavior and its impact on others.[24]

Apathy has been linked to tumors in the medial prefrontal cortex, which is functionally known to be associated with motivational aspects of behavior.[24] The anterior cingulate syndrome may be associated with apathy, akinetic mutism, and inability to respond to commands.

Other presenting symptoms of frontal lobe tumors include mania, classically described with right frontal, right anterior temporal, and orbitofrontal lesions.[17] Case reports detail patients who presented with an eating disorder in the form of anorexia nervosa, which was instead the initial symptom of a right frontal brain tumor.[25-27] Another unique presentation is cortical blindness (also known as Anton's syndrome), in which patients cannot see but deny blindness and confabulate by describing (often vividly) objects in their vicinity. While typically associated with occipital lesions, it can also occur with frontal lesions, including large anterior fossa meningiomas.[28]

Difficulties with personality and social behavior following damage to the frontal lobes can have devastating functional consequences resulting in reduced autonomy, unemployment, or divorce. Executive difficulties with organizing, initiating, directing, monitoring, and controlling interpersonal behavior can make it difficult for patients to function personally and professionally.[24]

The social effects of brain tumors on patients are currently understudied but may be of critical prognostic importance. One study examining the risk of separation or divorce after a diagnosis of brain tumor found that female gender and a marriage of shorter duration led to a higher likelihood of separation and divorce; there was also a trend toward higher risk of separation in patients with tumors localized to the frontal lobes. Furthermore, divorce resulted in a greater likelihood of treatment failure and probability of in-hospital death.[29]

Temporal Lobe Tumors

The temporal lobe is the second most common localization for a brain tumor. Medial temporal lobe tumors classically produce memory deficits. Tumors in the dominant (typically left) temporal lobe can produce a fluent aphasia. Tumors in the nondominant (typically right) temporal lobe may produce disruptions in discrimination of music or other nonspeech sounds as well as deficits in social cognition and emotional awareness such that patients have difficulty recognizing emotions appropriately.[30] Neuropsychiatric symptoms for temporal lobe tumors may be surprisingly similar to frontal lobe tumors. This is thought to be related to the microscopic infiltration of tumors across lobes, as well as reciprocal interactions between the white-matter tracts which connect brain regions.[20]

Adults with right hemisphere tumors have higher anxiety as compared to those with left hemisphere lesions.[9] Studies on the functional neuroanatomy of anxiety have found that the fear response has its basis in the amygdala, thalamus and hippocampus, as well as the cerebellar vermis.[31] During states of anxiety there is right greater than left activation in the frontal and temporal lobes and related mesial temporal lobe structures, and panic and severe anxiety are associated with dysfunction or injury in the right temporal lobe.[31] Similarly, psychopharmacological research on patients with anxiety disorders demonstrates

right greater than left temporal lobe benzodiazepine receptor binding.[31]

Other Symptom-Location Correlates

Depressive symptoms have been linked to dysfunction in extended neuronal networks involved in emotion, including cortical midline structures (medial orbitofrontal, prefrontal, and cingulate cortex) and subcortical limbic structures (striatum, thalamus, and amygdala).[32]

Clinical Presentation

Clinical signs and symptoms of primary brain tumors may be general or focal. General symptoms often occur secondary to increased ICP. Focal symptoms are due to tissue destruction or compression of specialized regions, as discussed above in the examples of frontal and temporal lobe tumors. For low-grade tumors, initial symptoms are often focal, progressing to generalized symptoms as the tumor increases in size and spreads, or if there are complications such as secondary hydrocephalus. General neurologic symptoms may progress to encephalopathy and dementia. Cognitive dysfunction is commonly present as part of the presentation.

An unrecognized brain tumor can present with psychiatric symptoms only, or psychiatric symptoms may arise during the course of the illness.[9] Indeed, over 50% of people with brain tumors experience psychiatric symptoms.[1] This is important to recognize and address, as both quality of life and adherence to treatment plans significantly deteriorate when depression and other mood disturbances are present. Poor treatment adherence is a significant risk factor for decreased quality of life and increased mortality.[33]

METASTATIC BRAIN TUMORS

Epidemiology

The CNS is a frequent target for metastases from systemic cancer. The most common location of CNS metastases is the brain parenchyma, followed by the leptomeningeal space. Metastases are the most common brain tumors and may occur up to 10 times more frequently than primary brain tumors in adults. They affect 9–17% of cancer patients in large population and autopsy-based studies.[34] Parenchymal metastases differ from leptomeningeal metastasis (LM) in clinical presentation, treatment modalities, and prognosis. However, superficial brain lesions may invade the subarachnoid space, and leptomeningeal disease may invade brain parenchyma, and thus combined presentations are not uncommon.

The exact incidence of brain metastases is unknown. Epidemiological studies have limitations because some brain metastases remain asymptomatic and are never diagnosed, and even symptomatic lesions may be overlooked in severely ill patients with systemic metastases elsewhere.[35] The reported prevalence of brain metastases has increased. This is partially due to increased identification of existing metastases given higher utilization of neuroimaging. For example, brain magnetic resonance imaging (MRI) is routinely performed as part of staging evaluations in lung cancer[36] and metastatic melanoma.[35] In addition, improved cancer treatments have lengthened overall survival but have also allowed for higher rates of CNS spread, given that many systemic chemotherapies do not effectively penetrate the blood-brain barrier (BBB); this may also contribute to an increased prevalence of brain metastases.

Pathophysiology

Brain metastases often result in cognitive deficits including attentional or memory impairment or lack of concentration, and emotional/behavioral disturbances ranging from personality changes to depression. The localization of metastases (frontal vs. temporal vs. occipital vs. parietal) often determines the specific neuropsychiatric symptoms, quite analogous to patterns described above for primary brain tumors. In adults, lung carcinomas, breast carcinomas, and malignant melanoma account for up to 75% of brain metastases.[37] Patients with lung cancer (especially small cell lung cancer [SCLC] and adenocarcinomas) make up about 50% of cases of brain metastasis.[38] Breast cancer accounts for about 15% of all brain metastasis,[38] with an increased risk in patients with estrogen receptor (ER) negative and human epidermal growth factor receptor (HER)-2/neu positive tumors. Melanoma accounts for 5–10% of cases,[39] and though it has a lower incidence than breast and lung metastasis, it has a very high likelihood of metastasis and about 50% of patients who die from melanoma will have brain metastasis.[40] Although any cancer may spread to the brain, the lowest rates are observed in prostate, ovarian, and thyroid cancer (incidence less than 1%).[41-43]

Most brain metastases occur in the cerebrum (approximately 80%), followed by the cerebellum (15%) and brainstem (5%). Metastases to the pineal gland, choroid plexus, and parasellar/sellar regions are less common. One study suggests that tumors arising in the pelvis such as prostate, uterine, or colorectal cancer have a special affinity for the cerebellum, although the reason is unclear.[42] The overall distribution of metastases corresponds roughly to the relative blood flow to each area of the brain given their hematogenous nature of dissemination through the arteries.[34] Common areas of metastasis are gray-white junctions, where there is a sudden luminal narrowing of vessels, as well as watershed areas of circulation, especially in the territory between the MCA and PCA.[34]

Clinical Presentation and Diagnosis

Approximately two-thirds of brain metastases become symptomatic in the course of the malignant disease.[41] Most of them are diagnosed in patients with already known systemic cancer (metachronous presentation) or found during diagnostic procedure of the malignant disease (synchronous presentation). The discovery of brain metastases before that of the underlying cancer (precocious presentation) is less common.

Any new neurologic manifestation occurring in a patient with cancer should raise the possibility of a metastatic brain tumor. Certain features such as headache, seizures, focal neurological signs or symptoms, cognitive and behavioral changes, and gait disturbance, are particularly common. MRI with contrast enhancement is the most commonly used modality in evaluating for the presence of brain metastases and, if present, for the accurate assessment of number and size of the tumors, their exact locations, and impact on nearby structures. Often the diagnosis of intracranial metastasis is made radiologically without histological confirmation. However, microscopic tissue diagnosis should be performed for brain mass(es) of uncertain etiology, especially when there is ambiguity in radiological features to exclude non-metastatic causes (e.g., abscess). In addition, excisional biopsy is indicated for a solitary lesion in an accessible area of the brain. For leptomeningeal carcinomatosis, detection of malignant cells on cytologic examination of the cerebrospinal fluid (CSF) is the diagnostic gold standard.[34]

Neuropsychiatric manifestations in patients with metastatic tumors are similar to those with primary tumors. Based on the location of a metastatic tumor and its effect on surrounding structures, the presentation may vary, similarly to primary brain tumors. Brain metastases are usually multifocal. Therefore the symptoms do not always localize to a specific brain region and patients may present with a variety of symptoms simultaneously.

LEPTOMENINGEAL METASTASIS

Leptomeningeal metastasis, leptomeningeal carcinomatosis, and carcinomatous meningitis are terms used interchangeably to designate the presence of metastatic tumors primarily involving the leptomeninges of the brain. This is a rare but devastating form of brain metastasis that usually confers a poor prognosis, with an average survival of 2–4 months despite treatment.

CASE VIGNETTE 28.1

A 58-year-old woman with metastatic breast cancer, in psychotherapy and medication management, who several years into her disease course sent an e-mail message about some psychodynamic issues contributing to anxiety and mentioning almost off-handedly headaches, nausea, and a "foggy thought process." At that point, the patient was on palliative chemotherapy and had systemic metastases as well as a known skull metastasis that was invading the dura, but no brain metastases. Four days after sending the message, she decompensated quite markedly and was hospitalized with hydrocephalus, which was found to be a result of leptomeningeal disease. She underwent a ventriculoperitoneal shunt which successfully palliated the headaches and nausea but did not have whole brain radiation because of her overall disease status and died somewhat abruptly a month later.

Epidemiology

The incidence of LM typically varies by primary tumor type, occurring in approximately 5–8% of patients with solid tumors and 5–15% of patients with hematologic malignancies.[44] Although nearly every type of tumor has been reported to metastasize to the leptomeninges, this is more common in some solid tumors including lung, breast, and melanoma. LM occurs in 5–8% of metastatic breast cancers,[45] 9–25% of all lung cancers (greater in SCLC),[46] and 6–18% of melanomas.[47] Overall, the incidence of LM may be increasing in the setting of improved systemic control and treatments that poorly penetrate the BBB, leading to longer survival and a reservoir of tumor cells in the CNS.[48–52] Progressive systemic disease is also observed in 60–70% of patients at the time of LM diagnosis.[53,54] In a large case series of 187 patients, including 150 patients with solid malignancies (primarily breast and lung cancers), 58% had concurrent or prior parenchymal brain involvement.[55] The median time from systemic cancer diagnosis to the diagnosis of LM ranges from 1.2 to 2.0 years in solid tumors and averages 11 months in hematologic malignancies.[53,55,56]

Clinical Presentation

LM involvement most commonly occurs in the basal cisterns of the brain, posterior fossa, and cauda equina.[57,58] Invasion of the leptomeninges can lead to local inflammation and impaired CSF resorption, which can then obstruct CSF flow and cause hydrocephalus and/or increased ICP. Signs and symptoms of LM depend on the location of involvement. Given the frequent multifocality, clinical presentation may be nonspecific, and the index of suspicion must be high. Common clinical findings are often attributable to cranial and spinal nerve dysfunction, increased ICP, or meningeal irritation. Cranial nerves VI, VII, and VIII are commonly affected, leading to diplopia, facial weakness, and changes in hearing, respectively. Spinal signs include dermatomal sensory loss, radicular pain, bowel and bladder dysfunction, and limb weakness. Other general symptoms include headache (which is often worse in the morning and while recumbent), nausea, vomiting, and changes in mental status. Involvement or compression of small vessels in the subarachnoid space may also lead to ischemic infarct.

Given the broad presenting features and frequently complex treatment histories, consideration should also be given to alternative diagnoses, including chronic infectious meningitis, autoimmune disorders (e.g., sarcoidosis), meningeal reaction to brain abscess, side effects of chemotherapy or radiation, paraneoplastic syndromes, and toxic-metabolic encephalopathy. In immunocompromised cancer patients, causes of infectious meningitis or encephalitis include bacterial (e.g., tuberculosis, listeriosis), fungal (e.g., *Cryptococcus*, candidiasis), or viral (e.g., cytomegalovirus, varicella zoster virus, Epstein-Barr virus, herpes simplex virus [HSV], and JC virus).

Of note, the symptomatic presentation of leptomeningeal disease can be either gradual or precipitous (see Case Vignette 28.2). It is important to remain vigilant in patients with active metastatic disease as this devastating complication can appear rapidly. However, response to treatment can vary and some

patients survive significantly longer.[44] Untreated, death occurs from progressive neurologic deterioration in 4–6 weeks.[54]

Primary tumor type also plays an important role. In one patient series, those with hematologic malignancies had slightly improved survival of 4.7 months when compared with 2.3 months for those with solid tumors.[55] Within solid tumors, breast cancer LM has a superior prognosis compared to other tumor types, with a median survival of 5–7 months.[55,59–62]

Diagnosis

The diagnosis of LM remains challenging, with no test sufficiently sensitive to rule out leptomeningeal involvement. MRI of the brain and spine is recommended if there is clinical suspicion and may reveal leptomeningeal enhancement, which is often irregular and nodular.[63] The sensitivity of MRI with gadolinium is approximately 70%, with specificity of 77–100% (higher for solid tumors than for hematologic malignancies).[64–66] In the presence of typical clinical features, an abnormal MRI is sufficient to make the diagnosis.[64] If it is safe to perform a lumbar puncture, it often reveals mild pleocytosis with elevated protein and hypoglycorrhachia. The use of CSF tumor markers has been limited by their low sensitivity and specificity as well as significant assay variability. However, these markers may support the diagnosis in the setting of an otherwise equivocal diagnostic evaluation.

PARANEOPLASTIC SYNDROMES

Epidemiology

Paraneoplastic limbic encephalitis (PLE) is a rare disorder characterized by personality changes, irritability, depression, seizures, memory loss, and sometimes dementia.[67] Corsellis et al. are credited with defining the term paraneoplastic limbic encephalitis[67,68]; however, autoimmune encephalitis was described in the literature dating back to Hermann Oppenheim in 1888.[69,70] In the 1960s, postmortem exams of patients with subacute encephalitis presenting with mood and behavioral changes revealed inflammatory changes that were most pronounced in the limbic structures (hippocampus and amygdala), resulting in a refinement of the term autoimmune encephalitis to the more specific limbic encephalitis in these cases.[68,69]

The prevalence of paraneoplastic syndromes depends on the type of cancer, and ranges from 1% in breast and ovarian cancers to 3–5% in SCLC and 20% in thymomas, although these may be underestimations of true prevalence rates.[71] Paraneoplastic encephalomyelitis refers to a syndrome involving multiple areas of the nervous system, which usually occurs in the setting of anti-Hu antibodies and lung cancer, and has been reported in 11% of patients with paraneoplastic syndromes.[72] The remainder of presentations are diverse in nature, including cerebellar degeneration, opsoclonus/myoclonus, retinal degeneration, sensory, autonomic, or motor neuropathy, myelitis, stiff person syndrome, or myasthenia gravis.

SCLC is the most commonly reported cancer associated with PLE, accounting for close to 50% of cases in the literature.[73] Other tumors associated with PLE include testicular tumors, other types of lung cancer, breast cancer, Hodgkin's disease, thymoma, ovarian teratoma, adenocarcinoma of the colon, esophageal carcinoma, chronic myeloid leukemia, plasma-cell dyscrasia, neuroblastoma, and malignancies of the ovary, prostate, mediastinum, kidney, and bladder.[73] PLE seems to be more common in females and individuals greater than 50 years old.[73]

Pathophysiology

Paraneoplastic syndromes are associated with cancer, but are caused by autoimmune processes rather than direct tumor invasion. Antigens in the CNS may resemble antigens found in malignancies (onconeural antigens). The recognition of an onconeural antigen outside the nervous system triggers an immune response that is toxic to CNS tissue when antibodies and cytotoxic T-cells cross the BBB and interact with neural cells expressing the same onconeural protein.[73]

The link between PLE incidence and certain tumors is not completely understood. Tumor genes responsible for producing onconeural antigens are not the result of mutations, and are present in many patients with malignancy who do not develop PLE. It is thought that PLE may result from differences in autoimmune responses, rather than differences in the tumors themselves.[73] By targeting ion channels, receptors or associated proteins, autoimmune antibodies interfere with synaptic transmission and neuronal plasticity.[69]

Antibodies associated with paraneoplastic disorders can be subcategorized based on the cellular locations of the antigens they recognize and whether the destruction is cellular or humoral in nature.[69] Antibody locations associated with autoimmune encephalitis can be divided into two main categories: those that target intracellular antigens and those with cell surface/synaptic-targeted antigens.[69,74]

Autoimmune encephalitis associated with antibodies targeted toward cell surface or synaptic proteins occurs more often in younger patients, is less often paraneoplastic, and generally responds favorably to immunotherapy, although exceptions can occur when diagnosis and treatment are delayed or when significant atrophy has occurred.[74] Cell-surface antibodies are often directly pathogenic, leading to reversible neurotransmitter receptor internalization and/or blockade.[74,75] Pathophysiology of autoimmune encephalitis caused by antibodies toward synaptic receptor antigens has been best studied in N-methyl-D-aspartate receptor (NMDAR) encephalitis (see *Anti-NMDAR* section later in this chapter). This condition serves as a prototype for understanding how a patient's IgG autoantibodies bind to the amino terminal domain of the GluN1 (obligatory) subunit, disrupting the association between NMDARs and the ephrin type B2 receptor and displacing NMDARs to the extra synaptic space, ultimately leading to their internalization.[74] This disrupts synaptic long-term potentiation, affecting memory and producing behavioral alterations in a largely reversible fashion.[74] Other antibodies with similar pathophysiology include those recognizing neuromuscular junction proteins, peripheral nerve membrane proteins, neuronal membrane proteins, and voltage-gated potassium channels.[69,76]

Another group of antibodies is directed against intracellular antigens.[69,76] Neurologic disorders with antibodies targeting intracellular antigens are more often paraneoplastic, occur in older patients, and respond poorly to immunotherapy.[74] Their pathogenic activity is thought to be mediated by CD8+ cytotoxic T-cell immunity, rather than by autoantibodies directly.[69,74,76,77] For example, patients with intracellularly targeted Purkinje cell cytoplasmic antibody (PCA-1) autoantibodies and paraneoplastic cerebellar degeneration have been demonstrated to have PCA-1 antigen-specific cytotoxic T lymphocytes and autopsies have revealed CD8+ cells in the CNS tissue.[74]

When presented on the cell surface, immune targeting of intracellular antigens can occur.[74] This type is characterized by infiltrates of oligoclonal T-cells in the CNS with deposits of paraneoplastic antibodies in T-cell dense areas.[69] Given the T-cell-mediated neural damage, treatment aimed at the humoral response is largely ineffective.[69] Indeed, these disorders are typically difficult to treat because irreversible parenchymal atrophy has occurred by the time of diagnosis and treatment.[74] An exception is glial fibrillary acidic protein (GFAP) autoimmune astrocytopathy, which despite being associated with an intracellular antigen, appears to be exquisitely responsive to glucocorticoids.[74]

On brain biopsy and postmortem histological exam, the neural tissue of a patient with PLE demonstrates inflammation and degeneration of the limbic gray matter, especially the hippocampi and the amygdalae. Further evidence of neuronal damage includes reactive paraneural gliosis, lipofuscin accumulation, and a large astrocyte presence.[73] Despite the historical designation of limbic encephalitis, inflammatory injury is rarely limited to limbic structures alone and the syndrome may progress to encephalomyelitis with dorsal root ganglionitis.[73]

In terms of the pathophysiology of PLE's neuropsychiatric symptoms, injury to specific structures in the limbic system can cause alterations in cognition and mood. For instance, injury to the amygdala can elevate emotionality and aggression. Lesions of the hypothalamus can increase or decrease appetite and sexual urge. Disruption of the hippocampus-amygdala circuit can interfere with concentration and memory storage.

Clinical Presentation

Paraneoplastic disorders may occur in the setting of a known cancer diagnosis.[71] However, in the majority of cases (60–70%) neuropsychiatric symptoms will precede a cancer diagnosis, sometimes by a period of a few years.[69,71]

Due to the variety of antibodies and brain regions they target, patients with paraneoplastic syndromes may present with a wide range of symptoms and syndromes. This includes cerebellar symptoms such as ataxia, seizures, visual impairment due to optic neuritis, hypothalamic symptoms such as sleep and appetite disturbances, and others described below. Within these, PLE is of particular significance within the field of neuropsychiatry given that its presentation may mimic other psychiatric disorders.

The PLE syndrome is typically characterized by mood disturbance, psychosis, cognitive impairment including memory dysfunction, sleep disturbance, irritability, or seizure activity (commonly complex partial seizures).[67,71] They may also experience sensory neuropathies, and dysfunctions in consciousness, behavior, and perception.[71] The symptoms develop over a course of days to weeks. Historically, the term "limbic encephalitis" was first used to describe patients with memory dysfunction in association with bronchogenic carcinoma. It was characterized as evolving over days to weeks to include psychiatric changes such as irritability, depression, hallucinations, personality disturbances, and cognitive changes.[71] Some symptoms may be more neurological in nature, such as sleep disturbances, confusion, or seizures, while others may more typically resemble psychiatric disorders such as delusional thought content, paranoid ideation, or obsessive-compulsive behavior.[71] Typical presentations consist of progressive confusion and deficits in short-term memory that worsen over days to weeks. Less commonly, patients may experience visual and auditory hallucinations, delusions, or paranoia.[73]

Even after a diagnosis of PLE is made and an underlying malignancy is identified, prognosis remains broadly variable, ranging from recovery of neurologic function to progression to coma and death.[73] Patients with antibodies to cell membrane antigens (NMDAR, VGKC) have been found to be significantly more likely to improve with treatment than those with antibodies to intraneuronal antigens.[73]

Most patients with a paraneoplastic syndrome usually display a subacute course and die a few months after the diagnosis as a result of the combined effects of the neurologic disability and cancer progression. Those that survive unfortunately may continue to have persistent deficits in memory, with some having severe deficits in learning and retention of new information, or remembering past events.[78]

Symptoms of CNS involvement outside of the limbic system (including brainstem abnormalities, cerebellar dysfunction, dorsal root ganglion dysfunction, or myelitis) are common in patients with PLE. These symptoms can be found in about 60% of patients with PLE.[67] Other studies have found that only 32% (6 of 19) patients had isolated limbic encephalitis.[79,80]

There are a number of paraneoplastic and autoantibody disorders of the peripheral nervous system (PNS).[76] These include myasthenia gravis, Lambert-Eaton myasthenic syndrome (LEMS), autoimmune autonomic neuropathy, Isaacs' syndrome, and inflammatory myopathy.[76]

Subacute cerebellar degeneration is one of the most common and characteristic paraneoplastic syndromes. It may present rather acutely with cerebellar signs, vomiting, and ataxia, with subsequent progression to dysarthria and wheelchair requirement. Patients with subacute cerebellar degeneration often require extensive full-time care. At times they may remain neurologically disabled even after the underlying cancer is in remission.

Paraneoplastic Syndromes with Intracellular Antigens

Autoantibodies involved in T-cell-mediated responses to intracellular or nuclear proteins include anti-Hu (ANNA-1), anti-Ma 1 and 2, anti-Yo, anti-Ri (ANNA-2), anti-CRMP-5 (collapsin response mediator protein type 5) antibodies, and others (Table 28-1).[68,72,74,76]

Anti-Hu/ANNA-1

Anti-Hu antibodies (type 1 antineuronal-nuclear antibodies) are most commonly associated with SCLC. They may also be associated with neuroblastoma and prostate cancer.[74] Anti-Hu antibodies recognize a family of RNA-binding proteins involved in normal neuronal development. These antibodies commonly present in patients in their 50s or 60s with a long history of smoking and complaints of painful sensory neuropathy with recent confusion and amnesia. Patients may present a wide variety of neurologic symptoms. They frequently have symptoms of confusion, memory disturbance, seizure activity, and psychosis. Some patients also have prominent mood and anxiety symptoms and nonspecific personality changes. Approximately half of patients with SCLC and PLE are anti-Hu antibody-positive and have a worse prognosis than those who are anti-Hu antibody-negative.[73] Median survival is 11 months to year, and the 3-year survival rate is only 20%.[72] Treatment of the tumor along with immunotherapy for the T-cell response can result in symptom stabilization and early intervention (within weeks of symptom onset) generally yields better results.[71]

Anti-Ma

Anti-Ma 1 and anti-Ma2/Ta antibodies may be found in patients with breast, colon, parotid, and non-SCLCs. Anti-Ma 2 antibodies may be also found in patients with germ cell testicular cancer.[74] Symptoms may include cognitive decline, hyperphagia, excessive daytime sleepiness, or cataplexy that develops over several months.[73] Common traits include severe short-term memory deficits. Less commonly, patients may exhibit signs of upper brainstem dysfunction. Symptoms may include visual dysfunction (diplopia, gaze abnormalities, nystagmus), gait disturbances, and hypokinesis. Depression, irritability, and hallucinations are relatively rare. CSF levels of hypocrenin have been demonstrated to be low in patients with anti-Ma encephalitis.

Patients with isolated anti-Ma antibodies may respond well to treatment of the tumor and immunotherapy. Approximately 30–50% of patients ultimately deteriorate neurologically with a death rate of 15% during the initial presentation, while one-third experience neurological improvement and 20–40% stabilize. The association of testicular cancer and anti-Ma2 limbic encephalitis in men <50 years old is so strong that studies suggest consideration of orchiectomy or testicular irradiation even if a tumor cannot be found. In one study, six patients with risk factors for testicular neoplasm and neurological deterioration underwent orchiectomy for questionable ultrasound findings in the absence of an identifiable tumor and all were found to have preinvasive malignant cells.[71]

Patients with anti-Ma2/Ta antibodies are usually men of younger age, present with limbic encephalitis, and are likely to have a testicular germ cell tumor. These types of tumors generally respond well to treatment with stabilization of the neurological syndrome and long-term survival. This presentation is in contrast to patients with anti-Ma antibodies, who can be of either sex, are usually middle aged, suffer from a range of tumors and neurological presentations, and do less well following tumor treatment.[81]

Anti-CV2/CRMP5

Anti-CV2 (aka anti-CRMP5) antibodies have been found in patients with PLE associated with an underlying SCLC or thymoma. CRMP localizes to neuronal cell bodies and axons in the mammalian CNS and is known to be involved in axon

TABLE 28-1 • Paraneoplastic Syndromes.

Syndromes Involving Antibodies to Intracellular Antigens

Antibody and Antigen	Patient Demographics	Commonly Associated Tumors	Neuropsychiatric Features
ANNA-1 (anti-Hu)	75% males, median age 63 years	Small cell lung cancer	Encephalomyelitis Sensory neuropathy/Neuronopathy Cerebellar degeneration Autonomic dysfunction
ANNA-2 (anti-Ri)	68% females, mean age 65 years	Lung, breast, and gynecologic cancers	Encephalomyelitis Cerebellar degeneration Opsoclonus-myoclonus
ANNA-3	Males and females, ages 8–83 years	Lung cancer	Multifocal Neuropathy Myelopathy Brainstem or limbic encephalitis
PNMA-1 (anti-Ma)	Males and females, middle aged	Diverse tumors, including lung, breast, colon and renal	Encephalitis Cerebellar ataxia Ophthalmoplegia Dementia
PNMA-2 (anti-Ma2 or anti-Ta)	Mostly males <45 years old (median age 34 years), fewer females (median age 64 years)	Germ cell tumors of the testis	Limbic encephalitis Brainstem encephalitis Cerebellar degeneration Neuropathy
PCA-1 (anti-Yo)	Almost all females, young adult to elderly	Breast and ovarian cancers	Cerebellar degeneration
PCA-2		Small cell cancers	Encephalitis Cerebellar degeneration Autonomic dysfunction Motor neuropathy
CRMP5 (anti-CV2)	Males and females, older adults	Small cell lung cancer, thymoma	Encephalomyelitis Sensory neuropathy/Neuronopathy Multifocal Dementia Ataxia Myelopathy Chorea Seizures Cranial neuropathies Peripheral neuropathy Retinopathy Uveitis
GAD-65	82% females, 33–80 years old	Neuroendocrine tumors	Limbic encephalitis Cerebellar degeneration Stiff person syndrome
Amphiphysin	60% males, mean age 64 years	Small cell lung cancer; breast and ovarian cancers	Encephalomyelitis Stiff person syndrome Cerebellar degeneration

Syndromes Involving Synaptic and Other Neuronal Surface Antibodies

Antibody and Antigen	Patient Demographics	Associated Tumors	Neuropsychiatric Features
NMDAR	80% females, mostly children, teens, young adults	Ovarian teratoma	Encephalitis Hallucinations Delusions Seizures Abnormal movements Coma Dysautonomia Respiratory arrest

TABLE 28-1 • Paraneoplastic Syndromes. (*Continued*)

Syndromes Involving Synaptic and Other Neuronal Surface Antibodies

Antibody and Antigen	Patient Demographics	Associated Tumors	Neuropsychiatric Features
AMPAR	90% females, adults to elderly	Lung, breast, and thymus cancers	Limbic encephalitis with prominent psychiatric features
GABA-B-R	60% males, mean age 62 years	Small cell lung cancer (50%), breast cancers, thymoma	Limbic encephalitis Severe seizures Opsocolonus-myoclonus Ataxia
GABA-A-R	5 of 6 males, median age 22 years	Hodgkin's lymphoma (1 of 6 high titer pts)	Status epilepticus or epilepsia partialis continua
LGI1	65% males, median age 60 years	Thymoma (<10%)	Encephalitis Fasciobrachial dystonic seizures Myoclonus (40%)
Caspr2	85% males, median age 60 years	Thymoma	Neuromyotonia Encephalitis Morvan's syndrome
GlyR	6 of 11 females, ages 5–69 years	Hodgkin's lymphoma (1 out of 11)	Stiff person syndrome PERM
mGluR5	15-year-old male, 46-year-old female	Hodgkin's lymphoma	Limbic encephalitis Ophelia syndrome
mGluR1	Males and females, 19–69 years	Hodgkin's lymphoma, prostate adenocarcinoma	Cerebellar degeneration
NDER (anti-Tr)	50% males, 12–73 years; 80% are males <45 years old	Hodgkin's lymphoma (90%)	Cerebellar degeneration

guidance and possibly synapse function. Both anti-CRMP5 and anti-CV2 antibodies recognize the CRMP5 antigen, and the presence of these antibodies may accompany anti-Hu antibodies in patients with SCLC. Presentation may include cerebellar ataxia and peripheral neuropathy in addition to symptoms of PLE. Notably, chorea characterized by involuntary movements often involving the face, optic neuritis, uveitis, and abnormalities of olfaction and taste occur in high frequencies with these antibodies.[71] Other notable symptoms in these patients include subacute dementia, personality changes, depression, mania, confusion, psychosis, and obsessive-compulsive behavior. Inflammation of the basal ganglia and their circuits may cause personality changes, obsessive-compulsive behavior, and cognitive decline.[76]

Because many patients have psychiatric changes and chorea, differentiating this disorder from Huntington's disease or Wilson's disease is important given the distinct approach to treatment and potential underlying tumor.[71] Outcomes are less clear for patients with anti-CV2/CRMP5 antibodies than for those with anti-Hu and anti-Ma2 antibodies. One study described improvement of chorea with tumor treatment, immunotherapy, and antipsychotics, with 50% of patients surviving 4–42 months after the onset of chorea.[71]

Anti-Amphiphysin
Anti-amphiphysin antibodies have been detected in patients with SCLC and breast cancer. Anti-amphiphysin antibodies have been implicated in cases of Stiff person syndrome, especially when it occurs comorbidly with PLE.[73] In these patients there is a strong association with female gender, breast cancer,

advanced age, and EMG abnormalities. The condition in these patients may respond to steroids and improve following cancer treatment.[82] Other disorders associated with these antibodies include cerebellar degeneration, myelopathy, peripheral neuropathy, and myoclonus.[74]

Anti-Yo/PCA-1
Anti-Yo (type-1 anti-Purkinje-cell) antibodies have been associated with paraneoplastic cerebellar degeneration (PCD).[73] This condition is often associated with breast and gynecological cancers but has also been found in the context of Hodgkin's lymphoma, SCLC, gastric cancer, esophageal cancer, prostate cancer, bladder cancer, and melanoma. Of note, there are multiple autoantibodies associated with PCD in addition to anti-Yo, namely anti-Hu, anti-Ri, anti-Tr, anti-voltage-gated calcium channel, anti-Ma, anti-Ta/Ma2, anti-collapsin receptor mediator protein 5/CV2, anti-mGluR1, anti-carbamylated protein VIII, anti-Zic family, and anti-ANNA3. Anti-Yo, however, is the most commonly identified antibody associated with PCD.

Anti-Yo antibodies target a cytoplasmic antigen in the Purkinje cells of the cerebellum, leading to extensive destruction of Purkinje cells. Patients typically present with cerebellar deficits that evolve over a period of weeks to months. Deficits include trunk and limb ataxia, dysmetria, dysarthria, nystagmus, diplopia, and vertigo, which often predates the cancer diagnosis. Nearly all patients reach a plateau in symptom severity within 6 months from the onset of symptoms. Most become wheelchair or bed bound. CSF examination may show lymphocytic pleocytosis, elevated protein, increased CSF IgG relative to serum, and oligoclonal banding. MRI is typically normal or shows subtle nonspecific changes. Cerebellar atrophy may be seen later in the course of illness. Diagnosis can be made by detection of anti-Yo in serum or CSF. Treatment of the malignancy does not reliably alter the course of the neurological syndrome. Patients with PCD have a poor prognosis with reduced survival time and little evidence of neurological improvement with current treatment strategies.[83]

Paraneoplastic Syndromes with Cell-Surface Antigens

Antibodies that attack cell membrane antigens have also been identified. These cell-surface antigens include voltage-gated potassium channels, NMDA glutamate receptors, alpha-amino-3-hydroxy-5-methyl-4-isoxazolepropionic acid (AMPA) receptors, gamma-aminobutyric acid type B (GABA-B) receptors, and others (Table 28-1).[68,74]

Voltage-Gated K Channels

VGKC-complex antibody encephalitis is caused by antibodies that target proteins associated with the VGKC complex: leucine-rich glioma inactivated 1 (LGI1) and contactin-associated protein-like 2 (CASPR2).[69,77] In these patients, pathological changes were observed in the medial temporal lobes with varying degrees of atrophy and cognitive outcomes.[69,84,85] In a study of 42 VGKC encephalitis patients, medial temporal lobe structures were uni- or bilaterally enlarged and hyperintense on T2/FLAIR images in 79% of patients, involving both the hippocampus and amygdala.[69,86] Almost 50% of patients developed hippocampal sclerosis.[69]

Antibodies against voltage-gated potassium channels are usually associated with non-PLE, but they can occur in the context of an underlying tumor (20% with SCLC or thymoma). This condition usually affects middle-aged or older patients, who develop severe verbal and visual memory deficits and confusion or disorientation. Seizures are common with symptoms such as faciobrachial dystonic jerking movements, but CSF pleocytosis is rare. Behavioral changes are frequent and often include apathy and irritability. Symptoms may occur with signs of autonomic dysfunction such as excess sweating and salivation. Visual hallucinations have been reported but seem to be rare. Limbic encephalitis caused by antibodies against voltage-gated potassium channels responds rapidly to immunotherapy. About 80% of patients improve neurologically and radiologically following prompt (within 2 months) treatment with high-dose steroids, IVIG, or plasma exchange. The majority of patients will still experience short-term memory deficits.[71]

Anti-NMDAR

NMDARs are ionotropic glutamate receptors with roles in synaptic transmission and plasticity and neuropsychiatric disease.[71] NMDARs have been proposed to play a pivotal role in executive functions and memory.[87] Encephalitis with antibodies against the NMDAR is among the most frequent forms of autoimmune encephalitis.[69,88] NMDAR encephalitis, first described in 2007, is the most common form of autoimmune encephalitis in those under 30.[74] While the exact prevalence is unknown, one study has estimated an incidence of 0.85 per million children per year in the United Kingdom.[89] Women are most commonly affected

with a median age of 21 years, but children as young as 2 months and adults as old as 85 years have been reported.

The hippocampus, which contains the highest density of NMDARs in the human brain, appears to be the most affected brain structure in NMDAR encephalitis.[69] Finke et al.[90] studied a sample of 40 patients recovering from anti-NMDAR encephalitis and found that patients with anti-NMDAR encephalitis had hippocampal subfield atrophy and impaired microstructural integrity of the hippocampus. However, all brain structures can be affected by the disease.

The clinical syndrome typically develops subacutely in stages which resolve in reverse order. Initially, neuropsychiatric manifestations develop and can be misinterpreted as evidence of a primary psychiatric condition, with approximately 75% of patients described with this disorder having been seen by a psychiatrist or admitted to a psychiatric unit. This initial presentation is followed by depressed level of consciousness alternating with episodes of agitation and catatonia. Patients then develop abnormal movements and autonomic dysfunction that may lead to hypoventilation, requiring medical ventilation.[74]

Patients with this condition are typically young women (75%) or children (40% younger than 18 years) with prominent psychiatric symptoms, including anxiety, agitation, bizarre behavior, delusional or paranoid thoughts, and auditory or visual hallucinations. In the pediatric population, patients may present with temper tantrums, behavioral changes, agitation, aggression, and progressive speech deterioration. About 50% of patients experience a viral prodrome-like illness. Patients rapidly deteriorate neurologically with seizures, decreased consciousness, progressing to a catatonic-like state with dyskinesias, autonomic instability, hypoventilation, and coma. Seizures are commonly seen, and the EEG is abnormal in many patients. The extreme delta brush pattern on EEG may be identified in NMDAR encephalitis.[74]

MRI findings are unreliable with approximately half of patients having no abnormalities and only 15% with specific signals in the medial temporal lobes.[71] Brain MRI can reveal nonspecific T2 hyperintense lesions in the frontal, parietal, or mesial temporal lobes and occasionally in the basal ganglia of one-third of patients.[69,74] PET imaging may show increased frontotemporal uptake, and decreased occipital uptake.[74]

NMDAR encephalitis was previously thought to be specifically associated with ovarian teratomas. The classical cases were typically young women presenting with encephalitis and dermoid cysts or teratomas of the ovary who tended to progress through a series of stages as described above.[73] As a result of advances in detection and recognition of this syndrome, about 50% of diagnoses of NMDAR encephalitis are now associated with teratomas, and many do not have an identifiable tumor. When identified, tumors should be removed without delay.[74] Rarely, NMDAR encephalitis is associated with carcinomas.

Patients with NMDAR encephalitis often recover with treatment, with nearly 50% making a full recovery following tumor resection and immunotherapy. In this regard, the presence of a tumor is a positive prognostic factor. Patients with tumor removal within 4 months of neuropsychiatric changes have better outcomes: immunotherapy and tumor removal leads to substantial improvement in 80% of patients when started early in disease.[69,91] Recovery from this condition is often slow, and it may take months for patients to return to their baseline behavioral and cognitive status.[71]

Anti-AMPA

The AMPA-type glutamate receptor mediates the majority of fast glutamatergic neurotransmission in the brain and plays a role in molecular mechanisms of learning and memory. In Anti-AMPA encephalitis, the GluR1 and GluR2 subunits of the AMPA receptor are targeted. AMPA receptors subsequently become internalized and redistributed away from the synapse. Almost all patients with anti-AMPA receptor encephalitis presented with isolated limbic symptoms: subacute memory loss (less than 8 weeks) and confusion. Other common symptoms include agitation, aggressive behavior, and behavioral changes. About 90% of reported cases were women, the median age is around 60 years, and 70% of patients had an associated tumor of the breast or lung, or thymoma. Patients who received cancer and immunotherapy treatments responded well with reduced cognitive and behavioral symptoms. However, 70% of patients experienced relapsing symptoms with deficits of short-term memory and persistent behavioral problems in the absence of tumor or tumor recurrence, suggesting that a persistent autoimmune disorder had been triggered.[71] Brain MRI may show T2/FLAIR hyperintensity in the mesial temporal lobes and cortical thickening; PET may show increased uptake in the temporal lobes.[74]

Anti-GABA-B

Anti-GABA-B receptors have been identified in patients with PLE and appear to be associated with lung and neuroendocrine cancer. Patients with these antibodies have presented with symptoms of limbic encephalitis, seizures, confusion, and severe memory abnormalities. Brain MRI may show T2 hyperintensity in the mesial temporal lobes; PET may show increased uptake in the temporal lobes.[68,74]

Assessment and Differential Diagnosis of Paraneoplastic Syndromes

Paraneoplastic syndromes should be considered when there is an acute onset of neurological or psychiatric symptoms and signs of inflammation in the CSF examination.[67]

Diagnosis of PLE is confirmed by pathological demonstration of limbic encephalitis with paraneoplastic antibodies, or by the combination of subacute onset of symptoms of short-term memory loss, seizures, or other psychiatric symptoms; a cancer diagnosis within 4 years of the onset of neuropsychiatric symptoms; exclusion of other etiologies of limbic dysfunction; and evidence of limbic encephalopathy on EEG, MRI, or CSF studies.[73]

When PLE is suspected, the following tests should be considered (i) MRI of the brain with and without contrast, (ii) paraneoplastic antibody testing of serum and CSF, (iii) CSF studies to rule out the presence of metastatic cells and demonstrate the presence of inflammatory abnormalities (oligoclonal bands, intrathecal synthesis of IgG, pleocytosis), and (iv) EEG studies, particularly in patients with an acute confusional state of unknown cause.

Brain PET imaging may be pursued, when available—although it lacks diagnostic specificity, it may be more sensitive than MRI in detecting abnormalities in autoimmune encephalitis. Regarding autoantibody testing, given the considerable overlap between autoimmune encephalitis syndromes, it may be important to test comprehensive panels.[74]

Imaging

In patients with PLE, unilateral or bilateral T2 hyperintense lesions in the medial temporal lobes, including the hippocampus, were observed in the majority of patients and accompanied by extralimbic cortical and subcortical alterations in up to 40%.[55,57,73,79–81] In 15–25% of patients, gadolinium contrast-enhancement was observed, indicating increased BBB permeability.[69] In a serial MRI study of patients with limbic encephalitis, swelling of medial temporal lobe structures was observed initially and followed by progressive atrophy, while hyperintensity persisted in most patients.[69,92] Post-inflammatory atrophy of the hippocampus contributes to persistent memory impairment and neurologic disability, representing a large part of the chronic disease burden.[69,93] These findings (progressive hippocampal gyrus volume loss upon repeat imaging) have been confirmed in other studies, which additionally note frequent findings of unilateral or bilateral medial temporal lobe hyperintensities on fluid-attenuated inversion recovery (FLAIR) images.[71]

18F-fluoro-2-deoxy-D-glucose (FDG)-positron emission tomography (PET) imaging significantly increases the sensitivity for abnormalities in limbic encephalitis and can show medial temporal lobe hypometabolism or hypermetabolism even in normally appearing temporal lobe structures on MRI.[69,94,95] FDG-PET often shows extralimbic abnormalities in the brainstem, cerebellum, or cerebral cortex, and seems to correlate more closely with clinical symptoms than MRI.[69,85]

The PLE syndromes more likely to present with features of limbic encephalitis and corresponding T2/FLAIR hyperintense signal alterations in the medial temporal lobes (e.g., hippocampus) include those with antibodies directed against LGI1, GABA-B receptors, AMPA receptors, GAD, and a subset of patients with CASPR2 antibodies. These syndromes are contrasted by frequently normal MRI in the NMDAR and DPPX encephalitis, extensive multifocal or widespread diffuse abnormalities in GABA-A receptor encephalitis, and basal ganglia lesions in dopamine D2R encephalitis.[69]

Despite the severity of the disease, routine structural MRI may be normal in the majority of patients with NMDAR encephalitis even in the acute disease stage. When changes are present, they are typically subtle and may include small white-matter lesions that do not correspond to the clinical syndrome. Some findings may overlap with other conditions; for example, HSV encephalitis may initially have a similar appearance to PLE on MRI. However, HSV encephalitis progresses to gross edema with mass effect and inflammation involving one or both inferior-medial temporal lobes, the inferior frontal lobes, and the cingulate gyrus.[73] Additionally, patients with HSV encephalitis may have gyral enhancement, and signs of hemorrhage are also common.[67] Thus, clinical routine imaging has only helped to exclude further differential diagnoses but has not allowed detection of disease-specific structural changes.[90]

Electroencephalography (EEG) may not be as useful for diagnosis of paraneoplastic syndrome, but is important to rule out seizures. Typical EEG shows background slowing of electrical activity or sharp-wave activity, or rarely a temporal lobe epileptic focus. Therefore the main utility of EEG is in assessing whether changes in the level of consciousness or behavior are related to temporal lobe seizures.[67]

CSF

CSF analysis is helpful for diagnosing PLE. Patients with PLE have normal glucose levels on lumbar puncture, however 75% of cases have an elevated protein level and 60% of cases have a predominance of mononuclear inflammatory cells.[73] Additionally, a negative cytological analysis for malignant cells in combination with the absence of meningeal enhancement on MRI helps to exclude leptomeningeal metastases. The detection of inflammatory abnormalities (pleocytosis, intrathecal synthesis of IgG, oligoclonal bands) supports the diagnosis of an inflammatory or immune-mediated neurological disorder. For example, the CSF of patients with PLE often shows a mild lymphocytic pleocytosis.[71] In a study by Gultekin et al.,[67] 64% of patients with PLE had one or more of these aforementioned abnormalities.

Differential Diagnosis

Despite the large number of patients reported, the diagnosis of PLE remains difficult. Presenting symptoms may be different from those considered typical of the disorder (short-term memory loss, seizures, and mood/behavioral changes).[67] Moreover, symptoms resembling PLE are frequent in cancer patients and may result from multiple different metastatic and non-metastatic complications.[55,83-86] For example, symptoms of cognitive and psychiatric dysfunction may be attributable to brain metastasis, treatment-induced side effects, or metabolic encephalopathies. Viral encephalopathies, including HSV and human herpesvirus (HHV)-6, and autoimmune conditions such as SLE and antiphospholipid syndrome, can also present with similar symptoms.[73]

Since symptoms of PLE mimic many of those seen in delirium, PLE will most likely enter the differential diagnosis in atypical cases (recurrent seizures, eye motility dysfunction, hypoventilation), those without an identifiable etiology commonly associated with delirium (infection, metabolic disturbance, intracranial process), or those that do not respond to treatments typically effective for delirium (neuroleptic administration).[67,73,95]

Several disorders may present with symptoms resembling PLE. These include systemic lupus erythematosus, Wernicke-Korsakoff encephalopathy with or without cancer, toxic effects of doxifluridine (an antineoplastic agent), and herpes simplex encephalitis.[67] As touched upon previously, patients with herpes simplex encephalitis usually develop acute or subacute mental confusion and seizures that often lead to stupor or coma. MRI findings and presence of RBCs in the CSF favor the diagnosis of herpes simplex encephalitis over PLE and a diagnosis of HSV can be confirmed by PCR analysis of the CSF or brain biopsy for the virus.[67]

This chapter describes conditions that are known to this date. There may be new paraneoplastic syndromes that are waiting to be discovered. If a patients symptoms do not seem to match the conditions being described, the reader may want to consider sending out for research testing.

Treatment of Paraneoplastic Syndromes

There is no definitive treatment available for paraneoplastic syndromes.[71] Combined efforts to eradicate the malignancy and suppress the immune reaction have been demonstrated to decrease morbidity and mortality.[73,87] Primary cancer treatments, including chemotherapy, radiation, and surgical removal of the tumor, help to remove the antigen source and optimize prognosis.[73,87] Immunosuppressive interventions, including the use of corticosteroids and cyclophosphamide, may help to minimize autoimmune response and neural inflammation. Studies of plasma-exchange and IVIG administration have not demonstrated significant efficacy, although these therapies are invariably still used in many circumstances. The exception to this rule is NMDAR encephalitis, for which every other day plasma exchange with albumin is a category I indication, with grade 1C levels of evidence for efficacy.[97] To reduce the risk of irreversible neuronal damage, it is recommended that treatment be instituted immediately after diagnosis.[73]

Unfortunately, there is a lack of information regarding management of neuropsychiatric symptoms caused by paraneoplastic syndromes. Management is limited to a relatively nonspecific, symptoms-based approach, often with limited success.[73]

There are a limited number of case reports describing the use of antipsychotic medications in patients with paraneoplastic syndromes. In one case report of PLE due to a mediastinal seminoma, haloperidol was administered to a patient with paranoid delusions, resulting in decreased severity of delusions.[73] However, the patient subsequently developed a dystonic reaction and haloperidol was discontinued.[73] In another case report, a patient with Hodgkin's lymphoma presented with symptoms of delirium including hypersomnolence, agitation, disorientation, paranoia, and visual hallucinations. These symptoms were unresponsive to treatment with haloperidol, olanzapine, quetiapine, or chlorpromazine.[73,98] Several case reports support the possible efficacy of ECT in the treatment of PLE-associated catatonia.[73]

NEUROPSYCHIATRIC SYMPTOMS ASSOCIATED WITH BRAIN TUMORS

Mood symptoms are common in patients with brain tumors. Many patients experience worsening depressive or anxiety symptoms as part of an adjustment disorder. Patients may experience depressed, anxious, or irritable mood, disappointment and frustration in the context of receiving bad news, loss of control, loss of independence, and physical or cognitive limitations.

Anxiety

Anxiety is one of the most commonly cited affective disturbances associated with cancer.[31] Approximately 62% of patients with brain tumors experience anxiety symptoms prior to surgery.[32] Patients with cancer may experience ruminations, fear of the unknown, fear of progression, and worry about what the next imaging study will show. Piil et al.[20] conducted a longitudinal study of patients with newly diagnosed high-grade gliomas and found that anxiety and emotional well-being improved over time for 1-year survivors; their data correlates emotional distress and anxiety with the postsurgical period.

A few studies have investigated the presence and characteristics of anxiety in patients with primary brain tumors. Arnold et al.[99] reported 48% of 363 patients with primary brain tumors had generalized anxiety disorder according to responses on a modified brief patient health questionnaire. In a study by Gregg et al.,[24] 71% of frontal tumor patients reported clinical levels of anxiety compared with 30.7% of non-frontal tumor patients as assessed by the HADS anxiety subscale. Interestingly, anxiety or panic attacks have been reported to be present before diagnosis of a brain tumor.[9] There have been reports of adult patients presenting with obsessional symptoms or specific phobias with brain tumors located in the frontal, temporal, or parietal regions of the brain.[9]

Depression

Major depressive disorder can affect up to 20% of brain tumor patients in the first 8 months after diagnosis.[21] While the prevalence of clinically significant depressive symptoms in patients with brain tumors is 15–44%,[9,32] depression often remains undiagnosed.[21]

Predictors of depression or anxiety in brain tumor patients may include female sex, lower WHO grade tumor, previous psychiatric history, and lower education level and these factors are independently associated with a higher incidence. Other predictors of depression may include frontal location and a family history of psychiatric illness.[7] Brain tumor histology and grade of malignancy can affect the production and release of biological factors that cause depressive symptoms.[20]

Patients with glioma have especially high rates of depression. For patients with high-grade gliomas, the prevalence of depression has been reported to be as high as 95% at a mean of 46 months following diagnosis.[100] Men with glioma have the highest risk of all cancer patients for psychiatric hospitalization in the year following glioma diagnosis. In these patients, depression is a strong risk factor for suicide and epilepsy.[9]

Depression has been associated with physical functional impairments, cognitive impairments, reduced quality of life, higher mortality, greater frequency of medical complications, and reduced work productivity.[9] Treating depression may reduce the risk of suicide and has been shown to reduce personal and/or family suffering.[21]

Mania

Satzer and Bond[1] reviewed case reports on mania in patients with brain tumors and found no evidence of correlation between tumor type and risk of mania. The majority (81%) of tumors were located in or produced mass effect on the frontal lobe, temporal lobe, or subcortical limbic structures. An additional 13% involved the pons, which contains serotonergic and noradrenergic cell bodies. There was a strong preponderance (~75%) of right-hemisphere involvement, while 6% were bilateral, 13% affected midline structures, and 6% the left hemisphere.[1]

Trauma/PTSD

Rates of severe PTSD symptomatology range from 1.4% to 17% in childhood cancer survivors and 9.8–44% in their parents.[99] Of note, rates of PTSD in childhood brain tumor survivors are considerably greater than other childhood cancer survivors, suggesting brain tumor survivors are at higher risk of developing PTSD.[101]

Cognitive Deficits

Cognitive deficits are common in patients with brain tumors, affecting 50–90% of patients.[3,5,23] These deficits are often present at the time of brain tumor diagnosis and persist as a long-term effect in brain tumor survivors.[5,23] Cognitive deficits are the major causes of disability for patients with brain tumors and have been noted to be the greatest source of burden for caregivers.[23,100] Cognitive impairments have been identified as independent predictors of shorter survival and worse health status.[23]

Most patients with brain tumors suffer from cognitive deficits involving language, memory, attention, executive functions, and speed of information processing.[102] Similarly, a systematic review of four studies in the past decade found that brain tumor survivors exhibited poorer cognitive performance on most measures in contrast to non-cancer control groups.[5] The cognitive deficits most reproducible across studies were in working memory, cognitive control and flexibility, cognitive processing speed, visual searching, planning and foresight, and general attention.[5]

Cognitive complaints are often associated with persistent fatigue and depressive symptoms, making it challenging to sort out whether the complaints of poor memory, attention, and difficulties with multitasking were related to brain dysfunction or were the manifestation of an uncontrolled mood disorder.[103] Patients undergoing chemotherapy tend to have a high degree of fatigue as a side effect of treatment, and patients with cancer have an increased risk of depression, anxiety, and other mood disorders, all of which can have a negative and interacting effect on cognitive function.[104]

Cognitive problems can be present before treatment and exacerbated by physiological distress and physical symptoms, compounding any cognitive effects of chemotherapy.[105–108]

Fatigue

Fatigue is frequently reported as the most troublesome factor affecting quality of life in brain tumor patients (more so than pain, nausea, or vomiting). Fatigue is associated with an adverse prognosis and is more commonly associated with high-grade than low-grade tumors.[109] Multiple factors may cause or contribute to fatigue in patients with brain tumors, including antiepileptic medications, radiation therapy, chemotherapy, anemia, depression, hypothyroidism, hypocortisolism, weight gain (related to inactivity and chronic steroid use), and sleep apnea. Usually, the sleep apnea is obstructive rather than central, but brainstem tumors can present with central sleep apnea. Sleep disturbances may also contribute to fatigue; there is a high prevalence and severity of both insomnia and drowsiness in brain tumor patients, with some evidence supporting increased risk for somnolence post-radiotherapy.[110] Treatment approaches toward managing fatigue in patient with brain cancer have limited clinical data and the principles are similar to managing cognitive deficits/chemobrain and these are discussed later in the chapter.

Seizures

Seizures are more commonly witnessed in association with low-grade gliomas than in higher-grade tumors or in brain metastases. Patients with low-grade gliomas have a better prognosis but may live for long periods of time with this significant comorbidity that invariably requires lifetime treatment with antiepileptics. Poorly controlled seizure disorders can have a particularly devastating psychological impact on patients, who may already have lost many of their social and occupational roles due to the burdens of treatment and are then additionally rendered unable to drive or to be alone with dependent children.

NEUROPSYCHIATRIC SIDE EFFECTS OF CANCER TREATMENTS

Radiotherapy

Whole brain radiation therapy (WBRT) involves 2–3 weeks of daily treatment during which the patient must lie very still for 20–30 minutes. This treatment modality is used in the setting of multiple metastatic brain lesions and active extracranial disease.

Many patients (perhaps over 60%) develop long-term learning or memory side effects which appear to be correlated with dose to the hippocampus or temporal lobes.[111] Given the low incidence of metastases in the hippocampus, hippocampal-sparing techniques are being investigated but have not yet been adopted as standard practice.[112] Late complications of WBRT include hearing loss (which may increase risk for delirium in the setting of other medical insults) and endocrinopathies especially hypothyroidism, hyperprolactinemia, and hypogonadism.

Stereotactic radiosurgery (SRS) involves one to five sessions of high-dose radiation (lasting an hour or more) to a targeted area of the brain. SRS tends to have fewer side effects compared to WBRT since it spares areas of normal brain and areas of the brain involved in neurogenesis, especially hippocampal and limbic areas. Acute side effects of SRS include headaches, nausea, vomiting, worsening of neurological deficits, and seizures. Over the long term, there is a small risk of radiation necrosis and cognitive deficits.

Due to the need for precise delivery of radiation, the patient's head must be completely immobilized during treatment, usually with a thermoplastic mask specifically molded to the patient's head and neck. The immobilization device is fixed to the table

---

CASE VIGNETTE 28.2

A 61-year-old woman with HER2-positive metastatic breast cancer status post whole brain radiation therapy completed 4 years prior to the brain MRI shown in Figure 28-1, as well as subsequent SRS to a right frontal lesion. Her clinical presentation was notable for marked cognitive slowing and mild frontal-executive dysfunction. At the time of this scan, her MoCA score was 26/30, and she was being treated with long-acting methylphenidate for fatigue and low-dose mirtazapine for depression. In subsequent years, she developed profound psychomotor slowing and frontal/executive dysfunction, ultimately meeting criteria for a subcortical dementia presumably due to prior whole brain radiotherapy exposure. She also has marked hearing impairment as a sequelae of whole brain radiation therapy.

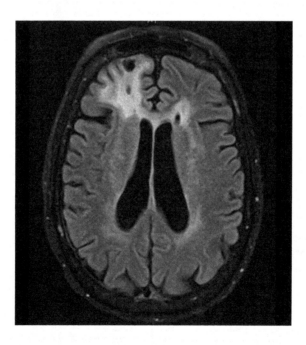

FIGURE 28-1. Brain MRI (T2 axial FLAIR sequence) showing gliosis in the right frontal lobe status postsurgical resection and stereotactic radiosurgery, as well as generalized atrophy.

to reduce patient motion. In this context it is not surprising that panic attacks, specific phobias (particularly claustrophobia), and even reactivation of PTSD may occur in the context of radiation treatments.[111] Sometimes difficulty tolerating the mask can result in treatment delays, interruptions, or even cessation; history of panic attacks and psychoactive medication use are risk factors associated with interruption of radiotherapy.[113]

Corticosteroids

Corticosteroids were first used in the late 1940s. Shortly after, case reports of mood disturbances, psychosis, and suicide associated with the use of corticosteroids started to appear in the literature.[114] Patients with brain tumors are commonly treated with steroids for cerebral edema and may be on steroids chronically. Corticosteroid administration has been associated with changes in the hippocampus and other brain regions.[114]

Neuropsychiatric symptoms from corticosteroids generally emerge soon after starting treatment and resolve within a few weeks of discontinuing the steroids.[115] Median onset is about 12 days after starting treatment. Fifty percent of symptoms resolve within 2 weeks and 90% resolve within 6 weeks of discontinuation.[115]

The risk of neuropsychiatric symptoms with corticosteroids is dose-dependent. There is a 20% incidence of psychiatric disturbances with prednisone doses >80 mg/day. Eighty milligrams of prednisone is equivalent to 12 mg of dexamethasone. Most patients with CNS tumors are on at least 16 mg of dexamethasone daily to treat significant symptomatic edema, and are therefore at high risk of psychiatric symptoms.[115] Past psychiatric history does not necessarily predict whether patients will experience psychiatric symptoms with corticosteroids. Some studies suggest that women may be at higher risk for psychiatric symptoms from corticosteroids, although the data remain mixed.[115]

Steroids most commonly cause affective symptoms. With short-term use, milder symptoms may include anxiety and insomnia, whereas more severe cases may present with hypomania or mania. Depression can be seen with long-term use.[115]

Cognitive deficits and psychosis may also occur in the context of corticosteroid use, but are less common.[115] Data from animal studies support a dose-dependent negative effect of corticosteroids on associative learning, spatial working memory, and long-term potentiation.[114] In humans, cognitive deficits have been observed in both clinical samples and healthy controls given corticosteroids. The most frequently reported cognitive changes associated with corticosteroid exposure involve declarative memory, which is thought to be a hippocampal-dependent process.[114] Concentration is also often impaired.

Treatment of Steroid-Related Psychiatric Complications

Atypical antipsychotics such as olanzapine and quetiapine are often used for insomnia, irritability, and mood lability. Other medications used for symptomatic management may include antidepressants and mood stabilizers. Removal or reduction of corticosteroid exposure can be helpful for reducing the severity of neuropsychiatric symptoms; however, gradual tapers are generally recommended. Patients can become steroid-dependent, and rapid tapers can contribute to worsening neuropsychiatric symptoms including rebound fatigue, depression, and irritability. These symptoms will typically subside within 2–8 weeks after discontinuation.[115]

Immunotherapy

Cancer immunotherapy refers to biological therapy targeted at activating the innate immune response to cancer.[116] Immunotherapies that increase the immune response against tumor cells are frequently associated with neurovegetative symptoms including fatigue, psychomotor slowing, and anorexia.[116,117] The symptoms appear to be closely related to the so-called "sickness behavior," caused by activation of inflammatory cytokines, which is commonly characterized by fatigue, anhedonia, low mood, social isolation, and irritability.[116,118] Sickness behavior is thought to be an adaptive response to promote healing and enhance survival by reducing energy expenditure and decreasing exploratory behavior. However, these symptoms can contribute to decreased quality of life and limit patients' ability to engage in and complete treatment.[116]

Interferons

The interferon family refers to a diverse group of cytokines with oncologic, immunoregulatory, and antiviral activity.[119,120] Interferon alpha (IFN-α) has been the most frequently studied immunotherapy treatment. IFN-α is a natural cytokine, with a synthetic version: IFN-α-2b. IFN-α and IFN-α-2b bind to IFN type I receptors, activating a signal transduction pathway leading to the expression of multiple genes responsible for the inhibition of tumor cell growth and proliferation.[114,119] IFN-α has been used to treat cancers including malignant melanoma and hairy cell leukemia.[116,122,123]

Common CNS side effects include headache, somnolence, cognitive slowing, and personality changes. Depression, mania, movement disorders, visual dysfunction, and other neuropsychiatric symptoms can also occur.[120] Neuropsychiatric side effects appear to be dose-related and are more common in patients who are elderly or who have underlying brain disease.[120] Symptoms generally resolve after discontinuation of the drug (Table 28-2).[120]

Interleukins

The interleukins (IL) are another family of cytokines with immunomodulatory and antineoplastic properties. IL-2 is utilized primarily in the treatment of metastatic melanoma and renal cell carcinoma. It is known to increase capillary permeability, which can lead to increased peritumoral edema and an elevation of ICP in patients with primary and metastatic brain tumors. Symptoms can include headache, nausea, vomiting, seizures, exacerbation of focal deficits, and somnolence. Other neuropsychiatric symptoms including depression, delusions, hallucinations, cognitive impairment, and focal neurologic deficits have also been noted. MRI may be normal or reveal multifocal regions of high signal abnormality on T2 images. In most cases, symptoms resolve after discontinuation of IL-2 (Table 28-2).[120]

Other Agents: Checkpoint Inhibitors and Chimeric Antigen Receptor (CAR) T-Cells

By blocking proteins that inhibit the host immune response, checkpoint inhibitors enhance the ability of the human immune system to recognize and target abnormal cells. Ipilimumab is a monoclonal antibody against cytotoxic T cell lymphocyte antigen (CTLA)-4, which limits the duration of T cell activity

TABLE 28-2 • CNS Side Effects of Monoclonal Antibodies and Immunotherapy Treatments.

Brentuximab	Progressive multifocal leukoencephalopathy (PML)
Blinatumomab	Seizures, encephalopathy, cerebellar symptoms
Rituximab	Headaches, myalgias, dizziness, PML
Chimeric antigen receptor (CAR) T-cell therapy	Headaches, encephalopathy, ischemia, seizures—related to inflammatory cytokines
Interferon-alpha	Depression, cognitive slowing; occasionally mania
Interleukin-2	Depression, cognitive impairment, psychosis
Bevacizumab	Ischemic stroke, intratumoral hemorrhage, posterior reversible leukoencephalopathy syndrome (PRES) (via hypertension)
Ipilimumab	Hypophysitis (up to 17%); rarely PRES
Pembrolizumab	Hypophysitis; rarely, PRES, limbic encephalitis, intracranial vasculitis

when it binds to ligands on antigen-presenting cells (APCs). Nivolumab and pembrolizumab are monoclonal antibodies against PD-1. Tumor cells express PD-1 ligands to evade antitumor immune responses, and therefore, PD-1 blockade may enhance activation of T cells with greater selectivity for tumor.

In CAR T-cell therapy, T cells are removed from the patient, genetically modified (usually by retroviral transduction), and then infused back into the patient as targeted treatments for leukemia/lymphoma.

Checkpoint inhibitors cause a variety of toxicities (rash, colitis, hepatitis) that may require treatment with steroids; most of the associated neuropsychiatric side effects are related to the concomitant steroid therapy, with the exception of hypophysitis, which may lead to adrenal insufficiency and depression/fatigue.[124]

CAR T-cell therapy is associated with cytokine release syndrome in 20–43% of patients, presenting with fatigue, fever, tachycardia, hypotension, nausea, capillary leak, and sometimes cardiac/hepatic/renal dysfunction. A subset of these patients will also have neurological toxicity including confusion, seizures, and aphasia. Although this is an emerging therapy, and more evidence is needed, these toxicities seem to be short-lived and not associated with permanent neurological sequelae (Table 28-2).[125]

Chemotherapy-Associated Cognitive Dysfunction

Epidemiology

Advances in cancer therapy, stemming from the development of novel chemotherapeutic agents and regimens, have contributed to decreased cancer recurrence and higher survival rates. This increased cancer survival, in turn, has led to increased awareness of chemotherapy adverse effects.[126,127] Normal cells, organs, and the CNS are susceptible to treatment toxicities, and chemotherapy-related cognitive dysfunction is recognized as a significant problem.[128,129] "Chemobrain" was a term originally used by breast cancer patients to describe a sense of mental "fogginess," or slowing down of cognitive processing from chemotherapy.[98,120-123]

This constellation of symptoms affects most cancer patients, with approximately 60–75% at some point experiencing mild cognitive deficits in memory, attention, psychomotor speed and executive functioning.[98,120-126] Long-term posttreatment cognitive changes persist only in a subgroup (17–34%) of cancer survivors.[111,129,130] Chemotherapy-related cognitive impairments can lead to significant challenges for patients as they try to resume day-to-day life.[111,137] Adjunctive medications including corticosteroids, antiepileptic medications, and immunosuppressive agents, may compound chemotherapy-related impairments in cognition.[109]

Pathophysiology

The etiology of chemotherapy-related cognitive dysfunction is being elucidated. It is thought to result from combined effects of direct damage to neural tissues and systemic causes.[118,136] Hypothesized mechanisms include repeated neuronal injury with inadequate repair, abnormal brain remodeling, neuro-endocrine-immunological changes, vascular injury, oxidative damage, inflammation, autoimmune responses, and chemotherapy-induced anemia.[129,130,138,139]

The BBB provides some protection from systemic chemotherapy,[111] however chemotherapy can affect the brain through direct or indirect toxicity leading to cognitive deficits.[125,130-134] Some cytotoxic drugs are unable to cross the BBB to cause direct damage, but are able to produce cognitive effects through systemic inflammation.[111] Other agents are able to gain access to the CNS and can directly contribute to toxicity.[128,129] Studies have described alterations in the BBB that allow increased access of cytotoxic agents to vulnerable neurons.[127] Those agents that cross the BBB concentrate their effects on cell proliferation.[144] Decreased cell proliferation and cell death appear to be especially pronounced in the hippocampus.[145] Thus, direct-acting agents impair cognitive performance especially for tasks that depend on the hippocampus.[145]

Optimal cognitive functioning relies on integrity of neuronal cells as well as cortical and subcortical structures interconnected by white-matter pathways forming a structural network.[146] Impairment to this structural network can have detrimental effects on cognition.[146] Functional and structural brain changes have been observed in patients exposed to chemotherapy.[125,138-142,157] Neuroimaging studies suggest that cognitive changes associated with chemotherapy correlate with structural changes in the frontal cortex and related white-matter tracts, which are implicated in executive and memory function.[127,151] Short-term cognitive changes after chemotherapy may also be attributable to temporary declines in neurogenesis in the hippocampus.[120,152,153] Chemotherapy-induced changes in white matter may also be caused by white-matter demyelination, especially with later-onset cognitive changes and persistent longer-term cognitive deficits.[124,144-147]

In long-term follow-up studies, the white- and gray-matter loss seen after termination of chemotherapy[141] partially returns to baseline, but persistent decrease in gray-matter volume predominantly in the frontal cortex leading to hypoactivation can be seen in some patients.[147–152] The mechanism of longitudinal recovery from cognitive deficits remains poorly characterized, and while remyelination can be seen, it is unclear whether this reflects axonal reorganization.[135]

Several risk factors for neurotoxicity with chemotherapy have been identified with the level of cognitive impairments correlating with the intensity of chemotherapy.[120,129] Significant risk factors include exposure to high-dose regimens, concurrent radiotherapy, intraarterial administration with BBB disruption, or intrathecal administration.[129] Older age may be linked to a higher vulnerability to chemotherapy treatment, slower recovery of white-matter damage, and less exposure to cognitive challenges stimulating recovery.[135,140,162]

Determining the biggest offenders among various chemotherapy agents is difficult because many agents are used in combination with other treatment modalities and medications. Certain agents such as methotrexate, platinum-based agents, and 5-fluorouracil are known to be particularly neurotoxic and have been shown to cause diffuse white-matter changes in neuroimaging (Table 28-3).[109,128] Cisplatin, carmustine, and cytarabine may be more toxic to white-matter progenitor and hippocampal stem cells.[109] Mice treated with cisplatin have been shown to have decreased white-matter integrity, reduced dendritic spine density and neuronal arborization, and cognitive dysfunction.[146] Cisplatin at both low and high concentrations has also been shown to regulate the exocytotic ability of cells, resulting in impaired neural communication at the neurotransmitter level.[146] Longer-term cognitive deficits (>20 years after treatment) are associated with cyclophosphamide, methotrexate, and fluorouracil.[120,156]

Psychological and medical factors, beyond chemotherapy exposure, can also contribute to cognitive problems.[131,138,140,163,164] Jung et al. conducted a prospective study of women treated for breast cancer and age-matched healthy controls; they found that the trajectory of fMRI-detected changes in neurocognitive executive network function from preadjuvant treatment to 1 year post-baseline was worse for women who received chemotherapy compared to controls. However, they also observed executive network abnormalities before any adjuvant treatment, suggesting that adverse neurocognitive outcomes are not entirely due to chemotherapy treatment.[163] An explanation for this finding is that neuroinefficiency prior to chemotherapy may be related to physiological distress after cancer diagnosis, proinflammatory responses to disease, surgery, or treatment-related symptoms such as fatigue.[105,106,108,163,165]

Inflammation/Cytokines

Chemotherapy and other cancer treatments can result in the production of various cytokines.[109] For example, many clinical studies have shown that chemotherapy increases levels of TNF alpha, IL-6, IL-8, IL-10, and MCP-1, and that these increases are correlated to cognitive dysfunction.[166] Research has established that circulating proinflammatory cytokines impair learning and memory.[109] Animal studies show that proinflammatory cytokines increase neurotransmitter metabolism, including noradrenaline, dopamine, and serotonin, which are central to

TABLE 28-3 • Neurological Side Effects of Chemotherapy Treatments.	
Vinca alkaloids (vinblastine, vincristine)	Peripheral neuropathy, autonomic neuropathy, seizures, SIADH
Small molecule inhibitors (axitinib, imatinib)	Peripheral neuropathy
Angiogenesis inhibitors (bevacizumab, sunitinib, regorafenib)	Somnolence, peripheral neuropathy
Platinums (carboplatin, cisplatin)	Peripheral neuropathy with sensory ataxia, lhermitte symptoms, ototoxicity
Antimetabolites (cytarabine, 5-fluorouracil, gemcitabine, fludarabine)	Headaches, cognitive difficulties, PRES, leukoencephalopathy
Alkylating agents (cyclophosphamide, melphalan, dacarbazine)	Encephalopathy, peripheral neuropathy
Intrathecal chemotherapy (methotrexate, cytarabine, thiotepa)	Aseptic meningitis, transverse myelopathy, encephalopathy

Source: Bradshaw and Linnoila[74]; Lancaster[190]; and Höftberger et al.[191]

the regulation of memory, learning, sleep, and mood.[109] Cancer patients who receive immunotherapy of IL-2 or interferon-alpha (IFN-α) experience cognitive dysfunction, depression, and fatigue.[166] Patients undergoing chemotherapy with taxanes or anthracycline containing regimens for breast, ovarian cancer, and Hodgkin's disease have statistically significant increases in IFN-α, IL-1β, IL-6, IL-8, IL-10, and MCP-1.[166]

The mechanisms by which peripheral cytokines exert their cognitive effects remain unclear. Recent studies demonstrate significant bidirectional communication between peripherally released cytokines and cytokines in the brain through (1) active transport into the brain across the BBB, (2) passive crossing through leaky regions in the BBB at circumventricular organs, and (3) stimulation of central cytokine release by peripheral cytokines via microglial cell production of proinflammatory cytokines and inflammatory mediators.[109] This communication between peripheral cytokines and cytokines inside the CNS may partly explain why cognitive dysfunction is not limited to patients with treatments directly targeting the brain.[109]

Cytokine changes may initiate alterations in neurotransmitter systems and neuronal integrity by inducing exocytotoxic glutamate receptor-mediated damage, altering monoaminergic systems (5-HT, DA, and NE), GAA, acetylcholine, neuropeptides, and nerve growth factors (BDNF), which are directly associated with cognitive function and neurodegenerative processes. Chemotherapeutic injury may also lead to overproduction of reactive oxygen species (ROS) and reactive nitrogen species (RNS) and produce further oxidative stress via the nitric oxide (NO) pathway.[166]

Genetic Effects

Chemotherapy may induce changes through DNA damage directly or through increased oxidative stress, leading to shortening of telomeres, accelerating cell aging, contributing to cytokine dysregulation, inhibiting hippocampal neurogenesis, or reducing brain vascularization and blood flow.[119,156–158]

There is some early evidence to support the role of epigenetic change in chemobrain. Learning and memory impairments following CMF (cyclophosphamide, methotrexate, 5-fluorouracil) chemotherapy were found to be associated with increased histone H3 acetylation and decreased DHAC (histone deacetylase) activity in the hippocampus. This chromatin remodeling leads to a decrease in neural cell proliferation in the hippocampus that might be the plausible mechanism that explains persistent cognitive dysfunction after chemotherapy, as the DNA methylation induced by cytokines is transient and reversed in 2 weeks after cytokines are removed from the environment.[166,170] It has been hypothesized that the administration of chemotherapy agents initiates a cascade of biologic changes, with short-lived alterations in the cytokine's milieu inducing persistent epigenetic alterations. These epigenetic changes eventually lead to changes in gene expression, altering metabolic activity and neuronal transmission, which are responsible for generating the subjective experience of cognition.[166]

An association between the development and persistence of chemotherapy-induced neuropsychological disorders and epigenetic changes following chemotherapy treatment was recently demonstrated in breast cancer patients. The transient methylation for a subset of genes seen after chemotherapy only persisted in patients who developed persistent neuropsychological symptoms.[166]

Genetic variability in genes that regulate neural repair and/or plasticity, such as apolipoprotein E4 and brain-derived neurotrophic factor (BDNF), genetic variability in genes that regulate neurotransmission, such as catechol-*O*-methyltransferase (COMT), or genetic variability in BBB transporters, such as protein P-glycoprotein, may increase an individual's vulnerability to chemotherapy-induced cognitive changes.[119,160–162] Small doses of chemotherapy can cause cell death and reduce cell division in brain structures crucial for cognition.[129,143] Other individual variables such as age and pretreatment cognitive reserve have also been associated with post-chemotherapy cognitive decline.[129,158]

Unfortunately data supporting these proposed mechanisms are limited.[129,169,171] Trying to understand the pathophysiology of chemotherapy-induced cognitive impairment has become a major challenge.[111] Considerable research is underway to identify biological mechanisms by which chemotherapy alters neural function.[163]

Most studies so far have been conducted on patients with breast cancer or lymphomas because these cancers tend to have the highest rates of long-term survival. Relatively little is known about cognitive side effects caused by treatments for cancers with poorer prognosis, such as pancreatic cancer.[111]

Clinical Presentation of Chemotherapy-Related Cognitive Dysfunction

Cognitive domains affected by "chemobrain" are variable across patients.[109] In general, the magnitude of impairment in cognitive functioning posttreatment is modest.[103] Chemotherapy-induced cognitive effects often include deficits in processing speed, executive functions, and working memory.[129,172] Multiple studies have reported subtle but significant impairments in memory, processing speed, and executive function among patients receiving chemotherapy in comparison to control subjects.[120] Typical concerns include memory lapses, difficulty concentrating, trouble remembering details (e.g., names, dates, telephone numbers), difficulty multitasking, slower processing speeds, and difficulty with word retrieval.[109] The symptoms of "chemobrain" consist of deficits in attention, learning, working memory and executive function, and an overall reduction in processing speed.[145] Many breast cancer survivors complain of increased difficulties with multitasking and slower mental processing time.[138,173] These cognitive deficits become more noticeable once cancer survivors try to resume normal activities and return to work, particularly for those in intellectually demanding occupations.[138,173]

Problems with working memory, concentration, and word finding can have a devastating effect on patients' personal and professional lives.[111] Cognitive symptoms can have a significant impact on daily functioning of an individual, resulting in changes to their health status, occupational performance, and well-being.[136] Cognitive symptoms may impact employment, finances, and relationships and may be a source of strain for patients and their families.[136,174] Chemobrain may affect cancer survivors' social relationships. Cancer survivors have reported withdrawing from social situations to avoid feelings of embarrassment about the effects of their chemobrain symptoms, thus causing changes in social relationships with family, friends, and colleagues.[138]

For most patients, cognitive impairment improves over a period of 6–9 months following systemic chemotherapy.[109] In many cases the symptoms resolve quickly when treatment is concluded, while some patients report long-term problems.[111] Cognitive deficits may persist >20 years after treatment (in particular with cyclophosphamide, methotrexate, and fluorouracil).[120,156]

There is currently no evidence on the most effective way to manage chemobrain symptoms and at what stage of treatment interventions should begin.[136] Clinically, we have found it useful to provide psychoeducation to patients and families about the mechanism of chemotherapy-induced cognitive dysfunction. One of the authors often shows patients a figure from a study depicting functional neuroimaging results during a working memory task in identical twins, one of whom had received chemotherapy for breast cancer, and the other of whom was cancer free. Both twins performed equally well on the executive function task, but the twin who received chemotherapy had to activate a much larger area of the brain in order to do so, potentially accounting for the experience of cognitive fatigue.[134] Pharmacological approaches toward management of chemobrain symptoms are discussed later in the chapter in treatment for cognitive symptoms section.

ASSESSMENT AND DIFFERENTIAL DIAGNOSIS OF NEUROPSYCHIATRIC SYMPTOMS IN CANCER PATIENTS

Assessment of Mood Symptoms

It is important to assess for the presence of neuropsychiatric illness in patients with brain tumors. The gold standard for diagnosing depression is a structured clinical interview conducted by a mental health specialist. However, routine use of screening instruments for depression and anxiety in patients with brain tumors may result in more effective detection and treatment intervention. Scales such as the PHQ-9 and GAD-7 with high sensitivity may be used for monitoring the course of reported mood symptoms. Significant depressive symptoms can be identified using rating scales that employ cutoff scores to estimate the likelihood of depression and are easy to administer[21]; for example, the Hospital Anxiety and Depression Scale (HADS) is considered to be a more accurate screening measure of depression in glioma, as it minimizes somatic symptoms.[24]

Assessment of Cognitive Symptoms

Both subjective (such as symptom report, self-report scales) and objective modes (such as Mini Mental State Examination [MMSE], Montreal Cognitive Assessment [MoCA]) of neuropsychological assessment are important. Objective assessments help patients and caregivers understand their current strengths and weaknesses and adjust to illness-induced limitations. Subjective complaints are valuable indicators of patients' general well-being and functioning.[23]

Cognitive deficits are not restricted to the brain area in which the tumor lesion is located (local damage) but are often related to global dysfunction of the brain with multifactorial origin due to tumor location, peritumoral invasion, and treatment neurotoxicity.[102] Given the association of cognitive function with age, education level, and gender, it is often difficult to identify the extent to which cognitive deficits are related to the brain tumor and treatment or to these demographic variables.[5]

Cognitive decline may be a reliable indicator of brain tumor progression, even before the tumor progression becomes evident on brain imaging studies.[23] Assessment of neuropsychological functioning before brain tumor treatment initiation and at subsequent treatment phases may be used as an indicator of disease severity and progression, among others.[23]

Patients with brain tumors will often underreport or overreport the extent of their cognitive difficulties, contributing to discrepancies between subjective complaints and objective findings.[23] In a study of 169 patients with low-grade gliomas, underreporting of symptoms was found to be more prevalent in patients with more severe objective impairment, while overreporting was associated with depression and other psychiatric symptoms.[23] Andrewes et al.[2] surveyed 32 post-surgery brain tumor patients and 29 patients following extracerebral surgery. Patients and care givers were asked to rate the patient's psychological well-being and their own level of distress. When compared with the control group, patients with brain tumors were more likely to underestimate their psychological problems, and the negative impact of changes to their emotional function, interpersonal relationships, cognition, and coping skills. It was thought that this may be due to reduced insight related to brain impairments, denial (a common coping mechanism used by oncology patients with a poor prognosis), or a combination of these factors. Underestimation of psychological and

interpersonal problems by brain tumor patients explained 35% of the variance in their care giver's anxiety.

Another study by Ownsworth et al. had contradictory results. They found that brain tumor patients tend to overestimate their functional impairments compared to their care givers. Of note, 40% of patients had been diagnosed with high-grade malignant tumors in this study, compared to 85% in the Andrewes et al.[2] study. This may suggest that patients with higher-grade malignant tumors associated with a poorer prognosis, shorter expected survival may present a greater decline of cognition and insight and greater degree of denial.[2]

It is important to evaluate for other potential causes of cognitive impairments. Laboratory evaluation should be requested and may include thyroid, vitamin B12, folate, hemoglobin A1c, and calcium tests.[137]

A variety of self-reporting tools have been used.[103] Patients should be formally screened for cognitive impairments using serial cognitive assessments, such as the MoCA. A score of <23 warrants attention by a neurologist, psychiatrist, or geriatric physician as this often indicates pathology beyond what would be expected with chemobrain; scores must also be interpreted in the context of baseline educational level and cognitive capacity.[137] Clinically, we find it extremely useful to perform a baseline MoCA in cancer patients and to repeat MoCA serially in order to monitor for progression of cognitive symptoms. Discussing MoCA findings and correlating them to brain lesion localization when applicable also help patients and families achieve a more integrated understanding of subjectively experienced cognitive deficits.

Referral for neuropsychological testing depends on the patient's functional or work status and degree of distress, as this testing is expensive, time consuming,[137] and access to formal testing may be limited in certain areas. Referrals are warranted for patients who have difficulties functioning at home or at work because of chemotherapy-related cognitive impairment.[137] Unfortunately, most neuropsychological evaluations involve tasks that may lack ecological validity.[135,175] There are few methods of measuring chemobrain symptoms using observable functional activities.[136] There is a need for a more ecologically valid method for testing and monitoring of neurocognitive function in cancer survivors complaining of cognitive changes.[138]

Neuropsychological Testing: It may support the need for pharmacological and nonpharmacological treatment, including cognitive rehabilitation or psychological support.[102] The reader may also wish to review the Chapter 7, *Neuropsychological Evaluation in Neuropsychiatry.*

Capacity Assessment: A large proportion of patients with brain tumors have impaired capacity to make treatment decisions and to provide consent for research clinical trials. This highlights the importance of early careful assessment of cognitive function in this population, especially given that most of these patients will experience physical decline and tumor progression.[20] Likewise, preoperative neuropsychological evaluation of brain tumor patients is clinically important when planning for rehabilitation, social adjustment, and return to work for the patients whose tumors are deemed curable.[23]

PHARMACOLOGICAL TREATMENTS FOR NEUROPSYCHIATRIC SYMPTOMS IN CANCER PATIENTS

Treatment of Emotional Symptoms

Depression

There are no randomized controlled trials evaluating the adequate treatment of depression in brain tumor patients. Interventions should consist of both psychotherapy and pharmacotherapy.[9] There is currently no high-quality evidence as to whether pharmacological treatments for depression in patients with brain tumors are effective—for instance, no studies have evaluated the benefit or harm of pharmacological treatment of depression in patients with a primary brain tumor.[21] Best practice would suggest that doctors treating depression in patients with brain tumors discuss the lack of evidence with the patient, document the discussion, and use their clinical judgment regarding whether to initiate a psychotropic medication. If pharmacological treatment is started, close follow up may help detect adverse effects. There is also a lack of evidence about the possible adverse effects of antidepressants specifically in patients with brain tumors, so physicians should be extra vigilant.

Antidepressants are nonetheless recommended based on expert consensus as first-line treatment for moderate-to-severe depression. The pharmacological classes of antidepressants are selective serotonin reuptake inhibitors (SSRIs), serotonin norepinephrine reuptake inhibitors (SNRIs), the tricyclic antidepressants (TCAs), monoamine oxidase inhibitors (MAOIs), and atypical antidepressants (mirtazapine, bupropion). Other drug classes including psychostimulants and acetylcholinesterase inhibitors have been proposed for use in patients with brain tumors. Antidepressants may reduce depressive symptoms in healthier patients, but in the physically ill a limited response to treatment and high relapse rates are common.[21]

Caudill et al.[176] conducted a retrospective cohort study of the frequency and toxicity of SSRI prescription among 160 glioblastoma patients presenting to a tertiary neuro-oncology service over a 10-year period. Being prescribed SSRIs was associated with improved survival at 2 years post-diagnosis. Patients being prescribed an SSRI reported similar levels of toxicities as those not on an SSRI. However, antidepressant prescription was uncontrolled and the study was not limited to depressed patients.[21]

Side effects of antidepressants should be considered. Antidepressants may lower the seizure threshold, impair memory, or contribute to fatigue.[21]

Anxiety

There is little controlled data on the treatment of anxiety in patients with brain tumors and metastases; treatment decisions are generally made based on clinical judgment and extrapolation of data from other medically ill populations. SSRIs, SNRIs, buspirone, and atypical agents (mirtazapine) are also considered first line for management of anxiety. It is advisable to avoid benzodiazepines because of the risk of delirium in patients with a poor cognitive substrate. Low-dose atypical antipsychotics and propranolol may be utilized instead for episodic anxiety. Bupropion is somewhat controversial because of its potential risk of lowering the seizure threshold, but low doses can be safe and effective in the absence of uncontrolled seizures.

Mania/Disinhibition/Aggression

Antipsychotics and benzodiazepines are effective for the emergency management of disinhibited, agitated, or aggressive behavior. Patients with brain lesions may be at higher risk of extrapyramidal symptoms, oversedation, and paradoxical disinhibition, and lower medication doses and close monitoring are warranted. Second-generation antipsychotics are preferred over first-generation antipsychotics because of their lower propensity for extrapyramidal side effects (EPS). Case series and reports suggest that second-generation antipsychotics and mood stabilizers (generally valproate over lithium in patients receiving chemotherapy, due to the risk of fluid shifts and consequent lithium toxicity) are effective in treating core manic symptoms; though to our knowledge there are no supportive RCTs. Further supporting the use of valproate, intriguing preclinical data suggest that valproate may inhibit the growth of GBM cells.[177] Combination treatment with mood stabilizers and atypical antipsychotics may be necessary for severe mania. ECT is also effective for severe or treatment-refractory mania, but neurological/neurosurgical consultation should be sought to ensure it is safe in the presence of brain disease.[1] Levetiracetam (often utilized for seizures in this population) may cause irritability and depression, which can be addressed by cross-tapering to lamotrigine or valproate depending on the clinical situation.

Treatments for Cognitive Symptoms

Pharmacologic therapies for chemotherapy-related cognitive impairment include stimulants such as methylphenidate and amphetamine compounds, modafinil, armodafinil, and donepezil.[137]

Recent placebo-controlled studies for methylphenidate, modafinil, and armodafinil in primary brain tumor patients have had negative results.[175-177] Similarly, a randomized double-blind placebo-controlled trial of the stimulant D-methylphenidate in breast cancer patients failed to demonstrate a benefit for this medication in the prevention and treatment of cognitive impairments.[109,180] A major limitation of this study is that it was underpowered. Despite these negative findings, clinicians often prescribe stimulants and modafinil, occasionally with some benefit, and therefore unless there are contraindications (such as structural heart disease in the case of stimulants) we recommend empirical trials of these agents. Of note, neuro-oncologists do not generally have major concerns about either agent lowering seizure threshold, so they can be utilized as long as seizures are presently well-controlled.

Modafinil is a stimulant medication approved by the FDA for treatment of narcolepsy, shift work sleep disorder, and excessive daytime sleepiness associated with obstructive sleep apnea. There is anecdotal evidence for its use in patients with chemobrain; however, no studies with cognition as a primary endpoint in patients with brain tumors have been published.[109] Clinical practice and literature support the use of modafinil as a first-line pharmacologic approach, although evidence is not compelling and the risk of side effects, drug interactions, and cost may limit the use of this medication on a broad scale.[137]

Some clinicians have employed donepezil based on positive open label phase 2 studies in both adults and children with brain tumors.[179,180] Unfortunately, a more recent phase 3 study was negative on the primary outcome, which involved delayed recall.[181] In this study, donepezil was administered 6 months after the completion of brain radiation, so there is ongoing interest in investigating it as prophylaxis for cognitive deficits.

A large randomized, placebo-controlled trial assessed memantine for prophylaxis of cognitive deficits in patients who were undergoing WBRT. It revealed that memantine slowed decline in multiple cognitive domains compared with placebo.[182] As a result, many radiation oncologists are administering memantine prior to WBRT.

NONPHARMACOLOGIC TREATMENTS FOR NEUROPSYCHIATRIC SYMPTOMS IN CANCER PATIENTS

Physical and psychological symptoms burden could be modified by evidence-based, targeted interventions such as cognitive-behavioral therapy to treat depressive and anxiety symptoms, and educational interventions for specific symptom management.[163,183,184] Cognitive-behavioral strategies may include relaxation training, enhancement of coping skills, sleep hygiene, and education.[109] Mindfulness, meditation, yoga, and relaxation breathing are used in a variety of treatment settings.[137]

Cognitive rehabilitation therapy delivered by an occupational therapist or speech-language pathologist can be helpful. Cognitive function may be improved with a multifaceted cognitive rehabilitation program, which includes computer-based attention retraining and compensatory skills training of attention, memory, and executive functioning.[3] This intervention is likely underutilized in patients with chemobrain and brain cancers despite its demonstrated efficacy in patients with brain injury and stroke. Physical and occupational therapists can play an important role in facilitating cognitive rehabilitation, helping patients return to work and to maintain their quality of life.[136] Executive function training may help to improve any co-occurring attention and working memory problems.[163,185,186] Cognitive rehabilitation can be particularly helpful for families because it often provides them with guidance on how to environmentally manage their loved one's deficits.

In studies of breast cancer survivors, brain fitness exercises improved objective (memory/processing speed) and subjective cognitive function.[185,187] EEG biofeedback improved subjective cognitive function, sleep, fatigue, anxiety/depression in a wait-list control trial.[188] In addition, socialization has been recommended by experts as cognitively protective.[137]

Summary and Key Points

- **Primary brain tumors** are uncommon (0.6% lifetime incidence) but present significant neuropsychiatric morbidity, in part due to their localizations which are most commonly in the frontal and temporal lobes. Low-grade tumors, while more indolent, are often complicated by seizure disorders; high-grade tumors confer a poor prognosis.
- **Metastatic brain tumors** have increased in prevalence as systemic cancer treatments improve and overall survival lengthens. Lung cancer, breast cancer, and melanoma are the most common causes of brain metastases. Neuropsychiatric morbidity is common, including depression, anxiety, fatigue, and cognitive deficits, and (less commonly) mania/psychosis sometimes related to steroid treatments.
- **Leptomeningeal disease** is a unique variant of metastatic brain cancer. It is an uncommon but devastating complication of systemic cancer which often confers a poor prognosis, which makes it important to be vigilant in patient with active metastatic disease.
- **Paraneoplastic syndromes** often precede a cancer diagnosis and thus their related neuropsychiatric symptoms can also precede a cancer diagnosis. They are heterogeneous in nature and difficult to treat.
- **Neuropsychiatric symptoms of brain tumors** such as anxiety, depression, mania, PTSD, cognitive dysfunction, and fatigue are common. They can cause significant distress when untreated and their impact can be significant. Early intervention and treatment can improve quality of life significantly for both patients and their care givers.
- **Neuropsychiatric side effects of cancer treatments** are also common. Whole brain radiation therapy can produce significant short-term memory deficits and cognitive slowing, including a dementia in long-term survivors. Chemotherapy may result in frontal-executive dysfunction, also informally called chemobrain, which is generally milder in nature. Antiepileptic drugs, steroids, and immunotherapies confer potential neuropsychiatric toxicities as well. Pharmacologic treatments include stimulants, modafinil, and antidepressants/mood stabilizers depending on the side effects and symptoms in question. Nonpharmacological treatments include cognitive rehabilitation therapy, exercise, and mindfulness meditation.
- **Assessment and evaluation** for neuropsychiatric complication is important and should be considered routine part of treatment for patients with brain tumors. Objective testing should be used to track trends in symptoms and is preferred over subjective assessment.
- **Pharmacological and behavioral treatment** approaches can help in management of symptoms.
- Cancer in general and brain cancer in particular is a devastating and often deadly illness, which affects not only the brain and its circuitry, but an individual's life, work, family, and identity. Our sincere hope is that improved knowledge of brain circuits, cytokines, genetic polymorphisms, and targeted cancer therapies will eventually ameliorate cancer-related complications afflicting the brain.

Multiple Choice Questions

1. For which medication does emerging data support efficacy in prophylaxis of cognitive deficits due to whole brain radiotherapy?
   a. Donepezil
   b. Memantine
   c. Methylphenidate
   d. Escitalopram
   e. Modafinil

2. Which antibody is typically associated with paraneoplastic syndromes in women with ovarian teratomas?
   a. Anti-AMPA
   b. Anti-Hu
   c. Anti-NMDAR
   d. Anti-Ro
   e. Anti-amphiphysin

3. What is the most common primary tumor location to metastasize to the brain?
   a. Breast carcinoma
   b. Prostate carcinoma
   c. Ovarian cancer
   d. Lung carcinoma
   e. Malignant melanoma

4. Which of the following tumor locations in the brain is most often associated with neuropsychiatric effects?
   a. Temporal lobe
   b. Occipital lobe
   c. Parietal lobe
   d. Hippocampus
   e. Frontal lobe

Multiple Choice Answers

1. **Answer: b**
   A large randomized, controlled placebo trial assessed memantine for prophylaxis of cognitive deficits in patients who were undergoing whole brain radiation therapy. That study revealed that memantine slowed decline in multiple cognitive domains compared with placebo,[182] and as a result, many radiation oncologists are now administering memantine prior to whole brain radiation therapy.

2. **Answer: c**
   The classical cases of NMDA receptor encephalitis are typically young women who present with encephalitis due to dermoid cysts or teratomas of the ovary and tend to progress through a series of stages: prodromal symptoms, a psychotic stage, unresponsiveness with hypoventilation, autonomic instability and dyskinesia, and eventual recovery or progression to death.[73]

3. **Answer: d**
   In adults, lung carcinomas such as SCLC and adenocarcinomas account for 50% of metastatic brain tumors. Breast cancers account for about 15% with a higher risk in ER negative, Her-2/neu positive tumors. Melanoma account for about 5–10% cases, and it has very high likelihood of metastasis.

4. **Answer: e**
   The frontal lobe is the most common location for brain tumors, and also associated with the greatest number of neuropsychiatric side effects.[24] Lesions in the frontal lobe can produce personality changes, apathy, executive dysfunction, apathy, and rarely even mania. They produce a great amount of distress in both patients and their caregivers, often due to associated lack of insight of the patient into these changes.

References

1. Satzer D, Bond DJ. Mania secondary to focal brain lesions: implications for understanding the functional neuroanatomy of bipolar disorder. *Bipolar Disord.* 2016;18(3):205-220.
2. Andrewes HE, Drummond KJ, Rosenthal M, et al. Awareness of psychological and relationship problems amongst brain tumour patients and its association with carer distress. *Psychooncology.* 2013;22(10):2200-2205.
3. Perkins A, Liu G. Primary brain tumors in adults: diagnosis and treatment. *Am Fam Physician.* 2016;93(3):211-217.
4. De Robles P, Fiest KM, Frolkis AD, et al. The worldwide incidence and prevalence of primary brain tumors: a systematic review and meta-analysis. *Neuro-Oncology.* 2015;17(6):776-783.
5. Gehrke A, Baisley M, Sonck A, et al. Neurocognitive deficits following primary brain tumor treatment: systematic review of a decade of comparative studies. *J Neurooncol.* 2013;115(2):135-142.
6. Belyi BI. Mental impairment in unilateral frontal tumours: role of the laterality of the lesion. *Int J Neurosci.* 1987;32(3-4):799-810.
7. Wellisch DK, Kaleita TA, Freeman D, et al. Predicting major depression in brain tumor patients. *Psychooncology.* 2002;11(3):230-238.

8. Irle E, Peper M, Wowra B, et al. Mood changes after surgery for tumors of the cerebral cortex. *Arch Neurol*. 1994;51(2):164-174.

9. Mainio A, Hakko H, Niemelä A, et al. Depression in relation to anxiety, obsessionality and phobia among neurosurgical patients with a primary brain tumor: a 1-year follow-up study. *Clin Neurol Neurosurg*. 2011;113(8):649-653.

10. Gathinji M, McGirt MJ, Attenello FJ, et al. Association of preoperative depression and survival after resection of malignant brain astrocytoma. *Surg Neurol*. 2009;71(3):299-303; discussion 303.

11. Litofsky NS, Farace E, Anderson F, et al. Depression in patients with high-grade glioma: results of the Glioma Outcomes Project. *Neurosurgery*. 2004;54(2):358-366; discussion 366-367.

12. Hahn CA, Dunn RH, Logue PE, et al. Prospective study of neuropsychologic testing and quality-of-life assessment of adults with primary malignant brain tumors. *Int J Radiat Oncol Biol Phys*. 2003;55(4):992-999.

13. Brown PD, Ballman KV, Rummans TA, et al. Prospective study of quality of life in adults with newly diagnosed high-grade gliomas. *J Neurooncol*. 2006;76(3):283-291.

14. Rooney AG, Carson A, Grant R. Depression in cerebral glioma patients: a systematic review of observational studies. *J Natl Cancer Inst*. 2011;103(1):61-76.

15. Jamieson RC, Wells CE. Manic psychosis in a patient with multiple metastatic brain tumors. *J Clin Psychiatry*. 1979;40(6):280-283.

16. Cummings JL, Mendez MF. Secondary mania with focal cerebrovascular lesions. *Am J Psychiatry*. 1984;141(9):1084-1087.

17. Starkstein S, Boston J, Robinson R. Mechanisms of mania after brain injury: 12 case reports and review of the literature. *J Nerv Ment Dis*. 1988;176(2):87-100.

18. Madhusoodanan S, Opler MG, Moise D, et al. Brain tumor location and psychiatric symptoms: is there any association? A meta-analysis of published case studies. *Expert Rev Neurother*. 2010;10(10):1529-1536.

19. Louis D, Perry A, Reifenberger G, et al. The 2016 World Health Organization classification of tumors of the central nervous system: a summary. *Acta Neuropathol (Berl)*. 2016;131(6):803-820.

20. Piil K, Jakobsen J, Christensen K, et al. Health-related quality of life in patients with high-grade gliomas: a quantitative longitudinal study. *J Neurooncol*. 2015;124(2):185-195.

21. Rooney A, Grant R. Pharmacological treatment of depression in patients with a primary brain tumour. *Cochrane Database Syst Rev*. 2010;3(3):CD006932.

22. Anic G, Madden M, Nabors L, et al. Reproductive factors and risk of primary brain tumors in women. *J Neurooncol*. 2014;118(2):297-304.

23. Pranckeviciene A, Deltuva VP, Tamasauskas A, et al. Association between psychological distress, subjective cognitive complaints and objective neuropsychological functioning in brain tumor patients. *Clin Neurol Neurosurg*. 2017;163:18-23.

24. Gregg N, Arber A, Ashkan K, et al. Neurobehavioural changes in patients following brain tumour: patients and relatives perspective. *Support Care Cancer*. 2014;22(11):2965-2972.

25. Chipkevitch E. Brain tumors and anorexia nervosa syndrome. *Brain Dev*. 1994;16(3):175-179.

26. Goddard E, Ashkan K, Farrimond S, et al. Right frontal lobe glioma presenting as anorexia nervosa: further evidence implicating dorsal anterior cingulate as an area of dysfunction. *Int J Eat Disord*. 2013;46(2):189-192.

27. Trummer M, Eustacchio S, Unger F, et al. Right hemispheric frontal lesions as a cause for anorexia nervosa: report of three cases. *Acta Neurochir (Wien)*. 2002;144(8):797-801.

28. Wessling H, Simosono CL, Escosa - Bage M, et al. Anton's syndrome due to a giant anterior fossa meningioma. The problem of routine use of advanced diagnostic imaging in psychiatric care. *Acta Neurochir (Wien)*. 2006;148(6):673-675.

29. Glantz MJ, Chamberlain MC, Liu Q, et al. Gender disparity in the rate of partner abandonment in patients with serious medical illness. *Cancer*. 2009;115(22):5237-5242.

30. Papagno C, Mattavelli G, Casarotti A, et al. Defective recognition and naming of famous people from voice in patients with unilateral temporal lobe tumours. *Neuropsychologia*. 2018;116(pt B):194-204.

31. Moitra E, Armstrong CL. Neural substrates for heightened anxiety in children with brain tumors. *Dev Neuropsychol*. 2013;38(5):337-351.

32. Richter A, Woernle CM, Krayenbühl N, et al. Affective symptoms and white matter changes in brain tumor patients. *World Neurosurg*. 2015;84(4):927-932.

33. Schrepf A, Lutgendorf SK, Pyter LM. Pre-treatment effects of peripheral tumors on brain and behavior: neuroinflammatory mechanisms in humans and rodents. *Brain Behav Immun*. 2015;49:1-17.

34. Takei H, Rouah E, Ishida Y. Brain metastasis: clinical characteristics, pathological findings and molecular subtyping for therapeutic implications. *Brain Tumor Pathol*. 2016;33(1):1-12.

35. Gavrilovic I, Posner J. Brain metastases: epidemiology and pathophysiology. *J Neurooncol*. 2005;75(1):5-14.

36. Shi AA, Digumarthy SR, Temel JS, et al. Does initial staging or tumor histology better identify asymptomatic brain metastases in patients with non-small cell lung cancer? *J Thorac Oncol*. 2006;1(3):205-210.

37. Nussbaum ES, Djalilian HR, Cho KH, et al. Brain metastases. Histology, multiplicity, surgery, and survival. *Cancer*. 1996;78(8):1781-1788.

38. Soffietti R, Cornu P, Delattre JY, et al. EFNS guidelines on diagnosis and treatment of brain metastases: report of an EFNS Task Force. *Eur J Neurol*. 2006;13(7):674-681.

39. Majer M, Samlowski W. Management of metastatic melanoma patients with brain metastases. *Curr Oncol Rep*. 2007;9(5):411-416.

40. Amer MH, Al-Sarraf M, Baker LH, et al. Malignant melanoma and central nervous system metastases: incidence, diagnosis, treatment and survival. *Cancer*. 1978;42(2):660-668.

41. Hjiyiannakis P, Jefferies S, Harmer CL. Brain metastases in patients with differentiated thyroid carcinoma. *Clin Oncol*. 1996;8(5):327-330.

42. Kolomainen DF, Larkin JMG, Badran M, et al. Epithelial ovarian cancer metastasizing to the brain: a late manifestation of the disease with an increasing incidence. *J Clin Oncol*. 2002;20(4):982-986.

43. Tremont-Lukats IW, Bobustuc G, Lagos GK, et al. Brain metastasis from prostate carcinoma. *Cancer*. 2003;98(2):363-368.

44. Beauchesne P. Intrathecal chemotherapy for treatment of leptomeningeal dissemination of metastatic tumours. *Lancet Oncol*. 2010;11(9):871-879.

45. Tsukada Y, Fouad A, Pickren JW, et al. Central nervous system metastasis from breast carcinoma. Autopsy study. *Cancer*. 1983;52(12):2349-2354.

46. Aroney RS, Dalley DN, Chan WK, et al. Meningeal carcinomatosis in small cell carcinoma of the lung. *Am J Med*. 1981;71(1):26-32.

47. Amer MH, Al-Sarraf M, Vaitkevicius VK. Clinical presentation, natural history and prognostic factors in advanced malignant melanoma. *Surg Gynecol Obstet*. 1979;149(5):687-692.

48. Frisk G, Svensson T, Bäcklund LM, et al. Incidence and time trends of brain metastases admissions among breast cancer patients in Sweden. *Br J Cancer*. 2012;106(11):1850-1853.

49. Kesari S, Batchelor T. Leptomeningeal metastases. *Neurol Clin.* 2003;21(1):25-66.

50. Fox BD, Cheung VJ, Patel AJ, et al. Epidemiology of metastatic brain tumors. *Neurosurg Clin North Am.* 2011;22(1):1-6.

51. Groves MD. New strategies in the management of leptomeningeal metastases. *Arch Neurol.* 2010;67(3):305-312.

52. Tosoni A, Franceschi E, Brandes AA. Chemotherapy in breast cancer patients with brain metastases: have new chemotherapic agents changed the clinical outcome? *Crit Rev Oncol Hematol.* 2008;68(3):212-221.

53. Balm M, Hammack J. Leptomeningeal carcinomatosis: presenting features and prognostic factors. *Arch Neurol.* 1996;53(7):626-632.

54. Wasserstrom WR, Glass JP, Posner JB. Diagnosis and treatment of leptomeningeal metastases from solid tumors: experience with 90 patients. *Cancer.* 1982;49(4):759-772.

55. Clarke JL, Perez HR, Jacks LM, et al. Leptomeningeal metastases in the MRI era. *Neurology.* 2010;74(18):1449-1454.

56. Waki F, Ando M, Takashima A, et al. Prognostic factors and clinical outcomes in patients with leptomeningeal metastasis from solid tumors. *J Neurooncol.* 2009;93(2):205-212.

57. Boyle R, Thomas M, Adams JH. Diffuse involvement of the leptomeninges by tumour—a clinical and pathological study of 63 cases. *Postgrad Med J.* 1980;56(653):149-158.

58. Olson ME, Chernik NL, Posner JB. Infiltration of the leptomeninges by systemic cancer: a clinical and pathologic study. *Arch Neurol.* 1974;30(2):122-137.

59. Herrlinger U, Förschler H, Küker W, et al. Leptomeningeal metastasis: survival and prognostic factors in 155 patients. *J Neurol Sci.* 2004;223(2):167-178.

60. Oechsle K, Lange-Brock V, Kruell A, et al. Prognostic factors and treatment options in patients with leptomeningeal metastases of different primary tumors: a retrospective analysis. *J Cancer Res Clin Oncol.* 2010;136(11):1729-1735.

61. Grant R, Naylor B, Greenberg HS, et al. Clinical outcome in aggressively treated meningeal carcinomatosis. *Arch Neurol.* 1994;51(5):457-461.

62. Chamberlain MC, Kormanik P. Carcinomatous meningitis secondary to breast cancer: combined-modality therapy. *Ann Neurol.* 1996;40(3):M8.

63. Collie DA, Brush JP, Lammie GA, et al. Imaging features of leptomeningeal metastases. *Clin Radiol.* 1999;54(11):765-771.

64. Freilich RJ, Krol G, DeAngelis LM. Neuroimaging and cerebrospinal fluid cytology in the diagnosis of leptomeningeal metastasis. *Ann Neurol.* 1995;38(1):51-57.

65. Straathof CS, de Bruin HG, Dippel DW, et al. The diagnostic accuracy of magnetic resonance imaging and cerebrospinal fluid cytology in leptomeningeal metastasis. *J Neurol.* 1999;246(9):810-814.

66. Chamberlain MC, Glantz M, Groves MD, et al. Diagnostic tools for neoplastic meningitis: detecting disease, identifying patient risk, and determining benefit of treatment. *Semin Oncol.* 2009;36(4 suppl 2):S35-S45.

67. Gultekin SH, Rosenfeld MR, Voltz R, et al. Paraneoplastic limbic encephalitis: neurological symptoms, immunological findings and tumour association in 50 patients. *Brain J Neurol.* 2000;123(pt 7):1481-1494.

68. Corsellis JA, Goldberg GJ, Norton AR. "Limbic encephalitis" and its association with carcinoma. *Brain J Neurol.* 1968;91(3):481-496.

69. Heine J, Prüss H, Bartsch T, et al. Imaging of autoimmune encephalitis—relevance for clinical practice and hippocampal function. *Neuroscience.* 2015;309:68-83.

70. Oppenheim H. *Lehrbuch der Nervenkrankheiten für Ärzte und Studierende.* Berlin: S. Karger; 1905. 2 v. (xiv, 1447 p.). Available at https://catalog.hathitrust.org/Record/011157599. Accessed November 27, 2018.

71. Kayser MS, Kohler CG, Dalmau J. Psychiatric manifestations of paraneoplastic disorders. *Am J Psychiatry.* 2010;167(9):1039-1050.

72. Ducray F, Graus F, Vigliani MC, et al. Delayed onset of a second paraneoplastic neurological syndrome in eight patients. *J Neurol Neurosurg Psychiatry.* 2010;81(8):937-939.

73. Foster AR, Caplan JP. Paraneoplastic limbic encephalitis. *Psychosomatics.* 2009;50(2):108-113.

74. Bradshaw MJ, Linnoila JJ. An overview of autoimmune and paraneoplastic encephalitides. *Semin Neurol.* 2018;38(3):330-343.

75. Lancaster E, Dalmau J. Neuronal autoantigens—pathogenesis, associated disorders and antibody testing. *Nat Rev Neurol.* 2012;8(7):380-390.

76. Lancaster E. Paraneoplastic disorders. *Contin Minneap Minn.* 2017;23(6, Neuro-oncology):1653-1679.

77. Irani SR, Gelfand JM, Bettcher BM, et al. Effect of rituximab in patients with leucine-rich, glioma-inactivated 1 antibody-associated encephalopathy. *JAMA Neurol.* 2014;71(7):896-900.

78. Dalmau J, Rosenfeld MR. Autoimmune encephalitis update. *Neuro-Oncology.* 2014;16(6):771-778.

79. Bakheit AM, Kennedy PG, Behan PO. Paraneoplastic limbic encephalitis: clinico-pathological correlations. *J Neurol Neurosurg Psychiatry.* 1990;53(12):1084-1088.

80. Berry E, Hampshire A, Rowe J, et al. The neural basis of effective memory therapy in a patient with limbic encephalitis. *J Neurol Neurosurg Psychiatry.* 2009;80(11):1202-1205.

81. Hoffman LA, Jarius S, Pellkofer HL, et al. Anti-Ma and anti-Ta associated paraneoplastic neurological syndromes: 22 newly diagnosed patients and review of previous cases. *J Neurol Neurosurg Psychiatry.* 2008;79(7):767-773.

82. Murinson B, Guarnaccia B. Stiff-person syndrome with amphiphysin antibodies: distinctive features of a rare disease. *Neurology.* 2008;71(24):1955-1958.

83. Key R, Root J. Anti-Yo mediated paraneoplastic cerebellar degeneration in the context of breast cancer: a case report and literature review. *Psychooncology.* 2013;22(9):2152-2155.

84. Vincent A, Buckley C, Schott JM, et al. Potassium channel antibody-associated encephalopathy: a potentially immunotherapy-responsive form of limbic encephalitis. *Brain J Neurol.* 2004;127(pt 3):701-712.

85. Ances BM, Vitaliani R, Taylor RA, et al. Treatment-responsive limbic encephalitis identified by neuropil antibodies: MRI and PET correlates. *Brain J Neurol.* 2005;128(pt 8):1764-1777.

86. Kotsenas AL, Watson RE, Pittock SJ, et al. MRI findings in autoimmune voltage-gated potassium channel complex encephalitis with seizures: one potential etiology for mesial temporal sclerosis. *AJNR Am J Neuroradiol.* 2014;35(1):84-89.

87. Finke C, Kopp UA, Prüss H, et al. Cognitive deficits following anti-NMDA receptor encephalitis. *J Neurol Neurosurg Psychiatry.* 2012;83(2):195-198.

88. Granerod J, Ambrose HE, Davies NW, et al. Causes of encephalitis and differences in their clinical presentations in England: a multicentre, population-based prospective study. *Lancet Infect Dis.* 2010;10(12):835-844.

89. Greene M, Lancaster E. Assessing the incidence of anti-NMDAR encephalitis. *Arch Dis Child.* 2015;100(6):512-513. doi:10.1136/archdischild-2014-307978.

90. Finke C, Kopp UA, Pajkert A, et al. Structural hippocampal damage following anti-N-methyl-D-aspartate receptor encephalitis. *Biol Psychiatry.* 2016;79(9):727-734.

91. Titulaer MJ, Höftberger R, Iizuka T, et al. Overlapping demyelinating syndromes and anti–N-methyl-D-aspartate receptor encephalitis. *Ann Neurol.* 2014;75(3):411-428.

92. Urbach H, Soeder BM, Jeub M, et al. Serial MRI of limbic encephalitis. *Neuroradiology.* 2006;48(6):380-386.

93. Bartsch T. *The Clinical Neurobiology of the Hippocampus: An Integrative View.* 1st ed. Oxford, UK: Oxford University Press; 2012. Available at http://nrs.harvard.edu/urn-3:hul.ebookbatch.GEN_batch:EDZ0000009295820160628. Accessed November 27, 2018.

94. Scheid R, Lincke T, Voltz R, et al. Serial 18F-fluoro-2-deoxy-D-glucose positron emission tomography and magnetic resonance imaging of paraneoplastic limbic encephalitis. *Arch Neurol.* 2004;61(11):1785-1789.

95. Basu S, Alavi A. Role of FDG-PET in the clinical management of paraneoplastic neurological syndrome: detection of the underlying malignancy and the brain PET-MRI correlates. *Mol Imaging Biol.* 2008;10(3):131-137.

96. Posner JB. *Neurologic Complications of Cancer.* Contemporary Neurology Series. Vol 45. Philadelphia, PA: FA Davis; 1995:xiv+482.

97. Schwartz J, Padmanabhan A, Aqui N, et al. Guidelines on the Use of Therapeutic Apheresis in Clinical Practice – Evidence-Based Approach from the Writing Committee of the American Society for Apheresis: The Seventh Special Issue. *J Clin Apheresis;* 2016;31:149-338

98. Kung S, Mueller PS, Geda YE, et al. Delirium resulting from paraneoplastic limbic encephalitis caused by Hodgkin's disease. *Psychosomatics.* 2002;43(6):498-501.

99. Arnold SD, Forman LM, Brigidi BD, et al. Evaluation and characterization of generalized anxiety and depression in patients with primary brain tumors. *Neuro-Oncology.* 2008;10(2):171-181.

100. Fox SW, Lyon D, Farace E. Symptom clusters in patients with high-grade glioma. *J Nurs Scholarsh.* 2007;39(1):61-67.

101. Bruce M, Gumley D, Isham L, et al. Post-traumatic stress symptoms in childhood brain tumour survivors and their parents. *Child Care Health Dev.* 2011;37(2):244-251.

102. Zucchella C, Bartolo M, Di Lorenzo C, et al. Cognitive impairment in primary brain tumors outpatients: a prospective cross-sectional survey. *J Neurooncol.* 2013;112(3):455-460.

103. Ganz PA. Doctor, will the treatment you are recommending cause chemobrain? *J Clin Oncol.* 2012;30(3):229-231.

104. Holmes D. Trying to unravel the mysteries of chemobrain. *Lancet Neurol.* 2013;12(6):533-534.

105. Askren MK, Jung M, Berman MG, et al. Neuromarkers of fatigue and cognitive complaints following chemotherapy for breast cancer: a prospective fMRI investigation. *Breast Cancer Res Treat.* 2014;147(2):445-455.

106. Berman MG, Askren MK, Jung M, et al. Pretreatment worry and neurocognitive responses in women with breast cancer. *Health Psychol.* 2014;33(3):222-231.

107. Ganz PA, Kwan L, Stanton AL, et al. Physical and psychosocial recovery in the year after primary treatment of breast cancer. *J Clin Oncol.* 2011;29(9):1101-1109.

108. Menning S, de Ruiter MB, Veltman DJ, et al. Multimodal MRI and cognitive function in patients with breast cancer prior to adjuvant treatment—the role of fatigue. *Neuroimage Clin.* 2015;7:547-554.

109. Asher A. Cognitive dysfunction among cancer survivors. *Am J Phys Med Rehabil.* 2011;90(5 suppl 1):S16-S26.

110. Jeon MS, Dhillon HM, Agar MR. Sleep disturbance of adults with a brain tumor and their family caregivers: a systematic review. *Neuro-Oncology.* 2017;19(8):1035-1046.

111. Holmes EG, Holmes JA, Park EM. Psychiatric care of the radiation oncology patient. *Psychosomatics.* 2017;58(5):457-465.

112. Oskan F, Ganswindt U, Belka C, et al. Primary non-small cell lung cancer in a transplanted lung treated with stereotactic body radiation therapy. *Strahlenther Onkol.* 2014;190(4):411-415.

113. Clover K, Oultram S, Adams C, et al. Disruption to radiation therapy sessions due to anxiety among patients receiving radiation therapy to the head and neck area can be predicted using patient self-report measures. *Psychooncology.* 2011;20(12):1334-1341.

114. Brown ES. Effects of glucocorticoids on mood, memory, and the hippocampus. *Ann N Y Acad Sci.* 2009;11791(1):41-55.

115. Bhangle S, Kramer N, Rosenstein E. Corticosteroid-induced neuropsychiatric disorders: review and contrast with neuropsychiatric lupus. *Rheumatol Int.* 2013;33(8):1923-1932.

116. Kovacs D, Kovacs P, Eszlari N, et al. Psychological side effects of immune therapies: symptoms and pathomechanism. *Curr Opin Pharmacol.* 2016;29(C):97-103.

117. Capuron L, Gumnick JF, Musselman DL, et al. Neurobehavioral effects of interferon-α in cancer patients: phenomenology and paroxetine responsiveness of symptom dimensions. *Neuropsychopharmacology.* 2002;26(5):643-652.

118. Dantzer R. Cytokine-induced sickness behaviour: a neuroimmune response to activation of innate immunity. *Eur J Pharmacol.* 2004;500(1):399-411.

119. Chelbi-Alix MK, Wietzerbin J. Interferon, a growing cytokine family: 50 years of interferon research. *Biochimie.* 2007;89(6-7):713-718.

120. Soffietti R, Trevisan E, Rudà R. Neurologic complications of chemotherapy and other newer and experimental approaches—Chapter 80. *Handb Clin Neurol.* 2014;121:1199-1218.

121. Sabel M, Sondak V. Is there a role for adjuvant high-dose interferon-α-2b in the management of melanoma? *Drugs.* 2003;63(11):1053-1058.

122. Alexandrescu T, Ichim E, Riordan H, et al. Immunotherapy for melanoma: current status and perspectives. *J Immunother.* 2010;33(6):570-590.

123. Pestka S. The interferons: 50 years after their discovery, there is much more to learn. *J Biol Chem.* 2007;282(28):20047-20051.

124. Luke JJ, Ott PA. PD-1 pathway inhibitors: the next generation of immunotherapy for advanced melanoma. *Oncotarget.* 2015;6(6):3479-3492.

125. Davila ML, Sadelain M. Biology and clinical application of CAR T cells for B cell malignancies. *Int J Hematol.* 2016;104(1):6-17.

126. Berger A, Shuster JL, Von Roenn JH. *Principles and Practice of Palliative Care and Supportive Oncology.* 4th ed. Philadelphia, PA: Wolters Kluwer Health/Lippincott Williams & Wilkins; 2013:xvii+942.

127. Wang X-M, Walitt B, Saligan L, et al. Chemobrain: a critical review and causal hypothesis of link between cytokines and epigenetic reprogramming associated with chemotherapy. *Cytokine.* 2015;72(1):86-96.

128. Meyers CA, Perry JR. *Cognition and Cancer.* Cambridge, NY: Cambridge University Press; 2008:xii+341.

129. Simó M, Rifà-Ros X, Rodriguez-Fornells A, et al. Chemobrain: a systematic review of structural and functional neuroimaging studies. *Neurosci Biobehav Rev.* 2013;37(8):1311-1321.

130. Ahles TA, Saykin AJ. Candidate mechanisms for chemotherapy-induced cognitive changes. *Nat Rev Cancer.* 2007;7(3):192-201.

131. Janelsins MC, Kesler SR, Ahles TA, et al. Prevalence, mechanisms, and management of cancer-related cognitive impairment. *Int Rev Psychiatry.* 2014;26(1):102-113.

132. Wefel JS, Kesler SR, Noll KR, et al. Clinical characteristics, pathophysiology, and management of noncentral nervous system cancer-related cognitive impairment in adults. *CA Cancer J Clin.* 2015;65(2):123-138.

133. Vodermaier A. Breast cancer treatment and cognitive function: the current state of evidence, underlying mechanisms and potential treatments. *Womens Health (Lond)*. 2009;5(5):503-516.

134. Feuerstein M. *Handbook of Cancer Survivorship*. New York, NY: Springer; 2007:xix+504.

135. Billiet T, Emsell L, Vandenbulcke M, et al. Recovery from chemotherapy-induced white matter changes in young breast cancer survivors? *Brain Imaging Behav*. 2018;12(1):64-77.

136. Player L, Mackenzie L, Willis K, et al. Women's experiences of cognitive changes or "chemobrain" following treatment for breast cancer: a role for occupational therapy? *Aust Occup Ther J*. 2014;61(4):230-240.

137. Baer W. Chemobrain: an opportunity in cancer survivorship to enhance patient wellness. *J Oncol Pract*. 2017;13(12):794-796.

138. Selamat M, Mackenzie L, Vardy J. Chemobrain experienced by breast cancer survivors: a meta-ethnography study investigating research and care implications. *PLoS One*. 2014;9(9):e108002.

139. Han R, Yang YM, Dietrich J, et al. Systemic 5-fluorouracil treatment causes a syndrome of delayed myelin destruction in the central nervous system. *J Biol*. 2008;7(4):12.

140. Ahles TA, Saykin AJ, McDonald BC, et al. Longitudinal assessment of cognitive changes associated with adjuvant treatment for breast cancer: impact of age and cognitive reserve. *J Clin Oncol*. 2010;28(29):4434-4440.

141. Vichaya EG, Chiu GS, Krukowski K, et al. Mechanisms of chemotherapy-induced behavioral toxicities. *Front Neurosci*. 2015;9:131.

142. Wefel JS, Schagen SB. Chemotherapy-related cognitive dysfunction. *Curr Neurol Neurosci Rep*. 2012;12(3):267-275.

143. Dietrich J, Prust M, Kaiser J. Chemotherapy, cognitive impairment and hippocampal toxicity. *Neuroscience*. 2015;309:224-232.

144. Skeel RT. *Handbook of Cancer Chemotherapy*. 7th ed. Philadelphia, PA: Lippincott Williams & Wilkins; 2007:xiv+817.

145. Nokia MS, Anderson ML, Shors TJ. Chemotherapy disrupts learning, neurogenesis and theta activity in the adult brain. *Eur J Neurosci*. 2012;36(11):3521-3530.

146. Amidi A, Hosseini SMH, Leemans A, et al. Changes in brain structural networks and cognitive functions in testicular cancer patients receiving cisplatin-based chemotherapy. *J Natl Cancer Inst*. 2017;109(12):9041-9044.

147. de Ruiter MB, Schagen SB. Functional MRI studies in non-CNS cancers. *Brain Imaging Behav*. 2013;7(4):388-408.

148. Deprez S, Vandenbulcke M, Peeters R, et al. Longitudinal assessment of chemotherapy-induced alterations in brain activation during multitasking and its relation with cognitive complaints. *J Clin Oncol*. 2014;32(19):2031-2038.

149. McDonald BC, Saykin AJ. Alterations in brain structure related to breast cancer and its treatment: chemotherapy and other considerations. *Brain Imaging Behav*. 2013;7(4):374-387.

150. Pomykala KL, de Ruiter MB, Deprez S, et al. Integrating imaging findings in evaluating the post-chemotherapy brain. *Brain Imaging Behav*. 2013;7(4):436-452.

151. Saykin AJ, de Ruiter MB, McDonald BC, et al. Neuroimaging biomarkers and cognitive function in non-CNS cancer and its treatment: current status and recommendations for future research. *Brain Imaging Behav*. 2013;7(4):363-373.

152. Deprez S, Amant F, Smeets A, et al. Longitudinal assessment of chemotherapy-induced structural changes in cerebral white matter and its correlation with impaired cognitive functioning. *J Clin Oncol*. 2012;30(3):274-281.

153. Wefel JS, Saleeba AK, Buzdar AU, et al. Acute and late onset cognitive dysfunction associated with chemotherapy in women with breast cancer. *Cancer*. 2010;116(14):3348-3356.

154. Kreukels BPC, van Dam FS, Ridderinkhof KR, et al. Persistent neurocognitive problems after adjuvant chemotherapy for breast cancer. *Clin Breast Cancer*. 2008;8(1):80-87.

155. Weis J, Poppelreuter M, Bartsch HH. Cognitive deficits as long-term side-effects of adjuvant therapy in breast cancer patients: "subjective" complaints and "objective" neuropsychological test results. *Psychooncology*. 2009;18(7):775-782.

156. Koppelmans V, de Ruiter MB, van der Lijn F, et al. Global and focal brain volume in long-term breast cancer survivors exposed to adjuvant chemotherapy. *Breast Cancer Res Treat*. 2012;132(3):1099-1106.

157. Inagaki M, Yoshikawa E, Matsuoka Y, et al. Smaller regional volumes of brain gray and white matter demonstrated in breast cancer survivors exposed to adjuvant chemotherapy. *Cancer*. 2007;109(1):146-156.

158. McDonald BC, Conroy SK, Ahles TA, et al. Gray matter reduction associated with systemic chemotherapy for breast cancer: a prospective MRI study. *Breast Cancer Res Treat*. 2010;123(3):819-828.

159. de Ruiter MB, Reneman L, Boogerd W, et al. Late effects of high-dose adjuvant chemotherapy on white and gray matter in breast cancer survivors: converging results from multimodal magnetic resonance imaging. *Hum Brain Mapp*. 2012;33(12):2971-2983.

160. Kesler SR, Kent JS, O'Hara R. Prefrontal cortex and executive function impairments in primary breast cancer. *Arch Neurol*. 2011;68(11):1447-1453.

161. Silverman DHS, Dy CJ, Castellon SA, et al. Altered frontocortical, cerebellar, and basal ganglia activity in adjuvant-treated breast cancer survivors 5-10 years after chemotherapy. *Breast Cancer Res Treat*. 2007;103(3):303-311.

162. Baltan S. Age-specific localization of NMDA receptors on oligodendrocytes dictates axon function recovery after ischemia. *Neuropharmacology*. 2016;110(pt B):626-632.

163. Jung M, Zhang M, Askren M, et al. Cognitive dysfunction and symptom burden in women treated for breast cancer: a prospective behavioral and fMRI analysis. *Brain Imaging Behav*. 2017;11(1):86-97.

164. Reuter-Lorenz PA, Cimprich B. Cognitive function and breast cancer: promise and potential insights from functional brain imaging. *Breast Cancer Res Treat*. 2013;137(1):33-43.

165. Wood LJ, Weymann K. Inflammation and neural signaling: etiologic mechanisms of the cancer treatment-related symptom cluster. *Curr Opin Support Palliat Care*. 2013;7(1):54-59.

166. Wang X-M, Walitt B, Saligan L, et al. Chemobrain: a critical review and causal hypothesis of link between cytokines and epigenetic reprogramming associated with chemotherapy. *Cytokine*. 2015;72(1):86-96.

167. von Zglinicki T, Martin-Ruiz CM. Telomeres as biomarkers for ageing and age-related diseases. *Curr Mol Med*. 2005;5(2):197-203.

168. de Visser KE, Eichten A, Coussens LM. Paradoxical roles of the immune system during cancer development. *Nat Rev Cancer*. 2006;6(1):24-37.

169. Seigers R, Fardell JE. Neurobiological basis of chemotherapy-induced cognitive impairment: a review of rodent research. *Neurosci Biobehav Rev*. 2011;35(3):729-741.

170. Lyon D, Elmore L, Aboalela N, et al. Potential epigenetic mechanism(s) associated with the persistence of psychoneurological symptoms in women receiving chemotherapy for breast cancer: a hypothesis. *Biol Res Nurs*. 2014;16(2):160-174.

171. Savitz J, Solms M, Ramesar R. The molecular genetics of cognition: dopamine, COMT and BDNF. *Genes Brain Behav*. 2006;5(4):311-328.

172. Jansen CE, Miaskowski C, Dodd M, et al. A metaanalysis of studies of the effects of cancer chemotherapy on various domains of cognitive function. *Cancer*. 2005;104(10):2222-2233.

173. Vardy J. Cognitive function in breast cancer survivors. *Cancer Treat Res.* 2009;151:387-419.

174. Boykoff N, Moieni M, Subramanian SK. Confronting chemo-brain: an in-depth look at survivors' reports of impact on work, social networks, and health care response. *J Cancer Surviv Res Pract.* 2009;3(4):223–-32.

175. Dhillon HM, Vardy J. "Chemo brain" and cognitive decline after cancer. *The Conversation.* Available at http://theconversation.com/chemo-brain-and-cognitive-decline-after-cancer-13199. Accessed November 27, 2018.

176. Caudill JS, Brown PD, Cerhan JH, Rummans TA. Selective Serotonin Reuptake Inhibitors, Glioblastoma Multiforme, and Impact on Toxicities and Overall Survival: The Mayo Clinic Experience. *Am J Clin* Oncol. 2011;34(4):385-87.

177. Tseng J-H, Chen C-Y, Chen P-C, et al. Valproic acid inhibits glioblastoma multiforme cell growth via paraoxonase 2 expression. *Oncotarget.* 2017;8(9):14666-14679.

178. Boele FW, Douw L, De Groot M, et al. The effect of modafinil on fatigue, cognitive functioning, and mood in primary brain tumor patients: a multicenter randomized controlled trial. *Neuro-Oncology.* 2013;15(10):1420-1428.

179. McCarthy BJ, Rankin KM, Aldape K, et al. Risk factors for oligodendroglial tumors: a pooled international study. *Neuro-Oncology.* 2011;13(2):242-250.

180. Lee EQ, Muzikansky A, Drappatz J, et al. A randomized, placebo-controlled pilot trial of armodafinil for fatigue in patients with gliomas undergoing radiotherapy. *Neuro-Oncology.* 2016;18(6):849-854.

181. Mar Fan HG, Clemons M, Xu W, et al. A randomised, placebo-controlled, double-blind trial of the effects of d-methylphenidate on fatigue and cognitive dysfunction in women undergoing adjuvant chemotherapy for breast cancer. *Support Care Cancer.* 2008;16(6):577-583.

182. Shaw EG, Rosdhal R, D'Agostino RB, et al. Phase II study of donepezil in irradiated brain tumor patients: effect on cognitive function, mood, and quality of life. *J Clin Oncol.* 2006;24(9):1415-1420.

183. Castellino SM, Tooze JA, Flowers L, et al. Toxicity and efficacy of the acetylcholinesterase (AChe) inhibitor donepezil in childhood brain tumor survivors: a pilot study. *Pediatr Blood Cancer.* 2012;59(3):540-547.

184. Rapp SR, Case LD, Peiffer A, et al. Donepezil for irradiated brain tumor survivors: a phase III randomized placebo-controlled clinical trial. *J Clin Oncol.* 2015;33(15):1653-1659.

185. Brown PD, Pugh S, Laack NN, et al. Memantine for the prevention of cognitive dysfunction in patients receiving whole-brain radiotherapy: a randomized, double-blind, placebo-controlled trial. *Neuro-Oncology.* 2013;15(10):1429-1437.

186. Covin R, Ouimet AJ, Seeds PM, et al. A meta-analysis of CBT for pathological worry among clients with GAD. *J Anxiety Disord.* 2008;22(1):108-116.

187. Given CW, Sikorskii A, Tamkus D, et al. Managing symptoms among patients with breast cancer during chemotherapy: results of a two-arm behavioral trial. *J Clin Oncol.* 2008;26(36):5855-5862.

188. Von Ah D, Carpenter J, Saykin A, et al. Advanced cognitive training for breast cancer survivors: a randomized controlled trial. *Breast Cancer Res Treat.* 2012;135(3):799-809.

189. Cimprich B, Ronis DL. An environmental intervention to restore attention in women with newly diagnosed breast cancer. *Cancer Nurs.* 2003;26(4):284-292; quiz 293-294.

190. Kesler S, Hadi Hosseini SM, Heckler C, et al. Cognitive training for improving executive function in chemotherapy-treated breast cancer survivors. *Clin Breast Cancer.* 2013;13(4):299-306.

191. Alvarez J, Meyer F, Granoff DL, et al. The effect of EEG biofeedback on reducing postcancer cognitive impairment. *Integr Cancer Ther.* 2013;12(6):475-487.

192. Ferguson RJ, McDonald BC, Saykin AJ, et al. Brain structure and function differences in monozygotic twins: possible effects of breast cancer chemotherapy. *J Clin Oncol.* 2007;25(25):3866-3870.

193. Lancaster E. Continuum: the paraneoplastic disorders. *Contin Minneap Minn.* 2015;21(20):452-475.

194. Höftberger R, Rosenfeld MR, Dalmau J. Update on neurological paraneoplastic syndromes. *Curr Opin Oncol.* 2015;27(6):489-495.

29

Neuropsychiatry of Epilepsy

Daniel Weisholtz · Rani Sarkis · Gaston Baslet

INTRODUCTION

In this chapter, we review the current state of knowledge regarding the various areas of overlap between the fields of epilepsy and psychiatry. After a brief discussion of the phenomenology, pathophysiology, and clinical approach to epilepsy in general, we discuss the various psychiatric and cognitive manifestations of epilepsy. Neuropsychiatric symptomatology in epilepsy can be broadly divided between *peri-ictal symptoms* and *interictal symptoms*. The former bear a direct temporal relationship to seizures while the latter do not. Lastly, we discuss the neuropsychiatric impact of epilepsy treatments and the special considerations necessary for psychopharmacological management in patients with epilepsy (PWE).

A HISTORICAL NOTE

A relationship between epilepsy and mental illness has been recognized since ancient times. The Hippocratic school in ancient Greece, who preferred natural explanations for disease over the supernatural ideas of the day, recognized the importance of the brain as a mediator of cognition and emotion, and of mental illness and epilepsy. A direct relationship between epilepsy and mental illness was also recognized, as evidenced by the Hippocratic statement that "Most melancholics usually also become epileptics, and epileptics melancholics. One or the other prevails according to where the disease leans: if toward the body, they become epileptics, if toward reason, melancholics."[1] Supernatural conceptions of epilepsy and mental illness were prevalent in ancient times, particularly among the nonmedical public, and ancient writers often failed to recognize a clear distinction between epilepsy and mental illness. This is exemplified by the concept of lunacy and the word "lunatic," colloquially (and pejoratively) used in modern English to refer to an individual with mental illness. The term derives from the Latin word "*lunaticus*" that likely referred initially to an individual with epilepsy, as can be seen by its usage in the Vulgate, the 5th-century Latin translation of the Bible, to refer to the epileptic child healed by Jesus (Matthew 17:15). While the Biblical perspective on epilepsy and mental illness is that both relate to demonic possession, both the Latin and original Greek versions of the word contain a prefix relating to the moon ("*luna-*" and "*selen-*," respectively), likely reflecting a notion during Roman times that the cyclical attacks characteristic of epilepsy are related to the cycles of the moon.

Christian views on the role of demonic possession became increasingly prominent during the Middle Ages, although the medical writers dissociated themselves from these views, often favoring natural explanations. However, an etiological role for cycles of the moon via natural mechanisms was considered by physicians in a manner akin to that in which the cycles of the moon affects the tides. The periodicity of symptomatology seen in bipolar disorder may have lent support to the lunar theory of mental illness. Because mental illness and epilepsy were considered mechanistically similar, there may have been little incentive to separate them nosologically, and the term "lunacy" came to refer to both conditions, although it eventually became associated more with mental illness than with epilepsy.

In the 16th and 17th centuries, increasing attention was paid to factors that preceded the onset of epileptic seizures and the belief that psychological factors such as sudden fear or excitement could cause epilepsy became widespread.[1] During the 18th and 19th centuries, PWE were housed in asylums together with the mentally ill, which led to an opportunity to study the overlap in symptomatology between the two groups of patients. (The term "Lunatic Asylum" was widely used until the 1870s in North America after which it was replaced by "Insane Asylum.") In the early 19th century, the French psychiatrist Jean-Étienne Dominique Esquirol (1772–1840) observed a temporal relationship between insanity and seizures. He described an "epileptic mania" that could occur before, after, or independently of seizures. This may have been the first description of what is now called postictal psychosis. Jean Pierre Falret (1794–1870) also described epileptic psychiatric phenomena, some of which were undoubtedly peri-ictal, including fits of despair, hallucinations, maniac agitation, incessant loquacity, and postictal behavioral disturbance characterized by violent acts such as suicide, homicide, and arson. Benedict Morel, another French psychiatrist, published cases in 1860 of paroxysmal behavioral disturbances, most of which involved criminal activities that he considered to be "epileptic equivalents." He characterized these behaviors as a subtle form of epilepsy called *épilepsie larvée* that could exist without typical epileptic seizures and be diagnosed by the "main symptoms of epileptic insanity." In the 1860s, it was theorized that "fright" and "moral" factors were major etiologies for epilepsy, which was, in some sense, still viewed as a behavioral disorder. These views are no longer considered valid, and they contributed to a stigmatized view of both epilepsy and mental illness that has persisted, to some extent, into the present day.

As scientific approaches helped to delineate the various neuropsychiatric diseases, epilepsy became clearly distinguished from other neuropsychiatric conditions. This was no doubt facilitated by the discovery of electroencephalography (EEG) by Richard Caton in 1875 and the subsequent discoveries by Gibbs, Gibbs, Davis, and Lennox in the 1930s that the epileptic spike, as seen on EEG, could be used as an epilepsy biomarker. EEG provided a diagnostic test that allowed epilepsy to be delineated from other behavioral disorders using biological criteria. Thus, the history of the neuropsychiatry of epilepsy is a history not of gradual recognition of the relationship between epilepsy and mental illness but a gradual conceptualization of epilepsy as an entity distinct from mental illness.

BASICS OF EPILEPSY

An epileptic seizure is defined as "a transient occurrence of signs and/or symptoms due to abnormal excessive or synchronous neuronal activity in the brain." A seizure is considered provoked if caused by a temporary and reversible factor (sudden metabolic changes, fever, alcohol withdrawal, etc.). Epilepsy is a disorder of the brain characterized by an enduring predisposition to generate unprovoked epileptic seizures. The current operational definition of epilepsy allows an individual to be diagnosed with epilepsy if he or she meets at least one of the following three criteria: (1) a history of two unprovoked seizures at least 24 hours apart, (2) a single unprovoked seizure but the probability of recurrence is deemed to be at least 60% (based on risk factors) over the next 10 years, or (3) the patient can be diagnosed with a clearly defined epilepsy syndrome.[2] The cumulative lifetime incidence of seizures is up to 10% while the cumulative risk of epilepsy is 1–4%.[3] Pathophysiologically, seizures are best conceptualized as the result of an imbalance between excitation and inhibition in the brain leading to abnormal excessive and synchronous firing of neurons. The main inhibitory neurotransmitter is gamma-aminobutyric acid (GABA) while glutamate is among the main excitatory neurotransmitters. Thus, defective GABAergic inhibition and/or excessive glutamatergic excitation can result in seizures.

Seizures can be broadly categorized as either *focal* or *generalized*. Seizures are considered focal if the onset is limited to a focus/region in one hemisphere. Generalized seizures, which involve both hemispheres of the brain simultaneously, can be considered secondary if they result from spread of epileptic activity from a unilateral focus to bilateral networks or can be considered primary if the bilateral networks are involved at the onset, driven by thalamocortical interactions. The symptoms experienced during a focal seizure depend on the area of brain involved at the onset and the manner in which the seizure spreads. For example, a seizure starting in the occipital lobe may produce visual hallucinations while a seizure in the temporal lobe may cause emotional/cognitive/auditory symptoms among others (see Figure 29-1 and section on ictal psychiatric symptoms). Focal seizures are further classified based on whether or not they lead to impaired awareness, and whether they have a motor or nonmotor onset.[4] If the symptom at the onset of the seizure is subjective, it is commonly referred to as an *aura*. Motor manifestations of seizures may be unilateral or bilateral and are considered *tonic* (or *dystonic*) if there is a sustained muscle contraction, *myoclonic* if there is a brief (less than 200 ms) contraction, and clonic if the contraction is repetitive and rhythmic. *Automatisms* are complex but purposeless automatic behaviors typically seen during focal unaware seizures that most commonly involve lip smacking, chewing, or fumbling movements of the hand, but can be quite varied in their manifestations. The most frequent type of focal epilepsy is *temporal lobe epilepsy* (TLE), which tends to be associated with focal seizures with impaired awareness (FIA), also referred to in prior classification schemes as *focal seizures with dyscognitive features* or *complex partial seizures*.

The most concerning seizure type is the *generalized tonic-clonic seizure* (GTC; also referred to in prior classification schemes as *grand mal*, *generalized convulsive seizure*, or *major motor seizure*) as it places the patient at the greatest risk for injury or death. This seizure type may be focal or generalized in onset, and is characterized by a tonic phase followed by a clonic phase. There is always loss of consciousness, and there may be upward deviation of the eyes and transient paralysis of respiratory musculature along with marked autonomic changes. The convulsion typically ends after 1–2 minutes but is usually followed by postictal lethargy and confusion.

Seizures with generalized onset include *GTC seizures*, *absence seizures*, *myoclonic seizures*, and a variety of other less common seizures types. Absence seizures (previously known as *petit mal*) occur mainly during childhood and are less frequent after puberty. They are characterized by the arrest or suspension of consciousness for 5–10 seconds. Parents may not notice the typical brief seizures in an otherwise healthy child, but teachers may report that the child stares absently for short intervals throughout the day. Without treatment, absence seizures can occur up to 70–100 times a day, and such frequent blackouts can significantly impact a child's academic performance. Absence seizures may sometimes be mistaken for inattention leading to concern for attention-deficit hyperactivity disorder (ADHD). However, absence seizures are the easiest seizure type to diagnose because of the pathognomonic EEG abnormality: a 3-Hz spike-and-wave pattern that is often elicited or accentuated when the child hyperventilates. On the other hand, while children with ADHD tend to have difficulties staying on task and completing their homework, episodes of inattention typically do not interrupt play, and are not associated with rhythmic blinking, twitches, or automatisms as can be seen with absence epilepsy.

Insula

Seizures characteristically present with laryngeal discomfort and a feeling of throat constriction. Contralateral paresthesias may follow this sensation. There is typically no loss of awareness. Insular seizures may also involve gustatory, olfactory, vestibular, and viscerosensory symptoms, autonomic symptoms, and even complex motor behaviors, and are often mistaken for temporal, frontal, or parietal lobe seizures.

Frontal Lobe

Dorsolateral – Seizures from primary motor cortex (M1) generally present with unilateral spreading clonic motor activity ("Jacksonian March") followed by speech arrest. Consciousness is preserved. With involvement of frontal eye fields, contralateral gaze deviation may be seen. Dorsolateral prefrontal cortex involvement may lead to more complex motor behaviors and/or forced thought.

Orbitofrontal – An aura of choking, nausea, or déjà vu is often present. Laughter or emotional defensive behaviors may be seen. Seizures most commonly begin with sudden behavioral arrest, staring, or loss of awareness that may be followed by head and eye deviation. Hyper-motor automatisms characterized by thrashing movements or automatisms of the temporal lobe type may be present.

Supplementary Sensorimotor Area (SSMA) – Seizures are often brief, during sleep or with preserved awareness if awake, and are characterized by asymmetric but bilateral tonic posturing of the limbs.

Anterior Cingulate Cortex – Seizures may begin with emotional or autonomic aura. Ictal vocalizations, either emotional cries, or verbal phrases are common. Motor manifestations are often complex body movements, at times flailing or violent. Facial or gestural automatisms may also be seen. Awareness may or may not be preserved. Postictal confusion or lethargy is typically minimal, but postictal aggression may be seen.

Parietal Lobe

Seizures often begin with contralateral somatosensory symptoms (numbness, tingling, pain, thermal sensations) in the face or extremities that may "march" to adjacent parts of the body based on functional organization of the primary somatosensory cortex. Ictal vertigo or visual symptoms may also be seen with involvement of parietotemporal cortex.

Occipital Lobe

Seizures are often characterized by visual hallucinations that are commonly described as multicolored and circular, although cases of other shapes, flashing lights, and shades or patterns are also possible. As the seizure progresses, these hallucinations may increase in number and/or size. Hallucinations are usually unilateral and in the temporal visual hemi-field contralateral to the origin of the seizure.

Temporal Lobe

Lateral (Neocortical) – The aura is typically characterized by auditory phenomena, aphasia, vertiginous symptoms, or visual distortions. Contralateral clonic movements are preceded by motionless staring and unresponsiveness. Contralateral dystonic posturing, body and head shifting, hyperventilation, and automatisms are also frequently seen.

Mesial (Limbic) – Mesial temporal seizures typically begin with an experiential or viscerosensory aura—anxiety/fear, déjà vu, and/or nausea are frequent. These symptoms may be followed by oral and/or manual automatisms, often with impaired awareness, particularly when involving the dominant hemisphere. Lateralization can be inferred by contralateral dystonic posturing, and ipsilateral automatisms. Aphasia suggests dominant lateralization, but if ictal speech, vomiting, and intermittent awareness are present, non-dominant hemisphere lateralization is suggested.

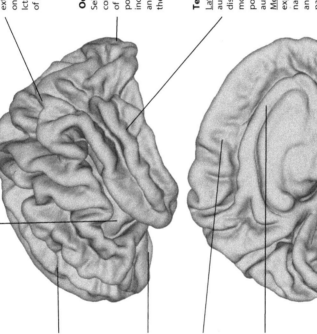

FIGURE 29–1. Characteristic symptoms of focal seizures depending on their localization. Symptoms may relate to the seizure onset zone and/or areas to which the seizure propagates. While propagation patterns vary, seizures tend to spread in characteristic ways along neural pathways.

Generalized epilepsy syndromes are characterized by generalized onset seizures such as GTC seizures, absence seizures, and myoclonic seizures and are generally felt to be due to genetic factors, although the causative gene is often not identified. They are often referred to as *idiopathic generalized epilepsy* or *genetic generalized epilepsy* (GGE). In contrast, focal epilepsy syndromes are often due to a localized structural abnormality, sometimes an acquired brain lesion. Among the common GGE syndromes are childhood absence epilepsy (CAE), characterized primarily by absence seizures during childhood that typically resolve in adulthood, and juvenile myoclonic epilepsy (JME), which usually begins in early adolescence and is characterized by myoclonic seizures, GTC seizures, and absence seizures. There are a variety of other generalized epilepsy syndromes as well. Providers should be careful to exclude GGE before prescribing certain antiepileptic drugs (AEDs) such as carbamazepine or phenytoin, which may worsen seizure control in GGE.

Clinical Evaluation and Management of a Patient with Seizures

The clinical workup of seizures starts with a careful history with specific questions directed at the patient and a witness. Ascertaining the first symptom experienced by the patient may help identify the seizure type and localize the seizure to a specific brain region. It is then important to determine whether there was any impairment in awareness and, if possible, to ascertain the progression and duration of symptoms over time as well as the behavior immediately after the seizure. A history of seizure triggers such as sleep deprivation, alcohol consumption, new medications, or a recent illness also needs to be obtained. This is then followed by a physical examination to look for focal neurologic signs. Neuroimaging is essential to evaluate for focal lesions such as tumors or strokes that may be the cause of the seizure. A magnetic resonance imaging (MRI) scan of the brain is favored over a computed tomography (CT) scan when possible, due to its higher resolution. In addition, an EEG is encouraged as it can aid in capturing a seizure or reveal a predisposition toward seizures by capturing interictal (in between seizures) epileptiform electrical activity such as spikes or sharp waves (also known as *interictal epileptiform discharges*). The duration of the EEG depends on the question being asked. Options include a routine 20–40 minute EEG, an ambulatory 1–7-day EEG, and an inpatient video EEG monitoring study which can last hours to days. Sphenoidal electrodes, placed transcutaneously inferior to the zygomatic arch, are sometimes used to increase diagnostic yield in suspected TLE due to their closer proximity to the mediobasal temporal dipole source.[5] However, their use remains controversial, as the nearly equivalent performance of noninvasive anterior temporal electrodes (T1 and T2) may not justify the discomfort produced by the sphenoidal electrodes.[6]

A lumbar puncture (LP) is usually not necessary as part of the first seizure evaluation, particularly if the patient recovers from the seizure and there are no persistent neurological deficits or neuroimaging abnormalities. However, if the seizure is accompanied by meningeal signs, or if imaging shows an abnormality concerning for encephalitis, LP should be performed to evaluate for meningitis/encephalitis. A seizure that occurs in the setting of fever may also necessitate an LP. An exception to this rule is the child with simple febrile seizures who is up to date on *Haemophilus influenzae* type b and *S. pneumonia* vaccines, as the incidence of bacterial meningitis is very low in this setting.[7]

It can sometimes be challenging to prove the diagnosis of epilepsy objectively, as it is not uncommon for initial testing to be normal. In such circumstances, the history is of paramount importance. A careful history (particularly when a witness if available) can often allow the clinician to distinguish an epileptic seizure from other types of episodes such as psychogenic non-epileptic seizures (PNES), panic attacks, convulsive syncope, cardiac arrhythmia, transient ischemic attack, attention lapse, narcolepsy, parasomnias, migraines, paroxysmal dyskinesias, or dissociative episodes (Table 29-1). When a patient has recurrent episodes, it is sometimes possible for a companion to record a video on a smartphone that can be shared with the physician.

Once there is compelling evidence of an unprovoked epileptic seizure, a decision then needs to be made about whether to start medications or not. Factors that place a patient at higher risk of recurrence include seizures occurring out of sleep, the presence of a cortical abnormality on brain imaging, and the presence of epileptiform discharges on EEG. An AED is recommended if a patient has experienced two or more unprovoked epileptic seizures at least 24 hours apart, or after one unprovoked seizure under certain circumstances where additional seizures are considered particularly likely.[8]

When seizures continue to occur despite adequate trials of at least two different AEDs, the epilepsy is considered refractory to medication, and epilepsy surgery must be considered. The most effective type of epilepsy surgery involves resection of the epileptogenic tissue, and this requires a workup to prove that the seizures originate from a single identifiable focus. This requires video EEG monitoring to record and characterize the

TABLE 29-1 • Seizure Differential Diagnosis.
• Syncope (can involve convulsive movements)
• Neurocardiogenic
• Cardiac arrhythmia
• Breath holding spell
• Migraine
• Transient ischemic attack (TIA)
• Paroxysmal dyskinesia
• Sandifer syndrome in infants
• Sleep disorder
• Narcolepsy
• NREM parasomnia
• REM behavior disorder
• Attention lapse
• Panic attack
• Dissociative episode
• Psychogenic non-epileptic seizure (PNES)
• Dissociative fugue
• Depersonalization
• Derealization

seizures electrographically. In some cases, additional imaging such as fluorodeoxyglucose positron emission tomography (FDG-PET) or ictal single-photon emission computed tomography (SPECT) may be utilized.

PERI-ICTAL NEUROPSYCHIATRIC SYMPTOMS

Seizures may be associated with a variety of transient psychiatric symptoms. The hallmark of these symptoms is a temporal relationship between symptom and seizure. While they may sometimes be mistaken for symptoms of idiopathic psychiatric illness, identification of their temporal relationship with seizures is of great importance, as it is likely to inform how they are managed. We use the term *peri-ictal* to refer to any definable temporal relationship between seizure and symptom. These can be further subdivided into *ictal* symptoms, *preictal* symptoms, and *postictal* symptoms. Ictal symptoms are symptoms of the seizure itself, while preictal symptoms occur before, and postictal symptoms occur after a seizure.

Ictal Neuropsychiatric Symptoms

Ictal psychiatric symptoms most commonly occur in the context of focal seizures and result from aberrant activation of a portion of the brain. Focal seizures tend to propagate via neural connections from an onset zone within the cerebral cortex or limbic system to additional brain regions. Much clinical attention is paid to the onset zone, as its ablation can sometimes cure the epilepsy. However, symptoms experienced during the seizure may relate either to seizure activity at the onset zone or to areas of propagation. The particular symptoms experienced during the early part of a seizure depend on the functional characteristics of the involved brain areas (Table 29-2). If enough of the brain becomes involved during the seizure, particularly when bilateral or left-lateralized, consciousness will be lost and psychiatric symptoms will no longer be experienced. Thus, psychiatric symptoms are typically noted when the seizure involves relatively small areas of brain tissue—at times too small for the seizure to be detected on scalp EEG. Because the loss of consciousness and motor symptoms that occur as a focal seizure spreads are usually more dramatic than the early subjective symptoms, they tend to be most notable to patients and clinicians and are typically thought of as the seizure itself, with early subjective ictal symptoms referred to as the *aura*. Seizure auras are most identifiable when they reliably precede "clear-cut" seizure symptoms, but auras can occur with considerably greater frequency than the more disabling seizure symptoms, reflecting the fact that many focal seizures do not propagate substantially enough to lead to dramatic symptoms. As a result, it is not uncommon for epilepsy to remain undiagnosed for a period of time despite recurrent auras, until a convulsion finally occurs leading to the appropriate medical evaluation.

Ictal Hallucinations

Ictal hallucinations from seizures in occipital cortex typically appear as elementary visual phenomena such as simple phosphenes or colored spheres, although other shapes can occur. They may flicker or change color or size as the seizure progresses, and

TABLE 29-2 • Ictal Psychiatric Symptoms.

Symptom	Proposed Localization
Elementary visual hallucinations (phosphenes, colored spheres)	Occipital lobe
Complex visual hallucinations	Occipitotemporal cortex, limbic structures
Visual distortions (micropsia, macropsia, metamorphopsia)	Visual association cortex (occipitotemporal, occipitoparietal)
Elementary auditory hallucinations (simple tones, buzzing sounds)	Transverse temporal gyri of Heschl
Complex auditory hallucinations (music, speech)	Lateral superior temporal cortex
Vertigo	Temporoparietal junction
Paresthesias, numbness, pain, thermal sensations	Contralateral parietal lobe somatosensory cortex
Sensation of a shrinking or swelling body part	Nondominant temporo-parieto-occipital junction
Out of body experience, autoscopy	Temporoparietal junction
Gastrointestinal sensations, autonomic symptoms (palpitations, piloerection, urinary urgency)	Insula or limbic structures such as cingulate cortex or amygdala
Olfactory hallucinations	Mesial temporal cortex
Gustatory hallucinations	Insula
Déjà vu or *jamais vu*, depersonalization, derealization	Hippocampus/Mesial temporal cortex
Fear	Amygdala
Ictal laughter (gelastic seizure)	Hypothalamus (hamartoma)
Forced thinking	Frontal lobe
Motor automatisms	Anterior cingulate cortex; may be a release phenomenon during temporal lobe seizures

they tend to occur in the visual field contralateral to the seizure focus.[9] Complex visual hallucinations (e.g., images of people or scenes) may be seen with involvement of occipitotemporal visual association areas, particularly when limbic structures are involved.[10] Visual distortions can also occur where images persist or duplicate (*palinopsia*), or objects appear to change in size (*micropsia* or *macropsia*) or shape (*metamorphopsia*). Ictal *autoscopy* has also been described, in which an individual has a hallucination of himself duplicated as if in a mirror.

Auditory ictal hallucinations typically occur with early involvement of the superior portion of the temporal lobe. Simple tones and buzzing sounds likely implicate the transverse temporal gyri of Heschl where primary auditory cortex resides. More complex auditory hallucinations of music or speech can occur with involvement of auditory association cortex in the lateral aspects of the superior temporal gyrus.[10] They are most commonly seen with neocortical TLE. Ictal auditory verbal hallucinations are rarely commanding or threatening and are generally brief and dream-like. As a result, they are rarely mistaken for the auditory hallucinations common in schizophrenia.

Vertigo can be experienced with involvement of the temporoparietal junction. Somatosensory ictal hallucinations typical occur in the setting of parietal lobe epilepsy and are usually experienced as paresthesias or numbness (but also sometimes pain or thermal sensations) localized to the contralateral region of the body represented by the portion of the somatotopic map involved in the seizure. Somatosensory distortions such as the sensation of a shrinking or swelling body part may implicate the nondominant temporo-parieto-occipital junction. Seizures in this region may also disrupt the mapping of visual input to extrapersonal space and can produce an out-of-body experience. This is distinct from autoscopy, which is a visual hallucination.

Gastrointestinal sensations and autonomic symptoms such as palpitations, piloerection, or urinary urgency can be experienced with involvement of the insula or limbic structures such as cingulate cortex or amygdala. Abdominal auras, often described as nausea or a rising epigastric sensation, are relatively common in patients with mesial TLE. Ictal olfactory and gustatory hallucinations can occur with seizures involving anteromesial limbic cortex and can be seen in mesial TLE, insular epilepsy, or orbitofrontal epilepsy. They are typically unpleasant and often described as a rotten or burning odor or metallic taste.

Experiential Auras and Other Ictal Psychiatric Manifestations

Some seizure auras involve subjective experiences that are not clearly hallucinatory and are sometimes referred to as *psychic* or *experiential auras*. Seizures from the mesial temporal lobe may produce abnormal feelings of increased or decreased familiarity (*déjà vu* or *jamais vu*, respectively). A more intense feeling of strangeness may be characterized as derealization or depersonalization.[11] These must be differentiated from psychogenic dissociative symptoms. Some PWE report a dream-like state that may be multimodal and can seem like a movie playing out in the person's mind. Such experiences likely involve limbic regions and widespread cortical networks. Auras may also take the form of emotional experience, the most common of which is *ictal fear*, a phenomenon linked to seizures involving the amygdala, particularly on the nondominant side. Ictal fear may mimic a panic attack but is usually considerably shorter and less severe (further discussed in section on differentiating Ictal Psychiatric Symptoms from Non-epileptic Psychiatric Symptoms). Ecstatic or mystical experiences are rarely reported, as are feelings of sexual arousal or orgasm, most often associated with right TLE. Inappropriate laughter may occur as part of a seizure (*gelastic* seizures) and is most typically associated with a hypothalamic hamartoma although it can also occur with other types of focal epilepsy. Wieser described a rage attack and a laughing fit each associated with prolonged runs of left peri-amygdalar epileptic activity.[12] Frontal lobe seizures, particularly when left-sided, may produce a phenomenon called *forced thinking* in which a stereotyped but irrelevant or intrusive phrase, thought, or sequence of thoughts seems to pop into the mind.[13] This must be differentiated from symptoms of obsessive-compulsive disorder (OCD).

Differentiating Ictal Psychiatric Symptoms from Non-Epileptic Psychiatric Symptoms

EEG can be helpful in diagnosing ictal psychiatric symptoms, particularly when electrographic seizures are seen to correlate with the patient's symptoms. However, a negative EEG study may not rule out an ictal etiology, even when an event is recorded, as scalp EEG has limited sensitivity for detecting focal seizures with preserved awareness. Seizures with small or deep foci may not be detectable without invasive (intracranial) electrodes. Thus, history and clinical observation are of great importance. Underlying risk factors and past medical history may influence the likelihood of one diagnosis or another. For example, a patient with a long history of well-characterized schizophrenia with prominent auditory and visual hallucinations now with new-onset olfactory hallucinations is unlikely to be experiencing ictal hallucinations. On the other hand, ictal hallucinations should be strongly suspected in a middle-aged patient with no past psychiatric history who experiences new-onset visual hallucinations and is discovered to have an occipital lobe tumor.

A seizure is typically a brief event with a discrete beginning and end, and usually lasts no more than a few minutes at a time. Thus, ictal psychiatric symptoms typically mirror this time course. Symptoms that are insidious in onset or chronic are unlikely to be ictal. Despite the variability of ictal manifestations across patients, individual patients tend to have highly stereotyped seizures that do not differ dramatically in nature from episode to episode. When a patient experiences a multitude of different types of paroxysmal symptoms, it is unlikely that they are all ictal. On the other hand, stereotyped brief paroxysmal neuropsychiatric symptoms that sometimes progress to loss of awareness are highly likely to be ictal (though the usual differential diagnoses such as syncope and psychogenic nonepileptic seizures must be considered).

A common diagnostic dilemma is the differentiation between ictal panic, a common symptom of amygdala seizures, and idiopathic panic attack. While a history of epilepsy increases the likelihood that the panic is ictal, PWE can experience non-epileptic panic attacks too. Ictal panic tends to be very brief (less than 30 seconds) and may progress to a loss of awareness or secondary bilateral tonic-clonic convulsion. It may be associated with other auras that typify mesial temporal lobe seizures such as visceral or olfactory sensations and déjà vu.[14] Ictal panic tends to be highly stereotyped and often occurs without an identifiable psychological trigger. On the other hand, panic attacks tend to last 5–20 minutes and can persist for hours.[15] Ictal panic also tends to be less intense than idiopathic panic attack and more stereotyped with regard to associated symptoms. Table 29-3 provides some of the features that can help distinguish panic disorder from focal epilepsy with ictal fear.

Psychiatric Symptoms during Nonconvulsive Status Epilepticus

Nonconvulsive status epilepticus (NCSE) is an unusual but not rare manifestation of epilepsy in which epileptic activity occurs recurrently or continuously for a prolonged period of time (typically diagnosed when longer than 30 minutes) resulting in persistent neuropsychiatric symptoms in the absence of overt motor activity. On EEG, NCSE is suggested when mental

TABLE 29-3 • Differentiating Features between Panic Disorder and Focal Epilepsy with Fear.

	Panic Disorder (Interictal)	Focal Seizure with Fear (Ictal)
Duration of attack	More than 5 minutes	Less than 2 minutes
Course of attack	Crescendo course that peaks within 10 minutes	Sudden onset and offset
Stereotypic presentation	Changes in symptoms may occur	Very stereotyped presentation
Consciousness during attack	Usually preserved during attack	These seizures are really supposed to be called focal impaired awareness seizures, not unaware seizures
Anticipatory anxiety	Common	Uncommon
Agoraphobia	Common	Very rare
Post-attack confusion	Very rare	Possible
Trigger	Possible, but unprovoked attacks also occur	Uncommon
Age of onset	20s–30s	Any age
Family history of panic disorder	Common	Uncommon

status alteration is accompanied by epileptic discharges at a frequency of >2.5 Hz or by a rhythmic pattern that evolves in space and time.[16] Incidence has been estimated at 1.5–18.5 cases per 100,000 per year.[17] NCSE may be focal or generalized. It is viewed as a neurological emergency, as it can often be reversed if treated promptly, but the untreated NCSE may cause neuronal damage and prolonged or permanent neurological deficits.[17] There must be a high index of suspicion for NCSE if there is no return to normal state of consciousness after a clear-cut seizure. Urgent EEG is warranted, and continuous EEG monitoring should be considered, if available.

Absence status epilepticus (ASE) is a form of NCSE characterized by a prolonged absence seizure, and typically manifests as a waking confusional state with minimal focal features, though there can be blinking or occasional myoclonus. There is often preserved ability to respond to simple commands, withdraw from pain, eat, drink, and walk. The patient may exhibit perplexity, bizarre automatic behavior, clumsiness, verbal or motor impersistence or perseveration, decreased spontaneity with either mutism, or poverty of speech. This suggests a frontal lobe syndrome. In fact, NCSE should be considered in the differential diagnosis for catatonia, as cases of ictal catatonia due to NCSE have been reported in the literature including characteristic features such as waxy flexibility.[18,19]

Focal NCSE most commonly occurs after convulsions or clusters of focal seizures or in the setting of acute brain injury. The typical clinical manifestation is stupor or coma, at times with subtle motor symptoms such as twitching, blinking, nystagmus, or gaze deviation. However, much like with seizure auras, a variety of different types of symptoms may be seen with well-localized NCSE depending on the localization. Manifestations may include hallucinations in all the varieties discussed above for focal seizures, catatonia, dysarthria, or aphasia. During focal status epilepticus of the frontal polar region, the patient may exhibit confabulation and hilarity, while during temporal lobe status epilepticus, the patient may show symptoms of fear, anxiety, irritability, or aggression. Rarely, delusional beliefs may manifest during focal NCSE, a phenomenon that may be referred to as *ictal psychosis*.[20] Symptoms may fluctuate as seizures start and stop. The NCSE diagnosis is likely to be missed in these settings if EEG is not employed. NCSE should be suspected and urgent EEG obtained if there is sudden-onset of persistent neuropsychiatric symptoms in a patient with a history of seizures and/or no preexisting relevant psychiatric history, unless an alternative explanation such as stroke or drug intoxication can be established. NCSE should also be strongly considered if there are ongoing symptoms suggestive of seizure such as intermittent unresponsiveness, gaze deviation, or automatisms.

Postictal Psychiatric Symptoms

The postictal period follows a clinical seizure. Symptoms during this period vary depending on seizure type. Minimal to no postictal symptoms are typical following absence seizures, myoclonic seizures, and many types of focal seizures. When focal postictal symptoms are prominent immediately after a focal seizure, it is common for the focality of the symptoms to reflect the seizure localization or lateralization such as focal weakness following a contralateral motor seizure (Todd's paresis) or aphasia following a focal seizure in the dominant hemisphere. After a GTC seizure, there is typically a brief period of stupor lasting no more than a few minutes, followed by a period of somnolence and confusion during which the patient is able to answer simple questions but may be disoriented and agitated and unable to form new long-term memories. When emergency services are called immediately after a convulsion is witnessed, it is quite common for the patient to regain consciousness before paramedics arrive but to note later that he has no recollection of the initial evaluation by paramedics or the trip to the hospital. Many focal impaired awareness seizures, such as those of a mesial temporal lobe origin, are associated with some degree of postictal confusion during the first few minutes, and persistent fatigue is commonly reported during the hours or days following a seizure.

Postictal Psychosis

Postictal confusion and lethargy almost always remit within the first hour following a seizure, but it is not uncommon for postictal psychiatric symptoms to persist for a considerably longer time. The best-studied example is *postictal psychosis* (PIP) which has been noted to occur in approximately 4% of patients with medication-resistant focal epilepsy.[21] PIP is most commonly seen in patients with longstanding medication-resistant epilepsy and usually occurs after a cluster of convulsive or FIA seizures. Classic descriptions involve a "lucid interval" of up to 72 hours after resolution of the immediate postictal state before the psychosis sets in, helping to distinguish it more clearly from ictal psychosis.[22,23] The lucid interval is a commonly described feature of PIP, though it is not always present. A "peri-ictal" form of psychosis has been described in which there is no clear separation between the postictal state and the onset of psychosis, and in which the distinction between ictal psychosis and PIP is more difficult to make.[21,24] This is contrasted with a "nuclear" or classic PIP in which the lucid interval is clearly present. Some authors have postulated that PIP, at least in some cases, may truly reflect an ictal rather than postictal phenomenon on the basis of case reports in which focal epileptiform activity in limbic brain regions has been seen on intracranial EEG to correlate with the psychotic symptoms in what otherwise appeared clinically as PIP.[20] PIP is characterized by hallucinations, delusions, and/or confusion with disorganized behavior and tends to be affect-laden, often with manic or hypomanic features.[25] Paranoia and grandiose or religious delusions are common.[26] Thus the episodes may sometimes resemble manic episodes. In fact, the term PIP is often used rather broadly in reference to a spectrum of postictal cognitive/behavioral abnormalities, some of which may not be considered psychotic by strict definitions of the term (Figure 29-2).[21] On the other hand, when PIP is distinguished from postictal mania (PIM) by strict criteria, some differences are seen: PIM may have a greater association with frontal lobe epilepsy than PIP and may last longer.[27] A set of criteria have been developed for defining PIP that is used by some research groups (Logsdail and Toone criteria, Table 29-4).[23] Bilateral independent ictal foci are a risk factor for PIP,[28,29] which may suggest that patients who have widely distributed neural network dysfunction are more prone to the condition.

It has been recognized that PIP and interictal psychosis (IIP) may occur in the same patient, and data have suggested that prior PIP is a risk factor for the subsequent development of IIP.[30,31] This does not necessarily mean that there is a causal relationship between PIP and IIP such that successfully treating or preventing PIP will prevent the development of IIP. The association between PIP and IIP may reflect the fact that a certain subset of PWE is vulnerable to psychosis under certain circumstances, and convulsions or seizure clusters may be a particularly potent provocation for a vulnerable individual.

Evaluation and Management of Postictal Psychosis

When a patient presents with persistently altered mentation following seizures, urgent EEG should be considered (ideally continuous video EEG monitoring) to exclude NCSE. Alternative diagnostic considerations include alternate psychosis (in which remission of seizures appears to lead to emergence of psychosis) and adverse drug effect, particularly if a new AED was recently added (see section on Psychiatric and Behavioral Adverse Effects of Antiepileptic Drugs below). There are no controlled trials studying treatment approaches to PIP. The episodes tend to abate on their own within a week or two, and pharmacological treatment may be unnecessary. If there are safety concerns, inpatient evaluation and treatment may be necessary—particularly if there is aggressive or grossly disorganized behavior. Some experts have reported that PIP can sometimes respond well to low doses of atypical antipsychotic drugs or benzodiazepines,[26] though this is not uniformly the case, and treatment may need to

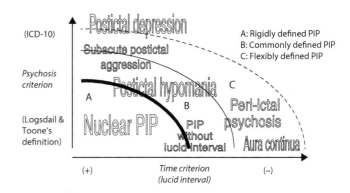

FIGURE 29-2. Spectrum of postictal psychosis (PIP) and related syndromes. The y-axis indicates the strictness of the psychosis criterion, with rigidly defined psychosis toward the origin. The x-axis indicates the degree of lucidity between end of seizure and beginning of psychiatric symptoms. Syndromes to the right side of the x-axis are continuous with the seizure and are presumed more likely to reflect ongoing ictal activity. (Reproduced with permission of the Cambridge University Press through PLSclear from Kanemoto K. Postictal psychoses: Established facts and new clinical questions. In: Trimble MR, Schmitz B, eds. *The Neuropsychiatry of Epilepsy*. 2nd ed. Cambridge University Press; 2011:67-79. Copyright © Cambridge University Press 2011.)

TABLE 29-4 • Logsdail and Toone Criteria for Postictal Psychosis.

- An episode of confusion or psychosis immediately after a seizure or emerging within a week of the return of apparently normal mental function.

- The episode has a minimum length of 24 hours and a maximum length of 3 months.

- The mental state during the episode is characterized by one or both of the following:
  - Clouding of consciousness, disorientation, or delirium
  - Delusions, hallucinations in clear consciousness

- There is no evidence of the following extraneous factors
  - Anticonvulsant toxicity based on drugs levels or physical exam
  - A previous history of interictal psychosis
  - EEG evidence of nonconvulsive status epilepticus
  - Recent head injury or alcohol or drug intoxication

be individualized. Because PIP is generally short-lived, patients may not require long-term pharmacotherapy for the psychosis, and short-term tapering of antipsychotic medications should be considered once the psychosis remits.

Other Postictal Psychiatric Symptoms

A variety of other nonpsychotic psychiatric symptoms can occur during the postictal period, although this has received relatively little attention in the literature. Kanner and colleagues[32] administered a survey to 100 patients with refractory partial epilepsy, and found that 74% of patients retrospectively reported at least one psychiatric symptom that either emerged de novo or worsened following at least 50% of their recent seizures. Among the symptoms reported, cognitive symptoms and neurovegetative symptoms such as excessive somnolence, loss of appetite, and loss of sexual interest were most common, reported by 82% and 62% of patients respectively, followed by symptoms of anxiety (45%) and depression (43%). The risk of postictal psychiatric symptoms was increased by a history of depression and anxiety, and 96% of the patients who endorsed interictal psychiatric symptoms reported worsening of their symptoms during the postictal period. Only 7% of patients reported postictal psychotic symptoms. A study of postictal psychiatric events in the epilepsy monitoring unit reported a rate of only 7.8%, most of which were psychotic events.[22] This may suggest that postictal psychotic symptoms are the ones most likely to come to clinical attention, while nonpsychotic symptoms may be more common but can be missed by clinicians unless they are specifically assessed for.

Preictal Psychiatric Symptoms

Some patients report prodromal symptoms during the minutes to days prior to a seizure that may herald its onset. These symptoms are generally considered preictal, as opposed to auras, which occur during the early seconds to minutes of a seizure and are considered to reflect the seizure onset. Among studies examining prevalence of seizure prodromes, a nonspecific "funny feeling" was most common (experienced by 10.4% of patients) while anxiety and irritability were also relatively common (experienced by 8.6% and 7.7%, respectively).[33] Preictal dysphoria and irritability may also be relatively commonplace, and a substantial percentage of patients with the interictal dysphoric disorder (discussed below) report a habitual relationship between affective symptoms and the peri-ictal period, with 22.6% of affective symptoms occurring before the seizure.[34] While patients' retrospective self-reports may be subject to recall bias and false attribution, at least one prospective study showed that preictal nervousness or mood worsening predicted an increased likelihood of seizure.[35] It is unclear to what extent the association between these symptoms and subsequent seizure reflects seizure prodrome versus seizure-provocation, since many patients report stress or intense emotions to be a precipitating factor for their seizures.[36]

INTERICTAL NEUROPSYCHIATRIC SYMPTOMS

Emotional, behavioral, and cognitive symptoms may appear independently of seizure occurrence in PWE. These interictal neuropsychiatric symptoms may occur transiently or chronically. In many cases, they resemble idiopathic psychiatric illnesses, but their prevalence among PWE is greater than would be expected by chance, and the manifestations may differ somewhat from what is typical in idiopathic psychiatric illnesses. In some sense, it may be appropriate to consider these to be comorbidities, in that, at least at the individual level, they may appear to be problems separate from the epilepsy. However, the statistical relationships between epilepsy and disorders of cognition, behavior, and emotion suggest that this variety of non-seizure symptoms may be considered part of the epilepsy syndrome itself. This has led to a conceptual definition of epilepsy that is not only characterized by the predisposition to recurrent seizures, but also "by the neurobiologic, cognitive, psychological, and social consequences of this condition."[37] In the sections that follow, we discuss interictal affective disturbances, anxiety, psychosis, and cognitive problems experienced by PWE.

Interictal Mood Disorders

Depressive disorders are common among PWE. Meta-analyses have shown a prevalence of depression (within the previous 12 months) in PWE of 13.2–36.5%.[38] Odds ratio (OR) of active depression in PWE relative to persons without epilepsy across 1,217,024 subjects in five studies was estimated at 2.77 (range of individual adjusted OR between 1.1 and 3.49), and overall OR for lifetime depression in 4195 subjects from three studies was 2.2 (range 1.48–3.96).[38] These numbers demonstrate that epilepsy confers an increased risk of depression. This is not solely explained by the presence of a chronic disease, as prevalence rates for depression are highest in epilepsy when compared against other chronic medical conditions (such as asthma, diabetes, migraines).[39]

Population-based cohort studies that compare incidence rates show that those individuals with depression were at higher risk of developing epilepsy and vice versa.[40,41] Current or past depression is also associated with poor seizure outcomes.[40] According to one study, depression was identified as the single most important predictor of quality of life in patients with recurring seizures.[42] Both neurobiological and psychosocial factors underlie the bidirectional risk between depression and epilepsy. Common neurobiological mechanisms that may predispose to both depression and epilepsy include a hyperactive hypothalamic-pituitary-adrenal (HPA) axis, neuronal and glial cell loss in frontal and mesial temporal structures, increased glutamatergic and decreased GABAergic and serotonergic activity, and neuroinflammatory changes.[43] Amygdalar kindling in rats is accelerated with chronic low-dose corticosteroid supplementation, akin to the physiological elevations in cortisol seen with chronic depression,[44] suggesting a possible mechanistic link between a hyperactive HPA axis and neuronal hyperexcitability and epilepsy.

TLE associated with structural brain lesions (e.g., hippocampal sclerosis) has been more strongly associated with depression than non-lesional or extratemporal epilepsy, although these findings have not been consistently replicated.[45,46] Depression is also common among patients with generalized epilepsy.[47] Some studies found no difference in rates of depression between patients with focal and generalized seizures[48,49] and one study showed more severe depression in TLE compared to generalized epilepsy.[50] The role of laterality in the development of depression is unclear, with some studies showing no relationship between side of seizure focus and history of depression[51,52] and other studies showing an association between depression and seizure focus on either side.[53,54]

On a psychosocial level, the fact that seizures are unpredictable, aversive events outside of the patient's control resembles the "learned helplessness" model of depression. In addition to this model, the burden of living with epilepsy leads to chronically increased stress influenced by associated injuries and symptoms (such as fatigue and cognitive complaints), lower academic achievement, lower socioeconomic and marital status, lack of independence, driving and vocational restrictions, social stigma, and lower self-esteem, all known to contribute to depression.[55]

DSM-5 criteria for depressive disorders, including major depressive disorder,[56] apply to PWE. Screening tools for major depressive disorder available in the public domain and validated in epilepsy include the Neurological Disorders Depression Inventory for Epilepsy (NDDI-E) and the Patient Health Questionnaire-9 (PHQ-9).[57,58] The NDDI-E is a six-item questionnaire that minimizes the contribution of confounding symptoms of depression that could be due to epilepsy itself or to effects of AEDs.[58] Mood syndromes specific to epilepsy populations have also been described, such as the *interictal dysphoric disorder*[59] or *dysthymic disorder of epilepsy*.[60] These constructs have not been validated in large-scale studies. The specific features of these phenotypic variations are listed in Table 29-5.[59,60] The assessment of depressive disorders in epilepsy should evaluate any temporal association to seizure occurrence, as this may reveal peri-ictal or postictal mood changes (discussed in prior section), any association to changes in AED regimen (discussed in subsequent section) or surgical interventions, and contributions from other substances or medical conditions.

PWE have an increased risk of death by suicide when compared to the general population (standardized mortality ratio of 3.5–5).[61,62] A large meta-analysis found increased risk for suicide in some specific epilepsy subgroups, including newly diagnosed epilepsy, tertiary care settings or epilepsy institutions, TLE, and post-epilepsy surgery cases including temporal lobectomy.[63] The risk of elevated suicide behaviors predates the formal diagnosis of epilepsy based on a large epidemiological study.[41]

Treatment of depression in epilepsy should be guided by the same principles used in primary depression with additional considerations including possible risk of lowered seizure threshold (discussed in section on Seizure Risk with Psychotropic Medication), possible pharmacokinetic interactions between psychotropic drugs and AEDs (discussed in section below), amplification of possible side effects given concomitant AEDs, the additional risk of suicide associated with epilepsy and its treatment, and the added psychosocial factors unique to this population. Despite lack of randomized controlled trials (RCTs) of selective serotonin reuptake inhibitors (SSRIs) in epilepsy, this class of antidepressants is safe and well-tolerated in PWE and SSRIs should be considered first-line agents in the psychopharmacological management of depression in this population. Those SSRIs with minimal effect on the CYP450 enzymes such as citalopram, escitalopram, and sertraline are preferred in patients taking hepatically metabolized AEDs in order to minimize pharmacokinetic interactions.[64]

RCTs of psychosocial interventions in epilepsy were included in a Cochrane review and consistently showed significant improvement in quality of life, the primary focus of the review. Depression outcomes were included in 11 studies, either as primary or secondary measures, and severity improved in most (7 out of 11) RCTs that evaluated cognitive behavioral (CBT) and/or mindfulness-based psychotherapies and self-management interventions.[65] Some of these interventions were delivered online[66] or by phone[67] circumventing some of the logistical limitations for PWE who are often unable to drive. Five out of nine studies that included seizure-related outcomes demonstrated significant improvement in at least one measure of seizure outcomes. The interventions that improved seizure outcomes were based on mindfulness and educational approaches,[65] demonstrating the transdiagnostic benefit of some of these treatments. Three other RCTs that specifically evaluated the efficacy of CBT in PWE, and not included in the Cochrane review cited above, showed no benefit in depression severity,[68-70] although two of those studies offered CBT with seizure-focused content, instead of depression-focused content. CBT focused on depression (rather than focused on seizure control) appears to result in reduced symptoms of depression.[71,72]

Electroconvulsive therapy (ECT) has proven to be a safe and effective treatment for depression in PWE, with induced seizure length no different from non-epilepsy populations. Potential challenges include inadequate seizure induction in the setting of AEDs or the risk of inducing spontaneous seizure activity, especially if AED doses are lowered to facilitate the planned seizure induction. Ongoing collaboration between the treating psychiatrist and neurologist is necessary to adjust AED doses to ensure the safety and efficacy of the treatment.[73]

Bipolar disorder and epilepsy share similarities, including a chronic course punctuated by episodes (mania and seizures, respectively), as well as a proposed involvement of kindling mechanisms, changes in neurotransmitters, abnormalities in voltage-gated ion channels and second messenger systems, and treatment response to AEDs.[74] Aside from peri-ictal and postictal mood changes (discussed above) and some specific phenotypic variations seen in epilepsy (see Table 29-5), classical bipolar disorder has been regarded as relatively uncommon in PWE.[75] This notion has been challenged by a prevalence of manic/hypomanic episodes of 15% in 117 PWE based on a structured interview.[76] Another community-based self-report questionnaire of 85,358 US adults demonstrated a 12.2% positive screen for past periods of hypomanic/manic symptoms in PWE. Hypomanic/manic symptoms were 1.6–2.2 times more common in PWE compared to patients with other chronic medical conditions and 6.6 times more common in PWE than in healthy adults.[77] There is limited understanding of the specific phenomenological features and therapeutic implications of interictal bipolar disorder.

Interictal Anxiety Disorders

Anxiety disorders as a group encompass a broad spectrum of specific disorders, which include generalized anxiety disorder

---

TABLE 29-5 • Interictal Mood Disorder Phenotypes Described in Epilepsy.

Interictal dysphoric disorder
- During a period of 12 months, 3 or more of the following symptoms (irrespective of symptom cluster) must be present:
  - Labile depressive symptoms (anergia, depressed mood, insomnia, pain);
  - Labile affective symptoms (fear, anxiety);
  - Specific symptoms (euphoric moods, paroxysmal irritability).
- Symptoms last few hours to several days and are interrupted by symptom-free periods.

Dysthymic disorder of epilepsy
- Chronic dysthymia.
- Frequently interrupted by periods of normal mood, irritability, anhedonia, fatigue, anxiety, low frustration tolerance, mood lability with bouts of crying.

TABLE 29-6 • Core Diagnostic Features of the Anxiety Disorders Most Frequently Studied in Epilepsy.

Generalized anxiety disorder (GAD)
- Excessive anxiety and worry almost daily for at least 6 months.
- Unable to control worry and one or more of the following: restlessness, muscle tension, irritability, easily fatigued, diminished concentration, and sleep disturbance.

Panic disorder
- Recurrent, unexpected panic attacks with persistent worry about future attacks or their consequences for at least 1 month after the initial attack.
- Panic attacks are discrete periods of intense fear that develop abruptly and reach peak within 10 minutes. A panic attack includes at least 4 of the following symptoms: palpitations, sweating, trembling, shortness of breath, sensation of choking, chest pain, abdominal discomfort, dizziness, derealization, fear of loss of control, fear of death, paresthesias, chills.

Agoraphobia
- Intense fear in response to two of the following situations: using public transportation, being in open spaces, being in enclosed spaces, standing in line or being in a crowd, being outside of the home alone.
- Avoidance of such situations or they are endured with severe distress.
- Concerns must persist for at least 6 months and occur virtually every time the individual encounters the place or situation.

Social anxiety disorder
- Fear or anxiety specific to social settings, grossly disproportionate to the situation, in which a person feels noticed, observed, or scrutinized.
- Fear that anxiety will be displayed and the person will be socially rejected.
- Avoidance of social situations or they are endured with severe distress.
- Concerns must persist for at least 6 months and social interactions consistently provoke distress.

Specific phobia
- Persistent unreasonable or excessive fear caused by a specific object or situation, or its anticipation. If exposed to the situation, a panic attack (in adults) or tantrum (in children) may occur.
- The person recognizes that the fear is excessive.
- Avoidance of such situations or they are endured with severe distress.
- The phobia has persisted for at least 6 months.

Obsessive-compulsive disorder (OCD)—reclassified in *DSM-5* within "obsessive compulsive and related disorders"
- Presence of obsessions, compulsions, or both, that are time-consuming (more than 1 hour a day) or cause distress or impairment.
- Obsessions are recurrent and persistent thoughts, urges, or impulses experienced as intrusive and unwanted, cause anxiety and distress and the person tries to ignore or suppress.
- Compulsions are repetitive behaviors performed in response to an obsession or rigidly following rules, aimed at neutralizing anxiety or preventing some unrealistic situation.

Post-traumatic stress disorder (PTSD)—reclassified in *DSM-5* within "trauma- and stressor-related disorders"
- Prior exposure to a traumatic event (actual or threatened; exposure can be direct or indirect).
- Symptoms of intrusion or reexperiencing (i.e., flashbacks, nightmares, intrusive memories), avoidance (i.e., of thoughts or people or situations connected to the trauma), negative mood or cognitions (i.e., distorted sense of blame for oneself related to the trauma), increased arousal (i.e., hypervigilance, being easily startled).

(GAD), panic disorder, and different types of phobias. In previous versions of the diagnostic classification of mental disorders (*DSM-IV* TR), OCD and post-traumatic stress disorder (PTSD) were classified as anxiety disorders, but these have been included in separate categories in *DSM-5*.[56] The core diagnostic features of the anxiety disorders most frequently studied in epilepsy are displayed in Table 29-6.[56] The common feature in these disorders is an exaggerated or inappropriate fear response.[78]

Although less studied than depression, anxiety disorders are very common in epilepsy. A population-based study of 36,984 individuals in Canada identified 253 with epilepsy.[79] Using a diagnostic interview, the prevalence (95% CI) of the following anxiety disorders was identified among the people with epilepsy: any lifetime anxiety disorder 22.8% (14.8–30.9), lifetime panic disorder and agoraphobia 6.6% (2.9–10.3), any anxiety disorder in the last 12 months 12.8% (6.0–19.7) and panic disorder and agoraphobia in the last 12 months 5.6% (1.9–9.2).[79]

Lifetime anxiety disorders were more likely in PWE than in the general population with an OR of 2.4 (1.5–3.8). Another population-based study of 7403 subjects from the United Kingdom, also using a psychiatric interview, identified 1.2% prevalence of epilepsy with the following prevalence (95% CI) for anxiety disorders and adjusted OR (95% CI): GAD 12.5% (7.6–20.1) and OR 2.6 (1.5–4.7), social anxiety disorder 6.0% (2.7–12.8) and OR 5.2 (2.1–13.1), specific phobias 1.8% (0.6–5.7) and OR 1.2 (0.3–4.5), agoraphobia 4.9% (2.7–11.4) and OR 3.2 (1.2–8.7), OCD 3.1% (1.5–6.3) and OR 1.8 (0.8–4.4), PTSD 4.9% (2.0–11.4) and OR 1.2 (0.5–2.9). While not all anxiety disorders had an elevated risk in epilepsy (specific phobia and OCD did not), the elevated risk of anxiety disorders was higher in epilepsy than in asthma and diabetes, two chronic medical conditions.[39] A population-based cohort study demonstrated that those individuals with anxiety were at higher risk of developing epilepsy, pointing out the bidirectional nature of both disorders.[41]

Neurobiological and psychosocial factors may explain the overlap between anxiety and epilepsy. While interictal anxiety disorders are most common in TLE, patients with generalized epilepsy are also at increased risk.[80] There is no conclusive evidence about the association between anxiety disorders and lateralization of epileptic focus in temporal lobe seizures.[81] The amygdala is associated with fear conditioning, and amygdalar kindling has been shown to increase anxiety behaviors in rats.[82] Many PWE who have ictal fear as a semiological feature of their seizures show amygdala atrophy in brain imaging studies.[83] On the other hand, increased amygdala size, especially on the right, has been demonstrated in patients with refractory focal epilepsy with interictal anxiety versus those without psychopathology.[84] These findings on amygdala size in ictal fear versus interictal anxiety from individual studies may seem contradictory, although they may signal a different effect of ictal versus interictal anxiety-related processes on brain structures. One hypothesis to explain the high rates of interictal anxiety in epilepsy stipulates that fear sensitization results from hyperexcitation of the fear circuitry due to long-term potentiation of excitatory amygdala efferents.[82] Changes in many neurotransmitters (serotonin, norepinephrine, and GABA) have been implicated in the interplay between epilepsy and anxiety. GABA plays a central role as GABAergic medications, such as valproic acid, barbiturates, and benzodiazepines can reduce both seizures and anxiety.[78,82] Polymorphism of a specific allele of the serotonin transporter gene was identified as an independent risk factor for anxiety in TLE.[85]

On a psychological level, reactions to the unpredictable nature of seizures, restrictions on regular life activities and resulting low self-esteem, stigmatization, and social rejection are important factors that can lead to anxiety.[80] Psychological mechanisms leading to the development of panic and anxiety symptoms in epilepsy include fear of seizure recurrence ("seizure phobia") and a sense of dispersed locus of control.[82]

Recognizing and treating anxiety in PWE is important. There is some evidence that increased levels of stress and anxiety can increase the frequency of seizures.[80] In addition, anxiety is known to have an independent negative effect on quality of life in epilepsy.[82] The assessment of anxiety in the context of epilepsy requires special attention to the temporal relationship between seizures and symptoms of anxiety. Recurrent panic attacks can be misdiagnosed as focal epilepsy (with ictal fear) and vice versa. Both share overlapping symptoms, can coexist, and have a possible common neurobiological substrate.[80] Table 29-3 and the subsection on ictal psychiatric symptoms provide distinguishing clinical features. One study showed that 33% of 12 patients with ictal fear also experienced interictal panic disorder,[86] although data from larger samples of patients with ictal fear is lacking.

The diagnostic criteria in *DSM-5*[56] are useful for the evaluation of interictal anxiety disorders. In addition to the temporal relationship to seizures, any contribution from AEDs, other medications, substances, or medical conditions needs to be considered during the evaluation of anxiety symptoms. Some AEDs can be associated with the development of anxiety (discussed in subsequent section). AED withdrawal can also lead to anxiety symptoms.[80] The Generalized Anxiety Disorder-7 (GAD-7) questionnaire has been validated in PWE and provides high

sensitivity and specificity at a cutoff of 6 (a lower cutoff than in primary care) for the detection of GAD in epilepsy.[87]

Treatment of interictal anxiety disorders should be guided by the same principles used in primary anxiety disorders with the same considerations outlined in the treatment of interictal depression regarding risk of lowered seizure threshold, pharmacokinetic interactions, augmentation of side effects, and psychosocial factors (see previous section). There are no RCTs of antidepressants in epilepsy that evaluate their efficacy in anxiety disorders. SSRIs are usually considered first-line agents, and selective norepinephrine reuptake inhibitors (SNRIs) are also frequently used in the treatment of most anxiety disorders. The prescription of benzodiazepines should be exercised with caution given potential sedating and cognitive effects, risk of dependence and, if used consistently and at high doses, a risk of withdrawal seizures with missed or decreased doses. The AED pregabalin has shown efficacy in primary GAD and therefore has been suggested as a reasonable treatment for interictal GAD.[88] Buspirone, a serotonergic agonist, may also be considered in patients with interictal GAD.

A Cochrane review on psychosocial interventions in PWE that reported on quality of life outcomes included five RCTs with anxiety severity measures as a secondary outcome.[65] Of those, only one RCT of mindfulness-based psychotherapy showed significant improvement in anxiety severity.[89] None of the reported interventions were specifically designed to address interictal anxiety disorders. Uncontrolled trials have demonstrated a benefit for CBT in reducing anxiety severity in PWE.[90] The broad-range applicability and efficacy of CBT across many primary anxiety disorders make this psychosocial intervention a reasonable and accessible treatment to offer in interictal anxiety disorders.

Interictal Psychosis

IIP may occur transiently, resembling a "brief psychotic disorder,"[56] or as a chronic schizophrenia-like illness.

Episodic Interictal Psychosis

Episodic interictal psychosis (EIP) should probably be distinguished from chronic IIP due to the better prognosis.[91] Possible causes for EIP include adverse drug reaction and forced normalization (discussed in section on Neuropsychiatric Adverse Effects of Epilepsy Treatment). A postictal psychotic episode may be mischaracterized as an IIP if the patient is unaware of the recent seizures or is not capable of providing a reliable history, and collateral history from the patient's family or caregivers may be necessary to determine the temporal relationship to the seizures.

Chronic Interictal Psychosis

Chronic interictal psychosis (CIP) occurs in 2–10% of PWE, and typically follows the onset of epilepsy by a decade or more.[91–93] The incidence is greater than would be expected by chance alone,[94] and in fact, epilepsy is associated with a 2–2.5-fold increased risk of schizophrenia and schizophrenia-like psychosis.[95,96] A history of febrile seizures progressing to epilepsy has been associated with a threefold increased risk of developing schizophrenia.[97] IIP has been most closely associated with TLE,[91] and in particular, left TLE, but this remains uncertain and controversial, and psychosis has been reported in association with generalized epilepsy as well as other focal epilepsies, most notably frontal lobe epilepsy.[98] Nevertheless, psychosis of any sort does appear to occur more often in patients with TLE than in patients with extratemporal epilepsy.[98] Functional and structural neuroimaging studies have tended to show predominantly left temporal dysfunction and volume loss, although this has been an inconsistent finding.[99]

Slater and Beard, in their early descriptions of chronic IIP of epilepsy, emphasized both its similarity to schizophrenia and its existence as a separate entity, by referring to it as schizophrenia-like psychosis of epilepsy (SLPE).[93,100] Patients who go on to develop SLPE may lack the premorbid schizoid personality traits sometimes seen in patients who subsequently develop schizophrenia,[100] and the illness itself may exhibit a greater degree of affective symptomatology and a lower likelihood of negative symptoms than is typical in schizophrenia.[101] Patients with SLPE may also be more responsive to lower doses of neuroleptics than patients with schizophrenia.[102] On the other hand, neuropsychological profiles are similar between patients with SLPE and schizophrenia,[103] and in many patients, the psychotic syndrome closely resembles schizophrenia, even including Schneider's first-rank symptoms.[101] Thus, while there may be some differences in psychopathology between patients with schizophrenia and those with SLPE, the distinctions are subtle and may not be apparent in an individual patient. Schizophrenia is increasingly recognized as a heterogeneous disorder that lies on a spectrum with other psychotic illnesses[104] and is neurobiologically characterized by frontolimbic dysfunction (see Chapter 11).

It is unclear what the causal relationship is between epilepsy and IIP. Because onset of epilepsy tends to precede the onset of psychosis by years, it is possible that excitotoxic injury or kindling from recurrent seizures alters neural circuitry in a way that leads to the development of psychosis. Another plausible explanation for the association between epilepsy and psychosis is that the psychotic illness and the epilepsy share a causal relationship with a third factor such as birth trauma, head injury, or some other developmental or genetic abnormality.[105] Epileptic seizures are manifestations of an underlying aberration of neural circuitry that may result from a wide variety of cerebral pathologies, some of which can be extremely subtle and difficult to identify without pathological tissue. Identification of neuropathological abnormalities in schizophrenia is even more difficult. Genetic risk factors are recognized for both epilepsy and for schizophrenia, although monogenetic inheritance is rare.[106] Nevertheless, a putative genetic link has been identified between epilepsy and psychosis[107] and several chromosomal loci have been linked with both conditions. The 15q11.2 BP1-BP2 microdeletion has been associated with both epilepsy and schizophrenia,[108] and the LGI gene loci overlap with loci that have been linked to schizophrenia.[105] It is likely that some pathologies that predispose patients to epileptic seizures (i.e., abnormalities in the structure and function of the neocortex and limbic system, and particularly those involving the temporal lobe) also play a role in the development of a psychotic illness. It has been proposed on the basis of rodent models that misguidance of mossy fiber projection in the hippocampus may be one cellular mechanism linking epilepsy and psychosis.[109]

Treatment of SLPE is similar to treatment of schizophrenia, though antipsychotic drugs such as clozapine that are known to lower the seizure threshold should be used with caution (see section below on treatment of psychiatric symptoms in PWE). Antipsychotic drugs side effects and their interactions with AEDs should also be considered (see Table 29-7).

Cognitive Problems Related to Epilepsy

PWE frequently have cognitive symptoms[110] that can adversely affect their quality of life. The pathophysiology of these symptoms is multifactorial and related to both fixed factors, factors related to disease course, and remediable factors.[111,112]

Fixed Factors
Location of the Epilepsy and the Presence or Absence of an Underlying Syndrome

In adults, TLE is the most common epilepsy subtype. Given its location and the involvement of hippocampal and parahippocampal structures, episodic memory is the cognitive function most impacted. In general, verbal memory is affected in epilepsy from the language-dominant temporal lobe, while visual memory is affected in epilepsy from the non-dominant temporal lobe, especially in the setting of atrophy or structural lesions. Patients are able to retrieve long-term memories while short-term material-specific (verbal/visual) memories are impaired. When the nondominant temporal lobe is involved, patients may experience difficulty with recognition of faces and facial expressions. Testing of temporal lobe functions by clinicians includes having the patient remember a word list or visuospatial information and testing the recognition of famous faces. It is also not uncommon for TLE patients to experience executive dysfunction as a result of the close interactions between the temporal lobe and the prefrontal cortices.

In frontal lobe epilepsy, symptoms related to frontal lobe dysfunction may arise. Depending on the type and extent of the pathology, there can be impairments in multitasking, working memory, sustained attention, response inhibition, and verbal fluency. Cognitive impairments in other types of epilepsies have been studied less, but one would expect attentional difficulties in parietal lobe epilepsies due to disruption of frontoparietal attention networks as well as verbal or visuospatial impairments depending on whether the dominant or nondominant hemisphere is involved. Patients with generalized epilepsy syndromes such as JME present with frontal-subcortical circuit dysfunction with difficulties retrieving information and sustaining attention. These deficits do not occur in isolation, and other cognitive domains are also impaired. There is evidence that visuospatial skills are the most spared.[113]

Coexisting Conditions

Epilepsy rarely occurs in isolation and PWE can also suffer from a number of comorbid neuropsychiatric conditions such as ADHD and autism spectrum disorder (ASD).

Children and adults with epilepsy have a high prevalence of comorbid ADHD. Studies focusing on children and adolescents have described rates as high as 32%, usually of the inattentive

TABLE 29-7 • Pharmacokinetic Interactions between Antiepileptic Drugs (AEDs) and Commonly Prescribed Psychotropic Drugs Metabolized by CYP450 System.

CYP450 Isoenzyme	Substrate (Most Significantly Eliminated by Isoenzyme)	Inhibitor (Moderate to Potent)	Inducer (Moderate to Potent)
CYP1A2	Fluvoxamine Duloxetine Asenapine Clozapine Olanzapine Carbamazepine	Fluvoxamine	Carbamazepine Phenytoin Phenobarbital Primidone
CYP2C9	Phenobarbital Phenytoin Primidone Valproic acid	Valproic acid Fluoxetine Fluvoxamine	Carbamazepine Phenytoin Phenobarbital Primidone
CYP2C19	Lacosamide Citalopram Escitalopram Phenytoin Phenobarbital Primidone Clobazam	Felbamate Fluoxetine Fluvoxamine	Carbamazepine Phenytoin Phenobarbital Primidone
CYP3A4	Carbamazepine Ethosuximide Clobazam Felbamate Perampanel Tiagabine Zonisamide Mirtazapine Reboxetine Trazodone Vilazidone Aripiprazole Brexipiprazole Lurasidone Quetiapine Risperidone	Fluoxetine Fluvoxamine	Carbamazepine Phenytoin Phenobarbital Primidone
CYP2B6	Sertraline Bupropion		Carbamazepine Phenytoin Phenobarbital Primidone

subtype.[114] Although there were initial concerns about the risk of seizures with stimulants, the data seems to suggest that they are safe to use in PWE. This is further discussed below.

Epilepsy and ASD have a bidirectional relationship with high rates of epilepsy in patients with ASD, and high risk of developing ASD in PWE, especially in the setting of developmental delay.[115] Patients with ASD also have high rates of epileptiform abnormalities on EEG even when there is no history of seizures, the clinical significance of which remains unclear.

Age of Onset of Epilepsy and Treatment

Childhood-onset epilepsy can have a significant adverse impact on a patient's neurodevelopmental course. Children with TLE prior to the age of 14 have reduced total brain volumes and intellectual status as compared to healthy controls or patients with a later disease onset.[116] There is a concern that these findings reflect the adverse impact of seizures during a critical period of neurodevelopment for the child.[117] Epilepsy surgery can lead to improved cognitive function in children, and evidence suggests that early surgical intervention in children may lead to better neurodevelopment outcome.[118] Thus, it is important to avoid delaying surgery in children with medication-resistant epilepsy who are candidates for potentially curative resection.

Educational Level and Gender

Women with TLE tend to have better verbal memory performance as compared to their male counterparts and are less susceptible to adverse cognitive sequelae from the surgical resection of the temporal lobe[119] possibly due to differences in connectivity and plasticity in the language dominant hemisphere. The concept of a cognitive reserve in epilepsy patients can also be applied. In the setting of a high educational level or complex vocation, patients are more resilient to the impact of refractory seizures and their cognitive functions are impacted less. However, these are the patients at higher risk of decline after epilepsy surgery, especially in the dominant hemisphere.

Factors Related to Disease Course

Epilepsy, when left unchecked for prolonged periods of time, can take its toll on the brain. In addition to the acute mortality risk of GTC seizures and status epilepticus (SE), the risk of a deleterious long-term cognitive impact is substantial. Over time, patterns of atrophy emerge in bilateral brain regions in patients with refractory epilepsy,[120] and there is evidence that a high GTC seizure burden is associated with a lower IQ. Persistent memory impairment and executive dysfunction can also be seen following a GTC longer than 5 minutes in duration.[121] Pathological analysis of surgical tissue in epilepsy patients reveals increased levels of tau pathology, similar to what can be seen in patients with recurrent concussions, and this is likely contributing to the cognitive impairment in these patients.[122]

Remediable Factors

Several remediable factors need to be assessed when evaluating PWE and cognitive complaints. The role of medication side effects and their impact on executive functions cannot be emphasized enough, especially in the setting of polytherapy (discussed later). Comorbid depression and anxiety disorders are also common and can have a direct impact on cognition if left untreated. Sleep disorders including obstructive sleep apnea are also remediable and comprise another therapeutic target with a high impact on cognitive outcomes.[123] The effect of interictal epileptiform discharges on cognition is controversial. There is compelling evidence from invasive surgical evaluations that the burden of these discharges directly disrupts cognitive functions such as information encoding and retrieval.[124] However, it is unclear whether the treatment of these discharges with medications improves outcomes, especially when the medications themselves may further contribute to the dysfunction.

Epilepsy and Dementia

Seizures are relatively common (up to 20%)[125] in patients with dementia (termed major neurocognitive disorder in the *DSM-5*) but were once thought to be a late complication of severe cortical atrophy after a prolonged course of a neurodegenerative disease. Over the past decade, however, evidence has suggested that seizures could represent the initial manifestation of a neurodegenerative illness and may precede cognitive deficits by a few years in a subset of patients.[126] In addition, Alzheimer's disease (AD) patients with seizures tend to have a more rapid cognitive decline over time as compared to those without.[127] Patients with AD have the highest cumulative incidence of seizures compared to other dementias, especially in the setting of early-onset disease. Lewy body disease patients develop seizures at a lower rate compared to AD, but are particularly susceptible to myoclonus.[128] Whether the treatment of seizures affects the dementia course remains to be seen.

The question of whether epilepsy in and of itself is a progressive neurodegenerative illness has not been definitively answered. There is evidence of cognitive decline over time in the setting of poorly controlled epilepsy, but neurodevelopmental

factors may be more significant determinants of cognitive dysfunction than neurodegeneration. Epilepsy has also been associated with elevated serum markers of vascular disease (CRP, lipoprotein A, lipids, homocysteine) and evidence of a higher burden of cerebral small vessel disease on neuroimaging.[129] These factors also contribute to the effects of the disease on cognition with aging.

Temporolimbic Personality

There has long been interest in the idea of a characteristic epileptic personality. In 1975, Waxman and Geschwind[130] described a set of five personality traits associated with TLE: hypergraphia, hyperreligiosity, hyposexuality, aggressiveness, and social viscosity, which they collectively referred to as the interictal behavioral syndrome of TLE. The behavioral characteristics of TLE patients were further specified by Bear and Fedio,[131] who identified 18 behavioral traits that they found to occur with increased frequency in patients with TLE as compared to healthy controls and patients with neuromuscular disease. There has been considerable controversy over the specificity of these particular traits for TLE.[132] Interictal behavioral aberrations are frequently noted in TLE patients, but there is considerable variability and likely many contributory factors. Determinants may include not only seizure and epilepsy-related neural network disturbance, but also the effects of AEDs, underlying brain lesions, and the social and cultural impact of living with epilepsy and its physical limitations and social stigma.

NEUROPSYCHIATRIC ADVERSE EFFECTS OF EPILEPSY TREATMENT

The mainstay of epilepsy treatment is pharmacological. A multitude of AEDs have emerged over the past 50 years. With few caveats, these drugs are relatively equivalent in terms of their efficacy at reducing the risk of seizure, but they vary considerably in terms of their side-effect profiles. Approximately 60% of patients achieve excellent seizure control with medication alone, but for the sizeable minority of patients with medication-refractory epilepsy, nonmedical treatments are often pursued. The most important of these is epilepsy surgery, which can, under the best of circumstances, cure an otherwise intractable epilepsy. Since epilepsy treatments affect brain function by design, it is not surprising that they are associated with a variety of neuropsychiatric adverse effects. While the full spectrum of side effects associated with epilepsy treatment is beyond the scope of this chapter, the cognitive and psychiatric adverse effects are reviewed below in some detail (Table 29-8).

Adverse Cognitive Effects of Antiepileptic Drugs

Because AEDs either affect inhibitory or excitatory mechanisms in the brain, it is to be expected that normal physiologic cognitive processes may be impacted by their use. In general, the cognitive side effects of AEDs are dose-dependent and reversible.[133] The speed of drug titration plays a role as

TABLE 29-8 • Antiepileptic Drugs with Higher and Lower Likelihoods of Psychiatric and Cognitive Side Effects.

Lower Likelihood of Psychiatric Side Effects	Higher Likelihood of Psychiatric Side Effects	Lower Likelihood of Cognitive Side Effects	Higher Likelihood of Cognitive Side Effects
Lamotrigine	Topiramate	Lamotrigine	Phenobarbital
Lacosamide	Zonisamide	Levetiracetam	Primidone
Eslicarbazepine	Levetiracetam	Lacosamide	Topiramate
Gabapentin	Perampanel	Gabapentin	Zonisamide
Pregabalin	Phenobarbital	Tiagabine	
Oxcarbazepine	Vigabatrin	Vigabatrin	
Carbamazepine		Rufinamide	
Valproic acid		Perampanel	
		Eslicarbazepine	

well as the use of polytherapy as opposed to monotherapy.[134] The exact nature of the side effects is not uniform across drugs and depends on their mechanisms of action and idiosyncratic properties. In general, the cognitive domain most impacted is that of executive functioning. GABAergic drugs such as benzodiazepines, phenobarbital, and primidone have some of the most common cognitive adverse side effects due to their impact on inhibitory cortical interneurons. Topiramate and zonisamide on the other hand seem to particularly affect language in addition to executive networks, as has been shown in functional MRI (fMRI) studies.[135] Valproic acid can impact cognition by causing a hyperammonemic encephalopathy or by chronically depleting folic acid, an essential vitamin for the generation of neurotransmitters. On the other hand, drugs with a favorable cognitive profile include lamotrigine, lacosamide, levetiracetam, and perampanel.[136]

Patient-related factors may also underlie the appearance of the cognitive adverse effects such as age, gender, and underlying epilepsy etiology. From a genetics perspective, there is an interest in the roles of Apoε4, COMT (catechol-O-methyltransferase), and BDNF (brain-derived neurotrophic factor) genetic variants and their impact on cognitive performance. Data in epilepsy have so far focused on Apoε4 with evidence for reduced memory performance in Apoε4 carriers with TLE especially with long disease duration as compared to noncarriers.[137] Strategies to prevent cognitive side effects include the selection of drugs with a better cognitive side-effect profile, the use of monotherapy and slow dose titration, and the use of the lowest effective dose. The choice of drug must also take into account its impact on mood and fatigue because of the effect of these symptoms on cognition. In some cases, the side effects may coincide with peak drug levels and the use of a sustained-release formulation could be a solution. Finally, in cases where the side effects are persistent and the drug cannot be changed, pharmacologic cognitive enhancement or a referral for cognitive therapy may help.[136]

Adverse Psychiatric and Behavioral Effects of Antiepileptic Drugs

Psychiatric and behavioral side effects of AEDs account for a significant portion of AED side effects, affecting 15–20% of adult PWE, contributing to poor adherence, AED discontinuation, and possibly to the substantial psychiatric morbidity in this patient population.[138] Thus, when evaluating PWE for psychiatric symptoms, attention should be paid to the potential role of AEDs, particularly when symptoms coincide with the start of a new AED with known psychiatric adverse effects. Depressive reactions are most closely associated with phenobarbital, vigabatrin, zonisamide, topiramate, and perampanel, while anxiety is associated with levetiracetam, topiramate, vigabatrin, felbamate, and lamotrigine. Felbamate and lamotrigine have generally positive psychiatric profiles but can be activating, increasing alertness, and in susceptible patients, this may increase anxiety level and can occasionally cause agitation. Agitation, irritability, anger, or hyperactivity have also been associated with levetiracetam, perampanel, zonisamide, topiramate, and several drugs that potentiate GABA such as phenobarbital, clobazam, and vigabatrin. This paradoxical effect of GABAergic medications, which are generally considered sedating and anxiolytic, may be particularly problematic in children with learning disabilities.[139] Psychosis is a more rare but troubling AED side effect that has been associated with zonisamide, topiramate, vigabatrin, and levetiracetam. Psychosis has also been associated with phenytoin in the setting of toxic drug levels and with ethosuximide in the setting of *forced normalization* of the EEG in patients with generalized epilepsy syndromes (see section on forced normalization below). In a study by Stephen and colleagues[140] that prospectively assessed for psychiatric adverse effects among 1058 patients treated for epilepsy with newer AEDs, depression was the most common psychiatric problem leading to discontinuation of the drug followed by irritable mood. Perampanel was associated with the highest rate of intolerable psychiatric adverse effects (16.7%); topiramate, zonisamide, levetiracetam with intermediate rates (7.6%, 7.4%, and 6.8%, respectively); and lacosamide and eslicarbazepine with the lowest rates (1.9% each). In general, medications that potentiate GABA or modulate AMPA glutamate receptor activity (levetiracetam, topiramate, perampanel) are associated with worse psychiatric profile than drugs that primarily act on sodium channels (e.g., carbamazepine, lacosamide, lamotrigine).

In 2008, the FDA issued a warning about an increased risk of suicidal ideation, suicide attempts, and completed suicides in patients taking AEDs. This was based on a meta-analysis of 199 randomized placebo-controlled trials of 11 AEDs. When

AEDs were examined collectively, there was a statistically significant increased risk of suicidality (suicidal ideation and suicidal behavior) for patients on AEDs (0.37%) compared to placebo (0.24%).[141] Among 27,863 patients taking AEDs and 16,029 patients taking placebo, there were 4 completed suicides and 30 suicide attempts in the drug arm and zero completed suicides and 8 suicide attempts in the placebo arm. Suicidal ideation occurred in 67 patients in the drug arm and 29 patients in the placebo arm. The FDA warning has sparked controversy and raised concerns that routinely counseling patients about this small risk may lead to excessive worry and may adversely affect medication adherence and thereby increase morbidity and potentially even mortality from uncontrolled epilepsy.[142] The purported class effect has been greeted with skepticism given the differing mechanisms of action among the drugs studied. When drugs were considered individually, only lamotrigine and topiramate showed a statistically significant increased risk. Valproic acid and gabapentin may actually have a protective effect against suicidality.[143] Individual studies have not shown concordant findings on which drugs pose the greatest risk. The association between lamotrigine and increased risk of suicidality in the FDA meta-analysis has been questioned given numerous studies showing a positive effect of this drug on mood. The interpretation of the meta-analysis is also limited by the fact that the adverse events in the trials were spontaneously reported and there was no systematic data collection on suicidality.[144] A prior history of a psychiatric disorder, and especially a history of a prior suicide attempt is a much greater risk factor for suicide attempt than AED use, and epilepsy is associated with an increased risk of psychiatric disorders and suicide-related behaviors both before and after epilepsy diagnosis.[41] Thus, a hypothetically increased risk of suicidality should not dissuade providers from prescribing needed AEDs, but AEDs should be carefully chosen in patients with other suicide risk factors. If a patient develops suicidal ideation soon after starting a new AED, prompt withdrawal of the drug should be strongly considered.

The risk of psychiatric and behavioral adverse effects of AEDs is not uniform across the population of PWE. Patients with a personal or family history of a psychiatric disorder, patients with intractable epilepsy, secondarily generalized seizures, absence seizures, and patients with developmental intellectual disorders are at increased risk for developing psychiatric and behavioral adverse effects from AEDs.[138–140] The nature of the preexisting psychiatric condition may contribute to the particular manifestations of the adverse drug effect. Temporal lobe involvement[145] or bilateral EEG abnormalities[146] may be risk factors for AED-induced psychosis. Seizure-freedom may also be a risk factor for psychosis, particularly with topiramate, ethosuximide, and vigabatrin,[147–149] a phenomenon known as *alternate psychosis* (discussed below).

When a patient develops new-onset psychiatric symptoms after starting or increasing the dose of an AED, alternate explanations should be considered before attributing the symptoms to the medication. PIP can sometimes be mistaken for an AED side effect if the seizure(s) that provoked it also prompted initiation of a new drug. New-onset psychosis after initiation of an AED may also be due to forced normalization/alternate psychosis. Destabilization of an underlying psychiatric disorder can potentially occur as a result of decreased levels of psychotropic medication if there is a pharmacokinetic interaction with the new AED. Lastly, patients with intellectual impairment may be incapable of verbally communicating physical discomfort, and physical adverse effects of AEDs such as dizziness or nausea may manifest with behavioral acting out in this population.

Adverse Cognitive Effects of Epilepsy Surgery

While the majority of epilepsy cases can be effectively managed with medication, approximately 40% of patients have medication-resistant epilepsy, in which seizures cannot be completely controlled with medication alone. A subset of these patients are candidates for epilepsy surgery in which the seizure focus is resected. Resection can be successful if the epileptogenic tissue can be well localized with a combination of ictal EEG recordings and neuroimaging techniques. The most common surgical procedure is anteromesial temporal lobectomy (ATL), in which several centimeters of lateral temporal neocortex is removed (often sparing the superior temporal gyrus), along with the temporal pole, and the mesial temporal structures including the hippocampus and amygdala back to the level of the quadrigeminal plate. With appropriate patient selection, temporal lobectomy can cure seizures or produce long-term remission in as many as 80% of patients with mesial TLE resulting in good psychosocial outcomes with improved quality of life. The surgery is generally well tolerated, but a variety of cognitive and psychiatric complications may occur.

From a cognitive standpoint, one of the most concerning outcomes is a decline in verbal memory after resection of the dominant temporal lobe.[150] A meta-analysis of surgeries involving the left temporal lobe revealed evidence of verbal memory decline in 44% of patients as compared to 20% on the right. Predictors of decline include absence of hippocampal sclerosis, good preoperative memory, later age of seizure onset, male sex, older age at operation, and preoperative depression.[119] In contrast, there is a risk of visual memory decline in 23% of right- and 21% of left-sided temporal lobectomies. Improvement in presurgical verbal memory functioning has also been described and can be seen in 7% of left- and 14% of right-sided resections. In general, larger resections tend to be associated with a higher risk of decline. There has been a shift toward more restricted surgeries in the dominant temporal lobe with the advent of selective ablation technologies such as laser ablation, although this technique is associated with a lower chance of complete seizure freedom.

Adverse Psychiatric Effects of Epilepsy Surgery

Psychiatric complications may appear for the first time after epilepsy surgery or an exacerbation of a preexisting psychiatric disorder may ensue. Depression and mood lability are often transient and usually occur in the first 3 months following surgery. De novo depression has been reported in 5–25% of patients following ATL, and some suicide cases have been reported. Patients with preoperative depression, poor postoperative seizure control, and older males are the highest risk groups for developing postoperative depression.[81] Following ATL, anxiety symptoms increase in 17–54% of patients, peaking at 1 month and decreasing at 3 months postoperatively. Preoperative mood and anxiety-disordered patients are more susceptible to postoperative anxiety. Interestingly, patients with ictal fear as part of their seizure semiology are at greater risk of postoperative anxiety and panic attacks despite becoming seizure free.[81] New-onset mania after ATL has been described in 3.9% of patients undergoing temporal lobectomy[151] with onset shortly after surgery (usually within the first year post-surgery), and symptoms are generally transient in duration (1–3 months).[81] Preoperative bitemporal abnormalities, poor postsurgical seizure control, and a history of preoperative PIP are possible risk factors for postsurgical mania.[81] There are rare reports of de novo obsessive-convulsive disorder and PNES following surgery. In summary, patients with preexisting psychopathology are at increased risk for psychiatric complications of ATL, and this risk is likely compounded by poor seizure outcome. Such patients should be closely monitored during the postoperative period.

Forced Normalization/Alternate Psychosis

In 1953, Heinrich Landolt described a group of PWE in which psychotic episodes occurred coincident with resolution of epileptic EEG abnormalities. This phenomenon could occur with a variety of AEDs and was termed "*forced normalization*" implying that the psychosis was provoked by the suppression of epileptic discharges with AEDs.[152,153] The related phenomenon of "*alternate psychosis*" was subsequently coined by Tellenbach to refer to the reciprocal relationship between abnormal mental states and seizures, which, unlike forced normalization, does not require EEG to be diagnosed. This could presumably occur with surgical treatment of epilepsy in addition to pharmacological treatment. The existence of this phenomenon has been controversial and there has been little research on it in recent years. A diagnosis of forced normalization or alternate psychosis might suggest a treatment strategy aimed at reducing AED dosage so as to allow a certain amount of epileptic activity or even occasional seizures to reduce the risk of psychosis (or to treat an existing psychosis), a strategy that is rarely carried out in practice. Since in some cases of ictal psychosis, seizure activity is detectable only with depth electrodes and may be associated with generalized attenuation or disappearance of interictal spikes on scalp EEG, it has been proposed that forced normalization may actually reflect ongoing seizure activity restricted to a deep focus.[20,82,154] If true, this would suggest an opposite treatment strategy.

TREATMENT OF PSYCHIATRIC SYMPTOMS IN PATIENTS WITH EPILEPSY

Seizure Risk with Psychotropic Medication

The choice of psychotropic medication in PWE should take into account the risk of inducing a seizure. Antidepressants have been described as having both anticonvulsant and proconvulsant properties according to different studies and reviews.[155,156] A meta-analysis that included several studies leading to FDA indications of psychotropic medications for psychiatric disorders (75,873 patients) examined the standardized incidence ratio of seizures (ratio between observed and expected number of subjects with seizures) as a side effect.[157] As a group, the examined antidepressants (SSRIs, SNRIs, bupropion, and atypical antidepressants) conferred protection against seizures compared to placebo, and this protection was more pronounced when bupropion immediate release was eliminated from the list of antidepressants. When examined in isolation, bupropion immediate release had a standardized incidence ratio for seizures of 1.58 (95%CI 1.03–2.32), which was statistically significant. In this same meta-analysis, antidepressants that carried FDA approval for OCD were examined separately (clomipramine, fluoxetine, sertraline, fluvoxamine). In this analysis, clomipramine also increased the incidence of seizures.[157] A review of other controlled trials and clinical studies of patients with depression without epilepsy shows that maprotiline, high doses of tricyclic antidepressants (TCAs; especially amitriptyline and clomipramine at more than 200 mg/day), and high doses of immediate-release bupropion (more than 450 mg/day) are associated with an increased risk of seizures.[64] Antidepressants with incident seizures in more than 10% of overdoses include imipramine, desipramine, nortriptyline, amoxapine, maprotiline, and bupropion.[158] Antidepressants with evidence of incident seizures in 5–10% of overdoses include citalopram, venlafaxine, amitryptiline, clomipramine, doxepin, trimipramine, and proptiptyline.[158] A review of a primary care database in the United Kingdom determined that exposure to all classes of antidepressants in 283,963 patients with depression increased the risk of seizures at a 5-year follow-up compared to no pharmacological treatment for depression, with all antidepressant classes and most of the 11 individual drugs (except sertraline, escitalopram, and mirtazapine) elevating the risk. Of note, 0.37% of the depressed subjects on antidepressants had an incident diagnosis of epilepsy/seizure at 5 years, so the overall incidence was low even in the exposed subgroup. This retrospective analysis of a primary care database does not control for clinical factors leading to choice of treatment (antidepressants or not), therefore these results should be taken with caution.[155] In sum, despite some conflicting data, SSRIs, SNRIs, and atypical antidepressants (i.e., mirtazapine, trazodone) are considered safe in terms of seizure risk by most analyses, with overdose elevating the risk with some specific agents.[156] Maprotiline and TCAs carry higher risk of seizure, particularly maprotiline and high doses of amitriptyline and clomipramine. Bupropion in its immediate release form and at high doses should be avoided in PWE and used with caution otherwise.

In the meta-analysis of studies leading to FDA approval of psychotropic medications, the included second-generation antipsychotics (SGAs) carried an elevated risk of incident seizures as a group. However, when clozapine and olanzapine were excluded from the analysis, SGAs no longer carried an elevated risk. Clozapine had a standardized incidence ratio for seizures

CASE VIGNETTE 29.1

A 34-year-old right-handed man has a long-standing history of chronic major depressive disorder (since adolescence), with one past suicide attempt in his early 20s and has only responded to fluoxetine after failed trials with a number of other antidepressants. He is also receiving long-term psychotherapy. He developed recurrent unprovoked focal seizures at age 30. He is otherwise healthy. His neuroimaging (brain MRI) shows left mesial temporal sclerosis with a concordant active interictal EEG (epileptiform abnormalities also in left temporal regions). He is first trialed on levetiracetam, which lowers his seizure frequency (from 2 to 4 per month to once every 2 months). Over the course of his first 6 months on levetiracetam, his chronic mood symptoms worsen and he describes elevated irritability and anxiety, passive suicidality reemerges, and his mood symptoms impact his performance at work. His neurologist and his psychiatrist discuss treatment options. Given his history of difficult-to-treat depression, it is decided to switch the AED. A cross-titration with lamotrigine renders improvement of the mood side effects but his seizure frequency escalates back to two per month despite therapeutic doses of lamotrigine. He develops a rash with lamotrigine once the dose reaches 400 mg/day, so the medication is discontinued. At this point, phenytoin is trialed, which initially provides improvement in seizure frequency. After 6 weeks on phenytoin at 400 mg total daily dose, he develops gait instability, slurred speech, dizziness, and nausea. His free phenytoin level is checked and it is 3.5 mcg/mL (ref: 1.0–2.5 mcg/mL). It is determined that fluoxetine was inhibiting the metabolism of phenytoin elevating it to toxic levels. A dose adjustment of phenytoin relieves the patient of phenytoin toxicity symptoms, while still preserving the therapeutic benefit of fluoxetine.

of 9.5, olanzapine had 2.5, and quetiapine 2.05.[157] A Taiwanese health claim database study of 288,397 new antipsychotic users provided an overall 1-year incident rate of seizures of 9.6 per 1000 person-years (uncommon but not rare), and first-generation antipsychotics (FGAs) were associated with a nonsignificant higher risk for seizures than SGAs.[159] A Spanish pharmacovigilance study comparing spontaneously reported seizures as side effects found that SGAs carried a higher risk of seizures than FGAs mainly, but not only due to clozapine.[160] This finding was also consistent with a WHO adverse drug reaction database report.[161] In a previous study, SGAs were related to more EEG abnormalities than FGAs in psychiatric inpatients (19.1% of patients on antipsychotics with EEG abnormalities vs. 13.3% of patients on no antipsychotics). The highest percentage of patients with EEG abnormalities were observed with clozapine and olanzapine.[162] Other controlled trials and open label studies show no increased risk of seizures with FGAs or SGAs except for clozapine's dose-related risk, highest at doses above 600 mg/day.[64] Risperidone and aripiprazole have been more extensively studied in ASD, a population known to have a higher risk of seizures, and they have been deemed safe in terms of seizure risk.[64] Except for clozapine and possibly olanzapine, seizure risk seems to be low with the use of antipsychotics in PWE.

Historically neurologists have been reluctant to prescribe psychostimulants in PWE. Data from double-blind placebo-controlled trials in PWE show that methylphenidate is safe in terms of seizure risk in children with well-controlled seizures and should be considered the first-line medication choice for treatment of ADHD when seizures are controlled.[163,164] In one randomized, controlled, cross-over study of OROS-methylphenidate, results seemed to suggest increasing risk of seizure with increasing doses of the stimulant.[165] Other studies show that methylphenidate at low doses is relatively safe in patients with active seizures.[166-168] Data from amphetamines and atomoxetine is mostly anecdotal in terms of seizure risk, therefore these drugs require close monitoring if prescribed after a failed trial of methylphenidate.[64] Other drugs used in ADHD such as guanfacine and clonidine have not been studied in PWE.

The evidence that lithium increases the risk of seizure is based on old case reports. The risk seems to be low even in the context of intoxication.[156]

Risk of epileptogenic potential at therapeutic doses and in overdose should be kept in mind by prescribing psychiatrists and neurologists when selecting a psychotropic agent. Low start doses and slow titration should be the rule for any psychotropic medication prescribed in PWE. The risk-benefit ratio of treating a psychiatric comorbidity should always be seriously considered, especially given the known risks of untreated psychiatric disorders in epilepsy and the safety data currently available.

Pharmacological Interactions

When prescribing psychotropic medications in PWE on AEDs, pharmacokinetic interactions should be considered. Some AEDs, such as carbamazepine, phenytoin, phenobarbital, and primidone are CYP450 enzyme inducers and could accelerate the metabolism of many psychotropic agents, minimizing their efficacy. Initial doses of the metabolized psychotropic should still be low and increases carefully monitored. Special attention should be placed when AEDs with inducing properties are discontinued, as this can suddenly lead to toxic levels of the metabolized psychotropic drug, particularly relevant in antipsychotics and TCAs. If guidelines are available, therapeutic drug monitoring can be considered and a dose correction may be offered. Some antidepressants are CYP450 enzyme inhibitors (such as fluoxetine and fluvoxamine) and could elevate AED blood levels leading to potential toxicity. Table 29-7 illustrates pharmacokinetic interactions between AEDs and psychotropic agents metabolized by the CYP450 enzyme system, including moderate to potent enzyme inducers and inhibitors.[169]

TABLE 29-9 • Positive Psychotropic Effects of Antiepileptic Drugs.

Antiepileptic Drug	Psychiatric Conditions Alleviated by Specific Antiepileptic Drugs
Barbiturates	• Barbiturate withdrawal • Benzodiazepine withdrawal • Alcohol withdrawal
Benzodiazepines	• Panic disorder, social anxiety disorder, and generalized anxiety disorder (FDA approved) • Insomnia (FDA approved) • Alcohol withdrawal • Benzodiazepine withdrawal • Catatonia • Acute agitation • Restless legs syndrome and other parasomnias
Phenytoin	• Neuropathic pain • Impulsive aggression
Valproic acid products	• Acute manic and mixed episodes in bipolar I disorder (FDA approved) • Migraine prophylaxis (FDA approved) • Maintenance in bipolar I disorder • Alcohol withdrawal • Borderline personality disorder • Impulsive aggression
Carbamazepine	• Acute manic episodes in bipolar I disorder (FDA approved) • Trigeminal neuralgia (FDA approved) • Maintenance in bipolar I disorder • Other neuropathic pain conditions • Alcohol withdrawal • Borderline personality disorder • Impulsive aggression
Oxcarbazepine	• Acute manic episodes • Impulsive aggression
Lamotrigine	• Maintenance in bipolar I disorder (FDA approved) • Acute depressive episodes in bipolar disorder • Borderline personality disorder (anger, affective instability)
Gabapentin	• Post-herpetic neuralgia (FDA approved) • Restless legs syndrome (FDA approved) • Insomnia • Social anxiety disorder and severe panic disorder • Alcohol dependence
Pregabalin	• Fibromyalgia (FDA approved) • Neuropathic pain associated with diabetic peripheral neuropathy (FDA approved) • Neuropathic pain associated with spinal cord injury (FDA approved) • Post-herpetic neuralgia (FDA approved) • Generalized anxiety disorder (approved in Europe) • Social anxiety disorder • Alcohol withdrawal
Topiramate	• Migraine prophylaxis (FDA approved) • Borderline personality disorder • Binge eating disorder • Alcohol dependence • Cocaine dependence • Pathological gambling • Tourette syndrome
Zonisamide	• Binge eating disorder

Potentiation of pharmacodynamic interactions should also be considered when combining AEDs with psychotropic medications. Examples include weight gain or movement abnormalities when combining SGAs with AEDs such as valproate or hyponatremia when combining an SSRI with carbamazepine, oxcarbazepine, or eslicarbazepine.[64]

Positive Psychotropic Effects of Antiepileptic Drugs

Most AEDs exert their antiepileptic effect via a number of mechanisms of action, with many drugs having more than one specific molecular target. Examples of the main (but not exclusive) mechanisms of action for some AEDs include modulation of voltage-dependent sodium channels (i.e., phenytoin, carbamazepine, oxcarbazepine, eslicarbazepine, valproic acid), calcium channels (i.e., gabapentin, pregabalin), GABAergic neurotransmission (i.e., barbiturates, benzodiazepines, tiagabine, vigabatrin), glutamatergic neurotransmission (i.e., felbamate, parampanel).[170,171] Many AEDs have such mixed profiles (i.e., topiramate, zonisamide, lamotrigine) that they are difficult to

classify based on their main mechanism of action.[171] In addition to their known mechanisms of action as anticonvulsants, some AEDs affect additional neurotransmitter systems that could be responsible for some of their psychotropic properties. For instance, AEDs with known psychotropic benefit, such as valproic acid, carbamazepine, and lamotrigine, cause an increase in serotonin.[172] The neurobiological basis of the psychotropic effects of AEDs is only superficially understood, and positive effects in animal models do not always translate into positive clinical trials results.[171]

The US FDA has approved valproic acid products and carbamazepine for the treatment of acute manic and mixed episodes in bipolar I disorder, and lamotrigine for treatment maintenance in bipolar I disorder. Pregabalin has been approved in Europe for the treatment of GAD.[171,172] A number of other AEDs have shown benefit in other neuropsychiatric conditions, besides epilepsy. Table 29-9 references some of the currently known non-epileptic positive psychotropic effects of AEDs based on FDA indications, data from positive double-blind, placebo-controlled trials and conventional practice.[171–173]

Summary and Key Points

- Neuropsychiatric symptoms are an important aspect of epilepsy and may include cognitive dysfunction, affective symptoms, anxiety, or psychosis.
- Neuropsychiatric symptoms may occur independently of seizures (interictal symptoms) or may occur in relation to a seizure or a seizure cluster. These peri-ictal symptoms are classified as preictal, ictal, or postictal depending on the temporal relationship to the seizure. Peri-ictal symptoms are, by definition, transitory, while interictal symptoms may be chronic or transitory. Chronic interictal symptoms may worsen peri-ictally.
- Seizure localization plays a role in the pathophysiology of neuropsychiatric symptoms. Psychopathology is most commonly associated with temporal lobe epilepsy.

- Treatment of epilepsy carries a risk of neuropsychiatric side effects that vary depending on the treatment. Risk may be reduced with careful drug choice.
- Use of psychotropic medication in patients with epilepsy carries some risk of seizure provocation and interactions with AEDs. On the other hand, certain AEDs have positive psychotropic properties, and may be useful both for seizure control and management of psychiatric symptoms.
- Neuropsychiatric symptoms should be addressed as part of the comprehensive care of patients with epilepsy. This may require interdisciplinary collaboration between neurologists, psychiatrists, psychologists, nurses, and social workers. An awareness of the neuropsychiatric aspects of epilepsy among the various providers can facilitate communication and collaboration and can help focus the treatment goal toward the overall well-being of the patient.

Multiple Choice Questions

1. Which of the following statements is true regarding the neurobiological mechanisms that explain predisposition to both depression and epilepsy?
   a. Amygdala kindling in rats is caused by corticosteroid supplementation equivalent to chronic physiological elevations seen in depression.
   b. Elevated serotonergic activity occurs in both disorders.
   c. Depression is more commonly seen in lesional epilepsy outside of the temporal lobe.
   d. Studies consistently show an association between depression and right-sided seizure focus.
   e. Higher incidence of depression in epilepsy is only detected years after the first seizure, according to large epidemiological studies.

2. A 35-year-old man with left temporal lobe epilepsy since childhood underwent an anterior temporal lobectomy. His seizures previously consisted of ictal fear followed by occasional secondary generalizations, and they were determined to originate from the left temporal lobe. After the surgery, he has continued to experience occasional "small seizures" characterized by ictal fear (a sudden fear sensation for 2 minutes that suddenly goes away, with no other associated symptom, and with complete preservation of awareness). He has not experienced secondary generalized seizures since the surgery 2 years ago. Independent of his seizures, he describes a long-term history of excessive worrying, frequent restlessness, muscle tension, and difficulty falling asleep due to his worries. The most likely diagnoses that explain his current symptoms are:

a. Panic disorder and generalized anxiety disorder.
b. Panic disorder explains both symptoms.
c. Focal seizures and interictal generalized anxiety disorder.
d. Focal seizures explain both symptoms.
e. Generalized anxiety disorder explains both symptoms.

3. A 49-year-old woman with a history of medication-resistant focal epilepsy since age 20 presents to the emergency department with worsened seizures. Typically, she experiences one to two seizures per month, beginning with an aura characterized by a rising epigastric sensation and dream-like vague auditory hallucinations followed within seconds by loss of awareness, oral and manual automatisms for 1–2 minutes, and then several hours of postictal fatigue. Her MRI shows left mesial temporal sclerosis. Baseline EEG shows frequent independent bitemporal sharp waves. She has been maintained on valproic acid, lamotrigine, and zonisamide. Now she arrives reporting a week of frequent auras every several hours, and three typical seizures with impaired awareness over the past 12 hours. In the ED, she is witnessed to have a typical seizure progressing to bilateral tonic-clonic convulsion. She is loaded with levetiracetam 1000 mg and maintained on levetiracetam 750 mg bid in addition to her other AEDs thereafter. Her mental status returns to normal within 30 minutes and she is monitored in the ED for 12 more hours during which she has no further seizures or auras, and she is discharged home on all four AEDs. She returns to the ED 3 days later, brought in by her husband due to altered mental status. No further seizures have been witnessed, but he notes that she was up all night boarding all the windows of their house and muttering that the devil was sending his minions to take their baby (although, in reality, their two children were teenagers). On the day of presentation, the patient reportedly resisted going to the hospital claiming that the doctors in the hospital are working with the devil. On exam, the patient is alert and communicative. There is no aphasia, and she follows simple instructions appropriately, but there is mild psychomotor agitation and she appears distracted by internal stimuli.

Which of the following represents the most likely possible explanations for the patient's mental status change?
a. AED side effect, forced normalization, postictal psychosis.
b. AED side effect, forced normalization, interictal psychosis.
c. AED non-adherence, postictal psychosis, brain tumor.
d. Brain tumor, stroke, nonconvulsive status epilepticus.
e. Schizophrenia, bipolar disorder, schizoaffective disorder.

4. Which is the most correct statement regarding the relationship between AEDs and suicidality?
a. AEDs should be avoided in patients with a history of suicidal ideation. There is an unacceptably high risk of suicide associated with AEDs.
b. AEDs may be cautiously prescribed to patients with a history of suicidal ideation, but if a patient with epilepsy develops suicidal ideation while on AEDs, all AEDs should be stopped immediately.
c. If a patient with epilepsy develops suicidality, lamotrigine and topiramate should be stopped, but other AEDs may be continued. Only lamotrigine and topiramate have been associated with increased risk of suicidality.
d. The risk of suicide due to AEDs is insignificant and should not be considered relevant. If a patient with epilepsy develops suicidality, the suicidality should be treated, but AEDs should be left unchanged.
e. The risk of suicide due to AEDs is small and must be balanced against the risk of AED discontinuation. Consideration should be given to removing AED(s) most likely to be contributing to the patient's suicidal ideation, and if necessary, adding an AED with a more benign psychiatric adverse effect profile.

Multiple Choice Answers

1. **Answer: a**
Amygdalar kindling in rats is accelerated with chronic low-dose corticosteroid supplementation, similar to the physiological elevations in cortisol seen with chronic depression. Decreased serotonergic activity is seen in both depression and epilepsy. Although not consistently replicated, depression has been more associated with lesional epilepsy with hippocampal sclerosis (mesial temporal sclerosis). Studies are not conclusive regarding laterality of seizure focus and its association with depression. Large epidemiological studies show an elevated incidence of depression even before onset of epilepsy.

2. **Answer: c**
Ictal fear is a common presentation in temporal lobe epilepsy. The description of the "small seizure" is more consistent with a focal seizure, with ictal fear as the main manifestation, rather than a panic attack, given duration, sudden onset and offset, and lack of other associated symptoms expected in panic attacks. Interictal generalized anxiety disorder can occur in epilepsy and may even start before the onset of seizures.

3. **Answer: a**
Acute onset of psychosis within days of a cluster of focal seizures with impaired awareness or convulsive seizures is typical of postictal psychosis. However, because of the recent introduction of levetiracetam, the possibility of levetiracetam-induced psychosis should be considered. Additionally, acute onset of psychosis following introduction of a new AED may be explained by forced normalization if there has been a significant reduction in interictal epileptiform activity on EEG. Interictal psychosis should not be diagnosed given the temporal association between the psychosis and a seizure cluster. AED non-adherence would not be expected to cause acute psychosis in the absence of another disorder

such as postictal psychosis. While stroke and brain tumor can occasionally cause psychosis, they are less likely explanations in this case, given the long-standing history of epilepsy and recent seizure cluster. Nonconvulsive status epilepticus is possible, but less likely given the initial return to normal mental status after treatment of her seizures and the absence of further seizures despite the mental status change. While schizophrenia, bipolar disorder, and schizoaffective disorder can be associated with psychotic episodes, these primary psychiatric diagnoses are less likely explanations for new-onset psychosis at age 49 in a patient with epilepsy, and the recent seizures and medication administration should raise suspicion for alternate possibilities.

4. Answer: e
The risk of suicide due to AEDs is small, but suicidality is a serious concern, and the potential role of AEDs should not be ignored. a and b are extreme statements that fail to take into account the risks of untreated epilepsy. If suicidality develops soon after introduction of a new AED, consideration should be given to the possibility that this drug may have contributed. It is also clear that certain AEDs, such as valproic acid and carbamazepine, have a more benign psychiatric adverse event profile than other AEDs such as levetiracetam and perampanel. While the FDA meta-analysis singled out topiramate and lamotrigine as specific drugs that may increase the risk of suicidality, they are not the only drugs that raise concern, and the primary finding of the FDA meta-analysis was a class effect of increased suicidality when multiple AEDs were considered collectively. Additionally, the association between lamotrigine and suicidality has been questioned, as numerous studies have shown this drug to have positive psychotropic properties.

References

1. Temkin O. *The Falling Sickness: A History of Epilepsy from the Greeks to the Beginnings of Modern Neurology*. Baltimore, MD: Johns Hopkins University Press; 2010.
2. Fisher RS, Acevedo C, Arzimanoglou A, et al. ILAE official report: a practical clinical definition of epilepsy. *Epilepsia*. 2014;55:475-482.
3. Hesdorffer DC, Logroscino G, Benn EK, Katri N, Cascino G, Hauser WA. Estimating risk for developing epilepsy: a population-based study in Rochester, Minnesota. *Neurology*. 2011;76(1):23-27.
4. Fisher RS, Cross JH, French JA, et al. Operational classification of seizure types by the International League Against Epilepsy: Position paper of the ILAE Commission for Classification and Terminology. *Epilepsia*. 2017;58:522-530.
5. Sperling MR, Guina L. The necessity for sphenoidal electrodes in the presurgical evaluation of temporal lobe epilepsy: pro position. *J Clin Neurophysiol*. 2003;20(5):299-304.
6. Blume WT. The necessity for sphenoidal electrodes in the presurgical evaluation of temporal lobe epilepsy: con position. *J Clin Neurophysiol*. 2003;20(5):305-310.
7. Oluwabusi T, Sood SK. Update on the management of simple febrile seizures: emphasis on minimal intervention. *Curr Opin Pediatr*. 2012;24(2):259-265.
8. Fisher RS, Acevedo C, Arzimanoglou A, et al. ILAE official report: a practical clinical definition of epilepsy. *Epilepsia*. 2014;55(4):475-482.
9. Adcock JE, Panayiotopoulos CP. Occipital lobe seizures and epilepsies. *J Clin Neurophysiol*. 2012;29(5):397-407.
10. Elliott B, Joyce E, Shorvon S. Delusions, illusions and hallucinations in epilepsy: 1. Elementary phenomena. *Epilepsy Res*. 2009;85(2-3):162-171.
11. Kasper BS, Kasper EM, Pauli E, Stefan H. Phenomenology of hallucinations, illusions, and delusions as part of seizure semiology. *Epilepsy Behav*. 2010;18(1-2):13-23.
12. Wieser HG. Depth recorded limbic seizures and psychopathology. *Neurosci Biobehav Rev*. 1983;7(3):427-440.
13. Mendez MF, Cherrier MM, Perryman KM. Epileptic forced thinking from left frontal lesions. *Neurology*. 1996;47(1):79-83.
14. Chong DJ, Dugan P, Investigators E. Ictal fear: associations with age, gender, and other experiential phenomena. *Epilepsy Behav*. 2016;62:153-158.
15. Kanner AM. Ictal panic and interictal panic attacks: diagnostic and therapeutic principles. *Neurol Clin*. 2011;29(1):163-175, ix.
16. Leitinger M, Beniczky S, Rohracher A, et al. Salzburg Consensus Criteria for Non-Convulsive Status Epilepticus—approach to clinical application. *Epilepsy Behav*. 2015;49:158-163.
17. Drislane FW. Presentation, evaluation, and treatment of nonconvulsive status epilepticus. *Epilepsy Behav*. 2000;1(5):301-314.
18. Kanemoto K, Miyamoto T, Abe R. Ictal catatonia as a manifestation of de novo absence status epilepticus following benzodiazepine withdrawal. *Seizure*. 1999;8(6):364-366.
19. Lim J, Yagnik P, Schraeder P, Wheeler S. Ictal catatonia as a manifestation of nonconvulsive status epilepticus. *J Neurol Neurosurg Psychiatry*. 1986;49(7):833-836.
20. Elliott B, Joyce E, Shorvon S. Delusions, illusions and hallucinations in epilepsy: 2. Complex phenomena and psychosis. *Epilepsy Res*. 2009;85(2-3):172-186.
21. Kanemoto K. Postictal psychoses: established facts and new clinical questions. In: Trimble MR, Schmitz B, eds. *The Neuropsychiatry of Epilepsy*. 2nd ed. Cambridge, UK: Cambridge University Press; 2011:67-79.
22. Kanner AM, Stagno S, Kotagal P, Morris HH. Postictal psychiatric events during prolonged video-electroencephalographic monitoring studies. *Arch Neurol*. 1996;53(3):258-263.
23. Logsdail SJ, Toone BK. Post-ictal psychoses. A clinical and phenomenological description. *Br J Psychiatry*. 1988;152:246-252.
24. Oshima T, Tadokoro Y, Kanemoto K. A prospective study of postictal psychoses with emphasis on the periictal type. *Epilepsia*. 2006;47(12):2131-2134.
25. Devinsky O, Abramson H, Alper K, et al. Postictal psychosis: a case control series of 20 patients and 150 controls. *Epilepsy Res*. 1995;20(3):247-253.
26. Trimble M, Kanner A, Schmitz B. Postictal psychosis. *Epilepsy Behav*. 2010;19(2):159-161.
27. Nishida T, Kudo T, Inoue Y, et al. Postictal mania versus postictal psychosis: differences in clinical features, epileptogenic zone, and brain functional changes during postictal period. *Epilepsia*. 2006;47(12):2104-2114.

28. Alper K, Kuzniecky R, Carlson C, et al. Postictal psychosis in partial epilepsy: a case-control study. *Ann Neurol.* 2008;63(5):602-610.

29. Kanner AM, Ostrovskaya A. Long-term significance of postictal psychotic episodes I. Are they predictive of bilateral ictal foci? *Epilepsy Behav.* 2008;12(1):150-153.

30. Kanner AM, Ostrovskaya A. Long-term significance of postictal psychotic episodes II. Are they predictive of interictal psychotic episodes? *Epilepsy Behav.* 2008;12(1):154-156.

31. Tarulli A, Devinsky O, Alper K. Progression of postictal to interictal psychosis. *Epilepsia.* 2001;42(11):1468-1471.

32. Kanner AM, Soto A, Gross-Kanner H. Prevalence and clinical characteristics of postictal psychiatric symptoms in partial epilepsy. *Neurology.* 2004;62(5):708-713.

33. Besag FMC, Vasey MJ. Prodrome in epilepsy. *Epilepsy Behav.* 2018;83:219-233.

34. Mula M, Jauch R, Cavanna A, et al. Interictal dysphoric disorder and periictal dysphoric symptoms in patients with epilepsy. *Epilepsia.* 2010;51(7):1139-1145.

35. Haut SR, Hall CB, Borkowski T, Tennen H, Lipton RB. Clinical features of the pre-ictal state: mood changes and premonitory symptoms. *Epilepsy Behav.* 2012;23(4):415-421.

36. Kotwas I, McGonigal A, Trebuchon A, et al. Self-control of epileptic seizures by nonpharmacological strategies. *Epilepsy Behav.* 2016;55:157-164.

37. Fisher RS, van Emde Boas W, Blume W, et al. Epileptic seizures and epilepsy: definitions proposed by the International League Against Epilepsy (ILAE) and the International Bureau for Epilepsy (IBE). *Epilepsia.* 2005;46(4):470-472.

38. Fiest KM, Dykeman J, Patten SB, et al. Depression in epilepsy: a systematic review and meta-analysis. *Neurology.* 2013;80(6):590-599.

39. Rai D, Kerr MP, McManus S, Jordanova V, Lewis G, Brugha TS. Epilepsy and psychiatric comorbidity: a nationally representative population-based study. *Epilepsia.* 2012;53(6):1095-1103.

40. Josephson CB, Lowerison M, Vallerand I, et al. Association of depression and treated depression with epilepsy and seizure outcomes: a multicohort analysis. *JAMA Neurology.* 2017;74(5):533-539.

41. Hesdorffer DC, Ishihara L, Mynepalli L, Webb DJ, Weil J, Hauser WA. Epilepsy, suicidality, and psychiatric disorders: a bidirectional association. *Ann Neurol.* 2012;72(2):184-191.

42. Boylan LS, Flint LA, Labovitz DL, Jackson SC, Starner K, Devinsky O. Depression but not seizure frequency predicts quality of life in treatment-resistant epilepsy. *Neurology.* 2004;62(2):258-261.

43. Kanner AM. Can neurobiological pathogenic mechanisms of depression facilitate the development of seizure disorders? *Lancet Neurol.* 2012;11(12):1093-1102.

44. Taher TR, Salzberg M, Morris MJ, Rees S, O'Brien TJ. Chronic low-dose corticosterone supplementation enhances acquired epileptogenesis in the rat amygdala kindling model of TLE. *Neuropsychopharmacology.* 2005;30(9):1610-1616.

45. Adams SJ, O'Brien TJ, Lloyd J, Kilpatrick CJ, Salzberg MR, Velakoulis D. Neuropsychiatric morbidity in focal epilepsy. *Br J Psychiatry.* 2008;192(6):464-469.

46. Sanchez-Gistau V, Sugranyes G, Bailles E, et al. Is major depressive disorder specifically associated with mesial temporal sclerosis? *Epilepsia.* 2012;53(2):386-392.

47. Cutting S, Lauchheimer A, Barr W, Devinsky O. Adult-onset idiopathic generalized epilepsy: clinical and behavioral features. *Epilepsia.* 2001;42(11):1395-1398.

48. Jones JE, Hermann BP, Barry JJ, Gilliam F, Kanner AM, Meador KJ. Clinical assessment of Axis I psychiatric morbidity in chronic epilepsy: a multicenter investigation. *J Neuropsychiatry Clin Neurosci.* 2005;17(2):172-179.

49. Manchanda R, Schaefer B, McLachlan RS, et al. Psychiatric disorders in candidates for surgery for epilepsy. *J Neurol Neurosurg Psychiatry.* 1996;61(1):82-89.

50. Sarkis RA, Pietras AC, Cheung A, Baslet G, Dworetzky B. Neuropsychological and psychiatric outcomes in poorly controlled idiopathic generalized epilepsy. *Epilepsy Behav.* 2013;28(3):370-373.

51. Inoue Y, Mihara T. Psychiatric disorders before and after surgery for epilepsy. *Epilepsia.* 2001;42(suppl 6):13-18.

52. Wrench J, Wilson SJ, Bladin PF. Mood disturbance before and after seizure surgery: a comparison of temporal and extratemporal resections. *Epilepsia.* 2004;45(5):534-543.

53. Glosser G, Zwil AS, Glosser DS, O'Connor MJ, Sperling MR. Psychiatric aspects of temporal lobe epilepsy before and after anterior temporal lobectomy. *J Neurol Neurosurg Psychiatry.* 2000;68(1):53-58.

54. Quigg M, Broshek DK, Heidal-Schiltz S, Maedgen JW, Bertram EH3rd. Depression in intractable partial epilepsy varies by laterality of focus and surgery. *Epilepsia.* 2003;44(3):419-424.

55. Hoppe C, Elger CE. Depression in epilepsy: a critical review from a clinical perspective. *Nat Rev Neurol.* 2011;7(8):462-472.

56. American Psychiatric Association. *Diagnostic and Statistical Manual of Mental Disorders: DSM-5.* Washington, DC: American Psychiatric Publishing, Inc.; 2013.

57. Fiest KM, Patten SB, Wiebe S, Bulloch AG, Maxwell CJ, Jette N. Validating screening tools for depression in epilepsy. *Epilepsia.* 2014;55(10):1642-1650.

58. Gilliam FG, Barry JJ, Hermann BP, Meador KJ, Vahle V, Kanner AM. Rapid detection of major depression in epilepsy: a multicentre study. *Lancet Neurol.* 2006;5(5):399-405.

59. Blumer D, Montouris G, Davies K. The interictal dysphoric disorder: recognition, pathogenesis, and treatment of the major psychiatric disorder of epilepsy. *Epilepsy Behav.* 2004;5(6):826-840.

60. Kanner AM. Depression in epilepsy: prevalence, clinical semiology, pathogenic mechanisms, and treatment. *Biological Psychiatry.* 2003;54(3):388-398.

61. Nilsson L, Tomson T, Farahmand BY, Diwan V, Persson PG. Cause-specific mortality in epilepsy: a cohort study of more than 9,000 patients once hospitalized for epilepsy. *Epilepsia.* 1997;38(10):1062-1068.

62. Rafnsson V, Olafsson E, Hauser WA, Gudmundsson G. Cause-specific mortality in adults with unprovoked seizures. A population-based incidence cohort study. *Neuroepidemiology.* 2001;20(4):232-236.

63. Bell GS, Gaitatzis A, Bell CL, Johnson AL, Sander JW. Suicide in people with epilepsy: how great is the risk? *Epilepsia.* 2009;50(8):1933-1942.

64. Mula M. Epilepsy and psychiatric comorbidities: drug selection. *Curr Treat Options Neurol.* 2017;19(12):44.

65. Michaelis R, Tang V, Wagner JL, et al. Cochrane systematic review and meta-analysis of the impact of psychological treatments for people with epilepsy on health-related quality of life. *Epilepsia.* 2018;59(2):315-332.

66. Schroder J, Bruckner K, Fischer A, et al. Efficacy of a psychological online intervention for depression in people with epilepsy: a randomized controlled trial. *Epilepsia.* 2014;55(12):2069-2076.

67. Thompson NJ, Walker ER, Obolensky N, et al. Distance delivery of mindfulness-based cognitive therapy for depression: project UPLIFT. *Epilepsy Behav.* 2010;19(3):247-254.

68. Davis GR, Armstrong HEJr, Donovan DM, Temkin NR. Cognitive-behavioral treatment of depressed affect among epileptics: preliminary findings. *J Clin Psychol.* 1984;40(4):930-935.

69. McLaughlin DP, McFarland K. A randomized trial of a group based cognitive behavior therapy program for older adults with epilepsy: the impact on seizure frequency, depression and psychosocial well-being. *J Behav Med.* 2011;34(3):201-207.

70. Tan SY, Bruni J. Cognitive-behavior therapy with adult patients with epilepsy: a controlled outcome study. *Epilepsia.* 1986;27(3):225-233.

71. Gandy M, Sharpe L, Nicholson Perry K, et al. Cognitive behaviour therapy to improve mood in people with epilepsy: a randomised controlled trial. *Cogn Behav Ther.* 2014;43(2):153-166.

72. Gandy M, Sharpe L, Perry KN. Cognitive behavior therapy for depression in people with epilepsy: a systematic review. *Epilepsia.* 2013;54(10):1725-1734.

73. Lunde ME, Lee EK, Rasmussen KG. Electroconvulsive therapy in patients with epilepsy. *Epilepsy Behav.* 2006;9(2):355-359.

74. Bostock ECS, Kirkby KC, Garry MI, Taylor BVM. Systematic review of cognitive function in euthymic bipolar disorder and pre-surgical temporal lobe epilepsy. *Front Psychiatry.* 2017;8:133.

75. Schmitz B. Depression and mania in patients with epilepsy. *Epilepsia.* 2005;46(suppl 4):45-49.

76. Mula M, Jauch R, Cavanna A, et al. Manic/hypomanic symptoms and quality of life measures in patients with epilepsy. *Seizure.* 2009;18(7):530-532.

77. Ettinger AB, Reed ML, Goldberg JF, Hirschfeld RM. Prevalence of bipolar symptoms in epilepsy vs other chronic health disorders. *Neurology.* 2005;65(4):535-540.

78. Josephson CB, Jette N. Psychiatric comorbidities in epilepsy. *Int Rev Psychiatry.* 2017;29(5):409-424.

79. Tellez-Zenteno JF, Patten SB, Jette N, Williams J, Wiebe S. Psychiatric comorbidity in epilepsy: a population-based analysis. *Epilepsia.* 2007;48(12):2336-2344.

80. Vazquez B, Devinsky O. Epilepsy and anxiety. *Epilepsy Behav.* 2003;4(suppl 4):S20-S25.

81. Foong J, Flugel D. Psychiatric outcome of surgery for temporal lobe epilepsy and presurgical considerations. *Epilepsy Res.* 2007;75(2-3):84-96.

82. Harden CL, Goldstein MA, Ettinger AB. Anxiety disorders in epilepsy. In: Ettinger AB, Kanner AM, eds. *Psychiatric Issues in Epilepsy: A Practical Guide to Diagnosis and Treatment.* 2nd ed. Philadelphia, PA: Lippincott Williams & Wilkins; 2007:248-263.

83. Cendes F, Andermann F, Gloor P, et al. Relationship between atrophy of the amygdala and ictal fear in temporal lobe epilepsy. *Brain.* 1994;117(pt 4):739-746.

84. Satishchandra P, Krishnamoorthy ES, van Elst LT, et al. Mesial temporal structures and comorbid anxiety in refractory partial epilepsy. *J Neuropsychiatry Clin Neurosci.* 2003;15(4):450-452.

85. Schenkel LC, Bragatti JA, Becker JA, et al. Serotonin gene polymorphisms and psychiatry comorbidities in temporal lobe epilepsy. *Epilepsy Res.* 2012;99(3):260-266.

86. Mintzer S, Lopez F. Comorbidity of ictal fear and panic disorder. *Epilepsy Behav.* 2002;3(4):330-337.

87. Seo JG, Cho YW, Lee SJ, et al. Validation of the generalized anxiety disorder-7 in people with epilepsy: a MEPSY study. *Epilepsy Behav.* 2014;35:59-63.

88. Mula M. Treatment of anxiety disorders in epilepsy: an evidence-based approach. *Epilepsia.* 2013;54(suppl 1):13-18.

89. Tang V, Poon WS, Kwan P. Mindfulness-based therapy for drug-resistant epilepsy: an assessor-blinded randomized trial. *Neurology.* 2015;85(13):1100-1107.

90. Munger Clary HM. Anxiety and epilepsy: what neurologists and epileptologists should know. *Curr Neurol Neurosci Rep.* 2014;14(5):445.

91. Kanemoto K, Tsuji T, Kawasaki J. Reexamination of interictal psychoses based on DSM IV psychosis classification and international epilepsy classification. *Epilepsia.* 2001;42(1):98-103.

92. Hyde TM, Weinberger DR. Seizures and schizophrenia. *Schizophr Bull.* 1997;23(4):611-622.

93. Beard AW, Slater E. The schizophrenic-like psychoses of epilepsy. *Proc R Soc Med.* 1962;55:311-316.

94. Sachdev P. Schizophrenia-like psychosis and epilepsy: the status of the association. *Am J Psychiatry.* 1998;155(3):325-336.

95. Qin P, Xu H, Laursen TM, Vestergaard M, Mortensen PB. Risk for schizophrenia and schizophrenia-like psychosis among patients with epilepsy: population based cohort study. *BMJ.* 2005;331(7507):23.

96. Bredkjaer SR, Mortensen PB, Parnas J. Epilepsy and non-organic non-affective psychosis. National epidemiologic study. *Br J Psychiatry.* 1998;172:235-238.

97. Vestergaard M, Pedersen CB, Christensen J, Madsen KM, Olsen J, Mortensen PB. Febrile seizures and risk of schizophrenia. *Schizophr Res.* 2005;73(2-3):343-349.

98. Kanemoto K, Tadokoro Y, Oshima T. Psychotic illness in patients with epilepsy. *Ther Adv Neurol Disord.* 2012;5(6):321-334.

99. Butler T, Weisholtz D, Isenberg N, et al. Neuroimaging of frontal-limbic dysfunction in schizophrenia and epilepsy-related psychosis: toward a convergent neurobiology. *Epilepsy Behav.* 2012;23(2):113-122.

100. Slater E, Beard AW, Glithero E. The schizophrenia-like psychoses of epilepsy. *Br J Psychiatry.* 1963;109:95-150.

101. Perez MM, Trimble MR. Epileptic psychosis—diagnostic comparison with process schizophrenia. *Br J Psychiatry.* 1980;137: 245-249.

102. Tadokoro Y, Oshima T, Kanemoto K. Interictal psychoses in comparison with schizophrenia—a prospective study. *Epilepsia.* 2007;48(12):2345-2351.

103. Mellers JD, Toone BK, Lishman WA. A neuropsychological comparison of schizophrenia and schizophrenia-like psychosis of epilepsy. *Psychol Med.* 2000;30(2):325-335.

104. Sadock BJ, Sadock VA, Kaplan HI. *Kaplan and Sadock's Comprehensive Textbook of Psychiatry.* Philadelphia, PA: Lippincott Williams & Wilkins; 2005.

105. Cascella NG, Schretlen DJ, Sawa A. Schizophrenia and epilepsy: is there a shared susceptibility? *Neurosci Res.* 2009;63(4):227-235.

106. Gallentine WB, Mikati MA. Genetic generalized epilepsies. *J Clin Neurophysiol.* 2012;29(5):408-419.

107. Clarke MC, Tanskanen A, Huttunen MO, Clancy M, Cotter DR, Cannon M. Evidence for shared susceptibility to epilepsy and psychosis: a population-based family study. *Biol Psychiatry.* 2012;71(9):836-839.

108. Cox DM, Butler MG. The 15q11.2 BP1-BP2 microdeletion syndrome: a review. *Int J Mol Sci.* 2015;16(2):4068-4082.

109. Nakahara S, Adachi M, Ito H, Matsumoto M, Tajinda K, van Erp TGM. Hippocampal pathophysiology: commonality shared by temporal lobe epilepsy and psychiatric disorders. *Neurosci J.* 2018;2018:4852359.

110. Thompson PJ, Corcoran R. Everyday memory failures in people with epilepsy. *Epilepsia.* 1992;33(suppl 6):S18-S20.

111. Wilson SJ, Baxendale S, Barr W, et al. Indications and expectations for neuropsychological assessment in routine epilepsy care: report of the ILAE Neuropsychology Task Force, Diagnostic Methods Commission, 2013-2017. *Epilepsia.* 2015;56(5):674-681.

112. Carreno M, Donaire A, Sanchez-Carpintero R. Cognitive disorders associated with epilepsy: diagnosis and treatment. *Neurologist.* 2008;14:S26-S34.

113. Loughman A, Bowden SC, D'Souza W. Cognitive functioning in idiopathic generalised epilepsies: a systematic review and meta-analysis. *Neurosci Biobehav Rev.* 2014;43:20-34.

114. Hermann B, Jones J, Dabbs K, et al. The frequency, complications and aetiology of ADHD in new onset paediatric epilepsy. *Brain.* 2007;130:3135-3148.

115. El Achkar CM, Spence SJ. Clinical characteristics of children and young adults with co-occurring autism spectrum disorder and epilepsy. *Epilepsy Behav.* 2015;47:183-190.

116. Hermann B, Seidenberg M, Bell B, et al. The neurodevelopmental impact of childhood-onset temporal lobe epilepsy on brain structure and function. *Epilepsia.* 2002;43:1062-1071.

117. Berg AT. Paediatric epilepsy surgery: making the best of a tough situation. *Brain.* 2015;138(pt 1):4-5.

118. Gallagher A, Jambaque I, Lassonde M. Cognitive outcome of surgery. *Handb Clin Neurol.* 2013;111:797-802.

119. Dulay MF, Busch RM. Prediction of neuropsychological outcome after resection of temporal and extratemporal seizure foci. *Neurosurg Focus.* 2012;32(3):E4.

120. Hermann B, Seidenberg M, Jones J. The neurobehavioural comorbidities of epilepsy: can a natural history be developed? *Lancet Neurol.* 2008;7:151-160.

121. Power KN, Gramstad A, Gilhus NE, Hufthammer KO, Engelsen BA. Cognitive dysfunction after generalized tonic-clonic status epilepticus in adults. *Acta Neurol Scand.* 2018;137:417-424.

122. Tai XY, Koepp M, Duncan JS, et al. Hyperphosphorylated tau in patients with refractory epilepsy correlates with cognitive decline: a study of temporal lobe resections. *Brain.* 2016;139:2441-2455.

123. Leeman-Markowski BA, Schachter SC. Treatment of cognitive deficits in epilepsy. *Neurol Clin.* 2016;34:183-204.

124. Horak PC, Meisenhelter S, Song Y, et al. Interictal epileptiform discharges impair word recall in multiple brain areas. *Epilepsia.* 2017;58:373-380.

125. Mendez M, Lim G. Seizures in elderly patients with dementia: epidemiology and management. *Drugs Aging.* 2003;20(11):791-803.

126. Sarkis RA, Dickerson BC, Cole AJ, Chemali ZN. Clinical and neurophysiologic characteristics of unprovoked seizures in patients diagnosed with dementia. *J Neuropsychiatry Clin Neurosci.* 2016;28:56-61.

127. Vossel KA, Tartaglia MC, Nygaard HB, Zeman AZ, Miller BL. Epileptic activity in Alzheimer's disease: causes and clinical relevance. *Lancet Neurol.* 2017;16:311-322.

128. Beagle AJ, Darwish SM, Ranasinghe KG, La AL, Karageorgiou E, Vossel KA. Relative incidence of seizures and myoclonus in Alzheimer's disease, dementia with lewy bodies, and frontotemporal dementia. *J Alzheimers Dis.* 2017;60:211-223.

129. Sillanpaa M, Anttinen A, Rinne JO, et al. Childhood-onset epilepsy five decades later. A prospective population-based cohort study. *Epilepsia.* 2015;56(11):1774-1783.

130. Waxman SG, Geschwind N. The interictal behavior syndrome of temporal lobe epilepsy. *Arch Gen Psychiatry.* 1975;32(12):1580-1586.

131. Bear DM, Fedio P. Quantitative analysis of interictal behavior in temporal lobe epilepsy. *Arch Neurol.* 1977;34(8):454-467.

132. Rodin E, Schmaltz S. The Bear-Fedio personality inventory and temporal lobe epilepsy. *Neurology.* 1984;34(5):591-596.

133. Eddy CM, Rickards HE, Cavanna AE. The cognitive impact of antiepileptic drugs. *Ther Adv Neurol Disord.* 2011;4:385-407.

134. Witt J-A, Elger CE, Helmstaedter C. Adverse cognitive effects of antiepileptic pharmacotherapy: each additional drug matters. *Eur Neuropsychopharmacol.* 2015;25:1954-1959.

135. Wandschneider B, Burdett J, Townsend L, et al. Effect of topiramate and zonisamide on fMRI cognitive networks. *Neurology.* 2017;88:1165-1171.

136. Witt J-A, Helmstaedter C. How can we overcome neuropsychological adverse effects of antiepileptic drugs? *Expert Opin Pharmacother.* 2017;18:551-554.

137. Busch RM, Najm I, Hermann BP, Eng C. Genetics of cognition in epilepsy. *Epilepsy Behav.* 2014;41:297-306.

138. Chen B, Choi H, Hirsch LJ, et al. Psychiatric and behavioral side effects of antiepileptic drugs in adults with epilepsy. *Epilepsy Behav.* 2017;76:24-31.

139. Eddy CM, Rickards HE, Cavanna AE. Behavioral adverse effects of antiepileptic drugs in epilepsy. *J Clin Psychopharmacol.* 2012;32(3):362-375.

140. Stephen LJ, Wishart A, Brodie MJ. Psychiatric side effects and antiepileptic drugs: observations from prospective audits. *Epilepsy Behav.* 2017;71(pt A):73-78.

141. *Statistical Review and Evaluation: Antiepileptic Drugs and Suicidality.* Silver Spring, MD: U.S. Food and Drug Administration, Center for Drug Evaluation and Research; 2008.

142. Britton JW, Shih JJ. Antiepileptic drugs and suicidality. *Drug Healthc Patient Saf.* 2010;2:181-189.

143. Ferrer P, Ballarin E, Sabate M, et al. Antiepileptic drugs and suicide: a systematic review of adverse effects. *Neuroepidemiology.* 2014;42(2):107-120.

144. Hesdorffer DC, Kanner AM. The FDA alert on suicidality and antiepileptic drugs: fire or false alarm? *Epilepsia.* 2009;50(5):978-986.

145. Chen Z, Lusicic A, O'Brien TJ, Velakoulis D, Adams SJ, Kwan P. Psychotic disorders induced by antiepileptic drugs in people with epilepsy. *Brain.* 2016;139(pt 10):2668-2678.

146. Trimble MR, Rusch N, Betts T, Crawford PM. Psychiatric symptoms after therapy with new antiepileptic drugs: psychopathological and seizure related variables. *Seizure.* 2000;9(4):249-254.

147. Mula M, Trimble MR. The importance of being seizure free: topiramate and psychopathology in epilepsy. *Epilepsy Behav.* 2003;4(4):430-434.

148. Thomas L, Trimble M, Schmitz B, Ring H. Vigabatrin and behaviour disorders: a retrospective survey. *Epilepsy Res.* 1996;25(1):21-27.

149. Wolf P, Inoue Y, Roder-Wanner UU, Tsai JJ. Psychiatric complications of absence therapy and their relation to alteration of sleep. *Epilepsia.* 1984;25(suppl 1):S56-S59.

150. Sherman EM, Wiebe S, Fay-McClymont TB, et al. Neuropsychological outcomes after epilepsy surgery: systematic review and pooled estimates. *Epilepsia.* 2011;52(5):857-869.

151. Carran MA, Kohler CG, O'Connor MJ, Bilker WB, Sperling MR. Mania following temporal lobectomy. *Neurology.* 2003;61(6):770-774.

152. Krishnamoorthy ES, Trimble MR, Sander JW, Kanner AM. Forced normalization at the interface between epilepsy and psychiatry. *Epilepsy Behav.* 2002;3(4):303-308.

153. Schmitz B. Chapter 13: The effects of antiepileptic drugs on behavior. In: Trimble MR, Schmitz B, eds. *The Neuropsychiatry of Epilepsy.* 2nd ed. Cambridge, NY: Cambridge University Press; 2011:vii, 225.

154. Wolf P. Acute behavioral symptomatology at disappearance of epileptiform EEG abnormality. Paradoxical or "forced" normalization. *Adv Neurol.* 1991;55:127-142.

155. Hill T, Coupland C, Morriss R, Arthur A, Moore M, Hippisley-Cox J. Antidepressant use and risk of epilepsy and seizures in people aged 20 to 64 years: cohort study using a primary care database. *BMC Psychiatry.* 2015;15:315.

156. Steinert T, Froscher W. Epileptic seizures under antidepressive drug treatment: systematic review. *Pharmacopsychiatry.* 2017;51(4):121-135.

157. Alper K, Schwartz KA, Kolts RL, Khan A. Seizure incidence in psychopharmacological clinical trials: an analysis of Food and Drug Administration (FDA) summary basis of approval reports. *Biol Psychiatry*. 2007;62(4):345-354.

158. Judge BS, Rentmeester LL. Antidepressant overdose-induced seizures. *Neurol Clin*. 2011;29(3):565-580.

159. Wu CS, Wang SC, Yeh IJ, Liu SK. Comparative risk of seizure with use of first- and second-generation antipsychotics in patients with schizophrenia and mood disorders. *J Clin Psychiatry*. 2016;77(5):e573-e579.

160. Lertxundi U, Hernandez R, Medrano J, Domingo-Echaburu S, Garcia M, Aguirre C. Antipsychotics and seizures: higher risk with atypicals? *Seizure*. 2013;22(2):141-143.

161. Kumlien E, Lundberg PO. Seizure risk associated with neuroactive drugs: data from the WHO adverse drug reactions database. *Seizure*. 2010;19(2):69-73.

162. Centorrino F, Price BH, Tuttle M, et al. EEG abnormalities during treatment with typical and atypical antipsychotics. *Am J Psychiatry*. 2002;159(1):109-115.

163. Feldman H, Crumrine P, Handen BL, Alvin R, Teodori J. Methylphenidate in children with seizures and attention-deficit disorder. *Am J Dis Child*. 1989;143(9):1081-1086.

164. Gross-Tsur V, Manor O, van der Meere J, Joseph A, Shalev RS. Epilepsy and attention deficit hyperactivity disorder: is methylphenidate safe and effective? *J Pediatr*. 1997;130(4):670-674.

165. Gonzalez-Heydrich J, Whitney J, Waber D, et al. Adaptive phase I study of OROS methylphenidate treatment of attention deficit hyperactivity disorder with epilepsy. *Epilepsy Behav*. 2010;18(3):229-237.

166. Gucuyener K, Erdemoglu AK, Senol S, Serdaroglu A, Soysal S, Kockar AI. Use of methylphenidate for attention-deficit hyperactivity disorder in patients with epilepsy or electroencephalographic abnormalities. *J Child Neurol*. 2003;18(2):109-112.

167. Santos K, Palmini A, Radziuk AL, et al. The impact of methylphenidate on seizure frequency and severity in children with attention-deficit-hyperactivity disorder and difficult-to-treat epilepsies. *Dev Med Child Neurol*. 2013;55(7):654-660.

168. Adams J, Alipio-Jocson V, Inoyama K, et al. Methylphenidate, cognition, and epilepsy: a 1-month open-label trial. *Epilepsia*. 2017;58(12):2124-2132.

169. Spina E, Pisani F, de Leon J. Clinically significant pharmacokinetic drug interactions of antiepileptic drugs with new antidepressants and new antipsychotics. *Pharmacol Res*. 2016;106:72-86.

170. Hanaya R, Arita K. The new antiepileptic drugs: their neuropharmacology and clinical indications. *Neurol Med Chir (Tokyo)*. 2016;56(5):205-220.

171. Mula M. Investigating psychotropic properties of antiepileptic drugs. *Expert Rev Neurother*. 2013;13(6):639-646.

172. Ettinger AB, Argoff CE. Use of antiepileptic drugs for nonepileptic conditions: psychiatric disorders and chronic pain. *Neurotherapeutics*. 2007;4(1):75-83.

173. Kaufman KR. Antiepileptic drugs in the treatment of psychiatric disorders. *Epilepsy Behav*. 2011;21(1):1-11.

30

Neuropsychiatry of Traumatic Brain Injury

Ginger Polich · Thomas W. McAllister

INTRODUCTION

Traumatic brain injury (TBI) is an exemplar of the advantages of a neuropsychiatric approach to the diagnosis and treatment of neurobehavioral disorders. The forces that act on the brain to cause neurotrauma typically result in a profile of regional brain damage that maps nicely onto the neuropsychiatric sequelae and functional distress commonly encountered by survivors of such injury. In turn, the effects of living with these neurobehavioral sequelae, including the meaning and the significance of being identified as "brain injured," influence the quality of life of the individual and their caregivers. Failure to appreciate these complex but predictable relationships impedes the proper assessment and treatment of the individual with a TBI. This chapter reviews the current knowledge of the neurobiological effects of TBI, with special emphasis on how these processes inform the understanding of the clinical presentation and treatment of a person with neurobehavioral complications of neurotrauma.

CLASSIFICATION AND EPIDEMIOLOGY

TBI is typically defined as a change in brain function occurring in response to an external force applied to the head.[1] Each year in the United States, approximately 3 million Americans sustain a TBI, with nearly 300,000 hospitalized and 56,000 dying on account of their injuries.[2] Two major risk factors associated with TBI include male gender and age in the following three brackets, >75 years, 15–24 years, and 0–4 years. The most common mechanisms of injury include falls, followed by motor vehicle accidents, being struck by or against an object, and violence.[2]

TBI severity is typically classified as mild, moderate, or severe based on the duration of loss of consciousness (LOC), post-traumatic amnesia (PTA)—defined as the time point at which individual becomes oriented and can once again form and recall new memories, and the highest Glasgow Coma Scale (GCS) within the first 24 hours after injury.[3,4] Table 30-1 uses these parameters to summarize the classification scheme for TBI.

Severe TBI is defined by LOC > 24 hours, GCS 3–8, and PTA >1 week. *Moderate* TBI is defined by LOC >30 min and <24 hours, GCS 9–12, and PTA lasting 24 hours–1 week. Cognitive, behavioral, and motor symptoms resulting from TBI tend to increase with increasing injury severity. Moderate-to-severe injuries are typically accompanied by focal and/or diffuse brain lesions that can be visualized on computed tomography (CT) or magnetic resonance imaging (MRI). Among a cohort of individuals hospitalized at acute care facilities after traumatic injury, more than 40% remained chronically disabled.[5] At present, more than 5.3 million Americans are estimated to live with some degree of disability related to a TBI.[6]

A *mild* TBI is defined as a traumatically induced event leading to an altered level of consciousness (e.g., being dazed, confused, having incomplete memory for the event) or focal neurologic deficit, with LOC <30 minutes, GCS 13–15, and PTA <24 hours.[7] Mild traumatic brain injuries are the most common form of TBI, accounting for 70–80% of cases. Mild TBI symptoms are generally short-lived, lasting on the order of days to weeks.[8] Neuroimaging findings on conventional imaging modalities such as CT or MRI are typically absent with mild TBI. If imaging abnormalities are present following mild TBI, the injury is typically referred to as a complicated mild TBI.[9]

There are several points worth making with respect to mild brain injury.[14] Mild brain injury is not a separate and distinct disease process from more severe injuries, but rather is best understood in the broader context of the entire spectrum of injury severity. With milder injuries, assessment of presence and duration of LOC and PTA, and accurate assessment of the GCS is often challenging in that these injuries may be unwitnessed, consciousness may not be impaired at the time of presentation to the Emergency Department, and clinicians often focus on evaluating serious injuries to other body regions. Injuries sustained in contact sports may not be recognized at the time of the event or may be underreported,[10] and approximately one-third of some athlete cohorts are diagnosed with concussion many hours or days after the event.[11]

TABLE 30-1 • Parameters of TBI Injury Severity.

	Mild TBI	Complicated Mild TBI	Moderate TBI	Severe TBI
Glasgow Coma Scale (GCS)	13–15	13–15	9–12	3–8
Loss of consciousness (LOC)	"Altered" or LOC <30 min	"Altered" or LOC <30 min and abnormality on neuroimaging	>30 min to <24 h	>24 h
Post-traumatic amnesia (PTA)	<24 h	<24 h	>24 h to <7 days	>7 days

The prognosis for those with mild TBI is better than that for moderate and severe injury. However, those with complicated mild TBI may represent a different group whose prognosis is similar to those with moderate TBI.[9,12,13] Thus, the combination of clinical signs and symptoms shortly after injury and initial radiological findings may be a better scheme for predicting outcome. The usual course of recovery is fairly rapid. Studies of cognitive testing 1 month and 3 months after mild TBI show progressive diminution of group differences in cognition, although when differences persist they are also usually in the domains of memory, attention, and processing speed.[14–16]

Studies of elite athletes with sport-related concussion (SRC)[17] suggest that for certain populations (young, healthy individuals highly motivated to return to play), the vast majority are symptom free and have returned to their previous baseline function within 7–10 days. However, recovery can take much longer for populations seen in Emergency Departments.[16] Furthermore even in the collegiate studies of SRC, approximately 10% of the athletes did not recover fully within the typical 1-week time frame.[17] The frequency and intensity of postconcussive symptoms generally improves with time, although this is not true for everyone.[18,19] Even 1 year after injury, several studies have suggested a surprisingly high rate of symptoms, especially in populations seen in Emergency Departments. Dikmen et al.[20] report that almost half of their hospitalized mild TBI group noted three or more symptoms that were new or worse since the injury. It is important to consider the effects of other system injuries, as well as the base rate of typical "postconcussive symptoms" in the general population when attributing persistent symptoms to brain injury.[20]

Certain factors appear to be associated with a poorer prognosis after mild TBI. For example, work in military populations suggest that the presence of comorbid psychiatric disorders such as depression and post-traumatic stress disorder (PTSD) may account for much of the distress in individuals who also suffered a mild TBI and have persistent symptoms.[21,22] Age at time of injury appears to play a role both in terms of symptoms and neuropsychological function.[23] Intuitively it would seem that repetitive injuries would be associated with persistent symptoms, and certainly studies of athletes playing contact sports would suggest that for some groups this holds true.[24] It is possible that specific genetic profiles contribute to response to neurotrauma and cognitive outcomes.[25–27]

The role that compensation seeking plays in outcome is controversial with a divided literature confounded by methodological concerns.[28–31] Litigation and compensation proceedings are typically highly adversarial and are associated with anxiety and distress.[32–34] Meta analyses[35,36] have suggested

that compensation is associated with higher symptom burden and distress over time. Carroll et al.[15] in the World Health Organization (WHO) report concluded that compensation and litigation were consistent predictors of delayed outcome.[15] The conclusion that desire for compensation causes the symptoms does not necessarily follow from a simple association. It is even possible that those with more severe injuries may be more likely to seek compensation. Furthermore, there are numerous reasons for apparent poor effort or negative response bias on tests of cognitive function, and malingering should not be immediately assumed. Inconsistent performance must be interpreted within the context of such factors as fatigue, medication effects, and medical or comorbid psychiatric conditions.

Is there a postconcussive syndrome? There is a good deal of confusion surrounding the use of this term. Some clinicians use it to describe any combination of one or more symptoms experienced at any time point after a mild TBI (see McAllister[14] for discussion). Others use the term to describe individuals who have persistent complaints after a mild TBI that they (or someone) attribute to that injury event. The issue is further confounded by the ICD-10 diagnosis of *postconcussion syndrome* and the DSM-IV provisional diagnosis of *postconcussional disorder* (PCD), as well as the observation that postconcussive symptoms are not specific to TBI and occur at high rates in the general population (e.g., see Iverson and Lange[37]). Furthermore, in Emergency Department populations, mild TBI does not predict "postconcussion syndrome" within a week of the injury.[38]

It may not be helpful to view the sequelae of TBI or mild TBI as a syndrome, but rather as a set of signs and symptoms that can be associated with an injury, depending on the profile of that injury and the person injured. In fact, it is not at all clear that there is a postconcussive "syndrome." For example, someone who experiences intermittent headache and dizziness for several months after a mild TBI may have a very different problem than an individual who presents 1–2 years after an astonishingly mild injury completely disabled by worsening complaints of poor memory, fatigue, chronic pain, and balance problems. If one considers multiple symptoms to be a syndrome with a common underlying mechanism (be it neural damage, depression, or compensation seeking), one tends to attribute multiple symptoms to a single etiology (i.e., "postconcussive syndrome") and look for treatments that will ameliorate the syndrome. If one views the symptoms as having many different mechanisms (albeit the same initiating event), then one tends to take a more careful look at the typology of each symptom and is better positioned to properly diagnose and treat the different sources of distress (e.g., dizziness related to labyrinthine trauma or headache due to cervical muscle strain). Common clinical experience suggests that individuals who experience multiple symptoms shortly after an injury can show improvement in all, some, or none of the symptoms over time, suggesting at the very least that the symptoms are not always tightly linked and can be uncoupled.

PATHOPHYSIOLOGY

As noted above, the application of force to the brain is a key element of the definition of TBI, and typically results in a predictable profile of regional brain injury. As such it is helpful to review key elements of the biomechanics of brain injury. Examples of external forces include the head striking or being struck by an object, rapid acceleration or deceleration of the brain, penetration of the brain by a foreign object, and exposure to forces associated with blasts as is more typical among military populations. The requirement of an external force acting on the brain separates TBI from other acquired brain injuries such as those due to cerebrovascular, neoplastic, or neurodegenerative conditions.

Two additional points are worth noting. Most definitions have distinguished *brain* injury from *head* injury, in which injury might be limited to the face or scalp. It is also helpful to distinguish between traumatic injuries involving penetration of the brain substance ("penetrating" or open injuries) and injuries that do not penetrate the brain (often referred to as closed injuries). Broadly speaking, the profile of injury associated with penetration of the brain substance will depend on the location and trajectory of the object involved. For example, the entrance location, trajectory, and size of a bullet that enters the head will largely predict the neurobehavioral sequelae. In these injuries, damage typically results from displacement or destruction of brain tissue by the projectile; fragmentation and deposition of bone or a projectile within brain tissue; or introduction of potential infectious material on the projectile.

Non-penetrating or closed injuries are better understood based on how the injury-producing biomechanical forces interact with the material properties of the brain substance as well as the brain's relationship to the bony structure (skull) in which it sits. The following discussion focuses primarily on closed or non-penetrating injuries. However, it is important to note that many injuries, particularly in the modern combat context, can be a combination of these different forces and injury types.

The brain sits within the bony skull suspended in spinal fluid and is partially tethered by the spinal cord. When either linear or rotational acceleration (or both) of the skull occur, the skull and brain move out of phase with each other, with inertia causing the brain's movement to lag behind the movement of the skull. This results in contact between the brain and the inner contours of the skull as well as the rigid fibrous contours of the falx cerebri, with subsequent deformation of brain tissue. Movement of the brain against the various ridges and bony protuberances of the anterior (frontal) and middle (temporal) fossae is particularly injurious to the temporal and frontal poles, the ventral anterior, medial, and lateral temporal cortices, and the frontal cortices,[39-41] with contusions in these regions a frequent result depending on the magnitude of the skull acceleration. Even relatively small displacement of brain tissue on the order of 5–7 mm can exceed tissue tolerance and lead to axonal and vascular injury.[42,43]

The planes between tissues of different densities and elasticities (e.g., the junction between gray and white matter), and at the rotational center of mass in the intracranial space (rostral brainstem) are particularly vulnerable. Also very susceptible to injury are axonal projections and small blood vessels within the brainstem, parasagittal white matter of the cerebrum, corpus callosum, and gray-white junctions of the cerebral cortex. Although this type of inertial injury usually is described as diffuse axonal injury (DAI), the term is somewhat misleading in that the actual pattern of injury is more accurately characterized as multifocal.[39,44] A few examples of common post-TBI radiographic findings including DAI are represented in Figure 30-1.

The above described forces initiate a complex set of events at the cellular and subcellular level that is only partially understood

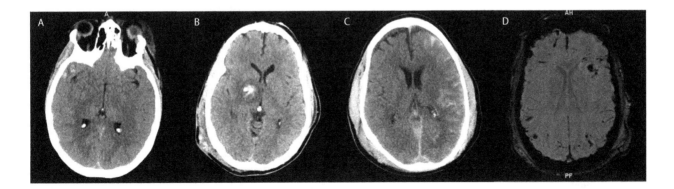

FIGURE 30-1. Examples of radiographic findings after TBI. **A.** A 25-year-old female with CT findings of a right anterior temporal contusion following a snowmobile accident. **B.** A 46-year-old male with traumatic right basal ganglia intracranial hemorrhage detected on CT following a motor vehicle accident. **C.** A 74-year-old male with CT findings of left > right traumatic subarachnoid hemorrhage following a fall down the stairs. **D.** A 60-year-old male with diffuse axonal injury detected on susceptibility-weighted MRI imaging after a motorcycle accident.

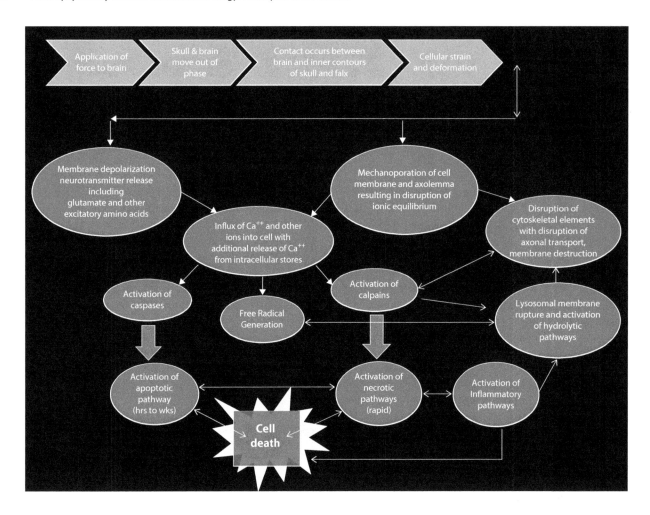

FIGURE 30-2. TBI-induced excitotoxic cascade.

(Figure 30-2).[45] Perturbation of Ca++ homeostasis appears to be of particular importance. At the time of injury, mechanical deformation of neurons is associated with a significant release of neurotransmitters. The release of glutamate and other excitatory amino acids drives an influx of extracellular Ca++ into the cell which can in turn release additional Ca++ from intracellular stores. This produces sufficient quantities of free intracellular Ca++ to initiate a host of intracellular reactions that can result in cytotoxic injury and eventually cell death.

Mechanical distortion of the neuron and its axon can damage its underlying structure and function. The ultimate fate of the cell membrane, axon, and neuron as a whole, appears related to the degree of distortion and other factors, with some cells repairing and resealing, and others progressing to further disruption and cell death. In addition to these processes, there is a growing appreciation for the role of additional factors in the cytotoxic cascades such as the generation of free radicals, and the disruption of lysosomal membranes with the subsequent release of hydrolytic enzymes into the intracellular environment.[45] Neuroinflammatory processes, including release of cytokines and/or activation of microglia, neutrophils, lymphocytes, and macrophages, have been implicated as possible pathophysiologic mechanisms underlying TBI as well.[46]

A variety of additional factors may complicate an injury including traumatic hematomas (e.g., subdural, epidural, subarachnoid, and intraparenchymal hematomas), focal or diffuse cerebral edema, elevated intracranial pressure, obstructive hydrocephalus, hypoxic-ischemic injury, and infection. Because TBI frequently occurs in the context of other injuries (polytrauma), medical complications such as volume depletion or blood loss, hypoperfusion, hypoxia, infection, and related problems can be seen and may increase post-traumatic mortality and morbidity.

Thus, in general terms the neuropathology of TBI includes a combination of multifocal and diffuse injury, damage that occurs at the time of the event (often referred to as "primary injury"), and additional damage ("secondary injury") that evolves over a variable period of time related to the elaborately choreographed injury cascades playing out at the cellular and subcellular level. Although each individual's injury is necessarily unique, there are certain brain regions that are particularly vulnerable to damage including the frontal cortex and subfrontal white matter, the deeper midline structures including the basal ganglia and diencephalon, the rostral brainstem, and the temporal lobes including the hippocampi.

Certain neurotransmitter systems, particularly the catecholaminergic[47] and cholinergic systems[48] can also be altered

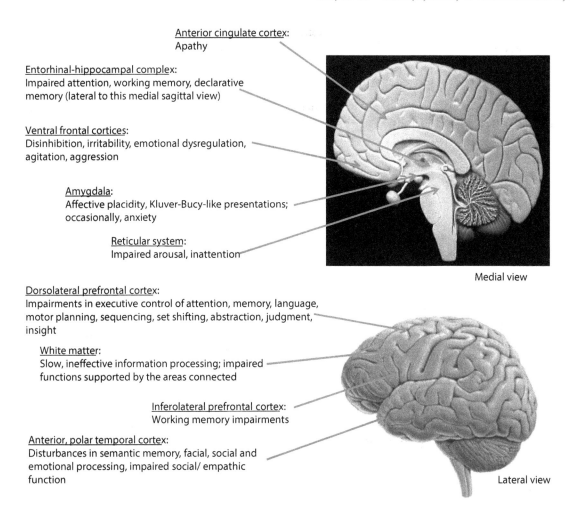

Anterior cingulate cortex:
Apathy

Entorhinal-hippocampal complex:
Impaired attention, working memory, declarative
memory (lateral to this medial sagittal view)

Ventral frontal cortices:
Disinhibition, irritability, emotional dysregulation,
agitation, aggression

Amygdala:
Affective placidity, Kluver-Bucy-like presentations;
occasionally, anxiety

Reticular system:
Impaired arousal, inattention

Medial view

Dorsolateral prefrontal cortex:
Impairments in executive control of attention, memory, language,
motor planning, sequencing, set shifting, abstraction, judgment,
insight

White matter:
Slow, ineffective information processing; impaired
functions supported by the areas connected

Inferolateral prefrontal cortex:
Working memory impairments

Anterior, polar temporal cortex:
Disturbances in semantic memory, facial, social and
emotional processing, impaired social/ empathic
function

Lateral view

FIGURE 30-3. Localization-based clinical phenomenon underlying brain-behavior relationships in traumatic brain injury. (Reproduced with permission from Barsky AJ, Silbersweig DA, Boland RJ. Depression and neurologic illness. In: *Depression in Medical Illness*. https://neurology. mhmedical.com. Copyright © McGraw Hill LLC. All rights reserved.)

in TBI. Strain across midbrain and pontine regions may impair catecholaminergic production and release through injury to the substantia nigra pars compacta, ventral tegmental area, and locus coeruleus.[49] Cholinergic nuclei projecting from the ventral forebrain and upper brainstem may be vulnerable to damage following traumatic biomechanical forces as well.[48] Both catecholaminergic and cholinergic systems play critical roles in a variety of behavioral homeostasis domains including arousal, cognition, reward behavior, and mood regulation. This profile of structural injury and neurochemical dysregulation occurs along a spectrum of injury severity, including "mild" injury.[50]

CLINICAL PRESENTATION

As noted above, the clinical presentation of the neuropsychiatric sequelae of TBI follows predictably from an understanding of the biomechanics of the typical injury, and the interaction of those factors with the physical properties of the brain and its relationship with the skull in which it sits. Figure 30-3 shows

examples of the possible cognitive and neurobehavioral sequelae resulting from damage to various neuroanatomical regions due to TBI.

However, as Sir Henry Symonds opined in 1937,[51] it is important to consider not only the injury, but the head that is injured. Failure to appreciate the myriad factors beyond injury biomechanics and the apparent injury profile that influence outcome will impede a full understanding of the individual with a brain injury. While numerous such factors exist, a few are worth highlighting.

Preexisting Psychiatric Illness

Individuals with TBI are not a random sample of the general population. Several studies of individuals with TBI have shown that this cohort has higher rates of pre-injury psychiatric illness (e.g., depression, anxiety, substance use disorder).[52] Not surprisingly, combining psychiatric vulnerability with TBI frequently results in a worsening or exacerbation of the underlying psychiatric disorder. This in turn can greatly complicate the rehabilitation and recovery from the injury, perhaps related to adverse impact on patient resilience or the ability to "bounce back" from adverse events such as trauma.[53]

Meaning of the Injury

All individuals have a variety of strengths and weaknesses that play critical roles in self-image and identity. If the profile of injury impairs domains that are highly valued by the individual, the impact of the injury may seem out of proportion to what one would otherwise expect. For example, an individual who depends on cognitive capacities for work, and takes pride in his/her ability to take on challenging demands, may be devastated by even small decrements in processing speed or memory, to a degree that someone whose work and sense of self is more tied to physical strength and appearance might not be.

Context of the Injury

The nature of the injury and the context of its occurrence often has a large impact on outcome. For example, the resolution of symptoms following a SRC is typically more rapid than recovery from other forms of mild TBI in patients of different ages and other etiologies recruited from Emergency Departments.[17,20] Again, there is a complex link to psychiatric illness here. It is not uncommon to encounter patients with a prior history of PTSD who were seemingly recovered or stable but when challenged with a seemingly mild TBI can experience a disabling recurrence of symptoms.

Psychosocial Supports and Network

A host of additional factors including physical disabilities, pain, speech and language impairment, loss of connectedness, and interaction associated with work or preferred activities can have profound effects on an individual's quality of life.[54] The strength and vitality of the network of relationships surrounding the injured individual, including family, intimate partner(s), friends, colleagues, and social networks can have a dramatic impact on quality of life and other outcome measures.[55]

In light of the above, the overarching approach to the evaluation and treatment of behavioral challenges in an individual with a TBI is best conceptualized as the integration of what is known about the neurobiology of TBI with a detailed knowledge of the specific injury profile of the individual, all in the context of the individual's pre-injury history, the context and meaning of the injury to the individual, and his/her network of strengths and supports. This can be conceptualized as a *neurobiopsychosocial* approach. Within this framework one can identify four broad categories of neuropsychiatric sequelae that commonly present in this population and will now be discussed: *dysexecutive syndromes, cognitive deficits, psychiatric disorders,* and *neurological and medical comorbidities.*

Dysexecutive and Other Neurobehavioral Syndromes

One of the most common concerns voiced by family/caregivers is personality change (e.g., "my spouse/child/partner is different than he/she was before"). Personality changes after TBI may reflect an exaggeration of pre-injury characteristics or present as a more fundamental alteration in how an individual conducts himself or herself in the world. Parsing of these complaints often reveals that the changes reflect dysexecutive syndromes usually attributable to damage to the frontal-subcortical circuits subserving complex human behavior.[41] The most common manifestations of personality change after TBI involve domains of higher-order cognition (i.e., executive cognitive function), social comportment, and motivated behavior. Often these categories overlap and a brain-injured individual can manifest varying degrees of one, two, or three of the domains at the same time.

Changes in Executive Cognitive Function

Executive cognitive functions are generally thought to be comprised of four broad components including response inhibition, interference inhibition, working memory, and cognitive flexibility.[56] A critical component of the substrate of these functions includes the dorsal-lateral prefrontal cortex and its related circuitry. Related to the injury vulnerability of this region, individuals with TBI are prone to experience challenges with problem solving, planning, sequencing, complex attention, and judgment.

Changes in Social Comportment

Social comportment encompasses a broad spectrum of human behaviors governing interactions with others in the context of expected social and group norms. Typically, individuals with TBI and their caregivers report challenges in several of the following areas, relevant to social comportment.

Impulsivity

Impulsivity commonly occurs after TBI. Behaviorally this can manifest in the form of verbal statements, actions, quick decisions, or poor judgment. Impulsivity can reflect impaired self-control capacities and/or one's inability to consider the full consequences of an action.[57] Impulsivity also shares characteristics with environmental dependency or stimulus boundedness —in which an individual responds to the most salient cue in the environment without regard for previously determined intentions.[58]

Irritability, Agitation, and Aggression

Irritability, agitation, and aggression are also common occurrences after TBI. Irritability has been described as episodic frustration and impatience, expressed to a degree that is out of proportion with the nature of a stimulus. Post-TBI irritability is estimated to occur in one- to two-thirds of individuals, with higher rates among those with more severe injuries.[59,60] Behaviorally, agitation can manifest in a variety of ways, and may include a state of irritability as well as motor restlessness, heightened emotional reactivity, and inappropriate behavior. Aggression typically refers to cases of agitation in which an individual wishes to cause harm to another person. Agitation and aggression are common in both the initial post-injury period as well as more chronically after TBI.[61,62] Injury to the frontal and temporal lobes, amygdala, and hippocampus, as well as alterations in monoaminergic neurotransmission have been associated with these behaviors.[63]

Affective Instability

Affective instability is also common after TBI, and has been referred to by many other names, including emotional lability, pseudobulbar affect (PBA), pathological laughing and crying, and emotional incontinence. These terms refer to exaggerated displays of emotion in response to seemingly trivial stimuli.[58] These displays are frequently stereotyped and perceived as involuntary. This is in contrast to expressions of affect, such as crying, that appropriately reflect a state of dysphoria among depressed individuals,[64,65] or individuals who simply have a lower baseline, pre-injury threshold for expressing emotions.[66] Estimates for emotional lability after TBI vary widely. Depending on choice of assessment tools and cut-off scores for reaching significance, the prevalence may range between 5.3%-to-48.2%.[64,65] Emotional expression and modulation are complex tasks. Recent studies have suggested a role for cortico-limbic-subcortico-thalamic-ponto-cerebellar networks modulated by multiple neurotransmitter systems, including serotonergic, dopaminergic, and glutaminergic networks.[67]

Awareness Deficits

Awareness deficits are another complication of TBI. Patients may deny any change to their capabilities or behavior following their injury, despite such changes being readily apparent to others. Awareness deficits occur in up to 45% of individuals with moderate-to-severe TBI and can be described across multiple dimensions, including one's acknowledgment of, emotional response to, and explanation for how a deficit arose, as well as the capacity to comprehend and predict its consequences.[68] Lack of awareness regarding deficits in cognition and behavior may be more frequent than lack of awareness of motor deficits.[57,69] Injury to frontal executive control systems responsible for self-awareness and self-monitoring,[57,58] as well as impaired functional connectivity between frontal-parietal control networks[70] have been implicated in such deficits.

Disorders of Motivation

Apathy is the predominant disorder of motivated behavior after TBI and is defined as a reduction in motivation and self-generated goal-directed behavior (lack of effort toward everyday activities) and cognition (lack of interest in new experiences or lack of concern for one's problems), typically accompanied by flat affect and blunted emotional reactivity not better explained by a depressed level of consciousness, cognitive impairment, or emotional distress.[71–73] In one study involving individuals with a history of severe TBI, apathy was the most common neuropsychiatric disturbance, with a prevalence rate of 42%.[74] More often than not, apathy presents in conjunction with depression.[75] In a cohort of individuals with TBI presenting to a neuropsychiatry clinic, ~60% demonstrated apathy comorbid with depression.[76] Deficits in motivated behavior have been associated with disrupted "reward" circuitry. Alterations in prefrontal and basal ganglia networks, cholinergic pathways of the anterior cingulate cortex, and mesolimbic dopaminergic pathways have been implicated in apathy.[72] In addition to being a source of distress to family/caregivers, apathy is associated with reduced participation in rehabilitation efforts and poor functional outcomes.[77,78]

Other Cognitive Deficits

Executive cognitive deficits have been described above. Additional deficits commonly reported after TBI include reduced processing speed, attention, working memory, memory and learning, as well as speech and language deficits.[35,79]

While these deficits can also occur across the spectrum of injury severity, individuals on the more severe end of the injury spectrum experience the most marked deficits.[80] While cognitive symptoms in the moderate-to-severe injury cohort typically improve over initial months to years, remaining deficits are often permanent.[81] Cognitive difficulties following mild TBI typically resolve completely within weeks to months,[15] though symptoms can be longer-lasting for a significant minority,[82] especially when in association with a variety of psychosocial factors.[35]

In addition to acute neurocognitive and neuropsychiatric changes, a history of TBI or exposure to multiple concussions or repetitive head-impact exposure in sports may increase the risk for neurodegenerative disorders later in life. Epidemiologic research suggests that TBI is a risk factor for Alzheimer's disease (AD).[83-85] In a recent systematic review and meta-analysis, Li et al.[86] reviewed 32 studies involving over 2 million individuals and found an elevated relative risk for both any dementia (RR=1.63) and for AD specifically (RR=1.51). Of interest, this elevated risk was not found in studies that included only those with a history of LOC (presumably a more severely injured group). While this might suggest that the increased relative risk is being driven by those with mild injury, from an epidemiologic perspective, it seems unlikely that a single incident of mild TBI or SRC predisposes one to a long-term risk of neurodegenerative disease, given what we know about the incidence of concussion in the general population.[85,87]

Sport-Related Concussion

SRC by virtually any definition is a mild TBI, though it is often considered to fall on the milder end of the mild TBI continuum. It has been recognized for some time that repetitive SRC and perhaps repetitive head impacts associated primarily with boxing,[88] but more recently with other contact sports, may be associated with a neurodegenerative condition referred to as chronic traumatic encephalopathy (CTE).[24,89] While a full discussion of this topic is beyond the scope of this chapter, publicity attending the deaths and neuropathological findings in several high-profile professional athletes[90–92] and class action lawsuits brought on behalf of former National Football League (NFL) and National Hockey League (NHL) players[93] have fueled concern in players, parents, legislatures, and sport-governing bodies. Questions are now being raised about how many concussions is too many: are some individuals more vulnerable to the effects of concussion and if so why; is concussion the proper metric of injury or should more attention be paid to the number and magnitude of repetitive head impacts; is mild TBI an exposure or an initiating event for long-term sequelae over the lifespan; and should certain sports such as football be banned.[87,94–96]

To date, the basis for the concerns consist of a growing but highly selective sample of athletes with a diverse array of neuropsychiatric symptoms who have died and then been autopsied by a single group. Recently formal neuropathological criteria were agreed to,[97] but there is a need for more population-based studies in order to ascertain the true risks inherent in contact sport participation. Currently CTE remains a pathological diagnosis though attempts are being made to operationalize clinical staging criteria for individuals with suspected CTE[98] and to determine if advanced neuroimaging techniques such as positron emission tomography using a tau protein ligand can be used for in vivo diagnosis.[99] With respect to exposure to repetitive head impacts, there is relatively little data available as of yet on which to base conclusions.

Psychiatric Disorders

Neuropsychiatric disorders after TBI are very common. In one prospective study of individuals with a history of moderate-to-severe TBI, 75.2% received a psychiatric diagnosis within 5 years of injury, with the majority of diagnoses occurring within the first post-injury year.[100] In another large systematic review, the long-term prevalence of psychiatric disorders after TBI was 54%, with depressive disorders observed in 43% and anxiety disorders in 36%.[101] Rates of neuropsychiatric diagnoses after mild brain injury tend to be slightly lower in comparison, but notably still exceed those of the general population. In a prospective study evaluating psychiatric illness following individuals with a history of mild TBI presenting to the hospital, 31% met criteria for a psychiatric diagnosis within the first post-injury year, with 22% reporting that they had never been diagnosed with a psychiatric condition before.[102]

Anxiety and mood disorders are the most common post-traumatic disorders,[100,102,103] and often co-occur.[104–106] In two large studies, more than two-thirds of psychiatric diagnoses in the first few post-injury years were new.[100,103] Nevertheless a premorbid psychiatric history remains one of the main risk factors, along with lower socioeconomic status, for developing a post-injury neuropsychiatric disorder.[107,108]

There is some evidence that psychiatric symptoms manifesting shortly after injury may be more closely tied to injury-related neurobiological factors (e.g., the profile of regional injury and disruption of key neurotransmitter pathways), whereas symptoms manifesting months later are more likely to be influenced by the psychological reaction to injury or disability.[109] Given that TBI generally represents a static, nonprogressive insult, after an initial period of adjustment lasting months to years, rates of new psychiatric symptoms would be expected to decrease. The literature generally supports this trend, though not across all diagnostic categories. For instance, one study demonstrated that while the frequency of post-TBI anxiety decreased over time, rates of depression remained relatively constant.[100]

In addition to being a major cause of psychological hardship, the development of a psychiatric disorder is associated with poorer psychosocial and functional outcomes such as lower vocational and relationship status, and reduced functional independence.[108,110,111] The most common neuropsychiatric disorders following TBI are discussed below.

Depression

Depression after TBI is common. Whereas the prevalence of depression in the general public is around 16%,[112] rates following TBI range from 15.6% to 61%.[113] Some of the more frequently reported risk factors for depression after TBI include female gender, history of major depressive disorder prior to injury or at the time of injury, lifetime alcohol dependence, and post-injury unemployment.[101,104,114] The relationship between injury severity and risk of depression is unclear.[115] Neurobiologically, depression after TBI has been associated with damage to specific neuroanatomic regions, including left prefrontal, ventrolateral, and dorsolateral regions.[105]

Accurately diagnosing depression after TBI can be challenging for a number of reasons. For one, following TBI, individuals often experience neurovegetative symptoms associated with a depressed mood such as fatigue, poor concentration, and sleep disturbance in the absence of depression.[113] In such cases, looking for the alternative indicators of depression such as rumination, self-criticism, and guilt may be necessary.[116] Some have suggested that the clinical manifestation of depression after TBI may differ from that in the general population, with irritability, anger, and aggression presenting more commonly than sadness or tearfulness.[116] Diagnosing depression in individuals with more severe TBI can be further challenged by cognitive limitations in insight, self-awareness, and memory. Reports from family members regarding anhedonia, irritability, or agitation may be helpful here.[58] The diagnostic utility of various psychometric depression scales has been evaluated for use in TBI, with the validity of the Patient Health Questionaire-9 (PHQ-9) and the Neurobehavioral Functioning Inventory-Depression noted by some.[116]

Mania

The literature on post-traumatic mania is limited. Prevalence estimates for episodic mania following TBI range from 1.7% to 9.0%.[117–119] Risk factors associated with the onset of mania after TBI are not clearly established. Post-traumatic mania has been variably, but not consistently, associated with injury severity. Some have suggested that the stress of injury or adjustment to disability may play a role in the emergence of symptoms.[120] Lesion localization may also contribute, with lesions of the temporal poles, orbitofrontal cortices, as well as right-sided limbic regions more broadly associated with mania.[118,120] Surprisingly, in two studies, a relationship between post-traumatic mania and personal or family psychiatric history was not observed.[118,121]

When mania does occur following TBI, increased irritability is reportedly a much more common mood complaint than euphoria.[118,121] That being said, caution must be made to not overdiagnose mania or hypomania following TBI, as irritability and other symptoms, such as affect dysregulation, impulsivity, and poor sleep may present in the absence of a mood disorder[119] due to more fundamental changes in social comportment or biologically mediated disruptions in circadian rhythms.

Treatment approaches would considerably differ in these cases, so an accurate diagnosis is important.

Anxiety Disorders

Anxiety is very common after TBI and can manifest as generalized anxiety disorder (GAD), panic disorder, social anxiety disorder, phobias, and obsessive-compulsive disorder (OCD).[122,123] Several factors might contribute to high rates of anxiety disorders following TBI. Neurobiologically, this may include injury to the prefrontal cortex, compromising top-down regulation and inhibition of circuits mediating fear and anxiety,[124] dysautonomia,[125,126] or pathological biochemical processes, such as excitotoxicity, oxidative stress, and chronic inflammation.[127] Psychosocial factors may include stress stemming from the traumatic circumstances during which a TBI was sustained as well as stress manifesting as one attempts to adjust to and cope with any lingering deficits.[128] One interesting feature regarding the relationship between TBI severity and anxiety is that the two may be inversely correlated in many cases,[122] with milder as opposed to more severe brain injuries associated with a greater likelihood of PTSD, social phobia, panic disorder, and agoraphobia.[102,117] The preservation of self-awareness and self-consciousness with milder injury may account for this trend.[129]

Generalized anxiety disorder is the most common anxiety disorder manifesting after TBI, though this may be due in part to its high frequency in the general population at large. In one outpatient TBI sample, 24% met criteria for GAD.[111] In other studies, lower rates in the range of 10% have been reported,[106,122] but these are still higher than base rates of GAD in the general population.[130] Given that GAD has been associated with stressful life events in the general population,[131] it is possible that in many cases, the stress of TBI and its psychosocial consequences may be a precipitating factor among those already genetically or environmentally predisposed to GAD.

Panic Disorder

Reported rates of panic disorder following TBI have ranged from ~6% to 14% across various studies,[103,132-134] representing a frequency substantially higher than that in the general population.[122] Various explanations have been raised to account for why this may be so. For one, following a traumatic injury sustained under traumatic circumstances, thoughts regarding recurrence of the event may precipitate a panic attack. Dysregulated sympathetic activity may play a role as well.[125,126] Furthermore following TBI, some persistent physical symptoms such as headache or dizziness could be misinterpreted as an indication of more serious injury, predisposing one to panic.[123]

Phobias

There is limited research on the rate of specific phobias manifesting after TBI, with estimates ranging between 0.8%[132] and 8.3%.[133] In many cases, some degree of fear following a traumatic accident would be appropriate, but for certain individuals the fear can become pathologic and disruptive to everyday functioning. The most common phobias for individuals sustaining injuries while in transit include travel or accident phobias.[123,135,136] These phobias may manifest as complete avoidance of driving or riding, driving only under optimal conditions,

excessive driving caution, or use of distraction, such as closing one's eyes when riding as a passenger.[136] Risk factors associated with phobic travel after an accident include female gender, being the passenger versus the driver (possibly due to perceived lack of control), or being a motorcyclist.[137] In addition to existing in isolation, accident phobias can also occur as one of the many symptoms constituting PTSD.

Social Anxiety Disorder

Rates of social anxiety following TBI are greater than those in the general population.[102] Factors at play here may include brain-based impairments in social cognition leading to greater interpersonal difficulty, self-consciousness emerging from acquired physical or cognitive disability, and/or social isolation following loss of social networks or employment after brain injury resulting in fewer opportunities for interpersonal engagement.[123]

Obsessive-Compulsive Disorder

Rates of OCD following TBI have been reported at ~3%, slightly higher than that in the general population.[122] Post-traumatic OCD has been observed across the spectrum of injury severity, with symptoms generally manifesting within the first few weeks to months after injury.[138] In one case series, some of the more common manifestations of OCD following TBI included obsessions about aggression, contamination, symmetry, somatic, and sexual themes; and cleaning, checking, and repeating behaviors.[138] The emergence of these symptoms may reflect a variety of factors. Neurobiological correlates have been suggested, with several case series associating post-traumatic OCD with lesions in the orbitofrontal and/or temporal cortices and subcortical structures such as the caudate.[138-140] The stress ensuing from the traumatic injury itself may be another important consideration —as a major life stressor is one of the primary environmental risks factors for OCD in the general population.[141] In some instances, it is also possible that a TBI may simply magnify one's premorbid inclinations—a previously organized or methodical person becoming rigidly organized following a brain injury. In other cases, cognitive impairment may drive OCD-like behaviors. Some researchers have associated checking behavior, for instance, with deficits in working memory, executive function, strategic processing, or capacity to "see the big picture."[142,143] As an example, after an action (e.g., turning off the stove), an individual may not feel confident of completion of the task, thus resorts to repeated checking.[144] Others have noted an association between components of impulsivity, such as urgency, and compulsive behaviors after TBI.[145]

Post-Traumatic Stress Disorder

Symptoms of post-traumatic stress exist along a continuum from normal stress reaction to acute stress disorder or PTSD. Reported rates of PTSD following TBI vary widely, from 1% to 50% across various studies,[146] with a prevalence that is inversely proportional to injury severity.[122] Neurobiological correlates here may involve disruption of central autonomic control centers by means of white matter injury to regions such as the uncinate fasciculus that links neocortical, subcortical, and limbic structures.[147]

Risk factors for developing PTSD after TBI include shorter PTA, memory of the traumatic event, and early post-traumatic symptoms.[114] For those with preserved recollection following TBI, some have postulated a role for altered medial prefrontal cortical capacity—disruption in one's ability to modulate fear during a traumatic experience increasing one's likelihood of PTSD. Despite prior claims to the contrary, PTSD can also occur in cases of severe injury, when recall of the event is limited or absent.[148] Several proposed mechanisms for this condition include fear conditioning, reconstruction of traumatic memories by means of photographs or stories told by others, as well as traumatic post-amnesia experiences such as one's recollection of time in the intensive care unit.[149]

In recent years, much has been written about the overlap between mild TBI and PTSD. When a mild TBI is sustained under traumatic circumstances it can be extraordinarily difficult to disentangle whether a particular symptom such as dizziness, cognitive slowing, poor sleep, or irritability more accurately reflects PTSD or brain injury. Misattribution and misdiagnosis are also quite common in these circumstances.[150,151]

Psychotic Disorders

Psychosis is a rare complication of TBI but can cause significant distress for individuals and caregivers.[152] Prevalence estimates for post-TBI psychosis range from 1% to 9%,[153] roughly three times that which occurs in the general population.[154] About half of these individuals will present with psychosis within the first year after injury and the majority within the first 5 years after TBI.[155] When the presentation of psychosis is delayed, it is unlikely that TBI is the only etiologic factor.[156] Some risk factors for post-traumatic psychosis include prior congenital neurological disorder, sustaining a head injury prior to adolescence, male gender, as well as frontal and temporal lesions.[153,155]

Post-TBI psychosis can manifest in numerous forms[153] and thus it is important to consider the full differential diagnosis prior to initiating treatment. Shortly after injury, psychotic symptoms may be seen in the context of post-injury delirium or post-traumatic confusion. This form of psychosis tends to be self-limited and spontaneously improve over time. Psychotic symptoms may also be seen in conjunction with mood disorders such as depression or mania. More challenging to diagnose are psychotic symptoms occurring in the setting of post-traumatic epilepsy. This can be seen in the peri-ictal period or postictal period, most commonly presenting in the setting of complex partial seizures.[157]

Post-traumatic psychosis can also manifest in a more pervasive form developing later on in the post-injury period.[156] Chronic, post-traumatic psychosis often presents as a delusional disorder (e.g., with bizarre somatic concerns, or a misidentification syndrome—which may reflect disruption of visual recognition circuits) or as a schizophrenia-like illness.[153,158] In contrast to primary schizophrenia, the schizophrenia-like illness emerging after TBI is characterized more often by positive symptoms of auditory and visual hallucinations than negative symptoms.[153,159] Evidence supporting an increased risk of schizophrenia following TBI among those genetically at risk also exists.[159-162]

Neurological and Medical Complications of TBI

The risk of neurologic complications following TBI is greatest within the first few weeks to months after injury, but can persist chronically as well. Any abrupt change in neurologic status should prompt evaluation for some of the more common post-TBI neurologic complications, including hyponatremia, extra- or intracranial infections (especially amongst those with a history of penetrating head injury, craniotomy, or craniectomy), hydrocephalus, or post-traumatic seizures. Other common medical comorbidities include neuroendocrine dysfunction and disordered sleep-wake cycles.

Hydrocephalus

Hydrocephalus is a concern after TBI and is seen most commonly in the context of a subarachnoid hemorrhage with intraventricular extension. In such cases, blood products in the ventricles obstruct CSF absorption, leading to a gradual buildup of fluid and ventricular enlargement. Clinical suspicion for hydrocephalus is raised in the setting of new onset ataxia, incontinence, and/or plateauing or worsening cognitive or functional progress in the post-acute period. A CT for further evaluation would be warranted in such cases.

Post-Traumatic Epilepsy

Post-traumatic epilepsy refers to recurrent seizures occurring in individuals with a history of TBI that cannot be attributed to another cause. Post-traumatic epilepsy occurs in 10–25% of individuals following a moderate-to-severe TBI,[163] and may arise in the immediate aftermath of a head injury, within the first few days, months, or years later. Risk factors associated with recurrent seizures after brain injury include seizures early after injury, chronic alcoholism, age >65 years old, brain contusions with SDH, higher injury severity, skull fracture, LOC, and amnesia >24 hours.[164-167] In one study of post-traumatic epilepsy, epileptic foci of activity were most common in the temporal (57%) and frontal lobes (35%), and less often observed in the parietal (3%) and occipital lobes (3%).[163] As is true with seizures from any origin, cognitive and affective changes are common. Temporal lobe seizures, for instance, may result in episodic fear or panic followed by postictal confusion or amnesia; whereas frontal lobe seizures can result in aggressive motor automatisms (thrashing, kicking) followed by postictal changes in mood, anger, or confusion.[167] On the whole, the presence of post-traumatic epilepsy has also been associated with increased rates of anxiety and depression.[168]

Neuroendocrine Dysfunction

Neuroendocrine function can be altered after TBI with repercussions for neuropsychiatric outcomes as well.[169] Neuroendocrine dysfunction is far more common after moderate-to-severe injury, but has on occasion also been documented after mild TBI.[170] In one prospective study of TBI across the spectrum of severity, deficiencies in at least one pituitary hormone was documented in 56% of patients at 3 months. By 12 months, fewer subjects (36%) were affected overall, and some new cases occurred. This study demonstrated that over time, some cases will spontaneously remit, and others will newly emerge.[171] After the 12-month post-injury mark, new cases of pituitary dysfunction are far less likely.

Growth hormone deficiency is the most common deficiency after TBI, followed by deficits in corticotropins, gonadotropins, and thyrotropins.[170,172] Several studies have suggested a relationship between growth hormone deficiencies and impaired attention and memory, mood, energy, and quality of life.[173–175] The literature on hormone replacement after TBI is sparse. A small handful of case reports have suggested that replacement of growth hormone can have beneficial results on neuropsychological test performance and measures of mood.[176–179] Low levels of testosterone have also been associated with lower mood and functional outcomes.[180] Testosterone supplementation after TBI is also an area of active interest and debate.[181] Current recommendations for post-TBI neuroendocrine testing include the following: fasting morning cortisol, thyroid-stimulating hormone, free T4, insulin-like growth factor (IGF-1), testosterone, as well as luteinizing- and follicle-stimulating hormone (for women) performed at 3–6 months after injury and again at 12 months.[172,182] If any results are abnormal, referral to neuroendocrinology or endocrinology should be made.

Sleep-Wake Cycle Dysregulation

Disruption of sleep architecture is another common issue following TBI.

Long-term sleep-wake cycle disturbances can result in poorer sleep quality, frequent nighttime awakenings, reduced sleep efficiency, increased 24-hour sleep need, and excessive daytime sleepiness.[183,184] Impaired sleep following TBI has been associated with decreased cognitive performance and capacity to perform activities of daily living.[185,186]

While the underlying mechanisms of sleep disturbance after TBI have not yet been well-established, there are likely a range of factors at play, including loss of wakefulness-promoting neurons in the hypothalamus and mesopontine tegmentum,[184,187] and dysfunction in sleep-regulating regions of the brain, such as the suprachiasmatic nucleus and pineal gland regulating melatonin release.[188,189] Here some early data have suggested that the exogenous melatonin supplementation can improve sleep quality[190] and daytime alertness.[191] Changes in mood and pain can also be disruptive to sleep.

Chronic Pain

Chronic pain, especially post-traumatic headache, is a common complaint after TBI.[192,193] In one systematic review of individuals with persistent symptoms after TBI, more than 40% of veterans and 50% of civilians reported chronic pain—for civilians, interestingly, mild TBI versus moderate-to-severe TBI was associated with much higher rates of pain.[192] Pain is a well-known confounder in cognitive and affective complaints.[193]

ASSESSMENT AND DIFFERENTIAL DIAGNOSIS

Assessment of a TBI case should begin with a comprehensive history and physical exam. As TBI is often a singular event with a distinct "before" and "after" profile, careful attention should be paid not only to the present condition and complaints but also to the individual's premorbid state. This may include a detailed discussion of premorbid personality and behavior, psychological status, cognitive, social, and occupational functioning.

Use of additional assessment tools and ancillary tests may also be useful. During psychological assessment, in addition to careful history-taking, some advocate for use of standardized scales, such as the PHQ-9[116] or Generalized Anxiety Disorder Screener (GAD-7) for the screening and tracking of depression and anxiety symptoms. For neurocognitive assessment, as a quick, in-office screen, the Montreal Cognitive Assessment or Mini-Mental Status Examination may be used. Such information, even if limited, can be very helpful when conceptualizing an individual's circumstances. In other cases, depending on injury severity and psychosocial context, referral for more extensive neuropsychological testing may be appropriate. For example, formalized testing may be useful when the individual is planning to return to work. Test results can help gauge the appropriateness of return to a given profession and provide useful information on specific neurocognitive deficits on which to focus in cognitive rehabilitation.

Ideally, during any TBI evaluation but especially in cases of moderate-to-severe injury, a clinician would have access to neuroimaging, such as a head CT or brain MRI. These visual representations can provide information regarding injury localization, lateralization, as well as whether the injury is more focal, multifocal, or diffuse. Such information can be very helpful when conceptualizing present complaints with respect to neuroanatomic injury profile as well as provide a very rough gauge regarding rehabilitative potential.

When an injury occurred remotely and no imaging is available, there may be times that ordering a new MRI scan may be appropriate—for example, when the extent of injury is unclear based on clinical history alone, obtaining an MRI that variably showed evidence of prior contusions, and/or DAI versus no evidence of structural damage would certainly change a clinician's conceptualization of the case. Ordering an MRI or repeating an MRI may also be appropriate in the presence of functional decline once other medical or neurologic causes have been ruled out. In addition to observing the evolution of prior structural damage, global atrophy can also be assessed.

Other ancillary assessments may include laboratory tests, including neuroendocrine screening as described in detail above. As also mentioned above, a history of TBI places individuals at elevated risk of developing post-traumatic epilepsy, which can initially manifest months to years after the original injury. If concern arises for seizure activity at any point following injury, a referral for electroencephalogram (EEG) is warranted.

TREATMENT

Treatment options for the neuropsychiatric sequelae of TBI are wide ranging and can include various pharmaceuticals, behavioral, and psychotherapeutic options.

Principles of Psychopharmacologic Treatment

To date, there is not a single medication approved by the Federal Drug Administration for the treatment of any post-TBI condition.[194] Instead, most guidelines follow the principle of "treatment-by-analogy," applying similar treatments approved for use in other disease entities—for instance treating inattention following

TBI as one would treat attention deficit disorder. However, certain principles are worth considering when prescribing psychotropic agents in this population. For example many clinicians advocate for a "start low, go slow" dosing approach, as individuals with TBI can vary considerably in their response to medications and be unusually sensitive to psychotropic drugs and their side effects, especially in the case of antipsychotics, dopaminergic agents, and anticholinergics.[80,82,195] A second principle is to "stay the course," meaning making sure that medications are trialed at adequate doses for adequate durations prior to discontinuation.[80,82,195] It is also important to keep in mind that brain injury and neurologic recovery are dynamic processes. A treatment that works very well in the acute or subacute aftermath of an injury may not be useful weeks or months later. As an example, while the neurostimulant amantadine may be acutely useful for poor arousal within the first few weeks after injury, as one recovers, it may become overactivating and worsen agitation. Psychotropic approaches to several of the more common TBI sequelae are reviewed briefly. Common pharmacologic approaches for treating TBI-related symptoms are summarized in Table 30-2.

Cognitive Complaints and Deficits

Treatment of cognitive complaints following TBI can be challenging.[80,196] Virtually all studies to date have involved cohorts of individuals across the injury spectrum and focused on altering catecholaminergic and cholinergic signaling mechanisms as mediators of vulnerable attentional and memory domains.[47,48]

A variety of stimulants and dopaminergic agents have been evaluated as treatment for post-TBI attentional impairments. Several studies,[166,197-199] including three randomized controlled trials (RCTs),[200-202] have shown methylphenidate to benefit post-TBI attentional impairments. However, a few other small studies on methylphenidate have been negative.[203,204] A single study on atomoxetine for attention was also negative.[205] The literature on amantadine for post-TBI attentional deficits is mixed, with one positive case series,[206] one positive small RCT,[207] and one negative small RCT.[208] Another RCT evaluating the utility of bromocriptine for attentional impairment was also negative.[209]

Arciniegas and colleagues have advanced the theory of the underlying role of cholinergic mechanisms with regards to attentional and memory deficits after TBI.[48] A limited number of small studies have suggested that cholinergic augmentation, generally through use of a cholinesterase inhibitor (e.g., physostigmine or donepezil), may improve TBI-induced memory deficits even in the late post-injury period.[210,211] Of note however in one of the most robust RCTs to date, use of rivastigmine demonstrated no effect over placebo across a spectrum of post-TBI memory impairments, though a significant benefit was found in a *post hoc* analysis involving those with more severely impacted memory performance.[212]

Irritability and Agitation

Various treatment strategies have been used for the management of irritability/agitation following TBI. Centrally acting beta-blockers, such as propranolol, are typically considered first line[213] on the basis of several small controlled studies.[61,214,215] Alpha-agonists such as clonidine are also frequently used, although data are not available to support their efficacy.

TABLE 30-2 • Common Pharmacologic Treatment Strategies for TBI-Related Symptoms.	
Cognitive deficits	Psychostimulants Dopaminergic agents Cholinergic agents
Agitation/ Irritability	Centrally acting beta-blockers Mood stabilizers Antipsychotics Antidepressants
Emotional lability	Selective serotonin reuptake inhibitors Serotonin and norepinephrine reuptake inhibitors Mood stabilizers Dextromethorphan/quinidine
Amotivation	Psychostimulants Dopaminergic agents Serotonergic agents
Depressive disorders	Selective serotonin reuptake inhibitors Serotonin and norepinephrine reuptake inhibitors Tricyclic antidepressants Psychostimulants
Mania	Mood stabilizers Antipsychotics
Anxiety disorders	Selective serotonin reuptake inhibitors Serotonin and norepinephrine reuptake inhibitors
Psychosis	Antipsychotics

Regarding use of antiepileptic drugs (AEDs) and mood stabilizers, benefit was indicated by a case series on valproic acid,[216] divalproex,[217] carbamazepine,[218] lithium,[219,220] as well as a single case study of lamotrigine.[221] Various antidepressants, including sertraline[222] and amitriptyline,[223] have also shown benefit.

More recently, amantadine has been evaluated specifically for the treatment of post-traumatic irritability and aggression. Amantadine is a N-methyl-D-aspartate (NMDA) receptor antagonist which also indirectly enhances dopamine neurotransmission. While an initial RCT on amantadine suggested benefit in treating post-TBI irritability,[224] a subsequent multisite RCT showed the medication to be no better than placebo.[225] In another RCT performed by the same group, amantadine showed potential in reducing post-TBI aggression.[226] While this medication is widely used in TBI, caution should be practiced with regards to its potential for lowering the seizure threshold and worsening anxiety, confusion, and even irritability when amantadine is prescribed at higher doses.

The utility of using typical and atypical antipsychotics in the treatment of post-TBI irritability and agitation has also been evaluated. Small studies on methotrimeprazine,[227] droperidol and haloperidol,[228] and loxapine[229] have shown benefit, as have studies on quetiapine,[230] clozapine[231] ziprasidone,[232] and aripiprazole.[233]

Despite this suggested benefit, there are many reasons to be cautious with use of antipsychotics after brain injury. Some of the adverse effects associated with these medications may be particularly problematic for those with TBI, including lowering of the seizure threshold, extrapyramidal effects, weight gain, and adverse cognitive effects. Regarding the latter, in one study on individuals with a history of TBI, tapering off antipsychotics resulted in improved cognition.[175]

Concerns have also been raised regarding the potential of antipsychotics to interfere with neurological recovery. Numerous animals models of brain injury suggest a deleterious effect of antipsychotics on neuroplasticity;[176–179] typical rather than atypical agents are more commonly implicated.[152,234] Human studies have further associated antipsychotic use in the early post-acute stage with prolonged PTA.[181,182] As an interesting counterpoint, with unclear relevance to TBI at this time, is that in the psychiatric literature, new data suggest a potential neuroprotective benefit of antipsychotics when used in the early treatment of psychotic spectrum disorders.[183]

Emotional Lability

Various medications have been used to treat emotional lability after brain injury. Selective serotonin reuptake inhibitors (SSRIs) are typically considered first-line treatment, with several small studies demonstrating efficacy with use of citalopram, fluoxetine, sertraline, and paroxetine.[235–238] A separate case study also suggested benefit with use of lamotrigine.[239] Other medications used to treat emotional lability in other neurologic conditions include tricyclic antidepressants (TCAs), noradrenergic reuptake inhibitors, and dopaminergic agents.[235] Recently the combination of dextromethorphan and quinidine (DM/Q) has also been evaluated for use following TBI.[240,241] DM acts as an uncompetitive NMDA receptor antagonist and sigma-1 receptor agonist, while Q increased DM bioavailability by blocking DM hepatic metabolism.[242] Though this drug shows some promise in early trials, further cost-effectiveness and efficacy studies are warranted.

Disorders of Motivation

The literature on pharmacologic treatments of apathy after TBI is sparse, and first-line approaches are typically behavioral rather than pharmacologic. Small studies have suggested benefit with use of stimulants such as methylphenidate,[243] dopaminergic agents such as amantadine or bromocriptine,[244,245] as well as serotonergic agents such as fluvoxamine and fluoxetine.[246]

Psychiatric Disorders

As noted above, there are no medications specifically approved by the FDA for use in neuropsychiatric sequelae of TBI. There is also no clear evidence that conventional medication approaches to disorders such as depression do not work, nor is there evidence that specific classes of agents or specific medications are more effective than others in treating psychiatric disorders in the context of a TBI. A brief sampling of this literature is provided.

Mood Disorders/Depression

Several studies evaluating the effectiveness of antidepressants to treat depression after TBI have been published, however the results are mixed. Positive results were observed in a small RCT

of sertraline,[247] a nonrandomized placebo run-in trial of sertraline,[248] an open-label study of fluoxetine,[249] and an open-label study of citalopram.[250] In the two largest double-blind RCTs using sertraline to treat major depression after TBI however, rates of improvement between experimental and control groups did not significant differ.[251,252] Notably in these studies both experimental and control groups improved at significant rates, suggesting a substantial role for placebo effects.[253] Very little data at this point exists on use of serotonin and norepinephrine reuptake inhibitors (SNRIs) following TBI, with a single, small uncontrolled study on milnacipran suggesting a benefit.[254] That being said, given the high frequency with which apathy is present in conjunction with depression after TBI,[76] SNRIs may be a very reasonable choice for treatment.

A small number of studies have also explored whether SSRIs, if administered soon after injury, could prevent the later onset of post-traumatic depression. In one study, subjects with new TBI were randomized to receive sertraline (n=48) versus placebo (n=46) and follow-up for 6 months or until the development of a mood disorder. The number needed to treat to prevent one new case of depression at 6 months after TBI was 5.9.[255] In another study, nondepressed moderate-to-severe TBI subjects who received sertraline (n=49) versus placebo (n=50) within 3 weeks after injury reported lower depressive symptoms at 3 months.[256] However in this same cohort, when sertraline or placebo were stopped after 3 months, there were no significant differences in depressive symptoms for the remainder of the year, suggesting that such an intervention does not have any lasting effects on the serotonergic system once the medication is stopped.[255]

Though serotonergic medications typically take several weeks to reach full effect, they are generally well tolerated. Sertraline, citalopram, and escitalopram may be preferred choices on the basis of their shorter half-lives and fewer anticholinergic effects; whereas fluoxetine and paroxetine may be less preferable given the greatest risk of drug-drug interactions via cytochrome P450 enzyme inhibition.[82,119] Another consideration with use of serotonergic agents is their effect on bleeding. Serotonin is a weak platelet activator and SSRIs can inhibit serotonin storage in platelets, increasing intracranial bleeding risk, especially within the first few weeks after injury and among those taking anticoagulants, though the overall absolute risk remains quite low.[257,258]

Fewer studies have evaluated the efficacy of TCAs following post-traumatic depression. While one small study showed benefit of desipramine in individuals with a history of severe TBI,[259] others have been less favorable. Based on a series of reviews, the overall consensus appears to be that TCAs treat depression after TBI less effectively than in the general population,[260] and that they are likely less effective than SSRIs.[261] TCAs may also be a less preferable treatment for depression after TBI given their less favorable side-effect profile, including anticholinergic effects (dry mouth, changes in bowel habits), sedation, and orthostatic hypotension. TCAs also carry a greater risk of cardiac arrhythmias and potential for lowering the seizure threshold, as has been documented in at least one study involving individuals with a history of severe TBI.[262]

Stimulants, including methylphenidate, have also been evaluated for treatment of depression following TBI. In one double blind RCT, involving 33 subjects with mild-to-moderate TBI and depression, methylphenidate, given over the course

A single 33-year-old male construction worker suffered a severe TBI in a motor vehicle accident 1 year prior to presentation. Neuroimaging shortly after the injury suggested a left frontal contusion and diffuse axonal injury. He recovered quite well overall, but has residual deficits in processing speed, attention, working memory, and executive function. He reports generalized apathy, low mood, feelings of sadness related to his loss of employment, and guilt over the burden his care has placed on others. He has no prior psychiatric history. He denies any changes in sleep or appetite. He has completed a course of cognitive rehabilitation in which he focused on learning compensatory strategies to help with memory and attention. He hopes to return to work someday, but has been unmotivated to initiate the steps required. He is interested in medications that could be helpful as part of his treatment.

Clinical considerations: The combination of persistent neurocognitive deficits along with low motivation and mood is a common clinical scenario following traumatic brain injury. It is important to try to determine whether this cluster of symptoms is due to depression, injury-induced apathy and cognitive deficits, or a combination of depression and injury-related deficits. While many of the symptoms suggest a depressive disorder, the normal sleep and appetite would be somewhat unusual. Additional information from family/caregivers may be helpful in sorting this out. In terms of treatment, cognitive rehabilitation is often a first-line treatment for attention and memory complaints, and psychotherapy is often considered for apathy and depressive symptoms. In addition, several pharmacologic strategies may be appropriate depending on his level of cognitive impairment and the availability of experienced therapists. If depression is thought to the overarching problem, then a trial of a conventional antidepressant such as an SSRI would be reasonable. If, as is often the case, the clinical impression is that he is suffering from a combination of depression and injury-induced cognitive and motivational deficits, it would still make sense to start with treatment of the depression and then to determine the residual level of cognitive and motivational deficits after resolution of the mood disorder. If these remain clinically significant, then one could consider starting a stimulant such as methylphenidate or dextroamphetamine/amphetamine, which may help with processing speed and attention. An alternative strategy would be to consider whether targeting mood symptoms with a potentially more activating antidepressant may be helpful, such as bupropion or venlafaxine, both of which can promote an increase in noradrenergic activity. Though monotherapy is preferred in most cases, dual treatment with both a stimulant and antidepressant may also be indicated in some circumstances.

of 30 weeks, was found to benefit depression symptoms.[263] Another double-blind, placebo-controlled study directly compared a 4-week trial of methylphenidate to sertraline among 20 patients with mild to moderate TBI and major depressive disorder. Methylphenidate here not only provided cognitive and fatigue-related benefit, but was also found to be as effective as sertraline in treating depressive symptoms.[247]

Mania

The literature on pharmacologic treatments for mania manifesting after TBI is very limited. While early studies suggested a benefit of lithium,[264,265] this medication is not frequently used presently due to its adverse side-effect profile, including tremor, ataxia, lethargy, and lowering of the seizure threshold.[119] Valproate and divalproex have shown benefit in a small number of cases,[266–268] as has quetiapine.[269,270] Given the limited available research, mania after TBI is typically treated similarly to mania in the general psychiatric population. Some have suggested consideration of valproic acid or quetiapine as initial options given their general efficacy and relatively more favorable side-effect profile.[119]

Anxiety

To date, no clinical trials have evaluated any specific treatments for anxiety disorders after TBI. Based on studies in the general psychiatric population, SSRIs and SNRIs are typically considered first line. Buspirone is another common treatment option, though common side effects such as light-headedness and dizziness can also be problematic for TBI patients. In many cases, psychotherapeutic and behavioral therapies are the most appropriate approach.

PTSD

As in the non-brain injured population, SSRIs and SNRIs are considered first-line agents for treating PTSD.[271] Prazosin is another agent often used for PTSD-related nightmares. While a prior meta-analysis suggested benefit in the treatment of nightmares and PTSD symptoms,[272] an even more recent large RCT was unable to demonstrate efficacy of prazosin over placebo.[273]

Use of benzodiazepines to treat anxiety after TBI carries all the risks they pose in the general population as well as some additional concerns for the TBI population. Regular use of benzodiazepines can lead to tolerance and dependency. Benzodiazepines can also cause sedation and adversely affect attention and memory capacities in both the short and long term.[274,275] By further dampening frontal function, these agents can also worsen behavioral disinhibition after TBI. In animal models, administration of benzodiazepines shortly after injury has been shown to delay or reduce neurorecovery,[276] though not all studies have noted this association[277] and it is not known whether this same effect is seen in humans.

Psychosis

Antipsychotics are first-line treatment for psychosis after brain injury. However antipsychotic use in individuals with TBI warrants caution given potential adverse effects on cognition, arousal, and lowering of the seizure threshold. As described above, psychosis can manifest in a variety of ways following TBI, as part of delirium, in conjunction with a mood disorder, in association with epilepsy, or more pervasively and chronically as a delusional disorder or schizophrenia-like illness.[153] Antipsychotics may be necessary post-acutely if a patient displays significant psychotic symptoms during PTA. Regarding psychosis in association with a mood disorder or seizure disorder, treatment of the primary underlying condition would be the most appropriate starting point, through use of antidepressants or AEDs. For chronic, pervasive psychosis, the appropriateness of antipsychotics depends on a number of factors. In some cases of delusional disorders, such as delusional misidentification syndromes, the dopamine-blocking properties of antipsychotics may not be of use, as these disorders may be best attributed to neuropsychological impairments in memory, executive function, and visuospatial processing, or a disconnection phenomenon (e.g., disrupted higher-order facial recognition, impaired sense of familiarity).[278] With schizophrenia-like illness, if psychotic symptoms cause distress or impair function, treatment with antipsychotics would in many cases be warranted.

Rehabilitative and Psychotherapeutic Interventions

Rehabilitative Therapies

For persisting cognitive complaints after TBI, cognitive rehabilitation delivered by speech and language pathologists or neuropsychologists is typically considered first-line treatment. The two principal approaches to cognitive rehabilitation after TBI include remediation and compensatory training. Remediation ("cognitive retraining") approaches are based on the theory that cognitive abilities can be improved by activating particular aspects of the cognitive process through graded mental exercise.[279-282] The techniques employed in a remediation approach often focus on drill and practice regimens within the specific cognitive domain or subdomain targeted by treatment. Compensatory training approaches focus on adapting to and compensating for cognitive impairment by capitalizing on remaining cognitive strengths and functional abilities. Compensatory approaches can include training in mnemonic strategies, self-monitoring, self-regulation, and therapist feedback.[281] To date, the majority of studies on cognitive rehabilitation after TBI involve individual rather than group-based work, with systematic reviews and meta-analyses suggesting strong scientific support for these approaches.[281] Some limited work suggests that augmenting cognitive rehabilitation with pharmacologic interventions (e.g., methylphenidate) may also be worth consideration.[283]

Psychotherapeutic Approaches

Psychotherapeutic approaches, particularly the use of syndrome-specific cognitive behavioral therapies, have gained popularity in the treatment of a variety of psychiatric syndromes including anxiety, depression, PTSD, and insomnia to mention only a few. Careful adherence to treatment fidelity with trained therapists has been associated with results similar to pharmacological interventions and may even be effective in individuals with severe mental disorders.[284] Most of these intervention studies today have evaluated individual, rather than group-based, psychotherapeutic modalities.[285-287] Given the concerns noted above of heightened vulnerability to common side effects associated with psychotropic agents in individuals with TBI, there may be some theoretical advantages to the use of psychotherapeutic techniques in this population. The literature on this is scarce, however.

Taylor and Koch[136] showed that systematic desensitization with or without graded imaginal exposure and mindfulness training could be effective for the treatment of accident-related phobias. A recent study in individuals with a history of depression and/or anxiety following TBI showed that an adapted CBT protocol resulted in significant reductions in anxiety and depression ratings as well as improvements in psychosocial functioning compared to waitlist controls.[285] Another study of individuals with TBI demonstrated that both CBT and supportive therapy were equally beneficial for treating depression, anxiety, and quality of life ratings.[286] An RCT comparing a psychotherapeutic telephone intervention (discussing concerns, providing psychoeducation, motivational interviewing, and facilitating problem-solving) to usual care delivered over the course of 9 months among individuals discharged from a rehabilitation unit showed decreased depression symptom severity 1 year later.[288] A randomized wait-list control study of CBT for individuals with mild-to-severe TBI with persistent PCS symptoms was found to positively benefit quality of life ratings, and after covarying for treatment duration were shown to affect symptom rating scores as well as measures of anxiety and fatigue.[289] Another study involving individuals with depression following mild-to-severe TBI compared CBT delivered by phone or in-person to usual care. After 16 weeks, those receiving CBT did not demonstrate statistically significant improvements in depression ratings based on the HAMD-17, however, in subsequent follow-up, those in the telephone group showed significant improvements on the SCL-20 at follow-up.[287] Whether combining behavioral therapy with psychopharmacologic augmentation as through use of d-cycloserine[290] remains to be determined.

When contemplating use of a psychotherapeutic intervention, it is worth considering the profile of the brain injury and how it might impact the delivery of the treatment. Many cognitive behavioral therapies rely on such functions as memory to learn and retain mnemonic strategies, sustained attention to complete homework assignments, the ability to generalize from one situation to another, and the ability to recognize cognitive distortions while inhibiting automatic responses and prioritizing and choosing alternate responses. These functions are the very higher order executive functions that may be impaired since the TBI. Thus, certain therapies may require adaptation to provide for a slower pace of acquisition, allowing more repetition, and patience on the part of both the individual and the therapist. Use of visual aids such as handouts, taking notes during appointments, and inclusion of a caregiver in the psychotherapy process may be some of the adaptations used.

Mindfulness-Based Therapies

Research into mindfulness after TBI is also growing. Several studies on mindfulness-based group interventions have shown benefit in improving quality of life, depression ratings, and mental fatigue.[291–296] A meta-analysis involving CBT or mindfulness-based cognitive therapy for individuals with depression following TBI identified three relevant studies, which collectively showed only a small and nonsignificant change in depression ratings.[297]

Exercise

Regular aerobic exercise has been evaluated as a potential modulator of mood and cognition, perhaps related to postulated changes in blood flow, growth factor release (brain-derived neurotrophic factor, vascular endothelial growth factor), and neuroplastic processes such as synaptogenesis, angiogenesis, and neurogenesis.[298] For those suffering from both subacute and chronic concussion symptoms, exercise is considered a cornerstone of treatment.[299] Numerous studies have demonstrated the utility of using aerobic exercise to treat depression and some anxiety disorders, with effect sizes in some cases comparable to those derived from cognitive therapy.[300–304] Many studies have also revealed an association between at least moderate levels of physical activity and improved cognitive functioning over the lifespan.[305–307] A handful of exercise studies involving individuals with a history of TBI demonstrated improvements in mood,[308,309] processing speed, and learning.[310,311]

Electroconvulsive Therapy (ECT) and Noninvasive Brain Stimulation

In cases where post-TBI depression is refractory to both psychopharmacologic and psychotherapeutic interventions, alternative approaches such as ECT and/or noninvasive brain stimulation may be considered. Seizure risk is of course a concern here. The sparse literature on ECT for depression after TBI is limited to three case reports of individuals with premorbid unipolar depression that severely worsened after TBI.[312] For all of these individuals,[313–315] ECT resulted in improvements in mood; significant adverse cognitive effects were not noted and in one case cognition even improved.[313] The application of noninvasive brain stimulation modalities, such as transcranial magnetic stimulation (TMS) or transcranial direct current stimulation (tDCS), are also presently an area of active investigation for post-traumatic depression.[316–318]

Summary and Key Points

- Traumatic brain injury is a significant worldwide public health problem that results in varying degrees of disability for affected individuals and their families, and a large economic cost to society.
- The neuropsychiatric sequelae of TBI are frequently the primary source of distress to injured individuals and their families.
- From a clinical perspective, neuropsychiatric sequelae follow predictably from an understanding of the profile of brain regions that are at greatest risk of damage from the biomechanical forces at play in most injuries, making TBI an exemplar of a neuropsychiatric disorder.
- Damage to the frontal and temporal cortices and subfrontal white matter tracts are associated with dysexecutive syndromes impacting social comportment, motivated behavior, and cognitive processes such as memory, processing speed, attention, judgment, and planning. Damage to these same brain regions puts individuals with TBI at heightened risk to develop a range of psychiatric conditions. These disorders are expressed through a variety of associated cognitive, speech/language, and medical sequelae of TBI, complicating the job of the clinician.
- The neuropsychiatric assessment of an individual with TBI should follow a logical progression of ascertaining what the individual was like prior to injury, what is the profile of the injury, and the "goodness of fit" between the current clinical presentation and the predicted presentation derived from knowledge of the pre-injury traits and the injury profile.
- While treatment approaches are based on paradigms similar to those used in the noninjured population, adjustments may need to be made in dose, titration intervals, pace of therapy, and other factors to account for the cognitive limitations and comorbid medical conditions of the individual.

Multiple Choice Questions

1. In TBI, secondary injury refers to:
   a. Diffuse axonal shearing of long white matter tracts
   b. The conglomerate of damage that cannot be visualized via conventional neuroimaging
   c. Transient changes in functional network connectivity which can subsequently evolve into more chronic, maladaptive neuroplastic changes
   d. Damage to the frontal poles, orbitofrontal cortices, anterior, lateral, and inferior temporal poles, regions abutting the bony protuberances of the skull base through contact mechanisms
   e. Delayed injury mediated by excitotoxicity, inflammatory cytokines, oxidative stress, cell apoptosis, necrosis, and diffuse edema

2. Which of the following is NOT consistently identified as a risk factor for post-traumatic anxiety or depression:
   a. Premorbid history of mood disorder
   b. Premorbid history of anxiety disorder

c. Mood or anxiety disorder at the time of injury

d. Greater injury severity

e. Lower socioeconomic status

3. Which of the following statements regarding treatment for depression after TBI is true?

a. Several RCTs at this point have demonstrated efficacy of SSRIs over placebo.

b. The risk of bleeding due to the platelet-activating effects of SSRIs severely limits their utility in TBI.

c. On the whole, TCAs appear to be of greater benefit than SSRIs.

d. Methylphenidate may not only be helpful for cognition and fatigue, but also for mood after TBI.

e. Cognitive deficits following moderate-severe TBI precludes the utility of psychotherapy in this population.

4. Concern that use of antipsychotics may interfere with post-traumatic neurorecovery is based on all of the following EXCEPT:

a. Data from the animal CNS injury models associating administration of these agents with decreased functional outcomes

b. Human rehabilitation studies showing decreased functional outcomes following use of these agents

c. Human studies associating use of these agents with prolonged PTA

d. Theoretical concerns regarding impaired cognition and learning following use of dopamine-blocking agents

e. The sedative nature of these agents, which could interfere with rehabilitation efforts

Multiple Choice Answers

1. Answer: e

In TBI, primary injury refers to injury resulting from direct biomechanical forces, such as contusions, intracranial bleeds, or diffuse axonal injury. Secondary injury refers to delayed insults resulting from complex neurochemical cascades, which may occur hours or even days after the initial impact. Secondary injury mechanisms may include excitotoxicity, inflammatory cytokines, oxidative stress, cell apoptosis, necrosis, and diffuse edema.

2. Answer: d

The relationship between injury severity and post-traumatic depression and anxiety is complex. Studies looking broadly across neuropsychiatric diagnostic categories suggest a positive correlation between injury severity and the prevalence of certain diagnostic categories, but not others.[100-102] PTSD, social phobia, panic disorder, and agoraphobia, for example, are more commonly associated with milder rather than more severe forms of TBI.[102,117]

3. Answer: d

Treatment of depression following TBI generally follows guidelines for treating depression in the general population.

Literature on the topic is sparse. While to date, the two largest RCTs on use of sertraline for post-traumatic depression were unable to show benefit beyond placebo,[251,252] SSRIs generally remain first-line treatment. Studies on TCAs generally show inferiority to SSRIs.[260,261] A few placebo-controlled studies have shown methylphenidate to be helpful in treating mood after TBI.[247,263] Psychotherapy has also been found to be of benefit across the spectrum of injury severity,[285,287,289] though may require a variety of adaptations (greater repetition, slower pace, use of visual aids, note-taking).

4. Answer: b

Use of antipsychotics in the TBI population, especially in the acute to subacute time frame, is frequently cautioned against for a variety of reasons, though evidence is limited. Theoretical risk of interference with neurorecovery has been raised, stemming in large part from animal data associating administration of antipsychotics with impaired functional outcomes after CNS lesions,[319-322] with typical agents potentially the more harmful.[152,234] Corresponding human data are far more limited with a small handful of studies associating antipsychotic use with prolonged PTA, but not with impaired functional outcomes overall.[323,324]

References

1. Menon DK, Schwab K, Wright DW, Maas AI. Position statement: definition of traumatic brain injury. *Arch Phys Med Rehabil.* 2010;91(11):1637-1640. Available at https://auth.elsevier.com/ShibAuth/institutionLogin?entityID=https://idp.eng.nhs.uk/openathens&appReturnURL=https%3A%2F%2Fwww.clinicalkey.com%2Fcontent%2FplayBy%2Fdoi%2F%3Fv%3D10.1016%2Fj.apmr.2010.05.017. Accessed June 30, 2019.

2. Rutland-Brown W, Langlois JA, Thomas KE, Xi YL. Incidence of traumatic brain injury in the United States, 2003. *J Head Trauma Rehabil.* 2006;21(6):544-548. doi:10.1097/00001199-200611000-00009

3. Nakase-Richardson R, Sherer M, Seel RT, et al. Utility of post-traumatic amnesia in predicting 1-year productivity following traumatic brain injury: comparison of the Russell and Mississippi PTA classification intervals. *J Neurol Neurosurg Psychiatry.* 2011;82(5):494-499. doi:10.1136/jnnp.2010.222489.

4. Malec JF, Brown AW, Leibson CL, et al. The Mayo classification system for traumatic brain injury severity. *J Neurotrauma.* 2007;24(9):1417-1424. doi:10.1089/neu.2006.0245.

5. Selassie AW, Zaloshnja E, Langlois J, Miller T, Jones P, Steiner C. Incidence of long-term disability following traumatic brain injury hospitalization, United States, 2003. *J Head Trauma Rehabil*. 2008;23(2):123-131. doi:10.1097/01.HTR.0000314531. 30401.39.

6. *Traumatic Brain Injury in the United States: A Report to Congress*; 1999. Available at https://www.cdc.gov/traumaticbraininjury/ pubs/tbi_report_to_congress.html. Accessed June 30, 2019.

7. Kay T, Harrington D, Adams R. Definition of mild traumatic brain injury: American Congress of Rehabilitation Medicine. *J Head Trauma Rehabil*. 1993;8:86-87.

8. Katz DI, Cohen SI, Alexander MP. Mild traumatic brain injury. *Handb Clin Neurol*. 2015;127:131-156. doi:10.1016/ B978-0-444-52892-6.00009-X

9. Iverson GL. Complicated vs uncomplicated mild traumatic brain injury: acute neuropsychological outcome. *Brain Inj*. 2006;20(13-14):1335-1344. doi:10.1080/02699050601082156

10. Pfister T, Pfister K, Hagel B, Ghali WA, Ronksley PE. The incidence of concussion in youth sports: a systematic review and meta-analysis. *Br J Sports Med*. 2016. doi:10.1136/bjsports-2015-094978

11. Duhaime A-C, Beckwith JG, Maerlender AC, et al. Spectrum of acute clinical characteristics of diagnosed concussions in college athletes wearing instrumented helmets. *J Neurosurg*. 2012. doi:10.3171/2012.8.jns112298

12. Williams DH, Levin HS, Eisenberg HM. Mild head injury classification. *Neurosurgery*. 1990:422-428.

13. Kashluba S, Hanks RA, Casey JE, Millis SR. Neuropsychologic and functional outcome after complicated mild traumatic brain injury. *Arch Phys Med Rehabil*. 2008. doi:10.1016/j. apmr.2007.12.029

14. McAllister T. Overview of mild brain injury. In: Silver J, McAllister T, Arciniegas D, eds. *Textbook of Traumatic Brain Injury*. 3rd ed. Washington, DC: American Psychiatric Association Publishing; 2019:583-607.

15. Carroll LJ, Cassidy JD, Peloso PM, et al. Prognosis for mild traumatic brain injury: results of the WHO Collaborating Centre Task Force on mild traumatic brain injury. *J Rehabil Med*. 2004;36(suppl 43):84-105. doi:10.1080/16501960410023859.

16. Heitger MH, Jones RD, Dalrymple-Alford JC, Frampton CM, Ardagh MW, Anderson TJ. Motor deficits and recovery during the first year following mild closed head injury. *Brain Inj*. 2006. doi:10.1080/02699050600676354

17. McCrea M, Guskiewicz KM, Marshall SW, et al. Acute effects and recovery time following concussion in collegiate football players: The NCAA concussion study. *J Am Med Assoc*. 2003;290(19):2556-2563. doi:10.1001/jama.290.19.2556.

18. McCullagh S, Ouchterlony D, Protzner A, Blair N, Feinstein A. Prediction of neuropsychiatric outcome following mild trauma brain injury: an examination of the Glasgow Coma Scale. *Brain Inj*. 2001. doi:10.1080/02699050010007353

19. Kraus J, Schaffer K, Ayers K, Stenehjem J, Shen H, Afifi AA. Physical complaints, medical service use, and social and employment changes following mild traumatic brain injury. *World Health*. 2005:239-256.

20. Dikmen S, Machamer J, Temkin N. Mild traumatic brain injury: longitudinal study of cognition, functional status, and post-traumatic symptoms. *J Neurotrauma*. 2017;34(8):1524-1530. doi:10.1089/neu.2016.4618

21. Schneiderman AI, Braver ER, Kang HK. Understanding sequelae of injury mechanisms and mild traumatic brain injury incurred during the conflicts in Iraq and Afghanistan: persistent postconcussive symptoms and posttraumatic stress disorder. *Am J Epidemiol*. 2008. doi:10.1093/aje/kwn068

22. Hoge C, McGurk D, Thomas J, Cox A, Engel C, Castro C. Mild traumatic brain injury in U.S. soldiers returning from Iraq. *N Engl J Med*. 2008:453-463.

23. Dikmen S, Machamer J, Temkin N. Mild head injury: facts and artifacts. *J Clin Exp Neuropsychol*. 2003. doi:10.1076/ jcen.23.6.729.1019.

24. McKee AC, Cantu RC, Nowinski CJ, et al. Chronic traumatic encephalopathy in athletes: progressive tauopathy after repetitive head injury. *J Neuropathol Exp Neurol*. 2009. doi:10.1097/ NEN.0b013e3181a9d503

25. McAllister TW, Flashman LA, Harker Rhodes C, et al. Single nucleotide polymorphisms in ANKK1 and the dopamine D2 receptor gene affect cognitive outcome shortly after traumatic brain injury: a replication and extension study. *Brain Inj*. 2008. doi:10.1080/02699050802263019

26. McAllister T, Flashman L, Rhodes C, et al. Two CHRM2 SNPs modulate working memory performance and anxiety shortly after mild/moderate TBI (MTBI). In: American Neuropsychiatric Association Meeting. 2005.

27. McAllister T. Genetic factors in traumatic brain injury. *Handb Clin Neurol*. 2015;128:723-739.

28. Miller H. Accident Neurosis. *Br Med J*. 1961. doi:10.1136/bmj. 1.5231.992.

29. Rutherford W. Postconcussive symptoms: relationship to acute neurological indices, individual differences, and circumstances of injury. In: Levin HS, Eisenberg HM, Benton AL, eds. *Mild Head Injury*. New York, NY: Oxford University Press; 1989: 217-228.

30. Keshavan MS, Channabasavanna SM, Narayana Reddy GN. Post-traumatic psychiatric disturbances: patterns and predictors of outcome. *Br J Psychiatry*. 1981. doi:10.1192/bjp.138.2.157.

31. Merskey H, Woodforde JM. Psychiatric sequelae of minor head injury. *Brain*. 1972. doi:10.1093/brain/95.3.521

32. Feinstein A, Ouchterlony D, Somerville J, Jardine A. The effects of litigation on symptom expression: a prospective study following mild traumatic brain injury. *Med Sci Law*. 2001. doi:10.1177/002580240104100206.

33. Paniak C, Reynolds S, Toller-Lobe G, Melnyk A, Nagy J, Schmidt D. A longitudinal study of the relationship between financial compensation and symptoms after treated mild traumatic brain injury. *J Clin Exp Neuropsychol*. 2003. doi:10.1076/ jcen.24.2.187.999.

34. Rees PM. Contemporary issues in mild traumatic brain injury. *Arch Phys Med Rehabil*. 2003. doi:10.1016/j.apmr.2003.03.001.

35. Belanger HG, Curtiss G, Demery JA, Lebowitz BK, Vanderploeg RD. Factors moderating neuropsychological outcomes following mild traumatic brain injury: a meta-analysis. *J Int Neuropsychol Soc*. 2005;11(3):215-227. doi:10.1017/S1355617705050277.

36. Binder LM, Rohling ML. Money matters: a meta-analytic review of the effects of financial incentives on recovery after closed-head injury. *Am J Psychiatry*. 1996. doi:10.1176/ajp.153.1.7.

37. Iverson GL, Lange RT. Examination of "postconcussion-like" symptoms in a healthy sample. *Appl Neuropsychol*. 2003. doi:10.1207/S15324826AN1003_02.

38. Meares S, Shores EA, Taylor AJ, et al. Mild traumatic brain injury does not predict acute postconcussion syndrome. *J Neurol Neurosurg Psychiatry*. 2008. doi:10.1136/jnnp.2007.126565

39. Bigler ED. Anterior and middle cranial fossa in traumatic brain injury: relevant neuroanatomy and neuropathology in the study of neuropsychological outcome. *Neuropsychology*. 2007;21(5):515-531. doi:10.1037/0894-4105.21.5.515.

40. Levin HS, Mendelsohn D, Lilly MA, et al. Magnetic resonance imaging in relation to functional outcome of pediatric closed head

injury: a test of the Ommaya-Gennarelli model. *Neurosurgery.* 1997;40(3):432-441. doi:10.1097/00006123-199703000-00002.

41. McAllister TW. Neurobiological consequences of traumatic brain injury. *Dialogues Clin Neurosci.* 2011;13(3):287-300.

42. Rowson B, Rowson S, Duma SM. Biomechanical forces involved in brain injury. In: Silver JM, McAllister TW, Arciniegas DC, eds. *Textbook of Traumatic Brain Injury.* (3rd ed. Washington, DC: American Psychiatric Press, Inc.; 2019.

43. Hardy WN, Mason MJ, Foster CD, et al. A study of the response of the human cadaver head to impact. *Stapp Car Crash J.* 2007;51:17-80. doi:10.1016/j.bbi.2008.05.010.

44. Meythaler JM, Depalma L, Devivo MJ, Guin-Renfroe S, Novack TA. Sertraline to improve arousal and alertness in severe traumatic brain injury secondary to motor vehicle crashes. *Brain Inj.* 2001;15(4):321-331. doi:10.1080/026990501750111274.

45. Frati A, Cerretani D, Fiaschi A, et al. Diffuse axonal injury and oxidative stress: a comprehensive review. *Int J Mol Sci.* 2017;18(12):2600. doi:10.3390/ijms18122600.

46. Simon DW, McGeachy MJ, Baylr H, Clark RSB, Loane DJ, Kochanek PM. The far-reaching scope of neuroinflammation after traumatic brain injury. *Nat Rev Neurol.* 2017. doi:10.1038/nrneurol.2017.13.

47. McAllister TW, Flashman LA, Sparling MB, Saykin AJ. Working memory deficits after traumatic brain injury: catecholaminergic mechanisms and prospects for treatment—a review. *Brain Inj.* 2004;18(4):331-350. doi:10.1080/02699050310001617370.

48. Arciniegas DB. The cholinergic hypothesis of cognitive impairment caused by traumatic brain injury. *Curr Psychiatry Rep.* 2003;5(5):391-399. doi:10.1007/s11920-003-0074-5.

49. Jenkins PO, Mehta MA, Sharp DJ. Catecholamines and cognition after traumatic brain injury. *Brain.* 2016;139(9):2345-2371. doi:10.1093/brain/aww128.

50. McAllister TW. Mild traumatic brain injury. In: Silver JM, McAllister TW, Yudofsky S, eds. *Textbook of Traumatic Brain Injury.* 2nd ed. Washington, DC: American Psychiatric Publishing, Inc.; 2011.

51. Symonds C. Mental disorder following head injury. *Proc R Soc Med.* 1937;3:1081-1092.

52. Whelan-Goodinson R, Ponsford JL, Schönberger M, Johnston L. Predictors of psychiatric disorders following traumatic brain injury. *J Head Trauma Rehabil.* 2010;25(5):320-329. doi:10.1097/HTR.0b013e3181c8f8e7.

53. Kreutzer JS, Marwitz JH, Sima AP, et al. Resilience following traumatic brain injury: a traumatic brain injury model systems study. *Arch Phys Med Rehabil.* 2016;97(5):708-713. doi:10.1016/j.apmr.2015.12.003.

54. Tomberg T, Toomela A, Pulver A, Tikk A. Coping strategies, social support, life orientation and health-related quality of life following traumatic brain injury. *Brain Inj.* 2005;19(14):1181-1190. doi:10.1080/02699050500150153.

55. Baker-Sparr C, Hart T, Bergquist T, et al. Internet and social media use after traumatic brain injury. *J Head Trauma Rehabil.* 2017:1. doi:10.1097/HTR.0000000000000305.

56. Diamond A. Executive functions. *Annu Rev Psychol.* 2013;64:135-156. doi:10.1146/annurev-psych-113011-143750.

57. Arnould A, Dromer E, Rochat L, Van der Linden M, Azouvi P. Neurobehavioral and self-awareness changes after traumatic brain injury: towards new multidimensional approaches. *Ann Phys Rehabil Med.* 2016;59(1):18-22. doi:10.1016/j.rehab.2015.09.002.

58. McAllister T. Emotional and behavioral sequelae of traumatic brain injury. In: *Brain Injury Medicine.* Zasler ND, Katz DI, Zafonte RD, eds. New York, NY: Demos Medical. 2013:1034-1052.

59. Deb S, Lyons I, Koutzoukis C. Neurobehavioural symptoms one year after a head injury. *Br J Psychiatry.* 1999;174:360-365. doi:10.1192/bjp.174.4.360.

60. McKinlay WW, Brooks DN, Bond MR, Martinage DP, Marshall MM. The short-term outcome of severe blunt head injury as reported by relatives of the injured persons. *J Neurol Neurosurg Psychiatry.* 1981;44(6):527-533. doi:10.1136/jnnp.44.6.527.

61. Brooke MM, Patterson DR, Questad KA, Cardenas D, Farrel-Roberts L. The treatment of agitation during initial hospitalization after traumatic brain injury. *Arch Phys Med Rehabil.* 1992;73(10):917-921. Available at http://www.ncbi.nlm.nih.gov/pubmed/1417466. Accessed February 2, 2017.

62. Baguley IJ, Cooper J, Felmingham K. Aggressive behavior following traumatic brain injury: how common is common? *J Head Trauma Rehabil.* 2006;21(1):45-56. doi:00001199-200601000-00005.

63. Lombard LA, Zafonte RD. Agitation after traumatic brain injury: considerations and treatment options. *Am J Phys Med Rehabil.* 2005;84(10):797-812. doi:10.1097/01.phm.0000179438.22235.08.

64. Work SS, Colamonico JA, Bradley WG, Kaye RE. Pseudobulbar affect: an under-recognized and under-treated neurological disorder. *Adv Ther.* 2011;28(7):586-601. doi:10.1007/s12325-011-0031-3.

65. Engelman W, Hammond FM, Malec JF. Diagnosing pseudobulbar affect in traumatic brain injury. *Neuropsychiatr Dis Treat.* 2014;10:1903-1910. doi:10.2147/NDT.S63304.

66. Green RL, McAllister TW, Bernat JL. A study of crying in medically and surgically hospitalized patients. *Am J Psychiatry.* 1987;144(4):442-447. doi:10.1176/ajp.144.4.442.

67. Rabins PV, Arciniegas DB. Pathophysiology of involuntary emotional expression disorder. *CNS Spectr.* 2007;12(4 suppl 5):17-22.

68. Flashman LA, McAllister TW. Lack of awareness and its impact in traumatic brain injury. *NeuroRehabilitation.* 2002;17:285-296.

69. Fahy TJ. Severe head injuries. *Science.* 1967;7:1958-1960.

70. Ham TE, Bonnelle V, Hellyer P, et al. The neural basis of impaired self-awareness after traumatic brain injury. *Brain.* 2014;137(2):586-597. doi:10.1093/brain/awt350.

71. Marin RS. Apathy: a neuropsychiatric syndrome. *J Neuropsychiatry Clin Neurosci.* 1991;3(3):243-254. doi:10.1176/jnp.3.3.243.

72. Levy R. Apathy: a pathology of goal-directed behaviour. A new concept of the clinic and pathophysiology of apathy. *Rev Neurol (Paris).* 2012;168(8-9):585-597. doi:10.1016/j.neurol.2012.05.003.

73. Starkstein SE, Leentjens AFG. The nosological position of apathy in clinical practice. *J Neurol Neurosurg Psychiatry.* 2008;79(10):1088-1092. doi:10.1136/jnnp.2007.136895.

74. Ciurli P, Formisano R, Bivona U, Cantagallo A, Angelelli P. Neuropsychiatric disorders in persons with severe traumatic brain injury: prevalence, phenomenology, and relationship with demographic, clinical, and functional features. *J Head Trauma Rehabil.* 2011;26(2):116-126. doi:10.1097/HTR.0b013e3181dedd0e.

75. Seel RT, Macciocchi S, Kreutzer JS, Kaelin D, Katz DI. Diagnosing major depression following moderate to severe traumatic brain injury—evidence-based recommendations for clinicians. *Eur Neurol Rev.* 2011;6(1):25-30.

76. Kant R, Duffy JD, Pivovarnik A. Prevalence of apathy following head injury. *Brain Inj.* 1998;12(1):87-92. doi:10.1080/026990598122908

77. van Reekum R, Stuss DT, Ostrander L. Apathy: why care? *J Neuropsychiatry Clin Neurosci.* 2005;17(1):7-19. doi:10.1176/jnp.17.1.7.

78. Starkstein SE, Pahissa J. Apathy following traumatic brain injury. *Psychiatr Clin North Am.* 2014;37(1):103-112. doi:10.1016/j.psc.2013.10.002.

79. Thomas DG, Collins MW, Saladino RA, Frank V, Raab J, Zuckerbraun NS. Identifying neurocognitive deficits in adolescents following concussion. *Acad Emerg Med.* 2011;18(3):246-254. doi:10.1111/j.1553-2712.2011.01015.x.

80. Wortzel HS, Arciniegas DB. Treatment of post-traumatic cognitive impairments. *Curr Treat Options Neurol.* 2012;14(5):493-508. doi:10.1007/s11940-012-0193-6.

81. Millis SR, Rosenthal M, Novack TA, et al. Long-term neuropsychological outcome after traumatic brain injury. *J Head Trauma Rehabil.* 2001;16(4):343-355. doi:10.1097/00001199-200108000-00005.

82. Arciniegas DB, Anderson CA, Topkoff J, McAllister TW. Mild traumatic brain injury: a neuropsychiatric approach to diagnosis, evaluation, and treatment. *Neuropsychiatr Dis Treat.* 2005; 1(4):311-327. Available at http://www.pubmedcentral.nih.gov/articlerender.fcgi?artid=2424119&tool=pmcentrez&rendertype=abstract. Accessed June 30, 2019.

83. Guo Z, Cupples LA, Kurz A, et al. Head injury and the risk of AD in the MIRAGE study. *Neurology.* 2000;54(6):1316-1323. doi:10.1212/WNL.54.6.1316.

84. Guskiewicz KM, Marshall SW, Bailes J, et al. Association between recurrent concussion and late-life cognitive impairment in retired professional football players. *Neurosurgery.* 2005;57(4). doi:10.1093/neurosurgery/57.4.719.

85. Laker SR. Concussion supplement epidemiology of concussion and mild traumatic brain injury. *PMRJ.* 2011;3:S354-S358. doi:10.1016/j.pmrj.2011.07.017.

86. Li W, Risacher SL, McAllister TW, Saykin AJ. Age at injury is associated with the long-term cognitive outcome of traumatic brain injuries. *Alzheimers Dement.* 2017. doi:10.1016/j.dadm.2017.01.008.

87. McAllister T, McCrea M. Long-term cognitive and neuropsychiatric consequences of repetitive concussion and head-impact exposure. *J Athl Train.* 2017;52(3):309-317. doi:10.4085/1062-6050-52.1.14.

88. Martland H. Punch drunk. *J Am Med Assoc.* 1928. doi:10.1001/jama.1928.02700150029009.

89. Omalu BI, TeKosky ST, Minster RL. Chronic traumatic encephalopathy in a National Football League player. *Neurosurgery.* 2005. doi:10.1227/01.NEU.0000249026.95877.F8.

90. Azad TD, Li A, Pendharkar A V., Veeravagu A, Grant GA. Junior Seau: an illustrative case of chronic traumatic encephalopathy and update on chronic sports-related head injury. *World Neurosurg.* 2016. doi:10.1016/j.wneu.2015.10.032.

91. Tierney M. Player who killed himself had brain disease. *New York Times;* 2012. Available at http://www.nytimes.com/2012/07/27/sports/football/ray-easterling-autopsy-found-signs-of-brain-disease-cte.html? Accessed November 15, 2019.

92. Schwarz A. Before suicide, Duerson said he wanted brain study. *New York Times;* 2011. Available at https://www.nytimes.com/2011/02/20/sports/football/20duerson.html. Accessed November 15, 2019.

93. Korngold C, Farrell HM, Fozdar M. The National Football League and chronic traumatic encephalopathy: legal implications. *J Am Acad Psychiatry Law.* 2013:430-436.

94. Guskiewicz KM, Marshall SW, Bailes J, et al. Recurrent concussion and risk of depression in retired professional football players. *Med Sci Sports Exerc.* 2007. doi:10.1249/mss.0b013e3180383da5.

95. Greenwald RM, Gwin JT, Chu JJ, Crisco JJ. Head impact severity measures for evaluating mild traumatic brain injury risk exposure. *Neurosurgery.* 2008. doi:10.1227/01.neu.0000318162.67472.ad.

96. Omalu B. Don't let kids play football. *New York Times.* Available at http://www.nytimes.com/2015/12/07/opinion/dont-let-kids-play-football.html? Published 2015. Accessed November 15, 2019.

97. McKee AC, Stein TD, Kiernan PT, Alvarez VE. The neuropathology of chronic traumatic encephalopathy. *Brain Pathol.* 2015;25:350-364. doi:10.1111/bpa.12248.

98. Montenigro PH, Baugh CM, Daneshvar DH, et al. Clinical subtypes of chronic traumatic encephalopathy: literature review and proposed research diagnostic criteria for traumatic encephalopathy syndrome. *Alzheimers Res Ther.* 2014. doi:10.1186/s13195-014-0068-z.

99. Stern RA, Adler CH, Chen K, et al. Tau positron-emission tomography in former National Football League players. *N Engl J Med.* 2019. doi:10.1056/NEJMoa1900757.

100. Alway Y, Gould KR, Johnston L, McKenzie D, Ponsford J. A prospective examination of Axis I psychiatric disorders in the first 5 years following moderate to severe traumatic brain injury. *Psychol Med.* 2016;46(6):1331-1341. doi:10.1017/S0033291715002986.

101. Scholten AC, Haagsma JA, Cnossen MC, Olff M, van Beeck EF, Polinder S. Prevalence of and risk factors for anxiety and depressive disorders after traumatic brain injury: a systematic review. *J Neurotrauma.* 2016;33(22):1969-1994. doi:10.1089/neu.2015.4252.

102. Bryant RA, O'Donnell ML, Creamer M, McFarlane AC, Clark CR, Silove D. The psychiatric sequelae of traumatic injury. *Am J Psychiatry.* 2010;167(3):312-320. doi:10.1176/appi.ajp.2009.09050617.

103. Whelan-Goodinson R, Ponsford J, Johnston L, Grant F. Psychiatric disorders following traumatic brain injury: their nature and frequency. *J Head Trauma Rehabil.* 2009;24(5):324-332. doi:10.1097/HTR.0b013e3181a712aa.

104. Bombardier CH, Fann JR, Temkin NR, Esselman PC, Barber J, Dikmen SS. Rates of major depressive disorder and clinical outcomes following traumatic brain injury. *JAMA.* 2010;303(19):1938-1945. doi:10.1001/jama.2010.599.

105. Jorge RE, Robinson RG, Moser D, Tateno A, Crespo-Facorro B, Arndt S. Major depression following traumatic brain injury. *Arch Gen Psychiatry.* 2004;61(1):42-50. doi:10.1001/archpsyc.61.1.42.

106. Jorge RE, Robinson RG, Starkstein SE, Arndt S V. Depression and anxiety following traumatic brain injury. *J Neuropsychiatry Clin Neurosci.* 1993;5(4):369-374. doi:10.1176/jnp.5.4.369.

107. Rogers JM, Read CA. Psychiatric comorbidity following traumatic brain injury. *Brain Inj.* 2007;21(13-14):1321-1333. doi:10.1080/02699050701765700.

108. Whelan-Goodinson R, Ponsford J, Schönberger M. Association between psychiatric state and outcome following traumatic brain injury. *J Rehabil Med.* 2008;40(10):850-857. doi:10.2340/16501977-0271.

109. Jorge RE, Robinson RG, Arndt SV, Forrester AW, Geisler F, Starkstein SE. Comparison between acute- and delayed-onset depression following traumatic brain injury. *J Neuropsychiatry Clin Neurosci.* 1993;5(1):43-49. Available at http://www.ncbi.nlm.nih.gov/pubmed/8428134. Accessed February 11, 2019.

110. Rapoport MJ, Mccullagh S, Streiner D, Feinstein A. The clinical significance of major depression following mild traumatic brain injury. *Psychosomatics.* 2003;44(1):31-37. doi:10.1176/appi.psy.44.1.31.

111. Fann JR, Katon WJ, Uomoto JM, Esselman PC. Psychiatric disorders and functional disability in outpatients with traumatic brain injuries. *Am J Psychiatry.* 1995;152:1493-1499. doi:10.1176/ajp.152.10.1493.

112. Kessler RC, Berglund P, Demler O, et al. The epidemiology of major depressive disorder: results from the National Comorbidity Survey Replication (NCS-R). *JAMA*. 2003;289(23):3095-3105. doi:10.1097/00132578-200310000-00002.

113. Kim E, Lauterbach EC, Reeve A, et al. Neuropsychiatric complications of traumatic brain injury: a critical review of the literature (a report by the ANPA committee on research). *J Neuropsychiatr*. 2007;19(2):106-127. doi:10.1176/appi.neuropsych.19.2.106.

114. Cnossen MC, Scholten AC, Lingsma HF, et al. Predictors of major depression and posttraumatic stress disorder following traumatic brain injury: a systematic review and meta-analysis. *J Neuropsychiatry Clin Neurosci*. 2017;29(3):206-224. doi:10.1176/appi.neuropsych.16090165.

115. Malec JF, Brown AW, Moessner AM, Stump TE, Monahan P. A preliminary model for posttraumatic brain injury depression. *Arch Phys Med Rehabil*. 2010;91(7):1087-1097. doi:10.1016/j.apmr.2010.04.002.

116. Seel RT, Macciocchi S, Kreutzer JS. Clinical considerations for the diagnosis of major depression after moderate to severe TBI. *J Head Trauma Rehabil*. 2010;25(2):99-112. doi:10.1097/HTR.0b013e3181ce3966.

117. Van Reekum R, Cohen T, Wong J. Can traumatic brain injury cause psychiatric disorders? *J Neuropsychiatry Clin Neurosci*. 2000;12(3):316-327. doi:10.1053/scnp.2000.9555.

118. Jorge RE, Robinson RG, Starkstein SE, Arndt SV, Forrester AW, Geisler FH. Secondary mania following traumatic brain injury. *Am J Psychiatry*. 1993;150(6):916-921. doi:10.1176/ajp.150.6.916.

119. Jorge RE, Arciniegas DB. Mood disorders after TBI. *Psychiatr Clin North Am*. 2014;37(1):13-29. doi:10.1016/j.psc.2013.11.005.

120. Starkstein SE, Pearlson GD, Boston J, Robinson RG. Mania after brain injury. A controlled study of causative factors. *Arch Neurol*. 1987;44(10):1069-1073. doi:10.1001/archneur.1987.00520220065019.

121. Shukla S, Cook BL, Mukherjee S, Godwin C, Miller MG. Mania following head trauma. *Am J Psychiatry*. 1987;144(1):93-96. Available at http://www.ncbi.nlm.nih.gov/entrez/query.fcgi?cmd=Retrieve&db=PubMed&dopt=Citation&list_uids=3799847. Accessed February 11, 2019.

122. Hiott DW, Labbate L. Anxiety disorders associated with traumatic brain injuries. *NeuroRehabilitation*. 2002;17(4):345-355. Available at http://iospress.metapress.com/content/3t9bgcdev52ue32h/. Accessed February 11, 2019.

123. Mallya S, Sutherland J, Pongracic S, Mainland B, Ornstein TJ. The manifestation of anxiety disorders after traumatic brain injury: a review. *J Neurotrauma*. 2015;32(7):411-421. doi:10.1089/neu.2014.3504.

124. Hoffman SW, Harrison C. The interaction between psychological health and traumatic brain injury: a neuroscience perspective. *Clin Neuropsychol*. 2009;23(8):1400-1415. doi:10.1080/13854040903369433.

125. Pertab JL, Merkley TL, Cramond AJ, Cramond K, Paxton H, Wu T. Concussion and the autonomic nervous system: an introduction to the field and the results of a systematic review. *NeuroRehabilitation*. 2018. doi:10.3233/NRE-172298.

126. Esterov D, Greenwald BD. Autonomic dysfunction after mild traumatic brain injury. *Brain Sci*. 2017. doi:10.3390/brainsci7080100.

127. Prasad KN, Bondy SC. Common biochemical defects linkage between post-traumatic stress disorders, mild traumatic brain injury (TBI) and penetrating TBI. *Brain Res*. 2015;1599:103-114. doi:10.1016/j.brainres.2014.12.038.

128. Fann J, Jakupcak M. Anxiety disorders. In: *Management of Adults with Traumatic Brain Injury*. Arciniegas DB, Zasler ND, Jaffee MS, Vanderploeg RD, eds.Washington D.C, U.S: American Psychiatric Publishing. 2013:195-212.

129. Fleming JM, Strong J, Ashton R. Cluster analysis of self-awareness levels in adults with traumatic brain injury and relationship to outcome. *J Head Trauma Rehabil*. 1998;13(5):39-51. doi:10.1097/00001199-199810000-00006.

130. Wittchen HU. Generalized anxiety disorder: prevalence, burden, and cost to society. *Depress Anxiety*. 2002;16(4):162-171. doi:10.1002/da.10065.

131. Moreno-Peral P, Conejo-Cerón S, Motrico E, et al. Risk factors for the onset of panic and generalised anxiety disorders in the general adult population: a systematic review of cohort studies. *J Affect Disord*. 2014;168:337-348. doi:10.1016/j.jad.2014.06.021.

132. Deb S, Lyons I, Koutzoukis C, Ali I, McCarthy G. Rate of psychiatric illness 1 year after traumatic brain injury. *Am J Psychiatry*. 1999;156(3):374-378. doi:10.1176/ajp.156.3.374.

133. Koponen S, Taiminen T, Portin R, et al. Axis I and II psychiatric disorders after traumatic brain injury: a 30-year follow-up study. *Am J Psychiatry*. 2002;159(8):1315-1321. doi:10.1176/appi.ajp.159.8.1315.

134. Hibbard M, Uysal S, Kepler K, Bogdany J, Silver J. Axis 1 psychopathology in individuals with traumatic brain injury. *J Head Trauma Rehabil*. 1998;13(4):24-39.

135. Munjack DJ. The onset of driving phobias. *J Behav Ther Exp Psychiatry*. 1984;15(4):305-308. doi:10.1016/0005-7916(84)90093-4.

136. Taylor S, Koch W. Anxiety disorders due to motor vehicle accidents: nature and treatment. *Clin Psychol Rev*. 1995;15(8):721-738.

137. Mayou R, Bryant B, Ehlers A. Prediction of psychological outcomes one year after a motor vehicle accident. *Am J Psychiatry*. 2001;158(8):1231-1238. doi:10.1176/appi.ajp.158.8.1231.

138. Berthier ML, Kulisevsky J, Gironell A, Lopez OL. Obsessive-compulsive disorder and traumatic brain injury: behavioral, cognitive, and neuroimaging findings. *Neuropsychiatry Neuropsychol Behav Neurol*. 2001;14(1):23-31.

139. Max JE, Smith WL, Lindgren SD, et al. Case study: obsessive-compulsive disorder after severe traumatic brain injury in an adolescent. *J Am Acad Child Adolesc Psychiatry*. 1995;34(1):45-49. doi:10.1097/00004583-199501000-00012.

140. Ogai M, Iyo M, Mori N, Takei N. A right orbitofrontal region and OCD symptoms: a case report. *Acta Psychiatr Scand*. 2005;111(1):74-76. doi:10.1111/j.1600-0447.2004.00395.x.

141. Fontenelle LF, Cocchi L, Harrison BJ, Miguel EC, Torres AR. Role of stressful and traumatic life events in obsessive–compulsive disorder. *Neuropsychiatry*. 2011;1(1):61-69. doi:10.2217/npy.10.1.

142. Harkin B, Kessler K. The role of working memory in compulsive checking and OCD: a systematic classification of 58 experimental findings. *Clin Psychol Rev*. 2011;31(6):1004-1021. doi:10.1016/j.cpr.2011.06.004.

143. Savage CR, Deckersbach T, Wilhelm S, et al. Strategic processing and episodic memory impairment in obsessive compulsive disorder. *Neuropsychology*. 2000;14(1):141-151. doi:10.1037//0894-4105.14.1.141.

144. Wood RL, Worthington A. Neurobehavioral abnormalities associated with executive dysfunction after traumatic brain injury. *Front Behav Neurosci*. 2017;11. doi:10.3389/fnbeh.2017.00195.

145. Rochat L, Beni C, Billieux J, Annoni JM, Van Der Linden M. How impulsivity relates to compulsive buying and the burden perceived by caregivers after moderate-to-severe traumatic brain injury. *Psychopathology*. 2011;44(3):158-164. doi:10.1159/000322454.

146. Tanev KS, Pentel KZ, Kredlow MA, Charney ME. PTSD and TBI co-morbidity: scope, clinical presentation and treatment options. *Brain Inj*. 2014;28(3):261-270. doi:10.3109/02699052.2013.sss873821.

147. Williamson JB, Heilman KM, Porges EC, Lamb DG, Porges SW. A possible mechanism for PTSD symptoms in patients with traumatic brain injury: central autonomic network disruption. *Front Neuroeng.* 2013. doi:10.3389/fneng.2013.00013.

148. McMillan TM, Williams WH, Bryant R. Post-traumatic stress disorder and traumatic brain injury: a review of causal mechanisms, assessment, and treatment. *Neuropsychol Rehabil.* 2003;13(1-2):149-164. doi:10.1080/09602010244000453.

149. Bryant R. Post-traumatic stress disorder vs traumatic brain injury. *Dialogues Clin Neurosci.* 2011;13(3):251-262.

150. McMillan TM. Errors in diagnosing post-traumatic stress disorder after traumatic brain injury. *Brain Inj.* 2001;15(1):39-46. doi:10.1080/02699050118030.

151. Sumpter RE, McMillan TM. Errors in self-report of post-traumatic stress disorder after severe traumatic brain injury. *Brain Inj.* 2006;20(1):93-99. doi:10.1080/02699050500394090.

152. Arciniegas DB, Harris SN, Brousseau KM. Psychosis following traumatic brain injury. *Int Rev Psychiatry.* 2003;15(4):328-340. doi:10.1080/09540260310001606719.

153. Fujii DE, Ahmed I. Psychotic disorder caused by traumatic brain injury. *Psychiatr Clin North Am.* 2014;37(1):113-124. doi:10.1016/j.psc.2013.11.006.

154. Batty RA, Rossell SL, Francis AJP, Ponsford J. Psychosis following traumatic brain injury. *Brain Impair.* 2013;14:21-41. doi:10.1017/BrImp.2013.10.

155. Fujii D, Ahmed I. Characteristics of psychotic disorder due to traumatic brain injury: an analysis of case studies in the literature. *J Neuropsychiatry Clin Neurosci.* 2002;14(2):130-140.

156. McAllister TW, Ferrell RB. Evaluation and treatment of psychosis after traumatic brain injury. *NeuroRehabilitation.* 2002;17(4):357-368. Available at http://www.ncbi.nlm.nih.gov/pubmed/12547983. Accessed February 11, 2019.

157. Clancy MJ, Clarke MC, Connor DJ, Cannon M, Cotter DR. The prevalence of psychosis in epilepsy: a systematic review and meta-analysis. *BMC Psychiatry.* 2014;14(1). doi:10.1186/1471-244X-14-75.

158. Hudson AJ, Grace GM. Misidentification syndromes related to face specific area in the fusiform gyrus. *J Neurol Neurosurg Psychiatry.* 2000;69(5):645-648. doi:10.1136/jnnp.69.5.645.

159. Stefan A, Mathe JF. What are the disruptive symptoms of behavioral disorders after traumatic brain injury? A systematic review leading to recommendations for good practices. *Ann Phys Rehabil Med.* 2016;59(1):5-17.

160. Molloy C, Conroy RM, Cotter DR, Cannon M. Is traumatic brain injury a risk factor for schizophrenia? A meta-analysis of case-controlled population-based studies. *Schizophr Bull.* 2011;37(6):1104-1110. doi:10.1093/schbul/sbr091.

161. Kim E. Does traumatic brain injury predispose individuals to develop schizophrenia? *Curr Opin Psychiatry.* 2008;21(3):286-289. doi:10.1097/YCO.0b013e3282fbcd21.

162. Malaspina D, Goetz RR, Friedman JH, et al. Traumatic brain injury and schizophrenia in members of schizophrenia and bipolar disorder pedigrees. *Am J Psychiatry.* 2001;158(3):440-446. doi:10.1176/appi.ajp.158.3.440.

163. Gupta PK, Sayed N, Ding K, et al. Subtypes of post-traumatic epilepsy: clinical, electrophysiological, and imaging features. *J Neurotrauma.* 2014;31(16):1439-1443. doi:10.1089/neu.2013.3221.

164. Annegers JF, Hauser WA, Coan SP, Rocca WA. A population-based study of seizures after traumatic brain injuries. *N Engl J Med.* 1998;338(1):20-24. doi:10.1056/NEJM199801013380104.

165. Frey LC. Epidemiology of posttraumatic epilepsy: a critical review. *Epilepsia.* 2003;44:11-17. doi:10.1046/j.1528-1157.44.s10.4.x.

166. Plenger PM, Dixon CE, Castillo RM, Frankowski RF, Yablon SA, Levin HS. Subacute methylphenidate treatment for moderate to moderately severe traumatic brain injury: a preliminary double-blind placebo-controlled study. *Arch Phys Med Rehabil.* 1996;77(6):536-540. doi:10.1016/S0003-9993(96)90291-9.

167. Yablon S, Towne A. Post-traumatic seizures and epilepsy. In: *Brain Injury Medicine.* Nathan D. Zasler ND, Douglas I. Katz DI, Zafonte RD, eds. New York, NY: Demos Medical. 2013:636-660.

168. Juengst SB, Wagner AK, Ritter AC, et al. Post-traumatic epilepsy associations with mental health outcomes in the first two years after moderate to severe TBI: a TBI model systems analysis. *Epilepsy Behav.* 2017;73:240-246. doi:10.1016/j.yebeh.2017.06.001.

169. Zihl J, Almeida OFX, Kopczak A, Stalla G. Neuropsychology of neuroendocrine dysregulation after traumatic brain injury. *J Clin Med.* 2015;4:1051-1062. doi:10.3390/jcm4051051.

170. Popovic V. GH Deficiency as the most common pituitary defect after TBI: clinical implications. *Pituitary.* 2005;8(3-4):239-243. doi:10.1007/s11102-006-6047-z.

171. Schneider HJ, Schneider M, Saller B, et al. Prevalence of anterior pituitary insufficiency 3 and 12 months after traumatic brain injury. *Eur J Endocrinol.* 2006;154(2):259-265. doi:10.1530/eje.1.02071.

172. Tanriverdi F, Schneider HJ, Aimaretti G, Masel BE, Casanueva FF, Kelestimur F. Pituitary dysfunction after traumatic brain injury: a clinical and pathophysiological approach. *Endocr Rev.* 2015;36(3):305-342. doi:10.1210/er.2014-1065.

173. Kelly DF, McArthur DL, Levin H, et al. Neurobehavioral and quality of life changes associated with growth hormone insufficiency after complicated mild, moderate, or severe traumatic brain injury. *J Neurotrauma.* 2006;23(6):928-942. doi:10.1089/neu.2006.23.928.

174. Moreau OK, Yollin E, Merlen E, Daveluy W, Rousseaux M. Lasting pituitary hormone deficiency after traumatic brain injury. *J Neurotrauma.* 2012;29(1):81-89. doi:10.1089/neu.2011.2048.

175. Popovic V, Pekic S, Pavlovic D, et al. Hypopituitarism as a consequence of traumatic brain injury (TBI) and its possible relation with cognitive disabilities and mental distress. *J Endocrinol Invest.* 2004;27(11):1048-1054. doi:10.1007/BF03345308.

176. Maric NP, Doknic M, Pavlovic D, et al. Psychiatric and neuropsychological changes in growth hormone-deficient patients after traumatic brain injury in response to growth hormone therapy. *J Endocrinol Invest.* 2010;33(11):770-775. doi:10.3275/7045.

177. High WM, Briones-Galang M, Clark JA, et al. Effect of growth hormone replacement therapy on cognition after traumatic brain injury. *J Neurotrauma.* 2010;27(9):1565-1575. doi:10.1089/neu.2009.1253.

178. Reimunde P, Quintana A, Castañón B, et al. Effects of growth hormone (GH) replacement and cognitive rehabilitation in patients with cognitive disorders after traumatic brain injury. *Brain Inj.* 2011;25(1):65-73. doi:10.3109/02699052.2010.536196.

179. Moreau OK, Cortet-Rudelli C, Yollin E, Merlen E, Daveluy W, Rousseaux M. Growth hormone replacement therapy in patients with traumatic brain injury. *J Neurotrauma.* 2013;30(11):998-1006. doi:10.1089/neu.2012.2705.

180. Barton DJ, Kumar RG, McCullough EH, et al. Persistent hypogonadotropic hypogonadism in men after severe traumatic brain injury: temporal hormone profiles and outcome prediction. *J Head Trauma Rehabil.* 2016;31(4):277-287. doi:10.1097/HTR.0000000000000188.

181. Seidel B, Lewis T, Kucer B. The decision to provide testosterone supplementation in patients with traumatic brain injury. *PM R.* 2013;5(11):985-986.

182. Quinn A, Agha A. Post-traumatic hypopituitarism—who should be screened, when, and how? *Front Endocrinol.* 2018;9(8):1-5.

183. Imbach LL, Büchele F, Valko PO, et al. Sleep-wake disorders persist 18 months after traumatic brain injury but remain underrecognized. *Neurology.* 2016;86(21):1945-1949. doi:10.1212/WNL.0000000000002697.

184. Grima NA, Ponsford JL, Pase MP. Sleep complications following traumatic brain injury. *Curr Opin Pulm Med.* 2017;23(6):493-499. doi:10.1097/MCP.0000000000000429.

185. Mahmood O, Rapport LJ, Hanks RA, Fichtenberg NL. Neuropsychological performance and sleep disturbance following traumatic brain injury. *J Head Trauma Rehabil.* 2004;19(5):378-390.

186. Duclos C, Beauregard M-P, Bottari C, Ouellet M-C, Gosselin N. The impact of poor sleep on cognition and activities of daily living after traumatic brain injury: a review. *Aust Occup Ther J.* 2015;62(1):2-12. doi:10.1111/1440-1630.12164.

187. Valko PO, Gavrilov YV, Yamamoto M, et al. Damage to arousal-promoting brainstem neurons with traumatic brain injury. *Sleep.* 2014:2014. doi:10.5665/sleep.5844.

188. Naseem M, Parvez S. Role of melatonin in traumatic brain injury and spinal cord injury. *Sci World J.* 2014:1-13.

189. Shekleton JA, Parcell DL, Redman JR, Phipps-Nelson J, Ponsford JL, Rajaratnam SMW. Sleep disturbance and melatonin levels following traumatic brain injury. *Neurology.* 2010. doi:10.1212/WNL.0b013e3181e0438b.

190. Grima NA, Rajaratnam SMW, Mansfield D, Sletten TL, Spitz G, Ponsford JL. Efficacy of melatonin for sleep disturbance following traumatic brain injury: a randomised controlled trial. *BMC Med.* 2018. doi:10.1186/s12916-017-0995-1.

191. Kemp S, Biswas R, Neumann V, Coughlan A. The value of melatonin for sleep disorders occurring post-head injury: a pilot RCT. *Brain Inj.* 2004. doi:10.1080/02699050410001671892.

192. Nampiaparampil DE. Prevalence of chronic pain after traumatic brain injury: a systematic review. *JAMA.* 2008;300(6):711-719.

193. Grandhi R, Tavakoli S, Ortega C, Simmonds MJ. A review of chronic pain and cognitive, mood, and motor dysfunction following mild traumatic brain injury: complex, comorbid, and/or overlapping conditions? *Brain Sci.* 2017;7(12):1-8.

194. Diaz-Arrastia R, Kochanek PM, Bergold P, et al. Pharmacotherapy of traumatic brain injury: state of the science and the road forward: Report of the Department of Defense Neurotrauma Pharmacology Workgroup. *J Neurotrauma.* 2014;31(2):135-158.

195. Hurley R, Taber K. Emotional disturbances following traumatic brain injury. *Curr Treat Options Neurol.* 2002;4(1):59-75.

196. Dougall D, Poole N, Agrawal N. Pharmacotherapy for chronic cognitive impairment in traumatic brain injury. *Cochrane Database Syst Rev.* 2015;2015(12). Available at: https://www.ncbi.nlm.nih.gov/pubmed/26624881.

197. Whyte J, Hart T, Schuster K, Fleming M, Polansky M, Coslett HB. Effects of methylphenidate on attentional function after traumatic brain injury. A randomized, placebo-controlled trial. *Am J Phys Med Rehabil.* 1997;76(6):440-450.

198. Kaelin DL, Cifu DX, Matthies B. Methylphenidate effect on attention deficit in the acutely brain-injured adult. *Arch Phys Med Rehabil.* 1996;77(1):6-9.

199. Kim Y-H, Ko M-H, Na S-Y, Park S-H, Kim K-W. Effects of single-dose methylphenidate on cognitive performance in patients with traumatic brain injury: a double-blind placebo-controlled study. *Clin Rehabil.* 2006;20(1):24-30.

200. Whyte J, Hart T, Vaccaro M, et al. Effects of methylphenidate on attention deficits after traumatic brain injury: a multidimensional, randomized, controlled trial. *Am J Phys Med Rehabil.* 2004;83(6):401-420.

201. Willmott C, Ponsford J. Efficacy of methylphenidate in the rehabilitation of attention following traumatic brain injury: a randomised, crossover, double blind, placebo controlled inpatient trial. *J Neurol Neurosurg Psychiatry.* 2009;80(5):552-557.

202. McAllister TW, Zafonte R, Jain S, et al. Randomized placebo-controlled trial of methylphenidate or galantamine for persistent emotional and cognitive symptoms associated with PTSD and/or traumatic brain injury. *Neuropsychopharmacology.* 2016;41(5):1191-1198.

203. Speech TJ, Rao SM, Osmon DC, Sperry LT. A double-blind controlled study of methylphenidate treatment in closed head injury. *Brain Inj.* 1993;7(4):333-338.

204. Dymowski AR, Ponsford JL, Owens JA, Olver JH, Ponsford M, Willmott C. The efficacy and safety of extended-release methylphenidate following traumatic brain injury: a randomised controlled pilot study. *Clin Rehabil.* 2016;31(6):733-741.

205. Ripley DL, Morey CE, Gerber D, et al. Atomoxetine for attention deficits following traumatic brain injury: results from a randomized controlled trial. *Brain Inj.* 2014;28(12):1514-1522.

206. Kraus MF, Maki PM. Effect of amantadine hydrochloride on symptoms of frontal lobe dysfunction in brain injury: case studies and review. *J Neuropsychiatry Clin Neurosci.* 1997;9(2):222-230.

207. Meythaler JM, Brunner RC, Johnson A, Novack TA. Amantadine to improve neurorecovery in traumatic brain injury-associated diffuse axonal injury: a pilot double-blind randomized trial. *J Head Trauma Rehabil.* 2002;17(4):300-313.

208. Schneider WN, Drew-Cates J, Wong TM, Dombovy ML. Cognitive and behavioural efficacy of amantadine in acute traumatic brain injury: an initial double-blind placebo-controlled study. *Brain Inj.* 1999;13(11):863-872.

209. Whyte J, Vaccaro M, Grieb-Neff P, Hart T, Polansky M, Coslett HB. The effects of bromocriptine on attention deficits after traumatic brain injury: a placebo-controlled pilot study. *Am J Phys Med Rehabil.* 2008;87(2):85-99.

210. Taverni JP, Seliger G, Lichtman SW. Donepezil medicated memory improvement in traumatic brain injury during post acute rehabilitation. *Brain Inj.* 1998;12(1):77-80.

211. Whelan FJ, Walker MS, Schultz SK. Donepezil in the treatment of cognitive dysfunction associated with traumatic brain injury. *Ann Clin Psychiatry.* 2000;12(3):131-135.

212. Silver JM, Koumaras B, Chen M, et al. Effects of rivastigmine on cognitive function in patients with traumatic brain injury. *Neurology.* 2006;67(5):748-755.

213. Fleminger S, Greenwood RR, Oliver DL. Pharmacological management for agitation and aggression in people with acquired brain injury. In: Fleminger S, ed. *Cochrane Database of Systematic Reviews.* Chichester, UK: John Wiley & Sons, Ltd; 2006:CD003299.

214. Greendyke RM, Kanter DR, Schuster DB, Verstreate S, Wootton J. Propranolol treatment of assaultive patients with organic brain disease. A double-blind crossover, placebo-controlled study. *J Nerv Ment Dis.* 1986;174(5):290-294.

215. Greendyke RM, Kanter DR. Therapeutic effects of pindolol on behavioral disturbances associated with organic brain disease: a double-blind study. *J Clin Psychiatry.* 1986;47(8):423-426.

216. Wroblewski B, Joseph A, Kupfer J, Kalliel K. Effectiveness of valproic acid on destructive and aggressive behaviours in patients with acquired brain injury. *Brain Inj.* 1997;11(1):37-48.

217. Chatham Showalter PE, Kimmel DN. Agitated symptom response to divalproex following acute brain injury. *J Neuropsychiatry Clin Neurosci.* 2000;12(3):395-397.

218. Chatham-Showalter PE. Carbamazepine for combativeness in acute traumatic brain injury. *J Neuropsychiatry Clin Neurosci.* 1996;8(1):96-99.

219. Glenn MB, Wroblewski B, Parziale J, Levine L, Whyte J, Rosenthal M. Lithium carbonate for aggressive behavior or affective instability in ten brain-injured patients. *Am J Phys Med Rehabil.* 1989;68(5):221-226.

220. Bellus SB, Stewart D, Vergo JG, Kost PP, Grace J, Barkstrom SR. The use of lithium in the treatment of aggressive behaviours with two brain-injured individuals in a state psychiatric hospital. *Brain Inj.* 1996;10(11):849-860.

221. Pachet A, Friesen S, Winkelaar D, Gray S. Beneficial behavioural effects of lamotrigine in traumatic brain injury. *Brain Inj.* 2003;17(8):715-722.

222. Kant R, Smith-Seemiller L, Zeiler D. Treatment of aggression and irritability after head injury. *Brain Inj.* 1998;12(8):661-666.

223. Mysiw WJ, Jackson RD, Corrigan JD. Amitriptyline for post-traumatic agitation. *Am J Phys Med Rehabil.* 1988;67(1):29-33.

224. Hammond FM, Bickett AK, Norton JH, Pershad R. Effectiveness of amantadine hydrochloride in the reduction of chronic traumatic brain injury irritability and aggression. *J Head Trauma Rehabil.* 2014;29(5):391-399.

225. Hammond FM, Sherer M, Malec JF, et al. Amantadine effect on perceptions of irritability after traumatic brain injury: results of the amantadine irritability multisite study. *J Neurotrauma.* 2015;32(16):1230-1238.

226. Hammond FM, Malec JF, Zafonte RD, et al. Potential impact of amantadine on aggression in chronic traumatic brain injury. *J Head Trauma Rehabil.* 2017;32(5):308-318.

227. Maryniak O, Manchanda R, Velani A. Methotrimeprazine in the treatment of agitation in acquired brain injury patients. *Brain Inj.* 2001;15(2):167-174.

228. Stanislav SW, Childs A. Evaluating the usage of droperidol in acutely agitated persons with brain injury. *Brain Inj.* 2000;14(3):261-265.

229. Krieger D, Hansen K, McDermott C, et al. Loxapine versus olanzapine in the treatment of delirium following traumatic brain injury. *NeuroRehabilitation.* 2003;18(3):205-208.

230. Kim E, Bijlani M. A pilot study of quetiapine treatment of aggression due to traumatic brain injury. *J Neuropsychiatry Clin Neurosci.* 2006;18(4):547-549.

231. Michals ML, Crismon ML, Roberts S, Childs A. Clozapine response and adverse effects in nine brain-injured patients. *J Clin Psychopharmacol.* 1993;13(3):198-203.

232. Noé E, Ferri J, Trénor C, Chirivella J. Efficacy of ziprasidone in controlling agitation during post-traumatic amnesia. *Behav Neurol.* 2007;18(1):7-11.

233. Umene-Nakano W, Yoshimura R, Okamoto T, Hori H, Nakamura J. Aripiprazole improves various cognitive and behavioral impairments after traumatic brain injury: a case report. *Gen Hosp Psychiatry.* 2013;35(1):e7-e9.

234. Wilson MS, Gibson CJ, Hamm RJ. Haloperidol, but not olanzapine, impairs cognitive performance after traumatic brain injury in rats. *Am J Phys Med Rehabil.* 2003;82(11):871-879.

235. Wortzel HS, Oster TJ, Anderson CA, Arciniegas DB. Pathological laughing and crying: epidemiology, pathophysiology and treatment. *CNS Drugs.* 2008;22(7):531-545.

236. Nahas Z, Arlinghaus KA, Kotrla KJ, Clearman RR, George MS. Rapid response of emotional incontinence to selective serotonin reuptake inhibitors. *J Neuropsychiatry Clin Neurosci.* 1998;10(4):453-455.

237. Müller U, Murai T, Bauer-Wittmund T, von Cramon DY. Paroxetine versus citalopram treatment of pathological crying after brain injury. *Brain Inj.* 1999;13(10):805-811.

238. Kaschka W, Meyer A, Schier K, Fröscher W. Treatment of pathological crying with citalopram. *Pharmacopsychiatry.* 2001;34(06):254-258.

239. Chahine LM, Chemali Z. Du rire aux larmes: pathological laughing and crying in patients with traumatic brain injury and treatment with lamotrigine. *Epilepsy Behav.* 2006;8(3):610-615.

240. Garcia-Baran D, Johnson TM, Wagner J, Shen J, Geers M. Therapeutic approach of a high functioning individual with traumatic brain injury and subsequent emotional volatility with features of pathological laughter and crying with dextromethorphan/quinidine. *Medicine (Baltimore).* 2016;95(12):e2886.

241. Hammond FM, Alexander DN, Cutler AJ, et al. PRISM II: an open-label study to assess effectiveness of dextromethorphan/quinidine for pseudobulbar affect in patients with dementia, stroke or traumatic brain injury. *BMC Neurol.* 2016;16(1):89.

242. Pioro EP. Review of dextromethorphan 20 mg/quinidine 10 mg (NUEDEXTA') for pseudobulbar affect. *Neurol Ther.* 2014;3(1):15-28.

243. Gualtieri CT, Evans RW. Stimulant treatment for the neurobehavioural sequelae of traumatic brain injury. *Brain Inj.* 1988;2(4):273-290.

244. Powell JH, al-Adawi S, Morgan J, Greenwood RJ. Motivational deficits after brain injury: effects of bromocriptine in 11 patients. *J Neurol Neurosurg Psychiatry.* 1996;60(4):416-421.

245. Van Reekum R, Bayley M, Garner S, et al. N of 1 study: amantadine for the amotivational syndrome in a patient with traumatic brain injury. *Brain Inj.* 1995;9(1):49-53.

246. Hoehn-Saric R, Lipsey JR, McLeod DR. Apathy and indifference in patients on fluvoxamine and fluoxetine. *J Clin Psychopharmacol.* 1990;10(5):343-345.

247. Lee H, Kim S-W, Kim J-M, Shin I-S, Yang S-J, Yoon J-S. Comparing effects of methylphenidate, sertraline and placebo on neuropsychiatric sequelae in patients with traumatic brain injury. *Hum Psychopharmacol.* 2005;20(2):97-104.

248. Fann JR, Uomoto JM, Katon WJ. Sertraline in the treatment of major depression following mild traumatic brain injury. *J Neuropsychiatry Clin Neurosci.* 2000;12(2):226-232.

249. Horsfield SA, Rosse RB, Tomasino V, Schwartz BL, Mastropaolo J, Deutsch SI. Fluoxetine's effects on cognitive performance in patients with traumatic brain injury. *Int J Psychiatry Med.* 2002;32(4):337-344.

250. Rapoport M, Chan F, Lanctot K, Herrmann N, McCullagh S, Feinstein A. An open-label study of citalopram for major depression following traumatic brain injury. *J Psychopharmacol.* 2008;22(8):860-864.

251. Ashman TA, Cantor JB, Gordon WA, et al. A randomized controlled trial of sertraline for the treatment of depression in persons with traumatic brain injury. *Arch Phys Med Rehabil.* 2009;90(5):733-740.

252. Fann JR, Bombardier CH, Temkin N, et al. Sertraline for major depression during the year following traumatic brain injury: a randomized controlled trial. *J Head Trauma Rehabil.* 2017;32(5):332-342.

253. Polich G, Iaccarino M, Kaptchuk T, Morales-Quezada L, Zaftone R. Placebo effects in traumatic brain injury. *J Neurotrauma.* 2018;35:1-8.

254. Kanetani K, Kimura M, Endo S. Therapeutic effects of milnacipran (serotonin noradrenalin reuptake inhibitor) on depression following mild and moderate traumatic brain injury. *J Nippon Med Sch.* 2003;70(4):313-320.

255. Jorge RE, Acion L, Burin DI, Robinson RG. Sertraline for preventing mood disorders following traumatic brain injury: a randomized clinical trial. *JAMA psychiatry.* 2016;73(10):1041-1047.

256. Novack TA, Baños JH, Brunner R, Renfroe S, Meythaler JM. Impact of early administration of sertraline on

depressive symptoms in the first year after traumatic brain injury. *J Neurotrauma.* 2009;26(11):1921-1928.

257. Hackam DG, Mrkobrada M. Selective serotonin reuptake inhibitors and brain hemorrhage: a meta-analysis. *Neurology.* 2012;79(18):1862-1865.

258. Renoux C, Vahey S, Dell'Aniello S, Boivin J-F. Association of selective serotonin reuptake inhibitors with the risk for spontaneous intracranial hemorrhage. *JAMA Neurol.* 2017;74(2):173.

259. Wroblewski BA, Joseph AB, Cornblatt RR. Antidepressant pharmacotherapy and the treatment of depression in patients with severe traumatic brain injury: a controlled, prospective study. *J Clin Psychiatry.* 1996;57(12):582-587.

260. Dinan TG, Mobayed M. Treatment resistance of depression after head injury: a preliminary study of amitriptyline response. *Acta Psychiatr Scand.* 1992;85(4):292-294.

261. Fann JR, Hart T, Schomer KG. Treatment for depression after traumatic brain injury: a systematic review. *J Neurotrauma.* 2009;26(12):2383-2402.

262. Wroblewski BA, McColgan K, Smith K, Whyte J, Singer WD. The incidence of seizures during tricyclic antidepressant drug treatment in a brain-injured population. *J Clin Pharmacol.* 1990;10(2):124-128.

263. Zhang W-T, Wang Y-F. Efficacy of methylphenidate for the treatment of mental sequelae after traumatic brain injury. *Medicine (Baltimore).* 2017;96(25):e6960.

264. Hale MS, Donaldson JO. Lithium carbonate in the treatment of organic brain syndrome. *J Nerv Ment Dis.* 1982;170(6):362-365.

265. Stewart JT, Hemsath RH. Bipolar illness following traumatic brain injury: treatment with lithium and carbamazepine. *J Clin Psychiatry.* 1988;49(2):74-75.

266. Pope HG, McElroy SL, Satlin A, Hudson JI, Keck PE, Kalish R. Head injury, bipolar disorder, and response to valproate. *Compr Psychiatry.* 1988;29(1):34-38.

267. Yassa R, Cvejic J. Valproate in the treatment of posttraumatic bipolar disorder in a psychogeriatric patient. *J Geriatr Psychiatry Neurol.* 1994;7(1):55-57.

268. Kim E, Humaran TJ. Divalproex in the management of neuropsychiatric complications of remote acquired brain injury. *J Neuropsychiatry Clin Neurosci.* 2002;14(2):202-205.

269. Daniels JP, Felde A. Quetiapine treatment for mania secondary to brain injury in 2 patients. *J Clin Psychiatry.* 2008;69(3):497-498.

270. Oster TJ, Anderson CA, Filley CM, Wortzel HS, Arciniegas DB. Quetiapine for mania due to traumatic brain injury. *CNS Spectr.* 2007;12(10):764-769.

271. Zhang W, Davidson JR. Post-traumatic stress disorder: an evaluation of existing pharmacotherapies and new strategies. *Expert Opin Pharmacother.* 2007;8(12):1861-1870.

272. Singh B, Hughes AJ, Mehta G, Erwin PJ, Parsaik AK. Efficacy of prazosin in posttraumatic stress disorder: a systematic review and meta-analysis. *Prim Care Companion CNS Disord.* 2016;18(4). Available at: https://www.ncbi.nlm.nih.gov/pubmed/27828694

273. Raskind MA, Peskind ER, Chow B, et al. Trial of prazosin for post-traumatic stress disorder in military veterans. *N Engl J Med.* 2018;378(6):507-517.

274. Barker MJ, Greenwood KM, Jackson M, Crowe SF. Persistence of cognitive effects after withdrawal from long-term benzodiazepine use: a meta-analysis. *Arch Clin Neuropsychol.* 2004;19(3):437-454.

275. Barker MJ, Greenwood KM, Jackson M, Crowe SF. Cognitive effects of long-term benzodiazepine use: a meta-analysis. *CNS Drugs.* 2004;18(1):37-48.

276. Schallert T, Hernandez TD, Barth TM. Recovery of function after brain damage: severe and chronic disruption by diazepam. *Brain Res.* 1986;379(1):104-111.

277. Cheng JP, Leary JB, O'Neil DA, et al. Spontaneous recovery of traumatic brain injury-induced functional deficits is not hindered by daily administration of lorazepam. *Behav Brain Res.* 2018;339:215-221.

278. Darby R, Prasad S. Lesion-related delusional misidentification syndromes: a comprehensive review of reported cases. *J Neuropsychiatry Clin Neurosci.* 2016;28(3):217-222.

279. Sohlberg MM, Avery J, Kennedy M, et al. Practice guidelines for direct attention training. *J Med Speech Lang Pathol.* 2003;11(3):xix-xxxix.

280. Tate RL. Beyond one-bun, two-shoe: recent advances in the psychological rehabilitation of memory disorders after acquired brain injury. *Brain Inj.* 1997;11(12):907-918.

281. Cicerone KD, Langenbahn DM, Braden C, et al. Evidence-based cognitive rehabilitation: updated review of the literature from 2003 through 2008. *Arch Phys Med Rehabil.* 2011;92(4):519-530.

282. Tate R, Kennedy M, Ponsford J, et al. INCOG recommendations for management of cognition following traumatic brain injury, Part III: executive function and self-awareness. *J Head Trauma Rehabil.* 2014;29(4):338-352.

283. McDonald BC, Flashman LA, Arciniegas DB, et al. Methylphenidate and memory and attention adaptation training for persistent cognitive symptoms after traumatic brain injury: a randomized, placebo-controlled trial. *Neuropsychopharmacology.* 2017;42(9):1766-1775.

284. Mueser KT, Glynn SM. Have the potential benefits of CBT for severe mental disorders been undersold? *World Psychiatry.* 2014;13(3):253-256.

285. Ponsford J, Lee NK, Wong D, et al. Efficacy of motivational interviewing and cognitive behavioral therapy for anxiety and depression symptoms following traumatic brain injury. *Psychol Med.* 2016;46(5):1079-1090.

286. Ashman T, Cantor JB, Tsaousides T, Spielman L, Gordon W. Comparison of cognitive behavioral therapy and supportive psychotherapy for the treatment of depression following traumatic brain injury: a randomized controlled trial. *J Head Trauma Rehabil.* 2014;29(6):467-478.

287. Fann JR, Bombardier CH, Vannoy S, et al. Telephone and in-person cognitive behavioral therapy for major depression after traumatic brain injury: a randomized controlled trial. *J Neurotrauma.* 2015;32(1):45-57.

288. Bombardier CH, Bell KR, Temkin NR, Fann JR, Hoffman J, Dikmen S. The efficacy of a scheduled telephone intervention for ameliorating depressive symptoms during the first year after traumatic brain injury. *J Head Trauma Rehabil.* 2009;24(4):230-238.

289. Potter SDS, Brown RG, Fleminger S. Randomised, waiting list controlled trial of cognitive-behavioural therapy for persistent postconcussional symptoms after predominantly mild-moderate traumatic brain injury. *J Neurol Neurosurg Psychiatry.* 2016;87(10):1075-1083.

290. Bontempo A, Panza KE, Bloch MH. D-cycloserine augmentation of behavioral therapy for the treatment of anxiety disorders: a meta-analysis. *J Clin Psychiatry.* 2012;73(4):533-537.

291. Bédard M, Felteau M, Mazmanian D, et al. Pilot evaluation of a mindfulness-based intervention to improve quality of life among individuals who sustained traumatic brain injuries. *Disabil Rehabil.* 2003;25(13):722-731.

292. Bedard M, Felteau M, Gibbons C, et al. A mindfulness-based intervention to improve quality of life among individuals who sustained traumatic brain injuries : one-year follow-up. *J Cogn Rehabil.* 2005;23(1):8-13.

293. Azulay J, Smart C, Mott T, Cicerone K. A pilot study examining the effect of mindfulness-based stress reduction on symptoms of

chronic mild traumatic brain injury/postconcussive syndrome. *J Head Trauma Rehabil.* 2013;28(4):323-331.

294. Johansson B, Bjuhr H, Rönnbäck L. Evaluation of an advanced mindfulness program following a mindfulness-based stress reduction program for participants suffering from mental fatigue after acquired brain injury. *Mindfulness (N Y).* 2015;6(2):227-233.

295. Johansson B, Bjuhr H, Rönnbäck L. Mindfulness-based stress reduction (MBSR) improves long-term mental fatigue after stroke or traumatic brain injury. *Brain Inj.* 2012;26(13-14):1621-1628.

296. McMillan T, Robertson IH, Brock D, Chorlton L. Brief mindfulness training for attentional problems after traumatic brain injury: a randomised control treatment trial. *Neuropsychol Rehabil.* 2002;12(2):117-125.

297. Liu Z-Q, Zeng X, Duan C-Y. Neuropsychological rehabilitation and psychotherapy of adult traumatic brain injury patients with depression: a systematic review and meta-analysis. *J Neurosurg Sci.* 2018;62(1):24-35.

298. Swain R, Berggren K, Kerr A, Patel A, Peplinski C, Sikorski A. On aerobic exercise and behavioral and neural plasticity. *Brain Sci.* 2012;2(4):709-744.

299. Leddy J, Hinds A, Sirica D, Willer B. The role of controlled exercise in concussion management. *PM R.* 2016;8(3 suppl):S91-S100.

300. Ströhle A. Physical activity, exercise, depression and anxiety disorders. *J Neural Transm.* 2009;116(6):777-784.

301. Asmundson GJG, Fetzner MG, Deboer LB, Powers MB, Otto MW, Smits JAJ. Let's get physical: a contemporary review of the anxiolytic effects of exercise for anxiety and its disorders. *Depress Anxiety.* 2013;30(4):362-373.

302. Cooney GM, Dwan K, Greig CA, et al. Exercise for depression. *Cochrane Database Syst Rev.* 2013;9(9):CD004366.

303. Lawlor DA, Hopker SW. The effectiveness of exercise as an intervention in the management of depression: systematic review and meta-regression analysis of randomised controlled trials. *BMJ.* 2001;322(7289):763-767.

304. Kvam S, Kleppe CL, Nordhus IH, Hovland A. Exercise as a treatment for depression: a meta-analysis. *J Affect Disord.* 2016;202:67-86.

305. Geda YE, Roberts RO, Knopman DS, et al. Physical exercise, aging, and mild cognitive impairment: a population-based study. *Arch Neurol.* 2010;67(1):80-86.

306. Middleton LE, Barnes DE, Lui L-Y, Yaffe K. Physical activity over the life course and its association with cognitive performance and impairment in old age. *J Am Geriatr Soc.* 2010;58(7):1322-1326.

307. Etgen T, Sander D, Huntgeburth U, Poppert H, Förstl H, Bickel H. Physical activity and incident cognitive impairment in elderly persons: the INVADE study. *Arch Intern Med.* 2010;170(2):186-193.

308. Gordon WA, Sliwinski M, Echo J, McLoughlin M, Sheerer M, Meili TE. The benefits of exercise in individuals with traumatic brain injury: a retrospective study. *J Head Trauma Rehabil.* 1998;13(4):58-67.

309. Weinstein AA, Chin LMK, Collins J, Goel D, Keyser RE, Chan L. Effect of aerobic exercise training on mood in people with traumatic brain injury. *J Head Trauma Rehabil.* 2017;32(3):E49-E56.

310. Grealy MA, Johnson DA, Rushton SK. Improving cognitive function after brain injury: the use of exercise and virtual reality. *Arch Phys Med Rehabil.* 1999;80(6):661-667.

311. Devine JM, Zafonte RD. Physical exercise and cognitive recovery in acquired brain injury: a review of the literature. *PM R.* 2009;1(6):560-575.

312. Srienc A, Narang P, Sarai S, Xiong Y, Lippmann S. Is electroconvulsive therapy a treatment for depression following traumatic brain injury? *Innov Clin Neurosci.* 2018;15(3-4):43-46.

313. Martino C, Krysko M, Petrides G, Tobias KG, Kellner CH. Cognitive tolerability of electroconvulsive therapy in a patient with a history of traumatic brain injury. *J ECT.* 2008;24(1):92-95.

314. Ruedrich SL, Chu CC, Moore SL. ECT for major depression in a patient with acute brain trauma. *Am J Psychiatry.* 1983;140(7):928-929.

315. Crow S, Meller W, Christenson G, Mackenzie T. Use of ECT after brain injury. *Convuls Ther.* 1996; 12(2):113-116.

316. Demirtas-Tatlidede A, Vahabzadeh-Hagh AM, Bernabeu M, Tormos JM, Pascual-Leone A. Noninvasive brain stimulation in traumatic brain injury. *J Head Trauma Rehabil.* 2012;27(4):274-292.

317. Fitzgerald PB, Hoy KE, Maller JJ, et al. Transcranial magnetic stimulation for depression after a traumatic brain injury: a case study. *J ECT.* 2011; 27(1):38-40.

318. Hoy KE, McQueen S, Elliot D, Herring SE, Maller JJ, Fitzgerald PB. A pilot investigation of repetitive transcranial magnetic stimulation for post-traumatic brain injury depression: safety, tolerability, and efficacy. *J Neurotrauma.* 2019;36(13):2092-2098.

319. Kline AE, Hoffman AN, Cheng JP, Zafonte RD, Massucci JL. Chronic administration of antipsychotics impede behavioral recovery after experimental traumatic brain injury. *Neurosci Lett.* 2008;448(3):263-267.

320. Feeney DM, Gonzalez A, Law WA. Amphetamine, haloperidol, and experience interact to affect rate of recovery after motor cortex injury. *Science.* 1982;217(27):855-857.

321. Phelps TI, Bondi CO, Ahmed RH, Olugbade YT, Kline AE. Divergent long-term consequences of chronic treatment with haloperidol, risperidone, and bromocriptine on traumatic brain injury–induced cognitive deficits. *J Neurotrauma.* 2015;32(8):590-597.

322. Hoffman AN, Cheng JP, Zafonte RD, Kline AE. Administration of haloperidol and risperidone after neurobehavioral testing hinders the recovery of traumatic brain injury-induced deficits. *Life Sci.* 2008;83(17-18):602-607.

323. Rao N, Jellinek HM, Woolston DC. Agitation in closed head injury: haloperidol effects on rehabilitation outcome. *Arch Phys Med Rehabil.* 1985;66(1):30-34. Available at http://www.ncbi.nlm.nih.gov/pubmed/3966865. Accessed February 2, 2017.

324. Mysiw WJ, Bogner JA, Corrigan JD, Fugate LP, Clinchot DM, Kadyan V. The impact of acute care medications on rehabilitation outcome after traumatic brain injury. *Brain Inj.* 2006;20(9):905-911.

31

Neuropsychiatry of Pain

Megan Dawson · Damien Miran · Victor Wang · Laura T. Safar

INTRODUCTION

Pain is a multidimensional experience and interacts with many aspects of an individual. In an attempt to standardize terminology, pain was defined by the International Association for the Study of Pain (IASP) in 1979[1] as "an unpleasant sensory and emotional experience associated with actual or potential tissue damage, or described in terms of such damage." In their note about this definition, it is stated that "pain is always subjective" and individuals learn through experience what it means to be in pain. An individual can experience pain in the absence of actual tissue damage, thus avoiding "tying the pain to the stimulus."[1] The potential interplay and overlap of mental health and pain is present in the 1979 definition of pain, but the relationship has become more explicit in terms of the comorbidity of pain and other psychiatric diagnoses, the possible common pathophysiology, and the bidirectional influence which pain and psychiatric conditions have over each other.[2] Updates to the 1979 definition have been suggested to incorporate the developmental, cognitive, and social aspects of how pain is perceived and treated[3,4] in line with biopsychosocial models used in mental health. The US Institute of Medicine in 2011 published a report calling for taking a comprehensive view of chronic pain as a biological, biobehavioral, and societal condition and promoting changes in pain education, research, and treatment, which include a focus on prevention, pain as a public health problem, and a multidisciplinary approach to treatment that involves psychiatry.[5]

This chapter will discuss the pathophysiology of pain and its clinical presentation, with a focus on the overlap of pain and psychiatric conditions such as depression, anxiety, and others. Specific pain clinical entities of interest to neuropsychiatry to be reviewed include fibromyalgia (FM), complex regional pain syndrome (CRPS), and somatic symptom disorder (SSD) with predominant pain. We will then discuss the general approach to the assessment and treatment of pain conditions, with an emphasis on the comorbid presentation of pain and psychiatric disorders.

EPIDEMIOLOGY

Chronic pain is defined as persistent or recurrent pain lasting longer than 3 months.[6] Reports on the lifetime prevalence of chronic pain in developed countries vary, but it is estimated to affect about 20% of the adult population.[7] In a study published in 2012, the estimated cost of chronic pain in the United States, including direct medical treatment costs and indirect costs due to lost productivity, was between 560 and 635 billion US dollars which exceeds the individual costs of heart disease, cancer, and diabetes.[5,7]

PATHOPHYSIOLOGY OF PAIN

Pain has always been an inherent part of medicine and is often the first sign of pathology that prompts a patient to present for medical care. The study of pain and the current body of evidence can describe how pain signals are transmitted to the brain. For example, how does the toe "tell" the brain that it was just slammed into the coffee table? How do the fingers tell the brain that the cup of coffee is just too hot?

Pain is a complex experience that depends on each individual's history and memories. However, the acute physiologic process in which pain is transmitted from the skin or organs to the spinal cord to the brain is the same, across humans and animals. This transmission of pain signals is called nociception.[8] Nociception has been defined as the detection of noxious stimuli that can cause tissue injury. Other basic terms that describe a malfunctioning sensory and pain system would include allodynia, defined as normally non-painful stimuli that is experienced as pain, and hyperalgesia, defined as a heightened sensation of pain, or experiencing more pain than normal for stimuli that are normally painful to begin with.[9,10]

The body senses these modalities through specialized nerve endings in the tissue where the sensory signal is transduced and encoded into action potentials of the primary afferent neuron, also called first-order neuron. The pain signal travels in ascending anatomical steps to the brain, where it is then decoded as "pain." The primary afferent, or first-order neuron, transmits the signal from the periphery to the spinal cord and synapses with the second-order neuron within the spinal cord. This second neuron then projects up to the thalamus, where the third-order neuron ultimately projects to different parts of the brain including the somatosensory cortex and limbic system (see Figure 31-1). Along the pathways, various modulatory mechanisms exist that can tune and affect the pain signal. This section will discuss with more detail the nociceptive aspect of pain. Discussion of the neuroanatomy and pathophysiology of visceral, muscle, and neuropathic pain exceed the scope of this chapter. Briefly, free nerve endings distributed through the muscle mediate muscle pain. Mechanical forces, ischemia, inflammation, and degeneration may cause muscle pain through stimulation of these nerve endings, which then project to the dorsal horn. The pain stimuli are transmitted primarily through the spinothalamic tract to several cortical and subcortical structures. Regarding visceral pain, the anterolateral fasciculus of the cord contains several slowly conducting systems of fibers. The conduction of diffuse, poorly localized visceral pain takes place via these slow-conducting pathways. The vagus nerve also carries visceral pain information.

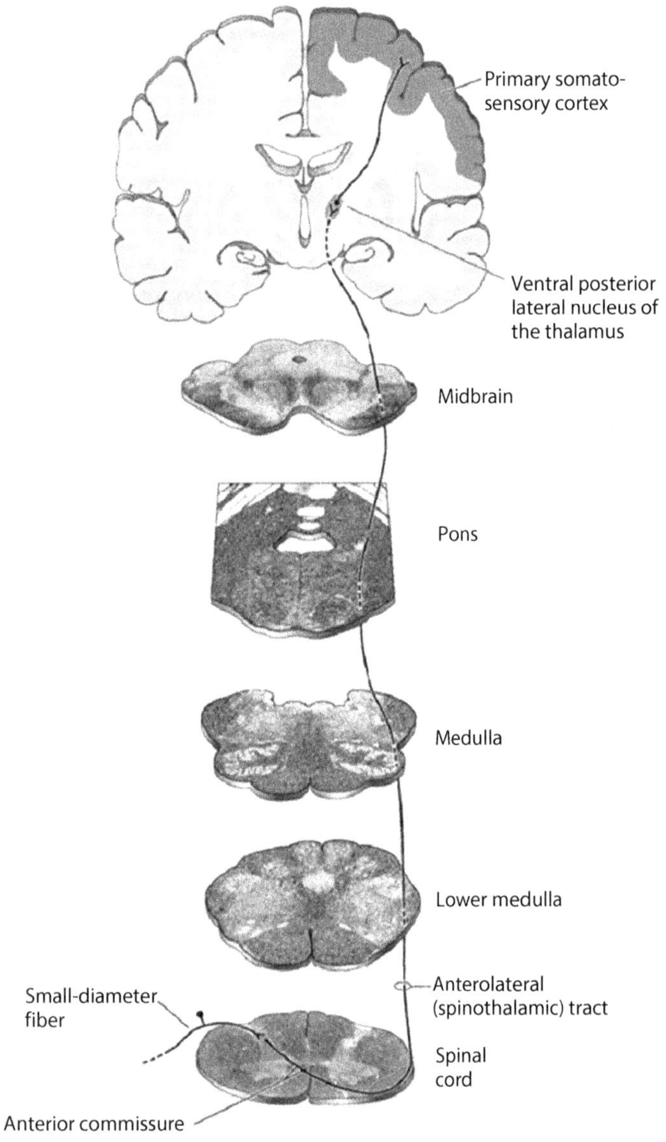

Primary Afferents: Receptor to Transduction and First-Order Neurons

In the somatosensory system, there are several different afferent fibers that carry sensory information from the periphery to the brain. These include A-fibers (subclassified into the subtypes alpha, beta, delta, and gamma), B-fibers, and C-fibers.[8,11] Primary afferent neurons are further classified by their conduction velocities, with A-fibers being the thickly myelinated and the fastest conducting, B-fibers being less myelinated and thus slower, and unmyelinated C-fibers being the thinnest and slowest. A-beta, A-delta, and C-fibers are the most relevant ones for this discussion, since they comprise the primary afferents for pain transmission. A-beta fibers are the fastest of these—they are myelinated, between 12 and 20 μm in diameter, and their conduction velocity is >25 m/s. A-delta fibers are smaller myelinated fibers, about 2–5 μm in diameter, and have conduction velocities of 5–25 m/s. Finally, the unmyelinated C-fibers are 0.2–1.5 μm in diameter, with conduction velocities below 2 m/s (Table 31-1).[12]

There are three modalities of nociception: temperature, pressure (mechanical), and chemical. These are sensed by the specialized nerve endings of the A-beta, A-delta, and C-fibers. All three types of nerve fibers have specialized nerve endings where sensation is transduced in the periphery. A-beta fibers have specialized nerve endings called Pacinian corpuscles that detect low-threshold stimulation like light touch,[13] and do play a role in nociception, though not as much as the A-delta and C-fibers.

On the other hand, A-delta fibers and C-fibers have specialized "free" nerve endings or nociceptors, which respond to different modalities of noxious stimuli. A-delta fibers are sensitive to both low- and high-threshold mechanical and thermal stimuli, whereas C-fibers are sensitive to high-threshold thermal, mechanical, and chemical stimuli. Noxious stimuli which come in contact with the skin, for example, will activate the specific nociceptor which then opens ion channels with subsequent depolarization of the cell membrane. When enough

FIGURE 31-1. Schematic of the anterolateral (spinothalamic) tract. It shows the first-order neuron, with its cell body in the dorsal root ganglion; the second-order neuron in the dorsal horn of the spinal cord; and the third-order neuron in the thalamus. (Reproduced with permission from Martin J. *Neuroanatomy Text and Atlas*. 4th ed. http://neurology.mhmedical. Copyright © McGraw Hill LLC. All rights reserved.

Labels in figure: Primary somato-sensory cortex; Ventral posterior lateral nucleus of the thalamus; Midbrain; Pons; Medulla; Lower medulla; Anterolateral (spinothalamic) tract; Spinal cord; Small-diameter fiber; Anterior commissure

TABLE 31-1 • Primary Afferent Neuron Axons.		
Fiber Type	**Conduction Velocity**	**Diameter**
A-beta (myelinated)	40–50 m/s	12–20 μm
A-delta (myelinated)	5–25 m/s	1–4 μm
C (unmyelinated)	<2 m/s	0.5–1.5 μm

channels are opened, an action potential is produced and conducted down the afferent axon. Increased channel openings would then increase action potential frequency. Using temperature as an example, there are several known receptors in the nerve ending that will activate ion channels when temperature rises or falls below a certain threshold.[13] For example, the TRPV1 receptor on the nerve ending opens ion channels when the temperature rises above around 43°C.[9,14] The TRPM8 receptor responds and opens ion channels when temperatures dip below about 25°C.[15,16] There are also specific channels that respond to a decrease in pH and other chemicals. In this way, the nervous system is able to deduce the respective pain modalities.

The cell bodies of the first-order neurons lie just outside the spinal cord, in the dorsal root ganglion. This is where the presynaptic neurotransmitters are synthesized, with the primary neurotransmitter being glutamate. Other peptides such as substance P are co-released at the synaptic cleft along with glutamate. There are several different types of glutamate receptors on the postsynaptic membrane, which then depolarize the second-order neuron.

Second-Order Neurons and Projections

The primary afferents, or first-order neurons, synapse onto the ipsilateral second-order neurons in the dorsal horn of the spinal cord in a preserved somatotopic fashion. In a cross-sectional view, the spinal cord is divided into anatomic layers called Rexed laminae I through X, where lamina I is the most superficial layer of the dorsal horn, lamina II is deeper, and

so on, all the way to lamina X at the central cord. The A-delta and C-fibers largely project to the second-order neurons in the outermost layers, laminae I and II. A-beta fibers end in layers III through V.[17,18] A-beta, A-delta, and C-fibers do trifurcate on entry to the spinal cord and travel both rostrally and caudally across multiple levels to synapse on second-order neurons in the superficial laminae (Figure 31-2). A-delta fibers trifurcate in the dorsal columns and C-fibers in the posterolateral tracts, also known as the tracts of Lissauer.

There are primarily two types of nociceptive second-order neurons that project to the brainstem and thalamus. The first type are called *nociceptive specific neurons*; they lie in the superficial laminae I and II and receive A-delta and C-afferents. Nociceptive-specific neurons respond only to specific noxious stimuli. The second type are called *wide dynamic range neurons*, and they lie deeper in laminae II–V.[19,20] They are so named because they respond to a wide range of somatosensory intensities as they receive input from all three different types of primary afferent fibers: A-beta, A-delta, and C. Wide dynamic range neurons have a graded response to stimuli as they can be activated by a range of sensory stimulation, ranging from light touch to higher threshold painful stimuli.

The axons of the second-order neurons then travel to the brain via the anterolateral system in the spinal cord. Several tracts within the anterolateral system carry information for crude touch, pain, and temperature. The primary tracts relevant for pain transmission include the spinothalamic and spinoreticular tracts, which have been described respectively as *direct* and *indirect* pathways. The spinothalamic tract fibers decussate,

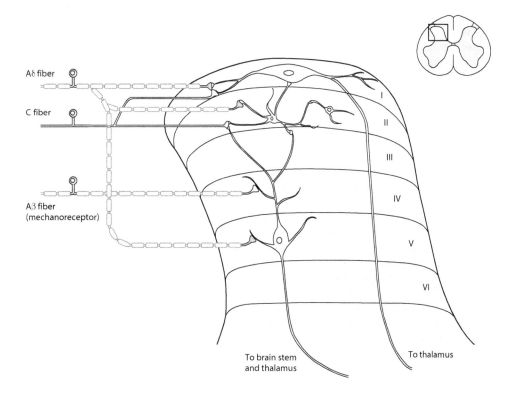

FIGURE 31-2. The first-order neurons synapse onto the ipsilateral second-order neurons in the dorsal horn of the spinal cord in a preserved somatotopic fashion. (Reproduced with permission from Kandel ER, Schwartz JH, Jessell TM, et al: Principles of Neural Science. 5th ed. https://neurology.mhmedical.com. Copyright © McGraw Hill LLC. All rights reserved.)

or cross to the opposite side of the spinal cord, near the level where the first-order neuron synapses. They then ascend the spinal cord in the contralateral side to eventually synapse onto third-order neurons in the ventral posterior nuclei of the thalamus. The spinoreticular fibers primarily run alongside the spinothalamic tract, but ipsilateral to the first- and second-order synapse. These fibers synapse onto the reticular formation in the brainstem which have extensive projections to the thalamus.[21] Other fibers synapse onto the periaqueductal gray (PAG), which may play a role in pain inhibition.

Third-Order Neurons and Modulation

The ventral posterior nuclei of the thalamus, mentioned above, include the ventral posterior lateral and ventral posterior medial nuclei. The third-order neurons in the thalamus then project to the somatosensory cortex. The pathway's organization is preserved anatomically along the contralateral spinothalamic tract and thalamus, with somatotopic cortical representation in the somatosensory cortex, referred to as the *sensory homunculus* in the postcentral gyrus.[22] This is the map-like representation of the body onto the brain, with a larger portion of the cortex devoted to sensation of the hands and face than the trunk and legs. This order is preserved in the spinal column as well (e.g., the nerves carrying signals from the hand run together and the nerves carrying foot information run together).

The third-order neurons in the thalamus also project to the anterior cingulate cortex and the inferior insular cortex. These are areas of the cortex associated with affect and emotion, awareness, and attention, which also play a role in the experience of pain.

The pain system is part of the somatosensory system that is organized into the different modalities of sensation (vibration, proprioception, pain, temperature). Information for the other modalities is transmitted in much the same way as pain, with first, second, and third-order neurons. The spinothalamic tract described above carries information for the pain and temperature modalities. The other modalities also start with specialized skin and stretch receptors in the periphery, which transduce vibration and proprioception into action potentials of the afferent fibers, mostly large myelinated A-delta fibers. These then enter the spinal cord and travel up the spinal cord in the dorsal columns ipsilaterally, and then cross, or decussate, at the medulla. This is known as the dorsal column-medial lemniscus pathway (Figure 31-3). The fibers then synapse onto the third-order neurons in the thalamus which eventually project to the somatosensory cortex.[21,23] This is the reason why, for instance, an injury to the spinal cord will cause ipsilateral loss of vibration and proprioceptive sense, and contralateral loss of pain and temperature below the level of the lesion.

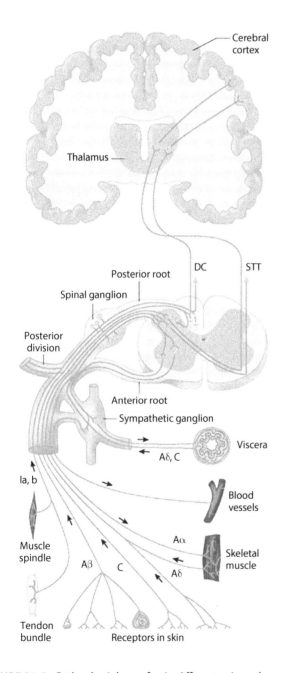

FIGURE 31-3. Pathophysiology of pain. Afferent pain pathways. (Reproduced with permission from Butterworth JF, Mackey DC, Wasnick JD. *Morgan & Mikhail's Clinical Anesthesiology.* 5th ed. https://accessmedicine.mhmedical.com/. Copyright © McGraw Hill LLC. All rights reserved.)

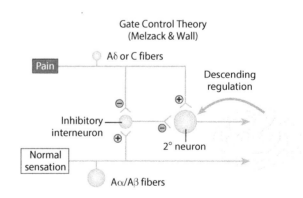

FIGURE 31-4. Gate control theory. (Reproduced with permission from O'Sullivan SB, Schmitz TJ, Fulk GD. *Physical Rehabilitation.* 6th ed. https://fadavispt.mhmedical.com/. Copyright © McGraw Hill LLC. All rights reserved.)

As mentioned earlier, the pathophysiology described above applies to nociceptive pain, defined as pain that results from actual tissue damage, or potentially tissue-damaging stimuli. A different mechanism that may activate the pain neural pathways is a direct lesion of the nervous system. Neuropathic pain is defined as pain caused by injury or disease of the somatosensory nervous system, for example by nerve trauma, or diabetic neuropathy. The pain is experienced in a neuroanatomically plausible body area, considering the nervous system lesion involved. The lesion or disease can typically be demonstrated, for example by imaging, biopsy, neurophysiological, or laboratory tests. Other negative or positive sensory signs (such as hypoesthesia, or paresthesias) compatible with the innervation territory of the lesioned nervous structure are typically present.[6]

Modulation of Pain Signals

Pain is a complex phenomenon, and its modulation can occur at any point along the pain pathways. Both sensation and pain can be modulated prior to the signal being recognized as "painful." At the most peripheral aspect, as discussed earlier, the TRPV1 sodium channel responds to temperatures greater than 43°C. This receptor also opens ion channels in response to capsaicin, the compound found in hot chili peppers. This is responsible for the burning sensation with chili peppers and modulates the system without thermal stimuli. The opposite phenomenon can occur with the TRPM8 receptor that responds to menthol in addition to cold temperatures and again, extending the experience of cold sensation.[16]

Modulation of the pain signal also occurs at the level of the spinal cord and higher. The pain signal can be modulated at the level of the spinal cord between the first order and second-order neurons. The gate control theory proposed by Melzack and Wall in 1965 is a simplified model of pain modulation.[24] The theory proposes that the system functions as a "gate" that can allow certain pain signals to travel to the brain through a non-noxious signal that can decrease the nociceptive input at the level of the spinal cord. The non-noxious signal enters the spinal cord and synapses on an inhibitory neuron, in addition to its terminal synapse on the second-order neuron. The inhibitory neuron then inhibits the signal from the pain transmission, dampening the pain signal on the way up to the brain (Figure 31-4). This has been the theory behind the fact that when an injury has occurred, rubbing the injured area can dull the pain. It is also an explanation for the use of transcutaneous electrical nerve stimulation (TENS) units, where non-painful stimulation of the skin can decrease pain at the same site.

Another alternative to explain the gate theory is through the summation of signals at the second-order neuron itself. As we discussed, wide dynamic range neurons are so-named because they receive input from different types of primary afferent fibers, including the low-threshold A-beta fibers. This means that a range of sensory stimulation, including non-noxious input, is detected by the wide dynamic range neurons, and thus their activity can be modulated with the summation of both noxious and non-noxious input at the level of these neurons. Some wide dynamic range neurons can be sensitized in their excitability

by repetitive input from C-fibers in a process termed "windup," which may be involved in development of hyperalgesia.[25]

The gate theory is probably the most well-known theory for modulation of the ascending pain signal. However, there is a large amount of ongoing research into descending modulation of pain. The most studied pathways are the PAG and rostral ventromedial medulla (RVM) pathways.[26,27] As previously discussed, the spinothalamic pathway projects to the anterior cingulate cortex and the limbic system. These cortical areas have projections to the PAG as well as the RVM. Stimulation of the PAG in animal models appears to have an analgesic effect without affecting other sensory modalities.[28,29] Additionally, opioids injected directly into the PAG produce analgesia in animal models[30,31] with some reports of reversal of this effect with naloxone administration.[32]

The PAG likely exerts its effects through extensive connections to the RVM which in turn has projections to the dorsal horn of the spinal cord. The RVM also receives input from thalamus, brainstem, and locus coeruleus.[33,34] The locus coeruleus is located in the pons and involved in attention and arousal. Stimulation of the RVM also has an analgesic effect as does injection of lidocaine and morphine. These have also reversed allodynia and hyperalgesia in animal models.

The modulation of pain by descending systems can be illustrated by the well-known phenomenon called stress-induced analgesia.[35] Stress-induced analgesia is the pain suppression response during a stressful situation. It is exhibited in the condition when an athlete can suffer an injury without realization until after a game, or when people who suffer a major injury after a motor vehicle accident don't notice the injury until the ambulance ride. Research suggests that this stress-induced analgesia involves the integration of several systems including the cortex, brainstem, and spinal cord. The endogenous opioid system has been shown to produce analgesia in a similar manner which is also reversed by naloxone in animal models. The endocannabinoid system may also play a role in modulating the descending pathway.[35-37]

Pain is a complex physiological manifestation crucial to the survival and preservation of biological systems. The complex pain pathways and their modulation take place in both bottom-up and top-down ways, at the levels of the peripheral and central nervous systems. How pain is perceived, however, differs across animal models and across individuals—depending on complex factors such as their neurobiological makeup, mood, memory, and prior experience.

CLINICAL PRESENTATION AND CLASSIFICATION

Pain can be both a symptom and a disease entity or disorder in it of itself, making it challenging to fit into a single classification system. The ACTTION-APS pain taxonomy (AAPT), a joint project of the US FDA and the American Pain Society aiming to develop an evidence-based, multidimensional taxonomy for pain, proposed five dimensions of pain. They include core criteria (i.e., specific diagnostic features of a pain condition), common features (i.e., features that further describe but are not required for diagnosis such as anatomical location and anticipated recovery), modulating factors/comorbidities (such as psychiatric conditions, medical conditions, and biopsychosocial factors), impact/functional consequences, and putative mechanisms.[38,39] The purpose of this taxonomy is to help further define and clarify various pain diagnoses for treatment and research, similar to the role of the *Diagnostic and Statistical Manual* (*DSM*) for psychiatry.[39]

Pain is commonly divided into acute and chronic pain—these are thought to differ in duration, function, and potentially in mechanism.[38,40] The American Academy of Pain Medicine defines acute pain as pain that is sudden in onset, time limited, and that typically serves a protective function, as it elicits behaviors to avoid potential or actual further injury.[38] Included in the core criteria for acute pain in the AAPT is an inciting event, as—unlike with chronic pain—there is usually a specific event that caused the pain.[38] Different time frames have been suggested for the duration of acute pain and the transition to chronic pain. An exact time cutoff may be artificial, given that acute and chronic pain may exist on a continuum.[38,41] But, at least for the International Classification of Diseases-11 (ICD-11) purposes, chronic pain is defined as pain lasting more than 3 months and further classified by etiology (i.e., cancer), pathophysiology (i.e., neuropathic vs. nociceptive), and location (i.e., abdominal, headache, etc.).[6]

There does seem to be a correlation between undertreated acute pain and the development of chronic pain which has further increased efforts to achieve adequate pain control in acute settings.[41,42] Outside of poorly treated acute pain, other risk factors for the development of chronic pain include poorly controlled postoperative pain, genetics, temperament, gender, as well as developmental and environmental factors such as trauma exposure, low socioeconomic status, obesity, low physical activity level, and other chronic, comorbid medical and psychiatric conditions.[5,43,44]

Given the subjective nature of both acute and chronic pain, measurements of pain tend to be based on patient-reported rating scales, such as the Visual Analog Scale, Verbal Analog Scale, Numerical Rating Scale, and Face Pain Scale, which have been validated in controlled settings.[45] However, the values resulting from these patient-reported scales should be considered in the context of the rest of the clinical information. For chronic pain especially, additional measures of physical and emotional functioning as well as the patient's overall sense of satisfaction and improvement with treatment have been suggested.[46]

CLINICAL INTERACTIONS BETWEEN PAIN AND SELECTED NEUROPSYCHIATRIC CONDITIONS

Pain and psychiatric disorders are frequently comorbid, and their relationship is complex and reciprocal: One condition may potentially cause or contribute to the development of the other, and vice versa.[47] Certainly, outcomes seem to improve if both conditions are diagnosed and treated.[47,48] The reason for the overlap between pain and psychiatric conditions is multifactorial, ranging from common neurochemical pathways (i.e., serotonin and norepinephrine) and shared symptoms (i.e., poor sleep secondary to pain vs. sleep disturbances due to

depression) to common personality/cognitive styles (i.e., catastrophic thinking in anxiety and pain).[49,50]

Pain and Depression

Perhaps the most commonly thought of comorbidity to pain is depression. Statistically, there have been wide ranges estimating that 10% to near 100% of patients with a chronic pain condition also have depression. This wide range owes to different criteria, methodology, and patient populations used,[49] though a more precise estimate using the Composite International Diagnostic Interview puts the comorbidity at 20%.[51] The wide variability in these values is due to different patient populations surveyed (i.e., community vs. clinic samples), different evaluation criteria used, different cutoffs for diagnostic criteria, and overlap in depression and pain symptoms—such as neurovegetative symptoms—which can skew screening results.[29,51,52] Regardless of the exact comorbidity, the rates of depression are higher in pain patients than in the general population. The mechanisms for this high comorbidity rate are not fully understood.[47,52] Several factors are likely involved, including the involvement of several shared neurotransmitters, the overlap of the neurocircuitry involved in both conditions, and shared cognitive and behavioral traits.[53] Serotonin, norepinephrine, GABA, opiate, and glutamate pathways are involved in both depression and pain, which may explain why some tricyclic antidepressants (TCAs) and serotonin and norepinephrine reuptake inhibitors (SNRIs) are effective in managing pain as well as depression.[53] Physical pain has both a sensory and an emotional dimension. The physical sensation of pain is primarily processed in the somatosensory cortices and the dorsal posterior insula. Neuroimaging studies have shown an overlap in several brain regions that are involved both in the emotional aspects of physical pain and in psychological pain or suffering—as is occurs in depression. These overlapping regions include the anterior insula, prefrontal cortex, anterior cingulate cortex, thalamus, amygdala, and hippocampus.[53] In terms of common psychological and behavioral features, catastrophic thinking, negative affect, poor sleep hygiene, and fear-based avoidance have been noted in both pain and depression, separately and concurrently.[53–55] The outcomes for patients with comorbid chronic pain and depression seem to be worse in terms of quality of life measures, functioning, and worsened symptoms outcomes for both conditions.[48] To this end, it is crucial to simultaneously address both conditions when treating these patients.[47]

Pain and Anxiety

Though it has received less attention than pain and depression, there is also a high prevalence of anxiety disorders in people with chronic pain. Estimates vary, but McWilliams et al.[51] found a 35% prevalence of anxiety disorders (this includes post-traumatic stress disorder [PTSD]) in chronic pain patients. As with depression, it seems plausible that the overlap may due to one condition predisposing an individual to the other, the two conditions mutually maintaining/exacerbating the other, and the presence of a common predisposition.[56]

The reported comorbidity rate of PTSD and chronic pain ranges widely from 0.69% to 50% depending on the type of chronic pain and patient population (i.e., Veterans) surveyed,[57] but even higher comorbidity has been reported.[58] As with anxiety and depression, potential explanations for the high comorbidity include common predisposing vulnerabilities, but there is also the possibility that the same event in an individual's life results in PTSD and chronic pain.[57]

The fear-avoidance model of chronic pain postulates that when pain is interpreted as threatening or even catastrophic, fear of pain develops which subsequently leads to avoidance behaviors, somatization, and subsequent disability and depression—which in turn maintain the pain.[59] This is largely similar to models described for the onset of anxiety disorders. This suggests that both anxiety and chronic pain may respond to common modalities of treatment such as cognitive-behavioral therapy.[59]

Personality Traits and Pain

There has been interest in looking for a "pain personality," that is, personality traits that seem to be common to chronic pain patients, as well as looking at specific personality disorders, such as borderline personality disorder, that may co-occur more often in chronic pain patients.[60,61] There does seem to be an increase in prevalence of personality disorders in chronic pain patients compared to the general population, and estimates have ranged from 31% to 81%.[61] Conrad et al.[62] reported that 41% of patients in a chronic pain sample had a comorbid personality disorder including paranoid, borderline, avoidant, and passive-aggressive personality disorders.

Certain personality traits may be commonly associated with chronic pain patients, including high scores in harm-avoidance and low scores in self-directedness.[62] On the Minnesota Multiphasic Personality Index (MMPI), patients with chronic pain may present with elevation in hypochondriasis and hysteria. However, these traits may be a consequence of chronic pain and not a part of the individual's premorbid personality.

Patients with trigeminal neuralgia and TMJ disorders also present with a high tendency to harm-avoidance and low scores in self-directedness. This could contribute to long-term disability and worse pain experience, due to pessimistic rumination about pain. Interestingly, low self-directedness seems to be a predictor of personality disorders in general, and in combination with high harm-avoidance is characteristic of cluster C personality disorders. Still, the directionality of this relationship is unclear: it is not certain if the personality disorder preceded the chronic pain condition or if the pain condition fostered a cluster C like personality.[60]

Pain and Suicide

Chronic pain is a risk factor for suicide and it is estimated that suicidal ideation and suicide are twice as likely in chronic pain patients than in the general population, making it important to screen for suicidal ideation in chronic pain patients and address modifiable risk factors.[63] Ratcliffe et al.[64] looked at suicidal ideation and suicide attempts in a national database and found that both were associated with having one or more chronic pain conditions (such as migraines, FM, back pain, or arthritis), and the risk of suicidal ideation and suicide attempts was increased even further if the patient had a comorbid psychiatric condition. Tang and Crane[65] identified several risk factors for suicidality in chronic pain patients including the type, intensity, and duration of the pain, insomnia due to pain, hopelessness and helplessness, catastrophizing and avoidance, desire to escape from pain, and deficits in problem solving. Racine et al.[66] found that the chronicity of pain had a higher association with suicidality than the intensity of the pain.

Pain and Malingering

The pain experience can be potentially exaggerated for secondary gain. Estimates of malingering with chronic pain for financial incentives range from 20% to 50%. There is much interest in developing tools to detect malingering in chronic pain, especially in regard to disability claims.[67] Current methods have focused on pain behavior signs (clinically observed verbal and nonverbal behavior), functional capacity evaluations (assessment of consistency of effort in testing), patient questionnaires (e.g., the Fake Bad Scale on the Minnesota Multiphasic Personality Inventory), and symptom validity tests (i.e., neurocognitive assessment to identify intentional poor performance) though there are limitations in all of these approaches.[68] Assessment of malingering in chronic pain is made difficult by several factors: chronic pain patients often have many nonspecific symptoms such as fatigue and poor sleep; physiologic mechanisms, such as pain amplification in the spinal cord, may cause a higher pain level than the expected for a given injury and the need to rule out other psychiatric conditions including factitious disorder, functional neurological symptom disorder and illness anxiety disorder.[68] Overall, a combination of different assessment tools should be used. Caution should be exercised in terms of doubting an individual's pain, especially without sufficient evidence of malingering, as this would likely result in poorer treatment outcomes.[68]

Pain and Insomnia

Sleep disturbances are very common in chronic pain patients, with an estimated comorbidity range of 50–80%, and a likely bidirectional relationship.[69] People with insomnia are more likely to develop chronic pain, though comorbid depression may also play a role in a subset of this group.[70] Finan et al.[71] found that while there is a likely bidirectional relationship, sleep seems to have a larger impact on pain, than pain on sleep. They report that poor sleep likely contributes to the propagation of pain by increasing pain sensitivity due to impairment of the pain modulation systems such as the endogenous opioid system. Patients with primary insomnia and those with insomnia related to pain share very similar phenomenological sleep features including the severity, long duration (i.e., greater than 90 months), and high frequency (i.e., 5–6 nights per week) of insomnia, extended sleep onset latency, and frequent awakenings, resulting in overall short total sleep time and quality.[72] Byers et al.[73] found that in patient with comorbid poor sleep and chronic pain, the cognitive and somatic levels of presleep arousal were the most important predictor of insomnia severity. Tang et al.[72] found considerable similarity between patients with primary insomnia and patients with chronic pain and insomnia including increased sleep anxiety and increased presleep somatic arousal, though the primary insomnia patients had more dysfunctional beliefs about their sleep and presleep cognitive arousal. They suggest that cognitive-behavioral therapy for insomnia (CBTi) may also be effective for patients with pain-related insomnia.[72] Please refer to Chapter 15, focused on sleep disorders, for further information about CBTi.

Pain and Cognition

Cognitive dysfunction in individuals with chronic pain commonly include difficulties in concentration, executive function, and information processing and occurs in at least 50% of patients with chronic pain.[74] Theories as to why cognitive dysfunction occurs in patients with chronic pain include the *limited resource theory*, which proposes that pain signals are preferentially processed over other information as pain represents a highly salient biological signal, and the *maladaptive plasticity theory*, which states that over time, persistent pain signals result in structural and neurotransmitter brain changes.[75] Secondary factors such as fatigue, insomnia, medications, and comorbid mood disorders also likely contribute to cognitive dysfunction in patients with chronic pain.[74] Intact cognition has a potentially beneficial role in endogenous pain modulation, and cognitive dysfunction may result in reduced effectiveness of CBT.[74] It is important to screen for cognitive dysfunction in chronic pain patients, provide psychoeducation, teach compensatory strategies and cognitive remediation, as part of a comprehensive pain treatment.[74] See Chapter 10, focused on psychosocial interventions, for possible adaptations to CBT when working with cognitively impaired individuals.

Pain and Addiction

The use of opioids to treat chronic pain has contributed to the current US opioid epidemic, raising much interest in evaluating their efficacy and effectiveness in treating chronic pain, how to predict which patients might become addicted, safe prescribing guidelines, and potential overlap in the neurobiology of pain and addictions.[76] Briefly, early small-scale studies in the 1980s and 1990s showed high efficacy and low rates of substance abuse for chronic pain patients who were prescribed opiates, prompting widespread use. However, larger-scale and longer-term studies show a much greater risk of opiate abuse (over 20% of patients) than estimated earlier, and a lack of efficacy of long-term opiates for chronic pain.[76] Chronic use of opiates results in tolerance, dependence, and hyperalgesia, as well as reductions in individuals' hedonic tone and ability to socialize, as seen in addictions.[76,77] Due to the commonalities between pain and addiction, neurobiological models of addiction are being used to better understand chronic pain.[77] Please refer to Chapter 14 for further discussion of the neuropsychiatry of addiction disorders.

SELECTED PAIN SYNDROMES AND DISORDERS

Fibromyalgia

Epidemiology

Estimates of the prevalence of FM vary but generally fall between 2% and 3% of the population, with a higher prevalence in women and an increasing prevalence with age.[78] Determining exact rates is difficult given changing diagnostic criteria as well as the varying assessment tools used in different settings.[79]

Pathophysiology

While the exact cause of FM and its associated symptoms have not been determined, it is generally considered to be a condition associated with central nervous system dysfunction.[40,80] Neurogenically derived inflammatory mechanisms occurring in the peripheral tissues, spinal cord, and brain, including a variety of neuropeptides, chemokines, and cytokines, have also been implicated.[81] The associated cognitive disturbances, sleep dysfunction, and systemic symptoms argue for this central nervous system implication. Multiple possible mechanisms have been proposed to explain FM symptoms. An inappropriate activation of the sympathetic nervous system and hyperactivity of the hypothalamic-pituitary-adrenal (HPA) axis have both been implicated.[82]

The role of genetic factors in the development and progression of FM is not certain. In general, such factors are thought to affect an individual's sensitivity to pain via increased transmission of nociception signals as well as by decreasing central inhibitory signals which would decrease response to a pain stimulus.[40] While multiple studies have been conducted to identify candidate genes that may be associated with individual development of chronic pain disorders, including FM, no clear causal genes have been identified.[40,83]

Clinical Presentation

FM is characterized by widespread, chronic pain. While the pain symptoms most typically manifest in muscles, joints can also be involved. Pain symptoms may be reported in specific locations described as trigger points although the reliability of using trigger points as part of the clinical diagnosis of FM has been questioned.[84,85] Specific concerns that have been raised include poor inter-rater reliability and lack of reliability when testing different muscle groups.[84] FM is frequently associated with neuropsychiatric manifestations including cognitive impairment and mood disturbances. The initial clinical presentation of FM often overlaps with other pain disorders as well as primary psychiatric illnesses. In addition to widespread pain, chronic fatigue is extremely common in patients with FM. Patients with FM often report waking from sleep not feeling rested and frequent disturbances in sleep overnight. The severity of fatigue does not seem to be correlated with the severity of cognitive impairment.[86] Cognitive impairments in FM are reported in multiple cognitive domains and most frequently include deficits in memory (both working memory and episodic memory), concentration, word fluency, and dual performance or task shifting.[87] These disturbances, especially inattentiveness, has been described as "fibrofog."[88] Studies found a strong correlation between cognitive complaints and concurrent anxiety and depressive symptoms.[86] Given this, it is important to consider ongoing psychiatric symptoms when evaluating cognitive complaints in patients with FM.

Walitt et al.[88] evaluated subjective cognitive appraisal, objective task performance, and brain activity during task performance in an effort to discriminate between how participants viewed their performance and the objective findings recorded.[88] This study demonstrated a disconnect between how participants with FM perceived their cognitive performance and the objective results of their performance, where "fibrofog" appeared to be better characterized by subjective rather than objective impairment. The exact cause of this discrepancy is not clear. Data related to brain activity during task performance did demonstrate a difference in task-related activation in fMRI between FM patients and controls. FM patients showed decreased activity in the right supra marginal gyrus/primary somatosensory cortex and posterior insula, right fusiform gyrus, right inferior parietal lobe, left inferior temporal cortex, and bilateral fusiform gyrus and occipital cortex.[88]

Diagnosis

The diagnosis of FM begins with a thorough gathering of history with an emphasis on history of pain symptoms. Physical examination involving inspection and palpation of affected areas helps to identify specific "trigger points" and to rule out other causes of symptoms including rheumatological conditions.[85,89]

In 1990 the American College of Rheumatology described classification criteria including the presence of widespread pain and identification of 11 of 18 possible defined tender points. The ACR revisited these findings in 2010 and sought to expand on those initial criteria and make the criteria more useful and practical in clinical settings. In that 2010 update, the authors used both the Widespread Pain Index (WPI) and Symptom Severity Scale (SS) in making a diagnosis. That update defined FM diagnostic criteria as a WPI of 7 or greater and a SS of 5 or more, or a WPI of 2–6 and SS of 9 or greater. Mood symptoms were not factored into the diagnosis due to concern that mood symptoms may be a result of FM symptoms and not a primary symptom of the illness itself.[90]

Treatment

Once a diagnosis of FM is made the patient should be provided with education explaining the diagnosis and setting expectations for treatment. Multidisciplinary and multimodal approaches to treatment should be pursued. Behavioral techniques to ensure appropriate sleep hygiene should be initiated, given potential for inadequate sleep to worsen cognitive complaints and fatigue. CBT may be helpful in restructuring maladaptive thinking patterns and providing patients with self-management tools, including mindfulness and relaxation techniques.[91]

Creating an exercise program has been found to be beneficial in managing FM symptoms over time. Multiple programs have been recommended including those focused on endurance training and strength training. Exercise programs may provide clinically significant effects on overall wellness, symptoms, and physical fitness.[92] Multiple specific exercise programs may be beneficial (varying in length of program; exercise intensity; and exercise goal, e.g., endurance or strength training) and should be tailored to individual patient preferences and capabilities.[92]

Medications for FM should be only used in conjunction with nonpharmacologic approaches. Antidepressants and anticonvulsants are typical first-line agents. Amitriptyline, duloxetine, and milnacipran are the best-studied antidepressants in this population.[93] These agents along with pregabalin are frequent initial treatment options.[93] Patient-specific factors should be considered when selecting an agent. Amitriptyline is preferred for patients with comorbid sleep disturbances while duloxetine may be preferable for patients with comorbid depressive disorder.[93] Studies suggest that only a minority of patients with FM find substantial symptom relief with medication options alone. Many other patients find little benefit from medication options or experience intolerable side effects while on the medication leading to medication discontinuation.[92]

Complex Regional Pain Syndrome

Epidemiology

CRPS is a chronic pain condition characterized by autonomic and inflammatory features.[94] It frequently develops following a specific injury to the body, most commonly a distal limb. The specific injuries that may give rise to CRPS vary. In retrospective studies the most common inciting events were fractures, followed by blunt traumatic injury, and surgical procedures.[95] While development following an injury is most common, CRPS may also develop spontaneously (with no identifiable incident event) in approximately 10% of patients.[96,97]

Recent population-based studies estimate that the incidence of CRPS ranges between 5.46 and 26.2 per 100,000 per year. Within the specific populations sampled the female:male ratio ranged between 3.4:1 and 4:1 with a higher incidence found in older women; one study specially found the 61–70-year-old female age group to have the highest incidence in the population sampled.[96,98]

Pathophysiology

The pathophysiology of CRPS is not yet fully understood. It is considered to be a multifactorial process involving both peripheral and central mechanisms. Contributions from various factors have been considered, including peripheral and central sensitization, autonomic changes, disturbances of the sympathetic nervous system, inflammatory and immune alterations, brain changes, and genetic and psychological factors.[94] Several theories have been proposed which may not be mutually exclusive. One suggests that CRPS is a disorder of inappropriate activity of the sympathetic nervous system.[95,99] The presence of sympathetic symptoms in CRPS and the benefits of interventions on this system support this theory. An alternative explanation suggests that local release of inflammatory cytokines following a traumatic injury may trigger peripheral nociceptors to increase release of neuropeptides leading to local edema, vascular changes, pain, and the trophic changes seen in CRPS.[95] Central maladaptive neuroplasticity has also been implicated in the pathogenesis of CRPS. Brain changes observed include a reduced representation of the affected limb in both primary and secondary somatosensory cortices and an increase in the somatosensory representation of the *unaffected* limb. Patients with CRPS showed reduced gray matter volume compared with healthy controls in brain regions underlying the affective component of pain (insula and cingulate cortex).[94,95,97,100]

Psychological factors have been repeatedly studied and suggested to play a role in CRPS pathophysiology, and this was the matter of controversy over the years due to conflicting findings. The conclusion from a comprehensive review and more recent, prospective studies suggests that there is no association between psychological factors and CRPS in terms of its causality.[101,102] However, psychological factors may have a role in modulating the syndrome's severity and functional impact.[103]

Clinical Presentation

The presentation of CRPS is often varied but generally includes pain, changes in sensation, changes in motor function, autonomic symptoms, and trophic changes in affected limbs. Patients with CRPS report pain in the extremities which is thought to be out of proportion to an inciting injury or lasting longer than would be expected for a given injury. Pain typically presents 4–6 weeks following an injury.[104] The quality of the pain varies and is frequently described as burning or stinging which may be constant or intermittent and exacerbated by movement, change in temperature, or stress.[100] Sensory changes include hyperalgesia, hyperesthesia, and allodynia.[100,104] Motor function may be affected by limited range of motion in a limb due to pain as well as decrease in strength in affected limbs. The autonomic changes in CRPS include changes in skin temperature, sweating, or edema.[100,104] Finally, trophic symptoms in CRPS include alterations in connective tissue with fibrosis of joints, skin atrophy, and changes in the growth rate of hair or nails.[100,103–105] It is important to evaluate for comorbid psychiatric comorbidities, as they may impact the individual's presentation and response to treatment.[103]

Diagnosis

The diagnostic criteria for CRPS has evolved over the last several decades as multiple consensus workshops attempted to formally describe this illness which historically was diagnosed using varying definitions.[100,106] Obtaining a thorough history and physical examination is crucial in making a diagnosis. A diagnosis of CRPS is considered in patients in which symptoms develop following a traumatic injury to a limb (although there may not be an identifiable injury); present symptoms can no longer be explained by the trauma temporally; and symptoms affect the distal extremity and extend past the trauma territory and the innervation territory where the trauma occurred.[104,106]

The diagnosis is made by applying the Budapest consensus criteria described by the IASP[94,100,104]:

- Continued pain which is considered to be disproportionate to inciting injury.
- At least one symptom in three of the following four categories:
  - Sensory: Reports of hyperesthesia and/or allodynia.
  - Vasomotor: Reports of temperature asymmetry and/or skin color changes and/or skin color asymmetry.
  - Sudomotor/Edema: Reports of edema and/or sweating changes and/or sweating asymmetry.

- Motor/Trophic: Reports of decreased range of motion and/or motor dysfunction (weakness, tremor, dystonia) and/or trophic changes (hair, nail, skin).
- Must display at least one sign at the time of evaluation in two or more of the following categories:
  - Sensory: Evidence of hyperalgesia (to pinprick) and/or allodynia (to light touch and/or temperature sensation and/or deep somatic pressure and/or joint movement).
  - Vasomotor: Evidence of temperature asymmetric (>1°C) and/or skin color changes and/or asymmetry.
  - Sudomotor/Edema: Evidence of edema and/or sweating changes and/or sweating asymmetry.
  - Motor/Trophic: Evidence of decreased range of motion and/or motor dysfunction (weakness, tremor, dystonia) and/or trophic changes (hair, nail, skin).
- There is no other diagnosis that better explains the signs and symptoms.

CRPS is further subdivided into two subtypes distinguished by the presence or absence of peripheral nerve injury. CRPS type I is diagnosed when there is no evidence of such injury while a diagnosis of CRPS type II is made when injury is present.[100,104]

Treatment

Nonpharmacological treatments should be emphasized when creating a treatment plan for CRPS, especially in the case of chronic CRPS, which is most likely to respond to an integrated multidisciplinary approach with medical, psychological, and physical and occupational therapy components. Physical and occupational therapy may decrease patient distress and improve overall function.[104] Patients should be educated that these therapies may increase pain symptoms temporarily but are ultimately important for recovery.[104]

With regards to pharmacological approaches, nonsteroidal anti-inflammatory drugs (NSAIDs) are typically a first-line choice for the treatment of CRPS. Specific agents to treat neuropathic pain may also provide benefit including anticonvulsants such as gabapentin and pregabalin as well as TCAs. Topical lidocaine or capsaicin may also provide benefit especially if combined with other agents. Glucocorticoids are typically more effective for acute CRPS.[107] Calcitonin has been studied in the treatment of CRPS but results thus far have been equivocal.[105,107] Bisphosphonates have been found to be effective but specific treatment strategies (e.g., optimum dose, frequency, and duration of treatment) are not clear.[107] Intrathecal baclofen and intravenous ketamine may be beneficial.[94]

SOMATIC SYMPTOM DISORDER WITH PREDOMINANT PAIN

Epidemiology

Somatic symptom disorder with predominant pain is the new designation for Pain Disorder in the *Diagnostic and Statistical Manual of Mental Disorders, Fifth Edition* (*DSM-5*).[108] Given the relatively recent introduction of the term somatic symptom disorder, information regarding its frequency is uncertain at this time. Most data used to determine the incidence and prevalence rates of SSD come from studies on its previous DSM nomenclature, Somatoform Disorders. Data suggest that the prevalence of somatoform disorders in the general population ranges between 4% and 6%.[109,110] This rate increases to near 17% in primary care patients.[111,112] The age of onset of SSD is unclear; studies suggest typical onset before 30 years old.[113] Females are more likely to have SSD with female:male ratios approaching 3:1.[113,114]

There is limited epidemiological information specifically about Pain Disorder, or SSD with predominant pain. A recent meta-analysis comprising 32 studies and more than 70,000 patients investigated the prevalence of somatoform disorders in primary care settings. It estimated the lifetime prevalence rate of chronic pain disorder as 9.2%.[115] Importantly, the presence of one medically unexplained and impairing pain symptom present for 6 months or longer was required for the diagnosis of chronic pain disorder. SSD with predominant pain does not require that symptoms be medically unexplained.[116,117] This discrepancy between the new and older diagnostic criteria adds to the difficulty of determining the exact prevalence rates of this relatively new diagnosis. A secondary analysis of nine population-based studies (total $n=28,377$) looked at reported burdensome symptoms,[114] without considering their status as "explained" or "unexplained." It found that the bothersome symptoms most commonly reported were back, joint, head, abdominal, and extremities pain. Other symptoms commonly reported were chest pain, dysuria, and diffuse pain. Pain symptoms were reported by 11–77% of respondents.[114] This study found that pain was the most frequent somatic symptom in patients diagnosed with SSD.

Pathophysiology

The pathophysiology of SSD, including SSD with predominant pain, is not fully known. It is considered to be the end result of the interaction of a complex set of biopsychosocial predisposing, precipitating, and perpetuating factors. SSD with predominant pain may develop following an organic injury leading to somatic symptoms and be further maintained by psychosocial factors including concurrent anxiety or depression, maladaptive coping, negative health habits, chronic stressors, over-attribution of physical symptoms to severe organic illness, and emotional distress related to symptoms.[118,119] One model suggests that somatosensory amplification, that is the tendency to experience benign bodily experiences as intrusive or noxious, leads to dysfunction in how an individual perceives somatic symptoms.[120] There are several known risk factors for the development of SSD. They include exposure to abnormal levels of illness in the family; comorbid psychiatric illness including depression and anxiety; and history of significant physical illness including chronic pain symptoms. A history of trauma including physical, emotional, or sexual abuse has been shown to be a strong risk factor for developing somatic disorders. This risk factor persists throughout life, according to a recent meta-analysis investigating the correlation between sexual abuse and lifetime diagnosis of SSD.[121,122]

Clinical Presentation

SSD with pain presents with a chronic history of one or more somatic symptoms that predominantly involve pain, and associated psychological distress related to these symptoms. This distress may take the form of excessive thoughts, behaviors, or anxiety related to the experienced pain. Somatic symptoms associated with SSD may include gastrointestinal symptoms (nausea, vomiting, diarrhea), neurologic symptoms (changes in sensation, paralysis), cardiopulmonary symptoms (palpitations, chest pain), and reproductive organ symptoms (erectile dysfunction).[114] As previously discussed, the most common pain symptoms reported include pain in the back, head, joints, abdomen, and extremities. Patients may also report dysuria, and diffuse pain.[114] Please see Chapter 13 "Functional Neurological Symptom Disorder" in this textbook, for a review of that disorder, which presents with altered voluntary motor or sensory function. SSD with predominant pain and FNSD are grouped, together with other disorders, in the "Somatic Symptom and Related Disorders" chapter in *DSM-5*. They appeared as *Pain Disorder* and *Conversion Disorder*, respectively, in the Somatoform Disorders chapter of *DSM-IV-TR*.

Assessment and Diagnosis

Prior to making a diagnosis of SSD with predominant pain it is important to investigate for other potential causes of the patient's pain symptoms. It is recommended that evidence-based approaches be used in this workup. The specifics of the medical evaluation and the ancillary tests required will vary depending on the presentation (e.g., low back pain vs. dysuria). While the evaluation should be thorough, it is important to consider that overly aggressive testing and examination may expose the patient to iatrogenesis and may create an expectation that a general medical condition will be found to explain the presenting symptoms.[123] As part of the evaluation, it is important to screen for psychiatric comorbidities, and for potential predisposing, precipitating, and perpetuating biopsychosocial risk factors.

According to the *DSM-5*, a diagnosis of SSD is made when one or more somatic symptoms that are distressing or result in significant disruption of daily life are present. The individual presents with excessive thoughts, feelings, and/or behaviors related to the somatic symptoms, and the state of being symptomatic is persistent. Somatic symptoms with pain, and associated psychosocial symptoms, must be present for 6 months to formally make the diagnosis. In SSD with predominant pain, the individual is particularly concerned about symptoms of pain that cause distress and functional impairment, and appear to be clearly in excess with respect to any physiological component. SSD with predominant pain can be further classified according to its current severity. Considering the (a) excessive thoughts about pain, (b) the emotional response—anxiety about pain, and (c) the excessive amount of time and energy devoted to physical symptoms, as follows:

- Mild—Only one feature is present (e.g., only excessive thoughts about pain).
- Moderate—Two or more of the features are present (e.g., both persistent thoughts and severe anxiety).
- Severe—Two or more of the features are present, plus the patient manifests either multiple somatic complaints, or one very severe somatic symptom.

Of note, a diagnosis of SDD does not require that the distressing symptoms, including pain symptoms, be without clear medical explanation.[116,117] The diagnosis of SDD may be found concurrently with other medical conditions, including a condition that is expected to cause the reported pain. Additionally, the presence of medically unexplained symptoms alone is not sufficient to diagnosis SDD.[124] The diagnosis requires that the patient be under significant distress with associated change in thoughts, feelings, and behaviors related to these symptoms.[124]

Treatment

Establishing a strong therapeutic alliance is helpful in engaging patients in treatment. Assessment for comorbid psychiatric illness or general medical illnesses is important to allow for management of these contributing factors. Exploration of other psychosocial stressors will also help guide and inform treatment.[119,125]

CASE VIGNETTE 31.1

Mrs. K is a 57-year-old married female referred to neuropsychiatric clinic by her multiple sclerosis (MS) neurologist for assessment of depression and chronic pain. The referring provider expressed concern that her affective state was impacting her complaints of pain, which she was misattributing to MS-related spasticity—resulting in a request for more medications to treat her physical pain.

Her major depressive episode started more than a year prior to assessment. She identified the death of her dog and the health decline and subsequent death of her father as precipitating factors. She presented with decreased interest, pleasure, energy, activity, appetite, sleep, and concentration. Her mood was depressed. She felt like a failure and worthless, as she was not able to take care of the house and her husband. She had suicidal thoughts without intent or plan. She had experienced mild depression in the past—it had never reached the current severity.

She also had chronic problems with pain. She presented with diffuse body pain for the past year and a half, involving arms and legs muscles, and multiple joints. She became more and more limited because of the pain. She tried a variety of medications without much benefit. She stated that at times her pain was 10/10. She was frustrated by the lack of resolution of her pain and its impact on her ability to function. At times, even shaking someone's hand was very painful, and she tried to avoid it. She had previous musculoskeletal problems over the years, particularly in her shoulders, and had undergone three shoulder surgeries in her right shoulder and one on the left, but was always able to recover. She also had a history of carpal tunnel syndrome on the left and was status post carpal tunnel release. She acknowledged the possible reciprocal influence between pain and depression, making each other worse. However, there was no question in her mind about the reality of her physical pain as a separate, nonpsychiatric entity that required medical diagnosis and treatment with medication—not at all related to her psychosocial stressors and only slightly, and perhaps, influenced by her emotional state. She presented with chronic fatigue and cognitive complaints, possibly with contributions from MS and her other medical problems, major depression, and her medications.

Her medical history included MS, question of polymyalgia rheumatica (PMR), question of fibromyalgia, sacroiliac joint problems, and history of chronic steroid use for her PMR.

She was on a complex medication regimen including several agents with potential CNS side effects: duloxetine 120 mg/day, amantadine 100 mg bid, cyclobenzaprine 5 mg qhs for spasticity, lorazepam 0.5 mg bid, diazepam 10 mg nightly, tramadol 50 mg bid, among other agents.

She had been taking duloxetine for about a year, prescribed by her primary care physician. It had been partially helpful for her pain and depression initially, but no longer seemed to be helping.

She was diagnosed as presenting with a Major Depression and Pain Disorder (DSM-IV-TR nomenclature for Somatic Symptom Disorder with predominant pain). Her treatment involved coordination with her primary care physician and neurologist, including centralization of her prescriptions within one medical system, gradual work on simplifying her medication regimen with reduction of the CNS depressants, and replacement of duloxetine with venlafaxine. She started psychotherapy. In addition to the losses she discussed initially, two important other factors were elicited as fundamental over the course of treatment: a long-term pattern of emotional abuse and neglect by her husband—with a complex marital dynamic, as in turn he was overwhelmed by her difficulties and was ignoring her as a way to cope with her issues—and a loss in her status in the family and mother role, as her children were young adults who left the house. Psychotherapeutic work included components of increasing insight about the above-mentioned factors and their influence on her emotions, thinking, and behavior; behavioral activation; marital counseling. Positive treatment outcomes included improvement of her depression, physical pain, and functional status; simplification of her medication list; improvement in the communication patterns between Mrs. K and her husband; increased insight about the impact of emotional factors in her physical symptoms; decreased frequency of medication-seeking behaviors from her providers; and decreased reliance on medications for symptom management.

When creating a treatment plan, patients should be educated regarding the diagnosis of SSD with predominant pain and expectations for management be outlined. Frequent, scheduled visits with primary care physicians help ensure patients feel their complaints are heard by providers. Brief physical examinations should be performed during visits, but invasive studies and procedures be limited to prevent iatrogenesis.

Referrals to specialists should also be made with caution to avoid alienating patients, creating an expectation that a general medical illness will be found to explain symptoms, and to avoid further iatrogenesis.[112,119,123] Referrals to psychiatric consultants should be integrated with primary care as much as possible to avoid patients feeling invalidated or abandoned by their primary providers.

An interdisciplinary approach with a focus on functional restoration and psychotherapy may be helpful.[126] Physical and occupational therapists may assist patients' work on rehabilitation goals, with graded steps and positive reinforcement of progress. Combined with psychotherapy, these rehabilitation strategies may help reshape patient's illness perceptions and reduce its functional impact. CBT has been demonstrated to be effective in patients with multiple somatic complaints whether or not organic illness has been identified. Antidepressants may be useful in treating mood and anxiety disorders and certain agents may be helpful in managing pain symptoms as well. Among antidepressants venlafaxine and duloxetine have been found to be the most effective especially with management of neuropathic pain.[119]

ASSESSMENT AND DIFFERENTIAL DIAGNOSIS OF PAIN

As with other clinical evaluations, the assessment of pain begins with a thorough gathering of history. A patient's self-report is the gold standard in assessing pain and cannot be substituted completely by objective findings or reports of proxy observers (e.g., clinical staff, family, etc.).[127] However, caution should be exercised and clinical judgment, as always, is paramount, as the patient's self-report may be colored by factors such as depression or substance abuse difficulties. Physiologic findings including heart rate, respiratory rate, blood pressure, palmar sweating, and transcutaneous oxygen and carbon dioxide pressures can be employed as a surrogate for assessing a patient's pain symptoms in specific circumstances,[128] but a lack of change in these areas does not mean that pain is not present. Additionally, the usefulness of these findings is limited to acute pain settings and not an appropriate gauge for chronic symptoms.

While a complete review of the elements to consider during a pain assessment is outside the scope of this chapter, there are basic principles to apply. During the interview phase of the assessment it is important to evaluate the onset and timing of symptoms, localization, aggravating and alleviating factors, quality and severity of the pain, and any associated signs and symptoms. Obtaining an initial assessment of pain prior to a procedure or change in treatment plan is crucial to monitor for post-procedural changes and to assess the effectiveness of a treatment plan.[129]

Multiple studies support employing a biopsychosocial model to best understand a patient's pain symptoms.[130] Given this, care must be taken to assess for a history of psychiatric illnesses and substance use disorders, as well as cultural, religious, and other personal factors that may impact the patient's pain perception, as well as treatment preference and adherence. These factors have been implicated both, in the perception of acute pain and in the progression from acute to chronic pain.[131,132] Eliciting patients' understanding about their pain symptoms and their expectations can help set appropriate expectations when creating a treatment plan.

While a patient's own description cannot be replaced, rating scales are useful to further characterize and quantify pain symptoms, to monitor symptoms over time, and to assess response to treatment. These tools must find a balance between thoroughness and brevity; brief assessments run the risk of oversimplifying a complex presentation while lengthy tools may limit their practical utility in clinical settings. Unidimensional tools, including the Numeric Rating Scale (NRS) promoted by the Veterans Health Administration's "Pain as the Fifth Vital Sign Toolkit" have not been found to improve pain outcomes and studies recommend against their use as the sole tool when creating a treatment plan.[133,134]

Multimodal rating scales may seek to answer more specific questions regarding a patient's presentation. Assessments may help identify the presence of pain and specific subtypes of pain including nociceptive and neuropathic pain, assess symptoms over time to monitor disease progression or treatment efficacy, and identify patients who are at risk for transitioning from acute pain to chronic pain. Multiple scales aim to assess for the presence of neuropathic pain including the Leeds Assessment of Neuropathic Symptoms and Signs (LANSS), the Neuropathic Pain Diagnostic Questionnaire (DN4), PainDETECT, the Neuropathic Pain Questionnaire (NPQ), and the ID Pain tool. The ID Pain tool may be useful to assess for the presence or absence of neuropathic pain in primary care setting, and the Neuropathic Pain Scale (NPS) and Neuropathic Pain Symptom Inventory (NPSI) may help characterize pain and measure individual response to treatment.[135] The Brief Pain Inventory (BPI) may be useful to monitor how pain impacts a patient's daily life and for ongoing monitoring of the effectiveness of a treatment plan when identifying and managing chronic pain in primary care settings.[136] Predicting those patients with acute pain who will go on to have chronic pain is challenging. For example with regards to low back pain, the STarT Back Tool (SBT) is a validated assessment that can be helpful to assess for the risk of this progression.[136,137] See Box 31-1 to review this scale's items. This nine-question tool includes five psychosocial subscale items: 1, 4, 7, 8, and 9. Patients scoring greater than or equal to 4 on this psychosocial subscale are categorized into the high-risk group for progression to chronic pain—this emphasizes the importance of psychosocial indicators when evaluating a patient's prognosis.[137] A recent review study found SBT scores at intake to be predictive of a patient's disability level 6 months later.[138] Additionally, SBT scores following 4 weeks of physical therapy were helpful in predicting disability scores 6 months later.[128]

Special considerations must be made in the assessment of pain in certain populations. Children may not cooperate with a lengthy questionnaire or all aspects of a physical exam so tools such as the Pediatric Pain Questionnaire (PPQ) incorporate input from the patient's parents and the medical team. The Adolescent Pediatric Pain Tool (APPT) may be more widely used than the PPQ and can be employed in multiple settings (e.g., schools, clinics, inpatient units).[135] In patients with cognitive dysfunction it can be challenging to obtain an accurate self-report, but this should still be attempted prior to enlisting the aid of proxy observers. Studies demonstrate that these observers may be able to accurately assess for the presence of pain but are less reliable when tasked with quantifying the severity of pain.[127]

When assessing pain, it is also important to consider possible psychiatric comorbidity. While it is acknowledged that biopsychosocial factors are important in evaluating pain and some assessment tools such as SBT incorporate psychosocial questions, not all pain assessment tools do so. It is also important to keep in mind the overlap of some symptoms between chronic pain and psychiatric conditions such as poor sleep, fatigue, and poor concentration which might cause a higher pain score when in fact the patient has a comorbid psychiatric condition such as depression. Furthermore, as pain is predominantly subjective, rating scales are potentially easy to exaggerate in the case of malingering.

TREATMENT OF PAIN

The treatment of pain is a vast topic, as the interventions will vary depending upon the type of pain—for example, acute versus chronic—its underlying cause, and other variables. For example, much has been written about managing postoperative pain and guidelines are frequently reviewed.[139] Given the large scope of this topic, we will briefly discuss here the pharmacologic and nonpharmacologic treatments of chronic pain, especially in the setting of its comorbidity with other psychiatric conditions.

INTERDISCIPLINARY APPROACH

As with psychiatric treatment, the management of pain is often more effective when addressed with an interdisciplinary team. Given the complexity of chronic pain (psychiatric comorbidity, social stressors, psychological and medical factors), frequent lack of full resolution of symptoms with medications, and potential benefits of nonpharmacological interventions (CBT, physical therapy), an interdisciplinary team approach is more likely to be effective.[5,140] An interdisciplinary team could include a pain physician, a nurse, a physical therapist, a psychologist, an occupational therapist, and alternative medicine practitioners.[5,140] Depending on the degree, severity, and complexity of the patient's clinical presentation, a psychiatrist may provide a consultation or follow the patient longitudinally in an integrated manner with the rest of the team. In addition to pain medication management, a pain physician can arrange invasive interventions including nerve blocks and stimulation therapies. Nerve blocks can be used for both diagnostic (i.e., help distinguish the cause of pain) and therapeutic purposes.[141] Some of the most common therapeutic nerve blocks include epidural steroid injections, facet joint nerve blocks, sympathetic blocks (i.e., celiac plexus, superior hypogastric), and intercostal and occipital nerve blocks.[141] Stimulation therapies are described further below. Unfortunately, interdisciplinary pain centers are not widely available in the United States for several reasons, including inconsistency in defining an interdisciplinary center, shortage of specialized professionals, and third-party payer systems that view interdisciplinary centers as too costly up front.[140]

PHARMACOLOGIC TREATMENT OF PAIN

Nonsteroidal Anti-Inflammatory Drugs and Acetaminophen

NSAIDs and acetaminophen are common, often over the counter, pain medications used for both acute and chronic pain conditions which are generally considered safe and effective.[142] Over the counter NSAIDs, which act by inhibiting COX-2, include aspirin, ibuprofen, and naproxen.[142]

Opiates

The use of opiates for acute pain is well established.[139] Mu, kappa, and delta opioid receptors reside in the periphery, the dorsal root ganglion, the spinal cord, and in supraspinal regions and are associated with pain modulation. However, their effectiveness for chronic pain that is not cancer related is much less clear.[143] Current meta-analyses suggest that there is insufficient evidence for their use for chronic non-cancer pain in terms of quality of life, function, and pain control outcomes, and that there is increased risk of harm in terms of overdose, dependence, opiate abuse, fractures, and myocardial infarction; however, in many of these areas, the strength of the findings were low.[143] Overall, if opiates are to be used to treat non-cancer chronic pain, patients must be selected and monitored carefully.[144] Patients should be screened for risk of substance abuse and the risks of chronic opiates for that patient should be weighed against potential benefits. There should be an ongoing conversation with the patient around the risks and benefits as well as the goals, expectations, and alternatives to long-term opiates.[144] Patients who elect to start long-term opiates for chronic pain should be then carefully monitored in terms of pain level, functionality, adverse events, and therapeutic goals. Urine drug screens may have a role, especially in those patients at risk for substance abuse.[144]

Tricyclic Antidepressants

TCAs including amitriptyline, nortriptyline, and desipramine have all been used to treat chronic pain conditions such as diabetic neuropathy, migraine headaches, and FM.[145] The dose range for chronic pain is typically lower than what is necessary to treat depression.[145]

Serotonin Norepinephrine Reuptake Inhibitors

SNRIs such as duloxetine and venlafaxine are effective for treating chronic pain, particularly neuropathic pain and FM, as well as anxiety and depression.[145,146] They are particularly helpful for those patients with comorbid chronic pain and depression.[48]

Anticonvulsants/Mood Stabilizers

Several antiepileptic medications are useful for treating pain including valproic acid to reduce migraine frequency, and carbamazepine for trigeminal neuralgia.[145] Gabapentin and pregabalin have been FDA approved for the treatment of diabetic neuropathic pain, postherpetic neuralgia, and FM.[145] However,

Goodman and Brett[147] note an increasing trend of prescribing gabapentin and pregabalin for all types of pain despite little evidence for their efficacy for off-label use. They suggest this trend shows providers' attempts to use alternatives to opiate medications for pain. Lithium has been used to treat cluster headaches but otherwise has limited use in pain.[145]

Ketamine

Ketamine is an NMDA antagonist anesthetic and analgesic agent that has been studied for cancer-related and non-cancer-related chronic pain. While there is some evidence of efficacy, further studies and clarification on the dose regimen and target patient population and diagnosis are needed. In addition, psychedelic side effects need to be monitored.[148,149] Ketamine is also currently being studied and used to treat major depression, typically at lower doses and shorter duration than when used to treat chronic pain.[150]

Cannabis

About 45–80% of patients seeking medical cannabis are doing so for pain. Tetrahydrocannabinol (THC) and CBD are the two cannabinoids of most medical relevance. THC is a psychoactive compound, and CBD is considered, with the information available at this point, to have less neuropsychiatric side effects. Studies have included either a combination of THC and CBD in varying ratios or stand-alone THC or CBD. The ideal ratio or doses for different disorders are not yet clear.[151]

There is some evidence supporting the use of cannabis for chronic neuropathic pain[152,153] but insufficient evidence in most other pain populations.[152] Evidence seems to support the use of cannabis for spasticity and symptoms of pain, excluding central neuropathic pain, in patients with multiple sclerosis (MS).[154,155] The use of cannabis may increase the risk for the development or worsening of psychotic disorders, cognitive dysfunction, anxiety disorders, mood disorders, and addiction disorders.[152,153,155] Cannabis preparations may also worsen physical symptoms, such as dizziness, fatigue, somnolence, and loss of balance.[156] However, ongoing research suggests that cannabidiol (CBD) may reduce psychiatric symptoms, for instance, of anxiety disorders. Further randomized controlled studies with larger samples are needed to confirm these preliminary observations.[157] Medical cannabinoids primarily exist in three forms: oral, oromucosal, and nasal spray. Oral versions may present a more favorable benefit to side-effects ratio, but this needs further confirmation.[154,158] In sum, data regarding the use of cannabis for treatment of chronic pain are still limited, and more research into the mechanisms of cannabis and its potential uses is needed.[159]

PSYCHOTHERAPY

CBT is both a safe and effective treatment for chronic pain.[160] While there is no single standard protocol for CBT for chronic pain, the focus is usually on the patient's beliefs about pain and the impact on behavior, as well as behavioral activation and cognitive restructuring.[160,161] While an effective treatment, many patients with chronic pain do not have access to CBT, and there is a need for more research on the most effective content and delivery for CBT.[161] Acceptance and commitment therapy (ACT) has also been studied for the use in chronic pain; it differs from CBT in that it focuses on the acceptance of pain rather than controlling the pain, mindfulness, and commitment to the individual's personal values.[162] Veehof et al.[162] in a meta-analysis of ACT found it to be about as effective as CBT for chronic pain, but more studies are needed.[162]

PHYSICAL ACTIVITY

Pain often results in patients limiting their physical activity due to discomfort and fear of worsening the pain. However, physical activity is unlikely to cause harm to chronic pain patients and can reduce pain and improve physical function.[163] Furthermore, physical activity is beneficial for reducing other chronic medical conditions that can be comorbid with chronic pain (i.e., diabetes, heart disease) as well as for mood, sleep, and cognitive function.[164] The sample size for most studies has been small and few had long-term follow up—further research is needed to strengthen this recommendation as well as to provide more specific recommendations about the type of physical activity and specific programs for different pain conditions.[163]

COMPLEMENTARY AND ALTERNATIVE MEDICINE (CAM)

CAM is becoming more popular in the United States—for instance, about 34% of the US adult population sought a CAM treatment in 2012.[165] The estimates of CAM use are even higher in patients with chronic conditions such as chronic pain, so it is important for providers to be aware and knowledgeable of these options.[166] Some common CAM therapies for chronic pain include massage, acupuncture, herbal and dietary supplements (i.e., capsaicinoids, devil's claw, willow bark extract), mind-body therapies (i.e., yoga, mindfulness, biofeedback), and whole-body cryotherapy.[166,167] Aside from herbal and dietary supplements, which have the potential to cause side effects and interact with conventional medications, CAM therapies for chronic pain are mostly safe and have some evidence for being helpful to chronic pain patients—in particular acupuncture, mind-body therapies, and massage.[166,167]

STIMULATION THERAPIES

Nerve stimulation therapies including TENS, spinal cord stimulation (SCS), deep brain stimulation (DBS), repetitive transcranial magnetic stimulation (rTMS), transcranial direct electrical stimulation (tDCS), and transcranial alternating current stimulation (tACS) at alpha frequency are currently being studied and used to treat chronic pain. The current evidence supporting their use is weak, and all warrant further investigation.[168-170] Briefly, TENS uses a small battery-powered device to deliver low-dose current through the skin to stimulate nerves and relieve pain. The stimulus can be varied in terms of duration and intensity and has been used for many pain conditions including diabetic neuropathy, post-stroke pain, cancer-related pain, surgical- or trauma-related nerve pain, and spinal cord injury. In a systematic review, Gibson et al.[168] found low-quality evidence that TENS is more effective at relieving pain than sham TENS and advised further study to clarify patient populations that TENS could help improve study design and outcome measures. SCS and DBS, while generally considered safe, are more invasive procedures, as stimulators are implanted in the central nervous system and therefore carry the risk of hardware malfunction (i.e., leads moving or breaking) and infection.[169] SCS delivers direct electric stimulation to the spinal cord to potentially suppress nerve hyperexcitability and to substitute paresthesias in the area of the pain; there is a weak recommendation for its use combined with conventional treatment.[169] DBS has been tried in various regions of the brain including the diencephalic periventricular gray area, the mesencephalic PAG area, and the thalamus, but the evidence for its efficacy is low quality and inconclusive at this time.[169] rTMS is a noninvasive and relatively safe procedure that uses magnetic pulses to stimulate the brain. Most studies have focused on stimulating the primary motor cortex for pain control, but some others stimulated the dorsolateral prefrontal cortex; there is a weak recommendation for the use of rTMS targeting the primary motor cortex to address neuropathic pain and FM.[169] tDCS is also a noninvasive and safe procedure; it uses weak electrical currents on the skin to modulate neuronal excitability by depolarizing or hyperpolarizing brain neurons. Currently the data are inconclusive as to its efficacy for management of pain disorders.[169] tACS is a noninvasive procedure that has been studied as a method to modify pain perception. Alpha activity, a type of oscillatory neural activity (8–13 Hz) has been implicated in pain experience, where higher alpha activity before a painful stimulus has been associated with lower reported pain.[170] Alpha tACS uses external electrodes placed on the scalp, over the somatosensory region, to modulate alpha activity.[170] A recent study exploring the effects of alpha tACS on the experience of pain showed that pain experience was significantly lower during alpha tACS compared with sham stimulation.[170] While this study had substantial limitations, alpha tACS might hold therapeutic promise for pain.

Summary and Key Points

- Chronic pain affects about 20% of the American adult population and costs the United States 560–635 billion dollars per year in health care costs and lost productivity.
- Pain is a complex physiological manifestation crucial to the survival and preservation of biological systems. Pain neuronal pathways can be modulated through both bottom-up and top-down mechanisms at the levels of the peripheral and central nervous systems.
- Pain perception differs across animal models and across individuals—depending on complex factors such as their neurobiological makeup, mood, memory, and prior experience.
- The comorbidity between pain and psychiatric conditions such as depression, anxiety, and insomnia is very common,

and both conditions need to be addressed as one can exacerbate the other.

■ There is overlap in the pathology of chronic pain and psychiatric comorbidities in terms of the neurotransmitters and neural circuitry involved, and the cognitive-emotional-behavioral characteristics of patients suffering from these conditions.

■ Treatment of chronic pain is ideally delivered through a multidisciplinary team approach. Therapeutic interventions include pharmacotherapy—which has significant overlap with pharmacotherapy of psychiatric conditions—and non-pharmacological management including psychotherapy, physical therapy, interventional strategies such as nerve blocks and stimulation therapies, and complementary and alternative medicine approaches.

Multiple Choice Questions

1. Possible reasons for the high comorbidity of chronic pain and depression include:
   a. Same neurotransmitters involved in both conditions, with acetylcholine having a fundamental role
   b. Shared cognitive patterns, including catastrophic thinking
   c. Shared neuropathways mostly modulated via the parietal-cerebellar-putamen circuit
   d. Shared behavioral styles, including a proactive, problem-solving stance when facing stressors
   e. Shared emotional styles, including a temperamental predisposition toward gratitude

2. Which option best describes the use of opiates to treat pain?
   a. Used to treat acute pain and chronic pain in the majority of patients
   b. Used to treat acute pain only
   c. Used to treat acute pain and to manage chronic pain only in a carefully selected and monitored minority of patients with this condition
   d. Used to treat acute pain and to manage chronic pain in a carefully selected and monitored majority of patients with this condition
   e. Used to treat chronic pain only

3. Which of the following is not an aspect of effective treatment of fibromyalgia?
   a. Patient education regarding the diagnosis
   b. Cognitive-behavioral therapy
   c. Chronic short-acting opioids
   d. Encouragement of appropriate sleep hygiene
   e. Exercise programs tailored to individual patient preferences

4. Which of the following symptoms is not typically found in patients with complex regional pain syndrome?
   a. Sensory disturbances such as hyperesthesia or allodynia
   b. Increased diaphoresis
   c. Changes in rate of nail growth
   d. Changes in bowel habits
   e. Limb pain exacerbated by movement

Multiple Choice Answers

1. Answer: b
The high comorbidity of depression and chronic pain is likely due to the overlap in cognitive-emotional-behavioral styles, including catastrophic thinking, negative affect, poor sleep hygiene, and fear-based avoidant behaviors; the overlap in neurotransmitters involved in pain and depression including serotonin, glutamate, GABA, and norepinephrine; and common brain areas involved including anterior insula, prefrontal cortex, anterior cingulate cortex, thalamus, amygdala, and hippocampus.

2. Answer: c
The use of opiates to address acute pain is well established. However, the use of opiates in the treatment of chronic pain is controversial. There is some evidence that for carefully selected patients, opiates maybe helpful for long-term pain management. However, these patients need to be carefully monitored for efficacy of treatment and risk of addiction/misuse, and they should be offered alternative treatments to opiates.

3. Answer: c
Multidisciplinary approaches to the treatment of fibromyalgia are considered to be most effective and may include CBT and work with physical therapists. Patients should be educated regarding their diagnosis to enhance their investment in treatment and be encouraged to maintain effective sleep hygiene in an effort to minimize cognitive symptoms. Opiates are not typically first-line treatments for fibromyalgia. Tricyclic antidepressants and anticonvulsants are generally considered to be first-line agents.

4. Answer: d
Complex regional pain syndrome (CRPS) is associated with symptoms in multiple categories including sensory disturbances; vasomotor changes (e.g., temperature asymmetry); sudomotor changes and edema; motor symptoms including decreased range of motion; and trophic changes including changes in rate of hair or nail growth. Changes in bowel habits are not included in the diagnostic criteria for CRPS and are not a typical part of initial presentation.

References

1. Merskey H, Albe-Fessard DG, Bonica JJ, et al. Pain terms: a list with definitions and notes on usage. *Pain.* 1979;6:247-252.

2. Elman I, Zubieta JK, Borsook D. The missing P in psychiatric training. *Arch Gen Psychiatry.* 2011;68(1):12-20.

3. Anand KJS, Craig KD. New perspectives on the definition of pain. *Pain.* 1996;67:3-6.

4. Williams A, Craig KD. Updating the definition of pain. *Pain.* 2016;157:2420-2423.

5. Pizzo PA, Clark NM, Carter-Pokras O; Institute of Medicine (US) Committee on Advancing Pain Research, Care, and Education. *Relieving Pain in America: A Blueprint for Transforming Prevention, Care, Education, and Research.* Washington, DC: The National Academies Press; 2011.

6. Treede RD, Rief W, Barke A, et al. A classification of chronic pain for ICD-11. *Pain.* 2015;156:1003-1007.

7. Gaskin DJ, Richard P. The economic cost of pain in the United States. *Pain.* 2012;8:715-724.

8. Raja SNMD, Meyer RAMS, Campbell JNMD. Peripheral mechanisms of somatic pain. *Anesthesiology.* 1988;68(4):571-590.

9. Cavalli E, Mammana S, Nicoletti F, Bramanti P, Mazzon E. The neuropathic pain: an overview of the current treatment and future therapeutic approaches. *Int J Immunopathol Pharmacol.* 2019;33:2058738419838383.

10. Liu M, Oh U, Wood JN. From transduction to pain sensation: defining genes, cells, and circuits. *Pain.* 2011;152(3 suppl):S16-S19.

11. Dubin AE, Patapoutian A. Nociceptors: the sensors of the pain pathway. *J Clin Invest.* 2010;120(11):3760-3772.

12. Ottestad E, Angst MS. Chapter 14—Nociceptive physiology. In: Hemmings HC, Egan TD, eds. *Pharmacology and Physiology for Anesthesia.* Philadelphia, PA: W.B. Saunders; 2013:235-252.

13. Viana F. Nociceptors: thermal allodynia and thermal pain. *Handb Clin Neurol.* 2018;156:103-119.

14. Caterina MJ, Pang Z. TRP: channels in skin biology and pathophysiology. *Pharmaceuticals (Basel).* 2016;9(4):1-28.

15. Khan A, Khan S, Kim YS. Insight of pain modulation: nociceptors sensitization and therapeutic targets. *Curr Drug Targets.* 2019;20(7):775-788.

16. Lin A-H, Liu M-H, Ko H-K, Perng D-W, Lee T-S, Kou YR. Menthol cigarette smoke induces more severe lung inflammation than non-menthol cigarette smoke does in mice with subchronic exposure—role of TRPM8. *Front Physiol.* 2018;9:1817.

17. Woolf CJ, Fitzgerald M. Somatotopic organization of cutaneous afferent terminals and dorsal horn neuronal receptive fields in the superficial and deep laminae of the rat lumbar spinal cord. *J Comp Neurol.* 1986;251(4):517-531.

18. Light AR, Perl ER. Differential termination of large-diameter and small-diameter primary afferent fibers in the spinal dorsal gray matter as indicated by labeling with horseradish peroxidase. *Neurosci Lett.* 1977;6(1):59-63.

19. Hanai F. C fiber responses of wide dynamic range neurons in the spinal dorsal horn. *Clin Orthop.* 1998;(349):256-267.

20. Svendsen F, Hole K, Tjølsen A. Long-term potentiation in single wide dynamic range neurons induced by noxious stimulation in intact and spinalized rats. In: *Progress in Brain Research.* Vol 129. Elsevier; 2000:153-161. Available at http://www.sciencedirect.com/science/article/pii/S0079612300290110. Accessed March 25, 2019.

21. Al-Chalabi M, Gupta S. Neuroanatomy, spinothalamic tract. In: *StatPearls.* Treasure Island, FL: StatPearls Publishing; 2019. Available at http://www.ncbi.nlm.nih.gov/books/NBK507824/. Accessed March 25, 2019.

22. Vierck CJ, Whitsel BL, Favorov OV, Brown AW, Tommerdahl M. The roles of primary somatosensory cortex in the coding of pain. *Pain.* 2013;154(3):334-344.

23. Navarro-Orozco D, Bollu PC. Neuroanatomy, medial lemniscus (Reils band, Reils ribbon). In: *StatPearls.* Treasure Island, FL: StatPearls Publishing; 2019. Available at http://www.ncbi.nlm.nih.gov/books/NBK526040/. Accessed March 25, 2019.

24. Melzack R, Wall PD. Pain mechanisms: a new theory. *Science.* 1965;150(3699):971-979.

25. Baranauskas G, Nistri A. Sensitization of pain pathways in the spinal cord: cellular mechanisms. *Prog Neurobiol.* 1998;54(3):349-365.

26. Basbaum AI, Clanton CH, Fields HL. Opiate and stimulus-produced analgesia: functional anatomy of a medullospinal pathway. *Proc Natl Acad Sci U S A.* 1976;73(12):4685-4688.

27. Lueptow LM, Fakira AK, Bobeck EN. The contribution of the descending pain modulatory pathway in opioid tolerance. *Front Neurosci.* 2018;12. Available at https://www.ncbi.nlm.nih.gov/pmc/articles/PMC6278175/. Accessed March 25, 2019.

28. Loyd DR, Morgan MM, Murphy AZ. Morphine preferentially activates the periaqueductal gray-rostral ventromedial medullary pathway in the male rat: a potential mechanism for sex differences in antinociception. *Neuroscience.* 2007;147(2):456-468.

29. Munn EM, Harte SE, Lagman A, Borszcz GS. Contribution of the periaqueductal gray to the suppression of pain affect produced by administration of morphine into the intralaminar thalamus of rat. *J Pain.* 2009;10(4):426-435.

30. Schoo SM, Bobeck EN, Morgan MM. Enhanced antinociception with repeated microinjections of apomorphine into the periaqueductal gray of male and female rats. *Behav Pharmacol.* 2017;1:234-240.

31. Li C, Sugam JA, Lowery-Gionta EG, et al. Mu opioid receptor modulation of dopamine neurons in the periaqueductal gray/dorsal raphe: a role in regulation of pain. *Neuropsychopharmacology.* 2016;41(8):2122-2132.

32. Besson JM, Chaouch A. Peripheral and spinal mechanisms of nociception. *Physiol Rev.* 1987;67(1):67-186.

33. Ossipov MH, Morimura K, Porreca F. Descending pain modulation and chronification of pain. *Curr Opin Support Palliat Care.* 2014;8(2):143-151.

34. Peyron C, Rampon C, Petit J-M, Luppi P-H. Sub-regions of the dorsal raphé nucleus receive different inputs from the brainstem. *Sleep Med.* 2018;49:53-63.

35. Butler RK, Finn DP. Stress-induced analgesia. *Prog Neurobiol.* 2009;88(3):184-202.

36. Woodhams SG, Chapman V, Finn DP, Hohmann AG, Neugebauer V. The cannabinoid system and pain. *Neuropharmacology.* 2017;124:105-120.

37. Hohmann AG, Suplita RL. Endocannabinoid mechanisms of pain modulation. *AAPS J.* 2006;8(4):E693-E708.

38. Kent ML, Tighe PJ, Belfer I, et al. The ACTTION-APS-AAPM pain taxonomy (AAAPT): multidimensional approach to classifying acute pain conditions. *J Pain.* 2017;18(5):479-489.

39. Fillingim RB, Bruehl S, Dworkin RH, et al. The ACTTION_American pain society pain taxonomy (AAPT): an evidence-based and multi-dimensional approach to classifying chronic pain conditions. *J Pain.* 2014;15(3):241-249.

40. Woolfe CJ. Central sensitization: implications for the diagnosis and treatment of pain. *Pain.* 2011;152:S2-S15.

41. Carr DB, Goudas LC. Acute pain. *Lancet.* 1999;353:2051-2058.

42. Sinatra R. Causes and consequences of inadequate management of acute pain. *Pain Med.* 2010;11:1859-1871.

43. Manhapra A, Becker WC. Pain and addiction. *Med Clin North Am.* 2018;102:745-763.

44. Tawfic Q, Kumar K, Pirani Z, Armstrong K. Prevention of chronic post-surgical pain: the importance of early identification of risk factors. *J Anesth.* 2017;31(2):424-431.

45. Ferreira-Valente MA, Pais-Ribeiro JL, Jensen MP. Validity of four pain intensity rating scales. *Pain.* 2011;152:2399-2404.

46. Dworkin RH, Turk DC, Farrar JT, et al. Core outcome measures for chronic pain clinical trials: IMMPACT recommendations. *Pain.* 2005;113:9-19.

47. Dersh J, Polatin PB, Gatchel RJ. Chronic pain and psychopathology: research findings and theoretical considerations. *Psychosom Med.* 2002;64:773-786.

48. Ishak WW, Wen RY, Naghdechi L, et al. Pain and depression: a systematic review. *Harvard Rev Psychiatry.* 2018. 26(6):352-363.

49. Howe CQ, Robinson JP, Sullivan MD. Psychiatric and psychological perspectives on chronic pain. *Phys Med Rehabil Clin North Am.* 2015;26:283-300.

50. Nicholson SE, Caplan JP, Williams DE, Stern TA. Comorbid pain, depression, and anxiety: multifaceted pathology allows for multifaceted treatment. *Harvard Rev Psychiatry.* 2009;17:407-420.

51. McWilliams LA, Cox BJ, Enns MW. Mood and anxiety disorders associated with chronic pain: an examination in a nationally representative sample. *Pain.* 2003;106:127-133.

52. Fishbane DA, Cutler R, Rosomoff HL, Rosomoff RS. Chronic pain-associated depression: antecedent or consequence of chronic pain? A review. *Clin J Pain.* 1997;13(2):116-137.

53. Goesling J, Clauw DJ, Hassett AL. Pain and depression: an integrative review of neurobiological and psychological factors. *Curr Psychiatry Rep.* 2013:15:421.

54. Richardson EJ, Ness TJ, Doleys DM, Banos JH, Cianfrini L, Richards JS. Depressive symptoms and pain evaluations among persons with chronic pain: catastrophizing, but not pain acceptance, shows significant effects. *Pain.* 2009;147:147-152.

55. Velly AM, Look JO, Carlson C, et al. The effect of catastrophizing and depression on chronic pain—a prospective cohort study of temporomandibular muscle and joint pain disorders. *Pain.* 2011;152:2377-2383.

56. Asmundson GJ, Katz J. Understanding the co-occurrence of anxiety disorders and chronic pain: state-of-the-art. *Depression Anxiety.* 2009;26:888-901.

57. Fishbain DA, Pulikal A, Lewis JE, Gao J. Chronic pain types differ in their reported prevalence of post-traumatic stress disorder (PTSD) and there is consistent evidence that chronic pain is associated with PTSD: an evidence-based structured systematic review. *Pain Med.* 2017;18:711-735.

58. Defrin R, Schreiber S, Ginzburg K. Paradoxical pain perception in posttraumatic stress disorder: the unique role of anxiety and depression. *J Pain.* 2015;16(10):961-970.

59. Vlaeyen JWS, Linton SJ. Fear-avoidance and its consequences in chronic musculoskeletal pain: a state of the art. *Pain.* 2000;85:317-332.

60. Gustin SM, Burke LA, Peck CC, Murray GM, Henderson LA. Pain and personality: do individuals with different forms of chronic pain exhibit a mutual personality? *Pain Pract.* 2016;16(4):486-494.

61. Kalira V, Treisman GJ, Clark MR. Borderline personality disorder and chronic pain: a practical approach to evaluation and treatment. *Curr Pain Headache Rep.* 2013;17:350.

62. Conrad R, Wegener I, Geiser F, Kleiman A. Temperament, character, and personality disorders in chronic pain. *Curr Pain Headache Rep.* 2013;17:318.

63. Racine M. Chronic pain and suicide risk: a comprehensive review. *Prog Neuropsychopharmacol Biol Psychiatry.* 2018;87:269-280.

64. Ratcliffe GE, Enns MW, Belik SL, Sareen J. Chronic pain conditions and suicidal ideation and suicide attempts: an epidemiologic perspective. *Clin J Pain.* 2008;24:204-210.

65. Tang NY, Crane C. Suicidality in chronic pain: a review of the prevalence, risk factors and psychological links. *Psychol Med.* 2006;36:575-586.

66. Racine M, Sanchez-Rodriguez E, Galan S, et al. Factors associated with suicidal ideation in patients with chronic non cancer pain. *Pain Med.* 2017;18:283-293.

67. Crighton AH, Wygant DB, Applegate KC, Umlauf RL, Granacher RP. Can brief measures effectively screen for pain and somatic malingering? Examination of the modified somatic perception questionnaire and pain disability index. *Spine J.* 2014;14:2042-2050.

68. Tuck NL, Johnson MH, Bean DJ. You'd better believe it: the conceptual and practical challenges of assessing malingering in patients with chronic pain. *J Pain.* 2019;20(2):133-145.

69. Cheatle MD, Foster S, Pinkett A, Lesneski M, Qu D, Dhingra L. Assessing and managing sleep disturbances in patients with chronic pain. *Sleep Med Clin.* 2016;11:531-541.

70. Generaal E, Vogelzangs N, Penninx BWJH, Dekker J. Insomnia, sleep duration, depressive symptoms and the onset of chronic multisite musculoskeletal pain. *Sleep.* 2017;40(1):1-10.

71. Finan PH, Goodin BR, Smith MT. The association of sleep and pain: an update and a path forward. *J Pain.* 2013;14(12):1539-1552.

72. Tang NKY, Goodchild CE, Hester J, Salkovskis PM. Pain-related insomnia versus primary insomnia. *Clin J Pain.* 2012;28(5):428-436.

73. Byers HD, Lichstein KL, Thorn BE. Cognitive processes in comorbid poor sleep and chronic pain. *J Behav Med.* 2016;39:233-240.

74. Baker KS, Georgiou-Karistianis N, Gibson SJ, Giummarra MJ. Optimizing cognitive function in persons with chronic pain. *Clin J Pain.* 2017;33(5):462-472.

75. Moriarty O, McGuire BE, Finn D. The effect of pain on cognitive function: a review of clinical and preclinical research. *Prog Neurobiol.* 2011;93:385-404.

76. Ballantyne JC. Opioids for the treatment of chronic pain: mistakes made, lessons learned, and future directions. *Anesth Analg.* 2017;125:1769-1778.

77. Elman I, Borsook D. Common brain mechanisms of chronic pain and addictions. *Neuron.* 2016;89(1):11-36.

78. Vincent A, Lahr BD, Wolfe F, et al. Prevalence of fibromyalgia: a population-based study in Olmsted County, Minnesota, utilizing the Rochester Epidemiology Project. *Arthritis Care Res (Hoboken).* 2013;65(5):786-792.

79. Jones GT, Atzeni F, Beasley M, Flüß E, Sarzi-Puttini P, MacFarlane GJ. The prevalence of fibromyalgia in the general population: a comparison of the American College of Rheumatology 1990, 2010, and modified 2010 classification criteria. *Arthritis Rheumatol.* 2015;67(2):568-575.

80. Kaye AD, Cornett EM, Hart B, et al. Novel pharmacological nonopioid therapies in chronic pain. *Curr Pain Headache Rep.* 2018;22:31.

81. Littlejohn G, Guymer E. Neurogenic inflammation in fibromyalgia. *Semin Immunopathol.* 2018;3:291-300.

82. Martinez-Lavin M, Lopez S, Medina M, Nava A. Use of the Leeds Assessment of Neuropathic Symptoms and Signs questionnaire in patients with fibromyalgia. *Semin Arthritis Rheum.* 2004;32(6):407-411.

83. Holliday KL, McBeth J. Recent advances in the understanding of genetic susceptibility to chronic pain and somatic symptoms. *Curr Rheumatol Rep.* 2011;13:521-527.

84. Lucas N, Macaskill P, Irwig L, Moran R, Bogduk N. Reliability of physical examination for diagnosis of myofascial trigger points. *Clin J Pain.* 2009;25(1):80-89.

85. Goldenberg DL. Fibromyalgia syndrome. An emerging but controversial condition. *JAMA.* 1987;257(20):2782-2787.

86. Suhr JA. Neuropsychological impairment in fibromyalgia: relation to depression, fatigue, and pain. *J Psychosom Res.* 2003;55: 321-329.

87. Bennett RM. Clinical manifestations and diagnosis of fibromyalgia. *Rheum Dis Clin North Am.* 2009;35;215-232.

88. Walitt B, Čeko M, Khatiwada M, et al. Characterizing "fibrofog": subjective appraisal, objective performance, and task-related brain activity during a working memory task. *Neuroimage Clin.* 2016;11:173.

89. Watson NF, Buchwald D, Goldberg J, Noonan C, Ellenbogen RG. Neurologic signs and symptoms in fibromyalgia. *Arthritis Rheum.* 2009;60(9):27.

90. Wolfe F, Clauw DJ, Fitzcharles MA, et al. Fibromyalgia criteria and severity scales for clinical and epidemiological studies: a modification of the ACR Preliminary Diagnostic Criteria for Fibromyalgia. *J Rheumatol.* 2011;38(6):1113-1122.

91. Baker N. Using cognitive behavior therapy and mindfulness techniques in the management of chronic pain in primary care. *Prim Care Clin Office Pract.* 2016;43:203-216.

92. Busch AJ, Webber SC, Richards RS, et al. Resistance exercise training for fibromyalgia. *Cochrane Database Syst Rev.* 2013;(12):CD010884. doi:10.1002/14651858.CD010884.

93. Hauser W, Wolfe F, Tolle T, Uceyler N, Sommer C. The role of antidepressants in the management of fibromyalgia syndrome: a systematic review and meta-analysis. *CNS Drugs.* 2012;26(4):297-307.

94. Bruehl S. Complex regional pain syndrome. *BMJ.* 2015;351:h2730.

95. Stephan O, Maihöfner C. Signs and symptoms in 1,043 patients with complex regional pain syndrome. *J Pain.* 2018;19(6):599-611.

96. Sandroni P, Benrud-larson LM, Mcclelland RL, Low PA. Complex regional pain syndrome type I: incidence and prevalence in Olmsted county, a population-based study. *Pain.* 2003;103(1-2):199-207.

97. Maihöfner C, Seifert F, Markovic K. Complex regional pain syndromes: new pathophysiological concepts and therapies. *Eur J Neurol.* 2010;17(5):649-660.

98. De mos M, De bruijn AG, Huygen FJ, Dieleman JP, Stricker BH, Sturkenboom MC. The incidence of complex regional pain syndrome: a population-based study. *Pain.* 2007;129(1-2):12-20.

99. Livingston WK. *Pain Mechanisms. A Physiological Interpretation of Causalgia and Related States.* New York, NY: Macmillan; 1943. Reprint by Plenum Press; 1976:83-84, 100-101, 209-210, 218, 221-226, 236-240.

100. Harden RN, Bruehl S, Stanton-Hicks M, Wilson PR. Proposed new diagnostic criteria for complex regional pain syndrome. *Pain Med.* 2007;8(4):326-331.

101. Beerthuizen A, van 't Spijker A, Huygen FJ, et al. Is there an association between psychological factors and the Complex Regional Pain Syndrome type 1 (CRPS1) in adults? A systematic review. *Pain.* 2009;145:52-59.

102. Beerthuizen A, Stronks DL, Huygen FJ, et al. The association between psychological factors and the development of complex regional pain syndrome type 1 (CRPS1)—a prospective multicenter study. *Eur J Pain.* 2011;15:971-975.

103. Bruehl S. An update on the pathophysiology of complex regional pain syndrome. *Anesthesiology.* 2010;113(3):713-725.

104. Birklein F, O'Neill D, Schlereth T. Complex regional pain syndrome: an optimistic perspective. *Neurology.* 2014;84(1): 89-96.

105. Kalita J, Vajpayee A, Misra UK. Comparison of prednisolone with piroxicam in complex regional pain syndrome following stroke: a randomized controlled trial. *QJM.* 2006;99:89.

106. Stanton-Hicks MD, Burton AW, Bruehl SP, et al. An updated interdisciplinary clinical pathway for CRPS: report of an expert panel. *Pain Pract.* 2002;2:1.

107. Perez RS, Zollinger PE, Dijkstra PU, et al. Evidence based guidelines for complex regional pain syndrome type 1. *BMC Neurol.* 2010;10:20.

108. American Psychiatric Association. *Diagnostic and Statistical Manual of Mental Disorders, Fifth Edition (DSM-5).* Arlington, VA: American Psychiatric Association; 2013.

109. Wittchen HU, Jacobi F, Rehm J, et al. The size and burden of mental disorders and other disorders of the brain in Europe 2010. *Eur Neuropsychopharmacol.* 2011;21(9):655-679.

110. Creed F, Barsky A. A systematic review of the epidemiology of somatization disorder and hypochondriasis. *J Psychosom Res.* 2004;56:391.

111. Kirmayer LJ, Robbins JM. Three forms of somatization in primary care: prevalence, co-occurrence, and sociodemographic characteristics. *J Nerv Ment Dis.* 1991;179:647.

112. Creed FH, Davies I, Jackson J, et al. The epidemiology of multiple somatic symptoms. *J Psychosom Res.* 2012;72:311-317.

113. Van Geelen SM, Rydelius PA, Hagquist C. Somatic symptoms and psychological concerns in a general adolescent population: exploring the relevance of DSM-5 somatic symptom disorder. *J Psychosom Res.* 2015;79(4):251-258.

114. Tomenson B, Essau C, Jacobi F, et al. Total somatic symptom score as a predictor of health outcome in somatic symptom disorders. *Br J Psychiatry.* 2013;203:373-380.

115. Haller H, Cramer H, Lauche R, Dobos G. Somatoform disorders and medically unexplained symptoms in primary care. *Dtsch Arztebl Int.* 2015;112:279-287.

116. Dimsdale JE. Somatic symptom disorder: an important change in DSM. *J Psychosom Res.* 2013;75:223-228.

117. Claase-van Dessel N, van der Wouden JC, Dekker J, et al. Clinical value of DSM IV and DSM 5 criteria for diagnosing the most prevalent somatoform disorders in patients with medically unexplained physical symptoms (MUPS). *J Psychosom Res.* 2016;82:4-10.

118. Henningsen P, Zipfel S, Herzog W. Management of functional somatic syndromes. *Lancet.* 2007;369:946-955.

119. Croicu C, Chwastiak L, Katon W. Approach to the patient with multiple somatic symptoms. *Med Clin North Am.* 2014;98:1079-1095.

120. Perez DL, Barsky AJ, Vago DR, et al. A neural circuit framework for somatosensory amplification in somatoform disorders. *J Neuropsychiatry Clin Neurosci.* 2015;27:e40-e50.

121. Paras ML, Murad MH, Chen LP, et al. Sexual abuse and lifetime diagnosis of somatic disorders: a systematic review and meta-analysis. *JAMA.* 2009;302(5):550.

122. Rief W, Broadbent E. Explaining medically unexplained symptoms-models and mechanisms. *Clin Psychol Rev.* 2007;27: 821-841.

123. Barsky A, Borus JF. Functional somatic syndromes. *Ann Intern Med.* 1999;130:910-921.

124. Ghanizadeh A, Firoozabadi A. A review of somatoform disorders in DSM-IV and somatic symptoms disorder in proposed DSM-5. *Psychiatria Danubina.* 2012;24(4):353-358.

125. Gordon-Elliott JS, Muskin PR. An approach to the patient with multiple physical symptoms or chronic disease. *Med Clin North Am*. 2010;94:1207-1216.

126. Tsui P, Deptula A, Yuan DY. Conversion disorder, functional neurological symptom disorder, and chronic pain: comorbidity, assessment, and treatment. *Curr Pain Headache Rep*. 2017;21(6):29.

127. Booker SQ, Herr KA. Assessment and measurement of pain in adults in later life. *Clin Geriatr Med*. 2016;32:677-692.

128. Ellison DL. Physiology of pain. *Crit Care Nurs Clin North Am*. 2017;29(4):397-406.

129. Miller RM, Kaiser RS. Psychological characteristics of chronic pain: a review of current evidence and assessment tools to enhance treatment. *Curr Pain Headache Rep*. 2018;22:22.

130. Dahlke LA, Sable JJ, Andrasik F. Behavioral therapy: emotion and pain, a common anatomical background. *Neurol Sci*. 2017;38(suppl 1):S157-S161.

131. Manhapra A, Becker WC. Pain and addiction: an integrative therapeutic approach. *Med Clin North Am*. 2018;102:745-763.

132. Sheng J, Liu S, Wang Y, Cui R, Zhang X. The link between depression and chronic pain: neural mechanisms in the brain. *Neural Plast*. 2017;2017:9724371.

133. Veterans Health Administration: Pain as the 5Th Vital Sign Toolkit. 2000. Available at http://www.va.gov/PAINMANAGEMENT/docs/Pain_As_the_5th_Vital_Sign_Toolkit.pdf. Accessed June 18, 2019.

134. Scher C, Meador L, Van Cleave JH, Reid MC. Moving beyond pain as the fifth vital sign and patient satisfaction scores to improve pain care in the 21st century. *Pain Manag Nurs*. 2018;19(2):125-129.

135. Morgan KJ, Anghelescu DL. A review of adult and pediatric neuropathic pain assessment tools. *Clin J Pain*. 2017;33:844-852.

136. Mills S, Torrance N, Smith BH. Identification and management of chronic pain in primary care: a review. *Curr Psychiatry Rep*. 2016;18:22.

137. Hill JC, Dunn KM, Lewis M, et al. A primary care back pain screening tool: identifying patient subgroups for initial treatment. *Arthritis Rheum*. 2008;59(2):632-641.

138. Beneciuk JM, George SZ. Pragmatic implementation of a stratified primary care model for low back pain management in outpatient physical therapy settings: two-phase, sequential preliminary study. *Phys Ther*. 2015;95:1120-1134.

139. Chou R, Gordon DB, Leon-Casasola OA, et al. Management of postoperative pain: a clinical practice guideline from the American Pain Society, the American Society of Regional Anesthesia and Pain Medicine and the American Society of Anesthesiologists' Committee on Regional Anesthesia, Executive Committee and Administrative Council. *J Pain*. 2016;17(2):131-157.

140. Gatchel RJ, McGeary DD, McGeary CA, Lippe B. Interdisciplinary chronic pain management. *Am Psychol*. 2014;69(2):119-130.

141. Hayek SM, Shah A. Nerve blocks for chronic pain. *Neurosurg Clin North Am*. 2014;25:809-817.

142. D'Arcy Y, McCarberg B. Managing patient pain: a focus on NSAID OTC formulations for relief of musculoskeletal and other common sources of pain. *J Fam Pract*. 2018;67(8 suppl):S67-S72.

143. Chou R, Turner JA, Devine EB, et al. The effectiveness and risk of long-term opioid therapy for chronic pain: a systematic review for a national institutes of health pathways to prevention workshop. *Ann Intern Med*. 2015;162(4):276-287.

144. Chou R, Fanciullo GJ, Fine PG, et al. Clinical guidelines for the use of chronic opioid therapy in chronic noncancer pain. *J Pain*. 2009;10(2):113-130.

145. Nicolson SE, Caplan JP, Williams DE, Stern TA. Comorbid pain, depression and anxiety: multifaceted pathology allows for multifaceted treatment. *Harv Rev Psychiatry*. 2009;17(6):407-420.

146. Aiyer R, Barkin RL, Bhatia A. Treatment of neuropathic pain with venlafaxine: a systematic review. *Pain Med*. 2017;18:1999-2012.

147. Goodman CW, Brett AS. Gabapentin and pregabalin for pain—is increased prescribing a cause for concern? *N Engl J Med*. 2017;377(5):411-414.

148. Michelet D, Brasher C, Horlin AL, et al. Ketamine for chronic non-cancer pain: a meta-analysis and trial sequential analysis of randomized controlled trials. *Eur J Pain*. 2018;22:632-646.

149. Maher DP, Chen L, Mao J. Intravenous ketamine infusions for neuropathic pain management: a promising therapy in need of optimization. *Anesth Analg*. 2017;124(2):661-674.

150. Schoevers RA, Chaves TV, Balukova SM, Rot MAH, Korekaas R. Oral ketamine for the treatment of pain and treatment-resistant depression. *Br J Psychiatry*. 2016;208:108-113.

151. Chohan H, Greenfield AL, Yadav V, Graves J. Use of cannabinoids for spasticity and pain management in MS. *Curr Treat Options Neurol*. 2016;18:1.

152. Nugent SM, Morasco BJ, O'Neil ME, et al. The effects of cannabis among adults with chronic pain and an overview of general harms. *Ann Intern Med*. 2017;167(5):319-332.

153. Andreae MH, Carter GM, Shaparin N, et al. Inhaled cannabis for chronic neuropathic pain: an individual patient data meta-analysis. *J Pain*. 2015;16(12):1221-1232.

154. Yadav V, Bever C, Bowen J, et al. Summary of evidence-based guideline: complementary and alternative medicine in MS. *Neurology*. 2014;82:1083-1092.

155. Hill KP. Medical marijuana for treatment of chronic pain and other medical and psychiatric problems: a clinical review. *JAMA*. 2015;313:2474-2483.

156. Whiting PF, Wolff RF, Deshpande S, et al. Cannabinoids for medical use: a systematic review and meta-analysis. *JAMA*. 2015;313:2456-2473.

157. Mandolini GM, Lazzaretti M, Pigoni A, et al. Pharmacological properties of cannabidiol in the treatment of psychiatric disorders: a critical overview. *Epidemiol Psychiatr Sci*. 2018;27(4):327-335.

158. Fernández Ó. THC:CBD in daily practice: available data from UK, Germany and Spain. *Eur Neurol*. 2016;75:1-3.

159. Aquino JPD, Ross DA. Cannabinoids and pain: weeding out undesired effects with a novel approach to analgesia. *Biol Psychiatry*. 2018;15(84):e67-e69.

160. Williams AC, Eccleston C, Morley S. Psychological therapies for the management of chronic pain (excluding headache) in adults. *Cochrane Database Syst Rev*. 2012;11:CD007407.

161. Ehde DM, Dillsworth TM, Turner JA. Cognitive-behavioral therapy for individuals with chronic pain. *Am Psychol*. 2014;69(2):153-166.

162. Veehof MM, Oskam MJ, Schreurs KMG, Bohlmeijer ET. Acceptance-based interventions for the treatment of chronic pain: a systematic review and meta-analysis. *Pain*. 2011;152:533-542.

163. Geenen LJ, Moore RA, Clarke C, Martin D, Colvin LA, Smith BH. Physical activity and exercise for chronic pain in adults: an overview of Cochrane reviews. *Cochrane Database Syst Rev*. 2017;1:CD011279.

164. Ambrose KR, Golightly YM. Physical exercise as a non-pharmacological treatment of chronic pain: why and when. *Best Pract Res Clin Rheumatol*. 2015;29(1):120-130.

165. Clarke TC, Black LI, Stussman BJ, Barnes PM, Nahin RL. Trends in the use of complementary health approaches among

adults: United States, 2002-2012. *Natl Health Stat Report.* 2015; 10(79):1-16.

166. Bauer BA, Tilburt JC, Sood A, Li GX, Wang SH. Complementary and alternative medicine therapies for chronic pain. *Chin J Integr Med.* 2016;22(6):402-411.

167. Thomas DA, Maslin B, Legler A, Springer E, Asgerally A, Vadivelu N. Role of alternative therapies for chronic pain syndromes. *Curr Pain Headache Rep.* 2016;20:29.

168. Gibson W, Wand BM, O'Connell NE. Transcutaneous electrical nerve stimulation (TENS) for neuropathic pain in adults (review). *Cochrane Database Syst Rev.* 2017;9:CD011976.

169. Cruccu G, Garcia-Larrea L, Hansson P, et al. EAN guidelines on central neurostimulation therapy in chronic pain conditions. *Eur J Neurol.* 2016;23:1489-1499.

170. Arensen LJ, Hugh-Jones S, Lloyd DM. Transcranial alternating current stimulation at alpha frequency reduces pain when the intensity of pain is uncertain. *J Pain.* 2018;19(7):807-818.

32

The Neuropsychiatry of Headache

Mia Minen · Benjamin Fuchs · Palak Patel

CASE VIGNETTE 32.1

A 35-year-old woman with a history of migraine presents to the office complaining of worsening headaches. She recently underwent an unexpected change in her job. She seems tearful and depressed. The clinician asks about her mood and she says, "Of course I am depressed. These headaches are preventing me from doing things I enjoy and are limiting my abilities at work. If you can stop them, my mood should improve." The health provider wonders: Is there a connection between depression and headaches? Which came first—the migraines or the depression? Does it even matter?

INTRODUCTION

Headaches are one of the most common disorders of the central nervous system (CNS). The International Classification of Headache Disorders (ICHD-3)[1] classifies headache disorders into two categories: (1) primary headache disorder and (2) secondary headache disorders. Secondary headache disorders only comprise about 10% of headache disorders[2] and result from known CNS pathology such as brain tumors, aneurysms, trauma, etc.[1] Table 32-1 illustrates many of the major causes of headache disorders. Taking a comprehensive history (Table 32-2) helps determine red flags, that is, whether there is significant concern for investigating a secondary headache. Table 32-3 demonstrates the red flags, potential differential diagnoses, and possible workups for some of these headache disorders. Of note, the Choosing Wisely Campaign specifically says, "Don't do imaging for uncomplicated headache. Imaging headache patients absent specific risk factors for structural disease is not likely to change management or improve outcome. Those patients with a significant likelihood of structural disease requiring immediate attention are detected by clinical screens that have been validated in many settings. Many studies and clinical practice guidelines concur. Also, incidental findings lead to additional medical procedures and expense that do not improve patient well-being."[3] Also, it is important to note that computerized tomography is good for looking for a bleed or a fracture, but it is not good for viewing the brain itself. Thus, in many cases of headache medicine, especially when there is not concern for a bleed, fracture, or herniation, magnetic resonance imaging is clearly preferred as it better visualizes the brain parenchyma and is without radiation (Figure 32-1).

Despite both patient and physician concern for having a secondary headache, the vast majority of headaches are primary headaches. The most common primary headache disorders are tension type headache and migraine. Migraine is the most common headache for which patients present for medical care.[4] Another primary headache is cluster headache (CH), and this is another extremely disabling headache disorder. In this chapter we focus on primary headache disorders such as migraine and CHs as these are the most common headache disorders with neuropsychiatric comorbidities.

EPIDEMIOLOGY

Migraine

Migraine is a chronic neurological disorder consisting of episodes of moderate-to-severe attacks. The diagnostic criteria can be found in Table 32-4, along with clinical pearls. There are two types of migraine: migraine with aura and migraine without aura. Migraine without aura is less common than migraine with aura.[2,5]

The Global Burden of Disease Study 2015 (GBD2015) ranked migraine as the second highest cause of disability among

TABLE 32-1 • Major Categories of Headache Disorders.

- Migraine
- Tension type
- Cluster and other trigeminal autonomic cephalgias
- Other primary headaches
- Primary stabbing, cough, exertional, thunderclap, associated with sexual activity, hypnic, hemicrania continua, new daily persistent
- Headache attributed to head and/or neck trauma
- Headache attributed to cranial or cervical vascular disorder-stroke, TIA, hemorrhage, unrupted vascular malformation, arteritis, carotid or carotid artery pain, venous thrombosis
- Headache attributed to nonvascular intracranial disorder—high or low CSF, noninfectious inflammatory disease, intracranial neoplasm, intrathecal injection, epileptic seizure, Chiari I malformation
- Headache attributed to a substance or its withdrawal
- Headache attributed to infection
- Headache attributed to disorder of hemostasis-hypoxia/hypercapnea, dialysis, arterial hypertension, hypothyroidism, fasting, cardiac cephalgia
- Headache or facial pain
- Headache attributed to psychiatric disorder
- Cranial neuralgias and central causes of facial pain

TABLE 32-2 • Points to Address When Taking a Headache History.

- Temporal profile
  - Age of onset, time to maximum intensity, frequency, time of day, duration, recurrence
- Headache features
  - Location, quality, and severity of the pain
- Associated signs and symptoms
  - Before headache, during headache, after headache
- Aggravating or precipitating factors
  - Trauma, medical conditions, triggers, activity, meds
- Relieving factors
  - Pharmacological and nonpharmacological
- Evaluation and treatment history
  - Physicians and other health care providers
- Psychosocial history
  - Substance use and occupational and personal life
- Psychological history
  - Sleep history and impact of the headache
- Patient's own diagnosis
- Family history

TABLE 32-3 • Red Flags, Differential Diagnoses, and Possible Workups for Headache.

Red Flag	Differential Diagnosis	Possible Workup
Headache beginning after 50 years of age	Temporal arteritis, mass lesion	Erythrocyte sedimentation rate, neuroimaging
Sudden onset of headache	Subarachnoid hemorrhage, pituitary apoplexy, hemorrhage into a mass lesion or vascular malformation, mass lesion (especially posterior fossa mass)	Neuroimaging; lumbar puncture if neuroimaging is negative*
Headaches increasing in frequency and severity	Mass lesion, subdural hematoma, medication overuse	Neuroimaging, drug screen
New-onset headache in a patient with risk factors for HIV infection or cancer	Meningitis (chronic or carcinomatous), brain abscess (including toxoplasmosis), metastasis	Neuroimaging; lumbar puncture if neuroimaging is negative*
Headache with signs of systemic illness (fever, stiff neck, rash)	Meningitis, encephalitis, Lyme disease, systemic infection, collagen vascular disease	Neuroimaging, lumbar puncture,† serology
Focal neurologic signs or symptoms of disease (other than typical aura)	Mass lesion, vascular malformation, stroke, collagen vascular disease	Neuroimaging, collagen vascular evaluation (including antiphospholipid antibodies)
Papilledema	Mass lesion, pseudotumor cerebri, meningitis	Neuroimaging, lumbar puncture†
Headache subsequent to head trauma	Intracranial hemorrhage, subdural hematoma, epidural hematoma, post-traumatic headache	Neuroimaging of brain, skull and, possibly, cervical spine

HIV, human immunodeficiency virus.
Lumbar puncture may follow a negative neuroimaging procedure if suspicion of hemorrhage, infection, or malignancy remains high.
†Suspicion of specific central nervous system infections (Lyme disease, syphilis, etc.) or intracranial hypertension (pseudotumor cerebri) warrants lumbar puncture with cerebrospinal fluid analysis and pressure measurement.
Adapted with permission from Newman LC, Lipton RB. Emergency department evaluation of headache. Neurol Clin. 1998;16:285-303. Elsevier. https://www.sciencedirect.com/journal/neurologic-clinics.

various neurological disorders in young women.[6] Migraine continues to be a significant public health problem in the United States affecting one out of every six Americans and one in five women over a 3-month period with a total prevalence of 15% (9.7% of males and 20.7% of females).[4] Migraine is most commonly observed in the age group of 45–64 (15.9%). There is a higher burden of disease in those who are unemployed, those with family income of <$35,000 annually, the elderly, and the disabled. In terms of financial burden, it accounts for about $20 billion annually.[4]

The annual incidence of chronic migraine among people with episodic migraine is 2.5–3% and is prevalent in about 2% of the population.[7-9] Risk factors that lead to chronification of episodic migraine include high baseline frequency, medication overuse, caffeine consumption, snoring, obesity, and inadequate treatment of migraine attacks.[7,10,11] Other factors that contribute to the development of chronic migraine include female sex,

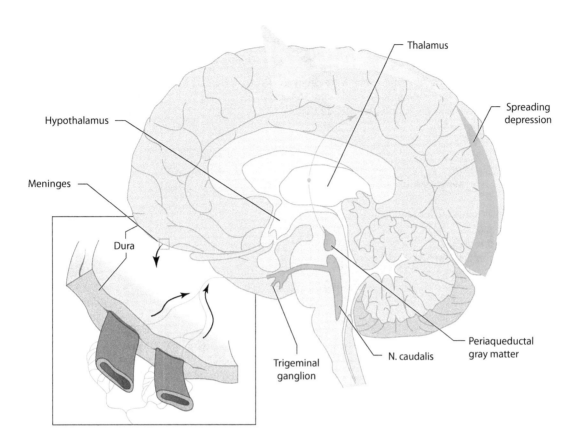

FIGURE 32-1. Central and peripheral nervous system sites proposed to be involved in migraine pathogenesis. (Reproduced with permission from Simon RP, Aminoff MJ, Greenberg DA. *Clinical Neurology,* 10e. http://accessmedicine.mhmedical.com. Copyright © McGraw Hill LLC. All rights reserved.)

genetic factors such as COMT gene polymorphisms, prenatal exposures to tobacco and alcohol, allodynia, head/neck injury, low education and socioeconomic status, depression, anxiety, stressful life events (such as marital status, residence and job changes, death of relatives or close friends), sleep apnea, and comorbid pain disorders.[7,12–21] Apart from the high utilization of health care resources, chronic migraine, if incompletely treated, can lead to reduced quality of life and it can negatively impact treatment outcomes.[22]

Cluster Headache

CH is a form of trigeminal-autonomic cephalgia characterized by unilateral headaches with autonomic symptoms ipsilateral to the pain, such as miosis, ptosis, lacrimation, and conjunctival injection.[23] It is a rare disorder occurring in about 0.1% of the global population.[24] It has a male predominance with age of onset between 21 and 30 years of age.[25] Cluster attacks occur more frequently in spring and autumn. Various risk factors for CH have been identified in epidemiology studies including cigarette smoking, head trauma, and a family history of headache.[26] Individuals with first-degree and second-degree relatives with CH have an increased risk compared to the general population. Several genetic association studies have identified some possible candidate genes for CH though not all of them were replicated and confirmed in subsequent studies.[23]

PSYCHIATRIC COMORBIDITIES IN MIGRAINE HEADACHES

Depression and Migraine

The unpredictable nature of migraine attacks predisposes patients to depression and anxiety. Thus, depression is the most commonly studied psychiatric comorbidity in patients with migraine. Several studies show that depression is 2.2 to 4 times more likely to occur in patients with migraine.[27] Also, rates of depression are higher in migraine with aura than migraine without aura.[28] Furthermore, the longitudinal studies show a bidirectional relationship between migraine and depression suggesting shared vulnerabilities.[29–31] Depression is a risk factor for migraine chronification as well as medication refractoriness, and so it should be treated as soon as it is identified in patients.[32,33]

Several mechanisms have been theorized to explain the comorbidity. Low central serotonergic levels have been proposed based on the response to 5HT agonists in migraine and selective serotonin reuptake inhibitors (SSRIs) in depression. Polymorphisms of the 5-HTT gene (which slow the production of serotonin transporter proteins) are associated with risk of depression and migraine. Hormonal changes (low estrogen levels) and hypothalamic-pituitary-adrenal (HPA) axis dysfunction from early stress sensitization are other putative mechanisms.[34]

TABLE 32-4 • Diagnostic Criteria and Pearls for Diagnosing Migraine and Cluster Headache.	

Migraine
A. At least five attacks fulfilling criteria B–D
B. Headache attacks lasting 4–72 hours (untreated or unsuccessfully treated) [If the patient falls asleep during the migraine and wakes up without it, duration of the attack is the time until awakening, in those less than age 18, time can be 2–72 hours.]
C. Headache has at least two of the following four characteristics:
  1. Unilateral location
  2. Pulsating quality
  3. Moderate or severe pain intensity
  4. Aggravation by or causing avoidance of routine physical activity (e.g., walking or climbing stairs)
D. During headache at least one of the following:
  1. Nausea and/or vomiting
  2. Photophobia and phonophobia
E. Not better accounted for by another ICHD-3 diagnosis.
Pearls:
  1. Note that in migraine, headaches do NOT have to be unilateral.
  2. Note that photophobia and phonophobia are not required to make a diagnosis if nausea and/or vomiting is present.
  3. There is a diagnosis called probable migraine for attacks fulfilling all but one of criteria A–D. In making a headache diagnosis, attacks that fulfil criteria for both tension type headache and probable migraine are generally coded as tension type headache. However, in patients who already have a migraine diagnosis, it is important to note for treatment purposes that mild migraine attacks, or attacks treated early, often do not have all characteristics necessary for a migraine attack diagnosis but they respond to specific migraine treatments.
  4. There are two types of migraine: migraine with aura and migraine without aura. Aura is defined as visual and/or sensory and/or speech/language symptoms (but no motor weakness) that gradually develop and are no more than 1 hour, it can be a mix of positive and/or negative features, e.g., flashing lights or loss of vision, tingling or numbness, and there is complete reversibility.
  5. There is a diagnosis of chronic migraine in which there is a headache occurring on 15 or more days/month for more than 3 months, and there are 8 days/month meeting migraine criteria.
	Cluster headache
	A. At least five attacks fulfilling criteria B–D
	B. Severe or very severe unilateral orbital, supraorbital, and/or temporal pain lasting 15–180 minutes (when untreated)
	C. Either or both of the following:
	  1. At least one of the following symptoms or signs, ipsilateral to the headache:
	    • Conjunctival injection and/or lacrimation
	    • Nasal congestion and/or rhinorrhea
	    • Eyelid edema
	    • Forehead and facial sweating
	    • Miosis and/or ptosis
	  2. A sense of restlessness or agitation
	D. Occurring with a frequency between one every other day and 8 per day
	E. Not better accounted for by another ICHD-3 diagnosis.
	Notes:
	1. There is chronic cluster headache: Cluster headache attacks occurring for 1 year or longer without remission, or with remission periods lasting less than 3 months.

Bipolar Disorder (BPD) and Migraine

Migraine prevalence in patients with BPD ranged from 25% to 54%.[35-37] Similar to depression, BPD and migraine may have a bidirectional relationship. Early studies of psychiatric comorbidities in migraine suggested that bipolar disorder 2 (BPD 2) is two to three times as likely to occur in people who have migraine with aura than people with migraine without aura.[38] The profile of people with migraine and comorbid BPD have been observed to share the following: female predominance, higher prevalence of BPD 2, early onset BPD with index episode of depression, increased prevalence of comorbid panic disorders, augmented risk of rapid cycling, and higher rate of attempted suicides.[35,36,39,40] Proposed underlying mechanisms for the link between migraine and BPD include serotonergic dysfunction and mutations of gene-coding calcium channels.[39]

Given the increased incidence of irritability and early depressive episodes in this population, it is important to correctly identify BPD and appropriately treat it with mood stabilizers rather than antidepressant monotherapy. Sodium valproate is a preferred medication because it is effective for migraine prevention and would help to improve overall treatment compliance and prevent medication overuse.[39]

Anxiety Disorders and Migraine

Anxiety disorders including generalized anxiety disorder (GAD) (18–67%), obsessive-compulsive disorder (OCD), and panic disorder (5–30%) are often comorbid in migraine.[34,41,42] Anxiety disorders are twice as prevalent as depression in patients with migraine.[34,43,44] Compared to people without migraine, people with migraine are at four to five times greater risk for GAD and OCD and three times increased risk for panic disorders.[42] In addition, about 67% of patients with GAD seem to have migraine, a threefold increased risk compared to individuals without GAD.[44] Thus, the overall relationship between migraine and anxiety disorder is also bidirectional.

A recent study also showed increased subthreshold levels of anxiety (19%) in the migraine population with reciprocal increased risk of migraine in patients with subthreshold anxiety by two- to threefold. It was suggested that subthreshold anxiety levels were associated with higher psychiatric comorbidity, conversion to depression, increased levels of suicidal ideations, psychological stress, and perceived pain.[44]

Panic disorder shares several common clinical characteristics with migraine: chronic disorders with episodic attacks, shared common symptoms (tingling/numbness, dizziness, palpitations),[45] greater functional impairments, inter-ictal anxiety, and absence of identifiable secondary pathology. Panic disorder tends to occur at a higher rate in people with migraine with aura than without and accrue negative impact in terms of increased frequency of attacks, disability, chronification, and medication overuse.[42]

Proposed shared mechanisms underlying panic disorder and migraine include low central serotonin and GABA leading to prolonged activation and sensitization of trigeminovascular nociceptive pathways, ovarian hormonal fluctuations, dysregulation of HPA axis, and interoceptive conditioning leading to increased fear and pain sensitivity.[42]

Abuse/Post-Traumatic Stress Disorder (PTSD) in Migraine

There is a high prevalence of all types of childhood abuse/neglect (emotional, physical, and sexual) in patients with migraine.[46] In one study, emotional abuse, emotional neglect, and/or sexual abuse were more strongly related to migraine than other types of headaches independent of comorbid depression and anxiety.[47] Childhood emotional abuse, in turn, is a risk factor for early onset of migraine, migraine chronification, increased disabilities, and allodynia.[48] HPA axis dysregulation from early stress has been theorized to cause increased stress reactivity and migraine.[49,50]

Recent studies in this field, however, have suggested that PTSD mediates the association of abuse to migraine. The odds of having PTSD in patients with migraine were higher than with trauma alone (2.3 vs. 1.17).[42] PTSD has a higher prevalence (14–25%) in migraineurs than in the general population (1–12%).[22] PTSD comorbidity further confers increased risk for chronification, greater disability, loss of work days, and difficulties developing and maintaining social relationships.[51,52] Conversely, PSTD itself increases the risk of migraine development.[53] This reciprocal association is currently explained by dysfunction in serotonergic, autonomic nervous system, and HPA axis.[54]

ADHD and Migraine

Data regarding comorbidity of ADHD and migraine are more limited. One study showed that the odds of having migraine in the ADHD population was 1.67 times higher than in the general population.[55] This higher prevalence was explained on the basis of greater comorbidity of psychiatric disorders, dopaminergic systems dysfunction, and mild cognitive impairment in the cohort of ADHD and migraine (during acute attacks) in the study. Dopaminergic dysregulation (speculated to be the underlying mechanism) is likely due to dopamine receptor gene polymorphisms (DRD2 in migraine and DRD4 in ADHD) and receptor hypersensitivity seen in these conditions.[56,57]

Substance Use Disorders and Migraine

It can be presumed that people with chronic migraine would be at an increased risk of prescription drug abuse due to poor pain control. Despite early studies showing an increased risk of substance use and addiction,[58,59] more recent studies have not confirmed these findings.[60] The National Comorbidity Survey Replication data showed no association between migraine and substance use disorder after adjusting for depression and PTSD.[53] Similarly, another study showed no difference in the prevalence of alcohol dependence between people with migraine and people without migraine.[61] Furthermore, people with migraine consumed less alcohol than the controls in another study.[62] This could be explained by the fact that alcohol is a trigger for migraine. However, in a recent cross-sectional study of 181 substance-dependent inpatients, alcohol dependence was associated with a threefold increased risk of migraine as compared to non-alcohol dependent patients.[63] These conflicting data suggest methodological differences between the studies and a need for longitudinal research to assess potential associations.

Personality Disorder (PD) and Migraine

Despite a well-known occurrence of psychiatric disorders in migraine patients, only a few studies have assessed psychopathological aspects in migraine patients. Personality traits were assessed using both dimensional and categorical scales in 20 patients with migraine. The most common personality traits in migraine patients were Cluster C type: obsessive compulsive (93.3%), anxious (60%), and dependent (23.3%).[64] Dimensionally, these patients also had traits consistent with neurosis; hypochondria (53.3%), depression (23.3%), and hysteria (33.3%) were the most common traits. No relation was observed between the personality traits and duration of chronic migraine.

PSYCHIATRIC DISORDERS IN CLUSTER HEADACHES

Depression and Anxiety in Cluster Headache

Depression is the most commonly studied psychiatric comorbidity in CH. The reported prevalence of depression in CHs varies from 6.3% to 43% in cross-sectional studies and from 4.6% to 56% in lifetime studies.[65] Anxiety has often been studied along with depression in CH due to their comorbidity and presumed role in migraine chronification.[65] The prevalence of anxiety disorders has ranged from 11.8% to 75.7% in cross-sectional and 19–24% in lifetime studies of CH patients. A recent cross-sectional study in young Dutch patients showed that CH (episodic as well as chronic CHs, who were attack free) patients had three times higher odds of depression.[66] In comparison to migraine, studies suggest a unidirectional relationship between CH and depression.[65]

Bipolar Disorder and Cluster Headache

BPD is not well studied in the CH population. Thus far, only one study by Robbins et al.[67] has evaluated for the presence of BPD among CH patients. Based on a combination of retrospective review, survey, and direct patient interviews of about 287 patients, BPD was found in 6.6% of overall patients (6.4% in episodic CH and 6.8% in chronic CH).

Suicide in Cluster Headache

CH is often called "suicide headache" based on the severity of headaches and suicidal tendencies that it invokes in the sufferers. Suicidal tendencies have been reported in 25–55% of CH patients[25,68,69] and 2% reported having attempted suicide.[25] A survey of 203 headache experts from multiple countries led investigators to estimate that primary headaches were associated with 1% of all reported suicides.[70] Of these headaches, 70–80% were associated with migraine and CHs. Individually, CH had the highest reported risk of suicide attempts and completed suicides in the patients. Prior psychiatric history was associated with the increased rates of suicides and physicians believed that these could have been prevented by more effective treatment.

Personality Disorders in Cluster Headache

As with migraine, a limited number of studies have assessed co-occurrence of PDs in CH patients. Earlier studies (from when hypochondrial and hysterical PDs were in the *DSM-I* and *II*) showed conflicting results with some studies suggesting higher rates of hypochondria and hysteria[71] among CH patients whereas others showed no correlation.[72] Piacentini recently conducted a cross-sectional survey of 26 inpatients with CH using Millon Clinical Multiaxial Inventory III for PD screening. PDs were observed in 92% of the study patients with the most common being obsessive-compulsive (OCPD) and histrionic personality types with comorbid anxiety (32%), depression (26%), and other somatoform disorders (15%).[73] Another study reported similar prevalence of OCPD (52.5%), anxious (47.5%), histrionic (45%), schizoid (42.5%), impulsive (32.5%), and paranoid (30%) traits in episodic CHs.[74] The presence of certain personality traits alter how pain is expressed and perceived in CH patients. For example, in histrionic patients, there may be an increased tendency to report physical symptoms as a way to seek more attention and release unconscious anxiety, whereas obsessive-compulsive patients may tend to rationalize pain.[73]

Shared Mechanism for Comorbidity between Psychiatric Disorders and Cluster Headaches

Several mechanisms have been theorized to explain the occurrence of psychiatric comorbidities in patients with CH. These include CNS serotonergic hypofunctioning (reduced 5-HT$_7$ reception function in hypothalamus), inflammation (elevation of inflammatory markers such as IL-2 and IL-1B in CH and psychiatric disorders such as depression and BPDs), and contribution of sleep disturbance.[65]

OVERVIEW OF NEUROIMAGING FOR MIGRAINE AND CLUSTER HEADACHE

Migraine

Neuroimaging studies in patients with migraine have identified structural and functional alterations in brain regions implicated in the sensory, affective, and cognitive processing of pain. People with migraine demonstrate volumetric abnormalities in the midbrain and periaqueductal gray,[75-77] somatosensory cortex,[78,79] insula and cingulate cortex,[79] as well as the cerebellum, temporal pole,[80,81] right parieto-occipital, and left frontoparietal regions.[82] A recent meta-analysis and systematic review further demonstrated that patients with migraine have decreased gray matter volume in several frontal regions, including inferior frontal, precentral, and anterior cingulate cortices.[83]

Importantly, certain structural brain changes—including decreased size of regions mediating affect[84] and increased size of primary somatosensory cortex—may be a consequence of recurrent migraine attacks.[79] Structural white matter changes and white matter hyperintensities[85] have also been demonstrated in people with migraine, with a positive association between the extent of white matter abnormalities and duration of migraine history.[86] Interestingly, patients with comorbid migraine and major depressive disorder demonstrate reductions in total brain volume that are not seen in those with either migraine or depression alone.[87] Still, despite these positive findings, other investigators have reported an absence of structural brain differences when comparing subgroups of individuals with migraine,[88] suggesting that more research is needed to further characterize specific patterns of brain abnormalities, including that which further stratifies people with migraine based on key demographics and clinical features.[89]

Beyond structural changes, migraine is increasingly understood as a disorder of brain function, and a growing body of evidence demonstrates abnormalities of functional connectivity and altered responses to sensory stimuli. Functional MRI (fMRI) studies in which individuals with migraine are exposed to painful stimuli reveal abnormal activation patterns that distinguish them from healthy controls, including increased activation of the dorsolateral prefrontal cortex, anterior cingulate cortex, temporal pole, lentiform nuclei, hippocampus/parahippocampus and primary somatosensory cortex, with a concomitant decrease in activation of the primary motor cortex, secondary somatosensory cortex, superior temporal gyrus, as well as brainstem regions including the pons and ventral medulla.[89,90] Collectively, these brain regions are thought to constitute functional circuits that subserve the cognitive, affective, and sensory-discriminatory aspects of pain processing, providing further evidence of distinct activation patterns that may differentiate individuals who experience migraine from those who do not.

People with migraine may also possess hypersensitivity to sensory stimuli. During a migraine attack, exposure to olfactory stimuli induces hyperactivation in the amygdala, insular cortex, pons, cerebellum, superior temporal gyrus, and temporal pole. During interictal periods (between migraine attacks), exposure to visual stimuli yields increased activation of primary and extrastriate visual cortices.[90] Functional connectivity studies in individuals with migraine help to further distinguish ictal versus interictal periods, revealing alterations in salience (insula, dorsal anterior cingulate cortex), sensory (somatosensory cortex), and default mode networks (mPFC,

ACC, precuneus, and pCC), as well as stronger functional connectivity between the pons and somatosensory cortex during migraine attacks.[91] People with migraine may also demonstrate altered brainstem and hypothalamic functional connectivity in the period immediately preceding an attack, potentially implicating these regions in the genesis of a migraine headache.[92] Resting state functional connectivity (rs-fc) patterns may possibly serve as imaging biomarkers to distinguish individuals with migraine from healthy controls based on differences in connectivity patterns in regions implicated in pain processing.[93]

Cluster Headache

In contrast to the migraine literature, neuroimaging investigations of structural brain abnormalities in CH have revealed more mixed findings. One early investigation in patients with CH demonstrated volumetric increases in the inferior posterior hypothalamus in comparison to healthy controls,[94] while more recent studies have shown gray matter volumetric changes in multiple brain regions,[95] including frontal regions implicated in pain modulation.[96]

Investigators have further sought to characterize functional changes associated with "in-bout" periods—referring to the days to months during which headache episodes cluster—versus "out-of-bout" periods—referring to the months to years without headache symptoms—as well as the transition between these two states. "In-bout" periods of episodic headaches may be characterized by deranged functional connectivity between the hypothalamus and "pain matrix" areas (including the insula, somatosensory cortex, and anterior and posterior cingulate cortices),[97] while the transition between "in-bout" and "out-of-bout" states may be characterized by functional abnormalities in the frontal top-down networks responsible for pain modulation.[98] The hypothalamus, in particular, has been further implicated in driving the circadian rhythmicity with which CHs present.[99] In the clinical context, it is important to distinguish "primary" CH from CH due to another neurologic condition (i.e., "secondary" CH), and MRI with high-resolution pituitary imaging is indicated given the incidence of pituitary gland lesions presenting with a CH phenotype.[23]

DISCUSSION OF TREATMENTS FOR MIGRAINE

Overview and Principles of Migraine Management

CASE VIGNETTE 32.2

A 28-year-old woman says, "Doctor-my migraines are so disabling! I am having nausea and vomiting. What are my treatment options? I am having to take my ibuprofen six times a month and it is not working. I have to leave work to lie down and sleep off these attacks. Once I had to go to the emergency department because the vomiting was so bad!"

The treatment of migraine is divided into abortive therapies (i.e., acute medications)—treatments to be initiated at the onset of migraine symptoms—and preventative therapies, which are intended to reduce the frequency and severity of episodic migraine and to enhance the patient's responsiveness to the treatment of acute attacks.[100] Choice of a particular abortive therapy is determined by the severity of the attack. Simple analgesics serve as first-line pharmacotherapy for migraine of mild-to-moderate severity, while medications such as triptans are for attacks that are moderate-to-severe. Further, in randomized controlled trials, the combination of a long-acting nonsteroidal anti-inflammatory drug (NSAID) and triptan is shown to be superior to NSAIDs or triptan alone.[101] Rescue medications, such as anti-dopaminergic agents like promethazine, may be used often in conjunction with first-line agents[102] if the attack fails to respond to the simple analgesic or triptan, or if in the patient's judgment there is a very low probability that the first-line treatment will work.[103] Some patients and providers may be hesitant to take prescription medications such as triptans, but triptans are actually over the counter in other countries like the United Kingdom and are considered fairly safe.[104]

A key component of migraine management is the use of headache diaries which track headache days, headache intensity, and the medications used. Use of a headache diary enables providers to assess the need for preventive treatment and the effectiveness of treatments initiated (so that improvements or lack of improvements of the trialed preventive medications can be assessed). This further allows providers to assess the frequency of abortive medications used in a given month and to monitor if concerned for medication overuse headache (MOH).[105]

Medication Treatment Options for Migraine

Medications shown to be effective for the treatment of acute migraine include acetaminophen, NSAIDs (including aspirin, ibuprofen, naproxen, and diclofenac), ergotamine derivatives, triptans and combination therapies, such as sumatriptan/naproxen.[106] Randomized clinical trials also have demonstrated a benefit in combining a triptan with an antiemetic agent, such as promethazine, for the treatment of acute migraine over triptan alone.[102] Importantly, medical providers must consider non-oral routes of administration when selecting the appropriate abortive therapy for patients who experience nausea and vomiting during an acute attack,[107] and also for those in whom oral medications do not work fast enough because people with migraine can also have delayed gastrointestinal motility.[108]

Migraine prophylaxis is indicated in patients whose attacks cause significant impact on their quality of life despite appropriate use of acute management therapies and lifestyle modifications. Typically, prophylaxis is indicated in patients with an average of four or more headache days per month. (It could be as low as two headache days per month if patients have contraindications or insufficient response to the abortive medications or as much as six if the attacks are not very disabling and readily respond to over-the-counter medications such as ibuprofen.) According to guidelines established by the Canadian Headache Society and the American Academy of Neurology (AAN) for the prophylaxis of episodic migraine, the medications for which there is the highest quality evidence include beta blockers (metoprolol, propranolol, timolol), and antiepileptics (topiramate, valproic acid). In addition, the AAN has made a Level A recommendation for the use of onabotulinumtoxinA (Botox) in managing chronic migraine.[109-111] It is important to note that in pediatrics, in a randomized controlled double-blind trial, there were no significant differences in decreasing headache days or headache-related disability in childhood and adolescent migraine with amitriptyline, topiramate, or placebo in a 24-week period. The active drugs were associated with higher rates of adverse events and the trial was terminated early because of non-inferiority.[112]

There are special treatment considerations in patients with migraine and psychiatric comorbidities. Table 32-5 demonstrates the pharmacologic treatment considerations for patients with migraine and psychiatric comorbidities. Of note, SSRIs have not been demonstrated to be efficacious in migraine prevention. Also, while the FDA issued a Black Box warning on the combined use of triptans and SSRIs or serotonin norepinephrine reuptake inhibitors (SNRIs), a recent study published found that the incidence of serotonin syndrome in those co-prescribed triptans and antidepressants was low: 19,017 patients were co-prescribed triptans and antidepressants during the study. Serotonin syndrome was suspected in 17 patients, 2 patients were classified as having definite serotonin syndrome and 5 patients were classified as having possible serotonin syndrome.[113] Thus, provided a patient is only on one other serotonergic medication at a standard dose, patients are still generally provided a triptan. Finally, there are new drugs recently approved by the FDA called the calcitonin gene related peptide (CGRP) antagonists.[114] These drugs will warrant further investigation to assess their response in patients with migraine and psychiatric comorbidities.

Behavioral Treatment Options for Migraine

There are three types of behavioral headache treatments with Level A evidence for migraine: relaxation, biofeedback, and cognitive-behavioral therapy (CBT).[115] These treatments

are effective (found to have a decrease in 50% of headache days), safe, well tolerated,[115] and have long-lasting effects.[116] Economically, they may have fewer costs compared to medications.[117] Furthermore, randomized controlled trials demonstrate that a combination of pharmacologic and behavioral interventions leads to improved outcomes in migraine prevention compared to monotherapy.[118,119]

Unfortunately, there is suboptimal adherence to behavioral therapy for migraine. In one study, only about half of those referred by a headache specialist for behavioral therapy

TABLE 32-5 • Pharmacological Treatments Used for Migraine Prevention and Psychiatric Comorbidities.

Treatment	Psychiatric Comorbidity Use	Migraine Prevention Effectiveness
Tricyclic antidepressants (TCAs), e.g., amitriptyline	Effective for depression at high doses, with more side effects	Effective for migraine prevention at low doses, with minimal side effects
Serotonin norepinephrine reuptake inhibitors (SNRIs), e.g., venlafaxine	Effective for depression and decreases anxiety	Only venlafaxine has grade B evidence of efficacy for migraine prevention
		However, the most recent Cochrane study did not find venlafaxine to be more effective than placebo for prevention of chronic migraines[145]
Selective serotonin reuptake inhibitors (SSRIs), e.g., fluoxetine	Effective for depression	According to the Cochrane review, SSRIs were not better than placebo for migraine prevention[145]
β-blockers, e.g., propranolol	Might help with anxiety, but might also worsen depression	Effective for migraine prevention
Anticonvulsants		
Topiramate	Might help with mood stabilization, but might also worsen depression	Effective for migraine prevention
Divalproex sodium	Might help with mood stabilization, bipolar disorder	Effective for migraine prevention

Source: Minen MT, Begasse De Dhaem O, Kroon Van Diest A, et al. Migraine and its psychiatric comorbidities. J Neurol Neurosurg Psychiatry. 2016;87:741-749. Reproduced with permission from BMJ Publishing Group Ltd.

initiated scheduling a first appointment.[120] Thus, it is important to familiarize oneself with these Level A evidence-based behavioral therapies and the common barriers to receiving the care, as providers who are knowledgeable about them are most likely to be the most effective in explaining, persuading, and referring patients for the treatment.[121] The behavioral therapy option should be presented to patients similar to how one would discuss the rationale for the pros and cons of medication therapies. Unfortunately, access to providers can be limited. However, providers can learn from a book titled *Headache: Advances in Psychotherapy (Evidence Based Practice)* about how to carry out behavioral therapies such as CBT for migraine.[122]

Neuromodulation Treatment for Migraine

Several noninvasive neuromodulation techniques, including transcranial magnetic stimulation (TMS), vagal nerve stimulation (VNS), and transcutaneous supraorbital neurostimulation, have been shown to be effective in patients with migraine. TMS is known to alter cortical excitability[123] and may inhibit cortical spreading depression in individuals with migraine.[124,125] Investigators have utilized single-pulse TMS and repetitive TMS for both migraine prophylaxis and acute treatment of migraine attacks. A randomized, double-blind, sham-controlled trial of patients with migraine with aura demonstrated that single-pulse TMS administered over the occiput is effective in the acute treatment of a migraine attack.[126] The more recent ESPOUSE Study—a multicenter, prospective, open label, observational trial—further demonstrated that single-pulse TMS administered over the occiput is effective for migraine prophylaxis as well.[127] Although studies investigating the efficacy of repetitive TMS (rTMS) for migraine prevention have yielded mixed results,[125,128,129] one retrospective analysis demonstrated that rTMS to the dorsolateral prefrontal cortex may be a useful therapeutic intervention for the management of patients with comorbid migraine and depression.[130]

VNS is thought to alter the activity of multiple brain regions involved in pain perception and processing.[124] This intervention has been shown to be effective for both the acute treatment[131] and prevention[132] of migraine headache, and is now cleared by the FDA for the acute treatment of migraine attacks. Transcutaneous supraorbital neurostimulation is another FDA-approved noninvasive technique by which nociceptive signals may be inhibited,[124] and a multicenter, double-blinded, randomized, sham-controlled trial showed this modality to be effective in the prevention of migraine attacks.[133]

These and other invasive neuromodulation techniques, such as occipital nerve stimulation (ONS), can be effective in the management of chronic migraine.[134] However, they are typically reserved for migraine patients who are refractory to previous pharmacologic and noninvasive therapeutics.[135] Other invasive modalities, such as sphenopalatine ganglion stimulation, may show promise in the management of refractory migraine; however, further research is warranted.[125,135]

CLUSTER HEADACHE TREATMENT

Similar to migraine headache, CH therapeutics are divided into abortive and preventative therapies. According to the latest American Headache Society (AHS) guidelines, the abortive therapies established as effective (Level A recommendation) for both episodic and chronic CH include subcutaneous sumatriptan, intranasal zolmitriptan, and high-flow oxygen. Although suboccipital steroid injection is currently the only prophylactic treatment with a Level A recommendation,[136] other commonly used maintenance therapies for the prevention of CH include verapamil and lithium (despite a Level C recommendation for each of these, respectively, in the latest AHS guidelines).

Furthermore, several invasive and noninvasive neurostimulation techniques have been applied to the treatment and prevention of CH. Positive findings have been reported in the use of noninvasive vagus nerve stimulation[137,138] as well as sphenopalatine ganglion stimulation.[139] Studies applying other neuromodulation techniques such as deep brain stimulation of the hypothalamus or ventral tegmental area have yielded mixed results.[140,141] Importantly, individuals with CH may also suffer from comorbid neuropsychiatric disorders, including recent evidence that this population is at a threefold increased risk for depression, highlighting the importance of adequate identification and intervention.[66]

FUTURE DIRECTIONS

Continued advancement in our understanding of migraine pathophysiology has paved the way for the development of novel therapeutics to target the specific pathways thought to give rise to migraine headache. CGRP antagonists, as mentioned above, represent an important example of these developments. Specifically, further study of CGRP—a vasoactive neuropeptide released during a migraine attack and implicated in the pathophysiology of migraine[142,143]—has led to the development of compounds designed to antagonize the effect of CGRP at its target receptor, and these drugs have recently been approved by the FDA as a treatment for patients with migraine. Similarly, further understanding of existing treatments, such as triptans, has led to the development of 5-hydroxytryptamine 1F receptor agonists, which bind specifically to the serotonin 1F receptor, and in so doing, may eliminate the vascular side effects seen with use of triptans.[144] Moreover, in addition to pharmacologic approaches, researchers may leverage increased understanding of the functional activation patterns characteristic of the migraine attack with the potential to utilize neuromodulation techniques to target specific circuits deranged during an acute migraine, such as alterations in thalamocortical circuitry as described above.[144] These developments in neuroimaging techniques and neurotherapeutic technologies highlight the potential for continued improvement in our understanding and treatment of headache disorders.

Summary and Key Points

- Individuals with migraine demonstrate alterations in the structure and function of brain regions implicated in the processing of pain.
- The treatment of migraine is subdivided into abortive (acute) medications, including NSAIDs, triptans, and combination pharmacotherapy (naproxen/sumatriptan), and prophylactic medications, including a large range of medication classes (various blood pressure, antiepileptic, and antidepressant categories as well as calcitonin gene related peptide antagonists).
- The presence of a comorbid psychiatric condition may guide the selection of migraine prophylactic medication. In some instances, the same medication may be used to treat both the migraine and the psychiatric conditions, for example, valproate for patients with bipolar disorder. However, the doses for the various conditions may be very different so separate treatments for migraine and the psychiatric condition are oftentimes indicated.
- Headache diaries are important tools to determine the effectiveness of a patient's abortive medications and whether migraine prophylaxis is indicated.
- Behavioral interventions, including relaxation, biofeedback, and cognitive-behavioral therapy are effective treatments for patients with migraine. They have Level A evidence when used alone, and well-designed studies show that behavioral therapies in addition to medication have not just an additive effect but rather a synergistic effect on headache outcomes.
- Cluster headache (CH) is a form of trigeminal-autonomic cephalgia characterized by unilateral headaches with autonomic symptoms ipsilateral to the pain, such as miosis, ptosis, lacrimation, and conjunctival injection. The attacks can be very disabling.
- Depression and anxiety are comorbid with cluster headache. In addition, suicidal tendencies have been reported in 25–55% of the CH patients.
- Level A treatments for cluster headache are subcutaneous sumatriptan, intranasal zolmitriptan, and high-flow oxygen for aborting attacks. Suboccipital steroid injections are used for preventing cluster headaches.

Multiple Choice Questions

1. A 21-year-old woman with no known past medical history presents to the clinic with 6 months of intermittent headaches. She describes seeing a bright spot in her visual field, and over several hours, develops a unilateral throbbing headache with associated nausea and vomiting. The patient occasionally needs to lie down in a dark, quiet room until her symptoms subside. You suspect she is suffering from migraines. What structural and/or functional brain abnormalities might you expect to find in this patient?
   a. Decreased activation of the dorsolateral prefrontal cortex in response to a painful stimulus
   b. Increased gray matter volume in inferior frontal and anterior cingulate cortices
   c. Normal functional connectivity involving the brainstem and hypothalamus
   d. Increased functional connectivity between the pons and somatosensory cortex during a migraine attack
   e. Multiple gray matter heterotopias in primary sensory cortex

2. A 40-year-old man with a history of tobacco use (20-pack-year smoker) presents with left unilateral, periorbital headaches with associated lacrimation and conjunctival injection of the left eye that occur multiple times per day for roughly 6 consecutive weeks, followed by months long headache-free periods. What is the most appropriate next step in the diagnosis and/or treatment of the suspected condition?
   a. Obtain serum ESR and CRP levels
   b. Prescribe sumatriptan to be taken as needed to abort the headaches
   c. Obtain serum prolactin levels

   d. Order a lumbar puncture to rule out a subarachnoid hemorrhage
   e. Order a brain MRI to rule out a potential secondary cause for headache

3. A 36-year-old woman is presenting to clinic for a follow-up appointment. She was recently diagnosed with mild episodic migraines and was instructed to create a headache diary with a plan to take ibuprofen as needed for recurrent headaches. She is now experiencing more frequent and disabling migraines (up to four a month), and while she is uninterested in taking a medicine every day to prevent these headaches, she asks if there is a better way to manage these attacks when they occur. What is the most appropriate next step?
   a. Instruct the patient to increase the dose of as needed ibuprofen
   b. Inform the patient that starting a prophylactic medication is the only appropriate next step in managing her migraines
   c. Start a combination long-acting NSAID like naproxen, and triptan to be taken as needed
   d. Prescribe promethazine to be taken as needed to abort acute migraine episodes
   e. Recommend transcranial magnetic stimulation for migraine prevention

4. A 31-year-old man with a history of episodic migraine was recently diagnosed with major depressive disorder. He typically takes naproxen as needed for his migraines with moderate effectiveness and is interested in starting a medication to help treat his depression. What is an appropriate next step in treating this patient?

a. Start a trial of low-dose citalopram, as studies have shown that SSRIs are better than placebo for migraine prevention.
b. Discuss with the patient the advantages and disadvantages of starting a trial of amitriptyline for both depression and migraine prophylaxis.
c. Switch naproxen to a combination naproxen-sumatriptan, as studies have shown that this combination adequately treats both depression and migraines.

d. Recommend discontinuing naproxen as this may have precipitated the patient's depression.
e. Instruct the patient to continue naproxen as needed and refer him to a psychotherapist who specializes in psychodynamic psychotherapy.

Multiple Choice Answers

1. Answer: d

Functional MRI studies have demonstrated that individuals who experience migraines may exhibit stronger functional connectivity between the pons and primary somatosensory cortex during migraine attacks, with specific activation of somatotopic areas representing the head and face,[80] suggesting that a migraine attack, itself, is characterized, in part, by abnormalities in systems responsible for sensory processing.

2. Answer: e

This patient presents with findings typical for episodic cluster headache. When a diagnosis of cluster headache is suspected,

it is important to obtain head imaging (ideally brain MRI) to rule out a potential secondary cause for the headache, such as underlying pituitary gland lesions.

3. Answer: c

Research has shown that the addition of an NSAID to the triptan helps prevent a migraine from recurring.

4. Answer: b

Patients who experience migraines and have comorbid mild unipolar depression may consider combined pharmacotherapy for both treatment of prevention and migraine prophylaxis.

References

1. Headache Classification Committee of the International Headache Society (IHS). The International Classification of Headache Disorders, 3rd edition. *Cephalalgia*. 2018;38(1):1-211.
2. Rasmussen BK, Jensen R, Schroll M, Olesen J. Epidemiology of headache in a general population—a prevalence study. *J Clin Epidemiol*. 1991;44(11):1147-1157.
3. American College of Radiology. 2017. Available at https://www.choosingwisely.org/clinician-lists/american-college-radiology-imaging-for-uncomplicated-headache/.
4. Burch R, Rizzoli P, Loder E. The prevalence and impact of migraine and severe headache in the United States: figures and trends from government health studies. *Headache*. 2018;(2):1-10.
5. David WD. Migraine. 2018;58(1):4-16.
6. Feigin VL, Abajobir AA, Abate KH, et al. Global, regional, and national burden of neurological disorders during 1990-2015: a systematic analysis for the Global Burden of Disease Study 2015. *Lancet Neurol*. 2017;16(11):877.
7. Lipton RB. Tracing transformation: chronic migraine classification, progression, and epidemiology. *Neurology*. 2009;72(5 suppl):3.
8. Natoli JL, Manack A, Dean B, et al. Global prevalence of chronic migraine: a systematic review. *Cephalalgia*. 2010;30(5):599-609.
9. Buse DC, Manack AN, Fanning KM, et al. Chronic migraine prevalence, disability, and sociodemographic factors: results from the American Migraine Prevalence and Prevention Study. *Headache*. 2012;52(10):1456-1470.
10. Lipton RB, Bigal ME. Migraine: epidemiology, impact, and risk factors for progression. *Headache*. 2005;45(suppl 1):S13.
11. Lipton R, Fanning K, Serrano D, Reed M, Cady R, Buse D. Ineffective acute treatment of episodic migraine is associated with new-onset chronic migraine. *Neurology*. 2015;84(7):688-695.
12. Couch JR, Bearss C. Chronic daily headache in the posttrauma syndrome: relation to extent of head injury. *Headache*. 2001;41(6):559-564.
13. Scher AI, Lipton RB, Stewart W. Risk factors for chronic daily headache. *Curr Pain Headache Rep*. 2002;(6):486-491.
14. Hagen K, Einarsen C, Zwart JA, Svebak S, Bovim G. The co-occurrence of headache and musculoskeletal symptoms amongst 51 050 adults in Norway. *Eur J Neurol*. 2002;(9):527-533.
15. Scher AI, Stewart WF, Lipton RB. Factors associated with the onset and remission of chronic daily headache in a population based study. *Pain*. 2003;106(1-2):81-89.
16. Scher AI, Lipton RB, Stewart W. Habitual snoring as a risk factor for chronic daily headache. *Neurology*. 2003;60(8):1366-1368.
17. Scher AI, Stewart WF, Lipton RB. Caffeine as a risk factor for chronic daily headache: a population based study. *Neurology*. 2004;63(11):2022-2027.
18. Lovati C, Amico D, Rosa S, et al. Allodynia in different forms of migraine. *Neurol Sci*. 2007;(28):S220-S221.
19. Scher A, Stewart WF, Buse D, Krantz DS, Lipton RB. Major life changes before and after the onset of chronic daily headache: a population-based study. *Cephalalgia*. 2008;28(8):868.
20. Bigal ME, Lipton RB. Migraine chronification. *Curr Neurol Neurosci Rep*. 2011;11(2):139-148.
21. Stark CD, Stark RJ. Sleep and chronic daily headache. *Curr Pain Headache Rep*. 2015;19(468):1-6.
22. Minen MT, Begasse De Dhaem O, Kroon Van Diest A, et al. Migraine and its psychiatric comorbidities. *Headache*. 2016;87:741-749.
23. Magis D, Pozo-Rosich P, Evers S, Wang SJ. Cluster headache. *Nat Rev*. 2018;4(2):1-17.
24. Russell MB. Epidemiology and genetics of cluster headache. *Lancet Neurol*. 2004;3(5):279-283.

25. Rozen TD, Fishman RS. Cluster headache in the United States of America: demographics, clinical characteristics, triggers, suicidality, and personal burden. *Headache*. 2012;52(1):99-113.

26. Case-control study on the epidemiology of cluster headache. I: Etiological factors and associated conditions. Italian Cooperative Study Group on the Epidemiology of Cluster Headache (ICECH). *Neuroepidemiology*. 1995;14(3):123-127.

27. Hamelsky SW, Lipton RB. Psychiatric comorbidity of migraine. *Headache*. 2006;46(9):1327-1333.

28. Oedegaard KJ, Neckelmann D, Mykletun A, et al. Migraine with and without aura: association with depression and anxiety disorder in a population-based study. The HUNT Study. *Cephalalgia*. 2006;26(1):1-6.

29. Breslau N, Davis GC, Schultz LR, Peterson EL. Joint 1994 Wolff Award presentation. Migraine and major depression: a longitudinal study. *Headache*. 1994;34(7):387-393.

30. Breslau N, Schultz LR, Stewart WF, Lipton RB, Lucia VC, Welch KM. Headache and major depression: is the association specific to migraine? *Neurology*. 2000;54(2):308-313.

31. Santos IS, Brunoni AR, Goulart AC, Griep RH, Lotufo PA, Benseñor IM. Negative life events and migraine: a cross-sectional analysis of the Brazilian Longitudinal Study of Adult Health (ELSA-Brasil) baseline data. *BMC Pub Health*. 2014;3(14):678.

32. Ashina S, Serrano D, Lipton RB, et al. Depression and risk of transformation of episodic to chronic migraine. *J Headache Pain*. 2012;13(8):615-624.

33. Peck KR, Smitherman TA, Baskin SM. Traditional and alternative treatments for depression: implications for migraine management. *Headache*. 2015;55(2):351-355.

34. Baskin SM, Smitherman TA. Migraine and psychiatric disorders: comorbidities, mechanisms, and clinical applications. *Neurol Sci*. 2009;30(suppl 1):61.

35. Mahmood T, Romans S, Silverstone T. Prevalence of migraine in bipolar disorder. *J Affect Disord*. 1999;52(1-3):239-241.

36. Dilsaver SC, Benazzi F, Oedegaard KJ, Fasmer OB, Akiskal KK, Akiskal HS. Migraine headache in affectively ill Latino adults of Mexican American origin is associated with bipolarity. *Prim Care Companion J Clin Psychiatry*. 2009;11(6):302-306.

37. Ortiz A, Cervantes P, Zlotnik G, et al. Cross-prevalence of migraine and bipolar disorder. *Bipolar Disord*. 2010;12(4):397-403.

38. Merikangas KR, Merikangas JR, Angst J. Headache syndromes and psychiatric disorders: association and familial transmission. *J Psychiatr Res*. 1993;27(2):197-210.

39. Fornaro M, Berardis DD, Pasquale CD, et al. Prevalence and clinical features associated to bipolar disorder-migraine comorbidity: a systematic review. *Compr Psychiatry*. 2015;56:1-16.

40. Gordon-Smith K, Forty L, Chan C, et al. Rapid cycling as a feature of bipolar disorder and comorbid migraine. *J Affect Disord*. 2015;175:320-324.

41. Senaratne R, Ameringen MV, Mancini C, Patterson B, Bennett M. The prevalence of migraine headaches in an anxiety disorders clinic sample. *CNS Neurosci Ther*. 2010;16(2):76-82.

42. Smitherman TA, Kolivas ED, Bailey JR. Panic disorder and migraine: comorbidity, mechanisms, and clinical implications. *Headache*. 2013;53(1):23-45.

43. Breslau N. Psychiatric comorbidity in migraine. *Cephalalgia*. 1998;18(suppl 22):61.

44. Lucchetti G, Peres MF, Lucchetti AL, Mercante JP, Guendler VZ, Zukerman E. Generalized anxiety disorder, subthreshold anxiety and anxiety symptoms in primary headache. *Psychiatry Clin Neurosci*. 2013;67(1):41-49.

45. Stewart WF, Linet MS, Celentano DD. Migraine headache and panic attacks. *Psychol Med*. 1989;51(5):559-569.

46. Tietjen GE, Peterlin BL. Childhood abuse and migraine: epidemiology, sex differences, and potential mechanisms. *Headache*. 2011;51(6):869-879.

47. Tietjen GE, Buse DC, Fanning KM, Serrano D, Reed ML, Lipton RB. Recalled maltreatment, migraine, and tension-type headache: results of the AMPP study. *Neurology*. 2015;84(2):132-140.

48. Tietjen GE, Brandes JL, Peterlin BL, et al. Childhood maltreatment and migraine (part II). Emotional abuse as a risk factor for headache chronification. *Headache*. 2010;50(1):32-41.

49. Kuhlman KR, Geiss EG, Vargas I, Lopez-Duran NL. Differential associations between childhood trauma subtypes and adolescent HPA-axis functioning. *Psychoneuroendocrinology*. 2015;54: 103-114.

50. Schreier HM, Enlow MB, Ritz T, Gennings C, Wright RJ. Childhood abuse is associated with increased hair cortisol levels among urban pregnant women. *J Epidemiol Community Health*. 2015;69(12):1169-1174.

51. Peterlin BL, Tietjen GE, Brandes JL, et al. Posttraumatic stress disorder in migraine. *Headache*. 2009;49(4):541-551.

52. Rao AS, Scher AI, Vieira RV, Merikangas KR, Metti AL, Peterlin BL. The impact of post-traumatic stress disorder on the burden of migraine: results from the National Comorbidity Survey-Replication. *Headache*. 2015;55(10):1323-1341.

53. Peterlin BL, Rosso AL, Sheftell FD, Libon DJ, Mossey JM, Merikangas KR. Post-traumatic stress disorder, drug abuse and migraine: new findings from the National Comorbidity Survey Replication (NCS-R). *Cephalalgia*. 2011;31(2):235-244.

54. Juang KD, Yang CY. Psychiatric comorbidity of chronic daily headache: focus on traumatic experiences in childhood, post-traumatic stress disorder and suicidality. *Curr Pain Headache Rep*. 2014;18(4):8.

55. Fasmer OB, Halmoy A, Oedegaard KJ, Haavik J. Adult attention deficit hyperactivity disorder is associated with migraine headaches. *Eur Arch Psychiatry Clin Neurosci*. 2011;261(8):595-602.

56. Peroutka SJ. Dopamine and migraine. *Am Acad Neurol*. 1997;49(3):650-656.

57. Nikolaidis A, Gray JR. ADHD and the DRD4 exon III 7-repeat polymorphism: an international meta-analysis. *Soc Cogn Affect Neurosci*. 2010;5(2-3):188-193.

58. Langemark M, Olesen J. Drug abuse in migraine patients. *Pain*. 1984;19(1):81-86.

59. Salomone JA, Thomas RW, Althoff JR, Watson WA. An evaluation of the role of the ED in the management of migraine headaches. *Am J Emerg Med*. 1994;12(2):134-137.

60. Swartz KL, Pratt LA, Armenian HK, Lee LC, Eaton WW. Mental disorders and the incidence of migraine headaches in a community sample: results from the Baltimore Epidemiologic Catchment area follow-up study. *Arch Gen Psychiatry*. 2000;57(10):945-950.

61. Jette N, Patten S, Williams J, Becker W, Wiebe S. Comorbidity of migraine and psychiatric disorders—a national population-based study. *Headache*. 2008;48(4):501-516.

62. Panconesi A. Alcohol and migraine: trigger factor, consumption, mechanisms. *A review*. *J Headache Pain*. 2008;9(1):19-27.

63. McDermott MJ, Tull MT, Gratz KL, Houle TT, Smitherman TA. Comorbidity of migraine and psychiatric disorders among substance-dependent inpatients. *Headache*. 2014;54(2):290-302.

64. Munoz I, Dominguez E, Hernandez MS, et al. Personality traits in patients with chronic migraine: a categorical and dimensional study in a series of 30 patients. *Rev Neurol*. 2015;61(2):49-56.

65. Robbins M. The psychiatric comorbidities of cluster headache. *Curr Pain Headache Rep*. 2013;17(2):1-8.

66. Louter M, Wilbrink L, Haan J, et al. Cluster headache and depression. *Neurology*. 2016;87(18):1899-1906.

67. Robbins L. The bipolar spectrum in migraine, cluster and chronic tension headache. *Eur Neurol Rev.* 2008;3(1):123.

68. Jurgens TP, Gaul C, Lindwurm A, et al. Impairment in episodic and chronic cluster headache. *Cephalalgia.* 2011;31(6):671-682.

69. Nesbitt AD, Goadsby PJ. Cluster headache. *BMJ.* 2012;344:e2407.

70. Trejo-Gabriel-Galan JM, Aicua-Rapún I, Cubo-Delgado E, Velasco-Bernal C. Suicide in primary headaches in 48 countries: a physician-survey based study. *Cephalgia.* 2018;38(4):798-803.

71. Harrison RH. Psychological testing in headache: a review. *Headache.* 1975;14(4):177-185.

72. Andrasik F, Blanchard EB, Arena JG, Teders SJ, Teevan RC, Rodichok LD. Psychological functioning in headache sufferers. *Psychosom Med.* 1982;44(2):171-182.

73. Piacentini SHMJ, Draghi L, Cecchini AP, Leone M. Personality disorders in cluster headache: a study using the Millon Clinical Multiaxial Inventory-III. *Neurol Sci.* 2017;38(suppl 1):S184.

74. Muñoz I, Hernández MS, Santos S, et al. Personality traits in patients with cluster headache: a comparison with migraine patients. *J Headache Pain.* 2016;17(1):1-5.

75. Chong CD, Plasencia JD, Frakes DH, Schwedt TJ. Structural alterations of the brainstem in migraine. *Neuroimage Clin.* 2016;13:223-227.

76. Ito K, Kudo M, Sasaki M, et al. Detection of changes in the periaqueductal gray matter of patients with episodic migraine using quantitative diffusion kurtosis imaging: preliminary findings. *Neuroradiology.* 2016;58(2):115-120.

77. Chen Z, Chen X, Liu M, Liu S, Ma L, Yu S. Volume expansion of periaqueductal gray in episodic migraine: a pilot MRI structural imaging study. *J Headache Pain.* 2017;18(1):83.

78. DaSilva AF, Granziera C, Snyder J, Hadjikhani N. Thickening in the somatosensory cortex of patients with migraine. *Neurology.* 2007;69(21):1990-1995.

79. Maleki N, Becerra L, Brawn J, Bigal M, Burstein R, Borsook D. Concurrent functional and structural cortical alterations in migraine. *Cephalalgia.* 2012;32(8):607-620.

80. Messina R, Rocca MA, Colombo B, et al. Structural brain abnormalities in patients with vestibular migraine. *J Neurol.* 2017;264(2):295-303.

81. Schwedt TJ, Berisha V, Chong CD. Temporal lobe cortical thickness correlations differentiate the migraine brain from the healthy brain. *PLoS One.* 2015;10(2):e0116687.

82. Chong CD, Starling AJ, Schwedt TJ. Interictal photosensitivity associates with altered brain structure in patients with episodic migraine. *Cephalalgia.* 2016;36(6):526-533.

83. Jia Z, Yu S. Grey matter alterations in migraine: a systematic review and meta-analysis. *Neuroimage Clin.* 2017;14:130-140.

84. Schmitz N, Admiraal-Behloul F, Arkink EB, et al. Attack frequency and disease duration as indicators for brain damage in migraine. *Headache.* 2008;48(7):1044-1055.

85. Hougaard A, Amin FM, Ashina M. Migraine and structural abnormalities in the brain. *Curr Opin Neurol.* 2014;27(3):309-314.

86. Chong CD, Schwedt TJ. Migraine affects white-matter tract integrity: a diffusion-tensor imaging study. *Cephalalgia.* 2015; 35(13):1162-1171.

87. Gudmundsson LS, Scher AI, Sigurdsson S, et al. Migraine, depression, and brain volume: the AGES-Reykjavik Study. *Neurology.* 2013;80(23):2138-2144.

88. Hougaard A, Amin FM, Arngrim N, et al. Sensory migraine aura is not associated with structural grey matter abnormalities. *Neuroimage Clin.* 2016;11:322-327.

89. Chong CD, Schwedt TJ, Dodick DW. Migraine: what imaging reveals. *Curr Neurol Neurosci Rep.* 2016;16(7):64.

90. Schwedt TJ, Chiang CC, Chong CD, Dodick DW. Functional MRI of migraine. *Lancet Neurol.* 2015;14(1):81-91.

91. Chong CD, Schwedt TJ, Hougaard A. Brain functional connectivity in headache disorders: a narrative review of MRI investigations. *J Cereb Blood Flow Metab.* 2019;39(4):650-669.

92. Meylakh N, Marciszewski KK, Di Pietro F, Macefield VG, Macey PM, Henderson LA. Deep in the brain: changes in subcortical function immediately preceding a migraine attack. *Hum Brain.* 2018;39(6):2651-2663.

93. Chong CD, Gaw N, Fu Y, Li J, Wu T, Schwedt TJ. Migraine classification using magnetic resonance imaging resting-state functional connectivity data. *Cephalalgia.* 2017;37(9):828-844.

94. May A, Ashburner J, Buchel C, et al. Correlation between structural and functional changes in brain in an idiopathic headache syndrome. *Nat Med.* 1999;5(7):836-838.

95. Absinta M, Rocca MA, Colombo B, Falini A, Comi G, Filippi M. Selective decreased grey matter volume of the pain-matrix network in cluster headache. *Cephalalgia.* 2012;32(2):109-115.

96. Yang FC, Chou KH, Fuh JL, et al. Altered gray matter volume in the frontal pain modulation network in patients with cluster headache. *Pain.* 2013;154(6):801-807.

97. Qiu E, Wang Y, Ma L, et al. Abnormal brain functional connectivity of the hypothalamus in cluster headaches. *PLoS One.* 2013;8(2):e57896.

98. Yang FC, Chou KH, Kuo CY, Lin YY, Lin CP, Wang SJ. The pathophysiology of episodic cluster headache: insights from recent neuroimaging research. *Cephalalgia.* 2018;38(5):970-983.

99. Holland PR, Barloese M, Fahrenkrug J. PACAP in hypothalamic regulation of sleep and circadian rhythm: importance for headache. *J Headache Pain.* 2018;19(1):20.

100. Loder E, Biondi D. General principles of migraine management: the changing role of prevention. *Headache.* 2005;45(suppl 1):S33-S47.

101. Brandes JL, Kudrow D, Stark SR, et al. Sumatriptan-naproxen for acute treatment of migraine: a randomized trial. *JAMA.* 2007;297(13):1443-1454.

102. Asadollahi S, Heidari K, Vafaee R, Forouzanfar MM, Amini A, Shahrami A. Promethazine plus sumatriptan in the treatment of migraine: a randomized clinical trial. *Headache.* 2014;54(1): 94-108.

103. Kelley NE, Tepper DE. Rescue therapy for acute migraine, part 2: neuroleptics, antihistamines, and others. *Headache.* 2012; 52(2):292-306.

104. Tfelt-Hansen P, Steiner TJ. Over-the-counter triptans for migraine: what are the implications? *CNS Drugs.* 2007;21(11):877-883.

105. Headache Classification Committee of the International Headache Society (IHS). The International Classification of Headache Disorders, 3rd edition (beta version). *Cephalalgia.* 2013;33(9):629-808.

106. Marmura MJ, Silberstein SD, Schwedt TJ. The acute treatment of migraine in adults: the American Headache Society evidence assessment of migraine pharmacotherapies. *Headache.* 2015;55(1):3-20.

107. Worthington I, Pringsheim T, Gawel MJ, et al. Canadian Headache Society guideline: acute drug therapy for migraine headache. *Can J Neurol Sci.* 2013;40(5 suppl 3):S1-S80.

108. Aurora SK, Kori SH, Barrodale P, McDonald SA, Haseley D. Gastric stasis in migraine: more than just a paroxysmal abnormality during a migraine attack. *Headache.* 2006;46(1):57-63.

109. Loder E, Burch R, Rizzoli P. The 2012 AHS/AAN guidelines for prevention of episodic migraine: a summary and comparison with other recent clinical practice guidelines. *Headache.* 2012;52(6):930-945.

110. Pringsheim T, Davenport W, Mackie G, et al. Canadian Headache Society guideline for migraine prophylaxis. *Can J Neurol Sci.* 2012;39(2 suppl 2):S1-S59.

111. Simpson DM, Hallett M, Ashman EJ, et al. Practice guideline update summary: botulinum neurotoxin for the treatment of blepharospasm, cervical dystonia, adult spasticity, and headache: Report of the Guideline Development Subcommittee of the American Academy of Neurology. *Neurology.* 2016;86(19): 1818-1826.

112. Powers SW, Coffey CS, Chamberlin LA, et al. Trial of amitriptyline, topiramate, and placebo for pediatric migraine. *N Engl J Med.* 2017;376(2):115-124.

113. Orlova Y, Rizzoli P, Loder E. Association of coprescription of triptan antimigraine drugs and selective serotonin reuptake inhibitor or selective norepinephrine reuptake inhibitor antidepressants with serotonin syndrome. *JAMA Neurol.* 2018;75(5):566-572.

114. Tepper SJ. History and review of anti-calcitonin gene-related peptide (CGRP) therapies: from translational research to treatment. *Headache.* 2018;58(suppl 3):238-275.

115. Campbell J, Penzien D, Wall E. Evidence-based guidelines for migraine headache: behavioral and physical treatments. 2000. doi: https://da7648.approby.com/m/df542e07c85a1669.pdf

116. Andrasik F, Blanchard EB, Neff DF, Rodichok LD. Biofeedback and relaxation training for chronic headache: a controlled comparison of booster treatments and regular contacts for long-term maintenance. *J Consult Clin Psychol.* 1984;52(4):609-615.

117. Schafer AM, Rains JC, Penzien DB, Groban L, Smitherman TA, Houle TT. Direct costs of preventive headache treatments: comparison of behavioral and pharmacologic approaches. *Headache.* 2011;51(6):985-991.

118. Powers SW, Kashikar-Zuck SM, Allen JR, et al. Cognitive behavioral therapy plus amitriptyline for chronic migraine in children and adolescents: a randomized clinical trial. *JAMA.* 2013;310(24):2622-2630.

119. Holroyd KA, Cottrell CK, O'Donnell FJ, et al. Effect of preventive (beta blocker) treatment, behavioural migraine management, or their combination on outcomes of optimised acute treatment in frequent migraine: randomised controlled trial. *BMJ.* 2010;341:c4871.

120. Minen MT, Azarchi S, Sobolev R, et al. Factors related to migraine patients' decisions to initiate behavioral migraine treatment following a headache specialist's recommendations: a prospective observational study. *Pain Med.* 2018;19(11):2274-2282.

121. Ernst MM, O'Brien HL, Powers SW. Cognitive-behavioral therapy: how medical providers can increase patient and family openness and access to evidence-based multimodal therapy for pediatric migraine. *Headache.* 2015;55(10):1382-1396.

122. Smitherman P, Penzien D, Rains J, Nicholson T, Houle H. *Headache: Advances in Psychotherapy—Evidence-Based Practice.* Oxford, UK: Hogrefe Publishing; 2013.

123. Kobayashi M, Pascual-Leone A. Transcranial magnetic stimulation in neurology. *Lancet Neurol.* 2003;2(3):145-156.

124. Starling A. Noninvasive neuromodulation in migraine and cluster headache. *Curr Opin Neurol.* 2018;31(3):268-273.

125. Schwedt TJ, Vargas B. Neurostimulation for treatment of migraine and cluster headache. *Pain Med.* 2015;16(9):1827-1834.

126. Lipton RB, Dodick DW, Silberstein SD, et al. Single-pulse transcranial magnetic stimulation for acute treatment of migraine with aura: a randomised, double-blind, parallel-group, sham-controlled trial. *Lancet Neurol.* 2010;9(4):373-380.

127. Starling AJ, Tepper SJ, Marmura MJ, et al. A multicenter, prospective, single arm, open label, observational study of sTMS for migraine prevention (ESPOUSE Study). *Cephalalgia.* 2018;38(6):1038-1048.

128. Lan L, Zhang X, Li X, Rong X, Peng Y. The efficacy of transcranial magnetic stimulation on migraine: a meta-analysis of randomized controlled trials. *J Headache Pain.* 2017;18(1).

129. Schoenen J, Roberta B, Magis D, Coppola G. Noninvasive neurostimulation methods for migraine therapy: the available evidence. *Cephalalgia.* 2016;36(12):1170-1180.

130. Kumar S, Singh S, Kumar N, Verma R. The effects of repetitive transcranial magnetic stimulation at dorsolateral prefrontal cortex in the treatment of migraine comorbid with depression: a retrospective open study. *Clin Psychopharmacol Neurosci.* 2018; 16(1):62-66.

131. Goadsby PJ, Grosberg BM, Mauskop A, Cady R, Simmons KA. Effect of noninvasive vagus nerve stimulation on acute migraine: an open-label pilot study. *Cephalalgia.* 2014;34(12):986.

132. Silberstein SD, Calhoun AH, Lipton RB, et al. Chronic migraine headache prevention with noninvasive vagus nerve stimulation: the EVENT study. *Neurology.* 2016;87(5):529-538.

133. Schoenen J, Vandersmissen B, Jeangette S, Herroelen L, Vandenheede M, Gerard P, et al. Migraine prevention with a supraorbital transcutaneous stimulator: a randomized controlled trial. *Neurology.* 2013;80(8):697-704.

134. Dodick DW, Silberstein SD, Reed KL, et al. Safety and efficacy of peripheral nerve stimulation of the occipital nerves for the management of chronic migraine: long-term results from a randomized, multicenter, double-blinded, controlled study. *Cephalalgia.* 2015;35(4):344-358.

135. Puledda F, Goadsby PJ. An update on non-pharmacological neuromodulation for the acute and preventive treatment of migraine. *Headache.* 2017;57(4):685-691.

136. Robbins MS, Starling AJ, Pringsheim TM, Becker WJ, Schwedt TJ. Treatment of cluster headache: the American Headache Society evidence-based guidelines. *Headache.* 2016;56(7):1093-1106.

137. Nesbitt AD, Marin JC, Tompkins E, Ruttledge MH, Goadsby PJ. Initial use of a novel noninvasive vagus nerve stimulator for cluster headache treatment. *Neurology.* 2015;84(12):1249-1253.

138. Gaul C, Diener HC, Silver N, et al. Non-invasive vagus nerve stimulation for PREVention and Acute treatment of chronic cluster headache (PREVA): a randomised controlled study. *Cephalalgia.* 2016;36(6):534-546.

139. Schoenen J, Jensen RH, Lanteri-Minet M, et al. Stimulation of the sphenopalatine ganglion (SPG) for cluster headache treatment. Pathway CH-1: a randomized, sham-controlled study. *Cephalalgia.* 2013;33(10):816-830.

140. Fontaine D, Lazorthes Y, Mertens P, et al. Safety and efficacy of deep brain stimulation in refractory cluster headache: a randomized placebo-controlled double-blind trial followed by a 1-year open extension. *J Headache Pain.* 2010;11(1):23-31.

141. Akram H, Miller S, Lagrata S, et al. Ventral tegmental area deep brain stimulation for refractory chronic cluster headache. *Neurology.* 2016;86(18):1676-1682.

142. Lambru G, Andreou AP, Guglielmetti M, Martelletti P. Emerging drugs for migraine treatment: an update. *Expert Opin Emerg Drugs.* 2018;23(4):301-318.

143. Charles A. The pathophysiology of migraine: implications for clinical management. *Lancet Neurol.* 2018;17(2):174-182.

144. Bohm PE, Stancampiano FF, Rozen TD. Migraine headache: updates and future developments. *Mayo Clin Proc.* 2018;93(11): 1648-1653.

145. Banzi R, Cusi C, Randazzo C, Sterzi R, Tedesco D, Moja L. Selective serotonin reuptake inhibitors (SSRIs) and serotonin-norepinephrine reuptake inhibitors (SNRIs) for the prevention of migraine in adults. *Cochrane Database Syst Rev.* 2015;4(4):CD002919. doi: 10.1002/14651858.CD002919.pub3.

Special Topics in Neuropsychiatry

Women's Neuropsychiatry

Kate Salama · Mary O'Neal · Margo Nathan · Leena Mittal

INTRODUCTION

Women's neurology and mental health are defined as the study of neurologic and psychiatric disorders approached through a sex-based lens. This chapter will discuss some of the sex-based differences in neurologic and psychiatric disorders. The specific concerns vary depending on the disorder, where the woman is in her reproductive cycle, and her psychosocial milieu. The neurologic diseases to be reviewed are those with significant sex differences in prevalence, clinical presentation, or management. They include systemic lupus erythematosus (SLE), migraine, epilepsy, anti-N-methyl-D-aspartate receptor (NMDAR) encephalitis, stroke, and Alzheimer's disease (AD). The psychiatric disorders to be discussed will include those that are related to, or influenced by, the reproductive events in a woman's life—including perimenstrual disorders, perinatal disorders, and perimenopausal disorders. We will focus on these periods of increased hormonal variability and discuss the relationship between sex hormones and serotonergic, dopaminergic, GABAergic, and glutamatergic transmission, and other neurobiological factors. While the focus of this chapter is on the *sex differences* in epidemiology, clinical features, pathophysiology, and treatment of many neurologic and psychiatric disorders, it is important to note that these same disorders are covered in detail in other chapters of this textbook. We direct the reader to the specific chapters, as appropriate, within each of the subtitles below.

AUTOIMMUNE DISEASE AND MULTIPLE SCLEROSIS

An autoimmune disorder occurs when the immune system mounts an attack against the body's own antigens, via a cell-mediated or autoantibodies-mediated mechanism, causing injury to host tissue. Autoimmune diseases affect approximately 8% of the population, and 78% of those affected are women.[1] This increased prevalence in women is likely related to the role of estrogens on both cell- and antibody-mediated immunity. In cell-mediated immunity, androgens and estrogens regulate the

Th1 (helper)/Th2 (suppressor) balance. These types of cell-mediated autoimmune diseases are improved when there is a decrease in type 1 cytokines, proinflammatory T cells, or when there is a rise in type 2 cytokines causing a suppression of inflammatory activity (corresponding to increased estrogens, as in pregnancy).[2]

Multiple sclerosis is an example of a cell-mediated autoimmune disorder in which shifts in cytokine types during pregnancy lead to fetal immunotolerance (the fetus represents a "foreign entity" to the maternal immune system; immunological tolerance during pregnancy protects against a maternal immune response directed at the paternal antigens expressed by the fetus). The result is that relapse rates typically improve during pregnancy with flares in the postpartum period.[3] Chapter 27, *Multiple Sclerosis,* reviews in detail the neuropsychiatric manifestations of this illness. In animal models, females generate more antibodies after vaccination compared to males.[4] This may explain why antibody-mediated autoimmune disorders such as SLE, Sjogren's syndrome, and neuromyelitis optica occur much more frequently in women. SLE will be described as an example of an autoimmune disorder in which there are significant sex differences.

SYSTEMIC LUPUS ERYTHEMATOSUS

Epidemiology

SLE is a chronic autoimmune and inflammatory disease with heterogenous manifestations. The prevalence of lupus in women is seven times greater than men.[5] The ethnicities most often afflicted include Hispanics, African Americans, and Asians.[6] The disease onset is usually in young adulthood intersecting with reproductive health for these women. The current preferred nomenclature to denote lupus involving the central nervous system is neuropsychiatric SLE, not lupus cerebritis which implies an inflammatory mechanism. Neurologic involvement is common with wide estimates of prevalence from 10% to 80%. This large range is due to the differences in the definition of neuropsychiatric lupus.[7,8]

Pathophysiology

The exact pathophysiology of lupus is unclear. The etiology of the disease is likely multifactorial with genetics, prior infections, and sex all playing a role. Many of the clinical manifestations are mediated directly or indirectly by antibody formation and the creation of immune complexes. Direct central neurologic involvement can be due to small vessel vasculopathy, cardioembolic stroke from Libman-Sacks endocarditis, as well as related to autoantibodies. SLE-associated vasculopathy may contribute to causing small vessel infarcts. The vasculopathy results from fibrinoid necrosis, thought to be related to perivascular accumulation of mononuclear cells, and not from a true "vasculitis." The presence of antiphospholipid antibodies causes a hypercoagulable state, increasing the risk of strokes—both arterial and venous, as well as placental infarction with miscarriages.[9] Lupus encephalitis has been associated with several autoantibodies. Anti-ribosomal P protein, anti-endothelial cell, and cross-reacting antibodies to excitatory NMDARs have been implicated in the psychiatric manifestations of lupus including psychosis and depression.[10-12] However, none of these antibodies are sensitive and specific enough to have clinically utility through testing their levels.

Neuropsychiatric Presentation

Headache, mood disorder, cognitive impairment, seizures, and stroke are the most common presentations of neuropsychiatric SLE. Headache alone is not clearly associated with lupus unless there are red flags such as associated neurologic signs/symptoms or elevated intracranial pressure. Similarly, there are conflicting reports about the causality of lupus in mood disorders. In contrast, studies have shown that psychosis is clearly related to disease activity and approximately 5% of patients with SLE can present with an organic psychotic disorder. The phenomenology of SLE-associated psychosis is similar to that of primary psychosis, including disorganized thinking, delusions, paranoia, or hallucinations among other symptoms.[13] Secondary psychosis related to steroids needs to be excluded.

Cognitive difficulties have been reported in 21–80% of lupus patients.[14,15] Impairments are most apparent on tests of psychomotor speed, complex attention, and memory. The mechanisms underlying cognitive dysfunction in lupus are likely multifactorial, related to vascular injury, autoantibodies, and inflammation. Seizures can occur in up to 11.2% of patients and can be focal, generalized, or provoked. Antiphospholipid antibodies levels and stroke were significantly correlated to seizures at SLE disease onset.[16] Please see the *Neuropsychiatry of Inflammatory, Autoimmune, and Infectious Disorders* chapter (Chapter 26) in this textbook for further information about the neuropsychiatry of SLE.

Diagnosis and Assessment

The American College of Rheumatology has formulated diagnostic criteria for SLE (see Table 33-1).[17] The assessment should be tailored to the clinical presentation. For example, a young woman presenting with stroke would need brain and vessel imaging, a cardiac ECHO, a 30-day event monitor to exclude

TABLE 33-1 • To Diagnose Lupus—4 Out of 11 Required.	
Criterion	**Definition**
Malar rash	Erythema over malar regions of the face
Discoid rash	Raised erythematous patches with keratotic scaling and follicular plugging
Photosensitivity	Skin reactivity to sunlight
Oral ulcers	Oral or nasopharyngeal ulceration, usually painless
Arthritis	Nonerosive arthritis with tenderness or swelling involving two or more joints
Serositis	Pericarditis or pleuritis
Renal dysfunction	Proteinuria or cellular casts
Neurologic disorder	Seizures or psychosis without any provocative factor
Hematologic abnormalities	Hemolytic anemia or leukopenia or lymphopenia or thrombocytopenia
ANA	Abnormal titer of ANA
Other positive serology	Presence of anti-double-stranded DNA, anti-Smith or antiphospholipid antibodies

Adapted from the American College of Rheumatology—SLE Diagnostic Criteria.

atrial fibrillation and a hypercoagulable evaluation. A young woman with new onset psychosis would be typically evaluated with a brain MRI, electroencephalogram, laboratory evaluations including a toxic screen, an ANA, and a paraneoplastic panel with consideration for cerebrospinal fluid analysis.

Sex-Specific Treatment Concerns

SLE confers significant maternal and fetal risks. The general recommendation is that women should have stable disease for 6 months prior to planning pregnancy. Table 33-2 illustrates the pregnancy category and breast-feeding ratings for the commonly used immunosuppressants to treat SLE.[18] A history of thrombotic complications is extremely important in preconception planning. Management of antiphospholipid antibody syndrome in pregnancy requires therapeutic enoxaparin sodium. Postpartum, warfarin can be initiated. Anti-Ro antibodies, if present, can cause neonatal lupus with the most serious problem related to complete heart block. Fortunately, this complication occurs in only 2% of women with this antibody, but careful pregnancy monitoring is warranted in this setting.[18] Lupus also confers substantive risks to the pregnancy including preterm labor, small for gestational age, increased risk of fetal loss, and eclampsia.[19]

MIGRAINE

Epidemiology

Migraine is three times more common in women than men. The difference in migraine prevalence begins at menarche and ends at menopause; it is primarily driven by migraine without aura.[20]

CASE VIGNETTE 33.1

Migraine

A 24-year-old woman presents with a 5-year history of unilateral throbbing headaches associated with nausea, vomiting, light and sound sensitivity. The headaches always start 2 days prior to her menses. She has tried multiple over-the-counter medications at the time of the headache. Her neurological exam is normal.

TABLE 33-2 • Lupus Medication—Pregnancy/Breast-Feeding Guidelines.

Drug	Pregnancy	Breast-Feeding
Nonsteroidal anti-inflammatories	Avoid after 30 weeks	Compatible
Glucocorticoids	Continue at lowest possible dose	Compatible
Azathioprine	Preferred immunosuppressant	Probably compatible
Cyclosporine	Unknown risk	Need to monitor for toxicity
Tacrolimus	Reasonable alternative to other more potent immunosuppressant	Not recommended
Rituximab	Unknown risk	Unknown risk
Cyclophosphamide	Avoid	Avoid
Hydroxychloroquine	Continue	Compatible
Methotrexate	Avoid	Avoid

Pathophysiology

The pathophysiology of the sex differences in migraine is thought to be related to changes in estrogen levels triggering activation of the trigeminal vascular system, inducing migraine in vulnerable individuals.[21] This interaction explains much of the known hormonal effects in female migraineurs. For instance, combined hormonal contraceptives (CHCs) (i.e., those containing both estrogen and progestin) may alter migraine frequency. Withdrawal from estrogen triggers menstrual migraine. Migraine in pregnancy (especially migraine without aura) is generally worst in the first trimester with a 77–83% remission by the second trimester when estrogen levels stabilize.[22–24] Postpartum is a common time for migraine recrudescence due to hormonal changes, sleep deprivation, and stress.

Sex-Specific Treatment Considerations

Combined Hormonal Contraceptives and Migraine

The influence of CHCs on migraine is unpredictable. They can cause migraine in susceptible individuals as well as increase or decrease migraine frequency and intensity. Migraine without aura is more hormonally driven than migraine with aura, and the type most influenced by CHCs.[25]

Migraineurs with aura have a small but real risk of stroke, especially when combined with other traditional stroke risk factors. For this reason, CHCs—due to their associated impact on coagulation—are generally avoided in women who have migraine with aura.[26] Women who have migraine without aura have no increased stroke risk.

Menstrual Migraine

For many women (particularly migraineurs without aura) their worst migraine is associated with menses. The predictability of menstrual migraine allows for several treatment strategies, such as *miniprophylaxis* by using either nonsteroidal anti-inflammatory medications or long-acting triptans to begin 1–2 days prior to the usual timing of the menstrual migraine. Another treatment strategy in migraine without aura is the use of CHC to avoid the estrogen withdrawal trigger.[27]

Migraine Treatment in Pregnancy

Migraines may worsen during the first trimester of pregnancy, but usually improve by the second trimester. This improvement is most common in migraineurs without aura and is driven by rising estrogen levels which plateau during the second trimester. This clinical scenario is less predictable for migraine with aura.

Prophylactic medication for migraine is usually avoided in pregnancy due to safety concerns as well as the fact that the headaches generally improve. Alternative treatments such as stress management, physical therapy, and occipital blocks are first line.[28] However, symptomatic medication is often needed. See Table 33-3 for safety information of commonly used symptomatic medication for migraine during pregnancy. See the *Headache* chapter (Chapter 32) in this textbook for a comprehensive discussion of the neuropsychiatry of migraine.

EPILEPSY

Epidemiology

The prevalence of epilepsy is higher in men than women. However, there are multiple concerns for women with epilepsy including hormonal effects on epilepsy, teratogenic risks of antiepileptic drugs (AEDs), interaction of AEDs with hormonal contraceptives, and management of AEDs during pregnancy.

Catamenial epilepsy

A 34-year-old woman is referred for evaluation for epilepsy. Seizures are described as beginning with a yawn; then she loses tone, followed by tonic posturing with arms flexed and legs extended. The seizures are 1–2 minutes in duration followed by a postictal confusion lasting up to 15 minutes.

She usually has one seizure a month typically at the onset of her menses. Her menses are regular. She is currently on levetiracetam 500 mg in the morning and 750 mg at night. Brain magnetic resonance imaging was normal.

TABLE 33-3 • Symptomatic Migraine Medication.		
Medication	**Level of Risk in Pregnancy***	**Hale Lactation Rating****
Acetaminophen	B	L1
Nonsteroidal anti-inflammatory drugs	B (D in 3rd trimester)	L1–L2
Metoclopramide	B	L2
Prochlorperazine	C	L3
Dihydroergotamine	X	L4
Magnesium	A (D)***	L1
Triptans	C	L3

*FDA pregnancy categories:

A: Adequate and well-controlled human studies have failed to demonstrate a risk to the fetus in the first trimester of pregnancy (and there is no risk in later trimesters).

B: Animal reproduction studies have failed to demonstrate a risk to the fetus and there are no adequate and well-controlled studies in pregnant women OR animal studies have shown an adverse effect, but adequate and well-controlled studies in pregnant women have failed to demonstrate a risk to the fetus in any trimester.

C: Animal reproduction studies have shown an adverse effect on the fetus and there are no adequate and well-controlled studies in humans, but potential benefits may warrant use of the drug in pregnant women despite potential risks.

D: There is positive evidence of human fetal risk based on adverse reaction data from investigational or marketing experience or studies in humans, but potential benefits may warrant use of the drug in pregnant women despite potential risks.

X: Studies in animals or humans have demonstrated fetal abnormalities and/or there is positive evidence of human fetal risk based on adverse reaction data from investigational or marketing experience, and the risks involved in use of the drug in pregnant women clearly outweigh potential benefits.

**Hale lactation ratings:

L1, Safest—Drug has been taken by many breast-feeding women without evidence of adverse effects in nursing infants OR controlled studies have failed to show evidence of risk.

L2, Safer—Drug has been studied in a limited number of breast-feeding women without evidence of adverse effects in nursing infants.

L3, Moderately Safe—Studies in breast-feeding women have shown evidence for mild non-threatening adverse effects OR there are no studies in breast-feeding women for a drug with possible adverse effects.

L4, Possibly Hazardous—Studies have shown evidence for risk to a nursing infant, but in some circumstances the drug may be used during breast-feeding.

L5, Contraindicated—Studies have shown significant risk to nursing infants. The drug should NOT be used during breast-feeding.

***New warning against continuous administration of IV Mg 5–7 days for preterm labor based on concern about bone abnormalities in the fetus suggesting rickets-like skeletal abnormalities in babies exposed to Mg in utero.*

Catamenial Epilepsy

Catamenial epilepsy refers to epilepsy that increases in relation to the menstrual cycle. This is particularly true of focal epilepsy. Using the definition of doubling the seizure frequency in relation to a part of the menstrual cycle, the prevalence of catamenial epilepsy is approximately one-third of women with focal epilepsy.[29] The increase in seizure frequency is related to the increase in estradiol, a proconvulsant, compared with progesterone, an anticonvulsant. Different patterns of catamenial epilepsy have been defined[28] in Table 33-4.

Treatment is best delineated for the C1 pattern, where there is a perimenstrual exacerbation. In these women, adjunctive medications such as progesterone lozenges, acetazolamide, and clobazam as well as increasing the AED dose around this part of the cycle may be effective.[30-32]

Contraception Interactions

Women with epilepsy need to plan pregnancy to optimize their outcome. Therefore, effective contraception is important. There are significant interactions between sex steroids and those anticonvulsants that induce hepatic enzymes (see Table 33-5). These interactions can both decrease contraception efficacy and alter AED levels. These interactions need to be considered when choosing an AED and the most appropriate contraceptive method.[33]

TABLE 33-4 • Patterns of Catamenial Epilepsy.[28]	
Catamenial Pattern	**Definition**
C1	Premenstrual seizure exacerbation
C2	Periovulatory exacerbation
C3	Seizure exacerbation in the luteal phase

TABLE 33-5 • Hepatic Enzyme-Inducing Antiepileptic Medication.[40]	
Strong Inducers	**Weak Inducers**
Phenobarbital, phenytoin, primidone, carbamazepine, oxcarbazepine	Topiramate, lamotrigine, felbamate, rufinamide

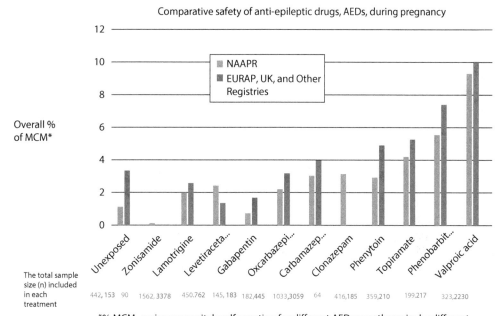

Comparative safety of anti-epileptic drugs, AEDs, during pregnancy

*% MCM- major congenital malformation for different AED monotherapies by different registries: NAAPR, North American AED Pregnancy Registry. The total sample size (n) included in each treatment is also presented; if n < 50, the information was not included
Slide courtesy of P. Voinescu, MD, PhD

FIGURE 33-1. Comparative safety of antiepileptic drugs (AEDs) during pregnancy. *% MCM, major congenital malformation for different AED monotherapies by different registries; NAAPR, North American AED Pregnancy Registry. The total sample size (n) included in each treatment is also presented; if n < 50, the information was not included. (Slide courtesy of P. Voinescu, MD, PhD.)

Teratogenic Risks of AEDs

The most important factor for choosing an AED is the type of epilepsy. In women of reproductive age further consideration needs to be given to the side effects of the AED in pregnancy, including major congenital malformations (MCMs) and long-term effects on fetal brain development. There has been considerable research in this area. Valproate is known to increase the risk of neural tube defects and have a long-term negative impact on cognitive outcomes of exposed children. Topiramate also has significant MCM risks causing cleft palate defects. In contrast, both lamotrigine and levetiracetam have proven to have excellent safety and cognitive outcomes. For many of the newer AEDs, there is not enough information to adequately address safety concerns.[34–37] (See Figure 33-1.)[38–40] Folate, 1–4 mg daily, should be prescribed for all women with epilepsy in their reproductive years given its known effect in decreasing neural tube defects.[41]

Management of AEDs during Pregnancy

The AED level varies according to hepatic and renal metabolism as well as the volume of distribution, all of which dramatically change in pregnancy. Best practice is to determine the therapeutic AED level before pregnancy, as a guide to the desired level to maintain during pregnancy. Monthly trough levels of the AED can be determined, with dosing aimed at preserving the previously determined therapeutic level. Postpartum doses of the AED need to be quickly decreased to the pre-pregnancy doses to prevent toxicity.[41] Please refer to the *Epilepsy* chapter (Chapter 29) in this textbook for a comprehensive discussion of the neuropsychiatric disorders that may present in this illness.

ANTI-NMDA RECEPTOR (ANTI-NMDAR) ENCEPHALITIS

Epidemiology

Anti-NMDAR encephalitis is the most common autoimmune encephalitis, with antibodies targeting the cell surface and synaptic proteins. The exact incidence is not known, but in one retrospective review anti-NMDAR encephalitis represented 1% of all young patients' admissions to the ICU.[42] Eighty percent of these patients are young women and two-third will have an associated ovarian teratoma.[43]

Pathophysiology

The main epitope targeted by the antibodies is on the cell surface which involves the N-terminal domain of the NR1/NR2 subunits of the NMDAR. It is postulated that there is tissue in the ovarian teratoma that stimulates the immune system to produce anti-NMDAR antibodies. These antibodies then enter the central nervous system, where they deplete cell-surface NMDARs on the NMDAR-rich neurons of the limbic system. It has been demonstrated that patients' antibodies can decrease the number of cell-surface hippocampal NMDARs, an effect that can be

Anti-NMDA receptor encephalitis

A 24-year-old woman in good health abruptly began having paranoid preoccupations. She became extremely agitated and could not sleep. She started having hallucinations, claiming that her mother's voice was coming from the TV. At that point, she was brought to the hospital. Initial exam showed temperature of 100.7°F; the rest of her vitals were normal. Her exam was notable for a confusional state, with affective lability and disinhibition (taking off her clothes); the rest of the neurologic exam was normal. A few days later, she became rigid, mute, and started posturing.

Routine labs, including a toxic screen, were normal. Brain MRI with gadolinium, brain MRA, head CT were negative. A lumbar puncture revealed lymphocytosis (48 WBC, 100% lymphocytes). ESR/CRP were mildly elevated. Herpes simplex virus PCR was initially ambiguous, so she received a 10-day course of IV acyclovir. An extensive infectious workup was performed, which was negative. EEGs were normal. Paraneoplastic panel results were negative. She underwent a transvaginal ultrasound and a pelvic MRI which were negative. Anti-NMDA-R antibodies were positive at 1:20, consistent with anti-NMDA-receptor encephalitis.

She received IV immunoglobulin for 3 days. Her symptoms, including confusion and behavioral changes, gradually normalized. She was discharged home on oral lorazepam with plans to start rituximab as therapy for anti-NMDAR encephalitis with no tumor identified.

reversed by antibody removal. Loss of these receptors leads to neuronal dysfunction, with changes in synaptic and neurocircuit function that in turn drive the behavioral changes.[44] This hypothesis is supported by the action of other NMDAR antagonists such as ketamine and phencyclidine which cause similar symptoms to anti-NMDAR encephalitis.

Clinical Presentation

Usually, there is a viral prodrome several weeks before the onset of neuropsychiatric manifestations. Most patients present with psychiatric symptoms such as agitation, delusional thoughts, and hallucinations.

Seizures of all types (generalized, focal with awareness unimpaired, and focal with impaired awareness) occur in 83% of patients. Almost all patients (96%) progress to develop a decreased level of arousal with catatonia associated with movement disorders, autonomic instability, and hypoventilation.[45]

Assessment and Differential Diagnosis

Spinal fluid analysis is very sensitive with 91% of patients showing a nonspecific lymphocytic pleocytosis. In contrast, brain MRI shows abnormalities 55% of the time and these are nonspecific FLAIR or T2 signal changes in one or several brain regions including mesial temporal lobes, cortex, basal ganglia, cerebellum, and brainstem.[45] The diagnosis is clinched by the findings of anti-NMDAR antibodies in cerebrospinal or serum. The differential diagnosis consists of other primary psychiatric conditions, causes of toxic metabolic encephalopathy, and other etiologies of encephalitis including infectious, autoimmune, and other paraneoplastic ones.

Given the high association with ovarian teratoma, all women suspected of anti-NMDAR encephalitis should have either a pelvic MRI, CT, or ultrasound.

Treatment

Treatment involves tumor removal if applicable and immunotherapy—intravenous immunoglobulin or corticosteroids are first line. Those patients that relapse (more common in patients with no

tumor or where tumor was not found in the initial evaluation) require ongoing immunosuppression. Recovery is good in 75% of cases, either with no deficits or substantial improvement with mild deficits. The median time from symptom presentation to initial signs of improvement is often prolonged—about 6 weeks.[46] Please refer to two chapters in this textbook: "Inflammatory, Autoimmune, and Infectious Disorders" (Chapter 26) and "Neuropsychiatric Complications of Cancer and Its Treatment" (Chapter 28) for a comprehensive discussion of autoimmune encephalitis.

STROKE IN WOMEN

Epidemiology

Within most age groups, women have a lower incidence of ischemic stroke (IS) than men; however, sex differences in IS incidence rates differ across the lifespan. The lifetime risk of stroke is higher in women (20%) compared to men (17%).[47] In addition, as women tend to be older when they have their stroke events, and women have a longer life expectancy than men, age-adjusted rates are misleading and underestimate the total burden of stroke in women. Stroke is the fourth leading cause of death in women.[48,49] Not only do women have more stroke events than men, but their functional outcomes are worse even after adjustment for baseline differences in age, pre-stroke function, and comorbidities.[50]

Risk Factors

Women have distinct risk factors for IS. These conditions include migraine with aura, hypercoagulability related to exogenous estrogen, pregnancy complications including hypercoagulability, hypertension, diabetes, and preeclampsia/eclampsia.[51–55]

A large body of literature supports that complications of pregnancy predict future cardiovascular risk decades later. For example, a woman with gestational diabetes has a 50% risk of developing diabetes within the next 5–10 years following her pregnancy.[56] Diabetes is a significant risk factor for stroke. Table 33-6[56–59] displays how pregnancy-related conditions alter the risk of IS.

Further, women have an increased risk of stroke compared with men related to atrial fibrillation (AF). Large cohort

TABLE 33-6 • Pregnancy-Related Complications and Stroke Risk.

Risk Factor	Risk of Future Ischemic Stroke
Preeclampsia	OR: 1.36–2.53
Gestational diabetes mellitus (DM)	50% risk of developing DM in 5–10 years; stroke risk unknown
Gestational hypertension	OR: 1.58–1.67

OR, odds ratio.

studies have confirmed an age-sex interaction in patients with AF, which suggests a higher risk of stroke in women ≥75 years with AF compared with men.[60] For example, in a study that included 100,802 patients with nonvalvular AF in Sweden, the incident risk of IS was greater in women than in men (6.2% vs. 4.2% per year).[61] Please refer to the *Stroke* chapter (Chapter 22) in this textbook for a comprehensive discussion of the neuropsychiatric disorders that may present in this illness.

ALZHEIMER'S DISEASE

Epidemiology

AD affects over 5.5 million Americans, and two-third of those affected are women.[62] It is known that the risk of AD doubles with each decade over age 60, and that women live longer than men. Some studies suggest that there may be a sex-specific risk, beyond the longevity factor.[63]

Pathophysiology

The apolipoprotein E4 (APOE4) allele is an important risk factor for sporadic AD. This allele plays an important role in reduced clearance of a beta amyloid. The risk of developing AD related to the APOE4 allele affects both genders. However, women who carry the APOE4 allele are more likely to develop mild cognitive impairment (MCI) than men. Further, women with either the *APOE3/3* or *APOE3/4* genotypes are more likely to develop AD compared to men.[64] In a meta-analysis of 27 independent research studies with 58,000 subjects, women and men with one copy of the APOE4 genotype did not show a difference in risk of AD across the lifespan of 55–85 years of age, but women were at increased risk between the ages of 65 and 75.[65]

Chromosomes are protected from degradation by telomeres, DNA structures that cap their ends. Telomere shortening has been associated with AD.[66] Women have longer telomeres compared to age-matched men. This fact appears to be estrogen driven. In a study looking at hormonal replacement in postmenopausal women who were APOE4 carriers versus those who did not carry the APOE4 allele, hormonal therapy prevented telomere shortening only in carriers—suggesting that in women at risk, estrogen may play a beneficial role.[67]

The Women's Health Initiative Memory study, WHIMS, showed that postmenopausal women treated with estrogen and progesterone had double the risk of dementia.[68] Subsequently, a few studies have suggested that there may be a therapeutic window for hormone replacement therapy (HRT). For instance,

in the Cache county study, women who used any type of HRT within 5 years of menopause had a 30% less risk of AD.[69,70]

Clinical Presentation—Sex Differences

Men with AD are more likely to have aggressive behavior and higher mortality than women. Women with AD are more likely to display affective symptoms, have greater disability, and have a longer survival.[71] Studies have shown that among individuals with AD, men outperform women in visuospatial, memory (both semantic and episodic), and language tasks, even after controlling for age, educational status, and severity of AD.[72] Further, women with two copies of the APOE4 allele compared to men with the same genotype are more likely to develop psychosis, delusions, and hallucinations during their illness.[73] This data suggest that women may have specific vulnerabilities as regards to AD symptomatology.

Assessment and Differential Diagnosis

Assessment for AD is the same for women and men. This includes a thorough neurologic exam, laboratory analysis, and brain imaging to exclude other causes of dementia. Brain imaging (MRI is the preferred modality) is important to look for structural mimics of dementia due to neurodegenerative disease such as tumor, stroke, and subdural hematoma as well as to assess patterns of atrophy that are suggestive of different types of neurodegenerative processes. For patients in whom the diagnosis is unclear, neuropsychological evaluation and CSF analysis (using beta-amyloid and tau proteins levels as biomarkers of Alzheimer's-type pathology) are helpful adjuncts.[74]

Treatment—Sex Differences

The acetylcholinesterase inhibitors (ChEIs) (FDA-approved for mild, moderate, and severe AD) and memantine (approved for moderate and severe AD) are used for the symptomatic treatment of AD. The randomized controlled trials to approve ChEIs and memantine recruited a larger number of female participants to reflect the female prevalence of AD.[75] There are a few studies showing a sex effect on treatment efficacy. For instance, women seem to respond better to ChEIs compared to men. The reason for this difference may be related to variants of the estrogen receptor gene which is reported to modulate AD susceptibility and disease course.[76] There are no studies that have investigated potential sex and gender differences in the safety and tolerability of the approved treatments.[76]

Take home points:

1. AD is more prevalent in women.
2. There are differential sex-specific risks associated with the APOE allele.
3. Telomere shortening is associated with AD and estrogen affects telomere length.
4. There may be a beneficial window where estrogen exposure improves cognition for women at risk for AD.

Please refer to the "Alzheimer's Disease" chapter (Chapter 21) in this textbook for a comprehensive discussion of the neuropsychiatric disorders that may present in this illness.

PERIMENSTRUAL PSYCHIATRIC DISORDERS

Puberty is initiated by the release of gonadotropin-releasing hormone from the hypothalamus that stimulates hormonal cascades and gonadal activation.[77] Menarche typically marks the near end of puberty in girls. Menstrual cycles occur in three phases: follicular, ovulatory, and luteal. During the follicular phase, FSH stimulates follicle development and maturation, which in turn produces estrogen to prepare the uterus for pregnancy. At ovulation, increased estrogen triggers a rise in LH from the pituitary, causing release of an egg from the follicle. The corpus luteum secretes progesterone and estrogen to continue to prepare for pregnancy. If the egg is not fertilized, estrogen and progesterone levels drop, and menses begin.[78] This is depicted in Figure 33-2.[79]

CASE VIGNETTE 33.4

Postpartum depression

A 32-year-old woman presents for her 6-week postpartum obstetric visit. She is tearful on interview and reports she has not been able to sleep, even when her baby is sleeping. She reports that her mood has been worsening since delivery and she is having a hard time bonding with the baby. She feels constantly anxious and agitated, worries that something bad will happen to the baby, and worries about leaving the home. She has become isolated from family and friends, and worries she is not a good mother. She reports one prior episode of depression in her early 20s for which she was treated to remission with sertraline.

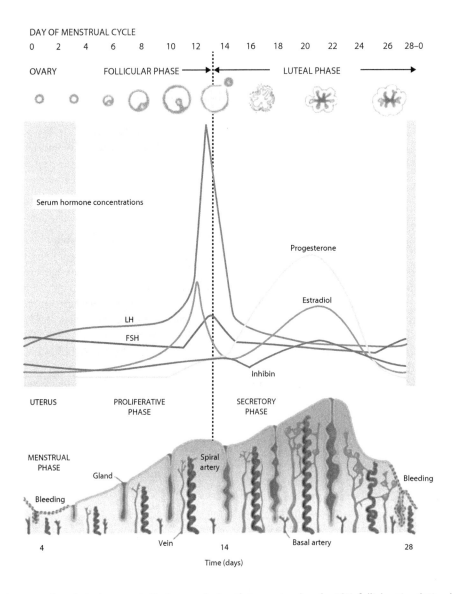

FIGURE 33-2. Ovarian, hormonal, and uterine events that occur during the menstrual cycle. FSH, follicle-stimulating hormone; LH, luteinizing hormone. (Rreproduced with permission from Kibble JD, Halsey CR. *Medical Physiology: The Big Picture.* https://accessmedicine.mhmedical.com. Copyright © McGraw Hill LLC. All rights reserved.)

One of the leading theories behind psychiatric disorders related to the menstrual cycle is that a subset of women has an abnormal brain response to the normal fluctuations in estradiol and progesterone. While the mechanism whereby fluctuations in steroid levels induce mood symptoms is unclear, it is thought that a change in steroid level could confer differential cellular effects compared with steady state.[80] Other researchers posit these disorders are related to withdrawal from allopregnanolone (ALLO), a progesterone metabolite.[81] Alternatively, these disorders may be caused by a deficit in the serotonin system and specifically the serotonin transporter, with complex estrogen-serotonin interactions that affect mood and cognition.[82,83] Some studies have also begun to demonstrate neurobiological functional differences in the premenstrual syndrome (PMS), such as abnormal spontaneous brain activity during the luteal phase in the precuneus, hippocampus, inferior temporal cortex, anterior cingulate cortex, and cerebellum, in women with PMS.[84]

The psychiatric disorders related to the hormonal fluctuations of the menstrual cycle include PMS, premenstrual dysphoric disorder (PMDD), and premenstrual exacerbation (PME) of an underlying psychiatric disorder.[85] These disorders are best diagnosed and distinguished by prospective tracking of mood symptoms throughout the menstrual cycle. These disorders indicate hormonal sensitivity and are a risk factor for perinatal and perimenopausal mood disorders. See Table 33-7 for a comparison of these disorders.

PRECONCEPTION PLANNING IN PSYCHIATRY

Patients with severe mental illness have increased risk for unplanned or unwanted pregnancies, are more likely to undergo an abortion, are at greater risk for violence, and have higher rates of substance abuse during pregnancy.[103] For these reasons, integrating mental health and family planning services enhances care for patients with psychiatric disorders.[104] In addition to the typical psychiatric assessment, a thorough sexual history, which includes sexual orientation, number of partners, contraceptive use, attitude toward becoming pregnant, alcohol and illicit substance use, OB/GYN history, and history of any traumatic life event should be gathered during initial meetings with patients and reassessed periodically. In addition, education on how to resist unwanted sexual advances, contraception, risks and benefits of pregnancy, management of mental illness during pregnancy, and how to advocate for condom use among male partners will help patients to make thoughtful decisions as it pertains to pregnancy and mental illness.[105] A simple way to begin this conversation is to ask patients if they would like to become pregnant in the next year. If they respond no, contraceptive methods should be discussed, and consistency should be emphasized. If they respond yes or are unsure, it is important to make family planning discussions part of the ongoing care and to discuss a psychiatric medication plan for pregnancy prior to conception.[106] This discussion, which unfortunately often does not occur, can be key to optimizing the chance for a healthy and desired pregnancy.

TABLE 33-7 • Premenstrual Disorders.

	PMS	PMDD	PME
Prevalence	20–30% of reproductive aged women[86]	1.2–8% of reproductive aged women[87]	2/3 of women with major depressive disorder[88]
Risk factors	White, obesity, metabolic syndrome, early life physical and sexual abuse[89-92]		
	Familial component, as concordance rates are higher among monozygotic twins[93,94]		
Presentation	Lability, irritability, depression, anxiety, feeling overwhelmed, physical symptoms such as breast tenderness, muscle pain, bloating		Can present as more severe depression, anxiety, manic or mixed states, or psychosis
	PMDD is a severe form of PMS and causes functional impairments[95]		
Time course	Symptoms present during luteal phase of most menstrual cycles, improve within few days of onset of menses, and become minimal or absent in week post menses; resolves during pregnancy and after menopause[95]		Worsening of preexisting mental health disorder during luteal phase
Treatment	Supportive therapy or CBT, diet rich in complex carbohydrates,[96] aerobic exercise,[97] calcium,[98] chasteberry[99]	SRI therapy[100]	Can increase dose of medication used for underlying disorder during luteal phase
		Continuous OCPs[101]	
		Most severe cases can consider leuprolide injections with TAH-BSO as last resort[95,102]	

PMDD, premenstrual dysphoric disorder; PME, premenstrual exacerbation of psychiatric illness; PMS, premenstrual syndrome.

PERINATAL PSYCHIATRIC DISORDERS

The perinatal period is defined as the time beginning at 22 weeks gestation and lasting 1 week after birth. Just as in the perimenstrual period, sensitivity to fluctuations in gonadal hormone levels can cause an exacerbation of mental health symptoms in the perinatal period, supported by evidence that women with perinatal depression have a different response to abrupt elevation or reduction of gonadal steroid levels compared to women without perinatal depression.[107] The leading theory behind worsening mood in the postpartum period is that the rapid changes in hormone concentrations at delivery, namely sharp drops in estrogen and progesterone levels, may lead to a serotonergic deficiency.[108] GABA signaling has also been implicated in the pathophysiology of postpartum depression and is a potential target for new treatments focused on this illness.

Brexanolone, a positive allosteric modulator of GABA type A receptors, was recently approved by the FDA as a novel treatment for moderate-to-severe postpartum depression.[109] In addition, the maternal hypothalamic-pituitary-adrenal (HPA) axis undergoes many changes during pregnancy, with a dramatic increase in cortisol levels by the third trimester. In the postpartum period, there is an increased risk for mood disorders if the HPA axis does not appropriately return to its pre-pregnancy state, marked by higher cortisol levels and ACTH levels.[110] Finally, a recent review of postpartum depression findings on neuroimaging demonstrates altered functional connectivity and activity changes in brain areas implicated in executive functioning and emotion and reward processing.[111] Please see Table 33-8 for a summary of perinatal and postpartum disorders.

To determine treatment during the perinatal period, an individualized risk versus benefit assessment is made, considering options for both nonpharmacologic and pharmacologic methods. It is important to consider current mental health symptoms, history and severity of mental health symptoms, history of coming off medication in the past, history of mental health during prior pregnancies, access to treatment, and patient preference. One of the biggest risk factors for decompensation in the postpartum period is the presence of symptoms during pregnancy, highlighting the importance of proactive planning and ongoing management of psychiatric disorders throughout pregnancy.

If mood symptoms are mild to moderate, psychotherapy is considered first-line treatment, with good evidence for cognitive-behavioral therapy and interpersonal therapy. If symptoms are moderate to severe, pharmacotherapy is typically appropriate.[106] Risks of medication must be balanced against risks of untreated illness, which can include preterm delivery, small for gestational age babies, other poor obstetric outcomes such as preeclampsia, and increased risk for postpartum illness. Postpartum depression and anxiety have been associated with poor maternal-infant attachment, elevated cortisol, and internalizing behavior in babies (characterized by crying or hanging onto you when you try to leave, getting upset when left with stranger, hanging on to you when with other people, and looking for you when you try to leave), and increased risk of mothers engaging in substance use.[108] The general principles of prescribing during pregnancy include minimizing exposures by limiting total number of medications and minimizing medication switches, using the lowest effective dose, selecting agents based on degree of placental crossing, and consideration of desire to breast-feed.

PERIMENOPAUSE AND MENTAL HEALTH

The menopause transition, triggered by diminished ovarian reserve and ending in cessation of menses, is another period of increased vulnerability for affective exacerbation in women. It is characterized by a gradual decline in estrogen and relatively long periods of estrogen unopposed by progesterone due to increasing frequency of anovulatory cycles, depicted in Figure 33-3.[123,124] Forty-five to 68% of perimenopausal women report elevated depressive symptoms compared with 28–31% of premenopausal women.[125] Being unmarried, having a high school education or less, experiencing financial hardship, having a history of depression, a history of perinatal mood episodes, and other adverse life events are risk factors for depression among perimenopausal women.[125,126] Severe PMS, poor sleep, and hot flashes also predict depression.[126]

Similar to perimenstrual and postpartum disorders, perimenopausal depressive symptoms are more likely to occur at times when estradiol, FSH, and LH variability are the highest, as estradiol fluctuation may adversely impact the serotonergic and noradrenergic systems to produce mood symptoms.[123,126] ALLO fluctuations, an effect of estradiol and progesterone fluctuations, are also implicated in perimenopausal depression in that they alter GABAergic modulation of the HPA axis and may sensitize women to stress and increase vulnerability to depressive symptoms.[127]

During perimenopause, classic depressive symptoms are seen in combination with menopause-specific symptoms like vasomotor symptoms, sleep and sexual disturbances, weight and energy changes, cognitive decline, and urinary symptoms. These challenges are often combined with psychological distress related to awareness of aging, body changes, health conditions, and decreased social support.[125]

Treatment can include cognitive-behavioral therapy and/or antidepressants, which show positive effects on mood as well as vasomotor symptoms, sleep, anxiety, and pain. While many SSRIs and SNRIs demonstrate efficacy in this population, selection of antidepressants should consider prior treatment response, drug–drug interactions, adverse effects such as weight gain or sleep disturbances, and efficacy for non-mood related menopause complaints like vasomotor symptoms.[125] Hormonal contraceptives dosed continuously may have benefits for irregular cycles, heavy bleeding, and vasomotor symptoms, but have not been well studied for perimenopausal depressive symptoms.[125,128] Estradiol has been shown to be more effective than placebo for perimenopausal women meeting criteria for MDD, but evidence is not sufficient to recommend estrogen-based therapy for preventing depression in asymptomatic women.[129] While estrogen augmentation may improve antidepressant response in perimenopausal women with major depressive disorder, it is also important to consider the potential complications and to collaborate with the treating gynecologist when making the decision to start HRT.[126]

CONCLUSION

Women's neurology and psychiatry focus on the sex differences in epidemiology, clinical features, pathophysiology, and treatment of many neurologic and psychiatric disorders. These sex differences arise from biological differences in neuroanatomy and neurochemistry, interactions between sex hormones and neurotransmitters, as well as from psychosocial determinants. There is a growing body of evidence supporting sex differences in brain function between males and females and within females across the menstrual cycle. This chapter also highlights the importance of preconception planning in psychiatry and neurology, in addition to developing an understanding of unique disease patterns in pregnancy and the postpartum, the safety profile of medications in pregnancy and during breast-feeding, and the way sex steroids may interact with medication metabolism and efficacy. To provide most effective patient care, it is critical to understand the influences of sex differences and reproductive life events on neuropsychiatric disease.

TABLE 33-8 • Perinatal and Postpartum Disorders.

Disorder	Prevalence	Presentation	Treatment
Major depressive disorder (MDD)	12% perinatal 30% postpartum[112]	MDD symptoms and prominent agitation with ruminative or obsessional thoughts.	• Psychotherapy • Antidepressants, serotonin reuptake inhibitors (SRIs), and TCAs • No increased risk for congenital malformations, except paroxetine which may increase risk for cardiac malformations. • Neonatal adaptation syndrome—mild and transient irritability, respiratory distress, tremors, feeding difficulties, sleep disturbances. Requires only supportive care and not shown to have long-term cognitive or developmental consequences. • Persistent pulmonary hypertension (PPHN): In 2006 studies showed association with AD use during pregnancy; in subsequent large studies the strength of the association has not been as strong, and absent for cases of severe PPHN.[106] • Neurodevelopmental outcomes: reassuring data, with recent large studies not showing an association between SSRIs and autism spectrum disorder.[113]
Generalized anxiety disorder	5%[114]	Worries center on having abnormal baby, pregnancy-related complications, weight gain, finances, cleanliness, and breast-feeding.[115]	
Obsessive-compulsive disorder	2%[114]	Obsessions focused on concern for baby, fear of contamination, fear of hurting the baby. Compulsions can include frequent checking of baby, frequent doctor's visits. Fear can lead to avoidance of newborn.[115]	
Bipolar disorder	Relapse rates range from 23% to 71% during pregnancy with much higher rates of relapse among those who discontinue their preconception psychotropics.[112,116] Postpartum, there is a 37–50% risk of developing a bipolar mood episode for women with known bipolar disorder.[116,118]	Depressive, manic, or mixed episodes.	• Lithium is the gold standard with evidence for postpartum psychosis prophylaxis if used in the third trimester.[116] • Risk for Ebstein's cardiac anomaly is 0.1–0.2% with first trimester exposure. A fetal echo can be checked at 16–18 weeks gestation.[106] • As the glomerular filtration rate increases during pregnancy, lithium dose may need to be increased in the 2nd and 3rd trimesters. • Therapeutic levels should be checked regularly. • Lithium dose should be held 24–48 hours prior to scheduled delivery or at onset of labor due to fluid shifts and reduced to pre-pregnancy dose over the first 2 weeks postpartum.[119] • Lamotrigine • Not thought to increase rates of congenital malformations or pregnancy complications.[120] • As estrogen increases the hepatic clearance rate, lamotrigine levels may drop as much as 50% during a pregnancy. Levels should be checked regularly and compared to pre-pregnancy level, with increase in dose made if clinically indicated. • After birth, dose should be immediately decreased by 25% if serum level is higher than baseline, and then tapered back to the pre-pregnancy dose within 2 weeks postpartum to avoid toxicity.[121] • Other treatment options for bipolar disorder during pregnancy include atypical antipsychotics and ECT. • Depakote contraindicated due to risk for neural tube defects. • Use benzodiazepines with caution due to neonatal abstinence syndrome.
Postpartum psychosis	Occurs in 1–2/1000 women. For those with bipolar disorder, there is a 20% risk of postpartum psychosis[117] and this risk increases to 30% for those with a history of postpartum psychosis.[116]	Prodromal symptoms typically start several days after delivery and escalate rapidly through postpartum day 10.[122] Presents with insomnia, mood symptoms, irritability, delusions, hallucinations, confusion.	• This is an emergency, due to increased risk of suicide and infanticide. • Typically requires psychiatric hospitalization. • Treatment with anti-manic agents and antipsychotics.

| | Menarche | | | | | | FMP (0) | | | |
Stage	−5	−4	−3b	−3a	−2	−1	+1a	+1b	+1c	+2
Terminology	Reproductive				Menopausal transition		Postmenopause			
	Early	Peak	Late		Early	Late	Early			Late
					Perimenopause					
Duration	Variable				Variable	1–3 years	2 years (1+1)		3–6 years	Remaining lifespan
Principal criteria										
Menstrual cycle	Variable to regular	Regular	Regular	Subtle changes in flow/length	Variable Length Persistent ≥7-day difference in length of consecutive cycles	Interval of amenorrhea of ≥60 days				
Supportive criteria										
Endocrine FSH AMH Inhibin B			Low Low	Variable* Low Low	↑ Variable* Low Low	↑ >25 IU/L** Low Low	↑ Variable Low Low	Stabilizes Very low Very low		
Antral follicle count			Low	Low	Low	Low	Very low	Very low		
Descriptive characteristics										
Symptoms						Vasomotor symptoms Likely	Vasomotor symptoms Most likely			Increasing symptoms of urogenital atrophy

*Blood draw on cycle days 2–5 ↑ = elevated.
**Approximate expected level based on assays using current international pituitary standard.

FIGURE 33-3. The Stages of Reproductive Aging Workshop +10 (STRAW +10) staging system for reproductive aging in women. AMH, anti-Müllerian hormone; FSH, follicle-stimulating hormone. (Reproduced with permission from SD Harlow, Gass M, Hall JE, et al. Executive summary of the Stages of Reproductive Aging Workshop 10: addressing the unfinished agenda of staging reproductive aging. *Menopause.* 2012; 14(2):387-395, https://journals.lww.com/menopausejournal. Copyright © 2012 The North American Menopause Society. https://www.menopause.org.)

Summary and Key Points

- Many neurological disorders have sex-specific differences in prevalence, clinical presentation, and management.
- Identifying and treating neurologic and psychiatric disorders in females across the life cycle require special consideration of the periods of hormonal flux, the influence of hormone-neurotransmitter interactions, the ways in which hormones affect autoimmune regulation, and the impact of how psychosocial factors contribute to disorders.
- For women in their reproductive years, there also needs to be an understanding about how the underlying disorder may affect pregnancy outcomes, and conversely, how pregnancy may affect the underlying disease.
- Further, during pregnancy and lactation, there are unique considerations around medication safety and medication response.

Multiple Choice Questions

1. Which of the following statements about SLE is not true?
   a. Lupus disease activity often worsens during pregnancy.
   b. Determining thrombotic complications is important in preconception planning.
   c. Warfarin is the drug of choice to treat antiphospholipid antibody syndrome during pregnancy.
   d. Women with lupus have an increased risk of eclampsia.
   e. It is recommended that women with lupus have stable disease for 6 months prior to planning pregnancy.

2. Which of the following conditions are sex-specific risk factors for ischemic stroke?
   a. Pregnancy
   b. Combined hormonal contraceptives
   c. Preeclampsia
   d. Migraine with aura
   e. All of the above

3. Which of the following is not a proposed mechanism for hormonally mediated mood symptoms?
   a. Sensitivity to normal hormonal fluctuations
   b. Low levels of estrogen
   c. Withdrawal from allopregnanolone
   d. Deficit in the serotonin system, specifically the serotonin transporter

4. Which of the following is not true about perinatal mood disorders?
   a. Postpartum psychosis is thought to be a type of schizophrenia.
   b. Postpartum OCD can lead to avoidance of the newborn.
   c. Postpartum blues typically resolve by 2 weeks postpartum.
   d. Up to 30% of women experience postpartum depression.

Multiple Choice Answers

1. **Answer: c**
   Warfarin is not usually used during pregnancy due to its teratogenic profile. Enoxaparin sodium is the drug of choice during pregnancy.

2. **Answer: e**
   All the above are sex-specific risk factors for ischemic stroke.

3. **Answer: b**
   It is not the absolute hormone level, but rather the fluctuation in levels, that are thought to contribute to mood symptoms.

4. **Answer: a**
   Bipolar disorder is the underlying psychiatric entity typically associated with postpartum psychosis. For those with bipolar disorder, there is a 20% risk of postpartum psychosis and this risk increases to 30% for those with a history of postpartum psychosis.

References

1. Fairweather D, Rose NR. Women and autoimmune diseases. *Emerg Infect Dis.* 2004;10(11):2005-2011.
2. González DA, Díaz BB, Rodríguez Pérez MC, et al. Sex hormones and autoimmunity. *Immunol Lett.* 2010;133(1):6-13.
3. Confavreux C, Hutchinson M, Hours MM, et al. Rate of pregnancy-related relapse in multiple sclerosis. *N Engl J Med.* 1998;339:285-291.
4. Weinstein Y, Ran S, Segal S. Sex-associated differences in the regulation of immune responses controlled by the MHC of the mouse. *J Immunol.* 1984;132(2):656-661.
5. Chakravarty EF, Bush TM, Manzi S, et al. Prevalence of adult systemic lupus erythematosus in California and Pennsylvania in 2000: estimates obtained using hospitalization data. *Arthritis Rheum.* 2007;56(6):2092.
6. Danchenko N, Satia JA, Anthony MS. Epidemiology of systemic lupus erythematosus: a comparison of worldwide disease burden. *Lupus.* 2006;15(5):308-318.
7. Wong KL, Woo EK, Yu YL, et al. Neurological manifestations of systemic lupus erythematosus: a prospective study. *Q J Med.* 1991;81(294):857-870.
8. Sibley JT, Olszynski WP, Decoteau WE, et al. The incidence and prognosis of central nervous system disease in systemic lupus erythematosus. *J Rheumatol.* 1992;19(1):47-52.
9. Toubi E, Khamashta MA, Panarra A, Hughes GR. Association of antiphospholipid antibodies with central nervous system disease in systemic lupus erythematosus. *Am J Med.* 1995;99(4):397-401.
10. Bonfa E, Golombek SJ, Kaufman LD, et al. Association between lupus psychosis and anti-ribosomal P protein antibodies. *N Engl J Med.* 1987;317(5):265-271.
11. Colasanti T, Delunardo F, Margutti P, et al. Autoantibodies involved in neuropsychiatric manifestations associated with systemic lupus erythematosus. *J Neuroimmunol.* 2009;212(1-2):3-9.
12. DeGiorgio LA, Konstantinov KN, Lee SC, et al. A subset of lupus anti-DNA antibodies cross-reacts with the NR2 glutamate receptor in systemic lupus erythematosus. *Nat Med.* 2001;7(11):1189-1193.

13. Appenzeller S, Cendes F, Costallat LT. Acute psychosis in systemic lupus erythematosus. *Rheumatol Int.* 2008;28(3):237-243.

14. Hanly IG, Fisk JD, Sherwood GJ, et al. Cognitive impairment in patients with systemic lupus erythematosus. *J Rheumatol.* 1992;19:562-567.

15. Ainala H, Loukkola J, Peltola J, Korpela M, Hietaharju A. The prevalence of neuropsychiatric syndromes in systemic lupus erythematosus. *Neurology.* 2001;57:496-500.

16. Appenzeller S, Cendes F, Costallat LT. Epileptic seizures in systemic lupus erythematosus. *Neurology.* 2004;63(10):1808-1812.

17. Tan EM, Cohen AS, Fries JF, et al. The 1982 revised criteria for the classification of systemic lupus erythematosus. *Arthritis Rheum.* 1982;25:1271-1277.

18. Lateef A, Petri M. Managing lupus patients during pregnancy. *Best Pract Res Clin Rheumatol.* 2013;27(3):435-447.

19. Clowse ME, Jamison M, Myers E, et al. A national study of the complications of lupus in pregnancy. *Am J Obstet Gynecol.* 2008;199(2):127.e1-6.

20. Lipton RB, Stewart WF, Diamond S, et al. Prevalence and burden of migraine in the United States: data from the American Migraine Study II. *Headache.* 2001;41(7):646-657.

21. Granella F, Sances G, Pucci E, et al. Migraine with aura and reproductive life events: a case control study. *Cephalalgia.* 2000;20(8):701-707.

22. Somerville BW. A study of migraine in pregnancy. *Neurol.* 1972;22:824-828.

23. Sances G, Granella F, Nappi RE, et al. Course of migraine during pregnancy and postpartum: a prospective study. *Cephalalgia.* 2003;23(3):197-205.

24. Kvisvik EV, Stovner LJ, Helde G, et al. Headache and migraine during pregnancy and puerperium: the MIGRA-study. *J Headache Pain.* 2011;12(4):443-451.

25. Johannes CB, Linet MS, Stewart WF, et al. Relationship of headache to phase of the menstrual cycle among young women: a daily diary study. *Neurology.* 1995;45:1076-1082.

26. MacGregor EA. Contraception and headache. *Headache.* 2013;53:247-276.

27. MacGregor EA. Migraine management during menstruation and menopause. *Continuum.* 2015;21:990-1003.

28. Marcus DA, Scharff L, Turk DC. Nonpharmacological management of headaches during pregnancy. *Psychosom Med.* 1995;57:527-535.

29. Herzog AG, Klein P, Ransil BJ. Three patterns of catamenial epilepsy. *Epilepsia.* 1997;38(10):1082-1088.

30. Harden C, Pennell P. Neuroendocrine considerations in the treatment of men and women with epilepsy. *Lancet Neurol.* 2013;12(1):72-83.

31. Mattson RH, Cramer JA, Caldwell BV, et al. Treatment of seizures with medroxyprogesterone acetate: preliminary report. *Neurology.* 1984;34(9):1255-1258.

32. Herzog AG, Fowler KM, Smithson SD, et al. Progesterone vs placebo therapy for women with epilepsy: a randomized clinical trial. *Neurology.* 2012;78(24):1959-1966.

33. Pennell P. Pregnancy, epilepsy, and women's issues. *Continuum.* 2013;19(3):697-714.

34. Harden CL, Meador KJ, Pennell PB, et al. Practice parameter update: management issues for women with epilepsy—focus on pregnancy (an evidence-based review): teratogenesis and perinatal outcomes: report of the Quality Standards Subcommittee and Therapeutics and Technology Assessment Subcommittee of the American Academy of Neurology and American Epilepsy Society. *Neurology.* 2009;73(2):133-141.

35. Meador KJ, Baker GA, Browning N, et al. Fetal antiepileptic drug exposure and cognitive outcomes at age 6 years (NEAD study): a prospective observational study. *Lancet Neurol.* 2013;12(3):244-252.

36. Pennell PB. Antiepileptic drugs during pregnancy: what is known and which AEDs seem to be safest? *Epilepsia.* 2008;49(suppl 9):43-55.

37. Tomson T, Battino D. Teratogenic effects of antiepileptic drugs. *Lancet Neurol.* 2012;11(9):803-813.

38. Hernández-Díaz S, Smith CR, Shen A, et al.; North American AED Pregnancy Registry. Comparative safety of antiepileptic drugs during pregnancy. *Neurology.* 2012;78(21):1692-1699.

39. Tomson T, Battino D. Teratogenic effects of antiepileptic drugs. *Lancet Neurol.* 2012;11(9):803-813.

40. Tomson T, Xue H, Battino D. Major congenital malformations in children of women with epilepsy. *Seizure.* 2015;28:46-50.

41. Harden CL, Pennell PB, Koppel BS, et al. Practice parameter update: management issues for women with epilepsy—focus on pregnancy (an evidence-based review): vitamin K, folic acid, blood levels, and breastfeeding: report of the quality standards subcommittee and therapeutics and technology assessment subcommittee of the American Academy of Neurology and American Epilepsy Society. *Neurology.* 2009;73(2):142-149.

42. Pruss H, Dalmau J, Harms L, et al. Retrospective analysis of anti-glutamate receptor (type NMDA) antibodies in patients with encephalitis of unknown origin. *Neurology.* 2010;75:1735-1739.

43. Dalmau J, Lancaster E, Martinez-Hernandez E, et al. Clinical experience and laboratory investigations in patients with anti-NMDAR encephalitis. *Lancet Neurol.* 2011;10(1):63-74.

44. Moscato EH, Jain A, Peng X, et al. Mechanisms underlying autoimmune synaptic encephalitis leading to disorders of memory, behavior and cognition: insights from molecular, cellular and synaptic studies. *Eur J Neurosci.* 2010;32(2):298-309.

45. Dalmau J, Gleichman AJ, Hughes EG, et al. Anti-NMDA-receptor encephalitis: case series and analysis of the effects of antibodies. *Lancet Neurol.* 2008;7(12):1091-1098.

46. Florance NR, Davis RL, Lam C, et al. Anti-N-methyl-D-aspartate receptor (NMDAR) encephalitis in children and adolescents. *Ann Neurol.* 2009;66(1):11-18.

47. Seshadri S, Beiser A, Kelly-Hayes M, et al. The lifetime risk of stroke: estimates from the Framingham Study. *Stroke.* 2006;37(2):345-350.

48. Leading causes of death in females: United States. Centers for Disease Control and Prevention. Available at cdc.gov/women/lcod/index.htm. Accessed January 28, 2018.

49. Leading causes of death in males: United States. Centers for Disease Control and Prevention. Available at cdc.gov/men/lcod/2013/index.htm. Accessed April 20, 2017.

50. Reeves MJ, Bushnell CD, Howard G, et al. Sex differences in stroke: epidemiology, clinical presentation, medical care, and outcomes. *Lancet Neurol.* 2008;7(10):915-926.

51. Li L, Schulz UG, Kuker W, Rothwell PM, Oxford Vascular S. Age-specific association of migraine with cryptogenic TIA and stroke: population-based study. *Neurology.* 2015;85(17):1444-1451.

52. Abanoz Y, Gulen Abanoz Y, Gunduz A, et al. Migraine as a risk factor for young patients with ischemic stroke: a case-control study. *Neurol Sci.* 2017;38(4):611-617.

53. Lidegaard O, Lokkegaard E, Jensen A, Skovlund CW, Keiding N. Thrombotic stroke and myocardial infarction with hormonal contraception. *N Engl J Med.* 2012;366(24):2257-2266.

54. Kittner SJ, Stern BJ, Feeser BR, et al. Pregnancy and the risk of stroke. *N Engl J Med.* 1996;335(11):768-774.

55. Steegers EA, von Dadelszen P, Duvekot JJ, Pijnenborg R. Pre-eclampsia. *Lancet.* 2010;376(9741):631-644.

56. Bushnell C, McCullough LD, Awad IA, et al. Guidelines for the prevention of stroke in women: a statement for healthcare professionals from the American Heart Association/American Stroke Association. *Stroke.* 2014;45(5):1545-1588.

57. McDonald SD, Malinowski A, Zhou Q, Yusuf S, Devereaux PJ. Cardiovascular sequelae of preeclampsia/eclampsia: a systematic review and meta-analyses. *Am Heart J.* 2008; 156:918-930.

58. Lykke JA, Langhoff-Roos J, Sibai BM, et al. Hypertensive pregnancy disorders and subsequent cardiovascular morbidity and type 2 diabetes mellitus in the mother. *Hypertension.* 2009;53:944-951.

59. Kestenbaum B, Seliger SL, Easterling TR, et al. Cardiovascular and thromboembolic events following hypertensive pregnancy. *Am J Kidney Dis.* 2003;42:982-989.

60. Fang MC, Singer DE, Chang Y, et al. Gender differences in the risk of ischemic stroke and peripheral embolism in atrial fibrillation-the anticoagulation and risk factors in atrial fibrillation (ATRIA) study. *Circulation.* 2005;112:1687-1691.

61. Leif F, Lina B, Mårten R, et al. Assessment of female sex as a risk factor in atrial fibrillation in Sweden: nationwide retrospective cohort study. *BMJ.* 2012;344:e3522

62. Alzheimer's Association. Alzheimer's disease facts and figures. *Alzheimers Dement.* 2017;13:325-373.

63. Gao S, Hendrie HC, Hall KS, Hui S. The relationships between age, sex, and the incidence of dementia and Alzheimer disease: a meta-analysis. *Arch Gen Psychiatry.* 1998;55:809-815.

64. Altmann A, Lu T, Henderson VW, Greicius MD. Sex modifies the APOE-related risk of developing Alzheimer disease. *Ann Neurol.* 2014;75(4):563-573.

65. Neu SC, Pa J, Kukull WA, et al. Apolipoprotein E genotype and sex risk factors for Alzheimer disease: a meta-analysis. *JAMA Neurol.* 2017;74(10):1178-1189.

66. Liu M, Huo YR, Wang J, et al. Telomere shortening in Alzheimer's disease patients. *Ann Clin Lab Sci.* 2016;46(3):260-265.

67. Jacobs EG, Kroenke C, Lin J, et al. Accelerated cell aging in female APOE-e4 carriers: implications for hormone therapy use. *PLoS One.* 2013;8(2):e54713.

68. Shumaker SA, Legault C, Rapp SR, et al. Estrogen plus progestin and the incidence of dementia and mild cognitive impairment in postmenopausal women: the Women's Health Initiative Memory Study: a randomized controlled trial. *JAMA.* 2003;289(20):2651-2662.

69. Carlson MC, Zandi PP, Plassman BL, et al. Hormone replacement therapy and reduced cognitive decline in older women: the Cache County Study. *Neurology.* 2001, 57(12) 2210-2216.

70. Zandi PP, Carlson MC, Plassman BL, et al.; Cache County Memory Study Investigators. Hormone replacement therapy and incidence of Alzheimer disease in older women: the Cache County Study. *JAMA.* 2002;288(17):2123-2129.

71. Sinforiani E, Citterio A, Zucchella C, et al. Impact of gender differences on the outcome of Alzheimer's disease. *Dement Geriatr Cogn Disord.* 2010;30:147-154.

72. Laws KR, Irvine K, Gale TM. Sex differences in cognitive impairment in Alzheimer's disease. *World J Psychiatry.* 2016;6(1):54-65.

73. Kim J, Fischer CE, Schweizer TA, Monoz DG. Gender and pathology-specific effect of apolipoprotein E genotype on psychosis in Alzheimer's disease. *Curr Alzheimer Res.* 2017;14(8):834-840.

74. Tapiola T, Alafuzoff I, Herukka SK, et al. Cerebrospinal fluid {beta}-amyloid 42 and tau proteins as biomarkers of Alzheimer-type pathologic changes in the brain. *Arch Neurol.* 2009;66(3):382-389.

75. Canevelli M, Quarata F, Remiddi F, et al. Sex and gender differences in the treatment of Alzheimer's disease: a systematic review of randomized controlled trials. *Pharmacol Res.* 2017;115:218-223.

76. Scacchi R, Gambina G, Broggio E, Corbo RM. Sex and ESR1 genotype may influence the response to treatment with donepezil and rivastigmine in patients with Alzheimer's disease. *Int J Geriatr Psychiatry.* 2014;29(6):610-615.

77. DiVall SA, Radovick S. Endocrinology of female puberty. *Curr Opin Endocrinol Diabetes Obes.* 2009;16(1):1-4.

78. Swerdloff RS, Odell WD. Hormonal mechanisms in the onset of puberty. *Postgrad Med J.* 1975;51:200-208.

79. Kibble JD, Halsey CR. Human menstrual cycle. In: *The Big Picture: Medical Physiology.* Weitz M, Kelly S, Davis K, eds. New York, NY: McGraw-Hill; 2009.

80. Schmidt PJ, Martinez PE, Nieman LK, et al. Premenstrual dysphoric disorder symptoms following ovarian suppression: triggered by change in ovarian steroid levels but not continuous stable levels. 2017;174(10):980-989.

81. Lovick T. SSRIs and the female brain- potential for utilizing steroid-stimulating properties to treat menstrual cycle-linked dysphorias. *J Psychopharmacol.* 2013;27(12):1180-1185.

82. Eriksson E. SSRIs probably counteract premenstrual syndrome by inhibiting the serotonin transporter. *J Psychopharmacol.* 2014;28(2):173-175.

83. Amin Z, Canli T, Epperson CN. Effect of estrogen-serotonin interactions on mood and cognition. *Behav Cogn Neurosci Rev.* 2005;4(1):43-58.

84. Liao H, Duan G, Liu P, et al. Altered fractional amplitude of low frequency fluctuation in premenstrual syndrome: a resting state fMRI study. *J Affect Disord.* 2017;218:41-48.

85. American Psychiatric Association. *Diagnostic and Statistical Manual of Mental Disorders.* 5th ed. Washington, DC: American Psychiatric Association; 2013.

86. Bornstein JE, Dean BB, Yonkers KA, Endicott J. Using the daily record of severity of problems as a screening instrument for premenstrual syndrome. *Obstet Gynecol.* 2007;109(5):1068-1075.

87. Qiao M, Huiyun Z, Huimin L, et al. Prevalence of premenstrual syndrome and premenstrual dysphoric disorder in a population-based sample in China. *Eur J Obstet Gynecol Reprod Biol.* 2012;162(1):83-86.

88. Kornstein SG, Harvey AT, Rush AJ, et al. Self-reported menstrual exacerbation of depressive symptoms in patients seeking treatment for major depression. *Psychol Med.* 2005;35(5):683-692.

89. Pilver CE, Kasi S, Desai R, Levy BR. Health advantage for black women: patterns in pre-menstrual dysphoric disorder. *Psychol Med.* 2011;41(8):1741.

90. Masho SW, Adera T, South-Paul J. Obesity as a risk factor for premenstrual syndrome. *J Psychosom Obstet Gynecol.* 2005;26(1):33-39.

91. Bertone-Johnson ER, Whitcomb BW, Missmer SA, Manson JE, Hankinson SE, Rich-Edwards JW. early life emotional, physical, and sexual abuse and the development of premenstrual syndrome: a longitudinal study. *J Womens Health.* 2014;23(9):729-739.

92. Hashemi S, Tehrani FR, Mohammadi N, et al. Comparison of metabolic and hormonal profiles of women with and without premenstrual syndrome: a community based cross-sectional study. *Int J Endocrinol Metab.* 2016;14(2):e28422.

93. Kendler KS, Silberg JL, Neale MC, Kessler RC, Heath AC, Eaves LJ. Genetic and environmental factors in the aetiology of menstrual, premenstrual and neurotic symptoms: a population-based twin study. *Psychol Med.* 1992;22(1):85-100.

94. Condon JT. The premenstrual syndrome: a twin study. *Br J Psychiatry.* 1993;162:481-486.

95. Yonkers KA, Simoni MK. Premenstrual disorders. *Am J Obstet Gynecol.* 2018;218(1):68-74.

96. Sayegh R, Schiff I, Wurtman J, Spiers P, McDermott J, Wurtman R. The effect of a carbohydrate-rich beverage on mood, appetite, and cognitive function in women with premenstrual syndrome. *Obstet Gynecol.* 1995;86(4):520-528.

97. Prior JC, Vigna Y, Sciarretta D, Alojado N, Schulzer M. Conditioning exercise decreases premenstrual symptoms: a prospective, controlled 6-month trial. *Fertil Steril.* 1987;47(3):402-408.

98. Shobeiri F, Araste FE, Ebrahimi R, Jenabi E. Effect of calcium on premenstrual syndrome: a double-blind randomized clinical trial. *Obstet Gynecol Sci.* 2017;60(1):100-105.

99. Verkaik S, Kamperman AM, Westrhenen RV, Schulte PFJ. The treatment of premenstrual syndrome with preparations of Vitex agnus castus: a systematic review and meta-analysis. *Am J Obstet Gynecol.* 2017;217(2):150-166.

100. Marjoribanks J, Brown J, O'Brien PM, Wyatt K. Selective serotonin reuptake inhibitors for premenstrual syndrome. *Cochrane Database Syst Rev.* 2013;(6):CD001396.

101. Yonkers KA, Brown C, Pearlstein TB, Foegh M, Sampson-Landers C, Rapkin A. Efficacy of a new low-dose oral contraceptive with drospirenone in premenstrual dysphoric disorder. *Obstet Gynecol.* 2005;106(3):492-501.

102. Muse KN, Cetal NS, Futterman LA, Yen SSC. The premenstrual syndrome—effects of medical ovariectomy. *N Engl J Med.* 1984;311:1345-1349.

103. Miller LJ, Finnerty M. Sexuality, pregnancy, and childrearing among women with schizophrenia-spectrum disorders. *Psychiatr Serv.* 1996;47:502-505.

104. Coverdale J, Roberts LW, Balon R, Beresin EV. Pedagogical implications of partnerships between psychiatry and obstetrics-gynecology in caring for patients with major mental disorders. *Acad Psychiatry.* 2015;39(4):430-436.

105. Coverdale J, Balon R, Beresin EV, et al. Family planning and the scope of the "reproductive psychiatry" curriculum. *Acad Psychiatry.* 2018;42:183-88.

106. Cohen LS, Wang B, Nonacs R, Viguera AC, Lemon EL, Freeman MP. Treatment of mood disorders during pregnancy and postpartum. *Psychiatr Clin N Am.* 2010;33:273-293.

107. Block M, Schmidt PJ, Danaceau M, Murphy J, Nieman L, Rubinow DR. Effects of gonadal steroids in women with a history of postpartum depression. *Am J Psychiatry.* 2000;157:924-930.

108. Mehta D, Newport DJ, Frishman G, et al. Early predictive biomarkers for postpartum depression point to a role for estrogen receptor signaling. *Psychol Med.* 2014;44:2309-2322.

109. Meltzer-Brody S, Colquhoun H, Riesenberg R, et al. Brexanolone injection in post-partum depression: two multicentre, double-blind, randomized, placebo-controlled, phase 3 trials. *Lancet.* 2018;392(10152):1058-1070.

110. Duthie L, Reynolds RM. Changes in the maternal hypothalamic-pituitary-adrenal axis in pregnancy and postpartum: influences on maternal and fetal outcomes. *Neuroendocrinology.* 2013;98:106-115.

111. Duan C, Cosgrove J, Deligiannidis KM. Understanding peripartum depression through neuroimaging: a review of structural and functional connectivity and molecular imaging research. *Curr Psychiatry Rep.* 2017;19:70.

112. Viguera AC, Tondo L, Koukopoulos AE, Reginaldi D, Lepri B, Baldessarini RJ. Episodes of mood disorders in 2,252 pregnancies and postpartum periods. *Am J Psychiatry.* 2011;168:1179-1185.

113. Zhou XH, Li YJ, Ou JJ, Li YM. Association between maternal antidepressant use during pregnancy and autism spectrum disorder: an updated meta-analysis. *Mol Autism.* 2018;9:21. doi: 10.1186/s13229-018-0207-7.

114. Nath S, Ryan EG, Trevillion K, et al. Prevalence and identification of anxiety disorders in pregnancy: the diagnostic accuracy of the two-item Generalised Anxiety Disorder scale (GAD-2). *BMJ Open.* 2018;8:e023766.

115. Williams KE, Koleva H. Identification and treatment of peripartum anxiety disorders. *Obstet Gynecol Clin N Am.* 2018;45:469-481.

116. Viguera AC, Whitfield T, Baldessarini RJ, et al. Risk of recurrence in women with bipolar disorder during pregnancy: prospective study of mood stabilizer discontinuation. *Am J Psychiatry.* 2007;164:1817-1824.

117. Wesseloo R, Kamperman AM, Munk-Olsen T, Pop VJ, Kushner SA, Bergink V. Risk of postpartum relapse in bipolar disorder and postpartum psychosis: a systematic review and meta-analysis. *Am J Psychiatry.* 2016;173:117-127.

118. Di Florio A, Forty L, Gordon-Smith K, et al. Perinatal episodes across the mood disorder spectrum. *JAMA Psychiatry.* 2013;70:168-175.

119. Newport DJ, Viguera AC, Beach AJ, et al. Lithium placental passage and obstetrical outcome: implications for clinical management during late pregnancy. *Am J Psychiatry.* 2005;162(11):2162-2170.

120. Hernandez-Diaz S, Smith CR, Shen A, et al. Comparative safety of antiepileptic drugs during pregnancy. *Neurology.* 2012;78(21):1692-1699.

121. Clark CT, Klein AM, Perel JM, et al. Lamotrigine dosing for pregnant patients with bipolar disorder. *Am J Psychiatry.* 2013;170(11):1240-1247.

122. Heron J, McGuinness M, Blackmore ER, Craddock N, Jones I. Early postpartum symptoms in puerperal psychosis. *Br J Obstet Gynaecol.* 2008;115(3):348-353.

123. Joffe H, Cohen LS. Estrogen, serotonin, and mood disturbance: where is the therapeutic bridge? *Biol Psychiatry.* 1998;44(9):798-811.

124. Harlow SD, et al. The Stages of Reproductive Aging Workshop. *Menopause.* 2012;14:387.

125. Maki PM, Kornstein SG, Joffe H, et al. Guidelines for the evaluation and treatment of perimenopausal depression: summary and recommendations. *J Womens Health*. 2019;28(2):117-134.

126. Freeman EW, Sammel MD, Lin H, Nelson DB. Associations of hormones and menopausal status with depressed mood in women with no history of depression. *Arch Gen Psychiatry*. 2006;63(4):375-382.

127. Gordon JL, Girdler SS, Meltzer-Brody SE, et al. Ovarian hormone fluctuation, neurosteroids and HPA axis dysregulation in perimenopausal depression: a novel heuristic model. *Am J Psychiatry*. 2015;172(3):227-236.

128. Miller TA, Allen RH, Kaunitz AM, Cwiak CA. Contraception for midlife women: a review. *Menopause*. 2018;25(7):817-827.

129. Gordon JL, Rubinow DR, Eisenlohr-Moul TA, Xia K, Schmidt PJ, Girdler SS. Efficacy of transdermal estradiol and micronized progesterone in the prevention of depressive symptoms in the menopause transition: a randomized clinical trial. *JAMA Psychiatry*. 2018;75(2):149-157.

34

Forensic Neuropsychiatry

Montgomery C. Brower

For as long as medicine has sought to diagnose and treat pathologies of thought, feeling, and behavior, society has turned to mental health professionals for insights into the perennial problems of crime and violence. The modern subspecialty of forensic psychiatry was pioneered in the United States by Dr. Isaac Ray, whose influential 1838 *Treatise on the Medical Jurisprudence of Insanity* argued for reform of the insanity defense based on advances in medical understanding of mental illness.[1] Today, as discoveries in clinical neuroscience have fostered the increasing integration of neurology and psychiatry in the diagnosis and treatment of mental illness, improved understanding of brain structural-functional relationships has also begun to influence the ways in which the criminal justice system views antisocial behavior. In the 2005 landmark case of *Roper v. Simmons*, for example, the U.S. Supreme Court ruled that capital punishment for crimes committed under the age of 18 is unconstitutional, based in part on advances in research concerning adolescent cognition and brain development.[2]

Neuropsychiatry can be viewed as a clinical approach to the patient that seeks to assess and treat psychopathology based on knowledge of structural-functional connections in the brain and of the clinical phenomenology of central nervous system disorders. When confronted with a pathological change in mental status or behavior, neuropsychiatry asks what might be called the classical neurological question: Could this be a disorder of the nervous system and, if so, where is the lesion? Forensic psychiatry is a psychiatric subspecialty that comprises two major domains of practice. First, as clinicians trained to work in secure hospitals and correctional settings, forensic psychiatrists have expertise in the care and treatment of patients involved with the criminal justice system. Second, as consultants and expert witnesses, forensic psychiatrists provide medical-legal opinions regarding mental health issues raised in the courts. Forensic neuropsychiatry, then, can be described as the application of a clinically integrated psychiatric and neurological approach to the care of patients in forensic mental health settings and to the performance of forensic psychiatric evaluations for the courts.

Neuropsychiatric and comorbid neurological conditions, ranging from neurodevelopmental disorders (NDDs), to sequelae of head injury, to neurodegenerative dementias, are highly prevalent in forensic mental health settings.[3-5] For clinicians practicing in prisons, jails, and forensic psychiatric hospitals, knowledge of the presentation and workup of neuropsychiatric disorders can prove invaluable, especially because correctional and other public-sector facilities often lack routine access to neurological consultation, neuroimaging, and other neurodiagnostic testing. Psychiatrists performing evaluations in the courts can expect to encounter criminal defendants or civil litigants presenting with conditions reflecting the full range of neuropathology. The ability to recognize the clinical manifestations of neuropsychiatric disorders and assess their relevance to medicolegal issues before the courts, therefore, can be essential to formulating and communicating accurate and useful expert opinions.

The evaluation of criminal and civil competencies, such as competence to stand trial or the need for guardianship, also routinely entails the assessment of cognitive capacities. Determining the nature and significance of cognitive impairments in competency-related abilities typically requires appreciation of the underlying neuropsychiatric disorder and its impact on function. In the civil litigation arena, assessment of psychiatric pathology and psychiatric disability claims (e.g., those involving mild traumatic brain injury [TBI]) may entail careful parsing of primary or preexisting disorders from psychiatric symptoms caused by a neurological disorder. Finally, neurobiological insights into the genesis of aggression and violence, as well as the neural basis for moral reasoning, may raise questions regarding the legal and philosophical assumptions that inform the criminal justice system as it judges and punishes those who offend against societal norms. Viewed from all of these clinical, evaluative, public health, and legal perspectives, neuropsychiatry can be seen to touch upon virtually every aspect of forensic psychiatric practice, although this chapter will mainly focus on neuropsychiatry in the criminal justice system.

HISTORICAL PRECEDENTS FOR NEUROPSYCHIATRY IN THE COURTS

In 1800, Thomas Erskine, the leading British jurist of his day and a noted defender of radicals and reformers, successfully used evidence of brain injury to win an insanity verdict in the landmark case of *Rex v. Hadfield*.[6] The defendant, James Hadfield, was charged with treason after he fired a missed shot at George III while the King was standing in the royal box at London's Drury Lane Theater. Hadfield, a veteran of the Napoleonic wars, had suffered multiple head injuries when he was sabered during a French cavalry charge in 1794. Thereafter, as multiple witnesses called by Erskine testified, Hadfield was prone to paranoid delusions and bizarre behavior. Two surgeons and a doctor called as expert witnesses testified as to the nature of Hadfield's head injuries and their role in causing his mental illness, including Hadfield's belief that his own death at the hands of the British government would bring about the Second Coming of Jesus Christ.

During the trial, Erskine was able to point dramatically to Hadfield's head, where a saber blow had removed a piece of the defendant's skull, leaving exposed brain covered with only a layer of dura and skin. Despite evidence that Hadfield had planned his attack on the King, Erskine successfully argued that Hadfield had acted in the grip of a delusion that impaired his ability to control his actions. "We are not here upon a case of insanity arising from the spiritual part of man, as it may be affected by hereditary taint—by intemperance, or by violent passions, the operations of which are various and uncertain," Erskine declared in yet another of his famous summations. "… [W]here a man has become insane from *violence to the brain, which permanently affects its structure*, however such a man may appear occasionally to others, his disease is *immovable*."[7] The judge found Erskine's evidence and arguments so legally persuasive that he stopped the trial, acquitted Hadfield, and ordered him psychiatrically detained. Hadfield was held for the rest of his life in Bethlehem Hospital (or Bedlam, as it was known), where he died of tuberculosis in 1841.

An insanity defense based on psychosis due to head trauma might well prevail in criminal court today, especially if judge and jury were presented with palpable evidence of a brain abnormality causing the relevant symptoms of mental illness. But the history of attempts to trace criminal behavior to specific brain abnormalities, or to other putative physiologic or genetic aberrations, argues for skepticism regarding comprehensive biological theories of criminality. The 1881 trial of Charles Guiteau, who shot and killed President James Garfield, featured a neurologist who testified for the defense that Guiteau suffered from "moral insanity," a diagnosis equivalent to the modern concept of psychopathy. During the trial, Guiteau was held at St. Elizabeth's psychiatric hospital in Washington, DC. The defense cited the theories of famed Italian criminologist and physician Cesare Lombroso, who asserted that criminality was inherited and could be identified by specific congenital physical defects.[8]

The trial was avidly followed in the public press as "expert" commentators peddled their analyses. A certain Professor A.E. Frew Mulley, for example, published a contemporary pamphlet on Guiteau (Figure 34-1), which claimed to offer "A Copious and

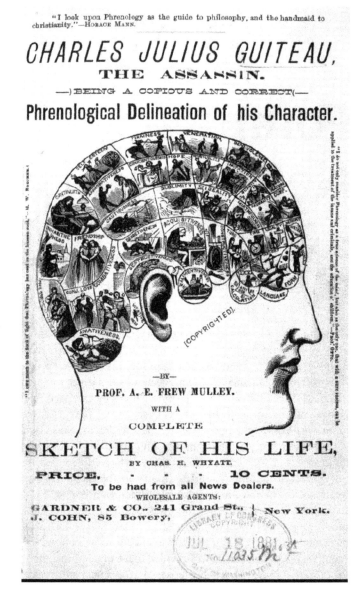

FIGURE 34-1. An 1881 phrenological pamphlet analyzing Charles Guiteau who assassinated President James Garfield. (Source: Library of Congress.)

Correct Phrenological Delineation of His Character." Although Guiteau likely had persecutory and grandiose delusions related to his conduct, he was, nevertheless, found guilty and executed. A later autopsy of his brain found a thickened dura mater and vascular changes, suggesting Guiteau may have had neurosyphilis, although contemporary reassessments have argued he more likely had schizophrenia and narcissistic personality traits.[9]

Despite the forensic failings of phrenology and Lambroso's theories of congenital criminality, the medical quest for neurobiological traits linked to violent and criminal behavior has continued down to the present day. In 1986, Dorothy Otnow Lewis, a psychiatrist, and Harold Pincus, a neurologist, published a case series reporting on the neuropsychiatric status of 15 death row inmates in the United States.[10] The authors conducted comprehensive clinical investigations, which included detailed histories and mental status examinations, and (where obtainable) record reviews and family interviews, as well as psychological and neuropsychological testing results. Lewis and Pincus subsequently reported on similar comprehensive evaluations of 14 juveniles facing execution.[11] Both the adult and juvenile offenders in these case series showed extensive indications of brain damage and dysfunction, evidenced by a range of findings, from histories of severe head injuries, to seizures, EEG, and brain CT scan abnormalities, to cognitive impairments and neurological soft signs. The subjects also showed common features in their psychosocial histories and psychopathology, leading the authors to suggest a triad of clinical features said to characterize murderers condemned to death row: a history of severe childhood physical and/or sexual abuse; paranoid psychotic spectrum symptoms; and clinical indications of brain damage or dysfunction.

The work of Lewis and Pincus has since been criticized for selection bias (the subjects in both studies were referred by their defense attorneys) and lack of controls (e.g., no comparisons with violent and nonviolent offenders not condemned to death row), and some studies have not fully corroborated their findings.[12] Their reports, however, led to the widespread introduction of neuropsychiatric evidence into death penalty proceedings and influenced public debate on capital punishment. The work of Lewis and Pincus also stimulated renewed interest in the prevalence of neuropsychiatric disorders in criminal justice populations and the hypothesized contribution of central nervous system dysfunction to violent crime.

EPIDEMIOLOGY OF NEUROPSYCHIATRIC DISORDERS IN FORENSIC MENTAL HEALTH SETTINGS

Studies of populations in correctional and forensic psychiatric facilities have typically found elevated rates of brain injury and central nervous system dysfunction. In a 1992 study of 50 randomly selected patients committed to a maximum-security state hospital for mentally ill offenders, 84% had at least one indicator of potential brain dysfunction, defined as any diagnosis of organic brain dysfunction, a history of head injury with loss of consciousness, a history of seizure activity, cognitive impairment, abnormal neurological findings, or abnormal neurodiagnostic testing results.[13] Most subjects (64%) had multiple indicators of neurological abnormalities, and subjects with a diagnosis or history of brain dysfunction were more likely to have been indicted for violent criminal charges. Of the 20 subjects charged with murder, manslaughter, or attempted murder, 30% had a diagnosis of *DSM-IIIR* organic brain disorder, while 67% of those found not guilty by reason of insanity and 63% of those found incompetent to stand trial had indicators of brain dysfunction.

Outside of specialized forensic mental health facilities, elevated rates of brain injury and cerebral dysfunction have also been observed in general correctional settings. A 2011 meta-analysis estimated the pooled prevalence for TBI in incarceration settings compared with estimates of TBI prevalence in the general population.[14] The authors found TBI prevalence rates in incarcerated populations averaging approximately 50%,

significantly higher than any of the range of estimates for the general population, where prevalence estimates run from 2% to 38.5% (the latter being from a large all-male sample, perhaps the most relevant comparison to incarcerated populations). Other survey studies have linked TBI in criminal offenders to higher rates of psychiatric disorders and substance abuse, as well as more repeat offending, more time served, and increased problems with anger and aggression.[4,15,16]

Studies of TBI prevalence in correctional settings have been criticized for lack of standardized, reliable definitions of head injury, overreliance on self-report data, absence of appropriate population comparison controls, and insufficient data concerning the degree of disability associated with reported TBI. These prevalence studies, moreover, are cross-sectional surveys, and do not resolve the question of whether TBI actually causes increased antisocial and aggressive behavior, or is simply an associated feature of criminal conduct.[17] Other criminogenic behaviors—such as propensity for risk-taking or increased substance abuse—could also contribute to an increased risk of sustaining a head injury, leading to elevated prevalence of reported TBI in correctional populations.

More recent community-based cohort studies of TBI and criminal offending have sought to control for such confounding factors. A 2015 Australian study assessed first-time criminal conviction rates in a retrospective cohort of subjects with a hospital-recorded TBI, compared with matched, unaffected community controls, while accounting for potential confounders of substance abuse, mental illness, social disadvantage, and Aboriginal background. Adjustment for these confounds lowered the risk of first-time offending associated with TBI, but the study still found males with TBI had a 1.58 times increased risk of any conviction, while females had a 1.52 times increased risk. The risk of a violent offense was increased 1.65 times in males and 1.73 times in females.[18] In contrast, a 2018 Canadian study found no increased risk of criminal conviction associated with TBI when adjusted for childhood disruptive behaviors and family social status (scored on such factors as parental education, employment level, and presence of both biological parents in the home). The study extracted prospective data regarding incidence of TBI and rates of criminal offending from two cohorts of male subjects who were recruited when they entered elementary school and then followed up to age 24. The authors concluded their results suggested "it was men who had been raised by single parents who were young and poorly educated with low prestige jobs, and who displayed conduct problems, behaviors that hurt other children, inattention, and hyperactivity through elementary school who were at increased risk to sustain a TBI in adulthood."[19]

Although the question of whether or how much TBI independently contributes to criminal behavior remains unsettled, these studies point to the importance of considering the complex ways in which neuropsychiatric disorders may interact with other psychological and social factors to engender antisocial and aggressive behavior. The observed high prevalence of TBI in correctional populations further highlights the need for an informed neuropsychiatric approach to assess and manage the cognitive, emotional, and behavioral sequelae of head injury among those confined to prisons and jails.

NEURODEVELOPMENTAL DISORDERS

Studies have also found elevated rates of NDDs in incarcerated populations. A 2017 Swedish consecutive cohort study, which used *DSM-IV* criteria to evaluate 270 male offenders age 18–25 convicted for "hands-on" violent offenses, found that most subjects met criteria for more than one neurodevelopmental diagnosis. Some 63% of subjects met lifetime criteria for childhood attention-deficit hyperactivity disorder (ADHD), while 43% had maintained an ADHD diagnosis into adulthood. Ten percent of the sample had an autism spectrum disorder (ASD), while 6% met criteria for Tourette syndrome. The study found 1% with intellectual disability (ID), and 22% with borderline intellectual functioning. Overall, the group of subjects with NDD had earlier onset antisocial behavior, more aggressive behavior, and lower school achievement than offenders without NDD.[20] A 2018 prevalence study of 390 male inmates found 25% with ADHD, 9% with ASD, and 9% with ID, with significantly higher rates of behavioral disturbance associated with ADHD and ID.[21]

With respect to high-functioning ASD in particular, characteristic clinic features may specifically contribute to an increased risk of behaviors that, while not deliberately antisocial in motivation or intent, may be construed as criminal conduct and result in charges. These clinical features include deficits in theory of mind, impaired executive function, and emotional dysregulation, leading to failure to appropriately perceive and respond to social cues, impulsivity, and temper outbursts.[22] A prospective study of adolescents and adults with ASD living in the community found that, over 12–18 months, approximately 16% were reported to have some police involvement, primarily for concerns about aggressive behavior. Correlates of police involvement included older age, a history of aggression, living outside the home, and having parents with greater caregiver and financial stress.[23]

Studies examining the impact of treatment further emphasize the importance of identifying NDDs in jail and prison populations. One Swedish registry study of over 25,000 patients diagnosed with ADHD showed that during periods when subjects were prescribed appropriate medication, the frequency of criminal offenses decreased 32% for men and 41% for women.[24] Another Swedish cohort study followed more than 22,000 released prisoners, finding that prescription of psychostimulants for ADHD was linked to reduced violent reoffending, with 42.8 fewer violent offenses per 1000 person-years following release to the community.[25]

SUBSTANCE ABUSE AND INTOXICATION STATES

The link between substance abuse and violent or other criminal offending is well established, and can involve both acute and chronic neuropsychiatric syndromes, ranging from frank intoxication, to substance-induced psychosis, to persistent cognitive impairment.[26] A 2018 survey of an urban emergency room in Switzerland found that 63% of patients presenting after committing a physical assault had used more than one drug, with 60% of those reporting alcohol co-use. The most recent survey data on substance use disorders in U.S. correctional settings show rates averaging over 70% among inmates with a mental health disorder and over 50% among those without a mental health condition.[27] The greatest risk for violence associated with mental illness is among those with co-occurring substance use disorders.[28]

Acute intoxication can contribute to aggression in both general and specific ways, depending on the substances involved. Alcohol, benzodiazepines, and other central nervous system depressants generally inhibit cerebral function in a dose-related progression from higher cortical to subcortical structures, beginning with prefrontal cortex. Intoxication from CNS depressants can thus affect frontal executive functions well before causing significant alternations in consciousness, leading to emotional disinhibition and impaired judgment and impulse control, which in turn increase the risk of aggression. In some cases, preexisting cerebral abnormalities, such as neurodevelopmental impairments or TBI, may conduce to pathological intoxication, with behavioral dyscontrol that exceeds the clinically expected level of impairment relative to dose. Chronic alcohol abuse can also cause degenerative brain changes with persisting cognitive impairment, taking the form of a frontal-subcortical dementia. In forensic mental health settings, the author has encountered such cases of alcohol-induced dementia presenting with irritability, affective lability, and paranoia, leading to anger dyscontrol and aggression.

Regarding more specific triggering of aggression, psychostimulants, primarily cocaine and amphetamines, are the most commonly implicated in acute intoxication.[25] The dopaminergic activating effects of cocaine and other psychostimulants can increase impulsivity, while psychotomimetic effects can induce paranoia, although personality and other risk factors appear to play a role in whether psychostimulant intoxication leads to aggression.[29] Over 50% of adult users of phencyclidine (PCP) reportedly present with a classic toxidrome characterized by violent agitation, nystagmus, tachycardia, hypertension, anesthesia, and analgesia, although some studies have found that many reported claims of PCP-induced aggression may be exaggerated or more causally related to prior risk factors for assaultive behavior.[30,31]

Personality factors, genetic, and other vulnerabilities also appear to play a significant role in substance-induced psychosis, with the greatest risk being associated with cocaine, amphetamines, cannabis, and alcohol.[32] The multifactorial nature of substance-induced psychosis is well illustrated by a young man charged with attempted murder who was evaluated by the author. The defendant had a history of social anxiety, depression, and ongoing heavy cannabis use since his early teens, as well as having schizotypal personality traits. While attending college, he additionally began frequent microdosing of psilocybin mushrooms, and became increasingly paranoid. Over several sleepless nights of abusing prescription psychostimulants to enhance his studying, he developed an acute paranoid psychosis with command auditory hallucinations to harm others, prompting him to assault and inflict multiple stab wounds on a random male victim. Although a rare event, this kind of case illustrates the complex mix of prior risk factors, chronic polysubstance use, and acute intoxication that may result in psychotically motivated aggression.

SEIZURE DISORDERS

Medical lore has long associated epilepsy with violence and criminality, and Lombroso went so far as to assert that most criminals were epileptic.[7,33] In a pair of classic surveys published some 50 years ago, however, British forensic psychiatrist John Gunn found that, while prison populations indeed showed a markedly higher prevalence of seizure disorders than the general population, prisoners with epilepsy were no more likely to have committed violent crimes than comparable non-epileptic offenders.[33] At about the same time as Gunn's observations, however, Bach-y-Rita and colleagues advanced the concept of the "episodic dyscontrol syndrome," based on a case series of 130 patients who presented seeking help for uncontrolled outbursts of property destruction and physical aggression toward others. Noting that a larger than expected number of these patients turned out to have temporal lobe epilepsy, the authors suggested that a subclinical form of temporal lobe discharge might underlie paroxysmal violent episodes in general.[34] The notional relationship between epilepsy and violence thus persisted, and made its way into the criminal courts as the "epilepsy defense."[35]

Although seizure activity may very rarely directly cause stereotyped violent behavior, such ictal aggression never involves multiple purposeful actions undertaken in a series. Seizure-related aggression more typically takes the form of a confused patient resisting physical restraint in the terminal or postictal phases of a seizure.[36] The presence of a seizure disorder, however, may indirectly contribute to aggressive behavior. Although often under-recognized as clinical manifestations of epilepsy, interictal and postictal psychotic syndromes can manifest with paranoid delusions leading to assaults against others. This author has also evaluated criminal defendants who presented with recurrent temper outbursts and aggressive dyscontrol associated with seizures and/or anterior temporal lesions involving the amygdala, and there exists a literature documenting similar cases.[36] Moreover, focal epilepsy may be a manifestation of more widespread brain injury or dysfunction, which itself may impair behavioral controls. In a neuroimaging study comparing temporal lobe epilepsy subjects with and without histories of interictal aggression, subjects with recurrent episode aggression had statistically significant frontal gray matter reductions.[37]

Gunn also noted that violent offenses were more likely to be committed by those with frontal lobe disorders, while Bach-y-Rita and colleagues recognized that, apart from any indications of temporal lobe epilepsy, their patients with episodic dyscontrol typically had what was then called "minimal brain dysfunction." This nosological concept was formerly applied to patients with neurodevelopmental deficits primarily affecting frontal executive functioning; it substantially overlaps with the contemporary diagnosis of ADHD. This clinically observed association between aggression and acquired or developmental frontal lobe dysfunction has proved to be the most enduring and fruitful insight into the neuropsychiatry of violent and criminal behavior.

FRONTAL LOBE INJURY AND "ACQUIRED SOCIOPATHY"

Reports highlighting the prevalence of neuropsychiatric disorders among violent offenders strongly suggest that the role of brain damage or dysfunction is a potentially important, and often overlooked, factor in violent and criminal behavior. The following case report illustrates how even forensically experienced clinicians may miss the importance of neurobehavioral pathology.

CASE VIGNETTE 34.1

A 27-year-old white male was committed to a maximum-security forensic psychiatric facility for evaluation of his criminal responsibility related to assault and battery charges, which he had incurred for alleged assaults on staff while in a state psychiatric hospital. The patient had an extensive history of childhood abuse and neglect, and had been effectively institutionalized since age 6, when he was placed in the custody of social services and assigned to foster and residential care. He had recurrent psychiatric hospitalizations starting in his preadolescent years, primarily for aggressive and disruptive behaviors. Early assessments showed a full-scale IQ of 112, with developmental learning difficulties, and he was diagnosed with ADHD. In adolescence, he was seen as having nascent narcissistic and antisocial personality traits, and by age 16, he was involved with the juvenile courts.

At age 19, while fleeing on foot across a highway following an attempted robbery, the patient was hit by a truck. Unconscious at the scene, he was emergently transported to the hospital, where he remained in a coma for 3 weeks. Regaining consciousness and recovering against expectations, he was referred to a rehabilitation facility, but then lost to follow-up. He subsequently began turning up in area emergency rooms, where he presented with mood complaints and suicidal ideation, leading to repeated psychiatric admissions. Records reflected multiple psychiatric hospitalizations with unclear diagnoses, ranging from mood and psychotic disorders, to unspecified impulse control disorder, to a personality disorder with antisocial and borderline traits.

During these hospitalizations, the patient was frequently threatening and assaultive toward staff and peers, and he was eventually committed to a state hospital. There, a well-regarded forensic psychiatrist was brought in to consult regarding the assessment and management of the patient's recurrent assaultive behavior. The consultant

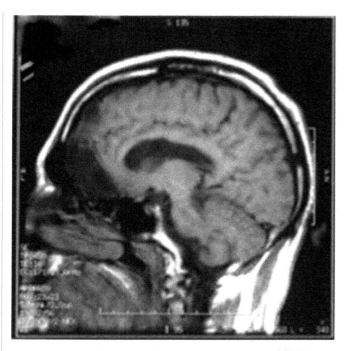

FIGURE 34-2. Sagittal view of an MRI brain scan of a 27-year-old man with recurrent aggression showing extensive orbitofrontal injury and tissue loss. (Courtesy of Dr. Montgomery C. Brower.)

opined that the patient had antisocial personality disorder, that mental health treatment would have no significant impact on his behavior, and that he should be referred to the criminal justice system. A clinical administrative decision was taken to press charges for the patient's assaults against staff, and the patient was brought into court, where his appointed defense counsel petitioned for a criminal responsibility evaluation.

When examined at the forensic facility, the patient presented as jocular and disinhibited, telling clinicians about his house in the suburbs and his garage full of high-performance cars, which he reported he had purchased with a settlement from a lawsuit. He was highly distractible and easily drawn to extraneous environmental stimuli, such as the sounds of neighboring voices or activities. Although he often engaged his listener with initially pleasant banter, his affect was labile, shifting into marked irritability whenever his immediate wishes were frustrated. Neuropsychological testing showed a full-scale IQ of 97, with minor impairments in attention, working memory, and higher executive functions.

Medical records of the young man's past hospitalization for head injury were obtained and a brain magnetic resonance imaging scan was performed. The MRI (Figure 34-2) showed extensive encephalomalacia and scarring involving the basal forebrain, with substantial loss of orbitofrontal, ventromedial, and anterior temporal cortex bilaterally.

This young man's extensive brain injury, sustained in his pedestrian-motor vehicle accident 8 years previously, recalls medical history's most famous head-injured patient, Phineas Gage. Wounded in 1897 by an explosively propelled iron tamping rod that passed through his left orbital skull and basal forebrain, Gage miraculously survived his injuries but underwent a marked personality change. In the famous medical account of his surgeon, John Harlow, Gage became "fitful, irreverent, indulging at times in the grossest profanity (which was not previously his custom), manifesting but little deference for his fellows, impatient of restraint or advice when it conflicts with his desires, at times pertinaciously obstinate, yet capricious and vacillating... Previous to his injury, he possessed a well-balanced mind, and was looked upon... as a shrewd, smart business man... [H]is mind was radically changed, so decidedly that... he was 'no longer Gage.'"[38]

This change in social comportment associated with inferior frontal brain damage has been dubbed "acquired sociopathy," because of trait similarities to the impulsive behavior, disregard of social norms, and lack of empathy or remorse that comprise key clinical features of the antisocial or psychopathic personality.[39] Case reports have also described subjects with childhood histories of frontal lobe injury who display antisocial behaviors as adults, associated with developmental deficits in social comportment and moral reasoning.[40] Studies of the developmental course of delinquent youth also find that, while most youths who engage in adolescent offending conduct will leave behind

their offending behaviors as they enter adulthood, the subset of delinquent youth who go on to follow a life-persistent criminal course are more likely to have early onset childhood aggressive behaviors and neurocognitive developmental abnormalities.[41] These lines of evidence all point to an association between recidivistic criminal offending and developmental or acquired brain abnormalities affecting frontal lobe function.

Human higher cognitive functions and socially cooperative behavior have long been linked to the evolutionary development of the brain's frontal lobes. This more highly developed prefrontal cortex does not function alone, but participates in a brain-wide network that includes connections with limbic structures (amygdala, hippocampus, anterior cingulum), the striatum, the thalamus, hypothalamus, brainstem, and cerebellum, as well as their associated white matter tracts. As characterized by Duffy and Campbell,[42] this prefrontal network prominently features three parallel, non-motor circuit loops connecting specific regions of prefrontal cortex with topographically matched loci in the striatum, pallidum, and thalamus. These circuits together underlie what Duffy and Campbell term the "metacognitive" functions needed for context-appropriate, goal-oriented behavior, including motivation, planning, self-regulation, and self-monitoring. Although a lesion anywhere along the extended brain prefrontal network can produce a clinical presentation of frontal lobe deficits, an acquired or developmental insult to these prefrontal circuit loops tends to produce one of three specific types of frontal network syndrome.

Damage or dysfunction in the dorsolateral prefrontal circuit loop produces a predominantly dysexecutive syndrome, characterized by problems with attention, concentration, working memory, and abstract conceptual abilities. The apathetic presentation is associated with the midline prefrontal circuit, where a lesion leads to a syndrome of amotivation, failure to initiate appropriately spontaneous speech and behavior, and passive indifference to social cuing. Dysfunction in the orbitofrontal circuit presents as a disinhibited syndrome, with prominent behavioral features of impulsivity, affective lability, loquacity, disregard for socially appropriate behavior, and impairments of insight and empathy. This structural-functional schema is a useful heuristic for characterizing patterns of frontal lobe impairment, however, in clinical practice these three classical frontal lobe syndromes may well present in incomplete or combined forms, depending on the nature and extent of the frontal network lesion involved.

Of the three frontal network syndromes, the disinhibited orbitofrontal type displays clinical features—such as impulsivity, superficial affect, and lack of empathy or remorse—most commonly associated with a criminal disposition. As reviewed in more detail below, a substantial research literature supports the association of orbitofrontal dysfunction with increased risk for antisocial and aggressive behavior. In contrast, the apathetic, amotivational[42] state associated with midline frontal lesions is unlikely to result in violating behavior or aggression directed at others. Other findings in the literature reviewed, however, suggest that dysexecutive impairments primarily associated with dorsolateral prefrontal network dysfunction may also play a role in the development of antisocial and aggressive behavior.

Attempts to establish a causal link between frontal lobe dysfunction and criminal behavior are further complicated by evidence for an extensive interaction between neuropathological, psychosocial, and environmental risk factors (as already reviewed above regarding the association between TBI and criminal behavior). Premorbid functioning, moreover, is a well-known factor affecting head injury outcomes. In the above case report of recurrent aggression associated with extensive basal forebrain injury, for example, the young man involved had a long-standing developmental history of disruptive and aggressive behaviors, along with multiple preexisting social and environmental risk factors for antisocial conduct, and was, ironically, in the act of committing a crime at the time he sustained his head injury. Subsequent to his head injury, he engaged in more frequent, impulsive, and reactive aggression, with assaultive behavior that was often disproportionate to the degree of provocation. But although the nature of this patient's aggressive behavior changed, it could not be solely attributed to his head injury, and the relative contribution of frontal lobe dysfunction versus his premorbid antisocial tendencies in such cases remains to be established.

THE CLINICAL CORRELATION OF FRONTAL LOBE DYSFUNCTION WITH AGGRESSION AND CRIME

Since the case reports of Lewis and Pincus, approximately three decades of studies have found clinical correlations between violent and criminal behavior and prefrontal abnormalities, beginning with observational studies and progressing to contemporary anatomical and functional neuroimaging studies. In 1995, Blake, Pincus, and Buckner reported on 31 cases of murderers referred for evaluation related to trial, sentencing, or clemency appeals. Sixty-four percent of their sample had evidence of frontal dysfunction on neurological examination, while 84% had abnormal neuropsychological testing, with half of those showing frontal dysfunction. The authors noted that minor irritants or frustration often triggered these defendants' homicidal acts, consistent with the hypothesis that disinhibition related to frontal lobe injury contributed to their violent crimes.[43] In noncriminal subjects, studies of aggression among patients committed to psychiatric hospitals have found that the presence of a frontal lobe lesion was the best single predictor of a patient engaging in a violent incident while hospitalized,[44] and that persistently violent patients have greater impairment on measures of frontal lobe functioning, associated with more problems following ward routine, managing social interactions, and maintaining temper control.[45]

Neurodegenerative disorders affecting frontal lobe function have also been associated with increased aggression and antisocial behavior. The degeneration of the basal ganglia in Huntington's disease (HD) impairs frontal subcortical network function, leading to progressive mood and behavioral disinhibition. In a Danish registry comparison of 221 HD subjects (99 males, 151 females) with 334 matched, first-degree relative non-HD controls, Jensen et al. found the crime rate among male HD subjects was significantly higher than controls, while no difference was found in female HD subjects. Male HD subjects committed more frequent thefts, minor sexual offenses, maltreatment of animals, illegal hunting, absences from military service, and drug offenses, but no serious violent offenses, such as murder, rape, or robbery. There was a striking difference in the incidence of drunk driving offenses, which occurred in over 14% of HD subjects compared with 2% of controls.[46]

Similarly disproportionate rates of antisocial behavior have been observed in association with frontotemporal dementia (FTD). In 1997, Miller et al.[47] published the pioneering study, comparing the frequency of antisocial behavior in 22 FTD subjects with 22 matched Alzheimer's disease (AD) subjects. Consistent with the clinical diagnoses of FTD versus AD, SPECT scans showed anterior frontotemporal and posterior temporal-parietal hypoperfusion respectively. Ten FTD subjects had engaged in antisocial behaviors as compared with one AD subject. FTD subjects had committed assault, indecent exposure, shoplifting, and hit-and-run collisions, in three cases leading to arrest.

Multiple studies have since confirmed the association of FTD and other frontal-predominant dementias with disproportionate rates of antisocial behavior. A 2015 chart review of 2397 patients seen at a tertiary referral dementia center found 8.5% of the total sample had a history of criminal behavior. Broken down by diagnosis, rates of offending behavior were 7.7% for AD, 20% for HD, 27% for semantic variant primary progressive aphasia, and 37.4% for behavioral variant FTD (bvFTD). Criminal behavior was associated with prefrontal dysfunction generally, and compared with AD patients, bvFTD patients were more likely to present with new onset antisocial behavior (14.4% vs. 2%), more likely to exhibit violence (6.4% vs. 2%), and showed more varied antisocial behavior, whereas AD subjects most frequently committed driving violations.[48] Although AD most commonly involves predominantly parieto-temporal pathology, particularly in the earlier stages, it should be borne in mind that AD patients may present with a frontal-variant form of the disease, which may produce behavioral impairments similar to FTD.

Other studies of FTD have focused more specifically on reports of increased rates of sexually inappropriate or sexual offending behavior. Mendez and Shapira reviewed hypersexuality (defined as increased sexual behavior distressing to others) in FTD versus AD patients. None of the AD patients in their sample engaged in hypersexual behavior, compared with 13% of the FTD patients, who were noted to have a dramatic increase in the frequency of sexual behavior, characterized by disinhibition and poor impulse control, more active seeking of sexual stimulation, a widening range of sexual interests, and sexual excitation to previously mundane or new stimuli.[49] Other researchers, however, caution that FTD frequently presents with *hypo*sexual behavior associated with progressive apathy, although episodes of sexual disinhibition may overlap with this more general diminishment in sexual interest and behavior.[50] Any new onset, out-of-character antisocial or sexually inappropriate behavior in a late-middle-aged or elderly person should prompt clinical suspicion of FTD, especially because bvFTD typically presents with changes in personality and social comportment, rather than cognitive or memory complaints.

The Vietnam Head Injury Study (VHIS) represents the most extensive modern effort to correlate aggression and violence with focal injury to specific frontal lobe regions.[51] Grafman et al. studied 279 Vietnam veterans with war-related penetrating head injuries presenting 10–15 years post injury, comparing them with 57 matched Vietnam veteran controls. In addition to gathering comprehensive clinical data, including neurological examination, neuropsychological testing, rehabilitation testing, speech and language testing, EEGs, evoked potentials, and heads CTs, the researchers obtained collateral reports from families and friends, who completed inventories and questionnaires resulting in a scaled score for aggressive and violent behavior.

Head-injured subjects had significantly higher violence scores compared with controls, and higher violence scores were significantly associated with focal ventromedial prefrontal and orbitofrontal injury. The nature of reported aggressive behavior was typically verbal confrontation, however, while physical assaults were less frequently reported and the study did not collect data on other antisocial or criminal behavior. The VHIS, however, was the first study to show a statistically significant correlation between increased aggression and specifically ventromedial/orbital prefrontal injury, consistent with the hypothesized association of the prefrontal disinhibition syndrome with increased risk for violent and criminal behavior.

FUNCTIONAL NEUROIMAGING STUDIES OF FRONTAL DYSFUNCTION, AGGRESSION, AND ANTISOCIAL BEHAVIOR

Beginning with the application of positron emission tomography (PET) scanning and progressing with the development of functional magnetic resonance imagining (fMRI), neuroimaging studies have led to increasingly specific findings about both the type of aggression associated with frontal lobe dysfunction, and the prefrontal cortical foci involved (Table 34-1). In an influential 1997 protocol, Raine et al. used fluorodeoxyglucose (FDG) PET to assess frontal metabolism in 22 subjects charged with murder who were referred for functional neuroimaging in connection with evaluations of criminal responsibility (insanity defense) and/or competence to stand trial. Compared with matched controls, the murderer group showed significantly decreased frontal metabolism during an activation task (the continuous performance task, where performance is vulnerable to prefrontal executive impairments of impulsivity and distractibility).[52] Like the death row case series of Lewis and Pincus, this study has been criticized for such shortcomings as selective referral of subjects by their attorneys and lack of nonviolent criminal controls.

In 1998, Raine and colleagues[53] extended this work based on Meloy's development of a typology distinguishing predatory versus affective violence. Predatory or instrumental violence is characterized by planned and deliberate use of physical aggression to achieve a specific aim, while affective or reactive violence features intense emotional arousal (typically anger or fear) in response to an immediate perceived provocation, triggering an aggressive outburst. Using FDG PET to compare 41 controls with 15 predatory murderers and 9 affective murderers, the study found that the affective violence group had decreased left and right hemisphere prefrontal activity and increased right hemisphere subcortical activity. The predatory violence group, by contrast, had prefrontal functioning equivalent to controls, but also had increased right subcortical activity. The authors hypothesized that excessive right subcortical activity predisposes to aggression, but that decreased frontal lobe function impairs the ability to inhibit affective violence, while intact frontal lobe functioning facilitates control of aggressive impulses, which may be then be directed to planned, instrumental ends.

While the studies by Raine and colleagues reported generalized frontal hypometabolism, subsequent functional neuroimaging studies have found more specific prefrontal foci associated with aggressive and antisocial behavior. In a 2001 study of subjects with FTD, results of single photon emission computerized tomography (SPECT) scans were correlated with subsequent blind ratings of antisocial behavior.[54] Among FTD subjects with predominantly right-sided frontal hypoperfusion on SPECT, 11 out of 12 showed antisocial behavior, while only 2 of 19 FTD subjects with predominantly left-sided hypoperfusion were rated as having antisocial behavior. Comparing FTD patients with AD patients, Mendez et al. found antisocial behavior in 57% of FTD patients compared with only 2.7% of AD subjects. In the FTD patients, antisocial behavior was associated with proportionately more right-sided frontotemporal hypoperfusion.[55] A 2006 SPECT study comparing 22 FTD patients with 76 age-matched, healthy controls found that, while FTD subjects showed the expected widespread frontal hypoperfusion, antisocial behavior in FTD subjects was specifically associated with decreased orbitofrontal perfusion.[56] There was no laterality difference reported in this study.

TABLE 34-1 • Functional Neuroimaging of Frontal Lobe Dysfunction in Antisocial Behavior.

Raine et al. (1994) FDG-PET	22 murderers c/w matched noncriminal controls	Murders showed decreased frontal activation
Raine et al. (1998) FDG-PET	15 predatory murderer and 9 affective murderer c/w 41 healthy, noncriminal controls	• Affective murderers showed decreased frontal activation • Predatory murderers equivalent to controls
Mychack et al. (2001) SPECT	41 subjects with FTD dementia	11 of 12 with right-sided FTD showed antisocial behavior c/w 2 of 19 with left-sided FTD
Mendez et al. (2005) PET/SPECT	28 FTD subjects c/w 28 AD subjects	• 57% of FTD showed antisocial behavior c/w 2.7% of AD • Antisocial behavior associated with right FTD hypoperfusion
Nakano et al. (2006) SPECT	22 FTD patients c/w 76 matched, healthy controls	FTD antisocial behavior correlated with orbitofrontal hypoperfusion
Yang and Raine (2009) Structural and functional neuroimaging	Meta-analysis of 43 studies pooling 789 antisocial subjects, 483 controls	Antisocial behavior associated with abnormalities of: • Right orbitofrontal • Left dorsolateral frontal • Right anterior cingulate
Alegria et al. (2016) fMRI	Meta-analysis of 24 studies pooling 338 youth w/ disruptive behavior, 298 controls	• Conducted disordered youth show rostro-dorsomedial anterior cingulate, fronto-cingulate, and ventral-striatal dysfunction • Psychopathic youth show ventromedial prefrontal/limbic dysfunction with dorsal/frontostriatal hyperfunctioning

AD, Alzheimer's disease; FTD, frontotemporal dementia.

In the past decade, sufficient neuroimaging data have accumulated to allow for meta-analyses. In 2009, Yang and Raine published pooled results from 43 structural and functional neuroimaging studies, which used a variety of brain morphometric and functional imaging modalities to examine antisocial,

violent, or psychopathic subjects. The cumulative data showed significantly reduced prefrontal cortical structure (e.g., volume, neural connectivity) and/or function (e.g., hemodynamic response, regional cerebral blood flow) associated with antisocial behavior, which specifically correlated with right orbitofrontal, right anterior cingulate, and left dorsolateral regions of prefrontal cortex. The authors calculated that the effect sizes for the contribution of decreased prefrontal function to antisocial behavior were in the moderate-to-large range.[57]

A 2017 meta-analysis tallied functional MRI studies examining disruptive behavior disorder in youths. Results identified two forms of antisocial behavior associated with two distinct types of frontal network dysfunction.[58] Youths with disruptive behavior that was characterized by impulsivity and failure to anticipate adverse consequences of their actions showed decreased function in rostro-dorsomedial anterior cingulate, fronto-cingulate, and ventral striatal areas—a pattern that was associated with impaired reward-based decision making. Youths with psychopathic personality traits, however, showed ventromedial prefrontal and limbic dysfunction, along with dorsal prefrontal and frontostriatal hyperfunctioning. These psychopathic youths showed decreased affective reactivity and empathy, yet with fully intact ability to plan antisocial behavior for instrumental purposes.

PREFRONTAL NETWORKS AND DEVELOPMENTAL PSYCHOPATHY

Cumulative research linking prefrontal dysfunction and antisocial behavior has prompted hypotheses that prefrontal network developmental abnormalities may explain the genesis of the psychopathic personality. Psychopathy is highly associated with recidivistic violence and criminal offending, and can be thought of as a virulent form of antisocial personality disorder, characterized by a habitual pattern of violating social and legal norms, present at least from early adolescence, coupled with a manipulative, emotionally superficial mode of relating to, and a marked lack of empathy, for others. Similarities between psychopathic personality traits and the behavioral syndrome of acquired sociopathy have led researchers to focus on ventromedial/orbitofrontal cortex and its connections in the search for a developmental lesion that could explain psychopathy.

In a study of patients with sociopathic personality changes following ventromedial frontal lobe injury, Damasio and colleagues[59] found that these subjects failed to show typical autonomic responses (as measured by skin conductance response, SCR) to socially meaningful stimuli. This lack of normative psycho-physiologic response to socially significant stimuli (e.g., pictures of people in distress) is a well-established phenomenon in psychopathic persons, and is thought to be associated with lack of empathy. Using an experimental paradigm known as the gambling task, the Damasio group further found that individuals with ventromedial prefrontal damage continued to make disadvantageous choices, even after they knew which choices were risky based on experience with the experimental task. In contrast, normal subjects would begin making advantageous choices based on a hunch even before they had explicitly learned the best strategy, and would also begin to generate an anticipatory SCR when facing a risky choice. Subjects with prefrontal decisional impairments, however, never developed this anticipatory SCR signaling risk.[60] This pattern of impulsively persisting in risky, short-term reward behavior, despite repeated experience with negative longer-term consequences, is a prominent feature of psychopathy.

Damasio posited that a key function of ventromedial prefrontal cortex is to lay down "somatic markers" that associate salient social stimuli and risk-reward learning with visceral autonomic signals, which then provide preconscious prompts for advantageous decision making. Thus, a developmental lesion in this prefrontal network could confer a tendency to recurrent poor judgment concerning the risks and rewards of antisocial conduct.

Research into the developmental impact of trauma on brain function also implicates prefrontal circuitry as a pathway whereby adverse childhood experience could contribute to later antisocial behavior. Early childhood trauma has been shown to alter functional connectivity between medial prefrontal cortex and the amygdala, suggesting that deficits in prefrontal regulation of emotion may lead to over expression of negative affect.[61] In a functional MRI study of male youths with disruptive behavior disorders and high levels of psychopathic traits, psychopathic youth showed diminished orbitofrontal response to reinforcement learning stimuli and rewards, along with decreased caudate response to reinforcement learning stimuli and overall lower amygdala response.[62] Such disruption in the functional integration of orbitofrontal cortex, caudate, and amygdala parallels functional alterations associated with childhood developmental trauma, particularly in males.[63] Thus, whether resulting from putative congenital abnormalities or from adverse environmental causes, alterations in brain function associated with antisocial behavior appear to converge on the prefrontal cortex and its limbic network connections, which mediate emotional regulation, response to socially significant stimuli, and the capacity to regulate behavior in anticipation of social rewards or punishment—all areas of deficit in the psychopathic personality.

BRAIN DYSFUNCTION, VIOLENCE, AND THE CRIMINAL JUSTICE SYSTEM

While the cumulative body of research reviewed above validates an increased risk of aggressive and antisocial behavior associated with prefrontal network dysfunction, the diagnosis of—for example—a frontal lobe tumor or a FTD does not equate with a predisposition for criminal offending. On this point, the overall data concerning violent crime and mental illness are instructive. Although the presence of a severe mental illness confers an increased risk of violence, this risk occurs in association with multiple interacting social and environmental factors that are generally linked with violence. Actual violent acts by mentally ill persons are largely associated with co-occurring substance abuse, and the proportion of all violent crime attributable to patients with severe mental illness is estimated to be only 5%.[64,65] Of note, there is no settled statistical estimate for the increased risk of violence associated with major mental illness itself.

Data are currently lacking to estimate rates of crime or violence attributable to neuropsychiatric disorders generally or to

prefrontal dysfunction specifically. Almost all of the research reviewed in this chapter consists of retrospective studies. The 1998 MacArthur Violence Risk Assessment Study,[27] which remains the most comprehensive and useful prospective study of violence risk in persons with psychiatric disorders, did not gather any data on neurocognitive or neurological abnormalities, or specific neuropsychiatric disorders. Meanwhile, research into the relationship between brain dysfunction, aggression, and crime has frequently been marred by failure to adequately control for the multiple developmental, psychosocial and environmental factors known to increase the risk for violent and criminal behavior, as well as by poorly defined measures of aggression or criminal offending. More recent study designs, however, have reflected increasing awareness of clinical forensic knowledge concerning the nature and genesis of violent and criminal offending, while advances in functional neuroimaging have further honed the findings gleaned from traditional lesion studies.

The research reviewed in this chapter points to two patterns of association between prefrontal cortical dysfunction and violence. One pattern associates prefrontal dysfunction and antisocial behavior with abnormalities of the dorsolateral prefrontal network, which are frequently developmental in nature. Here, the concern is with the broader risk of criminal offending, rather than with violent acts as such. Yang and Raine's[57] meta-analysis identified an association between antisocial behavior and abnormalities in specifically left dorsolateral prefrontal cortex, which is known to mediate classical executive functions. As characterized by Alegria and colleagues[58] developmental delays or abnormalities of dorsolateral prefrontal-anterior cingulate network function can impair the acquisition of self-restraint and the ability to defer gratification, leading to increased risk for conduct disorder in youth, reflecting impulsivity and failure to anticipate negative consequences. Such deficits in executive function are broadly associated with ADHD, but are also common in other NDDs, such as tic disorders, ASD, childhood lead toxicity, fetal alcohol or drug exposure, and intellectual developmental disability.

As described by Moffit,[41] a significant subset of adolescent delinquent behaviors may resolve with maturation of prefrontal cortex in early adulthood, when young people are also better situated to reap rewards from prosocial behaviors (such as access to income through employment). Patients with NDDs (as opposed to maturational delay) are likely to have more persistent impairments, but such syndromal neurodevelopmental deficits may still be amenable to social, educational, and clinical interventions (as suggested by studies linking psychostimulant treatment with reduced risk of criminal offending). Given the reported high prevalence of NDDs in correctional settings, early childhood intervention may decrease the risk of future offending, while effective diagnosis and treatment of adult inmates may reduce later reoffending and recidivism.

The second pattern of association implicates ventromedial/orbitofrontal dysfunction as a risk factor for violent and criminal behavior. The most robust data support a specific association of orbitofrontal network dysfunction with an increased risk of affective or reactive aggression. The clinical features of the orbitofrontal syndrome most closely fit the personality changes characterized as acquired sociopathy. Findings from the VHIS confirm increased aggression specifically associated with orbitofrontal lesions, and subsequent functional neuroimaging findings point to specifically right-sided orbitofrontal abnormalities. Given the right hemisphere's role in affective labeling and processing of social-emotional stimuli, an association of right orbitofrontal dysfunction with excessive aggression caused by affective lability or reactive impulsivity would make clinical sense.

Related prefrontal network abnormalities have been found in association with developmental forms of antisocial behavior, where orbitofrontal/ventromedial prefrontal and limbic dysfunctions are linked with decreased interpersonal affective reactivity and deficient empathy. The Yang and Raine[57] meta-analysis highlights an association between antisocial behavior and anterior cingulate abnormalities, which have also been linked to psychopathic traits of lack of empathy, shallow affect, impulsivity, and irresponsibility. Conversely, psychopaths typically show intact dorsolateral prefrontal functioning, or even hyperfunctioning, as noted by Alegria and colleagues[58] regarding psychopathic youth, consistent with the psychopathic person's intact ability to plan premeditated aggression for instrumental purposes. Based on his and others growing body of work on the neural correlates of psychopathy, Kiehl[66] traces the life-persistent violent and criminal offending of psychopaths to developmental deficits in a paralimbic prefrontal network that mediates attachment and related prosocial affects. Current work on the neural correlates of psychopathy has moved beyond regions of interest to examine brain-wide network activity. A recent large-scale, multicenter study examined whole-brain functional connectivity in a forensic sample of 985 psychopathic subjects. Consistent with the study's hypothesis, the affective and interpersonal deficits of psychopathy were correlated with aberrant functional connectivity in resting state networks involving the paralimbic system, including the insula, anterior and posterior cingulate cortex, amygdala, orbitofrontal cortex, and superior temporal gyrus.[67]

Given that criminogenic psychosocial and environmental factors likely interact with prefrontal impairments, much remains to be learned about the degree to which prefrontal dysfunction independently contributes to antisocial behavior. The current data, however, leave little doubt that neurobehavioral deficits play a role in some forms of violent and criminal offending. The extent to which current neuropsychiatric insights should influence jurisprudence and punishment remains controversial. Some neurobehavioral researchers have asserted that prefrontal neurocircuits constitute a brain network for moral behavior.[68] Fenwick[69] has noted that according to long-standing legal doctrine, "In order to be found guilty, a person must have a 'guilty mind.' It seems clear that the concept of a guilty mind belongs to a nonscientific era. There are clearly occasions when an act carried out will depend on a brain malfunction of which the person is not aware, or… of which he or she is aware, but cannot control." In most legal jurisdictions, lack of empathy and remorse are typically considered aggravating factors that worsen culpability for a criminal offense. Extrapolating from current research on the neural correlates of the psychopathic personality, however, some may argue that such deficits in affective and interpersonal behavior could one day be regarded

as clinical conditions that would be better addressed through treatment and early childhood intervention.

Current knowledge regarding clinical link between prefrontal dysfunction and antisocial behavior may already pose challenges to legal concepts of criminal responsibility. Mendez et al.[55] described 16 FTD subjects with new onset antisocial behavior who had all acted impulsively and without premeditation, although they were often aware that their behavior was socially inappropriate or wrong. Some states allow an insanity defense based on a mental condition that impairs behavioral controls, but many insanity statutes do not have such a volitional component, allowing a finding of lack of criminal responsibility only if the defendant's condition impairs his or her cognitive ability to understand the wrongfulness of the offending conduct. Under these statutes, a defendant with FTD that clearly caused a loss of ability to control antisocial impulses at the time of an alleged offense could nevertheless be found guilty.

Given the available evidence for a link between prefrontal network dysfunction and violence, defendants have increasingly sought to introduce claims of frontal lobe impairment into criminal proceedings, especially in the form of functional neuroimaging studies. Courts in some states with capital punishment have allowed findings from functional neuroimaging to be considered as potentially mitigating evidence during death penalty proceedings. The use of functional neuroimaging to evaluate psychopathology remains experimental, however, and attempts to admit functional neuroimaging evidence at trial as proof of lack of criminal responsibility face significant legal hurdles. In federal courts and the majority of states, current rules of evidence set specific legal criteria for the admission of expert theory or methodology in court. The criteria require that: the theory or method has been tested; subjected to peer review and publication; have a known error rate; have established standards controlling its operation; and have achieved widespread acceptance within the relevant scientific community. Current theories asserting a generalized association of neurobiological abnormality with violent or criminal behavior fall short of these legal requirements for admissibility in court. As Helen Mayberg,[70] a leading researcher in the functional neuroimaging of mood disorders, has cautioned, "Functional imaging methods have not reached the level of sophistication required to predict any neurological or psychiatric deficit, much less explain more esoteric behaviors such as lack of judgment or remorse." Although Mayberg penned this comment more than 20 years ago, it remains pertinent today, despite accelerating advances in functional neuroimaging technology and research.

Even as neuroimaging or other medical testing modalities eventually achieve diagnostic accuracy for specific neuropsychiatric disorders, in a legal context, such clinical data can serve only to confirm the presence or absence of specific neuropathology (analogous to an electroencephalogram, e.g., supporting the diagnosis of a seizure disorder). If a given disorder is shown to be present, such a clinical diagnosis does not, in itself, prove the impairment necessary to meet the legal standard for an insanity defense. "There is substantial controversy whether a test result … can be linked to a specific behavioral disorder," notes Ciccone. "Legal tests of insanity require a clear and direct link between the significant neurological and/or psychiatric pathological findings and the illegal act."[71]

Medical expert witnesses should be cautious when citing group statistical correlations between brain dysfunction and violence to support an argument for insanity in an individual defendant. While such evidence may help to show that a particular form of neurobehavioral pathology is relevant to a defendant's alleged conduct, the case must still be made that symptoms of a given neuropsychiatric disorder caused the legally necessary impairment in this particular individual at the time of this particular offense. Broad assertions that prefrontal network dysfunction, or any other form of brain-based pathology, explain a specific violent crime risk falling into the so-called G2I, or group-to-individual fallacy, in which a statistical correlation observed on average over a large sample of research subjects is construed as causation in the case of one individual, who may deviate significantly from the study sample average. As repeatedly noted throughout this chapter, violent and criminal acts are complex behaviors that appear to be influenced by multiple, interacting social, developmental, psychological, and (in some cases) neurobehavioral factors.

In the previously recounted case study of a 27-year-old man with orbitofrontal injury, for example, the patient's prefrontal deficits manifestly contributed to his recurrent, impulsive aggression following his head trauma. On the other hand, this young man clearly had a history and demonstrated propensity for antisocial behavior prior to his head injury, which itself resulted from criminal risk-taking behavior leading to his pedestrian-motor vehicle accident. A complete clinical account of his behavior must consider how all of these factors interacted to increase his risk of aggression. While this author has encountered many cases of brain injury causing impairments relevant to aggressive and antisocial behavior, in none of these cases has an acquired brain lesion by itself caused an otherwise psychologically healthy, socially functioning, and law-abiding individual to be transformed into a violent criminal. We cannot say (to paraphrase defense attorney Johnnie Cochran in the notorious 1994 celebrity murder trial of O.J. Simpson) that if a man has fits, you must acquit.

Even if forensic neuropsychiatry cannot currently provide—or wisely eschews—a comprehensive neurobehavioral explanation of violent and criminal behavior, rational application of knowledge concerning the relationship between brain dysfunction and antisocial behavior is clearly essential to the humane administration of criminal justice. Cumulative evidence for the prevalence and significance of neuropsychiatric disorders among those charged with violent offenses shows there is a "need for detailed clinical examinations of brain integrity in the majority of clinical forensic evaluations," as Martell asserts.[13] Such comprehensive forensic neuropsychiatric evaluation has not yet become the standard of care, and many forensic mental health systems lack the neurodiagnostic resources or clinical neuropsychiatric expertise to adequately identify and assess the nature and significance of brain dysfunction in criminal defendants referred for evaluations of competence to stand trial or criminal responsibility. Martell goes on to state, "Future research needs to explore the role of localized brain dysfunction in violent behavior and its interaction with other personal and environmental risk factors." We still lack such systematic, population-based data regarding the impact of neuropsychiatric disorders on the risk for violent crime.

Based on the most recent comprehensive survey data 45% of federal inmates, 56% of state prison inmates, and 64% of jail inmates had a recent history or current symptoms of a mental health problem.[27] Based on the research reviewed in this chapter, as well as the author's forensic mental health experience, many of these offenders will also have traumatic brain injuries, NDDs, or other neuropsychiatric disorders contributing to their psychiatric and behavioral morbidity. Faced with this massive public health crisis, forensic neuropsychiatry has an indispensable role to play in the understanding and melioration of criminal violence, as well as in addressing the burden of neuropsychiatric conditions afflicting those involved with the courts and the criminal justice system.

Summary and Key Points

- Cross-sectional and survey data find high rates of neuropsychiatric disorders in correctional and forensic mental health populations, but prospective data on rates of crime and violence associated with neuropsychiatric disorders are lacking.
- Studies of subjects with brain injury and neurodegenerative disorders find a consistent correlation between prefrontal network dysfunction and an increased risk of antisocial behavior. The strongest data find an increased risk of affective or reactive aggression associated with focal orbitofrontal brain injury or abnormality.
- Research on neural correlates of antisocial behavior has increasingly supported a link between the affective and interpersonal traits of the psychopathic personality and prefrontal paralimbic network abnormalities.

- Criminal violence is a complex behavior resulting from the interaction of psychosocial, environmental and, in some cases, neurobehavioral factors. The presence of frontal lobe dysfunction or any other neuropsychiatric condition does not equate with a criminal predisposition, and brain injury and central nervous system dysfunction do not offer a comprehensive explanation for the societal problem of violent and criminal behavior.
- Forensic mental health evaluations of criminal defendants should regularly include comprehensive clinical assessment for brain injury and central nervous system dysfunction, while future research should develop prospective data on the interaction of neurobehavioral disorders with other risk factors in the genesis of violent and criminal behavior.

Multiple Choice Questions

1. In 2005, the U.S. Supreme Court ruled the death penalty unconstitutional for juveniles. Based on research reviewed in this chapter, all of the following are true regarding juvenile offending behavior except:
   a. Conduct disordered youth show impaired reward-based decision making associated with decreased function in a network involving anterior cingulate, fronto-cingulate, and ventral striatal connections.
   b. Most adolescent offenders mature out of their delinquent behavior by early adulthood.
   c. Children with early frontal lobe injury may show lifelong developmental deficits in social comportment and moral reasoning associated with antisocial behavior.
   d. Youth with psychopathic personality traits show deficits in the capacity for planned or purposeful antisocial conduct, associated with decreased dorsolateral prefrontal function.
   e. In the 1980s, juveniles on death row were reported to show a clinical triad of severe childhood abuse, paranoid thinking, and brain abnormalities.

2. Studies of the association between traumatic brain injury (TBI) and criminal offending have found that:
   a. The prevalence of TBI in correctional settings is about 50% of that in the community.
   b. When adjusted for social and environmental risk factors, rates of criminal offending associated with TBI are uniformly elevated across studies.
   c. TBI is linked to higher rates of psychiatric and substance use disorders, more repeat offending, longer time served, and increased problems with anger and aggression.
   d. Researchers are in agreement on criteria for TBI severity and associated disability.

3. Regarding the association between prefrontal network dysfunction and antisocial behavior,
   a. The Vietnam Head Injury Study found an increased rate of arrests and criminal charges among subjects with focal frontal lobe lesions.
   b. Orbitofrontal abnormalities are linked to aggressive and antisocial behavior, while dorsolateral prefrontal dysfunction is not.
   c. Deficits in emotional reactivity are related to affective aggression in psychopathic persons.
   d. Frontal lobe disinhibition accounts for a large proportion of criminal violence.
   e. The clinical features of the orbitofrontal syndrome best fit the personality change after frontal lobe injury described as "acquired sociopathy."

4. Functional neuroimaging of frontal lobe function
   a. Is currently a reliable test of self-control related to legal tests of criminal responsibility.
   b. Has been used to evaluate affective versus predatory aggression in subjects who committed murder.
   c. Has found that antisocial behavior in frontotemporal dementia is associated with decreased left hemisphere blood flow.
   d. Can rule out Alzheimer's disease as a cause of prefrontal deficits.
   e. Has suggested that prefrontal network dysfunction is equivalent to the historical criminological concept of "moral insanity."

Multiple Choice Answers

1. **Answer: d**
   In a 2016 meta-analysis by Alegria et al., results of functional neuroimaging of studies of youth with psychopathic traits showed *increased* dorsolateral prefrontal functioning associated with the capacity to engage in premeditated offending behavior for instrumental purposes, while deficits in empathy and emotional reactivity were linked to ventromedial prefrontal/limbic dysfunction.

2. **Answer: c**
   Among incarcerated populations, TBI is linked to increased psychiatric morbidity, substance abuse, recidivism, and problems with institutional adaptation. Rates of TBI in incarcerated populations are estimated to be 50%, well above prevalence estimates for the community. TBI prevalence studies in correctional settings have been criticized for poorly defined clinical measures of head injury, and studies conflict regarding the role of TBI versus other criminogenic factors in offending behavior.

3. **Answer: e**
   The personality changes associated with orbitofrontal lesions best match the impulsivity, disregard for social norms, and lack of empathy described as the "acquired sociopathy" of frontal lobe injury. The Vietnam Head Injury Study did not report any data on arrests or criminal charges. Although focal orbitofrontal dysfunction has been associated with increased risk of aggression, developmental deficits in dorsolateral prefrontal network function have also been linked to antisocial behavior. Severe mental illness accounts for about 5% of all violent crime, but despite provocative claims, the actual rates of violence attributable to frontal lobe dysfunction are unknown.

4. Answer: b

Using FDG-PET to study a sample of murderers, Raine et al. found that frontal lobe hypofunction was associated with affective or reactive aggression, characterized by violent outbursts triggered by acute anger or fear. Functional neuroimaging remains a research modality that would likely not be admissible as evidence for legal insanity in a criminal trial. Functional neuroimaging studies have found *right*-hemisphere dysfunction associated with antisocial behavior in FTD, consistent with social-emotional disinhibition. Frontal-variant AD can present similarly to FTD. Based on the link between frontal lobe dysfunction and antisocial behavior, prefrontal neurocircuits have been hypothesized as a network for moral reasoning. Although the historical concept of "moral insanity" is similar to the contemporary clinical concept of the psychopathic personality, frontal lobe dysfunction does not equate with a general predisposition for violent or criminal offending.

References

1. Payne H, Luthe R. Isaac Ray and forensic psychiatry in the United States. *Forensic Sci Int*. 1980;15:115-127.
2. Sternberg L, Scott ES. Less guilty by reason of adolescence: developmental immaturity, diminished responsibility, and the juvenile death penalty. *Am Psychol*. 2003;12:1009-1018.
3. McCarthy J, Chaplin E, Underwood L, et al. Characteristics of prisoners with neurodevelopmental disorders and difficulties. *J Intellect Disabil Res*. 2016;60:201-206.
4. Durand E, Watier L, Fix M, Weiss JJ, Chevignard M, Pradat-Diehl P. Prevalence of traumatic brain injury and epilepsy among prisoners in France: results of the Fleury TBI study. *Brain Inj*. 2016;30:363-372.
5. Combalbert N, Valerie P, Claude F, Marine A, Morgan A, Brigitte G. Cognitive impairment, self-perceived health and quality of life of older prisoners. *Crim Behav Ment Health*. 2018;28:36-49.
6. Eigen JP. *James Hadfield (1771/2–1841)*. Oxford, UK: Oxford Dictionary of National Biography; 2018. Available at https://global.oup.com/academic/product/oxford-dictionary-of-national-biography-online-9780195221961?cc=us&lang=en&.
7. Resnick PO. Personal communication. American Academy of Psychiatry and the Law 2001 Forensic Psychiatry Review Course.
8. Lombroso C. *Criminal Man*. Gibson M, Rafter NH, trans. Durham, NC: Duke University Press; 2006.
9. Paulson G. Death of a president and his assassin: errors in their diagnosis and autopsies. *J Hist Neurosci*. 2006;15:77-91.
10. Lewis DO, Pincus JH, et al. Psychiatric, neurological and educational characteristics of 15 death row inmates in the United States. *Am J Psychiatry*. 1986;143:838-845.
11. Lewis DO, Pincus JH, et al. Neuropsychiatric, psychoeducational, and family characteristics of 14 juveniles condemned to death in the United States. *Am J Psychiatry*. 1988;145:584-589.
12. Frierson RL, Schwartz-Watts DM, Morgan DW, Malone TD. Capital versus non-capital murderers. *Am J Acad Psychiatry Law*. 1998;26:403-410.
13. Martell DA. Estimating the prevalence of organic brain dysfunction in maximum-security forensic psychiatric patients. *J Forensic Sci*. 1992;37:878-893.
14. Farrer TJ, Hedges DW. Prevalence of traumatic brain injury in incarcerated groups compared to the general population: a meta-analysis. *Prog Neuropsychopharmacol Bio Psychiatry*. 2011;35:390-394.
15. Williams WH, Mewse AJ, Tonks J, Mills S, Burgess CNW, Cordan G. Traumatic brain injury in a prison population: prevalence and risk of re-offending. *Brain Inj*. 2010;24:1184-1188.
16. Slaughter B, Fann JR, Ehde D. Traumatic brain injury in a county jail population: prevalence, neuropsychological functioning and psychiatric disorders. *Brain Inj*. 2003;17:731-741.
17. Mosti C, Coccaro EF. Mild traumatic brain injury and aggression, impulsivity, and history of other- and self-directed aggression. *J Neuropsychiatry Clin Neurosci*. 2018;30:220-227.
18. Schofield PW, Malacova E, Preen DB, et al. Does traumatic brain injury lead to criminality? A whole-population retrospective cohort study using linked data. *PLoS One*. 2015;10(7):e0132558.
19. Guberman GI, Robitaille MP, Larm P, et al. Are traumatic brain injuries associated with criminality after taking account of childhood family social status and disruptive behaviors? *J Neuropsychiatry Clin Neurosci*. 2019;31(2):123-131.
20. Billstedt E, Anckarsater H, Wallinius M, Hofvander B. Neurodevelopmental disorders in young violent offenders: overlap and background characteristics. *Psychiatry Res*. 2017;252:234-241.
21. Young S, Gonzalez RA, Mullens H, Mutch L, Malet-Lambert I, Gudjonsson GH. Neurodevelopmental disorders in prison inmates: comorbidity and combined associations with psychiatric symptoms and behavioral disturbances. *Psychiatry Res*. 2018;261:109-115.
22. Haskins BG, Silva JA. Asperger's disorder and criminal behavior: forensic psychiatric considerations. *J Am Acad Psychiatry Law*. 2006;34:374-384.
23. Tint A, Paluka AM, Bradley E, Weiss JA, Lunsky Y. Correlates of police involvement among adolescents and adults with autism spectrum disorder. *J Autism Dev Disord*. 2017;47:2639-2647.
24. Lichtenstein P, Halldner L, Zetterqvist J, et al. Medication for attention-deficit hyperactivity disorder and criminality. *N Engl J Med*. 2012;367:2006-2014.
25. Chang Z, Lichtenstein P, Långstrom N, Larsson H, Fazel S. Association between prescription of major psychotropic medications and violent reoffending after prison release. *JAMA*. 2016;316(17):1798-1807.
26. Lammers SM, Soe-Agnie SE, de Haan HA, Bakkum GAM, Pomp ER, Nijman HJM. Substance use and criminality: a review. *Tijdschr Psychiatr*. 2014;56:32-39.
27. Bureau of Justice Statistics 2016, NCJ 213600.
28. Steadman HJ, Mulvey EP, Monahan J, et al. Violence by people discharged from acute psychiatric inpatient facilities and by others in the same neighborhoods. *Arch Gen Psych*. 1998;55:393-401.
29. Hoaken PN, Stewart SH. Drugs of abuse and elicitation of human aggressive behavior. *Addict Behav*. 2003;28:1533-1554.
30. Bey T, Patel A. Phencyclidine intoxication and adverse effects: a clinical and pharmacological review of an illicit drug. *Calif J Emerg Med*. 2007;7:9-14.
31. Brecher M, Wang BW, Wong H, Morgan JP. Phencyclidine and violence: clinical and legal issues. *J Clin Psychopharmacol*. 1988;8:397-401.
32. Thirtalli J, Benegal V. Psychosis among substance users. *Curr Opin Psychiatry*. 2006;19:239-245.

33. Gunn J, Bonn J. Criminality and violence in epileptic prisoners. *Br J Psychiatry*. 1971;118:337-343.

34. Bach-y-Rita G, Lion JR, Climent CE, Ervin FR. Episodic dyscontrol: a study of 130 violent patients. *Am J Psychiatry*. 1971;127:1473-1478.

35. Treiman DM. Epilepsy and violence: medical and legal issues. *Epilepsia*. 1986;27(suppl 2):S77-S104.

36. Brower M, Price BH. Epilepsy and violence: when is the brain to blame? *Epilepsy Behav*. 2000;1(3):145-149.

37. Woerman FG, van Elst LT, Koepp M, et al. Reduction of frontal neocortical gray matter associated with affective aggression in patients with temporal lobe epilepsy: an objective voxel by voxel analysis of automatically segmented MRI. *J Neurol Neurosurg Psychiatry*. 2000;68:162-169.

38. Harlow JM. Recovery from the passage of an iron bar through the head. *Pub Mass Med Soc*. 1868;2:327-347.

39. Blumer D, Benson DF. Personality changes with frontal and temporal lobe lesions. In: Benson DF, Blumer D, eds. *Psychiatric Aspects of Neurological Disease*. New York, NY: Grune and Stratton; 1975:151-170.

40. Price BH, Daffner KR, Stowe RM, et al. The comportmental learning disabilities of early frontal lobe damage. *Brain*. 1990;113:1383-1393.

41. Moffitt TE. Adolescent-limited and life-course persistent antisocial behavior: a developmental taxonomy. *Psychol Rev*. 1993;100:674-701.

42. Duffy JD, Campbell JJ III. The regional prefrontal syndromes: a theoretical and clinical overview. *J Neuropsychiatry Clin Neurosci*. 1994;6:379-387.

43. Blake PY, Pincus JH, Buckner C. Neurologic abnormalities in murderers. *Neurology*. 1995;45:1641-1647.

44. Heinrichs RW. Frontal cerebral lesions and violent incidents in chronic neuropsychiatric patients. *Biol Psychiatry*. 1989;25:174-178.

45. Krakowski M, Czobor P. Violence in psychiatric patients: the role of psychosis, frontal lobe impairment, and ward turmoil. *Compr Psychiatry*. 1997;38:230-236.

46. Jensen P, Fenger K, Bolwig T, Sorensen SA. Crime in Huntington's disease: a study of registered offenses among patients, relatives, and controls. *J Neurol Neurosurg Psychiatry*. 1998;65:467-471.

47. Miller BL, Darby A, Benson DF, Cummings JL, Miller MH. Aggressive, socially disruptive and antisocial behavior in frontotemporal dementia. *Br J Psychiatry*. 1997;170:150-155.

48. Liljergren M, Nassan G, Temlett J, et al. Criminal behavior in frontotemporal dementia and Alzheimer's disease. *JAMA Neurol*. 2015;72:295-300.

49. Mendez MF, Shapira JS. Hypersexual behavior in frontotemporal dementia: a comparison with early-onset Alzheimer's disease. *Arch Sex Behav*. 2013;42:501-509.

50. Ahmed RM, Kaisik C, Irish M, Mioshi E, et al. Characterizing sexual behavior in frontotemporal dementia. *J Alzheimer Dis*. 2015;46:677-686.

51. Grafman J, Schwab D, Warden D, Pridgen A, Brown HR, Salazar AM. Frontal lobe injuries, violence and aggression: a report of the Vietnam Head Injury Study. *Neurology*. 1996;46:1231-1238.

52. Raine A, Buchsbaum M, LaCasse L. Brain abnormalities in murderers indicated by positron emission tomography. *Biol Psychiatry*. 1997;42:495-508.

53. Raine A, Meloy JR, Birhle S, Stoddard J, LaCasse L, Buchsbaum MS. Reduced prefrontal and increased subcortical brain functioning assessed using positron emission tomography in predatory and affective murderers. *Behav Sci Law*. 1998;16:319-332.

54. Mychack P, Kramer JH, Boone KB, Miller BL. The influence of right frontotemporal dysfunction on social behavior in frontotemporal dementia. *Neurology*. 2001;56 (suppl):S11-S15.

55. Mendez MF, Chen AK, Shapira JS, Miller BL. Acquired sociopathy and frontotemporal dementia. *Dement Geriatr Cogn Disord*. 2005;20:99-104.

56. Nakano S, Asada T, Yamashita F, et al. Relationship between antisocial behavior and regional cerebral blood flow in frontotemporal dementia. *NeuroImage*. 2006;32:301-306.

57. Yang Y, Raine A. Prefrontal structural and functional brain imaging findings in antisocial and psychopathic individuals: a meta-analysis. *Psychiatry Res*. 2009;174(2):81-88.

58. Alegria AA, Radua J, Rubia K. Meta-analysis of fMRI studies of disruptive behavior disorders. *Am J Psychiatry*. 2016;173:1119-1130.

59. Damasio AR, Tranel D, Damasio H. Individuals with sociopathic behavior caused by frontal damage fail to respond autonomically to social stimuli. *Behav Brain Res*. 1990;41:81-94.

60. Bechara A, Damasio H, Tranel D, Damasio AR. Deciding advantageously before knowing the advantageous strategy. *Science*. 1997;275:1293-1295.

61. Cisler JM. Childhood trauma and functional connectivity between amygdala and medial prefrontal cortex: a dynamic functional connectivity and large-scale network perspective. *Front Syst Neurosci*. 2017;11:29.

62. Finger EC, Marsh AA, Blair KS, et al. Disrupted reinforcement signaling in the orbitofrontal cortex and caudate in youths with conduct disorder or oppositional defiant disorder and a high level of psychopathic traits. *Am J Psychiatry*. 2011;168:152-162.

63. Helpman L, Zhu X, Suarez-Jimenez B, Lazarov A, Monk C, Neria Y. Sex differences in trauma-related pathology: a critical review of neuroimaging literature (2014-2017). *Current Psychiatry Rep*. 2017;19:104.

64. Stuart H. Violence and mental illness: an overview. *World Psychiatry*. 2003;2:121-124.

65. Fazel S, Grann M. The population impact of severe mental illness on violent crime. *Am J Psychiatry*. 2006;163:1397-1403.

66. Kiehl KA. A cognitive neuroscience perspective on psychopathy: evidence for paralimbic system dysfunction. *Psychiatry Res*. 2006;142:107-128.

67. Espinoza FA, Vergara VM, Reyes D, et al. Aberrant functional network connectivity in psychopathy from a large (N = 985) forensic sample. *Hum Brain Mapp*. 2018;39:2624-2634.

68. Mendez MF. What frontotemporal dementia reveals about the neurobiological basis of morality. *Med Hypotheses*. 2006;67:411-418.

69. Fenwick P. Brain, mind and behavior: some medicolegal aspects. *Br J Psychiatry*. 1993;163:565-573.

70. Mayberg H. Medico-legal inferences from functional neuroimaging evidence. *Semin Clin Neuropsychiatry*. 1996;1:195-201.

71. Ciccone JR. Murder, insanity and expert witnesses. *Arch Neurol*. 1992;49:608-611.

35

Holistic and Sustainable Management of Complex Neuropsychiatric Patients

Barry S. Fogel

Neuropsychiatric patients rarely have a single medical diagnosis. Even when they do, their disease may cause functional impairments that require adaptation and/or rehabilitation or entail a complex and demanding treatment regimen. The illness is likely to impact the patient's family and/or significant others, especially if it involves cognitive or sensory impairment; aggressive, self-injurious, psychotic, or otherwise risky or socially inappropriate behavior; or expensive treatment or care not covered by insurance. Consistent delivery of treatment to a patient might be difficult because of the patient's functional impairments or social and environmental issues, including challenges accessing health care and/or paying for treatments, and environmental hazards with disproportionate impact on patient's specific problems. Treatments for neuropsychiatric disorders sometimes have neuropsychiatric or general medical side effects. Finally, there often are illness-related educational, occupational, financial, and/or legal issues, which may be complicated by family conflicts about how best to deal with them.

Ideally, patients with neuropsychiatric disorders and accompanying comorbidities will receive treatment from a physician serving as a subspecialist in neuropsychiatry. The role might be filled by neuropsychiatrist, behavioral neurologist, or a general neurologist or psychiatrist with a one or more neuropsychiatric conditions as a focus of his/her practice. Geriatric and pediatric neurologists and psychiatrists often function as "brain/mind medicine" practitioners for a specific set of conditions, as do specialists in neurotrauma and stroke. For simplicity, any physician who works at the interface of psychiatry and neurology in their care for a patient with brain dysfunction will be referred to in this chapter as a neuropsychiatrist, with the understanding that most neuropsychiatric care is delivered by physicians who do not have neuropsychiatry as their primary specialty.

In approaching the care of complex patients, it is useful to acknowledge that clinical care is not delivered by physicians alone. Chronic neuropsychiatric conditions also frequently involve nonphysician health care professionals including physical, occupational, and speech therapists, social workers, and psychologists. However, even straightforward outpatient care of chronic conditions requires the involvement of pharmacists to fill prescriptions and answer patient's questions about medications, office staff to schedule appointments, technical and professional staff involved with diagnostic imaging and clinical laboratory tests, and people who handle coding of diagnoses and procedures, billing, claims processing, and payment. These individuals can facilitate and enable physicians' work, making it more efficient and more financially sustainable.

The neuropsychiatrist's role varies among cases, in a way that can be conceptualized in terms of his/her position on an organizational chart. A chief executive officer (CEO) has overall responsibility for deciding on strategy, assigning duties to others, evaluating results, and representing the team externally. A chief operating officer (COO) is responsible for organizing and overseeing the implementation of the strategic plan decided upon by the CEO. A chief strategy officer (CSO) is responsible for creating a strategic plan to be adopted in some form by the CEO and implemented by people who report to the CEO or COO. A team leader is responsible for coordinating the efforts of a group of people who implement *part* of the overall treatment plan. A consultant provides one-time or intermittent advice on strategy to professionals not on his/her own team; he/she is not directly responsible for execution of the recommendations. A team member provides a clinical service, communicates with other professionals, and may make suggestions to them, but usually does not have the role of assigning duties to others or coordinating their efforts.

Formally integrating different elements of a patient's treatment to address the full range of the presenting problems can improve the effectiveness and efficiency of care. This has been demonstrated in randomized controlled studies for specific combinations of comorbid conditions, such as depression comorbid with diabetes, coronary heart disease, or both.[1,2] It has also been found in retrospective observational studies comparing team-based care that includes integrated mental health service with care delivered in a traditional model of practice management. In one such study, outcomes of care for patients in 27 primary care practices offering team-based care were compared with outcomes for patients in 75 practices operating in the traditional model. The patients receiving team-based care had 23% fewer emergency department (ED) visits and 11% fewer hospital admissions, and system-wide cost savings were more than ten times greater than the incremental costs of team-based care.[3] Published comments on the study's findings emphasize that the cost savings realized by team-based care implied decreased revenues for the health care providers involved. Thus, physicians would have a financial incentive *not* to provide team-based care unless they were paid for the extra time and cost of the team-based model of care and/or rewarded financially for realized cost savings from hospitalizations and ED visits avoided.[4,5] Various models of "value-based payment" have been proposed as a longer-term solution to this paradox. Meantime, when an organization like an integrated care system or an accountable care organization (ACO) takes risk for the total cost of care, financial incentives favor team-based care for complex, high-cost patients.

For more severely impaired patients a common aim of neuropsychiatric care is to avoid the need for institutional care. For less impaired patients of school or working age, interventions to enable educational progress or consistent work performance should be a focus of treatment. For patients who are retired or with long-term disabilities, treatment aims to enable unpaid purposeful activity that keeps them mentally and physically active and makes life more meaningful and enjoyable. Such activity mitigates the suffering of chronic illness.

Neuropsychiatric illness does not necessarily imply proportional functional impairment, and functional impairment does not necessarily imply proportional disability and handicap. Holistic care involves addressing the diseases underlying the patient's illness, relieving symptoms or making them more bearable, and reducing the negative impact of the illness on functional performance and on the activities and relationships that make the patient's life meaningful.

Addressing the complete problem list of a neuropsychiatric patient almost always involves one or more clinical teams, each with a team leader. Ideally there is a "clinical CEO" who takes personal responsibility for overall leadership and coordination of care, though complex care often is given without overall leadership. When there is a clinical CEO, he/she will spend time on "behind the scenes" care coordination activities in addition to time and energy spent delivering direct, face-to-face care. Some of this work will be done by the CEO personally, and the remainder will be done by team members (e.g., nonphysicians, residents, and fellows in academic settings). If the requisite time and resources are not budgeted for the work, it will not be sustainable, and the clinicians involved will be at risk for burnout.

Typically, there are two sets of "players." The "patient-side players" comprise the patient, family, and significant others, and paid and volunteer caregivers, supporters, and advocates. There is usually a person among them who is the primary coordinator of care and primary liaison with health care professionals. The "clinical players" comprise the physicians and other health professionals involved in the patient's care, and representatives of organizations involved in hosting, supporting, and paying for care delivery. (In using this terminology there is no implication that "clinical players" are not "on the patient's side" in terms of

wishing the patient well, or that "patient-side players" always have the patient's best interests in mind. They apply to a situation in which transactions take place between a patient and those who share interests with him/her, and people in caregiving occupations and/or caregiving organizations.)

Clinicians involved in the care of complex neuropsychiatric patients include neurologists and psychiatrists, primary care physicians, specialists in the care of patients' general medical comorbidities, psychologists including neuropsychologists, therapists (PT, OT, SLP), social workers, and physician extenders (advanced practice nurses and physician assistants). Organizations with interests in complex neuropsychiatric cases include hospitals, clinics, community health and mental health centers, managed care organizations, and health insurance companies. Often financial or administrative responsibility for the care of a complex neuropsychiatric case will be divided between two organizations, one dealing with the "behavioral health" and the other with general medical care. This situation is referred to as a "carveout" of "mental health" or "behavioral health" services.

People with neuropsychiatric disorders and multiple comorbidities, and/or their families, often require the services of non-health care professionals such as lawyers and financial professionals. Those with fiduciary obligations to the patient (or the patient's guardian) are patient-side players. Others, like educational consultants, can be players on the patient side or on the clinical side, depending on circumstances.

The clinical players usually do not have a formally designated team leader. Sometimes it is assumed that the PCP (if there is one) will coordinate care across disciplines. Or, in the case of patients where one disease stands out as most important to overall health and function, people often assume that the physician specializing in that disease is the *de facto* team leader. When a patient is under treatment for metastatic cancer, the oncologist's plan for antineoplastic treatment takes precedence over other clinicians' plans to treat comorbidities that are not as life-threatening. People might assume that the oncologist will coordinate the efforts of non-oncologic specialists or at least make recommendations to them about how to harmonize their work with the patient's cancer treatment. However, an oncologist might not necessarily be aware of a patient's neuropsychiatric history and current therapies and their potential interactions and implications for treatment of the cancer. In a typical case seen by the author, a patient with complex partial epilepsy, PTSD, and a history of delayed diagnoses of both conditions was treated by a surgeon and oncologist for breast cancer. The trauma of mastectomy reactivated the patient's PTSD. The oncologist was slow to respond to the patient's complaints of post-mastectomy neuropathic pain and did not initially address the patient's fears of chemotherapy-related neuropathy. The patient reacted by leaving the hospital against medical advice and delaying her chemotherapy by several weeks.

PCPs might have limited knowledge of community resources for meeting the needs of patients with neuropsychiatric disorders, while front-line "case managers" employed by managed care organizations often have neither the authority nor the scope of knowledge to be comprehensive managers of a complex patient's care. Care management by a neuropsychiatrist working together with a nonphysician team member (e.g., neuropsychiatric nurse practitioner or neuropsychiatric social worker) and working closely with a patient-side representative may be a more effective option.

A challenge for neuropsychiatrists is providing care that is holistic and comprehensive but also *sustainable* over the long term. Most major neuropsychiatric disorders are either chronic or recurrent. In most parts of the United States there is a shortage of psychiatrists and of neurologists; physicians of both specialties are concentrated in and around metropolitan areas, and in smaller localities that have a highly educated and/or affluent population. For example, a 2011 study of the distribution of medical specialists by Hospital Referral Region, the median number of neurologists per 100,000 population was 3.3, but it ranged from 10.7 per 100,000 in Rochester, MN (home of the Mayo Clinic) to 1.5 per 100,000 in Oxford, MS. The median number of psychiatrists per 100,000 was 8.5, with 29.0 per 100,000 in San Francisco, CA and 3.5 per 100,000 in Oxford, MS.[6] At the beginning of 2020 there were 405 physicians certified by the United Council for Neurologic Subspecialties in behavioral neurology and neuropsychiatry.[7] This implies many smaller cities of the United States will have no physician certified in the subspecialty.

The shortage of neuropsychiatrists, combined with reimbursement structures in the United States that are biased against non-procedural specialties, makes them vulnerable to overwork and to eventual burnout. An American Academy of Neurology study found lower professional satisfaction among neurologists practicing in small cities or rural areas.[8]

To meet patients' needs for neuropsychiatric care, it is important to protect neuropsychiatrists from burnout and make sure that their practices—whether private or institutional—are financially and personally sustainable. Doing so will also make behavioral neurology and neuropsychiatry more attractive to medical students choosing their specialties, and to trainees in neurology or psychiatry considering fellowship training. This chapter describes strategies for care of complex neuropsychiatric patients that address common challenges to sustainability from the perspective of the neuropsychiatrist—unpredictable time demands, potentially preventable "emergencies," uncompensated time, poor coordination with other physicians of other specialties, difficulties negotiating with insurance companies and managed care organizations, and conflicts with concerned family members and other patient-side "players."

Holistic and sustainable neuropsychiatric care is based on fully identifying the patient's needs, setting goals and priorities, identifying the clinical and patient-side "players," identifying and empowering care managers, anticipating crises, and making full use of multidimensional quantitative measurements of disease activity, functional status, and relevant domains of symptomatology. Measurement should make use of technology whenever it will enhance the accuracy and utility of patient data without increasing clinician burden. Working with trusted professionals who address nonclinical aspects of patients' needs (e.g., legal, occupational, and educational) also is essential, and usually requires the deliberate development of local resources through reciprocal assistance.

Though doing all of this may seem overwhelming and impractical, it is more feasible if the neuropsychiatrist concentrates his or her ongoing care of patients on those with a small set of related diagnoses or conditions rather than on the full spectrum of neuropsychiatric disorders. For example, a clinician might concentrate on autism spectrum disorders (ASD) and their overlap with obsessive-compulsive disorder (OCD) and Tourette syndrome (TS), or on late complications of traumatic brain injury. While a neuropsychiatrist might evaluate patients with a broader range of problems, it is usually preferable for him/her to take a purely consultative role with most patients, if doing so is feasible within the environment of practice. To be most effective, consultation reports should include not only opinions about diagnoses and treatments, but also the neuropsychiatrist recommendations of a strategy for comprehensive treatment.

The complexity of neuropsychiatric care arises from the intersection of multiple considerations, outlined in Table 35-1.

Managing complexity begins with understanding who are the players on the patient's side, including the patient, friends, and family who care for or care about the patient, and others with a personal, financial, or legal interest in the patient's case. As the neuropsychiatrist comes to know who the key players are, he/she should develop an informal understanding about each one. What are his/her goals and expectations from care and treatment? What is his/her knowledge of the patient's condition and treatments? What is his/her level of proactive engagement with the patient's care? What is his/her level of executive cognitive function—organization, planning, self-control, and self-awareness? With which health care professionals does he/she communicate and, typically, under what circumstances? What is his/her role in medical decisions, on a continuum from minimal input to fully shared decision making? Clinicians should be clear about which people have the legal right to access a patient's medical records or be informed about the results of medical examinations and tests. Confidentiality concerns are especially great when issues of mental illness or substance use are involved. After defining who the relevant clinicians are in a case, the neuropsychiatrist should ensure that he/she has written permission of the patient (or the patient's legal representative) to share information with all of them. If a patient objects to sharing information with one or more of his/her physicians, exploring the reason sometimes yields new insights into the case.

For patients who will receive ongoing care, this is a gradual process rather than yet another burdensome requirement for a first visit. It can save time and stress for the neuropsychiatrist to know the key players and their interests and agendas early in the course of treatment, rather than find out later when treatment is disrupted by an interpersonal conflict. The patient or a family member or advocate usually can start the process by making a list of the people he/she thinks are most involved in the patient's care and/or concerned about its outcomes. Some of the questions can be put in the form of a questionnaire that a patient or family member can fill out while in the neuropsychiatrist's office, or that can be submitted via an online patient portal either before or after an initial appointment. Questionnaires can be tailored to the characteristics of patients in the practice such as educational level, cultural background, and preferred language.

In addition to the players "onstage" there usually are players "backstage" who function as "gatekeepers," controlling access to resources and payment for them: payers, utilization reviewers, pharmaceutical benefit managers, etc. Here they are included with the players on the clinical side. In fully integrated systems like the Veterans Health Administration system, Kaiser Permanente, and some countries' national health systems, backstage players are responsible for allocating limited resources (e.g., the time of salaried health professionals) rather than authorizing the payment of fees for individual services. Though details and incentives may differ among them, an important common element of private, public, and hybrid health care systems is that someone who is not on the front lines of care and does not personally know the patient must authorize the delivery of expensive treatments and services. Because neuropsychiatric conditions typically are complex and many neuropsychiatric syndromes are not well-known to nonspecialists, the neuropsychiatrist may face the challenge of either educating a "gatekeeper" about a patient's need for an expensive or unconventional treatment, or of appealing a case to someone with more advanced training and authority to approve such treatments.

The problem can be especially thorny when behavioral health services are carved out of general medical care and neuropsychiatric services are put into the behavioral health category. Behavioral health carveout plans often are designed so that initial diagnoses and treatment plans are made by nonphysicians who often would not have the knowledge and status to integrate patients' mental health care with management of their comorbid neurological and general medical and neurological diagnoses. For example, consider a young adult with poorly controlled partial complex seizures, an associated mood disorder in the bipolar spectrum, and occasional episodes of missed doses of antiepileptic drugs and/or inadequate sleep leading to generalized seizures and thence to hospitalization. Full control of the seizures and long-term mood stabilization might be possible with consistent adherence to medication. This might be accomplished by frequent, ongoing neuropsychiatric visits, some in person and some online; some with the neuropsychiatrist and some with a psychologist, nurse practitioner, or physician assistant on the neuropsychiatry team; combined with the use of mobile apps to continuously monitor treatment adherence and a bedside sleep monitor that continuously tracked the timing and duration of sleep. Patient visits might include exploration of the patient's difficulty with treatment adherence, education about epilepsy and bipolar disorder, teaching the importance of sleep and principles of sleep hygiene, supportive psychotherapy, and close monitoring of antiepileptic drug levels. When devices detected changes in sleep or medication adherence the issue would be addressed promptly with the patient before it presented as a seizure or as hypomania. The critical point is that behavior specifically related to controlling seizures (as well as preventing a relapse of hypomania) would be the main focus of mental health care.

If the strategy described were successful it would prevent hospitalizations and ED visits that could easily cost more than a year of neuropsychiatric services. However, a health plan might put the neuropsychiatric services in the "behavioral health" budget separate from the budget that would pay for an ED visit or hospitalization related to a generalized seizure. The carved-out behavioral health plan would be assuming the expense of neuropsychiatric treatment but would not receive credit for money saved by prevention of ED visits and hospitalizations. Typical behavioral health plans tend to minimize psychiatrists' involvement other than for medication management, and their guidelines for the number and duration of covered sessions might not fit the needs of a patient for substantial and frequent physician involvement until barriers to long-term treatment adherence were uncovered and addressed. They seldom are structured to support and pay for integrated care.

A care manager/gatekeeper at a behavioral health plan might not understand why a patient with complex partial seizures and bipolar disorder couldn't see a neurologist for his epilepsy once or twice a year, a psychiatrist two or three times annually for a 20-minute "med check," and perhaps receive time-limited psychotherapy from a master's level counselor at times of emotional distress. The power of fully integrated neurological, psychiatric, and psychological care would not be appreciated. Devices to directly monitor sleep and medication use probably would not be covered at all, despite their potential value.

Considerable—and uncompensated—effort by the neuropsychiatrist and/or his/her team members might be needed to get an optimal treatment plan authorized and paid for, and with some payers and health systems it might be impossible. But, if one of the neuropsychiatrist's specialties were epilepsy with major psychiatric comorbidity, it might be worthwhile for him/her to appeal the case to the highest level of the health plan, proposing that the total cost of care be prospectively tracked during a 12-month trial of the recommended treatment. With a few conspicuous successes, a neuropsychiatrist sometimes can establish relationships with more senior people at a health plan who will help get his/her patients get fast-tracked through the process of prior approvals and utilization reviews. Patients and families typically are deeply appreciative of their physicians making special efforts to get them coverage for effective and personalized treatment. In some cases a patient or family is willing and able to pay for an element of treatment that makes sense to them but their health plan won't cover. The one-time purchase of a device like a bedside sleep monitor is an example. In other contexts such as Medicaid managed care in some states of the United States, there is little flexibility permitted in treatment planning, and private practice providers of all specialties may be reluctant to take on new Medicaid patients because payments for services are so low. In this situation political advocacy, perhaps working together with a disease-oriented nonprofit organization, sometimes can reduce the clinician's sense of powerlessness even if it does not change policy in the near term.

A CASE EXAMPLE OF EVERYDAY COMPLEXITY

The following case illustrates how even an ordinary, uncomplicated neuropsychiatric case can have nontrivial complexity. In such a case there are several opportunities to improve the

TABLE 35-1 • Sources of Complexity in Neuropsychiatric Cases.

Categorical diagnoses
Syndromes without a categorical diagnosis
Symptoms
Results of biochemical, physiological, and microbiological tests done in the laboratory, at the point of care, at home
Data from mobile devices, wearables, and "invisibles" (location-based noncontact monitors)
Impairments in executive function, metacognition, and social cognition
Functional impairments (physical, instrumental, social, cognitive, sensory, communicative)
Physicians and other clinicians of various disciplines and specialties
Educational, social, occupational, financial, and legal implications of diagnoses and impairments
Psychotherapeutic treatments including those delivered online
Pharmacologic treatments
Nonpharmacologic somatic treatments including ECT, TMS, tDCS, tACS, DBS, VNS, tPBM, light therapy/chronotherapy, and TENS units
Adaptive devices such as tremor-modifying devices, communication aids, and advanced prostheses
Lifestyle and environmental issues related to diet, activity, sleep, and environmental exposures, including those related to occupation
Complementary, alternative, and integrative medicine interventions
Medical record systems, often full of uninformative cut-and-paste content, outdated medication lists, and irrelevant alerts
Living arrangements and settings of care
Concerned parties ("players") with different and sometimes conflicting agendas, including payers and care managers with goals of containing or shifting costs of care
Paid and unpaid caregivers with varying knowledge, skills, and intentions
Preferences and beliefs of patients and patient-side players
Culturally related views of illnesses and their treatments, including differences in idioms of distress across cultures
Stigma of neuropsychiatric illness, including self-stigma, anticipated stigma, public stigma, and institutional stigma

DBS, deep brain stimulation; ECT, electroconvulsive therapy; tACS, transcranial alternating current stimulation; tDCS, transcranial direct current stimulation; TENS, transcutaneous electrical nerve stimulation; TMS, transcranial magnetic stimulation; tPBM, transcranial photobiomodulation; VNS, vagus nerve stimulation.

patient's health outcomes and health-related quality of life by taking a comprehensive approach.

James T. is a 23-year-old single man with high-functioning ASD. His I.Q. is 110, and he has an associate degree from a junior college. He meets diagnostic criteria for TS and OCD. His tics include finger-snapping, throat-clearing, and occasional coprolalia. His most frequent compulsions are hand-washing and checking. He often feels anxious, especially when he makes efforts to suppress his tics and compulsions. He is a binge-drinker, drinking to intoxication two or three times per month. He has asthma for which he regularly takes an inhaled steroid, often requires a bronchodilator inhaler, and has needed systemic steroids several times for asthma exacerbations brought on by upper respiratory infections. He had two ED visits for asthma in the past winter and was hospitalized once for asthma when he was in his late teens. He is an only child. He lives with his parents who are now in their early 60s, and drives daily to his job as an office worker at an insurance company. His current medications are aripiprazole, fluvoxamine, and a fluticasone inhaler.

There are several ongoing problems. He sometimes is non-adherent to his medication regimen, and his symptoms rapidly worsen when this occurs. He has driven his car while intoxicated, though he has not had any crashes or arrests. He has been late to work several times because his compulsions delayed his drive to work, and he has twice been warned by his supervisor about his coprolalia disturbing other workers. He has had episodes of explosive anger, usually but not always after drinking alcohol, in which he has yelled and thrown objects, sometimes breaking them. He has never injured anyone during his anger outbursts. James has no close friends, but occasionally goes out to a bar or a movie with one of his junior college classmates. He is more comfortable with technology than with people and spends hours every day playing online games.

He agreed to a consultation with a neuropsychiatrist because he feels his medications are a hassle to take and don't give him enough relief from his anxiety, tics, and OCD symptoms to be worth the trouble. He would like to be more independent and less lonely and hopes someone can help him attain those goals. He feels that his father secretly blames him for his tics and behavioral issues.

His parents have many worries. James might drive while intoxicated and get into a crash or be arrested. He might get violently angry while outside the home and be violent with people, destroy others' property, get hurt in a fight, or get in trouble with the law. He might lose his job. His asthma might get out of control again. Most of all, they fear that their son will never "launch" as an independent adult.

IDENTIFYING THE PLAYERS, STRUCTURING CARE, SETTING GOALS, AND REDUCING RISK

The players in James' case include the patient and his parents, his primary care physician, and an educational consultant. James is moderately engaged but easily gets angry. His executive function fluctuates with his mood and alcohol use. *His mother* is highly engaged but not well-informed, knowing more about ASD and OCD than she does about TS, asthma, or alcohol use disorders. *His father* is disengaged; he doesn't like to think about his son's problems. He focuses on his job and delegates responsibility for his son's problems to his wife. The *PCP* knows much more about asthma than about neuropsychiatric disorders. His usual focus with his patients with chronic conditions is keeping them out of the hospital and the ED. The *educational consultant* was actively involved when James was in middle school, high school, and junior college, helped him prepare for employment with social skills training, and provided coaching during his job search and first month on the job. James last saw her 3 years ago. James's parents have high expectations of benefit from the neuropsychiatrist. They asked for a subspecialty referral from James's PCP after his mother heard about the neuropsychiatrist at a Tourette Syndrome Association meeting.

The *goals of treatment* are synchronous with the concerns of the different players. They are to keep James employed, to have him stop binge-drinking, to have him take his medications consistently, to avoid injuries and legal troubles, to build his social kills and his independence, to reduce the amount of time spent on compulsions and the number of days he is late to work, to reduce his vocal tics and coprolalia so he does not offend or disturb those around him, and to prevent ED visits and hospitalizations related to asthma.

The neuropsychiatrist, who has a special interest in high-functioning autistic adults and their common comorbidities, has decided upfront that he will directly manage the case as the "CEO." He has confirmed with the referring PCP that he will have this executive role. At the first visit, he introduces himself to the patient, explains that he has been asked by the PCP to coordinate and manage his care, and asks for his permission to talk regularly with his parents, his PCP, and any other involved professionals. He does a comprehensive neuropsychiatric assessment, after which he works collaboratively with the patient to reach an agreement about the goals of treatment discussed above. He reassures the patient that if giving up drinking makes him more anxious, he will help him deal with the anxiety. He asks for the patient's written consent to the goals of treatment and to his sharing information with other clinician and with his parents. Including the goals in the written consent isn't a legal requirement, but it implies *active agreement* rather than passive acceptance of the treatment plan.

Treatment begins with a focus on *risk mitigation*—a point the neuropsychiatrist emphasizes to the patient and his family. If James were seriously injured or were to injure another person in a fight or car crash, his future could be compromised forever. If he cannot commit himself to total abstinence from alcohol, he should carry a smartphone-linked alcohol breath tester and commit to not drive if his alcohol level is 40 mg/dL or higher. This level would probably allow him to have one standard drink, two drinks in 2 hours, or three drinks in 4 hours, but would be exceeded if he had more. Forty mg/dL is the legal limit in the United States for drivers of commercial vehicles, a more conservative limit than that for drivers of automobiles.[9]

If he cannot adhere to that standard his family should have an ignition interlock installed in his car. If he commits to complete abstinence, his blood levels of phosphatidylethanol (PEth) (or another alcohol biomarker) levels can be monitored to detect covert drinking.[10,11] The PCP should take care that James gets his influenza immunizations on time and other interventions directed at reducing asthma-related risk. If angry episodes persist despite cutting down on alcohol, an alpha-2 agonist (e.g.,

clonidine) should be considered for treating his tics; it might help with irritability and impulsiveness that underlie angry episodes. Clonidine would be given in an extended-release form to reduce adherence issues.

James's tics, his OCD symptoms, and anxiety and anger symptoms should be treated with appropriate forms of evidence-based behavior therapy. Internet-based (or smartphone-based) behavioral therapy can reinforce the benefits of conventional behavioral therapy or even substitute for it in some cases.[12-17] Using online or app-based behavior therapy would fit with James's enjoyment of online games and comfort with electronic devices.

The next step is *simplifying his drug treatment to facilitate adherence*. If James required medications just once a day at the same time, his mother could set them up each day and confirm that he takes them (or the medications could be ordered from an online pharmacy prepackaged in daily doses). For asthma he could take a once-daily inhaled steroid/long-acting beta agonist inhaler. For OCD he could take extended-release fluvoxamine once daily or take fluoxetine once a week if its efficacy for him were the same or better than that of fluvoxamine. Any new medication added should be one that is dosed once daily or less frequently.

If he made a commitment to long-term abstinence from alcohol, and daily naltrexone helped him stay sober, a monthly injection of naltrexone would be considered. If he started clonidine to help control anger outbursts and/or to reduce tics, he would begin with once-daily dosing of an extended-release preparation, and if the trial of clonidine were successful, a clonidine skin patch—changed once a week—would be an option to consider. His PCP would be promptly informed of all medication changes, and involved prospectively in decisions about his asthma medication.

An important step that closely follows the agreement about the goals of treatment is creating a panel of outcome measures that all players can use to "keep score" as changes in treatment are tried. The principle is to make measures valid, easy to use, and relevant to the patient's specific problem. Whenever possible, ratings of symptoms and signs should use questionnaires completed by the patient or by a family member rather than ones that require a clinician's direct involvement.

The panel might include the following measures, each corresponding to one of his problems.

Tourette Syndrome

The Parent Tic Questionnaire would be completed by the patient's mother once a month. This scale counts the number, frequency, and severity of various motor and vocal tics, takes 10–20 minutes to complete, does not require clinician involvement, and is highly correlated with the Yale Global Tic Severity Scale (Y-GTSS), the gold standard of clinician ratings that is the most common endpoint of clinical trials.[18,19] It is sensitive to clinically significant changes due to treatment, even when they are relatively small.[20] Additional options for efficiently rating tic severity and characterizing tic type are discussed in a review by Martino et al.[21] The patient himself would track the number of minutes he spends on weekday morning compulsions, and the number of days per month he is more than 5 minutes late to work.

Obsessive-Compulsive Disorder

Symptoms of OCD would be measured using the self-rated version of the Yale-Brown Obsessive-Compulsive Inventory (Y-BOCS).[22,23] At the outset of treatment, the patient's mother might be asked to review her son's answers to the questions and note if she thought her son was understating or overstating the severity of his symptoms. James would keep track of the number of days per month he was late to work because of compulsive behavior delaying his leaving the house to drive to work.

Asthma

Peak expiratory flow would be checked at home at least once a week, and daily during periods of higher risk for exacerbation (e.g., times of upper respiratory infection or high pollen count). This enables early detection of asthma exacerbations with a convenient and reliable home-based measure.[24] The patient would check his peak flow at the same time as he takes his once-daily inhaler.

Alcohol Use Disorder

Measurement would depend on whether James's goal was abstinence or harm reduction (avoiding driving or fighting when intoxicated). If his goal was abstinence, he would note each morning whether he had any alcohol the night before. The count of days of alcohol consumption would be another item on his monthly self-ratings, along with the self-rated version of the Y-BOCS and the Parent Tic Questionnaire. If there were reasons to doubt James's honesty about his drinking, a blood level of PEth would be checked monthly or as needed if his mother expressed a concern that he might be drinking secretly. If his goal was harm reduction, he would be asked to carry a smartphone-linked Breathalyzer on his keyring that would track his (estimated) blood alcohol level over time. Results would be recorded in his medical record monthly. He would agree to use the Breathalyzer any day on which he drank, in two situations at least: before getting into his car to drive, and after having his last drink on a single occasion. In the future, a wrist-worn transdermal alcohol sensor might be used to eliminate the need for self-reporting; at present such devices are not yet approved as consumer products.

Employment

James would be asked to share the semiannual reviews he receives from his supervisor.

Treatment sometimes can be made more effective by *enriching the team*. The *educational consultant who was helpful in the past would be reinvolved*, with the goal of increasing James's independence and social skills. The goals for James would be to make a friend, to have more leisure activity involving other people and not related to drinking, and to get more positive evaluation from his supervisor at work. James would be encouraged to join a social skills group, and with the consultant's encouragement might explore activity-based groups (e.g., bowling league, hiking club). His mother would be told about an education and support group for parents of autistic young adults

and encouraged to continue her connection with the Tourette Syndrome Association.

The neuropsychiatrist or a member of his/her team would meet once with the patient's father to better understand his relationship with his son, and his knowledge, beliefs, and expectations about his son's neuropsychiatric conditions. He would try to correct any major misconceptions and would assess the father's interest in knowing more about any of his son's problems. If the father were open to learning more, the neuropsychiatrist would make suggestions of books and online resources. These might include documents collected or created by the neuropsychiatrist and his/her team. The neuropsychiatrist would decide whether he or one of his staff should have the meeting with James's father. Depending on his personality, education, culture, social class, and prior experiences, a man might be more comfortable confiding concerns, doubts, personal details to a medical specialist or to a social worker, to a man or to a woman, to someone older or younger. The initial interviews with the patient and with his mother would inform the neuropsychiatrist's decision about who would best meet with the father.

Given the hours James already spends online every day, he would be told about online resources to help him with his neuropsychiatric issues and with his social isolation. This might include websites and social media pages for people with each of his conditions (with an example of each): ASD (www.autism-speaks.org; www.autism-society.org), TS (https://.tourette.org; www.ts-stories.org), OCD (www.beyondocd.org; https://iocdf.org), AUD (www.cdc.org); alcohol (www.healthline.com/health/best-alcoholism-blogs-of-the-year#1), and asthma (www.aafa.org/aafa-affiliated-asthma-allergy-support-groups/). The neuropsychiatrist and his/her team would recommend online resources with which they were personally familiar, and that had been checked for quality of information by them or by trusted colleagues. Each online resource would be one that neuropsychiatrist, his/her team members, and/or trusted colleagues had checked for the quality of their information.

ENHANCING SUSTAINABILITY

If the patient (or responsible family member, if the patient is too impaired to decide) commits to continue in treatment with the neuropsychiatrist, goals have been agreed upon, measures selected, and initial treatment initiated, the neuropsychiatrist can raise the issue of *sustainability*. He/she can explain to the patient and/or family that while implementing and maintaining an effective *long-term* plan of care and treatment surely will require ongoing time and effort, and occasional inconvenience, people involved in the patient's care should not be expected to be masochistically self-sacrificing or to put their own physical and mental health at risk from overwork. Demands on the patient for treatment adherence should not be unrealistic, either.

Burnout—whether of a family member, a paid caregiver, or a clinical professional, increases the risk of errors, emergencies, disruptions in care, and missed opportunities for improvement. One way to decrease burnout is to enlarge the group of people who are informed, concerned, engaged with helping the patient, and aligned with the treatment goals and plan. If family members or friends of the patient want to help but do not have the necessary knowledge or skills, the latter often can be developed. Organizations for family and friends of people with specific neuropsychiatric disorders offer online and in-person education. In the case of James, the Tourette Syndrome Association (www.tourette.org), the International OCD Foundation (www.iocdf.org), the Asperger/Autism Network (www.aane.org), or Autism Speaks (www.autismspeaks.org) all could be potential sources of education and support for the patient's parents.

A neuropsychiatrist should build an informal network of the various nonmedical professionals not already part of his/her practice or clinic, whose services his/her patients are likely to need. Patients in a neuropsychiatrist's practice will at various times require physical, occupational, and/or speech therapy; social work; financial planning; legal assistance; educational consultation or vocational rehabilitation. Developing resources in these areas is a process based on reciprocity and relationship-building. The neuropsychiatrist should identify professionals in the community and/or the health care system where he/she practices who are either already "neuro-aware" or open to learning more about the special issues of neuropsychiatric patients. He/she should let these professionals know about his/her special interests and expertise, and learn about theirs, offering to assist them with complex or difficult neuropsychiatric cases they encounter. Working with a professional of a different discipline on a common case—for example, working with a lawyer dealing with a mental competency issue in a person with a severe traumatic brain injury—helps the neuropsychiatrist understand the other professional's strengths and limitations, increases the knowledge and awareness of the other professional of neuropsychiatric issues, and builds a trusting connection.

Over time, a neuropsychiatrist can build a virtual multidisciplinary team that covers the range of issues likely to arise with patients in his/her practice. For example, a neuropsychiatrist might develop a professional relationship with a local estates-and-trusts lawyer who is knowledgeable about dementia-related issues and has empathy for patients with dementia and their families. The neuropsychiatrist would be a resource for that lawyer when legal situations required assessments of clients' decision-making capacities, or when there was a need for a retrospective review of a deceased person's medical records to form an expert opinion of testamentary capacity at the time a will was changed. The lawyer would be a resource for the neuropsychiatrist's patients with mild cognitive impairment. Neuropsychiatrists often encourage patients with newly diagnosed mild cognitive impairment to make sure their legal documents (e.g., will, durable power of attorney) are up-to-date at a time when there is no question about their competence or their judgment.

TAKING EXTRA TIME AND GETTING PAID FOR IT

Continually providing large amounts of uncompensated and/or unrecognized care is a recipe for professional burnout. Whether the neuropsychiatrist works on a fee-for-service basis or is salaried by a hospital or clinic, he/she should schedule complex patients for visits that include adequate "counseling

time" and should make liberal use of time-based Evaluation and Management (E&M) codes to document the time that was necessarily spent to deal with clinical complexity. Medicare guidelines for coding and documenting E&M visits specifically point out multiple comorbidities as a reason for using a higher code. Review of outcome measures with the patient and/or family, explanation of any abnormal test results and their implications, decisions about any modification of treatment, and introduction of new elements of the care plan all require additional time. These activities add to the time needed for taking an interim history, reviewing other providers' notes, checking interim laboratory data, physiologic data, psychological testing results and/or diagnostic images, and performing a neurological and mental status examination. Documentation of a personal assessment by the neuropsychiatrist of brain images, an EEG, and/or primary data from neuropsychological tests performed by another clinician would be supporting evidence of complexity of medical decision making to back up the use of a higher E&M code. Patient education and other dialogue can take longer than usual if a patient has impaired cognition or communication; when this rather than the complexity of content is a major reason for a longer-than-usual office visit, it should be noted in the medical record.

Medicare and many private health insurance plans pay for chronic care management (CCM) services that include making and updating strategic plans, communicating about plans to diverse players, and tracking interim data on symptoms and physiological data. Ongoing CCM services usually are delivered by nonphysician staff working under the physician's supervision. Remote patient monitoring using data captured by Bluetooth-connected blood pressure cuffs, scales, oximeters, spirometers, and wearable sleep and activity trackers is covered by another set of procedure codes that many (but not all) payers cover. Utilizing remote patient monitoring entails an obligation for the physician to respond to new data suggesting worsening of a patient's chronic condition. Some monitoring devices have built-in alerts. Often, a nonphysician team member is responsible for notifying the physician if there are significant changes in a patient's monitored data. Much of the documentation of remote patient monitoring is automated, and the remainder can be done most efficiently with the aid of templates in the electronic medical record (EMR). The physician should set appropriate expectations with patients regarding what monitoring can contribute to their treatment, the need to contact the physician or his/her coverage directly for new symptoms, and how long it might take the physician or his/her associates to respond to a change in status detected by monitoring. Because CCM services and remote monitoring are primarily done by nonphysician team members under the neuropsychiatrist's supervision, they can generate new revenue to offset losses from activities for which the neuropsychiatrist is not paid.

Complex neuropsychiatric patients often need clinical services between scheduled appointments. Additional appointments with nonphysician team members can fill some gaps, but they may be impractical (e.g., if the patient lives far away) or simply not substitutable, as when the purpose is adjustment of a complex medication regimen or adjustment of a medical device. Remote service can be delivered by telephone, secure text, or email with photographs or video clips attached, or by secure videoconferencing. The patient should receive the level of service necessary to optimally address the problem, and the time for the encounter should be on the neuropsychiatrist's schedule. In areas underserved by medical specialists, particularly rural areas, both public and private insurers usually pay for telemedicine visits. In metropolitan areas policies are more variable, but the trend is toward payment for telemedicine because it prevents more expensive urgent care and ED visits, and can prevent some hospitalizations.

Remote services, however delivered, should be tracked, documented, and billed even when they are not covered by insurance. In some contexts, patients or families can reasonably be asked to pay for uncovered services. In institutional contexts like clinics, hospital outpatient departments or group practices, tracking of uncompensated services can help in negotiating expectations for patient volume or clinician "productivity." When telephone calls with patients and responding to patients' emails and texts are unscheduled, unpaid, and unrecognized these activities will contribute to burnout, and undocumented communications with patients complicate care transitions and sometimes create professional liability risk.

A neuropsychiatrist should have time specifically allocated each day for telephone, email, text, or video interactions with patients he/she follows long term. Expectations can then be set with patients and families as to when text or email messages will be answered, when phone calls will be returned, and when a telemedicine visit might be scheduled. Physicians can always make good use of unexpected free time, while frequent interruptions and unscheduled overtime work are hard to sustain in the long term.

When negotiating with hospital or departmental management, or with payers, the point can be made that additional scheduled time for follow-up of complex patients—whether to educate patients and family more thoroughly when they are in the office, or to have more frequent remote check-ins between scheduled visits—can prevent hospitalizations and ED visits, and ultimately reduce the overall cost of care. Published studies like the ones cited above showing financial and clinical benefit from active care management have focused on patients with chronic diseases overall, or those with specific chronic diseases and comorbid depression. For specific neuropsychiatric populations like those with psychiatrically complicated epilepsy, stroke, TBI, neurodegenerative diseases, or neurodevelopmental disorders, the economic and clinical value of physician-directed care management can be demonstrated within a specific hospital, clinic, or health system by identifying a cohort of patients with high hospitalization rates and/or ED usage rates over the past year, and tracking their outcomes in the first year of active management of their complexity.

The neuropsychiatrist working in a specific organizational environment must "play the long game." It might be necessary to set up a special half-day clinic for complex high-risk patients in which longer visit durations and remote follow-ups are built in and contrast the ongoing outcomes of the patients in the special clinic with similar patients receiving treatment as usual. Neuropsychiatrists may feel it unfair that they must work hard to prove the seemingly obvious proposition that

more comprehensive, more frequent, and more attentive care to complex patients can prevent emergencies and yield better clinical outcomes without necessarily adding to the total cost of care. However, people unfamiliar with the specialty often don't appreciate at the outset that almost all neuropsychiatric care involves complexity and comorbidity, and that many neuropsychiatric disorders are associated with functional impairments that directly interfere with communication, organization, treatment adherence, and/or accurate perception and recall of events and symptoms. Brain dysfunctions of this kind affect the care of the patient's other psychiatric or general medical conditions—of which there usually are several. (In the case example, the patient had three psychiatric diagnoses [ASD, OCD, and AUD] plus a general medical condition [asthma].)

Someone on the neuropsychiatrist's team should keep current on Medicare and Medicaid regulations and typical private health plan guidelines concerning coding for E&M visits, telemedicine, chronic condition management, and remote monitoring. Getting reimbursement from payers for the unusually complex and/or frequent services needed by many neuropsychiatric patients requires meticulous attention to coding and documentation. Documentation templates and workflows that maximize nonphysician participation in documentation can be developed for the clinical scenarios the neuropsychiatrist most often encounters.

RELATIONS WITH OTHER MEDICAL SPECIALTIES

A neuropsychiatrist, either alone or with the aid of a team, is likely to see a complex patient more frequently than any of the specialists caring for the patient's other clinical problems. In the case example, the patient might be seen by his PCP once a year on a scheduled basis and as needed for acute illness, and he might have seen a pulmonologist once or twice a year, if at all—in a study of children and teenagers with asthma in New York City, only 19% were seen by a pulmonologist or allergist over a 5-year period.[25] Patients with diabetes, heart failure, epilepsy, and other chronic medical conditions often are managed by a primary care physician after initial consultation with a specialist on the diagnosis and recommended treatment; a patient will return to the specialist for a second consultation only if his/her symptoms worsen or there a new clinical issue develops. If a neuropsychiatrist recognizes during an in-person or remote encounter that the treatment of one of the patient's chronic medical conditions might require adjustment but there is no urgency, he/she should alert the colleague primarily managing that condition.

Depending on the scope of the neuropsychiatrist's knowledge and skill in general internal medicine, he/she might seek a "license" from a patient's PCP to make simple adjustments in a patient's treatment and notify the PCP after the fact. This option is attractive when a patient has a general medical condition that affects mental status or the symptoms or functional impact of a neurological disorder. If a patient under treatment for diabetes has had recent hypoglycemic episodes affecting his/her mental status, it would be appropriate for the neuropsychiatrist to suggest an immediate reduction in the dose of insulin or other antidiabetic drug, notify the PCP, and have a nonphysician team member (or engaged family member) help arrange and promote the patient's prompt follow-up with the PCP. If a patient with a history of small vessel strokes and associated mental status changes, on treatment for high blood pressure, had an unacceptably high BP in the neuropsychiatrist's office, the neuropsychiatrist might change the antihypertensive dose immediately, notify the PCP of the change, and have a team member or engaged family member assist the patient in regular monitoring of his/her BP at home between the neuropsychiatry appointment and the next PCP visit.

SPECIALIZING FOR SUSTAINABILITY

When the circumstances of his/her practice permit, a neuropsychiatrist should choose a limited set of related conditions for his/her work as a CEO of patient care. He/she might specialize in the comprehensive care of patients with Parkinson's disease, multiple sclerosis, epilepsy, autism/Asperger's syndrome, or late effects of TBI. He/she might see patients in consultation with many other neuropsychiatric conditions, but for those patients the goal would be to do a definitive diagnostic assessment, answer the specific questions of a consultee, and, if requested by the consultee or by the patient, recommend a treatment strategy that would be implemented by another physician or clinic. Primary care clinics with collaborative care or an integrated medical/behavioral health care model, comprehensive geriatric care programs, and clinics for children and adolescents with neurodevelopmental disorders are examples of providers that could assume ongoing responsibility for comprehensive care after a neuropsychiatrist confirmed diagnoses and suggested a long-term treatment strategy.

When the neuropsychiatrist plans to regularly assume the CEO role in managing complex cases of a specific category, he/she should develop and maintain especially broad and deep knowledge of conditions in that category. The ideal scope of knowledge for this "subsubspecialty" practice is described in Table 35-2; the listed items are specifically those related to the conditions on which the neuropsychiatrist focuses his/her CEO activities.

This specialized knowledge enables the neuropsychiatrist to fully address the concerns of the players in a case. It enhances efficiency, because the neuropsychiatrist immediately knows what additional services will be needed, who can provide them, and how to request them. It facilitates effective risk management and thus increases the likelihood that the costs of subspecialty care will be more than offset by crises and complications avoided. Familiarity with illness narratives facilitates the neuropsychiatrist's empathy—which can translate into greater trust, relief of patients' and families' anxiety, and more engagement of the patient and family in treatment. This translates into better communication, more accurate measurement and tracking of outcomes, earlier response to clinical problems, and better adherence to treatment.

TABLE 35-2 • Ideal Scope of Knowledge for "CEO" Neuropsychiatric Practice.
Local and regional epidemiology
Typical illness narratives, including variations related to local cultures and subcultures
Issues of stigma and common misconceptions
Usual comorbidities; how and by whom they are managed locally
Usual reasons for emergency care
Most common serious adverse outcomes, their causes, and preventive actions
Local supportive resources
Policies of payers, government agencies, and hospitals
Condition-specific coding and billing
Legal and risk management issues for the physician (e.g., mandatory reporting of driving impairment)
Legal and risk management issues for the patient and family (e.g., wills, trusts, advance directives)
Educational and occupational issues
Entitlements to services, supports, accommodations, disability payments, etc.
Clinically important lifestyle and environmental issues
Complementary, alternative, and integrative medicine interventions
Websites, organizations, and educational materials/programs offering valid information
Advocacy groups and philanthropies involved with the condition
Useful mobile device apps, wearable devices, and home-based technology
Clinical trials of new treatments for the conditions

THE GOALS OF TREATMENT

Comprehensive and holistic treatment of neuropsychiatric patients is distinguished by its goals—which are not limited to treating disease and managing symptoms. Broader and more humanistic goals for care facilitate greater engagement by patients, families, and other players—because everyone can relate to them even when the patient's disease is rare, hard to understand, and maybe even difficult to pronounce.

The goals for all patients include optimizing survival, function, and quality of life, and minimizing disability, pain, and suffering. For older patients, they include healthy adaptation to aging, delaying the onset of age-related impairments, and minimizing the impact of such impairments on quality of life. For children, adolescents, and young adult patients, they include promoting healthy physical, cognitive, and social development, education appropriate to the person's abilities and interests, and establishment in work or other meaningful activity. For all patients, comprehensive and holistic treatment aims to prevent illness and injury except when the assumption of risk is necessary for the attainment of a major life goal, and the patient knowingly and competently assumes the risk. Often, increasing safety and preventing future illnesses and injuries is a relatable next step for patients and families to take as they move beyond care that is narrowly focused on treating diseases and their symptoms.

Attaining the broad, ultimate goals of neuropsychiatric care requires a sustained effort by the patient, other players on the patient's side, and the clinical team; and sustained support for the process by the relevant health care system(s) and payer(s). Sustained effort by the patient's significant others requires optimizing their satisfaction, minimizing unnecessary or excessive burdens on individuals, and preventing and/or treating stress-related illness related to caregiving. Sustained effort by the clinical team requires preservation of their health, morale, and interest in their work. As previously discussed, financial sustainability of comprehensive and holistic care within a specific system may depend on showing that it enhances cost-effectiveness relative to treatment as usual.

A barrier to recognition of cost-effectiveness is when inpatient and outpatient care are separately managed, with discrete and unlinked budgets. To take a common example, hospitals and their inpatient staff may be rewarded for reducing rates of rehospitalization following episodes of acute care. If rehospitalization is prevented by increased effort and expense by an associated outpatient clinic, will the outpatient team share in the incentives or receive additional resources? It is well-established that integration of psychiatric and general medical care ("physical and behavioral health") can reduce overall costs of care and improve clinical outcomes, but under traditional fee-for-service payment, the practitioners involved in integrated care might be paid less for their time than they would delivering more limited and less coordinated services.[26] Medicare and other payers offer less money per hour of service for prolonged E&M visits and for psychotherapeutic services in contrast to briefer E&M visits and psychiatrist visits for medication management only. Table 35-3 shows 2019 national Medicare rates for E&M visits and for psychotherapy visits for established patients including a calculation of payment per hour.

Note that if visits are based on time, there is much better payment for evaluation and management—including patient and family counseling—than there is for psychotherapy alone. If psychotherapy is provided at the same visit as an E&M service, the services can be billed separately, and this can effectively raise the payment for psychotherapy. Taking overhead into account it would not be sustainable in most practices for a neuropsychiatrist to bill as a psychotherapist at appointments that were not also E&M visits. Typically, a nonphysician team member would provide psychotherapy sessions if frequent and numerous sessions were needed to implement the plan of care.

E&M codes can be based on time, if counseling, care coordination, patient education, and similar activities constitute more than half of the time spent with the patient. Otherwise they are based on the level of comprehensiveness of the history and examination, the level of risk, and the level of complexity of decision making. Well-designed documentation templates and team-based workflow enable the necessary support of level 4 and level 5 procedure codes to be recorded without excessive demand on the physician's time.

The key to establishing the applicability of a high-level E&M code without exhaustive documentation is providing support for complexity of decision making—a construct that combines problem complexity, data complexity, and risk level.[27] Obtaining the highest complexity code requires either high history complexity or high data complexity, or one of the two combined with high-risk decision making.

According to CMS criteria, all complex neuropsychiatric patients would involve at least moderate risk decision making, because they would have at least two chronic illnesses, and would be receiving prescription drug management. If they had acute neurologic symptoms or signs or major new psychiatric concerns (e.g., suicidal ideation) the risk level would be high. Medical decision making would virtually always be high complexity. CMS has a Medical Decision-Making point score system that gives points for problem complexity and points for data complexity; high complexity is a score of 4 or greater. When problem complexity is scored, there is one point for each established problem that is stable or improving, two points for each established problem that is worsening, and three points for any new problem. For data complexity one point is given for ordering *or* reviewing each of the following: clinical lab tests, imaging tests, and other tests (e.g., EEG, PFTs, EKG). An additional point is given for discussing a test result with the clinician who performed it (e.g., neuroradiologist, clinical neurophysiologist or neuropsychologist). Two points are given for personally reviewing diagnostic images or physiological data and two points for reviewing and summarizing old records.[28] Electronic record templates corresponding to the Medical Decision-Making scoring rules can reduce the time needed to document E&M visit complexity.

TABLE 35-3 • 2019 Medicare Rates for Outpatient E&M and Psychotherapy Services.				
HCPCS Code	Service	Typical Time in Minutes	Fee	Fee Per Hour
99212	E&M limited	10	$45.77	$274.62
99213	E&M low complexity	15	$75.32	$301.28
99214	E&M medium complexity	25	$110.28	$264.67
99215	E&M high complexity	40	$147.76	$221.64
90833	30 minutes psychotherapy with E&M billed on same day	30	$71.00	$142.00
90836	45 minutes psychotherapy with E&M billed on same day	45	$89.74	$119.65
90838	60 minutes psychotherapy with E&M billed on same day	60	$118.57	$118.57

Neuropsychiatrists and members of their teams might ask clinic and hospital administrators, and EMR technical support staff, for assistance in structuring and automating documentation, coding, and billing to obtain the fairest possible payment for providing comprehensive service to patients with neurological-psychiatric comorbidity. Well-designed and consistently implemented documentation and service coding strategies can financially sustain high-quality neuropsychiatric care better than pressuring physicians for ever-greater "productivity"—defined as seeing more patients for shorter visits.

Electronic medical record systems can at worst interfere with the implementation of a comprehensive and holistic care plan. Widely utilized EMR products by two vendors—Epic and Cerner—appear to give priority to documentation for billing compliance, risk management, calculation of standard quality measures, and implementation of evidence-based practice guidelines. Neither provides a convenient platform for individualized, comprehensive, consistent, and efficient care for complex, high-comorbidity patients. However, both systems allow for specialty-specific customization, for example, of templates for documenting specialty-specific E&M activities. Development and implementation of standard EMR enhancements for documenting strategy and management of common neuropsychiatric disorders is a near-term opportunity for making comprehensive and holistic care more efficient and sustainable. EMR modifications, and workflow changes to involve nonphysician team members more in documentation, can reduce physicians' paperwork and improve their morale. A report on EMR workflow modification by the Reliant Medical Group in Massachusetts describes who should do documentation, in order of preference: (1) the computer itself via keyboard macros; (2) the patient (or other patient-side players) using a patient portal or scannable forms; (3) a nurse or other nonphysician team member; and (4) the physician by speech recognition.[29]

A division of neuropsychiatry or behavioral neurology can develop subspecialty-specific templates and forms for the EMR that enable treatment goals and strategy to be recorded in a standard location. It can provide a dashboard framework and widgets for specific neuropsychiatric measures in the electronic record, so that the neuropsychiatrist can easily configure a patient-specific dashboard from easily accessed components. Standardized text can be written to introduce neuropsychiatric strategic plans and outcome dashboards to clinicians of other disciplines. Strategic plans can be stored with one-click access to them from the electronic record.

PATIENT AND FAMILY ENGAGEMENT

Engagement of patients—defined as having the interest, confidence, knowledge, and ability to take an active role in maintaining their health and managing their own health care—and similar engagement of family caregivers when a patient is unable to manage his/her own care is measurable with a well-validated instrument, the Patient Activation Measure (PAM).[30] The PAM is a scale with 10 items relating to patients' knowledge, attitudes, and confidence, each rated by the patient as strongly agree,

agree, disagree, or strongly disagree. Three exemplary items are: "Taking an active role in my own health care is the most important thing that affects my health"; "I know what each of my prescribed medications do"; and "I am confident that I can tell a doctor concerns I have even when he or she does not ask." A highly activated patient would know what each of his/her medications did, would be confident he/she could tell a doctor about concerns and even if not asked about them, and would be confident he/she could maintain healthy lifestyle changes even under stress. In populations of patients with chronic diseases, higher scores on the PAM are associated with significantly lower rates of hospitalization and ED use. When patients' care is managed by a family member, a caregiver-rated version of the scale has shown similar associations with outcomes. Highly engaged individuals will seek a physician's help; they may need education on the specific issues of the patient's case. Low-engagement players may need outreach, clinician-initiated contacts, and coaching or motivational interviewing to increase their level of engagement. If that doesn't work a trained professional or volunteer patient advocate can substitute for a patient or family caregiver.

Formal measurement of activation rarely is needed for neuropsychiatrists working with complex patients, as the patients' histories will reveal how engaged various players have been. However, in planning for the care of a *population* of neuropsychiatric patients (e.g., all patients in an epilepsy clinic or multiple sclerosis clinic with neuropsychiatric issues), screening patients and families with the PAM can aid in targeting outreach by clinic staff to improve population-level outcomes.

Motivational interviewing and groups for support and education are two ways to build engagement.[31,32] Distress over a specific event like an emergency hospitalization sometimes can be translated into increased engagement in the patient's care, and willingness to learn how to be more proactive in protecting the patient and mitigating risk. Similarly, distress over legal, financial, or relationship problems sometimes can drive increased engagement by the patient, his/her family and friends, or both.

CREATING A STRATEGIC PLAN FOR HOLISTIC AND SUSTAINABLE NEUROPSYCHIATRIC CARE

As discussed earlier in this chapter, an early step in the creation of a plan is identifying the players on the patient side and the clinician side, and the role, goals, and capabilities of each. Table 35-4 presents a list of questions that might be asked (or considered) by the neuropsychiatrist to establish the context for his/her work with a patient. With their answers in mind, he/she should decide at the first encounter what role and goals would best fit players' expectations, the patient's need, and the neuropsychiatrist's capabilities and limitations.

In the author's opinion, it usually is better to have a patient or family member or other advocate be the patient-side care coordinator rather than a professional case manager. Patients and those who care about them have much more time and energy for the job and usually have fewer distractions and competing priorities. And, a motivated and intelligent advocate can reasonably be expected to acquire substantial knowledge about the course, treatment, and complications of a handful of conditions even if he/she has no education in any clinical discipline. When considering who should be the patient-side care coordinator, the clinical CEO or strategist should consider the location, health, availability, intelligence, technological competence, motivation, communication skills and financial means

TABLE 35-4 • Context-Building Questions for the Neuropsychiatrist.
Can the players be grouped into teams, each with coordinated efforts?
For each group of players, whose opinion counts the most with the patient and family?
Who would be on the front line if the patient had an emergency? This might depend on the type of emergency.
What do different players expect from other players with respect to the patient's care?
What is the level of engagement, health-related knowledge, and executive function of the patient and of involved family or friends?
What are the relevant environmental and financial constraints on treatment?
Are there potential community resources not yet tapped?
What is the role of the neuropsychiatrist—CEO? Team leader? Strategic consultant? Provider of a diagnostic second opinion?
Do different players have the same understanding of the neuropsychiatrist's role?
Do different players have the same expectations regarding treatment, its goals, and its likely outcomes?
If there has been a recent, potentially preventable adverse event, ED visit, or hospitalization, what do various players think went wrong and how do they think it could have been prevented?
How does the patient (or other decision maker) weigh the avoidance or risk with preserving autonomy, continuing a specific activity, or pursuing a life goal?
Is a change in the setting of care under consideration?
Are additional therapies needed?
Should other clinical or nonclinical disciplines be involved?
What are the optimal channels for routine communication and for urgent communication?
If a medication needs to be changed, who will make the decision? Should more than one physician be involved?
Is a one-time group dialogue needed to get the principal players aligned with respect to goals, expectations, and processes? Could it be fit into an existing structure for team meetings or clinical rounds?
Who should be on a secure, patient-specific email distribution list?
Who should be the patient-side care coordinator? If there is someone with the engagement and executive function to do the job, what additional condition-specific or treatment-specific knowledge does he/she need to have to do it well?

of a potential choice. The person closest to the patient emotionally is not necessarily the best patient-side coordinator.

If the neuropsychiatrist is a treatment strategist or a CEO, he/she has the job of defining the goals of treatment. This task is best done in a collaborative manner with players from both the patient side and the clinical side. The patient must ultimately accept the goals of treatment, as must family members and other players who will be regularly involved in the patient's care. However, they might not fully understand or agree with all goals at the outset. Agreement on *initial* goals is essential, as it is part of the process of informed consent to initial treatments. Whether in the strategic consultant or leadership role, the neuropsychiatrist selects the initial panel of outcome measures and proposes a plan for frequency of measurement, who will complete the measures, and how they will be communicated to the neuropsychiatrist (or other designated team member).

A Clinical Time Budget Should Be Prepared

In addition to accounting for the professional time spent by clinicians of different disciplines, the strategist should estimate how frequently the team leader will need updates on the patient's status, how frequently a team member will need to have a scheduled in-person or remote visit with the patient, and how frequently there should be email, text, or other asynchronous communication with the patient. A specific team member should be identified as the person related to each line item in the time budget.

Legal and Financial Issues Should Be Identified

If the patient is a minor or has impaired decision-making capacity, there should be a person identified with legal authority to consent to medical procedures and to spend money on the patient's behalf. In cases of diminished capacity it is important to balance concerns of patient autonomy and best interests. If decision-making authority is not well-defined, one-time legal assistance might be needed to develop and document a structure for proxy decision making.

It should be clarified who is responsible for expenses related to the patient's care, what resources are available, and what limits apply. For people with severe disabilities or in need of supervision because of cognitive impairment or abnormal behavior, much of the care needed may not be covered by typical commercial health insurance, and its coverage by Medicaid and other public programs varies greatly among states. It is important to know the exact scope and limits of the insurance coverage the patient does have, and if the patient is uninsured, whether there is someone willing and able to pay the patient's medical bills. Regrettably, some systems of care for people with low income and/or poor insurance coverage pay for ED visits and hospitalizations but not the services needed to prevent those high-cost events.

Neuropsychiatrists and their team members can work by joining with patient advocacy groups, or by advising public officials, to address financial disincentives for providing comprehensive and holistic care that includes secondary prevention.

While advocacy takes time, it can protect clinicians against burnout by combatting the cynical detachment associated with passive acceptance of bad policy. As with many other of the suggestions in this chapter, advocacy is most feasible when it focuses on a specific clinical population and a policy issue—for example, lack of adequate state Medicaid coverage for a specific mental health or care management service, violations of mental health coverage parity laws, or unavailability of special education for ASD patients who do not meet criteria for mental retardation.

The "control panel" or "dashboard" of goals and outcome measures can either be a paper document, an electronic document that can be incorporated into an EMR, or a web page with discrete windows or widgets. There is a zone on the control panel for each specific problem (symptom, functional impairment, disease) or therapeutic objective. It contains one or more relevant measures of outcome (symptoms, function, laboratory tests, physiological data), information about when the measures were updated, what treatments are being given, and contact information for the people involved with that goal or outcome. The control panel approach is most feasible with EMR integration. Neuropsychiatrists working with a hospital, clinic, or large group practice will need administrative support for configuring specialty-specific tools within the EMR. Clinicians in small group or solo practice might seek technical support on record configuration from their EMR vendor. Initial dashboard design can be done using a standard office productivity application like Microsoft Excel.

The CEO or COO, with input from the patient, the PCP, and other players, should list the most likely serious, urgent, or emergent problems that might arise given the patient's overall diseases, conditions, impairments, living arrangements, and medical history. For these, the strategic plan would suggest how the problems might be prevented (or their risk reduced), how each problem might be identified quickly (using technology if helpful), and the planned response to early identification.

Once the targets of emergency prevention are selected, details of the response plans for potential emergencies often can be worked out and documented by a social worker or nurse rather than the neuropsychiatrist. However, both the neuropsychiatrist and the patient and/or patient's advocate must all agree on them. The process of explicit planning and consensus building can take time, but with complex neuropsychiatric patients the cost of that time usually is less than the cost of the hospitalizations and ED visits that are prevented, and the per-dollar improvement in patient's health-related quality of life can be greater than it is for many pharmacological treatments.

CHOICE OF OUTCOME MEASURES

When choosing a rating scale as an outcome measure, the neuropsychiatrist should consider the patient's primary diagnosis, the setting of care, the patient's baseline (to avoid floor and ceiling effects in measurement), and who would be most able to rate the item (e.g., symptom, syndrome, functional

capacity) most accurately and reliably. Potential measures are of five types.

- *Mental status rating scales* for cognition, mood, behavior, etc. Each scale should be selected so that the patient's score at baseline lies in the middle of the scale, permitting the detection of improvement and of decline. Self-rating questionnaires are acceptable only for those items of which the patient has adequate and accurate self-awareness. For cognition, tests should be used that are suitable for repeated measures rather than ones with answers that can be memorized over repeated administrations. The Stroop Test of response to conflicting stimuli, administered electronically via a smartphone or tablet, is an example of such a test. If the patient has comprehensive neuropsychological testing, the neuropsychologist can be asked for a suggestion of a suitable repeatable measure that focuses on areas where the patient has mid-range impairment at baseline.

- For depression or anxiety secondary to a primary neurological or general medical condition, it may be preferable to use a rating scale specifically adapted and validated for the patient's primary diagnoses. Two exemplary scales are the NDDI-E for depression in patients with epilepsy[33] and the Cornell Scale for Depression in Dementia.[34] Similarly, a psychometric analysis in patients with Parkinson's disease of three generic rating scales for anxiety showed that none met optimal criteria for reliability and validity,[35] and that a scale specific to PD—the Parkinson Anxiety Scale—performed better.[36]

- *Functional assessments* include assessments of basic activities of daily living (ADLs),[37] instrumental activities of daily living (IADLs),[38] and financial capacity (Financial Capacity Instrument).[39] Formal functional assessments can be combined with informal assessments of performance in daily life. For example, when the financial capacity of a patient with MCI or early dementia is a concern, the patient's checking account and credit card statements, and his/her checkbook, can be examined for errors and evidence of impaired judgment. Demonstration of problems in daily life can be more convincing to patients with impaired insight and families in denial than the results of neuropsychological tests indirectly related to the function at issue.

    Functional assessments can be based on patient self-report, informant report, or clinician observation. Differences between the self-reported function and clinician or informant assessments can reveal anosognosia or impaired metacognition (when patients' self-reports are unrealistically positive) or depressive, catastrophic thinking (when patients' self-reports are extremely negative relative to observed performance). Differences between clinicians' findings and reports of family informants can similarly reveal family members' tendencies to exaggerate or minimize illness-related impairments.

Informant-based questionnaires are an especially efficient way to profile the impairments of early-stage dementia and other neurocognitive disorders of mild-to-moderate severity. They can cover a broad range of functions, identifying deficits that can if needed be better characterized by specific testing. An exemplary instrument is the Activities of Daily Living

Questionnaire (ADLQ) developed by the Behavioral Neurology group at Northwestern.[40] Informants rate patients' performance on each function on a four-point scale ranging from intact performance (3) to complete incapacity (0). The questionnaire adapts to differences in culture, gender, and family norms by excluding from the summary score all items that were not part of the patient's life before becoming ill. The final score is the summary score as a percentage of the maximum possible score of 3 times the number of included items. Thus, if a man never cooked or did laundry, or if a woman never did household repairs or managed family finances, he/she would not be scored on those functions. Domains assessed are self-care activities (eating, dressing, bathing, elimination, taking medication, interest in personal appearance); household care (preparing meals, cooking, setting the table, housekeeping, home maintenance, home repairs, laundry); employment and recreation (employment, recreation, organizations, travel); shopping and money (food shopping, handling cash, managing finances); travel (public transportation, driving, mobility around the neighborhood, travel outside familiar environment); and communication (using the telephone, talking, understanding, reading, writing).

■ *Disease-specific rating scales,* such as those used for rating movement disorders: the UPDRS[41] for Parkinson's disease, the AIMS for tardive dyskinesia,[42] and the Y-GTSS for Tourette syndrome.[18]
■ *Disease-specific physiological or biochemical data,* provided by a laboratory, measured at the point of care (PoC), or tested at home. Home-based measures are ideal as they can be followed frequently without the inconvenience and expense of visiting a clinical laboratory. Examples include the measurement of oxygen saturation and peak flow for people with COPD or asthma, and measurement of blood glucose with a home glucometer.
■ *The patient's pattern of activity and sleep, measured with a wearable device.* The capabilities of wearable devices and PoC testing are rapidly improving and their prices are decreasing. Physiological and biochemical measures obtained at home or in an outpatient clinician's office will increasingly be used in control panels and early-detection strategies for risk mitigation and treatment monitoring.

DRIVING CARE WITH A DASHBOARD

A patient-specific multiproblem dashboard helps the CEO of care, or a team leader responsible for a subset of the patient's problems. determine whether the total effect of a treatment on function and health-related quality of life is positive and identify when the benefit for one condition is offset by worsening of another. For example, a specific antipsychotic might give improved mood stability in a patient with bipolar disorder, but at the cost of weight gain and a metabolic syndrome that could transition to Type II diabetes. If the neuropsychiatrist systematically reviews such issues, he/she might decide to switch antipsychotic drugs to one with lesser metabolic side effects, try to manage the bipolar disorder without an antipsychotic drug, or

treat the weight gain and metabolic problem by prescribing metformin and referring the patient to a group for help in modifying diet and exercise habits. Recognizing the issue is facilitated by having body weight, HbA1c, and rating scales for hypomanic and depressive symptoms displayed on the dashboard.

To fully implement the approach described here, the neuropsychiatrist (or other care strategist) should be familiar with several groups of measures, their applicability to the clinical populations he/she sees, their time and effort requirements, and their basic psychometric properties. Clinicians working with special populations defined by diagnosis, demographics, primary language and English proficiency, and/or specific cultural features may need to use alternatives to standard rating scales.

For rating symptoms, it often is adequate to use a simple 1–10 numerical scale or a visual analogue scale. One useful variation on the approach outlined is to have the patient rate *usual* symptom intensity and *worst* symptom intensity over a given time period like a day or a week. When the symptom is one like a tic or tinnitus that is noticeable but not necessarily distressing, three numerical or visual analogue ratings can be done, one for severity, one for associated distress/tolerability, and one for associated functional impairment. This is the approach taken by the well-known Abnormal Involuntary Movement Scale used to measure tardive dyskinesia in patients treated with dopamine antagonists.[42] Items 1–7 of the 10-item scale rate the severity of specific involuntary movements on a scale of 0–3; items 8–10 similarly rate the impact of the movement disorder overall on severity, distress, and impairment.

MOBILE DEVICES AND "CONNECTED HEALTH"

Wearable devices and smartphone or smartwatch apps that measure physiologic parameters can be used to monitor and/or promote adherence to a plan of treatment or behavior change, to assess the effect of a therapy, or to provide early warning of an acute event to enable risk mitigation. For example, sensors and mobile devices have been used clinically in Parkinson's disease to confirm diagnoses, detect dyskinesia and on-off phenomena, and aid in optimizing medication choice and dosage.[43-45] In patients with epilepsy, wearable devices can detect nonconvulsive as well as convulsive seizures and simultaneously monitor sympathetic activity and sleep, so that seizures can be related to sleep patterns and/or to stress. This can inform a treatment strategy that includes not only antiepileptic drugs but also to therapies involving sleep modification and biofeedback. They can warn parents of an impending seizure in a child with uncontrolled generalized epilepsy, helping them take action to reduce the risk of sudden death.[46-50] Systems that combine physiological measurements with electronic patient reported outcomes (ePROs) hold the promise of closer follow-up and more patient-centered care will require fewer face-to-face physician visits once a treatment strategy is created and implemented. Systems for managing specific diseases with ePROs and remote monitoring incorporate algorithms to detect clinically relevant signals and direct alerts initially to physicians or to nonphysician team members, depending on their nature and urgency.[51]

Other mobile devices are used to enhance safety for people with cognitive impairment. These include wireless emergency call systems, geographical locators, and home video monitoring for cognitively impaired people living alone. There has been rapid progress in the area of active driver assistance systems (ADAS)—electronics for automobiles that help drivers avoid crashes by assisting them with lane-keeping, obeying speed limits, and keeping a safe distance from other cars, and warning them if a pedestrian or cyclist is about to cross their path. Driver assistance systems also track driver behavior, enabling third parties to review drivers' performance. At present these technologies are mainly used for improving the safety of commercial fleets of trucks and buses. However, there is an obvious application to drivers with neurological diseases that affect—or can affect—driving performance. Many such drivers, such as those with amnestic MCI or early Parkinson's disease, may be able to drive safely under favorable conditions (familiar routes, fair weather, light traffic) but not under more demanding ones. Their capabilities to drive safely decline over time, sometimes without their awareness or acknowledgment of their problems. ADAS should make such drivers safer, while periodic review of actual driving behavior would aid in the decision of when a person should stop driving. Recorded evidence of dangerous driving behavior can be more persuasive to patients and their families than results of mental status tests or the results of a single road test. Road tests are too expensive to be repeated regularly, and they typically do not include especially challenging or unexpected driving situations. At the time of this writing, two options are widely available for consumer-focused ADAS and driver tracking. Safety technology like lane-keeping assistance and blind spot warnings are available as options or as standard equipment on most new cars. And, some automobile insurance companies (e.g., Allstate Insurance) offer discounts to drivers who permit tracking devices to be installed in their cars and monitored to assess their driving behavior.

Wearable and/or connected devices should be considered when treatment would be aided by knowing a physiological or behavioral variable that a patient could not self-report, when a patient has impaired memory and/or executive function that endangers personal safety or treatment adherence, when a major risk could be mitigated by an earlier warning of a potential problem, when a diagnostic question could be settled by timely measurement of a variable or recording of an event, or when feedback to a patient on the effects of a behavior change would meaningfully reinforce that change. That said, there are major open questions about the how "connected health" data should be integrated into clinical workflow while setting appropriate expectations with patients, maintaining privacy of health data, and not increasing demands for physicians' time and attention. Applications of connected devices to arrhythmia diagnosis and to COPD and asthma management have been studied, with literature showing both potential clinical value and significant implementation challenges.[52,53] A neuropsychiatrist initiating the use of connected devices in his/her practice should begin with a single clinical context and a single device that is relevant to a problem common in the practice. A single solution would be tested by the neuropsychiatrist's team on a series of patients before deciding to make it part of usual practice.

When a mobile or connected device is employed as part of a treatment plan, there should be clear responsibility for who will maintain the device, whether and how data will be recorded, and who will be responsible for tracking and/or reviewing the data. Making a device part of a formal treatment plan implies professional and legal responsibility. For example, if a patient with paroxysmal atrial fibrillation wears a device to detect episodes of atrial fibrillation and sends data to a clinician, the clinician has a professional obligation to respond to it. The clinician should make a clear and realistic statement to the patient—included in the medical record—about how rapidly a response might be expected.

KEEPING PATIENTS WORKING

If a patient is of working age (the upper end of the range is continually increasing), enabling a patient to keep working is a high priority unless the patient is truly ready to retire, or could not work even with all feasible accommodations. For many patients, work is a major source of meaning and purpose in life; for most others, earnings from work are essential to support their standard of living and quality of life. A focus on work—impediments, solutions to illness-related problems, and feasible adaptations of the patient's work tasks, work site, schedule, or other working conditions often can increase the engagement of patients and other players and bring them together in support of a treatment strategy. When there are several viable treatments, options should be preferred that have little or no risk of causing side effects that would interfere with the patient's work, and/or have early and significant benefits for symptoms that currently do interfere with the patient's work. For example, when a performing artist is treated for bipolar disorder, the clinician should avoid when possible treatments that often cause tremors or emotional blunting. The most persuasive argument for a payer to cover an expensive, disease-modifying treatment in a young adult with chronic migraine or a costly treatment for levodopa-induced dyskinesia in a patient might be related to work interference rather than to the patient's subjective distress.

Some occupations, from physicians to airline pilots and truck drivers, have rules and regulations that would disqualify people from working—or involve costly and burdensome monitoring—if they receive a certain diagnosis or treatment. It is important for the neuropsychiatrist to know such policies as they apply to the clinical populations that he/she treats, and to avoid treatment options that would *unnecessarily* disrupt the patients' work. For example, a commercial airline pilot in the United States can lose his/her certification for flying if he/she is treated for depression with any psychotropic medication other than one of four specific SSRIs, or if he/she receives a bipolar spectrum diagnosis of any kind. If a neuropsychiatrist were treating a pilot who had a mild depression that did not interfere with his flying performance and had no other illness-related impairments that would disqualify him, initial treatment should be nonpharmacologic. This would avoid triggering medication-related rules, as well as eliminate the possibility that an SSRI would cause drug-induced hypomanic symptoms, leading to a bipolar spectrum diagnosis that would end the pilot's career.

GUNS: A SPECIAL CONCERN FOR AMERICAN NEUROPSYCHIATRISTS

Neuropsychiatrists treating adults with neurodegenerative diseases often confront the issue of driving safety—when to tell a patient it is time to stop driving, and when to resort to family interventions or legal measures if a patient is an unsafe driver unwilling to relinquish his/her car keys. The problem is greatest when impairment of driving-relevant cognitive, motor, and/or sensory functions is compromised along with the patient's awareness of his/her impairments and their potential consequences. When the situation first arises, the patient would not meet criteria for legal incompetence, and might even be able to pass a road test under favorable circumstances.

In the United States, a similar issue concerns the ownership and use of firearms by people with dementia and other neuropsychiatric disorders.[54] While the issue is of obvious importance, an exploratory study of caregivers of people with dementia showed that fewer than half addressed the issue of guns in the home, and of those that did very few had discussed the issue of firearm safety with a health care provider.[55] Firearms account for half of all deaths by suicide in the United States and more than half in many specific states; in 2017, 23,854 Americans died of firearm suicide. The United States has the highest rate of firearm suicide and homicide among industrialized nations, and there is a significant correlation of regional rates of gun ownership and their rates of firearm suicide. Firearms are the most common method of suicide among people with dementia.[55] About 90% of suicide attempts with a firearm are lethal; no other common means of self-harm approaches the lethality of firearms. For this reason, restricting firearm access to people at high risk for impulsive self-harm will reduce their suicide mortality rate.[56]

People with a combination of general medical illness (especially with pain, cancer, functional decline), distressing emotional symptoms, and decreased impulse control are especially vulnerable to unplanned self-harm. Gun owners with impaired memory, executive function, and/or judgment are especially likely to leave loaded and unlocked firearms in places outside of their direct observation and control. Unsafely stored firearms cause many accidental deaths and severe injuries with young children at high risk for harm if they handle a loaded, unlocked firearm. For these reasons, a clinician caring for a neuropsychiatric patient should know whether he/she is a gun owner, and if so to know about where and how the patients' firearms and ammunition are stored. Optimal gun safety calls for a firearm not currently in use by a qualified person to be stored locked and unloaded, with ammunition stored separately from the gun. In a 2015 survey, approximately 30% of

gun owners kept at least one firearm loaded and unlocked.[57] Among gun-owning households with children, approximately 20% kept at least one firearm loaded and unlocked.[58] In households where children don't reside but visit periodically (e.g., those where the resident's young grandchildren live nearby) the rate is higher. Only a few states have a legal requirement that firearms be stored locked and unloaded, but the principles of safe gun storage are accepted by gun owners even when they are not legal requirements. Following those principles becomes potentially lifesaving when an unsafely-stored gun would be readily available to a young child, a moody and intoxicated teenager, or a neuropsychiatric patient experiencing physical and mental distress coupled with impairment in judgment and impulse control.

Recommendations for safe gun storage are made by physicians of many specialties, notably pediatricians, who routinely ask parents about firearms in the home that might get into the hands of a child. If the clinician is concerned that the need to unlock and load a firearm would be an insufficient deterrent to dangerous usage by a neuropsychiatric patient, there are more potent options. Ammunition might be stored separately from the firearm, in a locked container accessible only by someone other than the patient. Or, the firearm and ammunition might be stored outside of the person's home, for example, at a gun club or on the premises of a licensed firearm dealer who offered gun storage service. Having the gun kept by a friend or relative at a different location is another option, but one that is not always legal; it will depend on the type of weapon, state laws, and whether the criminal record of the person keeping the gun would allow him/her to legally own one.

For cultural reasons, firearm-related issues can be especially sensitive for some patients, but clinicians should not avoid them. This is especially the case when clinicians treat patients from populations with a high rate of gun ownership. These include military veterans, men over 50, residents of rural areas, and residents of states with a strong gun culture, including Alaska and the states of the Deep South, Greater Appalachia, and the Intermountain West. For example, an older veteran in rural Montana is likely a gun owner, so the question of gun safety should always be considered when such a patient presents with a neuropsychiatric disorder. Outside the United States, other countries with high rates of civilian gun ownership include Switzerland and the Nordic nations. In those countries, firearm suicide is a significant public health concern, and ensuring the safety of gun owners with neuropsychiatric disorders is a clinical challenge as it is in America.

When a neuropsychiatric patient at risk for causing harm with a gun is an enthusiastic and committed gun owner, the clinician's challenge is to raise the issue of gun safety without damaging the therapeutic relationship. Some suggestions can be offered to neuropsychiatrists who treat high-risk populations: First, asking standard questions about gun ownership and storage at the same time as questions are asked about driving, perhaps using a clinical note template, greatly increases the likelihood that the issue will be addressed and that patients will not be offended by the questions.[59] If the clinician is not a gun owner and does not have experience with guns, he/she might benefit from taking a course in gun safety and safe gun storage, and becoming familiar with gun culture and how gun owners use their weapons and think about them. He/she should be familiar with state laws pertinent to gun storage and to the circumstances under which law enforcement will temporarily remove a person's firearms from his/her home. He/she should visit a local licensed gun dealer, learn about trigger locks and gun safes, and discover whether there is a local firearm dealer who offers temporary storage of customers' firearms if they are unable to keep them safely at home. A gun owner might feel better about his/her gun being temporarily kept by gun dealer rather than by the police. The clinician can make comments that evidence his/her knowledge of firearms and convey the sense that he/she does not disapprove of gun ownership *per se*—that the issue at hand is purely clinical and is in no way political or moral. When talking with a patient, or (with the patient's consent) a family member or friend, the issue of gun ownership and storage should be framed in terms of gun safety and the importance of avoiding a tragic accident. Pointing out potential risks to young children and to teenagers can be an effective and face-saving way of raising the issue of gun safety with an older man who has enjoyed gun ownership most of his life.

If the gun-owning patient with episodic or fluctuating neuropsychiatric risk uses his/her guns for sport only rather than for self-defense, he/she may be open to their being kept unloaded and locked or in a gun safe, with a healthy and trusted family member or friend keeping the keys to the weapon, the safe, and the ammunition supply. If guns are used for self-defense at home, the clinician might explore alternative security measures. If a patient knows he/she is not doing well—suffering from depression or pain, drinking excessively, or using drugs that alter mental status, the clinician might propose that the patient's guns be stored away from home until his/her health improves.

If a patient will permit the issue of his/her use of guns to be discussed with a relative or friend, that person can be brought into the conversation and become an advocate for the proposed safety measures. The point can be made that having a gun in the home makes death by suicide significantly more likely. Because firearms cause such severe injuries, an impulsive act of self-harm using a firearm usually is fatal. The typical scenario for firearm suicide is not one in which a person with severe major depressive disorder plans his/her death and then executes the plan with a gun. It is one in which a person (usually a man) with a combination of negative emotions, general medical problems, financial or interpersonal issues, and perhaps an episodic user of alcohol or drugs becomes upset by an event, and issue, or a symptom, drinks alcohol or takes medication that impairs impulse control, and shoots himself. The risk of such a death increases when a person has a combination of personal and medical troubles, is lonely, and drinks to assuage negative emotions. If access to a loaded weapon requires the participation of a second person, an advance plan might provide that the second person not give the patient access to a loaded weapon (or to ammunition) if he/she has been drinking, is visibly upset, or

has had a recent change in medical status (e.g., increased pain, starting or stopping a medication, etc.).

A person vulnerable to transient abnormal mental states, such as one with complex partial epilepsy with postictal affective instability and executive impairment, or one with episodic binge-drinking, might use a gun in ways he/she would never consider in his/her usual state of mind. Helping a patient develop a harm-prevention plan, rather than insist that he/she immediately and permanently relinquish his/her gun, conveys respect and is less likely to offend a patient for whom gun ownership is linked to his/her feelings of security and self-esteem. If the patient has a progressive condition, he/she ultimately may lose access to a firearm, but if it occurs through the unfolding of a joint harm-reduction plan it might avoid the need for an adversarial legal proceeding.

A website, www.efsgv.org,[56] concerned with the prevention of gun violence and of firearm suicide in particular, provides convenient access to state-level statistics on gun ownership and gun suicide, state firearm laws (e.g., so-called Extreme Risk Laws), and potential interventions with gun owners at high risk for self-harm. When assessment of firearm-related risk is built into a neuropsychiatrist's clinical routine the details will vary according to the state or country in which the clinician practices and typical patterns of gun ownership and use among the patient groups most often seen. If the issue of gun safety is considered early in the course of a treatment relationship and is addressed prospectively and tactfully, legal action to remove a patient's guns should rarely be necessary.

CONSIDERING PREEXISTING BELIEFS AND BIASES

Patients and families may have beliefs and biases, sometimes based on religion or culture, sometimes based on personal or family experiences, and sometimes idiosyncratic, that cause them to privilege some goals of treatment over others, to stigmatize certain diagnoses, or to reject some treatments preemptively. For example, in some families, a child is expected to have some form of higher education without respect to his/her inclinations or cognitive capacities. Some will stigmatize depression but do not stigmatize a sleep disorder, chronic fatigue, or chronic pain. Some will stigmatize the profession of psychiatry and therefore will prefer to receive psychotropic medication from a PCP rather than a psychiatrist—or reject medication altogether. Some will see psychotherapy as the disclosure of shameful information to a potentially judgmental outsider, but might be willing consider using a psychotherapy smartphone app if they are confident about the security of their data. Some view mental illness as a spiritual problem rather than a medical one and would be more open to counseling by a clergyman than by a mental health professional.

Beliefs and biases like these can undermine the acceptance of diagnoses, engagement, and adherence to treatment if they are not identified and addressed in a timely way. Though desirable, accommodating patients' and families' preexisting preferences is isn't necessarily feasible. If optimal evidence-based treatment and the patient's and/or family's preferred treatment aren't the same, an initial goal is to find common ground with the patient and/or family and to establish trust and rapport that enables negotiation. Even if the choice of treatments is initially controversial, early agreement usually is possible on treatment goals, risks to be mitigated, functions to be preserved or enhanced if possible, and how the most important outcomes will be measured.

LIFESTYLE MEDICINE AND COMPLEMENTARY, ALTERNATIVE, AND INTEGRATIVE TREATMENTS

Patients who use complementary, alternative, and integrative medicine (CAIM) treatments often do not spontaneously tell their physicians about their use of these treatments. Herbal preparations and nutritional supplements in particular can have powerful therapeutic or adverse effects, and can interact with conventional prescribed therapies.[60,61] There are many reports of contamination of supplements with prohibited drugs, with most reports of contamination related to sexual performance enhancement, weight loss, or muscle-building supplements.[62] The United States Food and Drug Administration maintains a website with up-to-date information of reported cases of contaminated supplements.[63] However, many cases are not recognized or reported. Patients who choose to use a nutritional supplement or herbal preparation should be encouraged to obtain it from a source that conducts third-party testing of its products for potency and purity and has been certified as adhering to the FDA's Good Manufacturing Practices. A book by Gerbarg and colleagues[64] recommends sources for specific psychoactive supplements for which there is published evidence for efficacy and risk.

In developing a comprehensive, holistic treatment plan the neuropsychiatrist must know about the patient's engagement with CAIM. Opening a dialogue about CAIM use is aided by the clinician's knowing about the evidence for CAIM treatments for the conditions he/she most often sees. He/she can communicate openness to the patient's use of a CAIM treatment as long as the treatment has an evidence base, it is not substituting for a treatment of established efficacy and safety, it does not adversely interact with prescribed treatments, and the outcomes and adverse effects of the CAIM treatment are monitored systematically. In the author's experience, patients and families appreciate a physician's openness to the use of CAIM, especially if the physician offers to monitor the outcome of the CAIM treatment to assess whether it is safe and is offering enough benefit to justify its cost. Patient-initiated CAIM treatments rarely are covered by health insurance, while the physician's outcome monitoring usually would be.

If a patient wants to try a CAIM therapy whose efficacy has not been established for the patient's symptom or condition, the neuropsychiatrist (or member of his/her team) should first ensure that the patient is aware of FDA-approved, conventional options for treating it, that the patient has either not responded to conventional treatment, has not tolerated it, or has a valid reason for rejecting it . Then, if there is a reasonable

hypothesis for why the treatment might be helpful, if there is evidence for benefit from animal models or human case reports or open-label studies, and if there is a low probability of adverse effects on the patient's comorbidities and other treatments, the clinician could—but should not feel obliged to—offer to conduct an "N of 1 clinical trial" with systematic measurement of treatment outcomes and adverse effects if any. Such trials, which are increasingly used to assess the efficacy of personalized medical interventions including those of CAIM, typically use standardized periodic measurements of clinical outcomes during periods on and off the treatment of interest. When feasible, a placebo or sham treatment is used alternately with the active treatment of interest, and there is either a single- or double-blind design. Mobile devices often are used to make the collection of outcome data efficient enough to burden neither the patient nor the clinician. The N of 1 clinical trial is emerging as an important tool in validating personalized allopathic treatments as well as CAIM treatments and lifestyle interventions.[65-67]

Alternatively, the clinician should advise the patient to disclose any nonstandard treatment he/she is using or intends to use and ask the patient to describe his/her expectations for the treatment's effect and how he/she plans to evaluate whether the treatment has worked. After reviewing publications on the treatment, the clinician would inform the patient what he/she does and does not know about the treatment. He/she would plan to periodically assess the outcome targeted by the treatment and to screen for the potential adverse effects of greatest concern. In either case, the clinician should make clear that there is no assurance of benefit, and no guarantee that there will not be adverse effects.

The process of review and of planning an N of 1 trial or structured periodic monitoring takes time but a patient can experience it as a reflection of the clinician's care and concern, empathy, and openness. It may lead to better acceptance of conventional treatments in the future if the unconventional treatment is ineffective or not well-tolerated. If the clinician is concerned that risks outweigh benefits, he/she should convey his/her concern to the patient and document the conversation, indicating that the patient was not advised to use the alternative treatment, and that monitoring of its effects does not indicate the clinician's approval of the patient's choice.

With or without methods based on CAIM approaches, lifestyle modification is a powerful adjunct to conventional medications and therapies. Improvement in diet, exercise and sleep habits, reducing environmental hazards, and addressing home safety issues can improve outcomes across multiple domains, while increasing patient engagement and building trust. The value of lifestyle modification is self-evident in some cases, for example, the value of adequate sleep in people with epilepsy and of avoiding polluted air for people with asthma or COPD. Its value in treating depression is well-established.[68] Home safety assessments are a routine part of the care of frail older adults.

Summary and Key Points

■ Patients with neuropsychiatric disorders often have comorbidities and complicated treatment regimens. Their treatment often involves multiple "players" on both the patient side (patients, families, advocates, and other concerned parties) and the clinical side (physicians of various specialties and other clinicians of various disciplines, payers, and care managers). Aims of treatment comprise strictly biomedical ones and others related to function and well-being, educational and occupational concerns, and legal and financial issues. Prevention of adverse events is always relevant, and cost containment is a concern most of the time.

■ Systematically addressing this complexity of neuropsychiatric disorders can improve outcomes in an efficient way. Doing so involves identifying players and their agendas; identifying formal or informal team leaders and defining the responsibilities of each team member; explicitly establishing the goals and strategy of treatment; and creating a dashboard or control panel of outcome measures that is updated as treatment proceeds. Time is devoted to care coordination beyond the time required for face-to-face care delivery. Documentation of care is tailored to facilitate interdisciplinary collaboration and to support fair payment for time spent coordinating care and integrating its psychiatric and general medical components.

■ To make such care sustainable, the extra time spent by the neuropsychiatrist and by other team members must be recognized and either reimbursed or acknowledged in a way that reduces the team members' overall burden and stress. Making this happen requires dialogue between those who provide care and those who administer care settings and/or represent payers for care. It also involves limiting the range of conditions for which the neuropsychiatrist provides team leadership. Time required sometimes can be reduced by creating templates for documentation and standard strategies for managing common comorbidities, and training and empowering nonphysician team members to assume some of the responsibilities for continuity of care and early responses to adverse events and high-risk situations. Emerging technologies including point-of-care testing, mobile-wearable devices, and health apps may be useful as well.

■ Treatment planning should include consideration of lifestyle modification and complementary, integrative, and alternative medicine (CAIM). Patients' preexisting preferences and prejudices should be accommodated when feasible and challenged when necessary. Active engagement with people and organizations outside the usual scope of one's specialty practice—necessary for the best outcomes and for sustainability of practice—can enhance a neuropsychiatrist's effectiveness. It also helps combat burnout by frequently reminding the clinician of the distinctiveness and meaning of his/her work.

■ Health care in the United States and other high-income countries is undergoing rapid and disruptive changes related to new treatments, new technologies, increasing costs of care, and major demographic changes. Complex, high-comorbidity patients with issues of brain dysfunction affecting mood, cognition, and behavior are especially vulnerable to harm from disruption or disorganization of their care. Neuropsychiatrists are especially well qualified to protect complex patients from harm and help them benefit from potent new diagnostic and therapeutic technology. Doing so requires a proactive approach, engagement with nonclinicians, and advocacy for changes in policies and procedures. This requires additional investment of time and attention, but can nonetheless be more sustainable because the associated sense of agency and the evident benefits for some patients can protect against burnout and stimulate creative thinking about how to improve the quality and efficiency of care.

References

1. de Vries McClintock HF, Boyle KB, Rooney K, Bogner HR. Diabetes and depression care: a randomized controlled pilot trial. *Am J Health Behav.* 2016;40(4):503-513.
2. Katon WJ, Lin EH, Von Korff M, et al. Collaborative care for patients with depression and chronic illnesses. *N Engl J Med.* 2010;363(27):2611-2620.
3. Reiss-Brennan B, Brunisholz KD, Dredge C, et al. Association of integrated team-based care with health care quality, utilization, and cost. *JAMA.* 2016;316(8):826-834.
4. Schwenk TL. Integrated behavioral and primary care: what is the real cost? *JAMA.* 2016;316(8):822-823.
5. English AF. Team-based primary care with integrated mental health is associated with higher quality of care, lower usage and lower payments received by the delivery system. *Evid Based Med.* 2017;22(3):96.
6. Dartmouth Atlas Project. 2019. Available at www.dartmouthatlas.org. Accessed January 25, 2020.
7. United Council for Neurologic Subspecialties (UCNS). 2020. Available at www.ucns.org. Accessed January 25, 2020.
8. Teixeira-Poit SM, Halpern MT, Kane HL, Keating M, Olmsted M. Factors influencing professional life satisfaction among neurologists. *BMC Health Serv Res.* 2017;17(1):409.
9. Alcohol.org. An American Addictions Centers Resource. Available at www.alcohol.org. Accessed December 20, 2019.
10. Ulwelling W, Smith K. The PEth blood test in the security environment: what it is; why it is important; and interpretative guidelines. *J Forensic Sci.* 2018;63(6):1634-1640.
11. Luginbühl M, Weinmann W, Butzke I, Pfeifer P. Monitoring of direct alcohol markers in alcohol use disorder patients during withdrawal treatment and successive rehabilitation. *Drug Test Anal.* 2019;11(6):859-869.
12. Navarro-Haro MV, López-Del-Hoyo Y, Campos D, et al. Meditation experts try virtual reality mindfulness: a pilot study evaluation of the feasibility and acceptability of virtual reality to facilitate mindfulness practice in people attending a mindfulness conference. *PLoS One.* 2017;12(11):e0187777.

13. Mistler LA, Ben-Zeev D, Carpenter-Song E, Brunette MF, Friedman MJ. Mobile mindfulness intervention on an acute psychiatric unit: feasibility and acceptability study. *JMIR Ment Health*. 2017;4(3):e34.

14. Fennell AB, Benau EM, Atchley RA. A single session of meditation reduces of physiological indices of anger in both experienced and novice meditators. *Conscious Cogn*. 2016;40:54-66.

15. Conelea CA, Wellen B. Tic treatment goes tech: a review of TicHelper.com. *Cogn Behav Pract*. 2017;24(3):374-381.

16. Andersson E, Ljótsson B, Hedman E, et al. Internet-based cognitive behavior therapy for obsessive compulsive disorder: a pilot study. *BMC Psychiatry*. 2011;11:125.

17. Herbst N, Voderholzer U, Thiel N, et al. No talking, just writing! Efficacy of an Internet-based cognitive behavioral therapy with exposure and response prevention in obsessive compulsive disorder. *Psychother Psychosom*. 2014;83(3):165-175.

18. Leckman JF, Riddle MA, Hardin MT, et al. The Yale Global Tic Severity Scale: initial testing of a clinician-rated scale of tic severity. *J Am Acad Child Adolesc Psychiatry*. 1989;28(4):566-573.

19. McGuire JF, Piacentini J, Storch EA, et al. A multicenter examination and strategic revisions of the Yale Global Tic Severity Scale. *Neurology*. 2018;90(19):e1711-e1719.

20. Ricketts EJ, McGuire JF, Chang S, et al. Benchmarking treatment response in Tourette's disorder: a psychometric evaluation and signal detection analysis of the Parent Tic Questionnaire. *Behav Ther*. 2018;49(1):46-56.

21. Martino D, Pringsheim TM, Cavanna AE, et al. Systematic review of severity scales and screening instruments for tics: critique and recommendations. *Mov Disord*. 2017;32(3):467-473.

22. Goodman WK, Price LH, Rasmussen SA, et al. The Yale-Brown Obsessive-Compulsive Scale. II. Validity. *Arch Gen Psychiatry*. 1989;46(11):1012-1016.

23. Goodman WK, Price LH, Rasmussen SA, et al. The Yale-Brown Obsessive-Compulsive Scale. I. Development, use, and reliability. *Arch Gen Psychiatry*. 1989a;46(11):1006-1011.

24. Halpin D, Meltzer EO, Pisternick-Ruf W, Moroni-Zentgraf P, Engel M, Zaremba-Pechmann L. Peak expiratory flow as an endpoint for clinical trials in asthma: a comparison with FEV_1. *Respir Res*. 2019;20(1):159.

25. Warman KL, Silver EJ. Are inner-city children with asthma receiving specialty care as recommended in national asthma guidelines? *J Asthma*. 2018;55(5):517-524.

26. Floyd P. Integrating physical and behavioral health: a major step toward population health management. *Healthc Financ Manage*. 2016;70(1):64-71.

27. Medicare Learning Network. *Evaluation and Management Services*. Publication ICN 006764. Department of Health and Human Services, Center for Medicare and Medicaid Services. 2017. Available at https://www.cms.gov>downloads>eval-mgmt-serv-guide-ICN006764. Accessed November 8, 2019.

28. Pearls4Peers. 2018. Available at https://pearls4peers.com/2018/02/05/what-is-the-difference-between-moderate-and-high-complexity-medical-decision-making-under-the-centers-for-medicare-and-medicaid-services-cms-rule/. Accessed November 10, 2019.

29. Massachusetts Hospital Association. Changing the EHR from a liability to an asset to reduce physician burnout. The Reliant Medical Group story. 2019. Available at 19-04-22PR_Changing_EHR_PhysBurnout_0119_FINAL.pdf. Accessed November 10, 2019.

30. Hibbard JH, Stockard J, Mahoney ER, Tusler M. Development of the Patient Activation Measure (PAM): conceptualizing and measuring activation in patients and consumers. *Health Serv Res*. 2004;39(4 pt 1):1005-1026.

31. Tuccero D, Railey K, Briggs M, Hull SK. Behavioral health in prevention and chronic illness management: motivational interviewing. *Prim Care*. 2016;43(2):191-202.

32. Fisher L, Polonsky WH, Hessler D, Potter MB. A practical framework for encouraging and supporting positive behaviour change in diabetes. *Diabet Med*. 2017;34(12):1658-1666.

33. Gilliam FG, Barry JJ, Hermann BP, Meador KJ, Vahle V, Kanner AM. Rapid detection of major depression in epilepsy: a multicentre study. *Lancet Neurol*. 2006;5(5):399-405.

34. Alexopoulos GS, Abrams RC, Young RC, Shamoian CA. Cornell Scale for Depression in dementia. *Biol Psychiatry*. 1988;23(3):271-284.

35. Forjaz MJ, Martinez-Martin P, Dujardin K, et al. Rasch analysis of anxiety scales in Parkinson's disease. *J Psychosom Res*. 2013;74(5):414-419.

36. Leentjens AF, Dujardin K, Pontone GM, Starkstein SE, Weintraub D, Martinez-Martin P. The Parkinson Anxiety Scale (PAS): development and validation of a new anxiety scale. *Mov Disord*. 2014;29(8):1035-1043.

37. Katz S, Ford AB, Moskowitz RW, Jackson BA, Jaffe MW. Studies of illness in the aged: the index of ADL: a standardized measure of biological and psychosocial function. *JAMA*. 1963;185(12):914-919.

38. Lawton MP, Brody EM. Assessment of older people: self-maintaining and instrumental activities of daily living. *Gerontologist*. 1969;9 (3):179-186.

39. Marson DC, Sawrie SM, Snyder S, et al. Assessing financial capacity in patients with Alzheimer disease: a conceptual model and prototype instrument. *Arch Neurol*. 2000;57(6):877-884.

40. Johnson N, Barion A, Rademaker A, Rehkemper G, Weintraub S. The Activities of Daily Living Questionnaire: a validation study in patients with dementia. *Alzheimers Dis Assoc Disord*. 2004;18(4):223-230.

41. Fahn S, Elton R; Members of the UPDRS Development Committee. Unified Parkinson's Disease Rating Scale. In: Fahn S, Marsden CD, Calne DB, Goldstein M, eds. *Recent Developments in Parkinson's Disease*. Vol 2. Florham Park, NJ: Macmillan Health Care Information; 1987:153-163, 293-304. Available at http://www.mdvu.org/library/ratingscales/pd/. Accessed November 8, 2019.

42. Guy W. Abnormal Involuntary Movement Scale [AIMS]. National Institute of Mental Health Psychopharmacology Research Branch. ECDEU assessment manual for psychopharmacology, revised. Rockville, MD: U.S. National Institute of Health, Psychopharmacology Research Branch; 1976:534-537.

43. Monje MHG, Foffani G, Obeso J, Sánchez-Ferro Á. New sensor and wearable technologies to aid in the diagnosis and treatment monitoring of Parkinson's disease. *Ann Rev Biomed Eng*. 2019;4(21):111-143.

44. Galperin I, Hillel I, Del Din S, et al. Associations between daily-living physical activity and laboratory-based assessments of motor severity in patients with falls and Parkinson's disease. *Parkinsonism Relat Disord*. 2019;62:85-90.

45. Asakawa T, Sugiyama K, Nozaki T, et al. Can the latest computerized technologies revolutionize conventional assessment tools and therapies for a neurological disease? The example of Parkinson's disease. *Neurol Med Chir*. 2019;59(3):69-78.

46. Titgemeyer Y, Surges R, Altenmüller DM, et al. Can commercially available wearable EEG devices be used for diagnostic purposes? An explorative pilot study. *Epilepsy Behav*. 2020;103 (Pt A):106507.

47. Jeppesen J, Fuglsang-Frederiksen A, Johansen P, et al. Seizure detection based on heart rate variability using a wearable electrocardiography device. *Epilepsia*. 2019;60(10):2105-2113.

48. Thompson ME, Langer J, Kinfe M. Seizure detection watch improves quality of life for adolescents and their families. *Epilepsy Behav*. 2019;98(pt A):188-194.

49. Page RA. Technology-enabled seizure detection and reporting: the epilepsy network project. *Epilepsy Res*. 2019;153:85-87.

50. Bialer M, Johannessen SI, Koepp MJ, et al. A summary of data presented at the XIV conference on new antiepileptic drug and devices (EILAT XIV). *Epilepsy Res*. 2019;153:66-67.

51. Leviton A, Oppenheimer J, Chiujdea M, et al. Characteristics of future models of integrated outpatient care. *Healthcare (Basel)*. 2019;7(2):65.

52. Ip JE. Wearable devices for cardiac rhythm diagnosis and management. *JAMA*. 2019;321(4):337-338.

53. Goodridge D, Marciniuk D. Rural and remote care: overcoming the challenges of distance. *Chron Respir Dis*. 2016;13(2):192-203.

54. Greene E, Bornstein BH, Dietrich H. Granny, (don't) get your gun: competency issues in gun ownership by older adults. *Behav Sci Law*. 2007;25:405-423.

55. Betz ME, Rannel ML, Knoepke CE, et al. Dementia and firearms: an exploratory survey of caregiver needs. *J Gen Intern Med*. 2019;34(10):1984-1986.

56. EFSGV. The educational fund to stop gun violence. 2020. Available at www.efsgv.org. Accessed January 25, 2020.

57. Berrigan J, Azrael D, Hemenway D, Miller M. Firearms training and storage practices among US gun owners: a nationally representative study. *Inj Prev*. 2019;25(suppl 1):i31-i38.

58. Azrael D, Cohen J, Salhi C, Miller M. Firearm storage in gun-owning households with children: results of a 2015 national survey. *J Urban Health*. 2018;95(3):295-304.

59. LoConte NK, Gleason CE, Gunter-Hunt G, Carlsson CM, Siebers M. Standardized note template improves screening of firearm access and driving among veterans with dementia. *Am J Alzheimers Dis Other Dement*. 2008;23(4):313-318.

60. Trivedi R, Salvo MC. Utilization and safety of common over-the-counter dietary/nutritional supplements, herbal agents, and homeopathic compounds for disease prevention. *Med Clin North Am*. 2016;100(5):1089-1099.

61. Navarro VJ, Khan I, Björnsson E, Seeff LB, Serrano J, Hoofnagle JH. Liver injury from herbal and dietary supplements. *Hepatology*. 2017;65(1):363-373.

62. Mathews NM. Prohibited contaminants in dietary supplements. *Sports Health*. 2018;10(1):19-30.

63. FDA. 2019. Available at https://www.fda.gov/drugs/buying-using-medicine-safely/medication-health-fraud. Accessed November 8, 2019.

64. Gerbarg P, Muskin P, Brown R. *Complementary and Integrative Treatments in Psychiatric Practice*. Arlington, VA: American Psychiatric Association Publishing; 2017.

65. Lillie EO, Patay B, Diamant J, Issell B, Topol EJ, Schork NJ. The n-of-1 clinical trial: the ultimate strategy for individualizing medicine? *Pers Med*. 2011;8(2):161-173.

66. Moise N, Wood D, Cheung Y, et al. Patient preferences for personalized (N-of-1) trials: a conjoint analysis. *J Clin Epidemiol*. 2018;102:12-22.

67. Diezi L, Buclin T. N-of-1 trials or single-patient therapeutic tests: evidence-based tests to diagnose therapeutic efficacy. *Revue Médicale Suisse*. 2019;15(670):2058-2061.

68. Sarris J, O'Neil A, Coulson CE, Schweitzer I, Berk M. Lifestyle medicine for depression. *BMC Psychiatry*. 2014;14:107.

Integration of Neuropsychiatric Care in Primary Care and Other Medical Settings

36

Laura T. Safar · Tatenda Mahlanza · Hope Schwartz · Jane Erb

In this chapter, we discuss chronic disease management models, review their basic elements, and consider ways in which they may be adapted to neuropsychiatric care.

While having an extensive knowledge of neuropsychiatry is vital to patient care, implementing this knowledge through an effective and efficient model of care delivery is fundamental to increasing patients' access to such expertise.

The US system of health care delivery is most adept at caring for patients with episodic or acute illnesses. Chronic conditions, defined as those lasting more than 3 months and not self-limited,[1] are very difficult to manage in the current system due to its fragmented and largely hospital-centric design. Given the chronic nature of most neuropsychiatric conditions, it is essential that we focus our attention on how to optimize patient outcomes through our care delivery. This is especially the case given the rise in incidence of neuropsychiatric disorders with the aging population.

Chronic disease management principles have been recognized for several decades as leading to better outcomes than usual care in a variety of chronic diseases such as diabetes, cancer, and heart disease. Wagner, Von Korff, and colleagues[1,2] were instrumental in formalizing the concept of the collaborative chronic care model for nonpsychiatric illness management in primary care. Key components of their model include:

- Emphasizing the role of patients and their families in carrying out care
- Collaborating within the health care team to adhere to evidence-based treatment algorithms
- Ongoing symptom self-monitoring by patient and adjustment of care as indicated
- Close attention to and support for optimizing patient functioning in their communities

The importance of addressing the mental health needs of primary care patients was articulated as early as 1960 by the Cherokee Health Systems.[3] However, over the last 20 years, there has been an explosion of interest in applying chronic disease management principles to the mental health needs of the population. While largely driven by the chronic nature of most mental illness, other motivating factors include the inadequate supply of mental health clinicians and the common preference of patients to be managed by their primary care physicians (PCPs).[4] A variety of models integrating behavioral health into primary care have evolved. Features may include an on-site, "co-located" mental health clinician available to treat primary care patients directly, discuss cases during team meetings, or provide curbside consults during clinics. Figure 36-1 shows the range of integration models, and Figure 36-2 shows the collaborative care model (CCM) workflow.

CCM is now considered by many to be the most effective and efficient approach to integrating mental health care into primary care. One such model, IMPACT (improving mood and promoting access to collaborative treatment), has led to more than 80 randomized controlled trials (RCTs) providing evidence that the CCM compared to usual care improves mental and overall health outcomes and reduces functional impairment.[5] In most studies, it also leads to a decline in

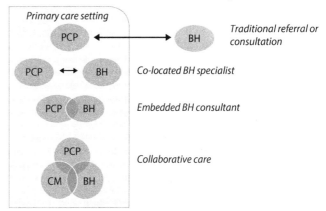

FIGURE 36-1. Levels of behavioral health integration.

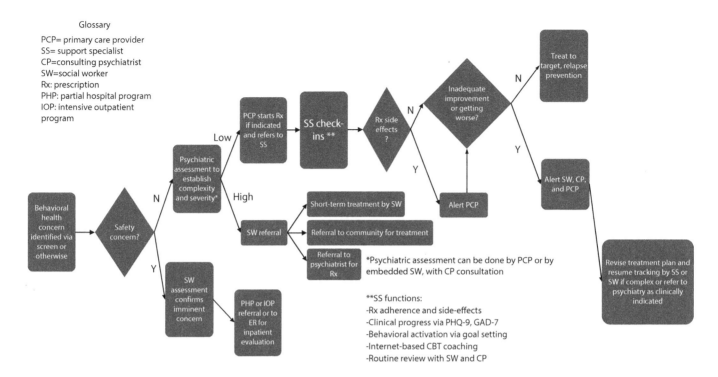

FIGURE 36-2. Illustration of the collaborative care workflow.

overall health care costs in the 2–4 years following implementation. This model has been studied in a variety of settings including socioeconomically and ethnically diverse populations ranging from adolescent to geriatric, in both fee-for-service and bundled payment systems. While IMPACT is the most evidence-based model to date, similar models have evolved concurrently and include the Intermountain Healthcare Integration Program and DIAMOND (Depression Improvement Across Minnesota-Offering a New Direction).[6,7] It is important to distinguish collaborative care from other models, such as co-located care, where mental health clinicians provide treatment as usual but are situated in primary care settings. In spite of increased communication and referral success fostered by co-located care, the IMPACT trial showed that the CCM remained superior to co-located care in outcomes, cost, and patient satisfaction.[8]

Factors thought to contribute to the success of CCMs of behavioral health care include:

1. Team-based care: In his HMS commencement address "Cowboys and Pit Crews," Atul Gawande, MD well summarizes the dilemma—traditionally delivered care is increasingly considered inadequate given the explosion of medical information that the clinician must have to provide the best possible care.[9] Electronic decision support systems can provide some assistance with applying evidence-based treatment standards, but ultimately this is insufficient. Rather, specialized "pit crews," teams that are embedded in practices and deployed when needed, allow for more efficient and higher quality care for complicated and/or chronic disease. Vital to this approach are the specific and well-honed skill sets of each team member that complement the others and serve a critical function in care delivery.

2. Seamless coordination of care: Given the teamwork necessary for collaborative care, assuring efficient communication, and minimizing redundant data collection are critical. This can be accomplished with a user-friendly electronic health record, which immediately captures care delivered by different team members at different times and locations.

3. Patient engagement: Research done in the field of motivational interviewing, a client-centered counseling approach that helps patients explore and resolve ambivalence as a way of eliciting behavior change, has underscored the importance of patients taking an active role in their care.[10] Without patient buy-in, adherence to treatment and outcomes suffer. Shared decision making is emphasized in CCMs and is slowly replacing paternalistic care.

4. Proactive, preventative care: As we become increasingly knowledgeable about chronic disease risk, primary prevention by addressing modifiable risk factors is key. For example, alcohol consumption is a well-studied risk factor for dementia.[11] CCMs allow for constructive inquiry and education about major preventable factors, conducted using motivational interviewing tools to optimize behavior change.

5. Systematic screening and measurement-based care: Given the importance of prevention and early detection, screening cannot be left to chance. For common conditions where early identification can prevent or modify the course of the disease, routine, predictable standards must be set and adhered to.

Cynthia is a 61-year-old divorced female, who reports symptoms of depression and anxiety during a visit with her primary care physician (PCP). Her 25-year-old son died suddenly, due to an acute medical illness. She is attending a bereavement group, but is still struggling with her symptoms. Her PHQ-9 score is 14. Her PCP prescribes escitalopram 5 mg/day and refers her to the clinic's care manager (CM).

The CM reaches Cynthia by phone. During the first phone visit she performs a routine psychiatric assessment including these items:

- Screening scales for depression, anxiety, and bipolar disorder: PHQ-9, GAD-7, Audit-C, and CIDI (Composite International Diagnostic Interview)
- Review of relevant history including past psychiatric history, use of alcohol and substances, family psychiatric history

Her scores at the time of that assessment were: PHQ-9=14; GAD-7=10; Audit-C=1. CIDI was fully negative, as Cynthia did not endorse any of the items as ever happening to her. She has no previous past psychiatric history, and she drinks minimal alcohol. She has one brother with history of anxiety and depression.

The first phone visit interventions and recommendations are:

- The CM prompts Cynthia to fill the escitalopram prescription, reviews instructions, and education about this medication.
- The CM reviews an iCBT (Internet-delivered cognitive-behavioral therapy) program available to patients of the practice, and the patient enrolls.
- She recommends continuing attendance to the bereavement group.
- She provides contact information of a grief counselor.

The CM continues reaching out to Cynthia by phone weekly to monitor on her progress and adherence to treatment recommendations. During phone follow-ups over the following 3 months, Cynthia has continued with all the interventions recommended. Her scores 3 months after the initial assessment are as follows: PHQ-9=7; GAD-7=5. Of note, she had a new loss (a brother died). She experienced sadness, but due to her active use of the skills learned during treatment she did not fall back into depression.

---

6. Systematic processes: Standardizing workflows with only essential variation improves the efficiency of systems.[12]

7. Use of patient registries: There are a variety of tools that can be useful in managing a patient population. Patient based registries improve the odds of not losing track of identified cases.

8. Rewarding prevention and positive health outcomes: Value-based payment systems (as opposed to payment for services rendered) are important, though complicated, to implement in a social structure unaccustomed to single-payer or universal health care. In the United States, accountable care arrangements are gradually replacing fee-for-service and are better aligned with chronic care management goals.[13]

9. Efficient resource utilization: Self-management and stepped care promote allocating our limited resources efficiently. Stepped care emphasizes implementing the most effective, least resource-intensive treatments first, and "stepping up" to more intensive specialist services only when first-line prevention or treatment fails.

10. Ease of appointments with one-stop care model: Patients can address different health care needs in the same setting.

11. Decreased stigma concerns: Access to psychiatric care in the primary care setting may help ease the concern of those patients who avoid mental health care appointments due to the unfortunate stigma still attached to psychiatric illness in sectors of our society.

The typical collaborative care team, for instance, as designed to address depression in primary care, includes a care manager, a consulting psychiatrist, and the PCP. They help the patient achieve symptom resolution and maintenance of remission through relapse prevention education and ongoing, active monitoring. The original IMPACT study[5,14] employed nurses or psychologists as care managers providing brief skill-building interventions through cognitive behavioral and/or problem-solving therapies. Variations on this model have evolved using nonclinician, trained care managers who work closely with non-MD clinicians such as psychologists or social workers and confer routinely with a consulting psychiatrist. While there is no direct, head-to-head comparative trial data, care management by trained and supervised nonclinicians seems to be similarly effective in our clinic's experience. Typically, the psychiatrist meets weekly with the care managers and the behavioral health team to review new and problematic cases, answer questions from PCPs, and provide educational in-services at the practice. In some settings, the psychiatrist might provide direct patient consultation in complex cases. These consultations can be comprehensive or focused, and in-person or telephonic. If a patient's needs exceed the management capacity of the PCP and the primary care-based behavioral health team, the individual is then referred to be treated in a psychiatric setting.

Woltmann and colleagues[15] published a rigorous review of collaborative care programs targeting mental health. There was ample evidence that collaborative care did not generally increase health care costs, and in many cases, overall health care costs declined over the course of 2–4 years.[16] Paired with very favorable patient outcomes and clinician satisfaction, collaborative care seems like a win-win. Despite the literature showing that cost does not increase and may actually decrease with the use of the CCM, institutions may be concerned about how to fund the reimbursement of team members for the work they do outside of the direct face-to-face contact with patients (i.e., case management, or curbside specialist consultations). In a traditional fee-for-service reimbursement environment this may represent an obstacle to implementing this model. Financial agreements between departments, with hospital administration, and/or with health care insurers may assist with funding this portion of team members' time. Collaborative care, on the other hand, fits well with the accountable care organization model—stepped and coordinated care are just two of the principles common to both. While most collaborative care has been implemented to address depression in primary care settings, there is evidence that at least some components of this model can be useful for more complex psychiatric illness such as bipolar disorder. Future trials involving treatment of other conditions and in other settings[17] will be critical.

THE COLLABORATIVE CARE MODEL IN NEUROPSYCHIATRY

The success of the CCM for the treatment of depression in the primary care setting necessitates consideration of its adaptation and use in other neuropsychiatric conditions. Implementation of CCMs could facilitate increased access to neuropsychiatric care for the large proportion of the population that seeks most of their medical care from their primary care practice due to patient preference,[4] limited availability of specialists, stigma, and other factors. As described above in the model of collaborative care for depression, care in specialty and subspecialty settings (psychiatry and neuropsychiatry, respectively) would still have a role in cases deemed too complex or challenging for the primary care setting.

When considering the adaptation of the CCM to neuropsychiatry, we can follow the five components of the original model (see Figure 36-3): patient, psychiatrist, care manager, intervention, and PCP in the primary care setting.

The Neuropsychiatric Patient

First, it is important to acknowledge that the CCM model as originally described and implemented already includes neuropsychiatric patients. The focus of the initial IMPACT study is late-life depression.[5,14] While patients with severe cognitive impairment were screened out,[5] many of these patients were medically complex, with multiple medical/neurological

comorbidities. The medically complex patient with psychiatric manifestations represents a typical subset of the population already treated in specialty neuropsychiatric clinics. Given the common difficulties and needs of neuropsychiatric patients, the CCM would benefit from several modifications to adequately serve this population:

- Awareness of atypical clinical presentations in neuropsychiatry. The presence of neurological disorders may modify the phenomenology of psychiatric syndromes. For instance, a patient with frontal lobe degeneration may show an atypical clinical presentation of depression with excessive disinhibition. Common differential diagnoses to consider in neuropsychiatric patients include apathy versus depression; pathological affect versus mood disorder; frontal disinhibition versus mania/other primary psychiatric reason for impulsivity; anosognosia versus denial; and aprosodia versus flat affect from depression.

- Analysis of pathogenesis. The CCM must consider, and adequately address, potential physiological contributions of neurological conditions to psychiatric presentation, for instance the contribution of Parkinson's disease pathophysiology to a depression syndrome.

- Adaptation of diagnostic and treatment algorithms. The algorithms followed by the collaborative care team should allow for flexibility in screening, assessment, and treatment, to address the variability of neuropsychiatric conditions and the contribution of underlying medical/neurological conditions. In most cases, addressing pathogenic factors should be part of the treatment of the presenting neuropsychiatric syndrome. Following the examples above: the treatment of Parkinson's disease with dopaminergic enhancers will likely improve the mood symptoms; a patient with depression and comorbid apathy may need a stimulant added to his antidepressant regimen.

- Response to treatment in the collaborative care setting. Due to brain lesions that increase their vulnerability to psychiatric disorders such as depression, neuropsychiatric patients may present increased rates of treatment-resistance or partial response. In addition, given the high prevalence of cognitive deficits, neuropsychiatric patients may not be able to fully engage in the intervention or treatment plan. See section "The Intervention—Modifications for Neuropsychiatry" that discusses proposed modifications to the CCM intervention for neuropsychiatric patients, such as those individuals with comorbid depression and cognitive dysfunction.

The Neuropsychiatric Patient with Alzheimer's Disease

The considerations above focus on the adaptation of the CCM for the care of neuropsychiatric patients with depression. The model can be also adapted for the treatment of other highly prevalent neuropsychiatric conditions such as Alzheimer's disease (AD). AD and related disorders affect nearly 6 million Americans.[18,19] A recent study by the Alzheimer's Association predicted that the total health care and long-term care costs for individuals diagnosed with dementia are projected to increase from $277 billion in 2018 to $1.1 trillion in 2050.[19] Many AD patients have comorbid medical and psychiatric conditions,

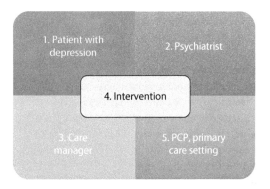

FIGURE 36-3. Components of the classic collaborative care model.

including depression, and thus would benefit from an interdisciplinary approach to care.[18] Over the past few decades, a focus on collaborative care has highlighted the ways in which interdisciplinary teams can impact how patients with dementia and their families navigate the progression of this chronic disease. CCMs that treat mental health and some neurodegenerative diseases like dementia can exist within primary care or specialized care settings. While these models have variability in implementation, many take interdisciplinary approaches, pairing an MD with a nurse or physician assistant who facilitates medical monitoring, while a social worker offers skills-based counseling, caregiver support, and resource management. Given the increasing incidence of AD and other dementias, and the availability of a growing body of literature applying the CCM specifically to this clinical area, we describe below these studies in some detail.

A 2015 Cochrane review[20] analyzed 13 RCTs of case management approaches offering integration of care and home support for 9615 people with dementia. The case management groups were significantly less likely to be institutionalized (admissions to residential or nursing homes) at 6 months and at 18 months. However, there was no difference in the number of hospital admissions at 6, 12, and 18 months and no significant effects on mortality. There was some evidence of reduced caregiver burden and depression, as well as increased caregiver well-being. Limited evidence indicated case management was more effective at reducing behavior disturbance in individuals with dementia. The case management intervention groups received significantly more community services, and there was some evidence that case management reduced the total cost of services at 12 months and the total per-patient expenditure over 3 years. Given the methodological heterogeneity between the studies, further research is necessary to understand which components of case management are associated with improvement in the various outcomes.

A 2017 RCT tested the effectiveness and safety of dementia care management (DCM), a model of collaborative care for the treatment of people with dementia and their caregivers in primary care.[21] DCM was administered in patients' homes by six nurses with specific qualifications in dementia care, supported by a computer-based intervention-management system (IMS). The nurses conducted an in-depth assessment of the 407 participants, and the IMS generated an individualized preliminary intervention task list. This list was reviewed in a weekly interdisciplinary case conference with a nurse, a neurologist or psychiatrist, a psychologist, and a pharmacist. The resulting list of intervention tasks was summarized in a semi-standardized informational letter, which was reviewed with the patient's PCP to establish a treatment plan. During the first 6 months, the nurse conducted six home visits carrying out the intervention tasks in close cooperation with the caregiver, the PCP, and health care and social service professionals. During the next 6 months, the study nurse monitored the completion of all intervention tasks. DCM significantly decreased behavioral and psychological symptoms of dementia and caregiver burden compared to usual care. Patients in the active group also had a higher chance of receiving anti-dementia drug treatment.

Substantial improvements in quality of care and quality of life were reported in an RCT investigating the effectiveness of a dementia guideline–based disease management program.[22] This program, led by care managers, was designed for 238 patient-caregiver pairs at nine intervention clinics for more than 12 months. The intervention was based on a chronic care model and included adherence to 23 dementia guideline recommendations, Internet-based caregiver self-management support, and provider education. The care managers performed in-home assessments, developed and initiated action plans, and reported to PCPs and designated health care and community agencies. Ongoing follow-up took place on an as-needed basis, and in-home reassessments took place every 6 months. Adherence to recommended guidelines was significantly higher in the intervention group than in the control group.[22] Overall quality of care, patient and caregiver quality of life, and social support were better in the intervention group than in the usual care group.

Callahan et al.[23] conducted a controlled clinical trial of 153 older adults with AD and their caregivers. The intervention, based on a CCM, consisted of comprehensive assessments and caregiver education and support. Intervention patients received 1 year of care management by an interdisciplinary, nurse practitioner led team. If appropriate, care managers facilitated access to PCPs and enrollment in Alzheimer's Association community programs. Patient progress was monitored through an Internet-based tracking system, and nonpharmacological protocols were applied as appropriate during each face-to-face visit. Care managers provided regular updates to the PCPs. Intervention patients had significantly fewer behavioral and psychological symptoms of dementia at 12 months and at 18 months, and were more likely to receive cholinesterase inhibitors and antidepressants. Their caregivers had significantly reduced distress and depression. There were no reliable group differences in death rates, hospitalization rates, nursing home placements, activities of daily living, or cognitive function.

LaMantia et al.[24] reported on the Aging Brain Care Medical Home (ABC MedHome), a population health management program based on a CCM for dementia and depression. The program served 1650 adult patients in Indiana, of which 77% had depression and 30% had dementia. The care team consisted of care coordinator assistants, the care coordinator, and a social worker. The study used an enhanced medical record software to track patient health outcomes, including hospital and emergency rooms visits. The team assessed the cognitive, behavioral, and psychological state of each patient and developed an individualized care plan which was reassessed and adjusted as necessary. For example, if a patient required hospitalization, the team provided hospitals with relevant information and devised a post-discharge care plan within 72 hours of hospital discharge. Throughout the follow-up period, the team supported the individual's PCP in management of comorbid conditions. There was a 50% reduction in depressive symptoms in 66% of the patient population with high depression scores. Stress symptoms were decreased by 50% in 51% of caregivers of individuals with dementia.

Maximizing Independence (MIND) at Home, a community-based, interdisciplinary, care coordination intervention was established to address the needs of 289 care recipient (CR) patients with dementia and mild cognitive impairment and their caregivers.[25] The care team consisted of informal caregivers (i.e., family members or other unpaid individuals) associated with a nurse and a geriatric psychiatrist. CR-caregiver dyads were randomized to the intervention or augmented usual care group. Intervention dyads received an individualized 18-month care coordination intervention delivered by nonclinical community workers. The intervention plan (MIND model) included referrals to dementia services within the community, caregiver dementia education and skill-building, and ongoing evaluation by an interdisciplinary team. There was a reduction in the total percent of unmet caregiver needs in both groups, with nonsignificant between-group differences. There were no significant differences between groups in most caregiver burden measures, depression, or QOL. There was a modest but clinically significant reduction in self-reported hours caregivers spent with the CR in the intervention group. The MIND care coordination model was also assessed by Samus et al.[26] to determine whether this intervention delays transition from home to a nursing care facility and reduces unmet needs in geriatric patients with memory disorders. Three hundred and three community-dwelling elders were randomized into the intervention group, which received an 18-month care plan based on the MIND model (described above) or a usual-care group. The intervention group demonstrated a significant delay in time to all-cause transitions from home. The adjusted hazard of leaving the home was decreased by 37% in the intervention group compared with the usual-care group. The intervention group had significant reductions in the proportion of unmet needs related to legal or advance care planning, as well as safety.

As evident from the studies described above, there is heterogeneity in existing interventions, study designs, sample size, and outcomes. However, a key component of the reviewed studies is the collaboration of team members. Galvin et al.[18] postulate that the successful execution of various team member roles is at the center of a thriving CCM. The usual roles of each team member are described as follows:

Physician: Makes initial diagnosis and initiates care plan, evaluates patient needs, and makes referrals to community resources.

Nurse practitioner (NP) or physician assistant (PA): Reevaluates the care plan, provides ongoing assessment and follow-up, coordinates care with other disciplines, and provides intervention education to patients and families. In some care models, the NP or PA may be responsible for initial diagnosis and initial care plan drafting.

Registered nurse (RN): In addition to performing routine vital signs and memory and cognitive function screenings, the RN provides patient and caregiver phone follow-up and assists with outpatient referrals. In models where there is no NP or PA, the RN also serves as the care coordinator or manager.

Social worker (SW): Provides patient and caregiver education and referrals to community resources, assists with transition to alternate care settings and provision of psychotherapy and counseling services.

Medical assistant: Coordinates paperwork for office visits and assists patients and their caregivers with completing paperwork and scheduling. Provides the care team with feedback on patient's compliance, may be responsible for conducting simple screening tests.

Neuropsychologist: Conducts and interprets neuropsychological testing, and may play an important role in initial diagnosis, provision of counselling and therapeutic services, and delivery of cognitive remediation or retraining programs.

Health educator: Completes surveys with patients and their families, maintains a library of health information for the care team and coordinates the distribution of educational materials for patients and caregivers.

Occupational and physical therapists: Provide home safety assessments, activities of daily living (ADL) evaluations, cognitive skills training, patient fall prevention and balance training, caregiver education, and driving evaluations.

Speech and language therapists: Can also provide cognitive skills training.

Cognitive Screening in the Primary Care Setting

Another key element, that may be common to the implementation of different CCMs in dementia, is the need for valid tools to screen for and diagnose cognitive disturbances that can be efficiently used by clinicians from the primary care team. The most widely studied cognitive screening instrument is the Mini-Mental State Examination (MMSE). A cut point of 23/24 or 24/25 (score considered "positive"/"negative") is appropriate for most populations.[27] It does have limitations, however—it can be considered too long to administer in busy primary care practices, and the score may be highly influenced by educational level and other sociodemographic variables. In addition, patients may have learned some of its items, given its frequent use.[28] Other screening instruments include Clock Drawing Test, Mini-Cog Test, Memory Impairment Screen (MIS), Abbreviated Mental Test (AMT), General Practitioner assessment of Cognition (GPCOG), Short Portable Mental Status Questionnaire, Free and Cued Selective Reminding Test, 7-Minute Screen, Telephone Interview for Cognitive Status, and Informant Questionnaire on Cognitive Decline in the Elderly.[27,28] The Montreal Cognitive Assessment (MoCA) has become widely used and can be helpful in the screening of mild cognitive impairment (MCI). Another screening instrument that, like the MMSE and MoCA, evaluates patients' performance in several domains (attention, memory, verbal fluency, language, visuospatial) is the Addenbrooke's Cognitive Examination-Revised (ACE-R). This test and its latest version, the ACE-III, are considered highly sensitive and specific for detecting dementia.[29]

The Neuropsychiatrist

What are possible roles for a neuropsychiatrist (or, as discussed below, the behavioral neurologist) in the workflow of the CCM? There may be situations where either the PCP or general psychiatrist embedded in the CCM may access the neuropsychiatrist for a curbside consultation, rather than referring a patient to specialty neuropsychiatry clinic. This increases access to subspecialty neuropsychiatric expertise in the primary care setting and reduces

---

BOX 36-1 Possible Roles of the Neuropsychiatrist in the CCM Algorithm

Consultant for relevant cases (e.g., depression + cognitive disorder + neurological illness)

Participation in CCM team meetings
Curbside consultations via phone or electronic medical record
Face-to-face consult with patient and feedback to primary team

Follow-up of patient in neuropsychiatric clinic and return to primary care team when stable.

---

wait time for patients seeking such services. There is also opportunity for the neuropsychiatrist to periodically participate in collaborative care team case conferences. For instance, cases that would benefit from a consult can be presented to the neuropsychiatrist monthly. The participation of the neuropsychiatrist in the CCM would result in the gradual development of a shared understanding of the principles relevant to the treatment of neuropsychiatric patients. Lastly, similar to the classic model of care delivery, the neuropsychiatrist can see a patient in a one-time, face-to-face consultation and refer back to the primary care practice for implementation and monitoring of their recommendations.

For patients where cognitive dysfunction or disorders are the main concern, the behavioral neurologist may assume the same roles assigned above to neuropsychiatrists, such as curbside consultant, consultant at periodic primary care team meetings or case conferences, and face-to-face consultant.

Care Manager and Additional Team Members

To facilitate timely access to consultations and referrals for neuropsychiatric patients, the collaborative care team would need to include—or work closely with—additional disciplines commonly utilized in neuropsychiatric care, including neuropsychologists and cognitive rehabilitation therapy (CRT) specialists. The nuclear CCM team members, and especially the care manager, would benefit from learning basic principles of CRT to use with patients. For instance, there is often a reciprocal influence between emotional and cognitive symptoms, so patients with co-occurring mood disorders and cognitive dysfunction will likely benefit from both evidence-based psychotherapies for mood and CRT. Because there can be a substantial overlap between these two interventions, care managers should be trained in basic CRT principles to help address these patients' needs efficiently and efficaciously.

The Intervention—Modifications for Neuropsychiatry

Modifications of the CCM in the neuropsychiatric context must account for limitations in patients' ability to participate in and respond to treatment plans including medical and mental health education, psychotherapy, and medication. Alongside emotional and behavioral disturbance, these patients often present

with cognitive dysfunction—this could take the form of memory problems, executive dysfunction, deficits in insight/awareness—that impacts engagement and adherence. Educational materials and psychotherapy instructions must be simple and clear, and repetition may be required to facilitate learning. Caregivers may also be included as coaches or facilitators. See Chapter 10, "Psychosocial Interventions in Neuropsychiatry," for detailed examples of the adaptation of psychosocial interventions for neuropsychiatric patients.

COLLABORATIVE CARE IN OTHER CLINICAL SETTINGS RELEVANT TO NEUROPSYCHIATRY

The potential list of relevant settings could be quite extensive. Given the high degree of collaboration between neuropsychiatrists and neurologists in the care of patients, we comment on the possible implementation of the CCM in neurology clinics. Lastly, we discuss its possible adaptation in inpatient settings.

Neurology Clinics

Many patients with neurological disorders, especially those without other prominent medical comorbidities, use their specialty neurology clinic as their primary source for medical care. For example, a young adult woman with MS, who otherwise is healthy, may not have ongoing contact with her designated PCP but will attend periodic visits at her MS center. This, in addition to the well-characterized elevated prevalence of psychiatric disorders in neurological illnesses makes the possibility of adapting the CCM to specialty neurology clinics very intriguing. A CCM would increase detection of psychiatric comorbidities through routine screening and provide a stepwise algorithm to address these patients' needs in the same setting as their neurological care.

Such adaptation would involve changes in the roles and routine practices of the relevant providers, and the addition of a care manager to the clinical team. Clinics should implement regular screening for the most prevalent psychiatric disorders in each neurological illness and use a standardized algorithm for a designated team member—likely the care manager—to respond to patients' intake data. The neurologist would take on a role analogous to that of the PCP in the primary care CCM and manage—along with other members of the collaborative care team—the more common psychiatric comorbidities. The neuropsychiatrist would take on the role of consultant and peer-educator, while also continuing to evaluate and treat more complex patients. The majority of patients seen in consultation, and brief follow-up if necessary, could be referred back to the collaborate care team and neurologist for management. The neuropsychologist, in addition to performing detailed neuropsychological evaluations, could deliver briefer cognitive screening tools and educate team members in their delivery and interpretation. A templated and customizable cognitive rehabilitation intervention, to be delivered by the care manager or other team member in a group workshop or one-to-one, would also be of benefit.

The literature addressing the implementation of the CCM in specialty clinics is nascent but promising. A literature review of models for treating depression in specialty medical settings showed that integrated care for depression can improve depression outcomes.[30] Six RCTs, one nonrandomized controlled trial, and two uncontrolled trials of integrated care for depression in oncology, infectious disease, and neurology clinics were assessed. Depression outcomes differed by comorbid diagnoses and/or specialty medical setting in which the integrated care model was implemented. There were significant reductions in depressive symptoms among patients receiving integrated care compared to usual care in most of the studies (seven out of nine), especially in oncology clinics. Results suggest that selecting specific components of the CCM for different patient populations could provide the most beneficial outcomes. In addition to helping patients and caregivers, the integration of mental health interventions in neurology clinics may assist the neurology care team too, as they may feel supported in addressing mental health disturbances that before—even in the cases when they identified them—felt they lacked the adequate tools to treat them.

Patten and colleagues[31] assessed the feasibility and effectiveness of implementing a depression management program in an MS clinic. Patients with a positive depression screen were referred to a case manager and offered depression management. After 6 months, patients in the intervention showed lower rates of major depression than controls, based on the Mini Neuropsychiatric Interview (MINI). The MS CARE model for chronic pain and depression in MS patients[32] employs a lead care manager (licensed clinical social worker) who coordinates all aspects of care, alongside a team of MS providers and consultants (psychologist, psychiatrist, and pain expert). The model uses systematic tracking strategies and telephone consultations to enhance existing comprehensive care provided to MS patients, with particular emphasis on equipping patients with evidence-based skills for self-managing pain and depression. The MS CARE model has been effective in reducing pain intensity and interference—a measure of the extent to which pain hinders engagement with physical, cognitive, emotional, cognitive, and recreational activities, as well as sleep and enjoyment in life,[33] fatigue, disability, and depression severity. The use of telephone consultations improved access to care and adherence to treatment plans.

Inpatient Medical and Neurological Services and Intensive Care Units

While the CCM has traditionally been employed in primary care and other outpatient settings, there is broad application potential for neuropsychiatric patients in inpatient and acute care settings. The need for psychiatric care in hospital inpatient settings is clear—patients with neuropsychiatric disorders are at higher risk for hospitalization, and research has shown that depression in admitted patients often goes undetected and untreated. A recent review of the literature found that 33% of hospital patients may be experiencing symptoms of depression, which is, in turn, associated with worse prognosis and functional outcomes, as well as higher rates of readmission.[34] The literature suggests that hospitalizations themselves, especially in acute and critical care settings, may have a long-lasting impact on emotional well-being after discharge. In particular, exposure to the physical and psychological stressors of treatment for a

critical medical condition—including invasive procedures and prolonged hospital stays—has been associated with long-lasting depression, anxiety, and PTSD.[35,36]

The CCM offers a potential tool for preventing and treating psychiatric comorbidities in medical and neurological admissions. In the inpatient setting, routine and standardized screening by a collaborative care team could identify patients with and at-risk for psychiatric conditions, resulting in faster response via a therapeutic algorithm and access to specialized care when needed. As in the specialty clinic-adapted CCM discussed above, the care manager could respond to initial intake data in order to coordinate an appropriate response from the care team. The patients' primary provider/hospitalist could manage the majority of cases, with the support of social workers and psychologists for education and supportive counseling where appropriate. For difficult cases involving complex neurological or medical comorbidities, neuropsychiatrists, consultation-liaison psychiatrists, and behavioral neurologists could be available for either curbside consults with the care team or face-to-face consultations with patients. Similar to the neuropsychiatrist's role in analogous models in other settings, neuropsychiatrists could efficiently provide their expertise in crafting a treatment plan and refer the patient back to the collaborative care team for follow-up and ongoing management. Care managers could continue to follow patients after discharge to monitor for the emergence of psychiatric symptoms related to the hospitalization.

The feasibility of implementing collaborative and integrated care in inpatient and acute care settings is well-studied. For example, the ThedaCare community health system, a network of 7 hospitals and 32 clinics in Wisconsin, used nurses as the primary care managers. Alongside a physician and pharmacist, the care managers participate in treatment planning with the patient and family within 90 minutes of hospital admission. Since piloting the program in its medical-surgical unit in 2007, ThedaCare has reported positive outcomes in patient satisfaction and length of stay.[37] Systematic implementation of multidisciplinary care has been associated with reduced health care utilization and cost in inpatient settings. Okere and colleagues[38] compared a pharmacist-hospitalist collaborative (PHC) model and multidisciplinary rounds (MDR) to standard care and found that patients in either intervention had reduced length of stay compared to patients receiving usual care, with no difference in all-cause readmission rates. In 100 patients hospitalized on an inpatient stroke unit, a novel collaborative model incorporated an advanced practice nurse as the care manager in collaboration with a hospitalist physician. Patients receiving daily care management from NPs had greater improvements in post-stroke medical outcomes and reported a more positive subjective experience of care.[39]

Limited research has considered the role of inpatient collaborative care on psychiatric outcomes. A trial comparing collaborative care to usual care in cardiac units studied 175 admitted patients with depression diagnosed by systematic screening. The study used a care manager to carry out a hospital-based depression intervention including education and treatment coordination. Patients receiving the intervention were significantly more likely to continue receiving appropriate psychiatric treatment upon discharge.[40] In the post-acute care setting, multidisciplinary care teams have been successfully utilized to mitigate the cognitive and psychological impact of an intensive care unit (ICU) stay. The Critical Care Recovery Center at Indiana University utilizes a team comprised of a nurse, social worker, critical care physician, neuropsychologist, and psychometrician. The model replicates the major features of a CCM (described above) including support for clinical decision making, reliable screening and assessments, longitudinal monitoring, and coordination of treatment resources.[35] In the context of inpatient care, rapid access to specialty psychiatric care through the incorporation of a neuropsychiatrist in the CCM has the potential to improve outcomes during hospitalization and after discharge.

Summary and Key Points

- Chronic disease management principles are well established in diabetes, cancer, and heart disease, among others. They include emphasis on the role of patients and families in treatment, collaboration among the health care team, standardized screening and evidence-based treatment, patient self-monitoring and treatment adjustment, and focus on patient functional status in the community.
- The benefits of collaborative care models (CCMs) in mental health care have been increasingly recognized given the chronic nature of mental illness and the shortage of mental health clinicians. The CCM integrates behavioral health resources into primary care, and has been shown to improve mental and overall health outcomes in over 80 RCTs.
- Important benefits of the CCM include coordinated team care, patient engagement, systematic screening, evidence-based treatment, standardized processes and workflows, preventive care, and effective resource utilization.
- Adapting the CCM to neuropsychiatry provides an opportunity to expand access to neuropsychiatric care. Important modifications to the original model for depression in primary care include awareness of atypical clinical presentations in neuropsychiatry, analysis and treatment of pathogenetic factors, adaptation of diagnostic and treatment algorithms, and addressing treatment-resistance and partial response.
- Heterogeneous case management approaches are well-studied in neurodegenerative diseases, including Alzheimer's disease and related dementias, and generally include a physician extender and social worker who supplement care provided by the MD. The literature on collaborative care interventions in these populations shows positive effects on patient's and caregiver's quality of life, behavioral and neuropsychiatric symptoms, and health care utilization.
- In an adapted CCM for neuropsychiatric patients, the neuropsychiatrist serves as a consultant for relevant cases through participating in CCM team meetings, curbside consultations via phone or EMR, and/or face-to-face consults with patients followed by referral back to the primary care team for ongoing management. The addition of cognitive rehabilitation therapy specialists and training is important to address co-occurring mood disorders and cognitive dysfunction in neuropsychiatric disorders. Additional considerations include increasing caregiver engagement in treatment and providing simple, clear patient education.
- Future directions: Further studies are needed to optimally adapt the CCM to serve the needs of neuropsychiatric patients. The CCM may also be adapted to neurology clinics, inpatient services, ICUs, where commonly occurring comorbid neuropsychiatric disorders should be routinely screened for and addressed. The limited literature studying team-based care in specialty clinics, inpatient units, and acute care shows promise in reducing health care utilization, psychiatric symptoms, and medical complications.

Multiple Choice Questions

1. Which of the following incorrectly describes the advantages of collaborative care models in behavioral health care?
   a. Stepped care decreases health care utilization by involving specialists to provide face-to-face care early on, when the patient has initial complaints of depression.
   b. Reducing variability in workflows improves early identification and efficient treatment.
   c. Increasing knowledge about preventive risk factors and accountable care arrangements are shifting the U.S. health care landscape to focus on prevention.
   d. Patient engagement in treatment plans and shared decision making lead to better outcomes and response to treatment.
   e. Access to teams of specialists in primary care promotes efficient and quality care for patients with complex medical and psychiatric illnesses.

2. Which of the following is not a component of the original CCM as studied in the IMPACT trial for depression in the primary care setting?
   a. Primary care physician
   b. Psychiatrist
   c. Care manager
   d. Patient with depression
   e. Caregiver or family member

3. Which of the following are important considerations to the CCM for neuropsychiatric patients?
   a. Relationship between pathophysiology and psychiatric symptoms in screening and treatment
   b. Atypical clinical presentations of psychiatric disorders due to neurological disorders

    c. Inability of neuropsychiatric patients, by definition, to engage in treatment plans without caregiver support

    d. a and b

    e. All of the above

4. Which of the following accurately describes an adaptation of the CCM beyond the primary care setting in the literature?

    a. The dementia care management model involved a computer-generated intervention plan carried out by nurses in collaboration with caregivers, PCPs, and social service professionals. Patients in the active group had decreased behavioral and psychological symptoms and decreased likelihood of receiving anti-dementia drug treatment.

    b. The Aging Brain Care Medical Home (ABC MedHome) utilized care coordinators, care coordinator assistants, and social workers to create and implement individualized care plans. There was a 50% reduction in depressive symptoms in the patients with lower baseline depression scores.

    c. The MS CARE model for chronic pain in MS patients employed a case manager who coordinated MS providers and consultants to systematically track outcomes and engaged patients to increase self-management of pain and depression. The use of telephone consultations increased adherence to treatment plans.

    d. Maximizing Independence at Home (MIND) paired patient-caregiver dyads with a nurse, geriatric psychiatrist, and nonclinical community workers in an intervention that included referrals to dementia services, caregiver education and skill-building, and ongoing evaluation by the interdisciplinary team. There were significant between-group (intervention vs. augmented usual care) differences in caregiver burden, depression, and quality of life.

    e. The ThedaCare Health System in Wisconsin utilizes a multidisciplinary team comprised of a physician, pharmacist, and care managers who participate in treatment planning with admitted patients within 90 minutes of admission. The model resulted in improved patient satisfaction with increased length of hospitalization.

Multiple Choice Answers

1. Answer: a

Stepped care involves implementing the most effective, least resource-intensive interventions first, and bringing in more intensive specialist treatment only when necessary. By promoting self-management and avoiding the use of expensive specialty care where possible, stepped care results in a more efficient allocation of limited health care resources.

2. Answer: e

While caregiver engagement is an important aspect of adapting the CCM to treat neuropsychiatric disorders, and has been part of later CCM versions, caregivers were not explicitly built into the initial CCM for depression in the primary care setting. The components of the original model are patient with depression seeking care in the primary care setting, psychiatrist providing support to the primary care provider and face-to-face consults as necessary, nurse or psychologist care managers who provide cognitive behavioral and problem-solving therapies, the primary care provider, and the intervention to change care delivery and bring together the members of the collaborative care team.

3. Answer: d

The CCM must consider and address the physiological contributions of neurological disorders to the clinical presentation. Addressing the underlying neurological pathology is an integral part of the treatment plan, as neurological and psychiatric symptoms are inextricably linked in many neuropsychiatric patients. Complex medical/neurological comorbidities may result in higher rates of treatment resistance or partial response, necessitating the involvement of a caregiver or family member in some, but not all, cases.

4. Answer: c

In the DCM model, patients in the active intervention were *more* likely to receive anti-dementia drug treatment. In ABC MedHome, depressive symptoms were reduced 50% in the patients with the *highest* depression scores. In the MIND intervention, between-group differences for caregivers were *not significant*. The ThedaCare intervention resulted in *decreased* length-of-stay in the inpatient hospitalization setting.

References

1. Von Korff M, Gruman J, Schaefer J, et al. Collaborative management of chronic illness. *Am Intern Med*. 1997;127:1097-1102.

2. Wagner EH, Austin BT, Von Korff M. Organizing care for patients with chronic illness. *Milbank Q*. 1996;74(4):511-544.

3. Agency for Healthcare Research and Quality. Case Example #7: Cherokee Health Systems. Rockville, MD: Agency for Healthcare Research and Quality. Available at http://www.ahrq.gov/ncepcr/primary-care-research/workforce-financing/case-example7.html.

4. Wun YT, Lam TP, Goldberg D, et al. Reasons for preferring a primary care physician for care if depressed. *Fam Med*. 2011;43(5):344-350.

5. Unützer J, Katon W, Callahan CM, et al. Collaborative care management of late-life depression in the primary care setting: a randomized controlled trial. *JAMA*. 2002;288(22):2836-2845.

6. Reiss-Brennan B, Kimberly DB, Carter D, et al. Association of integrated team-based care with health care quality, utilization, and cost. *JAMA*. 2016;8:826-834.

7. Rossom RC, Solberg LI, Parker ED, et al. A statewide effort to implement collaborative care for depression: reach and impact for all patients with depression. *Med Care.* 2016;54:992-997.

8. Unutzer J, Katon WJ, Fan MY, et al. Long-term cost effects of collaborative care for late-life depression. *Am J Manag Care.* 2008;2:95-100.

9. Gawande A. Cowboys and pit crews. *The New Yorker.* May 26, 2011.

10. Rubak S, Sandbæk A, Lauritzen T, Christensen B. Motivational interviewing: a systematic review and meta-analysis. *Br J Gen Pract.* 2005;55(513):305-312.

11. Anstey K, Mack H, Cherbuin N. Alcohol consumption as a risk factor for dementia and cognitive decline: meta-analysis of prospective studies. *Am J Geriatr Psychiatry.* 2009;7:542-555.

12. Fortney J, Unützer J, Wrenn G, et al. A tipping point for measurement-based care. *Psychiatr Serv.* 2017;68(2):179-188.

13. Goroll A, Schoenbaum S. Payment reform for primary care within the accountable care organization: a critical issue for health system reform. *JAMA.* 2012;308(6):577-578.

14. Hunkeler EM, Katon W, Tang L, et al. Long term outcomes from the IMPACT randomised trial for depressed elderly patients in primary care. *BMJ.* 2006;332:259-263.

15. Woltmann E, Grogan-Kaylor A, Perron B, et al. Comparative effectiveness of collaborative chronic care models for mental health conditions across primary, specialty, and behavioral health care settings: systematic review and meta-analysis. *Am J Psychiatry.* 2012;169:790-804.

16. Gilbody S, Bower P, Fletcher J, et al. Collaborative care for depression: a cumulative meta-analysis and review of longer-term outcomes. *Arch Intern Med.* 2006;166:2314-2321.

17. Erb J, Benedetto E, Cartreine J, et al. Delivering depression care: services and settings. In: Barsky AJ, Silbersweig DA, eds. *Depression in Medical Illness.* New York, NY: McGraw-Hill Education; 2017:360.

18. Galvin J, Valois L, Zweig Y. Collaborative transdisciplinary team approach for dementia care. *Neurodegener Dis Manag.* 2014;4(6):455-469.

19. Alzheimer's Association. Alzheimer's disease facts and figures. 2018. Chicago, IL: Alzheimer's Association. Available at https://www.alz.org/alzheimers-dementia/facts-figures.

20. Reilly S, Miranda-Castillo C, Malouf R, et al. Case management approaches to home support for people with dementia. *Cochrane Database Syst Rev.* 2015;1: CD008345.

21. Thyrian JR, Hertel J, Wucherer D, et al. Effectiveness and safety of dementia care management in primary care: a randomized clinical trial. *JAMA Psychiatry.* 2017;74(10):996-1004.

22. Vickrey B, Mittman B, Connor K, et al. The effect of a disease management intervention on quality and outcomes of dementia care. *Ann Intern Med.* 2006;145(10):713.

23. Callahan CM, Boustani MA, Unverzagt FW, et al. Effectiveness of collaborative care for older adults with Alzheimer disease in primary care: a randomized controlled trial. *JAMA.* 2006;295(18):2148-2157.

24. LaMantia M, Alder C, Callahan C, et al. The Aging Brain Care Medical Home: preliminary data. *J Am Geriatr Soc.* 2015;63(6):1209-1213.

25. Tanner J, Black B, Johnston D, et al. A randomized controlled trial of a community-based dementia care coordination intervention: Effects of MIND at home on caregiver outcomes. *Am J Geriatr Psychiatry.* 2015;23(4):391-402.

26. Samus Q, Johnston D, Black B, et al. A multidimensional home-based care coordination intervention for elders with memory disorders: the Maximizing Independence at Home (MIND) pilot randomized trial. *Am J Geriatr Psychiatry.* 2014;22(4):398-414.

27. Moyer VA. Screening for cognitive impairment in older adults: U.S. Preventive Services Task Force recommendation statement. *Ann Intern Med.* 2014;160(11):791-798.

28. Yokomizo JE, Sanz Simon S, Machado de Campos Bottino C. Cognitive screening for dementia in primary care: a systematic review. *Int Psychogeriatr.* 2014;26(11):1783-1804.

29. Abd Razak MA, Ahmad NA, Chan YY, et al. Validity of screening tools for dementia and mild cognitive impairment among the elderly in primary health care: a systematic review. *Public Health.* 2019;84-92.

30. Breland J, Mignogna J, Kiefer L, et al. Models for treating depression in specialty medical settings: a narrative review. *Gen Hosp Psychiatry.* 2015;37(4):315-322.

31. Patten S, Newman S, Becker M, et al. Disease management for depression in an MS clinic. *Int J Psychiatry Med.* 2007;37(4):459-473.

32. Drakulich A. Applying a collaborative care model to the treatment of chronic pain and depression. *Pract Pain Manag.* 2017;18:1.

33. Amtmann D, Cook KF, Jensen MP, et al. Development of a PROMIS item bank to measure pain interference. *Pain.* 2010;150:173-182.

34. IsHak WW, Collison K, Danovitch I, et al. Screening for depression in hospitalized medical patients. *J Hosp Med.* 2017;12(2):118-125.

35. Kahn BA, Lassiter S, Boustani MA. Critical care recovery center: an innovative collaborative care model for ICU survivors. *Am J Nurs.* 2015;115(3):24-31.

36. Rattray JE, Hull AM. Emotional outcome after intensive care: literature review. *J Adv Nurs.* 2008;64(1):2-13.

37. Toussaint J. Writing the new playbook for U.S. health care: lessons from Wisconsin. *Health Aff.* 2009;28(5):1343-1350.

38. Okere A, Renier C, Willemstein M. Comparison of a pharmacist-hospitalist collaborative model of inpatient care with multidisciplinary rounds in achieving quality measures. *AJHP.* 2016;73(4):216-224.

39. Wood JG. Collaborative care on the stroke unit: a cross-sectional outcomes study. *J Neurosci Nurs.* 2016;48(5):E2-E11.

40. Huffman JC, Mastromauro CA, Sowden GL, et al. A collaborative care depression management program for cardiac inpatients: depression characteristics and in-hospital outcomes. *Psychosomatics.* 2011;52(1):26-33.

37

Individualized Psychotherapy with the Neuropsychiatric Patient

Barbara Schildkrout

INTRODUCTION

The goal of medicine is to alleviate pain and suffering, and to that end, neuropsychiatry has focused on identifying pathology, establishing diagnostic criteria, and developing treatments. Yet many patients who are in distress have symptom constellations that do not meet the criteria for a defined neurological condition or *DSM* diagnosis. This chapter discusses presentations that fall outside the realm of current diagnostic categories, including dimensional symptoms, variations in neuropsychological functioning that may lead to difficulties even when within the range of normal, and problems that are traditionally considered to reside in the domain of psychology, although they emerge from the materiality of brain—internal mental conflicts, relationship difficulties, and maladaptive patterns of behavior.

While the care of all patients rests on a clinician's understanding of the patient as an individual, this is especially true when treating patients who do not meet criteria for diagnostic categories and, therefore, whose treatment is less prescribed. Designing and delivering treatments for an individual patient's specific health situation requires complex problem solving. The foundation for this personalized treatment within a clinician-patient relationship is an understanding of each patient as a whole person, including an appreciation for the patient's neuropsychological difficulties, personality and temperament, personal history, cultural background, family, and social situation. In addition, each person is more than the sum of parameters that are shared by all human beings; each person is unique in ways that are challenging to define scientifically. An awareness of the biological basis of individuality at every scale (from molecule and cell to personality and behavior) may help clinicians to conceptualize how individuals can be both similar and unique.

Even identical twins who begin with identical genomes have become different individuals by the time they are born.[1,2] While clinicians recognize that all patients begin life with certain inherent characteristics, the tendency of clinicians is to focus on postnatal forces that shape individuals from childhood through adulthood such as birth trauma, parental influence, nutrition,

toxic exposure, education, religious and cultural forces, socio-economic factors, and other life experiences including environmental enrichment, illness, loss, abuse, emotional and/or physical trauma, and therapy. Patients and their families are able to report about these factors and describe their experiences. From a practitioner's frame of reference, it is possible to assemble a large-scale narrative of how a person's life has unfolded, including how this particular individual has emerged from a unique life history. However, many aspects of individuality are largely established by the time of birth, as a result of genetic, epigenetic, developmental processes and also random (stochastic) molecular events.[2]

Because understanding the individual patient is fundamental to the psychotherapies and also to personalized medicine, the first portion of this chapter outlines some of the complex biological mechanisms that contribute to shaping individuality at the level of the brain; while the scientific study of brain-behavior differences between normal individuals is in its infancy, this discussion may serve as an introduction to this important area of investigation. The second portion of this chapter discusses elements of psychotherapy—with a focus on psychodynamic psychotherapy—with neuropsychiatric patients. Chapter 10 discusses cognitive-behavioral therapy and other psychosocial approaches in neuropsychiatry.

INDIVIDUALITY AND THE BRAIN

Introduction

While optimal clinical care rests on an appreciation of the patient's individuality, it has been difficult to define the scientific parameters by which normal human beings differ from one another. During the modern scientific era, psychiatrists, psychologists, social workers, and philosophers have utilized a variety of concepts in trying to define individual differences, including temperament, personality, intelligence, mechanisms of defense, multiple intelligences, and attachment theory.[1,3,4] For cognitive functions as well as for other specific spheres of mental activity, neuropsychologists have developed standardized tests and validated measures to help in describing particular elements that, taken together, contribute to a person's particular combination of strengths and weaknesses.

During this same historical timeframe, investigators in the neurosciences have focused more on commonalities of normal human behavior—motor and sensory functions, language, sleep and dreaming, executive functioning, and so on—in order to discern general principles of brain organization and function from which all human behaviors emerge.[5] Central to this ongoing endeavor has been the approach of utilizing "natural experiments" that arise when a patient presents with well-defined, focal pathology that reveals underlying brain organization. In many instances it has been possible to define what is different about a person who has a brain disorder, however, studying what makes healthy people different at a neurological level has been more challenging.

The Human Genome Project completed the first maps of the human genome in 2003, decoding the genetic material that distinguishes *Homo sapiens* from other species and individual human beings from one another. Since then, major advances in neuroimaging, nanotechnology, data analysis, genome editing, biological engineering such as optogenetics, and other techniques for molecular manipulation have made it possible for researchers to investigate the biology of individual cells, individual organisms, and individual brains over time, revealing more clearly the complex and dynamic origins of individual differences.[6]

For example, by using advancements in functional imaging and functional connectivity computation, some scientists have been able to distinguish individuals by their functional connectome patterns across scanning sessions and between task and rest conditions.[7] In addition, there have been studies of functional connectivity differences between normal human beings while reacting to real-world situations.[8] For instance, normal individuals display different degrees of trait-level paranoia. When listening to an ambiguous narrative while in an MRI scanner, subjects display patterns of functional connectivity that reflect differing degrees of paranoia; moreover, these patterns correlate with the degree of paranoia in the subjects' free recall of the narrative after the scanning session.[8] Even while remaining within the range of normal, these differences, nevertheless, may represent vulnerabilities in certain situations and may affect the trajectory of a person's life and relationships.

Biological Mechanisms Shaping Individuality

In addition to genetic endowment—which is unique to each individual except for monozygotic twins who share germinal DNA—numerous, nongenetic factors influence the trajectory of each individual's development from conception through adulthood and senescence. Some of the forces that contribute to individuality at the level of the cell, synapse, circuit, and large-scale, multisynaptic functional organization across the brain are briefly summarized in this section: stochastic events at the molecular level; embryonic development and neurogenesis; neuroplasticity; functional, wide-scale organization; and epigenetic processes.

Genetic Endowment

Although humans only differ from one another by substantially less than 1% of genetic material, differences in genetic inheritance of germ cell DNA are fundamental in determining the ways in which individuals are unique. In some instances, there may be a direct Mendelian relationship between a genetic variant and a trait or phenotype. However, more often variations in phenotype are a consequence of multiple small differences in a very large numbers of genes, with some rare variants making larger contributions. In addition, the regulation and expression or suppression of genes is crucial in influencing phenotype. Indeed, most genetic variation between individuals is found in regulatory rather than the protein-coding regions (the genes) of the genome. Studies have shown that even genes that code dominant Mendelian traits are not always expressed.[9]

Stochastic Molecular Events

At the level of the cell and the molecules within the cell, research has shown that single cells that are genetically identical and grown in the same environment nonetheless show variability in gene expression and large phenotypic variations.[6] At the level of an organism, it has been demonstrated that, even when genetically identical fruit flies are reared under identical conditions, up to 25% of the genes in the adult fruit flies are differentially expressed.[6]

The variations from individual to individual are believed to arise in part from the differences in randomly determined (stochastic) molecular events within the cell, even when those cells began as genetically identical. Stochastic molecular events are random; while the outcomes of any process involving stochastic molecular events may be studied, they cannot be predicted from readily measurable variables. One example would be a genetic mutation in which one base pair is altered in a DNA sequence. Clinically, it has been demonstrated that an early mutation of this kind in somatic (non-germ-line) cells in some instances may account for monozygotic twins who are discordant for psychiatric disorders.[10-12]

Another example of a stochastic molecular event is the influence of environmental factors on whether or not a gene is turned on. Gene regulation is complex and is influenced not only by inheritance but also by both the extracellular and the intracellular environment. One determining factor for gene expression is the binding of a transcription factor to the DNA promotor region for that gene. Transcription factors, present within the cell, are proteins that control when and how efficiently a gene is *transcribed* into messenger RNA that, in turn, is *translated* into a sequence of amino acids that make up other proteins (including the transcription factors themselves). If there are only a small number of transcription factor molecules for a particular gene within the cell nuclei, then, statistically, that gene will be turned on only occasionally and in different cells at different times.[6,13]

Once a particular gene is turned on in a cell, that cell begins development in a direction that is different from cells in which the gene has not been turned on (or in which the gene is turned on at a different point in development); these differences may be amplified by feedback mechanisms or environmental conditions in the complex dynamic system of the cell. One example of this is the process by which different organ systems develop.

All of the body's cells contain the same DNA; the differences between liver cells, a muscle cells, and neurons are determined by different sets of genes being turned on or silenced.

While stochastic molecular events may seem "chaotic," they generate the diversity upon which adaptation depends; the availability of diverse options allows for selection.[2] While stochastic events affect DNA in all cells, this chapter focuses on gene expression in the cells of the brain.

Embryonic Development of the Brain and Neurogenesis

Stochastic molecular events are fundamental to embryonic development, a complex dynamic process that is neither predetermined nor externally directed according to a set plan. While it is possible to predict that a brain will emerge by the end of embryonic development, each brain will be different in ways that cannot be predicted.

A simple outline of the embryonic development of the human brain and central nervous system includes the early establishment of the fundamental axes of the organism and the production of neural stem cells that migrate to different positions within the region that will become the brain. Between postconception weeks 3 and 6, approximately 100 billion neural stem cells are produced, and these are the source of all the cells that will make up the brain—glial cells and the different types of neurons. Once differentiated from the stem cells, neurons migrate to various positions in the developing brain and then synapse, each with 1000 or more other neurons. Over time, there is increasing specialization and stabilization of differentiated brain regions. By the end of gestation, the neocortex has been formed—a six-layered structure populated by numerous cell types—and the major neural networks as well as the area organization of the neocortex have been established.[14,15]

This process by which neural progenitor cells differentiate, migrate, and interconnect to form the brain and central nervous system is also notable for being one that is self-organizing. Each step sets the stage for steps that follow. Variations in gene expression are crucial to the unfolding process as they code for the proteins that are the active agents. Proteins (including transcription factors) act as signals to turn genes in other cells on or off; the nature of these signals depends upon the various concentrations and mixtures of these proteins that are present in the microenvironment of a cell.[14,15] In addition to this complex cascade of signals determined by protein gradients (the spatial distribution of a protein in gradually increasing or decreasing concentrations), other forces also contribute to the dynamic of embryonic brain development, including cellular competition for limited essential resources in the environment (such as neuron growth factor) and changing sensitivity to external influences as neurons mature. All of these as well as other intracellular and extracellular factors (including the central role of glial cells) influence a cell's fate (including possible death), axon growth, synapse formation, and system-wide organization—in short, the development of a unique brain. After birth, human brain development continues into adolescence and beyond, but neural stem cells only persist in two areas, the olfactory bulb and the hippocampus.[16] Hippocampal neurogenesis is important in memory formation early in life, and therefore may be central to an individual's conscious and nonconscious identity. It is not yet clear whether neurogenesis in the hippocampus continues throughout life.

Neuroplasticity

The term "neuroplasticity" refers to the ability of the brain to change in response to experience. In the 1940s, Donald Hebb postulated that when a neuron repeatedly fires at a synapse with another neuron, the connection between the two is strengthened.[17] This theory is often summarized by the phrase "cells that fire together, wire together." While this statement oversimplifies a complex process, it does capture a fundamental notion—structure and function are deeply linked. Hebbian theory focuses on synaptic plasticity, one aspect of neuroplasticity; it refers to alterations in the strength and efficiency of synaptic transmission in response to experience. When a postsynaptic neuron fires within a certain number of milliseconds of the presynaptic neuron, the connection between the two neurons is strengthened. When the timeframe is longer, the connection between the two neurons is weakened. The timeframes that are relevant vary from brain region to brain region.[18]

Synaptic plasticity is one element of neuroplasticity in which functional alterations in network transmission are accomplished by many different mechanisms, including active structural and metabolic changes in the dendritic spines, the timing and amount of neurotransmitter release, and the number and sensitivity of postsynaptic neuroreceptors. Neuroplasticity may be viewed over different timescales (from microseconds to years) and at different scales (from the individual synapse to a circuit or brain region). Changes in excitability of a neuronal circuit and the number of neuronal connections it makes leads to neural circuits being modified, strengthened or weakened, reshaped, and pruned which translates into brain regions shrinking, enlarging, or even brain functions shifting location. For example, researchers have demonstrated the topographic reorganization of somatosensory areas of the cortex following amputated digits or limbs.[19,20]

The effects of practice, learning, and experience also have been described.[21]

The complex mechanisms involved in neuroplasticity are being actively studied; gaps in understanding remain.[18] For example, on its own, the Hebbian mechanism for synaptic change cannot account for feedback about outcomes to the system when those outcomes occur on a more than millisecond timescale; one hypothesis that would allow for feedback suggests that additional signals change the neuroplastic responsivity of the circuit. Also, the important roles played by glial cells[22] and cell adhesion molecules are being elucidated.[23]

The synaptic organization of the brain is continuously being reworked as part of the ongoing processes of learning and instantiating of experience, compensating for areas of weakness, and reorganizing in response to injury. In addition, the networks that are actively engaged shift from moment to moment. By applying advanced computational approaches to functional connectivity data, it has been possible to describe large-scale, multisynaptic organizational networks in the brain; these brain-wide, self-organizing networks appear to be universal. However, of great importance to the topic of individuality is the observation that these networks vary to some extent from individual to individual in their strength, stability, and variability and may be reflective of the real-world capabilities of the different people.[24]

Epigenetics

Epigenetic mechanisms are another route by which experience changes an individual and, in this case, may affect offspring as well, although this has not been firmly established.[25] The term "epigenetics" refers to heritable molecular alterations and processes that influence gene expression without changing the DNA coding sequences themselves. Epigenetic effects in humans have been demonstrated through studies of the Dutch Hunger Winter, an approximately 5-month period of severe malnutrition (between 400 and 800 calories/day) that resulted from a German blockade of the Netherlands toward the end of World War II. Excellent medical record-keeping allowed for studies of children who were in utero at different stages of pregnancy during this Dutch famine. Long-term health effects were significant and independent of birth weight; they included increased incidence of type 2 diabetes, cardiovascular disease, schizophrenia, addiction, obesity, and accelerated cognitive aging.[26]

Early adverse life events such as abuse have been linked to later development of anxiety disorders, depression, and post-traumatic stress disorder. Other factors that have been linked to epigenetic alterations and risk for disease include toxic exposure, smoking, chronic disease, and overnutrition. These factors influence gene expression by altering the three-dimensional configuration of the DNA molecule; some configurations will make certain genes unavailable for transcription while others will make them more available for transcription as when regulatory regions are placed in closer proximity to coding regions. Changes in the three-dimensional configuration of DNA may be accomplished by the addition of methyl groups to the DNA molecule or by the alteration of histone groups around which DNA is coiled. Other epigenetic mechanisms involve alterations in noncoding RNAs, which lead to changes in gene expression. These molecular changes are part of normal biology, allowing for adaptation—providing a mechanism by which cells are responsive to the cellular environment.[25,27] Epigenetics lies at the intersection of gene and environment, including prenatal environment.[27]

The Fundamental Paradigm

The biological mechanisms that contribute to individuality (discussed above) may be better understood by placing them within the larger framework by which neuroscientists conceptualize the central nervous system. Any scientifically explanatory paradigm must account for the brain's capacity to reliably support essential aspects of biological functioning (such as body temperature, respiration, circadian rhythm) and stable aspects of behavior (such as language, vision, consciousness, and an enduring sense of self) while also being able to respond to changing conditions, both external (threat, novelty) and internal (hunger, fatigue), both momentary (loud noise) and longer term (learning). Any broad conceptualization of the brain also must account for millisecond-long pre-attentive processing (for sensory stimuli, shifts in attention) as well as, at the other end of the time spectrum, developmental changes that take place over

a lifetime. In other words, any fundamental paradigm must include mechanisms for continuity and reliability and for the maintenance of homeostasis, physiologic stability in the face of changing circumstances.

The reigning paradigm views the brain as a complex dynamical system—a system that is comprised of extraordinarily complex physical components (molecules, cells, simple and multisynaptic circuits, depending upon the scale at which it is viewed) that is in a state of constant change.[28] In addition, such a system is not organized by external forces and rules but is spontaneously self-organizing and nonlinear in its behavior; while it is possible to study complex dynamical systems (other examples: climate, chemistry, the stock market), the robust interplay of the physical elements that comprise the system, along with the role of randomness, make it impossible to predict precisely the outcomes of such a system. These outcomes are said to be emergent; they are novel, coherent, and not predictable from the properties of the component elements of the system (consider water resulting from the combination of two hydrogen atoms with one oxygen atom).

According to this fundamental paradigm, an individual is continuously changing at every scale in the interest of adaptation and is shaped by experience, including by the way one's life is lived—levels of stress, trauma, education, relationships.[29,30] Subjective experience, decision making, learning, creativity, indeed all human behaviors are viewed as emergent properties of brain. Individuality is also viewed as emergent.[2]

PSYCHOTHERAPY WITH THE INDIVIDUAL PATIENT

Introduction

At the heart of every diagnostic and treatment endeavor is the establishment of a therapeutic relationship in which the clinician gains an appreciation for the individual patient. This is foundational to effective clinical care. The relationship between the unique practitioner and the unique patient helps the diagnostic process itself by facilitating trust and aiding the clinician's grasp of the manner in which the patient communicates symptoms. It is important for clinicians to understand their patients' life circumstances, values, approaches to decision making, past experiences with health care systems, personal ideas about what causes disease, expectations regarding medical care, and also their fears and hopes.

It is within this context that the diagnostic process takes place, a process in which the neuropsychiatric practitioner has a dual role. As a clinician, part of the task is to focus on making a diagnosis, which involves determining whether the patient's difficulties fit into known disease categories. In other words, rather than highlighting how each person is unique, a diagnosis essentially describes how people with a particular disease are similar—for instance, their likely symptoms, clinical course, risk factors, and possible complications. While thinking diagnostically, which is to say categorically and in medical terms, the skilled clinician simultaneously needs to understand how a disease might manifest in this particular individual and how this specific patient might communicate his/her experience to the practitioner. This is especially relevant for neuropsychiatric illness, the manifestations of which result from an interaction between the patient's premorbid personality, cognition, and psychology, as well as the disease process and localization.

The practitioner-patient relationship also forms the foundation for individualization of treatment. There is much variation in the degree of personalization of treatment that is possible, some conditions allowing for more than others. While there may be only limited number of efficacious treatment choices for some diseases, for others there is the possibility of selecting which is best for the particular patient. Consider someone with the diagnosis of major depression. This patient has numerous available options for treatment, including combinations of the following, among others: numbers of antidepressant agents from a variety of different classes, rTMS, ECT, vagal nerve stimulation, bright light therapy, and psychosocial therapies utilizing many possible approaches. In designing a treatment strategy, the experienced clinician utilizes evidence-based approaches that are applied creatively for each patient: medication doses may be adjusted for those patients who are rapid-metabolizers; bright light therapy may be added when there is a seasonal patterns of symptom exacerbation; patients who are introspective may prefer insight-oriented psychotherapy to CBT; psychosocial considerations may make certain options unworkable, such as daily travel for rTMS.

The most highly personalized aspect of treatment is the clinician-patient interaction itself, whether this is as part of any practitioner-patient relationship or within a specific, evidenced-based psychotherapy framework. A particular clinician and a particular patient may interact in a wide variety of ways within the professional context; moment-to-moment flexibility is involved. A therapeutic relationship is the central aspect of virtually every clinical situation and a positive working relationship between the clinician and the patient contributes significantly to outcome, including by influencing compliance and placebo/nocebo effects on therapeutic outcome.[31,32]

The clinician's particular neuropsychological functioning is also a central aspect of the clinical encounter. Practitioners rely on both the conscious and nonconscious aspects of brain functioning to engage in careful observation, diagnosing, problem solving, and interacting therapeutically with the patient, the family, the care-team, and medical systems. The neuropsychological functioning of each practitioner is fundamental to performing the extraordinarily complex tasks involved in delivering competent health care. Some key factors include a clinician's ability to employ metacognition, to be self-reflective, and to utilize reactions to the patient (countertransference) as data.

Psychosocial Treatment

The dynamically oriented psychosocial therapies focus on a patient's subjective experiences, personal narrative, and sense of meaning—experiences that may not have been previously fully articulated by the patient. This can be considered as the most personal and individualized end of the treatment spectrum. See Chapter 10 for further review of psychosocial interventions in neuropsychiatry. In a psychosocial treatment, the clinician's therapeutic interactions are based on a complex understanding of the specific patient, including matters such as the patient's cultural background, personal beliefs and values, social supports, neuropsychological makeup, modes of communicating, and family history. While an understanding of the unique patient informs any practitioner-patient interaction, this understanding is a major focus of treatment in the office of a psychiatrist or psychotherapist.

In the psychosocial therapies a clinician may treat an individual patient, a patient with his/her significant other(s), or a group of patients. The treatment interactions occur within a carefully defined context—scheduled times, a defined length and frequency of sessions, and a place that is private, safe, and comfortable. Treatment approaches vary as they are based on different psychological models and clinical evidence, but each method aims to address maladaptive behavioral patterns and/or patient distress. For each patient, the treatment is individualized, some approaches offering more options for flexibility than others. For example, supportive therapy allows a broad range of possible therapeutic interactions while dialectical behavioral therapy utilizes a "manualized" approach. In practice, many clinicians utilize aspects of various treatment approaches, depending upon the patient and also the practitioner's own expertise.[33]

In contrast to the process by which a clinician gathers information in order to make a diagnosis, the psychosocial therapies as well as the interpersonal aspects of any clinical encounter call for a different way of observing, listening to, and thinking about the patient—the clinician tries to see the world through the patient's eyes, to understand the patient's worldview and ways of experiencing life events. The practitioner works to develop an understanding of the patient as an individual, including an empathic grasp of the patient's relationships, formative life events, and the meanings that these have to the patient. This process has been called the psychological formulation.

A crucial part of this formulation and of understanding the individual is taking into account the patient's neuropsychiatric functioning (including, e.g., executive functioning, social cognition, and fluid intelligence). Practitioners regularly think about the neuropsychological functioning of their patients when treating for a neurological or a major mental disorder, but consideration of neuropsychological functioning is also important with the population of patients who seek help but who have not been diagnosed with a neurological disease and who do not meet criteria for a mental disorder. Strengths and weaknesses in neuropsychological functioning comprise fundamental aspects of the patient's capabilities in dealing with life situations and, therefore, are key factors in understanding any patient's adaptive capacities.

All psychosocial therapies are based on certain foundational ideas, including the following:

- Every person is unique;
- The patient and the professional will work toward establishing a relationship of mutual trust;
- The patient is motivated to attend therapy sessions and wants something from the meetings; the patient's motivations may evolve over time;
- The patient and clinician discuss the goals of treatment as well as the plan for attaining those goals.

While the criteria listed above form the basis of any clinician-patient relationship, psychosocial therapy is distinct in certain respects. It is most often utilized for problems that involve the patient's patterns of behavior, subjective experiences, and/or interpersonal relationships. The individual patient is most often the subject of the treatment. The patient has the relevant information while the clinician has an approach, a framework, a methodology, and insights into the patient that the patient may not yet have. The patient and therapist are partners in the creative, problem-solving aspect of the treatment; solutions emerge from the content of the individual's life experiences and inner thoughts. Optimal treatment, therefore, requires the patient to have certain additional neuropsychological capacities.

In addition to life circumstances that allow for meetings or for an alternative treatment format (such as telepsychotherapy), the following additional neuropsychological, cognitive capabilities are needed for an individual to most effectively engage in a psychosocial treatment:

- An initial willingness to meet with a therapist (as opposed to being unwilling to consider the possibility of engaging in psychotherapy)
- With time, an awareness of having some kind of problem (as opposed to denial, externalization, anosognosia, or paranoia)
- Motivation to think about making changes and being open to learning new things about the self and others (in contrast to apathy, or lack of a sense of agency, or a fixed set of inflexible ideas)
- Ability to see the therapist as a potentially helpful person (rather than feeling distrust, paranoia, or grandiose and invulnerable, or disbelief in mental health problems and treatment)
- Willingness and ability to communicate with the therapist (in contrast to being secretive, distrustful, or having significant difficulties with communication)
- Trustworthy efforts toward honest communication (as opposed to manipulation)
- Some ability to be self-reflective (in contrast to lacking insight)
- Some types of psychosocial therapy also require
  - True psychological mindedness
  - Active curiosity about one's self
  - Robust capacity for insight

The focus of psychosocial treatment is at the highest levels of human neuropsychological functioning: putting feelings and thoughts into words; being self-reflective; generating meaning and narrative; relating to another human being in an open, honest manner; having one's verbal and nonverbal communications understood; being valued and cared about; and engaging in collaborative problem solving. When a patient does not have a neurological or psychiatric diagnosis, treatment requires that one learn who the patient is as a unique individual and then formulate an understanding of the patient's particular difficulties, taking into account the patient's neuropsychological functioning. Then, the task for the therapist is to guide the patients to discover new ways of understanding themselves and the problems that have been the focus of the treatment. Other therapies focus more on the acquisition of skills to modulate the response to events and emotions. All of these approaches may lead to new ways of thinking and behaving, with an eventual amelioration of the patient's difficulties.

The Patients

The patients who seek out the services of a neuropsychiatrist or other clinical neurosciences provider are individuals who are suffering in some way and who have framed their problem as neurological and/or psychiatric or as one that has a psychological component or consequence. They may have decided this on their own, with the urging of friends and family, or because they have been referred by another clinician. Some of these patients will have a diagnosable neuropsychiatric disorder; others will have no clearly diagnosable neurological disease and will not meet the full criteria for a mental disorder as defined by our current diagnostic systems, perhaps other than the less-specific adjustment disorder—having an unusually difficult time coping with an external stress.

Individualized psychotherapy may be helpful to patients who do have neuropsychiatric diagnoses and to their family members. Families of neuropsychiatric patients may benefit from psychotherapy for help in adapting to a family member's illness—understanding the basis for a patient's limitations or changed behavior, managing feelings about possible genetic implications, altered responsibilities and relationships within the family, amended expectations regarding the future. Many neuropsychiatric patients will lack fundamental capabilities that are needed for a traditional psychotherapeutic approach, including alertness, ability to be attentive, capacity for learning (memory), the ability to communicate through language (including sign), awareness of deficits, motivation, and emotional control. But many patients with neuropsychiatric disease will be able to utilize psychotherapy to help in adapting to deficits, managing symptoms and feelings about chronic illness, or dealing with life-threatening disease. For these patients, individualized treatment requires the clinician to engage the individual's strengths while maintaining awareness of the patient's areas of deficit. Other chapters in this textbook address specific treatment approaches for patients with neuropsychiatric disorders.

Those patients who seek consultation for neuropsychiatric symptoms but have no clear neuropsychiatric diagnosis also are in need of treatment that is tailored to the individual. These patients include the following (discussed more fully below):

- Patients who have a medical diagnosis that has not as yet been diagnosed/identified.
- Patients who do not meet criteria for a *DSM* diagnosis but have dimensional neuropsychiatric symptoms. Dimensional symptoms are those that are found in the population in varying degrees of severity.
- Individuals who have cognitive functioning that is "within the normal range," however, the patient's profile of abilities is a mismatch with his/her own aspirations and/or life circumstances.
- Individuals with relationship conflict, internal emotional turmoil, stressful, tragic, or traumatic life events and/or circumstances.

1. Patients who have a neuropsychiatric disturbance that has not yet been diagnosed.

CASE VIGNETTE 37.1

Just after his 60th birthday, John went to see a therapist for the first time in his life. His chief complaint was that he had been "feeling mildly depressed," and he assumed that his feelings about turning 60 were the cause. He had found himself focusing on regrets. Why had he become an accountant rather than pursuing a career that would have utilized his "creative, musical, and theatrical talents?" Why hadn't he "taken more risks" before settling down to marry and have children? He had been feeling bored with accounting and had been spending work hours on his cell phone, repeatedly checking the news and also watching pornography on his office computer. John had diminished interest in socializing or in attending concerts and theatrical performances, and he said that his wife had been complaining that he was increasingly impatient. The patient wanted to begin psychotherapy, hoping to come to terms with the

life choices he had made. After several months without improvement in his mood or level of motivation, John decided to try medication. The patient began to feel somewhat more positive after taking sertraline, and he elected to stop psychotherapy.

A year later, the patient's wife contacted the therapist with follow-up information. John had been asked to take a leave of absence from work because of declining work performance. He had repeatedly failed to return client phone calls, missed important filing deadlines, and had become argumentative with the administrative staff in the office. He was increasingly apathetic. Out-of-town friends had visited and found John to be "a changed person." At the urging of these friends, the patient had a thorough neurological workup and was diagnosed with early behavioral variant frontotemporal dementia.

Behavioral changes may be a consequence of normal development, personal growth, and/or life experiences, including trauma. An understanding of the individual patient helps in differentiating these situations from those in which the behavioral changes are a consequence of neuropsychiatric disease. When a patient exhibits changes that are inconsistent with long-standing patterns of behavior, this is referred to as a change in personality and signals the possible presence of a neuropsychiatric condition.

In any practice population, some patients will have neuropsychiatric condition that has not yet been diagnosed. In some instances, the patient is presenting very early in the course of a disease and the symptoms are subtle, intermittent, and/or too nonspecific to be diagnosed. In these cases, it only may be in retrospect, that the patient's symptoms are recognized to have been the very first signs of a particular disease. Consider, for example, depression, constipation, and fatigue that may be prodromal in Parkinson's disease. Another example is the subjective experience of "trouble with memory" that may be reported by patients well before neuropsychological testing documents any memory disturbance associated with the onset of dementia. Clinicians sometimes refer to individuals such as these as the "worried well," but this term fails to adequately value the patients' subjective experiences and anxiety-producing concerns. It is important for health care professionals to keep in mind the possibility that patients such as these might be presenting very early in the course of an emerging disease. Ongoing monitoring of these patients may be indicated.

Other patients may have a neuropsychiatric condition that is undiagnosed because the diagnosis, although possible to make, has been missed. Diagnostic errors are extremely common in all areas of medicine.[34] Rare diseases are apt to be misdiagnosed, but, more often, common diseases are missed when they present atypically. In patients who already have a neuropsychiatric disorder, the onset of a new disease may be missed if the patient's worsening state or latest symptoms are attributed mistakenly to the established diagnosis. An additional, significant source of misdiagnosis in the neuropsychiatric patient population is physician bias with patients who have psychiatric presentations or a history of mental illness. Especially prevalent is misattribution error or blaming the patient for his/her illness.[35] But neuropsychiatric patients also are vulnerable to other biases in clinical thinking that delay accurate diagnosis.[35]

Patients with covert, as yet undiagnosed disorders are not likely to robustly respond to psychosocial treatment alone. However, some relief may ensue from the treatment of secondary depression or anxiety while the underlying neuropsychiatric condition remains undiagnosed and untreated. Some patients may have diseases that medical science has not yet defined. When this is suspected, referral to the Undiagnosed Disease Network of the National Institutes of Health could be initiated.[36]

2. Patients who do not meet criteria for a *DSM* diagnosis but have dimensional neuropsychiatric symptoms.

CASE VIGNETTE 37.2

Emily was a 26-year-old, married, female graduate student who was ambitious and had succeeded at being accepted to a prestigious graduate program. Nonetheless, her chief complaint was "I feel like a failure." She also reported that she had been feeling some anxiety and that she didn't have her "usual morning zest."

During a year of individual psychotherapy, it was possible to discern a complex, layered set of factors that had led to the patient's anxiety and negative feelings about herself at the time of presentation. She did not meet criteria for a *DMS* disorder other than adjustment disorder.

Most clearly problematic was the state of the Emily's marriage. On the one hand, the patient felt she had a "wonderful husband" who was intelligent, witty, and warm, and also shared her interests and values. On the other hand, she felt "inexplicably unhappy" in the marriage and believed it was somehow her fault. Over time Emily began to recognize that a destructive interpersonal dynamic was taking place in which the husband was subtly devaluing her while his overt behavior was caring. "He needed me to be the ineffective one, so that he could be the strong one."

It was not difficult for the patient to take on this role in the psychological dynamic of her marriage. She had long-standing feelings of inadequacy. She had an identical twin who "had more friends than I did and who also was smarter and prettier." While school was easy for the Emily's twin, Emily had to work hard in order to do well. She drove herself to excel.

Emily never understood how she and her sister could be "identical" and yet so different from one another. Emily had always assumed that she must be "doing something wrong." Emily's twin sister had been born first and had weighed more than she had. Emily also reported that she initially had a low Apgar score.

Emily had neuropsychological testing only when she found herself falling behind in college courses that had long reading lists. The testing revealed that she had superior intelligence but also slowed reading speed and some difficulties in executive functioning.

Emily had been attracted to her husband in part because of his ability to "get things done," his organizational acumen, his efficiency, and his willingness to be of help to her when she was "running behind" or have trouble getting started on a project. He also took on certain tasks for the couple such as paying bills and keeping their social calendar. With time, however, Emily's husband began to resent this role. In addition, he was having difficulties in his career and began to buoy his self-esteem by casting himself as the effective one while viewing Emily as "lazy." This mirrored the way Emily felt about herself.

Even after having learned the results of her neuropsychological testing, Emily continued to berate herself for not reading faster, responding more promptly to emails, or keeping track of her keys. Given that she was someone who was able to grasp complex ideas and generate creative approaches to difficult problems, she could not grasp why she still failed to solve these "simple" problems in her own daily functioning.

Effective psychotherapy with Emily required an understanding of the specific psychological dynamics of her marriage as well as the childhood experiences that had set the stage for the patient to be vulnerable to this kind of couple's relationship. In addition, the therapist formulated that Emily's difficulties in reading and with executive functioning may have been the result of hypoxia at birth in the setting of unknown intrauterine factors that led to her having a lower birth weight than her sister. These likely formed a biological basis for why Emily had to work hard in order to excel at school—in contrast to her twin—and substantially contributed to shaping her sense of self. Emily did have areas of cognitive weakness, but she also had superior intelligence, determination, and stamina.

It took some time in therapy for Emily to accept the idea that there were some aspects of her cognitive functioning that she could not change, even with hard work; it took longer for her to accept that these limitations did not mean that she was lazy or inadequate, and that they certainly were not a "reason" to be treated badly by her husband. Emily's self-esteem improved, her anxiety lifted, and she turned her creative energies to her marriage. Emily persuaded her husband to engage with her in couple's therapy and to work on the problematic psychological dynamics in their relationship.

Studies of non-patient populations have found that nonclinical or subthreshold anxiety, depressive symptoms, psychotic symptoms, and manic symptoms occur at significant levels in the general population.[37] Furthermore, these traits are associated with documented dysfunction, meaning that they are not insignificant in terms of the life trajectories for the individuals involved.[38] Indeed, it is increasingly recognized that many mental symptoms occur in a dimensional pattern, that is, within a spectrum of severity, some individuals being severely affected while others are mildly affected. In addition, certain individual symptoms (such as auditory hallucinations), heretofore considered to be pathological by definition, may occur in the general population and may not represent serious pathology, particularly when they are not part of a constellation of symptoms that defines a *DSM* diagnosis.[39]

Given that many individuals have neuropsychiatric symptoms but do not meet criteria for a *DSM* diagnosis, and that *DSM* is not neuropsychiatrically based, clinicians need to adopt a nuanced, flexible, and individualized way of thinking about patients who fall outside diagnostic categories. Taking into account the patient as a whole person, symptoms may be viewed within the broader context of a patient's life, as part of a process of adaptation that may be more or less effective. Understanding neurobehavioral circuitry and processes also will help in conceptualizing and addressing conditions that are neurobiologically based.

3. The individual has cognitive strengths and weaknesses that are within the normal range in neuropsychological testing but have important functional impact.

Elspeth was a 38-year-old lawyer who presented for a consultation because "life wasn't turning out the way she had expected," and "someone" had told her that she might have autism spectrum disorder. She had been an outstanding student in high school, college, and then law school, after which she worked successfully for several years at a top law firm, mainly doing research for senior attorneys. But Elspeth had always dreamed of being her own boss, so she left the firm and started her own general law practice. The practice was never successful.

Elspeth was married to a software engineer and had one friend with whom she jogged and went to the movies. "I've always had one or maybe two friends that I would do things with, but we would never really *talk*." Elspeth said that she felt "unhappy and isolated" and didn't understand why she "hadn't been able to live up to my potential."

Neuropsychological testing revealed that Elspeth was very bright but had areas of relative weakness in social cognition and aspects of executive function, such as initiating. She did not meet criteria for autism spectrum disorder. These findings helped Elspeth to better understand the difficulties she had been having in attracting clients to her practice and keeping on top of her work without the structure that had been provided by school and the law firm at which she had worked. She also gained some insight into why she felt lonely.

Elspeth's professional aspirations did not match well with her cognitive profile. Also, she did not know how to engage at a deeper level with other people. Elspeth decided to pursue psychotherapy in order to work on how to chart a course forward.

Clinicians intuitively form an impression of their patients' abilities in various areas of neurocognitive functioning. Generally, formal neuropsychological testing is ordered when: there is a lack of clarity about whether a patient's behavioral difficulties might stem from an underlying deficit in some area of cognitive functioning; a significant cognitive problem is suspected; areas of cognitive weakness/strength need to be better defined or documented; obtaining a baseline measure of cognitive functioning is advisable.

Neuropsychological testing is a standard approach for measuring an individual's strengths and weaknesses in various areas of neuropsychological cognitive functioning (see Chapter 7). Neuropsychologists utilize specific test batteries that have been validated and standardized. There is wide variation in the population in all areas of neuropsychological cognitive functioning. Because "the normal range" is a statistical notion, having cognitive abilities that lie in this normal range does not rule out the possibility that the individual has neuropsychological difficulties that are a significant contributing factor in shaping their lives. Testing results are most useful when interpreted within the context of the patient's history, personal narrative, and current occupation or ecological context. At times the patient's problem may lie in a mismatch between the individual's strengths and weaknesses and the tasks and demands required within the environment.

While large discrepancies between verbal and performance IQs may be indicative of a learning disability, the vast majority of people are somewhat better in some cognitive realms than in others. This discrepancy can be problematic when individuals struggle with certain subjects in school or tasks in life and feel bewildered about the reason for this or judge themselves harshly. An individual with cognitive functioning in the normal range nonetheless may not have capacities that are required to attain wished-for goals; frustration or a sense of failure may result. Other individuals may be successful in one setting or situation but not in another.

When individualizing any treatment, it is important to keep in mind variations in the fundamental cognitive capabilities, including attention, social cognition, executive functioning, decision making, fluid intelligence, visuospatial skills, ability to utilize abstract thinking, memory, insight, judgment, and so on. Awareness of the patient's capabilities in these various areas will not only contribute to the clinician's understanding of the patient's difficulties but will also inform problem solving, guiding in the choice of interventions so as to build upon the patient's strengths and address or compensate for limitation(s). In addition, taking into account the nature of the patient's cognitive profile may facilitate a practitioner's interactions with the patient.

4. Individuals with relationship conflict, internal emotional turmoil, stressful, tragic, or traumatic life events and/or circumstances.

Human experience involves complex psychological challenges as one moves from childhood, through adulthood, and into advancing age. Each person is faced with the difficult task of creating a life that includes relationships, work, pleasure, and a sense of meaning. Inevitably, individuals will encounter difficulties, which may be external (such as traumatic loss) and/or internal (such as conflict about an important decision); at times, they may experience considerable distress and feel motivated to discuss their situation with a professional. Psychotherapy may be very helpful to these individuals.

CONCLUSION

Individuality is not a straightforward reflection of one's upbringing in concert with genetic endowment. We now understand that complex molecular and neurophysiological events are involved in the generation of unique human beings, though we do not yet fully understand these processes. Nonetheless, in grasping how deeply rooted individuality is in biological events, our appreciation for the depth of individual differences may be enhanced and thereby encourage clinical and research inquiry on this topic.

One of the challenges for neuropsychiatry has been to link psychological conceptualizations to the findings of neurologists and neuroscientists. Progress at this frontier of neurology and psychiatry has narrowed gaps in our thinking about constructs such as brain and mind, innate and learned, inherited and environmental. The study of individuality may provide an opportunity to further interrogate areas of overlap between the traditional domains of psychiatry and neurology.

Even with the current limitations of our knowledge in this arena, the implications of patient individuality in clinical practice are significant, informing thinking about problems that all neuropsychiatric clinicians face. Understanding of the patient as a unique individual is the basis of designing creative solutions with patients who are symptomatic but do not meet criteria for our standard diagnostic categories. In addition, at the molecular and cellular levels, practitioners regularly take into account molecular markers (e.g., on brain tumor cells) and genetic determinants of diseases such as Huntington's disease, neurofibromatosis, Wilson's disease, substance use/abuse, hemochromatosis; with more information it is possible to include genetic risk factors for disorders such as autism spectrum disorder, frontotemporal dementia, and Alzheimer's disease. At the level of the whole person, practitioners incorporate into their thinking the complex information about an individual patient's particular sociocultural environment, relational network, and neuropsychology; these will affect the patient's symptom experience and disease presentation, as well as treatment choice, compliance, and response to treatment.

Relationships rest upon our capacity to grasp the nature of individuality in one another; clinical care is centered upon this as well. And now it is gradually becoming possible to study individuality at a biological level. This capability may allow us to develop biomarkers for psychopathology; measures of the effectiveness of therapies; and it may allow the enhancement of neuropsychiatrically informed psychotherapy, and the improvement of treatment for neuropsychiatric conditions.

Summary and Key Points

- All human beings are remarkably similar, yet no two people are exactly alike. Understanding the neuropsychiatric uniqueness of each patient is important for designing and implementing personalized treatment.

- Our diagnostic categories do not capture the myriad variations in individuality that, in conjunction with personal circumstance, may be sources of human suffering; patients who lie outside the standard diagnostic categories require treatment that calls on clinicians to understand the person's neuropsychological individuality.

- Many patients do not meet criteria for a neurological disease or major mental disorder but may be suffering with dimensional symptoms; variations in neuropsychological functioning that interfere with personal goals; emotional problems related to internal conflicts, relationship difficulties, maladaptive patterns of behavior, and/or stressful circumstances.

- Individuality is present by the time of birth, having emerged after fertilization through cell division, neuronal differentiation, central nervous system formation, and the establishment of major neuronal networks. Beyond initial genetic endowment, some of the underlying mechanisms that are involved in the generation of individuality include stochastic molecular events, epigenetic forces, neurogenesis, and plasticity.

- Individuality has been difficult to study at the neurological level. Modern functional connectivity studies in humans may make it possible to help identify individuals by their functional connectome fingerprints and to study differences between individuals in real-life situations. Research in this arena may help us to better align theories about human behavior and brain function.

- Through understanding that individuality arises from complex biological forces, clinicians and researchers may begin to answer some fundamental questions that arise in all treatments: What is the nature of change? What can be changed? How and how much can it be changed?

Multiple Choice Questions

1. Which traits, typically thought to be associated with neuropsychiatric diagnoses, are distributed in the population in a dimensional fashion, with some people being minimally affected while others are more severely affected?
   a. Depression
   b. Social communication difficulties
   c. Psychotic/Schizotypal traits
   d. Only a and b
   e. All of the above

2. What are some basic requirements that would enable a patient to make use of psychosocial treatment?
   a. Good personal hygiene
   b. Awareness of having some sort of problem
   c. Viewing the clinician as a potentially helpful person
   d. b and c
   e. All of the above

3. When seeing a patient in psychosocial treatment it is important to keep in mind the possibility that the patient might have a medical diagnosis that has been missed. What factors

may contribute to a missed or delayed diagnosis?

a. The patient's medical condition exhibits a long prodromal period during which symptoms are nonspecific.

b. The patient has a common disease that is presenting in an atypical fashion.

c. The patient has a rare disease.

d. The patient has a long-term psychiatric condition, and the referring practitioner misattributed the patient's new symptoms to this mental disorder.

e. All of the above.

4. Which of the following factors contributes to individuality?

a. Germinal DNA in the fertilized ovum

b. The availability of transcription factors within the cells of the developing fetus

c. Early genetic mutations in fetal cells

d. a and c

e. All of the above

Multiple Choice Answers

1. **Answer: e**

Current systems for the diagnosis of neurodevelopmental and psychiatric disorders are categorical—patients either meet criteria or do not; however, many features of these disorders are distributed in the general population in a dimensional fashion, with some individuals only mildly affected. Depression, social communication difficulties, and psychotic/schizotypal traits are examples of traits that have been found to be dimensional.

2. **Answer: d**

There are a wide variety of psychosocial treatments, including CBT, but fundamental to them all is a therapeutic relationship that is focused on addressing a problem. The patient identifies some kind of difficulty and turns to the clinician as someone who might be helpful. In some psychosocial therapies the problem being addressed is a practical one, or an external circumstance (such as problem solving around financial matters); in other situations, the difficulty is more interpersonal (as with marital discord) or intrapsychic (such as self-hate). When a patient is able to think of the therapist as someone who has the skills and the motivation to be helpful, this sets the stage for the development of a therapeutic alliance in which the patient and therapist can work together toward agreed-upon goals. This trusting therapeutic relationship is often worked upon and developed early in treatment.

3. **Answer: e**

Diagnostic delays and errors are extremely common; many factors contribute to this problem. In treating patients who have long-standing symptoms that are nonspecific, practitioners need to be vigilant for the possible emergence of disease-defining signs and symptoms. While rare diseases may be missed because the clinician is unfamiliar with the condition, more often, common diseases are misdiagnosed when they present atypically. In addition, it is important to consider the possibility that a patient's diagnosis has been missed because the cognitive biases of a clinician have affected their diagnostic reasoning. Patients with a psychiatric history or with symptoms in the sphere of mental functioning are highly vulnerable to all forms of cognitive bias, especially to attribution error in which the patient is held responsible for his/her disease.

4. **Answer: e**

Many factors contribute to individuality. DNA that is inherited in the fertilized ovum is of prime importance. Two other factors that influence the course of individual development are early mutations in the DNA of fetal cells and the availability of transcription factors that determine whether and when genes are turned on.

References

1. Trofimova I, Robbins TW, Sulis WH, et al. Taxonomies of psychological individual differences: biological perspectives on millennia-long challenges. *Phil Trans R Soc B*. 2018;373 (1744):20170152.

2. Hiesinger PR, Hassan BA. The evolution of variability and robustness in neural development. *Trends Neurosci*. 2018;41(9):577-585.

3. Cloninger CR, Zwir I. What is the natural measurement unit of temperament: single traits or profiles?. *Phil Trans R Soc B*. 2018;373(1744):20170163.

4. Gardner H. *Frames of Mind: The Theory of Multiple Intelligences*. New York, NY: Basic Books. 2011.

5. Trimble MR. *The Intentional Brain: Motion, Emotion, and the Development of Modern Neuropsychiatry*. Baltimore, MD: JHU Press; 2016.

6. Honegger K, de Bivort B. Stochasticity, individuality and behavior. *Curr Biol*. 2018;28(1):R8-R12.

7. Finn ES, Shen X, Scheinost D, et al. Functional connectome fingerprinting: identifying individuals using patterns of brain connectivity. *Nat Neurosci*. 2015;18(11):1664.

8. Finn ES, Corlett PR, Chen G, et al. Trait paranoia shapes inter-subject synchrony in brain activity during an ambiguous social narrative. *Nat Commun*. 2018;9(1):2043.

9. Chen R, Shi L, Hakenberg J, et al. Analysis of 589,306 genomes identifies individuals resilient to severe Mendelian childhood diseases. *Nat Biotechnol*. 2016;34:531.

10. Insel TR. Brain somatic mutations: the dark matter of psychiatric genetics? *Mol Psychiatry*. 2014;19(2):156.

11. Nishioka M, Bundo M, Ueda J, et al. Identification of somatic mutations in monozygotic twins discordant for psychiatric disorders. *NPJ Schizophrenia*. 2018;4(1):7.

12. Li R, Montpetit A, Rousseau M, Wu SY, et al. Somatic point mutations occurring early in development: a monozygotic twin study. *J Med Genet*. 2014;51(1):28-34.

13. Bury-Moné S, Sclavi B. Stochasticity of gene expression as a motor of epigenetics in bacteria: from individual to collective behaviors. *Res Microbiol.* 2017;168(6):503-514.

14. Stiles J, Jernigan TL. The basics of brain development. *Neuropsychol Rev.* 2010;20(4):327-348.

15. Keunen K, Counsell SJ, Benders MJ. The emergence of functional architecture during early brain development. *NeuroImage.* 2017;160:2-14.

16. Bergmann O, Frisén J. Why adults need new brain cells. *Science.* 2013;340(6133):695-696.

17. Hebb DO. *The Organization of Behavior: A Neuropsychological Theory.* New York, NY: Lawrence Erlbaum; 1963.

18. Suvrathan A. Beyond STDP—towards diverse and functionally relevant plasticity rules. *Curr Opin Neurobiol.* 2019;54:12-19.

19. Merzenich MM, Nelson RJ, Stryker MP, Cynader MS, Schoppmann A, Zook JM. Somatosensory cortical map changes following digit amputation in adult monkeys. *J Comp Neurol.* 1984;224(4):591-605.

20. Ramachandran VS, Rogers-Ramachandran D. Phantom limbs and neural plasticity. *Arch Neurol.* 2000;57(3):317-320.

21. Woollett K, Maguire EA. Acquiring "the knowledge" of London's layout drives structural brain changes. *Curr Biol.* 2011;21(24):2109-2114.

22. Allen NJ, Lyons DA. Glia as architects of central nervous system formation and function. *Science.* 2018;362(6411):181-185.

23. Stachowicz K. The role of DSCAM in the regulation of synaptic plasticity: possible involvement in neuropsychiatric disorders. *Acta Neurobiol Exp.* 2018;78(3):210-219.

24. Liu J, Liao X, Xia M, et al. Chronnectome fingerprinting: identifying individuals and predicting higher cognitive functions using dynamic brain connectivity patterns. *Hum Brain Mapp.* 2018;39(2):902-915.

25. Huang B, Jiang C, Zhang R. Epigenetics: the language of the cell?. *Epigenomics.* 2014;6(1):73-88.

26. Roseboom TJ. Epidemiologic evidence for the developmental origins of health and disease: effects of prenatal undernutrition in humans. *J Endocrinol.* 2019;242(1):T135-T144.

27. Fraga MF, Ballestar E, Paz MF, et al. Epigenetic differences arise during the lifetime of monozygotic twins. *Proc Natl Acad Sci.* 2005;102(30):10604-10609.

28. Thelen E, Smith LB. *A Dynamic Systems Approach to the Development of Cognition and Action.* MIT Press; 1996.

29. Freund J, Brandmaier AM, Lewejohann L, et al. Emergence of individuality in genetically identical mice. *Science.* 2013;340(6133):756-759.

30. Vanderwal T, Eilbott J, Finn ES, et al. Individual differences in functional connectivity during naturalistic viewing conditions. *NeuroImage.* 2017;157:521-530.

31. Klinger R, Stuhlreyer J, Schwartz M, Schmitz J, Colloca L. Clinical use of placebo effects in patients with pain disorders. *Int Rev Neurobiol.* 2018;139:107.

32. Kelley JM, Lembo AJ, Ablon JS, et al. Patient and practitioner influences on the placebo effect in irritable bowel syndrome. *Psychosom Med.* 2009;71(7):789-797.

33. Ablon JS, Jones EE. On analytic process. *J Am Psychoanal Assoc.* 2005;53(2):541-568; discussion 569-578.

34. Ball J, Balogh E, Miller BT, eds. *Improving Diagnosis in Health Care.* Washington DC, USA: National Academies Press, 2015.

35. Croskerry P. The importance of cognitive errors in diagnosis and strategies to minimize them. *Acad Med.* 2003;78(8):775-780.

36. The Undiagnosed Diseases Network. Available at https://undiagnosed.hms.harvard.edu/. Accesed February 5,2020.

37. Evans DW, Lusk LG, Slane MM, et al. Dimensional assessment of schizotypal, psychotic, and other psychiatric traits in children and their parents: development and validation of the Childhood Oxford-Liverpool Inventory of Feelings and Experiences on a representative US sample. *J Child Psychol Psychiatry.* 2018;59(5):574-585.

38. Smith L, Reichenberg A, Rabinowitz J, et al. Psychiatric symptoms and related dysfunction in a general population sample. *Schizophr Res Cogn.* 2018;14:1-6.

39. Ford JM, Morris SE, Hoffman RE, et al. Studying hallucinations within the NIMH RDoC framework. *Schizophr Bull.* 2014;40(suppl_4):S295-S304.

38

Neuropsychiatry in Global Health

Diana M. Robinson · Nomi C. Levy-Carrick · Aaron L. Berkowitz · Stephanie L. Smith

INTRODUCTION

Neuropsychiatric conditions are common throughout the world and account for a substantial portion of the global burden of illness. Over the last decade, the burden of illness attributable to mental health, neurological, and substance use disorders, as measured in disability-adjusted life years (DALYs), has risen dramatically and exceeds the burden of illness attributable to cancer and cardiovascular disease.[1] DALYs have been one of the most prominent health metrics used to describe the global burden of mental, neurologic, and substance use disorders. The DALY includes both years lived with disability (YLDs) in addition to years of life lost (YLL).[2] Yet there are too few specialized psychiatric and neurologic providers to meet this burden. In many rural and resource-limited settings across the globe, the number of people with neuropsychiatric conditions who do not receive appropriate or adequate treatment for their disorder (defined as the treatment gap) can reach almost 90%.[3] There are many structural and operational challenges associated with mental health and neurologic care delivery, including a global scarcity of skilled psychiatric and neurologic practitioners, challenges in effective flow of medical services and goods from manufacturer to patient (defined as supply chain management), limited funding, sociocultural and stigma factors, and weak health systems in many places around the globe. Task sharing—moving care responsibilities from more specialized providers to less specialized health workers—has been increasingly emphasized as one key approach for addressing the global burden of mental disorders; however, this should be combined with improved funding, health system strengthening efforts and training, and engagement of specialized providers in task-shared systems of care. This chapter will provide an overview of the epidemiology and global burden of neuropsychiatric illness and the global neuropsychiatric treatment gap. It will then describe the challenges and potential solutions to effective global mental health service delivery, including current evidence on task-sharing approaches to neuropsychiatric care across the globe.

EPIDEMIOLOGY OF SELECTED NEUROPSYCHIATRIC DISORDERS

Community-based epidemiological studies have estimated that the lifetime prevalence rates of mental disorders in adults globally are 29.2%, and the 12-month prevalence rates of mental disorders are 17.6%.[4] In this chapter, the epidemiology of neuropsychiatric disorders will be reported by separating disorders into mental, neurological, and substance use disorders, as is consistent with international literature. Additionally, the epidemiology of neuropsychiatric disorders is commonly investigated in relation to the size of the economy of countries. The World Bank annually classifies national economies by gross national income (GNI), previously known as the gross national product (GDP), via the World Bank Atlas formula in billions of United States dollars (USD). For the 2019 fiscal year, low-income countries (LICs) were defined as <$995 GNI, lower middle-income countries were $996–3895 GNI, upper middle-income countries (UMICSs) were $3896–12,055 GNI, and high-income countries (HICs) were ≥$12,056 GNI.[5] The World Bank frequently combines low- and middle-income countries together (LMICs).

Mood Disorders: Major Depressive Disorder and Bipolar Disorder

The 12-month prevalence for depressive disorder, dysthymia, or bipolar disorder ranged from 1.1% to 9.7% across 17 countries including countries in the Americas (Columbia, Mexico, United States), Africa (Nigeria and South Africa), Eastern Mediterranean (Lebanon), Europe (Belgium, France, Germany, Israel, Italy, the Netherlands, Spain), and the Western Pacific Regions (China, Japan, and New Zealand).[6] Depression is also often comorbid with other mental disorders, and approximately half of people who have a history of depression have a comorbid anxiety disorder.[7] A review of epidemiological studies from 20 countries found that the 12-month prevalence of bipolar disorder was 0.84% and had an equal gender ratio.[8] In 2010, 33.8% of neuropsychiatric disorders were due to major depressive disorder, dysthymia, and bipolar disorder (24.5%, 4.3%, and 5.0%, respectively), and caused 3.4% of all-cause DALYs (2.5%, 0.4%, and 0.5%, respectively).[9]

Anxiety Disorders

Globally, the 12-month prevalence of anxiety disorders is 3.0%–19.0%, with specific phobia and social phobia accounting for the highest lifetime prevalence of anxiety disorders.[6] In 2010, 10.4% of neuropsychiatric disorders were due to anxiety disorders and caused 1.1% of all-cause DALYs.[9]

Stress-Related Disorders Including Post-Traumatic Stress Disorder (PTSD)

Trauma exposures are widespread. A recent WHO World Mental Health Survey Consortium of 24 countries (n = 68,894) identified at least one lifetime trauma exposure in over 70% of the population, and approximately 28% had four or more such experiences.[10] But not all those with exposures progress to meeting criteria for PTSD, with differential vulnerability based on age at time of trauma, gender, and history of prior traumas at time of exposure to subsequent trauma (particularly involving physical or sexual violence; OR 1.3–2.5).[10] In addition, mental disorders including PTSD in conflict settings was estimated as high as 22.1% in populations assessed during a recent WHO meta-analysis.[11] Of note, stress-related disorders such as PTSD were included in the "Anxiety Disorder" category until the release of the *Diagnostic and Statistical Manual of Mental Disorders*-Fifth Edition (*DSM-5*) in 2013. PTSD surveys have continued to use *DSM-IV* criteria, and this has confounded its discrete quantification as a contributor to global disability.[12,13]

Psychotic Disorders

In a study that included 73 primary investigations of psychosis in different countries around the world, the worldwide 12-month prevalence of psychosis was 0.4%, the point prevalence was 0.389%, and the median lifetime prevalence was 0.749%.[14] In 2010, 5.3% of neuropsychiatric disorders were due to schizophrenia, and caused 0.5% of all-cause DALYs and ~13,600,000 absolute DALYs.[9]

Autism, Attentional, and Disruptive Behavioral Disorders

There were an estimated 52 million global cases of autism spectrum disorders (ASDs) in 2010, with a prevalence of 0.76% or 1 in 132 people.[15] In 2010, 5.4% of neuropsychiatric disorders were due to autism, Asperger's syndrome, attention deficit-hyperactivity disorder (ADHD), and conduct disorder (1.6%, 1.4%, 0.2%, and 2.2%, respectively), and caused 0.52% of all-cause DALYs (0.2%, 0.1%, 0.02%, and 0.2%, respectively).[9]

Epilepsy

The median incidence per year of epilepsy is 0.0817% in LMICs and 0.045% in HICs.[16] In 2010, 6.8% of neuropsychiatric disorders were due to epilepsy, and caused 0.7% of all-cause DALYs

(0.2% and 0.1%, respectively).[9] Epilepsy is thought to be more common in LMICs due to endemic infectious diseases such as neurocysticercosis, high rates of accidents causing head trauma, higher rates of birth injuries, and differences in availability of prenatal and postnatal medical care.[9]

Cerebrovascular Disease

Cerebrovascular disease (stroke) is the second leading cause of death and disability worldwide,[17] causing 67.3% of mortality due to neurologic disorders and 47.3% of DALYs due to neurologic disorders.[18] Incidence rate, rate of DALYs lost, and mortality rate for stroke are all higher in LMICs.[19] In fact, the strongest predictor of stroke mortality and DALYs even after adjustment for cardiovascular risk factors is national per capita income.[20]

Dementia

Approximately 47 million people globally in 2015 carried a diagnosis of dementia such as Alzheimer's disease, vascular dementia, frontotemporal dementia, and Lewy body dementia,[21] with almost two-thirds of that total living in LMICs.[21] After the age of 65 years, the incidence of dementia is expected to double with every 5-year increment.[21] An estimated 76 million people will have dementia in 2030 and this figure is expected to increase to 145 million by 2050.[22] In 2010, 4.4% of neuropsychiatric disorders were due to Alzheimer's disease and other dementias and caused 0.5% of all-cause DALYs.[9]

Headaches

Headache disorders, including chronic migraines, chronic tension headaches, and chronic medication-overuse headaches have a global 12-month prevalence rate of 14.7% for migraines, 20.8% for tension headaches, and 7.1% for medication overuse headaches.[23,24] In 2010, 9.4% of neuropsychiatric disorders were due to migraines and tension headaches (8.7% and 0.7%, respectively), and caused 1.0% of all-cause DALYs (0.9% and 0.1%, respectively).[9]

Parkinson's Disease

In 2016, the global 12-month prevalence of Parkinson's disease was 1.6%.[25] The DALYs for Parkinson's disease in 2010 for women and men were 0.023% and 0.37%, respectively. The DALYs attributable to Parkinson's disease represent 0.1% of the total all-cause DALYs.[9]

Encephalitis

Encephalitis, or inflammation of brain, is associated with high morbidity and mortality. The differential is broad and includes bacterial, fungal, parasitic, viral, and autoimmune causes. The differential is even more broad in those who are immunocompromised versus immunocompetent. There are also regional differences in the burden of disease due to encephalitis, with India having the highest burden of disease. The global prevalence of encephalitis in 2015 was 0.06%. The DALYs attributable to encephalitis in 2015 were 0.12%.[26]

Substance Use Disorders

According to the United Nations World Drug Report, in 2015 approximately 29.5 million people, or 0.6% of the global adult population, had problematic substance use, substance dependence, or a substance use disorder (*DSM-IV* and *5* terminology for substance use that impairs functioning). An estimated 12 million people globally are intravenous drug users.[27] In 2010, 14.7% of neuropsychiatric disorders were due to substance use disorders (alcohol use disorders 6.9%, opioid dependence 3.6%, cocaine dependence 0.4%, amphetamine dependence 1.0%, cannabis dependence 0.8%, and other substance use disorders 2.0%) and caused 1.5% of all-cause DALYS (alcohol use disorders 0.7%, opioid dependence 0.4%, cocaine dependence 0.04%, amphetamine dependence 0.1%, cannabis dependence 0.1%, and other substance use disorders 0.2%).[9]

GLOBAL BURDEN OF NEUROPSYCHIATRIC DISORDERS

A substantial portion of the world's disease burden results from neuropsychiatric disorders. As methodology to estimate burden of illness has been refined to identify health problems which contribute to disability in addition to mortality, there has been increased focus on the impact of neuropsychiatric disorders in both HICs and LICs. Table 38-1 summarizes the leading global neuropsychiatric contributors to DALYs in 2005 and 2015. In 2005, the top 30 causes of DALYs worldwide included 6 neuropsychiatric conditions (Table 38-1—#3 cerebrovascular disease, #8 low back and neck pain, #17 depressive disorders, #19 self-harm, #23 migraines, and #24 meningitis).[1] By 2015, 8 neuropsychiatric conditions were among the 30 most common causes of DALYs (Table 38-1—#2 cerebrovascular disease, #4 low back and neck pain, #15 depressive disorders, #21 self-harm,

TABLE 38-2 • Most Prevalent Causes of Global Disability-Adjusted Life Years (DALYs) by Illness Group, 2010*.

Rank	Condition	% of Global DALYs
1	Cardiovascular and circulatory diseases	11.8
2	Infectious diseases (including diarrhea, lower respiratory tract infections, meningitis, and other common infectious diseases)	11.4
3	Neuropsychiatric disorders	10.4
4	Neonatal disorders	8.1
5	Neoplasms	7.6

Adapted from NIMH. Global leading categories of diseases/disorders. Available at https://www.nimh.nih.gov/health/statistics/global/global-leading-categories-of-diseases-disorders.shtml.

#23 migraines, #27 meningitis, #28 anxiety disorders, and #29 Alzheimer's disease).[1]

In 2010, the Global Burden of Illness Study estimated that neuropsychiatric disorders were the third most prevalent cause of global DALYs, accounting for 10.4% of the total all-cause DALYs (Table 38-2). Within this statistic, 7.4% are due to mental and behavioral health disorders and 3.0% are due to neurological disorders.[28] In 2010, DALYs for neuropsychiatric disorders were highest during the early- to mid-adulthood period from age 15 to 49 and accounted for 18.6% of total DALYs in this age group.[9] DALYs due to neurological disorders were highest in the elderly.[9] 51.9% of the neuropsychiatric disorder DALYs were in women and 48.1% were in men. The global burden of illnesses has important gender differences, with women accruing more DALYs in all neuropsychiatric disorders except for childhood mental disorders, schizophrenia, substance use disorders, and Parkinson's disease.[9] There are also regional differences, with the relative proportion of DALYs due to neuropsychiatric disorders making up 15.5% of total DALYs in HICs and 9.4% in LMICs. When accounting for the larger population of LMICs, the absolute DALYs for neuropsychiatric disorders is higher in LMICs than HICs.[9]

From 2006 to 2016 there was a 45% increase in the DALYs due to dementia, and from 2006 to 2016 there were also increases in the DALYs due to other neurological disorders including Parkinson's disease (+40%), motor neuron disease (+25%), and multiple sclerosis (+17%).[29]

Substance Use Disorders

Alcohol and substance use disorders continue to be a common cause of global morbidity and mortality. Approximately 5.1% of the global burden of disease and injury is attributable to alcohol, and alcohol is a major contributing factor of more than 200 diseases and injury conditions.[30] It is estimated that 70% of the negative health impact of substances is due to opioid use, making it the most harmful substance type.[27] Of the estimated 12 million people globally who use

TABLE 38-1 • Trends in Leading Neuropsychiatric Causes of Global Disability-Adjusted Life Years (DALYs), 2005 and 2015*.

2005		2015	
Rank	Condition	Rank	Condition
3	Cerebrovascular disease	2	Cerebrovascular disease
8	Low back and neck pain	4	Low back and neck pain
17	Depressive disorders	15	Depressive disorders
19	Self-harm	21	Self-harm
23	Migraine	23	Migraine
24	Meningitis	27	Meningitis
33	Anxiety disorders	28	Anxiety disorders
37	Alzheimer's disease	29	Alzheimer's disease

Adapted from GBD 2015 DALYs and HALE Collaborators. Global, regional, and national disability-adjusted life-years (DALYs) for 315 diseases and injuries and healthy life expectancy (HALE), 1990–2015: A systematic analysis for the Global Burden of Disease Study 2015. The Lancet. 2016;388:1603-1658.

intravenous drugs, 1.6 million of these people have HIV, 6.1 million have hepatitis C, and 1.3 million have both hepatitis C and HIV.[27] The opioid crisis in the United States has led to an enormous and growing public health crisis, with a 292% increase in the percentage of all deaths attributable to opioids from 0.4% to 1.5%.[31] While the opioid crisis has been documented extensively in the United States, the nonmedical use of prescription opioids is becoming a major public health problem around the world. Tramadol, a pharmaceutical opioid, is the main opioid of concern in countries in West and North Africa, as well as in the Near and Middle East. Heroin is the main opioid of abuse in Europe, with reports of nonmedical use of methadone, buprenorphine, and fentanyl.[32]

Comorbidity

The morbidity and mortality associated with neuropsychiatric disorders are compounded by comorbid noncommunicable and communicable diseases. Moreover, the landmark Adverse Childhood Experiences study demonstrated a dose-response relationship between number of adverse childhood events experienced and level of risk for poor health outcomes later in life.[33] This results in those with neuropsychiatric disorders living an average of 8–20 fewer years than the general population. People with neuropsychiatric disorders are disproportionately likely to die of noncommunicable illnesses such as cardiovascular disease, cancer, and pulmonary disease.[34] Mental illnesses play a bidirectional role with cardiovascular illness and independently have a negative impact on cardiovascular mortality: people with mental disorders are at higher risk for noncommunicable diseases and people with cardiovascular disease are at greater risk for depression.[36] Compared to the general population, people with depression have a three times higher rate of myocardial infarction.[36]

Communicable diseases also can influence the onset and course of psychiatric and neurologic illness. There are approximately 2 million people living with epilepsy due to neurocysticercosis, making it the most common preventable cause of epilepsy in the developing world.[37] Neurocysticercosis is the neurological infiltration of the larval form of *Taenia solium*, which is acquired by humans eating raw or undercooked pork containing the cysts or fecal-oral transmission of the *T. solium*. Other infectious causes of epilepsy include the mosquito-borne parasites *Plasmodium falciparum* and *Plasmodium vivax*, particularly in Sub-Saharan Africa, South East Asia, and Latin America. *P. falciparum* contributes to the majority of neurological complications associated with these parasites, including cerebral malaria. *P. vivax* is also a common cause of seizures and status epilepticus in children under the age of 5 years.[38] A systematic review of neurosyphilis infections in Africa described cases of neurosyphilis/meningovascular-induced strokes in adults in Morocco, Zambia, Malawi, Sudan, and Tanzania.[39] Finally, in tuberculosis-endemic areas such as Peru and Pakistan, patients receiving cycloserine for multidrug resistant tuberculosis (MDR-TB) were at high risk of psychiatric side effects of cycloserine such as psychosis in 12% of patients.[40,41]

CHALLENGES IN GLOBAL MENTAL HEALTH CARE DELIVERY

The large global burden of mental disorders demonstrates the imperative to scale-up and expand the world's capacity to implement successful mental and neurologic health care interventions. There are multiple challenges of neuropsychiatric care delivery, particularly in resource-limited settings, although these challenges exist across countries of all income levels.

Challenges of Mental Health Care Delivery

- Human resource limitations
- Financing
- Supply chain and diagnostic testing availability
- Centralized service delivery organization

Human Resource Limitations

The treatment gap is the number of people with a condition or disease who do not receive appropriate or adequate treatment for their disorder. It is calculated by the median and average rate of service utilization across studies for each disorder and takes into account the prevalence rate and population size of the country.[42] Median rates are used to reduce outliers skewing the results. However, while rates of mental health disorders show consistency worldwide, there is a treatment gap of more than 75% in many LMICs and 35–50% in HICs.[43] Forty-five percent of the world's population lives in a country with less than one psychiatrist per 100,000 people.[44] In a global WHO survey of the mental health workforce (including adult and child psychiatrists, other specialist medical doctors, nurses, psychologists, social workers, occupational therapists, and other paid mental health workers), there was an average of 9 mental health workers per 100,000 population, with large differences in mental health human resources by country income level: 71.7 per 100,000 in HICs, 20.6 in UMICs, 6.2 in lower middle income countries, and only 1.6 in LICs.[45] There are also few neurologists in many parts of the world, with 0.043 adult neurologists per 100,000 people in the African region, 0.1 adult neurologists per 100,000 people in the South East Asian region, 0.7 adult neurologists per 100,000 people in the region of the Americas, 0.8 adult neurologists per 100,000 people in the Eastern Mediterranean region, 1.2 adult neurologists per 100,000 people in the Western Pacific region, compared to 6.6 adult neurologists per 100,000 people in the European region.[46] In the United States in 2012 there were approximately 5.2 neurologists per 100,000 people—however, there is an uneven geographic distribution with shortages of neurologists in rural areas. For instance, there are approximately 1.8 neurologists per 100,000 people in Wyoming, compared to 12.1 in Massachusetts (which has a large number of academic medical centers).[47] The median number of mental health beds per 100,000 population ranges from <7 in LMICs to >50 in HICs. Disparities in child and adolescent services also exist, with the median number of child and adolescent beds ranging from 0.2 per 100,000 population in LMICs to >1.5 in HICs.[45]

Financing

There is a substantial gap between the burden attributable to neuropsychiatric illnesses and health budgets dedicated to mental health. Mental health spending encompasses mental health programs and service delivery at the community, primary care, or specialist/secondary care levels. In 2017, the WHO estimated that the global median mental health expenditure per capita was less than 2% of overall global median of domestic general government health expenditures (US$2.5 vs. $141). Global mental health expenditures also varied significantly by geographic region, with spending across the European and Americas regions more than 100 times the expenditures in the African and South East Asian regions.[45] There is a strong association between GNI per capita and total government mental health spending per capita. A number of countries at lower levels of national income are spending a larger proportion of total health spending on mental health, relative to some higher-income countries which devote only a small portion of their relatively large health budget to mental health[45]; however, almost a quarter of countries do not have a mental health budget.[48] In countries that do have a mental health budget, on average, the median is less than 2% of the overall health budget.[45] In LMICs more than 80% of the mental health budget goes to mental hospitals.[45]

Supply Chain and Diagnostic Testing Availability

The World Health Organization publishes an essential medicine list which includes recommendations for medications crucial for any health care system. It includes the most cost-effective, efficacious, and safe medicines for priority conditions (Table 38-3).[49] The list includes psychotropic medications for palliative care use, antiepileptic drugs (AEDs), anti-parkinsonism medications, antipsychotics, antidepressants, mood stabilizers, anxiolytics, and nicotine replacement therapy.[49]

Despite the WHO's recommendations, essential medications for neurologic and mental disorders are commonly unavailable in many places. For example, a study conducted in Mozambique found that only 46% of 24 public health facilities had at least one medication from each category of the recommended psychotropic medications, with thioridizine being the most available psychotropic medication.[50] The list includes mostly older medications (such as predominantly typical antipsychotic medications), which are generally less expensive but have a different side-effect profile compared with more recent psychotropic medications. In Mozambique, fluoxetine was only available at one quaternary care facility and no district warehouses.[50] Illness relapses from lack of access to treatment or interruptions in maintenance therapy can have long-term repercussions. Many people also do not have reliable or convenient access to pharmacies or medications, with individuals in high-income countries having more pharmacists per 10,000 people (HIC=7.61, LIC=0.60).[51] A US study showed that when people with mental health diagnoses did not have access to medications, 69% of people had adverse events compared with 40% of patients with no access problems.[52] The most common adverse events were increased side effects that interfered with functioning (23%), increases in suicidal ideation (22%), emergency room visits (20%), hospital admissions (11%), and becoming homeless (3%).[52]

Access to appropriate and effective diagnostic tests, including labs and neuroimaging, are limited in many places throughout the world. For example, around 90% of countries have fewer than two PET scanners, 46% have fewer than two MRI machines, and 30% have fewer than two CT scanners per million population. Overall, there are 0–8% of countries without any CT scanners, but there is significant regional variation, as 24% of countries without any CT scanners are in the Western Pacific region.[53] These machines are mostly located at tertiary-level medical hospitals but may be unavailable due to being out of order, having inadequate maintenance, being too expensive, or not having the trained available to operate the machine or interpret the results.

Centralized Service Delivery Organization

The organization of mental health service delivery affects treatment coverage for people with neuropsychiatric disorders.[54]

TABLE 38-3 • WHO Essential Medication List of Psychotropic Medications, 2017[*].

Category	Diseases	Medications
Palliative care		Amitriptyline, diazepam, fluoxetine, haloperidol
Anticonvulsants/ Antiepileptics		Carbamazepine, lamotrigine, diazepam, lorazepam, midazolam, phenobarbital, phenytoin, valproic acid
Antiparkinsonism medications		Biperiden, levodopa, carbidopa
Mental health and behavioral diseases	Psychotic disorders	Chlorpromazine, fluphenazine, haloperidol, risperidone
	Depressive disorders	Amitriptyline, fluoxetine
	Bipolar disorders	Carbamazepine, lithium carbonate, valproic acid
	Anxiety disorders	Diazepam
	Obsessive-compulsive disorders	Clomipramine
	Psychoactive substance use	Nicotine replacement therapy (chewing gum and transdermal patch)

[*]Adapted from WHO. WHO model list of essential medicines. 20th ed. Geneva, Switzerland: World Health Organization; 2017. Available at http://apps.who.int/iris/bitstream/handle/10665/273826/EML-20-eng.pdf?ua=1categories-of-diseases-disorders.shtml.

Despite over half of a century of efforts globally to decentralize mental and neurologic care from large psychiatric institutions to community-based services, the majority of mental health services in LMICs remain in tertiary psychiatric facilities in or near large cities.[55] In addition to reducing access to care, such institutions tend to consume a large proportion of scarce mental health resources, cost more than community-based care, isolate people from family and community support systems, and are associated with undignified life conditions, human-rights violations, and stigma.[56] Downsizing and/or eliminating psychiatric hospitals, while a public health and human rights recommendation for almost 50 years, is inextricably linked to the challenges of developing community mental health services, which requires significant political will, effective advocacy efforts, and material investments.[57] Thus, advocates strive to improve the quality and accessibility of psychiatric hospitals in tandem with increasing community mental health services.

ADDRESSING THE BURDEN

There are a number of key strategies to improve access to high-quality mental health and neurologic services across the globe. In this section, we highlight task-sharing and integration into care delivery platforms, improved policy and financing, professional education, and technology as strategies for reducing the global burden of mental disorders (Table 38-4).

Task Sharing and Integration into Care Delivery Platforms

Task sharing, or the movement of mental health and neurologic care to nonspecialists in the community or primary care setting instead of relying on specialist-delivered care, could improve access to mental health and neurologic care across the globe, and contribute to significant reductions in the treatment gap.[58] Task sharing requires the reimagining of the traditional model of specialists directly delivering mental health services, to specialists who engage in public mental health leadership, including supervision and consultation.[59] For example, a system of task sharing in global mental and neurologic care could include a collaborative, stepped approach using community health workers to identify people with neuropsychiatric illnesses in the community, perform basic mental health care, and refer to the primary care setting. Primary care practitioners can provide diagnosis and treatment including psychosocial approaches and medication management. If neuropsychiatric specialists are available, they can supervise and can provide recommendations or referrals for challenging cases.

Task sharing for mental health and neurologic care has been shown to be effective across a range of disorders, settings, and types of providers.[60-63] Major global initiatives have demonstrated efficacy in psychological treatments by nonspecialist providers for depression, anxiety, and substance use disorders.[64-71] For example, a stepped care intervention led by nonspecialist lay health workers was used in Chile for women with severe depression, which included a psychoeducational group intervention delivered by lay workers, structured and systemic follow-up,

TABLE 38-4 • Summary of Strategies to Address Global Burden.	
	Important Points
Task sharing and integration across care delivery platforms	• Involves shifting of tasks from more to less highly trained individuals, allowing all providers to work at the top of their scope of practice
	• Shown to be effective across a range of disorders, settings, and provider types
	• Requires reimagining the traditional model of specialists directly delivering mental health services, to specialists who engage in public mental health leadership, including supervision and consultation
	• Hub and spoke systems with universities or tertiary-care facilities have been effective at improving specialty service connections and supervision in rural, resource-limited areas
	• Collaborative and stepped care models, and integration of neuropsychiatric services into primary care settings, could increase access to services
Policy and financing	• The majority of mental health specific policies focus on mental health awareness, suicide prevention, and school-based mental health promotion
	• Effective policies for neuropsychiatric disorders include perinatal screening programs, preventing suicide by reducing access to lethal means, preventing head injuries, neurocysticercosis prevention, and cardiovascular risk factor management
	• Effective policies for alcohol use disorder include excise taxes to reduce the demand, restriction on sales/bar hours/days of sale, minimum legal age, and drunk driving countermeasures
Professional education	• Mental health training of nonspecialist clinicians should be increased in order to build capacity
	• A shift toward neuropsychiatry training for new postgraduate programs, and integration of neuropsychiatric training into psychiatry and neurology programs could improve clinical quality and access to care across the globe
	• Partnerships between established and newer programs can help build clinical and educational capacity
Digital technologies	• Digital technologies can include mobile phones, applications, and online platforms
	• Web-centered training can increase the reach and reduce costs for training different providers
	• Digital technologies can facilitate direct patient care, supervision, consultation between clinicians, and partnerships for collaboration

and referral to a physician for pharmacotherapy.[63] Task-shared interventions for treating serious mental disorders (schizophrenia, schizoaffective disorder, and bipolar disorder) have also been shown to be effective.[72,73]

Task-shared models of care have been successfully implemented in diverse settings and locations, including rural communities such as Haiti's Central Plateau region, rural Rwanda, and Pakistan's Rawalpindi district.[61,74,75] The MINAS study was conducted at 12 government-run primary health care facilities and 12 private general practitioner practices in Goa state, India.[60] Mobile clinics have been utilized to supplement clinic-based services in rural Haiti to provide mental health, substance use disorders, and neurologic care to patients, particularly those with epilepsy and depression.[76] The PRIME study of task-shared mental health care showed efficacy in task-shared interventions in a variety of settings including extremely under-resourced areas (Uganda and Ethiopia), a fragile political situation (Nepal), and LMICs with high socioeconomic inequality (India and South Africa).[77]

Task-shared interventions by different types of nonspecialist providers have also shown efficacy across disorders and settings. A single site study in Nepal's refugee camps found a rapid improvement in a nurse's accuracy in diagnosing epilepsy after a brief training intervention with a neurologist, and the high level of agreement between their diagnoses was maintained 1-year later.[78] A large, multisite study examined the acceptability and feasibility of task sharing of nonspecialist health workers to deliver mental health care in primary care settings in Ethiopia, India, Nepal, South Africa, and Uganda. The authors found that task sharing was perceived as acceptable and feasible in these countries as long as the following key conditions were met: (1) increased resources (human resources and access to medications), (2) ongoing supervision by mental health professionals at the community and primary care-levels, and (3) adequate training and compensation of health workers.[77] A perinatal depression intervention was led by community health workers with additional support from primary care doctors, midwives, and traditional birth attendants.[61] The MINAS study intervention was led by a combination of primary care physicians and nonspecialist workers (nurses, community health workers, and administrative staff) at government run primary health care facilities and private general practitioner clinics.[60] McLean et al. studied a pilot task-sharing training in rural Haiti. The program included a brief, structured group training of community health workers with and without an apprenticeship training and found that there was improved subjective clinical competency, increased confidence, and improved career advancement by adding an apprenticeship component.[74]

Integration of mental and neurologic care into existing care delivery platforms could also improve access to, and quality of, care for mental and neurologic disorders. Breuer et al. highlight that the key organizational barriers to mental health care in LMICs are difficulty in access, competing public health priorities, low investment in mental health services, a paucity of human resources, and resistance to decentralization. Local providers need connections with specialty services and supervision, and hub and spoke systems with university providers and other tertiary-care facilities have proven to be very helpful

in rural, resource-limited communities in the United States. Overlapping issues are addressed in Chapter 36, Integration of Neuropsychiatric Care in Primary Care and Other Medical Settings. Programs like ECHO (Extension for Community Healthcare Outcomes) is a telehealth system that potentially could serve as a template for such support and training.[79] Other countries have increased access to neuropsychiatric services by integrating them into primary care settings in Brazil, Chile, India, Iran, South Africa, Uganda, the United Kingdom, and the United States.[80] This has the dual benefits of providing a less stigmatizing treatment setting and increasing the availability of evidence-based treatments.

Improved Policy and Financing

The WHO recommends that countries adopt progressive policies that promote mental health and prevent mental disorders, reduce stigmatization, discrimination, and human rights violations, and that are responsive to specific vulnerable groups across the life span.[45]

The WHO estimates that 71% of countries have at least two functioning national mental health programs, with the majority of existing programs focused on mental health awareness (40%), suicide prevention (12%), and school-based mental health promotion (10%).[45] A systematic review of the evidence for building the capacity of policy development to strengthen mental health systems in LMICs found a small number of studies. The majority of the 14 studies meeting inclusion criteria used models of brief training combined with longer-term mentorship and/or establishing networks of support and consultation.[81] As part of the Programme for Improving Mental Health Care (PRIME) study, Breuer et al.[82] described a process of using theory of change (ToC) workshops to plan the development and evaluation of mental health care plans in resource-limited settings in five countries in Africa and South East Asia via collaborative community stakeholders' workshops. ToC appears to be a valuable method that can be used to develop and evaluate mental health care plans, particularly in resource-limited settings. It is important to strengthen the relevance and beneficence of policies to ensure they are comprehensive and address prevention, promotion, and treatment.

The global mental health expenditure per capita is low and varies significantly between regions. Globally, the primary sources of mental health financing are out-of-pocket expenditure by the patient or family, followed by taxes, social insurance, and private insurance.[45] A helpful step toward improving funding allocation to mental health services would be a benchmark of the ideal proportion of a national budget for neuropsychiatric health for countries to have as a guideline.

Policies for Neuropsychiatric Disorders Interventions

Policies for perinatal interventions to reduce causes of intellectual disability in children, such as congenital hypothyroidism, have strong evidence for effectiveness. Screening programs exist in more than 30 countries, including LMICs.[9] Interventions aimed at preventing suicide and self-harm, and policies and legislation that reduce access to lethal means of suicide— including pesticides and gun ownership—have evidence of effectiveness and cost-effectiveness (value for money).[9] After Sri Lanka banned pesticides in the 1990s, India conducted a cost-effectiveness study of banning pesticides to prevent self-harm and suicide. They specifically looked at ending access to endosulfan, a common pesticide which is highly lethal in intentional ingestions. The estimated cost of implementation of the ban and hospital treatment for self-harm cases was US$0.10 per capita, yielding a cost-effectiveness ratio of ~US$1000 per DALYs averted (YLL averted + YLD averted, where YLD averted =number of prevalent cases × disability weight × treatment coverage in the population).[83] The Assessing Cost-Effectiveness in Prevention project in Australia found that the estimated cost per healthy life year gained would be US$57000 for the cost-effectiveness of reducing access to lethal means by revised legislation for gun ownership.[84]

Policies for Neurologic Disorders Interventions

Population-based prevention interventions for targeting epilepsy risk factors (e.g., prevention of head injuries or neurocysticercosis) and management of cardiovascular risk factors (e.g., healthy diet, physical activity, and tobacco use cessation) have moderate evidence for effectiveness but no evidence of cost-effectiveness.[9] The mortality due to epilepsy can be reduced by targeting structural and metabolic epilepsy risk factors, such as by preventing head injuries by laws requiring motorcyclists to wear helmets, motorists to wear seat belts, and the enforcement of speed limits.[85] To reduce cardiovascular risk factors for neurologic disorders, in North America and Canada the TEAMcare study provided team-based care for diabetes, coronary artery disease, and depression via clinics and phone to promote self-care skills and encourage positive health behaviors.[86]

Policies for Substance Use Disorders Interventions

Policies that target reducing alcohol use disorder by decreasing access via excise taxes have strong evidence of effectiveness and cost-effectiveness.[9] Rehm et al. found that in countries with high levels of alcohol abuse (defined as >5% of adults), a 20–50% increase in alcohol taxes was highly cost-effective. They found that in LMICs in Central Asia, Europe, Latin America, the Caribbean, and Sub-Saharan Africa, the cost of preventing a DALY was US$200–400.[87] Interventions with strong evidence of effectiveness and no evidence of cost-effectiveness for alcohol use disorder include restriction on sales, minimum legal age, drunk driving countermeasures (cost US$236 per DALY averted), and limiting opening and closing hours and days of sale.[88]

Professional Training and Education

Improving professional education in mental and neurologic disorders will require a multipronged approach to improving psychiatry and neurology training and increasing mental health training of nonspecialist clinicians. Currently, education programs for nonspecialists in many countries include some degree of mental health and neurologic education: in 37 LMICs, 20% of countries reported the integration of the assessment and treatment protocols for mental disorder in primary care, 17% had some integration between primary care and mental health services, 27% had mental health retraining for primary

health care physicians, 13% had refresher programs for primary health care nurses, and 61% taught psychiatry and behavioral health topics in undergraduate courses.[89] However, mental health training of nonspecialist clinicians should be increased in order to build capacity for mental health service development across the globe. Tesfaye and colleagues[90] described an initiative to implement child psychiatry subspecialty training within a mental health graduate program for nonphysicians in Ethiopia. Students receive a 2-week child psychiatry course and a 4-week child psychiatry clinical internship as part of a 2-year Master of Science in Mental Health for nonphysicians in Ethiopia. The course and internship had good user acceptability, as defined as a trainee subjective rating of very good or excellent on a Likert scale at the end of the internship. Fricchione et al.[91] advocate for building capacity in global mental health by institutions in high-income countries partnering with institutions in low- and middle-income countries to create sustainable academic and research relationships. They suggest initial educational programs in mental and neurologic health for primary care physicians, with eventual expansion to educating specialized health professionals.[92] A partnership between the University of Toronto and Addis Ababa University in Ethiopia has fostered a collaborative psychiatry residency program that has increased the number of psychiatrists in Ethiopia by over 300% in 6 years from 11 to 34.[93] Given the broad scope of disorders that most specialist and nonspecialist providers encounter, improvements in training programs should also incorporate neuropsychiatric diagnostic skills. Proficiencies should include physical exam skills, treatment of high acuity psychiatric and neurologic patients, psychotherapeutic principles, as well as principles of collaborative care, supervision, and leadership and management skills. Integrating neurologic and mental health care into neuropsychiatric training is crucial not only to nascent postgraduate programs in psychiatry and neurology, but also programs in HICs where neurology and psychiatry are separate specialties with different training requirements. Individuals with more versatility in neuropsychiatric training will have greater capacity to expand access to care and bridge clinical gaps in task shared, decentralized medical systems, and also to adapt to transformations in care models in HICs, as delivery of care shifts from siloed tertiary care to more patient-oriented, value-based systems of care.

Growing appreciation for the widespread impact of trauma (from war, disaster, and intimate partners or sexual violence to structural racism, gender-bias, economic polarization, and food insecurity), along with other social determinants of health, also has resulted in an increased awareness of the need to address these variables explicitly in order to improve health equity.[93] The conceptual framework designated by the Substance Abuse and Mental Health Services Administration (SAMHSA) as "trauma-informed care" (TIC) strives for fully integrating knowledge about trauma into policies, procedures, and practices in order to resist triggering and retraumatization that can occur as individuals make efforts to access health care. It recognizes that providers treating these patients require an awareness of the potential for vicarious or secondary trauma and burnout, and strategies to manage them, in order to support an effective and consistent workforce.[94] The six principles of TIC include (1) physical and psychological safety, (2) trustworthiness and transparency, (3) collaboration and mutuality,(4) acknowledgment and incorporation of cultural, historical, and gender issues, (5) peer support, and (6) empowerment, voice, and choice. Helping those outside neuropsychiatric specialties feel equally empowered to engage population groups with comorbid psychiatric and substance use disorder histories is essential to address patient needs in a more collaborative and comprehensive manner. Collaboration with traditional and faith healers may be addressed within this framework as well.[95]

Digital Technology Strategies

Increases in digital technologies such as applications and online platforms can support mental and neurologic care delivery across the globe and provide opportunities for novel systems of care delivery. For example, web-centered training has been shown to be successful in training large numbers of therapists dispersed across a wide geographical area and mobile technology has been used effectively to deliver mental health services in rural India.[96,97] Additionally, with expansions in mobile phone ownership globally, there are greater opportunities to use applications for a variety of activities within a care delivery value chain such as self-help, symptom tracking, training and supervision, and quality improvement data collection. Technology, while it should not replace human interaction in health care, can be designed to increase human connection and empower specialists and nonspecialists to more effectively support mental and neurologic care. Telepsychiatry services can also facilitate direct patient care, consultation services between medical clinicians, and partnerships for collaboration clinically and on research endeavors. Although the use of digital technology for mental health care delivery is still nascent, it holds the potential to advance innovative models of neuropsychiatric care across the globe.

Summary and Key Points

- There is increasing global appreciation of the high burden of disease and impact of neuropsychiatric disorders.
- Significant challenges to addressing this burden exist, including inadequate human resources, low funding, and limited political will.
- Work remains to successfully implement potential solutions to effective global mental health service delivery including task sharing of mental and neurologic care, digital technological advances, and capacity building for nonspecialist and specialist clinicians and policy makers.
- Cross-disciplinary engagement and flexibility of health providers at different levels, health system strengthening, and public commitment to financing are crucial to developing innovative and sustainable solutions to reducing the burden of neuropsychiatric disorders across the globe.

Multiple Choice Questions

1. Which of the following neurologic conditions accounts for the largest percentage of global mortality and disability due to neurologic disorders?
   a. Epilepsy
   b. Stroke
   c. Head trauma
   d. Alzheimer's disease
   e. Parkinson's disease

2. Epilepsy is thought to be more common in lower-income countries due to which of the following?
   a. Higher rates of nervous system infection
   b. Lower access to pre- and perinatal care
   c. Higher rates of birth injuries
   d. Higher rates of head trauma
   e. All of the above

3. Global mental health delivery faces which of the following challenges?

   a. Lack of specialized services
   b. Limitations in financing
   c. Supply chain availability
   d. Access to diagnostic testing
   e. All of the above

4. The global burden of mental and neurologic disorders is high, yet there are too few specialized professionals to meet this need. Strategies for reducing the global burden of mental disorders include all of the following except:
   a. Task sharing of mental health care tasks to nonspecialist providers
   b. Increasing postgraduate neuropsychiatry training
   c. Increasing use of digital technologies for training, supervision, and consultation
   d. Implementing effective national prevention policies for mental and substance use disorders
   e. Moving community-based services into central neuropsychiatric facilities

Multiple Choice Answers

1. Answer: b

According to Global Burden of Disease Study 2015,[18] stroke accounted for 67.3% of the global burden of mortality due to neurologic disorders and 47.3% of global DALYs due to neurologic disorders.

2. Answer: e

In addition to genetic syndromes, epilepsy can result from any injury to the brain. Lower-income countries have higher rates of meningitis, lower access to pre- and perinatal care leading to higher incidence of in utero infection and birth trauma, and higher rates of head trauma due in part to poor road conditions and inadequate use of motorcycle helmets.

3. Answer: e

Global mental health delivery faces multiple challenges including lack of specialized services, limited financing, supply chain availability, and access to diagnostic testing.

4. Answer: e

Strategies for reducing the global burden of mental disorders include, but are not limited to, task sharing of mental health care tasks to nonspecialist providers, increasing postgraduate neuropsychiatry training, increasing use of digital technologies for training, supervision, and consultation, and implementing effective national prevention policies for mental and substance use disorders.

References

1. GBD 2015 DALYs and HALE Collaborators. Global, regional, and national disability-adjusted life-years (DALYs) for 315 diseases and injuries and healthy life expectancy (HALE), 1990–2015: a systematic analysis for the Global Burden of Disease Study 2015. *Lancet.* 2016;388:1603-1658.

2. Murray CJL, Lopez AD, World Health Organization, World Bank, Harvard School of Public Health. The global burden of disease: a comprehensive assessment of mortality and disability from diseases, injuries, and risk factors in 1990 and projected to 2020: summary. Geneva, Switzerland: World Health Organization; 1996. Available at http://apps.who.int/iris/handle/10665/41864.

3. Wang PS, Angermeyer M, Borges G, et al. Delay and failure in treatment seeking after first onset of mental disorders in the World Health Organization's World Mental Health Survey Initiative. *World Psychiatry.* 2007;6:177-185.

4. Steel Z, Marnane C, Iranpour C, et al. The global prevalence of common mental disorders: a systematic review and meta-analysis 1980–2013. *Int J Epidemiol.* 2014;43:476-493.

5. The World Bank Group. World Bank country and lending groups. Washington, DC: World Bank; 2019. Available at https://datahelpdesk.worldbank.org/knowledgebase/articles/906519-world-bank-country-and-lending-groups.

6. Kessler R, Aguilar-Gaxiola J, Alonso M, et al. Prevalence and severity of mental disorders in the World Mental Health Survey Initiative of Mental Disorders. In: Kessler R, Ustun T, eds. *The WHO World Mental Health Survey: Global Perspectives on the Epidemiology.* Cambridge: Cambridge University Press; 2008.

7. Kessler RC, Chiu WT, Demler O, et al. Prevalence, severity, and comorbidity of 12-month DSM-IV disorders in the National Comorbidity Survey Replication. *Arch Gen Psychiatry.* 2005;62:617-627.

8. Ferrari AJ, Baxter AJ, Whiteford HA. A systematic review of the global distribution and availability of prevalence data for bipolar disorder. *J Affect Disord.* 2011;134:1-13.

9. Patel V, Chisholm D, Dua T, Laxminarayan R, Medina-Mora ME, eds. *Mental, Neurological, and Substance Use Disorders: Disease Control Priorities.* Vol. 4. 3rd ed. Washington, DC: The World Bank; 2016.

10. Kessler RC, Aguilar-Gaxiola S, Alonso J, et al. Trauma and PTSD in the WHO World Mental Health Surveys. *Eur J Psychotraumatol.* 2017;8(suppl 5).

11. Charlson F, van Ommeren M, Flaxman A, Cornett J, Whiteford H, Saxena S. New WHO prevalence estimates of mental disorders in conflict settings: a systematic review and meta-analysis. *Lancet.* 2019;pii: S0140-6736:30934-1.

12. Alonso J, Liu Z, Evans-Lacko S, et al. Treatment gap for anxiety disorders is global: results of the World Mental Health surveys in 21 countries. *Depress Anxiety.* 2018;35:195-208.

13. NIMH. Global leading categories of diseases/disorders. Bethesda, MD: NIMH; 2018. Available at https://www.nimh.nih.gov/health/ statistics/global/global-leading-categories-of-diseases-disorders.shtml.

14. Moreno-Küstner B, Martín C, Pastor L. Prevalence of psychotic disorders and its association with methodological issues. A systematic review and meta-analyses. *PLoS One.* 2018;13:e0195687.

15. Baxter AJ, Brugha TS, Erskine HE, Scheurer RW, Vos T, Scott JG. The epidemiology and global burden of autism spectrum disorders. *Psychol Med.* 2015;45:601-613.

16. Ngugi AK, Kariuki SM, Bottomley C, Kleinschmidt I, Sander JW, Newton CR. Incidence of epilepsy: a systematic review and meta-analysis. *Neurology.* 2011;77:1005-1012.

17. GBD 2015 Mortality and Causes of Death Collaborators. Global, regional, and national life expectancy, all-cause mortality, and cause-specific mortality for 249 causes of death, 1980–2015: a systematic analysis for the Global Burden of Disease Study 2015. *Lancet.* 2016;388:1459-1544.

18. GBD 2015 Neurological Disorders Collaborator Group. Global, regional, and national burden of neurological disorders during 1990–2015: a systematic analysis for the Global Burden of Disease Study 2015. *Lancet Neurol.* 2017;16:877-897.

19. Feigin VL, Forouzanfar MH, Krishnamurthi R, et al. Global and regional burden of stroke during 1990–2010: findings from the Global Burden of Disease Study 2010. *Lancet.* 2014;383:245-254.

20. Johnston SC, Mendis S, Mathers CD. Global variation in stroke burden and mortality: estimates from monitoring, surveillance, and modelling. *Lancet Neurol.* 2009;8:345-354.

21. World Health Organization. *First World Health Organization Ministerial Conference on Global Action Against Dementia.* Geneva, Switzerland: World Health Organization; 2015.

22. Prince MJ, Wu F, Guo Y, et al. The burden of disease in older people and implications for health policy and practice. *Lancet.* 2015;385:549-562.

23. Murray CJL, Vos T, Lozano R, et al. Disability-adjusted life years (DALYs) for 291 diseases and injuries in 21 regions, 1990–2010: a systematic analysis for the Global Burden of Disease Study 2010. *Lancet.* 2012;380:2197-2223.

24. Mbewe E, Zairemthiama P, Paul R, Birbeck GL, Steiner TJ. The burden of primary headache disorders in Zambia: national estimates from a population-based door-to-door survey. *J Headache Pain.* 2015;16:513.

25. GBD 2016 Parkinson's Disease Collaborators. Global, regional, and national burden of Parkinson's disease, 1990–2016: a systematic analysis for the Global Burden of Disease Study 2016. *Lancet Neurol.* 2018;17:939-953.

26. GBD 2015 Neurological Disorders Collaborator Group. Global, regional, and national burden of neurological disorders during 1990–2015: a systematic analysis for the Global Burden of Disease Study 2015. *Lancet Neurol.* 2017;16:877-897.

27. United Nations Office on Drugs and Crime. World Drug Report 2017. Vienna, Austria: United Nations Office on Drugs and Crime; 2017. Available at http://www.unodc.org/wdr2017.

28. National Institute of Mental Health. Global individual mental and behavioral disorders. Bethesda, MD: National Institute of Mental Health; 2018. Available at https://www.nimh.nih.gov/health/statistics/global/global-individual-mental-and-behavioral-disorders.shtml.

29. GBD 2016 Causes of Death Collaborators. Global, regional, and national age-sex specific mortality for 264 causes of death, 1980–2016: a systematic analysis for the Global Burden of Disease Study 2016. *Lancet.* 2017;390:1151-1210.

30. World Health Organization. Global status on alcohol and health 2014. Geneva, Switzerland: World Health Organization; 2016. Available at http://apps.who.int/iris/bitstream/handle/10665/112736/9789240692763_eng.pdf;jsessionid=A6C264462D33A7A39D968857CF691C48?sequence=1.

31. Gomes T, Tadrous M, Mamdani MM, Paterson JM, Juurlink DN. The burden of opioid-related mortality in the United States. *JAMA Network Open.* 2018;1:e180217.

32. United Nations Office on Drugs and Crime. World Drug Report 2018. Vienna, Austria: United Nations Office on Drugs and Crime; 2018. Available at https://www.unodc.org/wdr2018/prelaunch/WDR18_Booklet_1_EXSUM.pdf.

33. Felitti VJ, Anda RF, Nordenberg D, et al. Relationship of childhood abuse and household dysfunction to many of the leading causes of death in adults. The Adverse Childhood Experiences (ACE) study. *Am J Prev Med.* 1998;14:245-258.

34. Druss BG, Zhao L, Von Esenwein S, Morrato EH, Marcus SC. Understanding excess mortality in persons with mental illness: 17-year follow up of a nationally representative US survey. *Med Care.* 2011;49:599-604.

35. Mensah GA, Collins PY. Understanding mental health for the prevention and control of cardiovascular diseases. *Glob Heart.* 2015;10:221-224.

36. Thombs BD, Bass EB, Ford DE, et al. Prevalence of depression in survivors of acute myocardial infarction. *J Gen Intern Med.* 2006;21:30-38.

37. Coyle CM, Mahanty S, Zunt JR, et al. Neurocysticercosis: neglected but not forgotten. *PLoS Negl Trop Dis.* 2012;6:e1500.

38. Singhi P. Infectious causes of seizures and epilepsy in the developing world. *Dev Med Child Neurol.* 2011;53:600-609.

39. Marks M, Jarvis JN, Howlett W, Mabey DCW. Neurosyphilis in Africa: a systematic review. *PLoS Negl Trop Dis.* 2017;11:e0005880.

40. Vega P, Sweetland A, Acha J, et al. Psychiatric issues in the management of patients with multidrug-resistant tuberculosis. *Int J Tuberc Lung Dis.* 2004;8:749-759.

41. Javaid A, Khan MA, Jan F, et al. Occurrence of adverse events in patient receiving community-based therapy for multidrug-resistant tuberculosis in Pakistan. *Tuberk Toraks.* 2018;66:16-25.

42. Kohn R, Saxena S, Levav I, Saraceno B. The treatment gap in mental health care. *Bull World Health Organ.* 2004;82:858-866.

43. World Health Organization. Mental disorders. Geneva, Switzerland: World Health Organization; 2018. Available at https://www.who.int/news-room/fact-sheets/detail/mental-disorders.

44. World Health Organization. Global mental health: how are we doing? Geneva, Switzerland: World Health Organization; 2015. Available at http://www.who.int/mental_health/evidence/atlas/interactive_infographic_2015.pdf.

45. World Health Organization. Mental Health Atlas 2017. Geneva, Switzerland: World Health Organization; 2018. Available at https://www.who.int/mental_health/evidence/atlas/mental_health_atlas_2017/en/.

46. World Health Organization. Atlas: country resources for neurological disorders, Second Edition. Geneva, Switzerland: World Health Organization; 2017. Available at http://apps.who.int/iris/bitstream/handle/10665/258947/9789241565509-eng.pdf;jsessionid=93D8D9E6E1C5EE8B67535C8ADD74E870?sequence=1.

47. Dall TM, Storm MV, Chakrabarti R, et al. Supply and demand analysis of the current and future US neurology workforce. *Neurology.* 2013;81:470-478.

48. World Health Organization. Mental Health Atlas 2011. Geneva, Switzerland: World Health Organization; 2011. Available at https://www.who.int/mental_health/publications/mental_health_atlas_2011/en/.

49. World Health Organization. World Health Organization model list of essential medicines. 20th ed. Geneva, Switzerland: World Health Organization; 2017. Available at http://apps.who.int/iris/bitstream/handle/10665/273826/EML-20-eng.pdf?ua=1.

50. Wagenaar BH, Stergachis A, Rao D, et al. The availability of essential medicines for mental healthcare in Sofala, Mozambique. *Glob Health Action.* 2015;8.

51. International Pharmaceutical Federation (FIP). Pharmacy at a glance 2015–2017. The Hague, The Netherlands: International Pharmaceutical Federation; 2017. Available at https://fip.org/files/fip/publications/2017-09-Pharmacy_at_a_Glance-2015-2017.pdf.

52. West JC, Wilk JE, Rae DS, et al. Medicaid prescription drug policies and medication access and continuity: findings from ten states. *Psychiatr Serv.* 2009;60:601-610.

53. World Health Organization. Global Atlas of medical devices: World Health Organization medical devices technical series. Geneva, Switzerland: World Health Organization; 2017. Available at http://apps.who.int/medicinedocs/documents/s23215en/s23215en.pdf.

54. World Health Organization. Organization of services for mental health: mental health policy and service guidance package. Geneva, Switzerland: World Health Organization; 2003. Available at https://www.who.int/mental_health/policy/services/essentialpackage1v2/en/.

55. World Health Organization. Mental Health Atlas 2005. Geneva, Switzerland: World Health Organization; 2005. Available at https://www.who.int/mental_health/evidence/mhatlas05/en/.

56. Saraceno B, van Ommeren M, Batniji R, et al. Barriers to improvement of mental health services in low-income and middle-income countries. *Lancet.* 2007;370:1164-1174.

57. World Health Organization. The development of comprehensive mental health services in the community. Copenhagen, Denmark: World Health Organization; 1973.

58. Patel V, Araya R, Chatterjee S, et al. Treatment and prevention of mental disorders in low-income and middle-income countries. *Lancet*. 2007;370:991-1005.

59. Lancet Global Mental Health Group, Chisholm D, Flisher AJ, et al. Scale up services for mental disorders: a call for action. *Lancet*. 2007;370:1241-1252.

60. Pereira B, Andrew G, Pednekar S, Kirkwood BR, Patel V. The integration of the treatment for common mental disorders in primary care: experiences of health care providers in the MANAS trial in Goa, India. *Int J Ment Health Syst*. 2011;5:26.

61. Rahman A. Challenges and opportunities in developing a psychological intervention for perinatal depression in rural Pakistan—a multi-method study. *Arch Womens Ment Health*. 2007;10:211-219.

62. Nyatsanza M, Schneider M, Davies T, Lund C. Filling the treatment gap: developing a task sharing counselling intervention for perinatal depression in Khayelitsha, South Africa. *BMC Psychiatry*. 2016;16:164.

63. Araya R, Rojas G, Fritsch R, et al. Treating depression in primary care in low-income women in Santiago, Chile: a randomised controlled trial. *Lancet*. 2003;361:995-1000.

64. Chibanda D, Verhey R, Munetsi E, Rusakaniko S, Cowan F, Lund C. Scaling up interventions for depression in sub-Saharan Africa: lessons from Zimbabwe. *Glob Ment Health (Camb)*. 2016;3:e13.

65. Sikander S, Lazarus A, Bangash O, et al. The effectiveness and cost-effectiveness of the peer-delivered Thinking Healthy Programme for perinatal depression in Pakistan and India: the SHARE study protocol for randomised controlled trials. *Trials*. 2015;16:534.

66. Eappen BS, Aguilar M, Ramos K, et al. Preparing to launch the "Thinking Healthy Programme" perinatal depression intervention in Urban Lima, Peru: experiences from the field. *Global Mental Health*. 2018;5:e41.

67. Dias A, Azariah F, Anderson SJ, et al. Effect of a lay counselor intervention on prevention of major depression in older adults living in low- and middle-income countries: a randomized clinical trial. *JAMA Psychiatry*. 2019;76:13-20.

68. Thirthalli J, Sivakumar PT, Gangadhar BN. Preventing late-life depression through task sharing: scope of translating evidence to practice in resource-scarce settings. *JAMA Psychiatry*. 2018;E1-E2.

69. Papas RK, Sidle JE, Gakinya BN, et al. Treatment outcomes of a stage 1 cognitive-behavioral trial to reduce alcohol use among human immunodeficiency virus-infected out-patients in western Kenya. *Addiction*. 2011;106:2156-2166.

70. Sorsdahl K, Myers B, Ward CL, et al. Adapting a blended motivational interviewing and problem-solving intervention to address risky substance use amongst South Africans. *Psychother Res*. 2015;25(4):435-444.

71. Nadkarni A, Weobong B, Weiss HA, et al. Counselling for Alcohol Problems (CAP), a lay counsellor-delivered brief psychological treatment for harmful drinking in men, in primary care in India: a randomised controlled trial. *Lancet*. 2017;389:186-195.

72. Hanlon C, Alem A, Medhin G, et al. Task sharing for the care of severe mental disorders in a low-income country (TaSCS): study protocol for a randomised, controlled, non-inferiority trial. *Trials*. 2016;17:76.

73. Chatterjee S, Pillai A, Jain S, Cohen A, Patel V. Outcomes of people with psychotic disorders in a community-based rehabilitation programme in rural India. *Br J Psychiatry*. 2009;195:433-439.

74. McLean KE, Kaiser BN, Hagaman AK, Wagenaar BH, Therosme TP, Kohrt BA. Task sharing in rural Haiti: qualitative assessment of a brief, structured training with and without apprenticeship supervision for community health workers. *Intervention (Amstelveen)*. 2015;13:135-155.

75. Smith S, Kayiteshonga Y, Misago C, et al. Integrating mental health care into primary care. *Intervention*. 2017;15:136-150.

76. Fils-Aimé JR, Grelotti DJ, Thérosmé T, et al. A mobile clinic approach to the delivery of community-based mental health services in rural Haiti. *PLoS One*. 2018;13:e0199313.

77. Mendenhall E, De Silva MJ, Hanlon C, et al. Acceptability and feasibility of using non-specialist health workers to deliver mental health care: stakeholder perceptions from the PRIME district sites in Ethiopia, India, Nepal, South Africa, and Uganda. *Soc Sci Med*. 2014;118:33-42.

78. Patterson V, Gautam N, Pant P. Training non-neurologists to diagnose epilepsy. *Seizure*. 2013;22:306-308.

79. Chaple MJ, Freese TE, Rutkowski BA, et al. Using ECHO clinics to promote capacity building in clinical supervision. *Am J Prev Med*. 2018;54:S275-S280.

80. WHO and WONCA. Integrating mental health into primary care: a global perspective. Geneva, Switzerland: WHO and WONCA; 2008. Available at https://www.who.int/mental_health/resources/mentalhealth_PHC_2008.pdf.

81. Keynejad R, Semrau M, Toynbee M, et al. Building the capacity of policy-makers and planners to strengthen mental health systems in low- and middle-income countries: a systematic review. *BMC Health Serv Res*. 2016;16:601.

82. Breuer E, De Silva MJ, Shidaye R, et al. Planning and evaluating mental health services in low- and middle-income countries using theory of change. *Br J Psychiatry*. 2016;208(suppl 56):s55-s62.

83. Nigam A, Reykar N, Majumder M, Chisholm D. Self-harm in India: cost-effectiveness analysis of a proposed pesticide ban. Working Paper No. 15. Disease Control Priorities; 2015.

84. Vos T, Carter R, Barendregt J, et al. Assessing Cost-Effectiveness in Prevention (ACE–Prevention): Final report. Melbourne: University of Queensland, Brisbane, and Deakin University; 2010.

85. World Health Organization. Global status report on road safety—time for action. Geneva, Switzerland: World Health Organization; 2009. Available at https://afro.who.int/publications/global-status-report-road-safety-time-action.

86. Katon W, Russo J, Lin EHB, et al. Cost-effectiveness of a multi-condition collaborative care intervention. *Arch Gen Psychiatry*. 2012;69.

87. Rehm J, Chisholm D, Room R, Lopez A. Alcohol. In: Jamison D, Breman J, Measham A, et al, eds. *Disease Control Priorities in Developing Countries*. 2nd ed. Washington, DC: World Bank and Oxford University Press; 2006:887-906.

88. Gureje O, Chisholm D, Kola L, Lasebikan V, Saxena S. Cost-effectiveness of an essential mental health intervention package in Nigeria. *World Psychiatry*. 2007;6:42-48.

89. Jacob KS, Sharan P, Mirza I, et al. Mental health systems in countries: where are we now? *Lancet*. 2007;370:1061-1077.

90. Tesfaye M, Abera M, Gruber-Frank C, Frank R. The development of a model of training in child psychiatry for non-physician clinicians in Ethiopia. *Child Adolesc Psychiatry Ment Health*. 2014;8:6.

91. Fricchione GL, Borba CPC, Alem A, Shibre T, Carney JR, Henderson DC. Capacity building in global mental health: professional training. *Harv Rev Psychiatry*. 2012;20(1):47-57.

92. Alem A, Pain C, Araya M, Hodges BD. Co-creating a psychiatric resident program with Ethiopians, for Ethiopians, in Ethiopia:

the Toronto Addis Ababa Psychiatry Project (TAAPP). *Acad Psychiatry*. 2010;34:424-432.

93. Levy-Carrick N, Lewis-O'Connor A, Rittenberg E, Manosalvas K, Stoklosa H, Silbersweig D. Promoting health equity through trauma-informed care: critical role for physicians in policy and program development. *Fam Community Health*. 2019;42:104-108.

94. U.S. Department of Health and Human Services. Trauma-informed approach and trauma-specific interventions. Rockville, MD: U.S. Department of Health and Human Services; 2014. Available at https://www.samhsa.gov/nctic/trauma-interventions.

95. van der Watt A, van de Water TT, Nortje G, Oladeji B, Seedat S, Gureje O, et al. The perceived effectiveness of traditional and faith healing in the treatment of mental illness: a systematic review of qualitative studies. *Soc Psychiatry Psychiatr Epidemiol*. 2018;53:555-566.

96. O'Connor M, Morgan KE, Bailey-Straebler S, Fairburn CG, Cooper Z. Increasing the availability of psychological treatments: a multinational study of a scalable method for training therapists. *J Med Internet Res*. 2018;20:e10386.

97. Maulik PK, Kallakuri S, Devarapalli S, Vadlamani VK, Jha V, Patel A. Increasing use of mental health services in remote areas using mobile technology: a pre–post evaluation of the SMART Mental Health project in rural India. *J Glob Health*. 2017;7:010408.

39

Neuropsychiatry and Behavioral Neurology: Future Directions

Laura T. Safar · David A. Silbersweig · Kirk R. Daffner

INTRODUCTION

Our textbook has evaluated advances in basic and clinical neuroscience and presented an integrated view of neuropsychiatry and behavioral neurology, with the ultimate goal of improving the care and reducing the suffering of those affected by neuropsychiatric disorders. Knowledge, practices, disciplines, and nosology involving the fields related to clinical neuroscience have undergone many iterations and classifications over the years. One important iteration has been the division of *neurology* and *psychiatry* into two separate disciplines that pay attention to different phenomena, pathogenic mechanisms, and treatment methods.[1,2] Table 39-1 provides an illustration of these differences, using a patient with multiple sclerosis and depression as an example. In other iterations of clinical neuroscience, the borders between fields are less distinct and there has been considerable overlap between psychiatry and neurology. For decades, researchers and clinicians have discussed intersection and commonalities between these fields. For centuries, philosophers have discussed the relationship between brain and mind, feelings and intellect, subjective experience and behavior.[3-5] The experience of patients is in agreement with an integrated view of neurology and psychiatry: Individuals with brain illness often suffer from combinations of motor, sensorial, autonomic, emotional, behavioral, and cognitive symptoms. It is not their priority to know which discipline "owns" their illness or their symptoms, other than to find appropriate care.

Neurology has long established itself as the medical specialty that contends with diseases of the nervous system, with *cognitive and behavioral neurology* as the subspecialty that focuses on the functional neurocircuitry of cognition and the ways in which to treat cognitive and behavioral manifestations of central nervous system disorders. *Psychiatry* has been a medical specialty with different orientations developing in parallel over time (see Table 39-2). In general, psychiatry has sustained a more integrative or bio-psycho-social view of human behavior. Neuropsychiatry focuses on a brain circuit-based understanding of disorders of emotion and behavior—including the neurological underpinnings of "psychiatric" conditions and the "psychiatric" aspects of "neurologic" conditions. A welcome challenge for the field of neuropsychiatry is to keep alive this integrative perspective, as knowledge about neurobiological pathogenesis and treatments continue to advance.

THE PRESENT TIME

Progress in basic and clinical research[8,9] and advances in technology, such as those observed in neuroimaging and computational sciences, have contributed to an exponential growth in the available knowledge about clinical neuroscience. As research tools and approaches used by psychiatry and neurology become increasingly similar, many of the distinctions between the fields are less relevant. Clinically, the field of psychiatry has been embracing the challenge and excitement of integrating neurobiological and psychosocial models.[10-12] The field of neurology has been increasingly paying attention to cognitive and emotional phenomena and the psychosocial impact of neurological illnesses.[13] Moreover, many of the "core" neurological diseases (e.g., Parkinson's disease [PD], multiple sclerosis [MS], amyotrophic lateral sclerosis [ALS]) that were considered to be disorders of sensory-motor function are now viewed as having major cognitive, emotional, and behavioral features. Nevertheless, most clinical training and practice in neurology and psychiatry remain relatively distinct regarding knowledge and skills sets.

Mastering the depth and breadth of available information at the interface is extremely difficult for any individual clinician. There are different ways in which to handle the seemingly overwhelming complexities of these fields. Some specialists have sought to define the scope of their role, for instance, deciding to take care of individuals with very specific neuropsychiatric illnesses (e.g., a subspecialization in movement disorders, or an even narrower field). Some of these clinicians have tried to care for all the manifestations of a certain illness, at least to some degree (e.g., motor, cognitive, and emotional symptoms associated with PD). Other specialists have limited their focus to specific dimensions of patients' difficulties, working with other

TABLE 39-1 • Neurology and Psychiatry as Different Disciplines*.

	Neurologic Focus	Psychiatric Focus
Phenomena	Physical (spasticity, paresthesia, visual changes, urinary frequency, etc.) and cognitive symptoms	Major depression syndrome: mood, interest/enjoyment, energy, activity, sleep, appetite, concentration, thought content, etc.
Assessment and diagnostic methods	History gathering, neurological exam, neuroimaging, lumbar puncture, Expanded Disability Status Scale (EDSS)	Emphasis on psychiatric interview/ history gathering; scales based on phenomenology, such as PHQ-9
Pathogenic mechanism	MS brain lesions disrupt the nervous system's normal anatomy and functioning	*Biological psychiatry:* disruption of neurotransmitters/ neurochemistry
		Psychosocial psychiatry: impact of MS on the individual's patterns of thinking, feeling, coping, and behaving, placed within the context of early experiences, and ongoing psychosocial stressors
Treatment	MS disease-modifying therapies, corticosteroids, and symptomatic treatments (e.g., baclofen)	Psychopharmacology and psychotherapy

Simplified for illustrative purposes. The table uses, as a case example, an individual with MS and Major Depression.

TABLE 39-2 • Psychiatric Subspecialties or Orientations— Their Focus and Relationship with the Brain*.

Psychiatric Subspecialty or Orientation	Main Focus	Discipline's Relationship with the Brain
Biological psychiatry	Phenomenology as related to neurotransmitters/ neurochemistry.	The brain plays a critical role, with the focus of the field on the chemical interactions between neurons and their impact on emotions, thoughts, and behaviors.
Psychosocial psychiatry	Psychological constructs including identity, self, coping strategies, defense mechanisms. Phenomenology a result of psychological makeup, impacted by early and ongoing experiences.	Reference to the brain is typically absent from the evaluation, clinical formulation, and treatment.
Neuropsychiatry	The neurobiological basis of psychiatric illnesses, with a focus on neurocircuitry. The emotional, behavioral, and cognitive manifestations of neurological illnesses and their treatment.[6]	The brain is the seat of the self. Identity, memories, emotions, and behaviors are encoded in/by the brain and result from the brain's anatomical/ network/functional makeup. This relationship applies to the individual's baseline or healthy functioning, as well as to disease manifestations and the effects of therapeutics.[7]

Simplified for illustrative purposes.

team members to provide the comprehensive care that individuals with neuropsychiatric illnesses need and deserve. Team-based care is becoming more widespread. This approach permits each clinician to keep up with the literature and master her/his field, while allowing patients to receive the most up-to-date, evidence-based care for the different aspects of their illnesses. The implementation of alternative models of clinical care delivery such as collaborative care and telehealth allows for more widespread access to advances in knowledge (see Chapters 36 and 38 in this textbook).

Increasingly over the last two decades, we have witnessed a rapid globalization of knowledge via electronic media (i.e., worldwide access to published articles and lectures through the Internet), telehealth practices and consultations, and increased availability of international educational, research, and clinical care collaborations. This has allowed for greater standardization of diagnostics and treatments. However, obstacles for this standardization exist, such as the administrative inertia of health care systems and economic factors such as uneven access to

specialists or expensive diagnostic methods and treatments in economically disadvantaged areas.

FUTURE DIRECTIONS

A critical question is whether neuropsychiatry and behavioral neurology will or should continue to be two separate fields, or become a single entity. This complex topic can be considered from different perspectives. A major unifying force affecting both disciplines is the growth of research that shares methods and increasingly focuses on common pathways underlying the pathogenesis (e.g., neuroinflammatory, genetic, developmental) of what have traditionally been viewed as psychiatric or neurologic diseases. This process has led to an expanding overlap between psychiatry and neurology in terms of the science elucidating causal mechanisms.

At the same time, there is a growing movement to divide each of these fields into smaller and smaller subspecialties that are creating their own separate vocabulary, certification, and narrow areas of expertise. From this perspective, there may be increasingly less overlap both *between* different components of neurology and psychiatry, and different components *within* neurology and psychiatry. Another way to describe these changes is to suggest that the variance within each of the subfields of psychiatry and neurology will be as great as, or greater than, the variance between the fields of psychiatry and neurology themselves. In short, the two fields may become indistinguishable not because we finally abandon arbitrary distinctions between psychiatric and neurologic disorders, but because within each of the fields, the many splintered parts will increasingly have less in common with the other parts. Note that the movement toward subspecialization and subsubspecialization is not specific to our field, but to medicine in general.

Even if this is an accurate picture of science's trajectory, it seems likely that the clinical symptomatology and types of patient interactions and interventions that animate the professional lives of clinicians and clinician-scientists in our field will continue to differ meaningfully across individuals. Some physicians will be more passionate about understanding and taking care of patients with emotional, psychological, or interpersonal dysfunction, while other physicians will be more engaged by patients with cognitive, behavioral, or motor dysfunction. To the extent that physicians will continue to be interested in different aspects of complex human function and behavior, and will have the associated areas of expertise, it is likely that distinctions between the fields of neuropsychiatry and behavioral neurology will be sustained.

Political, historical, and inertial forces also may align to help preserve the separate identities of the two fields. Psychiatry and neurology, the two medical specialties from which neuropsychiatry and behavioral neurology originate, each has its own rich traditions and history. As noted, each has focused on different aspects of mental life and different diseases of the nervous system. Each has its own professional organizations, departments, reimbursement mechanisms, and training programs. These factors lead to the expectation that neuropsychiatry and behavioral neurology are most likely to continue to exist as separate, but tightly linked subspecialties. While psychiatry and neurology departments may remain separate, the integration can be accomplished by creating interdisciplinary centers—such as our Center for Brain/Mind Medicine (CBMM) at Brigham and Women's Hospital—and "service lines" where both the psychiatric and neurological aspects of illnesses are addressed. Different models may fit better in different health care settings depending on the health centers' size, number of available subspecialists, and other factors.

A related question to consider is whether we envision the future of neuropsychiatry and behavioral neurology as one in which its practitioners will be experts in the neural underpinning of emotion, cognition, and behavior (i.e., how the brain works) that can be applied to a large range of human disorders (neurodegenerative, cerebrovascular, developmental, immune-mediated, primary psychiatric, etc.), or whether we see the future of our field as formed by practitioners whose work is mainly disease-centered (i.e., clinicians who have expertise in the neuropsychiatric/behavioral neurologic aspects of a specific disorder such as AD, MS, or Tourette syndrome (TS). Of course, the natural (neurally based) comorbidity among these conditions and the bidirectional interaction between experience and neurocircuits will always continue to require some degree of integrated expertise. At the CBMM, we come together as a large group of neuropsychiatrists, behavioral neurologists (and other relevant specialists such as neuropsychologists, social workers, and physiatrists) wearing both our "generalist" and "subspecialist" hats to participate in our weekly clinical teaching rounds where patients with a variety of illnesses are presented and discussed. Efforts are made to convey the patient's narrative and symptom profile, to identify neural networks that are dysfunctional, diseases that have a predilection for disrupting these networks, additional workup that is needed to narrow or confirm the differential diagnosis, and to highlight the range and combination of pharmacologic, behavioral, psychosocial, and supportive interventions that may improve function. While going through this process, clinicians rely on basic principles underlying neuropsychiatry and behavioral neurology, which provides a rich, shared language. Beyond enhancing care, this activity serves an important educational role, providing trainees with a truly integrated approach that transcends disciplines.

In addition to being part of our multidisciplinary center, many of us are also closely affiliated with programs or clinics focused on specific disorders (e.g., AD, MS, PD, epilepsy, TS, functional neurological disorders, etc.). In these settings, the neuropsychiatrist or behavioral neurologist contributes to a clinical community dedicated to the understanding and care of a particular disease area. Some experts would argue that the latter model represents the future of neuropsychiatry and behavioral neurology because it takes into account the rapid expansion of knowledge about individual diseases and the impossibility of maintaining expertise in multiple disorders. But these approaches are complementary, not mutually exclusive.

We would thus highlight the importance of supporting both approaches. A "generalist" subspecialty perspective in behavioral neurology and neuropsychiatry is critical for several reasons: educationally, for teaching foundational concepts to new trainees and to colleagues from other disciplines, and clinically, to take care of most patients in most health care settings, as the availability of sub-sub-specialists is currently limited to relatively few academic centers. In clinical research, a generalist perspective allows for an appreciation of the "big picture" and may facilitate the development of tools that can be helpful across diagnostic categories (e.g., an executive coaching program for individuals with dysexecutive syndromes arising from different disorders). At the same time, we also appreciate that a narrower focus allows for the advancement of research to develop more nuanced and specific knowledge about pathogenesis, clinical care, and therapeutic tools for a particular neuropsychiatric illness. Advances toward the "cures" for illnesses will most likely be achieved by groups that are laser focused.

Based on our experience at the CBMM, we would argue that there is considerable intellectual, clinical, and collegial value derived from separate, but allied disciplines bringing different perspectives to the table when considering the best way to understand and care for our complex patients. In the context of team-based care, team members complement each other, allowing all professionals to concentrate on what they do best, thus empowering each clinician to work at the top of their license. Multidisciplinary care allows a patient's predicament to be considered from a variety of perspectives, thus generating a comprehensive differential diagnosis and therapeutic plan. Members of one discipline often ask questions and have models that are distinct from those asked by colleagues originally trained in a different discipline. This process raises awareness of these issues in every member of the group, who begin to incorporate these questions and concerns in their own assessment and care of patients (who often need neurological and psychiatric interventions, as well as interventions from the other disciplines). A source of considerable pride at our center is that when visiting physicians attend our rounds, they often cannot discern whether the clinical fellow presenting a case had completed a psychiatry or neurology residency. Importantly, multidisciplinary care is most successfully practiced when institutional structures are created to ensure that the voices of each discipline will be heard, supported, and respected. Among the many colleagues with whom we practice interdisciplinary care, we appreciate the expertise of our neuroradiology and nuclear medicine colleagues and ongoing consultation with them, including at times when behavioral neurologists and neuropsychiatrists identify clinically pertinent neuroimaging findings that were not included in their original report.

In summary, rather than advocating for neuropsychiatry and behavioral neurology to become a homogenized "melting pot," we favor the metaphor of a tapestry of interwoven disciplines.

Keeping alive the foundational knowledge derived from the "forest" is particularly important, when we are focusing on the "trees." The intent of this chapter is to reflect upon and open up discussion about the direction our disciplines are headed regarding clinical care of individuals with neuropsychiatric disorders, and regarding research and education in the field of neuroscience. Some examples are outlined below, although this is not intended to be an all-inclusive list.

CLINICAL CARE

- Further development and more generalized use of alternative health care delivery models:
  - Team-based care, with a team-based body of knowledge, in which the group as a whole holds the knowledge about the various aspects of the illness and its treatment, and each individual provider only holds a part. Different iterations and submodels of team-based care in the primary care medical home include stepped-care and collaborative care. The inclusion of neuropsychiatry and behavioral neurology in the collaborative care model algorithm

would be helpful, particularly given the context of the aging population (see Chapter 36). Efficient screening for dementia can be integrated into the checkup, and neuropsychiatric evaluation can be facilitated.
  - Telehealth as a tool to increase access and limit the impact of geographic boundaries (other boundaries such as those involving financial resources continue to exist, especially with neuropsychiatric expertise being available only in a few centers).
  - Delivery of care electronically (e-psychotherapy, manualized care, self-help tools [apps]). In an era of increasing technology, the importance of human interactions and the value of the individual clinician in neuropsychiatry and cognitive neurology are critical.
- Advancement or development of computational approaches, for example, data-driven machine learning to identify potential diagnoses and appropriate treatments and to predict potential outcomes. This can include the use of passive sensing technology, such as real-time, remote monitoring of heart rate, voice affect, and steps number, that allows real-time, real-world evaluation of patients' functioning. Smartphone apps can facilitate this.
- Role changes: The specialist as a consultant guiding the selection and use of tools, as opposed to, or in addition to, directly delivering care in-office, visit to visit. Potentially positive aspects of this approach include the amplification of the clinician's therapeutic efficacy, mediated by the use of tools the patient will continue to employ between visits, and an increased sense of agency and responsibility the patient may have about his/her treatment. Potentially negative aspects include the "dilution" of the power of the therapeutic relationship and an excessive "mechanization" of care, especially if the appointments becomes solely centered on tools, gadgets, and resources.
- Individualized therapeutics based on a patient's biomarkers including genetic makeup, neurotransmitter and functional brain mapping, and illness-specific biomarkers.
- More widespread use of electronic medical records (EMRs), and augmented capacity to share information across different health care systems.

Challenges

- Access to effective clinical care seems to be an important challenge, a topic that exceeds the scope of this chapter. Even in industrialized, well-off economies such as in the United States, obstacles such as lack of parity in the payor system and the reimbursement model contribute to inequities in clinical care. It is important for neuropsychiatrists and behavioral neurologists to be mindful about issues of reimbursement and sustainability as they practice their profession and design/build services, including in the context of different health care systems, and ongoing movement toward health care redesign to include a population management model. Lack of parity and stigma around psychiatric illness continue to be challenges. Importantly, a neuropsychiatric approach can assist in overcoming stigma as it presents the psychiatric symptoms in the context of brain illness. See Chapter 4 for further discussion of this topic.

- The fragmentation of care among multiple team members necessitates a method to coordinate and hold a cohesive understanding of the patient's illness and treatment plan. The EMR provides a partial solution to this, but also adds complexities related to implementing and utilizing EMR technology, and concerns about protection of private information. There also is considerable risk for the perpetuation of errors, the "diffusion" of responsibility in such a system, and a need for clarity about who is the clinician "in charge" of the case. See Chapter 35 for further discussion, including concerns about the EMR.

- The practice of neuropsychiatry and behavioral neurology is labor intensive. Poor reimbursement for time spent with patients may discline trainees and practitioners from entering our fields. Given the growing need for neuropsychiatrists and behavioral neurologists, for example, to help care for our aging population, it is critical to advocate for a more equitable distribution of health care resources. As a field, we need to be able to articulate the value proposition of the services we uniquely offer, and advocate for changes in health policy and funding.

- Greater integration of neuropsychiatric expertise with neuroradiology and nuclear medicine, to facilitate increased recognition of subtle MRI or PET findings that may be present in neuropsychiatric disorders.

ADVANCEMENT OF KNOWLEDGE/RESEARCH

Current research trends in clinical neurosciences and other medical specialties that seem set to continue developing in the future include:

- Biologically based models of disorders to bring about taxonomical changes. Phenomenology or description-based diagnoses, such as schizophrenia, major depression, or catatonia, may be replaced or complemented by classifications based on mechanistic, intermediate-phenotype Research Domain Criteria (RDoC), and biomarker profiles (also see Chapter 11).[14,15]

- Research on common pathways of pathogenesis to contribute to an understanding of many illnesses (e.g., mechanisms involved in neuroinflammation, misfolded proteins, disorders of neural migration, genetic and epigenetic factors). Appreciation of critical mechanisms may result in therapeutics that reduce symptomatology in different illnesses that, for example, are mediated by neuroinflammatory mechanisms (e.g., SLE, MS, post-TBI dysfunction, poststroke depression).

- Big data: Access to data from large samples with the potential to increase the understanding of biological, environmental, and behavioral dimensions and their interactions, for multiple illnesses.

- Defining the genetic and epigenetic basis of neuropsychiatric disorders to facilitate the development of genetically based treatments.[16–19]

- Advances in neuroimaging, including functional neuroimaging, to assist in diagnosis and monitoring of illness progression and response to treatment, and the development of a circuit-based model of neuropsychiatric diseases, resulting in greater use of neuroimaging in neuropsychiatric clinical care.[18–22]

- Immunological, inflammatory, neurodegenerative, "omic," and other biomarkers to assist in diagnosis and monitoring of illness progression and response to treatment. Advances in the identification of new biomarkers and their greater use in neuropsychiatric clinical care, with growth of the "personalized medicine" approach in clinical neurosciences. These biomarkers can help specify the disease subgroups that will respond to certain interventions, can aid in early detection, and hopefully can bring about illness trajectory-altering interventions and ultimately prevention.

- Development of new treatments across specialty lines. An example would be illness-specific therapies for MS that address the immunological/inflammatory abnormalities and their effects on the myriad of symptoms involved in this illness, including depression and cognitive dysfunction.

- Sub-subspecialized clinical research in neurosciences (e.g., markers that predict response to deep brain stimulation in PD).

- Continued growth of the field of neuromodulatory and neuroplasticity-based techniques such as DBS, TMS, tDCS, and focused ultrasound.

Challenges

The expansion in the amount of research and the increasing fragmentation of research into narrow, illness-specific categories may bring delays in the transferability of knowledge across subspecialties caring for different disorders. In addition, expanding technologies and available treatments also mean increasing costs that create challenges at the system-level in terms of resource availability and access. Yet, advances in translation offer tremendous possibilities. Medical, academic, government, and industry sectors need to work together to support and disseminate innovation.

EDUCATION

Given the increasingly greater subspecialization in medicine, including in the fields of psychiatry and neurology in general, and neuropsychiatry and behavioral neurology in particular, a major goal of education should be to emphasize overarching principles that provide a framework for our fields and allow us to coherently add new information to our understanding of healthy and diseased brain functioning.

Several factors will contribute to the quality and accessibility of behavioral neurology/neuropsychiatric education. They include:

- Ease of access to information electronically and ease of mobility across the globe allow for faster and more widespread transmission of new knowledge to clinicians and patients.

- Formal education: Larger number of programs offering fellowship training in behavioral neurology and neuropsychiatry; larger influence of a behavioral neurologic/neuropsychiatric perspective in medical school, psychiatry and neurology residencies, and other training programs such as physiatry, medical psychiatry, and others. It is important to continue to work on attracting students to the fascinating, thriving fields of neuropsychiatry and behavioral neurology. There is a need to develop further the pedagogy and the curricula for the intersection area of neuropsychiatry and behavioral neurology, as well as an integrated neuropsychiatry and behavioral neurology curriculum that can be offered in the context of neurology and psychiatry residencies. In addition to the fellowship in behavioral neurology and neuropsychiatry, some centers offer *dual training*, where physicians can fully train in both psychiatry and neurology residencies—an alternative that can be important to individuals who prefer a broader exposure to the two disciplines. The development of formal training programs in child and adolescent neuropsychiatry is an important area that is ripe to grow in the near future.
- Continuing medical education (CME) programs in neuropsychiatry, such as the Harvard CME annual course offered by our group and other examples, facilitates an ongoing dissemination of neuropsychiatric knowledge for colleagues coming from a variety of professional backgrounds.
- Increase in the integration of knowledge. Models of illness that integrate knowledge from the social sciences and neurosciences rather than presenting dogmatically separate points of view. It is particularly important that trainees understand the bidirectional interaction of brain and environment in shaping behavior.
- Incorporation of training in procedures such as TMS into neuropsychiatric programs.
- Training of professionals with specific, task-focused skills (in the setting of a team-based delivery of care). Examples include genetic counselors, neuromodulation technicians, coaches for individuals with dysexecutive functioning, etc.

Challenges

The subspecialization of care makes the training of behavioral neurology and neuropsychiatry challenging. Clinical teachers must maintain up-to-date knowledge of relevant fields, and find creative ways to teach overarching principles as well as the most recent evidence-based advances in diagnostics and treatments. Of note, the widely available material online often includes scores of misinformation. This requires efficacious ways to direct trainees, colleagues, and patients to reliable sources and assist them in being discriminating.

CONCLUSION

We hope to have provided a description of current directions and convergence in neuropsychiatry and behavioral neurology that seem likely to continue to expand in the future. The chapter discusses some of the opportunities and challenges brought about by the growth and development of our fields. Our textbook offers an integrated view of these two disciplines, while acknowledging the richness of their individual contributions. Foundational principles of neuropsychiatry and behavioral neurology and a focus on the fundamental ethical principles of medical care must remain the guiding star to follow while navigating the waters of research, health systems, and technological advances.

References

1. Price BH, Adams RD, Coyle JT. Neurology and psychiatry: closing the great divide. *Neurology*. 2000;54:8-14.
2. Yudofsky SC, Hales RE. Neuropsychiatry and the future of neurology and psychiatry. *Am J Psychiatry*. 2002;159:8.
3. Arzy S, Danziger S. The science of neuropsychiatry: past, present, and future. *J Neuropsychiatry Clin Neurosci*. 2014;26:392-395.
4. Fitzgerald M. Do psychiatry and neurology need a close partnership or a merger? *B J Psych Bull*. 2015;39:105-107.
5. Trimble M. The intentional brain- a short history of neuropsychiatry. *CNS Spectr*. 2016;21:223-229.
6. Northoff G. Neuropsychiatry—an old discipline in a new gestalt bridging biological psychiatry, neuropsychology, and cognitive neurology. *Eur Arch Psychiatry Clin Neurosci*. 2008;258:226-238.
7. Ribeiro Porto P, Oliveira L, Mari J, et al. Does cognitive behavioral therapy change the brain? A systematic review of neuroimaging in anxiety disorders. *J Neuropsychiatry Clin Neurosci*. 2009;21:114-125.
8. Lodato MA, Woodworth MB, Lee S, et al. Somatic mutation in single human neurons tracks developmental and transcriptional history. *Science*. 2015;350:94-98.
9. Lisle BN, Hurley RA, Taber KH. Poststroke depression: contributions from network science. *J Neuropsychiatry Clin Neurosci*. 2018;30:256-261.
10. Silbersweig D. Integrating models of neurologic and psychiatric disease. *JAMA Neurol*. 2017;74(7):759-760.
11. Perez DL, Keshavan MS, Scharf JM. Bridging the great divide: what can neurology learn from psychiatry? *J Neuropsychiatry Clin Neurosci*. 2018;30:271-278.
12. Kovner R, Oler J, Kalin N. Cortico-limbic interactions mediate adaptive and maladaptive responses relevant to psychopathology. *Am J Psychiatry*. 2019;176:987-999.
13. Binzer S, McKay KA, Brenner P, et al. Disability worsening among persons with multiple sclerosis and depression—a Swedish cohort study. *Neurology*. 2019;93:e2216-e2223.
14. Insel TR. The NIHM Research Domain Criteria (RDoC) project: precision medicine for psychiatry. *Am J Psychiatry*. 2014;171:395-397.
15. Silbersweig DA, Loscalzo J. Precision psychiatry meets network medicine: network psychiatry. *JAMA Psychiatry*. 2017;74:665-666.
16. Le BD, Stein JL. Mapping causal pathways from genetics to neuropsychiatric disorders using genome-wide imaging genetics: current status and future directions. *Psychiatry Clin Neurosci*. 2019;73:357-369.
17. Sullivan PF, Agrawal A, Bulik CM, et al. Psychiatric genomics: an update and an agenda. *Am J Psychiatry*. 2018;175(1):15-27.
18. Van Erp TGM, Walton E, Hibar DP, et al. Cortical brain abnormalities in 4474 individuals with schizophrenia and 5098 control subjects via the Enhancing Neuro Imaging Genetics Through Meta Analysis (ENIGMA) consortium. *Biol Psychiatry*. 2018;84(9):644-654.

19. Breen G, Li Q, Roth BL. Translating genome-wide association findings into new therapeutics for psychiatry. *Nat Neurosci.* 2016;19(11):1392-1396.

20. Uddin LQ, Karlsgodt KH. Future directions for examination of brain networks in neurodevelopmental disorders. *J Clin Child Adolesc Psychol.* 2018;47(3):483-497.

21. Silbersweig DA, Rauch S. Neuroimaging in psychiatry: a quarter century of progress. *Harvard Rev Psychiatry.* 2017;25:195-197.

22. Etkin A. A reckoning and research agenda for neuroimaging in psychiatry. *Am J Psychiatry.* 2019;176:507-511.

Index

Page numbers followed by "t" denote tables.
Page numbers followed by "f" denote figures.

CPSIA information can be obtained
at www.ICGtesting.com
Printed in the USA
JSHW050915100423
39353JS00014B/6